# IAPSM's
# Textbook of
# COMMUNITY MEDICINE

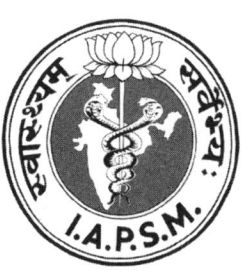

# IAPSM's Textbook of COMMUNITY MEDICINE

*As per the Competency-based Medical Education Curriculum (NMC)*

**THIRD EDITION**

### Editor-in-Chief

**AM Kadri**
State Health System Resource Centre
Gujarat, India

### Editors

**Rashmi Kundapur**
All India Institute of Medical Sciences
Telangana, India

**Amir Maroof Khan**
University College of Medical Sciences and
GTB Hospital, New Delhi, India

**Rakesh Kakkar**
All India Institute of Medical Sciences
Bhatinda, Punjab, India

**Ankit Sheth**
Indian Council of Medical Research (ICMR), National Institute
of Occupational Health (NIOH), Ahmedabad, Gujarat, India

**Nidhi Mangrola**
Kiran Medical College
Surat, Gujarat, India

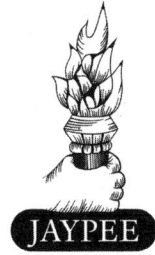

### JAYPEE BROTHERS MEDICAL PUBLISHERS
*The Health Sciences Publisher*

New Delhi | London

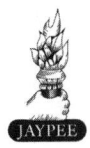

**Jaypee Brothers Medical Publishers (P) Ltd**

**Headquarters**
Jaypee Brothers Medical Publishers (P) Ltd
EMCA House, 23/23-B
Ansari Road, Daryaganj
New Delhi 110 002, India
Landline: +91-11-23272143, +91-11-23272703
+91-11-23282021, +91-11-23245672
Email: jaypee@jaypeebrothers.com

**Corporate Office**
Jaypee Brothers Medical Publishers (P) Ltd
4838/24, Ansari Road, Daryaganj
New Delhi 110 002, India
Phone: +91-11-43574357
Fax: +91-11-43574314
Email: jaypee@jaypeebrothers.com

**Overseas Office**
J.P. Medical Ltd
83 Victoria Street, London
SW1H 0HW (UK)
Phone: +44 20 3170 8910
Fax: +44 (0)20 3008 6180
Email: info@jpmedpub.com

Website: www.jaypeebrothers.com
Website: www.jaypeedigital.com

© 2024, Jaypee Brothers Medical Publishers

The views and opinions expressed in this book are solely those of the original contributor(s)/author(s) and do not necessarily represent those of editor(s) and publishers of the book.

All rights reserved. No part of this publication may be reproduced, stored or transmitted in any form or by any means, electronic, mechanical, photocopying, recording or otherwise, without the prior permission in writing of the publishers.

All brand names and product names used in this book are trade names, service marks, trademarks or registered trademarks of their respective owners. The publisher is not associated with any product or vendor mentioned in this book.

Medical knowledge and practice change constantly. This book is designed to provide accurate, authoritative information about the subject matter in question. However, readers are advised to check the most current information available on procedures included and check information from the manufacturer of each product to be administered, to verify the recommended dose, formula, method and duration of administration, adverse effects and contraindications. It is the responsibility of the practitioner to take all appropriate safety precautions. Neither the publisher nor the author(s)/editor(s) assume any liability for any injury and/or damage to persons or property arising from or related to use of material in this book.

This book is sold on the understanding that the publisher is not engaged in providing professional medical services. If such advice or services are required, the services of a competent medical professional should be sought.

Every effort has been made where necessary to contact holders of copyright to obtain permission to reproduce copyright material. If any have been inadvertently overlooked, the publisher will be pleased to make the necessary arrangements at the first opportunity.

**Inquiries for bulk sales may be solicited at:** jaypee@jaypeebrothers.com

*IAPSM's Textbook of Community Medicine*

*First Edition: 2019*
*Second Edition: 2021*
*Third Edition:* **2024**
ISBN: 978-93-5696-735-9

**Printed in India** at Rajkamal Electric Press, Kundli, Haryana.

# Editorial Support Team and Reviewers

## EDITORIAL SUPPORT TEAM

The Editorial Board express heartfelt gratitude to the dedicated members of the editorial support team for their commitment, invaluable contributions, and diligent efforts in shaping and refining third edition of this textbook.

**Bhargav Dave**
Nootan Medical College and Research Centre
Visnagar, Gujarat, India

**Nikita Savani**
Shantabaa Medical College and General Hospital, Amreli
Gujarat, India

**Manjula R**
S Nijalingappa Medical College,
Karnataka, India

**Roopa R Mendagudali**
Mahadevappa Rampure Medical College
Karnataka, India

**Anusha Rashmi**
KS Hegde Medical College
Karnataka, India

## REVIEWERS

The Editorial Board and Authors are grateful to the individuals listed below for their invaluable contributions as reviewers for various sections of this textbook. Their dedicated efforts and insightful feedback have played a crucial role in enhancing the quality and comprehensiveness of the content.

- A Bhagyalaxmi
- Anand Krishnan
- Anjali Mall
- AP Kulkarni *(Retired)*
- Ashwatha Narayan
- Bishan S Garg
- Deepak Saxena
- Devendra Gaur

- Dhrubajyoti Debnath
- Harivansh Chopra
- Lalit Sankhe
- Manju Toppo
- Najam Khalique
- Narayan Gaonkar
- Niraj Pandit
- PV Kotecha *(Retired)*

- Rajesh Kumar
- RB Jain
- Sairu Philip
- Sanjiv Kumar
- Sheetal Vyas
- Sonal Shah Parikh
- Sonu Goel
- Suneela Garg
- Uday Shankar Singh

# Contributors

**Abhay Srivastava**
Himalayan Institute of Medical Sciences
Swami Rama Himalayan University
Uttarakhand, India

**Abhik Sinha**
Indian Council of
Medical Research-National Institute of
Cholera and Enteric Diseases
Kolkata, West Bengal, India

**Abhimanyu Singh Chauhan**
Stichting Human Vaccine Project Europe
Amsterdam, The Netherlands

**Abhishek Mishra**
All India Institute of Medical Sciences
Bhubaneswar, Odisha, India

**Abhishek Singh**
SHKM Government Medical College
Mewat (Nuh), Haryana, India

**Abu Hasan Sarkar**
Public Health Expert, North East, India

**Afraz Jahan**
Kasturba Medical College
Manipal, Karnataka, India

**Akhil Dhanesh Goel**
All India Institute of Medical Sciences
Jodhpur, India

**Alka Kaware**
Indira Gandhi Government Medical College
Nagpur, Maharashtra, India

**AM Kadri**
State Health System Resource Centre
Gujarat, India

**Amir Maroof Khan**
University College of Medical Sciences and
Guru Teg Bahadur Hospital
Delhi, India

**Amit Kumar Mishra**
All India Institute of Medical Sciences
Raipur, Chhattisgarh, India

**Amit Sachdeva**
Indira Gandhi Medical College
Shimla, Himachal Pradesh, India

**Anand Krishnan**
All India Institute of Medical Sciences
New Delhi, India

**Anil J Purty**
Pondicherry Institute of Medical Sciences
Puducherry, India

**Animesh Jain**
Kasturba Medical College, Mangalore
Manipal Academy of Higher Education
Manipal, Karnataka, India

**Anjali Modi**
All India Institute of Medical Sciences
Rajkot, Gujarat, India

**Ankeeta Menona Jacob**
KS Hegde Medical Academy
Karnataka, India

**Ankit Sheth**
Indian Council of Medical Research-
National Institute of Occupational Health
Ahmedabad, Gujarat, India

**Anku Moni Saikia**
Dhubri Medical College
Dhubri, Assam, India

**Anmol Gupta**
Indira Gandhi Medical College
Shimla, Himachal Pradesh, India

**Anupam Banerjee**
Pandit Dindayal Upadhyay (PDU)
Medical College
Rajkot, Gujarat, India

**Anupam Parashar**
All India Institute of Medical Sciences
Himachal Pradesh, India

**Anusha Rashmi**
KS Hegde Medical Academy
Karnataka, India

**Arpit Prajapati**
GCS Medical College
Hospital and Research Centre
Ahmedabad, Gujarat, India

**Arundhathi B**
Government Medical College
Telangana, India

**Ashok Mishra** *(Retired)*
GR Medical College
Gwalior, Madhya Pradesh, India

**Ashwin Kumar**
SS Institute of Medical Sciences
and Research Centre
Karnataka, India

**Atul Trivedi**
BJ Medical College
Ahmedabad, India

**Ayesha Siddiqua Nawaz**
Women's Cancers, JHPIEGO
New Delhi, India

**Baridalyne Nongkynrih**
All India Institute of Medical Sciences
New Delhi, India

**Bhanu M**
Grassroots Research and Advocacy
Movement, Mysuru, India

**Bharatkumar M Gohel**
Pandit Dindayal Upadhyay
Government Medical College
Rajkot, Gujarat, India

**Bhargav Dave**
Narendra Modi Medical College
Ahmedabad, Gujarat, India

**Bhavana Laxmi Surity**
Government Medical College
Telangana, India

**Bhavani Kenche**
Osmania Medical College
Hyderabad, Telangana, India

**Bhavani Nivetha**
IQVIA, Bangaluru, India

**Bhavesh Modi**
All India Institute of Medical Sciences
Rajkot, Gujarat, India

**Bhavik Rana**
GMERS Medical College
Vadnagar, Gujarat, India

**Bhavna Seth**
Pulmonary and Critical Care Medicine
Johns Hopkins University Baltimore
Maryland, United States

**Bishan S Garg**
Mahatma Gandhi Institute of Medical
Sciences, Wardha, Maharashtra, India

**Bratati Banerjee**
Maulana Azad Medical College
New Delhi, India

**Chandresh Pandya**
Medical College, Baroda
Vadodara, Gujarat, India

**Charu Kohli**
Mannheim Business School, Germany

**Cherian Varghese**
Regional Advisor, NCD, WHO SEAR Office
New Delhi, India

**DS Dhadwal**
IG Medical College
Shimla, Himachal Pradesh, India

**DV Bala** *(Retired)*
NHL Municipal Medical College
Ahmedabad, Gujarat, India

**Darshan Mahyavanshi**
NAMO Medical Education and Research
Institute, UT of DNH and DD, India

**Deepshikha**
Himalayan Institute of Medical Sciences
Swami Rama Himalayan University
Dehradun, Uttarakhand, India

## Contributors

**Deepthi N Shanbhag**
St John's Medical College
Bengaluru, Karnataka, India

**Deepthi R**
ESICMC and PGIMSR
Bengaluru, Karnataka, India

**Devraj R**
Government Medical College
Thiruvananthapuram, Kerala, India

**Dhiraj Kumar Srivastava**
UP University of Medical Sciences
Uttar Pradesh, India

**Dibakar Haldar**
NRS Medical College
Kolkata, West Bengal, India

**Dinesh Kumar**
Pramukhswami Medical College
Karamsad, Gujarat, India

**Dipesh Zalavadiya**
GMERS Medical College
Junagadh, Gujarat, India

**Ekta Gupta**
Indian Council of Medical Research-
National Institute of Cancer Prevention and
Research, Noida, Uttar Pradesh, India

**Forhad Akhtar Zaman**
All India Institute of Medical Sciences
Guwahati, Assam, India

**G Rakesh Maiya**
St Peter's Medical College, Hospital and
Research Institute, Hosur, Tamil Nadu, India

**G Shiny Chrism Queen Nesan**
Saveetha Medical College and Hospital
Chennai, Tamil Nadu, India

**Gneyaa Bhatt**
GMERS Medical College
Ahmedabad, Gujarat, India

**Gowri Nambiar Sengupta**
CHEB, Directorate General Health Services
Ministry of Health and Family Welfare
New Delhi, India

**Gurmeet Kaur**
Lady Hardinge Medical College
Delhi, India

**Harsh Bakshi**
GMERS, Medical College Ahmedabad
Gujarat, India

**Harshal Ramesh Salve**
All India Institute of Medical Sciences
New Delhi, India

**Harshitha HN**
Sri Devaraj Urs Medical College
Karnataka, India

**Himanshu Negandhi**
Public Health Foundation of India
New Delhi, India

**Hitesh M Shah**
GMERS, Valsad, Gujarat, India

**Ipsa Mohapatra**
Kalinga Institute of Medical Sciences
Bhubaneswar, Odisha, India

**Jay K Sheth**
Narendra Modi Medical College
Ahmedabad, Gujarat, India

**Jayanthi Srikanth**
Kempegauda Institute of Medical Sciences
Bengaluru, Karnataka, India

**Jithin Daniel J**
Sree Mookambika Institute of Medical
Sciences, Tamil Nadu, India

**Jyothi Lakshmi Naga Vemuri**
Government Medical College
Nagarkurnool, Telangana, India

**Jyotiranjan Sahoo**
Institute of Medical Sciences and
Sum Hospital, Siksha 'O' Anusandhan
Bhubaneswar, Odisha, India

**Kalaiselvi**
All India Institute of Medical Sciences
Madurai, Tamil Nadu, India

**Kalpita Shringarpure**
Medical College Baroda
Vadodara, Gujarat, India

**Kapil Gandha**
MP Shah Govt Medical College
Jamnagar, Gujarat, India

**Kathiresan Jeyashree**
Indian Council of Medical Research-
National Institute of Epidemiology
Chennai, Tamil Nadu, India

**Kaushik Lodhiya**
GMERS Medical College
Junagadh, Gujarat, India

**Kaushik Mitra**
Burdwan Medical College
West Bengal, India

**Kedar Mehta**
GMERS Medical College
Vadodara, Gujarat, India

**Kumaril Goswami**
Gauhati Medical College and Hospital
Guwahati, Assam, India

*Late* **Shobha Mishra**
PDU Government Medical College
Rajkot, Gujarat, India

**Liaquat Roopesh Johnson**
Azeezia Institute of Medical Sciences and
Research, Kerala, India

**Madhur Verma**
All India Institute of Medical Sciences
Punjab, India

**Madhurjya Baruah**
Nagaon Medical College
Assam, India

**Malatesh Undi**
Karwar Institute of Medical Sciences
Karwar, Karnataka, India

**Manasa AR**
Rajarajeswari Medical College and Hospital
Bangaluru, Karnataka, India

**Manish Rana**
GMERS Medical College
Ahmedabad, Gujarat, India

**Manish Kumar Singh**
Dr Ram Manohar Lohia Institute of Medical
Sciences, Lucknow, Uttar Pradesh, India

**Manisha Gohel**
Pramukhswami Medical College
Karamsad, Gujarat, India

**Manjit Boruah**
Tinsukia Medical College
Assam, India

**Manju Toppo**
Gandhi Medical College
Bhopal, Madhya Pradesh, India

**Manjula R**
S Nijalingappa Medical College
Bagalkot, Karnataka, India

**Manoj Bansal**
GR Medical College
Gwalior, Madhya Pradesh, India

**Manoj Kumar Gupta**
All India Institute of Medical Sciences
Jodhpur, Rajasthan, India

**Manoj Talapalliwar**
Government Medical College
Akola, Maharashtra, India

**Manya Prasad**
Department of Clinical Research and
Epidemiology, Institute of Liver and Biliary
Sciences, New Delhi, India

**Mausumi Basu**
IPGMER, Kolkata, India

**Mihir Rupani**
Indian Council of Medical Research-
National Institute of Occupational Health,
Ahmedabad, Gujarat, India

**Mitasha Singh**
Dr Baba Saheb Ambedkar Medical College
and Hospital, New Delhi, India

**Mohua Moitra**
Baroda Medical College
Vadodara, Gujarat, India

**Muthukumar R**
Sri Ramachandra Medical College and
Research Institute
Chennai, Tamil Nadu, India

**NR Ramesh Masthi**
Kempegowda Institute of Medical Sciences
Bangalore, India

**Narayanan Namboothiri G**
MES Medical College, Kerala, India

**Neeraj Agarwal**
All India Institute of Medical Sciences
Hyderabad, Telangana, India

**Nidhi Mangrola**
Kiran Medical College, Surat, Gujarat, India

**Nilesh Fichadiya**
PDU Government Medical College
Rajkot, Gujarat, India

**Niravkumar Joshi**
Medical College Baroda
Vadodara, Gujarat, India

**Nirmal Kumar Mandal**
MJN Medical College and Hospital
West Bengal, India

**Nishanth Krishna K**
Father Muller Medical College
Mangaluru, Karnataka, India

**Nitu Kumari**
University College of Medical Sciences and
GTB Hospital, New Delhi, India

**Niyati Parmar**
Medical College Baroda
Vadodara, Gujarat, India

**P Amritha Krishna**
MVJ Medical College and Research Hospital
Bengaluru, Karnataka, India

**P Stalin**
Pondicherry Institute of Medical Sciences
Puducherry, India

**PV Kotecha** *(Retired)*
Medical College, Vadodara, Gujarat, India
At Present USA

**Palash Das**
Rampurhat Government Medical College
and Hospital, West Bengal, India

**Pankaj Bhardwaj**
School of Public Health AIIMS
Jodhpur, Rajasthan, India

**Pankaja Raghav**
All India Institute of Medical Sciences
Jodhpur, Rajasthan, India

**Paragkumar Chavda**
GMERS Medical College
Vadodara, Gujarat, India

**Paramita Sengupta**
All India Institute of Medical Sciences
Kalyani, Nadia, West Bengal, India

**Paras Agarwal**
Senior Consultant Diabetologist, Max
Healthcare Ltd

**Pooja Goyal**
ESIC Medical College and Hospital
Faridabad, Haryana, India

**Poonam Sancheti**
BJGMC Pune, Maharashtra, India

**Pracheth R**
National Institute of Mental Health and
Neuro Sciences (NIMHANS), Institute of
National Importance
Bengaluru, Karnataka, India

**Pradeep Aggarwal**
All India Institute of Medical Sciences
Rishikesh, Uttarkahnd, India

**Pradeep Kumar**
Dr MK Shah Medical College
Ahmedabad, Gujarat, India

**Pragti Chhabra**
University College of Medical Sciences
Delhi, India

**Prakash Patel**
Surat Municipal Institute of Medical
Education and Research (SMIMER)
Surat, Gujarat, India

**Pranab Chatterjee**
BJGMC Pune, Maharashtra, India

**Pranay Jadav**
GMERS Medical College
Himmatnagar, Gujarat, India

**Praveen Kulkarni**
JSS Medical College, JSS Academy of Higher
Education and Research
Mysuru, Karnataka, India

**Preetam Mahajan**
JIPMER karaikal, Puducherry, India

**Prince Alex Abraham**
Mount Zion Medical College
Adoor, Kerala, India

**Priscilla Kayina**
Jawaharlal Nehru Institute of Medical
Sciences, Imphal, Manipur, India

**Priya Arora**
Army College of Medical Sciences
New Delhi, India

**Priyesh Marskole**
Governmet Medical College
Khandwa, Madhya Pradesh, India

**RB Jain**
World College of Medical Sciences and
Research, Jhajjar, Haryana, India

**Rachana AR**
Karwar Institute of Medical Sciences
Karwar, Karnataka, India

**Radha Valaulikar**
World Diabetes Foundation (WDF) NCD
Project, Piramal Swasthya Management and
Research Institute

**Rahul Hegde**
Nitte (Deemed to be University)
KS Hegde Medical Academy
Mangaluru, Karnataka, India

**Rajesh Chudasama**
PDU Government Medical College
Rajkot, Gujarat, India

**Rajesh Kumar Konduru**
Pondicherry Institute of Medical Sciences
Pondicherry, India

**Rakesh Kakkar**
All India Institute of Medical Sciences
Bathinda, Punjab, India

**Ramya MP**
Kempegauda Institute of Medical Sciences
Mangalagiri, Andhra Pradesh, India

**Rashmi Kundapur**
All India Institute of Medical Sciences
Telangana, India

**Rashmi Sharma**
GMERS Medical College
Ahmedabad, Gujarat, India

**Ravikumar**
MRMC, Kalaburagi, Karnataka, India

**Ravish HS**
Kempegowda Institute of Medical Sciences
Bengaluru, Karnataka, India

**Ravneet Kaur**
All India Institute of Medical Sciences
New Delhi, India

**Ritesh Singh**
All India Institute of Medical Sciences
Kalyani, West Bengal, India

**Ritika Tiwari**
York St John University (London Campus),
London, United Kingdom

**Rivu Basu**
All India Institute of Hygiene and Public
Health, Kolkata, India

**Rizwan Suliankatchi Abdulkader**
ICMR-National Institute of Epidemiology
Chennai, Tamil Nadu, India

**Rohit Ram**
MP Shah government Medical College
Jamnagar, Gujarat, India

**Roopa Shivashankar**
ICMR-HQ, New Delhi, India

**Ruchi Juyal**
Himalayan Institute of Medical Sciences
Swami Rama Himalayan University
Dehradun, Uttarakhand, India

**Rupsa Banerjee**
International Institute of Health
Management Research
Delhi, India

## Contributors

**Saikat Bhattacharya**
NRS Medical College, Kolkata, India

**Sandeep Kumar Panigrahi**
Institute of Medical Sciences and
Sum Hospital, Siksha 'O' Anusandhan,
Bhubaneswar, Odisha, India

**Sanjana SN**
Digital Health Manager and Founding
Member at Eka Care
Bengaluru, Karnataka, India

**Sanjay Zodpey**
Public Health Foundation of India and
Indian Institute of Public Health
New Delhi, India

**Sanjib Bandyopadhyay**
Burdwan Medical College
West Bengal, India

**Santosh K Yatnatti**
BLMK ICS R&I Hub Project Manager
University of Bedfordshire
United Kingdom

**Sarmila Mallik**
Tamralipto GMCH, Medinipur
West Bengal, India

**Sasmita Mungi**
GR Medical College
Gwalior, Madhya Pradesh, India

**Saurabh Kumar**
KLE JGMMMC
KLE Academy of Higher Education
and Research
Karnataka, India

**Saurabh Sharma**
ICMR-National Institute of Medical Statistics
New Delhi, India

**Senkadhirdasan**
Mahatma Gandhi Medical College and
Research Institute, Puducherry, India

**Shailee Vyas**
Government Medical College
Surat, Gujarat, India

**Shaili Vyas**
Himalayan Institute of Medical Sciences
SRHU, Dehradun, Uttarakhand, India

**Shalini Pradeep**
Ramaiah International Medical School
Bengaluru, Karnataka, India

**Shalini Sundaram**
Rajendra Institute of Medical Sciences
Ranchi, Jharkhand, India

**Sharon Baisal**
MOSC Medical College
Kochi, Kerala, India

**Shashi Kumar M**
ESI PGIMSR and ESIC Medical College and
ODC (EZ), Joka, Kolkata, India

**Shikha Jain**
BJ Medical College
Ahmedabad, Gujarat, India

**Shreyaswi Sathyanath M**
AJ Institute of Medical Sciences and
Research Center
Mangaluru, Karnataka, India

**Shubha Davalagi**
JJM Medical College
Karnataka, India

**Shveta Lukhmana**
Vardhman Mahavir Medical College and
Safdarjang Hospital, New Delhi, India

**Sudhir Prabhu H**
Father Muller Medical College
Mangaluru, Karnataka, India

**Sukamal Bisoi**
Deben Mahata Government Medical
College, West Bengal, India

**Sumanth MM**
Mysore Medical College and Research
Institute, Mysuru, Karnataka, India

**Sumit Aggarwal**
Division of Descriptive Research, Indian
Council of Medical Research Headquaters
New Delhi, India

**Sumit Malhotra**
All India Institute of Medical Sciences
New Delhi, India

**Sunil Kumar D**
JSS Medical College, JSS Academy of Higher
Education and Research
Mysuru, Karnataka, India

**Swetha Rajeshwari**
All India Institute of Hygiene and Public
Health, Kolkata, India

**Teeku Sinha**
Government Medical College
Chhattisgarh, India

**Tulika Goswami**
Assam Medical College
Assam, India

**Tushar Manohar Rane**
Chief of Field Office, UNICEF

**Umed Patel**
PDU Government Medical College
Rajkot, Gujarat, India

**Vaidehi S Gohil**
Dr MK Shah Medical College and Research
Centre, Ahmedabad, Gujarat, India

**Varghese Iybu Chacko**
Azeezia Institute of Medical Sciences and
Research, Kollam, Kerala, India

**Vartika Saxena**
All India Institute of Medical Sciences
Rishikesh, Uttarakhand, India

**Veena Kumari**
Communication for Development (C4D)
Specialist, UNICEF,
West Bengal Feld Office, India

**Velavan A**
Pondicherry Institute of Medical Sciences
Puducherry, India

**Venkatarao Epari**
Institute of Medical Sciences & Sum
Hospital, Siksha 'O' Anusandhan
Bhubaneswar, Odisha, India

**Venu Shah**
GCS Medical College, Hospital and Research
Centre, Ahmedabad, Gujarat, India

**Vidisha Vallabh**
Himalayan Institute of Medical Sciences
Swami Rama Himalayan University
Dehradun, Uttarakhand, India

**Vidya R**
Akash Institute of Medical Sciences and
Research Centre,
Bengaluru, Karnataka, India

**Vikas Doshi**
Government Medical College
Vadodara, Gujarat, India

**Vinayak J Kempaller**
Ministry of Health and Family Welfare
Bagalkot, Karnataka, India

**Viral Dave**
GCS Medical College, Hospital and Research
Centre, Ahmedabad, Gujarat, India

**Yogita Bavaskar**
Government Medical College
Maharashtra, India

**Zinia T Nujum**
Government Medical College
Kollam, Kerala, India

**(Brig) Zile Singh** *(Retired)*
AFMC, Pune
PIMS, Puducherry, India

# Foreword

The discipline of Community Medicine is vital for Health Promotion and Disease Prevention. Learning in Community Medicine develops an insight about factors influencing health of individuals in general and the community at large. It also gives us an insight about how diseases spread in the community. While conventional disciplines of medicine talk about the actions required to be taken after the occurrence of diseases, Community Medicine focuses on preventing diseases and promoting health. It gives an idea of burden of disease in the community and talks about methods and techniques to reduce them. This makes Community Medicine unique among all disciplines of medical science.

Teaching and learning in Community Medicine requires the understanding of various disciplines of medical science. Hence, its learning and practices are multidisciplinary. Understanding of social factors, nutrition, and environmental health is the base of Community Medicine and skills to apply tools of epidemiology, biostatistics, health management, behavioral, and social sciences are fundamental for practices of Community Medicine. While the application of knowledge of Community Medicine is useful for individuals, it is also very much required for organizing primary, preventive, and promotive healthcare services for the community.

There has been a long-standing demand for Textbook of Community Medicine which can articulate community medicine in real spirit rather than just being a pile of information on topics related to Community Medicine. Indian Association of Preventive and Social Medicine (IAPSM), an apex professional organization of experts in Preventive and Social Medicine/Community Medicine, has come up with an aim to bridge this gap. A group of teachers, researchers, and practitioners have joined hands to prepare an *IAPSM's Textbook in Community Medicine*. Previous two editions of this textbook were out and well-received among undergraduates, postgraduates, teachers, and professionals of Community Medicine/Preventive and Social Medicine/Public Health. Third edition of the book is a continuation of this journey.

As a National President and Editor in Chief of this textbook, it is my honor to write Foreword for third edition of this textbook. The third edition is built on experiences from the previous two editions. It will continue to help its readers to decipher and describe community/public health, develop solutions to address community/public health problems, and contribute to developing relevant skills in Community Medicine.

As an association, IAPSM is committed for developing good understandings about discipline in the medical students. Editorial teams as well contributors are working hard for the same. Finally, I appeal to all readers of this book to give their suggestions, helping us in making this textbook better.

**Prof (Dr) AM Kadri**
National President
Indian Association of Preventive and Social Medicine (IAPSM)
2023-24

# Preface to the Third Edition

Being a Secretary General of Indian Association of Preventive and Social Medicine (IAPSM), it gives me immense pleasure to pen this Preface for the third edition of *IAPSM's Textbook of Community Medicine*. It is a result of efforts done by large number of Community Medicine faculties, researchers, and public health experts to reshape the discipline according to modern day scenario and give it a desired direction for teaching, learning, and practices. It is written with the goal and specific objectives, specially required for Indian Medical Graduate (IMG) with topics explained very comprehensively and in a manner which fulfills all the necessary criteria to become a competent medical undergraduate.

After COVID-era, more focus is shifted toward preventive and management aspects of community health. The recent recommendations by the National Medical Commission (NMC) advocating for the inclusion of the Family Adoption Programme (FAP), electives, and an extended internship duration in Community Medicine underscore a broader approach to holistic healthcare. Also, in the modern day, every medical practitioner requires knowledge about epidemiology of diseases, biostatistics as well as research methodology, so relevance of learning Community Medicine has increased enormously in present era.

The success of the previously released two editions, well-received by both undergraduate and postgraduate students, teachers, and professionals of Community Medicine, speaks to their effectiveness. These editions incorporated competency linkages with each topic, aligning with the competency-based curriculum designed for undergraduates. The sequential flow of topics, starting from the basics of health to core and allied sciences, simplifies the understanding for undergraduates as it corresponds with the chronology of their study period. The textbook then delves into community health problems, providing in-depth knowledge about prevailing disease conditions and their management plans. The subsequent sections focus on community health management, covering a comprehensive range of topics in a need-based and chronological manner. I personally thank each faculty for making a lot of effort and coming up with such a comprehensive book.

The third edition is one step further and in the line of progress with the previous two editions incorporating all valuable suggestions from experts and readers with the inclusion of newer updates in Community Medicine. We invite you to share your valuable feedback and suggestions at iapsmtextbook2023@gmail.com, contributing to the ongoing efforts to enhance and develop this textbook in the future.

**Purushottam Giri**
Secretary General
Indian Association of Preventive and Social Medicine (IAPSM)
(2022-25)

# Preface to the First Edition

*IAPSM's Textbook of Community Medicine* is an attempt by the Indian Association of Preventive and Social Medicine (IAPSM) to reshape the discipline and give it a desired direction for teaching, learning and practices.

The goal and specific objectives as envisaged by the Medical Council of India (MCI) for Indian medical graduates, has placed a very important role and responsibility to the subject 'Community Medicine' in the undergraduate medical curriculum. A textbook for undergraduate students is an effective tool to realize these important roles.

This textbook of community medicine subject for undergraduate medical students is prepared with the aim to provide a comprehensive information about all topics relevant to undergraduate medical students with their expected roles as medical graduates.

Preparation of first edition of this book has gone through a long period of three years. IAPSM has carried out wide consultations with students to stalwarts in the field of community medicine to understand the issues affecting the practice of teaching and training and its needs. We have reviewed published literature on issues and have included the suggestions received from the vast experience of IAPSM members in teaching the various topics in community medicine. The syllabus was prepared by the following guiding principles:

- The goals, objectives and specific objectives for community medicine as per the Graduate Medical Education Regulation, 1997, MCI are to be used to decide about topics and subtopics.
- Removing of unnecessary details in topics that are not relevant to MBBS graduates.
- Emphasis is to be given to the topics which are relevant to current need and role of medical graduates.
- Flow of the topics and subtopics are to be logical and progressive, i.e. from basic level to applied levels.

Based on the above principles, many obsolete topics and unnecessary details are removed. Newer topics as per the current needs are incorporated. Also, applications in community medicine practice is emphasized keeping focus on the Indian health situation and healthcare system. This will also keep the future health professional of India well informed about country's health conditions and the ongoing preventive and promotive efforts by the government. This will help in understanding their roles and responsibilities instead of practicing curative medicine in isolation.

In this textbook, the chapters and topics are grouped in five sections. The topics progress from the development of basic understanding of the individual health and disease to understanding the community health and dynamics of diseases/health problems in the community. It further provides the understanding of principles and methods to manage health of the community through healthcare delivery system. Lastly, it describes 'How the health of people of India is being managed'.

This textbook is the result of collective efforts of IAPSM members who are experts in the field of community medicine. This is the first edition and there is a scope of improvement. While presenting the first edition of this textbook, we are committed to improve its quality further in the subsequent editions. This can be possible only, when we would receive feedback from respected teachers and importantly from the students.

The IAPSM is eager to have your valuable feedback/suggestions for improving this textbook. Please do give them through academia.iapsm@gmail.com.

**AM Kadri**
Editor-in-Chief and Secretary General
IAPSM

# Acknowledgments

**SPECIAL ACKNOWLEDGMENT**

We extend a special acknowledgment to the esteemed past presidents of IAPSM, under whose tenures the IAPSM's Textbook was conceptualized, developed, and met with success. Their visionary leadership has been instrumental in shaping the journey of *IAPSM's Textbook of Community Medicine*.

| **Ashok Mishra** | **Ratan Srivastava** | **Anil Purty** | **Sanjay Zodpey** | **Suneela Garg** | **Harivansh Chopra** |
|---|---|---|---|---|---|
| Past IAPSM President (2016-17) | Past IAPSM President (2017-18) | Past IAPSM President (2018-19) | Past IAPSM President (2020-21) | Past IAPSM President (2021-22) | Past IAPSM President (2022-23) |

We also express our heartfelt thanks to our senior IAPSM members for their continuous support and guidance in advancing the goals and mission of IAPSM's textbook.

| | | |
|---|---|---|
| **A Bhagyalaxmi** | **Bishan S Garg** | **Rajesh Kumar** |
| **AK Bhardwaj** | **Chitranjan Roy** | **Sanjiv Kumar** |
| **AP Kulkarni** *(Retired)* | **Farooq Ahmed** *(Retired)* | **SK Rasania** |
| **Abraham Joseph** | **Mohan Doibale** | |
| **Anand Krishnan** | **Pradeep Kumar** | **VK Srivastava** |
| **Ashok Kumar Jindal** | **PB Verma** *(Retired)* | **(Brig) Zile Singh** *(Retired)* |

I am very grateful to the whole team of M/s Jaypee Brothers Medical Publishers (P) Ltd, New Delhi, India, who helped and guided me, Shri Jitendar P Vij (Group Chairman), Mr Ankit Vij (Managing Director), Mr MS Mani (Group President), Dr Madhu Choudhary (Director–Educational Publishing), Ms Pooja Bhandari [Director–Production (Books and Journals)], Ms Sunita Katla (Executive Assistant to Group Chairman and Publishing Manager), Mr Ajay Kumar Sharma [Deputy General Manager (Books and Journals)], Ms Samina Khan (Executive Assistant to Director–Educational Publishing), Dr Aditya Tayal (Team Lead–UG Publishing), Mr Rajesh Sharma (Production Coordinator), Ms Seema Dogra (Cover Visualizer), Ms Neelam Kakriya and Mr Rabindra Kumar (Proofreaders), Mr Dinesh Bhardwaj (Typesetter), Mr Rajesh Gurkundi (Graphic Designer) and their team members, for all their support to work in this project and make it a success. Without their cooperation, I could not have completed this project.

# Contents

## COLOR PLATES

## PROLOGUE

1. **Story of the Upstream** .................................. 3
   AM Kadri
2. **Community Medicine: An Introduction** ..................... 6
   Core Committee IAPSM

## SECTION 1: BASICS OF HEALTH AND DISEASE

3. **Concept of Health and Disease** ........................... 13
   Anmol Gupta, Anupam Parashar, DS Dhadwal, Amit Sachdeva
4. **Nutrition and Health** .................................. 25
   Zinia T Nujum
5. **Physical Activity, Exercise, and Health** ................. 52
   Yogita Bavaskar, Manisha Gohel, Abhay Srivastava
   Saurabh Sharma, Santosh K Yatnatti
6. **Sociology and Health** .................................. 60
   Paramita Sengupta
7. **Environment and Health** ................................ 71
   A. Air and Health   71
   Radha Valaulikar, Muthukumar R
   B. Water and Health   84
   P Stalin, Velavan A, Anil J Purty
   C. Sanitation and Health   93
   P Stalin, Velavan A, Anil J Purty
   D. Temperature and Health   100
   Vinayak J Kempaller, G Rakesh Maiya, Shiny Chrism Queen Nesan
   E. Noise and Health   106
   NR Ramesh Masthi, Manasa AR
   F. Light and Health   109
   NR Ramesh Masthi, Afraz Jahan
   G. Healthy House and Surrounding   111
   Sumanth MM, Praveen Kulkarni, Bhavani Nivetha
   H. Medical Entomology   115
   Ipsa Mohapatra

## SECTION 2: CORE AND ALLIED SCIENCES

8. **Preventive Medicine** ................................... 133
   Vartika Saxena, Rakesh Kakkar, Senkadhirdasan
9. **Basics of Epidemiology** ................................ 150
   Nirmal Kumar Mandal, Teeku Sinha, Sarmila Mallik
10. **Epidemiological and Research Studies** .................. 164
    Shikha Jain
11. **Research Methodology and Biostatistics** ............... 182
    Paragkumar Chavda, Mihir Rupani, Kalpita Shringarpure, Kedar Mehta
12. **Population Science** ................................... 216
    Chandresh Pandya, Paragkumar Chavda, Vikas Doshi
13. **Social Medicine** ...................................... 226
    Late Shobha Mishra, Shalini Sundaram
    Kalpita Shringarpure, Niyati Parmar
14. **Health Communication** ................................. 232
    Tulika Goswami, Tushar Manohar Rane
    Abu Hasan Sarkar, Veena Kumari, Manjit Boruah

## SECTION 3: COMMUNITY HEALTH PROBLEMS AND VULNERABLE GROUPS

15. **History and Important Events in Community Health** ..... 243
    Devraj R, Bishan S Garg
16. **General Epidemiology of Infectious Diseases and its Prevention and Control** ..... 248
    Pankaj Bhardwaj, Akhil Dhanesh Goel
17. **Specific Epidemiology of Infectious Diseases** ........ 260
    A. Epidemiology of Airborne Diseases and its Prevention and Control   260
    General Epidemiology of Airborne Diseases and General Principles of Prevention and Control   260
    Malatesh Undi, Vidya R
    Epidemiology of Acute Respiratory Infections and its Prevention and Control   264
    Rajesh Kumar Konduru, Anil J Purty, Preetam Mahajan
    Amit Kumar Mishra, Kalaiselvi
    Epidemiology of Chickenpox and its Prevention and Control   272
    Shalini Pradeep
    Epidemiology of Measles and its Prevention and Control   276
    Rachana AR, Prince Alex Abraham
    Epidemiology of Mumps and its Prevention and Control   282
    Deepthi N Shanbhag
    Epidemiology of Rubella and its Prevention and Control   286
    Ravish HS, Nitu Kumari, Ramya MP

**Epidemiology of Influenza and its Prevention and Control**  289
*Rajesh Kumar Konduru, Anil J Purty, Preetam Mahajan, Amit Kumar Mishra, Kalaiselvi*

**Seasonal Influenza**  297

**Severe Acute Respiratory Syndrome**  305

**Epidemiology of Tuberculosis and its Prevention and Control**  306
*Ritesh Singh*

**Epidemiology of Diphtheria and its Prevention and Control**  320
*Ayesha Siddiqua Nawaz, Ashwin Kumar*

**Epidemiology of Whooping Cough and its Prevention and Control**  325
*Swetha Rajeshwari, Ravikumar*

**Epidemiology of Meningococcal Meningitis and its Prevention and Control**  329
*Jayanthi Srikanth*

**Other Airborne Diseases of Community Health Importance**  332
*Shubha Davalagi, Sanjana SN*

**Inhalational Anthrax (Woolsorter's Disease)**  332

**Pneumonic Plague**  335

**B. Epidemiology of Intestinal (Waterborne and Foodborne) Diseases and its Prevention and Control**  338

**General Epidemiology of Waterborne Diseases and General Principles of its Prevention and Control**  338
*Bhavani Kenche, Jyothi Lakshmi Naga Vemuri, Arundhathi B, Bhavana Laxmi Surity*

**General Epidemiology of Intestinal (Foodborne) Diseases and General Principles of its Prevention and Control**  341
*Abhishek Singh*

**Epidemiology of Poliomyelitis and its Prevention and Control**  352
*Bhavani Kenche, Jyothi Lakshmi Naga Vemuri, Arundhathi B, Bhavana Laxmi Surity*

**Epidemiology of Cholera and its Prevention and Control**  359
*Bhavani Kenche, Jyothi Lakshmi Naga Vemuri, Arundhathi B Bhavana Laxmi Surity*

**Epidemiology of Acute Diarrheal Diseases and its Prevention and Control**  365
*Bhavani Kenche, Jyothi Lakshmi Naga Vemuri, Arundhathi B, Bhavana Laxmi Surity*

**Epidemiology of Salmonellosis and Typhoid Fever and its Prevention and Control**  370
*Abhishek Singh*

**Epidemiology of Shigellosis and its Prevention and Control**  375
*Abhishek Singh*

**Epidemiology of Viral Hepatitis (A and E) and its Prevention and Control**  376
*Abhishek Singh*

**Epidemiology of Campylobacteriosis and its Prevention and Control**  380
*Abhishek Singh*

**Epidemiology of Escherichia Coli Infection and its Prevention and Control**  382
*Abhishek Singh*

**C. Epidemiology of Soil Helminths and its Prevention and Control**
*Manoj Bansal, Dhiraj Kumar Srivastava, Ashok Mishra, Roopa M*

**Epidemiology of Dracunculiasis and its Prevention and Control**  385

**Epidemiology of Amoebiasis and its Prevention and Control**  387
*Dhiraj Kumar Srivastava*

**Epidemiology of Giardiasis and its Prevention and Control**  390

**Epidemiology of Ascariasis and its Prevention and Control**  392

**Epidemiology of Trichuriasis and its Prevention and Control**  394

**Epidemiology of Ancylostomiasis and its Prevention and Control**  396

**D. Epidemiology of Zoonotic Diseases and its Prevention and Control**  400
*Mohua Moitra, Shailee Vyas*
**Rabies Part:** *Ashok Mishra, Sasmita Mungi, Manoj Bansal, Priyesh Marskole*

**E. Epidemiology of Vector-Borne Diseases and its Prevention and Control**  420
*Rashmi Sharma*

**F. Epidemiology of Blood-Borne Diseases and its Prevention and Control**  459
*Abhik Sinha, Palash Das, Sukamal Bisoi, Dibakar Haldar*

**G. Epidemiology of Contact Diseases and its Prevention and Control**  471

**Epidemiology of HIV and its Prevention and Control**  471
*Mausumi Basu, Abhik Sinha, Mohua Moitra, Sukamal Bisoi*

**Epidemiology of Sexually Transmitted Diseases and its Prevention and Control**  485
*Abhishek Mishra, Neeraj Agarwal*

**Epidemiology of Leprosy and its Prevention and Control**  492
*Anku Moni Saikia, Kumaril Goswami*

**Epidemiology of Trachoma and its Prevention and Control**  501
*Anku Moni Saikia, Kumaril Goswami*

**Epidemiology of Tetanus and its Prevention and Control**  505
*Anku Moni Saikia, Kumaril Goswami*

**H. Epidemic Prone Diseases and Investigating the Outbreaks**  513
*Atul Trivedi, Rohit Ram*

I. Emerging and Re-Emerging Diseases of Global Importance  523

General Epidemiology of Emerging and Re-emerging Diseases and Public Health Action  523
*Venkatrao Epari, Jyotiranjan Sahoo*

Specific Epidemiology of Emerging Diseases  526
*Madhur Verma*

Coronavirus Induced Disease (COVID-19)  532
*Forhad Akhtar Zaman*

**18. General Epidemiology of Noncommunicable Diseases and its Prevention and Control ............... 536**
*Dinesh Kumar*

**19. Specific Epidemiology of Noncommunicable Diseases ................................................................. 541**

A. Epidemiology of Hypertension and Stroke and its Prevention and Control  541

Epidemiology and Prevention of Hypertension  541
*Anusha Rashmi, P Amritha Krishna, Varghese Iybu Chacko*

Epidemiology and Prevention of Stroke  546
*Anusha Rashmi, Varghese Iybu Chacko, P Amritha Krishna*

B. Epidemiology of Cardiovascular Diseases and its Prevention and Control  549

Epidemiology of Cardiovascular Diseases—Ischemic Heart Disease  549
*Ankeeta Menona Jacob, Nishanth Krishna K*

Epidemiology of Cardiovascular Diseases—Rheumatic Heart Disease  556
*Ekta Gupta*

C. Epidemiology of Diabetes Mellitus and its Prevention and Control  562
*Bhanu M*

D. Epidemiology of Cancer and its Prevention and Control  570
*DV Bala, Animesh Jain, Pracheth R*

E. Epidemiology of Injuries, Accidents and its Prevention and Control  587
*Shreyaswi Sathyanath M, Narayanan Namboothiri G, Jithin Daniel J*

F. Blindness  599
*Deepthi R, Manjula R, Shashi Kumar M*

G. Epidemiology of Chronic Obstructive Pulmonary Disease (COPD) and its Prevention and Control  604
*Sandeep Kumar Panigrahi, Venkatarao Epari*

**20. Primary Health Care Approach to Noncommunicable Diseases ................................... 609**
*Baridalyne Nongkynrih, Cherian Varghese*

**21. Screening for Noncommunicable Diseases ........... 617**
*Rizwan Suliankatchi Abdulkader, Kathiresan Jeyashree*

**22. Noncommunicable Disease Surveillance .............. 624**
*Roopa Shivashankar*

**23. Epidemiology of Nutrition and Food-related Diseases and its Prevention and Control ............... 628**

Epidemiology of Nutrition-Related Diseases and its Prevention  628
*Amir Maroof Khan, Paras Agarwal, Shveta Lukhmana, Charu Kohli*

Epidemiology of Food-Related Diseases and its Prevention  648
*Abhishek Singh*

**24. Reproductive Health and Family Welfare ............... 656**
*Pooja Goyal, Mitasha Singh, Shveta Lukhmana*

**25. Maternal Health ...................................................... 674**
*Pragti Chhabra*

**26. Child Health ............................................................ 685**
*Ravneet Kaur, Akhil Dhanesh Goel*

**27. Adolescent Health .................................................. 704**
*Shaili Vyas, Deepshikha, Rakesh Kakkar*

**28. Geriatric Health ...................................................... 711**
*Rakesh Kakkar, Gouri Sen Gupta*

**29. Occupational Health .............................................. 717**
*Pankaja Raghav, Manoj Kumar Gupta, Ankit Sheth*

**30. Mental Health ......................................................... 740**
*Harshal Ramesh Salve*

**31. Urban Health, Rural Health and Tribal Health ........ 746**

Urban Health  746
*Manish Rana, Harsh Bakshi, Anjali Modi, Priscilla Kayina, Gneyaa Bhatt, Madhurjya Baruah*

Rural Health  750

Tribal Health  752

**32. Traveler's Health ..................................................... 758**
*Yogita Bavaskar, Sumit Aggarwal, Alka Kaware, Manoj Talapalliwar, Poonam Sancheti*

**33. Genetics and Health ............................................... 764**
*Manju Toppo*

**34. Special Topics ......................................................... 773**

A. Climate Change and Health  773
*Praveen Kulkarni, Sunil Kumar D*

B. Disaster Management  778
*Jyotiranjan Sahoo, Venkatarao Epari*

C. Hospital-Acquired Infections and its Prevention and Control  783
*Jay K Sheth*

D. Biomedical Waste and its Management  788
*Ashok Mishra, Manoj Bansal, Sasmita Mungi, Priyesh Marskole*

E. Bioterrorism  794
*Ashok Mishra, Priyesh Marskole, Manoj Bansal, Sasmita Mungi*

## SECTION 4: COMMUNITY HEALTH MANAGEMENT

35. **Great Achievements in Community Medicine** ........ 803
    *Liaquat Roopesh Johnson*

36. **Global Health Situation** ............................................. 815
    *Prakash Patel*

37. **Community Health** ..................................................... 821
    *Manish Kumar Singh*

38. **Managing Community Health** ................................. 830
    *AM Kadri, Ankit Sheth, Anupam Banerjee*

39. **Healthcare Delivery System Across Nations** ........... 848
    *Rashmi Kundapur, Harshitha HN, Rahul Hegde*

40. **Human Resources for Health** ................................... 854
    *Sanjay Zodpey, Ritika Tiwari, Himanshu Negandhi*

41. **Health Financing** ........................................................ 859
    *Rashmi Kundapur, Sharon Baisal*

42. **Health Management** .................................................. 863
    A. Basics of Management   863
    *Bhavesh Modi, Rashmi Kundapur, Sudhir Prabhu H, Shreyaswi Sathyanath M, Manjula R, Pranay Jadav, Kapil Gandha*
    B. Health Planning   874
    *AM Kadri, Ankit Sheth, Nidhi Mangrola, Rajesh Chudasama, Bhavesh Modi*
    C. Managerial Skills   880
    *Rivu Basu, Sanjib Bandyopadhyay, Kaushik Mitra, Saikat Bhattacharya, Bhavesh Modi*
    D. Monitoring and Evaluation
    *Sumit Malhotra, Manya Prasad*
    E. Logistics and Finance Management   893
    *Kapil Gandha, Umed Patel, Niravkumar Joshi, Bhavesh Modi*

43. **International Healthcare Agencies** ......................... 899
    *Viral Dave, Venu Shah, Arpit Prajapati*

44. **Special Topics** ............................................................. 907
    A. International Classification of Diseases   907
    *Vaidehi S Gohil*
    B. Quality in Healthcare   911
    *Ruchi Juyal, Vidisha Vallabh*

    C. Health Economics   916
    *Abhik Sinha, Sukamal Bisoi*
    D. Health System Research   919
    *Pranab Chatterjee, Bhavna Seth, Abhimanyu Singh Chauhan*

## SECTION 5: MANAGING COMMUNITY HEALTH IN INDIA

45. **Health Situation in India** ........................................... 925
    *Prakash Patel*

46. **Indian Healthcare System** ........................................ 928
    *Kaushik Lodhiya, Dipesh Zalavadiya*

47. **Health Policies and Programs in India** ................... 953
    *Bratati Banerjee, Rupsa Banerjee, Bhargav Dave, Nidhi Mangrola, Ankit Sheth*

48. **Monitoring and Evaluation System in India** ......... 1034
    *Kedar Mehta, Paragkumar Chavda*

49. **Health Legislations in India** ................................... 1040
    *Priya Arora, Gurmeet Kaur*

50. **Indian Healthcare Agencies** ................................... 1058
    *Viral Dave, Venu Shah, Bhavik Rana, Arpit Prajapati*

51. **Special Topics** ........................................................... 1064
    A. Village Health and Nutrition Day: Planning and Preparedness   1064
    *Bharatkumar M Gohel*
    B. Cold Chain Management   1068
    *Hitesh M Shah, Darshan Mahyavanshi*
    C. Adverse Events Following Immunization and its Management at Community Level   1074
    *Nilesh Fichadiya, RB Jain*
    D. Medical Certification of Cause of Death, Maternal Death Surveillance and Response, Child Death Review   1079
    *Sudhir Prabhu H, Saurabh Kumar*
    E. Use of Information Technology in Community Health Care   1083
    *Pradeep Aggarwal, Rakesh Kakkar*
    F. Essential Medicines   1088
    *Anusha Rashmi*

*Index*                                                                1093

# Competency Table

## SUMMARY OF COMPETENCY CODES FOR COMMUNITY MEDICINE AS PER COMPETENCY-BASED MEDICAL EDUCATION (NMC)

| Code | Competency | Chapter Number |
|---|---|---|
| **Topic: Concept of Health and Disease** | | |
| CM1.1 | Define and describe the concept of Public Health (Community Medicine) | 2, 38 |
| CM1.2 | Define health; describe the concept of holistic health including concept of spiritual health and the relativeness and determinants of health | 3 |
| CM1.3 | Describe the characteristics of agent, host and environmental factors in health and disease and the multi factorial etiology of disease | 3 |
| CM1.4 | Describe and discuss the natural history of disease | 3, 8 |
| CM1.5 | Describe the application of interventions at various levels of prevention | 8 |
| CM1.6 | Describe and discuss the concepts, the principles of Health promotion and Education, IEC and Behavioral change communication (BCC) | 14 |
| CM1.7 | Enumerate and describe health indicators | 9, 37 |
| CM1.8 | Describe the Demographic profile of India and discuss its impact on health | 12 |
| CM1.9 | Demonstrate the role of effective Communication skills in health in a simulated environment | 14 |
| **Topic: Relationship of Social and Behavioral to Health and Disease** | | |
| CM2.1 | Describe the steps and perform clinico-socio-cultural and demographic assessment of the individual, family and community | 6 |
| CM2.2 | Describe the socio-cultural factors, family (types), its role in health and disease and demonstrate in a simulated environment the correct assessment of socio-economic status | 6 |
| CM2.3 | Describe and demonstrate in a simulated environment the assessment of barriers to good health and health seeking behavior | 6 |
| CM2.4 | Describe social psychology, community behavior and community relationship and their impact on health and disease | 6 |
| CM2.5 | Describe poverty and social security measures and its relationship to health and disease | 13 |
| **Topic: Environmental Health Problems** | | |
| CM3.1 | Describe the health hazards of air, water, noise, radiation and pollution | 7A, 7B, 7E, 34A |
| CM3.2 | Describe concepts of safe and wholesome water, sanitary sources of water, water purification processes, water quality standards, concepts of water conservation and rainwater harvesting | 7B |
| CM3.3 | Describe the etiology and basis of water borne diseases/jaundice/hepatitis/ diarrheal diseases | 17B |
| CM3.4 | Describe the concept of solid waste, human excreta and sewage disposal | 7C |
| CM3.5 | Describe the standards of housing and the effect of housing on health | 7G |

| | | |
|---|---|---|
| CM3.6 | Describe the role of vectors in the causation of diseases. Also discuss National Vector Borne Disease Control Program | 7H, 47 |
| CM3.7 | Identify and describe the identifying features and life cycles of vectors of Public Health importance and their control measures | 7H |
| CM3.8 | Describe the mode of action, application cycle of commonly used insecticides and rodenticides | 7H |
| **Topic: Principles of Health Promotion and Education** | | |
| CM4.1 | Describe various methods of health education with their advantages and limitations | 14 |
| CM4.2 | Describe the methods of organizing health promotion and education and counselling activities at individual family and community settings | 14 |
| CM4.3 | Demonstrate and describe the steps in evaluation of health promotion and education program | 48 |
| **Topic: Nutrition** | | |
| CM5.1 | Describe the common sources of various nutrients and special nutritional requirements according to age, sex, activity, physiological conditions | 4 |
| CM5.2 | Describe and demonstrate the correct method of performing a nutritional assessment of individuals, families and the community by using the appropriate method | 23 |
| CM5.3 | Define and describe common nutrition related health disorders (including macro-PEM, Micro-iron, Zn, iodine vitamin A), their control and management | 23 |
| CM5.4 | Plan and recommend a suitable diet for the individuals and families based on local availability of foods and economic status, etc. in a simulated environment | 4 |
| CM5.5 | Describe the methods of nutritional surveillance, principles of nutritional education and rehabilitation in the context of socio-cultural factors | 23 |
| CM5.6 | Enumerate and discuss the National Nutrition Policy, important national nutritional Programs including the Integrated Child Development Services Scheme (ICDS), etc. | 47 |
| CM5.7 | Describe food hygiene | 17B |
| CM5.8 | Describe and discuss the importance and methods of food fortification and effects of additives and adulteration | 23 |
| **Topic: Basic Statistics and its Applications** | | |
| CM6.1 | Formulate a research question for a study | 11 |
| CM6.2 | Describe and discuss the principles and demonstrate the methods of collection, classification, analysis, interpretation and presentation of statistical data | 11 |
| CM6.3 | Describe, discuss and demonstrate the application of elementary statistical methods including test of significance in various study designs | 11 |
| CM6.4 | Enumerate, discuss and demonstrate Common sampling techniques, simple statistical methods, frequency distribution, measures of central tendency and dispersion | 11 |
| **Topic: Epidemiology** | | |
| CM7.1 | Define Epidemiology and describe and enumerate the principles, concepts and uses | 9 |
| CM7.2 | Enumerate, describe and discuss the modes of transmission and measures for prevention and control of communicable and non-communicable diseases | 16, 17, 18, 19 |
| CM7.3 | Enumerate, describe and discuss the sources of epidemiological data | 11 |
| CM7.4 | Define, calculate and interpret morbidity and mortality indicators based on given set of data | 9 |

## Competency Table

| | | |
|---|---|---|
| CM7.5 | Enumerate, define, describe and discuss epidemiological study designs | 10 |
| CM7.6 | Enumerate and evaluate the need of screening tests | 8 |
| CM7.7 | Describe and demonstrate the steps in the Investigation of an epidemic of communicable disease and describe the principles of control measures | 17H |
| CM7.8 | Describe the principles of association, causation and biases in epidemiological studies | 10 |
| CM7.9 | Describe and demonstrate the application of computers in epidemiology | 11, 51E |
| **Topic: Epidemiology of Communicable and Non-communicable Diseases** | | |
| CM8.1 | Describe and discuss the epidemiological and control measures including the use of essential laboratory tests at the primary care level for communicable diseases | 16, 17, 32 |
| CM8.2 | Describe and discuss the epidemiological and control measures including the use of essential laboratory tests at the primary care level for non-communicable diseases (diabetes, Hypertension, Stroke, obesity and cancer etc.) | 18, 19, 21 |
| CM8.3 | Enumerate and describe disease specific National Health Programs including their prevention and treatment of a case | 47 |
| CM8.4 | Describe the principles and enumerate the measures to control a disease epidemic | 17B, 17H |
| CM8.5 | Describe and discuss the principles of planning, implementing and evaluating control measures for disease at community level bearing in mind the public health importance of the disease | 17B, 20, 48 |
| CM8.6 | Educate and train health workers in disease surveillance, control and treatment and health education | 17E, 22 |
| CM8.7 | Describe the principles of management of information systems | 48, 51E |
| **Topic: Demography and Vital Statistics** | | |
| CM9.1 | Define and describe the principles of Demography, Demographic cycle, Vital statistics | 12 |
| CM9.2 | Define, calculate and interpret demographic indices including birth rate, death rate, fertility rates | 12 |
| CM9.3 | Enumerate and describe the causes of declining sex ratio and its social and health implications | 12 |
| CM9.4 | Enumerate and describe the causes and consequences of population explosion and population dynamics of India. | 12, 24 |
| CM9.5 | Describe the methods of population control | 24 |
| CM9.6 | Describe the National Population Policy | 47 |
| CM9.7 | Enumerate the sources of vital statistics including census, SRS, NFHS, NSSO, etc. | 12, 48 |
| **Topic: Reproductive Maternal and Child Health** | | |
| CM10.1 | Describe the current status of Reproductive, maternal, newborn and Child Health | 24, 25, 26, 45 |
| CM10.2 | Enumerate and describe the methods of screening high risk groups and common health problems | 21, 25, 26 |
| CM10.3 | Describe local customs and practices during pregnancy, childbirth, lactation and child feeding practices | 25, 26 |
| CM10.4 | Describe the reproductive, maternal, newborn & child health (RMCH); child survival and safe motherhood interventions | 47 |
| CM10.5 | Describe Universal Immunization Program; Integrated Management of Neonatal and Childhood Illness (IMNCI) and other existing Programs. | 26, 47 |
| CM10.6 | Enumerate and describe various family planning methods, their advantages and shortcomings | 24 |

| | | |
|---|---|---|
| CM10.7 | Enumerate and describe the basis and principles of the Family Welfare Program including the organization, technical and operational aspects | 47 |
| CM10.8 | Describe the physiology, clinical management and principles of adolescent health including ARSH | 27 |
| **Topic: Occupational Health** | | |
| CM11.1 | Enumerate and describe the presenting features of patients with occupational illness including agriculture | 29 |
| CM11.2 | Describe the role, benefits and functioning of the employee's state insurance scheme | 49 |
| CM11.3 | Enumerate and describe specific occupational health hazards, their risk factors and preventive measures | 29 |
| CM11.4 | Describe the principles of ergonomics in health preservation | 29 |
| CM11.5 | Describe occupational disorders of health professionals and their prevention & management | 34C |
| **Topic: Geriatric Services** | | |
| CM12.1 | Define and describe the concept of Geriatric services | 28 |
| CM12.2 | Describe health problems of aged population | 28 |
| CM12.3 | Describe the prevention of health problems of aged population | 28 |
| CM12.4 | Describe National program for elderly | 47 |
| **Topic: Disaster Management** | | |
| CM13.1 | Define and describe the concept of Disaster management | 34B |
| CM13.2 | Describe disaster management cycle | 34B |
| CM13.3 | Describe man-made disasters in the world and in India | 34B |
| CM13.4 | Describe the details of the National Disaster management Authority | 34B |
| **Topic: Hospital Waste Management** | | |
| CM14.1 | Define and classify hospital waste | 34D |
| CM14.2 | Describe various methods of treatment of hospital waste | 34D |
| CM14.3 | Describe laws related to hospital waste management | 34D |
| **Topic: Mental Health** | | |
| CM15.1 | Define and describe the concept of mental Health | 30 |
| CM15.2 | Describe warning signals of mental health disorder | 30 |
| CM15.3 | Describe National Mental Health program | 47 |
| **Topic: Health Planning and Management** | | |
| CM16.1 | Define and describe the concept of Health planning | 42 |
| CM16.2 | Describe planning cycle | 42 |
| CM16.3 | Describe Health management techniques | 42 |
| CM16.4 | Describe health planning in India and National policies related to health and health planning | 47 |

| | | |
|---|---|---|
| **Topic: Health Care of the Community** | | |
| CM17.1 | Define and describe the concept of health care to community | 37 |
| CM17.2 | Describe community diagnosis | 9, 37, 38 |
| CM17.3 | Describe primary health care, its components and principles | 38 |
| CM17.4 | Describe National policies related to health and health planning and millennium development goals | 38, 47 |
| CM17.5 | Describe health care delivery in India | 46 |
| **Topic: International Health** | | |
| CM18.1 | Define and describe the concept of international health | 32, 43 |
| CM18.2 | Describe roles of various international health agencies | 43 |
| **Topic: Essential Medicine** | | |
| CM19.1 | Define and describe the concept of Essential Medicine List (EML) | 51F |
| CM19.2 | Describe roles of essential medicine in primary health care | 51F |
| CM19.3 | Describe counterfeit medicine and its prevention | 51F |
| **Topic: Recent Advances in Community Medicine** | | |
| CM20.1 | List important public health events of last five years | 17I |
| CM20.2 | Describe various issues during outbreaks and their prevention | 35 |
| CM20.3 | Describe any event important to Health of the Community | 35 |

# PLATE 1

**Punjabi Bagh, New Delhi**

| Day | Subindex | | | | | | | | | AQI |
|---|---|---|---|---|---|---|---|---|---|---|
| | CO (min) | CO (max) | $O_3$ (min) | $O_3$ (max) | $NO_2$ | $NH_3$ | $SO_2$ | PM2.5 | PM10 | |
| 10–Nov–13 | 41 | 96 | 13 | 64 | 67 | 12 | 12 | 371 | 294 | 371 |
| 11–Nov–13 | 52 | 105 | 22 | 68 | 76 | 9 | 15 | 320 | 272 | 320 |
| 12–Nov–13 | 44 | 114 | 15 | 76 | 93 | 11 | 12 | 384 | 390 | 390 |
| 13–Nov–13 | 43 | 114 | 9 | 79 | 91 | 13 | 15 | 407 | 406 | 407 |
| 14–Nov–13 | 37 | 110 | 11 | 68 | 90 | 10 | 13 | 335 | 306 | 335 |

PM10 and PM2.5 = particulate matter less than 10 microns and 2.5 microns respectively

**Fig. 7A.4:** Subindices of air quality index.

| Good (0–50) | Satisfactory (51–100) | Moderately polluted (101–200) | Poor (201–300) | Very poor (301–400) | Severe (> 400) |

**Fig. 7A.5:** Color categories of air quality index.

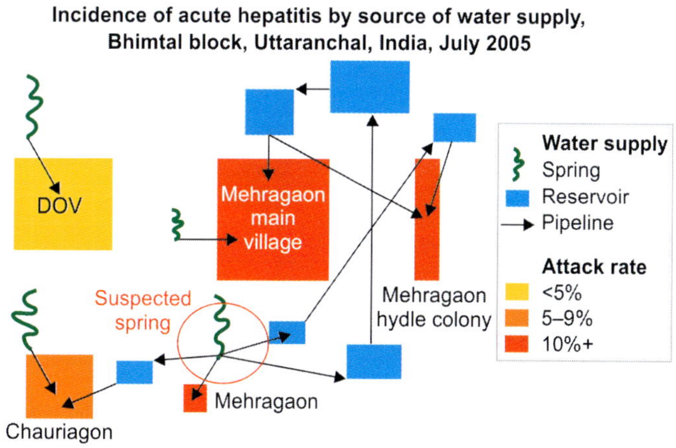

### Incidence of acute hepatitis by source of water supply, Bhimtal block, Uttaranchal, India, July 2005

**Water supply**
- Spring
- Reservoir
- Pipeline

**Attack rate**
- <5%
- 5–9%
- 10%+

DOV, Mehragaon main village, Suspected spring, Mehragaon hydle colony, Mehragaon, Chauriagon

**Fig. 10.6:** Classic example of place distribution of a disease outbreak in India.

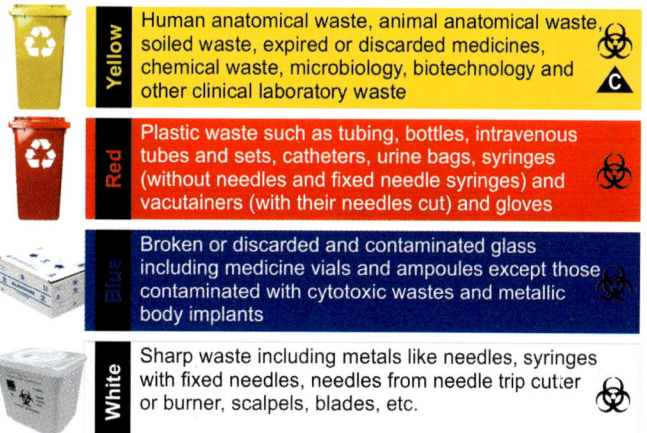

**Yellow:** Human anatomical waste, animal anatomical waste, soiled waste, expired or discarded medicines, chemical waste, microbiology, biotechnology and other clinical laboratory waste

**Red:** Plastic waste such as tubing, bottles, intravenous tubes and sets, catheters, urine bags, syringes (without needles and fixed needle syringes) and vacutainers (with their needles cut) and gloves

**Blue:** Broken or discarded and contaminated glass including medicine vials and ampoules except those contaminated with cytotoxic wastes and metallic body implants

**White:** Sharp waste including metals like needles, syringes with fixed needles, needles from needle trip cutter or burner, scalpels, blades, etc.

**Fig. 34D.1:** Segregation of biomedical waste as per BMW Rules 2016.

# PLATE 2

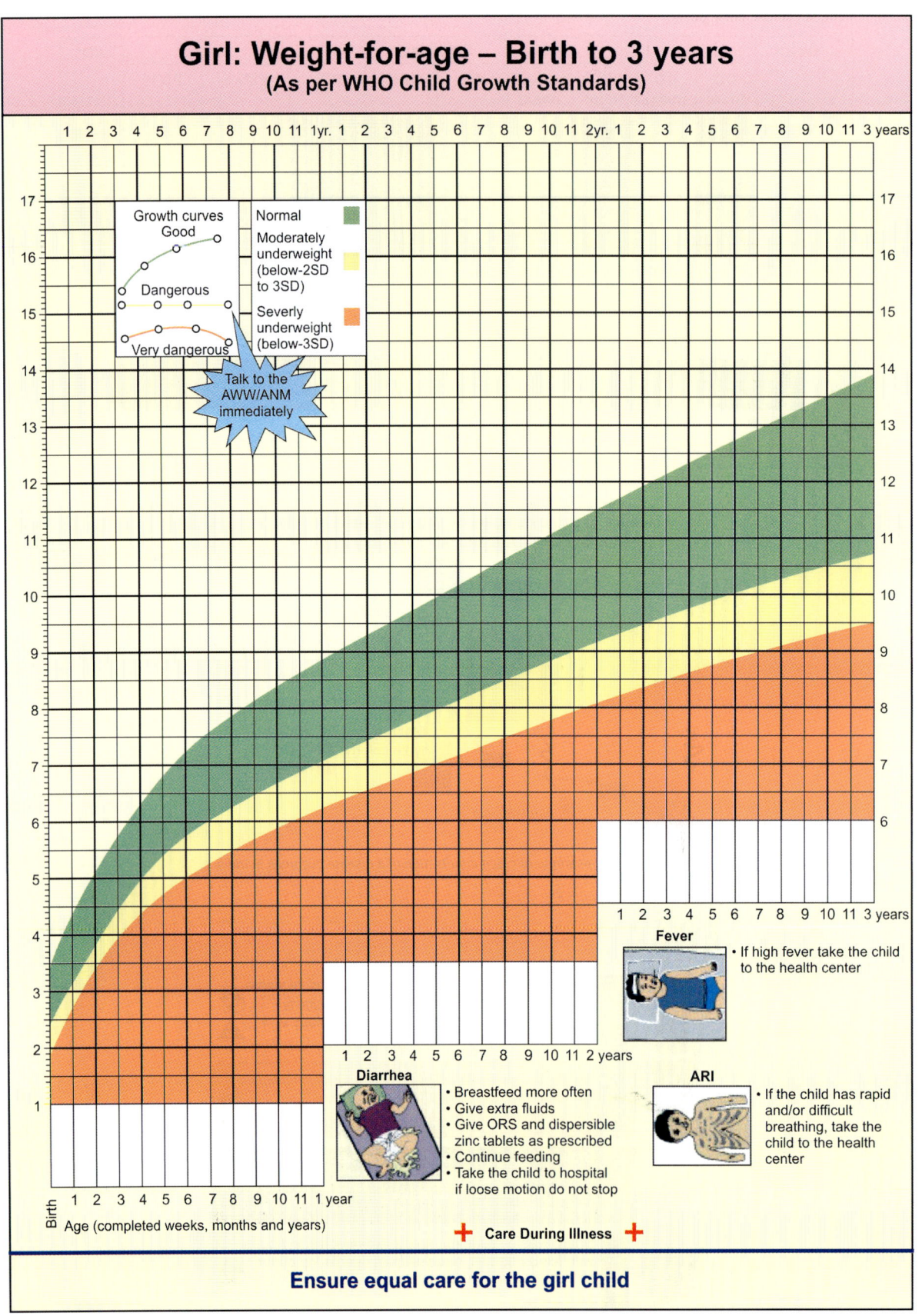

Fig. 26.9A

# PLATE 3

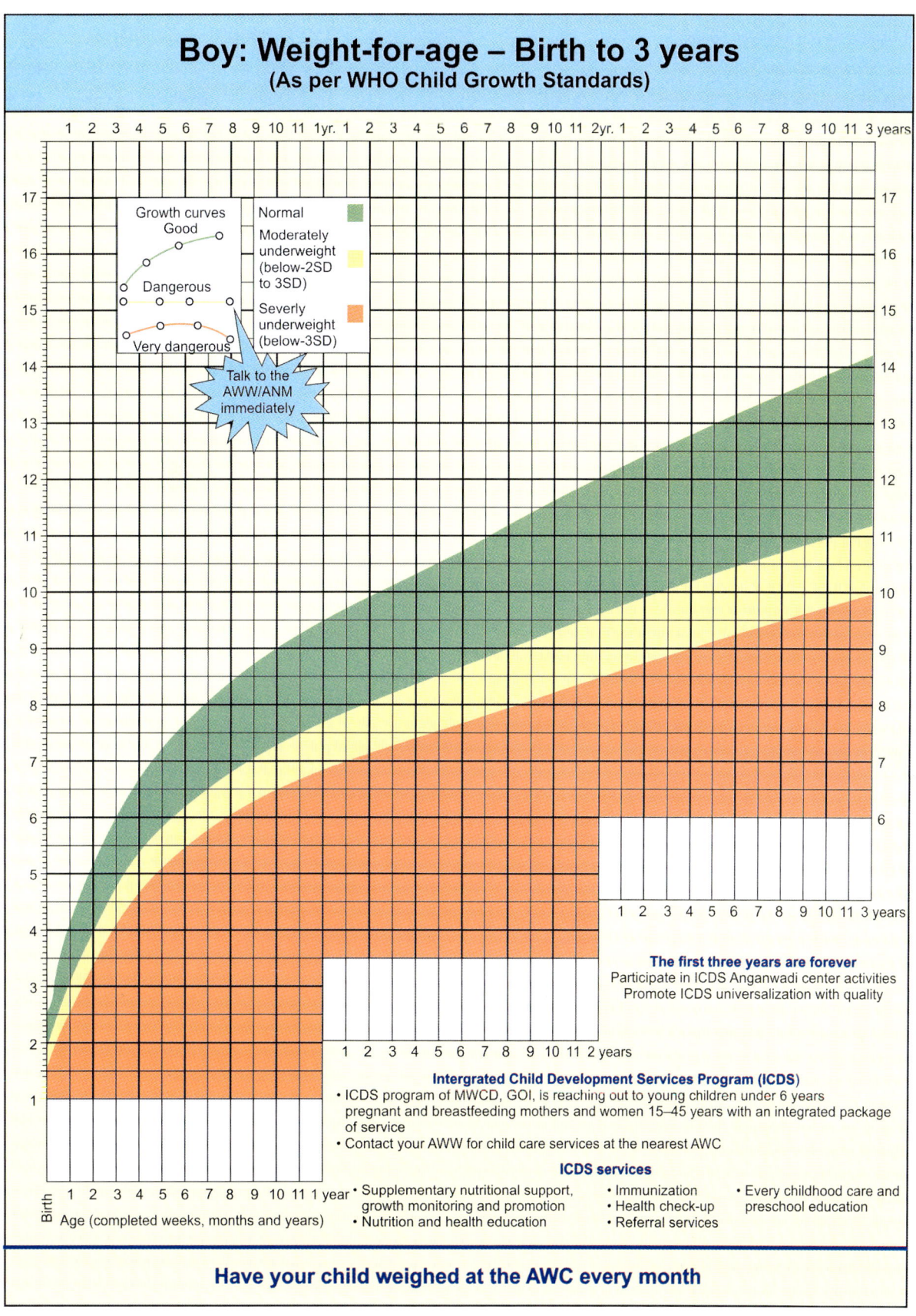

**Fig. 26.9B**

**Figs. 26.9A and B:** Growth chart.

# PLATE 4

**Table 38.7:** Performance of SDG3 by indicators, India.

**SDG3—Good health and well-being**

| Indicator | Value | Year | Dashboard | Trend |
|---|---|---|---|---|
| Maternal mortality rate (per 100,000 live births) | 102.7 | 2020 | 🟡 | ↑ |
| Neonatal mortality rate (per 1,000 live births) | 19.1 | 2021 | 🔴 | ↑ |
| Mortality rate, under-5 (per 1,000 live births) | 30.6 | 2021 | 🟡 | ↑ |
| Incidence of tuberculosis (per 100,000 population) | 210.0 | 2021 | 🔴 | → |
| New HIV infections (per 1,000 uninfected population) | 0.1 | 2021 | 🟢 | ↑ |
| Age-standardized death rate due to cardiovascular disease, cancer, diabetes, or chronic respiratory disease in adults aged 30–70 years | 21.9 | 2019 | 🟠 | → |
| Age-standardized death rate attributable to household air pollution and ambient air pollution (per 100,000 population) | 139.3 | 2019 | 🟠 | ⚫ |
| Traffic deaths (per 100,000 population) | 15.6 | 2019 | 🟠 | → |
| Life expectancy at birth (years) | 70.8 | 2019 | 🟠 | ↗ |
| Adolescent fertility rate (births per 1,000 females aged 15–19) | 12.2 | 2018 | 🟢 | ⚫ |
| Births attended by skilled health personnel (%) | 89.4 | 2021 | 🔴 | ↑ |
| Surviving Infants who received 2 WHO-recommended vaccines (%) | 85 | 2021 | 🟡 | → |
| Universal health coverage (UHC) index of service coverage (worst 0–100 best) | 61 | 2019 | 🟠 | ↗ |
| Subjective well-being (average ladder score, worst 0–10 best) | 3.9 | 2022 | 🔴 | ↓ |

Dashboards: 🟢 SDG achieved  🟡 Challenges remain  🟠 Significant challenges remain  🔴 Major challenges remain  ⚫ Information unavailable

Trends: ↑ On track or maintaining SDG achievement  ↗ Moderately improving  → Stagnating  ↓ Decreasing  •• Trend information unavailable

# Prologue

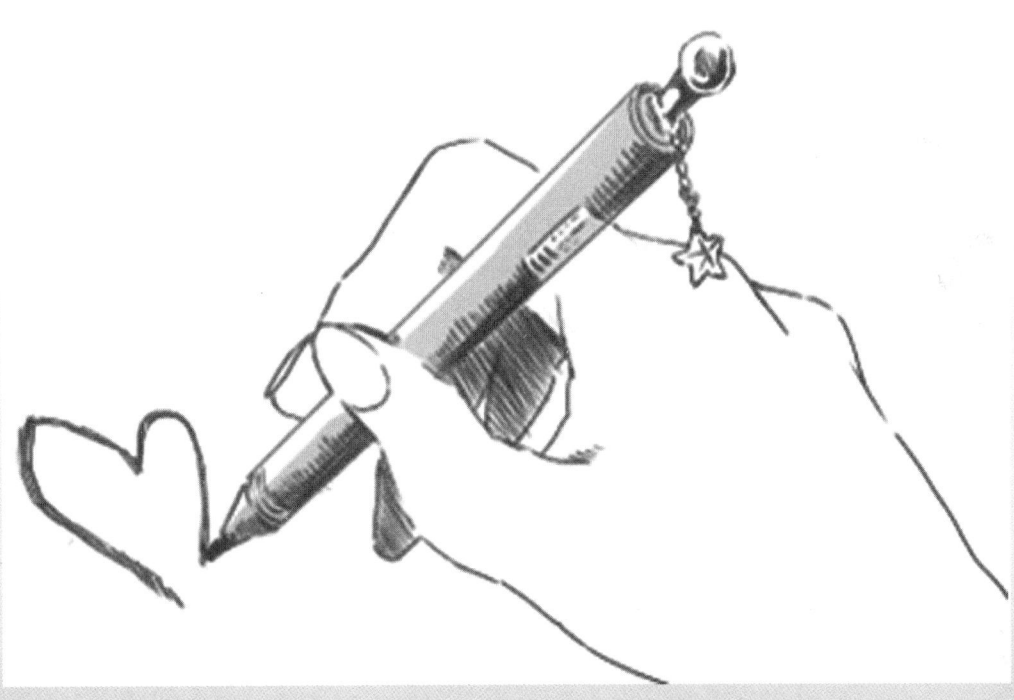

# SECTION OUTLINE

1. Story of the Upstream
2. Community Medicine: An Introduction

# CHAPTER 1

# Story of the Upstream

*AM Kadri*

This is a story of small country, blessed with numerous beautiful mountains and rivers. A story about villages and towns with people living happily with blessed nature all around.

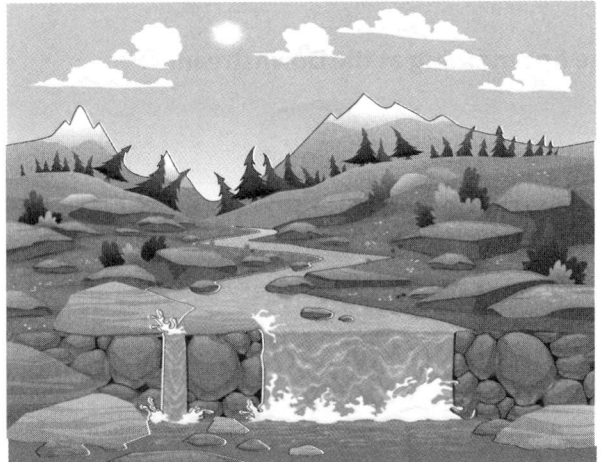

### At the Downstream...

One day, few people living in a village situated at downstream of a river, were going to their farms. They saw a person drowning in the river. One of them, who happened to be a good swimmer immediately jumped into river and whisked him out. They were happy for their good deed.

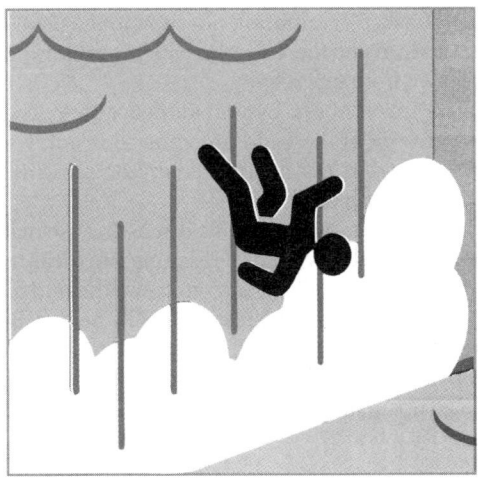

After a few days, these villagers again saw someone drowning in the river, while they were going to their farms. One of the villagers, again a good swimmer, jumped in, to save them. Soon he realized that not one, but three persons were drowning, of whom, he could save only two. One unfortunate was drowned into deep of water. Still villagers were happy that at least they could save two of them.

After few days, the incident got repeated. Villagers again found few more persons were getting drowned. This time, more villagers jumped in the river to save the people. In spite of greater rescuing efforts by villagers, they could not save all lives. The villagers mourned the loss of lives, and were satisfied that at least they could save few lives, if not all.

Over the time, such incidences continued to recur and the villagers used to put all their hard efforts to save as many people as they could during each such recurrence.

### The Story Continued...

The leaders and government of that country come to know about such frequent unfortunate incidents in that village and soon the authorities swung into action. A team of qualified and trained rescuers were deployed at the riverbank and with their help, the rate of saving lives improved.

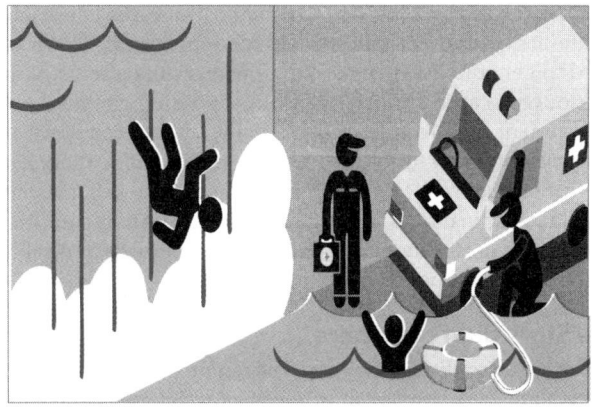

All were happy, government, leaders, people, including those who were saved.

Yet, few casualties continued, and especially during the monsoons, when the torrent of river was getting wild, deaths due to drowning, escalated. To reduce these losses, the government deployed more well equipped teams, provided equipment and other aids to facilitate rescuing.

## Some Other Places at Downstream in the Country...

This was not happening in isolation. Many other villages situated at the downstream frequently reported similar cases of mishap, demanding scaling up of efforts across all such places by the government.

## Efforts Escalated up...

With escalating of efforts, the government soon learnt that apart from drowning, many people got injured and many survivors were developing disabilities or illnesses due to the trauma underwent during drowning. Following this, the rescue operations were now having added facilities of ambulance and services of a qualified medical team and established medical care centers near rescue sites to attend to all possible medical eventualities.

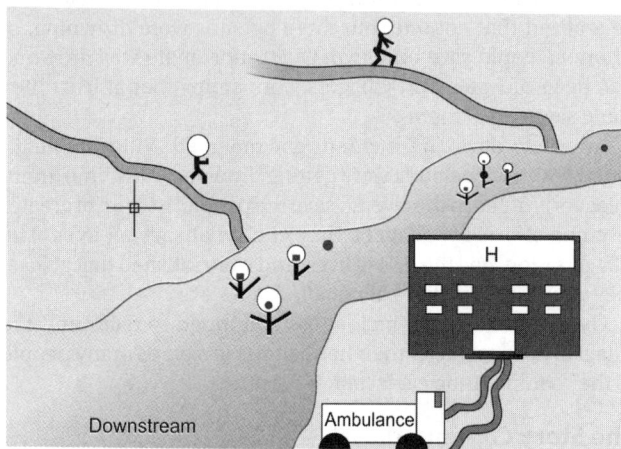

With the increase in the frequency and number of drowning cases, there was a lack in the availability of qualified/trained rescuers as well as medical/paramedical personnel. Hence, institutes and training centers were established to prepare a trained cadre of medical/para medical personnel. Soon, to improve the quality of rescue and medical care, the latest state-of-the-art equipment and devices were procured. There was need to generate finances to fund these arrangements. Being a resource scarce country, to meet the rising expenses, the government mobilized funds internally, by slashing down the budget earmarked for other activities such as education, road and infrastructure development, citizen welfare schemes, etc. With increase in efforts and resource allocations they could save more lives if not all and better managed the injured and disabled which they could not do in the past.

## The Story didn't end here....

The situation continued for years. The requirement of budget kept on escalating year by year affecting the developmental activities of the country. It was worrisome situation, but government was deep in the rescuing and managing the injured. Government was riding high in applauding self for establishing a well operational system, equipped with advanced equipment and modern methods in managing these casualties at downstream.

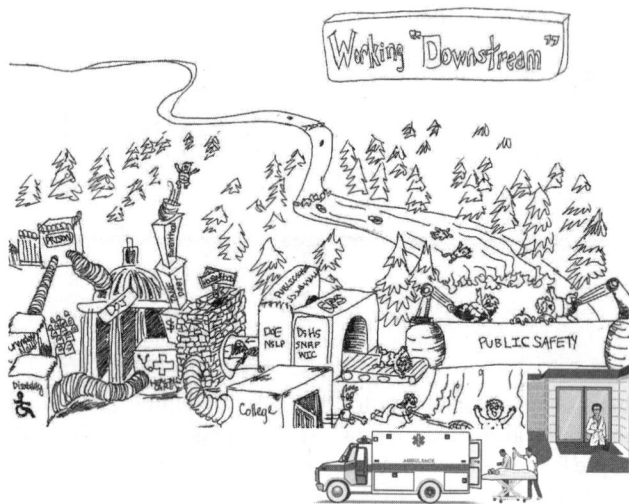

## One fine morning at the Downstream...

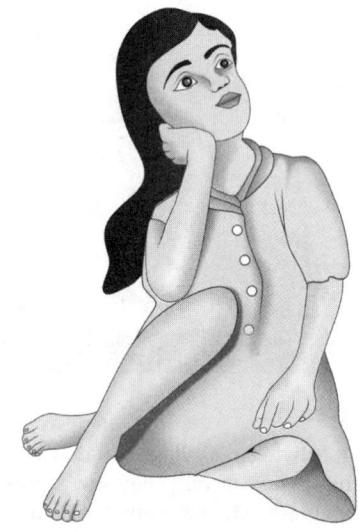

One child playing near river bank every day, curiously watching the rescue operation and management of injured people by medical team, asked an innocent question to the team engaged in it, "What is wrong up there so as to which, so many people are drowning down from upstream?"

They were taken aback by the sudden query. They stood speechless in front of the child for some time and went away quietly. Engrossed in rescue and rehabilitation work, such a thought had never occurred to them.

Most of the team members, while discussing the matter over dinner time, opined that quality rescuing, medical relief and rehabilitation were the definite ways to casualties and dismissed the child's query, as a useless question by silly person. But few of them were not in agreement with them.

Moved by the child's reflective question, few of the members decided to go upstream and get answer for it.

# Chapter 1: Story of the Upstream

## The Journey to Upstream...

The cynics tried to dissuade the visiting team, many got mad at them, some warned them, while the rest told not to waste time. They even warned them, if they would derelict their duties of rescuing and medical care, it would be disservice to the country and harming the interest of people. But without getting distracted by these arguments the team of small moved up. They were determined to be focused in reaching to the root of the problem. They visited few places upstream and found...

There were many small villages at upstream and people living there had to cross rivers daily for routine requirements like, visiting their farms, home purchase, attending schools trade related activities, etc. There were very few bridges and many were in old, dilapidated and dangerous condition. Many of villagers fell down while crossing these broken bridges. At few places bridge like arrangements were made by tying ropes between two banks. Also at many places; there were no bridges. In such cases, villagers were crossing rivers from 'identified points'. Few of them were using unstable raft like structures to cross the river. Peoples lipped from the rocks or lost balance and hence suffered fall into the river. There were also cases of the rafts getting upturned. Those who needed to venture out more frequently to tend to the daily needs and the old and infirm, pregnant women and kids were more at risk. Incidents of drowning were increasing during rainy seasons due to increase in the winds and flow of the water.

They also found more or less, the similar conditions prevailed in all upstream locates, wherever frequent drowning of people was reported.

## Working at the Upstream

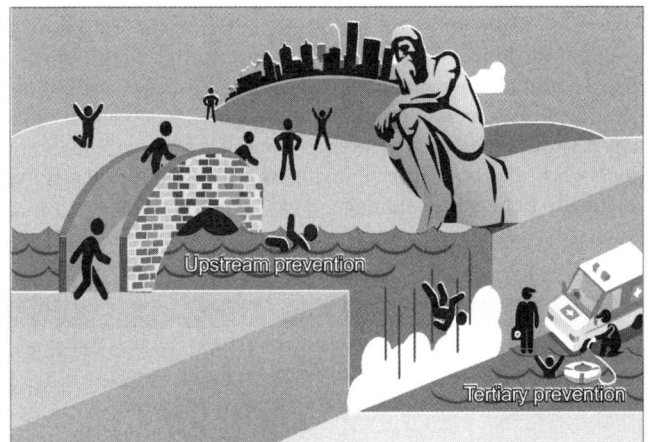

The group of like minded people initiated awareness generation programmes, motivating people to use safety precautions while crossing rivers and avoid the use of dilapidated bridges and risky short cuts to cross the river. They identified the 'danger' points and marked them with placards, to prevent people from venturing into river especially during rainy seasons. They held dialogues with the government authorities and convinced them to repair the broken bridges and spend on building new bridges to meet the routine requirement to villagers living at upstream areas.

## Fruits of Works at Upstream

Next year, as much as 90% reduction was recorded in the cases for drowning in villages at downstream. Encouraged by the positive results, the authorities built bridges at upstream on as many rivers as it could. With increased transportation and diligence on the part of the people in villages upstream, all the rescue and medical centres at downstream reported reduction in load of drowning, injuries and death. The need to create more rescue and medical care centres and buy costlier equipment was no more a priority. Instead, the money saved was used for other development activities to increase the happiness and prosperity quotient of the country.

**This happened only after 'SOMEONE' decided to look and act at the 'UPSTREAM'.**

Post script Nuggets: Refocusing at upstream

**Richest of rich countries cannot afford to keep on building hospitals ignoring the factors leading to increase in diseases and early deaths.**

*******

**Clinical care at hospital is like working at the downstream, while Community health care is about working at the upstream for prevention of diseases and early deaths.**

**Dr AM Kadri**
*Editor-in-chief*
(Adapted from a story told by Irving Zola, a medical sociologist, as cited by McKinlay, John B in "A case for refocusing upstream: The political economy of illness." In Conrad and Kern, The Sociology of Health and Illness: Critical Perspectives.)

*******

# CHAPTER 2

# Community Medicine: An Introduction

*Core Committee IAPSM*

## CONCEPT

Around 10,000 years ago seeds of civilization were sown. As a result, human beings became more organized, disciplined, and dependent on each other. Humans got connected with each other and were known as a community, i.e. a group of people living together and sharing possessions and responsibilities. Human thinking gradually became more community oriented. Individualistic issues like water, food, shelter, education, trade to law and order started to be viewed in community context. Systems developed for progress and protection norms, rules and guidelines, and formal and informal institutions. This evolution continued with advancement of knowledge and technology. Medical science also evolved in its outlook from only curing individuals to providing community care. Community medicine as a specialized branch of medical science is the outcome of this quest.

## DEFINITION AND SCOPE OF COMMUNITY MEDICINE

Community medicine, public health, and preventive and social medicine have a common goal of improving health of the community. Indian Association of Preventive and Social Medicine (IAPSM) has defined community medicine as *"a science and art of promoting health, preventing diseases and prolonging life by range of interventions (promotive, preventive, curative, rehabilitative, and palliative) in close partnership or association with healthcare delivery system and with active community participation and intersectoral coordination".*

Individual's health is largely related not only with its biological constitution, but is also influenced by other determinants such as environment, nutrition, social factors, as well as behavior and healthcare services. These determinants become more relevant when they are linked to the health of entire community. The scope of community medicine includes working in partnership with other stakeholders with the aim of *"improving the health of people living in a defined community".* The interventions could be applied in community, workplace or hospital.

## COMMUNITY MEDICINE PRACTICE: A MULTIDISCIPLINARY APPROACH

Community medicine practitioners require to act beyond the medical domain/health sector and should have an understanding about other related disciplines. IAPSM has categorized various subdisciplines related to community medicine in three groups **(Table 2.1)**.

Need and relevance as well as level of understanding and skills required in both the categories are described below.

### Core Disciplines

#### Epidemiology

Epidemiology is defined as *"the study of the distribution and determinants of health-related states or events in specified populations, and the application of this study to the control of health problem"*. Community medicine specialists use epidemiological skills to know the community health needs, disease burden, identify risk factors, association and attribution in health outcomes, dynamics of disease transmission, and assess the effectiveness of interventions. Clinical epidemiology deals with diagnostic, prognostic, and therapeutic decisions relating to patient care management.

**Table 2.1:** Subdisciplines related to community medicine.

| Category | Subdisciplines |
|---|---|
| A. Core disciplines | Epidemiology, basic clinical sciences, and healthcare delivery system including primary healthcare |
| B. Critically allied disciplines | Biostatistics, social and behavioral sciences, environmental health, health management, and public health nutrition |
| C. Other related disciplines | Occupational health, medical entomology, health economics, public health engineering, research methodology, public health laws and ethics, documentation and communication, information technology, health informatics and health technology assessment, etc. |

### Basic Clinical Science

Community medicine specialists are expected to be experts in primary healthcare and require to be equipped with skills in providing basic clinical care. Involvement in basic clinical care helps community medicine specialists in developing better epidemiological understanding of health problems and greater skills for their effective community management.

### Healthcare Delivery System

Community medicine experts work in partnership or close association with the healthcare delivery system. A good understanding of the availability, accessibility, affordability, acceptability, and organization and functioning of healthcare delivery system (both public and private); along with good understanding of healthcare providers and their role in managing community health. Primary healthcare, including universal healthcare are important approaches for delivering preventive, promotive, and primary clinical care. Also, various health programs and schemes covering community at a large or specific groups of the community are important areas under healthcare delivery system.

## Critically Allied Disciplines

### Health Management

Community-based interventions are applied on large scale and require higher resources in terms of finance, equipment, materials, and human resource with varied capacity and skills. If these resources are not properly managed (planned, organized, monitored, and evaluated) and the team members are not properly led (directed, supervised, monitored, and motivated), their effectiveness and efficiency will be hampered. Hence, community medicine practitioners should have a good understanding of management science and its application in healthcare setting.

### Social and Behavioral Sciences

Health and social development are interdependent. Effective community and health action can happen only when social and cultural aspects of the community are recognized and respected. Various social determinants such as nutrition, safe drinking water, shelter, and proper sanitation are well-established factors affecting health outcomes. All these factors are indirectly influenced by economic conditions, educational level, politico-legal environment, social support and security mechanism in the society, peace and harmony, political stability, etc. Community medicine specialists should facilitate in improvement of these social determinants through intersectoral coordination and policy advocacy with various stakeholders including policy makers at local, state, and national level.

Human behavior influences the risk of occurrence of the diseases. Health literacy, custom, and culture influence health-related belief and behaviors of the community. Discouraging unhealthy habits and promoting healthy behavior are two important aspects of community medicine practice. To achieve this, community medicine practitioners are required to equip themselves with knowledge of the factors influencing the individual and community health behavior and apply communication skills for behavior change in the community.

### Environmental Health

The importance of environmental factors in human health has been recognized since antiquity. Hippocrates (1950), in his classical writing *"On airs, waters and places"* emphasized the relevance of environment to human health. Health of the people is greatly influenced by environment surrounding them. Environment is home for numerous pathogens and vectors, where they can stay, grow, and multiply. Thus, they can facilitate the transmission of pathogen/disease from one person to another. Besides this, pollution of air, water, and soil can have adverse impact on health. Meteorological parameters such as temperature, humidity, air velocity, etc. impact the health directly by affecting the comfort zone and indirectly by influencing survival, multiplication, and transmission of pathogens or vectors.

Community medicine specialists identify the adverse environmental factors and act accordingly with other related departments such as public health engineering, water supply and sanitation, animal husbandry and pollution control board, etc. to protect the health of the community against ill effects of pollutants, pathogens, and vectors.

### Biostatistics

Statistics is defined as *"a method of collecting, organizing, analyzing, and interpreting the numerical data".* Biostatistics deals with data relating to living organism and other health sciences. Biostatistics along with research methodology is an important allied discipline for community medicine and is concerned with identifying health needs/issues and factors influencing the health. It helps to define the limits of normality [blood pressure, serum creatinine, height, body mass index (BMI), etc.] of various parameters of human body. Central tendency, standard deviation, test of significance, correlation, regression, mathematical modeling, etc. are some of the key statistics principles and methods used in community medicine practice.

### Public Health Nutrition

Nutrition is a major determinant of health. Nutritional needs of young children are as important as their emotional and social needs. Nutrition behavior regarding food selection, preparation and consumption is the product of culture, education, economics, food availability, social strata, family position, and health status. There exists a strong association between family income and the growth and cognitive development of children. Improved nutrition and environmental conditions can modify the effects of early undernutrition. Community medicine expert identifies nutrition-related knowledge, habits, and nutritional status of the community and carries out the following functions:
- Increasing awareness about nutrition and inculcating healthy dietary habits.

- Facilitating improvement of nutritional status by coordination with various sectors concerned with food production, distribution, supplementation, fortification, and food safety.
- Nutritional assessment and surveillance, screening of vulnerable population, and nutritional rehabilitation.

### Other Related Disciplines

There are many other disciplines which are related with community medicine practice as shown in **Table 2.1**. List of related disciplines may vary as per the prevailing community health issues and it may change from time to time. Community medicine experts need to acquire conceptual knowledge and understanding of these disciplines to discharge their functions effectively.

## FUNCTIONS OF COMMUNITY MEDICINE SPECIALIST

Whereas, conventional clinical specialist's role is confined to a hospital, the scope of a community medicine specialist extends from a clinic to the community to provide preventive, promotive, curative, rehabilitative, and palliative healthcare. He performs his duties in various capacities and combinations of one or more of these at a time as a clinician, epidemiologist, researcher, team leader, health consultant/manager, and an effective communicator as shown in **Figure 2.1**. He should be committed to professional excellence, be ethical, responsive, and accountable to patients and community.

Specific duties and responsibilities of a community medicine specialist are as follows:
- ***Identify and prioritize health needs of the defined community***: Identifying the health needs and knowing the magnitude of a problem forms the first step in community medicine practice. Once community health needs and health problems are identified and prioritized based on their impact on health of the community, only selective health needs and problems can be dealt at a time due to availability of limited resources. Knowledge and skills of epidemiological methods, research methodology, and biostatistics are essential in identifying and prioritizing health needs.
- ***Identify the (direct and indirect) determinants influencing health and diseases***: Health and disease are multifactorial in nature and have several determinants other than biological or medical factors contributing directly or indirectly to the chain of causation. To prevent the occurrence of disease and promote health, community medicine practitioners are required to identify various determinants influencing health outcomes.
- ***Prioritize and undertake the interventions to address the health needs and health determinants of the defined community***: Once a community diagnosis is made, i.e. identification and prioritization of health needs, health problems, and determinants; the next step is to undertake appropriate interventions to promote health, prevent diseases, disabilities, and deaths. This calls for expertise and experience in community medicine practice to understand the complexity of health issues, their relative importance, cost-effectiveness, feasibility, and decide the best possible interventions at various levels in the community.
- ***Plan and organize healthcare delivery services to address health needs through community mobilization to achieve community empowerment***: Community medicine practitioners should participate with other stakeholders in planning, organizing, and successful delivery of healthcare services to address health needs of the community. To achieve the optimum results of community-based health interventions, the community should be mobilized and empowered through their full participation at every stage of health planning and management with the ultimate aim of "*putting people's health in their hands*".
- ***Lead the health team and provide community-oriented primary healthcare***: Healthcare delivery to a community is a team work. The health team is invariably led by a community medicine specialist with good leadership skills for effective delivery of healthcare.
- ***Advocate for equitable, quality, accessible, cost-effective, and appropriate healthcare services as basis to achieve universal health coverage (UHC)***: Specialist in community medicine should play a key role in public healthcare. Being conversant with both medical and social issues, he is in a unique position to advocate for important health-related issues. Hence, he must use his advocacy skills to access policy makers for providing equitable, high quality, cost-effective, and relevant healthcare services by allocation of adequate resources for primary healthcare to achieve UHC. IAPSM strongly supports the concept of UHC.
- ***Conduct health system research to evaluate health services and recommend measures to improve their effectiveness and efficiencies***: Health system research is an important tool for assessing the effectiveness and efficiency of any health

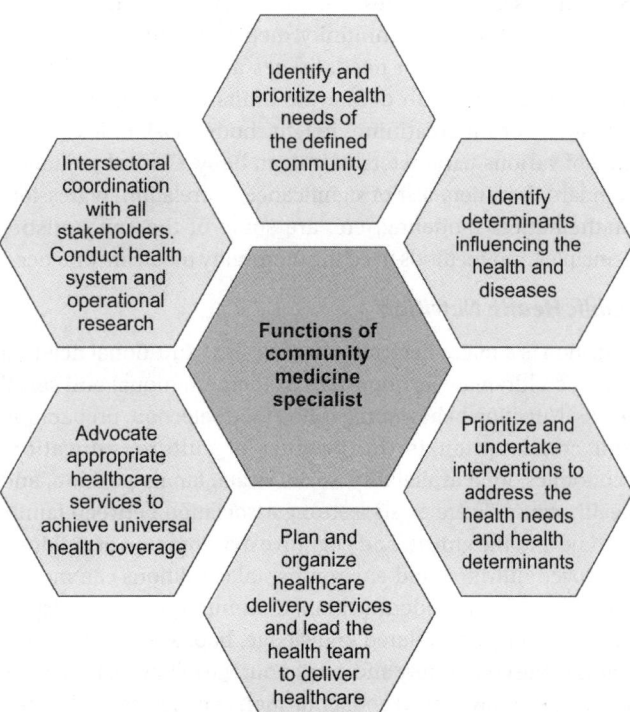

**Fig. 2.1:** Functions of community medicine specialist.

program or services. Community medicine experts identify need for operational research related to the health services/programs and help in designing, execution, evaluation, and making suitable recommendations for achieving optimum health outcomes.
- ***Understand the role of other sectors which influence health and work with them to improve health status of community***: Community medicine specialists need to understand the role of other sectors which influence health of the community. They should identify the key sectors/stakeholders for each health needs and services and develop plan to establish coordination mechanism with them based on mutual respect and trust.

## COMPETENCIES FOR COMMUNITY MEDICINE PRACTICE

*"Competencies are abilities and attributes that are essential to effective healthcare delivery."* Community medicine practitioners should possess the following competencies to discharge their functions effectively **(Fig. 2.2)**:

- ***Clinical competency***: *"A competent community medicine specialist should also be a good clinician."*
  - He should be able to diagnose the common illnesses in general practice and manage them effectively with minimum available resources.
  - He should identify additional healthcare needs of a patient with disability.
  - He should be well informed of the presence and location of hospital facilities including specialized services of curative and rehabilitative nature and make judicious use of these facilities/services.
  - He should understand clearly the integrated approach to meet the need of individual, his family, and the community.
- ***Teaching/training competency***:
  - Training in community medicine should be community based and in close association with local health systems to enable understanding of community health issues and acquisition of skills to manage the same.
  - Assess the learning needs of any given group (students, paramedical staff or community).
  - Formulate learning objectives.
  - Plan curriculum and prepare curriculum materials.
  - Select and implement appropriate learning methods.
  - Evaluate learning experiences.
- ***Public health management competency***:
  - Identify and prioritize social, economic, environmental, biological, and emotional determinants of health in a given case and take them in to account while planning therapeutic, rehabilitative, preventive, and promotive measures/strategies.
  - Identify groups which require special attention (elderly, adolescents, gender, the poor and other marginalized groups, and persons with disability) including those facing occupational hazards.
  - Initiate, implement, and supervise national health programs effectively and responsibly.
  - Identify threats to the environment and anticipate, prepare for, and respond to disasters.
  - Plan health manpower development.
  - Manage logistics and materials effectively.
  - Assess costs and carry out program budgeting.
  - Monitor and assure quality in program implementation.
  - Manage health information system and respond appropriately to the information gathered.
  - Understand and implement public health laws.
  - Establish surveillance system and respond to public health threats efficiently.
- ***Research competency***:
  - Acquire a spirit of scientific enquiry and orientation to the principles of research methodology and epidemiology.
  - Critically evaluate data, identify gaps in knowledge, and formulate research questions.
  - Design and implement epidemiological and health systems research studies.
  - Analyze data and present findings.
  - Effectively communicate findings and public health information.
  - Apply ethical principles to the collection, maintenance, use, and dissemination of data and information.
- ***Leadership competency***:
  - Interact and communicate effectively with people from diverse backgrounds, ages, and preferences to promote healthy behavior through community participation.
  - Explain scientific information to public, decision makers, and opinion leaders.
  - Facilitate intersectoral coordination.
  - Promote and establish partnerships.

## CONCLUSION

Community medicine deals with managing health of the community in close association with healthcare delivery system and various other health-related institutions. Its scope includes promoting health, preventing diseases, and prolonging the quality and life of the people. Community medicine practices

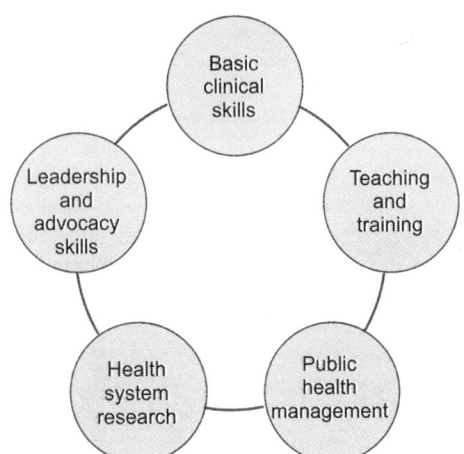

**Fig. 2.2:** Competencies of community medicine practitioners.

multidisciplinary approach and is concerned with identifying and prioritizing health needs of the community, conducting operational research, and organizing comprehensive healthcare services with community participation.

**Core Committee IAPSM**
*Dr AM Kadri, Dr Anand Krishnan, Dr Anil J Purty,
Dr Bishan S Garg, Dr PV Kotecha,
Dr Pradeep Kumar, Dr (Brig) Zile Singh*

## SUGGESTED READING

1. Antonisamy B, Premkumar PS, Christoper S. Role of biostatistics in health sciences. Principles and Practice of Biostatistics, 1st edition. Gurgaon, Haryana, India: Elsevier; 2017.
2. Canoy D. A dictionary of epidemiology, 6th edition. Oxford: Oxford University Press; 2015.
3. Chen CJ. Environmental health issues in public health. In: Detels R, Gulliford M, Karim QA, Tan CC (Eds). Oxford Textbook of Global Public Health, 6th edition. USA: Oxford University Press; 2015. p. 823.
4. Frank GC. Healthy eating in early life—infants and preschoolers. Community Nutrition, 2nd edition. Sudbury, Canada: Jones and Bartlett Publishers; 2008. p. 298.
5. Garg BS, Zodpey S. Status Paper on Public Health Courses in India. New Delhi: WHO India Country Office; 2006. pp. 34-5.
6. Joseph A, Kadri AM, Krishnan A, et al. IAPSM declaration 2018: Definition, role, scope of community medicine and functions of community medicine specialists. Indian J Community Med. 2018;43:120-1.
7. Kumar P, Prahlad A. Sociology in health: The Indian scenario. In: Mariados P (Ed). Health, Illness and Society in the New Millennium, 1st edition. New Delhi: Viva Books Private Limited; 2004. p. 7.
8. MCI. (2000). Postgraduate Medical Education Regulations, 2000. [online] Available from https://www.mciindia.org/documents/rulesAndRegulations/Postgraduate-Medical-Education-Regulations-2000.pdf.

# SECTION 1

# Basics of Health and Disease

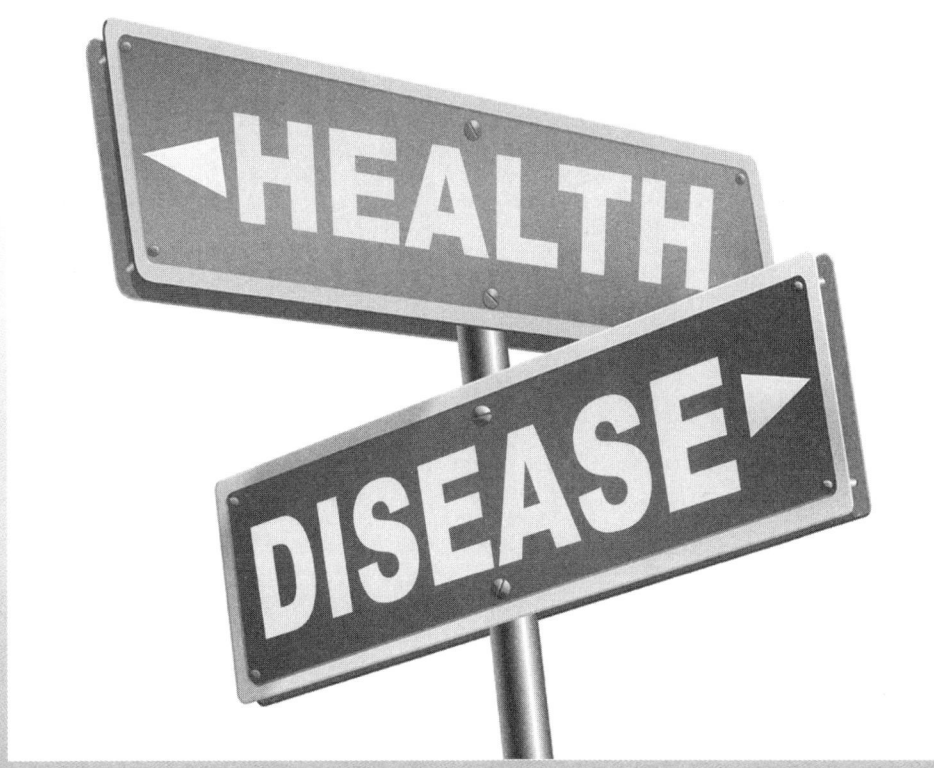

*Health and diseases are not about your genes and biology. Your lifestyle, your environment, many other determinants decide about your path towards 'Health' or 'Diseases'.*

# SECTION OUTLINE

3. Concept of Health and Disease
4. Nutrition and Health
5. Physical Activity, Exercise, and Health
6. Sociology and Health
7. Environment and Health

# CHAPTER 3

# Concept of Health and Disease

*Anmol Gupta, Anupam Parashar, DS Dhadwal, Amit Sachdeva*

*"Although health is one of the most important of all goods relating to our body, it is nevertheless the one that we consider and enjoy the least. When we have the best health, we even do not think of it."*

| | |
|---|---|
| CM1.2 | Define health; describe the concept of holistic health including concept of spiritual health and the relativeness and determinants of health |
| CM1.3 | Describe the characteristics of agent, host and environmental factors in health and disease and the multi-factorial etiology of disease |
| CM1.4 | Describe and discuss the natural history of disease |

## INTRODUCTION

Health is now considered to be one of the most precious goods in our life and it is also considered as an integral component of the overall socioeconomic development of any country. Good health is central to living a long, prosperous and active life for any member of the society. Therefore, health should be protected and enhanced as much as possible we can. The maintenance and promotion of health are achieved through different combination of physical, mental, and social factors, together sometimes referred to as the "health triangle".

The Greek, Democritus in the 5th century BC, said that "without health, nothing is of any use, not money or anything else". Koos (1954) recognized the complex and mysterious nature of health in his utterance that "health is imponderable".

The concept of health is multidimensional, complex, elusive and subject to various interpretations. An understanding of each and every concept of health is very important because they constitute an essential component of every field of medical science. The conceptualization of health gives an ability to open the door for self-assessments aimed at improving human health and also create an opportunity for every person to feel healthy.

Individuals' ideas of the concept of health and illness have a high impact on their health attitudes and behavior; still, there has not been an absolute consensus on the definitions of health, disease and illness. Health can mean different things to different people in the entire world. To some, it may mean freedom from any sickness or disease while to some it may mean harmonious functioning of all body systems of the body. As there is no single yardstick for measuring the health of an individual, the current definitions of health are a fusion of various perspectives, often presents a complex definition like the WHO's definition of health.

## CONCEPT OF HEALTH: BIOLOGICAL TO HOLISTIC HEALTH

### INTRODUCTION

In this world of continuous change, newer concepts of health are bound to emerge based on the new patterns of thought. Health has developed gradually as a concept from an individual concern to a worldwide social goal, and it holds within itself the whole quality of life. Various concepts of health are:
- Biomedical
- Ecological
- Psychosocial
- Holistic.

### Biomedical Concept

According to this Biomedical Concept, health has been viewed as an "absence of disease". "Biomedical Concept" has the basis in the "germ theory of disease" as germs are supposed to cause disease. This concept views:

| Human body | As | Machine |
|---|---|---|
| Disease | As | Consequence of the breakdown of this machine |
| Doctor's task | Is | To repair the machine |

#### Limitations

- This concept had minimized the role of environmental, social, psychological and cultural determinants of health.
- This concept found to be inadequate in solving some of the significant health problems of mankind (e.g. malnutrition, chronic diseases, accidents, drug abuse, mental illness, environmental pollution, population explosion, etc.).

## Ecological Concept

According to this concept, health is a dynamic equilibrium between man and his environment while disease is maladjustment of the human organisms with their environment.

This ecological concept raises two issues namely "imperfect man" and "imperfect environment".

It is a proven fact that improvement in human adaptation to their natural environments can lead to longer life expectancies and a better quality of life even if modern health delivery services are absent. This concept supports the importance of clean air, safe water, clean atmosphere, etc. to protect the human being from exposure to unhealthy factors.

## Psychosocial Concept

According to this concept, Health is not only a biomedical phenomenon, but it is also influenced by social, psychological, cultural, economic, political factors, etc.

## Holistic Concept

There is a famous saying that "health implies a sound mind, in a sound body, in a sound family, in a sound environment". This holistic concept is the combination of all the above concepts. It has been defined as a multidimensional process involving the health and well-being of the person in the context of his environment. It recognizes the strength of social, economic, political, and environmental influences on health.

The holistic concept implies that all sectors of society influence the health of an individual particularly agriculture, animal husbandry, food industry, education, housing, public works, communication, and other sectors.

Holistic Concept = Biomedical + Ecological + Psychosocial Concept.

## WHO DEFINITION OF HEALTH

"Health is a state of complete physical, mental, and social well-being and not merely the absence of disease or infirmity".

—**Constitution of the World Health Organization, July 1946**

In recent years this statement has been amplified to include the ability to lead a "socially and economically productive life."

In this definition, WHO has projected three different dimensions of health namely physical, social and mental which are closely associated.

*Strength*: Concept of health as defined by WHO is broad and also positive in its implications. It sets out the standard of "positive health".

*Criticism*: Health cannot be defined as a "state" at all, but must be seen as a process of continuous acclimatization to the changing demands of living. It is a dynamic concept. It assists or aid people live well, work well and enjoy well with themselves.

## Positive Health

Positive health is the scientific study of health assets. Hippocrates was the composer of the concept of "positive health", which depended on the primary human constitution (which we consider today as genetics), diet, and exercise. He thought that balanced diet and exercise were essential for good health and that environmental changes had a profound effect on the mind and body of a person, resulting in different types of diseases during the winter (respiratory tract diseases like acute respiratory infection, asthma) and summer (digestive tract diseases like diarrhea, vomiting, etc.)

So, positive health describes the health as a state beyond the mere absence of disease and predicts increased longevity, decreased expenditures on health, healthy aging, and better prognosis while illness. In short, it conceptualizes health in all its form; Biologically, Psychologically and Socially.

## DIMENSIONS OF HEALTH

Health is described as multidimensional. The WHO definition considers three specific dimensions namely the physical, the mental, and the social. Many more dimensions are also cited like spiritual, emotional, vocational, and political dimensions. As our knowledge grows day by day, these lists may be expanding.

Various dimensions of health (**Fig. 3.1.**):
- Physical dimension
- Mental dimension
- Social dimension
- Spiritual dimension
- Emotional dimension
- Vocational dimension.

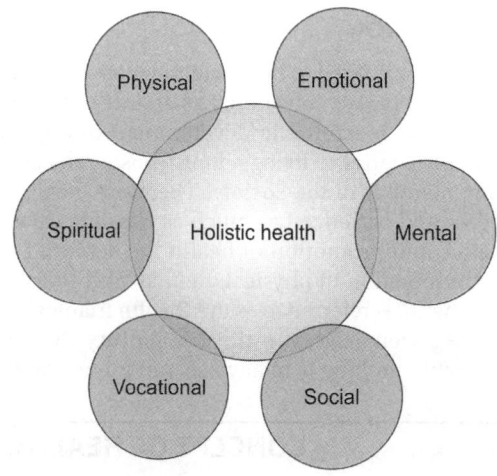

**Fig. 3.1:** Various dimensions of health.

## Physical Dimension

In the 5th century BC, Pindar defined the health as a "harmonious functioning of all the organs". He highlights the physical dimension of health, the physical body, and the overall functionality, along with the feeling of comfort and absence of pain. Even today, his definition bears importance as a prerequisite for the overall health and wellness of an individual.

The state of physical health signifies the notion of "perfect functioning" of the human body. The physical health of a person can be determined by "a good complexion, a clean skin, bright eyes, lustrous hair with a body well dressed with firm flesh, not too obese, a sweet breath, a good appetite, sound sleep, regular activity of bowels and bladder and smooth easy coordination of all bodily movements. All the organs of the body are of ideal size and function "normally", all the special senses are intact, pulse rate, blood pressure, and exercise tolerance capacity are all within the range of "normality" for the individuals' age and gender.

### *Evaluation of Physical Health*

- Self-assessment
- Standardized questionnaires
- Clinical examination
- Anthropometric measurements
- Nutrition and dietary assessment
- Biochemical and laboratory investigations.

## Mental Dimension

Mental health is defined as "a state of balance between the individual and the surrounding world, a state of harmony between oneself and other individuals, a coexistence between the realities of the self and that of other people and with that of the environment". The mental health of any person can be determined by self-satisfaction, self-confidence, no conflict within himself and others, happy, calm, and cheerful personality, well adjustment with others, good understanding, self-control and not govern by fear, anger, love, jealousy, guilt or worries.

## Social Dimension

It is defined as the "quantity and quality of an individual's interpersonal ties and the extent of involvement with the community". Social health is well rooted in "positive material environment" and "positive human environment" of the individual.

In general, this dimension signifies the abilities as those of making a friendship that are satisfying and long lasting, of taking responsibilities as per one's capacities, of finding satisfaction, success, happiness in the attainment of day-to-day tasks, of living effectively with others and showing socially considered behavior.

## Spiritual Dimension

It is a recent concept in health. The spiritual dimension plays a significant role in motivating people's achievement in all aspects of life. Having compassion, the capacity for love and forgiveness, selflessness, joy and fulfillment help one to enjoy spiritual health. All our religious faith, values, beliefs, principles, and morals define our spirituality. Spiritual health may help to resolve both internal as well as external conflicts.

## Emotional Dimension

This dimension focuses on awareness and acceptance of stressors and feelings both positive and negative. Emotional well-being incorporates the ability to manage one's feelings and related behaviors, cope effectively with stress and adapt to any change. Mental health can be seen as "knowing" or "cognition" while emotional health relates to "feeling". Nowadays with newer advances in neurosciences and psychology, more importance is given to EQ (Emotional Quotient) than the IQ (Intelligence Quotient).

## Vocational Dimension

Vocational dimension relates to growth and happiness in one's work. As a vocationally well person seeks jobs that give personal satisfaction, enrichment, self-realization, and enhanced self-esteem.

## Other Dimensions of Health

These are:
- Philosophical dimension
- Cultural dimension
- Socioeconomic dimension
- Environmental dimension
- Educational dimension
- Nutritional dimension
- Curative dimension
- Preventive dimension.

# SPECTRUM OF HEALTH

The health of an individual is not static, it is a dynamic phenomenon and a process of continuous change. It is always influenced by the various factors making the individual survive in this globe. The health of a person always lies along a continuum and there is no single cut-off point. At any given point of time, the health of individual changes in a range of spectrum varying from the highest point corresponds to the WHO definition of "positive health" to the lowest point of "death". A person may attain the maximum levels of health today which may be minimum tomorrow.

Different stages of Spectrum of Health are positive health, better health, freedom from sickness, unrecognized sickness, mild sickness, severe sickness, and death **(Fig. 3.2)**. This transition of health from one level to other level is so gradual that it is hard to say when one level ends and when the other level begins. It is just a matter of judgment. It is only in acute cases or under exceptional conditions; there is a sudden decline from the state of positive health to the state of death. For example, one person can rush from the condition of "positive health" into the "sickness" as in case of any acute illness like vomiting or diarrhea. Any intervention including rest, replacing fluids, medicines will help in supporting the body's capacity to self-heal and the person may either again go to the stage of "better health" to "positive health" or may go to "severe sickness" and "death" in the absence of any desired intervention.

In other acute situations like acute heart failure, a heart attack, severe acute asthma, a diabetic crisis (hypoglycemia or diabetic ketoacidosis ) and so on, medical treatments including drugs or surgical procedures can make the difference in any stage of the spectrum of health depending upon the treatment. Any attempt to attain this state of positive health indicates that there is an improvement in the "quality of life" of a person. There are degrees or levels of health in this spectrum. As long as we are alive, there is some degree of health in us.

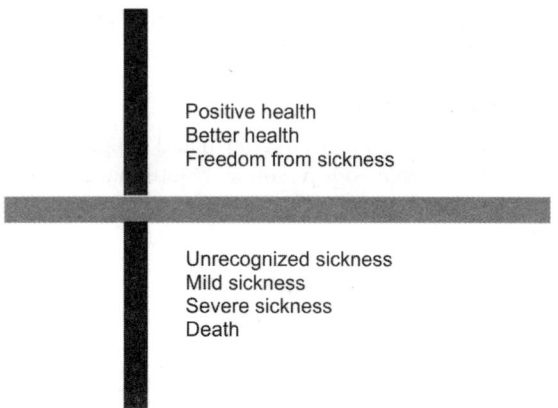

Fig. 3.2: Spectrum of health.

## DETERMINANTS OF HEALTH

Health is a state of dynamic equilibrium or adjustment between man and his environment.

Determinants of health are defined as the range of behavioral, biological, socioeconomic, and environmental factors that influence the health status of individuals or populations. The important determinants are shown in **Figure 3.3**.

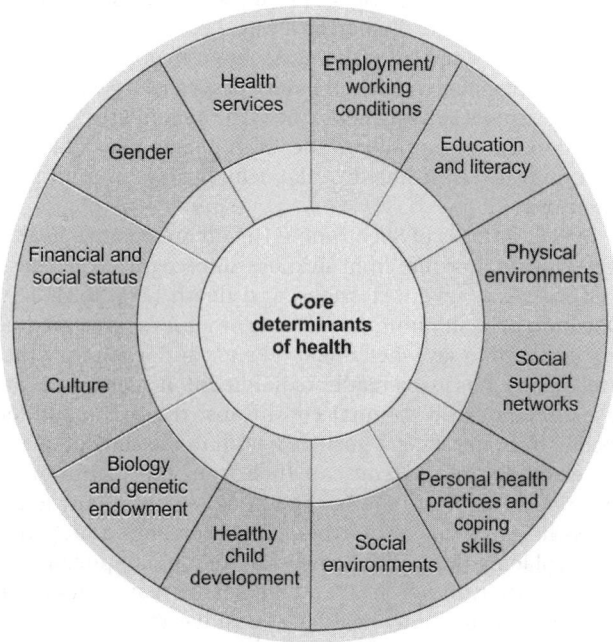

Fig. 3.3: Determinants of health.

### Biological Determinants

The physical and mental traits of every individual are to some extent decided by the nature of his genes at the time of conception. Many diseases have a direct relationship with the heredity. The state of health, therefore, depends partly on the genetic constitution of a person. This genetic constitution can never be altered after the conception. Thus from the genetic standpoint, health may be defined as that "state of the individual which is based upon the absence from the genetic constitution of such genes as correspond to character that take the form of any severe defect or derangement and to the absence of any aberration in respect of the total amount of chromosomal material in the karyotype. From the presence in the genetic constitution of the genes that correspond to the standard characterization and the presence of a normal karyotype".

Many diseases that result from the defective genetic constitution are chromosomal disorders, sickle cell anemia, inborn errors of metabolism, phenylketonuria, mental retardation, some types of diabetes, etc. Nowadays, advances in medical genetics (genetic screening, genetic counseling, and gene therapy) offers hope for the prevention and treatment of a broad-spectrum of diseases.

### Behavioral and Sociocultural Determinants

Behavioral and sociocultural factors are customs, lifestyles and values that characterize a society. The health of the individual depends upon the lifestyle of the person. It comprises all the day-to-day activities of the individual. For example, if an individual quits smoking, his or her risk of developing heart disease is significantly reduced.

The achievement of optimum health requires the adoption of healthy lifestyles. There are many lifestyle factors like adequate nutrition, enough sleep, Yoga exercises, meditation, sufficient physical activity, and others that can promote the health of individual. Lifestyles are learned through social interaction with parents, peer groups, friends, sibling, school teachers, and mass media. Many current health problems like (coronary heart disease, obesity, lung cancer and drug addiction) are strongly associated with lifestyle changes.

### Environmental Determinants

The health status of the individual also depends upon the internal environment of the man himself as well as the external environment. The internal environment refers to every part of the body system while the external environment is the aggregation of all external conditions and circumstances which affect the development and life of an individual. The external environment includes physical, biological, and social components as a whole. Generally speaking, environmental health risks include problems with air quality, water quality, food quality and safety, waste disposal, hazardous substances, unsafe public spaces and housing conditions.

### Socioeconomic Determinants

Socioeconomic status is also an important factor on which the health status depends. The countries with the lowest socioeconomic status find higher mortality rates in comparison to the countries with the higher socioeconomic status. The critical socioeconomic factors influencing the healthcare are education, occupation and income of the individual.

### Political Determinants

Health also depends upon the country's political system. Decisions concerning resource allocation, manpower policy, choice of appropriate technology and the extent to which health services are made available and accessible to different segments of the society are examples of the manner in which the political system can shape community health services.

The health sector in Syria, currently in the midst of a civil and political war, now faces destruction from on-going violence due to political instability which affects the access to healthcare, to medicines and essentials of health as well as the destruction of health infrastructure.

The percentage of gross national product (GNP) spent on health is a quantitative indicator of political commitment. The WHO has set the target of at least 5% expenditure of each country's GNP on healthcare. However, India spends about 2% of its GNP on health and family welfare.

## Health Services

It is the sum total of services available for the better health. It means all those personal and community services, including medical care, directed toward the protection and promotion of the health of the community. So the health status is not only influenced by the physical and social environment, but also by the quality and availability of health services. Barriers in accessing health services include lack of availability, high cost, lack of insurance coverage, limited language access and many others.

These barriers to access health services lead to unmet health needs, delays in receiving appropriate care, inability to get preventive services and hospitalizations that could have been prevented.

## CONCEPT OF WELL-BEING

It has two components:
1. Objective components: Standard of living
2. Subjective component: Quality of life.

### Standard of Living

Refers to the usual scale of our expenditure, the goods we consume, the services we enjoy, and other comforts of modern living.

Standard of living (WHO) includes:
- Income and occupation
- Standards of housing, sanitation, and nutrition
- Level of provision of health, educational, recreational, and other services.

Standard of living depends on "per Capita GNP".

> **Note**
> Gross national product includes the gross income generated within the country as well as the net income received from abroad.

### Quality of Life

The condition of life of person is determined by the combination of the effects of the complete range of factors such as those determining health, happiness (including comfort in the physical environment and the satisfying occupation), education, social and intellectual attainments, freedom of action, justice and freedom of expression. It is a composite measure of physical, mental and social well-being as perceived by each or group of individuals. There are various indices to measure the quality of life:
- Physical quality of life index (PQLI)
- Human development index (HDI)
- Human poverty index (HPI)
- Gender-related development index (GDI)
- Gender empowerment measure (GEM).

### *Physical Quality of Life Index*

The quality of life can be evaluated by a composite index called "physical quality of life index" which consolidates three indicators, viz.
1. Infant mortality rate (IMR)
2. Life expectancy at the age of 1 year
3. Literacy

The composite index is calculated by taking the average of all the three indicators, giving equal weight to each of them. Per capita gross national product (GNP), a measure of economic growth, is not taken into consideration. It measures results of socioeconomic and political policies and seeks to complement GNP. PQLI value ranges from 0 to 100 (0 = worst performance and 100 = best performance). Ultimate objective is to attain a PQLI of 100. PQLI is applicable for international and national comparison. PQLI of India is 65.

### *Human Development Index*

Human development index is also a composite index. It combines indicators representing three dimensions:
1. *Longevity:* Life expectancy at birth
2. *Knowledge:* Expected years of schooling and mean years of schooling
3. *Income:* Gross national income (GNI) per capita in purchasing power parity (PPP) in US dollars.

Human development index is the geometric mean of indices for each of the three dimensions, with equal weightage to all. Its value ranges between 0 and 1. It allows for international comparison. Countries are also classified on basis of HDI as developed (HDI ≥0.8), developing (HDI 0.5–0.799), and underdeveloped country (HDI < 0.5) (UNDP, Human Development Report, 2019).

> **Note**
> **Gross domestic product**: The gross income generated within the country, excluding the net income received from abroad. The World's Top 10 economies concerning nominal GDP are United States, China, Japan, Germany, United Kingdom, India, France, Brazil, Italy, and Canada.
> - HDI of India is 0.633 (rank 132 out of 189 countries) (Human Development Report, UNDP, 2021)
> - India comes in the medium human development category
> - Switzerland has HDI of 0.962 which is ranked 1st (Human Development Report, UNDP, 2021)
> - From South Asian region India ranked 3rd after Sri Lanka and Maldives.

The difference between HDI and PQLI is shown in **Table 3.1**.

**Table 3.1:** Difference between HDI and PQLI.

|  | HDI | PQLI |
|---|---|---|
| Components | Longevity—life expectancy at birth | Life expectancy at 1 year age |
|  | Income (gross domestic product per capita in purchasing power parity US$) | Infant mortality rate |
|  | Knowledge (mean years of schooling—gross enrolment ratio and literacy rate) | Literacy rate |
| Range | 0–1 | 0–100 |
| Value of India | 0.633 | 65 |

(HDI: human development index; PQLI: physical quality of life index)

### Human Poverty Index

Human poverty index was introduced in 1997 by the United Nations Development Program (UNDP). HPI measures: deprivation in the basic dimensions of human development (longevity, knowledge, standard of living/income). HPI is complementary to the human development index.

### Multidimensional Poverty Index (UNDP, Human Development Report, 2019)

It identifies how people are being left behind across three key dimensions: health, education, and standard of living. It comprises 10 indicators. People who are deprived of at least one-third of these weighted indicators fall into the category of multidimensionally poor. The global multidimensional poverty index (MPI), revised and updated in September 2018, now covers 105 countries in total, which are home to 77% of the world's population. In 2015–16, more than 364 million people were poor as per MPI in India.

*PQLI, HDI, and MDPI are further explained in detail in Chapter 37: Community Health.*

## CONCEPT OF DISEASE

(Dis = opposite, Ease = comfort; health)

### INTRODUCTION

Like health, the concept of disease is also not very well defined. Many people define it in different ways. With the progress of civilization from the ancient to modern man, the concept of diseases also evolved by stages from supernatural and deistic in origin to the natural and "multifactorial" causation.

An adequate definition of disease is yet to be found. The Oxford English Dictionary defines disease as, "a condition of the body or, some part or organ of the body in which its functions are disturbed or deranged". Webster defines disease as "a discomfort, a condition in which bodily health is seriously attacked, deranged or impaired; a departure from the state of health, an alternation of human body interrupting the performance of the vital function". From the ecological point of view, the disease is "a maladjustment of the human organism to the environment" while according to the sociological point of view disease is considered "a social phenomenon that occurred in all societies anywhere in the world" and defined in terms of the particular cultural forces prevalent in that society.

### LIMITATION OF THESE DEFINITIONS

These definitions do not give the specific criterions by which one can decide when a particular disease state will begin. Also, these definitions do not measure the extent of disease.

World Health Organization has defined health but not disease, because of the following reasons:
- Disease has got varying shades and spectrum from subclinical state to the severe illness.
- The onset of disease may be acute (as in food poisoning) or insidious (as in mental illness, rheumatoid arthritis). Sometimes, the diseased person may look apparently healthy but may be spreading infection to others (as in carrier state of typhoid fever). The same pathogen sometimes causes more than one disease (e.g. streptococci). The same disease sometimes caused by more than one organism (e.g. diarrhea). The course of the disease may be short or prolonged.
- It is challenging to demarcate between a normal and abnormal state in some disease like in hypertension, diabetes, mental illness, etc. The endpoint or outcome of the disease is variable, i.e. recovery, disability or death.

### DIFFERENCE BETWEEN DISEASE, ILLNESS, AND SICKNESS

The difference has been shown in **Table 3.2**.

### THEORIES OF DISEASE CAUSATION

#### Old Theories

Till the end of the 18th century, various theories were in vogue, e.g.:
- Supernatural theory of disease (e.g. curse of God; an evil eye).

**Table 3.2:** Difference between disease, illness, and sickness.

| Sr. no. | Disease | Illness | Sickness |
|---|---|---|---|
| 1. | "Disease" literally means "without ease" (uneasiness)— when something is wrong with bodily function | "Illness" refers not only to the presence of a specific disease, but also to the individual's perceptions and behavior in response to the disease, as well as the impact of that disease on the psychosocial environment | "Sickness" refers to a state of social dysfunction |
| 2. | Disease is a physiological/psychological dysfunction of the body | Illness is a subjective feeling of the person who feels aware of not being well | Sickness is a role that the individual assumes when he/she become ill (inability to perform his "Social Role") |

- The Ayurveda considers that the disease is due to an imbalance of the "tridoshas". These are vata (air), pitta (bile), and kapha (mucus).
- The Chinese medicine believes that the disease is caused due to an imbalance of male principle (Yang) and female principle (Yin).

## Germ Theory of Disease

The discoveries in microbiology in the 18th century became a turning point in the etiological concept of disease. —**Louis Pasteur** (1860) demonstrated the presence of bacteria in the air and Robert Koch (1877) showed that bacteria caused anthrax. These discoveries of Pasteur and Koch confirmed the germ theory of disease.

*Koch's postulates* must be fulfilled before any microorganism is considered as "the necessary cause" for any disease. The postulates are:
- The organism must be continuously associated with the lesions of the disease.
- Isolating the organism from the lesions should be possible.
- Inoculation of the isolated organism into the experimental animal should reproduce the lesions of the disease.
- It should be possible to reisolate the organisms in pure culture from the lesions produced in experimental animals.

Thus, the emphasis has shifted from empirical causes (like bad air as a cause in malaria) of old theories to microbes of germ theory. The concept of Germ Theory gained momentum during the 19th and the early part of 20th century. The concept of cause embodied in the germ theory of disease is generally referred to as a one-to-one relationship between causal agent and disease.

The disease model accordingly is:

Disease agent—Man—Disease

However, later in the 20th century, it was recognized that a disease is rarely caused by a single agent alone but depends upon many contributory factors. There are factors relating to the host and environment which are equally important to determine the occurrence of disease. That demanded a broader concept of disease causation that synthesized the fundamental factors of agent, host, and environment (*Epidemiological triad*).

### Limitations of Germ Theory

We know that only some people develop tuberculosis after exposure to tubercle bacilli and not all. Similarly, not everyone exposed to beta-hemolytic streptococci develops acute rheumatic fever while some people do not suffer from the disease even though they harbor the pathogens in the body (as in healthy carriers of typhoid).

## Theory of Multifactorial Causation

After the doctrine of a one-to-one relationship between cause and disease had been shown to be unjustifiable, even for microbial diseases like tuberculosis, leprosy, the theory of multifactorial causation was given by Pettenkofer of Munich (1818-1901). This theory de-emphasizes the "Germ theory" (or single cause idea).

Modern epidemiology has also contributed significantly to our present day understanding of the multifactorial causation of disease. Nowadays, the epidemiologists are looking beyond the "germ theory" of disease into the total life situation of the patient and the community in search of multiple (or risk) factors of disease. This new theory includes all facets of the communicable disease model, and to make it more relevant and useful with regard to today's diseases, conditions, disorders, defects, injuries, and deaths. This theory has taken into account all the behavior, lifestyle factors, environmental causes, culture, physiological factors, ecological elements, and physical factors.

As a result of advances in public health, it is now well recognized that many diseases are neither caused by an organism nor could they be prevented by the traditional methods of isolation, immunization or improvements in sanitation. These diseases are predisposed by many factors (social, economic, cultural, genetic, and psychological) contributing to its occurrence, especially in the case of "modern diseases" of civilization like coronary heart disease, various types of cancer, many types of diabetes, chronic obstructive pulmonary disease (COPD), mental illness, etc.

It is now known that most of these factors (excess of fat and salt intake, smoking, lack of physical exercise, junk foods, and obesity) are so much linked to lifestyle and human behavior that they are considered as "risk-factors", in the web of causation of the disease. The multiple factors in the web of causation of coronary heart disease are smoking, high blood pressure, high cholesterol, obesity lack of exercise, type A personality, etc. (*See* **Fig. 3.11**).

The term agent is now replaced by causative factors, which signifies the need to identify multiple causes or the etiologic factors of disease, disability, injury, and death. The objective of knowing the multiple factors of disease is to quantify and prioritize them for modification or amelioration to prevent or control the disease. Thus, the multifactorial theory offers multiple approaches to the prevention and control of various diseases.

## NATURAL HISTORY OF THE DISEASE

While discussing the "concept of disease", it is evident that the disease is nothing but a "process". The term "natural history of disease" is applied to the course of the disease process in man. This natural history of disease comprises of two phases:
1. *Prepathogenesis* (i.e. the process in the environment)
2. *Pathogenesis* (i.e. the process in man).

> **Note**
> Cohort studies best establish the natural history of the disease.

### Prepathogenesis Phase

The prepathogenesis period refers to the preliminary period of any disease. A man is always in the midst of the disease; potentially, we are in the prepathogenesis period of many diseases like typhoid, jaundice, and so on. The disease process starts only when the agent, host, and environment interact. These three factors are referred to sometimes as an ecological triad. Under optimal conditions, the interaction between these three results in disease. In the beginning of any disease, the signs and symptoms may not be clear-cut, but it becomes clear as the disease advances and takes its course.

### Epidemiological Triad

Many models of disease causation have been proposed. Among them, the simplest is the epidemiological triad or triangle, the traditional model for the infectious disease. The triad consists of an external agent, a susceptible host, and an environment that brings the host and agent together **(Fig. 3.4)**. According to this model, disease occurs when the equilibrium between agent, host, and environment is disturbed. Thus, this model explains that some persons do not suffer from the disease even though they harbor the pathogens for that disease because equilibrium is established between the causative agent and the host.

The triangle in **Figure 3.4** is based on the communicable or infectious diseases model. It is useful in showing the interaction as well as the interdependence of various factors used in the investigation of diseases and epidemics (i.e. agent, host, environment and time).

***Agent:*** The disease "agent" may be defined as a substance, living or nonliving or a force, tangible or intangible, the excessive presence or relative lack of which is the immediate cause of a particular disease. The disease agents are categorized into five broad groups in **Figure 3.5**.

- **Biological agents:** Viruses, bacteria, rickettsia, fungi, protozoa, metazoan, helminths, and arthropods. These agents have some "host-related" biological features.
  - *Infectivity*: This is the ability of an infectious agent to invade and multiply (produce infection) in a host.
  - *Pathogenicity*: This is the ability to induce clinically apparent illness.
  - *Virulence*: This is defined as the proportion of clinical cases resulting in severe clinical manifestations (including sequelae like death).

> **Note**
> The case fatality rate is one way of measuring virulence.

- **Nutritive agents:** These are proteins, fats, carbohydrates, vitamins, minerals, and water. Any excess or deficiency of these nutritive elements may result in nutritional disorders. Some of the current nutritional problems are protein-energy malnutrition (PEM), anemia, goiter, obesity, and vitamin deficiencies like scurvy, rickets, etc.
- **Physical agents:** Excessive heat, cold, humidity, noise, atmospheric pressure, radiation, electricity, sound, etc.
- **Chemical agents:** It includes both endogenous and exogenous agents inside and outside the body. They are mainly of two types:
  1. *Endogenous*: These chemicals are produced in the body as a result of derangement of function, e.g. urea (uremia), serum bilirubin (jaundice), glucose (diabetes) ketones (ketosis), uric acid (gout), calcium carbonate/calcium oxalate (kidney stones), etc.
  2. *Exogenous*: These agents arise outside of a human host, e.g. allergens, metals, fumes, dust, gases, insecticides, etc. These may be acquired by inhalation, ingestion or inoculation.
- **Mechanical agents:** These are chronic friction or other mechanical forces like injury, sprain, accidents, etc. resulting in crushing, tearing, sprains, dislocations and fractures, and even death.

***Host:*** In the disease process, the human host factor is very complex. In epidemiological terms, the human host is referred to as "Soil" and the disease as "Seed". The host contribution to disease is first through his inherent or genetic characteristics, all of which must be considered while considering the natural history of the disease. The association of any particular disease with a specific set of host factors frequently provides an insight into the cause of any disease. These are age, sex, race, genetics, nutrition, occupation, immunity status, customs and habits, human behavior, and psychological factors. In some situations like in tuberculosis, host factors play a significant role in determining the outcome of an individual's exposure to infection.

The host factors may be classified as **(Fig. 3.6)**:
- Demographic characteristics such as age, gender, race, ethnicity, etc.
- Biological characteristics such as genetic factors; biochemical levels of the blood (e.g. fasting blood sugar, serum cholesterol); blood groups and enzymes; cellular constituents of the blood, immunological factors, and physiological function of

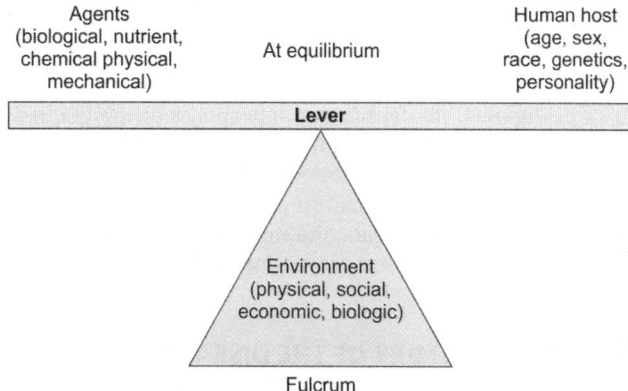

**Fig. 3.4:** Epidemiological triad.

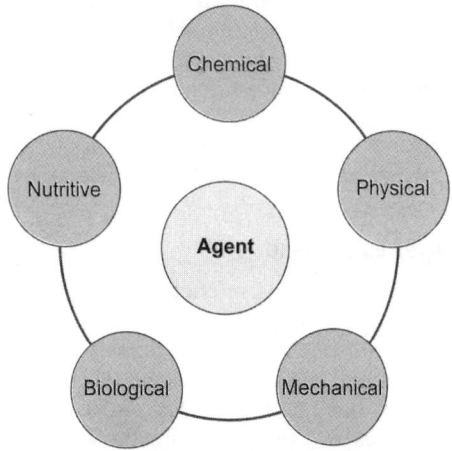

**Fig. 3.5:** Five groups of agents.

## Chapter 3: Concept of Health and Disease

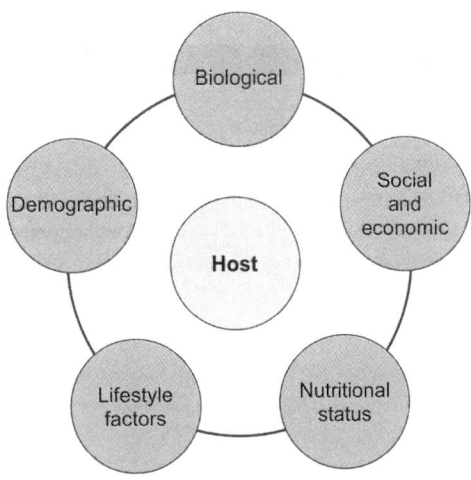

Fig. 3.6: Characteristics of hosts.

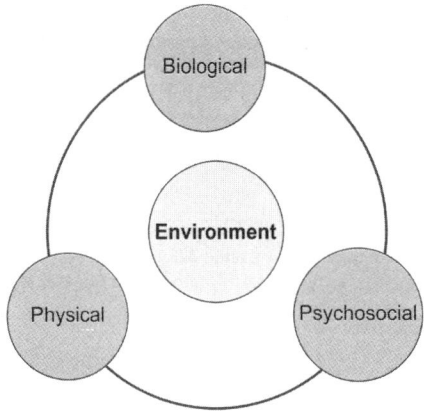

Fig. 3.7: Classification of environment.

different organ systems of the body (e.g. blood pressure, forced expiratory ventilation), etc.
- Social and economic characteristics such as education, income, occupation, marital status, etc.
- Nutritional status: Underweight, overweight, obese, and malnourished.
- Lifestyle factors such as physical exercise, use of alcohol, drugs, and smoking, multiple sexual partnerships, etc.

*Environment:* The environment is the surroundings or conditions within a host or external to it in the community that can cause or allow the disease transmission. The relationship between environment and disease is very complex as millions of people suffer by the diseases originating in the environment. These are classified into the physical, biological, and psychosocial environment **(Fig. 3.7)**.
- *Physical environment*: It is applied to nonliving things and physical factors (e.g. air, water, soil, housing, climate, geography, heat, light, noise, debris, radiation, etc.)
- *Biological environment*: It is the universe of living things which surrounds the man, including man himself, viruses, and other microbial agents, insects, rodents, animals, and plants.
- *Psychosocial environment*: These include cultural values, customs, habits, beliefs, attitudes, morals, religion, education, lifestyles, community life, health services, and social and political organization.

A harmonious adjustment to the environment enables man to enjoy health and happiness, whereas maladjustment may not only cause illness but may also deprive a man of taking adequate action against the disease **(Fig. 3.8)**.

*Time:* Time accounts for incubation period, the life expectancy of the host or the pathogen and duration of the course of illness or condition. Time also includes severity of illness till the person is infected or until towards the disease causes death or passes the threshold of danger toward recovery from disease. Delays in time from infection to the start of symptoms, duration of illness, and threshold of an epidemic in a community are various essential time elements about disease to occur.

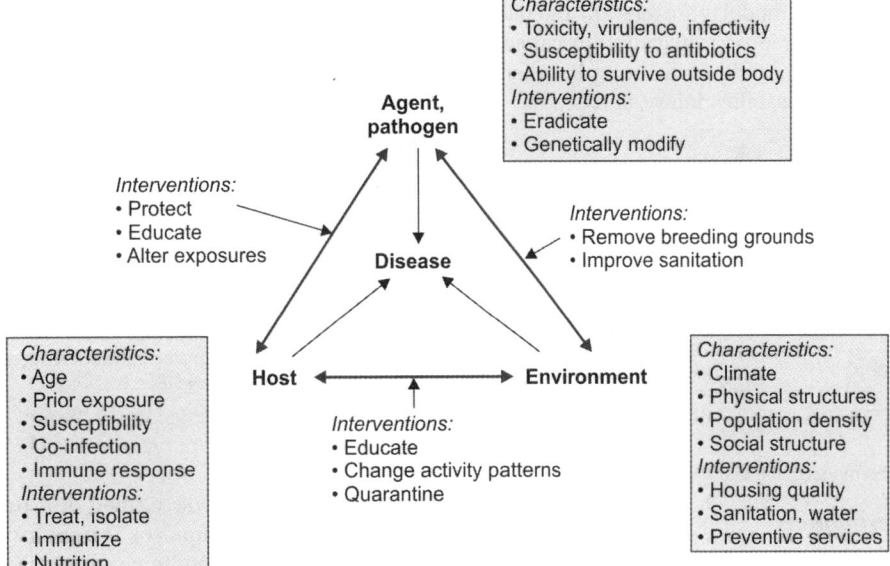

**Fig. 3.8:** Characteristics of agent, host, and environment.

**Table 3.3:** Prominent risk factors for noncommunicable and communicable diseases.

| Disease category | Disease | Risk factors |
| --- | --- | --- |
| Noncommunicable diseases | Coronary heart disease | Smoking, high blood pressure, high cholesterol, obesity, lack of exercise, type A personality |
| | Lung cancer | Smoking, ionizing radiation, asbestos dust, air pollution, and work-site hazards |
| | Diabetes | Obesity, lack of exercise and excessive food consumption |
| | Stroke | High blood-pressure, elevated cholesterol level, and smoking |
| | Vehicular accidents | Alcohol, nonuse of seat belts, excessive speed, roadway design, and automobile design |
| Communicable diseases | Hepatitis A/E, tuberculosis, flu, sexually transmitted diseases, etc. | Lack of safe water, inadequate excreta disposal facilities, poor hygiene, poor living conditions, and unsafe food |

**Table 3.4:** Examples of various risk factors.

| | |
| --- | --- |
| Additive | Smoking and occupational exposure (shoe, leather, rubber, dye, and chemical industries) for bladder cancer |
| Synergistic | Smoking with other risk factors such as hypertension and high blood cholesterol |
| Indeed causative | Smoking for lung cancer |
| Merely contributory to the undesired outcome | Lack of physical exercise for coronary heart disease |
| Only predictive statistically | Illiteracy for perinatal mortality |
| Modifiable | Smoking, hypertension, high serum cholesterol level, physical activity, obesity, etc. |
| Nonmodifiable | Age, sex, race, family history, and genetic factors |
| Individual risk factors | Age, sex, smoking, hypertension |
| Community risk factors | Presence of malaria, air pollution, substandard housing, poor water supply, inadequate healthcare services, etc. |

The overall GOAL of epidemiology is to provide information about the factors or events that result in breaking one of the legs of the triangle, thereby disrupting the equilibrium between agent, host, and environment.

### Advance Model of the Triangle of Epidemiology

As we know, infectious diseases are no longer the leading cause of death in many industrialized nations, so a more advanced model of the triangle of epidemiology has been proposed **(Fig. 3.9)**. This model includes not only all facets of the communicable disease model but also all relevant factors concerning today's diseases conditions, disorders, defects, injuries, and deaths. All the factors including behavior, lifestyle, environment, ecology, physical factors, and chronic diseases are taken into account to make the model more relevant and useful.

In this model, the term agent is replaced with causative factors, which implies the need to identify multiple causes of etiological factors of disease, disability, injury, and death.

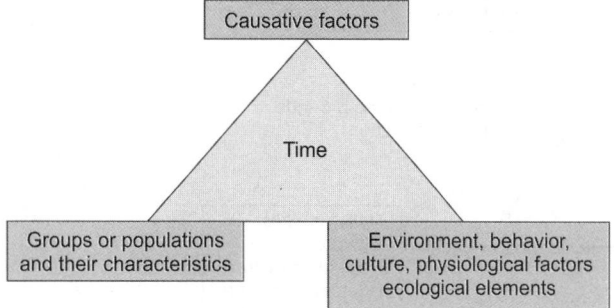

**Fig. 3.9:** Advanced model of the triangle of epidemiology.

### Risk Factors or Determinants

In many situations, where the disease "agent" is either unidentified or not established firmly, the etiology of the disease generally discussed regarding "risk factors" **(Tables 3.3 and 3.4)**. The term "risk factors" has mainly two aspects:
1. It is an attribute or exposure that is significantly associated with the occurrence of a disease.
2. It is a determinant that can be modified by intervention, thereby decreasing the possibility of occurrence of disease.

Risk factors are observable or identifiable before the disease they predict. Risk factors are often suggestive, but absolute proof of cause-and-effect relationship between a risk factor and disease usually lacks. This means the presence of a risk factor does not assure that the disease will occur, and in its absence, the disease will not occur.

The degree of risk indirectly indicates the need for promotive and preventive health services. Epidemiological methods (e.g. case–control and cohort studies) help to identify risk factors and estimate the degree of risk, i.e. smoking as a risk for lung cancer; high serum cholesterol and high blood pressure as risk factors for coronary heart disease.

> **Note**
> **Applied aspect**
> - Within a few months of quitting smoking, coughing and shortness of breath decrease.
> - Within 1 year of quitting smoking; the person's risk of heart attack and angina is about half that of a smoker.
> - Fifteen years after quitting, the risk of heart attack and angina is the same as that of a nonsmoker.
> - Quitting smoking after a heart attack reduces the chances of having another heart attack by 50%.

### Risk Groups

"Risk approach" was developed and promoted by WHO to identify the "risk groups" or "target groups" or "vulnerable groups" (e.g. at-risk mothers, at-risk infants, at-risk families, chronically ill, handicapped, elderly) in the population by

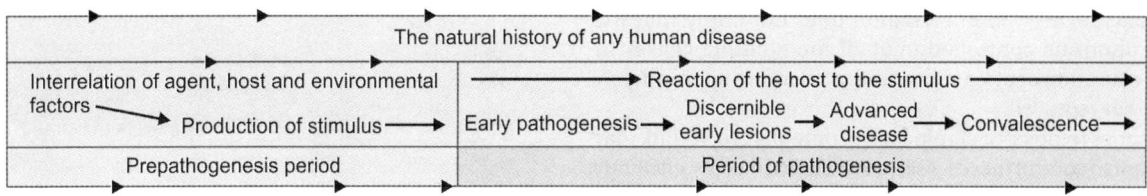

**Fig. 3.10:** Natural history of the disease.

certain well-defined criteria and direct appropriate action to them at priority basis.

The underlying concept for this approach is "something for all, but more for those who are in need—in proportion to their need". This approach is a managerial device for increasing the efficiency of healthcare services within the limits of existing resources.

Modern epidemiology is concerned with the identification of risk factors and high-risk groups in the population as the resources are very scarce and identification of those at risk is imperative to define priorities and points to those who need them most.

*Guidelines for defining "at-risk" groups:*
- *Biological situation*: Age group like infants (low birth weight), toddlers, elderly; sex like females in the reproductive age period; physiological state like pregnancy, cholesterol level, high blood pressure; genetic factors like family history of genetic disorders; other health conditions like a disease, physical functioning, and unhealthy behavior.
- *Physical situation*: Rural, urban slums, living conditions like overcrowding, environment—like water supply, proximity to industries; sociocultural and cultural situation—like social class, ethnic and cultural group, family disruption, education, housing, customs, habits, and behavior (e.g. smoking, lack of exercise, over-eating, drug addicts), access to health services, and lifestyles and attitudes.

## Pathogenesis Period

It is the second phase of the disease in man. The phase of pathogenesis begins when the causative disease agent enters the human being. After entering, irrespective of the route, disease agent goes to the site of election, lodges there, gets adapted, multiplies, reaches an optimum number, disturbs the structure and function of that organ, and produces changes in the blood and tissue fluid.

Then the disease progresses through a period of incubation and later into early and late pathogenesis. After the onset of clinical features, the outcome of the disease may be complete recovery, chronicity, disability or death of the individual. This phase is modified by intervention measures such as immunization and chemotherapy.

A host's reaction to infection with a disease agent may result in a clinical case, subclinical case or becomes carrier (as in diphtheria, typhoid).

In chronic diseases (e.g. diabetes, coronary heart disease, hypertension, COPD, cancer), the early pathogenesis phase is referred to as a presymptomatic phase (i.e. no manifest disease). The pathological changes are essentially below the level of the "clinical horizon". The clinical stage begins when recognizable signs or symptoms appear. By the time signs and symptoms appear, the disease phase is already well advanced into the late pathogenesis phase.

> **Note**
> The period between the successful entrance of the organism and the onset of the first symptom is called "incubation period". Secondary and tertiary levels of prevention are possible during the "period of pathogenesis". Screening of the disease may improve prognosis and increase survival at this stage.

Understanding about the natural history of any disease is essential as it gives the necessary framework to the pathogenic chain of events for that disease, and for the application of preventive measures at different phases of the disease process **(Fig. 3.10)**. *The levels of prevention and modes of intervention are discussed in Chapter 8: Preventive Medicine.*

## Web of Causation

MacMahon and Pugh gave this model of disease causation in their book "Epidemiologic Principles and Methods". This model is basically for the study of noncommunicable disease, where the disease agent is often not recognized, but the disease is an outcome of the interaction of multiple factors. The "web of causation" considers all the predisposing risk factors of any type and their complex interrelationship with each other.

For example, the multiple predisposing factors in the web of causation of coronary heart disease are excess of smoking, high blood pressure, high cholesterol, obesity, lack of exercise, type A personality, etc. So these are considered as "risk-factors", in the web of causation of the disease **(Fig. 3.11)**.

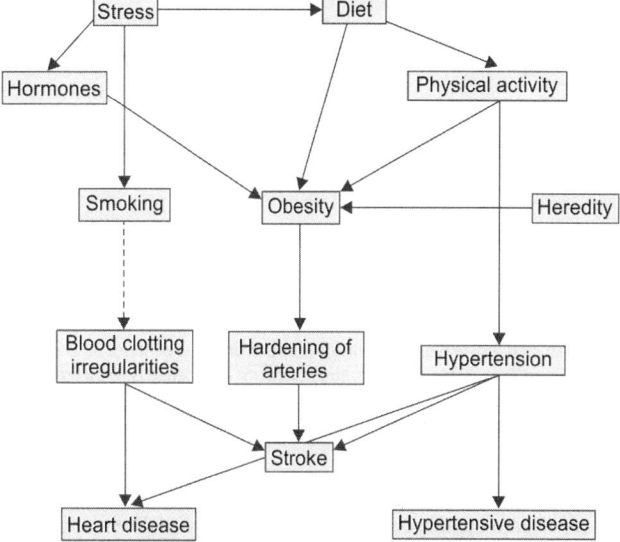

**Fig. 3.11:** The web of causation of disease.

This model shows a variety of possible interventions that could be taken which might reduce the occurrence of coronary heart disease. The web of causation does not imply that the disease cannot be controlled until all the multiple causes or chains of causation or at least a number of them are appropriately controlled or removed.

Sometimes removal or elimination of only one crucial link may be sufficient to control the disease, provided that link is sufficiently important in the pathogenesis process. In a multifactorial event, therefore, individual factors do not have equal weight age. The relative importance of these factors may be expressed concerning "relative risk".

> **Note**
> "Silent epidemic" of the century: Alzheimer's disease
> Modern epidemic: Coronary heart disease

## SPECTRUM OF DISEASE

It is a graphic representation of variations in the manifestations of the disease. It is like the spectrum of light where the colors of light varying from one end to the other, but not easy to determine where one color ends and the other begins. At one end of the disease spectrum are subclinical infections which are not ordinarily identified, and at the other end are fatal illnesses. In the middle of the spectrums lie illnesses ranging from mild to severe degree of severity **(Fig. 3.12)**.

These different manifestations are the result of individuals' different states of immunity and receptivity. The sequence of events in the spectrum of disease can be interrupted by early diagnosis and treatment or by preventive measures which if introduced at a specific point will prevent the further development of the disease.

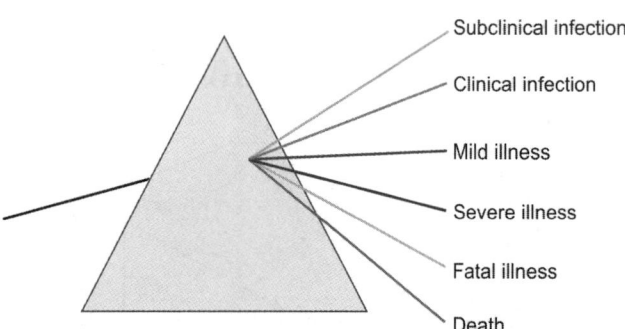

**Fig. 3.12:** Spectrum of disease.

> **Note**
> - Leprosy is an excellent example of the spectrum of disease.
> - Rabies is a disease not having the spectrum of severity.
> - In communicable diseases, the spectrum of disease is referred to as the "gradient of infection".

### Iceberg Phenomenon of Disease

It is a concept closely related to the spectrum of disease. Disease in a community may be compared to an iceberg. When a piece of ice is allowed to float on water, only a small portion is visible, and a significant portion is submerged in the water **(Fig. 3.13)**.

*Floating tip*: What physician sees in the community (clinical cases)

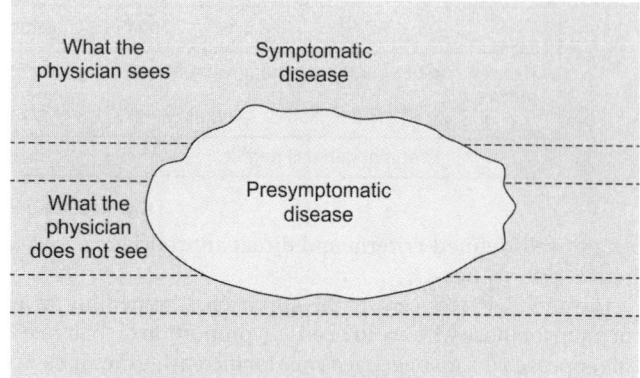

**Fig. 3.13:** Iceberg phenomenon of disease.

*Large submerged portion*: The hidden mass of disease (latent, in-apparent, presymptomatic and undiagnosed cases, and carriers) which are all responsible for the constant prevalence of the disease in the community.

*The line of demarcation (water surface)*: Is demarcation between apparent and in-apparent infections.

*Water surrounding iceberg*: Healthy population.

In some diseases like hypertension, diabetes, anemia, malnutrition, mental illness, the unknown morbidity (i.e. the submerged portion of the iceberg) far exceeds the known morbidity. Epidemiologist is concerned with a "hidden portion of an iceberg" whereas clinician is concerned with "tip of the iceberg".

> **Note**
> - Screening is done for a hidden portion of iceberg whereas diagnosis is made from the tip of the iceberg.
> - Iceberg phenomenon of disease is not shown by: rabies, tetanus, measles, and rubella.

This chapter deals with basic concept of health, well-being and disease. ***Different indicators of health are further discussed in Chapter 9: Basics of Epidemiology. Concept of control and prevention as well as modes of intervention are discussed with further details in Chapter 8: Preventive Medicine.***

## SUMMARY

Health and disease are among the fundamental experiences of human life. The global scientific and economic limitations of medicine have made the concepts of health and disease a central topic in theory as well as in practice. This chapter describes in detail about the various concepts of health and disease, dimensions and determinants of health, spectrum of health and disease, various indices of quality of life, natural history of disease, epidemiological triad and iceberg phenomenon. Understanding of these concepts of health and disease is very important because they influence the thinking of medical graduates, helping them to broaden their vision about holistic and comprehensive health care.

## SUGGESTED READING

1. Detels R, Beaglehole R, Lansang MA, et al. Oxford Textbook of Public Health, 5th edition. Oxford University Press; 2015. pp. 56-88.
2. MacMahon B, Pugh TF. Epidemiology: Principles and Methods, 1st edition. Little, Brown; 1970. pp. 72-8.

# CHAPTER 4

# Nutrition and Health

*Zinia T Nujum*

| CM5.1 | Describe the common sources of various nutrients and special nutritional requirements according to age, sex, activity, physiological conditions |
|---|---|
| CM5.4 | Plan and recommend a suitable diet for the individuals and families based on local availability of foods and economic status, etc., in a simulated environment |

## INTRODUCTION

### Role of Nutrition in Health—Why Study?

Nutrition is an essential requirement of human being to stay healthy. Food consumption determines the nutrition and health of the population. Food consumption is in turn influenced by the production, distribution of foods, purchasing power of the individual, and related policies of the country and state. Food provides nutrients and non-nutrient phytochemicals required for health. Since people consume food and not nutrients, it is important to understand nutrition in the language of food instead of nutrients. Therefore, the focus is now on a food-based approach to nutrition for optimal health. The mouth is considered as the gateway to our body, the food we eat decides ultimately our identity and immunity. Therefore, it determines ourselves and our health.

## DEFINING SOME IMPORTANT CONCEPTS

### Food

According to the Prevention of Food Adulteration Act, 1954 (PFA, now replaced with the Food Safety and Standards Act, 2006), food is defined as, "Any article used as food or drink for human consumption other than drugs and water and includes any article which is used for the preparation or is part of the composition of human food, flavoring matter or condiments and any article which the Central Government may notify in the official gazette as food".

So, it is the use by humans/function which defines food more than its structure. We determine our food choices. This is called food preference. Thereby, we determine our health.

### Health

Health is defined as the state of complete physical, mental, and social well-being and not merely the absence of disease or infirmity.

### Nutrients

Nutrients are specific dietary constituents in the diet, which may be organic and inorganic complexes. It is a chemical factor (active ingredient) present in food item, which determines the quality of food and in turn the health of the individual. There are about 50 different nutrients in food. Each nutrient has a specific role to perform in the body. In particular, food provides more than one nutrient. To keep us healthy the food we eat should be such that it provides all nutrients in adequate quantity and quality.

### *Macronutrients and Micronutrients*

Macronutrients are those nutrients which are needed in high quantities by the body. The macronutrients that food gives are carbohydrates, proteins, and fats. Macronutrients are also called the **proximate principles**. Micronutrients are those nutrients which are required only in small quantities. Vitamins and minerals are micronutrients.

### Diet

Kinds of food on which a person or group lives. **Dietetics** is the practical application of principles of nutrition for well and sick persons.

### Nutrition

It is that branch of science, which deals with the study of a dynamic process, in which the consumed food is utilized for nourishing the body.

## CLASSIFICATION OF FOODS

Foods are classified on the basis of origin, chemical composition, major function, nutritive value, etc. The most important classification to understand as health professional is the classification based on nutritive value.

### Classification by Origin

- Foods of animal origin
- Foods of vegetable origin.

### Classification by Chemical Composition

- Carbohydrate
- Protein

- Fat
- Vitamins
- Minerals.

## Classification by Predominant Function

- Body-building—milk, meat, egg, poultry, pulses
- Energy-giving-cereals, sugars, roots and tubers, fats and oils
- Protective foods—vegetables, fruits, and milk.

## Classification by Nutritive Value

- Cereals and millets
- Pulses
- Vegetables and fruits
- Animal foods
- Nuts and oilseeds
- Fats and oils
- Sugar and jaggery
- Condiments and spices

## BALANCED DIET

A balanced diet is defined as one which contains a variety of foods in such quantities and proportions that the need for energy, carbohydrates, proteins, fats, vitamins, minerals, and other nutrients is adequately met for maintaining health, vitality and general well-being and also makes a small provision for extra nutrients to withstand a short duration of leanness. Carbohydrate sources should constitute around 60% of total calories in a balanced diet. Around 20% energy should be from proteins and remaining 20% from visible and invisible fat.

The other nutrients mentioned in the definition include dietary fiber, antioxidants, and phytochemicals. These also have a role in providing positive health to the individual. Antioxidants and phytochemicals protect the body from free radical damage. The spices that are commonly used in India like ginger, garlic, cumin, and turmeric are rich in antioxidants. We will learn more about these towards the end of this section. Eating a balanced diet is required to keep a person healthy. A balanced diet contains all the essential nutrients in the required quantities. Each nutrient has a special function to perform in our body, so providing this balance of the variety is essential to promote health and maintain well-being.

## What Constitutes Adequate Quantities?

### Dietary Reference Intakes—Definitions

#### Adequate Intake (AI)

It is the recommended average daily intake level based on observed or experimentally determined approximations or estimates of nutrient intake by a group (or groups) of apparently healthy people, that are assumed to be adequate. It is used when a recommended dietary allowance (RDA) cannot be ascertained. In the Indian context, this is referred to as acceptable intake.

#### Tolerable Upper Intake Level

The highest average daily nutrient intake level that is likely to pose no risk of adverse health effects for almost all individuals in the general population. As intake increases above the upper intake level (UL), the potential risk of adverse effects increases.

#### Estimated Average Requirement

The average daily nutrient intake level estimated to meet the requirement of half of the healthy individuals in a particular life stage and gender group is called the average nutrient requirement (ANR). This value is called estimated average requirement (EAR) when it is derived on the basis of available scientific knowledge. For nutrients where such evidence is not there, the term average intake (AI) is used.

#### Recommended Dietary Allowance

Recommended dietary allowance (RDA) is the average daily dietary nutrient intake level sufficient to meet the nutrient requirement of nearly all (97.5%) healthy individuals in a particular life stage and gender group.

**The equations used to calculate the RDA are as follows:** If the standard deviation (SD) of the EAR is available and the requirement for the nutrient is symmetrically distributed, the RDA is set at two SD above the EAR. Thus, RDA = EAR + 2 SD (EAR). If data about variability in requirements are insufficient to calculate an SD, we assume that RDA is 20% more than EAR. Thus, RDA = 1.2 EAR. This level of intake of RDA statistically represents 97.5% of the requirements of the population. It also implies that at a particular RDA intake level, it would cause a harmful nutrient deficiency in just 2.5%.

**The formulation of RDA:** Nutrition Advisory Committee of Indian Research Fund Association (IRFA), which is now known as Indian Council of Medical Research (ICMR) formulated RDA for Indians first in 1944, based on the recommendations given by the Health Committee of League of Nations in the year 1937. This was revised by the same committee in 1960. The most recent revision took place in 2020 by the expert group of National Institute of Nutrition (NIN), based on international reports and researches from India.

The recommended level is based on the bioavailability of nutrients. Bioavailability of a nutrient will depend on the amount that is absorbed and utilized. RDA is recommended considering the bioavailability and also a safety margin. This safety margin will take care of the individual variations and the dietary cooking practices. The important determinants of RDA are age, physical activity, and physiological state. RDA is actually the suggested averages for a day. Daily intake of food and the corresponding nutrients will vary depending on the availability and many other factors. This average is to be achieved over a time period.

### General Principles for Arriving at Nutrient Requirements

Various principles have been employed to arrive at the nutrient requirements. Some of these are the dietary intake, growth assessment, nutrient balance, factorial approach, nutrient turnover, and depletion and repletion studies. Factorial approach is used for calculation of energy requirement. In this method, the nutrients required for sleep, rest, occupational and non-occupational activity are calculated. Nutrient turnover method uses isotopically labeled nutrients to determine the requirements of some nutrients like vitamins A, C, iron and vitamin $B_{12}$. Depletion and repletion studies are used for finding the requirement of water-soluble vitamins.

## Dietary Goals—Prudent Diet

The recommendation by Indian Council of Medical Research for dietary goals are as below:

### Dietary Goals—ICMR

- Not more than 20% of total energy should be from fat source.
- Saturated fat should not constitute 10% of total energy.
- Protein should provide 15–20% of total energy intake.
- The consumption of refined carbohydrates should be restricted.
- The consumption of carbohydrates rich in natural fiber should be encouraged.
- Salt consumption should be less than 5 g/day.
- Alcohol and fat have to be restricted.
- Junk foods like colas and ketchups that provide empty calories (calories are provided, but no nutrients) are to be avoided.

**Table 4.1** for the recommended proportions.

Table 4.1: Proportions of nutrients.

| Dietary factor | Goal (% of total energy, unless otherwise stated) |
|---|---|
| Total fat | 15–30% |
| Saturated fatty acids | <10% |
| Polyunsaturated fatty acids (PUFAs) | 6–10% |
| n-6 polyunsaturated fatty acids (PUFAs) | 5–8% |
| n-3 polyunsaturated fatty acids (PUFAs) | 1–2% |
| Trans fatty acids | <1% |
| Monounsaturated fatty acids[a] | By difference |
| Total carbohydrates[b] | 55–75% |
| Free sugars[c] | <10% |
| Protein | 10–15%[d] |
| Cholesterol | <300 mg per day |
| Sodium chloride (sodium)[e] | <5 g per day (<2 g per day) |
| Fruits and vegetables | 400 g per day |
| Total dietary fiber | From foods |
| Nonstarch polysaccharides (NP) | From foods |

[a]This is calculated as: total fat − (saturated fatty acids + polyunsaturated fatty acids + trans fatty acids).
[b]The percentage of total energy available after taking into account that consumed as protein and fat, hence the wide range.
[c]The term "free sugars" refers to all monosaccharides and disaccharides added to foods by the manufacturer, cook or consumer, plus sugars naturally present in honey, syrups and fruit juices.
[d]The suggested range should be seen in the light of the Joint WHO/FAO/UNU Expert Consultation on Protein and Amino Acid Requirements in Human Nutrition, held in Geneva from 9 to 16 April 2002.
[e]Salt should be iodized appropriately. The need to adjust salt iodization, depending on observed sodium intake and surveillance of iodine status of the population, should be recognized.

## ENERGY—REQUIREMENTS AND SOURCES

### How Much Energy Do We Need?

Energy requirement was considered to be that level of intake which balances the energy expenditure required to keep the person healthy on a long-term and at the same time economically and socially productive. If an individual's intake is much less than required for the energy expenditure, it results in either burning extra fat or reducing body weight or an adaptation of the metabolic processes to maintain weight. Similarly, an excess energy intake can result in obesity. The approach currently used to find energy requirement is based on energy expenditure and this is considered a more rational approach. Energy expenditure depends on several factors like age, gender, physical activity at work and leisure, and body build of the person. For the purpose of calculating requirements based on these factors, reference woman and a reference man have been defined **(Box 4.1)**. Examples of occupations that are referred to as sedentary, moderate, and heavy are listed in **Table 4.2**. Energy expenditure should also meet a child's requirement for growth, pregnant and lactating women's need for the developing fetus and secretion of milk.

> **Box 4.1: Criteria for Indian Reference woman and man.**
> **Reference woman (for a change, we will learn the woman first):**
> - 19–39 years of age
> - Non-pregnant non-lactating (NPNL)
> - Weighs 55 kg with a height of 1.62 m and a BMI of 20.95 kg/m$^2$
> - Free from disease and physically fit for active work
> - On working day, 8 hours in occupation involving moderate activity
> While not at work, 8 hours in bed. 4–6 hours in sitting and moving about, 2 hours in walking and in active recreation or household duties.
> **Reference man:**
> - 19–39 years of age and weight 65 kg
> - Height of 1.77 m with a BMI of 20.75 kg/m$^2$
> - Free from disease and physically fit for active work
> - On working day, 8 hours in occupation involving moderate activity
> While not at work, 8 hours in bed, 4–6 hours in sitting and moving about 2 hours in walking and in active recreation or household duties.

Table 4.2: Examples of sedentary, moderate, and heavy worker.

| Work | Examples |
|---|---|
| Sedentary | Teacher, Tailor, Barber, Priest, Executive, Peon, Retired personnel, Shoemaker, Housewife, Maid, Nurse, Doctor, Clerk, Shopkeeper, Manager, Goldsmith |
| Moderate | Potter, Basket maker, Carpenter, Mason, Electrician, Fitter, Welder, Fisherman, Coolie worker, Site supervisor, Postman |
| Heavy | Stonecutter, Blacksmith, Mine worker, Wood cutter, Farm laborer, Army soldier |

### Methods used for Finding the Energy Expenditures

The earlier committee used 5% reduction in basal metabolic rate (BMR) from FAO/WHO/UNU equations and higher PAL values for deriving energy requirements for adults. Whereas, 2020 ICMR committee proposed a reduction in the BMR to 10% and 9% for males and females respectively with simultaneous reduction in PAL values. The physical activity ratio (PAR) is expressed as follows:

Physical Activity Ratio (PAR) =

$$\frac{\text{Energy cost of an activity per minute}}{\text{Energy cost of basal metabolism per minute}}$$

The PAR is unit-less. The aggregate of the PAR values of all the activities done in a day gives the physical activity level (PAL). It is the ratio of the energy expenditure for 24 hours and the BMR over 24 hours. The PAR of different activities is shown in **Table 4.3A** and the PAL values in **Table 4.3B**.

**Table 4.3A:** PAR of different activities obtained from single study or averaged across studies.

| Activity | Average PAR | |
|---|---|---|
| | Male | Female |
| Sleeping | 1.0 | 1.0 |
| Sitting quietly | 1.2 | 1.2 |
| Reading | 1.3 | 1.5 |
| Standing | 1.4 | 1.5 |
| Dressing | 2.4 | 3.3 |
| Walking slowly | 2.8 | 3.0 |
| Walking briskly | 3.8 | 3.8 |
| Cycling | 5.6 | 3.6 |
| Running—sprint | 8.2 | 8.3 |
| Running—long distance | 6.3 | 6.6 |
| Basketball | 7.0 | 7.7 |
| Football | 8.0 | – |
| Swimming | 9.0 | – |

(PAR: physical activity ratio)

**Table 4.3B:** PAL values proposed by ICMR Expert Group of 2020, 2010, 1989 compared to the figures proposed by FAO/WHO/UNU Consultation, 2004.

| Level of activity | ICMR 1989 | ICMR 2009 | ICMR 2020 | FAO/WHO/UNU |
|---|---|---|---|---|
| Sedentary work | 1.60 | 1.53 | 1.40 | 1.40–1.69 |
| Moderate work | 1.90 | 1.80 | 1.80 | 1.70–1.99 |
| Heavy work | 2.50 | 2.30 | 2.30 | 2.0–2.40* |

*PAL of more than 2.4 is difficult to maintain over prolonged periods.
(FAO/WHO/UNU: Food and Agriculture Organization of the United Nations/World Health Organization/United Nations University; ICMR: Indian Council of Medical Research; PAL: physical activity level)

The total energy requirement or the total energy expenditure (TEE) is calculated based on a multiplication of basal metabolic rate (BMR) to physical activity level (PAL): TEE = BMR × PAL.

## Units of Energy

Joule has been adopted as unit of energy by the International Union of Sciences and International Union of Nutritional Sciences (IUNS). These units are defined as follows:
- **Joule**, a physical unit of energy, is defined as the energy required to move 1 kg of mass by 1 meter by a force of 1 Newton acting on it (1 Newton is the force needed to accelerate 1 kg mass by 1 meter per sec).
- **Kilocalories (kcal)** was the unit of energy used for a long time. kcal is defined as the heat required to raise the temperature of 1 kg of water by 1°C from 14.5°C to 15.5°C. The unit kcal is still popularly used. Both units are used in defining human energy requirement.
- The relationship between the two units of energy is as follows:
  - 1 kcal = 4.184 KJ (Kilojoule)
  - 1 KJ = 0.239 kcal
  - 1000 kcal = 4184 KJ = 4.18 MJ (Mega joule), 1 MJ = 239 kcal

## Source of Energy

The metabolizable energy (ME) from different foods is shown below:

| Nutrient | kcal/g |
|---|---|
| Carbohydrate | 4 |
| Protein | 4 |
| Fat | 9 |
| Dietary fiber | 2 |

## Requirements of Energy in Pregnancy

In pregnancy additional nutrients are required for the fetal growth, increase in BMR and body weight. An Indian woman weighing 55 kg prior to pregnancy with a weight gain of 10–12 kg will require 350 kcal/day in addition to the normal requirement.

## Requirements of Energy during Lactation

The additional requirement during the first 6 months of exclusive breastfeeding is 600 kcal/day. It is reduced to 520 kcal/day in the next 6 months for partial breastfeeding. The requirement depends on the amount of breast milk.

The summary of energy requirements of Indians is shown in **Table 4.4**.

**Table 4.4:** Energy requirements of Indians at different ages (ICMR NIN Expert Group 2020).

| Age Group | Category | Body weights | (kcal/d)[a] |
|---|---|---|---|
| Men | Sedentary work | 65.0 | 2,110 |
| | Moderate work | 65.0 | 2,710 |
| | Heavy work | 65.0 | 3,470 |
| Women | Sedentary work | 55.0 | 1,660 |
| | Moderate work | 55.0 | 2,130 |
| | Heavy work | 55.0 | 2,720 |
| | Pregnant | 55.0 + GWG[b] | +350 |
| | Lactating (0–6 months) | 55.0 | +600 |
| | Lactating (7–12 months) | | +520 |
| Infants | 0–6 months | 5.8 | 530 |
| | 6–12 months | 8.5 | 660 |
| Children[c] | 1–3 years | 12.9 | 1,110 |
| | 4–6 years | 18.3 | 1,360 |
| | 7–9 years | 25.3 | 1,700 |
| Boys | 10–12 years | 34.9 | 2,220 |
| Girls | 10–12 years | 36.4 | 2,060 |
| Boys | 13–15 years | 50.5 | 2,860 |
| Girls | 13–15 years | 49.6 | 2,400 |
| Boys | 16–18 years | 64.4 | 3,320 |
| Girls | 16–18 years | 55.7 | 2,500 |

[a]Rounded off to the nearest 10 kcal/d
[b]GWG—Gestational Weight Gain. Energy need in pregnancy should be adjusted for actual bodyweight, observed weight gain and activity pattern for the population.
[c]Energy needs of children have been computed for reference children which were assumed to have a moderate daily physical activity level.

# MACRONUTRIENTS

## Carbohydrates—Requirement and Sources

Carbohydrates (CHO) are a major and vital source of energy in the diet. The quantity and quality of CHO are important to maintain appropriate health and have been indicated to substantially impact nutrition related chronic disorders/non-communicable diseases (NCDs). Carbohydrates are made up of three components: fiber, starch, and sugar. Fiber and starch are complex carbs, while sugar is a simple carbohydrate **(Table 4.5)**.

CHO are the major source of easily available energy in human diets comprising more than 60-78% of total energy intake, particularly in India. CHO is important to maintain glycemic homeostasis and gastrointestinal integrity and function. The major dietary sources of CHO are sugars, cereals and millets, roots and tubers, pulses and legumes and to a limited extent from vegetables, fruits and dairy.

The nature and type of dietary CHO is more critical rather than the quantity of CHO for desired health effects. CHO from whole grains, legumes, vegetables and whole fruits are associated with reduced risk of type-2 diabetes mellitus and cardiovascular disease. "Free sugars or Added sugars" refers to all monosaccharides and disaccharides added to foods and beverages by the manufacturer, cook or consumer, as well as to sugars naturally present in honey, syrups, fruit juices and fruit juice concentrates. The World Health Organization in 2003 recommended that not more than 10% of total energy should be from free sugars/added sugars with a goal to reduce or prevent diet-related chronic diseases.

The estimated average requirement (EAR) for CHO has been reported to be 100 g/day for ages 1 year and above with a Recommended Dietary Allowance (RDA) of 130 g/day. The RDA for CHO for pregnant women is set at 175 g/day and for lactating women it is set at 200 g/day. For children below 1 year of age, an Adequate Intake (AI) value is suggested. For the children below 6 months of age, AI is 55 g/day. For children 7-12 months of age, the AI is 95 g/day.

### Glycemic Index

The glycemic index is a value assigned to foods based on how slowly or how quickly those foods cause increases in blood glucose levels.

The glycemic index (GI) of foods is categorized into three groups: a GI value below 55 is defined as low, 56 to 69 as moderate and 70 and above as high. Glycemic load (GL) considers the GI and the total amount of available CHO present in the food consumed (GL = GI/100 × CHO content). GL value is categorized as low (≤10), moderate (10-19) and high (≥20).

*Note:* **Glycemic index is further explained under therapeutic diet at the end of this chapter.**

## Proteins

The proteins needed by the body are synthesized using the amino acids from dietary proteins. Body synthesis proteins that are either structural, or function as enzymes, or other nitrogenous compounds in the body. Proteins form the basic structural and functional unit of life. The sites where the body proteins are found include muscle, bone, cartilage, and skin. Structurally, proteins are made up of a variety of amino acids to form complex molecules. Children require dietary proteins during growth for the synthesis of new proteins in tissues. In adults they are required for substituting the broken-down proteins. Synthesis of fetal, placental and other body proteins demands extra protein requirement in pregnancy. Extra proteins are also necessary during lactation to meet the need of production of proteins of the breast milk.

The amino acids which cannot be synthesized by our body need to be obtained from the diet and are called essential amino acids. Proteins are a source of energy besides other functions mentioned earlier. 4 kcal is obtained from 1 g of protein as metabolizable energy. Animal proteins obtained from fish, milk, eggs, and meat are thought to be of high quality, since they have all the essential amino acids in the required quantities. Egg protein is considered as a reference protein. Plant or vegetable proteins obtained from foods like pulses and legumes are considered to have a lower quality. They have a lower content of essential amino acids. Essential amino acids (see the list in **Table 4.6**) are also called indispensable amino acids (IAA).

**Table 4.5:** Types of carbohydrates.

| Type | Type of carbohydrate | Source |
|---|---|---|
| Simple | Glucose and fructose | Fruits, vegetables, and honey |
| | Sucrose | Sugar |
| | Lactose | Milk |
| Complex | Starch | Cereals, millets, pulses, and root vegetables |
| | Glycogen | Animal foods |
| | Cellulose (dietary fiber) | Vegetables and whole grains |
| | Gums and Pectin (dietary fiber) | Vegetables, fruits, and cereals |

**Table 4.6:** Requirement of amino acids and proteins in adults.

| Amino acid | FAO/WHO/UNU 2007 | | FAO/WHO/UNU 1985 | |
|---|---|---|---|---|
| | mg/kg/d | mg/g protein | mg/kg/d | mg/g protein |
| Histidine | 10 | 15 | 8–12 | 15 |
| Isoleucine | 20 | 30 | 10 | 15 |
| Leucine | 39 | 59 | 14 | 21 |
| Lysine | 30 | 45 | 12 | 18 |
| Methionine | 10 | 16 | – | – |
| Cysteine | 4 | 6 | – | – |
| Methionine + Cysteine | 15 | 22 | 13 | 20 |
| Threonine | 15 | 23 | 7 | 11 |
| Phenylalanine + Tyrosine | 25 | 38 | 14 | 21 |
| Tryptophan | 4 | 6 | 3.5 | 5.0 |
| Valine | 26 | 39 | 10 | 15 |
| Total EAA | 184 | 277 | 93.5 | 141 |
| Total protein | 0.66 g/kg/d | | 0.60 g/kg/d | |
| Safe level of protein (Mean + 1.96 × SD) | 0.83 g/kg/d | | 0.77 g/kg/d | |

Safe level of protein is the requirement from a mixed or single dietary protein. (EAA: essential amino acids; FAO/WHO/UNU: Food and Agriculture Organization of the United Nations/World Health Organization/United Nations University)

## Supplementary Action of Protein

The essential amino acid which is deficient in a food is called the limiting amino acid. In pulses and legumes, the limiting amino acid is methionine and in cereals it is lysine and threonine.

Cereals and pulses, used in combination (for example; rice and dal in India) provides the amino acids which are essential and complement each other for improving the quality proteins. This is known as supplementary action of protein. Cereal and pulses are usually combined in a 5:1 proportion to achieve this supplementary action. Pulses contain 20–25% protein and are called poor man's meat. A still more important source is cereals with a protein content of 8–13%. Since, they are taken in bulk, cereals form the main source of protein in diet. They account for 50% of the total intake of proteins. The amino acid content is only one factor that determines the protein quality. Digestibility, absorption, and utilization are the others, e.g. the protein digestibility is decreased by the presence of high content of dietary fiber in vegetables.

## Quantitative Assessment of Protein Quality

The assessment of protein quality can be done by the following methods:

- **Digestibility coefficient** = Nitrogen absorbed/Nitrogen intake × 100
- **Biological value** = Nitrogen retained/Nitrogen absorbed × 100
- **Net protein utilization (NPU)** = Nitrogen retained/Nitrogen intake × 100; or DC × BV
- **Amino acid score** = (mg/g of limiting amino acid in the test protein)/(mg/g of the particular amino acid in reference protein) × 100. It is the percentage of the limiting amino acid present in the food compared to the reference protein.
- **Protein digestibility corrected amino acid score** = Protein digestibility × amino acid score

Mixed vegetarian diet has a protein digestibility of 85%. The efficiency of protein utilization is obtained from the PDCAAS value. BV is related to its amino acid score. BV cannot be more than 100. The quantity of protein to meet the safe requirement will be equal to the safe level of protein divided by the PDCAAS value.

> **Exercise:** Find the amino acid score (lysine score) of wheat, if the amount of lysine in wheat is 27 mg/g of protein and reference protein contains 45 mg/g of protein.
> Did you get the answer as 60%—very good.

## Protein Energy Ratio

For the dietary proteins to be used effectively for protein synthesis and other functions of proteins in the body, adequate amount of energy has to be obtained from carbohydrates and fats. Thus, the protein and energy requirement may be preferably considered together. The protein requirement can be expressed as ratio of protein energy to the total dietary energy requirement (PE ratio). This PE ratio will be different across age categories and in adults involved in different activities **(Table 4.7)**. It can be seen from the table that protein requirements are not related to activity, but energy requirement depends on activity. By increasing activity, the PE ratio decreases. Diets with a high PE ratio of more than 15% are not recommended. Some elderly and pregnant women use commercial high protein supplements. This is not generally recommended.

Human protein requirements can be determined by several methods. The method that is recommended by the 1985 and 2007 FAO/WHO/UNU (Food and Agriculture Organization of the United Nations/World Health Organization/United Nations University) is the nitrogen balance method. The requirement of protein is determined by the protein quality. Previously, it was recommended as 0.60 mg/kg/day. In 2007, it has been revised as 0.66 mg/kg/day. This is when the median nitrogen required is 105 mg of N/kg/day. The earlier recommendation of safe requirement of protein was 0.77 mg/kg/day. Now, it has been raised as 0.83 mg/kg/day (*refer* **Table 4.6**). These changes have resulted from the evidence that has cumulated based on available N balance studies. The requirement of protein for adult male is 54 g and adult female is 46 g. The extra requirement of protein during the first 6 months of lactation is 16.9 g and the next 6 months is 13.2 g (ICMR-NIN Expert Group 2020) **(Table 4.8)**.

**Table 4.7:** Protein energy ratio (ICMR-NIN Expert Group 2020).

| Group | Protein requirement (g/kg/d[a]) | Energy requirement (kcal/kg/d) | PE ratio of requirement | PE ratio after adjusting for PDCAAS** |
|---|---|---|---|---|
| **Preschool children[b]** | | | | |
| 1–5 years | 0.95 | 79 | 4.8 | 5.9 |
| **School children[b]** | | | | |
| 6–10 years | 0.91 | 68 | 5.4 | 6.6 |
| **Adolescents[b]** | | | | |
| 11–17 years (boys) | 0.88 | 56 | 6.3 | 7.4 |
| 11–17 years (girls) | 0.86 | 51 | 6.7 | 8.1 |
| **Adults** | | | | |
| Men (sedentary) | 0.83 | 32 | 10.4 | 10.3 |
| Women (sedentary) | 0.83 | 30 | 11.1 | 11.2 |
| Men (moderate active) | 0.83 | 39 | 8.5 | 8.7 |
| Women (moderate active) | 0.83 | 37 | 9.0 | 9.6 |

PE Ratio = Protein energy ratio; these values refer to the requirement
[a]Safe requirement of high-quality protein
[b]Assuming moderately active children and adolescents
**PDCAAS: protein digestibility-corrected amino acid score

## Fats

Oil, butter, ghee, and vanaspati form the visible dietary fats. Besides this, they are also obtained from food as invisible fat. Fats provide 9 kcal/g. These are rich sources of energy. Other important function of fat is the transportation and absorption of fat-soluble vitamins. Therefore, they need to be consumed in adequate quantities. Dietary fats have fatty acids of different kinds in different proportions. Choice of the right kind of fats and oils enable the body to obtain the sufficient polyunsaturated fatty acids and the essential fatty acids. The level of cholesterol and triglyceride in

**Table 4.8:** Requirement of protein in adults (ICMR-NIN Expert Group 2020).

| | Body weight (kg) | RDA (g/kg/d) | Daily additional requirement (g) | RDA (g/d) |
|---|---|---|---|---|
| Adult Men | 65 | 0.83 | – | 54 |
| Adult Women | 55 | 0.83 | – | 45.7 |
| **Pregnant Women** | 55 + GWG | | | |
| 2nd trimester | | | 9.5 | 55.2 |
| 3rd trimester | | | 22 | 67.7 |
| **Lactating Women** | 55 | | | |
| (0–6 months) | | | 16.9 | 62.6 |
| (7–12 months) | | | 13.2 | 58.9 |

(GWG—gestational weight gain)
For people consuming cereal-based diet with low quality protein, the protein requirements are 1 g/kg per day.
*Note:* The cereal-legume-milk composition of the diet should be 3:1:2.5 for good protein quality.

the blood is determined by the dietary intake of fat. Fat in diet promotes satiety and gives flavor, texture, and taste to food.

Lipids can be simple, compound, or derived. Triglycerides are simple lipids. Fats are a type of lipid, which are triglycerides, with three fatty acids bound to a molecule of glycerol. Phospholipids are compound lipids and cholesterol is a derived lipid. 99% of fat in the body are seen as triglycerides.

Cooking oils which are in the liquid state and solid fats which are in the solid state are together called fats. Excessive fat in diet can elevate the blood lipids, promote atherosclerosis, and increase risk of obesity, cardiovascular disease, and malignancy.

Fats such as cooking oil, ghee, and vanaspathi are called visible fat. Most foods have fat as an integral component in them. This is known as invisible fat. For example, rice has 2–3% of fat in it (invisible fat) and it contributes to 15–30 g of fat in an average Indian diet. Fat present in processed foods is also not seen. It is referred to as hidden fats. For example, when we eat French fries, we do not see the visible fat which has gone into its preparation besides the invisible fat of the food item.

Fats should be consumed in moderation **(Table 4.9A)**. 15–30% of total calories comes from dietary fat.

Fats are made up of fatty acids. These may be saturated, mono or polyunsaturated. Animal foods are the predominant source of saturated fatty acids. Fats obtained from plant sources are usually unsaturated. An exception is coconut oil which contains 92% saturated fatty acids. Body can synthesize saturated fatty acids during the catabolism of carbohydrates and proteins. Lauric acid, palmitic acid, and stearic acid are examples of saturated fatty acids (SFA). The number of chains of carbon atoms in most of the SFA is even, ranging from 4 to 24. Those with less than 10 are classified as small, 12–14 as medium and 16–24 as long chain fatty acids. Short and medium chain fatty acids are good for infants and young children since they can be easily digested and absorbed. They are, however, not good for adults since they are highly atherogenic. SFAs should not contribute to more than 10% of the energy intake.

Unsaturated fatty acids are primarily derived from vegetable sources **(Table 4.9B)**. The body can synthesize monounsaturated fatty acids, but it cannot synthesize polyunsaturated fatty acids. Oleic acid is an example of monounsaturated fatty acid. Linoleic, arachidonic, eicosapentaenoic, and docosahexaenoic acid are polyunsaturated fatty acids. These polyunsaturated fatty acids have to be obtained from the diet and are called essential fatty acids. Unsaturated fatty acids have double bonds which can either be cis or trans, based on the location in relation to the acyl chain. When the double bond is in the trans configuration, the fatty acids are called trans fatty acids (TFA). PUFAs belong to n-6 series or n-3 series based on the location of the double bond in relation to the methyl end. Linoleic acid has 18 carbon atoms and has two double bonds. The first double bond is located in the sixth position from the methyl end, so it is written as 18:2n-6. Likewise, alpha linoleic acid (ALA) can be written as 18:3n-3. The current human diets have high contents of LA but low contents of ALA.

The type of fatty acid present in different foods are shown in **Table 4.9B**.

**Table 4.9A:** Recommendations for dietary fat intake in Indians (ICMR NIN Expert Group 2020).

| Age/Gender/physiological groups | Physical activity | Minimum level of Total fat (% E) | Fat from foods other than visible fats % E | Visible fat %E | Visible fat g/p/d |
|---|---|---|---|---|---|
| **Adult Men** | Sedentary | 20 | 10 | 10 | 25 |
| | Moderate | | | | 30 |
| | Heavy | | | | 40 |
| **Adult Women** | Sedentary | 20 | 10 | 10 | 20 |
| | Moderate | | | | 25 |
| | Heavy | | | | 30 |
| | Pregnant women | 20 | 10 | 10 | 30 |
| | Lactating women | | | | 30 |
| **Infants** | 0–6 months | 40–60 | Human milk | | |
| | 6–24 months | 35 | 10 | 25 | 25 |
| **Children** | 3–6 years | 25 | 10 | 15 | 25 |
| | 7–9 years | | | | 30 |
| **Boys** | 10–12 years | | | | 35 |
| | 13–15 years | | | | 45 |
| | 16–18 years | | | | 50 |
| **Girls** | 10–12 years | | | | 35 |
| | 13–15 years | | | | 40 |
| | 16–18 years | | | | 35 |

**Table 4.9B:** Types of fatty acids from different sources.

| Saturated | Monounsaturated | Polyunsaturated | | |
|---|---|---|---|---|
| • Coconut<br>• Palm kernel<br>• Ghee/butter<br>• Vanaspati | • Red palm oil<br>• Palmolein<br>• Groundnut<br>• Rice bran<br>• Sesame<br>• Olive Oil | Linoleic (n–6) | | Linolenic (n–3) |
| | | Low | Red palm oil, palmolein, olive oil | Rapeseed, mustard, soya bean |
| | | Moderate | Groundnut, rice bran, sesame | |
| | | High | Safflower, sunflower, cottonseed, corn, soya bean | |

Long chain n-3 fatty acids are obtained from fish and fish oils which are more biologically active and healthier than n-3 fatty acids derived from plant foods.

Dietary fat may also contain small quantities of tocopherols (rice bran oil), tocotrienols (palm oil), sterols, lignans (sesame oil), and oryzanol (rice bran oil). These have antioxidant properties and some of these help in reducing cholesterol. Refining of oils modifies the composition of these substances, e.g. while refining palm oil, carotenes are lost.

Cholesterol is a derived lipid. It can be synthesized in the body. Therefore, it is not considered as an essential dietary component. Cholesterol is present only in foods of animal origin. Egg yolk and organ meats like liver, kidney and brain are rich sources of cholesterol. It is also obtained from milk, meat, shrimp, and prawn. Cholesterol is a component of all cells and play an important role in formation of brain and nerve tissue. It is a precursor of vitamin D. Dietary cholesterol consumption should be kept at below 300 mg/day.

It is beneficial to replace some of the visible oils in diet with whole nuts and legumes because along with fat we also get protein, fiber, vitamins, and minerals.

### *Vanaspathi Ghee*

It is prepared by the hydrogenation of vegetable oils. It becomes solid and is used as a substitute for ghee. Since, it is resistant to oxidation, the keeping quality improves. The chemical change that occurs is the conversion of unsaturated fatty acids to saturated fatty acid and formation of transfat. This product is considered unhealthy and its use should be restricted. Not more than 2% of the energy should come from trans fatty acids.

### *Refined Oils*

Refining is usually done by treatment with steam, alkali, etc. Refining and deodorization of raw oils is done mainly to remove the free fatty acids and rancid materials which may be present in them. Refining does not bring about any change in the unsaturated fatty acid content of the oil. It only improves the quality and taste of oils. Refined oils are costly.

> **Note**
> - Take only adequate quantities of fat
> - Whole nuts can be substituted for some of the visible and invisible fats
> - High fat, SFA, and cholesterol containing animal foods may be taken only moderately
> - Use of ghee and butter for cooking as oil should be limited
> - In case of dairy products, it is better to choose low fat dairy products instead of whole, like skimmed milk
> - As a source of linoleic acid, it would be good to use legumes, fenugreek, mustard, and green leafy vegetables.
> - Prefer fish over meat and poultry
> - Organ meats like liver, brain, and kidney should be avoided
> - The number of eggs consumed should be restricted to three in a week
> - Consumption of the white of egg gives good quality protein and is encouraged
> - Hydrogenated oils like vanaspati is used for the preparation of bakery and processed foods. Its use is not recommended
> - The use of oils which have been reheated should be avoided
> - Variety of foods in moderation and in adequate proportions shall provide the optimum mix of fatty acids in diet.

## MICRONUTRIENTS

### Vitamins

Vitamins are essential micronutrients because they cannot be synthesized in the body. Beta-carotene is a provitamin which can be converted to vitamin A in the body. Vitamins may be water-soluble or fat-soluble. Fat-soluble vitamins are vitamin A, D, E, and K. They can be stored in the body. However, water soluble vitamins namely B and C are excreted in the urine. So they have to be taken daily. Water-soluble vitamins are easily destroyed by heating, cooking, and processing.

### *Fat-soluble Vitamins*

#### *Vitamin A*

In plant foods, vitamin A is present as beta carotene and in animal foods, it is present as retinol. Carotene is converted into retinol in the intestine, which is then absorbed and stored in the liver as retinol-palmitate.

**Functions:** Vitamin A helps in the synthesis of a pigment called "Rhodopsin". It occurs in the part of the eye called the retina. This pigment is essential for the normal vision, especially in the dim-light for dark adaptation. Thus, vitamin A is indispensable for normal vision.
- The integrity of the skin and mucous membrane of the conjunctiva, cornea, respiratory, alimentary, and urinary system is kept by the help of this vitamin.
- It promotes skeletal growth.
- It increases the immune response and is considered to have an anti-infective role.
- The vitamin also protects against some cancers like carcinoma of bronchus.

**Sources:** Vitamin A is found in both animal and plant foods. Animal sources (as retinol) are—meat, liver, fish, egg-yolk, milk, cheese, butter, and ghee. Richest source is fish liver oil (cod liver oil and shark liver oil).

**Vegetable sources (as β-carotene):** Cheapest source is green leafy vegetables, e.g. spinach and amaranth. Darker the green color of the vegetables, higher the carotene content. Richest source is red palm oil. Other sources are yellow fruits like mango and papaya. Some roots like carrots are also rich in β-carotene.

**Requirements:** Adult males require 1000 µg/day of vitamin A, while adult females require 840 µg/day of vitamin A **(Tables 4.10A and B)**.

#### *Vitamin D*

Vitamin D exists in two forms, vitamin $D_2$ and $D_3$. Vitamin $D_2$ also called calciferol and vitamin $D_3$ also referred as cholecalciferol are the two forms. Chemically, these are steroids. D2 is formed by the irradiation of ergosterol in the plants and is not obtained from the diet. $D_3$ is the naturally occurring vitamin D, obtained from animal fats and fish liver oils. When 7-dehydrocholesterol which is present as provitamin under the skin is exposed to ultraviolet rays of the sun, vitamin D is synthesized naturally. It is then stored in the liver and fat depots.

**Functions:** Vitamin D helps the absorption of calcium and phosphorus. It helps in the mineralization, i.e. calcification of bones and their hardening.

**Sources:** Vegetable foods do not contain this vitamin. If skin is exposed to UV rays of sun, adequate amounts of vitamin D can be synthesized in the body. Fish liver oil, butter, milk, ghee, and egg-yolk are rich sources of vitamin D.

**Requirements:** Since exposure to sunlight at least 5 minutes/day enables the synthesis the required amounts of vitamin D in the body, it is now considered more a pro-hormone than a vitamin. Traditional Indian diet gives only 10% of the requirement. WHO recommends the intake of 200 IU (5 μg)/day. In conditions of minimal sun exposure, the daily requirement is retained at 600 IU/day (ICMR-NIN Expert Group 2020). In several countries foods like milk and vegetable oils are fortified with vitamin D.

### *Vitamin E (Alpha Tocopherol) and Vitamin K*

Vitamin E is present in the invisible fat of plant foods and vegetable oils, consumed by Indians in adequate quantities. So, deficiency of this vitamin is rare. Dietary tocopherols are considered as supplementing antioxidants. The requirement is related to the need of antioxidants provided by the essential fatty acid in the diet. For one gram of essential fatty acid 0.8 mg is required. The daily requirement may be 8–10 mg based on the oil consumed.

Vitamin K deficiency is also very rarely encountered in India. Vitamin K has an important role to play in blood clotting and in the bone matrix formation and its turnover. Very little is known about the vitamin K content of Indian foods. The WHO/FAO recommendation of RDA is 55 μg of vitamin K per day.

### *Water-soluble Vitamins*

### *Thiamine ($B_1$)*

**Functions:** The function of thiamine in the body is mainly as coenzyme thiamine pyrophosphate (TPP). TPP is involved in carbohydrate and lipid metabolism.

**Dietary sources:** The important dietary sources of thiamine include cereals, nuts, green leafy vegetables, liver, organ meat, and eggs. Around 50% of the vitamin is lost during Indian methods of cooking and processing of raw foods, since it is water soluble.

**Requirement:** Thiamine can be stored in the body only in small quantities. Therefore, regular intake of thiamine in food is necessary. Absorption is poor if it is taken in large quantities together. The requirement is dependent on the calorie intake because this vitamin is essential for energy utilization. Minimum requirement is 1.4–2 mg irrespective of the calorie consumed. During pregnancy and the first 6 months of lactation an additional 0.6 mg and 0.7 mg is required respectively. The additional requirement reduces to 0.7 mg for the next 6 months of lactation. Compared to the recommendations of the FAO/WHO, this amount is low, since the secretion of thiamine in breast milk of Indian women is low **(Tables 4.10A and B)**.

### *Riboflavin ($B_2$)*

**Functions:** Riboflavin and its derivatives are cofactors for enzymes required for oxidation–reduction reactions. The vitamin itself has antioxidant activity. Riboflavin has a role in the metabolism of some vitamins like $B_6$, niacin, and vitamin K.

**Source:** Flesh foods, poultry, dairy products, legumes, nuts, and green leafy vegetables are rich sources of the vitamin. Riboflavin is heat stable but light labile. Indian cooking practices can lead to around 20% loss of riboflavin. Germination increases the riboflavin content of pulses and cereals.

**Requirements:** The minimum recommended intake is 2 mg/day irrespective of the calorie consumption. Additional requirements in pregnancy and lactation are similar to that of thiamine **(Tables 4.10A and B)**.

### *Niacin ($B_3$)*

The term niacin is used for nicotinic acid and nicotinamide. Niacinamide is a part of coenzymes that are necessary in glycolysis. During the synthesis of the essential amino acid tryptophan, niacin is produced. If tryptophan is consumed in the diet adequately, it is enough to satisfy the need for niacin. The efficiency of conversion of tryptophan to niacin depends on the amount of calorie and protein in food. About 60 mg tryptophan is considered equivalent to 1 mg niacin.

**Sources:** Usually animal foods are the predominant source of niacin, but in India, cereals also form a satisfactory source of the vitamin. However, in maize it is present in an unavailable or bound form. Compared to other B vitamins, niacin is more stable. The loss of the vitamin in cooking is also less and it is thought to be 25%.

**Requirement:** 14 mg and 11 mg are the requirements for sedentary male and female per day respectively **(Tables 4.10A and B)**.

### *Pantothenic Acid $B_5$*

It is required for the synthesis of corticosteroids in the body. The requirement of pantothenic acid is 10 mg/day. It is present in all foods. It is excreted at the rate of 3 mg/day in the urine.

### *Vitamin $B_6$*

Vitamin $B_6$ includes pyridoxal, pyridoxamine, pyridoxine, and their phosphorylated compounds. This vitamin is essential for gluconeogenesis and synthesis of neurotransmitters. The enzymes aminotransferases, decarboxylases, and side chain cleaving enzymes have pyridoxal phosphate as their coenzyme. Vitamin $B_6$ is essential for the functioning of immune system, nucleic acid, and homocysteine metabolism.

**Sources:** The rich sources of vitamin $B_6$ are egg, fish, meat, nuts, and wheat. Cereals, banana, and potato also provide the vitamin in moderate quantities. In plant foods, the predominant form of the vitamin is pyridoxine whereas in animal foods it is pyridoxal and pyridoxamine. Pyridoxine is not lost during the process of cooking, while pyridoxal and pyridoxamine are lost.

**Requirement:** The requirement of pyridoxine depends on the protein content in diet. The requirement is placed at 1.9 mg/day for sedentary adults. Pregnant women show deficiency of pyridoxine, unless given high doses of pyridoxine. An additional 0.4 mg is recommended for pregnant women. During lactation an extra amount of 0.26 mg of vitamin $B_6$ in first 6 months and 0.17 mg in next 6 months of vitamin $B_6$ is required **(Tables 4.10A and B)**.

**Table 4.10A:** Recommended dietary allowance of micronutrients (ICMR-NIN Expert Group 2020).

| Group | Particulars | Vitamin A (µg/day) | Thiamin (mg/day) | Riboflavin (mg/day) | Niacin equivalent (mg/day) | Pyridoxine (mg/day) | Ascorbic acid (mg/day) | Dietary folate (µg/day) | Vitamin $B_{12}$ µg/day | Magnesium (mg/day) | Zinc (mg/day) |
|---|---|---|---|---|---|---|---|---|---|---|---|
| Man | Sedentary work | 1000 | 1.4 | 2.0 | 14 | 1.9 | 80 | 300 | 2.5 | 385 | 17 |
| | Moderate work | | 1.8 | 2.5 | 18 | 2.4 | | | | | |
| | Heavy work | | 2.3 | 3.2 | 23 | 3.1 | | | | | |
| Woman | Sedentary work | 840 | 1.4 | 1.9 | 11 | 1.9 | 65 | 220 | 2.5 | 325 | 13.2 |
| | Moderate work | | 1.7 | 2.4 | 14 | 1.9 | | | | | |
| | Heavy work | | 2.2 | 3.1 | 18 | 2.4 | | | | | |
| | Pregnant woman | 900 | 2.0 | 2.7 | +2.5 | 2.3 | +15 | 570 | +0.25 | 385 | 14.5 |
| | Lactation 0–6 months | 950 | 2.1 | 3.0 | +5 | +0.26 | +50 | 330 | +1.0 | 325 | 14 |
| | 7–12 months | | 2.1 | 2.9 | +5 | +0.17 | | | | | |
| Infants | 0–6 months | 350 | 0.2 | 0.4 | 2 | 0.1 | 20 | 25 | 1.2 | 30 | - |
| | 6–12 months | 350 | 0.4 | 0.6 | 5 | 0.6 | -27 | 85 | 1.2 | 75 | 2.5 |
| Children | 1–3 years | 390 | 0.7 | 0.9 | 7 | 0.9 | 27 | 110 | 1.2 | 135 | 3.0 |
| | 4–6 years | 510 | 0.9 | 1.3 | 9 | 1.2 | 32 | 135 | 1.2 | 155 | 4.5 |
| | 7–9 years | 630 | 1.1 | 1.6 | 11 | 1.5 | 43 | 170 | 2.5 | 215 | 5.9 |
| Boys | 10–12 years | 770 | 1.5 | 2.1 | 15 | 2.0 | 54 | 220 | 2.5 | 270 | 8.5 |
| Girls | 10–12 years | 790 | 1.4 | 1.9 | 14 | 1.9 | 52 | 225 | | 255 | 8.5 |
| Boys | 13–15 years | 930 | 1.9 | 2.7 | 19 | 2.6 | 72 | 285 | | 355 | 14.3 |
| Girls | 13–15 years | 890 | 1.6 | 2.2 | 16 | 2.2 | 66 | 245 | | 325 | 12.8 |
| Boys | 16–18 years | 1000 | 2.2 | 3.1 | 22 | 3.0 | 82 | 340 | | 405 | 17.6 |
| Girls | 16–18 years | 860 | 1.7 | 2.3 | 17 | 2.3 | 68 | 270 | | 335 | 14.2 |

**Table 4.10B:** Micronutrients from different source (All values are for 100 g edible portion).

| Micronutrients | Cereals[a] | Pulses[b] | Leafy Vegetables[c] | Other vegetables | Roots and Tubers[d] | Fruits[e] | Milk (Buffalo)[f] | Milk (Cow)[f] | Egg | Chicken | Mutton |
|---|---|---|---|---|---|---|---|---|---|---|---|
| Iron (mg) | 3.00 | 5 | 8.5 | 2.12 | 0.6 | 0.56 | 0.2 | 0.2 | 1.82 | 1.5 | 1.3 |
| Zinc (mg) | 2.16 | 2.1 | 0.2 | 0.3 | 0.3 | 0.11 | 0.4 | 0.3 | 1.2 | 1.7 | 3 |
| Vitamin A (µg) | 2.43 | 8.6 | 259.1 | 22.4 | 70.0 | 32.36 | 49.8 | 58.3 | 198 | 21.4 | 9 |
| Riboflavin (mg) | 0.15 | 0.14 | 0.1 | 0.07 | 0.0 | 0.01 | 0.13 | 0.11 | 0.2 | 0.09 | 0.16 |
| Dietary folate (µg) | 24.03 | 127.7 | 16.7 | 24.4 | 31.3 | 17.61 | 8.6 | 7 | 49.3 | 9.3 | 6.4 |
| Vitamin $B_{12}$ (µg) | Nil | Nil | Nil | Nil | Nil | Nil | 1.5 | 1.5 | 1.8 | NA | 2.8 |

[a]Mean values of nutrients from commonly consumed cereals (67% weightage) such as rice and wheat were taken and 33% weightage was also given to millets such as Bajra, Jowar, Maiz and Ragi.
[b]Mean values of nutrients from Lentils, Tur dal, Bengal gram, Black gram, Cowpea, Green gram, Peas, Rajmah, Red gram and Soya bean were considered.
[c]Carotenoid conversion to retinol equivalents.
[d]Mean values of nutrients from Beetroot, Carrot, Colocasia, Onion, Radish, Tapioca and Yam were considered.
[e]Mean values of nutrients from Amla, Apple, Banana, Cherries, Grapes, Guava, Jack fruit, Lemon, Lichi, Mango, Melon, Orange, Papaya, Pine apple, Pomegranate, Sapota, Custard apple, Strawberry were considered.
[f]Good source of bioavailable calcium.
NA, Not available; NR, Not reported

*Folic Acid*

Folic acid provides carbon atoms for the synthesis of metabolites in the body including nucleic acid.

Folic acid can be obtained from a variety of plant and animal foods. Rich sources of folic acid are leafy vegetables, fruits, and yeasts. Cereals and pulses also provide moderate amounts of the vitamin. Pulses give twice as more than cereals. The vitamin may be found in the free form or as conjugated form as polyglutamates. The absorption of folic acid is inhibited by fibers in diet. From a habitual Indian diet 50% of the vitamin is absorbed.

**Requirement:** The current recommended allowance is 220 µg for adult woman and 300 µg for adult man per day. Of this, only 50–70 µg folic acid/day is obtained from an Indian diet. So 50–60% of the diets are deficient in this vitamin. During pregnancy and lactation an additional amount of 350 and 100 µg are required, respectively **(Table 4.10A)**.

*Vitamin $B_{12}$*

Like folic acid, this vitamin also is part of several coenzymes. Vitamin $B_{12}$ also catalysis similar metabolic reactions as folic acid.

**Sources:** Vitamin $B_{12}$ present in nature is almost completely synthesized by microorganisms. Although microflora in the large intestine can synthesize the vitamin, it is very little to meet the body needs. Egg, milk, meat, and liver are the richest sources of the vitamin. The vitamin is generally absent in plant foods. In them the vitamin may get in as a result of contamination due to pollution and unhygienic practices. This could be the reason why vegetarians do not manifest deficiency of the vitamin in spite of not taking animal foods.

**Requirement:** The recommended intake is 2.5 µg/day for adults with addition of 0.25 and 1 µg during pregnancy and lactation.

### Vitamin C (Ascorbic Acid)

Many animals can synthesize this six carbon lactone from glucose. However, humans cannot do this. It is a reducing agent, antioxidant, and an electron donor. Ascorbic acid prevents the formation of potentially mutagenic N-nitroso compounds. Gastric cancer risk can be reduced by high intake of vitamin C. Ascorbic acid may protect the oxidation of low-density lipoprotein in the blood.

**Sources:** Citrus fruits, tomatoes, berries, and green vegetables are good sources of vitamin C **(Table 4.11)**. Potato has low content of ascorbic acid, but since it is used in plenty by certain population, it forms a major source of vitamin C for them. More than 75% of the vitamin is destroyed during cooking.

**Requirements:** Satisfactory levels of vitamin C can be maintained by an intake of 30–35 mg/day. The recommended dietary intake is twice this amount, 65 mg/day for woman and 80 mg/day for man, considering the fact that 50% of the vitamin is lost in cooking. 15 mg/day is required extra by pregnant women. The requirement in lactation is additional 50 mg/day but it may vary based on the amount of vitamin C secreted in breast milk **(Table 4.10A)**.

## Minerals

Minerals are inorganic compounds needed by the body. Calcium, magnesium, phosphorus, potassium, sodium, and sulfur are the important macrominerals while copper, cobalt, chromium fluorine, iron, iodine, molybdenum, selenium, and zinc are the important microminerals.

### Iron

According to the National Nutrition Monitoring Bureau (NNMB) in most states in India, the iron intake is less than 50% of the RDA. Iron is an important mineral required for the synthesis of hemoglobin. Its deficiency can lead to anemia, improper mental functioning, susceptibility to infections, and poor learning in children. Children and women of the productive age are more vulnerable to this deficiency. The body has iron stores and the absorption of iron from the diet is inversely related to the iron stores. The iron stores in Indians are less compared to their counterparts in the developed countries. Iron absorption is only 5% except in adult women where it can be up to 10%.

**Sources:** Animal foods like fish, meat, and poultry are good sources. Plant sources of iron include dried foods like dates, jaggery, and legumes. The bioavailability of iron from plant foods which is generally low can be enhanced by consuming Vitamin C rich foods like citrus fruits, guava, and gooseberry. Beverages like tea inhibit iron absorption. So it is not advisable to have tea along with a meal.

**Requirements:** In adult males, the daily iron is required to replace the basal iron lost through desquamated gastrointestinal cells, bile, urine and sweat. Additionally, in females, iron is also lost during menstruation. The RDA for iron is given in **Table 4.12**. The RDA values are adjusted for lower intestinal absorption rate (8%) of iron.

### Iodine

The micronutrient iodine is essential for producing thyroid hormone. 20 mg of iodine is present in the body and 80% of it is found in the thyroid gland.

**Sources and requirement:** Food forms the source of 90% of iodine while water provides the remaining 10%. When 10 g of iodized salt is consumed containing 15 ppm of iodine, 150 µg of iodine is obtained which is adequate to meet once daily requirements if completely absorbed. However, there is loss of about 30% during cooking and only 70% of the remaining is absorbed. So, the iodine from the food sources are required to

**Table 4.11:** Vitamin C content of common food groups.

| Food | Vitamin C (mg/100 g) |
| --- | --- |
| Cereals | 0 |
| Pulses and legumes | 0–3 |
| Leafy vegetables | 60–250 |
| Roots and tubers | 10–40 |
| Other vegetables | 20–80 |
| Nuts and oilseeds | 0–7 |
| Condiments and spices | 0–50 |
| Fruits | 45–600 |
| Fish | 10–30 |
| Meat and poultry | 2–20 |
| Milk and milk products | 1–6 |

**Table 4.12:** Iron requirements (ICMR-NIN Expert Group 2020).

| Group | Body weight (kg) | RDA (mg/day) |
| --- | --- | --- |
| Adult man | 65 | 19 |
| Adult woman | 55 | 29 |
| Pregnant woman | 55 +10 | 40 |
| Lactating woman | 22 | 23 |
| Infants 0–6 months | 5.4 | – |
| Infants 6–12 months | 8.4 | 3 |
| Children 1–3 years | 12.9 | 8 |
| Children 4–6 years | 18.0 | 11 |
| Children 7–9 years | 25.1 | 15 |
| **Adolescents (boys)** | | |
| 10–12 years | 34.3 | 16 |
| 13–15 years | 47.6 | 22 |
| 16–18 years | 55.4 | 26 |
| **Adolescents (girls)** | | |
| 10–12 years | 35.0 | 28 |
| 13–15 years | 46.6 | 30 |
| 16–18 years | 52.1 | 32 |

(RDA: recommended dietary allowance)

Table 4.13: Iodine from food sources.

| Food groups | Mean iodine contents (μg/kg weight) |
|---|---|
| Sea fish | 832 |
| Fresh water fish | 30 |
| Vegetables | 29 |
| Meat | 50 |
| Eggs | 93 |
| Legumes | 29 |
| Fruits | 18 |

meet daily needs (**Table 4.13**). The excess iodine after absorption is excreted as urinary iodine (UIE), and its levels reflect the iodine intake. It is expected to be in the range of 100–200 μg if the intake is adequate. The reports of a survey show that many districts of India did not have the required amounts of UIE. In pregnancy and lactation, the requirement is increased to 250 μg/day and 280 μg/day respectively.

### Calcium and Phosphorous

Calcium and phosphorous have functions that are linked to each other and therefore their requirement is being considered together. Calcium is found mainly in the bone. It is major mineral and an adult man having a weight of 65 kg, will have 1 kg of this element. Calcium is an important element required for bone formation, neuromuscular excitation, blood coagulation, and membrane permeability. When the calcium in the diet is insufficient, the calcium in the bone helps to maintain the blood levels. This bone turnover and calcium absorption and excretion are regulated by hormones like Vitamin D, parathormone (PTH), thyrocalcitonin, and other steroids in the body. Daily around 700 mg of calcium is lost in urine, stools, bile, and sweat.

**Source:** Milk is a major resource of calcium. It can provide up to 1 g of calcium among individuals who consume milk in large quantities. Ragi is another important source of calcium. Cereals and leafy vegetables also provide calcium in low amounts. The absorption of calcium from cereals is inhibited by the phytates. Oxalates in leafy vegetables also inhibit calcium absorption.

**Requirement:** The intake of calcium is recommended at 1000 mg/day for adults, 1000 mg/day for pregnant women and additional 200 mg/day for lactating women. Adolescent boys and girls require 850 mg of calcium/day. Elemental Ca:P ratio is 1:1, except in infancy. In infants the ratio of Ca:P is 1:1.5. A loss of 30 mg/day of calcium occurs in postmenopausal women in urine. Therefore, an extra 200 mg/day is required to be taken by them.

### Magnesium

Like calcium, magnesium is also found mostly in bones. It is also found in muscle, soft tissue, and extracellular fluid. An adult has 20–25 g of magnesium in the body. It maintains the electrical potential in membranes and nerves. Plant foods form a major source of magnesium because it is part of chlorophyll. Generally, up to 50% of magnesium is absorbed. Since magnesium is widely distributed in foods, deficiency of this element is unlikely unless there are some malabsorption diseases in the individual.

**Requirement:** The requirement of magnesium is 325 mg/day for adult woman and 385 mg/day for adult man (*refer* **Table 4.10A**).

### Zinc

Zinc is an essential element. It is known to reduce the incidence and severity of childhood illnesses like pneumonia and diarrheal diseases. During diarrheal episodes' zinc supplementation is recommended. Zinc is also found to have a role in reducing morbidity and mortality of children. In undernourished children zinc promotes weight gain. Zinc is a constituent of enzymes required for DNA and RNA synthesis. It is also part of skeletal, muscle, and soft tissue.

**Source:** Animal sources of zinc are flesh, liver, fish, and milk. Among plant foods, grains, pulses, and nuts provide zinc. Milling and other processing methods reduce the zinc in plant foods.

**Requirement:** The RDA for zinc adult man and woman is set at 17 and 13 mg/day respectively (**refer Tables 4.10A and B**).

### Sodium

Sodium is responsible for maintaining the water balance and blood pressure. Common salt is the most important source of this element. It contains 40% of sodium and 60% of chloride. Salt in food enhances the taste and flavor. It is also used as a preservative. Indians consumes 5–30 g of salt/day. About 40% of families in India take more than 10 g/day. The taste of salt is an acquired habit. So if restricted from a young age, its consumption can be reduced. It is seen that even with minimal amounts of sodium the body is able to maintain this equilibrium due to powerful inbuilt mechanisms in the body. The requirement of the element depends on the loss. The sweat loss in turn depends on climatic conditions and physical activity. But even with a loss of 3 liters of sweat in 6 hours, the sodium requirement is not beyond 8 g/day. Besides sweat, sodium is also lost through feces and urine. Salt is high in sun dried foods, papads, pickles, canned, and processed foods. Restricting the consumption of these foods can help to maintain the sodium levels in the required range. Cereals, pulses, vegetables, milk, sea foods, and animal foods have sodium as a natural ingredient in them.

## Antioxidants

Oxidation is a ubiquitous chemical reaction. During this process electrons are transferred from one compound to another. Many diseases like cancer and heart disease can be attributed to the oxidation of molecules such as DNA and lipids, both of which are required for normal life function. Antioxidants provide electron density to compounds likely to undergo oxidation, thus preventing them from losing electrons.

### Categories

Antioxidants can be natural or synthetic. Natural antioxidants are obtained from fruits, vegetables, grains, and meat. Synthetic antioxidants are manufactured in laboratories. These are generally used for the preservation of foods.

Natural antioxidants are found in natural sources like fruits, vegetables, meat, etc., vitamin C, vitamin E, vitamin A, polyphenols including flavonoids, anthocyanins, lycopene, and coenzyme Q10 (ubiquitin).

## *Biologic and Cellular Effects of Antioxidants*

Though vitamin C is one of the most commonly consumed antioxidants, there have been no definitive cellular mechanism found to elucidate its effects on cancer and heart disease. But it is thought to have an impact on these diseases. Vitamin C prevents common cold.

Vitamin E from the liver is delivered to the adipose tissue where it prevents oxidation. Similarly, carotenoids, vitamin A in particular also passed through liver and deposited in adipose tissue, whereby they inhibit oxidation of fat. Additionally, carotenoids have same regulatory function in cells, but no conclusive evidence. Vitamin A is useful in prevention of lung cancer.

Lycopene has a definitive role in preventing the cellular process that leads to cancer. Lycopene binds to IGF-1, one of the main growth factors that leads cells to become cancerous by binding with IGF-1, lycopene inhibits the ability to communicate with cells by binding to its membrane surface proteins. This lack of communication prevents or slows down cell cycle, reducing risk of cancer.

All polyphenols (including anthocyanins and flavonoids) have shown evidence in preventing oxidation of LDL molecules. When LDL is oxidized, it is converted to plaque. This accumulates in the inner surface of arteries. This results in higher risk of heart disease. Polyphenols prevent the buildup of plaques. Some flavonoids prevent oxidation of enzymes, thus preserving their proper function.

Coenzyme Q10 alleviates hypertension and prevents ischemic heart disease.

The antioxidants of importance and the foods from it are obtained as shown in **Table 4.14**.

## Dietary Fiber

Dietary fiber is the part of plant food that remains after digestion and absorption in the intestine. It includes polysaccharides, oligosaccharides, lignin, and organic acids like butyric acid and polyols like sorbitol. They are regarded as "unavailable carbohydrates". Dietary fiber has important functions in the body as a laxative. It increases the bulk of stool and also makes it soft. Dietary fiber is also found to reduce the blood cholesterol and sugar levels. Dietary fiber gets fermented in the intestine by microbes and this results in release of energy. So dietary fiber is also now considered as a source of metabolizable energy. Animal foods do not contain dietary fiber.

## *Types and Source*

Based on solubility dietary fiber can be classified as soluble and insoluble. Water-soluble fiber is present in legumes, oats, fruits, barley, beans, soyabean, plum, banana, apple, broccoli, carrots, onion, and potato. Water-insoluble fiber is present in whole grain, wheat, corn bran, nuts, seeds, cauliflower, and tomato. Foods with low, moderate, and heavy dietary fiber content is shown in **Table 4.15** and the dietary fiber content of different food groups is shown in **Table 4.16**.

## *Beneficial Effects on Health*

High intake of dietary fibers reduces the risk of CHD by 29% compared to those with low intake. It is also seen to reduce risk of ischemic stroke by 26%. Fiber has a hypocholesteremic effect. Soluble fiber, 2–10 g/d is associated with significant decreases in total cholesterol. It reduces LDL levels by binding with bile acids in the small intestine, which gets excreted. Fermentation of fibers occur in the large intestine which releases short chain fatty acids which can alter the cholesterol synthesis and thereby reduce cholesterol levels. According to the Finnish study there is a 62% reduction in the progression of prediabetes to diabetes during a four-year period among those in the category of highest dietary consumption compared to the lowest. Dietary fiber also reduces blood pressure and body weight. In the context of the rising incidence of non-communicable disease the role of dietary fiber in diet needs to be emphasized.

**Table 4.14:** Antioxidants.

| Compound | Source |
|---|---|
| Vitamin C | Most fruits particularly citrus, some vegetables like tomatoes |
| Vitamin E | Cereal grains, broccoli, brussels sprouts, tomatoes, cooking oil (olive, sunflower, safflower), almonds, hazelnuts |
| Beta carotene | Vegetables, spinach, tomatoes, carrots, sweet potato, papaya |
| Flavonoids | Potatoes, tomatoes, lettuce, onion, chocolates, grapes, red wine, black tea |
| Anthocyanins | High content in red wine, green tea |
| Polyphenols | Red/purple fruits, grape wine |
| Lycopene | Tomato, papaya, watermelon, grapefruit, guava |
| CoQ | Wheat, bean, fish, organ meat |

**Table 4.15:** Foods with low, moderate and high dietary fiber.

| Low fiber foods | Moderate fiber foods | High fiber foods |
|---|---|---|
| Milled rice, Refined wheat flour | Whole wheat flour, Brown bread | Rice bran |
| Green gram dal | Field beans, red gram dal | Bengal gram, Whole rajmah, peas |
| Bottle guard, ash gourd, cucumber, tomato | Brinjal, cauliflower | Drumstick, Colocasia |
| Green leafy vegetables—spinach, lettuce | Fenugreek, cabbage | Amaranth |
| Fruit juices, canned fruits | Apple, Orange | Guava, Papaya |

**Table 4.16:** Dietary fiber in food groups.

| Food group | TDF (total dietary fiber) | Soluble (% of TDF) |
|---|---|---|
| Cereals | 4.11–12.48 | 22.4–22.7 |
| Pulses | 8.23–15.30 | 20.5 |
| Vegetables | 2.5–6.3 | 27–30 |
| Roots and tubers | 1.7–2.5 | 30–34 |
| Green leafy vegetables | 2.5–4.0 | 22–28 |
| Fruits | 1.1–3.2 | 28–45 |

Optimal function of gut associated lymphatic tissue (GALT) which has an important role in immunity, depends on dietary constituents especially probiotics. Most probiotics are non-fermentable dietary fiber which are fermented in the colon. Inulin and oligofructose stimulate the growth of lactobacillus and bifidobacteria.

Fiber has no metabolic effects, but too much fiber can decrease absorption of valuable micronutrients.

### Recommended Intake

Children >1 year—14 g/1000 kcal; Adults—40 g/2000 kcal.

### Phytochemicals

Functional foods are the foods which contain bioactive ingredients known to enhance the health of human being. The active ingredient in these functional foods is called nutraceuticals. These are also called neutraceuticals. They may be extracted and provided as a food supplement. Examples of phytochemicals are lycopene in tomatoes, allicin in garlic, and isoflavones in soyabeans. Other examples are shown in the **Table 4.17**.

**Table 4.17:** Phytochemicals in foods.

| Phytochemical | Food |
|---|---|
| Sulforaphanes, indoles, carotenoids | Broccoli, cabbage, cauliflower |
| Isoflavones, saponin | Soyabean |
| Lycopene, carotenoids | Tomato |
| Beta-glucans, saponins, terpenoids, phytic acid | Oats, wheat, barley |
| Allicin, flavonoids, organosulfur compounds | Garlic |

> We do not eat nutrients, we eat food, so we need to relate our foods to the nutrients.
>
> Our life today is stressed by the choices we have to make and food is no exception. An educated health professional should not be guided by the looks and perceived taste of food but by the wisdom gained by the knowledge on the nutritive value of foods to make healthy choices for the community.
>
> We should remember at the same time that there are communities which do not have the luxury of these choices. Let us enable them also to create their own rainbow.

## FOOD GROUPS

All foods can be categorized into six major groups based on nutrients they share in common as—(1) Cereals and millets, (2) Pulses and legumes, (3) Vegetables and fruits, (4) Animal food, (5) Oils and fats, and (6) Nuts and oilseeds.

### Cereals and Millets

Cereals like wheat, rice, and maize are the most common staple food in most countries including India and hence are grown in greater quantities across the world. Cereals are the edible components of the grain of cultivated grass. It is composed of endosperm, germ, and bran. It is processed by milling during which the outer bran is removed to varying extents. Nutritive quality depends on the amount of bran removed as it is concentrated with fiber, vitamins, and minerals. Millets are grains of small seeded grasses that are eaten without removing the outer layer. Commonly consumed millets in India are jowar, bajra, ragi, and kodri. Cereals and millets form the major source of dietary protein and carbohydrate, since they are consumed in large quantities. They are also a rich source of dietary fiber, minerals, and B group of vitamins. A balanced diet of a sedentary male should contain around 360 g of cereals and millets and that of a sedentary female 270 g per day.

The nutritive value of few common cereals and millets are shown in **Table 4.18**.

### Wheat

It contains more protein than any other cereal (12%), but is deficient in lysine. When milled, whole wheat flour (100%) is sieved and about 5% bran is sieved off, resulting in 95% extraction flour known as "atta". It is used for making *chapati, roti, naan*, etc. On further refining, 90% extraction flour is obtained which is known as *maida* or all-purpose flour. It is used for making bread, cakes, biscuits, etc. Highly refined flour is poorer in proteins, dietary fiber, minerals, and vitamins; hence, it is fortified with calcium and thiamine to make up for the loss. While semolina (suji) is prepared from the outer part of wheat, it is richer in minerals and vitamins. Wheat flour contains gluten which is a sticky protein that makes the dough spongy and stretchable which can cause sensitivity in some persons especially those with celiac disease. Maida is rich and suji is poor in gluten.

**Table 4.18:** Nutritive value of cereals and millets.

| Item | Energy (kcal) | Protein (g) | Fat (g) | Minerals (g) | Crude fiber (g) | Carbohydrate (g) | Calcium (mg) | Phosphorus (mg) | Iron (mg) | Carotene (µg) | Vitamins (mg) $B_1$ | $B_2$ | $B_3$ |
|---|---|---|---|---|---|---|---|---|---|---|---|---|---|
| Ragi | 328 | 7.3 | 1.3 | 2.7 | 3.6 | 72 | 344 | 283 | 3.9 | 42 | 0.42 | 0.19 | 1.1 |
| Barley | 336 | 11.5 | 1.3 | 1.2 | 3.9 | 69.5 | 26 | 215 | 1.6 | 10 | 0.47 | 0.2 | 5.4 |
| Maize | 342 | 11.1 | 3.6 | 1.5 | 0.7 | 66.2 | 10 | 348 | 2.3 | 90 | 0.42 | 0.1 | 1.8 |
| Jowar | 344 | 10.4 | 1.9 | 1.6 | 1.6 | 76.0 | 25 | 222 | 4.1 | 47 | 0.37 | 0.13 | 3.1 |
| Rice raw | 345 | 6.8 | 0.5 | 0.6 | 0.2 | 78.2 | 10 | 160 | 0.7 | 0 | 0.06 | 0.06 | 1.9 |
| Rice parboiled | 346 | 6.4 | 0.4 | 0.7 | 0.2 | 79 | 9 | 143 | 1 | - | 0.21 | 0.05 | 3.8 |
| Wheat | 346 | 11.8 | 1.5 | 1.5 | 1.2 | 71.2 | 41 | 306 | 5.3 | 64 | 0.45 | 0.17 | 5.5 |
| Bajra | 361 | 11.6 | 5.0 | 2.3 | 1.2 | 67.5 | 42 | 296 | 8 | 132 | 0.33 | 0.25 | 2.3 |

> **Exercise:** Try to list out the foods that you eat which are made predominantly from wheat. You can discuss with your friends from other states to find out their wheat delicacies. Here is a list to which you can keep adding. Which of these do you think are healthy and why? Do this exercise after you read each paragraph in this section and enjoy your learning.

## Rice

The grain consists of three parts—embryo, endocarp, and pericarp. The pericarp and embryo contain most of the protein, fat, minerals, and vitamins. The endocarp mainly contains starch. The protein content of rice is 6–8.5%. Though rice contains lesser protein than wheat quantitatively, qualitatively rice protein is considered better than wheat protein as it is rich in cysteine and methionine and also contain lysine in small quantities. The nutrient value of rice depends on the way or extent to which the husk is removed. Hard milling removes a good part of pericarp along with husk which results in a reduced nutrient value. Under milling and hand pounding are less damaging. Nutrient loss can be minimized by parboiling of rice.

### Washing and cooking

The rice grain is subjected to further loss of essential nutrients during the process of washing and cooking. Washing in large quantities of water would remove upto 60% of the water-soluble vitamins and minerals. The practice of cooking rice in large quantities of water and draining away the excess of water at the end of cooking leads to further loss of B-group vitamins. Thus, the combined effect of washing and cooking may affect seriously the nutritive value of rice. It is therefore best to cook rice in just enough water (about 2 measures of water for 1 measure of rice).

### Maize/Corn/Bhutta

It is an important source of energy, proteins, and also fairly rich in fat. The yellow variety of maize is a good source of carotenoids. Maize lacks lysine and tryptophan, but is rich in leucine which further interferes with the conversion of tryptophan to niacin. So pellagra, due to niacin deficiency, may be found in areas where maize is the staple food. The quality of maize protein has been improved by the opaque 2 gene institution into maize.

***Nutritive losses:*** Milling is the process of grinding and refining of cereals, and polishing makes the rice smooth, shiny, and whiter. But these processes result in loss of nutrients including fiber and protein. Subsequent washing and draining of water from cooked cereals like rice adds to the losses during milling and processing specially the water-soluble vitamins.

***Preventing nutritive losses:*** The nutrient losses mentioned above can be prevented by different methods. One such method is parboiling.

**Parboiling:** This is a method of preserving the nutritive value of rice by partially boiling in the husk. It is practiced since time immemorial. Basic steps of parboiling includes soaking, steaming, and drying. It is done at household and commercial level. Central Food Technological Research Institute (CFTRI) advocates the hot soaking process. It consists of soaking the rice in hot water at 70° C for 3–4 hours, followed by draining off the water, steaming for 10 minutes, and drying. After this it is either hand pounded at household level or milled at the commercial level. There are different methods for parboiling, but minimum expenditure of energy is for the short soaking tempering process. However, this process, imparts an off flavor and a pale hue to the rice, which is unacceptable to some. Parboiled rice takes longer cooking time for required softness.

**Advantages of parboiling:** By the process of parboiling the germ gets firmly fixed to grain. This prevents losses during milling and pounding. The vitamins like thiamine and other nutrients are driven from the outer layers into the inner layers so that these nutrients are not lost during milling and pounding. Also during the process, starch in the cereal is gelatinized which makes it hard. This enables it to be stored better, for longer durations and makes it resistant to insects.

### Millets

The commonly consumed millets are jowar (sorghum) used by people of Maharashtra, bajra (pearl millet), used by people of Rajasthan and ragi, used throughout the country especially as a weaning food. The outer layer of millets are not usually removed like cereals. Millets provide 350 calories, 8–14 g of protein and minerals like calcium. Ragi is especially rich in calcium, providing 344 mg of calcium/100 g of the millet.

***Jowar*** *(sorghum/kafir corn/milo)* is generally consumed by people of Maharashtra, Madhya Pradesh, and Andhra Pradesh. Jowar ki roti, jowar ki bhakar, dhapate are examples of food items made from jowar. It is rich in iron (4.1 mg/100 g) and protein (9–14%) but deficient in the amino acids, lysine, and threonine. The excess leucine present in jowar interferes with conversion of tryptophan to niacin.

***Bajra*** (pearl millet) is used commonly in Rajasthan, Gujarat, and some parts of Maharashtra. Some examples of bajra recipes are bajra ki khichdi and bajra ki khatti raabdi. It is also used to make flour for preparing chapatis. It is a rich source of iron (8 mg/100 g), protein (10–14%), and vitamins like beta carotene, riboflavin, niacin, folic acid, and minerals like calcium.

***Ragi*** is a cheap millet widely used in all parts of India, mostly in Andhra Pradesh and Karnataka. Its flour is used for making porridge, which forms a nutritious complementary food during weaning. Ragi is also a rich source of calcium **(Table 4.18)**.

> **Exercise:** Discuss among yourselves the common cereals and millets that you use. Look at the picture (food pyramid) and try to identify the cereals and millets. Make your own collection of pictures of cereals and millets and stick in your record book. Repeat this exercise after you finish each food group.

## Pulses

Pulses and legumes are an important component of Indian diet. Commonly used pulses are red gram, green gram, lentil, Bengal gram, and peas. Pulses are the major source from which we get protein, especially in vegetarian diet. Since they are cheap and easily available they are considered as the poor man's meat.

Table 4.19: Nutritive value of pulses and legumes.

| Item | Energy (kcal) | Protein (g) | Fat (g) | Moisture (g) | Minerals (g) | Crude fiber (g) | Carbohydrate (g) | Calcium (mg) | Phosphorus (mg) | Iron (mg) | Carotene (µg) | Vitamins (mg) | | | | |
|---|---|---|---|---|---|---|---|---|---|---|---|---|---|---|---|---|
| | | | | | | | | | | | | $B_1$ | $B_2$ | $B_3$ | FA | C |
| Bengal gram | 360 | 17.1 | 5.3 | 9.8 | 3.0 | 3.9 | 60.9 | 202 | 302 | 4.6 | 189 | 0.39 | 0.15 | 0.9 | 186 | 3 |
| Peas dry | 315 | 19.7 | 1.1 | 16.0 | 2.2 | 4.5 | 56.5 | 75 | 298 | 7.0 | 39 | 0.4 | 0.19 | 3.4 | 7.5 | 0 |
| Horse gram | 321 | 22.2 | 0.5 | 11.8 | 3.2 | 5.3 | 57.2 | 287 | 311 | 6.7 | 71 | 0.42 | 0.2 | 1.5 | – | – |
| Red gram | 335 | 22.3 | 1.7 | 13.4 | 3.5 | 1.5 | 57.6 | 73 | 304 | 2.7 | 132 | 0.45 | 0.19 | 2.9 | 103 | 0 |
| Rajmah | 346 | 22.9 | 1.3 | 12.0 | 3.2 | 4.8 | 60.6 | 260 | 410 | 5.1 | – | | | | | |
| Black gram | 347 | 24.0 | 1.4 | 10.9 | 3.2 | 0.9 | 59.6 | 154 | 385 | 3.8 | 38 | 0.42 | 0.2 | 2.0 | 132 | 0 |
| Green gram | 334 | 24.0 | 1.3 | 10.4 | 3.5 | 4.1 | 56.7 | 124 | 326 | 4.4 | 94 | 0.47 | 0 | 2.1 | – | – |

## Nutritive Value

Pulses provide 350 kcal of energy and 20–25 g of protein/100 g. The highest protein content among pulses is in soyabean (43 g/100 g). The protein in pulses is, however, poor in cysteine and methionine. But it is rich in lysine, which is deficient in cereals. It also provides vitamins like vitamin B, minerals like calcium, and iron.

Nutritive value of pulses can be increased by germination. This is done by soaking the pulse in water for about 24 hours followed by wrapping the drained pulses in a piece of thin damp cloth and leaving it aside for few more hours. Germination increases the vitamin C and B content and complex proteins are broken down to simpler amino acids. There is cell multiplication and therefore the quantity increases. Cooking time is also decreased after germination.

Fermentation is another method of increasing the nutritive value. It makes the pulses more digestible and increases the vitamin B content. The nutritive value of common pulses and legumes is summarized in **Table 4.19**.

The recommended intake of pulses per day for a vegetarian is 60 g and for a nonvegetarian is 30 g.

> **Exercise:** Pulses are known as the poor man's meat. Go to the market today and try to find out the cost of 100 g of different pulses, different types of meat, fish, and egg. Make a table of cost/100 g of each item, protein content/100 g and cost/g of protein. Draw this table in your record book.

## Vegetables and Fruits

Vegetables and fruits are a storehouse of micronutrients, phytonutrients, and fiber. Their liberal consumption prevents micronutrient malnutrition and chronic diseases like cardiovascular disease and cancers. Since most of the fruits and vegetables provide low calories, diets rich in fruits and vegetables helps in reducing obesity. However, some fruits like bananas, and roots and tubers have high calories **(Tables 4.20 and 4.21)**.

| Our food rainbow | | |
|---|---|---|
| Color | Food | Phytochemical |
| Red | Tomato | Lycopene |
| Yellow | Green pumpkin, papaya | Zeaxanthin |
| Red | Purple beet root | Anthocyanins |
| Orange | Pumpkin, papaya, mango | Beta carotene |
| Orange-yellow | Apricots, apple, cherry, tomatoes, oranges | Flavonoids |
| Green | Green leafy vegetables, cabbage | Glucosinolates |
| White | Garlic, onion | Allyl sulfides |

Fresh fruits are superior to fruit juices. Locally available, seasonal fruits and vegetables belonging to a variety of groups and colors (rainbow colors—VIBGYOR) are to be chosen. Care should be taken to minimize cooking losses. A healthy adult requires 300 g of vegetables and 100 g of fruits/day. Vegetables

Table 4.20A: Nutritive value of roots and tubers.

| Item | Energy (kcal) | Protein (g) | Fat (g) | Minerals (g) | Moisture (g) | Crude fiber (g) | Carbohydrate (g) | Calcium (mg) | Phosphorus (mg) | Iron (mg) | Carotene (µg) | Vitamins (mg) | | | | | |
|---|---|---|---|---|---|---|---|---|---|---|---|---|---|---|---|---|---|
| | | | | | | | | | | | | $B_1$ | $B_2$ | $B_3$ | $B_6$ | FA | C |
| Beetroot | 43 | 1.7 | 0.1 | 0.8 | 87.5 | 0.9 | 8.8 | 18 | 55 | 1.2 | 0 | 0.4 | 0.9 | 0.4 | – | – | 10 |
| Carrot | 48 | 0.9 | 0.2 | 1.1 | 86 | 1.2 | 10.6 | 80 | 530 | 1 | 1890 | 0.04 | 0.02 | 0.6 | – | 15 | 3 |
| Onion big | 50 | 1.2 | 0.1 | 0.4 | 86.6 | 0.6 | 11.1 | 47 | 50 | 0.5 | | 0.08 | 0.01 | 0.4 | – | 6 | 11 |
| Onion small | 59 | 1.8 | 0.1 | 0.6 | 84.3 | 0.6 | 12.6 | 40 | 60 | 0.46 | 15 | 0.08 | 0.02 | 0.5 | – | – | 2 |
| Potato | 97 | 1.6 | 0.1 | 0.6 | 74.7 | 0.4 | 22.6 | 10 | 40 | 0.48 | 4 | 0.1 | 0.01 | 1.2 | – | 7 | 17 |
| Colocasia | 97 | 3.0 | 0.1 | 1.7 | 73.1 | 1 | 21.1 | 40 | 140 | 0.4 | 24 | 0.09 | 0.03 | 0.4 | – | 54 | 0 |
| Yam | 110 | 2.5 | 0.3 | 1.4 | 70.4 | 1 | 24.4 | 0 | 74 | 1 | 565 | 0.19 | 0.47 | 1.0 | – | – | 1 |
| Sweet potato | 120 | 1.2 | 0.0 | 1 | 68.5 | 0.8 | 28.2 | 46 | 50 | 0.2 | 6 | 0.06 | 0.04 | 0.7 | – | – | 24 |
| Tapioca | 157 | 0.0 | 0.2 | 1 | 59.4 | 0.6 | 38.1 | 50 | 40 | 0.9 | – | 0.05 | 0.1 | 0.3 | – | – | 25 |
| Arrowroot flour | 334 | 0.2 | 0.1 | 0.1 | 16.5 | – | 83.1 | 10 | 20 | | | | | | | | |

**Table 4.20B:** Nutritive value of condiments and spices.

| Item | Moisture (g) | Protein (g) | Fat (g) | Minerals (g) | Crude fiber (g) | Carbohydrate (g) | Energy (kcal) | Calcium (mg) | Phosphorus (mg) | Iron (mg) | Carotene (µg) | Vitamins | | | | | |
|---|---|---|---|---|---|---|---|---|---|---|---|---|---|---|---|---|---|
| | | | | | | | | | | | | $B_1$ | $B_2$ | $B_3$ | $B_6$ | FA | C |
| | | | | | | | | | | | | (mg) | | | | | |
| Asafoetida | 16 | 4 | 1.1 | 7 | 4.1 | 67.8 | 297 | 690 | 50 | 39.4 | 4 | 0 | 0.04 | 0.3 | - | - | - |
| Cardamom | 20 | 102 | 2.2 | 5.4 | 20.1 | 42.1 | 229 | 130 | 160 | 4.6 | 0 | 0.2 | 0.17 | 0.8 | - | - | - |
| Chillies (dry) | 10 | 15.9 | 6.2 | 6.1 | 30.2 | 31.6 | 246 | 160 | 370 | 2.3 | 345 | 0.9 | 0.4 | 9.5 | - | - | 50 |
| Chillies (green) | 85.7 | 2.9 | 0.6 | 1 | 6.8 | 3 | 29 | 30 | 80 | 4.4 | 175 | 0.19 | 0.39 | 0.43 | - | 29 | 111 |
| Cloves dry | 25.2 | 5.2 | 8.9 | 5.2 | 9.5 | 46 | 286 | 740 | 100 | 11.7 | 253 | 0.08 | 0.13 | - | - | - | - |
| Coriander | 11.2 | 14.1 | 16.1 | 4.4 | 32.6 | 21.6 | 288 | 630 | 393 | 7.1 | 942 | 0.22 | 0.35 | 1.1 | - | 32 | - |
| Cumin seed | 11.9 | 18.7 | 15 | 5.8 | 12 | 36.6 | 356 | 1080 | 511 | 11.7 | 522 | 0.55 | 0.36 | 2.6 | - | - | - |
| Fenugreek | 13.7 | 26.2 | 5.8 | 3 | 7.2 | 44.1 | 333 | 160 | 370 | 6.5 | 96 | 0.34 | 0.29 | 1.1 | - | 84 | - |
| Garlic | 62 | 6.3 | 0.1 | 1 | 0.8 | 29.8 | 145 | 30 | 310 | 1.2 | 0 | 0.06 | 0.23 | 0.4 | - | - | 13 |
| Ginger fresh | 80.9 | 2.3 | 0.9 | 1.2 | 2.4 | 12.3 | 67 | 20 | 60 | 3.5 | 40 | 0.006 | 0.03 | 0.6 | - | - | 6 |
| Mustard | 8.5 | 20 | 39.7 | 4.2 | 1.8 | 23.8 | 541 | 490 | 700 | 7.9 | 162 | 0.65 | 0.26 | 4.0 | - | - | - |
| Pepper | 18.2 | 11.5 | 6.8 | 4.4 | 14.9 | 49.2 | 304 | 460 | 198 | 14 | 1080 | 0.09 | 0.14 | 0.14 | - | - | - |
| Tamarind pulp | 20.9 | 3.1 | 0.1 | 2.9 | 5.6 | 67.4 | 283 | 170 | 110 | 17 | 60 | - | 0.07 | 0.7 | - | - | 3 |
| Turmeric | 13.1 | 6.3 | 5.1 | 3.5 | 2.6 | 69.4 | 349 | 150 | 282 | 67.8 | 30 | 0.03 | 0 | 2.3 | - | 18 | 0 |

**Table 4.21:** Nutritive value of fruits.

| Item | Energy (kcal) | Protein (g) | Fat (g) | Minerals (g) | Moisture (g) | Crude fiber (g) | Carbohydrate (g) | Calcium (mg) | Phosphorus (mg) | Iron (mg) | Carotene (µg) | Vitamins (mg) | | | | | |
|---|---|---|---|---|---|---|---|---|---|---|---|---|---|---|---|---|---|
| | | | | | | | | | | | | $B_1$ | $B_2$ | $B_3$ | $B_6$ | FA | C |
| Watermelon | 18 | 0.6 | 0.16 | | 95 | 0.78 | 3 | 4.3 | 8 | 0.22 | 4,300 | 0.02 | 0.02 | 0.3 | 0.07 | 5.5 | 11 |
| Tomato | 20 | 0.9 | 0.2 | 0.5 | 94 | 0.8 | 3.6 | 48 | 20 | 0.5 | 351 | 0.12 | 0.06 | 0.4 | - | 30 | 27 |
| Strawberry | 25 | 1.0 | 0.56 | | 92 | 0.25 | 3.4 | 15 | 6 | 0.36 | 218 | 0.06 | 0.1 | 0.48 | 0.9 | 8.9 | 50 |
| Star fruit | 26 | 0.8 | 0.94 | | 91 | 2.81 | 4.5 | 4.9 | 11 | 0.45 | 15 | 0.08 | 0.02 | 0.34 | 0.06 | 8.4 | 33 |
| Papaya | 32 | 0.6 | 0.1 | 0.5 | 90.8 | 0.8 | 7.2 | 17 | 13 | 0.5 | 666 | 0.04 | 0.25 | 0.2 | - | - | 57 |
| Pineapple | 46 | 0.4 | 0.1 | 0.4 | 87.8 | 0.5 | 10.8 | 20 | 9 | 2.4 | 18 | 0.2 | 0.12 | 0.1 | - | - | 39 |
| Orange | 48 | 0.7 | 0.2 | 0.3 | 87.6 | 0.3 | 10.9 | 26 | 20 | 0.3 | 1,104 | - | - | - | - | - | 30 |
| Guava | 51 | 0.9 | 0.3 | 0.7 | 81.7 | 5.2 | 11.2 | 10 | 28 | 0.27 | 0 | 0.03 | 0.03 | 0.4 | - | - | 212 |
| Lemon | 57 | 1.0 | 0.9 | 0.3 | 85.2 | 1.7 | 11.1 | 70 | 10 | 0.26 | 0 | 0.02 | 0.01 | 0.1 | - | - | 39 |
| Grapes | 58 | 0.6 | 0.4 | 0.9 | 82.2 | 2.8 | 13.1 | 20 | 23 | 0.5 | 3 | 0.04 | 0.03 | 0.02 | - | - | 1 |
| Amla | 58 | 0.5 | 0.1 | 0.5 | 81.8 | 3.4 | 13. | 50 | 20 | 1.2 | 9 | 0.43 | 0.01 | 0.2 | - | - | 600 |
| Lime | 59 | 1.5 | 1 | 0.7 | 84.6 | 1.3 | 10.9 | 90 | 20 | 0.3 | 15 | 0.02 | 0.03 | 0.1 | - | - | 63 |
| Apple | 59 | 0.2 | 0.5 | 0.3 | 84.6 | 1.0 | 13.4 | 10 | 14 | 0.6 | - | - | - | - | - | - | 1 |
| Pomegranate | 65 | 1.6 | 0.1 | 0.7 | 78 | 5.1 | 14.5 | 10 | 70 | 1.8 | 0 | 0.06 | 0.1 | 0.3 | - | - | 16 |
| Mango ripe | 74 | 0.6 | 0.4 | 0.4 | 81 | 0.7 | 16.9 | 14 | 16 | 1.3 | 2,743 | 0.08 | 0.09 | 0.9 | - | - | 16 |
| Jackfruit | 88 | 1.9 | 0.1 | 0.9 | 76.2 | 1.1 | 19.8 | 20 | 41 | 0.56 | 175 | 0.03 | 0.13 | 0.4 | - | - | 7 |
| Sitaphal | 104 | 1.6 | 0.4 | 0.9 | 70.5 | 3.1 | 23.5 | 17 | 47 | 4.3 | 0 | 0.07 | 0.17 | 1.3 | - | - | 37 |
| Banana | 116 | 1.2 | 0.3 | 0.8 | 70.1 | 0.4 | 27.2 | 17 | 36 | 0.36 | 78 | 0.05 | 0.08 | 0.5 | | | 7 |
| Dates fresh | 144 | 1.2 | 0.4 | 1.7 | 59.2 | 3.7 | 33.8 | 22 | 38 | 0.96 | | | | | | | |
| Dates dry | 317 | 2.5 | 0.4 | 2.1 | 15.3 | 3.9 | 75.8 | 10 | 50 | 7.3 | 6 | 0.01 | 0.02 | 0.9 | | | 3 |

belonging to three categories namely green leafy vegetables (50 g), roots and tubers (50 g), and other vegetables (200 g) should be included. During pregnancy an additional 50 g of GLV is recommended.

> **Exercise:** Search the internet and try to add to the colors of your food rainbow.

## Animal Foods

Animal foods include meat, fish, eggs, poultry, milk, and milk products.

### Meat

It is a good source of protein. 100 g of meat gives around 20 g of protein. It is qualitatively as good as that of other animal

**Table 4.22:** Nutritive value of different varieties of meat and fish.

| Name of food stuffs | Energy kcal | protein (g) | Fat (g) | Carbohydrate (g) | Minerals (g) | Vitamin A (kJ) | Thiamine (mg) | Moisture (g) |
|---|---|---|---|---|---|---|---|---|
| Fish (pomfret) | 87 | 17.0 | 1.3 | 1.8 | 1.5 | - | - | 78.4 |
| Fowl | 109 | 25.9 | 0.6 | - | 1.3 | - | | 72.2 |
| Beef (muscle) | 114 | 22.6 | 2.6 | - | 1.0 | 18 | 0.15 | 74.3 |
| Pork (muscle) | 114 | 18.7 | 4.4 | - | 1.0 | 0 | 0.54 | 77.4 |
| Liver, sheep | 150 | 19.3 | 7.5 | 1.3 | 1.5 | 690 | 0.36 | 70.4 |
| Mutton (muscle) | 194 | 18.5 | 13.3 | - | 1.3 | 9 | 0.18 | 71.5 |

foods like egg, since it contains the essential amino acids. Animal foods are also rich in vitamins like nicotinic acid and minerals like phosphorous, iron, and zinc. It is, however, a poor source of calcium. The heme iron present in meat has high bioavailability. Meat has high content of fat especially saturated fatty acids, due to which its consumption has to be restricted. In a healthy diet low fat chicken meat is preferred to mutton and beef **(Table 4.22)**.

## Fish

Fish consumption is of high value in the diet, especially with the current emphasis on intake of omega three polyunsaturated fatty acid. Fish is also a good source of easily digestible protein (15–25 g/100 g) with high biological value. It is a good source of vitamin A and D. Iodine can be obtained from sea foods.

## Milk and Milk Products

Milk forms the sole food for babies under 6 months. It is rich source of vitamins and minerals. The amount of vitamin C in fresh milk is 2 mg/100 mL, which decreases on heating. Vitamin A and D is also high in milk. Milk is rich in calcium (1,200 mg per liter of cow's milk) and phosphorus. It is, however, poor in nicotinic acid and iron. Milk is a source of good quality protein (3–4 g/100 mL). Milk proteins like lactalbumin, lactoglobulin, and casein are easily digestible. They are rich in tryptophan and cysteine. Milk fat is a rich source of oleic and linoleic acid. Of the 30 types of sugars available in milk, lactose is the most important. As a source of energy milk provides about 67 kcal of energy/100 mL.

Curd is a common ingredient of Indian diets. It is a milk derivative and its nutritive value is the same as the milk source from which it is derived. Lactobacilli act on lactose in milk and breaks it down to lactic acid.

The fats derived from milk include cream, butter, and ghee. Cream is obtained by centrifugation of unboiled milk. The fat extracted from buttermilk is butter and ghee is the clear fat obtained by boiling butter. Cream has nutritive value in between whole milk and butter. Butter has only 80% fat and 100 g butter yields about 729 kcal, while ghee is 100% fat and yield 900 kcal.

## Skimmed and Toned Milk

Skimmed milk is the type of milk recommended for those with conditions requiring low fat consumption, because fat has been removed from this milk. By adding skimmed milk, skimmed milk powder, and water to buffalo milk, toned milk is obtained. It is then pasteurized and bottled to get milk which is very similar to cow's milk. Advantages of toned milk are the reduced fat content, toning up of the nonfat solids, and increased quantity of milk. This makes it more widely available at low cost.

> **Note**
> Milk can be made available in the powdered form, by the process of condensation, evaporation, and homogenization. It is tinned with or without the addition of sugar. Sugar acts as a preservative. Up to 50% sugar may be present in tinned milk. It may be reconstituted by adding seven volumes of water or as per the instructions of the manufacturer.

The nutritive value of milk and milk products is shown in **Table 4.23**.

In a balanced diet 300 mL of milk and milk products are recommended/day.

> **Exercise:** How much of milk and milk products did you consume yesterday (24-hour recall). Was it adequate/inadequate/excess?

## Eggs

Eggs have a high nutritive value, but it lacks carbohydrates and vitamin C. An egg provides about 70 kcal, 6 g protein, 6 g of fat, and 250 mg of cholesterol. Egg white is a rich source of high-quality protein with an NPU of 100. Egg protein is considered the standard to which other proteins are compared. Egg is also rich in riboflavin. The yolk contains fat, minerals like calcium, phosphorous and vitamins, especially A and D. Fat is finely-emulsified and hence easily assimilated. One egg weigh 60–70 g. Two eggs without shell weighs 100 g.

Nutritive value of egg is given in **Table 4.24**.

## Oils/Fats

### Choice of Cooking Oils

Choice of cooking oil should be such that a ratio of polyunsaturated to saturated fatty acids is maintained at 0.8–1.0. The ratio of linoleic to alpha linoleic acid should also be preferably 5–10, which can be achieved by taking more fish, sea foods, legumes, and GLV. **Box 4.2** for the choice of cooking oils. The risk of CHD is modified significantly by this choice. The goals to be achieved in this regard have been set by the WHO/FAO.

**Table 4.23:** Nutritive value of milk and milk products.

| Item | Energy (kcal) | Protein (g) | Fat (g) | Minerals (g) | Moisture (g) | Crude fiber (g) | Carbo-hydrate (g) | Calcium (mg) | Phosphorus (mg) | Iron (mg) | Carotene (µg) | Vitamins B$_1$ (mg) | B$_2$ (mg) | B$_3$ (mg) | B$_6$ (mg) | FA (mg) | C (mg) |
|---|---|---|---|---|---|---|---|---|---|---|---|---|---|---|---|---|---|
| Milk human | 65 | 1.1 | 3.4 | 0.1 | 88 | - | 7.4 | 28 | 11 | - | 41 | 0.02 | 0.02 | - | - | 1.3 | 3 |
| Milk (cow) | 67 | 3.2 | 4.1 | 0.8 | 87.5 | - | 4.4 | 120 | 90 | 0.2 | 53 | 0.05 | 0.19 | 0.1 | - | 8.5 | 1 |
| Curd (cow) | 60 | 3.1 | 4 | 0.8 | 89.1 | - | 3 | 149 | 93 | 0.2 | 31 | 0.05 | 0.16 | 0.1 | 1 | 12.5 | 1 |
| Cheese | 348 | 24.1 | 25.1 | 4.2 | 40.3 | - | 6.3 | 790 | 520 | 2.1 | 82 | - | - | - | - | - | - |
| Skimmed milk powder | 357 | 38 | 0.1 | 6.8 | 4.1 | - | 51 | 1,370 | 1,000 | 1.4 | 0 | 0.45 | 1.64 | 1 | - | - | 5 |
| Whole milk powder | 496 | 25.8 | 26.7 | 6 | 3.5 | - | 38 | 950 | 730 | 0.6 | 420 | 0.31 | 1.36 | 0.8 | - | - | 4 |
| Butter | 729 | - | 81 | 2,5 | 19 | - | - | - | - | - | 960 | - | - | - | - | - | - |
| Ghee | 900 | - | 100 | - | - | - | - | - | - | - | - | - | - | - | - | - | - |

**Table 4.24:** Nutritive value of egg (per 100 g).

| | Energy (kcal) | Protein (g) | Fat (g) | Iron (mg) | Carotene (mg) | Thiamine (mg) | Riboflavin (mg) | Niacin (mg) | Phosphorous (mg) | Calcium (mg) |
|---|---|---|---|---|---|---|---|---|---|---|
| Egg hen | 173 | 13.3 | 13.3 | 2.1 | 420 | 0.1 | 0.40 | 0.1 | 220 | 60 |
| Egg duck | 181 | 13.5 | 13.7 | 2.5 | 405 | 0.12 | 0.26 | 0.2 | 260 | 70 |

---

**Box 4.2: Cooking oil combinations recommended.**
- Groundnut/sesame/rice bran + mustard
- Groundnut /sesame/rice bran + canola
- Groundnut/sesame/rice bran + soyabean
- Palmolein + soya bean
- Safflower/sunflower + palmolein + mustard
- Sunflower/safflower + palmolein/olive
- Safflower/sunflower + groundnut/sesame/rice bran.

## Nuts and Oilseeds

Groundnut, cashew nut, walnut, pistachio, coconut, mustard, and sesame seeds belong to this food group. Nuts and oilseeds contain high amounts of fat, protein, vitamin B, and iron. Peanut contains 14 mg of iron/100 g. After oil extraction, the resultant cake can be used for making foods, as it has a high content of protein. Improper storage of peanuts can result in growth of aspergillus which produces aflatoxin.

Groundnut is regarded as the king of nuts because it is nutrient rich and is also cheap. It has high amount of fat (40%), high protein (25.3%), and niacin (20 mg/100 g). It is also readily available in most Indian states. Hence, it is part of a low-cost nutritious diet in our national program menus. It is consumed as such in boiled, fried, or steamed form. Powdered or ground form is used in curries. It is a very popular and nutritious sweet when combined with jaggery.

## Sugar and Jaggery

Sugar is present naturally in fruits, vegetables, milk, and honey. The most common form of sugar that is consumed is sucrose. Refined sugar or table sugar provide empty calories with no added nutritive value. Most processed foods from bakery cakes, pastries, ice-creams, and chocolates contain very high sugar levels. Excess intake of sugar can lead to obesity, hyperlipidemia in adults, and caries tooth in children. Jaggery is considered healthier alternative for sweetening foods. Besides calories, jaggery also provides iron and carotene.

# THE BALANCE OF FOOD GROUPS

## Concept of Food Pyramid and Food Plate

Food pyramid and food plate are pictorial/visual depictions which highlight the relative proportion of the food groups to be incorporated in the diet. Food pyramid is a time old concept, representing the five food groups, namely:
1. Cereals and millets
2. Vegetables (root and tubers, green leafy vegetables, and other vegetables) and fruits
3. Pulses and legumes
4. Animal foods
5. Sugar and jaggery, oils and fat, nuts and oilseeds.

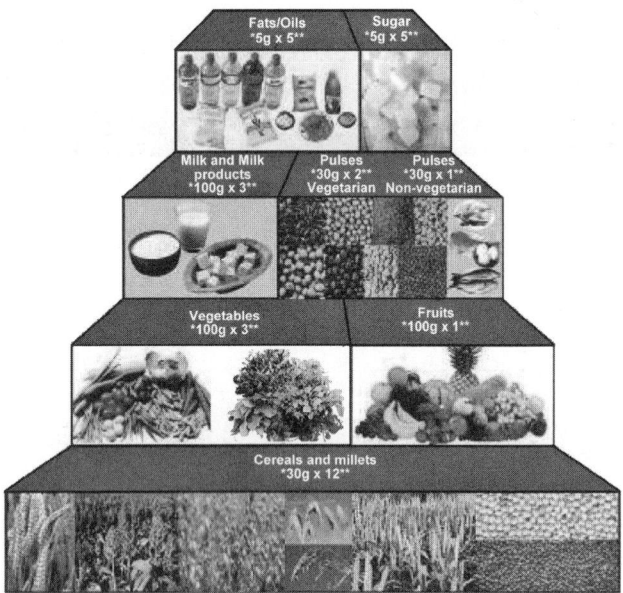

**Fig. 4.1:** Balanced diet for a sedentary woman and man (*portion size, **no. of portions).
*Source:* Krishnaswamy K, Sesikeran B. Dietary Guidelines for Indians—A Manual, 2nd edition. Hyderabad: National Institute of Nutrition; 2011.

**Table 4.25:** Balance of food groups for the different types of work (Dietary guidelines for Indians, ICMR-NIN 2011).

| Food items | g/portion* | No. of portions for different type of work ||||||
|---|---|---|---|---|---|---|---|
| | | Sedentary || Moderate || Heavy ||
| | | Man | Woman | Man | Woman | Man | Woman |
| Cereals and millets | 30 | 12.5 | 9 | 15 | 11 | 20 | 16 |
| Pulses | 30 | 2.5 | 2 | 3 | 2.5 | 4 | 3 |
| Milk and milk products | 100 mL | 3 | 3 | 3 | 3 | 3 | 3 |
| Roots and tubers | 100 | 0.5 | 0.5 | 0.5 | 0.5 | 0.5 | 0.5 |
| Green leafy vegetables | 100 | 0.5 | 0.5 | 0.5 | 0.5 | 0.5 | 0.5 |
| Other vegetables | 100 | 2 | 2 | 2 | 2 | 2 | 2 |
| Fruits | 100 | 1 | 1 | 1 | 1 | 1 | 1 |
| Sugar | 5 | 5 | 4 | 6 | 6 | 11 | 9 |
| Fat | 5 | 5 | 4 | 6 | 5 | 8 | 6 |

*To calculate the day's requirement of above-mentioned food groups for an individual, multiply grams per portion with number of portions.

The base of the pyramid is formed by the cereals and millets which has to be taken in good amounts. Next part of the pyramid is vegetables and fruits which can be taken liberally. The portion above this is formed by two food groups namely pulses and animal foods which have to be taken moderately and the last section is for the sugar, jaggery, fats, and oils which have to be consumed only sparingly **(Fig. 4.1)**.

Food plate is a recent concept which makes us realize the importance of variety of food groups in the plate from which we eat every day and the relative proportion to be given for each food group. Groups in food plate includes fruits, vegetables, grains, protein, and dairy. The term protein in the plate stands for animal foods excluding milk. Pulses are considered as a part of the grains.

It is more understandable to the common man and hence has been widely popularized.

The Barilla Center for Food and Nutrition has come up with a new model which addresses health diet and environmental impact. This model has two pyramids, the first is the familiar food pyramid and the other is inverted and reclassifies foods according to their environmental impact, with most damaging foods placed at the top **(Fig. 4.2)**.

## Change in Requirements of Food Quantity of the Food Groups for Different Category

The balanced diet for males and females doing sedentary, moderate, and heavy work in terms of portions is given in **Table 4.25**.

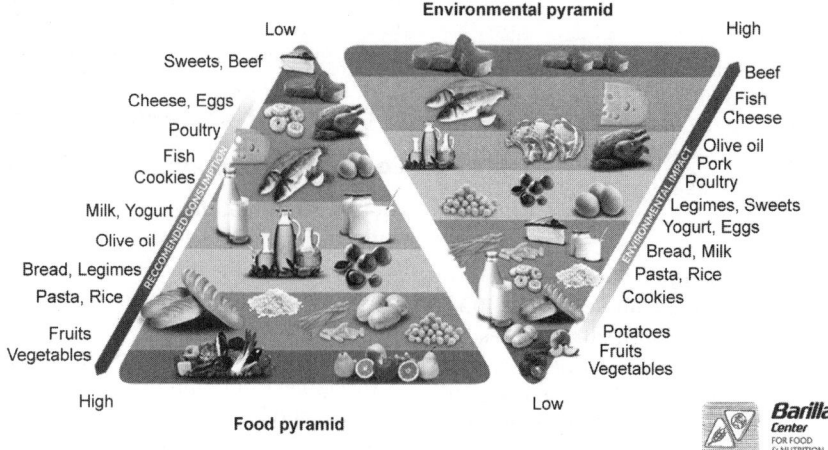

**Fig. 4.2:** Double pyramid model (2015).
*Source:* Barilla Center for Food and Nutrition (BCFN).

**Table 4.26:** Changes required in representation of food groups for different physiological states.

| Category | Change from adults |
|---|---|
| Elderly man | Reduce 3 portions (90 g) of cereals and millets (requirement reduced to 9 portions) and add a serving of fruit (100 g) |
| Elderly woman | Reduce 2 portions (60 g) of cereals and millets (requirement reduced to 7 portions) and add one portion of fruit (100 g) |
| Pregnant woman | Half a portion of green leafy vegetable (50 g)—total 100 g<br>One portion of fruit (100 g)—total 200 g<br>Two portions of milk (200 mL)—total 500 mL<br>Two portions of fat/oil (10 g)—total 30 g |
| Lactating woman (up to 6 months) | One portion of cereals (30 g)<br>Two portions of pulses (60 g)<br>Half a portion of green leafy vegetable (50 g)<br>One portion of fruit (100 g)<br>Two portions of milk (200 mL)<br>Two portions of fat/oil (10 g)<br>Or<br>One portion of cereals + two portions of pulses + the additional requirement of a pregnant woman |
| 6–12 months postpartum | Diet gradually brought back to normal |

## Balanced Diet for Different Types of Work

The changes in diet to be brought about for elderly men and women and pregnant and lactating women are shown in **Table 4.26**.

Let us do some exercises to understand some of the principles we learned.

> **Exercise:** Calculate the total calories, proteins and fat you consumed by a 24-hour recall of the foods you consumed yesterday. Find the difference from RDA for your age, sex, and activity level. How could this be modified to suit your RDA?

## Steps for Analyzing the Adequacy of Diet—Worked Out Example

### Calculation of Adequacy of a Diet

There are different methods to assess whether the diet followed is balanced and in accordance with RDA. One such simple method used is called the 24-hour recall method. It is used for assessing the nutritional status of an individual. *Other methods are discussed in detail in Chapter 23: Epidemiology of Nutrition and Food-related Diseases and its Prevention and Control.*

In the 24-hour recall method, the individual is asked to tell about the foods that he/she has consumed the last day over 24 hours.

### Sample Meal Plan for Adult Man (Sedentary)

| Meal Time | Food Group | Raw | Cooked Recipe | Servings Amount |
|---|---|---|---|---|
| Breakfast | Milk | 100 mL | Milk | ½ cup |
|  | Sugar | 15 g | Tea or coffee | 2 cups<br>1 cup |
|  | Cereals | 70 g | Breakfast item |  |
|  | Pulses | 20 g |  |  |

*Contd...*

| Meal Time | Food Group | Raw | Cooked Recipe | Servings Amount |
|---|---|---|---|---|
| Lunch | Cereals | 120 g | Rice | 2 cups |
|  |  |  | Phulkas | 2 Nos. |
|  | Pulses | 20 g | Dal | ½ cup |
|  | Vegetables | 150 g | Veg curry | ¾ cup |
|  | Vegetables | 50 g | Veg salad | 7-8 slices |
|  | Milk | 100 mL | Curd | ½ cup |
| Afternoon Tea | Cereals | 50 g | Snack |  |
|  | Milk | 50 mL | Tea | 1 cup |
|  | Sugar | 10 g |  |  |
| Dinner | Cereals | 120 g | Rice | 2 cups |
|  |  |  | Phulkas | 2 Nos. |
|  | Pulses | 20 g | Dal | ½ cup |
|  | Vegetables | 150 g | Veg curry | ¾ cup |
|  | Milk (curd) | 50 mL |  | ½ cup |
|  | Vegetables | 50 g | Veg Raita |  |
|  | Fruit | 100 g | Seasonal | 1 medium |

1 Cup = 200 mL

*Note:* For Non-Vegetarians - Substitute one pulse portion with one portion of egg/meat/chicken/fish

Use 25 g visible fat and <5 g salt during preparation of meal per day.

Breakfast Items: Idli – 4 Nos. /Dosa – 3 Nos. /Upma – 1-1/2 Cup /Bread – 4 Slices/Porridge – 2 Cups/Corn flakes with milk – 2 Cups.

Snacks: Poha – 1 Cup/Toast – 2 Slices/Dhokla – 4 Nos/Sandwiches – 2/Biscuits – 5

> Well started is half done. Let the first 1,000 days of life give you the beacon for the next 100 years.

## NUTRITION THROUGH THE LIFECYCLE

### Pregnancy and Lactation Period is Special for a Woman and She Requires Some Special Foods too

Pregnancy and lactation are special physiological situations that need specific attention due to increase in demand of most nutrients. Nutritional problems like low birth weight and maternal mortality are related to this problem. The additional requirements depend on the BMI, prepregnancy, and weight gain, besides other factors.

The extra requirement of calories in pregnancy is 350 calories. Protein requirement also increases during all trimesters of pregnancy. Iron is needed in additional amounts for erythropoieis, iodine for the mental development, calcium for bones, teeth and milk production, and vitamin A for better survival of child. Folic acid reduces the risk of congenital malformation and improves birth weight.

A variety of foods needs to be consumed. Seasonal locally available fruits and vegetables including GLV have to be taken. The dietary pattern need not be changed if it is already balanced. The quantity and frequency of food consumption may have to be changed slightly to meet the additional requirements. In order to improve the bioavailability of iron in foods, Vitamin C from citrus fruits and fermented and sprouted pulses can be taken. 200 mL milk should be consumed in addition **(Box 4.2)**. If the consumption is adequate, the weight gain in pregnancy will be around 10–12 kg. Taking adequate fiber is essential to prevent constipation (25 g/1,000 kcal). 8–12 glasses of water have to be taken. Salt should be restricted to 5 g/day. Beverages like coffee should be curtailed as it has adverse effects on the fetus. Besides regular health checkup, adequate rest, avoiding smoking, tobacco chewing, and consumption of alcohol are critical for the proper growth and development of the fetus.

## Exclusive Breastfeeding for First 6 Months of Life

All the essential nutrients required by the baby during the first 6 months of life are obtained through breast milk. These nutrients especially the protein, fat, vitamins, and minerals are of good quality. The quality can be further improved by providing the mother with supplements of certain nutrients. The nutrients in breast milk can be easily digested and absorbed by the baby. The milk secreted in the first few hours is called colostrum. It should be given to the baby as it is rich in protein, vitamins, minerals, growth factors, enzymes, and antibodies. Apart from these, breast milk also contains a bifidus factor that promotes the natural gut flora. This along with the low pH of the flora created by the breast milk plays an important role in protection from infections. Breast-milk has immunoglobulins (IgA), lactoferrin, lactoperoxidase, and complements which protect the infant from several infections. Antibodies to some viruses are found in breast milk, which protect the gut mucosa. Breast-feeding also protects infants from vulnerability to allergic reactions. It is a good laxative as well. Breastfeeding also promotes the cognitive development of the baby, since breast milk has high content of docosahexaenoic acid. Women who breastfeed have lower fertility and therefore it enhances spacing. Both mother and baby get a lot of emotional satisfaction and bonding through the process of breastfeeding. There is evidence to suggest that breastfeeding has some long-term benefits in the form of protection from autoimmune disease, inflammatory bowel disorders, obesity and related diseases like cancers. So no mother and baby shall be deprived of all these advantages of breastfeeding.

The quality of breast milk keeps improving over the first few days after delivery and is best at 6 months. An average Indian woman secretes 750 mL of milk per day during the first 6 months. It reduces to 600 mL/day in the next 6 months. Breastfeeding has to be initiated as soon as possible after child birth. Exclusive breastfeeding is recommended for 6 months. After this, complementary feeding can be started. Breastfeeding should still be continued up to 2 years. Demand feeding is to be done.

Additional water is not required for an exclusively breastfed baby in the first 6 months. Feeding water can reduce the demand for breast milk and increases the risk of diarrheal diseases.

It is important that a lactating mother is adequately nourished for good quality milk.

The quality of breast milk depends on the mother's nutrition and diet. Although even malnourished mothers are able to breastfeed adequately, severe malnourishment can compromise breastfeeding. The quality of protein is less affected than fat by the maternal diet. Maternal diet also influences the quality of the water-soluble vitamins and vitamin A. Trace elements content in milk, however does not depend on the quality of maternal diet.

Postpartum is a period in which the mother undergoes a lot of emotional and mental instability. It is important for the family to provide adequate support to keep her stable and give adequate rest for better feeding. Preparation of the breast prior to initiation of breastfeeding is necessary. Nipple retraction has to be looked for in the antenatal period itself and corrected. Working mothers can provide their babies with expressed breast milk which can be hygienically kept for up to 8 hours and provided by the caretaker.

## Complementary or Supplementary Feeding after 6 Months

After 6 months, mothers' milk is inadequate to meet the nutritional requirements of the baby, so along with breast milk other foods are given which are called complementary or supplementary foods. These have to be nutritionally adequate, hygienically prepared to prevent malnutrition and infections and must be semisolid in consistency. The baby must be fed frequently (3–4 times/day is advised). Cereal-pulse-nut combination with added sugar/jaggery forms most of the complementary foods. Vegetables and fruits can also be introduced as juice which has to be thoroughly washed and steamed before use. Later on cooked and mashed semisolid vegetables can be given. Even green leafy vegetables can be introduced this way. Cooked and mashed egg yolk, fish, meat soups, and minced meat later on can also be introduced. Only one new food should be introduced a day. Amylase rich foods (ARF) like germinated and powdered cereal flour can be added to the complementary foods to reduce bulk and make it energy dense.

## Childhood and Adolescent Nutrition

Childhood and adolescent periods are stages of rapid growth and development. An infant weight should be doubled by 5 months and tripled by a year if adequately nourished. An adolescent should gain 1.5–3 kg weight and increase in height by 6–7 cm very year, if nutrition is proper. Tissues and organs especially reproductive undergo important changes during this time. Hormonal changes and sexual maturation occurs. Emotional immaturity and instability also marks this period. Adolescent growth spurt starts at around 10–12 years in girls and 2 years later in boys. The menstruation related needs of the girls make the nutrient requirement/unit weight for them more than boys. Formation of critical bone mass with adequate mineral density, fat and muscle mass depends on the nutrient intake during these years. Taking adequate calcium in the form of milk and other calcium rich foods to get at least 600–800 mg/day is important.

Oil intake of 25–50 g according to the age group is recommended. Care should be taken to avoid excess consumption of salt especially if there is a family history of CHD. Substance abuse also has to be avoided. These would form primary prevention strategies. Engaging in regular physical activity is also essential.

## Nourishing Our Elderly is Important

Due to changes in elderly like the reduction of lean mass, basal metabolic rate, and physical activity, the amount of calories required reduces. Elderly are more susceptible to infections. They have to consume food adequately and exercise regularly to maintain good quality life. Macronutrients and micronutrients need to be consumed adequately. Vitamins, minerals, and antioxidants play a role in minimizing the degenerative changes. Chronic diseases of elderly namely diabetes, hypertension, and cardiovascular diseases are all diet related. The lack of variety in diet and reduced intake of micronutrient result in their deficiency.

After 40 years, the energy needs reduce by 5% for every decade of life till the age of 60. After 60 years, the requirements of energy reduce 10% every decade. Generally, food intake decreases but the protein requirement does not change. So, if the quantity of food taken is reduced, it is likely that the protein requirement may not be met. So, it is advisable to increase the physical activity and increase the energy requirements, so that protein intake also increases. Another way of dealing with meeting the protein need is increasing the quality of protein. High protein diets and the use of commercially available high protein supplements are not recommended. Dietary fat can be kept to the minimum in view of most chronic diseases in elderly. In sedentary elderly 30% of energy (in more physically active elderly 35%) of energy can come from fat. The contribution of saturated fat to the total energy should not exceed 8%. For a sedentary elderly male three portions of cereals and millets can be reduced and two portions for an elderly female. One portion of fruit can be added extra (*refer* **Table 4.26**). Cardiovascular risk can be reduced by 30%, if the vegetable and fruit intake is increased by two portions. The micronutrient requirements do not change but again since the intake reduces, and the total calorie requirement is less, extra care needs to be taken to prevent micronutrient deficiency.

## Maternal, Infant, Young Child Nutrition

Improved nutrition during pregnancy, lactation, and early childhood is important to avoid micronutrient deficiencies, for both mothers and children. Hence the concept of Infant and Young Child Nutrition/Infant and Young Child Feeding (IYCN/IYCF) was introduced in 2002 during the 55th World Health Assembly. IYCN forms the foundation for growth, development, health, and well-being. ICYF is also a critical component of the 1000 days' approach to improve child health. The first 1000 days included 270 days in-utero and 730 post-natal days (up to 2 years - young child). The term maternal has also been added to the IYCN nutrition. Maternal, Infant, Young Child Nutrition (MIYCN) targets the reduction of stunting, anemia, low birth weight, overweight, improving breastfeeding practices, and reducing wasting. The nutrition of the mother enables primordial prevention of malnutrition in the infant and young child. During the intrauterine period, a single cell embryo transforms into a 3 kg fetus. By 2 years the child can master the environment, body growth is 20%, height 50%, and brain growth 75–80% of an adult.

Good maternal nutrition during pregnancy and lactation improves the birth outcomes and growth of children. It reduces the risk of pregnancy-related health complications. For this, nutrition-related education and counseling need to be given to the mother.

World Health Organization recommends initiation of breastfeeding within the first hour of delivery. It has to be continued as exclusive breastfeeding for the first 6 months of life. Timely and appropriate complementary feeding should be started but breastfeeding has to be continued until 2 years. This is because exclusive breastfeeding reduces infant morbidity and mortality from common infections, such as diarrhea or pneumonia and also indirectly reduces anemia by preventing the inhibitory effects of inflammation on iron absorption, mobilization, and, consequently, red blood cell production.

Complementary feeding starts at 6 months of age when breast milk alone cannot meet the nutritional requirements of an infant, and other foods and liquids are needed with the breast milk. The guiding principles of complementary feeding include—(1) giving amounts of food that increase with the age of the child; (2) ensuring the food has the right consistency, nutrient, and energy density; and (3) ensuring the caregiver practices responsive feeding. Ensuring dietary diversity in these early months of life when growth is rapid helps avoid micronutrient deficiency. Additionally, fluid intake should meet the daily requirements, micronutrient fortified foods should be used when available, and food and fluid should not be restricted during or after illness.

## SOCIOCULTURAL ASPECTS OF NUTRITION

### Healthy Cooking Practices

Cooking makes the food more digestible and palatable as certain foods cannot be chewed and eaten raw. Besides, changing the texture, it also improves the appearance, flavor, and taste of food. But in the process, we should preserve the most important function of food to provide the required nutrients.

### *Precooking Procedures*

Prior to cooking, some of the procedures done are washing, cutting, fermenting, and germination. Fermentation and germination of seeds are two important precooking practices which are part of Indian culture, which improves the nutritive value.

### *Washing and Cutting*

Food items like grains and vegetables are subjected to repeated washing to remove pesticides, parasites, and other extraneous substances. But too much washing can lead to loss of nutrients. Washing vegetables after cutting is not advisable as it can lead to loss of water-soluble vitamins. Care should be taken not to keep the vegetables soaked in water for long. When vegetables are cut into small pieces, it is more likely that vitamins will be lost because a greater surface area is exposed to oxidation. Water that has been used for soaking washed grains or cut vegetables can be put to use during cooking.

**Do's and Don'ts related to cooking practices**

*Don'ts*
- Do not wash food grains repeatedly before cooking
- Do not wash vegetables after cutting
- Do not soak the cut vegetables in water for long periods
- Do not waste the excess water leftover after cooking
- Do not use baking soda while cooking pulses and vegetables
- Do not reheat the left over oil repeatedly
- Do not rinse meat and eggs before cooking

*Do's*
- Use only sufficient water for cooking
- Cook foods in vessels covered with lids
- Prefer pressure/steam cooking to deep frying/roasting
- Encourage consumption of sprouted/fermented foods
- Cook only the quantity that is required so as to avoid leftover food and reheating
- Cut away any damaged or bruised areas of fruits and vegetables
- Immediately refrigerate any fresh-cut items, like salad or fruit
- Wash your hands after handling raw meat to prevent cross-contamination.

## Some Indian Food Beliefs and Taboos

Food habits that we acquire during our childhood persist through to adulthood. These are passed on from the elders in our family. Hence, it is important to understand "why our children eat, what they eat". Food beliefs vary with community. These may be harmless or harmful to health.

It is a sad truth that most food beliefs are related to women and children and are detrimental to their health. Some exaggerate benefits of foods without any scientific basis. These constitute food fads. In addition, the concept of hot and cold foods is widely prevalent. Sugar, jaggery, groundnuts, fried foods, and eggs are considered as hot foods while apple, curd, milk, and GLV are regarded as cold foods. People believe that papaya consumption can lead to abortion and pregnant women are deprived of the nourishment from this fruit, because of this belief. Taking only vegetarian food, is also part of the religious belief, but this can result in Vitamin B deficiency, if other foods which can provide it, like milk, are not consumed. Dietary restrictions are practiced during infections like measles, chickenpox, and some communicable diseases, which may result in malnutrition.

Boiling leads to loss of nutrients that are water and heat labile. Shallow frying is preferred to deep frying because the quantity of oil consumed will be lesser. When oil is used, care must be taken to use just the required quantity. Reuse of left over oil can be carcinogenic. Used oil must not be mixed with fresh oil. It may be used for seasoning. It is better to wash vegetables before cutting to retain its nutritive value. Vegetables have to be cooked in minimum water and put in low flame, covered with lid. Cooking rice in excess water and draining it off produces a loss of nutrients.

Microwave cooking and reheating are considered healthy. Care should be taken not to keep frozen food in microwave. The food kept in microwave needs to be kept for sufficient time so that it is thoroughly cooked. Improper timing can leave the inner parts of the food cold during reheating.

## APPLIED NUTRITION

We are building more and more star hotels, so are we building more and more multispecialty hospitals. What is that we are in pursuit of? Is it the Health or the Disease?

**Note**

*Nutritional disorders (malnutrition—undernutrition and overnutrition, low birth weight, micronutrient deficiency), Assessment of nutritional status and Nutritional surveillance and other applied aspects like Food fortification, Food additives, Food preservatives, Food adulteration, Food toxicants are discussed in detail in Chapter 23: Epidemiology of Nutrition and Food-related Diseases and its Prevention and Control.*

## Therapeutic Diet

### Diabetes

The aim of dietary therapy or prescribing a therapeutic diet for a diabetic patient is the following:
- To keep the blood glucose values under control (premeal blood glucose <120 mg/dL, bedtime blood glucose <140 mg/dL, HbA1C <7%)
- Maintain a normal body weight
- Meet energy needs in a timely manner
- Provide optimum level of nutrients
- Achieve a desirable lipid profile (LDL <100 mg/dL, HDL >45 mg/dL, triglycerides <200 mg/dL).

***Energy:*** Permissible calorie intake/kg body weight can be roughly obtained using the guideline in table below:

|  | Sedentary (calorie/kg) | Moderate (calorie/kg) | Heavy (calorie/kg) |
| --- | --- | --- | --- |
| Obese | 20 | 25 | 30 |
| Normal | 30 | 35 | 40 |
| Underweight | 35 | 40 | 45 |

Therefore, if a diabetic is obese, weighing 70 kg and he is a moderate worker, his calorie requirement would be only 1,750 calories.

***Carbohydrate:*** Simple sugars and sugar containing sweet dishes like cakes and pastries have to be avoided. Complex sugars like cereals, vegetables, and fruits are to be consumed. Food with low glycemic index (0–55) and moderate glycemic index (56–69) are to be preferred over foods with high glycemic index (70 or more). Factors influencing the glycemic index (GI) of food are the types of starch, physical entrapment, viscosity of fiber, sugar, protein, fat content, acid content, and state of cooking. Nowadays, the concept of glycemic load is considered. It reflects both the quality and the quantity of dietary carbohydrate.

Glycemic load = (GI/100) × Carbohydrate in grams/serving

Glycemic load is used for controlling the portions of food. Low glycemic index foods allow for larger portions while regulating the glycemic load.

**Glycemic index of food items:**

| Value | Food item |
| --- | --- |
| 100% | Glucose |
| 80–90% | Corn flakes, potato mashed, carrot, honey |
| 70–79% | Polished rice, wheat bread |

*Contd...*

*Contd...*

| Value | Food item |
|---|---|
| 60–69% | Brown rice, banana |
| 50–59% | Peas |
| 40–49% | Beans |
| <40% | Legumes, peanut |

**Fruits that can be consumed in prescribed amounts/day**

| | |
|---|---|
| Apple | 1 small/1/2 medium |
| Guava | 1 medium |
| Orange | 1 medium |
| Papaya | 1/3 medium or 3 slices |
| Pineapple | 2–3 slices |
| Pear | 1 medium |
| Watermelon | 2–3 slices |
| Pomegranate | 1/3rd medium |
| Grapes | 12 |

***Fat:*** Not more than 20% of the total energy should be from fat and not >10% from saturated fat. Use of PUFA should be promoted. Preferred oils are olive oil, rice bran oil, sunflower, and groundnut oil.

***Dietary fiber:*** Foods rich in dietary fiber is to be promoted.

Meal pattern should include three major meals and two minor meals. Small frequent meals are advised over heavy meals. Breakfast has to be consumed within an hour of rising. It should be rich in complex carbohydrate and protein. Lunch should include protein. Dinner should be light, low in carbohydrate. It is good to have regular fixed timings for food. Those on oral hypoglycemic agents/insulin should take it an hour before food.

## Cardiovascular Disease including Hypertension

The energy requirement should be calculated according to the body mass index of the patient.

Fat intake should be restricted. It should form only 15% of the total energy and saturated fat <7%. Unsaturated fatty acids, especially PUFA is preferred and the cholesterol in diet is to be reduced.

## Cholesterol Content of Foods/100 g

| | |
|---|---|
| Meat, chicken, fish | 100 mg |
| Liver, kidney | 300 mg |
| Brain | >200 mg |
| Egg yolk | 250 g |
| Egg white | zero |
| Milk whole | 40 mg/glass |
| Ice cream | 50 mg/small cup |
| Butter | 35 mg/table spoon |
| Fish oil | 500 mg |
| Veg oil | zero |
| Nuts and oil seeds | zero |

Salt has to be restricted, especially if hypertensive. A gradual stepwise approach is to be adopted for this. To start with, added salt, processed food, and foods rich in salt like papads, pickles are avoided. Salt is restricted to 5 g/day initially (mild salt restriction). Moderate salt restriction (2.5– 5 g/day) and severe restriction (<2.5 g/day) are advised in patients if necessary.

***Low salt diet:*** This is a diet that includes not more than 1.5–2.4 mg of salt per day. Hence, soups, fried items, salted crisps, and nuts are to be avoided. Salt is not added to cooking. Pepper, herbs, and spices are used as alternatives. Processed foods are also cut down. Home cooked foods are to be consumed and bottled beverages are to be avoided.

> ***DASH diet (dietary adjustment to stop hypertension):*** This is a diet that is rich in fruits, vegetables, low fat, or no fat dairy products. It also includes grains, lean meat, fish and poultry, nuts and beans. It lowers cholesterol and makes it easy to lose weight.

## Renal Diseases

### Acute Renal Failure

In acute renal failure, there is water retention and reduced urine output. Hypertension may also coexist. So the intake of fluid, sodium and potassium in the diet has to be restricted. Protein of good quality should be provided. Salt is restricted till edema clears. The amount of fluid to be consumed will depend on the urine output of the previous day. Usually the volume will be the amount of insensible loss (400 mL/m$^2$) added to the previous days' urine output. Calories can be taken as normal for the age. Fruits with high potassium content should be restricted.

### Nephrotic Syndrome

A high protein diet is advised as there is loss of protein from the body. A child should receive 1.5 to 2 g/kg of proteins. Patients with persistent proteinuria are prone to malnutrition and should receive 2–2.5 g/kg/day. Carbohydrates are best given as complex forms. Salt has to be restricted if there is edema. A modest reduction (1–2 g/day) is advised in presence of marked edema. No added salt should be given. Snacks containing high salt also should be avoided. Corticosteroids given as part of treatment may stimulate appetite and result in weight gain. So physical activity should be advised to prevent weight gain.

### Urinary Tract Infection

Plenty of fluids and a high fiber diet are advised.

### Chronic Kidney Disease

Dietary restrictions include, salt, phosphate, potassium, fluid, and protein. Diabetes and hypertension should be controlled.

Excess proteins can be harmful leading to increased urea production and can accelerate the disease process. Predialysis protein requirement is 0.8–1.0 g/kg/day. Hemodialysis and peritoneal dialysis patients should be given high protein diet (1.2 g/kg/day), because there is loss of protein during dialysis.

Hemodialysis patients should be given high calories of 30–35 cal/kg. Peritoneal dialysis patients gain calories from the peritoneal dialysis fluid, so dietary calories can be restricted. Predialysis, they also may be given 30–35 cal/kg.

Malnutrition is common in patients with renal failure with an incidence of 20–30%. This is because of uremia, anemia, depression, meals missed due to treatment, and dietary restrictions.

Low salt diet is advised. Diet should also be low in potassium. Fruits and vegetables rich in potassium should be restricted. For example, banana and spinach. Other potassium rich foods include herbs, raisins, coco, pistachio, apricots, fish, beans, figs. Vegetables low in potassium are cucumber, raw cabbage, and lettuce. Fruits like lemons, apples, and grapes are also low in potassium. Potassium levels are moderate in broccoli, cauliflower, mushroom, carrots, turnip greens, and celery. Potatoes should always be boiled. Milk consumption should be limited. Target potassium levels in dialysis and predialysis patient should be 3.5-5.5 mmol/day. The target phosphate levels in hemodialysis and peritoneal dialysis patients is less than 1.7 mmol/day and in predialysis patients is less than 1.5 mmol/day. For this a low phosphate diet is recommended. Phosphates are high in high protein foods like dairy products, tinned fish, shell fish, chocolate, and nuts. Phosphate binders if taken, should be taken 20 minutes before meals containing protein. Parathormone levels are to be monitored and Vitamin D supplementation should be given if required.

### Renal Stones
In those with oxalate stones, restrict high oxalate food items such as cocoa drinks, chocolate, candies, black tea, coffee, spinach, asparagus, celery, parsley and tomatoes, almonds, peanuts, cashews, walnuts, beetroot, strawberries, soya products, wheat bran, rice bran, sweet potato, and yam.

### Uric Acid Stones
Restrict meat, chicken, and sea food.

### Cysteine Stones
Restriction of methionine containing foods, peanut, broccoli, pistachio, popcorn, mushroom, cauliflower, potatoes, spinach, green peas, kidney beans, and black beans.

## Gastrointestinal Problems

### Peptic Ulcer
Adequate protein is required for tissue healing but not in excess as it can increase stimulation of gastric secretion. This means that adequate carbohydrate should be given for energy, so that proteins can be spared for tissue healing.

Moderate amounts of fat should also be taken as it helps to suppress gastric secretion and motility. If cardiovascular disease is a concern, reduction of saturated fat and cholesterol is indicated.

Meals and snacks should be taken at regular intervals and in small proportions.

Individual needs should be considered and flexible program has to be tailored.

### Irritable Bowel Syndrome
Dietary measures for optimal nutrition and regular bowel motility must be followed. There should be additional amounts of bulk foods in the diet such as fruits, vegetables, and whole grains. However, during periods of diarrhea and flatulence, fiber content of the diet should be reduced. Supportive therapy to reduce stress factors is also required.

### Constipation
More dietary fiber, fruits, dried fruits, and fluid intake should be included in the diet.

### Diarrhea
The cause of diarrhea should be identified. If there is lactose intolerance, lactose has to be avoided. Milk treated with lactase enzyme, lactose hydrolyzed milk, and soya milk products are recommended.

### Inflammatory Bowel Disease
Diet that supports tissue healing should be given. Nutritional deficiency states should be avoided.

### Food Allergies
Elimination diets are given and family education is required to eliminate the suspected allergen from food.

### Phenylketonuria
Low protein and phenylalanine free diet should be given. Avoid foods such as milk and dairy products, meat, fish, chicken, and eggs.

### Galactosemia
Galactose free diet should be taken.

## Liver Diseases

### Hepatitis
Adequate protein should be given for liver cell regeneration. Also provide lipotropic agents such as methionine and choline for conversion of fat to lipoprotein and removal from the liver. High carbohydrate should be given to restore the glycogen stores 300-400 g/day. Adequate calories from carbohydrates spare the protein for vital tissue regeneration. Energy required is high 2500-3000 kcal/day for tissue regeneration. Meals may be given in liquid form or blended form, if required.

### Cirrhosis
Protein is given according to the tolerance. Low sodium diet is given; if there are esophageal varices, soft textured food is to be given.

In hepatic encephalopathy, low protein diet is given.

### Gallbladder Disease
Intake of fats to be limited. Restrict calorie for weight reduction and restrict cholesterol.

### Cancer
The guidelines for nutritional therapy for cancer patients, should meet their nutritional needs.

Because of the hypermetabolic state of disease process and the tissue healing requirements, cancer patients require great amounts of energy in their diet. Of the total dietary energy sufficient proportion should come from carbohydrates to spare the protein for vital tissue synthesis. Healthy well-nourished individuals may require around 2,000 kcal/day, whereas malnourished individuals may require 3,000-4,000 kcal, depending on the degree of malnutrition and body trauma.

Protein requirement is increased. A well-nourished individual may require 80-100 g/day whereas a malnourished individual may require 100–200 g/day to restore positive nitrogen balance.

Optimum intake at least to meet the RDA is recommended.

Adequate fluids are required for two reasons. One reason is to replace the GI losses caused by infection and fever and the second is to help the kidneys dispose the metabolic breakdown products from the destroyed cancer cell as well as from the toxic drugs used in treatment. For example, some drugs like cyclophosphamide require as much as 2–3 L of forced fluids daily to prevent hemorrhagic cystitis.

## SUGGESTED READING

1. Brown L, Rosner B, Willett WW, et al. Cholesterol-lowering effects of dietary fiber: A meta-analysis. Am J Clin Nutr. 1999;69(1):30-42. [online] Available from https://doi.org/10.1093/ajcn/69.1.30.
2. Dietary fiber: Importance of function as well as amount. Lancet. 1992;340(8828):1133-4.
3. Dietary Reference Intakes: Applications in Dietary Assessment Institute of Medicine, National academic press, Washington, DC. (2000). [online] Available from http://www.nap.edu.
4. Dillard CJ, German JB. Phytochemicals: Nutraceuticals and human health. J Sci Food Agric. 2000;80(12):1744-56.
5. Elizabeth KE. Nutrition and Child Development, 5th edition. New Delhi: Paras Medical Publishers; 2001.
6. Gopalan C, Rama Sastri BV, Balasubramanian SC. (2017). Nutritive Value of Indian Foods. Hyderabad: Institute of Nutrition, Indian Council of Medical Research. [online] Available from http://www.eeb.cornell.edu/biogeo/nanc/Food_Feed/table%201%20gopalan%20et%20al%201989.pdf.
7. Gopalan C. The current National nutrition scene: Areas of concern. NFI Bulletin. 2008;29(4):1-8.
8. ICMR-National Institute of Nutrition, Govt. of India. Recommended Dietary Allowances & Estimated Average Requirements for Indians—2020 A SHORT REPORT; 2020.
9. Krishnaswamy K, Sesikeran B. Dietary Guidelines for Indians—A Manual, 2nd edition. Hyderabad: National Institute of Nutrition; 2011.
10. Kumar V, Singh J, Chauhan N, et al. Process of paddy parboiling and their effects on rice, A Review. Journal of Pharmacognosy and Phytochemistry. 2018;SP1:1727-34.
11. Mann J, Truswell AS. Essentials of Human Nutrition, 3rd edition. New York: Oxford University Press; 2007.
12. Narasinga Rao BS. Dietary fiber in Indian diets and its nutritional significance. Bulletin of Nutrition Foundation of India. 1988;9(4):1-4.
13. National Institute of Nutrition, Indian Council of Medical Research. (2003). NNMB Technical Report No. 22. National Nutrition Monitoring Bureau (NNMB). Prevalence of micronutrient deficiencies. Hyderabad, India.
14. National Institute of Nutrition, Indian Council of Medical Research. (2009). A Report of the Expert Group of the Indian Council of Medical Research. Nutrient requirements and recommended dietary allowances for Indians. Hyderabad, India.
15. Report from the commission to the European Parliament and the Council regarding trans fats in foods and in the overall diet of the union population. SWD 268 final Brussels, 3.12.2015 COM. 619 final. (2015). [online] Available from https://ec.europa.eu/food/sites/food/files/safety/docs/fs_labeling-nutrition_trans-fats-report_en.pdf.
16. The Prevention of Food Adulteration Act; (1954).
17. Williams SR. Essentials of Nutrition and Diet Therapy, 5th edition. St Louis, Missouri: Moshy College, Publishing; 1990.
18. World Health Organization. (2003). WHO/FAO Expert Group on Diet, Nutrition and the Prevention of Chronic Diseases. WHO Technical Report Series, No. 916 (TRS 916). [online] Available from http://apps.who.int/iris/bitstream/handle/10665/42665/WHO_TRS_916.pdf;jsessionid=CABB49FDDC99074A6ABBD075953CF542?sequence=1.
19. World Health Organization and Food and Agriculture Organization of the United Nations. Vitamin and mineral requirements in human nutrition, 2nd edition;2004.

# CHAPTER 5

# Physical Activity, Exercise, and Health

*Yogita Bavaskar, Manisha Gohel, Abhay Srivastava, Saurabh Sharma, Santosh K Yatnatti*

*Take care of your body, it's the only place you have to live.*
—Jim Rohn

## CONCEPT

Physical inactivity is a fourth leading risk factors of death worldwide. Insufficient physical activity is one of the important risk factors for noncommunicable diseases (NCDs) such as cardiovascular diseases, stroke, hypertension, cancer and diabetes. Physical activity benefits in various ways to improve health and well-being of individual. Still, world is becoming less and less active. Urbanization and mechanization have led to changes in pattern of work at workplaces, passive modes of transportation, increase in screen time, all contributing to sedentary lifestyle and increase in physical inactivity all over the world. In various surveys done globally, it is seen that 23% of adults and 81% school-going adolescents are not physically active enough (Physical activity fact sheets, WHO, 2018).

Physical activity and exercise are one of the most important strategies for health promotion. Motivating people to move more and incorporate physically active lifestyle is a key strategy for reducing the burden of NCDs, as articulated in WHO's *Global Action Plan for the Prevention and Control of NCDs 2013–2020*. The plan calls for a 10% reduction in physical inactivity by 2025, which contributes to achieving the Sustainable Development Goals (SDGs).

The recommendations are provided for the minimum amounts of activity for all age groups for maintenance of health and prevention of disease. Olympic games started in 1896 were one of the ways to emphasize the importance of physical activity and to motivate the individuals to undertake sports as a hobby.

### Note

**An interesting read**

Sitting is the new smoking: In a study published in the Lancet by Ekelund et al. in 2016, he stated that sitting for long period/low physical activity leads to 59% more risk of mortality which is similar to that of smoking. Based on this study lot of infographical messages were circulated in social media. Sitting was associated with cancers, cardiac disease, and diabetes mellitus. And it was compared as a slow poison as that of smoking. Later, Ekelund published another meta-analysis stating 1 hour of moderate intensity physical activity eliminates ill effects of 8 hours of inactivity.

### Physical Activity and Exercise Definition

Physical activity and exercise both involve voluntary movement of muscles that burn calories. Physical activity is defined as *"any bodily movement produced by skeletal muscles that requires energy expenditure"* including activities undertaken while working, doing household chores, traveling and engaging in recreation, e.g. sports, gardening, walking, etc. While "exercise", which is one of the categories of physical activities, is *"specifically planned, structured, repetitive and aims to improve or maintain one or more components of physical fitness"*, e.g. aerobics class, weight training or practicing Yoga.

## PHYSICAL ACTIVITY, EXERCISE, AND RELATIONSHIP WITH HEALTH

*Regular and adequate levels of physical activity*:
1. Helps to achieve and maintain ideal body weight and healthier body composition. Exercise increases lean muscle and bone mass and reduce fat contents of the body.
2. Reduce resting blood pressure thereby protect against hypertension as well as brings about reduction of blood pressure in hypertensive patients.
3. Increases insulin sensitivity and peripheral utilization of glucose, thus protects against metabolic syndrome (syndrome X) and non-insulin-dependent diabetes mellitus (NIDDM). It reduces type 2 diabetes risk by 33–50%. Exercise also is a modality of treatment in diabetic patients.
4. Mobilizes dangerous visceral fat thus protects against dyslipidemia, ischemic heart disease (IHD), NIDDM.
5. Alters lipid profile in healthier way. The HDL levels increases and LDL, triglycerides and total cholesterol level reduces in persons who exercise regularly.
6. Protects against cardiovascular diseases by reducing blood pressure, improving lipid profile and reducing visceral fat. Also, exercise causes cardio protective effect by increasing stroke volume, reducing oxygen demand of myocardial muscle and opening up of collateral blood vessels in myocardium.

7. Reduces the risk of number of cancers especially colon cancer and breast cancer.
8. Weight-bearing activities, such as running, skipping or weight training, increase bone strength. So helpful in prevention of osteoporosis.
9. Tones up the muscles and increase flexibility so improves balance and reduces the chances of falls especially in elderly. Helps to build and maintain healthy bones, muscles, and joints.
10. Shown beneficial effects in treatment and prevention of anxiety and depression. Exercise brings about elevation in mood and feelings of well-being. This effect is believed to be caused by release of beta endorphin.
11. Helpful to arthritic patients by reducing joint swelling and pain associated with arthritis. Stretching exercise improves range of motion in persons with disability. Exercise helps to reduce backache and other type of muscular pain.
12. In children, physical activity helps to develop motor skills, improves cognitive development, enhance bone and muscular development.

> **Note**
> **Health benefits of physical activity**
> - Helps to achieve ideal body weight
> - Protects against hypertension, dyslipidemia, IHD, NIDDM, cardiovascular diseases, colon and breast cancer
> - Increases insulin sensitivity thus helpful in management of diabetes mellitus
> - Improves bone strength, muscle tone, and flexibility of joints
> - Helps in prevention of anxiety and depression. Improves mental health.

## TYPES OF PHYSICAL EXERCISE

There are four main types of exercise.
1. Aerobic/endurance/cardio
2. Anaerobic/strength training
3. Balance
4. Stretching/flexibility training.

Though they are described as separate categories there is no watertight compartment, as some activities may be classified in more than one category. For example, many aerobic exercises also help to build strength. Like skipping is an endurance exercise but also helps to build strength.

1. *Endurance/aerobic exercise*: Aerobic in literal sense means "derived from air and, aerobic metabolism is used to meet the energy demand of contracting muscle. Movement of the major skeletal muscles of the body is done in a rhythmic and sustained manner.
   *Benefits*:
   - Strengthening of the cardiovascular system by increasing cardiac output and perfusion. It also facilitates increased aeration in lungs by increasing respiratory capacities and tone of respiratory muscles. This leads to improved circulation efficiency and reduction in the blood pressure by lowering the peripheral resistance.
   - Improves the mental health. Exercise causes release of β-endorphins and some other mediators, which elevates mood, gives the feeling of well-being so is useful in reducing stress and alleviating anxiety and depression.
   - Reduction of risk factors for lifestyle diseases like cardiovascular problems, obesity, dementia, Alzheimer's disease, and diabetes.
   
   *For example*: Brisk walking, jogging, cycling, dancing, swimming, and playing tennis/basketball.

2. *Strength/anaerobic training*: Anaerobic exercise is a type of exercise which is of severe intensity due to which the oxygen supply is unable to flush out the excess lactate from muscle cells. Unlike aerobic exercise it is independent of oxygenation for muscular contraction. It is used by athletes in sports where endurance is not needed but speed and power are required in short spurt and also by body builders for increasing muscle mass. In this, muscles are made to work against a resistance. So, it is also known as resistance training. The resistance can be external weights or dumbbells used in weight lifting or biceps muscle strengthening. Or it may be own body weight, as in push-ups and sit-ups, for example, lifting weights, using anaerobic band, jumping rope, and running.
   *Benefits*:
   - This type of exercise produces an impact or tension force on the bones that promotes bone growth and strength. They help in improving muscle strength and bone mass.
   - Long-term beneficial effects on cardiovascular system such as improvement of the strength of the heart muscles, relaxation of endothelial vascular system resulting in vasodilation and lowering of blood pressure.
   - It also leads to secretion of natriuretic peptides that have anticoagulant and antiproliferative properties.
   
   Anaerobic exercises favorably alter body's lipid profile.

3. *Balance*: Balance exercises helps to prevent falls especially helpful in elderly. Exercises which improve balance are:
   - Standing on one leg at a time
   - Walking heel to toe in a straight line
   - Tai-chi exercise.

4. *Stretching*: Stretching is one of the common forms of exercise used by athletes, for rehabilitation of patient's post-trauma or surgery and in elderly.
   
   *For example*: Shoulder and upper arm stretch, calf stretch, and stretching in yogasana.
   *Benefits*:
   - *Flexibility and range of motion (ROM)*
   - *Stretching as warm up exercise*: Stretching as part of a warm up before exercise reduces stiffness and increase range of movement during exercise. The type of stretching used by sportsmen depends upon the need of their sport. Generally, static stretching is useful for athletes requiring flexibility for their sports (e.g. gymnastics, dance, etc.) on the other hand they are detrimental to athletes who require muscular strength in their performance.
   - *Rehabilitation*: Stretching is a usually advised during rehabilitation after soft tissue injuries or after orthopedic surgeries.
   - *Posture correction*: Performing the stretches like chest stretch, twisting lumbar stretch, shoulder back to forward fold, etc. help in loosening the tight muscles and maintaining a good posture. Energy expenditure on various physical activities are shown in **Table 5.1**.

**Table 5.1:** Energy expenditure* on various physical activities.

| Activity | Kcal/hr | Activity | Kcal/hr |
|---|---|---|---|
| Cleaning/Mopping | 210 | Shuttle | 348 |
| Gardening | 300 | Table tennis | 245 |
| Watching TV | 86 | Tennis | 392 |
| Cycling | | Valley ball | 180 |
| 15 (km/hr) | 360 | Dancing | 372 |
| Running | | Fishing | 222 |
| 12 (km/hr) | 750 | Shopping | 204 |
| 10 (km/hr) | 655 | Typing | 108 |
| 8 (km/hr) | 522 | Sleeping | 57 |
| 6 (km/hr) | 353 | Standing | 132 |
| Walking 4 (km/hr) | 160 | Sitting | 86 |

*Approx, energy expenditure for 60 kg reference man. Individuals with higher body weight will be spending more calories than those with lower body weight. Reference woman (50 kg) will be spending 5% less calories.
*Source:* Dietary guidelines for Indians, NIN, ICMR 2010.

## EXERCISE REGIMES FOR GENERAL WELL-BEING, FITNESS, AND WEIGHT LOSS

Regular exercise is the key to both physical and mental health. Exercise is for everyone and one can start being physical active at any age and stage of life. The best part is there are many ways to become physically active. One can set aside a time for exercise or can incorporate activity in day-to-day life. The choice will depend on individual, based on interest, lifestyle, underlying health condition and budget. It should be emphasized that structured exercise program as well as lifestyle modifications, both are equally important.

The first step to be physically active is to inculcate "physically active lifestyle" as a part of day-to-day life.

> **Ways to adopt physically active lifestyle**
> - Whenever possible, walk rather than using vehicle to reach to destination.
> - Climb stairs instead of using lifts/elevators.
> - Park your vehicle farthest and walk briskly to the destination.
> - Avoid taking much help for household chores. Get your glass of water yourself than asking a maid.
> - In office, walk up to the colleague for any communication instead of calling on phone or e-mail.
> - Take a small activity break after every 30 minutes sedentary work at office.
> - Incorporate the physical activity in your routine like walk briskly while you are talking on mobile. Practice balance by standing on one leg when waiting in a queue.
> - Lift 1/2 kg grocery packets as a weight for muscle strengthening when working in kitchen.
> - Exercise on stationary bike or treadmill or do skipping while watching television. Multitask your activities in this manner if one is not able to take separate time out for exercise.
> - Inculcate recreational activities which help you to be physically active, like swimming, playing badminton or taking a pet to walk and reduce the screen time.

## Recommended Levels of Physical Activity for Health

World Health Organizations (WHOs) publication on *Global recommendations on physical activity for health* has given guidelines for 3 age groups, 5–17 years, 18–64 years, and 65 years and above. The guidelines are applicable to most of the individuals irrespective of sex, ethnicity or income level. These recommendations can be applied to persons with chronic diseases such as hypertension or diabetes. In case of medical conditions related to mobility and in disability, adjustments can be done based on their exercise capacity. Pregnant, postpartum women and persons with cardiac events should take medical advice before following these recommendations. Physical activity here includes both planned and unplanned exercise (e.g. recreational activity/activity at workplace).

> **For 5–17 years old:**
> - Children and young people aged 5–17 years old should get involved in at least 60 minutes of moderate- to vigorous-intensity physical activity daily.
> - Physical activity done above 60 minutes daily will provide additional health benefits.
> - Most of daily physical activity should be aerobic. As it is a growing age, vigorous-intensity activities which will strengthen muscle and bone, should be incorporated, at least 3 times per week.

> **For adults aged 18–64 years and for Older adults—65 years old and above:**
> - Adults aged 18–64 years should get involved in at least 150 minutes of moderate-intensity aerobic physical activity throughout the week or do at least 75 minutes of vigorous-intensity aerobic physical activity throughout the week or an equivalent combination of moderate- and vigorous-intensity activity.
> - Aerobic activity should be performed in bouts of at least 10 minutes duration.
> - For additional health benefits duration of moderate-intensity aerobic physical activity can be increased to 300 minutes or 150 minutes of vigorous-intensity aerobic per week.
> - Muscle-strengthening activities involving major muscle groups should be done on 2 or more days a week.
>
> **For older adults—65 years old and above:**
> - In addition to above recommendations, elderly in this age group, with poor mobility, should perform physical activity to enhance balance and prevent falls on 3 or more days per week.
> - If adults of this age group cannot do the recommended amounts of physical activity due to health conditions, they should try to be as physically active as they can be.

*Source*: Global recommendations on physical activity for health WHO.

> Various combinations to get the equivalent of 150 minutes (2.5 hours) of moderate-intensity aerobic physical activity a week plus muscle-strengthening activities:
> - Thirty minutes of brisk walking (moderate intensity) on 5 days, exercising with anaerobic bands (muscle strengthening) on 2 days
> - Twenty-five minutes of running (vigorous intensity) on 3 days, lifting weights on 2 days (muscle strengthening)
> - Thirty minutes of brisk walking on 2 days, 60 minutes (1 hour) of social dancing (moderate intensity) on 1 evening, 30 minutes of swimming (moderate intensity) on 1 evening, heavy gardening muscle strengthening) on 2 days
> - Thirty minutes of an aerobic dance class on 1 morning (vigorous intensity), 30 minutes of running on 1 day (vigorous intensity), 30 minutes of brisk walking on 1 day (moderate intensity), calisthenics such as sit-ups, push-ups) on 3 days (muscle strengthening)
> - Thirty minutes of cycling to and from work on 3 days (moderate intensity), playing badminton for 60 minutes on 1 day (moderate intensity), using weight machines on 2 days (muscle strengthening on 2 days)

- Forty-five minutes of doubles tennis on 2 days (moderate intensity), lifting weights after work on 1 day (muscle strengthening), hiking vigorously for 30 minutes and rock climbing (muscle strengthening) on 1 day.

*Source*: 2008 Physical Activity Guidelines for Americans (content modified).

**Note**

**Tips to get active:**
- Incorporate physically active lifestyle.
- Children less than 17 years should do 60 minutes of moderate-intensity activity daily.
- Adults should perform 150 minutes of moderate-intensity exercise per week and muscle strengthening exercise on 2 days a week. Add stretching exercises to improve balance.
- Structured exercise program should include all; aerobic, anaerobic as well as flexibility exercises.
- Exercise more to get additional benefits.
- Exercise can be accumulated. Perform in spells and then sum up.
- It is never too late to start exercising and be physically active.

### Exercise for Weight Loss

*Energy balance*: Energy balance is said to be achieved when energy input balances energy output in the body. A person gets energy from the food and drinks consumed and energy expenditure occurs on metabolic processes (BMR and thermic energy of food) and physical activity.

**Note**

**Energy balance**
Energy consumed through food = BMR (Energy expenditure on maintenance of metabolism) + TEE (Energy utilized for digestion of food) + Energy required for physical activity.

Basal metabolic rate is responsible for 45–70% daily energy expenditure. BMR of a person is dependent on his muscle mass or body composition and varies according to age and sex. TEE accounts for around 10% of daily energy expenditure and it is fairly constant. Therefore, energy expenditure through physical activity is the most variable component of TEE. And it can be controlled by an individual. Physical activity consists of both incidental and planned activity occurring throughout the day.

A change in energy input or output results in disruption of energy balance either positive or negative. Positive energy balance results in excess calories which get deposited as fats and increase in body weight and negative energy balance results in less than required calories, removal of fat from the body and weight loss.

Thus, if weight loss is to be achieved one should be in a negative energy balance, i.e. energy input should be reduced by diet control or diet modification (calories restricted diet) and energy output should be increased by increasing the physical activity. Aerobic exercise, which causes more calorie expenditure, is ideal for weight loss. As BMR is dependent on muscle mass, muscle strengthening/weight bearing exercise will also help by increasing muscle mass of the body. Also they will help by improving the muscle tone and thereby preventing laxity-related bulkiness. Aerobic exercises like brisk walking, skipping, cycling or jogging reduce all body fat, while specific exercises like crunches, lunges, squats, dips, planks, and *surya asana* (Sun salutations) are designed to target specific body parts and muscle groups for toning them. Consistency is the key for weight loss. Planning the most appropriate sustainable structured exercise plan and sticking to it will result in desired weight loss. It is necessary to continue exercise routine beyond weight loss to maintain the results achieved.

## YOGA AND HEALTH

### Introduction

Yoga is the most valuable and precious gift of the Indian civilization to the world. It is an applied science, a systematized discipline to bring harmony between man and nature. It is a holistic approach to health and well-being. The word yoga originates from the Sanskrit root "Yuj" meaning to unite, to join, to harness, to yoke, to contact, or to connect.

**Note**

**What is yoga?**
It is the union of the "Jeevatma (individual soul)" with the "Paramatma (universal soul)".
According to Maharishi Patanjali, yoga is "**Chitta vritti nirodha**" means yoga is the stoppage of mind fluctuations.
According to the Bhagavad Gita:
- Yoga is the calmness of mind.
- Yoga is the art of performing an action.
- Yoga is the destroyer of mystery.

**The ultimate aim of yoga is self-realization, i.e. moksha.**

United Nations General Assembly (UNGA) accepted 21st June as "International Day of Yoga", which was resolution set by 177 co-sponsoring countries with consensus, proposed by the Honorable Prime Minister of India Shri Narendra Modi on December 11, 2014.

### History of Yoga

Yoga is the ancient tradition which originated in India, trace to be seen in the pre-Vedic period (2700 BC.). Lord Shiva is considered to be the first yogi (Adiyogi) and the first guru. *Vedas* and *Upanishad* contain the oldest known yogic teaching and, gem concepts of yoga, respectively.

***Ashtanga yoga:*** The first systemic presentation of yoga was done by the great Maharishi Patanjali, known as Patanjali's yoga sutras between 3rd and 6th Century BC. Yoga was established as a specific discipline with "eight-limbed paths" by Maharishi Patanjali, which contains the steps and stages towards obtaining enlightenment (samadhi) **(Table 5.2)**.

### Asanas (Yogasanas)

Patanjali defines Asana as "Sthira Sukham Asanam" means asana is a posture which is stable and comfortable. Asanas (yogasanas) can be broadly classified into two categories: (1) meditative, and (2) cultural (physical). Meditative yogasanas prepare the individual for sitting for a long time with comfort and without being fatigued. Yogasanas are again classified into

**Table 5.2:** Ashtanga yoga; eight limbs.

| Sr. No. | Eight limbs | | | | | |
|---|---|---|---|---|---|---|
| 1. | Yamas (five) | **Ahimsa:** Nonviolence | **Satya:** Truth | **Asteya:** Non-stealing | **Brahmacharya:** Sexual abstinence | **Aparigraha:** Non-possession |
| 2. | Niyamas (five) | **Shaucha:** Physical and mental purity | **Santosha:** Contentment | **Tapa:** Austerity | **Svadhyaya:** Study of the self | **Ishvara pranidhana:** Devotion to God |
| | **Hatha yoga: External limb/practices (Bahirangs)** | | | | | |
| 3. | **Asana** | Physical postures | | | | |
| 4. | Pranayama | Breath control | | | | |
| 5. | Pratyahara | Withdrawal of mind from the senses | | | | |
| | **Raja yoga: Internal limbs/practices (Antarangs)** | | | | | |
| 6. | Dharna | Concentration | | | | |
| 7. | Dhyana | Meditation | | | | |
| 8. | Samadhi | The state of super consciousness and perfect equability (divine communion). | | | | |

standing, sitting, prone and supine position asanas. It should be practiced under the guidance of yoga teacher/expert.

**Advantages of asanas**
- Rebuild, purify, and toughen the psychological and physiological structure.
- Improve coordination between nerves (nervous system), muscles and organs and improve sensory functions.
- Improve the function of cardiac, respiratory, digestive, excretory, endocrine, reproductive, and skeletomuscular muscles.
- Sharpen the intellect and enhance the memory.
- Provide the exercise necessary to the body while reducing physical and mental stress.
- Prepare an individual to deal with the modern-day lifestyles' problems.
- Create harmony between the body and mind and establish a sense of well-being through perfect health.

**Difference between asanas and physical exercise (Table 5.3).**

**Table 5.3:** Difference between asanas and physical exercise.

| S. No. | Asanas | Physical exercise |
|---|---|---|
| 1. | It improves physical and mental health and also expands spiritual consciousness | It improves physical health and creates a strong muscular physique but they fail to create spiritual consciousness |
| 2. | It can be practiced by the old and infirm as well | It may be suitable for healthy and youthful persons only |
| 3. | There is rhythmic breathing, body movement and relaxation which calm the mind and increase the flexibility of the body | There is no rhythmic breathing and relaxation but violent muscle movements, which produces large quantities of lactic acid in muscle fibers causing fatigue |
| 4. | It stimulates the parasympathetic nervous system, so feeling of being fresh and rejuvenate after performing asanas | It stimulates the sympathetic nervous system which consumes energy, produces heat in the body, and leads to tiredness |
| 5. | It improves mental faculties, concentration and memory | It increases adrenaline secretion which stimulates the mind |

**Note**

**Asanas:**
- Signify series of scientific postures uttered as physical movements, not just an exercise
- Impact on the deep control-centers of the body
- Stimulate and conserve energy rather than consume it
- Bring harmony to the tri-fold abode of spirit: the mind, the body, and the heart.

## Pranayama: Precept of Breath Control

Prana means "breath" and ayama means "regulation" or control; thus, pranayama indicates the regulation and control of the breathing process. The air that we breath contains gases, such as oxygen, hydrogen, and nitrogen and a very important component, which is subtle and intangible in nature, called "prana" or "vital life force". The respiratory process can be deliberately controlled, partly or totally through pranayama even though it is an involuntary process which is a basis of the precept of pranayama. A normal breathing has three phases, inhalation, exhalation and pauses after exhalation. Pranayama involves three elements: Puraka (inhalation), Kumbhaka (retention), and rechaka (exhalation). The diaphragm should be utilized efficiently to get more oxygen which is known as "yogic breathing". Yogic breathing practices increase the levels of leptin, a hormone produced by fat tissue which signals the brain to inhibit hunger. There are 250 types of pranayama and each has its own advantages.

**Advantages of pranayama**
- Balances the three doshas, vata, pitta, and kapha.
- Keeps the breathing process and all organs at the normal functional level; improve blood circulation, reduce blood pressure, enhances the lung capacity, improves the function of the digestive system, relaxation to the nervous system.
- Gives protection against falling and graying of hair, wrinkles on the face, poor eyesight, weak memory, etc. and delays the aging process.
- Increases oxygen supply to the brain.
- Eliminates negative thinking and nurtures positive thinking, energy, and self-confidence in the regular practitioner of pranayama.

- Purifies the body and enhances the psychological efficiency of the mind.
- Attainment of spiritual power (kundalini awakening) through purification, penetration, and awakening of chakras (energy centers).
- Reduction of all the diseases at the gross and the subtle body.

## Meditation (Dhyana)

Meditation is an act of constant observation. Meditation practices typically involve breath observation, concentration on the object of choice and non-judgmental awareness of thoughts. These practices entail training the senses and the mind to dissociate from the object and stand apart as a witness. Meditation stimulates the parasympathetic nervous system which leads to the mind and body relaxation.

The benefits of meditation are: Control blood pressure, improve blood circulation, normalize heart rate, slow down the respiration and decrease anxiety. It develops positive emotions and helps to eliminate negative emotions like anxiety, depression, etc. It keeps the mind peaceful and quiet. It enhances memory, clarity, and willpower. It revitalizes the whole body and ultimately leads to self-realization.

## Mitahara/Yogic Diet

Mitahara is a Sanskrit word which is originated from Mita (moderate) and Ahara (diet) which together mean moderate diet/balance diet. Mitahara means the diet which is nutritious, sweet, lubricating, one's liking and fills only half of the stomach. Rest half of the stomach should be filled up with water and air, for circulation. An individual should eat only when one feels hungry and never overeat. The yogic diet is a balanced, vegetarian diet that fulfills all the nutritional needs for mind-body balance. Tenets of a yogic diet are: Eating the right food, in the right quantity, with the right attitude and at the right time.

There are three types, Sattvic, Rajasic, and Tamasic diet according to Bhagavad Gita. Sattvic diet is also referred to as yogic diet. Sattvic diet is natural, unprocessed, fresh, and free from any additives or preservatives and in its natural form as possible. It comprises of cereals (whole grains), pulses, lentils, nuts and seeds, fresh fruit and vegetables, ghee and pure organic milk.

## Role of Yoga in Health

Health is closely related to the lifestyle of an individual. Principles of yoga help individual to embrace a lifestyle which is effective in reducing stress and enhancing overall health and wellness of an individual. Yoga is the finest lifestyle which has potential in the prevention, treatment, and restoration of prevalent lifestyle disorders.

Application of yoga (yogasanas, pranayama, meditation, etc.) for the treatment of illness and diseases are known as therapeutic yoga. Therapeutic yoga includes teaching different yoga practices as therapy which may reduce or improve the health situations, pain, agony, etc. in terms of physical, mental or spiritual dimensions of health. A study on the evaluation of the therapeutic effects of yoga of selected articles findings found that yogic practices enhance and recover cardiovascular and respiratory function, increase muscles strength, and flexibility of the body. It is helpful in de-addiction, improving mental health and sleep disorders, reduction of stress and anxiety, and alleviate chronic pain. It improves all over the quality of life and well-being of an individual. The yoga therapy works through activation of the parasympathetic system and its associate anti-stress mechanism. It activates the hypothalamic-pituitary-adrenal axis and recovers metabolic and psychological functions, improves glucose tolerance and lipid metabolism. The study reported that pranayama produces the positive effect on the cardiovascular and autonomic system, while no such effects by fast breathing. A randomized controlled study revealed that practicing yoga for a year helped significant improvements in the ideal body weight and body density. Yoga is simple and effective, considered as an additional beneficial therapy for type II diabetes mellitus and also attenuates the negative relationship between body weight and waist circumference. A regular practice of yoga helps in increasing gamma-aminobutyric acid (GABA) level in a practitioners' brain and hence improves mental health. Yoga has positive health effects in geriatric and child population.

## HEALTH PROMOTION AND PHYSICAL EXERCISES

According to WHO, health promotion is the process of enabling people to enhance, improve and have control over their own health. Lifestyle modifications including physical activity is an important health promotion strategy.

There are various methods, in which health promotion of physical exercise could be initiated:
1. Community wide campaigns through all the available means of communication. For example, Celebration of International Yoga Day every year on 21st of June.
2. Using prompts or behavioral change messages as a means of change in lifestyle. For example, next to the lifts prompts like use stairs instead of lift can be helpful.
3. Separate cycle lanes for the people interested in cycling. This will encourage more people to involve in cycling. For example, in the Netherlands there are separate biking lanes and the number of bikes is more than the population of Netherlands.
4. Specific or individual based behavior change lifestyle. For example, arthritis program, wherein specialized exercises are designed for elderly with arthritis.
5. Strengthening the existing school-based physical education.
6. Innovations in urban development and planning. For example, encourage events by residents of cities to come up with plans for physical activity friendly towns or cities.
7. Robust travel and transportation policies and practices. For example, encouraging more public transportation, safety measures for walkers and bicycle riders.

Exercises in special medical conditions with possible benefits is discussed in **Table 5.4**.

### Cautions to be Taken during Exercise
- High intensity exercise should be discouraged.
- The person should always warm up slowly and steadily.
- During the exercise frequent rest periods should be given so that a person will not overexert themselves.

**Table 5.4:** Exercises in special medical conditions with possible benefits.

| Disease | Effective exercises |
|---|---|
| Arthritis | • Aerobic exercises have limited role. Anaerobic exercises are more effective only after weight reduction is achieved<br>• Aquatic exercise are also helpful |
| Cancer | Aerobic and anaerobic exercises improve overall quality of life |
| Chronic obstructive pulmonary disease | Aerobic and anaerobic exercises are effective if combined together |
| Chronic renal failure | Aerobic and anaerobic exercises when combined help in reducing cardiovascular and metabolic risk factors |
| Cognitive impairment | Both aerobic and anaerobic exercises are effective in cognitive impairment |
| Congestive heart failure | Resistant exercises are more tolerable when compared to aerobic exercises as there is more chances of dyspnea |
| Coronary artery disease | Both aerobic and anaerobic exercises are cardio-protective in nature |
| Depression | For moderate and major depression combination of high intensity aerobic and resistant exercises are beneficial |
| Disability | Type of exercises will depend on the underlying disease condition |
| Hypertension | Both aerobic and anaerobic exercises help to reduce both systolic and diastolic blood pressure. However, the difference in reduction of blood pressure is large if weight reduction is done |
| Obesity | Anaerobic exercises are more beneficial for weight loss when compared to aerobic exercises |
| Osteoporosis | High impact anaerobic exercises are more beneficial |
| Peripheral vascular disease | • Balance training help in preventing falls<br>• The anaerobic exercises should be limited up to the level of pain tolerance |
| Stroke | Aerobic, anaerobic and treadmill exercises are beneficial, however the mechanism is unknown |
| Type 2 diabetes | Anaerobic exercises are more effective and protective |

- Do not exercise after a large meal, there should be a minimum of 2 hours gap after having a large meal.
- Avoid extreme climatic conditions as the body may have to put extra effort and extra stress.
- If an individual is under medications, kindly ask for the same and check their heart rate and blood pressure before starting the exercise.
- If the person is having a systolic blood pressure more than 180 mm Hg and or diastolic blood pressure more than 110 mm Hg then the person should not do any exercises until the blood pressure is controlled using medications.
- Avoid isometric exercises for patients with high blood pressure.
- Do not encourage the person to hold the weight or resistant exercise in one spot or above their heads as it can increase blood pressure to dangerous limits.
- These are the signs of emergency while doing the exercises:
  - Chest pain
  - Difficulty in breathing
  - Dizziness
  - Irregular heart beat
- Special care should be given to the patients suffering from heart diseases in the form of individualized exercises based on their physical status. Once the patient is stable in their parameters we can shift them to group exercises under supervision.

## Common Exercise-induced Injuries

- *Rotator cuff injuries*: Occurs due to over exertion of rotator cuff activity.
- *Iliotibial band injuries:* Occurs due to over use of aerobic exercises like running, cycling, etc.
- *Plantar fasciitis:* Occurs due to inflammation of the plantar fascia.
- *Shin splints*: Occurs due to overuse of lower limbs and leads to leg injuries, which are collectively referred as shin splints.

**General symptoms of all exercise-related injuries:** Pain, weakness in the affected area, and loss or limited range of motion in the affected area.

### Self-care in Exercise-related Injuries

- Analgesics and muscle relaxants will help in reducing various types of pain and inflammation.
- Keep ice pack on the injured part multiple times a day based on the severity.
- Give adequate rest to injured area.
- Strengthen the injured muscles with the help of physiotherapist to prevent the injury in future.

## SUGGESTED READING

1. American College of Sports Medicine, Chodzko-Zajko WJ, Proctor DN, et al. American College of Sports Medicine position stand. Exercise and physical activity for older adults. Med Sci Sports Exerc. 2009;41(7):1510-30.
2. Basavaraddi IV. 1st June, International Day of Yoga, Common Yoga Protocol, 3rd Edition. New Delhi: Ministry of AYUSH, Govt. of India; 2017.
3. CDC. (2011). The CDC Guide to Strategies to Increase Physical Activity in the Community. [online]. Available from https://www.cdc.gov/obesity/downloads/PA_2011_WEB.pdf.
4. Certification of Yoga Professionals Official Guidebook for level I & level II. Delhi: Excel Books; 2016.
5. Chronic Diseases and Exercise. [online]. Available from http://www.aahf.info/pdf/SN_Training_clients_with_Heart_Disease.pdf.
6. Cooper KH. Aerobics (revised, reissue edition). New York, Toronto: Bantam Books; 1983, 1968.
7. Ekelund U, Steene-Johannessen J, Brown WJ, et al. Does physical activity attenuate, or even eliminate, the detrimental association of sitting time with mortality? A harmonised meta-analysis of data from more than 1 million men and women. Lancet. 2016;388:1302-10.
8. Health Plus. Common Exercise Induced Injuries: Stretches and Exercises for Prevention and Treatment. [online]. Available from https://

9. Jake W. (2011). "Aerobic Vs. Anaerobic Fitness". [online]. Available from livestrong.com.
10. Miles L. Physical activity and health. Br Nutr Bull. 2007;32:314-63.
11. Muni SR. Classical Hatha Yoga, second edition. India, Gujarat, Vadodara: Life Mission Publications; 2011.
12. Patel NK, Newstead AH, Ferrer RL. The effects of yoga on physical functioning and health related quality of life in older adults: a systematic review and meta-analysis. J Altern Complement Med. 2012;18(10): 902-17.
13. Ross A, Thomas S. The health benefits of yoga and exercise: a review of comparison studies. 2010;16(1):3-12.
14. Sengupta P. Health Impacts of Yoga and Pranayama: A State-of- the-Art Review. Int J Prev Med. 2012;3(7):444-58. [online]. Available from https://www.ncbi.nlm.nih.gov/pmc/articles/PMC3415184.
15. World Health Organization. (2010). Global recommendations on physical activity for health WHO. [online]. Available from http://www.who.int/dietphysicalactivity/global-PA-recs-2010.pdf.
16. World Health Organization. (2018). Physical Activity. [online]. Available from http://www.who.int/news-room/fact-sheets/detail/ physical-activity.

Also referenced: www.vumc.org/health-wellness/files/health-wellness/public_files//hpCommonExerciseInducedInjuries.pdf.

# CHAPTER 6

# Sociology and Health

*Paramita Sengupta*

| | |
|---|---|
| CM2.1 | Describe the steps and perform clinico-socio-cultural and demographic assessment of the individual, family and community |
| CM2.2 | Describe the socio-cultural factors, family (types), its role in health and disease and demonstrate in a simulated environment the correct assessment of socio-economic status |
| CM2.3 | Describe and demonstrate in a simulated environment the assessment of barriers to good health and health seeking behavior |
| CM2.4 | Describe social psychology, community behavior and community relationship and their impact on health and disease |

## CONCEPT AND ITS RELATIONSHIP WITH HEALTH

Different social classes even within the same society enjoy different dimensions of health and disease. Certain "health-related behaviors" like alcoholism, cigarette smoking, exercise and food, which are the key determinants of health, are influenced by the type of the social environment. Understanding the social science and its influence on health and diseases can help in improving the health of an individual and community as a health.

## MEDICAL SOCIOLOGY

Medical sociology is the study of the effects of social and cultural factors on health and medicine. Around 1950s, when for the first time the study of doctor–patient relationship was studied as a social system, medical sociology was conceptualized. Medical sociology generally deals with social aspects of health and illness, social role of health establishments and organizations as well as the relationship of healthcare delivery to other social systems and also the social conduct of health personnel and consumers of health. It essentially includes community organization, responsibilities of community for health and development, healthcare delivery, community participation in health programmers, doctor–patient relationship and the social factors in the prevalence, incidence, etiology and interpretation of disease. Family is the basic unit of a society and medical sociology deals with family-based health care by home visits to the family. The social problems approach to health care recognizes that advances in medical knowledge and technology may create as well as solve human problems. Social medicine is a scientific, interdisciplinary branch of medicine which studies the effect of environment on health. It is a broad term which encompasses genetics, public health, and health equity.

Poor lifestyle and social conditions have an impact on health. Illness can be prevented, and costs can be saved by targeting the determinants of health like housing, education, income, poverty, transport, health care, and environmental and genetic influences. Medical sociology has following perspectives:
- Observing the pattern of diseases among the various social groups.
- Explaining the response of people for diseases according to their cultural perspectives.
- Description of how a society manages and treats a disease.
- Investigation of support given by the society to the medical institution to help treat the sick and their rehabilitation.

Social medicine is a scientific, interdisciplinary branch of medicine which helps us to understand how different socio-economic conditions impact the determinants of health, leading to a healthier society. Social medicine studies means—man as a social being in relation to the environment.

### Social Sciences

Social science deals with the study of society and the way people relate to each other and the group. Social science includes economics, political science and international relations, sociology, social psychology, and anthropology. The last three, i.e., the social psychology, anthropology and sociology are included in the behavioral sciences.

### Sociology

It is concerned with social interaction, social groups and social behavior. It tells us about the way in which human groups and social relationships form and influence people's behavior with one another. Sociology deals with the development, structure, functioning and interaction, as well as collective behavior of human society. Sociology derives its name from a Latin word, Socius (for society) and a Greek word, logos (study), meaning "the study of companionship."

## MILESTONES OF SOCIOLOGY

Sociology, founded in 1838 by a French philosopher named Auguste Comte, is a major discipline in the social sciences. Comte believed in the study of social dynamics, or social change and argued that a proper study of social behavior would lead to more rational human interactions. He found the Law of Three Stages in which the society was divided into three different stages: Theological, metaphysical, and positive. The theological stage discusses the superstitious nature of human beings, in the metaphysical stage human beings begin to shed their superstitious nature and in the positive stage human beings finally attribute reason and science behind the occurrence of natural phenomena and world events. Comte, otherwise considered as the Father of Sociology, named the scientific study of social patterns as positivism.

## Social Structures

Social structure is the pattern of relationships and bonds between people and social institutions in a society. Social structure is any group of people who come together or are put together for any purpose. This could range from a family to a household, marriage and kinship, custom and law, belief and meaning, workplace structure, social stratification and class, community and city, employment and leisure. The state, social policy, welfare, law, etiquette, religion, culture, government and education are all parts of the complex mechanism by which a social structure exists and persists. Social activism is a proactive involvement to modify the existing social structures and bring about a change in the society.

## Social Process

The process of how the social structure is built and sustained is known as the social process. The important social processes are socialization, acculturation and social controls.

### Socialization

It is a process of transfer of civilization including culture, beliefs, traditional practices, general codes of conduct, healthy habits, etc., from parents to the children. Socialization is thus acquiring culture and norms of the family and becoming a member of society. Socialization is a process of inducting the individuals into the society wherein an individual learns the habits, attitudes, values and beliefs of the social group, he belongs to. It plays a major role in help-seeking behaviors. An example of socialization is children going to school.

### Acculturation

Culture contact leading to culture exchanges is known as acculturation. When two people or groups of people with different cultural backgrounds mingle, there is exchange of culture both ways. This is known as acculturation. Local and global travel and even migration leads to acculturation. It even affects the health of both, the new entrant population as well as the host population group.

### Social Change

Social change refers to any significant alteration in social structure, social order, values, customs, traditions, norms, cultural heritage, code of conduct, standards, attitudes, style of living, dressing and way of conducting oneself in the society. Social change is of two types—Evolutionary and Revolutionary. Industrialization creates changes in social institutions.

### Social Controls

Social controls are the constraints and restrictions imposed on social behavior. There are two types of social controls, formal and informal. Formal controls are the laws and enactments, rules and regulations. Informal controls though are not laws but they serve as pressures exerted on individuals for desired behavior.

### Social Order

Every society has a set of rules and regulations which helps maintain its sanctity. Social order regarding social sciences alludes to a set of social structures, institutions and practices which help maintain methods to relate and behave.

### Social Activism

To bring about social change there must be diversification of business practices, government or business policies which can be achieved by promotion and counseling. A good social activist should understand and have in-depth knowledge of the cause to be able to communicate the needs with the policy makers and creating awareness with the help of media. Its main aim should be to create an impact and help improve quality of living in the society.

## Social Pathology

The study of social problems in the society is dealt with by social pathology. These can be grouped in three categories: (1) social constraints, (2) social evils, and (3) social deviance.

### Social Constraints

These are the restrictions or impediments, which prevent the growth and prosperity of the community, leading to increased morbidity and mortality. These are poverty, illiteracy, ignorance, migration, industrialization and urbanization.

### Social Evils

The various social evils are: smoking and drinking, caste and casteism, gender bias and discrimination, prostitution and STDs, child neglect and abuse, child labor, crime and corruption, and stress.

### Social Deviants

Social deviants consist of a group of persons who come into conflict with law who exhibit social deviant behavior, may be due to mental or physical traumas, poverty, breakdown of societal control and unemployment. These include people involved in alcohol and substance use, beggars, street children, juvenile delinquents, sex workers, suiciders, etc. Petty criminal activities help them meet their needs and sustain.

## Social Defense

It is inclusive of preventive, therapeutic and rehabilitative services that help protect the society from anti-social or criminal elements. It is focused on the marginalized groups which need social protection of some sort. For example, the provision of juvenile homes for delinquents, the old age homes, de-addiction centers, etc.

## Sociometry

It is a quantitative method for measuring social relationships. It can also be defined as a technique to measure the interpersonal connection between two people. It provides an effective structure and tools for use both in small group interactions and in interpersonal dynamics.

## SOCIAL DETERMINANTS OF HEALTH

Social determinants of health (SDOH) are the social factors that relate to health outcomes. These are the conditions in the environments, where people are born, live, learn, work, play, worship, and age that affect a wide range of health, functioning, and quality-of-life outcomes and risks. Social determinants include income, education, social status, social networks and social support, social norms, custom and culture, etc. Accessibility, inequality, opportunity and differences in these factors in various societal groups, families or individual result in to health status and outcome of that particular group, family or an individual.

Some social determinant which deserve special mention are shown in **Figures 6.1 to 6.4**.

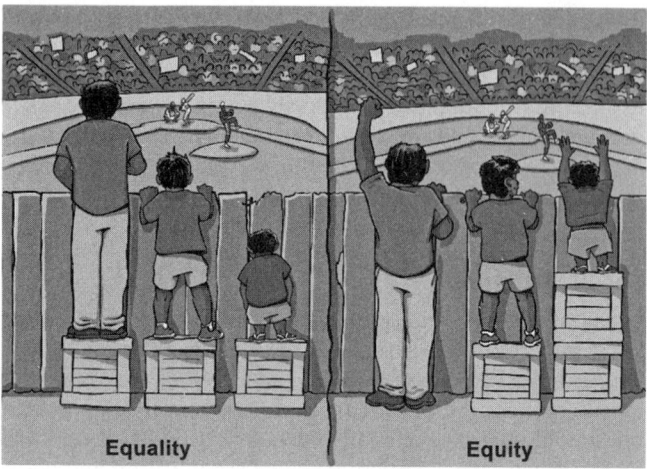

Fig. 6.1: Equality and equity.

### Education

Social factors such as education and literacy also influence health outcomes. Higher education not only improves the chances of attainment of a better job opportunity but also a better quality of life. Opportunities leading to improvement of socioeconomic conditions increase the capacity for better decision-making regarding one's health and better health-related behaviors.

### Poverty

Poverty and insufficiency of health services leave a considerable percentage of the population with limited access to basic healthcare facilities. There is much social discrimination against the poor. They are mostly engaged in labor, have less awareness of their social and economic rights, and stay in substandard houses/slums. This makes them vulnerable to many diseases. Being unrepresented and powerless, they are harassed and humiliated by society at large, which also lower their self-esteem. Low-income countries and poor people are exploited by their wealthier counterparts on whom they are economically dependent.

### Social Status

Socio-economic status or social class is an important determinant of one's health as it influences the incidence and prevalence of various health conditions and also accessibility, acceptability and actual utilization of various available health facilities.

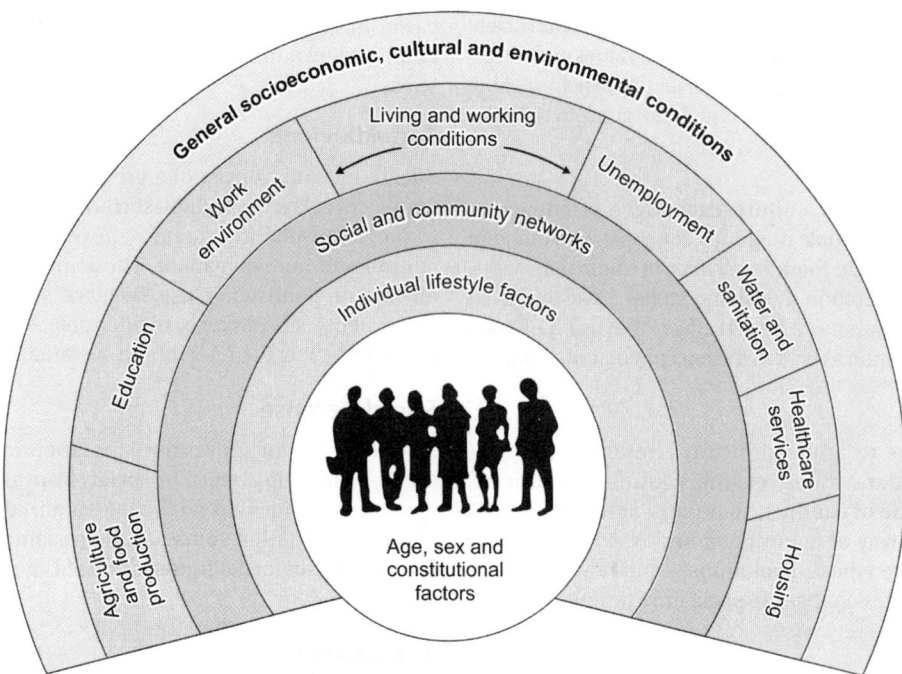

Fig. 6.2: Social determinants of health.

## Chapter 6: Sociology and Health

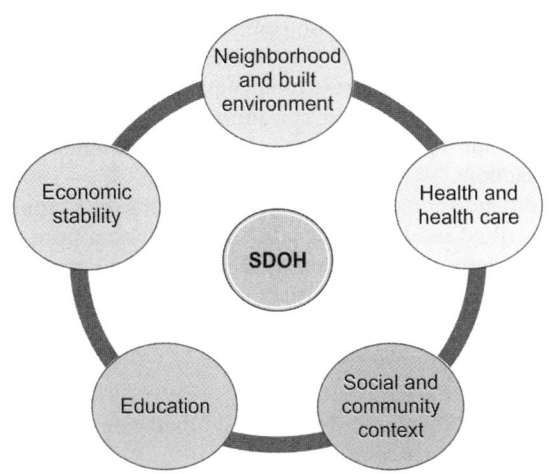

Fig. 6.3: Social determinants of health (SDOH) (Healthy People 2020).

People at the bottom of our social ladder are at a greater risk of serious illness and premature death as compared to those near the top. McKeown observed that class, income level and living environment influence health and disease. He hypothesized that the growth in population in the industrialized world from the late 1700s to the present is not due to life-saving advancements in medicine or public health but due to public health improvements in living standards, especially improvement in diet and nutritional status. McKeown thus made renewed emphasis on the social determinants of disease as the cause of morbidity and mortality.

### Gender

The terms, gender and sex are often used interchangeably, but they carry two distinct interpretations. Sex is the biological trait that categorizes a person into either male or female while gender is a social attribute. Society creates some gender norms which are considered appropriate for one sex. Children perceive the difference in the societal expectations from boys and girls at a very young age. Gender socialization occurs through family, by reading our religious scriptures, education, peer groups and mass media. For example, an aggressive behavior is considered a sign of masculinity for boys whereas girls are expected to be passive and obedient and that they should shoulder domestic responsibilities. Men also enjoy more freedom in the society and are even paid more than women for similar work. Moreover, women face various exploitations (rape, incest, female feticide, dowry, etc.) which affect their health, even then women generally live longer than men. Sexism refers to prejudiced beliefs that value one sex over another. In 2014, the Supreme Court of India created the third gender distinct from the traditional ones, i.e., males and females.

### Urbanization and Industrialization

India has witnessed a rapid economic growth in the last two decades leading to a rapid growth of industrial and service sectors, which in turn has led to an increased urbanization. In the last decade in India, the growth of urban population represents the 2-3-4-5 syndrome. India's average annual growth rate is that of 2%, where urban India grew at rate of 3%, mega cities at a rate of 4%, and a 5-6% rise in the slum population. Urban areas have over 30% of Indians, and it is projected to show a growth to 40%, or around 59 crore people, by 2030. The absence of affordable housing can be foreseen as a major factor for the growth of slums in the urban areas of the country. As per Census 2011, as many as 2,613 towns of India have reported the presence of about 33,510 slums of which 13,761 were notified and 19,749

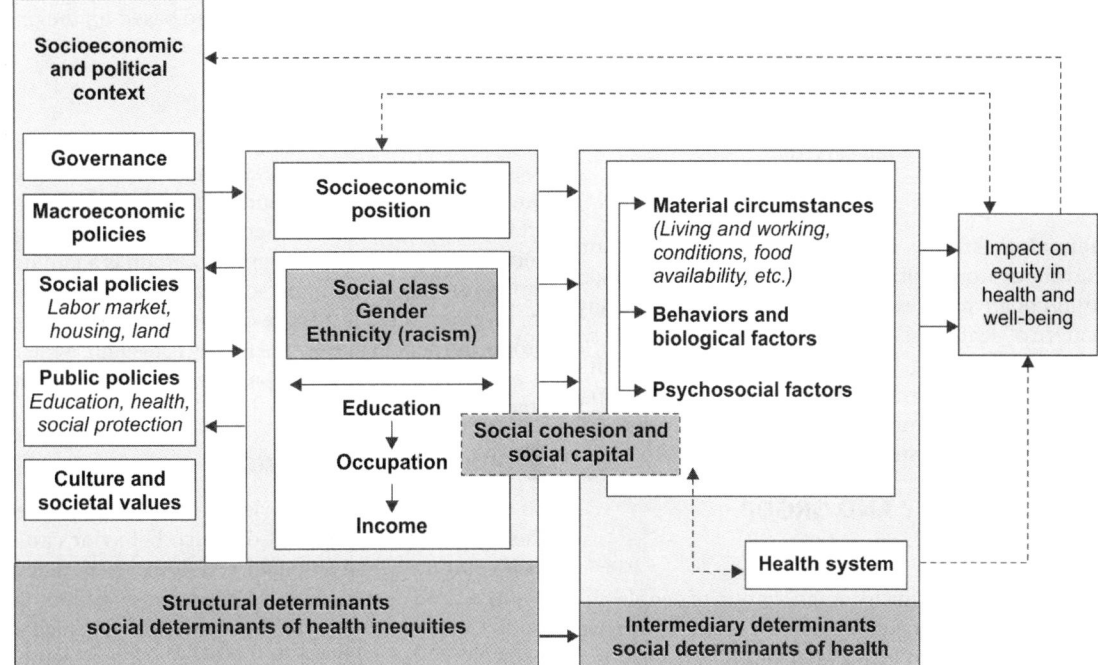

Fig. 6.4: Conceptual Framework of Social Determinant of Health (WHO).

were non-notified. Increased urbanization in India is likely to increase urban poverty.

### Migration

Migration has been an important part of existence for rural poor who go to cities/towns in search of employment. The migrant moves to a new place either as a result of positive attraction or simply to escape from the old. The economic and socio-political causes vary from one migration stream to another, but with a similar psychosocial and health effect. The acute sense of uprootedness, frustration of expectation, difficulties of adjustment, and a restriction of the social field lead to increase in psychosomatic diseases and sometimes to deviant behavior. Moreover, the migrant population has poor access to healthcare services, due to inadequate health staffing and the exclusion of migrant pockets from primary healthcare services. Distance to available services, lack of knowledge about such services, or having special needs can be listed as few of the significant barriers in accessing healthcare or services.

### Health Equity

Components that make sure that health equity is possible are:
- Equal opportunity for everyone—availability of health facility
- Equal access for the population irrespective of their financial status to help them stay healthy.

Health equity can also be defined as "the absence of systematic disparities in healthcare services between economically different social groups that have various levels of social advantages or disadvantages". The accessibility of health, welfare and development services, availability of educational and employment opportunities is unequally distributed between different sections of a society and hence the quality of life also varies. Material conditions, behavioral changes, and psychological support available—these three components show a difference in different subgroups which makes them vulnerable to poor health. Prevalent social inequalities prove to be a deterrent in providing prompt and quality healthcare and even in its utilization. This in turn causes an inequality in health promotion, prevention of disease, its treatment, recovery and survival.

### Social Epidemiology

Social epidemiology studies the effect of social factors on individual and population health and is based on the assumption that distribution of advantages and disadvantages in a society affects the pattern of health and disease distribution in a society. Social epidemiology deals with the mechanisms by which health is influenced by social structures, institutions, and relationships. A major focus of social epidemiology is to identify the origins of health disparities and devise strategies to eliminate them.

## COMMUNITY, SOCIETY AND GROUP

### Community

Community is a sociological unit in which a group of people live in the same place for satisfying their day-to-day needs or have a characteristic or interests in common. Community creates a sense of attachment and belonging, and offers a common sense of identity. The beneficial contribution of a community is that it helps to build a strong and vibrant society.

Community is a process of engaging and connecting with others. Different types of community exist, having unique characteristics, purpose, membership requirements, and type of interactions.

Ferdinand Tönnies is credited with the notion of 'Community'. He described modern society to be in transition from village to urban settings and other early sociologists extended this notion of community. Tönnies distinguished two types of communities, a simple village community (Gemeinschaft) and those with complex social relationships in urban environments (Gesellschaft).

Brint classified communities into four broad types based on:
1. Relationship: Geographic or choice.
2. Reason for interaction: Activity or belief.
3. Location of other members: Concentrated or dispersed in space.
4. Amount of interaction: Frequent or in frequent.

### Society

A society is a group of people involved in persistent social interaction living in a definable community, typically subject to the same political authority and sharing a common culture. Sociologist Gerhard Lenski (1924) classified societies into three main types: Preindustrial, Industrial and Postindustrial. Examples of Preindustrial is Hunter-Gatherer (small rural societies dependent on human labor), Pastoral (domestication of animals), Horticultural (cultivation of plants), Agricultural (farming) and Feudal. Feudal societies operate on a strict hierarchical system of power based around land ownership and protection. Industrial societies are based on production of material goods and Postindustrial societies (otherwise called information or digital societies) are based on the production of information and services.

### Group

Group refers to a gathering of at least two people who work together and share a sense of identity, aligned to the group. Groups are of two types, primary and secondary. Primary group play a vital role in our lives, serve emotional needs and impact on our socialization. Example of a primary group is a family. Secondary groups are larger and impersonal, and are more task-oriented. In an in-group there is a sense of belongingness to, and in an out-group, the person may have a feeling of disdain. A reference group is a group that people compare themselves to, and it provides a standard of measurement.

## COLLECTIVE BEHAVIOR

To understand health behavior of individuals, we need to study their collective behavior. Collective behavior can be defined as a voluntary, goal-oriented action that occurs in a relatively disorganized situation, in which society's predominant social norms and values cease to govern individual behavior. Collective behavior is the behavior that takes place between two or more people and can be organized as well as unorganized. The different forms of collective behavior are: crowd, mob, audience, riots, fads and fashion, panic and crazes, rumors and mass hysteria.

## Crowds

Crowds are temporary gatherings of people for a common short-term or long-term purpose. People in crowds are prone to being swept up in group emotions and lose their ability to make rational decisions. A crowd turning violent is called a mob. People come together in crowds often having an animal like behavior, stimulating and go adding one another into movement. The group-mind is mostly irrational and dangerous. Casual crowds, conventional crowds, protest crowds, expressive crowds and acting crowds are the common types. They mostly have no thinking capacity and blindly follow the leader.

# CUSTOMS AND CULTURES

## Customs

Customs refers to the usual behavior of people as per the traditions of the particular group or place. Knowing about customs and cultures is important for a medical graduate, as India has a diverse cultural background where there needs to be a transition in the "one-size-fits-all" approach, to a more patient-centered approach. The latter approach suiting patient's unique perspectives improves patient satisfaction by better quality of care, and improves health outcomes, thus making cross-cultural care an important topic in health professionals' curricula.

## Values

Values are set standards for determining what is good and just in a society as per their cultural practices. Values are deeply embedded and critical for transmitting and teaching a culture's beliefs. Beliefs are the convictions that people hold to be true.

## Norms

Norms are defined as a guide or an expectation of a behavior, a set of behaviors pre-defined and agreed upon by a society as good, right, and important, according to which members of the society are supposed to behave. Formal norms are established written rules, suiting most of the people in the society. Norms can be classified further into either **mores** or **folkways**. The moral views and principles of a group are embodied by Mores (mor-ays), violating which can lead to serious consequences. Many mores are also legally protected with laws or other formal norms. Folk ways are also norms, but they do not have any moral under pinnings. Folk ways show the appropriate behavior in the daily practices in a culture, for example, they suggest whether shaking hands or kissing on the cheek is proper practice when greeting another person.

## Culture

Tylor defines culture as "that complex whole which includes knowledge, belief, art, morals, law, custom, and any other capabilities and habits acquired by man as a member of society." Culture is a learned behavior acquired through generations. It consists of customs, traditions, beliefs, and laws of family or community, by which groups of people define themselves, thus following the society's shared values and contribute to society. Cultural practices can affect health, for example, the practice of giving prelacteal feeds comes in the process of exclusive breast-feeding. Similarly, in some cultures, there is a practice of writing 'Om' on the tongue of the newborn by his paternal aunt, which unnecessarily delays in breastfeeding.

**Household:** A group of people living in the same house and sharing the kitchen is called a household. A family differs from household in that all the members in household may not be related by blood, for example, a fulltime maid working in the house is a part of the household.

# FAMILY

The word "family" has been taken from the Roman word, "famulus", meaning a servant. Family refers to a group of individuals who are tied by "kinship" (related by blood, adoption or marriage) and share the same kitchen and common purse.

The family forms the basic unit of social organization in which members interact with each other in their respective social roles of husband and wife, mother and father, brother and sister creating a common culture. A variety of educational, demographic, economic and legal factors affect the structure of a family in India.

A family cycle consists of five phases:
1. *Phase of formation:* Starts with marriage and ends with the birth of first child.
2. *Phase of expansion:* A stage of growth starting with the birth of first child to birth of successive children.
3. *Phase of completion:* This phase is completed with the birth of the last child.
4. *Phase of contraction:* This phase is characterized by marriage of female children or son leaving the house for job.
5. *Phase of dissolution:* This phase starts with the death of one of the parents.

## Types of Family

Sociologists identify different types of families based on how one enters into them. A family of orientation refers to the family into which a person is born. A family of procreation describes one that is formed through marriage.

Based on size or structure family can be classified into two main types:
1. *Nuclear or primary family:* Consists of two generations consisting of parents and their own or adopted children living in the same household. In this type of family, child-rearing responsibilities solely rely on husband and wife as no grandparents or uncle and aunts are present. The relationship between husband and wife is more intimate as compared to joint family.
2. *Joint family:* This may be three generation family, or lateral extended family. Here all responsibilities are shared among all family members which provides a greater economic and social security to family. It also provides economic and social security to the old, and the unemployed.

Based on marriage family can be classified into three major types:
1. *Polygamous or polygynous family:* Family where a man has multiple simultaneous wives
2. *Polyandrous family:* Family where a woman has multiple simultaneous husbands
3. *Monogamous family:* Family consists of a husband and his wife. Under this type of family system neither husband nor wife is allowed to have more than one spouse at a time.

Based on the nature of residence family can be classified into three main forms:
1. Family of matriarchal residence
2. Family of patriarchal residence
3. Family of changing residence

Based on the nature of authority family can be classified into two main types:
1. *Matriarchal:* A family headed by a female, found among the Nairs of Malabar, the Khasis and Garos of Meghalaya
2. *Patriarchal:* A family headed by a male

Based on ancestry or descent family can be classified into two main types:
1. *Matrilineal family:* Descent through mother (family name through mother), matrilocal residence system (husband lives in wife's residence), and inheritance of parental property by daughter.
2. *Patrilineal family:* Sons inherit property from their fathers; children and wives take the father's surname.

Based on the nature of relations family can be classified into two main types:
1. Conjugal family is a nuclear family that may consist of a married couple and their children (by birth or adoption)
2. Consanguine family is a family that extends beyond the conjugal family. In addition to the married couple and their children, this family consists of grandparents, aunts, uncles or cousins, all living in the same household.

**Symmetrical family** in which couples share domestic work between themselves.

**Reconstituted family** in which one or both partners were previously married or partnered, with children from previous marriages or partnerships.

**Cohabitation**—a household comprising of two people who live together, without marriage on a long-term basis in a relationship.

**Broken family**—these are families where parents are separated or divorced. Children live with one of the parents, or many a time they are looked after by one of the grandparents due to death of one or both the parents.

**Problem families**—problem families are troubled families who lag behind the rest of the community. There are usually many children who may be feeble-minded, quality of life is lower than expected and parents are unable to meet the physical and emotional needs of their children. They usually require care, supervision and support for their well-being as they are socially defective. Problem families commonly belong to the lower social classes.

**New family**—this is a family of less than 10 years duration and consists of parents and children. This concept is important in family planning studies.

**Redefining of family:** People related by marriage, birth, consanguinity or legal adoption, who share a common kitchen and financial resources on a regular basis. A new family classification has been framed as under:

| Type | Name | Description |
|---|---|---|
| I | Proton | Single individual staying alone |
| II | Electron | No married couple or one parent family |
| III | Nuclear | Single married couple with/without their children |
| IV | Atom | Nuclear family with any other family member(s) but no other married couple |
| V | Molecular | Two married couples of any different generations (vertical levels) with/without unmarried people of any other generation |
| VI | Joint | Two or more married couples of a single generation (horizontal level) or three or more couples if multiple generations (vertical levels) |
| VII | Quasi | The prefix "quasi-" can be added to any of the previous types (III onward), for a couple who are sharing kitchen and financial resources as a married couple but not legally married |

## Functions of Family

- Provision of a home
- Provision of economic security
- Imparting knowledge and life skills
- Provision of emotional and social support
- Provision of social status
- Socialization
- Reproduction

## Role of Family in Health and Illness

- *Child-rearing:* Family takes care of the young so that they become responsible adults and perpetuate the family.
- *Socialization:* Socialize the "stream of newborn barbarians" process whereby individuals develop qualities essential for functional affectivity in the society. Schools and religious places play an important role in introducing the child to adult childhood.
- *Personality formation:* Capacity of an individual to with stand stress and strain is determined by the early experiences in the family. Family acts as a buffer against certain bad influences and help in laying foundation of physical, mental and social health of the child.
- *Care of dependent adults:* Family takes care of the sick and injured, of pregnant women and children, elders and adolescents and of the handicapped. Attitude of society to pregnant and child-bearing may have an important bearing on the infant deaths, maternal morbidity and mortality.
- *Stabilization of adult personality:* Family is like a "shock absorber" to the stress and strains of daily life like injury, illness, deaths, emotional turmoil, and economic insecurity. A family helps in alleviating stress and helps in stabilization of personality in meeting their emotional needs.

- *Family susceptibility to disease:* Some diseases have a genetic predisposition. They are—hemophilia, hypertension, color blindness, diabetes, schizophrenia, congenital malformations.
- *Role of family in stress:* The family helps an individual in coping up with stress. Any change in the family situations is a stressor (divorce, a child leaving home for studies or after marriage, pregnancy, change in job, graduation, visit to a tourist place).

If there is an increasing demand in the ability to cope stress, it becomes a threat to the physical and emotional well-being of all other members of the family. The way in which the family perceives the stressor explains the values and previous experiences of the family in meeting the crisis.

## APPLICATION IN HEALTH PROMOTION

Habit is habit, and not to be flung out of the window, but coaxed down the stairs a step at a time. —*Mark Twain*

Health promotion can be defined as the process of empowering people to adopt healthy lifestyles and be able to control their own behavior and manage their own health by education, counseling, and support mechanisms. For example, health education and counseling to promote physical activity, improve nutrition, or reduce the use of tobacco, alcohol, or drugs.

### Individual Care and Community Care

Social and cultural factors of the community play an important role in the way the community looks at health and illness and hence shaping of individual behaviors and habits. Health providers have to understand this so that their health promotion activities are effective. An understanding of how health provider or health system's actions are perceived by the community where they work, cultural interactions with environment, socioeconomic conditions, will of the local leaders or politicians, is important for health promotion in the community. A community-led approach to health supports vulnerable communities which experience poor health outcomes to identify social factors affecting their health and impact their well-being. It also helps in identifying and implementing solutions. To improve the efficacy of health promotion programs the following four questions can be raised for application in health promotion:
1. Is functioning enhanced?
2. Is longevity increased?
3. Is super-health achieved?
4. Are there any ill-effects of these programs?

There are five models of health promotion.

### *Ecological Model*

This model has emerged from developments in many disciplines, some of them being public health, sociology, psychology. According to this model, health is shaped by many environmental subsystems including the physical and social environments like family, community, workplace, beliefs, traditions, etc. Effective interventions must influence multiple levels which address not only individual behaviors and their cognitive determinants but also the multiple social contexts that shape behaviors. Ecological model is a framework for integrating and conceptualizing the dynamic interrelations among various personal and environmental factors on human behavior.

### *Social Cognitive Theory*

Cognition refers to both awareness and judgment, i.e., people gain understandings of themselves and their environments. Reciprocal and dynamic relationships between environment, personal factors, and attributes of health behavior bring about change. A unique feature of this model is the emphasis of social influence on external and internal social reinforcement.

### *Health Belief Model*

People will adopt recommended health behaviors if they perceive that their susceptibility to the disease, how threatening and severe the disease is, and the benefits of cure outweighs their perceived barriers to action (the cost to the individual; convenience, time, pain).

### *Stages of Change Model (Transtheoretical Model)*

Change is a continuous process. In adopting healthy behaviors or eliminating unhealthy ones there are five levels of change, e.g., precontemplation, contemplation, preparation, action, and maintenance.

### *Theory of Reasoned Action/Planned Behavior*

A person's behavior is determined by his intentions, which are determined by his attitude towards the behavior and his beliefs regarding other people's attitude.

## SOCIAL STRATIFICATION: SOCIAL STATUS, SOCIAL CLASS AND HEALTH

### Social Stratification

Stratification refers to a system wherein there is difference in availability and access to resources according to the person's socioeconomic status. Here, a hierarchy is created among the members of society based on either caste or wealth or class. Referring to social status is in respect to social standing or socioeconomic status of the family. A social class is part of the strata whose members objectively share characteristics which can be lifestyle, income, or ownership of productive wealth. Social stratification refers to a society divided into different layers or strata where occupants have unequal access to social opportunities and rewards. People at the top of strata enjoy power and prestige which are not usually available to other members of society. Social stratifications can be used to predict patterns of mortality and morbidity.

### Caste System

One of the most common ways in which Indian society has been stratified is caste. Occupation, social interaction, power, and education of a person are governed by his belonging to a caste. The caste system brings inequality as no extra achievement can change one's caste position. The caste system initially was created to divide people on the basis of their occupation into four main categories: Brahmins (teaching and preaching), Kshatriya (kingship and war), Vaishya (business), and Shudra (laborer). Later it became a means on which society was divided into different strata and socioeconomic status.

## Social Mobility

Social mobility is the change over a course of time of socioeconomic class of an individual/family after attainment of literacy/educational status, better occupation and enhanced income. This movement can be in either direction, from lower socioeconomic class to higher and vice versa, and is known as social mobility.

## Socioeconomic Status Scales

"Social class or socioeconomic status (SES) is the strongest predictor of health, disease causation, and longevity in medical sociology."

Socioeconomic status (SES) is a measure of the social standing of the individual or his family in the society and has an impact on his health, family life, knowledge and educational attainment, diet, lifestyle, etc. SES tells us about the health status of any country. The accessibility, affordability, acceptability, utilization of health-care services depend on his SES, and hence is an important factor affecting the health condition of an individual or a family. This reflects the affordability of health services, necessities and purchasing power of the same.

Attempts have been made to classify different sections of society according to their SES. Different scales have been developed for use in community-based research in India.

Conventionally, income is a core SES indicator and some SES measures are solely based on per capita family income such as 'Prasad's scale', that evolved in 1961 for use in both urban and rural areas, and later modified in 1970. However, considering high level of unreliability, including the unwillingness of people to discuss about income, social scientists consider "consumption" or "expenditure" as better markers of SES than income. Composite SES indices are used that usually incorporate education and occupation along with income to reflect three distinct and interrelated dimensions of class, status, and power of social hierarchy. Kuppuswamy's scale developed in 1976 for urban areas has combined education, occupation, and income of head of household in his composite SES scale. Udai Pareekh's scale added caste and family type and created a new scale with a total of nine indicators, to be used for rural areas only. Tiwari's scale used seven profiles (housing, material possession, education, occupation, economic profile, cultivated land, and social profile) in his scale. Other indices such as multidimensional poverty index (MPI) and unsatisfied basic needs (UBN), which are based on different economic theories, are capable of identifying non-income factors associated with social inequalities.

## Modified BG Prasad Classification

Consumer Price Index for industrial workers (CPI-IW) and linking factors between the base years are the essential components for calculating the SES. The base year of price index numbers is revised at regular intervals, reflecting the changes in the population's consumption pattern. Linking factors are used to convert the CPI from the new base to the old base. The first

Table 6.1: Modified BG Prasad classification. For BG Prasad Scale, using CPI-IW, October 2023, which is 138.4 (base year 2016) (latest AICPI-IW can be obtained from www.labourbureau.gov.in) and calculated using online scale from (scaleupdate. weebly.com).

| Social-economic Classes | Per capita income of family monthly (1961) | Per capita income of family (October 2023, CPI-IW of 138.4) |
|---|---|---|
| I | ≥100 and above | ≥9096 |
| II | 50–99 | 4549–9095 |
| III | 30–49 | 2728–4548 |
| IV | 15–29 | 1365–2727 |
| V | 14 and below | <1364 |

base year for CPI is 1960. Taking the base of CPI for 1960 as 100 and it got modified in 1982, 2001, and 2016. The linking factors for 1982, 2001, and 2016 were 4.93, 4.63, and 2.88, respectively.

CPI-IW is updated regularly every month based on retail prices of various commodities. A multiplying factors is used to link CPI-IW of any current month with last base year, i.e. 2016.

Multiplying factor = Current index value for October 2023 (=138.4)/Base index value in 2016 (= 100) = 1.38.

Current income value (shown in **Table 6.1**) = Multiplying factor (1.38) × [Old income value × Linking factor between 1960 and 1982 series (4.93) × Linking factor between 1982 and 2001 series (4.63) × Linking factor between 2001 and 2016 series (2.88)].

### Kuppuswamy Classification

It is used for urban area. It was first published in the year 1981 and recently updated in the year 2022. Kuppuswamy scale score is based on the assessment of three criteria: Education level of the head of family (HOF), Occupation of the HOF, and Income per month **(Table 6.2)**.

### Udai Pareekh Classification

Pareekh's socioeconomic scale is used for rural areas. It takes into consideration caste, occupation, education, land-holding, social participation, family size, housing and farm power and material possession **(Table 6.3)**.

### Newer Ways of Measuring SES

A newer and more objective way of measuring SES is wealth index (WI) where construction materials of dwelling houses and household assets are combined through data reduction using statistical procedure of Principal Component Analysis (PCA) and Factor Analysis (FA) methods to come up with a summary [wealth index (WI) usually in quintiles]. Related asset information is usually extracted from household survey or census data. The WI is thus a composite and relative measure of households' SES. The WI has been constructed from national household surveys such as Demographic Health Surveys (DHS) in 56 countries and the National Family and Health Survey (NFHS) in India.

## Below Poverty Line Families

The poverty line was originally fixed in terms of income/food requirements in 1977 by the Planning Commission of India. BPL

Table 6.2: Kuppuswamy's method of social classification of an individual (urban areas). (income updated according to 2022) (Link: https://www.researchgate.net/publication/361601731).

| # | Education of head of family | Score | Occupation of head of family | Score | Family Income (INR) | Score |
|---|---|---|---|---|---|---|
| 1 | Profession or honours | 7 | Legislators, Senior Officials and Managers | 10 | ≥ 1,84,376 | 12 |
| 2 | Graduate | 6 | Professionals | 9 | 92,191–1,84,370 | 10 |
| 3 | Intermediate or diploma | 5 | Technicians and Associate Professionals | 8 | 68967–92185 | 6 |
| 4 | High school certificate | 4 | Clerks | 7 | 46095–68961 | 4 |
| 5 | Middle school certificate | 3 | Skilled worker and Shop and Market Sales Workers | 6 | 27654–46089 | 3 |
| 6 | Primary school certificate | 2 | Skilled Agricultural and Fishery Workers | 5 | 9232–27648 | 2 |
| 7 | Illiterate | 1 | Craft and Related Trade Workers | 4 | ≤9226 | 1 |
| - | - | - | Plant and Machine operators and Assemblers | 3 | - | - |
| - | - | - | Elementary occupation | 2 | - | - |
| - | - | - | Unemployed | 1 | - | - |

| Total score | Social class |
|---|---|
| 26 – 29 | I (upper) |
| 16 – 25 | II (upper middle) |
| 11 – 15 | III (lower middle) |
| 5 – 10 | IV (upper lower) |
| <5 | V (lower) |

Table 6.3: Udai Pareekh's scale.

| Components | Score |
|---|---|
| a. Caste | |
| ➤ Scheduled caste | 1 |
| ➤ Lower caste | 2 |
| ➤ Artisan caste | 3 |
| ➤ Agriculture caste | 4 |
| ➤ Prestige caste | 5 |
| ➤ Dominant caste | 6 |
| b. Occupation | |
| ➤ None | 0 |
| ➤ Laborer | 1 |
| ➤ Caste occupation | 2 |
| ➤ Business | 3 |
| ➤ Independent profession | 4 |
| ➤ Cultivation | 5 |
| ➤ Service | 6 |
| c. Education | |
| ➤ Illiterate | 0 |
| ➤ Can read only | 1 |
| ➤ Can read and write | 2 |
| ➤ Primary | 3 |
| ➤ Middle | 4 |
| ➤ High school | 5 |
| ➤ Graduate and above | 6 |
| d. Land | |
| ➤ No land | 0 |
| ➤ Less than 1 acre | 1 |
| ➤ 1–5 acre | 2 |
| ➤ 5–10 acre | 3 |
| ➤ 10–15 acre | 4 |
| ➤ 15–20 acre | 5 |
| ➤ 20 and above | 6 |
| e. Social participation | |
| ➤ None | 0 |
| ➤ Member of an organization (like Panchayat member, Nambardar, etc. | 1 |
| ➤ Member of more than one organization | 2 |
| ➤ Office holder in such organization | 3 |
| ➤ Wider public leader | 6 |
| f. Family member | |
| ➤ Up to 5 | 2 |
| ➤ Above 5 | 1 |
| g. House | |
| ➤ No house | 1 |
| ➤ Kutcha house | 2 |
| ➤ Mixed house | 3 |
| ➤ Pucca house | 4 |
| ➤ Mansion | 6 |
| h. Farm power | |
| ➤ No draught (buffalo/cows) animal | 1 |
| ➤ 1–2 draught animals | 2 |
| ➤ 3–4 draught animals | 3 |
| ➤ 5–6 draught animals or tractor | 6 |
| i. Material possession | |
| ➤ Bullock cart | 1 |
| ➤ Circle | 1 |
| ➤ Radio | 1 |
| ➤ Chairs | 1 |
| ➤ Improved agriculture equipment | 2 |
| ➤ None | 0 |

**Socioeconomic class**

| Total scores | Grading |
|---|---|
| Score more than 43 (Upper) | I |
| Score 33–42 (Upper middle) | II |
| Score 24–32 (Lower middle) | III |
| Score 13–23 (Upper lower) | IV |
| Score less than 13 (Lower lower) | V |

is defined as a cut-off line of per capita monthly income, below which it is not possible to purchase food as to obtain minimum desirable limit of energy. The calorie standard for a typical individual in rural areas is 2400 kilocalories and 2100 kilocalories in urban areas. BPL families fall below the socioeconomic class V of BG Prasad's classification. Internationally, an income of less than $1.90 per day per head of purchasing power parity is defined as extreme poverty. In India those individuals earning less than ₹32 a day in rural areas and ₹47 in urban areas, are considered to be BPL (Rangarajan Committee 2014). India had 30% of its population (224 million) living below poverty line in 2013 (World Bank Report, 2016). Income-based poverty line is to provide basic food requirements and no other essentials such as health care and education.

***BPL population in India:***
- 22% (Tendulkar Committee 2011–12)
- 29.5% (Rangarajan Committee 2014)

***Social challenges, social problems diagnosis and social interventions are discussed in Chapter 13: Social Medicine.***

## SUGGESTED READING

1. Appelbaum RP, Chambliss WJ. Sociology: A Brief Introduction. New York: Longman;1977.
2. BC Campus. (2017). Society and Social Interaction-Introduction to Sociology [online]. Available from: https://opentextbc.ca/ introduction to sociology/.../chapter4-society-and-social-interactio.
3. BC Campus. Culture: Introduction to Sociology. [online] Available from: https://opentextbc.ca/ introduction to sociology/chapter/chapter3-culture.
4. Bergner M. Measurement of health status. Med Care. 1985;23:696-704.
5. Braveman P, Gruskin S. Defining equity in health. J Epidemiol Community Health, 2003;57(4):254-8.
6. Brennan Ramirez LK, Baker EA, Metzler M. Promoting Health Equity: are source to help communities address social determinants of health. Atlanta: U.S. Department of Health and Human Services/Centers for Disease Control and Prevention; 2008.
7. Brint S. Gemein schaftre visited : acritique and reconstruction of the community concept. Sociological Theory. 2001;19(1):1-23.
8. Commission on Social Determinants of Health (CSDH). (2008). Closing the gap in a generation: Health equity through action on the social determinants of health. Final report of the Commission on Social Determinants of Health. 2008, World Health Organization: Geneva. [online] Available from: http://www.who.int/social_determinants/final_report/csdh_finalreport_2008.pdf.
9. Douglas H. Types of Community. In: AnheierHK, Toepler S, ListR (Eds). International Encyclopedia of Civil Society. New York: Springer; 2010. pp. 539-44.
10. Emanuel EJ, Dubler NN. Preserving the physician care to the urban poor in India. JAMA. 1995;273(4):323–9.
11. Fred NK. Behavioral Research: A Conceptual Approach. New York: Holt, Rinehart & Winston;1979.
12. Government of India. Construction and maintenance of index numbers. [online] Available form:http://www.labourbureau.nic.in.
13. Modugu HR, Kumar M, Kumar A, et al. State and socio-demographic group variation in OOP expenditure, borrowings and Janani Suraksha Yojana (JSY) programme use for birth deliveries in India. BMC Public Health. 2012;12:1048.
14. Moreno JL. Sociometry, Experimental Method, and the Science of Society. Ambler, PA: Beacon House;1951.
15. Prasad BG. Social classification of Indian families. J Indian Med Assoc. 1961;37:250-1.
16. Sharma R. Revised Kuppuswamy's Socioeconomic Status Scale: Explained and updated. Indian Paediatr. 2017;54:867-70
17. Sharma R. The family and family structure classification redefined for the current times. 2013;2(4):306-10.
18. The National Sample Survey Organization (NSSO) (2012). Government of India. Report no. 561.
19. Urban Health and Resource Center. Improving access of health care to the urban poor in India. [online] Available from: http://www. uhrc.in/module-ContentExpress-display-ceid-92.html.
20. US Department of Health and Human Services. Centers for Disease Control and Prevention. (2002). Theories and models frequently used in health promotion. Physical activity evaluation handbook (Appendix 3). [online] Available from: http://www.cdc.gov/nccdphp/dnpa/physical/handbook/pdf/handbook.pdf.

# CHAPTER 7

# Environment and Health

## A. AIR AND HEALTH

*Radha Valaulikar, Muthukumar R*

**CM3.1** Describe the health hazards of air, noise, radiation

Air is an important component of the environment. It has a bearing not only on human health, but also on the country's economy. In this chapter, we are going to look at various air parameters that have a bearing on health and the ways to measure them. We shall try to understand the impact of air on human health and understand the approach to manage the adverse effects.

## VENTILATION

### INTRODUCTION

Indoor air quality in a building is mainly maintained by ventilation. Lack of ventilation leads to numerous problems like air pollution and increased humidity. However, if there is an excess of ventilation, there will be discomfort inside the building due to indoor cooling.

**Effects of inadequate ventilation on health of the community:**
- Higher chances of spread of airborne diseases.
- Poor indoor air quality which leads to fatigue, hypersensitivity, headaches, and sinus congestion.
- *Sick building syndrome*: The symptoms include irritation of eyes, nose, headache, fatigue, and a susceptibility to colds and flu. Symptoms tend to be less severe away from workplace.
- Poor ventilation may lead to dampness in rooms leading to rats and insect infestation.
- Excessive and irritating workplace odors cause discomfort and affect concentration.
- Extremely poor ventilation can even lead to high levels of carbon dioxide, and low levels of oxygen can cause fatigue and affect concentration. This can happen in large gatherings of people in ill ventilated spaces.

### TYPES OF VENTILATION

There are three types of ventilation: (1) Natural, (2) mechanical and (3) hybrid or mixed-mode.

### Natural Ventilation

Natural forces (e.g. winds and thermal buoyancy force due to indoor and outdoor air density differences) drive outdoor air through purpose-built, building envelope openings. Purpose-built openings include windows, doors, and trickle ventilators. **Cross ventilation** is said to exist when doors or windows are on the opposite sides facing each other in the room thus facilitating air exchanges. Cross ventilation is preferable and helps in maintaining adequate ventilation of a room.

### Mechanical Ventilation

Mechanical fans and air conditioners drive mechanical ventilation. These can either be installed directly in windows or walls, or installed in air ducts for supplying air into, or exhausting air from, a room. The types of mechanical ventilation used depend on climate. There are three types of mechanical ventilation systems:

a. *Positive pressure system/plenum ventilation:* The room is in positive pressure and the room air is leaked out through envelope leakages or other openings. Through this system, airborne particles originating in the room (e.g. germs, contaminants) can be filtered out. In medical settings, this can protect hospital staff and patients from infections and disease, e.g. operation theatres, IVF labs.

b. *Negative pressure system*: The room is in negative pressure, and the room air is compensated by "sucking" air from outside. For a room with locally generated pollutants, such as a bathroom, toilet or kitchen, the negative pressure system is often used. In hospital facilities, this can be used to isolate patients with infectious conditions to protect others from risk of exposure.

c. *Balanced mechanical ventilation system:* A system where air supplies and exhausts have been adjusted to introduce fresh outdoor air into the home at the same rate as the stale indoor air is exhausted from the home.

## Hybrid or Mixed-mode Ventilation

Hybrid (mixed-mode) ventilation is a mix of both natural and artificial ventilation. It relies on natural driving forces to provide the desired (design) flow rate. It uses mechanical ventilation when the natural ventilation flow rate is too low. For example, homes, conference rooms.

## NORMS AND STANDARDS FOR ADEQUATE VENTILATION

### House

*Norms for maintaining cross ventilation, adequate floor space and cubic space for a house are elaborated in Table 7A.1.*

It should be noted that windows and doors should be kept open to facilitate ventilation. If they are kept closed permanently, it is functionally equivalent to having no doors or windows.

The living rooms and the kitchen area should be given special attention with respect to ventilation.

*This is further discussed in details in Chapter 7G: Healthy House and Surrounding.*

**Table 7A.1:** Standards of ventilation.

| Parameter | Reference value |
|---|---|
| Air changes required per hour | 2–3 in living room and 4–6 in working room |
| Floor area | • 100 sq ft for single person, 120 sq ft for more than one person<br>• Floor area in living rooms per person should not be less than 50 sq ft |
| Cubic space | 500 cubic ft per capita, preferably 1000 cubic ft |
| Windows | • At least 2 windows per living room with at least one of them should open directly to an open space<br>• Windows should be at a height not more than 3 ft from ground<br>• Window area should be one-fifth of floor area<br>• Doors and windows combined should be two-fifth of the floor area |

### Large Halls or Auditoria

Large halls or auditoria have exhaust fans in walls higher up near the roof which help upper layers of vitiated air to escape.

*Occupational situation:* As per Model rules under the Factories Act 1948, the amount of ventilating openings in a work-room should not be less than 15% of the floor area and location should be able to afford a continued supply of fresh air.

*Hospitals:* Natural ventilation can be applied to areas except where controlled ventilation is required but air supply and removal cannot be controlled. Hence the ideal mode of ventilation for hospitals especially for infection control is mechanical (when resources are available) which in turn has subtypes as shown in **Table 7A.2**.

**Table 7A.2:** Ideal mode of ventilation in hospitals.

| Type of ventilation | Mechanical ventilation | Mechanical negative pressure ventilation | Mechanical HEPA filtered pressure ventilation |
|---|---|---|---|
| Areas where it is required | • Intensive care units<br>• Neonatal unit<br>• Endoscopy units<br>• General wards | • Burns unit<br>• Bronchoscopy unit<br>• TB hospitals<br>• Isolation rooms<br>• Laboratories<br>• Bathroom and toilets | Bone marrow transplant—during early periods of bone marrow suppression |

## SUMMARY

- Inadequate ventilation leads to poor indoor air quality, fatigue, and lack of concentration.
- Three types of ventilation are: natural, mechanical and hybrid or mixed. The three types of mechanical ventilation systems are positive pressure ventilation, negative pressure ventilation and *Balanced mechanical ventilation systems*.
- Air changes required per hour in living room is 2–3 and in working room is 4–6.
- Ideal floor area is 100 sq ft for single person.
- Cubic space recommended is 500 cubic feet per capita.

## SUGGESTED READING

1. Atkinson J, Chartier Y, Pessoa-Silva CL, et al. (2009). Natural ventilation for infection control in health-care settings. [Online] WHO Publication/Guidelines. Geneva: World Health Organization; 2009 Available from http://www.who.int/water_sanitation_health/publications/natural_ventilation/en/.
2. Industrial ventilation. A manual of Recommended Practice. AJPH. 1998.
3. Model Building Bye-Laws 2016. [Internet] Town and Country Planning Organisation Ministry of Urban Development. Available from: http://www.indiaenvironmentportal.org.in/files/file/ MODEL%20BUILDING%20BYE%20LAWS-2016.pdf.
4. National Building Code of India 2016 (Volume 1). [Internet] Bureau of Indian Standards. Available from: https://ia800601.us.archive. org/13/items/nationalbuilding01/in.gov.nbc.2016.vol1.digital.pdf.
5. National Building Code of India 2016 (Volume 2). [Internet] Bureau of Indian Standards. Available from: https://ia800601.us.archive. org/11/items/nationalbuilding02/in.gov.nbc.2016.vol2.digital.pdf.

---

# AIR PRESSURE AND HEALTH

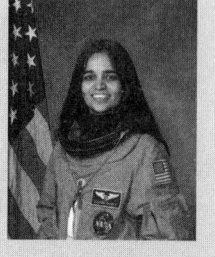

A bulky pressure suit painted orange is an essential in any astronaut's picture. It is a pressure shell that protects their body during lift off and landing. Why is such a suit needed? What changes occur as we ascend up and descend down a high altitude? What are the risks faced by mountaineers as they ascend up? This section will help you understand various implications of air pressure on health.

## INTRODUCTION

Millions of people today travel to high altitude areas for recreation or adventure sports whereas several others are inducted to high altitude areas for occupational pursuits such as the military and border roads. The terrestrial environment at high altitudes is unconducive for health of unacclimatized travelers due to several stressors that are characteristic of such areas. In this chapter, we will discuss the effects of altitude and pressure on health and their prevention.

# EFFECTS OF ATMOSPHERIC PRESSURE ON HEALTH

## High Altitude

The illnesses that affect unacclimatized individuals after a recent ascent to high altitude are collectively called as high-altitude illnesses. At higher altitudes, partial pressure of oxygen is decreased which leads to increased respiration rate, increase in concentration of hemoglobin and increased cardiac output. The physiological definition of high altitude is a height of over 2,700 m (9,000 ft) above sea level because the clinical symptoms and signs of hypoxia become recognizable at an alveolar partial pressure of oxygen ($P_aO_2$) level as low as 60 mm Hg found at that height. **(Box 7A.1)**. This can cause several pathological presentations, including high altitude pulmonary edema, high altitude cerebral edema, and the milder, but much more common, acute mountain sickness (also referred to as altitude illness or altitude sickness). High altitude pulmonary edema and high-altitude cerebral edema are both life-threatening emergencies requiring immediate treatment, with a descent to lower altitude (or higher-pressure artificial environment) as quickly as can be safely arranged and executed. The hallmark of acute mountain sickness is a headache, with other symptoms including nausea, vomiting, loss of appetite, fatigue/malaise (particularly at rest), sleep disturbance, and dizziness/lightheadedness. Acute mountain sickness symptoms can begin after only a few hours and typically present the first day at a given altitude, resolving after one to three days, even without treatment, as the body adjusts physiologically (acclimates) to the lower oxygen levels.

**Risk groups for high altitude illnesses:** Persons who have recently arrived at a high-altitude location from a visit to a low-lying area such as for recreation, occupation, pilgrimage and sports.

---

**Box 7A.1: Stressors at high altitude (HA).**

**Hypobaric hypoxia:** Barometric pressure reduces with altitude thereby causing a reduction in the partial pressure of oxygen in ambient, inspired, and alveolar air.
**Low environmental temperature:** The environmental temperature falls by 1°C per 150 m gain in altitude. High wind velocity at HA adds to the low temperature due to a "wind chill factor".
**Low absolute humidity in the atmosphere:** This increases the insensible water loss from the body and predisposes to dehydration.

---

## Low Altitude

As one descends below the sea level, there occurs increase in the barometric pressure. With increase in the pressure, the gases in the air gets dissolved in blood and tissues. The most commonly encountered hyperbaric situation is hyperbaric oxygen and the effects and complications of high oxygen concentrations are tracheobronchitis, acute lung injury, hypertension and seizures. Hyperbaric nitrogen toxicity manifests as muscular tremors, loss of coordination, memory deficits, confusion and psychosis. The effects of increased pressure are most commonly observed by underwater divers, miners and caisson workers.

# MEASUREMENT OF ATMOSPHERIC PRESSURE

- A measurement of 760 mm of mercury (Hg), also called 1 atmosphere of pressure is the atmospheric pressure at sea level. Atmospheric pressure is inversely proportional to altitude, for every 33 ft depth below sea level the pressure increases by one atmosphere.
- The instrument used to measure atmospheric pressure is called barometer.

## Types of Barometers

- Of various types of barometers, the mercury barometer is more accurate than aneroid barometer.
- The aneroid barometer is more useful in the field to measure atmospheric pressure fluctuations, but requires constant calibration and recalibration with a mercury barometer to prevent erroneous measurements.
- The Indian Meteorological Department uses the Kew-Pattern station barometer. This barometer gives a continuous measurement of the atmospheric pressure over a 24 hour period, which is called as the barograph.
- There are also micro-barographs that give a more accurate reading by recording the minimal fluctuations in atmospheric pressure.

---

**Application of the knowledge of air pressure in health care**
- Identifying high-risk groups that may experience health effects due to air pressure, e.g. high altitude climbers, space shuttles
- Providing and designing personal protective equipment to high-risk groups
- Allowing time for "acclimatization" during scaling up and scaling down in different air pressure zones.

---

# SUGGESTED READING

1. Basnyat B, Murdoch DR. High altitude illness. Lancet. 2003;361:1967-74.
2. Gabry AL, Ledoux X, Mozzi CM, et al. High altitude pulmonary oedema at moderate altitude (below 2400m, 7870 ft): a series of 52 patients. Chest. 2003;123:49-53.
3. Government of India. Instructions to observers at the surface observations. Part 1. Indian Meteorological Department. Manager of Publications. New Delhi. 1954.

# HUMIDITY

## INTRODUCTION

A heat wave is a period where there is unusually hot weather, sometimes with high humidity. One such calamity happened in India in May 2015. There were 2,500 deaths reported in various parts of India over a month.

Humidity is the main driving force behind most of the weather aspects like rains, storm and even hurricane. It is difficult to forecast the weather exactly without knowing the humidity in the atmospheric layers. The feeling of comfort inside the closed rooms is mainly due to decreased humidity and that is why it is an important component controlled by an Air conditioner other than temperature.

The highest ever recorded temperature in the world so far is 134°F at Death valley, California. With the on-going global warming, it is projected that by latter part of this century, most parts of India will reach an alarming temperature of 170 °F. Now we will see in detail how this humidity is important to health and the different ways it is measured.

## TERMINOLOGIES

***Humidity***: Atmospheric humidity or the moisture content of air is contributed from large water bodies. Moisture is also added to air by living animals and plants due to their constant discharge of water vapor from the lungs or leaves.

***Absolute humidity:*** It is the amount of water vapor per unit weight or volume of air expressed as grams per liter or grams per cubic meter ($g/m^3$), and is measured by absorption hygrometers.

***Relative humidity:*** It describes the moisture content of air at any given temperature as a percentage of the maximum possible moisture content, i.e. the ratio of amount of water vapor actually present in the air to the amount that would be present where the air is saturated with moisture expressed as a percentage out of 100.

$$RH = \frac{\text{Water vapor content}}{\text{Water vapor capacity}}$$

***Dew point:*** The dew point is the temperature the air needs to be cooled to (at constant pressure) in order to achieve a relative humidity (RH) of 100%. It is a better indicator of comfort than just humidity.

## HUMIDITY AND HEALTH

Both the low **(Table 7A.3)** and high humidity **(Table 7A.4)** have effects on our health since the primary mechanism by which human body temperature is regulated is by evaporative cooling. Normal relative humidity range is 40–50%.

### Humidifier

Humidifier adds moisture to the air to prevent dryness in our body.

***Types of humidifier:*** Central humidifiers, evaporators, impeller humidifiers, steam vaporizers, and ultrasonic humidifiers.

**Table 7A.3:** Effect of low humidity.

| Organ | Effect of low humidity | Reason |
|---|---|---|
| Eyes | Irritation | Rapid evaporation of tears removes protective barrier |
| Nasal passage | Dry, painful sinuses | Rapid evaporation of moisture causes mucus membrane to dry and leads to painful sinuses and also pathway for pathogens to bloodstream. This explains why flu is so prevalent during the fall and winter |
| Throat | Sore throat | |
| Skin | Dry, scaly and itchy | Reduced moisture leads to small cracks in skin |

**Table 7A.4:** Categories of heat index and effects of high humidity

| Category | Classification | Heat Index/ Apparent temperature | Heat syndrome |
|---|---|---|---|
| I | Extremely hot | 130°F or higher (54°C or Higher) | Heatstroke or sunstroke *imminent* |
| II | Very hot | 105–130°F (41–54°C) | Sunstroke, heat cramps, or heat exhaustion *likely*, heatstroke possible with long exposure and physical activity |
| III | Hot | 90–105°F (32–41°C) | Sunstroke, heat cramps, and heat exhaustion *possible* with prolonged exposure and physical activity |
| IV | Very warm | 80°F–90°F (27°C–32°C) | Fatigue *possible* with prolonged exposure and physical activity |

### Heat Index or Humidex

Heat index (HI) combines "relative humidity" and "air temperature" to find an "apparent temperature"—what the air temperature "feels like" to the average person for various combinations of air temperature and relative humidity. It is categorized as in **Table 7A.4**.

## MEASURING HUMIDITY

The common instruments that obtain humidity are the psychrometer and hygrometer.

### Which Instrument to Choose? Psychrometer or Hygrometer?

This depends on the needs. If accuracy is the most important thing (e.g. meteorologists) then Psychrometer is required but for convenience and faster processing, hygrometer can be used.

***Mason's hygrometer:*** This is used in most of the meteorological stations. It has a Stevenson's screen with a dry bulb thermometer and a wet bulb thermometer placed adjacent to each other **(Fig. 7A.1)**. The ambient air temperature is measured by the dry bulb thermometer, and the wet bulb thermometer measures air temperature under the effect of evaporation of water from a muslin cloth.

In dry conditions, rate of evaporation is faster and the wet bulb thermometer would show a higher reading. Equal readings

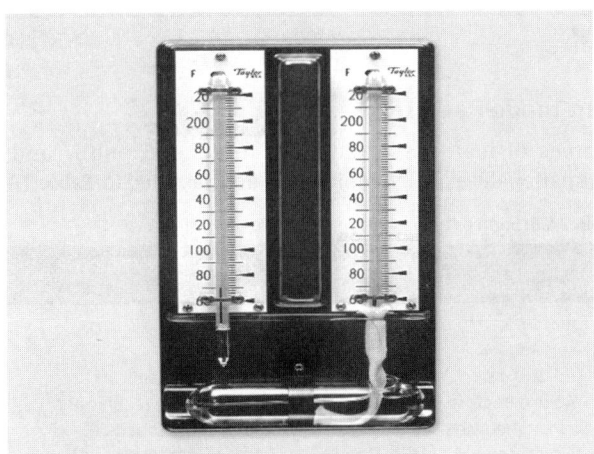

Fig. 7A.1: Mason's hygrometer.
Source: https://www.sciencesource.com/archive/Mason-s-Hygrometer-SS2586031.html.

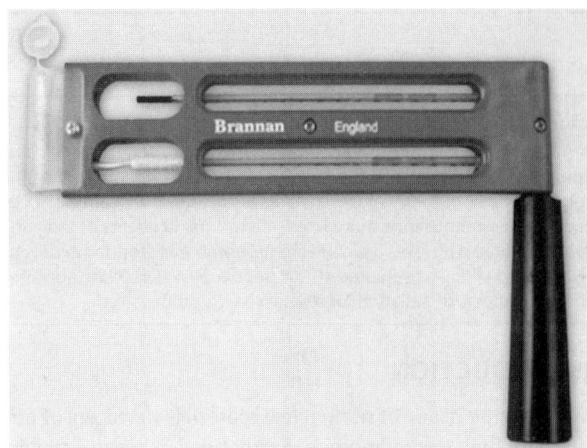

Fig. 7A.2: Sling psychrometer.
Source: https://www.sciencesource.com/archive/Mason-s-Hygrometer-SS2586031.html)

of wet and dry bulb thermometers can be found in a saturated atmosphere. Higher the level of atmospheric moisture, higher is the difference between the readings of wet and dry bulb thermometers, which is called as wet bulb depressions.

The relative humidity and dew point can be estimated by looking into the hygrometric tables with the readings taken from Stevenson's screen.

It must be noted that the air in the immediate surrounding of the wet bulb thermometer is more humid and it will, therefore, give higher-than-actual readings. This is corrected by setting the air around the wet bulb thermometer in motion, by rotating the two thermometers. This is the principle behind the sling psychrometer described below.

***Sling psychrometer:*** Also known as the whirling psychrometer, this instrument has a metal strip on which the dry and wet bulb thermometers are fixed. This metal strip is attached to a wooden frame with a handle on one side that serves as a pivot **(Fig. 7A.2)**. On this pivot, the frame rotates and thus the metal strip spins in the air. A small cylindrical container has water at room temperature which moistens a cotton wick and keeps the bulb of one thermometer wet.

The user goes outside in the sun, with his/her back against the sun, holds the instrument by the handle with dominant hand and whirls it at a rate of 2 to 3 revolutions per second, making a total of 120 to 180 revolutions per minute. The whirling is repeated till two same wet bulb readings are obtained. The readings of dry and wet bulb thermometers are now recorded. These two readings are read against the standard charts for measurement of relative humidity.

The ***Assman's psychrometer*** employs a modified technique by using a motor to whirl the thermometers and driving in air using a clockwork fan. This improves the accuracy of measurement.

***Electrical hygrometer*** consists of a flat plate coated with a film of carbon. An electric current is sent across the plate. As water vapor is absorbed, the electrical resistance of the carbon coating changes. These changes are translated into relative humidity.

This instrument is commonly used in the Radiosonde (attached to helium or hydrogen balloon), which gathers atmospheric data at various levels above the earth.

> **Application of knowledge of humidity in health care**
> Low relative humidity can pose various problems in health care setting especially in an operating theater, it will make the air to draw moisture from all available sources in the room, in fact even from any body tissue exposed during surgery. This leads to scab formation from coagulated blood during surgery. This along with the events mentioned in **Tables 7A.3 and 7A.4** can be prevented by applying knowledge about humidity.

## THERMAL COMFORT

Thermal comfort is a subjective feeling which is dependent on factors other than the temperature. Humidity and air movement too can play a role in it. Air movement is also called as the cooling power of air. It is measured by an instrument called Kata thermometer. An index which considers these three factors, i.e. temperature, humidity, and air movement is called 'Effective temperature'. Further when 'radiant' heat is considered in addition to these three, the index generated is 'Corrected Effective Temperature'. ***This concept is further explained in detail in Chapter 7D: Temperature and Health.***

## SUMMARY

- **Absolute humidity** is the amount of water vapor per unit weight or volume of air expressed in $g/m^3$.
- **Relative humidity** describes the moisture content of air at any given temperature as a percentage of the maximum possible moisture content.
- **Dew point** is the temperature at which the excessive moisture precipitates if the air is cooled.
- Air temperature is inversely proportional to relative humidity (at constant water vapor content).
- **Heat index (HI) or humidex** combines 'air temperature' with 'relative humidity' to determine an **apparent temperature**.
- Humidity can be measured by **psychrometer or hygrometer.**

## SUGGESTED READING

1. Ahrens CD. Meteorology Today, 8th edition. Belmont, CA: Thomson/Brooks/Cole; 2007.
2. India Meteorological Department—Meteorological data.
3. Indian Institute of Tropical Meteorology publications.

# RADIATION

> **Historical fact**
> On August 6, 1945, during World War II, America dropped world's first deployed atomic bomb over the Japanese city of Hiroshima. The resulting explosion wiped out 90% of the city and resulted in the death of 80,000 people; several thousands more later suffered the ill effects of radiation exposure. Three days later, a second atomic bomb was dropped in the city of Nagasaki, killing an estimated 40,000 people. Survivors of the bombing suffered ill effects of radiation for several years after the attack.

## INTRODUCTION

Ever increasing usage of radioactive materials in variety of fields comes with high cost of increased radiation accidents especially when the radiation protection guidelines are not followed properly. In March 2010, a Gamma unit containing Cobalt 60 pencils was planned to be disposed after non-usage since 1985 in Delhi. The unit's residual radioactivity was miscalculated and sold to scrap dealers in Mayapuri scrap market in Delhi. The cobalt pencils along with other scrap were kept in a crowded shop in the market and remained as continuous source of radiation exposure without the workers' knowledge. Eventually, it lead to acute radiation syndrome in four people and the one who received the highest dose died due to acute respiratory distress syndrome and multi-organ failure.

Many minor radiation exposure incidents have happened in India because of noncompliance to radiation protection measures. In this chapter we will see the different sources and effects of radiation followed by the protective measures.

## SOURCES OF RADIATION EXPOSURE

Broadly sources can be classified as: Natural background radiation (82%) and man-made radiation (18%).

### Natural Background Radiation

It comes from three sources: Cosmic radiation, terrestrial radiation, and internal radiation.

#### Cosmic Radiation

All living things present on earth are continuously exposed to radiation from space. Charged particles from the sun and stars meet with the atmosphere and magnetic field around the earth to generate a burst of radiation, especially beta and gamma radiation.

#### Terrestrial Radiation

Radioactive material is also present in the water, soil and vegetation. Minute levels of thorium, uranium and their decay products are there everywhere. Few of these are consumed with food and water, while others, like radon, are inhaled.

#### Internal Radiation

Apart from the above two natural sources, we also have radioactive carbon-14, potassium-40, lead-210, and other isotopes in our body from birth.

### Man-made Radiation

Sources of man-made radiation in general public and in occupationally exposed individuals are classified in **Table 7A.5**.

**Table 7A.5:** Sources of man-made radiation.

| Among general public | Among occupationally exposed individuals |
|---|---|
| • Tobacco<br>• Televisions<br>• Medical X-rays<br>• Smoke detectors<br>• Nuclear medicine<br>• Major isotopes: I-131, Tc-99m, Co-60, Ir-192, Cs-137 | • Radiography<br>• X-ray technicians<br>• Nuclear power plant<br>• Nuclear medicine technicians<br>• Major isotopes: Cobalt-60, cesium-137, americium-241 |

## TYPES OF RADIATION

*Ionizing radiation*: Electromagnetic (X-ray, gamma rays) and corpuscular (alpha-particles, beta-particles).

*Nonionizing radiation:* Ultraviolet radiation, visible light, infrared radiation, microwave radiation and radiofrequency radiation.

- *In order of penetrating power:* Nonionizing radiation < gamma < X-ray < beta < alpha
- *In order of wavelength:* nonionizing radiation > gamma > X-ray > beta > alpha

The annual limit of radiation is summed up in **Table 7A.6**.

**Table 7A.6:** Annual limit of radiation.

| Organ | Annual limit of radiation |
|---|---|
| Whole body (sum of external and internal dose) | 5 rems |
| Extremity<br>Skin of whole body<br>Maximum exposed organ (sum of external and internal dose) | 50 rems |
| Lens of the eye | 15 rems |

## UNITS OF RADIATION

The units of radiation are given in **Table 7A.7** with definition.

**Table 7A.7:** Units of radiation.

| Previously used units | Corresponding newer International System of Units (SI) | How they are related? |
|---|---|---|
| Curie | Becquerel | 1 Curie = $3.7 \times 10^{10}$ disintegrations/second<br>1 Becquerel = 1 disintegration/second<br>1 Becquerel = $2.7 \times 10^{-11}$ Curie |
| Roentgen | Coulomb per kg | 1 Roentgen = $2.58 \times 10^{-4}$ Coulomb/kg |
| RAD | Gray | 1 RAD = 0.01 Gray<br>1 Gray = 100 RADs |
| REM | Sievert | 1 REM = 0.01 Sievert<br>1 Sievert = 100 REM |

***Becquerel:*** The activity of a radioactive material is the number of nuclear disintegration per unit of time. The unit of activity is becquerel and formerly it was curie.

***Roentgen:*** It is the unit of exposure. One roentgen is that amount of X-ray or gamma radiation that will deposit enough energy to strip about two billion electrons from their orbits (called one electrostatic unit) in 1 mL of dry air. This is now replaced by the SI unit Coulomb per kg.

***RAD (Radiation absorbed dose):*** RAD is a measure of the absorbed dose per gram of body tissue or material. ***Gray*** is the SI unit of absorbed dose. 1 Gray is equal to 1 Joule of energy deposited in one kilogram of matter.

***REM:*** Term for dose equivalence and equals the biological damage that would be caused by 1 RAD of dose. It is the product of the absorbed dose and the modifying factors. ***Sievert*** is the SI unit of dose equivalent. In the same way as converting from the absorbed dose (RAD) to the dose equivalent (REM) involved the use of quality factors, the conversion of gray to sievert uses quality factors.

The REM is numerically equal to the dose in RADs multiplied by a quality factor, which accounts for the difference in the amount of biological damage caused by the different types of radiation. That is, the damage from 1 RAD deposited by beta-radiation is less than that caused by 1 RAD of alpha-radiation.

## EFFECTS OF RADIATION ON HEALTH

When human body is exposed to the radiation it causes the change in DNA of cell and tissue of human and all these effect on body are called biological effect of radiation. Biological effects are of two types:
1. Somatic: Deterministic and stochastic effect
2. Hereditary effects

### Somatic Effect

#### *Deterministic Effects of Radiation*

Deterministic effects are also called non-stochastic effect. These effects depend on time of exposure, doses, type of radiation. It has a threshold of doses below which the effect does not occur. The threshold may be varied from person to person. Deterministic effects are those responses which increase in severity with increased dose.

Deterministic effect includes **(Table 7A.8)**.
- Acute radiation sickness
- Chronic radiation sickness
- Systemic-involving various organs of the body.

#### *Stochastic Effect*

Stochastic effect is those effect which occur when a person receives a high dose of radiation. These effects have an increase probability of occurrence with increased dose. There is no threshold dose below which is certain that a stochastic effect cannot occur. Severity does not depend on magnitude of absorbed doses; these effects occur by chance usually without any threshold level of dose.

Table 7A.8: Deterministic effects of radiation.

| System | Effects |
|---|---|
| Hematopoietic system | Low platelets, granulocytes |
| Gastrointestinal system | Nausea, vomiting, diarrhea |
| Lung | Radiation pneumonitis |
| Thyroid | Acute radiation thyroiditis, hypothyroidism |
| Skin | Erythema, desquamation |
| Eye | Cataract |
| Gonads | Sterility |
| Embryo | Embryonal death, congenital malformation |
| Central nervous system | Death |
| Effects of acute exposure | Nausea, vomiting, headache, pyrexia, diarrhea |
| Effects of chronic exposure | Influenza type syndrome, fever, diarrhea, vomiting |

**Somatic stochastic effect:** These effects of radiation limited to expose individual and they are distinguished from genetic effect. Long term exposure of radiation in individuals may induce cancer like Ca. breast, Ca. thyroid, leukemia, etc.

### Hereditary Effect

The radiation damages the genetic material in reproductive cell and by the result of which these effects are transmitted from generation to generation. Radiation induced material to an individual gene and DNA that can contribute to the birth of defective descendants like Color blindness, Down's syndrome.

### *Exposure of the Gonads and the Blood-forming Organs*

The maximum permissible total dose accumulated in the gonads and the blood forming organs at any age over 18 years is:

$$D = 5(N - 18)$$

where, D is tissue dose in REMs and N is age in years **(Table 7A.9)**.

Table 7A.9: Maximum permissible dose.

| Organs | Maximum permissible dose (in REMs) during any period of 13 consecutive weeks |
|---|---|
| Gonads and the blood-forming organs | 3 |
| Internal organs other than the thyroid, the gonads and the blood-forming organs | 4 |
| Skin, thyroid and bone | 8 |
| Hands and forearms, feet and ankles | 20 |

## PROTECTION AGAINST RADIATION EXPOSURE

### Protection against External Infrared Radiation

It works on **"the principle of time, distance and shielding"**: Keeping the exposure as short as possible, keep as far as possible and wherever possible place shielding between the source and employee.

**Lead aprons:** Lead aprons should contain 0.5-mm-thick lead lining. The protective fabric in the apron is made from lead-

**Table 7A.10:** Do's and Dont's during a radiation emergency.

| Do's | Dont's |
|---|---|
| 1. Go indoors. Stay inside | 1. Do not panic |
| 2. Switch on the radio/television and look out for public announcements from your local authority | 2. Do not believe in rumors. Only rely on authentic sources of information. |
| 3. Close doors/windows | 3. Do not stay outside/or go outside |
| 4. Cover all the consumables and take only such covered items | 4. Avoid taking water from open wells/ponds; avoid consumption of exposed crops and vegetables |
| 5. Provide cooperation to local authorities | 5. Do not ignore any orders of the district or civil defense authorities |
| 6. Discuss on radiation safety among children and family members, to reduce their fear of radiation | |

infused rubber as lead is the most efficient material for stopping X-ray and gamma radiation. They can attenuate over 90% of 80 kVp radiation.

### Protection against External Contamination

Use of protective clothing prevents contamination of skin. Exposure time also needs to be limited.

### Protection against Internal Irradiation

Use of fume cupboards or glove boxes as containment may help in protection.

### Application of Knowledge of Radiation in Health Care

The knowledge of radiation and its effects on health can be useful in prevention of radiation hazard in following ways:
- Providing shielding and training on radiation protection for potentially exposed workers **(Table 7A.10)**
- Evaluation of potentially exposed workplaces like radiology department in health care setting
- Regulating the safety measures:
  – To display appropriate signs
  – To check the correct use of shielding
  – To measure dose rate behind shielding
  – To calculate shielding thicknesses (Lead apron should be at least 0.5 mm thick)
  – To write a protocol describing any measures to take in case of incident.

## SUMMARY

- Natural or background radiation arises from three sources: cosmic, terrestrial and internal radiation.
- Sources of man-made radiation can result in radiation exposures in general public as well as in those exposed by virtue of their occupation.
- The two types of radiation are ionizing radiation (X-ray, gamma rays, alpha particles and beta-particles) and nonionizing radiation (UV, visible light, IR radiation, microwave and radiofrequency radiation).
- Effects of radiation can be classified into somatic (deterministic and stochastic) effects and hereditary effects.
- Protection against external irradiation works on the principle of time, distance and shielding.

## SUGGESTED READING

1. Baxter PJ, Aw TC, Cockcroft A, et al. Hunter's diseases of occupations. London: CRC Press; 2010.
2. Dose standards and methods for protection against radiation and contamination [Internet] US Nuclear Regulatory Commission Technical Training Center. Available from: https://www.nrc.gov/reading-rm/basic-ref/students/for-educators/08.pdf.
3. Do's and Dont's. Nuclear-radiological emergency. [Internet] National Disaster Management Authority. Available from: https://ndma.gov.in/en/nuclear-do-s-dont-s
4. ICRP publication 103. 2007 recommendations.
5. International Commission on Radiological Protection (1958). Recommendations of the International Commission on Radiological Protection. [online] Available from http://journals.sagepub.com/doi/pdf/10.1016/S0074-27402880016-X.
6. Nuclear Recycle Group. Radioactive waste management at a glance. Mumbai: Bhabha Atomic Research Center; 2012.

# AIR POLLUTION

> **Historical fact**
> The city of London witnessed "a dark period" from 5 to 9 November 1952 as one of the worst events of air pollution in global history hit the city. This was the Great Smog of London, which combined fog with smoke, which together with temperature inversion resulted in dense layer of "smog" in the city. It not only disrupted traffic, hampered visibility and marred the flora and fauna but also caused health effects on the population and affected the economy. Air pollution resulting from industrial revolution took its toll on one and all in the city.

## INTRODUCTION

Air pollution refers to presence of molecules of chemical or biological origin in the air in levels that pose a risk to health and environment **(Fig. 7A.3)**.

Air pollution—both indoor and outdoor—is widely recognized as a risk factor for various diseases in all age groups, ranging from respiratory diseases to cancers, from cardiovascular diseases to adverse pregnancy outcomes. It is also shown to reduce the average lifespan thus contributing to DALYs. Several countries, including India, are making efforts to contain the level of air pollutants through various policy and public health measures. As students of Community Medicine, understanding the role of air pollution in health is of great importance. How does air pollution affect human health? How can we, as community health professionals, interpret measurements of air pollution? What is the role of air pollution in managing disease and promoting health? These are some of the critical questions that are addressed in this section.

# Chapter 7: Environment and Health

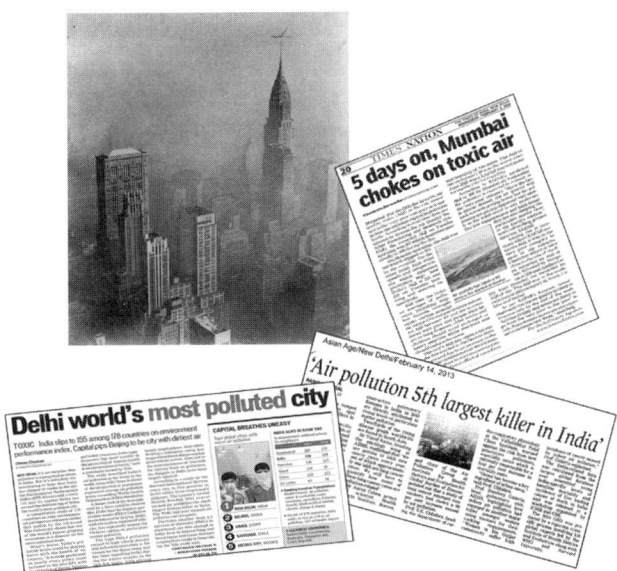

Fig. 7A.3: Air pollution, a global concern

## PROBLEM STATEMENT (WHO FACT-SHEETS FOR AMBIENT AND HOUSEHOLD AIR QUALITY AND HEALTH, 2022)

- In 2019, 99% of world population lived in places where guidelines of air quality as prescribed by WHO were not met.
- There were 4.2 million premature deaths worldwide in 2019 due to outdoor air pollution in urban and rural areas combined, around 89% of which were in South East Asia and Western Pacific regions. The combined effects of ambient air pollution and household air pollution are associated with 6.7 million premature deaths annually.
- India is home to 13 of the 20 most polluted cities in the world as documented by WHO.
- The 2020 State of Global Air Report showed that between 2010–2019, the exposure to outdoor air pollution and related deaths in India has significantly increased while with major investments in clean energy for cooking, household air pollution has shown decline.
- Indoor smoke poses serious risk for around 3 billion people who use biomass, kerosene fuels, and coal as their domestic fuels.

## AIR POLLUTANTS AND THEIR SOURCES

The chemicals or compounds that lower the quality of air are referred to as air pollutants.

These may be solid (e.g. particulate matter) or gaseous (e.g. sulfur dioxide, carbon monoxide).

A *primary pollutant* is an air pollutant which is directly emitted into the air from a source.
- The source can be natural or anthropogenic (influenced by man). Natural sources include volcanic eruptions, windblown dust, sandstorms, etc. Anthropogenic sources include industrial processes, vehicular emissions, burning of fossil fuels, passive smoking.
- Examples of primary pollutants include:
  - Sulfur dioxide ($SO_2$) from processing of mineral ores containing sulfur
  - Nitrogen oxide (NO) from diesel engines
  - Carbon monoxide (CO) from burning of biomass fuels
  - Particulate matter originating from soil dust or automobile exhausts, and
  - Volatile organic compounds (VOCs) from paints and coatings, chlorofluorocarbons from refrigerators and cleaning products, fossil fuel combustion and tobacco products.

A *secondary pollutant* is an air pollutant which is formed within the air by physical or chemical interaction of other compounds or primary pollutants.

Examples include ozone, nitrogen dioxide, sulfur trioxide, and secondary particulate matter.

> **Importance in community health**
> Levels of primary pollutants can be controlled to a great extent by controlling their emissions from respective sources or by reducing the sources. Control of levels of secondary pollutants requires understanding and interrupting of chemical and physical reactions that lead to their formation.

### Smog

Smog is a combination of *smoke + fog*. The term was first used to describe discoloration of air as a result of coal burning during the industrial revolution. However, in modern context it refers to a complex combination of primary and secondary air pollutants that cause the air to turn yellow or brown.

> **Importance in community health**
> Smog is more common around urban areas and is associated with respiratory illnesses and poor visibility.

*Temperature inversion:* Generally, warm air is found closer to earth's surface and it becomes cooler as we go upwards in the atmosphere. In a phenomenon known as 'temperature inversion', due to the topographic and atmospheric factors, a layer of warm air traps cool air near the Earth's surface. This inversion of the usual pattern keeps the smog and other pollutants close to earth's surface.

### Acid Rain

Air pollutants like $SO_2$ and NO cause pH changes in the atmosphere, causing water molecules to be formed that are of pH less than the normal. This phenomenon is called acid rain. Acid rain has destructive effect on crops, buildings, flora and fauna.

## TYPES OF AIR POLLUTION

Air pollution can be broadly classified as outdoor air pollution and indoor air pollution.

### Sources of Outdoor Air Pollution (Flowchart 7A.1)

**High-risk groups:** As a result of exposure to high concentration of air pollutants, traffic police, filling station workers, construction workers, pedestrians.

Flowchart 7A.1: Sources of outdoor air pollution.

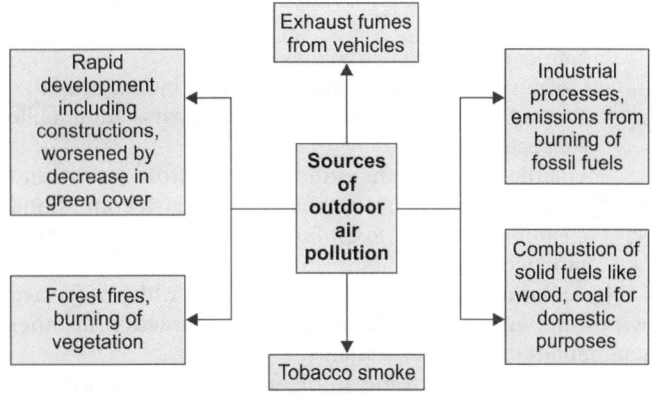

## Sources of Indoor Air Pollution

The sources of indoor air pollutants are shown in **Flowchart 7A.2**. Poor air conditioning systems and improper ventilation worsens indoor pollution.

- In many poor households in developing countries, the domestic fuel used is wood and fodder. The houses are small and poorly constructed and the kitchens lack a smoke vent or a chimney. This causes air pollutants such as carbon monoxide, nitrogen dioxide and suspended particles to be released in large quantities and be concentrated in a small, enclosed area.

Flowchart 7A.2: Sources of indoor air pollution.

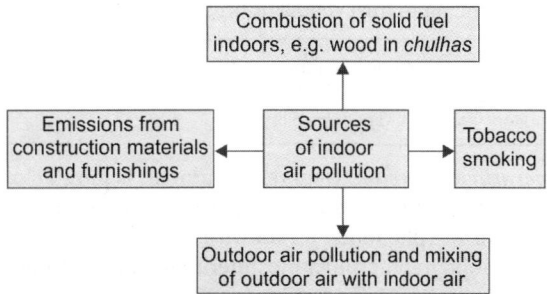

- Dust emissions from lead-based paints and asbestos and radon released from building materials have also been incriminated in indoor air pollution.
- Radon is a colorless and an odorless gas that is emitted from natural breakdown of uranium in soil and rock. Because of its radioactive nature, this indoor air pollutant is incriminated in cancers.

**High-risk groups:** Women and children under the age of 5 years constitute high-risk groups as they spend more time near the site of burning of solid fuel in kitchen.

## HEALTH EFFECTS OF AIR POLLUTION

The health effects of air pollution can be classified as:
- Effects on respiratory system
- Effects on cardiovascular system
- Effects on pregnancy and its outcomes
- Carcinogenic effects
- Other effects.

Let us list each of these briefly (Flowcharts 7A.3 to 7A.6).

Flowchart 7A.3: Effects of air pollution on respiratory system.

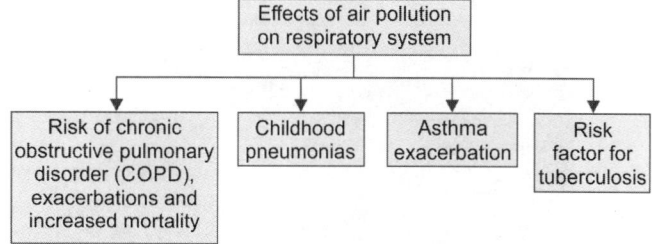

Flowchart 7A.4: Effects of air pollution on cardiovascular system.

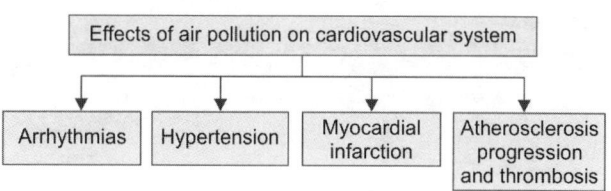

Flowchart 7A.5: Effects of air pollution on pregnancy and its outcomes.

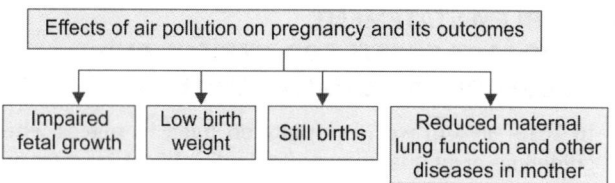

Flowchart 7A.6: Carcinogenic effects of air pollution.

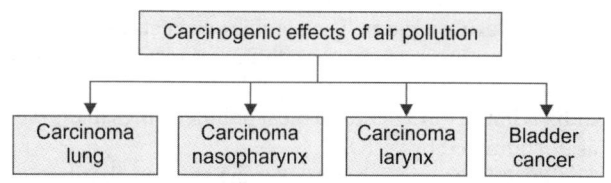

## Effects on Respiratory System

- Ultrafine particles (diameters < 100 nm) are known to inhibit phagocytosis in the lungs.
- Ultrafine and transition metal compounds of $PM_{10}$ (particulate matter 10 micrometers or less in diameter) increase the oxidative stress in lungs by generating free radicals.
- Air pollutants cause ciliostasis and destroy alveolar macrophages thereby make the airways prone to invasion by organisms.
- Children's lungs are more vulnerable to polluted air as the epithelial lining of the respiratory tract is more permeable and airways are also smaller than adult airways.
- As children breathe twice as fast as adults, they inhale more air per unit of body weight in comparison to adults.

## Effects on Cardiovascular System

- $PM_{2.5}$ (particulate matter 2.5 micrometers or less in diameter) hampers the autonomic nerve reflexes, thus inducing cardiac automaticity, conduction and repolarization, causing arrhythmias.

- Inflammation in the lungs also results in systemic inflammation, resulting in increased thrombosis which increases the risk of myocardial infarction. Endothelial dysfunction may cause plaque to rupture from already atherosclerosed vessels.
- Some air pollutants increase vascular tone, thereby causing or worsening hypertension.

### Effects on Pregnancy and its Outcomes

- Exposure to cooking smoke and tobacco smoke (both active and passive) increase blood levels of carbon monoxide (CO) and particulate matter in mother's blood.
- This results in reduced oxygen delivery to placenta, causing harmful effects on the fetus.
- Reduced maternal lung function and other lung diseases in the mother also affects fetal development.

### Carcinogenic Effects

- Among all pollutants, polycyclic aromatic hydrocarbons (PAH) and Benzo-a-pyrene include some of the most dangerous carcinogens that have mutagenic potential among outdoor air pollutants.
- Among indoor air pollutants, environmental tobacco smoke (ETS) and radon are the major sources of cancer risk.
- Levels of the carcinogenic pollutant in air are directly proportional to their mutagenic potency. Also, occupational exposure, as described earlier, predisposes individuals to the risk of cancer from air pollutants.

### Other Effects of Air Pollution

In addition to direct health effects on the body, air pollution also has several indirect effects.

These include:
- Reduction in life expectancy
- School absenteeism
- Disruption in physical and cognitive development in children
- Sick workforce
- Climate change
- Poor visibility from smog leading to road traffic accidents and crimes
- Reduction in the economic value of crops, expensive cleaning of cultural heritage, reduces plant biodiversity and affects other ecosystem services, such as clean water, recreational activities, etc.

## MEASURING AIR POLLUTION: NATIONAL AIR QUALITY INDEX

### Air Quality Index

Levels of air pollution in a region reflect not only potential risks to health status of citizens but also mitigation efforts of the country. Citizens need to be well-informed about both these. Keeping this in mind, the Central Pollution Control Board (Ministry of Environment, Forests and Climate Change), Government of India provides a composite index called the National Air Quality Index (AQI). The index is unique to each area for which it is calculated.

### Computing Air Quality Index

Air quality index transforms weighted values of individual air pollution related parameters (e.g. $SO_2$, CO, visibility, etc.) into a single number. Eight parameters (PM10, PM2.5, $NO_2$, $SO_2$, CO, $O_3$, $NH_3$, and Pb) having short-term standards are factored in to generate a near real-time AQI.

The sub-indices for individual pollutants at a monitoring location are calculated using its 24-hourly average concentration value (8-hourly in case of CO and $O_3$) and health breakpoint concentration range. The worst subindex is the AQI for that location **(Fig. 7A.4)**.

### Interpretation of Air Quality Index

The AQI has six categories with elegant color scheme, as shown in **Figure 7A.5**. Each of these categories is decided based on ambient concentration values of air pollutants and their likely health impacts (known as health breakpoints). While green color indicates that adverse health effects at that AQI level are unlikely,

**Punjabi Bagh, New Delhi**

| Day | Subindex | | | | | | | | | AQI |
|---|---|---|---|---|---|---|---|---|---|---|
| | CO (min) | CO (max) | $O_3$ (min) | $O_3$ (max) | $NO_2$ | $NH_3$ | $SO_2$ | PM2.5 | PM10 | |
| 10–Nov–13 | 41 | 96 | 13 | 64 | 67 | 12 | 12 | 371 | 294 | 371 |
| 11–Nov–13 | 52 | 105 | 22 | 68 | 76 | 9 | 15 | 320 | 272 | 320 |
| 12–Nov–13 | 44 | 114 | 15 | 76 | 93 | 11 | 12 | 384 | 390 | 390 |
| 13–Nov–13 | 43 | 114 | 9 | 79 | 91 | 13 | 15 | 407 | 406 | 407 |
| 14–Nov–13 | 37 | 110 | 11 | 68 | 90 | 10 | 13 | 335 | 306 | 335 |

PM10 and PM2.5 = particulate matter less than 10 microns and 2.5 microns respectively

**Fig. 7A.4:** Subindices of air quality index. *(For color version, see Plate 1)*

| Good (0–50) | Satisfactory (51–100) | Moderately polluted (101–200) | Poor (201–300) | Very poor (301–400) | Severe (> 400) |
|---|---|---|---|---|---|

**Fig. 7A.5:** Color categories of air quality index. *(For color version, see Plate 1)*

dark red is a warning of severe health effects with other colors ranging in between.

## Air Quality Monitoring

At present, continuous air quality monitoring stations from 10 cities are connected to the web-based system. Continuous monitoring systems are operated by various State Pollution Control Boards (SPCBs). It is planned to strengthen the network of monitoring systems in all 46 cities having population more than a million and 20 State Capitals, and networking them to the central AQI portal, in phased manner.

Importance of AQI in Community Health:

1. **Monitoring of National Air Monitoring Programme**: To see if the objectives of the program are met through adequate air pollution control.
2. **Ranking of locations**: To assist in comparing air quality conditions at different locations/cities.
3. **Trend analysis**: To determine change in air quality (degradation or improvement) which have occurred over a specified period.
4. **Enforcement of standards**: To determine extent to which the legislative standards and existing criteria are being adhered.
5. **Resource allocation**: To assist administrators in allocating funds and determining priorities.
6. **Public information**: To inform the public about environmental conditions (state of environment).
7. **Scientific research**: As a means for reducing a large set of data to a comprehendible form that gives better insight to the researcher while conducting a study of some environmental phenomena.

## PREVENTION AND CONTROL OF AIR POLLUTION

Prevention and control of air pollution go hand-in-hand **(Table 7A.11)**. The following are some of the modern concepts in prevention and control of air pollution, explained with suitable examples.

## National Air Quality Monitoring Programme

The Central Pollution Control Board in India is executing a nation-wide program of ambient air quality monitoring known as National Air Quality Monitoring Programme (NAMP). The network consists of 683 operating stations covering 300 cities/towns across India. Under this program, air quality monitoring is being carried out with the help of Central Pollution Control Board; State Pollution Control Boards; Pollution Control Committees; National Environmental Engineering Research Institute (NEERI), Nagpur.

Table 7A.11: Strategies of prevention and control of air pollution.

| Sr. No. | Concept | Meaning | Examples |
|---|---|---|---|
| 1. | Environmental audit | A management tool that provides a comprehensive assessment of an industry, process involved, flow of material and functioning of waste disposal mechanisms | An environmental audit on pollution of river Ganga found that air pollution was above permissible limit. Based on this report, the Supreme Court directed certain industries to raise the height of their chimneys and construction of ash ponds for dry fly ash disposal |
| 2. | Industrial pollution control | Cleaner production and waste minimization by adopting processes that are cost-effective yet produce minimum hazardous waste in industries (control at source) | • Using low sulfur fuels and liquid petroleum gas (LPG) or liquefied natural gas (LNG) instead of coal<br>• Certification, periodic checking and maintenance of machinery used |
| 3. | Vehicular pollution control | Using improved automobile technology, better quality fuel, improved systems of traffic management | • Phasing out of >15-year old commercial vehicles, which are grossly fuel inefficient and high polluters in Delhi in 1998<br>• Running vehicles of public transport on CNG<br>• The Odd-Even formula for running cars on roads on alternate days in Delhi to reduce vehicular traffic<br>• PUC certification also known as the 'pollution control certificate', validates that a particular vehicle is safe to be driven and poses no threat to the environment as its carbon emission level is well within the standard set by the Government of India |
| 4. | Dilution | Reducing the concentration of air pollutants by cleaning property of vegetation | Having "green belts" (tree plantation) in between industrial and residential areas |
| 5. | Zoning and mapping for siting of industries | Spatial planning for location of industries such that the effects caused by air pollution due to them are minimized | Use of Geographic Information Systems (GIS) to map out areas where industries can be located; their distance from habitation and environmentally sensitive zones like forests and national parks |
| 6. | Legislative actions | Law and enforcement to reduce air pollution | • The Air (Prevention and Control of Pollution) Act, 1981<br>• The Environment (Protection) Act, 1986 |
| 7. | Framework for monitoring air quality | Laying down a framework for monitoring air quality, setting alerts and giving authority to supervisory bodies to take action | • Ministry of Environment and Forests has set up Central Pollution Control Board which in turn has State Pollution Control Boards under it<br>• Development of a composite AQI |
| 8. | Innovations in air pollution control | Use of existing knowledge and technology to develop innovative solutions to monitor/control air pollution | • The 'SAFAR' (System of Air quality weather Forecasting and Research) mobile app by Indian Institute of Meteorology, Pune<br>• Scrubber systems in chimneys, incinerators, etc. that remove or neutralize harmful gases before they are emitted |

## APPLICATION OF THE KNOWLEDGE OF AIR POLLUTION IN HEALTHCARE

- Prevention of air pollution in the community (both outdoor and indoor) before level of pollutants rises to potentially harmful levels
- Screening of high-risk groups for effects of air pollution on health
- Providing protective measures like masks to those at risk
- Suggesting engineering measures at homes and workplaces as holistic approach to disease management and prevention
- Implications in tobacco control strategies in preventing of health effects due to direct and passive smoke in those exposed
- In undertaking awareness and advocacy campaigns.

## SUMMARY

- ❖ Air pollution is an issue of grave concern, not just in households but also at state, regional, national and global level.
- ❖ Air pollutants may be primary or secondary, solid or gaseous. Major ones include PM10, PM2.5, $NO_2$, $SO_2$, CO, $O_3$, $NH_3$, and lead.
- ❖ The two major types of air pollution are outdoor and indoor air pollution. Persons with underlying respiratory and cardiovascular diseases, the elderly and the traffic police constitute high-risk groups for outdoor air pollution, whereas women and children under the age of 5 years constitute high-risk groups for indoor air pollution.
- ❖ Air pollution has wide variety of effects on health such as those on respiratory and cardiovascular system, effects on maternal and child health, carcinogenic effects and effects on country's economy.
- ❖ The air quality index (AQI) is an area-specific, real time composite index developed by the Central Pollution Control Board (Ministry of Environment, Forests and Climate Change) that helps to assess air pollution levels and serves as an alarm in indicating harmful levels of pollutants for human health.
- ❖ Air pollution can be prevented and controlled by a multipronged approach.
- ❖ The National Air Quality Monitoring Programme (NAMP) of India lays down guidelines for ambient air quality and a monitoring framework for air pollution in India.

## SUGGESTED READING

1. Government of India. (2017). About NAMP. Central Pollution Control Board (IN). [online]. Ministry of Environment, Forest & Climate Change. Available from http://cpcb.nic.in/about-namp/.
2. Government of India. National Air Quality Index. New Delhi: Central Pollution Control Board. Ministry of Environment, Forests & Climate Change. 2014.
3. Mabahwi NAB, Leh OLH, Omar D. Human health and wellbeing: Human health effect of air pollution. Procedia-Social and Behavioral Sciences. 2014;153:221-9.
4. UNICEF. Clear the air for children. United Nations Children's Fund. 2017.
5. World Health Organization. (2018). Ambient (outdoor) air quality and health. Fact Sheet. [online]. Available from http://www.who.int/en/news-room/fact-sheets/detail/ambient-(outdoor)-air-quality-and-health.
6. World Health Organization. (2018). Household air pollution and health. Fact Sheet. [online]. Available from http://www.who.int/en/news-room/fact-sheets/detail/household-air-pollution-and-health.

## B. WATER AND HEALTH

*P Stalin, Velavan A, Anil J Purty*

**CM3.1** Describe the health hazards of water

**CM3.2** Describe concepts of safe and wholesome water, sanitary sources of water, water purification processes, water quality standards, concepts of water conservation and rainwater harvesting

### Case Study

*A Primary Health Center (PHC) has reported that 11 individuals were diagnosed and treated for acute diarrheal disease from village A in the last 2 days. Next month, the important annual public festival is scheduled in this village which has a population of 1,500 and primarily depends for their drinking water from two tube wells connected to two overhead water tanks with a capacity of 30,000 L each. During the 3 days of festivities, over 6,000 individuals from neighboring villages and nearby town are expected to visit this village. The Block Development Officer (BDO) is concerned about the possibility of water-borne diarrheal disease during the festival and urgently requires a plan of action.*
*i. What immediate steps need to be undertaken to prevent the spread of acute diarrheal disease?*
*ii. Describe the steps that you would recommend to ensure safe drinking water supply during the festival.*
*Answers:*
*i. In order to break the chain of transmission, isolation and effective treatment of the individuals with diarrheal diseases should be followed.*
*ii. Water sources should be tested for microbiological contamination. After assessing the chlorine demand, water should be disinfected by chlorination. Efforts should be taken to prevent leakage and contamination of water distribution system. Hygienic practices should be followed while storing the drinking water.*

### Historical fact

On 31 August 1854, a major cholera outbreak occurred in Soho, London city. Within 19 days, 500 people had died. After initial survey, the public water pump on Broad Street at Cambridge Street was identified as the source of outbreak by John Snow **(Fig. 7B.1)**. Snow also mapped the locations of individual water pumps and houses of the city. The number of cholera cases in and around the Broad Street pump was much higher compared to other areas. After showing his survey report regarding illness and deaths to the authorities in Soho, the handle of water pump on Broad Street was removed. This led to decline in cholera cases and deaths.

### INTRODUCTION

*"Thousands have lived without love, not one without water"*
—**WH Auden**

Human beings need clean water, basic sanitation, and proper hygiene for their survival and development. In 2010, water and sanitation are recognized as human rights by the UN General Assembly that is "essential for the full enjoyment of life and all human rights". Today, improved sanitation facilities and water sources are not available to about 2.4 billion people and 663 million people, respectively. Diseases due to poor quality of

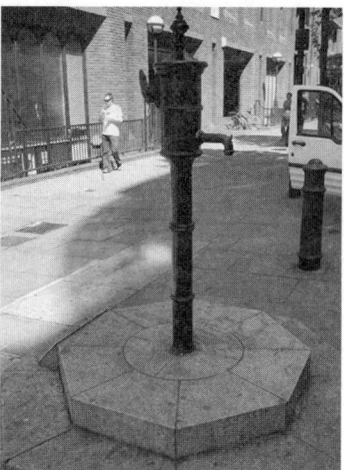

**Fig. 7B.1:** Water pump in Broad Street, London.
*Source:* Soho M. (2016). The Museum of Soho's Blog: Soho and the Cholera Outbreak of 1854. [online] Available from http://mosoho.blogspot.com/2016/06/soho-and-cholera-outbreak-of-1854.html.

water and inadequate sanitation are one of the leading causes of death among young children (UNICEF, Strategy for Water, Sanitation and Hygiene, 2016–2030).

Most of these deaths are preventable by providing safe water and sanitation. This lead to a new strategy called water, sanitation, and hygiene (WASH). They are grouped together due to their interdependent nature. For example, there is possibility of contamination of water sources without sanitary latrine; basic hygiene practices cannot be followed without adequate quality of water.

In 2015, safely managed drinking water service was used by 71% of the World population. 89% of the global population (6.5 billion people) used improved source within 30 minutes of round trip to collect water, 26 crores people spent more than 30 minutes per round trip to collect water from an improved source (WHO and UNICEF, Progress on Drinking Water, Sanitation and Hygiene: 2017 Update and SDG baseline). According to the National Family Health Survey—5 in India, 95.9% of the households are availing water from improved drinking water sources.

### SAFE AND WHOLESOME WATER

Water used by human for consumption should be safe and wholesome. It should be pleasant to taste, colorless and odorless, free from pathogenic agents and harmful chemical substances and usable for domestic purposes.

### USES AND REQUIREMENT OF WATER

Domestic use of water can be classified into four categories such as:
1. Consumption (drinking and cooking),
2. Hygiene (bathing and laundry),

3. Amenity (gardening and cleaning vehicles), and
4. Production (animal watering, brewing, etc.).

The daily requirements of drinking water for adults and children are 1.5–2 L and 1 L per person, respectively. Domestic consumption under normal condition in an Indian city is taken as 150 LPCD (i.e. liters per capita per day) for urban areas and 55 LPCD for rural areas (National Water Academy, Department of Water Resources, Ministry of Jal Shakti). Water is used for various other purposes like industry, agriculture, electricity generation, etc.

## SOURCES OF DRINKING WATER (FIG. 7B.2)

An "improved drinking water source" is one that by the nature of its construction adequately protects the source from outside contamination, in particular from fecal matter. According to the World Health Organization (WHO) and United Nations International Children's Emergency Fund (UNICEF) Joint Monitoring Programme for WASH, drinking water facilities are classified as shown in **Table 7B.1**.

### Surface Water

Surface water gets water directly from rainfall. It is easily accessible and relatively soft but the risk of contamination is high due to pollution from human and animals. Water in lakes, ponds, and rivers are consumed by large number of people either directly or through piped water distribution system after proper treatment. If they drink directly without purification, it can lead to many water-borne diseases.

**Table 7B.1:** WHO/UNICEF JMP for WASH: Classification of drinking water facilities.

| Service | Definition |
|---|---|
| Safely managed | Drinking water from an improved water source that is located on premises, available when needed, and free from fecal and priority chemical contamination |
| Basic | Drinking water from an improved source, provided collection time is not more than 30 minutes for a round trip, including queuing |
| Limited | Drinking water from an improved source for which collection time exceeds 30 minutes for a round trip, including queuing |
| Unimproved | Drinking water from an unprotected dug well or unprotected spring |
| Surface water | Drinking water directly from a river, dam, lake, pond, stream, canal, or irrigation canal |

*Note:* Improved sources include: piped water, boreholes or tube wells, protected dug wells, protected springs, rainwater, and packaged or delivered water.

(JMP: Joint Monitoring Program; UNICEF: United Nations International Children's Emergency Fund; WASH: water, sanitation, and hygiene; WHO: World Health Organization)

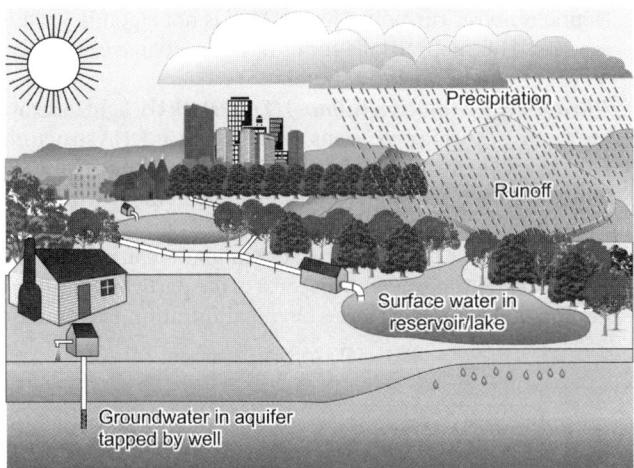

**Fig. 7B.2:** Sources of drinking water.
*Source:* AqualifeUSA. (2006). What You Need to Know About Drinking Water! [online] Available from http://aqualifeusa.com/eng/water_health.htm.

### Groundwater

Groundwater levels are determined by the amount of rainfall. The risk of contamination is very low in groundwater but the hardness is higher compared to surface water. Therefore, softening of water may be required in some places to make it suitable for drinking. It is also difficult and expensive to access the groundwater through construction of boreholes, tube wells, and dug wells, etc. **(Fig. 7B.3)**. Groundwater is usually retrieved manually using

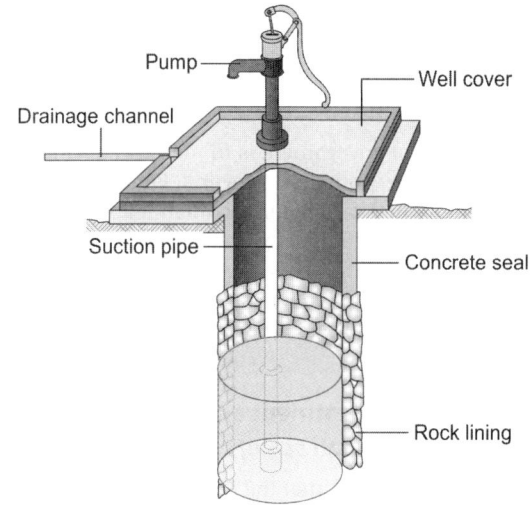

**Fig. 7B.3:** Protected dug well.
*Source:* Bruni M, Spuhler D. (2002). Dug Wells. [online] Available from https://sswm.info/water-nutrient-cycle/water-sources/hardwares/groundwater-sources/dug-wells.

bucket and rope/hand pump or mechanically using electric motor pumps. In springs, water emerges to the surface from the underground naturally.

## WATER–RELATED DISEASES

According to Bradley (1977), there are four categories of diseases related to water:
1. ***Water-borne***: Due to consumption of contaminated water (e.g. diarrhea, hepatitis A, cholera, typhoid, and guinea worm).
2. ***Water-washed***: Due to poor personal hygiene resulting from nonavailability of adequate water (e.g. diarrhea, typhoid, trachoma, and skin and eye infections).
3. ***Water-based***: Caused by an intermediate host dwelling in water (e.g. guinea worm, schistosomiasis).

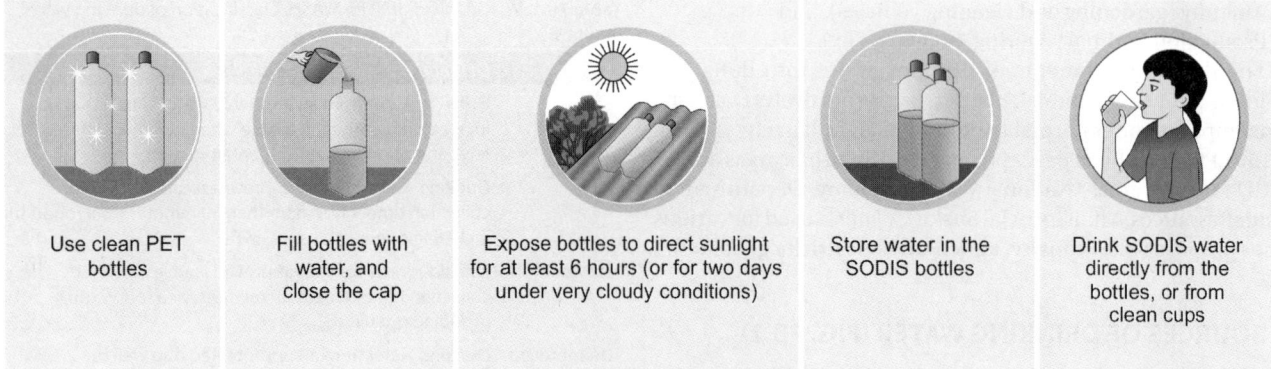

**Fig. 7B.4:** Solar water disinfection (SODIS).

4. **Water-related**: Diseases transmitted by vectors breeding in water (e.g. filarial, chikungunya, malaria, and dengue fever).

> **Note**
> In 18th century, there was a greater number of typhus outbreaks caused by *Rickettsia prowazekii* among the prisoners in London which was transmitted by the feces of infected louses. Poor personal hygiene due to lack of water required for bathing, cleaning, etc. contributed to the spread of epidemic typhus, also known as jail fever.

## WATER TREATMENT

The primary aim of government is to identify sustainable and accessible safe water source. However, it is not possible many times due to microbial and chemical contamination which could potentially affect the health of the individuals. Water treatment technologies should be simple, affordable, and easy to operate and maintain. Successful implementation of these technologies mainly depends on the availability of resources and community participation.

### Household Water Treatment and Safe Storage (Purification on a small scale)

Many studies have found that the household water treatment and safe storage (HWTS) methods are useful in improving the quality of household water and thereby reducing the incidence of infectious diseases among the household members.

- **Boiling**: Boiling is a common method of disinfecting water at the household level. It has been recommended for many years that boiling water at 100°C for 15–20 minutes is an effective method used to kill all types of pathogens such as bacterial spores and protozoan cysts which cannot be killed by chemical disinfection and viruses that cannot be mechanically removed by microfiltration. However, the latest WHO guidelines now recommend holding the water at boiling level for 1 minute at sea level and for 3 minutes at higher altitudes to make it safe for drinking. The WHO recommends that bringing water to a rolling boil is an indirect indication of achievement of temperature required for disinfection. High cost related to fuel in boiling and the change in taste of the boiled water are two common disadvantages of boiling water.
- **Chlorination**: Chlorination can be used for disinfection at the household level also. At doses of a few mg/L and contact time of about 30 minutes, free chlorine can inactivate more than 99.999% of enteric pathogens excluding *Cryptosporidium* and *Mycobacterium* species. Bleaching powder, chlorine solution, high test hypochlorite (HTH), chlorine tablets (0.5 mg for 20 L), and iodine (two drops for 2 L) are the different chemical forms of water disinfection available in the market.
- **Solar water disinfection (SODIS)**: SODIS is an appropriate method for treating drinking water mostly in developing nations **(Fig. 7B.4)**. It uses solar radiation [ultraviolet A (UVA) and thermal components] to kill pathogenic microorganisms especially bacteria and viruses. Water-filled bottles are placed in sunlight for at least 6 hours. Water with high turbidity [>30 Nephelometric Turbidity Unit (NTU)] is not suitable for this method. This method kills germs but does not have any effect on the chemical quality of water.
- **Ultraviolet irradiation (lamps) (Fig. 7B.5):** UV light destroys the disease causing pathogens by damaging its DNA structure. Flow chamber through which water flows is exposed to the UV lamp. It is always better to combine these methods with other forms of filtration like reverse osmosis (RO), granular activated carbon (GAC) so that chemical contaminants can be reduced.
- **Filtration**: Filtration removes most of the particles and some microbes from water. In mechanical filtration, suspended

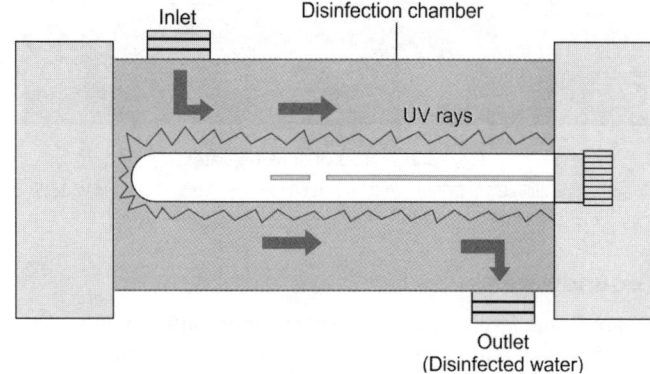

**Fig. 7B.5:** Schematic diagram of ultraviolet (UV) irradiation lamp.
*Source:* All about water filters. (2017). Ultraviolet Light Treatment. [online] Available from http://www.watairwatercoolers.com/images/uv_water_cooler.jpg.

# Chapter 7: Environment and Health

## Community-based Water Supply and Treatment (Purification on a Large Scale)

In many villages and towns of our country, houses do not have their own individual water source. They are dependent on central water supplies. The main source of water for such central water supplies is surface waters such as ponds, lakes, and rivers, etc. Groundwater is also used in many places through bore wells. There is a potential risk of contamination to these water sources especially surface waters. Therefore, before storing the water at central water tanks and distributing through pipelines to individual houses, it needs to be treated and contaminants should be removed safely.

Community-based water treatment plants are used at centralized locations in the community to provide safe water which are maintained by the government or private agencies. Coagulation, sedimentation, filtration, and disinfection are the different methods used together in many water treatment plants. Usually, coagulants such as aluminum or iron salts are added to water to initiate reactions, which bind the dissolved suspended particles together. These larger particles sediment down quickly and the water moves on to the next step of filtration. During the filtration, particulate matters are removed by forcing the water to pass through porous media such as sand, gravel, and charcoal. There are two types of sand filtration, the "biological" or "slow sand" filters and the "rapid sand" or "mechanical" filters **(Table 7B.2)**.

### Slow Sand Filter

- Essentially it consists of a layer of supernatant water above the sand bed, whose depth varies from 1 meter to 1.5 meter. It provides a constant head of water so as to overcome the resistance of the filter bed and thereby promote the downward flow of water through the sand bed; and secondly, it provides waiting period of some hours (3 to 12 hours, depending upon the filtration velocity) for the raw water to undergo partial purification by sedimentation, oxidation and particle agglomeration. The thickness of the sand bed is about 1 meter with "effective diameter" between 0.2 and 0.3 mm. The sand bed is supported by a layer of graded gravel 30–40 cm deep

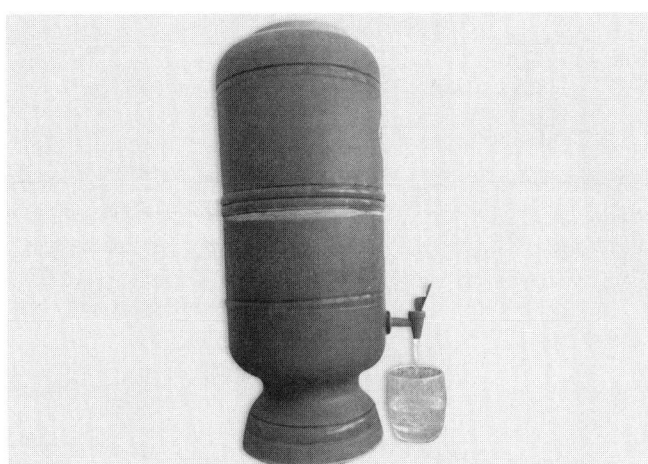

**Fig. 7B.6:** Pot-type ceramic filter.
*Source:* Wikimedia. (2018). Ceramic water filter. [online] Available from https://commons.wikimedia.org/wiki/File:Ceramic_water_filter.jpg#filehistory.

solids (including microbes) are removed physically from water using a porous media. The size of the pores is smaller than the target contaminant. Porous rock, sand, clothes, and unglazed ceramics are some of the common media used for filtration. Nonelectrical pot and candle-type ceramic filters are suitable for use in developing countries due to its simplicity, low cost, and effectiveness at removing bacteria and the larger protozoans **(Figs. 7B.6 and 7B.7)**. However, the disadvantages are ineffectiveness against viruses and low flow rate. Electrical filters with advanced membranes for microfiltration, ultrafiltration, nanofiltration, and reverse osmosis (RO) are also used, but their usage in low-income settings is minimal due to high cost and complex technology.

- ***Safe storage***: Households with no access to piped water supply usually store water. During the process of water collection, transport, and storage in the home, it can be contaminated due to poor hand hygiene and the practices of dipping the small vessels into large-mouth water containers. Safe storage can be ensured by the provision of a lid and withdrawal of water using a small vessel with handle.

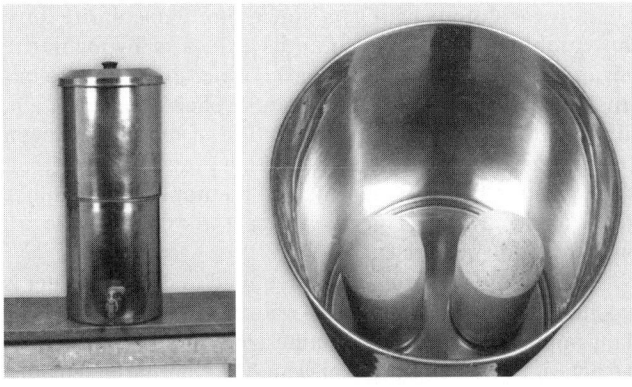

**Fig. 7B.7:** Candle-type ceramic filter.
*Source:* The choice sanitary wares. (2017). Water Candle Filters. [online] Available from http://choicesanitary.com.ng/water-candle-filters.

**Table 7B.2:** Comparisons between Rapid and Slow sand filter.

|  |  | Rapid sand filter | Slow sand filter |
|---|---|---|---|
| 1. | Space | Occupies very little space | Occupies large area |
| 2. | Rate of filtration | 200 mgad | 2–3 mgad |
| 3. | Effective size of sand | 0.4–0.7 mm | 0.2–0.3 mm |
| 4. | Preliminary treatment | Chemical coagulation and sedimentation | Plain sedimentation |
| 5. | Washing | By backwashing | By scrapping the sand bed |
| 6. | Operation | Highly skilled | Less skilled |
| 7. | Loss of head allowed | 6–8 feet (2–2.5 m) | 4 feet (1.5 m) |
| 8. | Removal of turbidity | Good | Good |
| 9. | Removal of color | Good | Fair |
| 10. | Removal of bacteria | 98–99% | 99.9–99.99% |

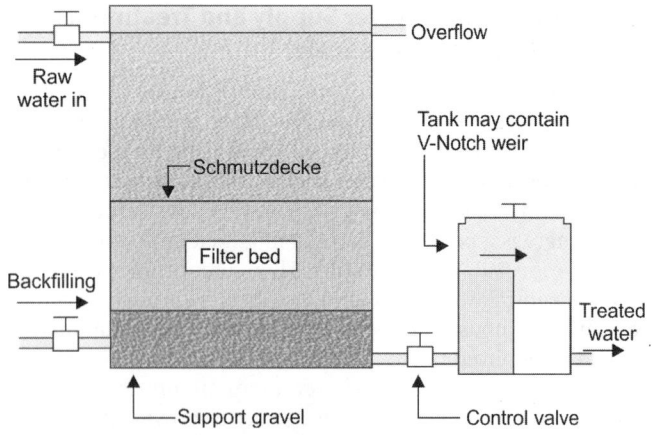

Fig. 7B.8: Slow sand filter.

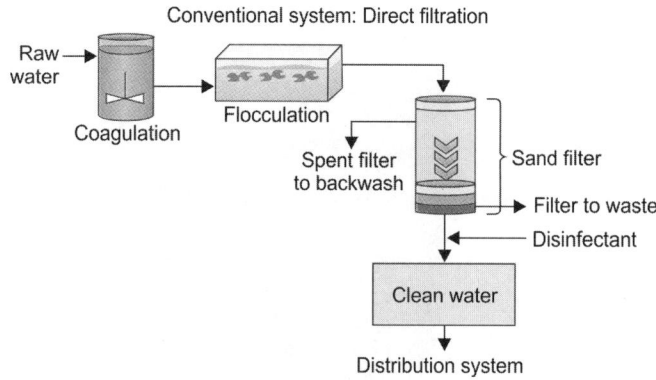

Fig 7B.9: Rapid sand filter.

which also prevents the fine grains being carried into the drainage pipes (Fig. 7B.8). The surface of the sand bed gets covered with a slimy growth known as "Schmutzdecke", vital layer, zoogleal layer or biological layer. This layer is slimy and gelatinous and consists of threadlike algae and numerous forms of life including plankton, diatoms and bacteria. The vital layer is the "heart" of the slow sand filter. It removes organic matter, holds back bacteria and oxidizes ammoniacal nitrogen into nitrates and helps in yielding a bacteria-free water.

- At the bottom of the filter bed is the under-drainage system. It consists of porous or perforated pipes which serve the dual purpose of providing an outlet for filtered water, and supporting the filter medium above. The filter is equipped with certain valves and devices which are incorporated in the outlet-pipe system.
- Normally, the filter may run for weeks or even months without cleaning. When the bed resistance increases to such an extent that the regulating valve has to be kept fully open, it is time to clean the filter bed, since any further increase in resistance is bound to reduce the filtration rate. At this stage, the supernatant water is drained off, and the sand bed is cleaned by "scraping" off the top portion of the sand layer to a depth of 1 or 2 cm.

### Rapid Sand Filter

- Rapid sand filters are of two types, the gravity type (e.g. Paterson's filter) and the pressure type (e.g. Candy's filter). The steps involved in the purification of water by rapid sand filters are shown in **Figure 7B.9**.
- Sand is the filtering medium. The "effective size" of the sand particles is between 0.4–0.7 mm. The depth of the sand bed is usually about 1 metre. Below the sand bed is a layer of graded gravel, 30 to 40 cm deep. The gravel supports the sand bed and permits the filtered water to move freely towards the under-drains. The depth of the water on the top of the sand bed is 1.0 to 1.5 m. The under-drains at the bottom of the filter beds collect the filtered water. The rate of filtration is 5–15 $m^3/m^2/$hour.
- As filtration proceeds, the "alum-floc" not removed by sedimentation is held back on the sand bed. It forms a slimy layer comparable to the zoogleal layer in the slow sand filters. It adsorbs bacteria from the water and effects purification. Oxidation of ammonia also takes place during the passage of water through the filters. As filtration proceeds, the suspended impurities and bacteria clog the filters. The filters soon become dirty and begin to lose their efficiency. When the "loss of head" approaches 7–8 feet, filtration is stopped and the filters are subjected to a washing process known as "backwashing", in which the flow of water is reversed through the sand bed. It dislodges the impurities and cleans up the sand bed.

### Chlorination

It is a widely used disinfection method in forms of chlorine gas, chloramines, or perchloron. It can kill all microorganisms except viruses and spores. It also helps in oxidizing iron, hydrogen sulfide, etc.

Any type of chlorine that is added to water during the treatment process will result in the formation of hypochlorous acid (HOCl) and hypochlorite ions (OCl$^-$), which are the main disinfecting compounds in chlorinated water. Of the two, hypochlorous acid is the most effective. The amount of each compound present in the water is dependent on the pH level of the water prior to addition of chlorine. At lower pH levels, the hypochlorous acid will dominate. When the pH value exceeds 8.5, chlorine is unreliable as a disinfectant because about 90% of the hypochlorous acid gets ionized to hypochlorite ions. The combination of hypochlorous acid and hypochlorite ions makes up what is called 'free chorine.' Free chlorine has a high oxidation potential and is a more effective disinfectant. Combined chlorine is the combination of organic nitrogen compounds and chloramines, which are produced as a result of the reaction between chlorine and ammonia. Chloramines are not as effective at disinfecting water as free chlorine due to a lower oxidation potential.

The amount of chlorine that is required to disinfect water is dependent on the impurities in the water that needs to be treated. Many impurities in the water require a large amount of chlorine to react with all the impurities present. The chlorine added must first react with all the impurities in the water before a chlorine residual is present. The amount of chlorine that is required to satisfy all the impurities is termed the 'chlorine demand'. This can also be thought of as the amount of chlorine needed before residual chlorine can be produced. Once the chlorine demand has been met, breakpoint chlorination has occurred. After the breakpoint, any additional chlorine added will result in a free chlorine residual proportional to the amount of chlorine added. Thus, residual chlorine is the difference between the amount of chlorine added and the chlorine demand. Most water treatment plants will add chlorine beyond the breakpoint to provide a margin of safety against subsequent microbial contamination such as may occur during storage and distribution. The minimum recommended concentration of residual chlorine is 0.5 mg/L.

The amount of chlorine required to disinfect the water is known as chlorine demand which can be estimated using Horrock's apparatus. It contains six white cups, one black cup, two metal spoons, seven glass stirring rods, one special pipette, two droppers, starch iodide indicator solution, and instruction folder. Prepare stock solution by initially making a thin paste of 2 g of bleaching powder with little water in the black cup, then add more water up to the circular mark with vigorous stirring. All six white cups shall be filled with water to be tested just 1 cm below the brim. Using the special pipette, add one drop of stock solution in the first cup, two drops in the second cup, and so on. Stir it with a separate rod. After half an hour, add three drops of starch iodide indicator to all the white cups and stir again. Note the first cup which shows blue color. If the fourth cup shows blue color, then 8 g of bleaching powder is required to disinfect 455 L of water. Orthotoluidine (OT) test is used to determine the presence of free and combined chlorine in drinking water. Yellow color is produced by adding 0.1 mL of the reagent to 1 mL of water. The intensity of the color indicates the concentration of the chlorine. OT test gives higher chorine values as its reading is influenced by the presence of iron, manganese, nitrates, etc. in water. Orthotoluidine arsenite (OTA) test overcomes this error and gives better results. Both OT and OTA test gives both free as well as combined chlorine residuals' value in water.

# HARDNESS OF WATER

Dissolved polyvalent metallic ions, mainly calcium and magnesium cations are responsible for hardness. It can also lead to deposition of precipitates in containers. Hardness is also indirectly measured by the reaction between soap and water. Hard water needs more soap to form lather. Water containing calcium carbonate at concentrations below 60 mg/L is generally considered as soft; 60–120 mg/L, moderately hard; 120–180 mg/L, hard; and more than 180 mg/L, very hard.

## Effects of Hardness on Health

Excess calcium and magnesium intake can potentially harm the people who are at risk of developing milk-alkali syndrome and renal insufficiency, respectively. High magnesium intake may cause diarrhea due to its laxative effect. Exposure to hard water could be a risk factor for eczema. The reported association between hardness of water and cardiovascular diseases has been found to be inconclusive.

## Household Treatment for Hardness

Water softener devices are used at the point of water entry in households to remove hardness (calcium, magnesium) and iron from water using ion-exchange method. Softening reduces scaling in pipes, fixtures, and water heaters and improves laundry and washing characteristics at the cost of increasing the sodium (and chloride) content of the drinking-water. Point-of-use RO and distilling devices remove virtually all the minerals from the input water. It is important to use RO water filters only for the water which is hard and suffers from high level of chemical contents. This is because RO leads to wastage of water, i.e. for 1 gallon of drinking water delivered, 4 gallons of water are wasted. Therefore, unnecessary use of RO should be strictly avoided.

# DRINKING WATER QUALITY CRITERIA AND STANDARDS

Access to safe drinking-water is essential to health, a basic human right and a component of effective policy for health protection. The importance of water, sanitation and hygiene for health and development has been reflected in the outcomes of a series of international policy forums. This includes, most recently, the adoption of the Sustainable Development Goals by countries, in 2015, which include a target and indicator on safe drinking-water. Further, the United Nations (UN) General Assembly declared in 2010 that safe and clean drinking-water and sanitation is a human right, essential to the full enjoyment of life and all other human rights. The World Health Organization (WHO) published four editions of the Guidelines for drinking-water quality (in 1983–1984, 1993–1997, 2004, and 2011), as successors to the previous WHO International standards for drinking water, which were published in 1958, 1963 and 1971. The first addendum to the fourth edition was published in 2016. The Guidelines provide the recommendations of WHO for managing the risk from exposure to hazards, such as waste, air, food and consumer products.

The guidelines for drinking water quality recommended by WHO relate to following variables:
 I. Acceptability aspects
 II. Microbiological aspects
 III. Chemical aspects
 IV. Radiological aspects.
 I. **Acceptability aspects:** Physical parameters such as color, odor, taste, and turbidity determine the acceptability of drinking water. Inorganic constituent like pH of water, total dissolved solutes, hardness of water and amount of chlorides, ammonia, iron, sodium, sulfate and dissolved oxygen also determine the acceptability of drinking water. Acceptable limits for each parameter are given in **Table 7B.3**. It is recommended that the acceptable limit is to be implemented. Values in excess of those mentioned under "acceptable" render the water not suitable, but still may be tolerated in the absence of an alternative source but up to the limits indicated under "permissible limit in the absence of alternate source", above which the sources will have to be rejected.
 II. **Microbiological aspects:**
    a. Bacteriological indicators used for assessing water quality are *Escherichia coli* or thermotolerant coliform bacteria. They shall not be detectable in any 100 mL sample in all water intended for drinking **(Table 7B.4)**. Immediate investigative actions shall be taken if either *Escherichia*

**Table 7B.3:** Acceptability parameters of drinking water.

| Characteristic | Requirement (acceptable limit) |
| --- | --- |
| Color, Hazen units, maximum | 5 |
| Odor | Agreeable |
| Taste | Agreeable |
| Turbidity, nephelometric turbidity unit (NTU), maximum | 1 |
| Temperature | Cool water (palatable) |
| pH value | 6.5–8.5 |
| Total dissolved solids, mg/L, maximum | 500 |
| Hardness (Calcium ion) | 100–300 mg/liter |
| Chlorides | 200 mg/liter |
| Sodium | 200 mg/liter |
| Manganese | <0.1 mg/liter |

**Table 7B.4:** Bacteriological quality of drinking water.

| Organisms | Requirements |
| --- | --- |
| **All water intended for drinking:** | |
| *Escherichia coli* or thermotolerant coliform bacteria | Shall not be detectable in any 100 mL sample |
| **Treated water entering the distribution system:** | |
| *Escherichia coli* or thermotolerant coliform bacteria | Shall not be detectable in any 100 mL sample |
| Total coliform bacteria | Shall not be detectable in any 100 mL sample |
| **Treated water in the distribution system:** | |
| *Escherichia coli* or thermotolerant coliform bacteria | Shall not be detectable in any 100 mL sample |
| Total coliform bacteria | Shall not be detectable in any 100 mL sample |

*coli* or total coliform bacteria are detected. Total coliform bacteria are not acceptable indicators in tropical areas where many bacteria of no sanitary significance occur in almost all untreated supplies. The minimum action in the case of total coliform bacteria is repeat sampling; if these bacteria are detected in the repeat sample, the cause shall be determined by immediate further investigation.

Fecal streptococci regularly occur in feces, but in much smaller numbers than *E.coli;* in doubtful cases, the finding of fecal streptococci in water is regarded as important confirmatory evidence of recent feces pollution of water. Streptococci are highly resistant to drying and may be valuable for routine control testing after laying new mains or repairs in distribution systems or for detecting pollution by surface run-off to ground or surface waters.

*Cl. perfringens* also occur regularly in feces, though generally in much smaller numbers than *E.coli*. The spores are capable of surviving in water for a longer time than organisms of the coliform group, and usually resist chlorination at the doses normally used in waterworks practice. The presence of spores of *Cl. perfringens* in a natural water suggests that fecal contamination has occurred, and their presence, in the absence of the coliform group, suggests that fecal contamination occurred at some remote time. Its presence in filtered supplies may indicate deficiency in filtration practice.

b. Virological aspects : It is recommended that, to be acceptable, drinking-water should be free from any viruses infectious for man. Disinfection with 0.5 mg/L of free chlorine residual after contact period of at least 30 minutes at a pH of 8.0 is sufficient to inactivate virus. This free chlorine residual is to be insisted in all disinfected supplies in areas suspected of endemicity of hepatitis A to take care of the safety of the supply from the virus point of view, which incidentally takes care of safety from the bacteriologic point of view as well.

c. Biological aspects: Drinking-water should not contain any pathogenic intestinal protozoa like *Entamoeba histolytica, Giardia spp.* and *rarely, Balantidium coli.* which can be introduced into water supply through human or, in some instances, animal fecal contamination. Helminths like *Dracunculus medinensis* (guinea worm) and the human schistosomes, are primarily hazards of unpiped water supplies. Free living organisms like fungi, algae, etc. may cause interference in the operation of water-treatment process, color, turbidity, taste and odor of finished water.

III. **Chemical aspects:** Chemical substances of drinking water can be classified as undesirable substances, toxic substances, and residues of pesticides. Chemicals of public health importance and their maximum acceptable limits are provided in **Table 7B.5**. Toxic and carcinogenic nature of many chemicals may lead to health problems after chronic exposure.

IV. **Radiological aspects:** Radioactive materials in drinking water can lead to health problems especially cancer. Therefore, it should be within safe limits which is less than 0.1 Bq/L and less than 1.0 Bq/L for alpha and beta emitters, respectively.

## SURVEILLANCE OF DRINKING WATER QUALITY

Drinking water supply surveillance is "the continuous and vigilant public health assessment and review of the safety and acceptability of drinking water supplies" (WHO, 1976). Surveillance should not be restricted only to quality but also quantity, affordability, accessibility, and continuity. Quality surveillance includes inspection of the water resources and its distribution system, collection and testing of water samples for contamination using standard methods, and reporting of findings and ensuring follow-up action.

### Sanitary Inspections

It is the first step undertaken in water quality surveillance. The purpose of sanitary inspection is to identify the potential sources of water contamination at water sources, treatment plants, water distribution system, and household containers and to take corrective actions accordingly. Potential sources of contamination may include pit latrine located near a dug well, leaks in water supply pipes, and contamination of unprotected springs by animals, etc.

**Table 7B.5:** Chemical parameters of drinking water.

| Characteristic | Requirement (acceptable limit) (mg/mL, maximum) |
|---|---|
| *Undesirable substances* | |
| Aluminum (Al) | 0.03 |
| Ammonia (N) | 0.5 |
| Barium (Ba) | 0.7 |
| Boron (B) | 0.5 |
| Chloride (Cl) | 250 |
| Copper (Cu) | 0.05 |
| Fluoride (F) | 1.0 |
| Iron (Fe) | 0.3 |
| Manganese (Mn) | 0.1 |
| Nitrate ($NO_3$) | 45 |
| Selenium (Se) | 0.01 |
| Sulfate ($SO_4$) | 200 |
| Sulfide ($H_2S$) | 0.05 |
| Zinc (Zn) | 5 |
| *Toxic substances* | |
| Arsenic (As) | 0.01 |
| Chromium (Cr) | 0.05 |
| Cadmium (Cd) | 0.003 |
| Lead (Pb) | 0.01 |
| Molybdenum (Mo) | 0.07 |
| Nickel (Ni) | 0.02 |
| Mercury (Hg) | 0.001 |
| Pesticides (µg/L) | |
| Aldrin/dieldrin | 0.03 |
| Beta-/delta-HCH | 0.04 |
| Chlorpyrifos | 30 |
| DDT | 1 |
| Endosulfan (alpha, beta, and sulfate) | 0.4 |
| Lindane | 2 |
| Malathion | 190 |
| Methyl parathion | 0.3 |

(DDT: dichlorodiphenyltrichloroethane; HCH: hexachlorocyclohexane)

## Collection of Water Samples

***Tap/pump:*** Firstly, any things attached to tap/pump should be removed and outlet to be cleaned with a dry and clean cloth and sterilize it using flame. After allowing the initial water to flow out for 1 minute, collect the sample in a sterile bottle.

***Well/storage tank:*** Sterile bottle attached to a string is lowered into the well/tank and immersed into it below the surface without disturbing the sediments. If there is delay (>6 hours) in transport to the laboratory for quality assessment, store the sample at 5°C.

## Feedback and Remedial Measures

Remedial measures should be taken based on the data collected through sanitary inspection and water quality assessment from collected samples. These remedial measures can be broadly classified as (a) environmental (i.e. control of land-use around sources or reducing pollution discharges), (b) engineering (i.e. design and construction of treatment plants), and educational interventions (i.e. proper purification, storage, and handling).

# WATER POLLUTION

Water pollution is defined as the contamination of water bodies such as surface water, groundwater, and marine water with toxic chemicals, radiological and biological agents in quantities that exceed what is naturally found in the water and may pose a threat to human health and/or the environment.

Water is polluted from various sources such as:
1. *Industry:* The effluents from industries and factories usually comprises of chemical and radiological pollutants that are discharged into surface water bodies such as lakes, rivers, etc.;
2. *Agriculture:* The residues of pesticides and fertilizers used in farming and agriculture sectors usually pollute the groundwater and surface water through monsoon runoff; and
3. *Human waste:* The sewage excreted from houses if not properly treated before disposing, can contaminate the water distribution system through leakage. Some places, they are directly discharged into drinking water reservoirs such as ponds, lakes, and rivers.

In order to prevent and control water pollution, removal of the toxic pollutants from industrial effluents through specialized treatment, usage of alternate nonchemical pest control methods in agriculture, and proper treatment and disposal of human excreta should be followed.

Under the water act (prevention and control of pollution) 1974, the central and state boards were formed to implement the policies and provide technical assistance regarding the prevention and control of water pollution, specifically with regard to maintaining and restoring wholesomeness of water in the country.

# WATER CONSERVATION

Water is a finite resource and cannot be replaced/duplicated. Only 2.7% of the water on earth is fresh. Rainfall is highly unevenly distributed over time and space in various parts of the country. Increased demand in coastal areas is threatening the freshwater aquifers with seawater intrusion. Therefore, it is very essential to conserve water in order to meet the inevitable emergency of shortage of drinking water in near future.

Government agencies and community should work together to fully utilize the monsoon rainwater and store it by creating new storage sites and renovating and repairing the existing water bodies.

Due to industrialization and urbanization, there is a continuous decrease in uncovered areas which in turn reduces the percolation of rain waters to the ground. In order to overcome this loss in recharge of groundwater, roof rainwater harvesting should be made mandatory through legislation in all public as well as private buildings particularly in urban and semiurban areas. In addition, there is a need to promote harvesting of rainwater in open fields located at both public and private premises **(Fig. 7B.10)**.

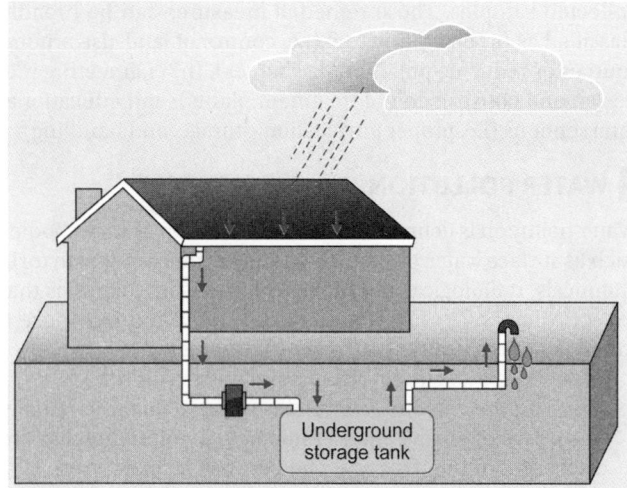

**Fig. 7B.10:** Rainwater harvesting.
*Source:* Hydroscapes. (1998). Rainwater harvesting. [online] Available from https://hydroscapespa.com/rainwater-harvesting.php.

Public campaigns should be conducted to create awareness about the necessity of water conservation and common tips can be shared with the people to save water at house, public, and industrial areas, etc.

Some of the common tips for domestic use are given here:
- Avoiding/minimizing use of shower/bath tub in bathroom
- Using smaller drinking glasses to avoid wastage
- Planting of native and/or drought tolerant grasses
- Washing vehicles less often, or using commercial car wash that recycles water.

Water is a scarce resource. It is everyone's responsibility to conserve water and minimize the wastage. For good health, water should be safe and wholesome without any contamination. All measures should be taken to prevent the pollution besides following various purification methods at household and community level to achieve the water quality standards.

## SUMMARY

- Drinking water should be safe, wholesome, free from pathogens and harmful chemicals.
- Diarrhea, hepatitis A, trachoma, schistosomiasis and malaria are some of the water related diseases.
- Surface water is more contaminated than ground water and it requires treatment before consumption.
- Water can be treated at household level using boiling, chlorination, filtration and reverse osmosis methods.
- Coagulation, flocculation, sedimentation, filtration and chlorination are the key techniques used for community based water treatment.
- Drinking water quality are assessed using criteria and standards based on physical, bacteriological and chemical parameters.
- Continuous surveillance of drinking water sources is essential to ensure the good water quality.

## SUGGESTED READING

1. Bradley D. Health aspects of water supplies in tropical countries. In: Feachem R, McGarry M, Mara D (Eds). Water, Wastes and Health in Hot Climates. Chichester: John Wiley and Sons; 1977. pp. 3-17.
2. Bureau of Indian Standards (BIS). (2012). Indian Standard Drinking Water—Specification (Second Revision).
3. Centers for Disease Control and Prevention (CDC). (2012). Ceramic filtration: Safe Water System.
4. Ministry of Drinking Water and Sanitation. (2011). Handbook on Drinking Water Treatment Technologies.
5. Ministry of Water Resources. (2005). General Guidelines for Water Audit and Water Conservation.
6. World Health Organization (WHO), United Nations International Children's Emergency Fund (UNICEF). (2017). Progress on Drinking Water, Sanitation and Hygiene: 2017 Update and SDG Baselines.
7. World Health Organization (WHO). (2011). Hardness in Drinking-water: Background document for development of WHO Guidelines for Drinking-water Quality.
8. World Health Organization (WHO). (2012). Considerations for Policy Development and Scaling-Up Household Water Treatment and Safe Storage with Communicable Disease Prevention Efforts.
9. World Health Organization (WHO). (2012). Rapid Assessment of Drinking-water Quality: A Handbook for Implementation.
10. World Health Organization (WHO). (2017). Guidelines for Drinking-water Quality: Fourth Edition.

# C. SANITATION AND HEALTH

*P Stalin, Velavan A, Anil J Purty*

**CM3.4** Describe the concept of solid waste, human excreta and sewage disposal

### Case Study

A mega temple festival is celebrated annually in Mayilam village located in Villupuram district of Tamil Nadu. During this occasion, thousands of people from nearby villages gather near the temple and do their rituals for seven days.
i. Enlist the preventive sanitation measures to be taken before the temple festival?
ii. What possible environmental hazards can happen in the absence of adequate preventive sanitation measures?

**Answers**
i. Adequate number of trench latrines, hand washing stations near food stalls and litter containers for garbage disposal should be established.
ii. Contamination of water sources with human excreta, emergence of breeding sites for vectors and street dog menace fed by garbage, etc.

## INTRODUCTION

*"Sanitation is more important than independence"*
—**Mahatma Gandhi**

One of the marked advances in public health, the "Great sanitary awakening" occurred in 19th century when filth was identified as both a cause and vehicle of transmission of disease. Edwin Chadwick, a lawyer from London and secretary of the "Poor law commission" in 1838 is a remarkable name in sanitary reform movement. His report on the sanitary conditions of the laboring population of Great Britain identified that "sanitation" has a key role in controlling diseases and recommended public health engineering measures such as construction of drainage networks is vital for the health of the population. Similarly "Report of the Massachusetts Sanitary Commission" by Lemuel Shattuck from United States published in 1850 identified cleanliness as a central component of social reforms. Thus, sanitation modified the way society thought about health and protecting health became a social responsibility.

Sanitation, hygiene, and safe water are essential elements for good health. "Sanitation refers to the provision of facilities and services for the safe disposal of human urine and feces and maintenance of hygienic conditions, through services such as garbage collection and wastewater disposal". Improved sanitation facilities refer to ensured methods of separation of human excreta from human contact. Providing a clean environment and disrupting the chain of transmission promotes the health of the community. Diarrheal diseases, cholera, typhoid, hepatitis A, and polio are transmitted mainly due to poor sanitation and it accounts for about 10% of the global burden of the disease.

## ACCESS TO SANITATION

- More than 35% of the global population have no access to improved sanitation.
- According to WHO and UNICEF statistics, South Asia (33%), sub-Saharan Africa (33%), and Eastern Asia (65%) had the lowest coverage of improved sanitation in 2006.
- About 7 out of 10 people in rural areas lacked access to improved sanitation.
- In India, about 594 million (approximately 50%) people practice open defecation and 44% of mothers dispose their children's feces in the open, which poses high-risk of contamination of water.
  - Improved sanitation facilities are available only to 31% of population while in rural areas, it is just 21%.
  - Public health association states that only 53% of population washes hands with soap after defecation and only 11% of rural families practice safe disposal of child's stool.
  - The WASH (Water, Sanitation and Hygiene) interventions like hand washing with soap and sanitation can reduce the morbidity due to diarrheal diseases by 44% and 36%, respectively.

(*Source:* UNICEF, Water Environment and Sanitation Report, 2018.)

## IMPACT OF SANITATION ON HEALTH

- In developing countries, every year about 801,000 children under 5 years die due to diarrheal diseases.
- Lack of water and sanitation facilities for hygiene, unsafe drinking water are responsible for about 88% of deaths due to diarrheal diseases.
- It also contributes to malnutrition in children.
- Many of the neglected tropical diseases (NTDs) such as trachoma, guinea worm disease, Buruli ulcer, and schistosomiasis are water and/or hygiene related and affects millions of population worldwide.
- More than 1 billion people are affected by soil transmitted helminths which is a result of inadequate sanitation.

Recognizing the importance of access to safe drinking water and sanitation, UN declared it as a human right and requested for international efforts to provide the same.

(*Source:* European Commission, Excreta Disposal—Emergency Sanitation, 2018.)

## TYPES OF WASTES

- ***Broad classification***:
  - *Controlled waste*: Wastes that are generated from households (municipal solid waste), commercials firms and industries, and from construction and demolition debris.
  - *Noncontrolled waste* includes agricultural waste and wastes generated from mines, quarries, and dredging operations.
- ***Based on their type and sources of generation***:
  - *Municipal solid wastes*: Solid wastes that are managed by any municipality/local administration which includes household garbage, rubbish materials, construction and demolition wastes, sanitation residues, etc.

- *Garbage:* Organic refuse resulting from the preparation of food, and decayed and spoiled food from any source.
- *Rubbish:* All inorganic refuse matter such as glass, paper, cloth or wood.
- *Sullage:* Domestic wastewater resulting from food preparation, personal washing, washing of cooking and eating utensils and clothes other than that which comes from toilet.
- *Sewage:* It includes human wastes (i.e. feces and urine) as well as wastewater from various sources.
- *Biomedical wastes*: Solid or liquid wastes which are generated either as intermediate or end products during diagnosis, treatment, and research activities of health sector.
- *Industrial wastes*: Solid and liquid wastes that are generated by various industries like petroleum, chemical, coal, etc. from their manufacturing and processing units.
- *Agricultural wastes*: Wastes that are generated from farming activities.
- *Fishery wastes*: Wastes generated from fishing industry.
- *Radioactive wastes*: Wastes which contain radioactive materials, usually produced as byproducts of nuclear processes.

- **Based on their property of disintegration**:
  - *Biodegradable wastes*: Wastes that get degraded (e.g. paper, wood, food, etc.)
  - *Nonbiodegradable wastes*: Wastes that do not get degraded (e.g. plastics, metals, etc.).

- **Based on their effect on environment and human health**:
  - *Hazardous wastes*: Wastes that are generated commercially, industrially, and agriculturally which are unsafe to environment or living being and have any of the properties like ignitability, corrosivity, reactivity, and toxicity.
  - *Nonhazardous wastes*: Wastes that do not pose any risk to environment or living being and do not have any of the above mentioned properties.

## SOLID WASTE MANAGEMENT

Urbanization has led to a multifaceted challenge to the environment management due to increase in population, industrialization, changing lifestyle, increasing economic activities, and introduction of newer technologies (e-wastes). The process of generation, collection, processing, transport, and disposal of waste is called waste management. It is important as it impacts on the health of the public as well as the environment. The main sources of solid wastes include domestic waste, commercial waste, street refuse, industrial waste, agricultural and animal waste, and mining waste.

### Impact of Solid Wastes on Environment and Health

Anything discarded by an individual, household, industrial firm, or an organization is considered as "waste". Hence, it is a complex mixture of substances and some of which are hazardous to health. Wastes, directly by itself and by the consequence of managing it, have the potential to affect health and environment. Poor management of waste has direct and indirect implications. Directly, it affects the environment leading to pollution of air, water, and soil and has long-term impact on health. Indirectly, it affects the growth and economy of a country. The following hazards are caused by inadequate management of solid wastes:

- Contamination of surface and groundwater supplies due to indiscriminate dumping of waste resulting in waterborne diseases.
- Clogging of drains and creating stagnant water which can be potential breeding sites for mosquitoes that can propagate malaria, filarial disease, dengue, etc.
- Generation of greenhouse gases from the decomposing organic wastes in landfills.
- Sanitary workers are at the risk of direct contact injury when there is co-disposal of medical and hazardous wastes along with municipal solid waste.
- Risk of fire arises from the heaps of garbage dumped especially from the smoke if the garbage has plastics and other chemicals.
- Air pollution is caused through persistent emissions of organic substances that pollute the environment and due to heavy metals.
- People living in the vicinity of sanitary landfills are at the risk of exposure to pollutants through inhalation, contact with polluted water or soil, and by consumption of contaminated products and water. Uncontrolled, illegal landfills are of great concern in this regard.
- Proximity to landfills and exposure to emissions from incinerator have been linked to health issues like cancer, congenital anomalies, low birth weight, and respiratory illness has been established through research.

### Methods of Waste Management

- ***Recycling***: The materials are recovered from products after their use by the consumers and subjected to recycling.
- ***Composting***: The process by which biodegradable organic matter is subjected to aerobic digestion.
- ***Sewage treatment***: Treatment of raw sewage water to produce a nontoxic effluent and a semisolid sludge. The effluent is discharged into seawater or river while the sludge is incinerated or disposed in landfill.
- ***Incineration***: The process of combustion of waste to reduce the volume and sent for disposal.
- ***Landfill***: It includes deposition of waste in a special designated area. Modern sites consist of a preconstructed "cell" lined with an impermeable layer and protective mechanism to minimize emissions.

The key advantages and disadvantages of individual methods are listed here in **Table 7C.1**.

### Solid Waste Management in Urban and Rural Areas (Fig. 7C.1)

#### Solid Waste Management in Urban Areas

Diverse kinds of waste materials are generated in urban areas and the major constituents are putrescible organic matter. The ideal arrangement for collection of solid waste in an urban area would be door to door collection by a team of waste handlers which is then sorted out to separate the hazardous and recyclable wastes.

## Chapter 7: Environment and Health

**Table 7C.1:** Waste management options—key advantages and disadvantages.

| Methods | Advantages | Disadvantages |
|---|---|---|
| Recycling | • Conservation of resources<br>• Supply of raw materials to industry<br>• Reduction of waste disposed to landfill and incineration | • Diverse range of processes<br>• Emissions from recycling process |
| Composting | • Reduction of waste to dispose to landfill and incineration<br>• Recovery of useful organic matter for use as soil amendment | • Bioaerosols: Organic dust containing bacteria or fungal spores<br>• Emits volatile organic compounds<br>• Potential pathway from use on land for contaminants to enter food chain |
| Sewage treatment | Safe disposal of human waste | Discharges may contain organic compounds, endocrine disrupting compounds, heavy metals, and pathogenic microorganisms |
| Incineration | • Protects sources of potable water supply<br>• Reduces weight and volume of waste | • Odor nuisance<br>• Produces hazardous solid waste |
| Landfill | Cheap disposal method | • Water pollution from leachate and runoff<br>• Air pollution from anaerobic decomposition of organic matter to produce methane, carbon dioxide, nitrogen, sulfur, and volatile organic compounds |

Sorting is done at household level, at municipal bin, central sorting facility, and at disposal sites. Proper storage of waste and educating people on this aspect are essential before giving it for collection. Waste should be collected on daily basis and can be stored in secondary waste storage depots before they are taken to the final disposal site. Final disposal is done by sanitary landfill, incineration, and composting depending on the availability of land, labor, and local conditions.

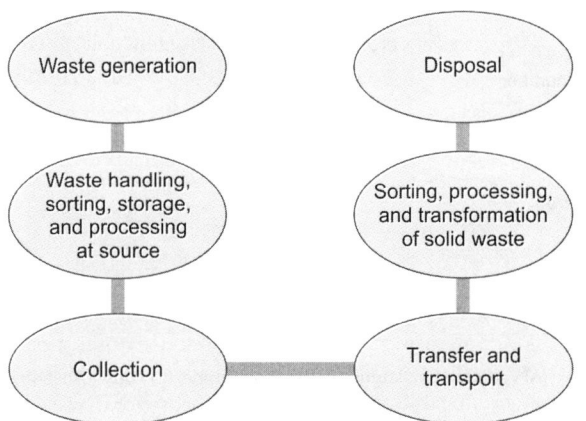

**Fig. 7C.1:** Waste management process.

### Solid Waste Management in Rural Areas

Wastes generated in rural areas are relatively lesser in quantity and predominantly organic matter from households and agricultural wastes. Since, there is no organized system of collection and disposal of wastes in rural areas, it is temporarily stored in pits and bins before final disposal outside the village by burning or dumping. The local self-governance or Panchayati Raj Institutions are responsible for the waste management in rural areas.

## EXCRETA DISPOSAL

### Community Health Importance

Safe disposal of excreta is an important element for prevention of contamination of environment, water, and food and thus, prevent spread of a wide range of feco-orally transmitted diseases. This barrier between excreta and the environment is known as the "sanitation barrier" **(Fig. 7C.2)**. Unsafe or inadequate disposal of excreta contaminate the soil and water sources and provide breeding sites for houseflies. Diseases such as diarrhea, dysentery, typhoid, cholera, hookworm, schistosomiasis, etc. are examples of feco-oral diseases. Lack of hygiene involving food and hands is a major cause of disease transmission even in places where facilities for safe disposal of excreta is available. Improvement in health is related not only to the availability of sanitation facilities but it should also address the social and cultural needs of the community at an affordable cost. Children less than 5 years, malnourished children, and elderly are at high-risk of acquiring diarrheal diseases.

### Open Defecation and Sanitation Practices

The Joint Monitoring Program by WHO and UNICEF estimated the safely managed sanitation services in 2015 and it was found that

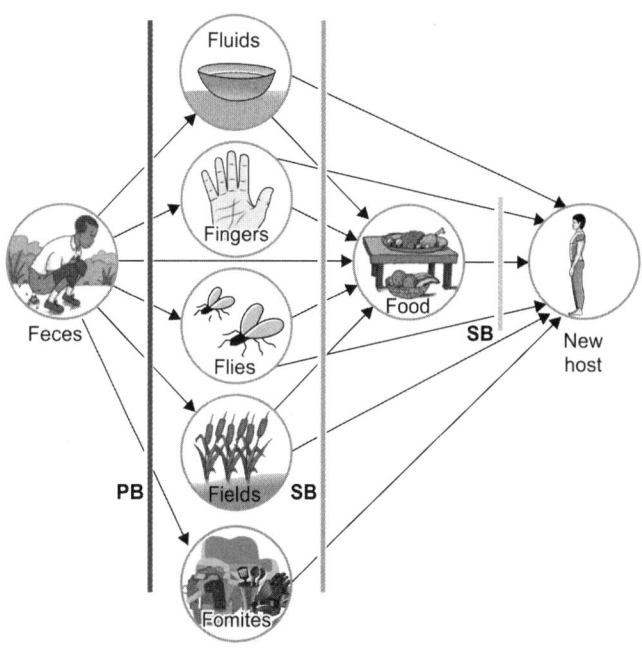

**Fig. 7C.2:** Transmission of disease from feces.
(PB: primary barrier; SB: secondary barrier)

## Section 1: Basics of Health and Disease

**Table 7C.2:** WHO/UNICEF JMP for WASH: Classification of sanitation services.

| Service level | Definition |
|---|---|
| Safely managed | Use of improved facilities that are not shared with other households and where excreta are safely disposed off in situ or transported and treated of site |
| Basic | Use of improved facilities that are not shared with other households |
| Limited | Use of improved facilities shared between two or more households |
| Unimproved | Use of pit latrines without a slab or platform, hanging latrines, or bucket latrines |
| Open defecation | Disposal of human wastes in fields, forests, bushes, open bodies of water, beaches or other open spaces, or with solid waste |

*Note:* Improved facilities include flush/pour flush to piped sewer systems, septic tanks or pit latrines, ventilated improved pit latrines, and composting toilets or pit latrines with slabs.

(JMP: Joint Monitoring Programme; UNICEF: United Nations International Children's Emergency Fund; WASH: water, sanitation, and hygiene; WHO: World Health Organization)

40% of the world's population used a *safely managed* sanitation service which includes safe disposal of excreta or treating it off site and 68% used at least a *basic* sanitation service **(Table 7C.2)**. However, 892 million people worldwide practiced open defecation and 2.3 billion people still lacked basic sanitation services.

## Methods of Excreta Disposal

### Unsewered Areas

- ***Service type latrines (conservancy system):***
  - Night soil is removed by a human agency using a bucket. Disposal may be done through dumping, composting, or burial by shallow trenching. This method is considered insanitary and undignified.
  - It was recommended by the Environmental Hygiene Committee, in 1949, that service type latrines must be replaced by sanitary latrines.
  - The founder of Sulabh International, Dr Bindeshwar Pathak, revolutionized the sewage disposal to eliminate human carriage of night soil and replacing them by low-cost sanitary latrines.

- ***Nonservice type (sanitary latrines):***
  - *Borehole latrine*: Most appropriate method in situations where large numbers are required to be constructed rapidly and where there is difficulty to excavate. It lasts for about 2 years for a small family.
  - *Dug well or pit latrine*: It is a cheap and quick way of constructing latrines wherein pits of 2 m depth is made and covered by a slab with a squat. It does not require water to operate.
  - *Water seal/pour flush-type of latrines*: It is a hygienic method of excreta disposal. It functions on the principle of a "water seal" where the water acts as a hygienic seal and helps remove excreta to a wet or dry disposal system. Pour flush latrines use a latrine pan with a shallow U-bend which retains the water (water seal). Different models were developed by Planning, Research and Action Institute (PRAI), Lucknow, Research-cum-Action (RCA) project of Ministry of Health, and Sulabh Shauchalaya.
  - *Septic tank*: Septic tank is final safe disposal system attached to different types latrines, but it itself is not actually a sanitary latrine. It is designed to collect and treat excreta from many water-seal latrines.
  - *Aqua privy*: Aqua privies are latrines constructed directly above a septic tank. They are appropriate in places where pit latrines are unacceptable **(Figs. 7C.3A to D)**.

- ***Latrine suitable for camps and temporary use:***
  - *Shallow trench latrine* **(Fig. 7C.4)**: Shallow (1-foot depth) and parallel trenches are dug with a gap of at least 60 cm between them and earth removed is used to cover the excreta by each user. Plastic sheets, bamboo mats are used as walls for privacy.
  - *Deep trench latrine* **(Fig. 7C.5)**: Trenches up to 6 m length and 2–3 m depth are dug providing six cubicles so that it is used by 100 people for few months.
  - Pit latrine
  - Borehole latrine.

### Sewered Areas

**Water carriage system and sewage treatment:** The human excreta and wastewater are carried away by a network of

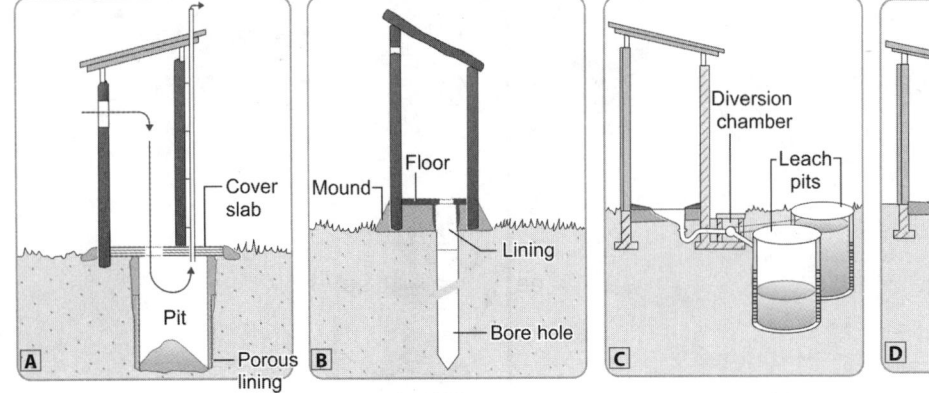

**Figs. 7C.3A to D:** Schematic diagram showing different types of latrines and septic tank: (A) Ventilated pit latrine; (B) Borehole latrine; (C) Pour flush latrine; (D) Septic tank.

*Source:* World Health Organization, IRC Water and Sanitation Centre. (2003). Linking technology choice with operation and maintenance in the context of community water supply and sanitation: A reference document for planners and project staff. [online] Available from https://www.who.int/water_sanitation_health/hygiene/ om/wsh9241562153.pdf.

# Chapter 7: Environment and Health

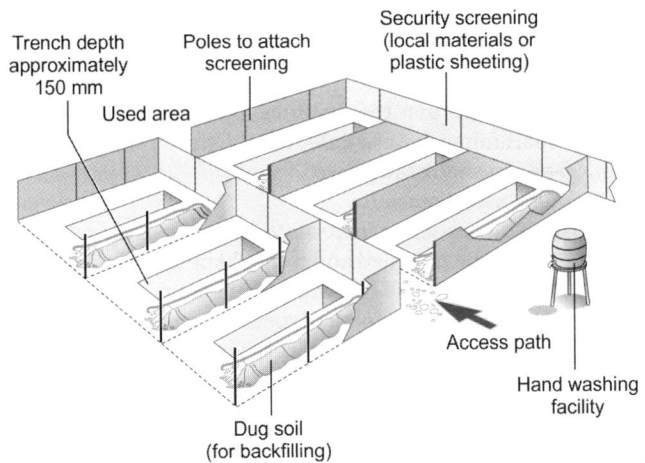

Fig. 7C.4: Shallow trench latrine.

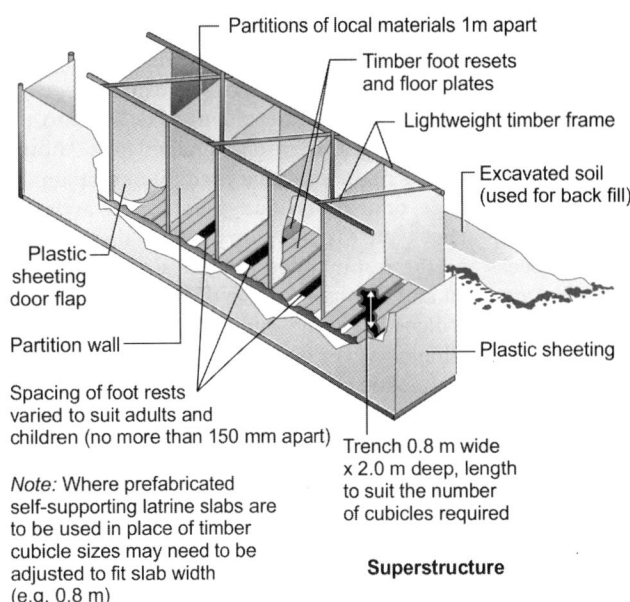

Fig. 7C.5: Deep trench latrine.

underground pipes called sewers to the ultimate disposal site. Laying down such a system is infrastructure and capital intensive. However, it is the ideal system of sewage disposal in large cities.

### Sewage Treatment Plant

Modern sewage treatment plants are based on biological principles of sewage purification, where the purification is brought about by the action of *anaerobic* and aerobic bacteria. **Figure 7C.6** shows the flow diagram of a modern sewage treatment plant.

The treatment of sewage may be divided into two stages:

***Primary treatment:*** The solids are separated from the sewage partly by screening and partly by sedimentation and subjected to anaerobic digestion which is the first stage in purification. The sewage spends about 6–8 hours in the tank. Nearly 50–70 % of the solids settle down under the influence of gravity and coliform organisms are reduced by 30 to 40 per cent. The organic matter which settles down is called *sludge* and is removed by mechanically operated devices, without disturbing the operation in the tank. While this is going on, a small amount of biological action also takes place in which the microorganisms present in the sewage attack complex organic solids and break them down into simpler soluble substances and ammonia. A certain amount of fat and grease rise to the surface to form scum which is removed from time to time and disposed of. When the sewage contains organic trade wastes, it is treated with chemicals such as lime, aluminum sulfate and ferrous sulfate. Addition of one of these chemicals precipitates the animal protein material quickly.

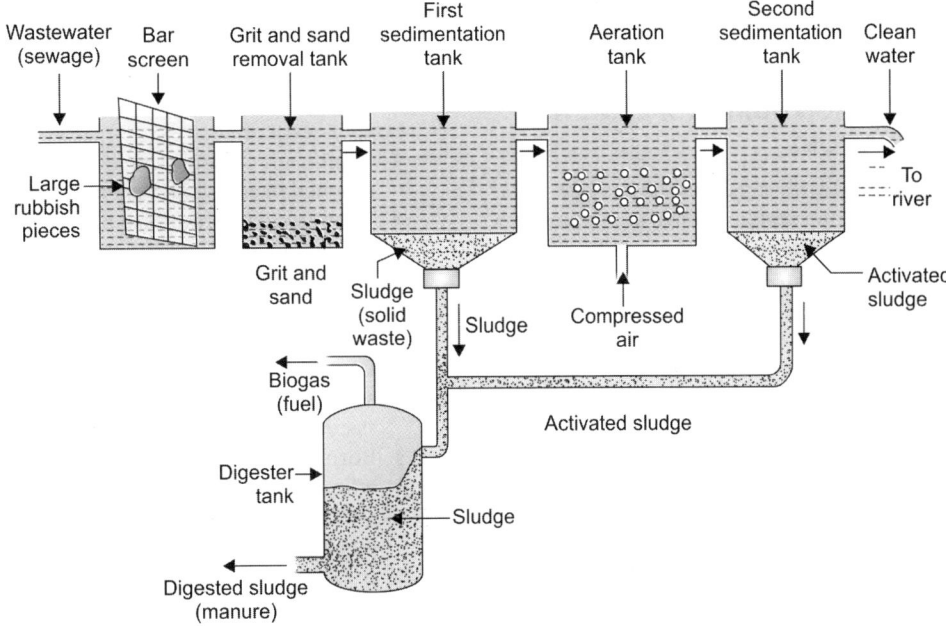

Fig. 7C.6: Sewage treatment plant.

*Secondary treatment:* The effluent is subjected to aerobic oxidation by trickling filter method or activated sludge process which is the second stage in purification. The oxidized sewage from the trickling filter or aeration chamber is led into the secondary sedimentation tank where it is detained for 2-3 hours. The sludge that collects in the secondary sedimentation tank is called 'aerated sludge' or activated sludge. Part of the activated sludge is pumped back into the "aeration tanks" in the activated sludge process and the rest pumped into the sludge digestion tanks for treatment and disposal. Sludge disposal can be done by anaerobic auto digestion in the sludge digester or by sea or land disposal. Methane gas is a by product of sludge digestion and can be used for heating and lighting purposes.

## SANITARY WASTE DISPOSAL

"Sanitary waste" refers to those wastes comprising of used diapers, napkins, tampons, condoms, incontinence sheets, sanitary towel, and any other similar waste.

In India, the problems related to sanitary waste disposal have become an important concern as the plastic component of the disposable sanitary napkins is not degradable and can cause environmental hazards. Lack of proper waste management services in many areas worsens the situation. Another issue regarding sanitary waste is its categorization as it is covered by both solid waste management rules and biomedical waste management rules. A study conducted in 2011, estimated that among the 335 million menstruating women, only 12% of them have access to disposable sanitary napkins.

### Sanitary Waste Disposal Methods

The Menstrual Hygiene Management (MHM) guidelines 2015 defines "safe disposal" as methods by which destruction of sanitary waste is done without human contact and with minimal environmental pollution while throwing away used cloth or other waste into field, pond, and river is termed as "unsafe disposal". Incinerators, deep burial, composting, and pit burning are some methods used for disposal of sanitary wastes.

## MANAGING SANITATION DURING SPECIAL AND EMERGENCY SITUATIONS

Disease outbreak associated with mass gatherings like fairs, festivals, and camps is a common problem which is encountered frequently. The festive organizers and the public health department have the responsibility to ensure safe provision of food, water, and toilet facilities at mass gatherings. In case of emergency situations like floods and other natural disasters, interventions should aim at preventing transmission of feco-oral diseases, contamination of water resources, development of breeding sites, etc.

- *Special event sanitation*: In case of fairs and festivals, proper planning should be done to ensure adequate number of toilets, hand washing stations and litter containers.
  - **Toilet and hand washing facilities:**
    - Adequate number required should be estimated based on previous year attendance
    - Hand washing junctions should be in conjunction with toilet facilities and provided with soaps and disposable towels
    - To ensure that the facilities are cleaned regularly, a maintenance schedule should be set and supplies replenished as required.
  - **Solid waste disposal:**
    - Adequate number of receptacles for garbage and refuse should be provided and it should be in close proximity to food stalls and high movement areas
    - As part of maintenance, specific schedules should be set up for emptying the garbage containers and this should be mentioned by the concerned authorities.
  - **Liquid waste disposal**:
    - Disposal of liquid waste from portable toilets, hand washing facilities, and food stalls should be done in an approved manner
    - For large events, sewage pump out truck should be available onsite to service the portable toilets when needed.
- *Sanitation in emergency situations*: Excreta disposal is a key element in any emergency sanitation program. Implementing agency should not only focus on the quantity of toilets but also on their quality and usage.
  - **Immediate measures**: These measures are designed for use in initial stages of emergency.
    - Clearing of scattered excreta after application of lime to a safe disposal site like pit with workers using appropriate personal protective tools
    - Controlled open defecation in initial stages in places where contamination of water resources is not possible
    - Constructing shallow trench latrines
    - Deep trench latrines are constructed during immediate stage of emergency if appropriate resources are available
    - Shallow family latrines are appropriate in certain situations where people are keen to have their own latrines.
  - **Longer-term measures:**
    - Simple pit latrines are the most common method adopted in emergency scenario
    - Deep trench latrines are the choice when communal latrines are to be constructed
    - A ventilated improved pit latrine (VIP latrine) is an improvised pit latrine with a vent pipe to remove odorous gases from the pit
    - Pour flush latrines which use water to act as a hygienic seal and help to remove excreta to a wet or dry disposal system
    - Borehole latrines are more appropriate in places where boring and drilling machines are readily available and large number of latrine needs to be constructed
    - In sites with existing sewerage system, toilet blocks can be directly constructed over them.

## TOTAL SANITATION CAMPAIGN OR NIRMAL BHARAT ABHIYAN

In the year 1999, Total Sanitation Campaign (TSC) was introduced by the Indian Government to improve sanitation coverage throughout the country, particularly in rural areas. It aimed at motivating rural households to construct low-cost toilet facilities and encouraging their use. It also focused on information and education to create public demand for sanitation facilities, especially in schools. Though the campaign achieved some progress, it suffered a setback due to lack of priority and its ineffective utilization of resources. It was renamed Nirmal Bharat Abhiyan (NBA) in 2012 and relaunched as Swachh Bharat Abhiyan in 2014. ***This is further explained in detail in Chapter 47: Health Policies and Programs in India.***

## SUMMARY

- Sanitation refers to the provision of facilities and services for the safe disposal of human urine and feces and maintenance of hygienic conditions, through services such as garbage collection and waste water disposal.
- Impact of inadequate management of solid waste includes contamination of ground and surface water, stagnation of water which forms breeding sites for vectors, generation of greenhouse gases from organic wastes, risk of fire from garbage heaps and posing of health risk to sanitary workers and people living in the vicinity of sanitary landfills.
- Recycling, composting, sewage treatment, incineration and landfill are some of the methods of solid waste management.
- Unsafe or inadequate disposal of excreta contaminate the soil and water sources resulting in feco-oral diseases.
- In unsewered areas, excreta disposal methods include use of bore hole latrine, pit latrine, water seal latrine, septic tank and aqua privy. In sewered areas excreta disposal is done through underground sewers.
- For camps and other temporary uses, shallow and deep trench latrines are used.
- "Sanitary waste" refers to those wastes comprising of used diapers, napkins, tampons, condoms, incontinence sheets, sanitary towel, and any other similar waste.

## SUGGESTED READING

1. Centers for Disease Control and Prevention (CDC). (2016). Global WASH Fast Facts.
2. Central Pollution Control Board. (2018). Guidelines for Management of Sanitary Waste: As per Solid Waste Management Rules, 2016.
3. ENVIS Centre on Hygiene, Sanitation, Sewage Treatment Systems and Technology. (2018). Nirmal Bharat Abhiyan.
4. Mara D, Lane J, Scott B, et al. Sanitation and health. PLoS Med. 2010;7(11):e1000363.
5. Ministry of Drinking Water and Sanitation. (2018). Swachh Bharat Mission—Gramin.
6. PwC. (2018). Waste Management in India: Shifting Gears.
7. Rushton L. Health hazards and waste management. Br Med Bull. 2003;68(1):183-97.
8. World Health Organization (WHO). (2015). Waste and human health: Evidence and needs.
9. World Health Organization (WHO). (2018). Sanitation.

# D. TEMPERATURE AND HEALTH

*Vinayak J Kempaller, G Rakesh Maiya, Shiny Chrism Queen Nesan*

## INTRODUCTION

Temperature variation poses a major, and largely unfamiliar, challenge which is all because of man made activities. Overall, temperature change can affect human health and lifestyle including biodiversity directly and indirectly through changes in the ranges of disease vectors, Ambient Air Quality, water-borne pathogens, water quality, and food availability and quality which leads to an unnotified, unrecognized mortality and morbidity and healthcare expenditure.

## EFFECTS OF HEAT AND COLD ON HEALTH

Let us now try to look at the spectrum of effects of temperature on health through **Flowcharts 7D.1 and 7D.2**.

## THERMAL COMFORT AND INDICES

Thermal comfort is a term used by the American Society of Heating, Refrigerating and Air-Conditioning Engineers, an international body. It is defined as "the state of mind in humans that expresses satisfaction with the surrounding environment" (ANSI/ASHRAE Standard 55). Maintaining this standard of thermal comfort for occupants of buildings or other enclosures is one of the important goals of HVAC (heating, ventilation, and air conditioning) design engineers. Thermal comfort is affected by heat conduction, convection, radiation, and evaporative heat loss. It is maintained when the heat generated by human metabolism can dissipate, thus maintaining thermal equilibrium with the surroundings. It has been long recognized that the sensation of feeling hot or cold is not just dependent on air temperature alone. The combination of high temperature and high relative humidity serves to reduce thermal comfort and indoor air quality. Thus, the thermal comfort is a criterion or a phenomenon that interferes with the metabolism, physiology and psychology of the human beings and it involves in creating an impact on their health as well as it affects the heat exchange between the human body and the external environment. It must be noted that the psychological parameters in terms of individual expectation and satisfaction also play a major role, that affects thermal comfort and human health. Management in thermal comfort will improve the morale and productivity among workers who work in extreme temperatures, which will in turn improve human health and safety.

The major factors which determine the heat illnesses are also known as 'indices of thermal comfort' or 'indices of heat stress'. These are as follows:

1. Ambient air temperature measured by dry bulb thermometer (DBT).
2. Relative humidity measured by both Wet bulb thermometer (WBT) and dry bulb thermometer (DBT).
3. Mean radiant temperature (MRT) measured by globe thermometer (GT).
4. Speed of air measured by anemometer or kata thermometer.

Based on the combination of these parameters, certain indices of environmental heat illnesses are developed. These are as follows:

**Thermal indices**
- Air temperature
- Air temperature and humidity
- Cooling power
- Effective temperature (ET)
- Corrected effective temperature (CET)
- Discomfort index (DI)
- Predicted four hourly sweat rate (P4SR)

**Flowchart 7D.1:** Effect of heat on health.

Effect of heat on health
- Rashes, heat cramps, heat edema, dehydration, heat syncope
- Heat stroke: Rise of body temperature above 105°F, associated with delirium, convulsions, coma and even death
- Worsening of pre-existing respiratory and cardiovascular complications; stroke; increased no. of hospitalizations

**Flowchart 7D.2:** Effect of cold on health.

Effect of cold on health
- Frostnip—involvement of ear lobes, nose tips, toes, and superficial layers
- Frostbite: Freezing of skin as well as of underlying tissues. Hands, feet and face are most commonly affected. Trench foot
- Hypothermia: Core temperature below 35°C or 95°F. Can be mild, moderate or severe
- Trench foot: It is caused by prolonged exposure to a cold temperature that is usually above freezing and damp

1. **Air temperature:** An index of thermal comfort, but later realized as an inadequate index.
2. **Air temperature and humidity:** Even this was found to be an unsatisfactory index to evaluate thermal comfort.
3. **Cooling power:** Air temperature, humidity and air movement were considered together and expressed as "cooling power" of the air. These indices along with mean radiant heat are used by Bulgarian standards to evaluate thermal comfort.
4. **Effective temperature (ET):** A combination of effect of temperature, humidity and air movement on a subjective feeling of warmth or cold felt by the human body at a given DBT of air, when RH is 100% and the air is almost still and humans are ordinarily clothed. The numerical value of effective temperature is that of the temperature of still, saturated air which will induce the same sensation of warmth or cold as that experienced in the given conditions.
5. **Corrected effective temperature (CET):** It deals with all the four factors namely, air temperature, humidity, velocity and mean radiant heat. CET is an index preferred for outdoor setting. CET value up to 27 degree Celsius is considered comfortable, 28 degree Celsius as very hot and above 30 degree Celsius in intolerable.
6. **Discomfort index (DI) (Oxford Index or Wet dry index):** It is based on DBT and WBT and calculated as DI (WD) = 0.85WBT + 0.15DBT. It is interpreted as <22 degree Celsius is comfortable, 22–24 degree Celsius is mild sensation of heat especially during physical work, 24–28 degree Celsius is moderate difficulty in doing physical work and >28 degree Celsius is high-risk of heat stress especially during physical work.
7. **Predicted four hourly sweat rate (P4SR):** The amount of sweat secreted which can be considered as allowable as a physiological normal reaction of acclimatized and fit individual when exposed to the heat for 4 hours. Three liters of sweat is considered as the upper limit of comfort zone, moderate heat stress when it is between 3 to 4.5 liters which can be just tolerable and severe heat stress when it is more than 4.5 liters and which is intolerable.

## EFFECTS OF HEAT STRESS AND ITS PREVENTION

Heat is a kind of energy. It is produced by endogenous or exogenous process like convection and radiation and heat loss occurs by convection, radiation and evaporation. It is influenced by environmental conditions like temperature, humidity, wind speed and body surface area. For proper working of the body, it is essential for maintaining the core temperature of the body within a small range of ±1°C over and below the core temperature of the body that is 37°C. Continual exchange of heat between environment and body is needed to achieve this. The amount of heat exchange and the rate at which it is exchanged is based on:
a. Total metabolic heat produced (ranges from 80 watts during rest to approximately 500 watts during moderate working).
b. Heat gained from the environment (Increase of 17.5 watt per increase of 1°C of environment).

> The amount of heat exchanged and the rate at which it happens is based on:
> - Total metabolic heat produced.
> - Heat gained from the environment.

The quantity of heat exchanged is primarily a role of sweat evaporation. Other forms are convection, conduction and radiation. Human beings feel comfortable when this exchange process is sufficiently supported by the surrounding thermal environment.

### Heat Stress

Due to climate change there is global warming which in turn is increasing the environmental temperature. This causes thermal discomfort and several issues related to heat such as heat stroke, heat exhaustion, heat cramps and heat rashes. All these together is grouped as effects of heat stress. It happens when the means of controlling internal temperature of the body fails. High radiant heat sources, air temperature, rigorous physical activity or high humidity have prominent chances for causing heat stress. At risk people are those who are directly exposed to the sun such as farmers, soldiers, athletes, travelers and people who work in open field. According to several studies done, insidious and chronic exposure to high temperature for longer periods can result in several health hazards. It affects human being's health directly thus reducing his working capacity and effect his socio-economic status and economic development.

Heat concern of workplace had come in the "4th Intergovernmental Panel on Climate Change (IPCC)"(2005-07). 5th report of assessment of IPCC (2013-15) suggested that if the warming levels are to be at 4°C then the cost of heat may cross 2 trillion USD globally by 2030 and also there might be a reduction of output globally by 20% by the 2nd half of the century. India recorded the maximum ever temperature in the month of May in 2016 in Phalodi, a town in Rajasthan (51°C). Increased vulnerability of workers in India to the changing climatic conditions have significant implications for organizations and policy makers.

The various heat related health issues are **(Table 7D.1)**:

> - "Heat Rash"
> - "Heat Cramps"
> - "Heat Exhaustion"
> - "Heat Stroke"

### Heat Rash

It is the most common health issue when working in hot environments. It is an irritation of skin due to excess sweating in humid and hot condition of weather. On examination it is a cluster of small blisters. Common place of occurrence is neck, upper chest, groin, elbow creases and under the breasts.

Providing cooler and less humid environment is the most appropriate treatment. It should be kept dry and to increase the comfort powder can be applied. Ointments and creams should not be applied on it. Proper care should be taken to prevent from skin getting warm or moisty as it worsens the rash.

**Table 7D.1:** Difference between signs, symptoms and treatments of heat exhaustion and heat stroke.

| Heat exhaustion/heat stroke | |
|---|---|
| Normal core body temperature –37°C or 98.6°F | |
| Heat exhaustion –38°C to 40°C or 100.4°F to 104°F | |
| Heat stroke ≥41°C or 105.8°F | |
| **Signs and symptoms** | |
| **Heat exhaustion** | **Heat stroke** |
| Listless | Reduced level of consciousness |
| Weak | Irritable |
| Dizzy | Muscular pain |
| Rapid pulse | Rapid pulse |
| Low blood pressure | High blood pressure |
| Nausea | Nausea |
| Vomiting | Vomiting |
| Mental status—Normal | Mental status—Confused |
| Behavior—Normal | Behavior—Irritated |
| | Hot, dry, red skin |
| | Death |
| **Treatment** | |
| Lay person down and elevate legs | Moving person to a cool and well-ventilated area |
| Ensure normal breathing | Checking for breathing, circulation and pulse |
| If thirsty give water to drink | If possible, covering the person with cold water or ice packs for reducing the temperature of the body |
| Get to hospital if needed | Give water to drink |
| Report the incident to the supervisor | Monitor vital signs |
| | Get person to hospital |
| | Report the incident to the supervisor |

## Heat Cramps

This is also due to excessive heat conditions in the environment. Due to loss of body fluid and salts due to sweating there will be muscle pains usually of legs and arms. It usually affects people who sweat a lot while doing strenuous work. It could also be an indication of heat exhaustion.

Every 15–20 minutes they should have water and/or electrolyte replacement liquids like ORS. Salt tablets should be avoided. The person should be taken to emergency room or clinic if he is suffering from heart problems or he is taking diet which is low in sodium or in-case even after an hour the cramps do not settle.

## Heat Exhaustion

It is the response of the body to an excessive loss of salt and water, mostly due to excessive sweating. Elderly people, people with raised blood pressure and people who do work in hot surroundings will be having higher chances of suffering from heat exhaustion. Headache, vomiting sensation, giddiness, weakness, irritability, thirstiness, excessive sweating, tachycardia, weak pulse, low blood pressure, decreased urine output and temperature of the body more than 100° Fahrenheit are considered as the symptoms and sign.

Treatment includes shifting the heat exhausted patients to a cooler area and giving them plenty of liquids. Cold compression to head, neck and face should be given to cool the person. Or the person is asked to rinse his/her neck, face and head with cold water. Unnecessary clothing including shoes and socks should be removed. Frequent sips of cool water should be encouraged. Person with signs and symptoms should be taken to emergency room or clinic for medical evaluation and treatment. It is advisable for someone to stay with the person until help arrives. Usually recovery is fast.

## Heat Stroke

It is the most grievous health illness due to excessive heat. Also called as heat hyperpyrexia. It is a medical emergency that can cause permanent disability or death of the person if treatment is not given immediately. Outstanding features are:

a. Absence of sweating
b. High body temperature.

It happens when there is a failure of body's temperature regulating system in hypothalamus because of which there is rapid increase in body's temperature along with sweating mechanism failure and as a consequence the body does not cool down. Within 10–15 minutes body temperature can raise to 106°F or more.

The signs are confusion, hot and dry skin, very high temperature, breathing is rapid and can become acidotic or Cheyne-Stokes type later, seizures and loss of consciousness.

The person should be taken to emergency room immediately. Meanwhile the person should be sprayed cool water and fanning should be done to circulate the air to speed cooling. Unnecessary clothing should be removed. He/she should be kept in a shady and cool area. Cold wet cloth or ice should be placed on the body or the clothing should be soaked using water which is cold. Thirst should be quenched by giving enough cold water.

## Heat Stress Indices

At the time of early 20th century there were numerous attempts to investigate the heat stress effect on productivity. But none could withstand criticism. Mackworth was the first to conduct genuine scientific studies on heat stress effects on human performance at the Medical Research Council (MRC), Applied Psychology unit located in Cambridge, followed by the study of Pepler at the MRC's Tropical Research unit located in Singapore.

There has been active research during 20th and 21st century regarding the conditions that will give rise to thermal comfort and regarding the grading of heat stress. The result of which was numerous theories trying to explain the thermal comfort. Apart from scientific merit, these studies were done to identify the safety levels and to enhance the productivity.

Heat stress index is an overall value which incorporates the effects of base line parametric quantity in any human thermal surroundings in such a way that its values will change with the thermic strain felt by the person. It is the measurement of stress put on human beings by raised grades of moisture and temperature. The more the heat index, one feels the hotter the weather, as the sweat does not evaporate readily and cools the skin.

Widely used heat indices are:
a. Wet Bulb Globe Temperature (WBGT)
b. Dry Bulb Thermometer

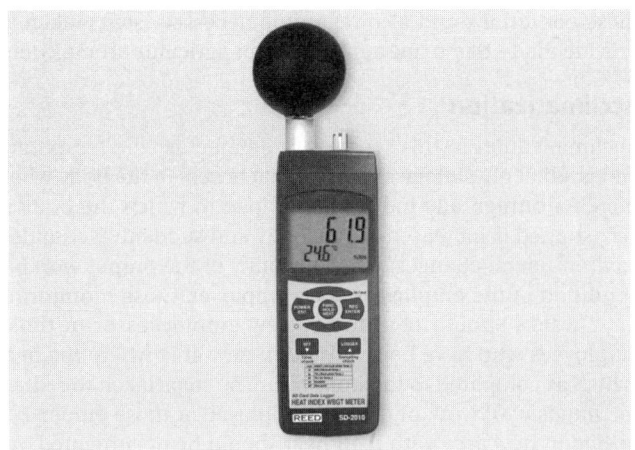

Fig. 7D.1: Wet bulb globe temperature.

c. Kata Thermometer
d. Heat Index (HI)
e. Humidex
f. Universal Thermal Climate Index (UTCI)

### Wet Bulb Globe Temperature (Fig. 7D.1)

It is considered as the most common method for assessing the work place heat stress. It is also used to advice sports organizations on the suitability of holding events or practice sessions during hot days. It was developed by Yaglou and Minard for controlling the outbreak of the heat illnesses among training camps of US Army and Marine Corps. In 1972, the "US National Institute for Occupational Safety and Health (NIOSH)" accepted this as the heat stress index for industrial use. It has been used widely for assessing occupational health risks, physiological impacts on work capacity and discomfort at different levels of metabolic rates. Threshold limit value has been given for exposure, alert and ceiling limits. These at given metabolic rates define what should be the proportion of working hours and rest time and they have been considered in the context of climate change. For heat radiation measurements WBGT introduced the global temperature Tg which measures effect of radiation and wind speed on man. It uses an instrument consisting of a black globe fitted with an internal temperature sensor. The Tg sensor considers the human body to be like the black globe which absorbs all the radiation.

WBGT (expressed in temperature units) is estimated as follows:

For indoor use, WBGT = 0.3 GT + 0.7 WB and
for outdoor use, WBGT = 0.2 GT + 0.7 WB + 0.1 DB

where WB = Natural wet bulb temperature; GT = Globe thermometer temperature (°C) whereas DB = Dry bulb temperature (°C).

### Dry Bulb Thermometer (Fig. 7D.2)

It is useful in measuring ambient air temperature.

### Kata Thermometer (Fig. 7D.3)

Used to measure air velocities less than 0.5 m/s.

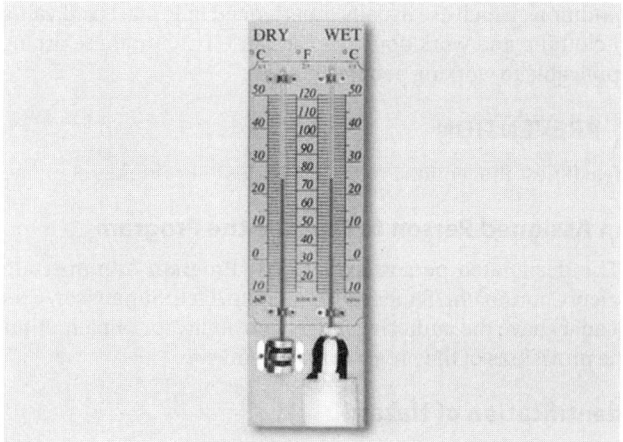

Fig. 7D.2: Dry bulb thermometer.

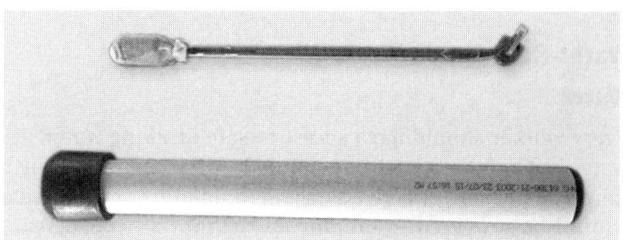

Fig. 7D.3: Kata thermometer.

### Heat Index

The heat index (HI) is an index that combines air temperature and relative humidity to posit a human-perceived equivalent temperature, as how hot it would feel if the humidity were some other value. The result is also known as the "felt air temperature", "apparent temperature", "real feel" or "feels like". For example, when the temperature is 32°C (90°F) with 70% relative humidity, the heat index is 41°C (106°F). Point of reference for ambient conditions is absolute humidity with dew point of 14°C.

### Humidex

Used in Canada for general public heat stress assessment. Temperature and water vapor is combined as one parameter to reflect the perceived temperature. It uses a dew point of 7°C as a base.

### Universal Thermal Climate Index (UCTI)

Developed in a European program that is Co-operation in Science and Technological Research (COST) Action. Around 730 working group aimed at preparing guidance for the public on heat and cold stress within the same index. Equivalent temperature is the main concept of UCTI and is based on energy balance equation. The results calculated based on the formula represent heat stress for indoor condition or in full shade outdoor condition. The advantage of UTCI is that it is based on the latest knowledge in the field of physics, biometeorology and physiology integrated together. UTCI- Fiala model has been validated in almost all terrains with extremes of temperature and humidity. Further, it was not validated at high humidity and high temperatures, the conditions which are usually experienced in India. Fixed values of clothing and work done are used in UTCI and these are not applicable to working people in India.

## PREVENTION

Heat Illness Prevention Program includes following key elements.

### An Assigned Person to Oversee the Program

"The designated person or persons (Program Administrator Safety Coordinator/Supervisor/Foreman/Field Supervisor/Crew Leader) have the authority and responsibility for implementing the provisions of the program at the worksite."

### Identification of Hazard

Heat-wave early warnings are designed to reduce the avoidable human health consequences from heat waves through timely notification of prevention measures to vulnerable populations.

### Water-Rest-Shade Message

#### Water

Every worker should have access to safe drinking water. The water level of the containers should be checked from time to time as a part of "Effective Replenishment Procedure". Water should be provided to employees without any cost. Water containers should be located at the proximity to the working place for encouraging frequent drinking. Bottled water or personal water containers should be made available, if the field terrain does not allow for water being placed in close proximity. Water should be placed in multiple locations if employees are employed across large areas. Sanitary condition should be maintained where water is kept.

The importance of drinking water and place where water coolers are placed should be reminded to the employees as and when possible every day.

#### Tailgate Meeting

When the temperature exceeds 80°F, employees should be gathered and told about prominence of drinking water, number and schedule of water and rest breaks and the signs and symptoms of heat stress.

Auditory devices like air horns or whistles should be used to remind worker to consume water. If the temperature ≥95°F, workers should be encouraged to consume lot of water and remind them of their right to take a rest and the number of water breaks should be increased. Supervisors should remind workers.

#### Shade

If the temperature is ≥80°F, shade structures should be kept as near as possible to the workers. Otherwise it should be given promptly as and when required.

Enough shade structures with ample amount of space without any adjustments should be available for all employees even during meal period. The employees are reminded of shade locations and should be encouraged to take rest break under shade regularly. If there is no feasible or safe area to provide shade a note should be made informing employees regarding these conditions and also regarding necessary steps taken to provide shade. Same rule applies for non-agricultural employers.

### Acclimatization

Acclimatization in this scenario is defined as "the temporary and gradual physiological change that occurs in the body when the environmentally induced heat load to which the body is accustomed is increased significantly and suddenly by sudden environmental changes." Responsibility of the proper working condition of the employees is on employer. Close monitoring for 2 weeks should be done of new employees or of those employees who have been posted in new area where the heat is high as compared to their old area. The steps taken to reduce the intensity of work of the new employee or those employees posted in new area with high heat should be documented. All the employees should be monitored closely during a heat wave and should be checked for signs and symptoms of heat illness.

### Modifying the Work Schedules

During a heat wave or heat spike, the workday should be cut short during heat wave and should be rescheduled or if not possible then should be ceased for the day.

### Training

Training should be given in the language that employees understand. A separate record should be maintained by the employer regarding the date and timing of the trainings, persons who attended trainings and the subjects covered. It should be given to supervisors and employees.

### Monitoring and Checking for Signs and Symptoms

Provision should be made for employees to contact supervisor whenever necessary. As it may not be possible for an employee in distress to call for help on his or her own, employees should be contacted at frequent intervals during the complete shift. In the absence of the supervisor an alternate designated person should be made responsible. Immediate actions should be taken based on the severity of the disease if any employee with heat illness or if any employee reports of symptoms of heat illness.

### Emergency Planning and Response

In order to avoid any delay of emergency medical services the employees and the foremen should be given a map of the jobsite containing clear directions. It is necessary to assign a qualified and trained person at the jobsite. Whenever an employee shows the symptoms of possible heat illness, he/she should be taken to cool place and made comfortable along with calling emergence service responders to ensure that the heat illness does not progress. These written emergency procedures are included in detail in the training of employees and supervisors.

### General Principles Applicable to Heat–Health Action Plan

- Using existing systems and linking them to general emergency response system
- Adopting a long-term approach

- Being broad
- Communicating effectively
- Ensuring that heat-wave responses does not increase the problem of climate change
- Evaluating.

### Core Elements of Heat-Health Action Plan

Eight core elements have been identified from the existing heat-health action plan that are most important for implementation of Heat-Health Action Plan successfully:
1. Agreeing for a lead body.
2. A heat-related health information plan regarding what communication given to whom.
3. Timely and accurate alert systems.
4. Special care of vulnerable population.
5. Medium and short-term strategies to reduce indoor heat exposure.
6. Staff training and planning, physical environment and appropriate health care to keep the health and social care system prepared.
7. Real-time surveillance and evaluation.
8. Long-term urban planning by addressing building design, energy and transport policies which will ultimately reduce the exposure to heat.

## COLD AND HEALTH

### Hypothermia

Hypothermia means the body temperature has fallen below 35°C or about 95°F, which is potentially fatal and serious condition. Hypothermia occurs infrequently in day-to-day life, accidents, extreme weather events, substance abuse, environmental, behavioral and individual risk factors and high-risk populations (homeless people, geriatric age group).

### Frost Nip and Frost Bite

These two conditions can physically damage bits of our body. Frost nip happens when part of our body becomes so cold that the blood flow slows because that area is losing too much heat and is starting to be sacrificed. The nose, ears, cheeks, fingers and toes are first one to get affected. It can by pale color as there is little or no blood circulation through it.

### Frost Bite

A serious situation where ice crystals form inside body cells killing them in the process. Superficial frostbite is manageable or recoverable, though can be intensely painful whereas deep frost bite can lead to the loss of fingers, toes and even parts of limbs.

*Immersion foot/trench foot*: It mainly occurs, when the feet are wet for long periods of time in conjunction with temperatures less than 10°C.

### Low Body Temperature Effects on Human Health (≤95°F/35°C)

The associations between exposure to cold conditions on human health are increasingly being shown by epidemiologic studies, data contributing to a wide range of public health outcomes.

It is a common documentation that especially among geriatric age group, known to have arthritis get worse in winter season. Signs and symptoms of joint stiffness, rheumatoid arthritis, osteoarthritis, are influenced by low temperatures. The impacts of temperature variations localized mainly to the smaller joints have shown to increase pain and stiffness at lower temperatures and get improved at higher temperatures. Exposure to cold can alter the human body and its physiological pathways in number of ways, while also interacting with pre-existing health conditions and communicable and non- communicable chronic diseases. On exposure to cold temperatures blood vessels becomes constricted, blood becomes more viscous leading to increase cardiac workload and ultimately to myocardial infarction. Increased amount of cardiovascular events with decreased temperature is found more among women than men.

Differences in geographical variations, general population health conditions, awareness toward temperature-related health outcomes and accessibility of health care, potentially contribute in concurrence and increase in the prevalence of these mortality and morbidities.

### Management of Cold Weather

Extra care to vulnerable population, wear layers of clothing, protection of extremities, respiratory tract protection, usage of insulating or heating materials that are touched, wind shelters, work place organization, places where cold or heat exposure can be interrupted, health communication on management of cold weather, and knowing the weather forecast and climate change before traveling to particular region.

## SUGGESTED READING

1. Allnutt MF, Allan JR. The effects of core temperature elevation and thermal sensation on performance. Ergonomics.1973;16:189-96.
2. Barnett AG, Dobson AJ, McElduff P, et al. Cold periods and coronary events: An analysis of populations world wide. J Epidemiol Community Health. 2005;59(7):551-7.
3. Biswas G, Bhattacharya A, Ali M, et al. Assessment of heat stress on open field workers at four Indian coastal stations. 2016;5(3):2998- 3003.
4. Center for Disease Control and Prevention (CDC). (2009). "Extreme Heat: A Prevention Guide to Promote Your Personal Health and Safety".
5. Dash SK, Dey S, Salunke P, et al. Comparative study of heat indices in India based on observed and model simulated data. Current World Environment.2017;12(3):504-20.
6. Department of Industrial Relation, State of California. (2018). Employer Sample Procedures for Heat Illness Prevention.
7. Environmental Health Perspectives. 2015;123(11).
8. Epstein Y, Moran DS. Thermal comfort and the heat stress indices. Industrial Health. 2006;44:388-98.
9. Net Zero Energy Building. Thermal comfort. Available at http://www.nzeb.in/knowledge-centre/passive-design/thermal-comfort/.
10. Parson K. Human thermal environments. 2nd edition. Taylor & Francis publisher;2003. pp258-92.
11. Shapiro Y, Epstein Y. Environmental physiology and indoor climate—thermoregulation and thermal comfort. Energy Build 1984;7:29-34.
12. Smedley J, Dick F, Sadhra S. Oxford handbook of occupational health. 2nd edition. Oxford: Oxford Medical Publications;2013. pp. 30-5.
13. World Health Organization. (2016). Ambient Air Quality and Health.
14. World Health Organization. HEAT–HEALTHACTIONPLANS.

# E. NOISE AND HEALTH

*NR Ramesh Masthi, Manasa AR*

**CM3.1** Describe the health hazards of air, noise, radiation

> A Dolby music truck used for festival celebration was parked near our house. The heavy dose of bass that blasted from the truck towards our house made me stressful, annoyed, and aggressive. Similarly, while attending a colleague's marriage in Bengaluru, the drums were beaten so loudly that it caused anxiety and momentary loss of hearing.

## INTRODUCTION

Noise pollution is an emerging public health problem worldwide including India. Rapid urbanization, migration, deforestation, and changing lifestyles have all contributed to the crisis of noise pollution. The magnitude of the problem is not known and epidemiological studies need to be undertaken to find out the prevalence in India.

## DEFINITION

Any sound that is undesired or interferes with one's hearing of something is noise.

## CAUSES

Noise pollution can be categorized based on:

### Environmental Causes

Sounds occurring naturally such as, lightning and thunderstorms, cyclones and tornadoes, landslides, earthquakes, volcanic eruptions, waterfalls and sounds produced by certain animals.

### Human Causes

**A list of human causes can be as follows:**

*Vehicular noise:* Bus, cars, trains, bikes, aircrafts, etc.
*Industrial noise:* Mining, heavy industries, office machines, etc.
*Commercialization of residential areas*: Garages, Crushing, Printing Press, Dyeing/Tinting machines, etc.
*Household noise:* Radio, television, instrumentation, kitchen noise like mixers and grinders, etc. and other noises like crying, shouting, scolding, etc.
*Construction activities:* Flyovers, roads, apartments, etc.
*Events related to politics:* Election campaigns, protests, demonstrations, slogans, processions, and rallies.
*Hospitals:* Noise from oxygen cylinders, pulling of trolleys, wheelchairs, sounds from disinfection plants, loud talks among patients and relatives, noises due to announcements over speakers, grieving following death.
*Fireworks and other reasons:* Siren, theft alarms of vehicles, machines tools, air horn, megaphone, electrical equipment, etc.

## PROPERTIES OF NOISE

*Loudness or intensity*: Loudness or intensity depends upon the amplitude of the vibrations which initiated the noise. It is measured in decibels (dB). In a quiet environment, decibels in the range of 20 is whisper, 60 is normal conversation and at 80 the sound is considered physically painful.

*Frequency*: It is denoted as Hertz (Hz). The human ear can hear frequencies from about 20 to 20,000 Hz. The range of vibrations below 20 Hz are infra-audible and those above 20,000 Hz are ultrasonic.

## PERMISSIBLE EXPOSURE LIMIT

The Permissible Exposure Limit (PEL) for noise is **90 dBA**, measured as an eight-hour time-weighted average (TWA). Any noise in excess of this PEL is known to be harmful to human health **(Tables 7E.1 to 7E.3)**.

**Table 7E.1:** Permissible noise exposures.

| Duration in hours per day and allowable sound level in dBA | |
|---|---|
| Duration per day (hours) | Sound level (dBA, slow response) |
| 8 | 90 |
| 6 | 92 |
| 4 | 95 |
| 2 | 100 |
| 1 | 105 |
| ½ (30 minutes) | 110 |
| ¼ (15 minutes) | 115 |

**Table 7E.2:** Acceptable noise level.

| At various places | | Sound level (dB) |
|---|---|---|
| Residential | Bedroom | 25 |
| | Living room | 40 |
| Commercial | Office | 35–45 |
| | Conference | 40–45 |
| | Restaurants | 40–60 |
| Industrial | Workshop | 40–60 |
| | Laboratory | 40–50 |
| Educational | Classroom | 30–40 |
| | Library | 35–40 |
| Hospital | Wards | 20–35 |

**Table 7E.3:** Sound levels of some noises.

| Source of noise | Sound level (dB) |
|---|---|
| Whisper | 20 |
| Speech, 2–3 people | 73 |
| Speech on radio | 80 |
| Music on radio | 85 |
| Children shouting | 79 |
| Children crying | 80 |
| Vacuum cleaner | 76 |
| Piano | 86 |
| Jet take-off | 150 |

## INSTRUMENTS FOR NOISE MEASUREMENT

- Sound level meters **(Fig. 7E.1)**
- Noise dosimeters **(Fig. 7E.2)**
- *Auxiliary equipment:* For measuring non-steady noise exposures, such as, intermittent or impulse noise, an integrating sound level meter is most appropriate.

## METHODS FOR NOISE MEASUREMENT

*The survey method:* Easy to carry out, in the shortest possible time and with a limited number of measuring points.

*The engineering method:* Speech interference levels (SILs) can be calculated. Helps in noise abatement programs and estimation of the auditory and non-auditory effects of noise.

*The precision method:* Useful in complex situations, where thorough description of the noise problem is needed.

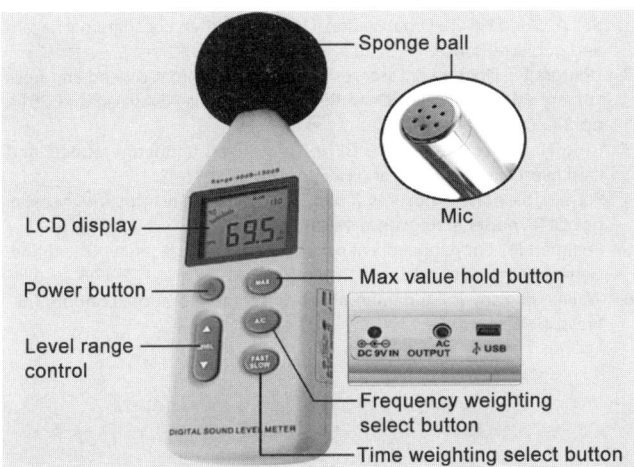

**Fig. 7E.1:** Sound level meters.
*Source:* Digital Sound level meter. Available from: https://www.gainexpress.com/products/slm-814cd-digital-sound-level-meter-decibel-logger-40-130db-usb-cd. [online].

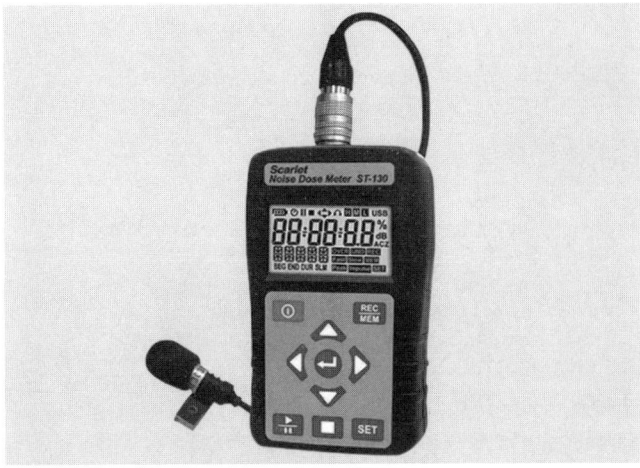

**Fig. 7E.2:** Noise dosimeter.
*Source:* Noise dosimeter. Available from: https://www.indiamart.com/proddetail/noise-dosimeter-17162750112.html. [online].

## TYPES OF NOISE EXPOSURE

- *Continuous noise:* The noise of boilers in a power house, ventilation fans.
- *Intermittent noise:* Observed in factories.
- *Impulse noise:* Due to gunfire and metal stamping.

## HEALTH EFFECTS OF NOISE

*Auditory effects* observed are Tinnitus, auditory fatigue and deafness/hearing loss. Auditory fatigue occurs at 90 dB/4000Hz. Two types of hearing loss are recognized: (1) Acoustic trauma: When the noise exposure exceeds 160 dB, the tympanic membrane can rupture and lead to permanent hearing loss and (2) Noise-induced hearing loss (NIHL). The NIHL may be either occupational hearing impairment or nonoccupational hearing impairment. When there is specific exposure to noise for long period of time, there can be temporary loss of hearing which lasts for 24 hours and then it is resolved. While, repeated exposure of noise above 100 dB can lead to damage to the structures of inner ear and can lead to permanent hearing loss.

*Nonauditory effects* Nonauditory effects like interference in day-to-day communication, annoyance, constant exposure to noise can lead to irritability and lack of concentration and reduced work efficiency. Exposure to high decibels of noise have been known to induce hypertension, vasoconstriction, and other cardiovascular diseases. Chronic noise exposure has also been linked with increased incidence of diabetes. Noise hinders sleep, thus causing insomnia. In the absence of adequate sleep, the person develops irritability, anger or neurosis. Excessive noise is also associated with decrease in the production of digestive juices. Exposure to noise of 180 decibels intensity or more may also result in death in humans. Due to loud velocity of sound, there are chances of abortion, intrauterine fetal death and developmental anomalies in newborns and infants.

## NOISE POLLUTION IN INDIA

Based on the recent findings of Central Pollution Control Board, the level of noise in the country was found to be the highest in Mumbai, followed by Lucknow, Hyderabad and Delhi.

In India, noise of more than 75 decibels (measured up to 1 meter distance from the source of the sound) is banned from 10 pm to 6 am. On violation of these rules, the convicted persons can face a fine of 1 lakh or a prison sentence for up to five years, under Sections 290 and 291 of the Indian Penal Code, under the Environment Protection Act, 1986.

## MEASURES TO CONTROL NOISE POLLUTION

### Preventive Measures

The individuals and industries should abide by the rules framed by the government relating to pollution control by establishing new industries away from residential or urban settlements, encouraging use of ear-plugs among industrial workers, installation of newer generation machines, regular maintenance of the silencers of vehicles. Similarly musical instruments and loudspeakers need to be periodically serviced. Motor engines and other machines that produce noise should be replaced with less noise producing machines. Vehicles producing loud noise should not be allowed in residential areas.

Changing the road surface, limiting the speed of vehicles, banning heavy duty vehicles, traffic control measures that reduce braking and acceleration, erecting noise barriers, and changing tyre pattern and tread design can curb roadway noise. The Supreme Court of India in October, 2018 has delivered a judgement on regulation and bursting of firecrackers during festivals. According to the judgement, firecrackers can be burst between 8 pm to 10 pm and in a few states, during the morning hours. All the above measures will lead to significant reduction in noise pollution.

### Remedial Measures

If prevention is not feasible, at least remedial steps should be taken to control noise pollution. These measures help in extenuating the damage to the environment due to noise pollution. Trees are good sound absorbers, hence noise pollution in the surrounding environment can be reduced by afforestation. Noise standard norms have been stipulated by the Ministry of Environment and Forests (MoEF) for usage of fireworks during celebrations, for example, prohibition of firecrackers that produce sound of 125 dB or more, up to four meters from the point of source.

Noise pollution produced by loudspeaker, marriage band, musical instruments, scooter, car, bus horns, disc jockey and public functions are banned from 10 pm to 6 am. Those not complying with these laws should be dealt with strictly.

### Awareness Building

It is important to create awareness among the general public regarding the causes of environmental noise pollution and its prevention. Awareness program covering the entire country needs to be conducted. Few commercial organizations and non-governmental organizations are taking up the responsibility of the development and maintenance of parks in urban areas. Prompt reporting of any incidence of the violations of the prescribed limits of sound should be done. The law-enforcement agencies should take stringent measures against all those willfully producing noise pollution.

## SUMMARY

Noise is defined as any unwanted sound. The sources are natural and human sources. The properties of sound are loudness and intensity. The sound is measured in decibels. Any sound above 90 dB for a period of more than eight hours is harmful. The health effects of noise are categorized into auditory and non-auditory effects. The measures to control noise pollution are preventive, remedial, and awareness building.

## SUGGESTED READING

1. Bell A, World Health Organization. (1966). Noise: an occupational hazard and public nuisance.
2. Dhingra PL, Dhingra S. Diseases of ear, nose & throat & head and neck surgery. 6th edition. New Delhi: Reed Elsevier India Private Limited; 2014. pp. 34-36.
3. Ising H, Babisch W, Kruppa B. Noise-induced endocrine effects and cardiovascular risk. Noise and Health. 1999;1(4):37-48.
4. Permissible noise exposures. [online]. Available from: https://www.osha.gov/SLTC/noisehearingconservation/pel.html.
5. Stellman JM. Encyclopaedia of occupational health & safety. 4th edition. Geneva: International Labour Organization; 1998. pp. 47.3-47.6.
6. Walker JR, Fahy F. Fundamentals of noise and vibration. London: CRC Press; 1998.

# F. LIGHT AND HEALTH

*NR Ramesh Masthi, Afraz Jahan*

> A worker in an ill-lit laboratory with inadequate natural lighting was finding it difficult to work throughout the day. An advertisement billboard with flashing colors was causing nuisance and disturbed sleep to residents

## INTRODUCTION

Light pollution, a consequence of industrialization, has become a serious issue facing humanity, the magnitude of which is still unknown. The major sources of light pollution include streetlights, building lighting, advertising, offices, factories, and illuminated sporting venues.

## LIGHT

Light refers to visible light responsible for the sense of sight. Wavelength of visible light ranges from of 400–700 nanometers (nm) and lies between the infrared rays (with longer wavelength) and the ultraviolet rays (with shorter wavelength).

### Types

Light can be classified into two types: (1) Natural light, and (2) artificial light.

### Natural Lighting

Natural light is from the Sun which can be distinguished into two types: *Sunlight*, direct ray of light and *Daylight*, scattered light reflected from the sky. Natural light constantly changes in terms of intensity, color, direction, focus, and efficacy, as it depends on the position of the Sun, seasonal weather patterns and various other factors.

Natural lighting can be improved by increasing the height of the windows to match that of the ceiling. This will improve the uniformity of indirect lighting. To avoid glare caused by over exposure of natural light, mechanical shading devices can be used.

### Artificial Lighting

Any light source produced by means of electricity is an artificial light. There are three types of artificial light:

1. ***Incandescence***: It is the visible radiations emitted when solids or liquids are heated to temperatures above 1000 kelvin.
   *Examples:* Incandescent lamps used for domestic purposes; halogen lamps used in automotive headlamps, spotlights and floodlights.
2. ***Electric discharge***: Radiations emitted due to excited atoms and molecules when an electric current is passed through a gas is electric discharge. Sodium and mercury are the common metals used.
   *Examples:* Mercury vapor lamps, fluorescent bulbs and tubes—used at homes and offices; metal halide lamps—used in parking lots, sports arenas, factories and retail stores; low pressure and high-pressure sodium lamps—used for industrial purposes and street lighting.
3. ***Light-emitting diodes (LEDs)***: Electric current is passed through the crystalline structure of a semiconductor material and electric energy is transformed to radiant energy.
   *Examples:* Exit signs, brake lights on automobiles, traffic signals, indicator lights and supplementary lighting.

> *Conditions required for visual comfort are* uniform lighting, no glare, sufficient contrast, acceptable colors.

### Units of Illumination

Light is measured by the following:

***Luminous flux:*** Luminous energy emitted per unit of time by a light source. Unit used to measure luminous flux is lumen (lm).

***Luminous intensity:*** Luminous flux emitted in a given direction by a light that is not equally distributed. Unit used to measure it is candela (cd).

***Level of illumination:*** Level of illumination of a source of one square meter when it receives a luminous flux of one lumen. Unit used to measure level of illumination is lux (=$lm/m^2$).

The recommended level of illumination for various activities have been described in **Figure 7F.1**.

## BIOLOGICAL EFFECTS OF LIGHT

Bright colors generate a comfortable and calm effect, while dark colors tend to generate depressing effect. The ultraviolet radiation in sunlight is the principal source of vitamin $D_3$ but overexposure is harmful as it is also a mutagen. Melatonin synthesis and normal circadian rhythm is maintained by exposure to light. It is also known to reduce the risk of seasonal affective disorder. Sunlight when uniformly distributed at home acts as a natural disinfectant. Ultraviolet rays and infrared rays have therapeutic uses.

## LIGHT POLLUTION

The International Dark-Sky Association (IDA) defines light pollution also known as photo pollution as "the inappropriate or excessive use of artificial lighting." Light pollution is increasing at the rate of 2.2% covering more and more of Earth's surface every year. Light pollution is an outcome of the excessive use of artificial light at night. This "loss of night" poses a significant health risk to humanity and is impinging on the habitat of nocturnal animals. India is losing its night more than three times faster than the global average. Between 2012 and 2016, India's area exposed to light pollution grew by three times.

### Types of Light Pollution

***Light Trespass***: Illumination by artificial light more than the intended area is known as light trespass.

***Light clutter:*** It is the excessive collection of a group of lights. This grouping of lights often causes confusion, distraction and

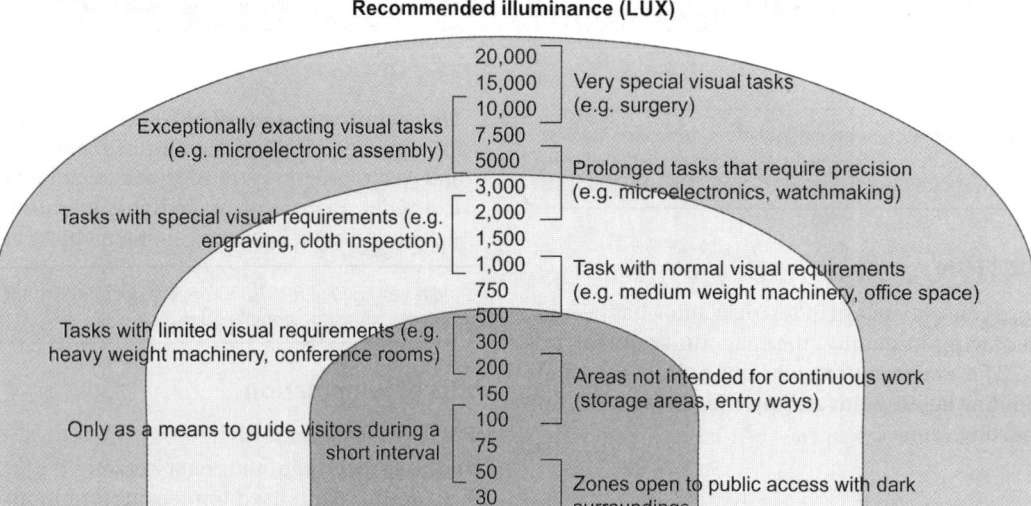

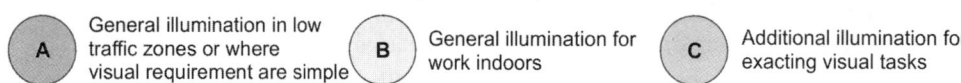

**Fig. 7F.1:** Levels of illumination as a function of task performed.
*Source:* Encyclopedia of occupational health and safety.

may potentially cause accidents. For example, Badly designed street lights, brightly lit advertising surrounds the roadways.

## Harmful Effects of Light

*Glare*: It is the effect produced when a radiant source of light is present in the visual field, resulting in reduced capacity to differentiate objects.
- ***Blinding glare***: It is the glare caused by gazing at the Sun. It leads to permanent or temporary visual defects like sunburn, snow blindness, and solar retinopathy.
- ***Disability glare***: This glare is caused by approaching car lights or scattering of light in fog. It considerably decreases contrast and visual capability causing momentary blindness leading to accidents.
- ***Discomfort glare***: This is a continuous exposure to a bright light source and can cause fatigue over extended periods.

Exposure to sun over a long period of time is harmful and associated with the skin aging, skin cancer, and immune suppression. Cataracts and macular degeneration are also a side effect of long-term exposure to sun. Long-term excessive use of computer/mobile screen can lead to eye fatigue, eyestrain, blurred vision, and headaches. Excessive use of smartphones or devices at bedtime can lead to delayed sleep or insomnia and disrupted circadian rhythm. People working in night shifts over extended period of time are prone to eye problems, insomnia, and other health hazards.

## Prevention of Light Pollution

Light pollution can be easily reduced by efficient use of lights. The following measures may be used to decrease light pollution. Direct illumination toward the ground to decrease light scatter, exchange high-wattage bulbs for dimmer ones and replacing halogen car lamps with traditional ones to prevent glare. Judicious use of lights at household level and avoidance of unnecessary lighting. Spreading awareness about light pollution, and its harmful effects to friends and family.

## SUMMARY

Light is referred to as visible light responsible for the sense of sight. There are two types of lighting: (1) Natural, and (2) artificial. Light pollution is defined as the inappropriate or excessive use of artificial lighting. It is of two types: (1) Light trespass, and (2) light clutter. Light pollution causes different kinds of health hazards, and unless preventive measures are taken, it can prove detrimental to health of people.

## SUGGESTED READING

1. BenyaJ, Heschong L, McGowan T, et al. Advanced lighting guidelines. Lighting Design Considerations. 2001.
2. Business Standard. (2017). Light pollution: India losing its night at over 3 times world average. [online]. Available from: https://www.business-standard.com/article/current-affairs/ light-pollution-india-losing-its-night-at-over-3-times-world- average-117120300415_1.html.
3. International Dark Sky Association. What is light pollution. (2018) [online]. Available from:http://www.darksky.org/light-pollution.
4. Kozeis N. Impact of computer use on children's vision. Hippokratia. 2009;13(4):230-1.
5. Lucas RM, Repacholi MH, McMichael AJ. Is the current public health message on UV exposure correct? Bull World Health Organ. 2006;84(6):485-91.
6. Mead MN. Benefits of sunlight: a bright spot for human health. Environ Health Perspect. 2008;116(4):A160-A167.
7. Sihota R, Tandon R. Parsons Diseases of the Eye, 22nd edition. New Delhi: Elsevier; 2015. p. 41.
8. Stellman JM. Lighting. Encyclopedia of occupational health and safety, 4th edition. Geneva: International Labor Organization; 1998. pp. 46.2-18.

# G. HEALTHY HOUSE AND SURROUNDING

*Sumanth MM, Praveen Kulkarni, Bhavani Nivetha*

**CM3.5** Describe the standards of housing and the effect of housing on health

## WHY YOU NEED TO KNOW ABOUT HOUSING?

We may think as doctors what is the need to know about house? It is just a physical structure in which we live, provides us place to rest. But, it is something more than that, it may be a nonliving object but it is something that comes to life when people live in it. So it is an emotional comfort which takes care of our psychological well-being, a physical structure that provides place to carry out our life with our family. It is something which will help in taking care of our basic needs like food, water, and livelihood. A good house will lead to a healthy and happy individual that leads to a healthy family which produces healthy community hence a healthy nation. Now, public health experts do not view house as just a physical structure, it is the place for us to intervene to ensure a healthy nation.

**Activity to be done:**
Visit few different types of houses in different setting (urban/rural/big/small kutcha/pucca, etc.), including your own and observe every part/aspect of house and reflect upon role of housing in health and disease.

## INTRODUCTION

World Health Organization (WHO) states that the quality of housing impacts health. The housing environment has a direct effect on the physical, mental, and social dimensions of health of the people living in it. We spend an estimated two-thirds of our life within the home and its immediate surroundings. Children, the elderly and the disabled or those with a chronic disease spent most of their time within their home. The term "Housing" encompasses various aspects like land, public facilities, access to employment, and to other services, as well as the structure itself, but not just that.

A WHO Expert Group (1961) prefers to use the term "Residential Environment" which is defined as the physical structure that man uses and the Environs of the structure including all necessary services, facilities, equipment and devices needed or desired for the physical and mental health and the social well-being of the family and the individual.

The health of each occupant is potentially at risk from an insanitary or otherwise unhealthy housing environment. One in six urban Indians lives in slum housing that is cramped, poorly ventilated, unclean, and "unfit for human habitation", according to the country's first complete census of its vast slum population. The United Nation Centre in Human Settlement (habitat) estimates that throughout World, over 1 billion people live in inadequate housing, with an excess of 100 million people living in conditions classified as homelessness. Hence, housing has been rightly included in Sustainable Development Goals on health (SDG 3) and sustainable cities (SDG 11).

> **Note**
> **Problem of housing**
> Nationwide, more than one-third of slum homes surveyed had no indoor toilets and 64% were not connected to sewerage systems. About half of the households lived in only one room or shared with another family. However, 70% had televisions and 64% had mobile phones (Rahman M, The Guardian, 2013).

## HEALTHFUL HOUSING

1. Should provide physical protection.
2. Should provide sanitary conditions for cooking, eating, washing, and excretory functions.
3. Should be designed, constructed, maintained, and used in such a manner that the spread of communicable diseases are prevented.
4. Should provide protection from hazards of exposure to noise and air pollution.
5. Should be free from unsafe physical arrangements (due to construction or maintenance) and toxic or harmful materials.
6. Should encourage personal and community development, promote social relationships, regard for ecological principles, and by these means should promote mental health.

### Factors Affecting Healthful Housing

- Per capita floor space
- Family income
- Family size and composition
- Standard of living
- Lifestyle
- Stage in lifecycle
- Education and cultural factors
- Cultural diversity
- Climate
- Social tradition.

## HOUSING STANDARDS

With the changing lifestyle and urbanization, the concept of housing is also changing. Housing is a broader concept now, it is no longer just concerned about the physical structure, it depends on a wide range of factors as mentioned above. So it is difficult to form a set of rigid uniform standards addressing all the aspects of housing. However minimum standards of housing is still maintained with a aim of trying to maintain at least a minimum set of standards in majority of the houses built. As there is cultural and regional variations, the standards also has to be formed varying with region to region.

The standards in India are those recommended by the Environmental Hygiene Committee (1947), which are as follows:
- **Site**:
  - It should be elevated from surroundings in order to protect from floodwater.
  - The site should independently open to a street of sufficient width. The street should not contain any breeding places

for mosquitoes and flies, and also free from nuisances such as dust, bad odor, smoke, noise, and traffic.
- It should have sufficient privacy.
- It should be in pleasing surroundings.
- The foundation for the site should be built upon the soil which is dry and safe. "Made-soil", i.e. ground that is formed by dumping refuse is not suitable for building purposes for 25 years. The water beneath the soil should be at least 10 feet from surface.

- *Set back*: Open space around the house is called "set back". It is to provide adequate lighting and ventilation without obstruction of air and light. In urban areas, the built-up area may be up to two-thirds of the total area.
- *Floor*: The floor should be of concrete or any other impermeable rat proof material (pucca) and satisfy the following criteria:
  - Can be easily washed and kept clean and dry. Mud floors are not recommended as it breaks up easily.
  - Free from cracks and crevices to prevent the breeding of insects and harborage of dust.
  - Should be damp-proof.
  - The height of the plinth should be 2–3 feet (0.6–1 meter).
- *Walls*:
  - The walls should have a low heat and transmittance capacity, i.e. should not absorb heat and conduct the same. It should have a minimum heat transmittance coefficient of 0–35 British Thermal units per square feet per hour per 1°F difference of temperature and the sound insulation value of external walls should be 55 dB and internal value should be 35–45 dB.
  - It should be smooth, easy to clean, weather resistant, not easily damaged, and unsuitable for the harborage of rats or vermins.
  - Should be raised sufficient to ensure privacy. These standards can be attained by 9-inch brick wall which is plastered smooth and colored cream or white.
- *Roof*: The height of the roof should not be less than 10 feet (3 m) in the absence of air-conditioning for comfort. The roof should have a low heat transmittance coefficient not more than 0–30.
- *Rooms*: There should be at least two living rooms. The number and area of rooms should be increased according to size of family, so that the recommended floor space per person is available.
  - *Floor area*: The living room should have a floor area of at least 120 sq ft, if it is to be occupied by more than one person and at least 100 sq ft for a single person. The floor area available in living rooms per person should never be less than 50 sq ft.
  - *Cubic space*: Unless means are provided for mechanical replacement of air the height of rooms should be such as to give an air space of at least 500 cubic feet per capita, preferably 1,000 cubic feet.
- *Windows*:
  - Each living room should have at least two windows, of which one should open directly into an open space. This norm can be relaxed if there is adequate ventilation and artificial lighting inside the room.
  - The windows should be placed at least at a height of more than 3 feet (1 m) above the ground in living rooms.
  - The area of the window should be one-fifth of the floor area. Total area of doors and windows should be two-fifth of the floor area.
- *Lighting*: The daylight factor should exceed 1% overhalf the floor area. The room is said to be adequately lighted, when one can read or write in the center of the hall without the help of artificial light during day time. But, the house should have sufficient artificial lighting in all parts to supplement natural lighting.
- *Kitchen*: Every house must have a separate kitchen. The kitchen must be protected against dust and smoke; away from the privy; should have adequate lighting; should have proper space for storing food, fuel, and provisions; clean fuel like LPG should be used, provision of exhaust in the form of chimneys, should have water supply and a sink for washing utensils and adequate drainage facility. The kitchen floor must be impervious.
- *Privy*: A sanitary privy is a necessity in every house; it should belong exclusively to it and readily accessible and equipped with water carriage systems or septic tanks.
- *Garbage and refuse*: Refuse should be collected by segregation as dry and wet waste in a container closed with a lid. These should be removed from the dwelling at least daily and disposed off in a sanitary manner.
- *Bathing and washing*: The house should have facilities for bathing and washing belonging exclusively to it fitted with proper privacy and drainage.
- *Water supply*: The house should have a safe and adequate water supply available at all times.

## Some Points for Rural Housing Standards

All the standards mentioned for urban housing should be applied for rural housing as well, certain standards are specially mentioned taking into consideration of rural environment, which is as follows:

- Two-roomed house on a dry site with separate access giving sufficient security
- It should have a separate kitchen with a paved platform for washing utensil and a sanitary privy
- Windows should form at least 10% of the floor area
- Separate and adequate accommodation for animals and implements associated with rural occupants
- The built up area should not exceed one-third of the total area in-order to ensure setback
- The source of water should be within a reach of 400 meters.

## PROBLEMS EXPERIENCED IN A POOR HOUSING

### Direct and Indirect Health Effects

- *Site*: It causes frequent flooding during disasters, noise and air pollution, unpleasant smell, accident, and thefts in poorly maintained areas.
- *Ventilation and lighting condition*: Poor ventilation and lighting causes accidents inside the household, poor sunlight penetration which cause both physiological and psychological distress, and darkness inside the house promote mosquito and rodent breeding which leads to communicable diseases.

- ***Floors***: Rodent breeding and dust collection causing communicable diseases like leptospirosis, dust collection in homes with children may lead to pica and hence worm infestations. If the cracks are little bigger there can be collection of water and vector breeding can occur.
- ***Walls***: Houses made with high quality materials throughout, including the floor, roof, and exterior walls, are called pucca houses. Houses made from mud, thatch, or other low-quality materials are called kutcha houses. Dampness in walls can cause unpleasant smell and fungal growth. It can also cause economic loss as damp walls tend to get destroyed soon. Cracks and crevices can serve as breeding or resting grounds for mosquitoes, flies, cockroach, sandfly, ticks, bugs which can lead to spread of diseases like, gastroenteritis, amoebiasis, malaria, dengue, etc.
- ***Roof***: Pucca houses are the safe and healthy option, kutcha and semi-pucca houses can cause various health implications, a thatched or tiled roof can cause leakage during rains, asbestos roofs increase the temperature inside the house during summers and can lead to heat exhaustion.
- ***Rooms and floor space***: Lack of adequate rooms and floor space leads to overcrowding. **Overcrowding** refers to the situation in which more people are living within a single dwelling than there is space for, so that movement is restricted, privacy compromised, hygiene impossible, rest and sleep difficult. Overcrowding can result in following health problems:
  - Diseases spread by transmission of infectious pathogens spread by droplet/or aerosols like tuberculosis, influenza, measles, and other respiratory infections.
  - The sharing of beds and close contacts of clothes among family members increase the risk of transmission of skin infections like scabies, etc.
  - It also affects psychosocial health leading to irritability, frustration, lack of sleep, anxiety, interpersonal violence, and mental disorders.
  - Adolescent girls and boys need privacy and in the absence of which their overall personality development may be affected. The accepted standards with respect to overcrowding are as described in **Table 7G.1**.

**Table 7G.1:** Grading of overcrowding.

| Based on person per room | Based on floor space area | Based on sex separation |
|---|---|---|
| Acceptable norm is—1 room—2 persons<br>2 rooms —3 persons<br>3 rooms—5 persons<br>4 rooms—7 persons<br>5 or more rooms—10 (additional 2 for each room) | Accepted standards are:<br>• 110 sq ft or more—2 persons<br>• 90–100 sq ft—1½ persons<br>• 70–90 sq ft—1 person<br>• 50–70 sq ft—½ person<br>• Under 50 sq ft—nil | Overcrowding is considered to exist if 2 persons over 9 years of age, not husband and wife, of opposite sexes are obliged to sleep in the same room |

*Note*: A baby under 12 months is not counted; children between 1 to 10 counted as half a unit.

- ***Kitchen***: The lack of proper storage of raw and cooked food can cause food poisoning outbreak in the family and pest infestations in the raw foods; improper disposal of waste can cause a bad odor and flies and mosquito breeding; Lack of clean fuel and exhaust contributes to indoor air pollution and predispose the individuals to chronic bronchitis and asthma.
- ***Toilets***: A sanitary latrine is a requirement in every house. Sanitary latrines are very effective in preventing diseases spread by water, soil, insects, and dirty hands. Provision of flush, either pour or cistern flush is important to effectively clean the toilet.
- ***Water supply***: Unsafe water can cause outbreak of water-borne diseases like cholera, amoebiasis, viral enteritis, bacterial diarrhea, and dysentery. Irregular supply of water causes individuals to store the water which can result in vector breeding. Access to water should be optimal. In many communities, access to water is a health risk. No access to water is when more than 1 km distance or more than 30 minutes of round trip is needed to bring water, and the quantity of water is less than 5 liters per capita per day. Basic access to water is when 20 liters per capita per day is available and it is within 1 km or less than 30 minutes of round trip.

## WHO HOUSING AND HEALTH GUIDELINES 2018

World Health Organization has recently released its Housing and Health guidelines. It summarizes the available evidence relating health to household crowding, low indoor air temperature and insulation, high indoor temperatures, injury hazards, and housing accessibility. This presents a roadmap for the future steps to be taken in healthy housing. A new addition is housing accessibility. As aging population increases globally with increasing life spans and reducing morbidities, accessibility to the house and its various sections will gain more prominence.

## GOVERNMENT POLICIES TO PROVIDE HOUSING FACILITIES

Government of India has been taking active steps to provide good housing conditions to all Indians. The Ministry of Housing and Urban Poverty alleviation, the Ministry of Housing and Urban Affairs, and the Ministry of Rural Development are mainly responsible for tackling the housing problem in the country.

Housing policies of the Government of India have come a long way since the 1950s **(Table 7G.2)**.

**Table 7G.2:** Housing policies of the Government of India.

| Phase I (1950–60s) | Phase II (Early 1970s–1980s) | Phase III (Mid 1980s–Early 2000s) | Phase IV (Early 2000s onward) |
|---|---|---|---|
| National building organization and housing boards at state level | National level Housing and Urban Development Corporation (HUDCO) in 1970 | Various 5 years plans to address all the aspects of housing and National Housing Bank | Indira Awas Yojana and Pradhan Mantri Awas Yojana |

### Phase I (1950–60s)—Mainly Focused on Housing for all and Slum Clearance

National Building Organization was created in 1954 to facilitate building construction activity. Town and Country Planning Organization came into existence in 1962 to facilitate spatial planning activities across the country. At the state level, various housing boards were created during the same period. The main objective of these housing boards was to take up housing activities for all the sections of society with a special focus on lower income groups.

### Phase II (Early 1970s–Mid 1980s)

With a vision of "controlled and well-directed growth" of the housing sector, the government created a national level Housing and Urban Development Corporation (HUDCO) in 1970. At its inception, HUDCO was envisaged as an institution which will work as the government's nodal agency in promoting "sustainable habitat development to enhance the quality of life".

### Phase III (Mid 1980s–Early 2000s)

In this period, the central government's focus shifted to facilitating the financing activities for housing rather than providing it physically on ground, as was the norm before. The Seventh Plan admitted that "The most crucial need for housing development…[is to establish] a proper and diversified institutional structure for housing finance…". To serve this purpose, the National Housing Bank (NHB) was created in 1987. Parallel to the creation of NHB, commercial banks and other housing finance institutions were directed by the government to participate on a larger scale in housing finance activities.

### Phase IV (Early 2000s Onwards)

By now, the government had comfortably placed itself in the role of facilitator of housing activities and has started looking for ways to attract private sector investment in this sector. Two main programs are working in this regard as described here.

#### *Indira Awaas Yojana and Pradhan Mantri Awas Yojana*

Indira Awaas Yojana was started as a part of rural employment scheme to provide housing for below poverty line people in 1984. Due to series of gaps identified in the implementation of IAY (Indira Awas Yojana) the government has restructured it into Pradhan Mantri Awas Yojana with an ambitious aim to provide "Housing for all" by 2022.

#### *Benefits in Pradhan Mantri Awas Yojana*

- *Urban*: Benefits through the following program verticals:
  - Slum rehabilitation of slum dwellers with participation of private developers using land as a resource with private participation for providing houses to eligible slum dwellers.
  - Promotion of affordable housing for weaker section through credit linked subsidy—beneficiaries of economically weaker section (EWS) and low income group (LIG) and middle income group (MIG) seeking housing loans from Banks, Housing Finance Companies and other such institutions would be eligible for an interest subsidy at the rate of 6.5% for tenure of 15 years or during tenure of loan whichever is lower.
  - For EWS/LIG groups beneficiaries should not own a pucca house anywhere and combined income of family unit should be less than 6 lakhs a year.
  - For MIG the beneficiaries should not own a pucca house anywhere and combined income of family should be less than 18 lakhs a year.
  - Affordable housing in partnership with public and private sectors—will provide financial assistance to EWS houses being built with different partnerships by States/UTs/Cities.
  - Subsidy for beneficiary-led individual house construction or enhancement—assistance to individual eligible families belonging to EWS categories to either construct new houses or enhance existing houses on their own to cover the beneficiaries, who are not able to take advantage of other components of the mission. Such families may avail central assistance of 1.50 lakhs.
- *Rural—Pradhan Mantri Awas Yojana Gramin*: The beneficiaries are eligible for a pucca house with basic amenities. The minimum size of the house has been increased to 25 sq m (from 20 sq m) with hygienic cooking space. Beneficiaries are those living without house or in a kutcha house, these beneficiaries are not based on below poverty line status but are segregated from socioeconomic and caste census of 2011 as it captures specific housing deprivations.

The toilet facilities for all these households are addressed through Swachh Bharat Abhiyan programs.

---

**Some case studies revealing impacts of healthy housing**

*Housing, insulation, and health study in New Zealand*
Collected information on the standard of 1,350 houses across New Zealand and the health of the occupants. Insulation was installed to the houses by random allocation and the results revealed that self-reported health improved significantly for people living in insulated houses.

*Housing and vector-borne disease control*
Housing improvements have been used as preventive strategies for vector-borne diseases such as Chagas disease, dengue fever, and leishmaniasis. In Latin America, infestation by vectors of Chagas disease has been mitigated through better plastering of walls, concrete floors, tiled roofs, and improved hygiene and sanitation.

*Healthy homes—des moines case study*
Reducing pediatric asthma through home improvements and education, $150,000 worth of repairs were completed, 42 homes were repaired, $17,000 in supplies were given to families and 6.2 more asthma-free days per month for children was achieved. They demonstrated the feasibility of implementing a housing initiative to impact a health outcome.

---

## SUGGESTED READING

1. Housing Act 1985. London: H.M.S.O.; 1986.ch.68.sec 324-26.
2. Planning Commission of India. (2010). Housing.
3. Pradhan Mantri Awas Yojana (scheme guideline). Ministry of Housing & Urban Poverty Alleviation Government of India. 2016. pp. 2-9.
4. Ranson RP. Guidelines for Healthy Housing. Copenhagen, Denmark: WHO Regional Office for Europe;1988.
5. Report of the Environmental Hygiene Committee. Shimla: Government of India press; 2018.
6. Tiwari P, J Rao. (2016). Housing Markets and Housing Policies in India. ADBI Working Paper. Tokyo: Asian Development Bank Institute.
7. UN HABITAT. UN Habitat's Global reports on Human settlements. (2011).
8. World Health Organization. (2018). Case studies of healthy, sustainable housing.
9. World Health Organization. (2018). Housing and health.
10. World Health Organization. (2018). The Build Health Challenge.

# H. MEDICAL ENTOMOLOGY

*Ipsa Mohapatra*

CM3.6 Describe the role of vectors in the causation of diseases
CM3.7 Identify and describe the identifying features and life cycles of vectors of Public Health importance and their control measures
CM3.8 Describe the mode of action, application cycle of commonly used insecticides and rodenticides

## INTRODUCTION

***Entomology:*** It is derived from two Greek words "ENTOMON" meaning insect and "LOGOS" meaning study. It is the "branch of science dealing with study of insects". It is a science that deals with the study of arthropods in general, and incorporates sciences like zoology, biology, parasitology and microbiology.

***Medical Entomology***: This is a branch of entomology which deals with arthropods which affect the health and well-being of man and vertebrate animals. In other words, medical entomology is the medical science directly concerned with vectors that affect human and animal health.

The name **Arthropoda** is derived from two Greek words: "*Arthro*" means jointed and "*Poda*" means legs. Arthropods are invertebrate animals with jointed-legs and identified by their peculiar characteristics, presence of chitinous exoskeleton.

They affect human health—directly and indirectly.

Directly they are responsible for various conditions like, bites and stings by bees, wasps and ants can cause erythema, hemorrhage, wheals, urticaria or eczema; injury to stratum corneum by itch mites causes intense itching at night; flies cause myiasis.

Indirectly, arthropods act as vectors for transmission of communicable diseases like, malaria, filaria, dengue, JE, kala-azar, etc.

To control these diseases, we need to have knowledge about the lifecycle, habits, habitats and diseases transmitted by these vectors.

## ARTHROPODS OF MEDICAL IMPORTANCE

The arthropods of medical importance are given in **Table 7H.1**.

## ARTHROPOD BORNE DISEASES

Arthropods are responsible for transmission of innumerable diseases. Some of the important arthropod borne diseases is listed in **Table 7H.2** along with their vectors, causative organisms and reservoir hosts.

## CHARACTERISTICS OF ARTHROPOD

The distinctive features of the arthropods are given in **Table 7H.3**.

## PREVENTION AND CONTROL OF ARTHROPODS

The general principles include the following methods:
- Environmental control
- Chemical control
- Biological control

**Table 7H.1:** Arthropods of medical importance.

| Class insecta | Class arachnida | Class crustacea |
|---|---|---|
| 1. *Mosquitoes:*<br>➤ Anophelines<br>➤ Culicines (Culex and Aedes)<br>➤ Mansonia | 1. *Ticks:*<br>➤ Hard ticks<br>➤ Soft ticks | 1. *Cyclops* |
| 2. *Flies:*<br>➤ Houseflies<br>➤ Sandflies<br>➤ Tsetse flies<br>➤ Blackflies | 2. *Mites:*<br>➤ Trombiculid mite (Chiggers mite, Red bug)<br>➤ Itch mite<br>➤ House dust mite | |
| 3. *Human Lice:*<br>➤ Head and body<br>➤ Lice; crab lice | | |
| 4. *Fleas:*<br>➤ Rat fleas<br>➤ Sand' fleas | | |
| 5. *Reduviid bugs* | | |

**Table 7H.2:** Important arthropod borne diseases.

| Disease | Vector | Causal organism | Reservoir |
|---|---|---|---|
| **I. Mosquito borne diseases** | | | |
| Malaria | Anopheles species | Plasmodium species | Man |
| Filariasis | Culex quinquefasciatus Aedes niveus group Mansonoides species | W. bancrofti (nocturnal, periodic) | Man |
| | | W. bancrofti (diurnal sub-periodic) | Man |
| | | Brugia malayi | Man, primate |
| Chikungunya | Aedes species | Arbovirus group A | Man |
| Dengue fever and DHF | Aedes species | Arbovirus group B | Man |
| Yellow fever | Aedes species | Arbovirus group B | Man/monkeys |
| Japanese encephalitis | Culex vishnui group (C. tritaeniorhynchus) | Arbovirus group B | Mammals/birds |
| **II. Sandfly borne diseases** | | | |
| Leishmaniasis Visceral (Kala-azar) | Phlebotomus argentipes | Leishmania donovani | Man/mammals |
| Cutaneous (Oriental sore) | P. papatasi | L. tropica | Man/mammals |
| Espundia | P. sergenti | L. braziliensis | Man/mammals |
| Sandfly fever | P. sergenti, P. papatasi | Virus | Man |
| **III. Fly borne diseases** | | | |
| Bacillary dysentery | M. domestica | Shigella | Man |
| Amoebic dysentery | M. domestica | E. histolytica | Man |
| Gastroenteritis | M. domestica | Specific/nonspecific organisms | Man/animals |
| Typhoid | M. domestica | Salmonella typhi | Man |

*(Contd...)*

(Contd...)

| Disease | Vector | Causal organism | Reservoir |
|---|---|---|---|
| Paratyphoid | M. domestica | Paratyphoid A and B | Man |
| Cholera | M. domestica | Vibrio cholera | Man |
| Poliomyelitis | M. domestica | Virus | Man |
| Viral hepatitis (Type A) | M. domestica | Hepatitis A virus | Man |
| Trachoma | M. domestica | C. trachomatis | Man |
| Yaws | M. domestica | T. pertenue | Man |
| **IV. Rat Flea borne diseases** | | | |
| Plague (Bubonic) | Xenopsylla species | Yersinia pestis | Rodents |
| Endemic/Murine Typhus | Xenopsylla species | R. typhi | Rodents/domestic animal |
| Chiggerosis (Jigger) | Tungapenetrans (chigoe) | – | – |
| Dipylidium caninum | Ctenocephalides felis/canis | Dipylidium caninum | Dogs, cats, wild |
| Hymenolepis diminuta | X. cheopis/N. fasciatus | Hymenolepis diminuta | Carnivores |
| H. nana | X. cheopis/C. canis/Pulex irritans | H. nana | Rats, mice |
| **V. Louse borne diseases** | | | |
| Epidemic typhus | Pediculus humanus | R. prowazekii | Man |
| Epidemic relapsing fever | Pediculus humanus | Borrelia recurrentis | Man |
| Trench fever | Pediculus humanus | Bartonella quintana | Man/animals |
| Dermatitis | Pediculus humanus/capitis | Secondary organisms | Man |
| **VI. Tick borne diseases** | | | |
| Kyasanur forest disease (KFD) | Hard ticks species | Arbovirus group B | Monkeys/birds |
| Tick typhus | Hard ticks species | R. conorii | Dogs |
| Tularaemia | Hard ticks species | P. tularensis | Rabbits/rodents/cattle |
| Relapsing fever | Soft tick | B. duttoni | Rats |
| **VII. Mite borne diseases** | | | |
| Scrub typhus | L. deliense | Orientia tsutsugamushi | Rodents |
| Rickettsial pox | Liponyssoides sanguineus* | R. akari | Rodents* |
| Scabies | S. scabei | – | Man |
| **VIII. Cyclops transmitted diseases** | | | |
| Dracontiasis | Cyclops species | D. medinensis | Man |
| Fish tape worm | Cyclops species | D. latum | Fish |
| **IX. Reduviid bugs** | | | |
| Chagas disease | Reduviid/Cone-nosed | T. cruzi | Domestic animals/man |
| **X. Tsetse flies** | | | |
| Trypanosomiasis | Glossina species | T. gambiense and T. rhodesiense | Wild animals/cattle/man |

*It is a species of mite that infests Mus Musculus (house mouse). Causes 'rodent mite dermatitis'.

**Table 7H.3:** Characteristics of arthropods.

| Class | Body divisions | Legs | Antennae | Wings | Where found |
|---|---|---|---|---|---|
| Insecta | Head, thorax and abdomen | 3 pairs | 1 pair | 1 or 2 pairs, some are wingless | On land |
| Arachnida | Cephalothorax and abdomen (no differentiation in some) | 4 pairs | None | None | On land |
| Crustacea | Cephalothorax and abdomen | 5 pairs | 3 pairs | None | In water |

- Genetic control
- Others.

## Environmental Control

Is one of the best approaches for their control. Environmental manipulation is done by elimination (source reduction) of the specific breeding habitat, for example, drainage of marshy areas, destruction of burrow pits for controlling malaria; filling up of ditches; planned management of water supply with the provision of piped water; proper disposal of wastes; keeping the surroundings of the house clean, etc. Health education of the community, political support being the essential prerequisites.

## Chemical Control

Is one of the most effective and cost-efficient methods of vector control. There is availability of a wide range of insecticides of the organochlorine, organo-phosphorus and carbamate group. Due to the dangers of insecticidal resistance, coupled with environmental pollution, these should be used judiciously.

### Classification of Insecticides

Insecticides may be classified in many ways based on mode of entry, target stage, chemical composition and mode of action. However, the most common classification used is based on chemical composition. According to this classification, the insecticides are classified in the following categories as presented in **Flowchart 7H.1**.

### Natural insecticides

- *Pyrethrum:* Pyrethrum extract is obtained from the dried heads of the flower *Chrysanthemum cinerariaefolium* and contains the active ingredients pyrethrins I and II, constituting 1 to 2% of the total weight of the raw pyrethrum. Pyrethrum is characterized by rapid knockdown action on arthropods even when used in very low dilution. It is very unstable in light and air and has practically no residual effect. This makes repeated applications necessary. Pyrethrum is available as 2% extract, which needs 20 times dilution to make it 0.1% solution, which is actually used for spraying. Using a 0.4 mm or lower calibre nozzle, 50 to 100 mL of pyrethrum solution in kerosene oil is sprayed per 100 m$^3$ of space. Addition of an Organophosphorus insecticide to pyrethrum formulation is a common commercial practice for obtaining a better effect. It is one of the main insecticidal constituents in aerosol dispensers and also an insecticide of choice for ULV sprays. Pyrethrum is perhaps the most

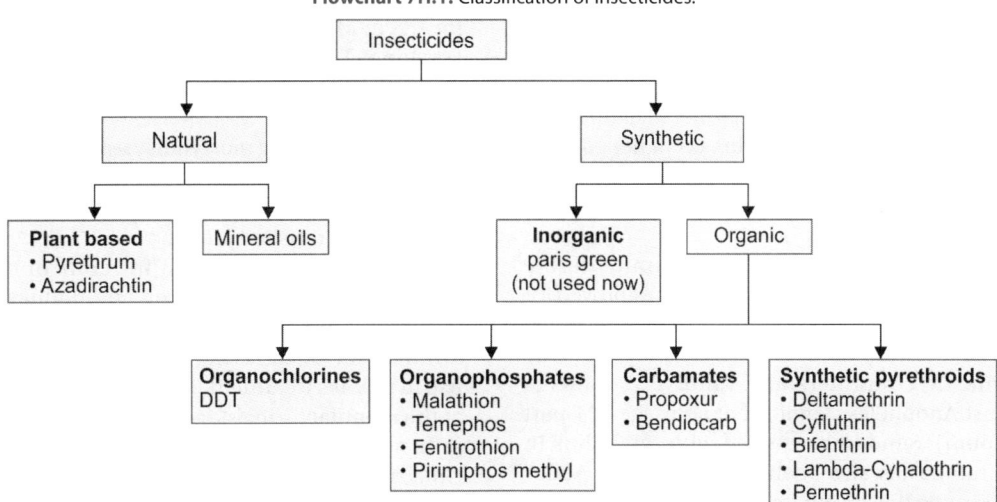

Flowchart 7H.1: Classification of insecticides.

acceptable insecticide for use in cook houses, dining halls and other food preparation areas.
- *Azadirachtin (Neem):* The active ingredient Azadirachtin is obtained from the seed of neem plant Azadirachta indica. It acts by inhibiting egg development, molting of larvae, antifeedant action, sterilizing action and also repellent action. It has been variously formulated for mosquito larval and adult control in the form of liquid and cream formulations. Neem products contain up to 3% Azadirachtin. It also used in shampoo for lice control.
- *Mineral oils:* Petroleum products such as kerosene oil, diesel oil, petrol, and crude engine oil have been used as mosquito larvicides for many years. These oils work by forming a film on the surface of water, which cuts off the air supply to the larvae. The oil can also enter and block the trachea of the larvae, act as a stomach poison, and lower the surface tension of the water, making it difficult for the larvae to float.
Malariol is a synthetic larvicide that is more effective and easier to use than petroleum products. Malariol is applied directly to water bodies at a rate of 10 liters per 500 linear meters. It is effective against both Anopheline and Culicine larvae, which are the two main types of mosquitoes that transmit malaria.

**Synthetic insecticides:** Mosquito larvicides can be organic or inorganic. The only inorganic compound that was used in vector control was Paris green, which is a copper-arsenite compound. Paris green acts as a stomach poison when ingested by mosquito larvae. However, it is no longer widely used due to its toxicity to humans and the environment. Organic mosquito larvicides fall into four major groups: organochlorines, organophosphates, carbamates, and synthetic pyrethroids. Organophosphates are a more recent group of insecticides that are generally more effective and less toxic than organochlorines.

Modern day synthetic insecticides are available in a variety of formulations, including emulsifiable concentrates (EC), suspension concentrates (SC), wettable powders (WP), aqueous suspensions (AS), emulsions in water, granules, water dispersible granules, water soluble granules, dust powders, aerosols, and poisonous baits. The choice of formulation depends on the specific application and the target pest.

- *Organochlorine compounds:* Organochlorine insecticides are contact poisons that act on the nervous system. They are stored in body fat and can be found in milk, urine, and sweat. They have variable residual action and are toxic to humans and animals. The most important organochlorine insecticide used in public health is DDT. DDT is currently used for indoor residual spray (IRS) in the North Eastern states of India only. A deposit of 1 g of DDT per square meter of wall and ceiling surface area up to a height of 3.5 meters in all dwellings, applied at 10–12-week intervals, effectively controls mosquitoes and other insects that rest on treated surfaces. The use of DDT in agriculture was withdrawn in India in 1989. It is now restricted for public health programs only, except in the North East where it is still used for IRS.
- *Organophosphorus compounds:* These are derivatives of phosphoric acid that act by inhibiting the activity of cholinesterase. This enzyme is responsible for breaking down acetylcholine, a neurotransmitter that is essential for nerve signalling. When cholinesterase is inhibited, acetylcholine builds up in the nervous system and causes overstimulation, leading to death of the insect. They are also relatively short-lived in the environment, which makes them less harmful to non-target organisms. However, organophosphate insecticides can be toxic to humans and animals if not used properly. Some of the most common organophosphate insecticides used in public health are malathion, temephos, fenthion, DDVP-2,2-dichlorovinyl dimethyl phosphate and fenoxycarb.

*Malathion* is one of the least toxic compounds in this class. It is a broad-spectrum insecticide, meaning that it is effective against a wide range of insects, including mosquitoes, houseflies, cockroaches, bedbugs, and lice. Malathion is available in a variety of formulations, including technical grade (95%), water dispersible powder (WDP), emulsifiable concentrate (EC), and dust. Malathion is used for a variety of purposes, including indoor residual spraying (IRS), ultra-low volume (ULV) spraying, and space spraying. IRS is the application of insecticide to the interior walls and ceilings of homes and other buildings to kill mosquitoes and other insects that rest on these surfaces. ULV spraying is the application of insecticide in very fine droplets that can stay suspended in the air for long periods of time. Space spraying is the application of insecticide in a mist to kill mosquitoes and other insects in the air.

The dosage of malathion used for IRS is 2 g/m². Malathion has also been used very widely during outbreaks of dengue and Japanese encephalitis (JE) as an anti-adult mosquito measure. However, resistance to malathion has been reported in a large number of vectors.

*Temephos (Abate)* is available as a 50% emulsifiable concentrate (EC). It is the only insecticide that is approved for use in potable water. Temephos is a low-toxicity insecticide that has been successfully used to control mosquito larvae in wells, domestic containers and sand. Temephos is effective against Anopheles stephensi at a dosage of 1 part per million (ppm). Sand impregnated with temephos in a 1% concentration has also been used to control Aedes aegypti, the mosquito that transmits dengue and yellow fever. Temephos has also been used to eradicate guinea worm disease in India.

> **Note**
> Fenthion, a larvicidal is now banned as per government rules.

- *Carbamates:* These compounds are derived from carbamic acid and resemble organophosphorus compounds in their mode of action. Some of the preparations produce a rapid knockdown effect like that of pyrethrum. The inhibition of Acetylcholine esterase is reversible with Carbamates and hence these compounds are less toxic. Some of the compounds in common use are Propoxur, Carbaryl and Bendiocarb.

  *Propoxur (Baygon/Blattanex)* is considered as the least toxic Carbamate compound for man and domestic animals. It has a flushing out effect and therefore is mostly used for cockroach and bedbug control. It is also used in bait formulations against houseflies and cockroaches.

  *Bendiocarb* is an alternative insecticide for IRS. It is available as 80% WP. For IRS, it is recommended @ 200 mg/m². Two rounds of spray are recommended for effective control against malaria.

- *Synthetic pyrethroids:* These are synthetic derivatives or analogues of natural Pyrethrum. These are broad spectrum, highly potent with quick knock down action and long residual life. Synthetic pyrethroids are many times more effective than the previously available insecticides. Their relative safety to man and higher animals, their efficient biodegradability together with their higher target specific toxicity makes them very attractive materials for integrated vector control. The commonly available products are Permethrin, Allethrin, Phenothrin, Cypermethrin, Cyfluthrin, Deltamethrin and Bifenthrin. Being broad spectrum, these insecticides are being used for vector control as residual spray, space spray and topical application as well as for treatment of clothing.

  *Deltamethrin* is one of the most widely used Synthetic pyrethroid molecule in the field of vector control. It is available in many formulations for various vector control strategies viz. SC 2.5% (Flow) formulation for treatment of bednet and routine household pest control activity; 2.5% WP formulation for IRS in Malathion resistant areas and 1.25 ULV for space spraying. The target dose (for Indoor Residual Spray) is generally 20 mg of a.i. (active ingredient) per square meter of surface area.

  *Cyfluthrin* is the next most widely used molecule. It is available as 0.5% EW formulation for treatment of bednets; 5% EC for household use and 10% WP for use as indoor residual spray in Malathion resistant areas.

  *Permethrin* is widely used for control of lice, scabies and for treatment of clothing and bednets. The product is formulated in varying concentration as Shampoo formulation for use as anti-lice treatment and 5% cream for use in scabies treatment. Bed nets treated with Permethrin at the manufacturing stage itself are available as Pretreated or Long-Lasting Nets (LLNs).

- *Other synthetic pyrethroids used in public health:* There is a large range of molecules used in the field of Public health besides the ones listed above. These molecules are Allethrin, Resmethrin, Phenothrin, Cypermethrin, Imiprothrin, Bifenthrin, Cyhalothrin, Cyphenothrin, etc. These are all available as WP, EC or Aerosol formulations for use against pests like cockroaches, houseflies and mosquitoes.

### Newer group of insecticides

- *Phenyl pyrazoles:* Fipronil is the only member of this class of insecticide. Fipronil acts by antagonizing the effect of GABA. It is available as 0.3% Gel for use against cockroach as a crack and crevice treatment. It is a systemic material with contact and stomach activity. It has a unique action called 'cascade effect' which is evident due to necrophagy seen in cockroaches. When cockroaches consume the insecticide bait, they are killed; these dead cockroaches when consumed by other cockroaches bring about the death of these cockroaches and this goes on for about two months or so, thus obviating the need to retreat the area at lesser intervals.

- *Neonicotinoids:* Imidacloprid is the sole member from this class. It acts by causing irreversible blockage of postsynaptic acetylcholine receptors. Imidacloprid is a systemic insecticide, having notable contact and stomach action. It is available as 2.15% Gel for use against cockroaches and as bait for use against houseflies, where it is formulated with housefly pheromone—Muscalure.

## Biological Control

Is given more emphasis to minimize the risks due to insecticides usage. The use of larvivorous fish especially *Gambusia* is well known in mosquito control. Fungi [e.g. genus *Coelomomyces*] are also known to be pathogenic to mosquitoes. Other biological agents (e.g. bacteria, fungi, nematodes, protozoa and viruses) are under research for their use.

## Genetic Control

Techniques of genetic control of mosquitoes, such as sterile male technique, cytoplasmic incompatibility and chromosomal translocations. New and innovative methods are being sought for pest control. These are: (a) insect growth regulators (b) chemosterilants, and (c) sex attractants or pheromones.

### Others

#### Personal Protection
Physical barriers between a vertebrate and arthropods, chemical barriers that repel arthropods from actual biting; and arthropod toxicants that are applied directly to or within a vertebrate, e.g. insecticide treated bed nets worldwide for the control of malaria and leishmaniasis.

#### Barrier Zones and Quarantines
An area free from certain vectors, either naturally or as a consequence of control programs, may need protection from invasion.

#### Integrated Vector Control Approach
Is preferred in the present trend for vector control; this approach combines two or more methods so as to obtain maximum results and also avoids the excessive use of any one method (thereby issues due to resistance are avoided).

## ARTHROPODS OF PUBLIC HEALTH IMPORTANCE

The phylum arthropoda consists of five classes, of which three are important in terms of public health aspects:
1. Class Insecta
2. Class Arachnida
3. Class Crustacea.

## CLASS INSECTA

### Mosquito
- **General description:** It is the most important group among insects, in aspects of human health, in disease transmission. The body of a mosquito consists of head, thorax and abdomen. *Anopheles* has various species. *A. culicifacies* is a vector in the rural areas of North, South and central India. *A. stephensi* is a vector in the urban areas. *A. minimus* is found in the NE states. *A. fluviatilis* along the foothills of the Himalayan range and in irrigation channels. *A. dirus* in the deep forests in the NE region, and *A. Sundaicus* in the Andaman and Nicobar islands.
  *Culex* are also called "nuisance mosquitoes". It has various species. Culex fatigans, causing bancroftian filariasis is found around dwellings. Culex vishnui group (*Culex tritaeniorhynchus, Culex vishnui* and *Culex pseudovishnui*) are the chief vectors of JE in different parts of India.
  *Aedes* distinguished by white stripes on a black body; also referred to as "tiger mosquitoes", because of the striped or banded character of their legs. Important among them being *Aedes aegypti, Aedes vittatus* and *Aedes albopictus*.
- **Life cycle of mosquito:** The mosquito passes through four distinct stages: egg, larvae, pupa and adult **(Figs. 7H.1 and 7H.2)**. Metamorphosis is complete.

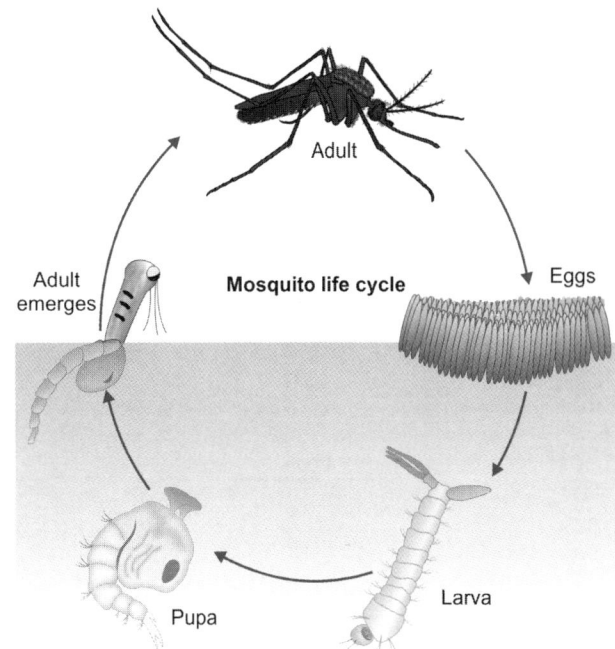

**Fig. 7H.1:** Life cycle of mosquito.

1. *Eggs*: Are laid on the surface of water, 100–250 at a time. Under favorable conditions, the egg stage of mosquitoes lasts for 1–2 days.
2. *Larvae*: Are free swimming creatures with an elongated body divisible into head, thorax and abdomen. It feeds on algae, bacteria and vegetable matter and passes through four stages of growth called "instars" with moulting between each stage. The larval stage occupies 5–7 days.
3. *Pupa*: Is comma-shaped in appearance, with a large rounded cephalothorax and a narrow abdomen. Two small respiratory tubes or trumpets project from the upper surface of the thorax. The pupa represents the resting stage in the life history of the mosquito; it does not feed but prefers to stay quiet at the water surface. When the pupa is disturbed it swims rapidly downwards. The pupal stage lasts for 1–2 days.
4. *Adult*: After development is complete, the pupal skin splits along the back and the adult mosquito or imago emerges. It rests for a while on the pupal skin to allow its wings to expand and harden and then flies away. Under favorable conditions of temperature and food supply the life cycle from the egg to adult is complete in 7–10 days. Normally, the adult mosquito lives for about 2 weeks. The males are generally short-lived.

- **Classification and characteristics:** The three important groups of mosquitoes in India which are related to disease transmission are the *Anopheles, Culex and Aedes* **(Table 7H.4)**.

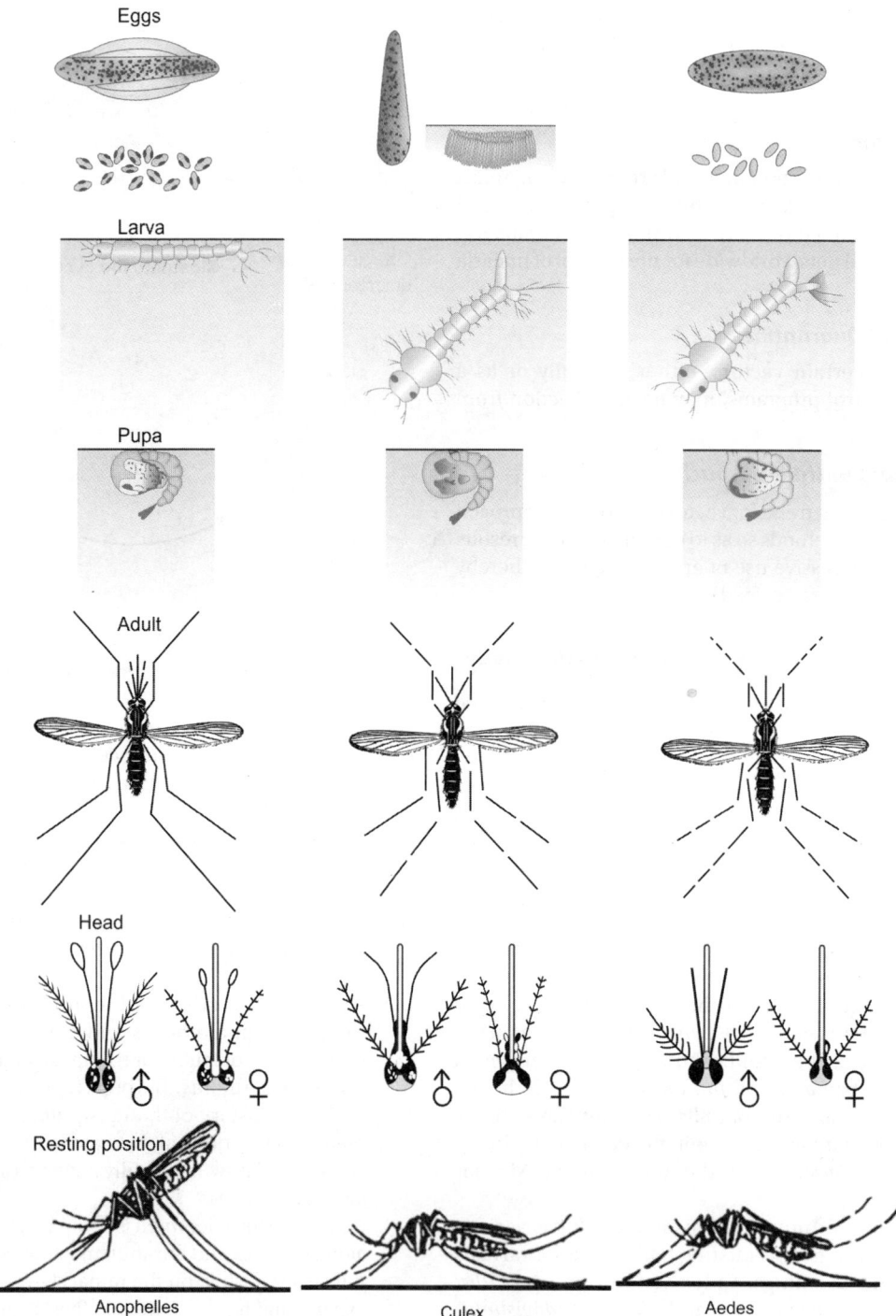

Fig. 7H.2: Identification of different types of mosquitoes and their larva.

## *Anopheles*

*Anopheles culicifacies* is the main vector of malaria. It is a small to medium sized mosquito; with around 45 species in India.

### Feeding habits
- It is both anthrophilic (human blood) and zoophilic (animal blood)
- Females are hematophagous, males live on plant juices
- When high densities build up relatively large numbers feed on men.

**Resting habits**: Rests during daytime in human dwellings and cattle sheds.

**Breeding places**: Breeds in rainwater pools and puddles, burrow pits, river bed pools, irrigation channels, seepages, rice fields, wells, pond margins, sluggish streams with sandy margins.

**Table 7H.4:** Differentiation between Anopheles, Culex and Aedes.

| Mosquito | Anopheles | Culex | Aedes |
|---|---|---|---|
| Eggs | • Eggs are laid singly<br>• The eggs are boat-shaped and possess lateral floats | • Eggs laid in small clusters or rafts<br>• The eggs do not possess lateral floats | • Eggs laid singly<br>• The eggs are cigar-shaped and do not possess lateral floats |
| Larvae | • Floats horizontally in the water<br>• Have no siphon tube at the tip of its abdomen<br>• Palmate hairs present on abdominal segments | • Are suspended in water with their heads downward<br>• Have siphon tube at the tip of its abdomen<br>• No palmate hairs | • Are suspended in water with their heads downward<br>• Have siphon tube at the tip of its abdomen<br>• No palmate hairs |
| Pupae | • Siphon tube is broad and short | • Siphon tube is long and narrow | • Siphon tube is long and narrow |
| Adult | • Wings spotted<br>• Palpi long in both species<br>• When at rest, inclined at an angle to surface | • Wings unspotted<br>• Palpi short in females<br>• When at rest, the body exhibits a hunch back | • Wings unspotted<br>• Palpi short in females<br>• When at rest, the body exhibits a hunch back |

- They prefer clean water for breeding
- Extensive breeding is generally encountered following monsoon rains.

**Biting time**: Biting time of each vector species is determined by its generic character but can be readily influenced by environmental conditions.

Most of the vectors, including *Anopheles culicifacies*, start biting soon after dusk. Therefore, biting starts much earlier in winter than in summer but the peak time varies from species to species.

**Dispersal**: Anopheles adult mosquitoes have an average flight range of 0.75–1.5 km.

**Life span:**
- On an average have a life span of 1 month
- Hibernating mosquitoes may live for six months or even longer.

## Culex

**Feeding habits:**
- Female sucks human blood (anthrophilic)
- They are principally cattle feeders, though human and pig feeding are also recorded in some areas.
- Vector is mainly exophagic (outdoor feeding)

**Resting habits:** These vectors are primarily outdoor resting in vegetation and other shaded places but in summer may also rest in indoors.

**Breeding places:**
- Breeds in association with human habitations and is the domestic pest mosquitoes, preferring polluted waters, such as sewage and sullage water collections including cesspools, cesspits, drains and septic tanks.
- In the absence of such type of water collections, they can breed in comparatively clean water collections also.
- *Culex vishnui* subgroup is found very commonly and breeds in water with luxuriant vegetation, mainly in paddy fields and the abundance is related to rice cultivation, shallow ditches and pools.

**Biting time:** Very active during dusk and night.

**Dispersal:** Flight range is one to three kilometers.

**Life span:** Average lifespan of 21 days.

### Aedes Aegypti

It is a small, black mosquito with white stripes and is approximately 5 mm in size. It takes about 7 to 8 days to develop the virus in its body and transmit the disease.

**Feeding habits:**
- Day biter
- Mainly feeds on human beings in domestic and peridomestic situations
- Bites repeatedly.

**Resting habits:**
- Rests in the domestic and peridomestic situations
- Rests in the dark corners of the houses, on hanging objects like clothes, umbrella, etc. or under the furniture.

**Breeding places:**
- *Aedes aegypti* mosquito breeds in any type of man-made containers or storage containers having even a small quantity of water
- Eggs of *Aedes aegypti* can live without water for more than one year.

**Biting time:**
- Bite throughout the day
- Vigorous in biting and can bite many persons.

**Dispersal**: Flight range is usually 400 meters.

## Medical Importance/Diseases Transmitted by Mosquito

The various mosquito borne-diseases are summarized in **Table 7H.2**.

## Application in Diseases Prevention and Control

The various methods of mosquito control may be classified as:
- *Anti-larval measures:*
  - Environmental control
  - Chemical control
  - Biological control.
- *Anti-adult measures:*
  - Residual sprays
  - Space sprays
  - Genetic control.

- *Protection against mosquito bites:*
  - Mosquito net
  - Screening
  - Repellents.

Integrated vector management under National Vector Borne Disease Control Program (NVBDCP) by insecticide residual spray, larvicides, by biological and environmental control is currently being used.

### Anti-larval Measures
- **Environmental control**: By eliminating their breeding places "source reduction". Their breeding places should be filled by appropriate engineering measures.
- **Chemical control**: The application of mineral oil like diesel oil, fuel oil, kerosene, various fractions of crude oils and special oils (e.g. mosquito larvicidal oil)—cuts off the air supply to the mosquito larvae and pupa. It has disadvantages like it needs weekly administration, renders water unfit for drinking and kills fish. Use chemical larvicides like abate in potable water.

  Paris green or copper acetoarsenite is an emerald green, microcrystalline powder practically insoluble in water and is a stomach poison; kills mainly the *Anopheles* larvae because they are surface-feeders.
- **Biological control**: Use of larvivorous fish—*Gambusia affinis* and *Lebister reticulates*—in ornamental tanks, fountains, etc.

### Anti-adult Measures
- **Residual sprays**: Use of indoor residual spray (IRS) with insecticides **(Table 7H.5)** recommended under the program, aerosol space spray during day time and malathion fogging during outbreaks.
- **Space sprays**: Are sprayed into the atmosphere in the form of a mist or fog to kill insects. The common space sprays are pyrethrum extract and malathion and fenitrothion for ultra low volume (ULV) fogging.
- **Genetic control**: Such as sterile male technique, cytoplasmic incompatibility, chromosomal translocations, sex distortion, and gene replacement are in research phase.

### Protection Against Mosquito Bites
- **Mosquito net**: Use of bed nets treated with insecticide. The size of the openings in the net should not exceed 0.0475 inch in diameter. The number of holes in one square inch is usually 150.
- **Screening**: Of the houses with wire mesh. Screening of buildings with copper or bronze gauze having 16 meshes to the inch is recommended. The aperture should not be larger than 0.0475 inch. Screening of buildings is costly but gives excellent results.

**Table 7H.5:** Insecticides used as residual spray applications.

| Insecticide | Dosage in g/sqm | Average duration of effectiveness (in months) |
|---|---|---|
| DDT | 1–2 | 6–12 |
| Lindane | 0.5 | 3 |
| Malathion | 2 | 3 |
| OMS-33 | 2 | 3 |

- **Repellents**: Effective are indalone, dimethyl phthalate, dimethyl carbate, ethyl hexanediol; Repellents are used mainly for application on the skin, and their chief advantage is quick application.
- **Personal prophylactic measures by individuals/communities**: Use of mosquito repellent creams, liquids, coils, mats, etc.; wearing clothes that cover maximum surface area of the body.

### Environmental Management
- Detection (coolers, flower vases, discarded tins, broken bottles, tyres, plastic containers, etc.) and elimination of mosquito breeding sources
- Management of roof tops, porticos and sunshades
- Proper covering of stored water
- Reliable water supply
- Observation of weekly dry day.

### Vector Surveillance in Case of Dengue Fever
- **Larval surveys:** For larval surveys, the basic sampling unit is the house or premise, which is systematically searched for water holding containers. Containers are examined for the presence of mosquito larvae and pupae. Depending on the objective of the survey, the search may be terminated as soon as *Aedes* larvae are found, or it may be continued until all containers have been examined. The collection of specimens for laboratory examination is necessary to confirm the species. Four indices that are commonly used to monitor *Aedes aegypti* infection levels are:
  - *House index (HI)*: Percentage of houses infested with larvae and/or pupae.
  - *Container index (CI)*: Percentage of water-holding containers infested with larvae or pupae.
  - *Breteau index (BI)*: Number of positive containers per 100 houses inspected.
  - *Pupa index (PI)*: Number of pupae per 100 houses inspected.

### Legislative Measures
Suitable laws and byelaws should be enacted and implemented for regulating storage/utilization of water by communities, various agencies and avoidance of mosquitogenic conditions at construction sites, factories.
- **Model civic byelaws**: Under this act fine/punishment is imparted, if breeding is detected. These measures are being strictly enforced by Mumbai, Navi Mumbai, Chandigarh and Delhi Municipal Corporations.
- **Building Construction Regulation Act**: Building byelaws should be made for appropriate overhead/under ground tanks, mosquito proof buildings, designs of sunshades, porticos, etc. for not allowing stagnation of water vis-a-vis breeding of mosquitoes. In Mumbai, prior to any construction activity, the owners/builders deposit a fee for controlling mosquitogenic conditions at site by the Municipal Corporation.
- **Environmental Health Act (HIA)**: Suitable byelaws should be made for the proper disposal/storage of junk, discarded tins, old tyres and other debris, which can withhold rain water.

- **Health Impact Assessments**: Appropriate legislation should be formulated for mandatory HIA prior to any development projects/major constructions.

### Health Education

Impart knowledge to common people regarding the disease and vector through various media sources like TV, radio, cinema slides, etc.

### Community Participation

Sensitizing and involving the community for detection of *Aedes* breeding places and their elimination.

> **Mansonides (mansonia mosquito)**
> - Mosquito is identified by speckled wings and legs
> - Breeds on aquatic plants *Pistia stratiotes*
> - *M. uniformis* and *M. annulifera* transmit *Brugia malayi* infection of filariasis in India
> - For control of vector, removal of *Pistia* plant is recommended.

> **Hibernation**
> Mosquitoes are known to hibernate in the adult stage when the environmental conditions are not favorable. Severe winters are tided over by hibernation.

> **Aedes aegypti index** is defined as "the ratio, expressed as percentage, between the number of houses in a limited well-defined area on the premises of which actual breeding of *Aedes aegypti* are found, and the total number of houses examined in that area". This index is kept at zero at all ports.

> **Note**
> **Remote sensing in vector control:** Remote sensing data acquired in the visible and infrared regions of the electromagnetic spectrum are sensitive to subtle differences in vegetation and water, so they provide a potential tool for surveying large areas to identify vector habitats and direct control measures and is
> - Likely to become a rapid epidemiological tool for surveillance of vector borne diseases
> - Coupled with Geographical Information System, it will play a key role in stratification of malarious area.

## House Flies

- *General description*: Belongs to order Diptera; have many species of which *Musca domestica* is most common. Adult fly is about 6-9 mm in length and has labile proboscis which can be retracted and projected. Has restless nature, is an intermittent feeder and vomits and defecates very often. Its indiscriminate feeding habits are highly conducive for spread of pathogenic organisms. They act as mechanical carriers and propagate disease germs on their hair, bristles, wings, footpads and proboscis. Fly can deposit its eggs on wounds and causes myiasis (infection with the larva of the fly).
- *Life cycle of fly* are egg, larva, pupa and adult **(Fig. 7H.3)**, with complete metamorphosis. Life span of adult fly is 15-25 days.
- *Medical importance/diseases transmitted by house flies:* Flies act as vectors in mechanical transmission of many diseases (refer **Table 7H.2**).

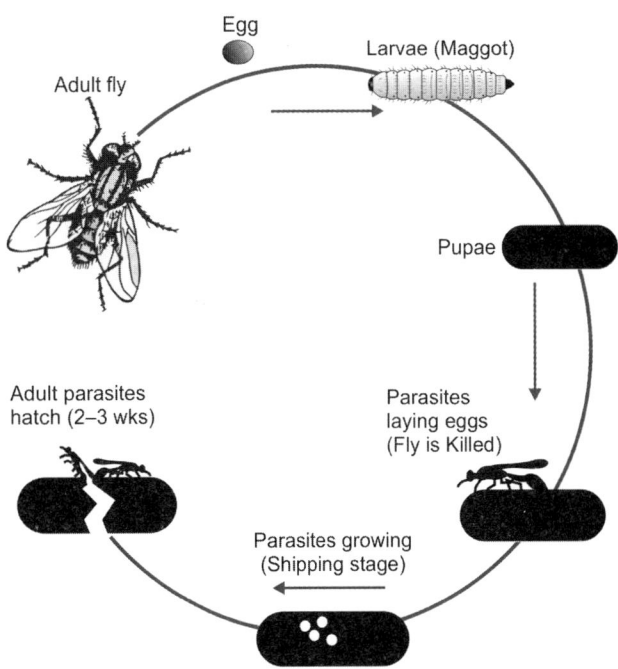

**Fig. 7H.3:** Life cycle of housefly.

- *Application in diseases prevention and control*
  - **Environmental control (control of breeding)**: As it is difficult to eliminate flies totally, our aim should be to reduce their population. This can be achieved by elimination of breeding places, proper disposal of refuse garbage and animal excreta. Gobar gas plant installation can be done for effective disposal of animal and human excreta. Promoting sanitary latrines and safe composting of garbage and refuse are other measures.
  - **Control of adult flies:**
    - *Residual spray:* With malathion and synthetic pyrethroids on resting and breeding sites. Pyrethrum 0.1% is useful for destruction of adult flies. Sticky fly paper is also used.
    - *Physical control:* Light traps (electrocutors) can be used in public eating places.
    - **Fly proofing**: Fly-proof containers and cupboards can be used; food can be covered with proper fly mesh. Doors and windows can be covered with mesh.

> - Vomit drop: The fly vomits frequently. The "vomit drop" is often a culture of disease agents
> - Flies transmit disease in the following ways: (1) Mechanical transmission, (2) Vomit drop, and (3) Defecation
> - Also called "porters of infection".

## Sand Flies

- *General description*: Belong to genus *Phlebotomus*. Important species are *P. argentipes*, *P. papatasi*, *P. sergenti* and *P. braziliensis*. Sandflies are small insects, about one-fourth of a mosquito. The length of a sandfly body ranges from 1.5 mm to 3.5 mm.

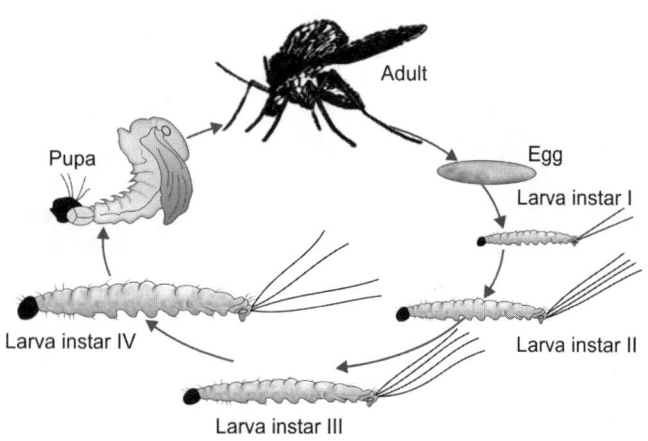

**Fig. 7H.4:** Life cycle of sandfly.

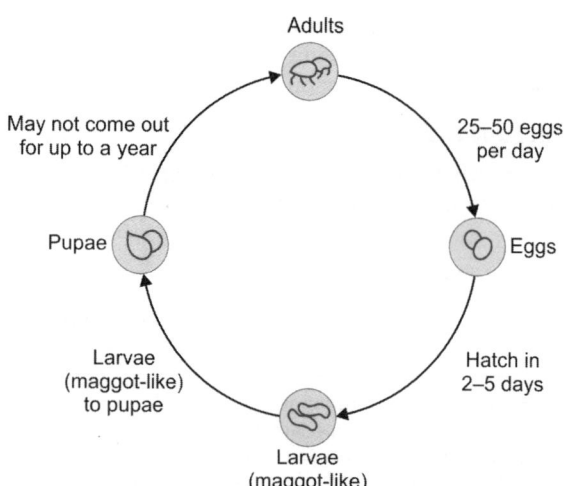

**Fig. 7H.5:** Life cycle of flea.

Adult is a small fuzzy, delicately proportionate fly with erect large wings. The entire body including wings is heavily clothed with long hairs. Adult lives for about 15 days. Even though winged, sandflies do not fly; they hop from one place to another. Only females bite. Males have claspers.

- *Life cycle* consists of egg, four instars of larvae, pupa and adult **(Fig. 7H.4)**. The whole cycle takes more than a month; however, duration depends on temperature and other ecological conditions. They prefer high relative humidity, warm temperature, high subsoil water and abundance of vegetation. Sandflies breed in favorable micro-climatic conditions in places with high organic matter that serve as food for larvae. These are ecologically sensitive insects, fragile and cannot withstand desiccation.
- *Medical importance/diseases transmitted by sandflies*: Sandfly of genus *Phlebotomus argentipes* are the only known vectors of kala-azar in India **(Table 7H.2)**.
- *Application in diseases prevention and control*: Sandflies transmit *Leishmania donovani* from man to man; man being the only reservoir of kala-azar. Sandflies feed on cattle, goats and man.
  - **Source control**: Abolition of breeding places, sealing the cracks, crevices and holes, frequent removal of animal dung from stable and cattle sheds and maintaining proper sanitation, location of cattle sheds and poultry away from human habitations.
  - **Anti-adult measures**: Residual spraying with DDT. Lindane is also sprayed once in 3 months.
  - **Personal protection**: Proper clothing-long trousers with socks, tops drawn over the trouser cuffs. Repellents can also be used. Lizards and spiders are natural predators of sandflies.

## Fleas

- *General description*: Belong to order *Siphonaptera*. Adult flea is a blood-sucking ectoparasite; wingless, small (1.5–6 mm) and its body is laterally compressed; cuticle is strongly chitinized.
- *Types of fleas*
  - From a thousand different species, of fleas around 37 found in India. The fleas causing diseases are:
    ♦ Rat fleas *(Oriental): Xenopsylla cheopis, Xenopsylla astia, Xenopsylla braziliensis*
    ♦ Rat fleas *(Temperate zone): Nosopsylla fasciatus*
    ♦ Human fleas: *Pulex irritans*
    ♦ Dog and cat fleas: *Ctenocephalus canis, Ctenocephalus fells*
    ♦ Sand fleas *(Jigger or chigoe fleas): Tunga penetrans*
- *Life cycle*: Egg, larvae, pupa and adult complete metamorphosis **(Fig. 7H.5)**, taking around 2–4 weeks. The adult flea can jump about 3–4 inches from ground. Both sexes suck blood. Average life span is 4 weeks.
- *Diseases transmitted by fleas (refer Table 7H.2)*
  X. cheopis is the most efficient vector in transmission of disease.
- *Application in diseases prevention and control:*
  - **Insecticidal control:**
    ♦ About 10% dust of DDT on rodents
    ♦ *Indoor residual spray:* At the lower one meter of the walls with diazion or malathion
    ♦ *Patch dusting of grain birds, rat runs and furniture*: With 2% diazion, 5% malathion or 2% carbaryl
    ♦ *Dusting of pet:* Dogs and cats.
  - **Repellents:** Diethyltoluamide, benzyl benzoate are used as flea repellents.
  - **Rodent control measures**: Indirectly reduce the rat flea numbers (mentioned in section "Rodents").

> **Flea indices:** Are useful indicators to predict a plague outbreak in an endemic area.
> **The following indices are used in flea surveys:**
> - **General flea index**: It is the average number of fleas of all species per rodent.
> - **Specific flea index** (X.cheopis index; X.astia index, etc.): It is the average number of fleas of each species, found per rodent.
> - **Percentage incidence of flea species**: It is the percentage of fleas of each species, found per rodent.

- **Rodent infestation rate**: It is the percentage of rodents infested with the various flea species.
  **Blocked fleas** (Fleas which ingest plague bacilli, become blocked due to the multiplication of plague bacilli in their proventriculus or stomach) **play a great role in the spread of plague**.

## Lice

- *General description*: Belong to order *Anoplura*. These are parasites on mammals. Belong to genus *Pediculus*. The important species of human lice are *P. capitis*, *P. corporis* and *P. pubis*. They are ectoparasites and live exclusively on human blood. Lice infestation is called "Pediculosis".
- *Characteristics*: The body of lice is elongated and divided into head, thorax and abdomen, have three pairs of legs with strong claws.
- *Life cycle* takes an average period of 15–16 days; with egg, three larval stages and adult (**Fig. 7H.6**); and incomplete metamorphosis. Average life span is 34 days.
- *Diseases transmitted by lice*: Only body louse is a vector for disease epidemic typhus, trench fever and relapsing fever (refer **Table 7H.2**). Both male and female transmit the disease.
- *Application in diseases prevention and control*
  - **Good personal hygiene**: Like regular bathing and washing of clothes.
  - **Steam disinfection**: Of clothing and sun drying of clothing.
  - **Dusting**: 10% DDT powder is used to dust garments of lousy individuals. Second application may be needed after 10 days.

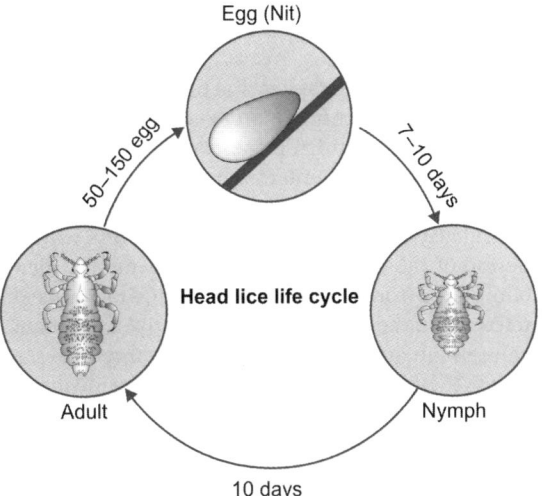

Fig. 7H.6: Life cycle of lice.

  - **Anti-lice shampoos**: Fenitrothion (0.2-0.4%), deltamethrin shampoo (0.03%).
  - **Health education** of the people about spread of vector due to overcrowding and hence its avoidance; importance of personal hygiene.

> **Note**
> **Vagabond's disease**: The lice bites are associated with local pigmentation of skin and there is associated hardening of skin too.

## CLASS ARACHNIDA

### Ticks

- *General description*: Belong to order Acarina; are all bloodsucking ectoparasites of vertebrate animals. It takes about 2 to 4 months to complete its life cycle (**Fig. 7H.7**); and it is completed on 2 to 3 hosts.
- *Classification and characteristics:* Ticks are of two kinds: hard ticks (*ixodidae*) and soft ticks (*argasidae*) (**Fig. 7H.8**). The differences are discussed in **Table 7H.6**.

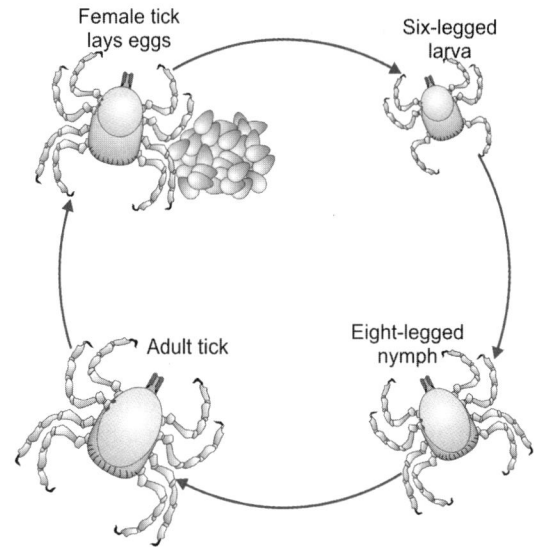

Fig. 7H.7: Life cycle of tick.

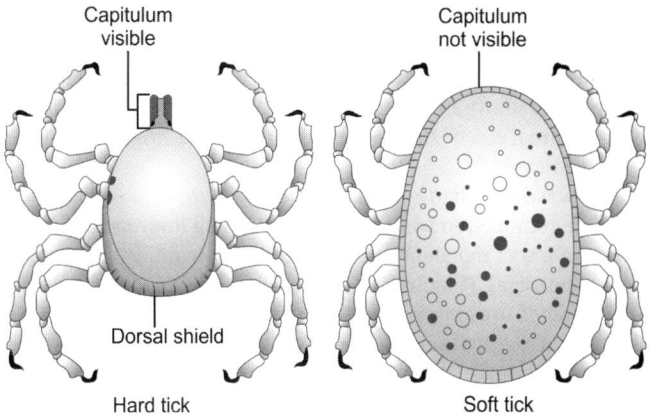

Fig. 7H.8: Difference between hard and soft tick.

The body of a tick is oval in shape and is not distinctly separated into head, thorax and abdomen. They have four pairs of legs, and no antennae. The hard ticks are covered on their dorsal surface by a chitinous shield, called scutum. The males are generally smaller than females.

- *Diseases transmitted by hard tick and soft tick*: The pathogens of all the diseases (refer **Table 7H.2**) transmitted by the infected ticks (except Q-fever), are found in feces, saliva and coxal fluid (is secreted by the coxal glands,

Table 7H.6: Differences between hard tick and soft tick.

| Tick | Hard, or "scutate", ticks (Ixodidae) | Soft, or "non-scutate", ticks (Argasidae) |
|---|---|---|
| Scutum (hard dorsal shield) | Present | Absent, body often wrinkled |
| Mouthparts | Terminal | Not at extreme anterior end of body, but rather subterminal (ventral) |
| Sexual dimorphism | Apparent as scutum covers entire dorsal surface of male, but only anterior third (approximately) of unengorged female | Not pronounced because of absence of scutum |
| Feeding habits | Feed both night and day and cannot stand starvation | Feed at night and can withstand starvation for several months |
| Host infestation characteristics | Always found on their hosts | Hide in cracks and crevices during the day and emerge at night to feed on the host |
| Species in India infecting cattle and dogs | *Dermacentor*, *Haemophysalis*, *Hyalomma*, *Rhipecephalus* and *Boophilus* | *Ornithodorus moubata* |

*Source*: science.marshall.edu/joy/PDF/MedEnt/HardSoftTicks.pdf

located between first and second legs) of the ticks. In case of Q-fever, man gets infection through inhalation of dry feces of the infected tick.

- *Prevention and control*
  - **Insecticidal control**: DDT, chlordane, dieldrin, lindane, Malathion and toxaphane at rates of 1 to 2 Lbs per acre give effective control. Either dusting or spray formulations can be employed. Animals like dogs may be freed of ticks by treating them with insecticidal sprays or dusts. The premises which they frequent should be treated with insecticides.
  - **Environmental control:** Cracks and crevices in ground particularly near buildings and paths should be sealed. Animal hosts such as wild rodents and dogs should be reduced.
  - **Personal protection measures:** Workers should be encouraged to wear protective clothing impregnated with an insect repellent (indalone, diethyltoluamide and benzyl benzoate). Persons working in tick-infested areas should be trained to examine themselves for ticks both during the lunch hour and at the end of work and to remove promptly any ticks found.

## Mites

### Itch Mite (Sarcoptes scabiei or Acarus scabiei)

- Extremely small, globular arthropod just visible to the naked eye
- Causes scabies
- Essential to treat all members of the affected household simultaneously whether or not they appear to be infested
- Treatment of the person is by a good scrub with soap and hot water; using either-benzyl benzoate, 0.5 to 1.0% strength of gamma-HCH (lindane), 5% solution of tetmosol or sulfur ointment (2.5–10%).

### Trombiculid Mite

These are spider-like arthropods. The important species are *Leptotrombidium deliense* and *L. akamushi* which are vectors of scrub typhus in Asia and South Pacific.

## CLASS CRUSTACEA

Form a large, diverse arthropod group with animals as crabs, lobsters shrimp, etc. Cyclops is of medical importance. Their body is divided into cephalothorax and abdomen, have five pairs of legs and two pairs of antennae.

### Cyclops

Cyclops belongs to the family Cyclopidae. They are found in stagnant bodies of fresh water. The disease is transmitted to humans when they drink water containing infected cyclops.

- *General description:* Cyclops is just visible (0.5–2 mm) to the naked eye; recognized by their typical jerky mode of swimming. They feed on plankton and other small aquatic organisms. Average lifespan of a cyclop is three months.
  - **Transmission:** Larvae of the guinea worm enter the human body when people drink water contaminated with cyclops containing infective larvae. In the stomach, the cyclops are digested and the larvae can then move around freely. They subsequently try to penetrate the thin intestinal wall. If successful, they end up in the connective tissues of the abdomen and thorax, where they develop into adult worms, mating after three months. When mature, the female moves towards the surface. About a year after the infection begins, the female is ready to emerge from the body to reproduce by releasing up to three million larvaes. In order to emerge, the female produces toxic substances that break down the overlying skin causing painful blisters and ulcers. The worm partly emerges and releases larvae, frequently when the affected person enters water, for example, to collect drinking-water. Hundreds of thousands of small larvae are released every time the person enters water over a period of 1–3 weeks. The worm subsequently dies and is eliminated from the body over a period of 3–8 weeks. The released larvae are not directly infective to humans. They can remain active in water for about three days and die unless they are swallowed by a cyclop. Inside the cyclops, the guinea-worm larvae develop over a period of about two weeks into a larval stage that is infective to humans.
- *Medical importance/diseases transmitted:*
  - **Guinea worm disease:** Cyclops act as an intermediate host of Dracunculiasis or guinea worm disease. Man acquires infestation by drinking water containing infected cyclops.
  - Cyclops mediates also as one of the intermediate hosts of fish tape worm, *Diphyllobothrium latum* infestation. The disease is rare in India.
- *Application in diseases prevention and control:* There is no natural immunity against guinea worm and no effective drugs or vaccines are available to prevent or treat the disease. The main aim in dealing with infected people is to prevent and treat secondary infections (abscesses, tetanus,

septicemia) and arthritis. The only available treatment is to extract the worm. This has to be done very slowly to prevent the worm from breaking. Only a few centimeters can be pulled out each day.

- **Installation of safe drinking-water supplies:** Communities may consider installing bore holes with pumps, piped water systems, or wells with concrete rims to prevent run-off water from draining back. Abolition of step wells and provision of sanitary wells. Effective prevention and control of dracunculiasis requires the education of community members.
- **Filtration** of drinking-water using woven cotton cloth (0.15 mm pore size) can be used.
- **Boiling** of drinking-water at 60°C is a simple and effective method for killing cyclops in drinking-water. However, it is time-consuming.
- **Chemical control:** Cyclops can be killed by treating water sources with chlorine (5 ppm), lime (4 g in 1 gallon of water) and temephos (an insecticide that is safe in drinking-water if used at the correct dosage of 1 mg/L).
- **Biological control:** Small fish, e.g. barbel fish and gambusia fish have been found to feed on cyclops.

> - Cyclops are also called water fleas
> - Live cyclops have been observed within 30 minutes of a dry pond being filled with water
> - Cyclops are the intermediate hosts of guinea worm, *Dracunculus medinensis*, a parasite that causes guinea-worm disease or dracunculiasis. The disease has been eradicated from India in 2000.

## INTEGRATED VECTOR CONTROL

### General Principles for Prevention and Control of Arthropod Diseases

#### Integrated Vector Management

- **The concept:** Integrated vector management (IVM) is a rational decision-making process for the optimal use of resources for vector control. The approach seeks to improve the efficacy, cost-effectiveness, ecological soundness and sustainability of disease-vector control.
  The ultimate **goal** is to prevent the transmission of vector-borne diseases such as malaria, dengue, Japanese encephalitis, leishmaniasis, schistosomiasis and Chagas disease.
- **Rationale:** Driving forces behind a growing interest in IVM include the need to overcome challenges experienced with conventional single-intervention approaches to vector control as well as recent opportunities for promoting multisectoral approaches to human health.
- **Operational strategy:** The Global Strategic Framework for IVM notes that IVM requires the establishment of principles, decision-making criteria and procedures, together with time frames and targets. The Framework identifies the following as five key elements for the successful implementation of IVM (Fig. 7H.9):
  - *Advocacy, social mobilization and legislation*: Promotion and embedding of IVM principles in the development

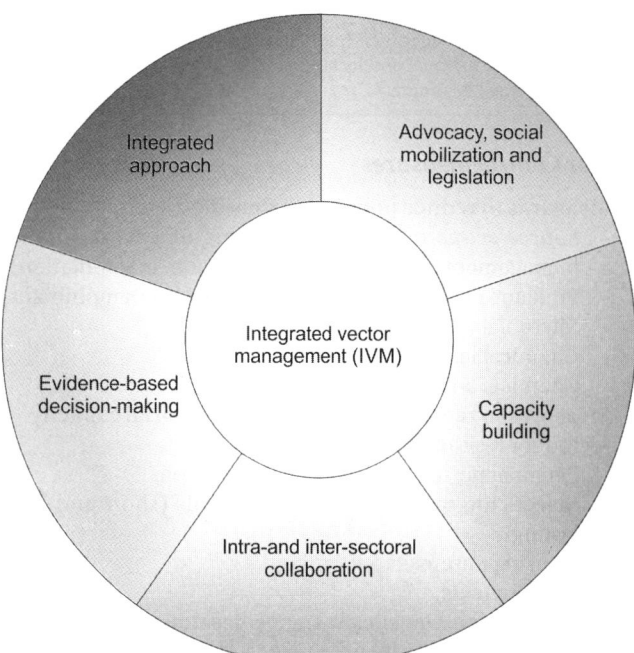

**Fig. 7H.9:** Integrated vector management.

policies of all relevant agencies, organizations and civil society; establishment or strengthening of regulatory and legislative controls for public health and pesticide management; empowerment of communities.
- *Collaboration within the health sector and with other sectors*: Consideration of all options for collaboration within and between public and private sectors; strengthening channels of communication among policy makers, vector-borne disease control program managers and other IVM partners.
- *Integrated approach*: Ensure rational use of available resources through a multidisease control approach, integration of nonchemical and chemical vector control methods, and integration with other disease control measures, such as active and passive case detection and treatment.
- *Evidence-based decision-making*: Adaptation of strategies and interventions to local vector ecology, epidemiology and resources, guided by operational research and subject to routine monitoring and evaluation.
- *Capacity-building*: Development of essential physical infrastructure, financial resources and adequate human resources at local and national levels to manage IVM programs based on needs assessments.

> **Main strategies for IVM:**
> - Collaboration within the health sector and with other sectors through the optimal use of resources, planning, monitoring and decision-making.
> - Integration of nonchemical and chemical vector control methods and integration with other disease control measures.
> - Evidence-based decision making guided by operational research and entomological and epidemiological surveillance and evaluation.

- Development of adequate human resources, training and career structures at national and local level to promote capacity building and manage IVM programs.

## Vector Control Measures

- **Measures to reduce population densities**
  - *Source reduction*: Different forms of environmental management (engineering, modification, manipulation)
  - Predator-prey systems (fish, predator insects, amphibians)
  - Microbial toxins
  - Chemical larviciding
  - Chemical adulticiding (e.g. fogging).
- **Measures to reduce vector longevity/vectorial capacity**
  - Indoor residual spraying
  - Personal personal/community protection.
  - Insecticide treated nets and materials (short and long lasting)
  - Housing improvement
- **Zooprophylaxis**
- **In the pipeline:** Genetically engineered mosquitoes.

## Modern Methods

- Genetic control of mosquitoes
- Sterile male technique of mosquitoes
- Cytoplasmic incompatibility (in mosquitoes)
- Chromosomal translocations
- Insect growth regulators
- Chemosterilants
- Sex attractants or pheromones.

## RODENTS

The word 'Rodent' has been derived from "rodere", which means to gnaw; classified into two distinct groups:

1. **Domestic rodents**: The black rat *(Rattus rattus,* the Norway rat; *R. norvegicus)* and the house mouse*(Mus musculus)* which are of chief public health concern **(Fig. 7H.10)**.

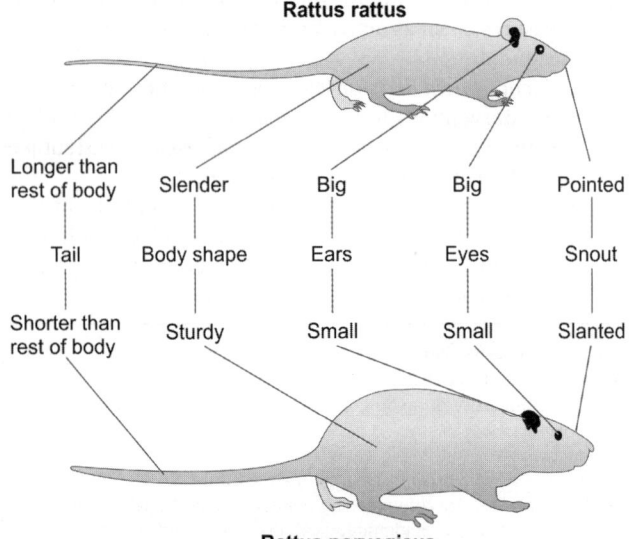

Fig. 7H.10: Rodents.

2. **Wild rodents**: Common in India are *Tateraindica, Bandicota bengalensis (Gunomyskok), B.indica, Millardia meltada, M. gleadowi* and *Mus booduga*. In India, *Tateraindica* has been found to be the natural reservoir of plague.
   - **Diseases transmitted:** The mode of transmission may be directly through rat bite (e.g. rat bite fever); some through contamination of food or water (e.g. salmonellosis, leptospirosis) and some through rat fleas (e.g. plague and typhus) **(Table 7H.7)**.

Table 7H.7: Diseases transmitted by Rodents.

| Disease | Vector | Agent |
|---|---|---|
| Plague | Flea/*Mode of spread-direct contact with infected animal | Bacteria *(Yersinia pestis)* |
| Tularemia | *Mode of spread- handling infected animal carcasses, eating or drinking contaminated food or water, breathing in the infected bacteria | Bacteria *(Francisella tularensis)* |
| Salmonellosis | *Mode of spread- water and food contaminated with urine from infected animals | Bacteria *(Salmonella species)* |
| Lassa fever | *Mode of spread- direct contact with rodents or their urine and droppings | Lassa virus |
| Hemorrhagic fever | *Mode of spread- breathing in the dust that is contaminated with rodent urine or droppings, direct contact with rodents or their urine and droppings | Virus |
| Encephalitis | *Mode of spread- breathing in the dust that is contaminated with rodent urine or droppings, direct contact with rodents or their urine and droppings | Virus |
| Scrub typhus | Trombiculid mite | Rickettsial |
| Murine typhus | Flea | Rickettsial |
| Rickettsial pox | Mouse mite | Rickettsial |
| *Hymenolepis diminuta* | *Mode of spread—water and food contaminated with urine from infected animals | Parasitic |
| *Cutaneous leishmaniasis* | Sandfly/*mode of spread—by species of burrowing rats is under investigation | Parasitic |
| Amoebiasis | *Mode of spread—water and food contaminated with urine from infected animals | Parasitic |
| Trichinosis | *Mode of spread—water and food contaminated with urine from infected animals | Parasitic |
| Chagas disease | *Mode of spread—water and food contaminated with urine from infected animals | Parasitic |
| Rat bite fever | *Mode of spread—bite or scratch from an infected rodent | Bacteria *(Spirillum minus)* |
| Leptospirosis | *Mode of spread—water and food contaminated with urine from infected animals | Spirochete *(leptospiraictero haemorrhagia)* |

*Direct transmission by rodents or through contaminated water, food or animal.

- **Application in diseases prevention and control:** The anti-rodent measures are:
  - **Eliminating the hiding and nesting sites** is best method of prevention is to deny rodents a place to live/nest and food to eat.
  - **Sanitation measures:** Proper storage, collection and disposal of garbage, proper storage of food—stuffs, construction of rat-proof buildings, godowns and warehouses, and elimination of rat burrows by blocking them with concrete.
  - **Trapping** of rats causes temporary reduction in the number of commensal rodents. It is recommended that the number of traps laid should be at least 5% of the human population. The 'wonder trap' developed by the Haffkine Institute, Mumbai is credited to trap as many as 25 rats at a time. The traps are usually baited with indigenous foods of the locality. The various types of traps are: *Cage traps, sherman traps, trigger or snap traps, break back traps.*
  - **Rodenticides** are of two main types—single-dose (acute) and multiple-dose (cumulative). The former are lethal to the rat after a single feeding, while the latter require repeated feedings over a period of 3 more days. The commonly used single-dose (acute) poisons are *Barium carbonate* and *zinc phosphide* recommended for large scale use against rats.

The *multiple-dose* (cumulative) poisons are warfarin, diphacinone, coumafuryl and pindone.
- **Fumigation** is an effective method of destroying, both rats and rat fleas. The fumigants used are calcium cyanide, carbon disulfide, methyl bromide, sulfur dioxide, etc.
- **Chemosterilants** are chemicals that can cause temporary or permanent sterility in either sex or both sexes. Rodent chemosterilants are still in the experimental stage.

**Note**
- Rodents are the largest order of mammals with over 2,000 living species placed in about 30 families
- Rodents range in size from 5 g (pygmy mice) to over 70 kg (capybaras)
- The incisors of the rodents keep growing and to keep them in check, the rodents gnaw continuously.

## SUGGESTED READING

1. Dhaar GM, Robbani I. Foundations of community medicine. 1st edition. Elsevier; 2006.
2. Goddard J, Zhou L. Physician's guide to arthropods of medical importance, 5th edition; Florida: CRC Press; 2007.
3. How to identify Culex Anopheles and Aedes mosquitoes and their larvae.
4. Malaria. National Vector Borne Disease Control Programme.

# SECTION 2

# Core and Allied Sciences

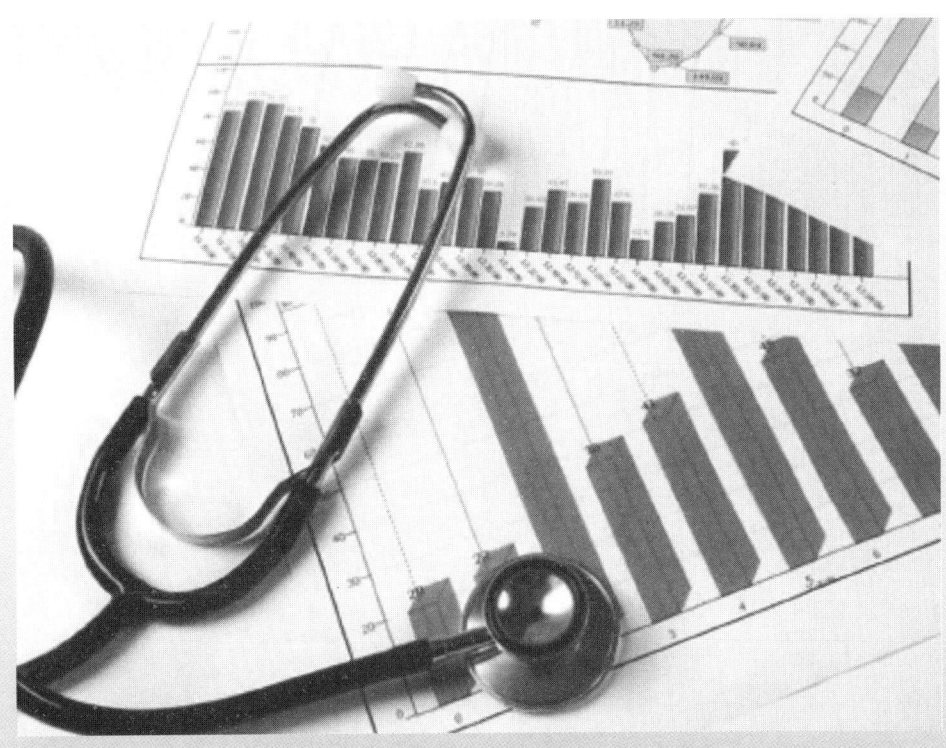

*If you want to know health of community, you need to travel many learning roads of different disciplines.*

# SECTION OUTLINE

8. Preventive Medicine
9. Basics of Epidemiology
10. Epidemiological and Research Studies
11. Research Methodology and Biostatistics
12. Population Science
13. Social Medicine
14. Health Communication

# CHAPTER 8

# Preventive Medicine

*Vartika Saxena, Rakesh Kakkar, Senkadhirdasan*

*The aim of medicine is to prevent disease and prolong life; the ideal of medicine is to eliminate the need of a physician.*
—**William J Mayo** *(1861–1939) in National Education Association: Proceedings and Addresses, 66:163, 1928*

| | |
|---|---|
| CM1.4 | Describe and discuss the natural history of disease |
| CM1.5 | Describe the application of interventions at various levels of prevention |
| CM7.6 | Enumerate and evaluate the need of screening tests |

## INTRODUCTION

Leavell and Clark defined preventive medicine as "the science and art of preventing diseases, prolonging life and promoting physical and mental health and improving efficiency." In essence and principle, it embodies "all medicine that seeks to alter the course of diseases or to better patient's physiological status," thus including all measures that protect, promote, and maintain health and well-being and prevent disease, disability, and death. It helps in managing the health of the individuals, communities and defined population.

Main aim of preventive medicine is to achieve a diseases free state, which can be attained either by stopping occurrence of a disease or by halting a disease progress and deterring resulting complications after its onset. Preventive medicine can be practiced by governmental agencies, healthcare physicians and also by individuals themselves. In present scenario when different countries of world are facing ever increasing challenge of non-communicable diseases (NCDs) like diabetes, cancer, cardiovascular diseases, etc., over and above existing communicable diseases [diarrhea, malaria, dengue tuberculosis (TB), etc.], it becomes very important and essential that preventive strategies are practiced at wider scale against these diseases for saving lives of people, prolonging disease free life span and minimizing cost for disease management.

## PREVENTION IS NOT ONLY BETTER, BUT ALSO CHEAPER THAN CURE

There are different ways of preventing diseases and promoting health. Suppose, if we want to reduce mortality among mothers and children, this can be achieved by taking adequate care of pregnant women, conducting delivery by trained personnel, ensuring breastfeeding, early identification of any risk factor in newborn baby, or by timely referral. All these are examples of different methods of preventing maternal or child mortality. There are several Accredited Social Health Activist (ASHA) under National Health Mission who are actually practicing it. The story given below is a success story of one of such worker.

> **A Success Story of ASHA from Uttarakhand**
>
> *National Rural Health Mission (NRHM) (2005–2012) was launched by Ministry of Health and Family Welfare, Government of India with the objective to address the health needs of rural population, especially the vulnerable section of the society. Under this scheme, deployment of ASHA has been identified as one of the key strategy for wider coverage of services. It was considered that ASHA will be the first port of call for any health related demand of deprived sections of population, especially for women and children, who find it difficult to access health services.*
>
>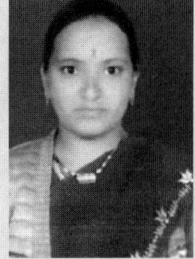
> **Mrs Champa Kunwar**
>
> *Uttarakhand state has 13 districts and 95 blocks, spread out in three distinct zone as per altitude, viz., Foothill region, Middle Himalayan region, and Upper Himalayan region. Gram sabha Hadwad is located in the remotest area of Block Kapkot; district Bageshwar in Upper Himalayan region of the state. Mrs Champa Kunwar, aged 40 years; wife of Shri (late) Mohan Singh, is ASHA from Hadwad village. She is educated up to high school and working as ASHA since 2006 in the village.*
>
> *Hadwad village was a backward village with complete lack of health services and health awareness among people. Champa, after completing ASHA training in the year 2007, took it as a challenge to change the situation of her village. She started house-to-house visit for meeting people. She has informed everyone about health services available in the nearby Public Health Center (PHC) and Community Health Center (CHC). She has motivated villagers to come forward to avail health services and adopt healthy lifestyle. She has been so consistent in her efforts that people of her village got encouraged to adopt healthy practices and started coming forward for availing health services from CHC and PHC. With her constant persuasion in 1 year period, 10 sanitary toilets were constructed, 50 immunization, 54 institutional deliveries and five home deliveries were successfully conducted. Further, her counseling resulted in eight couples adopting permanent method of sterilization and five couples started using spacing methods. She has also collected 30 slides for malaria testing, she has also provided Directly Observed Treatment, Short-course (DOTS) for Tuberculosis to two patients and motivated three elderly of the village for cataract operation. She is constantly putting her untiring*

*efforts for women empowerment by encouraging them to participate in panchayat activities on issues concerning them. She is a member of Village Health and Sanitation Committee and regularly voices issues pertaining to her village.*

*She has got state award as one of the Best ASHA from district Bageshwar. The way Mrs Champa has rendered her services for Hadwad village, she has become symbol of ideal ASHA as envisaged by the NRHM planners.*

Source: Saxena V. A success story of ASHA from Uttarakhand. Indian Journal of Community and Family Medicine. 2015;1(2):95.

For further understanding of prevention, it is important to recognize that disease and health are not two water tight compartments, health of an individual is a dynamic phenomenon and a process of continuous change.

Different stages in spectrum of health are positive health, better health, freedom from sickness, unrecognized sickness, mild sickness, severe sickness, and death **(Fig. 8.1)**.

Strategies of disease prevention and control should be applied according to health status of individual in disease spectrum. **Figure 8.2** explains that person can be in comfort zone (overweight person) without realizing that he can slip to zone of poor health (obesity) if appropriate health measures (diet control, exercise, etc.) are not being timely taken. If he follows healthy habits, he may enjoy benefits of good health (normal weight).

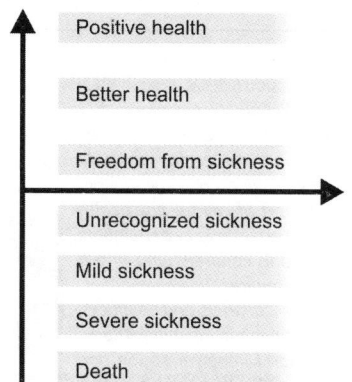

**Fig. 8.1:** Spectrum of health and disease.

Disease spectrum is basically a concept at community level with noticeable and imperative inferences for clinical medicine in it. If healthcare providers are not conscious of wide-spectrum of disease, the less severe form will not alert them for chances of impending severe form of cases or the cases in which diseases are not yet precipitated. If doctor sees one case of diarrhea in a family, and if he is aware of the concept of spectrum of disease he should also suspect there could be other family members who might be harboring infectious agent in their body though disease symptoms are not yet precipitated. Then doctor may give appropriate advice to rest of the family members. So understanding of spectrum of disease helps in practicing prevention. Similarly, spectrum of coronary heart disease is wide and ranges from no signs, symptoms, or disability to overwhelming chest pain and disability. The key identified variants in the spectrum of coronary heart disease ranges from asymptomatic, angina, arrhythmia, heart failure to myocardial infarction (heart attack). It is important for community physician to understand this spectrum to intervene appropriately and halt progression of disease at early stage.

The disease spectrum is mainly a community-based concept, while natural history of disease is largely a concept relating to individuals. Understanding of natural history of disease is important for understanding level of prevention and mode of interventions.

## NATURAL HISTORY OF DISEASE

Although covered in *Chapter 3: Concept of Health and Disease*, to reiterate, the natural history of disease is the continuous advancement of the biological development of disease in an individual from the moment that it is initiated by exposure to the underlying agents. Do the exercise in **Box 8.1** (activity 1) before reading further.

> **Box 8.1: Activity 1**
>
> Students should have discussion in small groups about possible outcomes in an individual exposed to a causal agent. The causal agents could be tubercle bacilli, excess salt intake, exposure to pollution in traffic, smoking, etc. **Figure 8.3** provides ideas for discussion.

There are two main stages in natural history of a disease **(Fig. 8.4)**:
1. Prepathogenesis
2. Pathogenesis.

### Prepathogenesis Period

In this stage, disease agent/risk factors (bacteria/virus/fungus/excessive salt intake, etc.) are present in population. In this

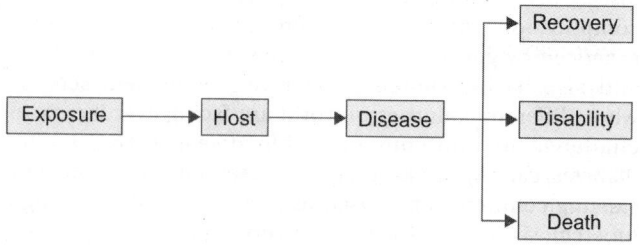

**Fig. 8.3:** Graphical presentation of natural history of disease.

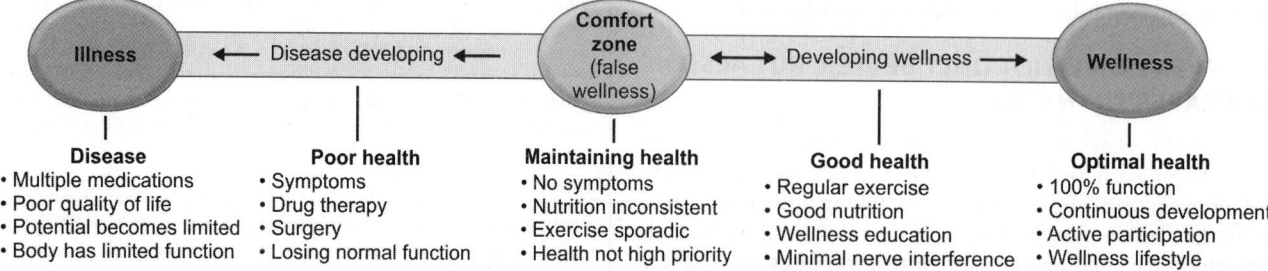

**Fig. 8.2:** Concept of illness and wellness and health status.

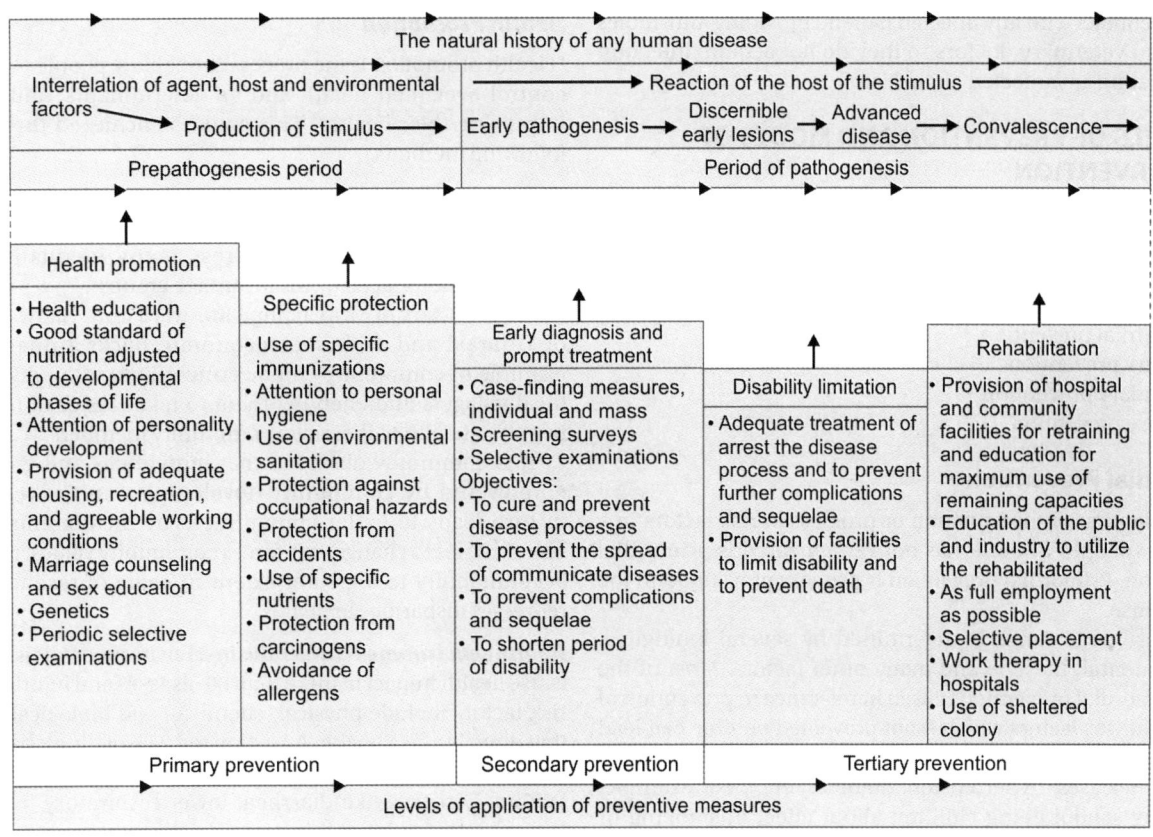

Fig. 8.4: Natural history of disease with level of prevention.

stage person has no sign and symptoms of disease but is susceptible to disease. So he is in comfort zone of spectrum of health. At this stage, if there is a susceptible host, and environment is suitable, infection may be acquired or disease process may start and person will move to subclinical stage or pathogenesis period.

## Pathogenesis Period

### Subclinical Stage

In this stage, early pathological changes happen but there is no overt expression of signs and symptoms. Disease remains in subclinical form. Still person is in comfort zone but regressing toward poor health. This is early pathogenesis. If treatment is not taken by patient till this stage, then patient will move to stage III.

### Clinical Stage

In this stage, overt signs and symptoms of disease appear in the individual. This is clinical phase of natural history of disease.

### Outcome Stage

This is late pathogenesis; in this stage, individual faces final outcome of the disease in terms of recovery, death, or disability. In certain cases, disease establishes itself in chronic form.

The knowledge of natural history of disease helps us to understand that there are several points during progression of disease when it can be intervened to bring favorable outcome.

The point at which we do intervention is level of prevention and method commonly used is known as mode of intervention, which will be discussed subsequently.

## STRATEGIES OF PREVENTION

Prevention includes all measures from general measures of health promotion (hygiene and sanitation practices) to specific measures of disease prevention and disability limitation like immunization, prophylactic therapies, starting early treatment, providing support for rehabilitation, etc.

These interventions can be applied to whole population of defined area or to a certain specific groups, based on this criteria there are two preventive strategies are discussed here:

### Population/Mass Strategies

When we apply certain techniques for all the members of given population is known as population strategy. Example—in a medical institute educating all the faculty, staff and students about hand hygiene practices to prevent cross infection, providing iodized salt in public distribution system for reducing dietary deficiency of iodine, etc.

### High-risk Strategy

These are the techniques applied to certain group of population whom we know that they are at high-risk of acquiring disease/ health condition. For example, ensuring hepatitis B vaccination for medical students to prevent acquiring hepatitis B if they come in contact with any infected patient. Providing anti-rabies vaccine to veterinary doctors so they do not acquire infection while treating any infected animal, etc.

## LEVELS OF PREVENTION AND MODES OF INTERVENTION

***Levels of prevention:*** Levels of prevention are defined by considering the point of time when interventions are applied for halting occurrence or progression of disease or its risk factors; classically, there are four levels of prevention:
1. Primordial prevention
2. Primary prevention
3. Secondary prevention
4. Tertiary prevention

### Primordial Prevention

The prevention of the initiation or progress of risk factors in a region or people where it has not yet appeared is primordial prevention. Primordial prevention is primary prevention in the purest sense.

Disease occurrence is determined by several biological, environmental, lifestyle and many other factors. Most of the time primordial prevention is used in reference to prevention of those behavior factors which if not prevented on time can lead to emergence of risk factors which can lead to lifestyle diseases (cardiac diseases, hypertension, diabetes, etc.). For example, educating school going children about effect of smoking or alcohol at their early age would deter them from acquiring habit of smoking or alcoholism (risk factors for lifestyle diseases), teaching yoga and meditation to young children is also method of primordial prevention as it will help them to handle various challenges of life easily and will not build up stress among them which could be a potential risk factor for hypertension, diabetes, cancer, etc.

We can apply strategies of mass education (group education) or individual education for primordial prevention.

This is usually applied in susceptible stage in the natural history of diseases which will prevent people progressing in subclinical stage.

### Primary Prevention

Efforts or interventions done before the commencement of disease to remove the likelihood of disease in future.

When methods of prevention are applied before person has acquired infection or pathogenesis starts, then it is known as primary prevention. This ends the possibility that disease will ever occur. For example, giving measles vaccine to an infant so that chances of measles are minimized. Wearing personal protective devices (mask or gloves) for prevention of acquiring infection while handling patients are methods of primary prevention. In primary prevention, all those measures are included which will halt the emergence of diseases even if the person is exposed or living in the environment where disease agent exists.

There are two interventions for primary prevention:
1. Health promotion
2. Specific protection

### *Health Promotion*

"Health promotion is the process of enabling people to increase control over their health and its determinants, and thereby improving their health." This could be achieved through the following methods.

#### *Community Development Approach for Health Promotion*

Community development is a concept that has become very popular strategy to address many inequalities and discriminations faced by disadvantage groups.

Success story of Mrs Champa Kunward from Hadwad village of Uttarakhand with socioeconomic backwardness, is an example of community empowerment by health education to local villagers and enabling them to take charge of their own health or health of their own community members.

It is commonly observed that individuals and groups are empowered by community development initiatives, which in turn leads to better commitment by the community and beneficiaries to change, reinforces community values, promotes accountability to a greater extent in using of resources, and redresses disparities in health.

***Healthy environments and housing:*** Environmental risks factors cause health impact in more than 80 diseases and injuries. These risk factors include physical, chemical, and biological hazards that directly affect health. An estimated 24% of the global disease burden and 23% of all deaths can be attributed to environmental factors. Diseases like diarrhea, lower respiratory infections, "other" unintentional injuries (workplace hazards, radiation, and industrial accidents), road traffic accident, chronic obstructive pulmonary disease (COPD), and vector borne disease like malaria, dengue, etc. can be averted with ensuring healthy environment and housing conditions. For example, ensuring proper roads with adequate transport facilities can decrease road traffic accidents, adequately ventilated houses will reduce chances of respiratory diseases, availability of safe drinking water will reduce diarrheal diseases, worm infestation, etc. (Pruss-Ustun A, et al., WHO, 2018).

***Health education:*** Health literacy—health education is very crucial for promotion, maintenance, and restoration of health. Health education can play vital role in reducing the disease incidence and spread from person to person in case of communicable disease like TB, measles, chickenpox, etc. In case of NCDs, health education on causes and consequences of diabetes, hypertension, cardiac diseases, mental conditions would help in persons taking appropriate measures to avoid risk factors of disease. For example, if one knows high salt intake can lead to hypertension, this knowledge is helpful in reducing high salt intake and would reduce chances of developing hypertension.

***Healthy behavior and lifestyles:*** Certain lifestyle and behavioral factors like regular physical activity, healthy diet, sleep, disciplined life, ability to manage and coping challenges of life through meditation and yoga are certain behaviors important for preventing NCDs.

### *Specific Protection*

Preventing the disease by specific intervention includes applying specific techniques or tools to halt emergence of specified disease or risk factor. This could be achieved through several methods like vaccination, pre- and post-exposure prophylaxis, specific measures for preventing road traffic injuries, etc., as described below.

***Immunization:*** It is a process whereby an individual is protected against an infectious disease usually by the administration of a vaccine. Vaccines augments the body's own immunity system thus providing protection to an individual against subsequent infection or disease. It is one of the most cost-effective health investments, with proven strategies that make it accessible to even the most hard-to-reach and vulnerable populations.

Immunization is one such activity which helped to abolish smallpox from the world and polio from several countries of the world.

***Usage of pre- and post-exposure prophylaxis:*** Pre- and post-exposure prophylaxis are methods of specific protection so that disease does not precipitate after accidental exposure of infectious agent. This prophylaxis could be in the form of vaccines, immunoglobulin, or medicines. When treatment is given before exposure to infectious agent then it is known as pre-exposure prophylaxis and when treatment is given after exposure to infectious agent it is known as post-exposure prophylaxis. Human immunodeficiency virus (HIV), hepatitis B, and rabies are few diseases in which pre- and post-exposure prophylaxis can be given. Pre-exposure prophylaxis is mostly given to those personnel who work in high-risk situation, e.g., veterinarians, laboratory workers dealing with rabies vaccine, etc., are at high-risk for rabies, so should be given pre-exposure prophylaxis against rabies. High-risk persons for hepatitis B who should receive pre-exposure prophylaxis are the persons having high-risk sexual behavior, injecting drug users, persons requiring frequent blood donation or blood products.

***Protection against accidents:*** Taking all the measures for preventing road traffic accidents like wearing seat belt, following particular speed limit and rules of driving are methods of specific protection for avoiding accidents.

***Prevention of NCDs:*** NCDs can be avoided by keeping weight within normal limit, taking cholesterol and other saturated fats within limits of recommended daily allowance, etc.

***Herd immunity:*** The transmission chain of the infectious agent is broken by protecting an adequate proportion of susceptible individuals. Thus, the risk of disease in the unimmunized children is also reduced, this phenomenon is called herd immunity. This is how people can be protected even without being vaccinated by herd effect of immunization. But enormous quantity of the population needs to be vaccinated for effective herd immunity effect **(Fig. 8.5)**.

## Secondary Prevention

Secondary prevention includes all actions which halt the progress of a disease at its incipient stage and prevent complications.

It is a process of stopping progression of diseases as early as possible, so that complication and adverse outcomes can be minimized. Early detection of the disease and its prompt treatment are the main interventions of secondary prevention. If we search

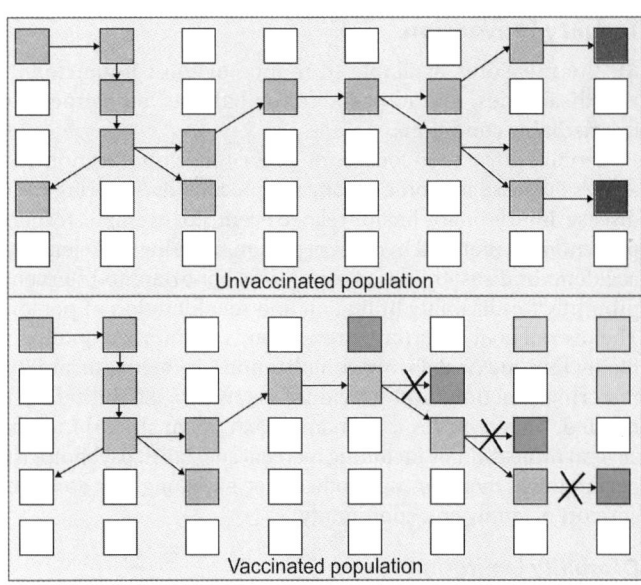

**Fig. 8.5:** Concept of herd immunity for prevention of infection.

People are shown in squares. Infectious agents spread between the people in light blue, although they do not get severe disease. When the infection reaches people who are highly susceptible (dark blue) they get the disease and can be very sick or die.

In the lower panel, the people in dark gray have been vaccinated. This now protects those in light gray as well, who had previously got the infection and possibly the disease. Although the figure only shows a few people being vaccinated, in reality many people have to be vaccinated for herd immunity to work.

*Source:* Oxford Vaccine Group, Department of Paediatrics, Clinical Vaccine Research and Immunisation Education htpps://www.ovg.ac.uk/images/site-logos/primary- logo.

for disease cases in community or in apparently healthy-looking population, then there are chances that we can pick up cases which are in very early stage of diseases development and can refer them for prompt treatment. This will increase chances of their full recovery, this is secondary prevention.

Process of early identification of cases from apparently healthy population is known as screening which is one of the important tools of secondary prevention. For example, if we measure blood pressure of all the members of community in a village, we can come to know who all are hypertensive, even if they themselves are not aware of the status and then we can treat them appropriately. This is known as secondary prevention. Details of screening you will study subsequently.

Secondary prevention can also be achieved if surveillance is done religiously. Surveillance is the continuous scrutiny of the factors that determine the occurrence and spread of diseases and other conditions of ill health which are pertinent of effective control. This is most important tool for averting epidemics. You will study in detail about it in subsequent section.

> **Note**
> **Important points to be remembered**
> - Primordial and primary prevention is prevention in purest sense.
> - Health education, health promotion, and specific protection are most important methods of primary prevention.
> - Immunization is most cost-effective tool for disease prevention.
> - Screening and surveillance are important tools for secondary prevention.

## Tertiary Prevention

All the measures available to reduce or limit impairments and disabilities, and to promote the patients' adjustment to irremediable conditions.

Tertiary prevention focuses on preventing complication and adverse disease outcome among people already suffering from disease, injury, or any health-related event. For example, tertiary prevention is required in cases of person suffering from leprosy, accident, or disaster. In such cases, it is important to intervene promptly for disability limitation and rehabilitation of person. The overall goal of tertiary prevention is to improve quality of life by limiting or delaying complications, reducing disability, restoring function, and providing means for rehabilitation if needed. This requires a team approach, team should include several professionals including medical specialist, psychologist, occupational therapist, physiotherapist, etc. along with constant support of family and community.

### Disability Limitation

When a patient reports late in the pathogenesis phase, the mode of intervention is disability limitation. The objective of this intervention is to prevent or halt the transition of the disease process from impairment to handicap. The intervention in disability will often be social or environmental as well as medical. While impairment which is the earliest stage has a large medical component, disability and handicap which are later stages have large social and environmental components in terms of dependence and social cost.

> **Definitions: Impairment, Disability, Handicap**
> The Disability Discrimination Act (DDA) defines a "disabled person as someone who has a physical or mental impairment that has a substantial and long-term adverse effect on his or her ability to carry out normal day-to-day activities. The adverse effect is substantial and long-term (meaning it has lasted for 12 months, or is likely to last for more than 12 months or for the rest of the person's life)."
> *Definitions* of International Classification of Impairments, Disabilities, and Handicaps (ICIDH) as given by World Health Organization in 1980 draws a three-fold distinction between impairment, disability, and handicap **(Fig. 8.6)**.
> *Impairment* "is any loss or abnormality of psychological, physiological, or anatomical structure or function."
> *Disability* "is any restriction or lack (resulting from an impairment) of ability to perform an activity in the manner or within the range considered normal for a human being."
> *Handicap* "is a disadvantage for a given individual, resulting from an impairment or a disability, that prevents the fulfillment of a role that is considered normal (depending on age, sex, and social and cultural factors) for that individual."
> Handicap is a situation when a disabled person is not able to perform his function because of unsupportive environment. Unsupportive environment could be because of cultural, physical, or social barriers. This can also be because unavailability of appropriate medical or rehabilitation facilities.

### Disability Prevention

Another concept is "disability prevention". It relates to all the levels of prevention: (a) reducing the occurrence of impairment, (b) disability limitation by appropriate treatment (secondary prevention), and (c) preventing the transition of disability into handicap (tertiary prevention). The major causes of disabling impairments in the developing countries are communicable diseases, malnutrition, low quality of perinatal care and accidents. These are responsible for about 70% of cases of disability in developing countries. Primary prevention is the most effective way of dealing with the disability problem in developing countries.

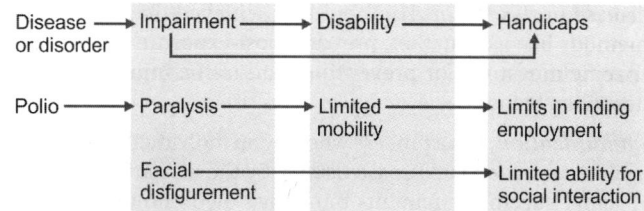

**Fig. 8.6:** Impairment, disability, and handicap in case of polio.

### Rehabilitation

Rehabilitation is a scientific method which is aimed at recovery of a person from disability. Disability could be because of any congenital problem or acquired due to injury or habit. Rehabilitation helps a person to achieve his near normal function so at least a person is not handicapped and can return to his normal functional state. All the efforts for preventing handicaps require robust mechanism of rehabilitation process.

Most of the time rehabilitation is slow and steady process and involves multidisciplinary team.

In recent days, there has been much emphasis on community-based rehabilitation (CBR) which is more effective and sustainable than hospital-based rehabilitation. There are different types of rehabilitation available for different types of disabilities. Some of them are listed below:

***Neurological rehabilitation:*** In this type of rehabilitation, patients suffering from stroke, neuromuscular disease, certain types of head trauma, and spinal cord injury are treated. It aims at making the patient self-dependent. It helps create a positive thinking in patient. The patient is treated so that he leads an improved life physically, emotionally, and socially.

***Cardiac rehabilitation:*** It is designed to help those people who have heart problems. Heart patients are educated to live a healthy life and reduce stress for the proper functioning of the heart.

***Drug/alcohol rehabilitation:*** It involves programs that are designed to make an addict/alcoholic free from the addiction. These programs usually adopt family-based approach in which all the family members are involved to support the patient for getting rid of their habit. In severe cases, patients are hospitalized also for detoxification.

***Physical rehabilitation:*** It is for those people whose lifestyle has changed after they have gone through a serious illness, surgery, or accident. In such cases, therapist introduces programs to improve the mobility and functioning of the injured body part of the patient. Proper exercise program is designed to improve the functioning of physical body. Often this requires physiotherapy also along with emotional support of family members.

***Vocational rehabilitation:*** It is designed to help those people who find it difficult to get employment or retain it after they have gone through certain situation that caused mental physical disability in them. This includes appropriate training of vocation which person can easily perform in the given physical condition. For example, after loosing lower limbs a traffic police man can be re-employed as clerk in the office after required training.

Besides rehabilitation programs mentioned above, social and psychological rehabilitation are integral part of any of the above program for restoring person's confidence, dignity, and relationships.

***Community-based rehabilitation:*** CBR is a multi-sectoral approach was initiated by WHO in 1978 in an effort to enhance the quality of life for people with disabilities and their families to meet their basic needs. CBR is implemented through the combined efforts of government and non-government organizations on health, education, vocational, social, and other services.

***Palliative care:*** Special care which improves the quality of life of patients and also of their families who encounters the problem associated with fatal illness, through the prevention and relief of suffering by means of early identification and impeccable assessment and treatment of pain and other problems, physical, psychosocial, and spiritual.

Multidisciplinary team may include doctors, nurses, registered dieticians, pharmacists, chaplains, psychologists, and social workers. They provide holistic care to the patient and family or caregiver focusing on physical, emotional, social, and spiritual issues. In India, with increasing life expectancy and increasing number of chronic illnesses importance of palliative care is increasing. However, country is still in very initial phase of providing palliative care services. So this explains various methods of tertiary prevention which includes approaches for disability limitation, rehabilitation, and palliative care.

Recently, higher level of prevention has also been suggested by the Belgian general practitioner Marc Jamoulle and Ronald, this is called quaternary prevention which is defined as "action taken to identify patient at risk of over medicalization to protect him from new medical invasion, and to suggest him interventions ethically acceptable." These are set of health activities to mitigate or avoid the consequences of unnecessary or excessive intervention of the health system.

The summary of levels of prevention and mode of intervention has been listed in **Table 8.1**.

> **Approach for prevention of stroke in community**
> ***Primordial prevention:*** Inculcating healthy dietary and exercise practices, e.g., low salt intake, regular exercise/yoga/meditation, healthy school and home atmosphere, so that children do not develop habit of smoking or drinking alcohol.
> ***Primary prevention:*** Early detection of hypertension, diabetes, and hyperlipidemia through regular health checkups and starting both nonpharmacological (weight control activities, deaddiction activities, destressing activities) and pharmacological intervention to prevent further risks.
> ***Secondary prevention:*** Identification of patient with transient ischemic attack/stroke with previous history of hypertension, patient and family members of patients having potential risk factors for stroke must be made aware to recognize early sign and symptoms of stroke. So that it can be detected early within 1 hour of golden period. Appropriate management of patient should be done as soon as possible.
> ***Tertiary prevention:*** Patient and his relative must be educated to avoid recurrence of stroke by ensuring regular medication and supportive therapy to patient. Paralyzed patients may require physical, mental, social and vocational rehabilitation to be able to come back to normal life.

## Quaternary Prevention

It is a new concept which is defined as "steps taken to prevent, decrease, and/or alleviate the harm caused by health activities." Health activities can also cause harm. So quaternary prevention focuses on avoidance of unnecessary medical activity, keeping in mind the medical principal of "First do no harm." Examples of quaternary prevention includes avoidance of unnecessary antibiotics, avoidance of invasive clinical procedures when they are not required.

## DISEASE: CONTROL, ELIMINATION, ERADICATION, AND EXTINCTION (FIGS. 8.7 AND 8.8)

### Control

As described above, disease control refers to reduction of disease incidence, prevalence, morbidity or mortality to a locally acceptable level as a result of deliberate efforts and continued intervention. Control of communicable diseases depends on a healthy environment (clean water, adequate sanitation, vector control, shelter), immunization, and health workers trained in early diagnosis and treatment. For example, control of diarrheal diseases emphasizes on maintenance of hygiene and sanitation with safe water supplies, control of dengue emphasizes on vector control measures, etc.

**Table 8.1:** Levels of prevention and mode of intervention.

| Stage of disease | No disease or risk factors | Pre-pathogenesis stage (risk factors but no disease) | Early-stage disease | | Late stage of disease | |
| --- | --- | --- | --- | --- | --- | --- |
| Level of prevention | Primordial | Primary | Secondary | | Tertiary | |
| Target population | Not yet susceptible to disease | Susceptible | Asymptomatic | | Symptomatic | |
| Goals | Reduce risk and determinants of risk factors | Reduce incidence | Reduce prevalence/consequences | | Reduce complications/limit disability | |
| Modes of intervention | Individual and mass education | Health promotion | Specific protection | Early diagnosis and treatment | Disability limitation | Rehabilitation |

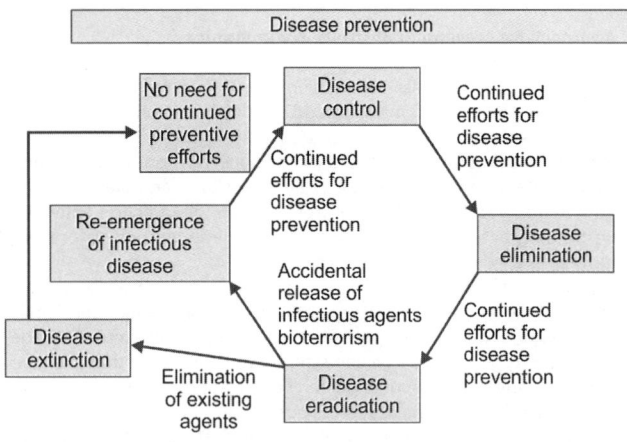

Fig. 8.7: Disease prevention.

## Elimination of Disease

Reduction of incidence of a disease in a defined geographic area to a predetermined very low level or to a zero level with continued intervention is known as elimination. For example, Guinea worm (2000), Leprosy (2005), Maternal and Neonatal Tetanus (2016) and Yaws (2016) have been eliminated from India.

## Elimination of Infections

Reduction of the incidence of infection to a very low level, or, zero level by a specific agent in a defined geographical area as a result of deliberate efforts: Continued measures to prevent re-establishment of transmission are required. Example—measles and poliomyelitis.

Elimination of lymphatic filariasis and kala-azar (in endemic pockets) was targeted in the latest National Health Policy by 2017.

> **Note**
> **Criteria for elimination**
> - Maternal and neonatal tetanus cases have been brought to less than one case per 1000 live births in all 675 districts of India in the year 2016.
> - Leprosy cases brought to below 1/10,000 population at national level in the year 2005.
> - Elimination of Lymphatic Filariasis (LF) is to achieve <1% microfilaria rate (Mf rate) in the endemic areas.
> - The definition for kala-azar elimination as a public health problem is to achieve annual incidence of less than one case per 10,000 population at block level.
> - For elimination of Malaria the goal is to achieve zero indigenous cases of Malaria in the country by 2030.

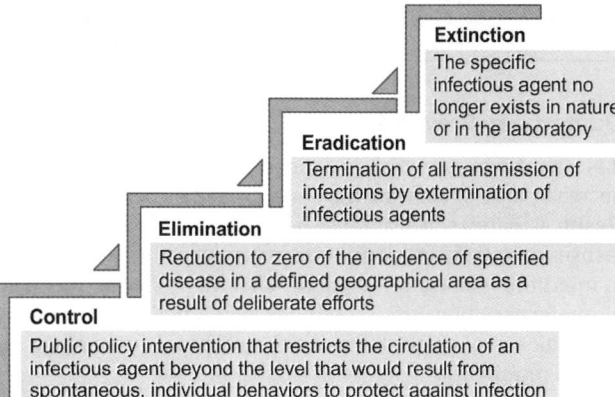

Fig. 8.8: Graphical presentation of control elimination, eradication, and extinction.

*Government of India runs several diseases control programs like* National Vector Borne Disease Control Programme (NVBDCP), prevention and control of vector borne diseases, viz., malaria, JE, dengue, kala-azar, chikungunya, and lymphatic filariasis, National Iodine Deficiency Disorders Control Programme (NIDDCP), National Tuberculosis Elimination Programme (NTEP), etc.

> **Control of cholera**
> Cholera is used as an example because the disease remains endemic in many parts of Africa, Asia, and Latin America. In the early 1990s, cholera epidemics affected millions of people in Africa and Latin America. Its prevention and control in emergencies provide examples of general approaches to be adopted with other epidemics.
> "Healthy" cholera carriers (i.e., people carrying *Vibrio cholerae* with no manifest disease) are now common in the general population of many developing countries. Although most cases of cholera are mild and treatable with simple measures, the disease can rapidly progress and result in death from dehydration. It can also spread easily where there is rudimentary sanitation and crowding, as in a refugee camp. It is therefore important to plan ahead in order to prevent cholera by the proper management of the water supply, sanitation, and food hygiene in camps. Although cholera can be treated, it cannot be controlled by vaccinations or by mass chemotherapy, but only by redoubling efforts to safeguard water supplies; maintaining a high free residual chlorine level (preferably 0.4–0.5 mg/L) in water supplies; disposing of feces properly so as not to contaminate water or food; encouraging hand washing with soap; and encouraging hygienic preparation and storage of food. The role of hygiene education in its control measures is critical.

## Eradication

Eradication is permanent reduction to zero of the worldwide incidence of infection caused by a specific agent as a result of deliberate efforts. If eradication is achieved there is no longer need for intervention measures. It is sometimes confused with elimination, which describes either the reduction of an infectious disease's prevalence in a regional population to zero, or the reduction of the global prevalence to a negligible amount. So far eradicated disease is smallpox. Polio has been eliminated from most of the countries of world except from two countries, i.e., Afghanistan and Pakistan. The World Health Organization (WHO) South-East Asia Region, home to a quarter of the world's population, was certified polio-free in 2014 by an independent commission under the WHO certification process. India is one of the country in this region out of total 11 countries.

Conceptually, elimination is a regional phenomenon, whereas eradication is global phenomena. In elimination, we aim at bringing down the number of cases to such a low level that its transmission stops. In eradication, we try to exterminate the disease agent from population so it is no longer a threat to a population that is why we can stop preventive measures after eradication.

Selection of infectious diseases for eradication is based on rigorous criteria, as both biological and technical features determine whether a pathogenic organism is (at least potentially) eradicable. The following are important criteria for eradication:
- The targeted organism must not have a nonhuman reservoir. Sufficient information on the lifecycle and transmission

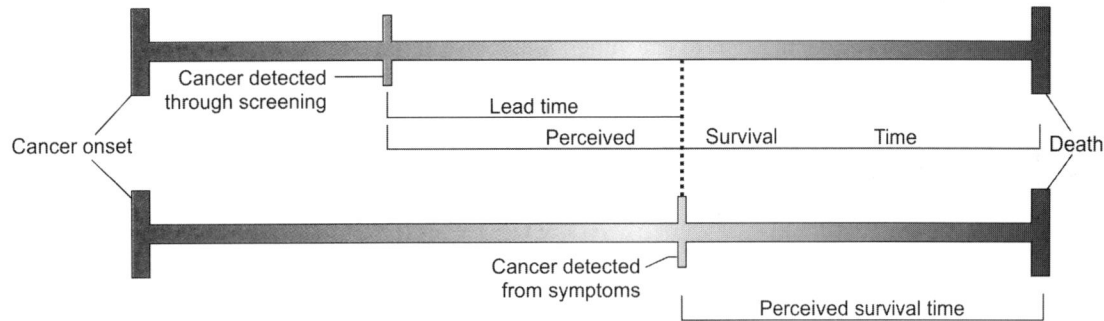

**Fig. 8.9:** Concept of lead time and gain in survival duration with screening.

dynamics is available at the time an eradication initiative is programmed.
- An efficient and practical intervention (such as a vaccine or antibiotic) must be available to interrupt transmission of the infective agent.
- The disease to be eradicated should be clearly identifiable, and an accurate diagnostic tool should exist.
- Disease should not be infective/communicable in its subclinical form.
- Economic considerations, as well as societal and political support and commitment, are other crucial factors that determine eradication feasibility.

## Extinction

Extinction is a status when specific infectious agent no longer exists in nature or in the laboratory. So far there is no such disease that exists. Even after eradication, disease agent is kept in laboratory of Centers for Disease Control (CDC) for combating future threats of re-emergence of disease; like smallpox virus is still maintained in two laboratories. Recently, Smallpox Eradication Advisory Group has concluded that the risk of accidental release from these laboratories could not be reduced to zero. It is therefore recommended that smallpox surveillance be continued and that an international stockpile of smallpox vaccine be maintained.

> **Points to Remember**
> - Tertiary prevention focuses on preventing complication and adverse disease outcome
> - Maternal and Neonatal Tetanus (2016), Yaws (2016), and Leprosy (2005) have been eliminated from India
> - Two diseases, namely, kala-azar and lymphatic filariasis (in endemic pockets) have been targeted for elimination
> - Elimination is a regional phenomenon, whereas eradication is global phenomenon
> - So far eradicated disease is smallpox.

## CONCEPT OF SCREENING

The US Commission on Chronic Illness, defined screening as: "The presumptive identification of unrecognized disease or defect by the applications of tests, examinations or other procedures which can be applied rapidly." or

"Screening is a process of searching unidentified diseases, defect or any condition of ill health by means of rapidly applied simple tests, examination or other procedures in apparently healthy-looking individuals."

Screening tests sort out apparently healthy persons who probably have a disease from those who probably do not have disease. Screening is the use of tests to help diagnose diseases (or their precursor conditions) in an earlier phase of their natural history or at the less severe end of the spectrum than is achieved in routine clinical practice. This helps in gaining sometime by making the diagnosis at early stage. This is known as lead time. It is an important factor when evaluating the effectiveness of a specific test (**Fig. 8.9**). For example, usually carcinoma cervix remains asymptomatic in its early stage. In later stages, it presents with symptoms of *abnormal bleeding*, such as *bleeding between menstrual periods*, after sex, after a *pelvic* exam, or after *menopause*. So, if patient comes with these symptoms, its already late and survival of patient will remain shorter. If we do Pap smear screening, it is possible we can diagnose many such cases at their very early stage when treatment can completely cure patient for longer survival.

> **Note**
> **Lead time**
> It is the length of time between the detection of a disease based on new, experimental criteria (screening) and its usual time of diagnosis based on clinical presentation or traditional criteria. It is the time between early diagnosis with screening and the time in which diagnosis would have been made without screening.

The main aim of screening is to reverse, halt, or slow the progression of disease more effectively than would normally happen. Screening is also done to protect society, even though the individual may not benefit. Screening of potential immigrants at the point at which a visa is issued or at the port of entry (for both contagious and chronic diseases) is an example. National AIDS Control Organization (NACO) conducts anonymous screening of pregnant women attending antenatal clinics to analyze trend of HIV infection in the country. The most extreme example of screening is the practice of triage (to sort) which we conduct when there is mass causality, when those unlikely to survive wounds are left untreated.

It is also important to understand that while we do screening, the method/procedure/instrument used for identifying cases should be very simple, easy to handle, inexpensive and should be accepted by community otherwise purpose of screening program will be defeated. Screening tests are not necessarily final test for making confirmatory diagnosis of disease.

Once a person comes positive for screening test, we apply another test to confirm diagnosis, that test is known as diagnostic test. Those tests which have highest level of efficacy in diagnosing a disease are known as tests of gold standard. Some of screening tests and their gold standards are listed in **Table 8.2**.

Table 8.2: List of screening tests and their corresponding gold standards.

| Disease or condition | Screening tests | Gold standard |
|---|---|---|
| Urinary tract infection | Urine microscopy | Urine culture |
| Hypertension | Blood pressure (Korotkoff sounds) | Intra-arterial measurement of pressures |
| Myocardial infarction | ECG or cardiac enzymes | Cardiac biopsy (at autopsy) |
| Breast cancer | Mammography | Biopsy |
| Celiac disease | IgG- and IgA-antigliadin antibodies, IgA-endomysial antibodies, and intestinal permeability | Small bowel biopsy |

(ECG: electrocardiography; IgA: immunoglobulin A; IgG: immunoglobulin G)

## Screening and Diagnostic Tests

A screening test is not intended to be a diagnostic test. It is only an initial examination. Those who are found to have positive test results are referred to a physician for further diagnostic work-up and treatment. Screening and diagnostic tests may be contrasted as in **Table 8.3**.

However, there are some tests which are used both for screening and diagnosis, e.g., test for anemia and glucose tolerance test. Different criteria apply to both screening and diagnosis.

## Scope of Screening

Screening is very useful for identifying undetected cases (prescriptive screening), which is its most common use. Screening can also be conducted to control spread of infection (prospective screening). Screening tools are applied to detect potentially infectious cases (immigrants from countries harboring diseases), e.g., screening for cases of fever at airport during global epidemic of H1N1. It can also be conducted

Table 8.3: Screening and diagnostic tests.

| Screening test | Diagnostic test |
|---|---|
| Done on apparently healthy | Done on those with indications or sick |
| Applied to groups | Applied to single patients |
| Test results are arbitrary and final | Diagnosis is not final but modified with new evidence every time |
| Based on one criterion or cut-off point | Based on evaluation of a number of symptoms, signs (e.g., diabetes) and laboratory findings |
| Not a basis for treatment | Used as a basis for treatment |
| Less accurate | More accurate |
| Less expensive | More expensive |
| The initiative comes from the investigator or agency providing care | The initiative comes from a patient with a complaint |

for health education of community as "knowing is believing" once people know that certain diseases exist among their community members, it becomes easier to educate them about their method of prevention. It can also be done for research purposes to provide estimates of prevalence of disease and other parameters **(Figs. 8.10 and 8.11)**.

## Types of Screening

Screening can be of three types based on the population group on which it is applied.
1. ***Mass screening:*** When screening is conducted for whole population or its subsection it is known as mass screening.

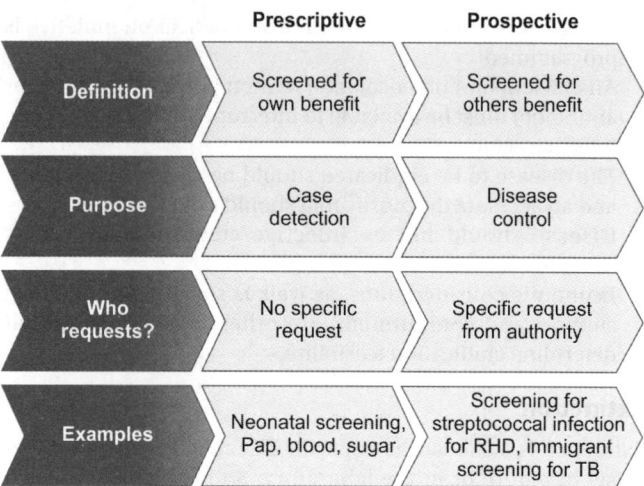

Fig. 8.10: Difference between prescriptive and prospective screening. (RHD: rheumatic heart disease; TB: tuberculosis)

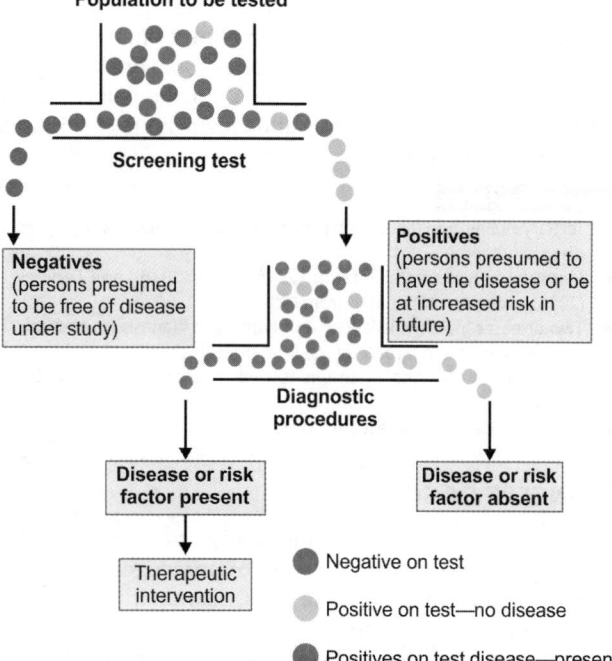

Fig. 8.11: Conceptual framework of test results versus real disease/health status.

For example, measuring blood pressure of all members of defined population and identifying hypertensive among them or measuring blood pressure among all adult males of defined population and identifying hypertensive among them is mass screening. Other examples of population screening are clinical breast examination of all adult women for breast cancer, checking all infants for hearing problems, etc.

2. *High-risk/selective screening:* When we conduct screening in a group which is at high-risk of developing disease in question then it is known as high-risk screening. Risk status for particular disease can be decided based on past epidemiological research which indicate which sub-group of population is at higher risk for developing disease in question. For example, we know people having high stress level are at higher risk of developing hypertension, so screening of senior professionals in an institute would constitute high-risk screening. Other examples of high-risk screening are mammography for women more than 40 years of age, retinal examination of diabetics, etc.

3. *Multiphasic screening:* When two or more screening tests are applied together to assess particular disease status then it is known as multiphasic screening. For example, undernourishment can be assessed through physical examination and blood investigation (e.g., blood hemoglobin level) of a person, if these two methods are applied together to identify undernourished cases then it is known as multiphasic screening. Apparently multiphasic screening seems to provide much better results; however, it should be carefully considered as it can require extra resources and may decrease population compliance.

## Criteria for Screening

Selection of diseases for screening and screening tool to be used for identifying diseases cases should be based on the criteria in **Table 8.4**.

## Properties of Screening Test

Tests which are applied for screening program must be consistent or reliable and valid. These are the most important properties of screening tests.

***Consistency/reliability:*** This is the ability of test to give same results if repeated with keeping other factors same.

***Validity of test:*** Validity of test is assessment of its accuracy to measure what it is supposed to measure.

**Table 8.4:** Criteria of selection of disease for screening and its screening tools.

| Sr. no. | Criteria for selecting disease | Criteria for selecting screening test/procedure/tool |
|---|---|---|
| 1. | It should be an important public health problem with relatively higher prevalence | It should be acceptable to people on whom applied. For example, test requiring very long time, cumbersome procedures will be unacceptable |
| 2. | Its pathogenesis should be understood so that one should have clear idea of early asymptomatic phase (duration between infection and appearance of disease sign and symptoms) | Test should be able to show consistency in its results. In other words, test results/measurement (height/weight/blood pressure) must be reproducible/repeatable |
| 3. | There should be a method/tool available to recognize disease in early asymptomatic phase | Test should give valid (accurate) results. It should be able to distinguish between disease and non-disease cases accurately |
| 4. | There should be availability of tool for confirmation of disease and its appropriate treatment. Screening program must be offered to those in need | |
| 5. | Existence of a prior evidence that early detection reduces morbidity and/or mortality | |
| 6. | There should be an agreed-on policy on when and at what levels to treat | |
| 7. | Expected benefits of early detection are cost-effective | |

**Figure 8.12** shows four possible situations. In the first one, we are hitting the target consistently, but we are missing the center of the target. That is, we are consistently and systematically measuring the wrong value for all respondents. This measure is reliable, but not valid (it is consistent but wrong). The second shows hits that are randomly spread across the target. We seldom hit the center of the target but, on average, we are getting the right answer for the group (but not very well for individuals). In this case, we get a valid group estimate, but we are inconsistent. Here, we can clearly see that reliability is directly related to the variability of what we measure. The third scenario shows a case where hits are spread across the target and we are consistently missing the

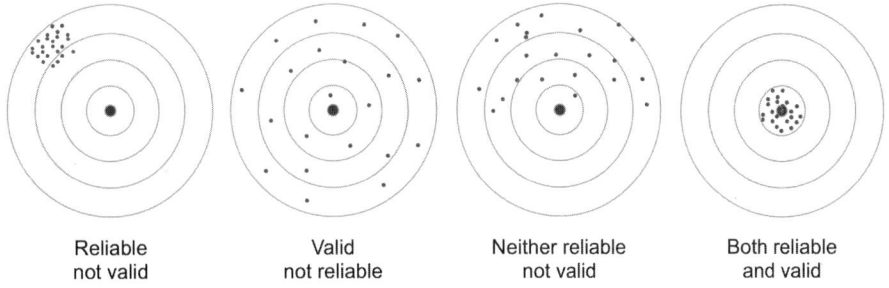

Reliable not valid    Valid not reliable    Neither reliable not valid    Both reliable and valid

**Fig. 8.12:** Four possible situations of explaining reliability and validity (*see* text for explanation).

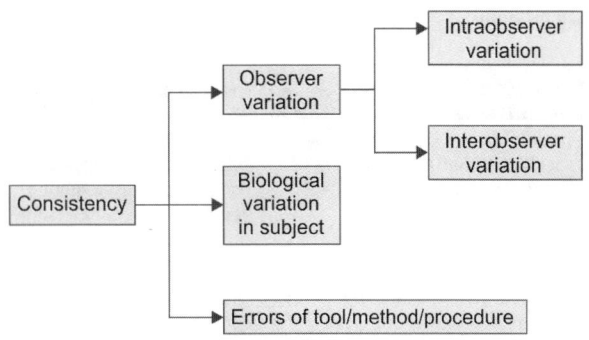

**Fig. 8.13:** Factors affecting consistency of test results.

center. Your measure in this case is neither reliable nor valid. Finally, we see the "Robin Hood" scenario—we consistently hit the center of the target. This measure is both reliable and valid.

### Consistency/Reliability of Test Results

This is the property of test to able to repeat same results if measurement is done in similar conditions. Consistency of test results may vary because of the following factors **(Fig. 8.13)**:

***Observer variation:*** Observer can make mistake in measurement. If he is measuring height of a same person three times, he may report different readings all three times, this error is known as intraobserver variation. It can be minimized by taking average of all readings. Sometimes if two different observers take same measurement in same person there is possibility of giving different results. For example, two doctors can report blood pressure of same person different at same point of time. Same X-ray picture seen by two different doctors may result in identifying different findings. This type of error is interobserver variation. This can be minimized by ensuring high standard of training and skills to them and standardizing the criteria/procedure for measuring or making conclusion.

***Biological variation in subjects:*** As many of body parameters follow diurnal rhythm so there could be difference in measurement if measured during different time of the day. For example, blood pressure, hormonal levels, blood sugar can show variation in their level if measured in same person at different time of the day. Sometimes change in emotional status of responder can also result in recording varied response.

It is also an important observation that if repeat questions are asked person avoids giving answers with extreme values (very negative or very positive), they would just tell that things are fair/average/better. If a person has taken pain killer then his tendency would to answer that pain has reduced. There is also a phenomenon that if some extreme values are observed (very negative or very positive), they tend to regress to mean during repeat measurements.

***Error of tool/methods/procedures:*** There is possibility that instrument is malfunctioning, it is not properly calibrated or some wrong reagents are used which can give misleading results.

### Validity of Test

Validity of test is assessment of its accuracy to measure what it is supposed to measure. In other words, validity of a diagnostic or screening test is ability of test to differentiate diseased cases from non-disease cases. To be valid in true sense, a test should be highly sensitive as well as specific. Quantitatively, the validity of a diagnostic or screening test is the proportion of all test results that are correct, as decided by comparison gold standard, which is generally accepted as correct.

***Sensitivity and specificity:*** Basics of sensitivity and specificity can be understood by analyzing a $2 \times 2$ table with a case scenario comprising a disease with only dichotomous condition (disease present or disease absent) and a test with only dichotomous outcome (test positive or test negative) **(Table 8.5)**.

**Table 8.5:** Status of test results versus real occurrence of disease.

| Test results | Test results of a disease | |
|---|---|---|
| | Present | Absent |
| Present | True positive (A) | False positive (B) |
| Absent | False negative (C) | True negative (D) |

Under ideal conditions, ideal test will have 100% sensitivity and specificity. **Table 8.5** shows a test which classifies individuals into two possible outcome groups—(1) individuals with positive test result, i.e., having the disease (true positives, [A]) and (2) individuals having a negative test result, i.e., without the disease (true negatives, [D]), but this is only hypothetical scenario. In real world, no such test exists. In fact, the outcome of most tests include positive results in disease-free individuals (false positives, [B]) and negative results in people with that actually have the disease (false negatives, [C]).

Sensitivity is defined as the proportion of individuals with a disease that have a positive test result. **Table 8.5** shows the total number of diseased individuals is represented by the sum of cells A and C; the number of positive test results for this group is represented in cell A. Thus, for this standard $2 \times 2$ table, sensitivity is defined as:

$$\text{Sensitivity} = \frac{A}{(A + C)} \quad (1)$$

It is usually expressed in per cent value such as 80%, which mean the proportion of test positive among diseased subject is 80 out of 100.

Similarly, specificity is defined as the test of ability to correctly identify a healthy or nondiseased subjects (B + D) as test negative (D) and is, therefore, represented by the following formula:

$$\text{Sensitivity} = \frac{D}{(B + D)} \quad (2)$$

It should also be noted that for a test with dichotomous results, the accuracy of the test is calculated based on the following formula (ability of test to give you all correct results: =

Accuracy = sensitivity + specificity

$$\text{Accuracy} = \frac{\text{True positive (TP) + true negative (TN)}}{\text{TP + FP + FN + TN}}$$

$$= \frac{(A + D)}{(A + B + C + D)} \quad (2)$$

Accuracy is the proportion of true results, either true positive or true negative in a population. In addition to the equation shown above, accuracy can be determined from sensitivity and specificity where prevalence is known.

**Accuracy = (sensitivity) × (prevalence) + (specificity) × (1 − prevalence).**

*Sensitivity and specificity of few tests are given in Table 8.6.*

**Table 8.6:** Sensitivity and specificity of few tests.

| Diseases | Tests | Sensitivity | Specificity |
| --- | --- | --- | --- |
| Ca cervix | Pap smear | 55.4% | 96.8% |
| Typhoid | WIDAL | 72% | 87% |
|  | Typhi dot | 96% | 89.5% |
| HIV | ELISA | 77.5% | 99.3% |
|  | Western blot | 99.7% | 98.5% |
| Ca breast | Mammography | 75–90% | 90–95% |
| CBNAAT | Pulmonary TB | 95.7% | 99.3% |

### Predictive Value

Though sensitivity and specificity are useful measures for evaluating test validity, they are less helpful from a clinical point of view where disease prevalence in population is unknown. The validity of a test can also be expressed as the extent to which being categorized as positive or negative actually predicts the presence of the disease, i.e., the ability of a test to predict disease among those who are test positive and non-disease who are test negative. Positive predictive value (PPV) and negative predictive value (NPV) help clinicians to understand if a patient who has come to their clinic with positive (or negative) test report, what is the probability that this patient actually has (or does not have) disease?

Suppose if a man is positive on the screening test and asks what is his chance of having the disease once all the tests are done, what can we advise? Similarly, what do we advise if the test is negative on the screening test? This can be answered by calculating PPV and NPV.

Now, considering **Table 8.5** again, it is the proportion of those with a positive test who have the disease. It is the probability that a subject has the disease given that the subject has a positive screening test result.

$$PPV = \frac{A}{(A + B)} \quad (4)$$

Positive predictive value depends on sensitivity, specificity, and prevalence of diseases in the population. For a given sensitivity and specificity, the PPV increases as the prevalence of disease increase in the population.

Similarly, NPV can be defined as the proportion of individuals with a negative test result that are actually do not have disease:

$$NPV = \frac{D}{(C + D)} \quad (5)$$

In more general terms, the PPV is the probability that someone with a positive test result actually has the disease. The NPV describes how likely it is that a patient with a negative test result is truly unaffected.

An ideal test would have both a PPV and NPV of 100%; however, tests with such optimal performance characteristics are rare in clinical practice.

Sensitivity and specificity are inherent property of any test; however, PPV and NPV values change with prevalence of disease in community. This concept is further explained with yield of test.

> **Activity 2—calculating sensitivity and specificity**
> Five hundred patients known to have a particular disease were screened with a new test. Five hundred controls without this disease were also screened. Of the 500 patients, 473 had a positive test. Of the healthy group without the disease, seven had a positive test. Create a 2 × 2 table and discuss the inference.
> Calculate sensitivity and specificity of the test. Is this a good performance? What are the implications for those wrongly classified by the test?
> **Answer**
> - Sensitivity—94.6%
> - Specificity—98.6%
> - This test will correctly identify most people who have the disease and also correctly identify most people who are disease-free. About one person in 20 who does have the disease will be misclassified as disease free and hence wrongly reassured.
> However, fewer people without disease will be misclassified as having the disease.
> - This is reassuring from a population perspective, but it is not exactly the information of direct interest to individuals and their doctors who want to know the implications of their individual results; this is given by predictive powers as follows:
> Predictive power of a positive test is a/(a+b) = 473/480 = 98.5%
> Predictive power of negative test is d/(c+d) = 493/520 = 94.8%.
> In other words, only 1 or 2% of those testing positive will have this result overturned by the definitive test. More of those with a negative test, however, will have this result overturned. This excellent performance is, however, a result of the artificial nature of the population, in which 50% have the disease.

### Yield of a Test

One factor that influences the feasibility of a screening program is the *yield*, i.e., the number of cases detected. This can be estimated from the PPV.

The PPV of a test, or the yield, is very dependent on the prevalence of the disease in the population being tested. The higher the prevalence of disease is in the population being screened, the higher the PPVs (and the yield). Consequently, the primary means of increasing the yield of a screening program is to target the test to groups of people who are at higher risk of developing the disease.

To illustrate the effect of prevalence on PPV, consider the yield that would be obtained for HIV testing in three different settings. Serological testing for HIV is *extremely* sensitive (100%) and specific (99.5%), but the PPV of HIV testing will vary markedly depending on the prevalence of preclinical disease in the population being tested. The examples below show how drastically the predicative value varies among three groups of test subjects.

These three scenarios all illustrate the consequences of HIV testing using a test that is 100% sensitive and 99.5% specific. All three show the effects of screening 100,000 subjects. The only thing that is different among these three populations is the prevalence of previously undiagnosed HIV.

### Screening Program A
The first scenario explains the yield if the screening program was conducted in male blood donors, in whom the prevalence of disease is only 0.01%. Even with 100% sensitivity and 95% specificity, the PPV (yield) is only 1.9% **(Table 8.7)**.

**Table 8.7:** HIV screening in a population with HIV prevalence of male blood donors.

| Test | Truly HIV+ | Truly HIV– | Total |
|---|---|---|---|
| Screen test + | 20 | 1,020 | 1,040 |
| Screen test – | 0 | 1,98,960 | 1,98,960 |
| Total | 20 | 1,99,980 | 2,00,000 |

Prevalence is 20/200,000 = 0.01%
Positive predictive value = 20/1040 = 0.019, or 1.9%

### Screening Program B
The second scenario illustrates the yield if the screening program was conducted in males in a RTI/STI clinic, in whom the prevalence of disease is 4%. With the same sensitivity and specificity, the PPV (yield) is 89% **(Table 8.8)**.

**Table 8.8:** HIV screening in a population of males visiting RTI/STI clinic.

| Test | Truly HIV+ | Truly HIV– | Total |
|---|---|---|---|
| Screen test + | 2,000 | 240 | 2,240 |
| Screen test – | 0 | 47,760 | 47,760 |
| Total | 2,000 | 48,000 | 50,000 |

Prevalence in males visiting RTI/STI clinic = 2,000/50,000 = 0.04, or 4%
Positive predictive value = 2,000/2,240 = 0.89, or 89%

### Screening Program C
This third scenario illustrates the yield if the screening program were conducted in users of intravenous drugs, in whom the prevalence of disease is 20%. With the same sensitivity and specificity, the PPV (yield) is 98% **(Table 8.9)**.

Prevalence of HIV in these IV drug users = 2000/10,000 = 0.20, or 20%
Positive predictive value = 2,000/2,040 = 0.98, or 98%

**Table 8.9:** HIV screening in a population of male intravenous drug users.

| Test | Truly HIV+ | Truly HIV– | Total |
|---|---|---|---|
| Screen test + | 2,000 | 40 | 2,040 |
| Screen test – | 0 | 7,960 | 7,960 |
| Total | 2,000 | 8,000 | 10,000 |

So, if we have limited resources for screening, and we want to increase chances of getting cases, one should target a subset of the population that is likely to have a higher prevalence of disease, and avoid screening that subsets who have low prevalence of diseased.

### Combination of Tests: Simultaneous (Parallel) versus Sequential (Series) Tests

When two or more screening tests are performed concomitantly, then it is parallel testing, parallel testing results into increased sensitivity. When second test is conducted after getting the result of first test, then it is known as sequential (series) testing, this increases the specificity of test results **(Table 8.10)**.

**Table 8.10:** Parallel testing versus serial testing.

| Testing strategy | Parallel testing | Serial testing |
|---|---|---|
| Procedure | Two screening tests performed at the same time and the results are subsequently combined | Second screening test is performed only if the result of the first screening test is positive |
| Effect | Higher sensitivity but lower specificity | Improves specificity at the cost of lower sensitivity |
| Example | In suspected HIV cases are screened with three parallel ELISA test, even single positive is considered HIV positive | In breast cancer screening those who come positive on clinical examination are subjected to mammography and those positive on mammography are subjected to histological examination. This results into higher specificity, i.e., it identifies all true negatives. |

(HIV, human immunodeficiency virus)

*Combined sensitivity and specificity can be achieved through following formulas:*

---
**Sensitivity and specificity in serial and parallel testing**
Sensitivity (series) = sensitivity test 1 × sensitivity test 2
Sensitivity (parallel) = 1 – (1 – sensitivity test 1) × (1 – sensitivity test 2)
Specificity (series) = 1 – (1 – specificity test 1) × (1 – specificity test 2)
Specificity (parallel) = specificity test 1 × specificity test 2

---

## Use in Community Medicine Practices

Sensitive tests are commonly used as screening test as they bring out more number of cases which are suspected to have disease. While specific tests are used as diagnostic test as they have ability to weed out those who do not have disease. ELISA is a sensitive test performed to identify HIV positive cases, however Western blot testing which is highly specific test is performed to confirm the diagnosis. So if a patient has come positive for diagnostic test there are very negligible chances that he will not have disease.

**Points to Remember**
- Positive predictive value of a test, or the yield, is very dependent on the prevalence of the disease in the population being tested
- Higher the prevalence of disease is in the population being screened, higher will be the positive predictive values (and the yield)
- Sensitive tests are commonly used as screening test
- Specific tests are used as diagnostic tests
- Serial testing is performed only if the result of the first screening test is positive.

## SURVEILLANCE

In attempt to diagnose diseases at early stage, we do certain activities like measuring and scrutiny of certain indicators related with health parameters, nutritional parameters, environmental parameters to be able to detect any change happening in trend, thereby can predict future occurrence of certain disease or health related event. This process is known as surveillance. The term "surveillance," derived from the French roots, *sur* (over) and *veiller* (to watch).

**For example:** Continuous monitoring of air pollution detected dangerous suspended particulate matter (SPM) levels during winter season in Delhi and people were advised to use protective measures to avoid respiratory diseases. So the purpose of surveillance is to detect change in trend or distribution in order to initiate investigation or control measures.

Surveillance has been defined as *"the continuous scrutiny of the factors that determine the occurrence and spread of diseases and other conditions of ill health which are pertinent of effective control."*

The use of health surveillance is mainly to estimate the prevalence of the health problems in a community, the natural history of a disease, to detect the disease epidemics, to generate the hypotheses in research, and to facilitate emergency planning.

Surveillance is considered the best weapon to avert epidemics.

Globally, the public health surveillance program is coordinated by the WHO. In 1965, the Director General of the WHO established the epidemiological surveillance unit in WHO's Division of Communicable Diseases.

> **An interesting read**
> John Snow (1813–1858), an anesthesiologist, is famous for his investigations into the causes of the 19th century cholera epidemics and is also known as the father of modern epidemiology. In 1849, Snow mapped cholera cases in London and identified the source of the outbreak as the public water pump on Broad Street (now Broadwick Street). Using a dot map, he illustrated the cluster of cholera cases around the pump. Snow's work is a good illustration of collection, analysis, interpretation, and dissemination of data leading to public health intervention.

*Source:* D Bachom's Father of Modern Epidemiology, Old News, 2005;16(8):8–10.

## Uses of Public Health Surveillance

The World Bank described six uses of public health surveillance.
1. Recognize cases or clusters of cases to trigger interventions to prevent transmission or reduce morbidity and mortality.
2. Assess the public health impact of health events or determine and measure trends.
3. Demonstrate the need for public health intervention programs and resources, and allocate resources during public health planning.
4. Monitor effectiveness of prevention and control measures and intervention strategies.
5. Identify high-risk population groups or geographic areas to target interventions and guide analytic studies.
6. Develop hypotheses that lead to analytic studies about risk factors for disease causation, propagation, or progression.

Surveillance can be conducted at the following levels:
- ***Individual surveillance:*** This is conducted for all infected cases till they become noninfectious thereby not able to spread the diseases. This is conducted potentially for those diseases which have very high fatality.
- ***Local population surveillance:*** Surveillance of malaria, sexual practices in defined population, etc.
- ***National population surveillance:*** For polio, as India has already eradicated it while its neighboring country is still harboring its virus.
- ***International surveillance:*** WHO routinely conduct surveillance of diseases of public health importance, so that nations can be timely warned if the disease trends changes indicating potential threat epidemic.
- Diseases under international surveillance are Anthrax, Avian influenza, Crimean-Congo hemorrhagic fever, Dengue hemorrhagic fever, Ebola virus disease, Hepatitis, Severe acute respiratory syndrome, Smallpox, Tularemia, Yellow fever, etc.

## Types of Surveillance

### Active Surveillance

Active surveillance is used when there is an indication that something unusual is occurring or disease is highly contagious, fatal or in the process of elimination or eradication. In this process, criteria are established for reporting disease (or its absence), risk factors or health events, but those maintaining the surveillance system (health authorities) initiate reporting.

Using the example from above—if a health department receives a case report for measles, a serious vaccine-preventable disease, active surveillance will be triggered. In active surveillane community practitioners will actively search for other cases using a standard case definition, will call doctors' offices for any cases, will follow-up to find additional cases among those exposed and will ensure checking laboratories.

Active surveillance can also take the form of regular outreach to potential reporters, to stimulate the reporting of specific diseases or injuries. Active surveillance is a means of validating the representative nature of passive reports and providing a more complete reporting of health events. Its major disadvantage is its high use of resources. For this reason, when it is used, it is for a limited time period.

Active surveillance presently conducted for polio cases and its importance will remain till polio is eradicated. Other examples of active surveillance are Domiciliary Fortnightly visits for Malaria cases in NVBDCP, Project Nikshaya for active TB surveillance.

In active surveillance, health functionaries or any designated person visits community and collect data on predefined indicators.

### Passive Surveillance

In **passive surveillance**, criteria are established for reporting diseases, risk factors, or health-related events. Health practitioners are notified of the requirements and they report events as they come to their attention. This is the more common type of surveillance.

For example, a physician sees a patient, diagnose measles, and then initiates a case report by contacting the local health department and providing the details as required for a case of measles. Here, the local health department relies on the physician to report the case.

Passive surveillance is simple to conduct, and in most cases, once the procedures are established (who to report to, case definition, laboratory confirmation) it is not a huge burden on the reporter. However, passive reporting is vulnerable to incompleteness, e.g., malaria, leprosy, etc.

### Sentinel Surveillance

A sentinel surveillance system is used when high-quality data are needed about a particular disease that cannot be obtained through a passive system. Selected reporting units such as hospitals, with a high probability of seeing cases of the disease in question, good laboratory facilities and experienced well-qualified staff, can identify and notify on certain diseases. Whereas most passive surveillance systems receive data from as many health workers or health facilities as possible, a sentinel system deliberately involves only a limited network of carefully selected reporting sites. For example, a network of large hospitals might be used to collect high-quality data on various diseases and their causative organisms, such as invasive bacterial disease caused by *Haemophilus influenzae* type b, meningococcus or pneumococcus.

Data collected in a well-designed sentinel system can be used to signal trends, identify outbreaks and monitor the burden of disease in a community, providing a rapid, economical alternative to other surveillance methods. Because sentinel surveillance is conducted only in selected locations, however, it may not be as effective for detecting rare diseases or diseases that occur outside the catchment areas of the sentinel sites.

### Behavioral Surveillance

It is a surveillance tool designed to track trends in HIV-related knowledge, attitudes, and behaviors in populations at risk of HIV and sexually transmitted infections (STIs). Behavioral surveillance is defined as ongoing systematic collection, analysis, and interpretation of behavioral data relevant to understanding trends in the transmission of HIV and STIs. In low-level and concentrated HIV epidemics, surveillance systems for HIV should rely to the large extent on behavioral data as they help us to understand the potential dynamics of HIV and STI epidemics.

### Nutritional Surveillance

Nutritional surveillance is an important tool for identifying existing system for collecting information on the current and future magnitude, distribution, and causes of malnutrition in populations—with emphasis on protein-energy malnutrition in order to assist governments and international agencies in policy formulation, program planning, management, and evaluation. Attention to be given to situations of acute food shortages as well as chronic malnutrition.

Nutritional surveillance process includes routine collection and compilation of data to know about the details of nutrition related disease. Initially it was presumed that there are some diseases which occur due to nutritional deficiencies (e.g. anemia, rickets, and osteoporosis) but later it was noticed that it includes wide range of morbidities (e.g. obesity, hypertension, cancers, coronary heart disease, and dental caries). ***Nutritional surveillance is further discussed in Chapter 23: Epidemiology of Nutrition and Food-related Diseases and its Prevention and Control.***

### Surveillance in Practice

There are three parallel systems of surveillance:
1. *Syndromic surveillance:* It is conducted by field/community workers based on predefined symptoms. So this helps in finding out suspected cases from community. Example: For RTI and STI cases we conduct syndromic surveillance.
2. *Presumptive surveillance:* All the suspected cases are referred to medical officers for confirmation. Doctor confirms the case based on sign and symptoms. This is presumptive surveillance gives idea of probable cases.
3. *Laboratory surveillance:* Probable cases are subjected to laboratory investigations for confirmation. Then finally we know confirmed cases. This system is in practice in India under Integrated Diseases Surveillance Project.

### Vertical Surveillance versus Integrated Surveillance

Surveillance when used for specific disease or injury, vertical surveillance systems can be used. Information obtained by this can be then used for specific disease control program.

Similarly, surveillance by integrated approach foresees a collective system for numerous diseases using common structure, processes, and personnel. Through proper coordination more proficient and economical system develops, as it allows utilizing existing resources and capacity. Thus, it promotes the optimum use of health resources. Integrated Disease Surveillance Programme (IDSP) launched by World Bank in 2004 is the example of integrated surveillance. ***It is discussed in detail in Chapter 47: Health Policies and Programs in India.***

## SUMMARY

This chapter provides understanding of concept of prevention with its practical applicability in community for prevention of disease and securing optimum health. This chapter explains various levels of prevention, viz.—(1) **primordial prevention**, (2) **primary prevention**, (3) **secondary prevention**, (4) **tertiary prevention**, and (5) also the latest **quaternary prevention**. It further discusses various interventions required for each level of prevention which includes Health Promotion and Specific Protection for primary prevention, early detection of the disease and its prompt treatment for secondary prevention, Rehabilitation and palliative care for tertiary prevention. This chapter gives in-depth understanding of primordial prevention and its importance in current disease scenario.

*Disease prevention* covers measures not only to prevent the occurrence of disease but also to arrest its progress and reduce its consequences once established. *Disease Control, Elimination, Eradication, and Extinction* are very well explained in the chapter which mainly aim at reducing disease incidence, disease transmission, its financial burden on the community, and its morbidity and mortality.

*Screening* is one subtopic of chapter which is useful to understand the process of searching unidentified diseases, defect or any condition of ill health by means of rapidly applied simple tests, examination or other procedures in apparently healthy looking individuals. Understanding of types of screening and criteria for screening will be useful for planning any screening program. This section also explains *sensitivity, specificity, positive predictive value (PPV), and negative predictive value (NPV)* of the test and their importance for knowing the chances of real occurrence of disease and how these value changes with the change in prevalence of the disease.

Another section of chapter is **Surveillance**, which is defined as continuous scrutiny of the factors that determine the occurrence and spread of diseases and other conditions of ill health for their effective control. This section will give you knowledge of *Active surveillance, Passive surveillance, Sentinel surveillance, Nutritional surveillance*, etc., which play a major role in further disease prevention and important for disease eradication.

## SUGGESTED READING

1. American College of Preventive Medicine. Preventive medicine. Available from: www.acpm.org/page/preventive medicine.
2. Benenson AS. Control of Communicable Diseases in Man, 13th edition; American Public Health Association (APHA), New York; 1981.
3. Brachman PS. Public health surveillance. In: Brachman PS, Abrutyn E (Eds). Bacterial Infections of Humans: Epidemiology and Control. New York, NY: Springer; 2009.
4. Centers for Disease Control and Prevention. The Pink Book: Course Textbook. Epidemiology and Prevention of Vaccine-Preventable Diseases, 13th edition; 2015.
5. Community-based rehabilitation: CBR guidelines. World Health Organization 2010.
6. Disease Control Priorities Project. Public Health Surveillance—The Best Weapon to Avert Epidemics 2008.
7. Dowdle W, Cochi SL (Eds). Disease Eradication in the 21st Century. Implications for Global Health. Cambridge, MA: The MIT Press; 2011.
8. Dowdle WR. The principles of disease elimination and eradication. Bull World Health Organ. 1998;76(Suppl 2):23-5.
9. Fenner F, Henderson DA, Arita I, et al. Potential sources for a return of smallpox. In: Smallpox and its eradication. Geneva: World Health Organization; 1988;20:1321-44.
10. Ferrini R, Mannino E, Ramsdell E, et al. Screening mammography for breast cancer: American College of Preventive Medicine Practice Policy Statement. Am J Prevet Med. 1996;12(5):340-41.
11. Garcia-Albreu A, Halperin W, Danel I. Public Health Surveillance Toolkit: A guide for busy task managers. Washington, DC: World Bank; 2002.
12. Glaser AN. High-yield, Biostatistics Epidemiology and Public Health, 4th edition. Wolters Kluwer Health/Lippincott Williams & Wilkins, 2014.
13. Government of India. Handbook for Vaccine and Cold Chain Handlers, 2nd edition. New Delhi: Ministry of Health and Family Welfare; 2016.
14. Govt of India. National Health Policy 2017. Ministry of Health and Family Welfare; 2017.
15. Johnson LR, Heymann DL. Encyclopedia of Life Support Systems (EOLSS) Ramsey, Isle of Man: Eolss Publishers; 2004. Public Health Surveillance. Raska K. National and international surveillance of communicable diseases. WHO Chronicle. 1966;20(9):315-21.
16. Leavell HR, Clark EG. The science and art of preventing disease, prolonging life, and promoting physical and mental health and efficiency. Preventive Medicine for the Doctor in his Community: Krieger Publishing Company; 1979.
17. Mayrand MH, Franco ED, Rodrigues I, et al. Canadian Cervical Cancer Screening Trial Study Group. Human papillomavirus DNA versus Papanicolaou screening tests for cervical cancer. N Engl J Med. 2007;357(16):1579-88.
18. Pandve HT. Quaternary prevention: Need of the hour. J Family Med Prim Care. 2014;3.4:309-10.
19. Petersen AR. Community development in health promotion: empowerment or regulation? Aust J Public Health. 1994;18(2):213.
20. Prüss-Üstün A, Wolf J, Corvalán CF, et al. Maria Purificación. Preventing disease through healthy environments: A global assessment of the burden of disease from environmental risks. 2016. World Health Organization.
21. Rutherford GW. Principles and practices of public health surveillance. Am J Epidemiol. 2001;154(4):385-6.
22. Sergeant and Perkins. Epidemiology for field veterinarians: An introduction. Wallingford, UK: CABI; 2016, pp. 98-102.
23. Sharma SK, Kohli M, Yadav RN, et al. Evaluating the diagnostic accuracy of Xpert MTB/RIF assay in pulmonary tuberculosis. Goletti D (Ed). PLoS ONE. 2015;10(10):e0141011.
24. The persons with disabilities (equal opportunities, protection of rights and full participation) act, 1995 published in part ii, section 1 of the extraordinary gazette of India Ministry of Law, Justice and Company Affairs (Legislative Department), New Delhi, 1st January, 1996.
25. Thrusfield. Veterinary epidemiology, 2nd edition. Oxford, UK: Blackwell Science Ltd.; 1995. pp. 279-80.
26. WHO. Current strategies for Human Rabies Pre and Post-Exposure Prophylaxis, 3rd September, 2010.
27. WHO. Expanded Programme on Immunization, Report and working papers, 1978; 31st session of the WHO reg. Committee, Mongolia, 1978, SEARO.
28. WHO. International Classification of Impairments, Disabilities, and Handicaps, A Manual of Classification Relating to the Consequences of disease. Published in accordance with resolution WHA29. 35 of the Twenty-ninth World Health Assembly, May 1976.
29. WHO Definition of Palliative Care for Children. Available from: http://www.who.int/cancer/palliative/definition/en.
30. Wilson JMG. Principles and practice of screening for disease. Geneva: WHO; 1968.

# CHAPTER 9

# Basics of Epidemiology

*Nirmal Kumar Mandal, Teeku Sinha, Sarmila Mallik*

| | |
|---|---|
| CM7.1 | Define epidemiology and describe and enumerate the principles, concepts and uses |
| CM7.4 | Define, calculate and interpret morbidity and mortality indicators based on given set of data |
| CM17.2 | Describe community diagnosis |

## INTRODUCTION

Epidemiology is the foundation of public health. It was first expressed over 2,000 years ago by Hippocrates and other, that environment causes and influences the existences of disease. Effort to quantify disease and deaths in population began in 1662 when John Graunt published analysis of birth and deaths in London. He was the first person who quantified patterns of birth, death, and disease occurrence, noting male-female disparities, high infant mortality, urban-rural differences, and seasonal variations. However, the distribution of disease in specific population was first measured to any great extent in the 19th century. James Lind, a naval surgeon in 1747 conducted a planned trial on 12 sailors suffering from scurvy, and found visible good effect of oranges and lemons to cure it. John Snow (1813–1858), a renowned anesthesiologist of his time is popularly known as the father of modern epidemiology for his historical investigation on cholera epidemic in London. First he described the occurrence of mortality due to cholera and its distribution. He then compared mortality experience of the people according to their drinking water sources to identify offending source. In a second experiment in Broad Street, first time in the history of medicine, he developed a spot map to see whether there was clustering of cholera deaths around any pump and identified Broad Street pump as a source of contaminated water, and removed its handle to control epidemic. In 1839, William Farr, a physician, systematized the collection, analysis and reporting of medical statistics in office of registrar general for England and Wales. Farr is considered as the father of modern vital statistics and surveillance. He developed many of the basic practices used today in vital statistics and disease classification. He compared mortality and patterns of cause of deaths in population according to characteristics of individuals, place of residence, etc. Thus, human race has been trying to answer the question on occurrence of the disease, pattern of its distribution, factors causing it and its remedial measures by use of contemporary knowledge and skills. As a part of such constant attempts, science of epidemiology evolved. Epidemiology started as "a branch of medical science which treats epidemics." Now concept has been expanding over the time. In 1960, MacMahon defined epidemiology as "the study of distribution and determinants of disease frequency in man." In the past 90 years, the definition has broadened from concern with communicable disease epidemics to include all phenomena related to health in populations. Chronic diseases have now overtaken infectious diseases as the major global health problem even in developing countries. Concept of epidemiology is currently used to examine the role of biomarkers at molecular level and genetic variation as determinants of health and diseases. Now epidemiology is not only concerned about disease only, but any health-related states and events like risk factors, risk behavior, etc., came under purview of epidemiology. Its knowledge is applied to generate much of the information required by public health professionals to plan, implement, and evaluate effective interventions to prevent disease and promote health.

> **Note**
> The Scientific study of disease at different levels:
> - Submolecular or molecular level: Cell biology, genetics, biochemistry, immunology
> - Tissue or organ level: Anatomic pathology
> - Level of individual patients: Clinical medicine
> - Level of populations: Epidemiology.

## CONCEPT AND DEFINITION

In 2001, John Last, in the dictionary of Epidemiology, has defined epidemiology as "The study of the distribution and determinants of health-related states or events in specified population, and application of this study to the control of health problems."

*(Word "Epidemiology" is derived from three Greek roots: Epi = upon, demos = people or population and Logos = study. Thus, epidemiology means study on community or population)*

Epidemiology has been defined by many authors in different times. A short list is given below:

- **Frost (1927):** The Science of mass phenomenon of infectious diseases. An inductive science concerned not merely with describing the distribution of disease, but equally or more with fitting it into a consistent philosophy.
- **Greenwood (1934):** Study of disease, any disease, as a mass phenomenon.
- **Lilienfeld (1957):** The study of the distribution of a disease or a physiological condition in human population and of the factors that influence the distribution.
- **Morris (1964):** The study of health and disease of population.
- **Taylor (1967):** The study of health or ill-health in a defined population.
- **Maxcy:** That field of medical science which is concerned with the relationship of various factors and conditions which determine the frequencies and distributions of an infectious process, a disease, or a physiologic state in human community.
- **Porta MA (2008):** The study of the occurrence and distribution of health-related events, states, and processes in specified populations, including the study of the determinants influencing such processes, and the application of this knowledge to control relevant health problems.

The definition of epidemiology (JM Last) uses few important terms which reflect some of the principles of the discipline:

***Study:*** It includes methods of scientific inquiry like surveillance, observation, hypothesis testing, analytic research and experiments.

***Distribution:*** Distribution refers to *frequency and pattern* of health-related events in community. Frequency means numbers reflecting magnitude of the problems and expressed in terms of rate, ratio and proportions. Pattern refers to the distribution of events in the community in terms of place, person and time.

***Determinants:*** Why and how such events are occurring? These are the factors that influence the occurrence of disease and health-related events like biological, chemical, physical, social, cultural, economic and genetic and behavioral factors.

***Health-related states and events:*** Diseases, accidents, death, lifestyle, heath seeking behavior, etc.

***Specified populations:*** Epidemiology concerns about collective health of a community like population in a block or districts, occupational groups, vulnerable groups, etc.

***Application to prevention and control (the aims of public health):*** Epidemiology describes disease occurrence and its etiology for *directing public heath action* to promote, protect, and restore health.

## CLINICAL APPROACH AND EPIDEMIOLOGICAL APPROACH

In clinical medicine, a patient with specific symptoms and signs goes to a physician who examines the patient, makes a provisional diagnosis, does some investigations, reaches a confirmed diagnosis and finally treats the patient and makes follow-up advices during convalescent period. An epidemiologist, on the other hand, goes to the community, makes a study or survey to know the magnitude of a health problem, its distribution in the community in terms of place, person and time, identifies the contributing risk factors, and finally assists in planning, implementing, monitoring and evaluating, preventive and remedial measures **(Table 9.1)**.

Both clinician and epidemiologist play very important role in disease control. In fact, role of the both approaches supplement, each other covering all phases of natural history of diseases. A clinician uses the concept of epidemiology while predicting about prognosis of a disease, and an epidemiologist uses clinical approach while examining and treating a patient at field level.

**Table 9.1:** The differences between clinical and epidemiological approaches.

| Clinical approach | Epidemiological approach |
|---|---|
| Individual approach | Community or group approach |
| Patients goes to clinician | Epidemiologist goes to community |
| Process starts with signs and symptoms of a patient like episode of fever | Process starts with health problem in a community like fever outbreak |
| Concerned about only ill persons | Concerned about both ill and healthy persons |
| Physician examines a patient clinically | Epidemiologist conducts a study or survey |
| Physician investigates to diagnose the disease of a patient | Epidemiologist uses epidemiological indicators to reach community diagnosis |
| Physician treats the patient, e.g. treatment of malaria with antimalarial drugs; treatment of appendicitis with surgical procedure like appendectomy, etc. | Epidemiologist suggests community health measure like safe water supply, immunization of children, active surveillance for diseases, etc. |
| Physician follows-up and assesses the patient | Epidemiologist evaluates community health measure (program) and observes change in health status of the community |

## AIMS AND OBJECTIVES OF EPIDEMIOLOGY

Aim of epidemiology is to eliminate or reduce health problem and its consequences in a community. To achieve this, there are specific objectives of epidemiology as follows:
- To assess magnitude of health problems, e.g., frequency of diseases
- To understand distribution pattern of health problems in terms of place, person and time

> **Place:** Where did it happen? Geographic variation, urban, rural differences.
> **Person:** Who were the persons affected? Personal and demographic factors like age, sex, occupation, religion, etc.
> **Time:** When did it occur? Seasonality, daily occurrence like epidemic.

- To identify etiological factors contributing to the occurrence of such health problems
- To identify remedial or preventive measures
- To provide data essential for the planning, implementation, evaluation of services for prevention, control and treatment of health problems.

Ultimate aim is to lead effective action:
- To reduce or eliminate the health problems and its consequences.
- To prevent its occurrence in future.

## USES OF EPIDEMIOLOGY

There are wide ranges of application of epidemiology in public health and clinical medicine. They are:

- **Study of history of health of population:** Studying past history of rise and fall of diseases and health related events like lifestyle help to understand the trend of health phenomena over time. This knowledge helps in making future trend of health problems.
- **Study of natural history of diseases:** Epidemiological approach helps to study normal course of a disease starting from prepathogenesis phase through pathogenesis phase to outcome (recovery, disability or death). It is required to complete the clinical picture and outcomes of both communicable and noncommunicable diseases (observational epidemiology).
- **Investigation of outbreak of disease:** Epidemiological concept is very frequently used to investigate outbreak of disease like food poisoning, measles outbreak, outbreak of water-borne diseases, etc. (application of both descriptive and analytical epidemiology).
- **Studying the occurrence and distribution of any health problem:** Descriptive epidemiology is useful to measure magnitude (burden) of health problems in a community, and its distribution by place, person and time.
- **Making community diagnosis:** Identification and quantification of current health problems and risk factors prevalent in the community, and assessment of available resources are required to prioritize appropriate interventions.
- **Identification of syndromes:** Studying the occurrence of clinical phenomena and its distribution in the community help epidemiologist to identify disease syndromes.
- **Estimating individual risk and chances:** Based on the group experience of many patients in the community, individual risks on disease, injury and defect and its prognosis can be estimated.
- **Studying the risk or causal factors (determinants) of a health problem:** We can identify etiological agents or risk factors of diseases by using analytical approach of epidemiology.
- **Studying the efficacy of preventive, promotive, and curative measure:** Experimental epidemiology helps us to know efficacy of a measure, preventive, promotive or curative, at hospital or in community setting.
- **Surveillance of diseases and community health interventions:** Surveillance of diseases such as acute flaccid paralysis (AFP) surveillance for poliomyelitis includes the entire process of collecting, analyzing, interpreting, and reporting data. This is considered important for interventions aiming at preventing disease and promoting heath. They are based on the epidemiological principles and methods.
- **Prediction about future disease trend:** An epidemiologist can develop predictive model to comment on future trend of the disease by appropriate use of epidemiological approach and statistical methods.
- **Evaluation of health programs:** Use of epidemiology is not restricted to identifying disease occurrence or its treatment, its use is now extended to program evaluation and health services research. Epidemiological approach is used to evaluate the effectiveness and efficiency of health services such as the efficiency of safe water supply to control diarrheal diseases.
- **Conduction of health services research:** The epidemiological principles and methods are used effectively in health services research.

> **Points to Remember**
> 1. Epidemiology is the study of distribution (pattern and frequency) and determinants of health-related events, specified populations and used for preventive action
> 2. The clinical medicine is based on epidemiological data. So, the approach in clinical disease is through epidemiology
> 3. Epidemiology is used to study the disease history in population, to study natural history of the disease, investigation of risk factors and epidemic, study the efficiency of surveillance, understand the prediction or trend to involve the preventive measures and to evaluate health programs.

## COMMUNITY HEALTH PROBLEM

These are the health problems, which affects the normal functioning and development of community by way of imposing burden by affecting large number of people, reducing their contributions to the community due to sickness or disability, or premature deaths. Health status and health problem are the prerequisite for planning healthcare services in any country. Knowledge of the disease burden in populations is essential for health authorities, who have to prioritize the areas to use limited resources to the best possible effect for prevention and control of the diseases.

### Vulnerable Groups

There are many groups who are more vulnerable to risk of morbidity and mortality. These groups need to be identified so that appropriate timely action can be taken:

- Pregnant and lactating mothers
- Under-five children
- Adolescents
- Elderly people (geriatric population)
- People living in tribal, hilly and riverine belts (difficulty to access areas)
- Migrant laborers and street children.

### Communicable and Noncommunicable Diseases

- **Communicable diseases:** Among the communicable diseases prevalent in India, tuberculosis (TB), gastrointestinal (GI) infections, vector-borne diseases (VBDs) and HIV contribute as the leading causes of morbidity and mortality. The year 2022 marks a milestone year for TB surveillance efforts in India, with 13% increase in case notification rate (172 cases per lakh population) as compared to 2021 (India TB Report 2023). The disease burden due to malaria is declining slowly in India and we are optimistic about elimination of malaria by 2030. However, dengue is posing a great public health challenge in recent years with recurrent outbreaks. In 2022, a total of 2,33,251 cases with 303 deaths have been reported (NVBDCP report).
- **Noncommunicable diseases:** India will be the diabetic capital of the world in coming years. Due to changes in lifestyle, dietary habits and behavioral risk factors, there is silent migration of Indian population towards affliction

with noncommunicable diseases like hypertension, stroke, ischemic heart disease and hypertension. As per NFHS-5 data, 21.3% of women and 24% of men aged 15–49 have hypertension. About 13.5% of women and 15.6% of men have random blood glucose levels greater than 140 mg/dL. Obesity is considered as risk factor for these diseases and key indicators of NFHS-5 revealed that 24% of women and 22.9% of men are overweight or obese. Cancer, blindness and accidents are also remarkable causes of morbidity, mortality and disability in India.

## Malnutrition

Under-five children, pregnant and lactating mothers are the most vulnerable group for malnutrition in India. As per NFHS-5, 35.5% of children less than 5 years are stunted (short for their age); 19.3% are wasted (thin for their height); 32.1% are underweight (thin for their age). Not only under fives, 18.7% of women and 16.2% of men are also having below normal BMI. Poor infant and young child feeding (IYCF) practices are considered as key factors behind malnutrition of these under 5 children.

***Initial breastfeeding:*** About two-fifths (42%) of children born in the last 5 years were breastfed within 1 hour of birth, as recommended.

***Exclusive breastfeeding***: 64% of children less than 6 months are exclusively breastfed (NFHS-5, 2019-21).

***Anemia and other nutritional deficiency:*** A great majority of Indian population is suffering from anemia as revealed by NFHS-5 key indicators; 67.1% of children aged 6–59 months and 52.2% pregnant mothers have anemia (hemoglobin levels below 11.0 g/dL). Other prevalent nutritional problems are vitamin A deficiency among under five children, goiter and iodine deficiency disorder (IDD). Moreover as like noncommunicable diseases (NCDs), we cannot ignore the recent alarming trend of obesity and overweight among Indian population.

## Environmental Health Problem and Related Issues

Safe water and sanitation are basic needs of the community. Census 2011 reports that 22% of rural households have their drinking water source beyond 500 meters. Water quality has also emerged to be a growing concern due to bacterial contamination as well as arsenic and fluoride toxicity. About 39% of households have no facility of sanitation, which means that the household members practice open defecation. Prevalence of diarrhea and other GIT diseases and viral hepatitis are closely associated with unsafe water and poor sanitation. Both outdoor and indoor air pollution have already emerged to be a serious public health concern especially in urban areas of India. Only 58.6% of households use clean fuel for cooking. Prevention and control of acute respiratory infections (ARI) among under-fives, bronchial asthma and cancers in adult population caused as a menace of air pollution is an area of great concern to the public health policy makers and implementers (NFHS-5).

## Reproductive and Child Health Problems

***Maternal health:*** NFHS key indicators revealed rise of antenatal care (ANC) from 51.2% (NFHS-5) to 58.1% (NFHS-5) of women had at least 4 ANC visits. Institutional delivery had also improved markedly from 39% in NFHS-3 to 79% in NFHS-5 and at present according to NFHS-5, it is 88.6%; but maternal malnutrition and anemia, poor quality and inadequacy of antenatal and postnatal care are big challenges to reduce maternal mortality and morbidity in India. Teenage pregnancy with its complications and unsafe abortions are also other contributory factors. Maternal mortality ratio (MMR) has also declined considerably from 212/100,000 live births (2007–09) to 97/1,00,000 live births currently (Special bulletin on Maternal Mortality in India, SRS, November, 2022) although interstate and rural urban variations still exist. There is still a long path ahead as India is committed to achieve MMR less than 70/100,000 live births as per UN target of Sustainable Development Goals by 2030.

***Child health:*** ARI and diarrhea are found to be the leading causes of under-five mortality in India. NFHS-5 data revealed symptoms of ARI and diarrhea among under-five children in the period of 2 weeks prior to the survey as 2.8% and 7.3% respectively. Out of which 60.6% of children with diarrhea received oral rehydration therapy (ORT), as recommended. Key indicators also revealed that only 54% of children received any service from an anganwadi center under Integrated Child Development Service (ICDS); 48% received food supplements. Low birth weight, malnutrition, low immunization coverage and poor Infant and Young Child Feeding (IYCF) practices also contribute to high infant and child mortality and morbidity in India. About 58% of under-five deaths occur within first-1 month of life. India had remarkable success in decreasing under-five mortality to 36 per 1000 live births and infant mortality rate to 28 per 1000 live births as per SRS 2020 Report (published in May 2022), but still neonatal deaths are a major concern and thrust area.

## Population Growth

India is contributing 17.5% of total population of the world, while occupying only 2.4% of global land mass. Moreover, adverse child sex ratio is also a big threat to the girl children. Early age of marriage and child birth, decreased spacing between pregnancies, low contraceptive use rate and unmet need of family planning are the major factors behind the population explosion in India. At present 9.4% (NFHS-5) currently married women have an unmet need for family planning, which was 14% during the survey of NFHS-3. Modern contraceptive use by currently married women has remained unchanged, at around 50%, between NFHS-3, 4 and 5. In spite of availability of basket of choices under family planning methods, female sterilization is still the most popular contraceptive method, used by 37.9% of currently married women. Commitment on the part of the government and huge investment on family planning have helped a decline of total fertility rate (TFR) to 2.0 (NFHS-5).

## Health Problems of Adolescents and School Age Children

Adolescents and school age children are vulnerable to develop anemia, malnutrition (both under and over nutrition) and IDD. Behavioral health problems are also major health problems among this age group, especially among school dropouts and orphans. It is revealed from NFHS-5 key indicators that among children under age 18, 5% are orphans (one or both parents are dead) and 3% are not living with a biological parent. Regarding school attendance, the net attendance ratio falls from 78% in primary school to 68% in middle, secondary, and higher secondary school.

### Health Problems of the Elderly

The geriatric population in India has increased from 7.7% in 2001 census to nearly 8.14% as per census 2011 report. This population group has high burden NCDs, chronic as well as multiple health problems leading to disability. In spite of growing proportion of this geriatric age group, there is lack of dedicated health infrastructure and specialist and trained manpower in India.

### Behavioral Health Problems

An estimated 1 million of Indians die annually due to tobacco related diseases. According to NFHS-5, 8.9% of women and 38.0% of men age 15 years and above consume any kind of tobacco.

*Use of alcohol:* 18.8% of men and 1.3% of women aged 15 years and above drink alcohol, as revealed by NHFS-5, 2019-21 key indicators. As per the report of ICMR, nearly 50% of cancers in male and 25% in females and more than 80% of oral cancers are attributed to tobacco use. A majority of lung and cardiovascular diseases are also directly caused by tobacco use.

*Sexually transmitted infections (STIs):* 12% of women and 9% of men aged 15–49 who have ever had sex reported having an STI and/or symptoms of an STI in the 12 months preceding the survey, as obvious from NFHS-5 data. We cannot ignore the recent trend of alarming use of internet and mobile with its associated health hazards.

### Poor Coverage of Healthcare

India has developed a wide network of primary healthcare infrastructure to provide health services to 72% of population living in rural areas, but still it is not accessible to a wide range of population living in difficult to reach areas, especially in hilly and tribal areas. Many times they cannot enjoy the benefits of modern medicine and become compelled to depend on indigenous medicine, traditional healers or registered medical practitioners. Moreover, the present disease-oriented hospital based healthcare services are mostly concentrated in urban areas; still the out of pocket expenditure is huge for people with poor socioeconomic status. So, the present healthcare delivery system is inadequate, as well as not equitable.

## COMMUNITY DIAGNOSIS (MEASURING COMMUNITY HEALTH)

### Concept and Purpose

A community is defined as a cluster of people with at least one characteristic such as geographic location, occupation, ethnicity, housing condition, exposure to similar risk factor, etc. World Health Organization (WHO) defines community diagnosis as "a quantitative and qualitative description of the health of citizens and the factors which influence their health including the population's perception of their own health. It identifies problems, proposes areas for improvement, and stimulates action."

So, the main purpose of the community diagnosis is to assess the health status or health problems of a community, its determinants of health, and whether the community has achieved the level of health which has been envisaged by the health policy or programs. In short it is to assess where the community stands now; where it wants to reach; and how it will get there?

This basic principle of community diagnosis has been applied in many developing countries to identify the ways to improve the health status under scarce resources.

Types of community diagnosis:
- **Comprehensive:** To gather general information about community like demographic, sociocultural, economic, health-related information, resources available.
- **Problem based:** To gather information responding to a particular problem and to address its solution.

### Concept about Epidemiological Parameters

Epidemiologists are always interested to know the magnitude of the health problem in a community. We also need to assess trend of a disease over the time or compare the health status of two different communities or districts or states. But how will we do it? Some epidemiological parameters or units of measurement are necessary to comprehend the magnitude of the health problems **(Table 9.2)**.

**Table 9.2:** Category of epidemiological parameters.

| Category | Parameter | Units of measurement |
|---|---|---|
| Morbidity (disease, injury and disability) | • Incidence rate<br>• Incidence density (person-time incidence rate)<br>• Point prevalence<br>• Period prevalence | • Rate<br>• Rate<br><br>• Proportion<br>• Proportion |
| Mortality (death) | • Crude death rate<br>• Case-fatality rate<br>• Cause-specific death rate<br>• Age-specific death rate<br>• Proportional mortality rate<br>• Standardized mortality ratio | • Rate<br>• Proportion<br>• Rate<br>• Rate<br>• Proportion<br>• Ratio |

Let us see an example:

Twenty persons of village A and 10 persons of village B were affected with diarrhea in the month of June 2018. It seems apparently that the case load is twice in village A than village B. But when we find out the population of the two villages, i.e., 2,000 in village A and 1,000 in village B, the case load stands to be 10/1,000 population for each village. So there is no difference in case load, though apparently it looks like. So, knowing only frequency will not help, but denominator population is necessary for comparison.

Measurement of cases or events in relation to denominator population will produce some epidemiological parameters which will help the epidemiologists for making comparisons. In epidemiology, we are all more concerned with denominator population of a community.

## Units of Measurement: Rate, Ratio, Proportion

In epidemiology, rate, ratio and proportion are very frequently used as units of measurement. They compare a part of the population to another part or to total population. Basic form of these measures is same, one numerator (upper part), one denominator (lower part) and one multiplier.

**Ratio:** Ratio is a comparison of two values, when they are independent to each other, and numerator is not a part of denominator. If X is numerator and Y is denominator, they are independent to each other and X is not a part of Y, then X:Y or X/Y is a ratio. This fraction can be multiplied by 1,100, 1,000, and so on.

*Uses of ratio:* As descriptive measure, we calculate sex ratio, dependency ratio, doctor-population ratio, etc. As analytical measures it is used to compare occurrence of diseases, injuries, disabilities between two groups. Examples are relative risk, odds ratio, and so on.

> **Example: Calculation of ratio**
> **Sex ratio:** In a medical college, 150 students got admitted in a year, of them 100 were males and 50 were females. So, sex ratio was female:male = 50:100 or $\frac{50}{100}$ or 500 females per 1,000 males.
> **Interpretation:** Enrolment of female students in the medical college in that year is half of the male students.

**Proportion:** When numerator is a part of denominator, it is expressed as proportion. If X is numerator and (X+Y) is denominator, and X is a part of (X + Y). So, proportion will be $\frac{X}{X+Y}$. Proportion can be expressed as a fraction or a percentage.

*Uses:*
- It is used as a common descriptive measure in different fields. For example, proportion of students in a class, proportion of the children between 12 months and 23 months fully immunized, proportional mortality rate.
- Proportions can be used to measure amount of disease attributable to a risk factors.

> **Example: Calculation of proportion**
> Proportion of female students admitted in a medical college (see example of ratio above):
> Proportion of female students = $\frac{\text{No. of female students}}{\text{Total students both female and male}} = \frac{50}{150} = 0.33$ or 33%

**Rate:** In epidemiology, a rate is a measure of the frequency with which an event occurs in a defined population over a specified period of time. In calculating rate, we require numerator, denominator, multiplier and time specification. Numerators are events like number of deaths, number of patients, number of episodes, etc. Population at risk, mid-year population, and person-time are used as denominator. Multiplier depends on proportion of numerator with respect to denominator. It may be 100, 1,000, 10,000 or 100,000. Time specification is very important and it makes difference between rate and proportion.

It may be point of time (day) or period of time (months, years, 5 years, etc.). Examples of rates are given as health-related epidemiological parameters.

*Uses:*
- Comparison of an observed rate with national rate or national target
- Comparison between rates of two different populations
- Comparison of rates of same population over a period of time.

### Directly Health-related Epidemiological Parameters

**(1) Morbidity-related parameters:** Incidence, prevalence, disability.

Incidence and prevalence are two important measures of health information and can be expressed as numbers or a calculated rate (incident cases, prevalent cases or incidence rate, prevalence rate).

### Incidence

Incidence measures number of new cases, episodes or events in a specified population at a given period of time, usually 1 year. It is the most basic and appropriate measure of disease frequency. It measures the rate at which new events occur in the population.

Incidence rate is calculated as number of new cases at a given period of time with reference to the population at risk.

$$\text{Incidence rate} = \frac{\text{New cases occurring in a given period}}{\text{Population at risk during the same time period}} \times 1{,}000$$

> **Example: Calculation of incidence rate**
> In a kala-azar endemic district, estimated mid-year population in 2014 was 1,850,000; new reported cases of kala-azar were 200 in that
> Incidence rate = $\frac{200}{1{,}850{,}000} \times 1{,}000 = 0.108$ per 1000 population.

*Numerator:* new cases (events)

*Denominator:* Population at risk. Population at risk is those who are susceptible to the particular disease. For cervical cancer, population at risk is women, not men. From practical point of view, population as on 1st July (mid-year population) of the community is taken as denominator.

*Time period:* It will differ from disease to disease, commonly 1 year, but may be week, month, even 5 years. It is necessary to follow-up the entire population at risk throughout the specified period of time.

*Multiplier:* Commonly 1,000, depending on number of cases with reference to denominator population, 10,000, 100,000 may be used.

### Incidence in Special Situations

**Incidence density:** When population at risk cannot be followed evenly through entire time period, person-time like person-month, person-year is used as denominator. Incidence density is particularly used where chance of occurrence of episode of a disease in a person is more than once during the period of follow-up.

$$\text{Incidence density} = \frac{\text{Number of new events}}{\text{Person-time}} \times 100$$

It is explained in a schematic **Figure 9.1**. Ten under-fives are followed up for a period of 2 years to identify episode of ARI among them. During that period 15 episodes of ARI are noted by investigator.

Total child-months follow-up = 6 + 12 + 8 + 18 + 12 + 24 + 18 + 12 + 16 + 24 = 150

Incidence density = (15/150) × 100 = 10 episodes per 100 child-months

This means if 50 children are followed up for 2 months, or 10 children are followed for 10 months, 10 episodes of ARI are likely to occur.

*Attack rate*: In case of short-term fluctuation of disease like outbreak, attack rare is used instead of incidence rate; it is expressed in percentage. It measures the severity of disease outbreak.

$$\text{Attack rate} = \frac{\text{Number of new cases}}{\text{Number of persons exposed during the outbreak}} \times 100$$

*Secondary attack rate*: It measures the number of new cases developing among susceptible within incubation period after they are exposed to a primary case:

> **Example: Calculation of secondary attack rate**
> One relative with fever and few vesicular rashes (chickenpox) visited the residence of a joint family of 12 members. Two members of this family had history of chickenpox in the past. Seven members developed same symptoms within a period of 3 weeks. As two adult members had history of past attack, so they had natural immunity against chickenpox. Therefore, susceptible family members are 10. Secondary attack rate = 7/10 × 100 = 70%.

$$\text{Secondary attack rate} = \frac{\text{Number of new cases within the range of incubation period}}{\text{No. of susceptibles exposed to primary case}} \times 100$$

### Prevalence

Prevalence is of two types: Point prevalence and period prevalence.
1. *Point prevalence* measures total number of existing cases, episodes or events, both new and old, in a specified population at a given point of time. It is the proportion of population who are cases at a given point of time.
2. *Period prevalence* measures total number of cases, episodes or events, both new and old, in a specified population in a period of time.

Incidence and prevalence are illustrated in **Figure 9.2**.

Out of 10 cases with reference of year 2017, P1, P2, P8 and P10 are old cases (detected in 2016), continuing their illness in 2017. P3, P5, P6, P7, P9 are new cases for the year 2017 (incidence cases). P4 has no relation with 2017. So, period prevalence for 2017 is 9

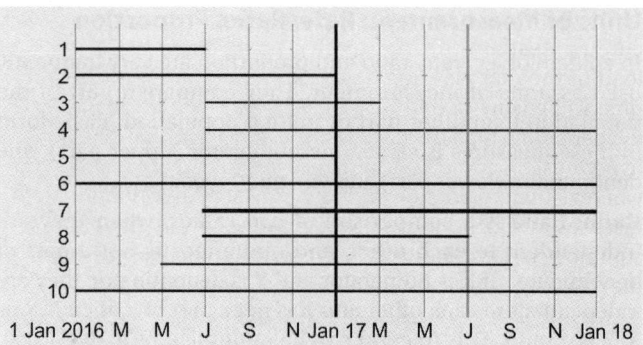

**Fig. 9.1:** Follow-up period of 10 under-five children starting from 1st January 2016 to 31st December 2017.

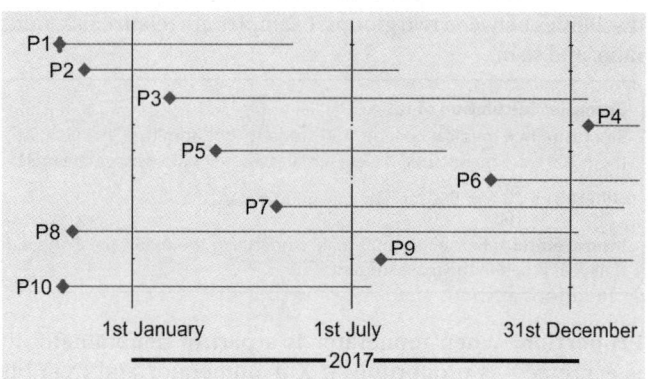

**Fig. 9.2:** Schematic presentation of incidence and prevalence.

(4 old cases + 5 new cases), and incidence is 5. Point prevalence of the disease on 1st January, 1st July and 31st December are 4, 6 and 5, respectively.

*Prevalence rate:*

$$\text{Point prevalence} = \frac{\text{Existing cases (both new and old) at a point of time}}{\text{Total population at risk}} \times 100$$

$$\text{Period prevalence} = \frac{\text{Total number of cases (both new and old) in a period of time}}{\text{Mid-interval population}} \times 100$$

> **Example: Calculation of point prevalence rate**
> A cross-sectional study conducted among urban adults showed that out of 500 subjects, 30 were suffering from diabetes mellitus.
> *Prevalence of diabetes mellitus* = 30/500 × 100 = 6%

Factors contributing to increase in prevalence:
- Longer duration of illness
- Increase in incidence
- Prolonged life without cure from the disease
- In-migration of cases
- Increase in diagnostic facilities.

Incident cases entering prevalent pool remain there until cure or death. Point prevalence might underestimate total load of the diseases. Repeated observations over a period of time will ensure better measure of it (period prevalence). Low incidence and high prevalence are found in chronic diseases like hypertension, diabetes, where recovery and death rates are low; whereas high incidence and low prevalence is found in acute diseases of short duration with rapid recovery like influenza, common cold, etc. **Table 9.3** will help the students to understand the differences between incidence and prevalence.

Table 9.3: Difference between incidence and prevalence.

|  | Incidence | Prevalence |
|---|---|---|
| Numerator | New case | Existing cases (both new and old) |
| Denominator | Population at risk/ under observation | Population at risk/mid-interval population |
| Time | Specified period of time | A point of time/specified period of time |
| Mostly applicable in | Short-duration cases | Chronic cases |
| Indicates | Chances of new events to occur | Magnitude of problem |
| Study design for estimation | Longitudinal | Cross-sectional |
| Use | Study of disease causation | Study of disease burden |

Relation between incidence and prevalence is expressed with following formula:

Prevalence (P) = Incidence (I) × average duration of disease (D)

**Figure 9.3** will help student to understand the relationship between point prevalence and incidence.

If incidence of a disease in a locality is 2 per week, and average duration of the disease is 2 weeks (presumed to be fixed), then at any point of time we can expect 2 × 2 = 4 cases (point prevalence).

## Disability Rate

Epidemiologist is concerned to measure disease, death as well as disability. Disability results from impairment and leads to handicap. Poliomyelitis (disease) causes paralysis of leg (impairment), which leads to inability to walk (disability). As a result of disability, the individual fails to discharge his or her social role which is normal for his age, sex or social position. In this example, inability to walk leads to unemployment (handicap).

Due to increased survival, number of elderly people increases. Many of them live with disability, which is thus, becoming more important in public health. It is difficult to measure incidence or prevalence of disability. A single measure, **Disability Adjusted Life Years (DALYs)** comprising of effect of early death and that of disabling diseases is popularly used.

DALY is a combination of YLL (years of lost life) and YLD (years lost to disability).

$$DALY = YLL + YLD$$

One DALY Means One Lost Year of Healthy Life

Years of lost life is measured with respect to life expectancy at birth of a standard population (world's longest surviving population, Japan). If a male Indian dies at the age of 50 years, his YLL will be 80 years (life expectancy at birth of standard population) minus 50 years, i.e., 30 years.

Years lost to disability can be calculated by multiplying duration of the disease or injury with weighting factor (indicating severity of the disease or injury). If weighting factor of a disease is 0.25 and duration of suffering is 10 years, then his YLD will be 10 × 0.25 = 2.5 years.

$$DALY = YLL + YLD = (80 - 50) + (10*0.25) = 32.5$$

**Quality-adjusted life year (QALY)** is the measure of life expectancy corrected for loss of quality of life caused by diseases and disabilities. QALY for a year of normal health is 1, whereas for a year of complete functional impairment (i.e. death) is zero. QALY measures the number of years of quality life added by an intervention. It is used to analyze cost-effectiveness of clinical/public health interventions. It can be used to compare interventions that prolong life but compromise the quality of life (e.g. chemotherapy for cancer) with an intervention that improves quality of life but does not prolong life (e.g. palliative pain management). While DALY gives negative impact on community due to a specific disease or disability in terms of life years lost, QALY gives life years added to the community due to specific interventions.

**(2) Mortality-related parameters:** India has routine system for collecting mortality data. They are very important sources for epidemiologist to study different aspects of deaths including its distribution by place, person and time, causes of death and trend over the time. Mortality data have some limitation including incomplete and irregular reporting and lack of uniformity limiting its comparison. Absence of cause of death or its incomplete entry makes mortality data less valid. Like many other countries, India has dearth of accurate, complete and regular data on death. For International comparison, International Classification of diseases (10 revision), popularly known ICD-10 is used to classify diseases and cause of death. Accurate cause of death is a priority area in public health.

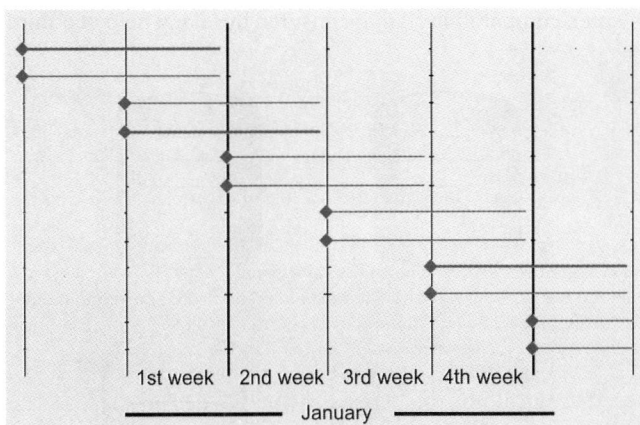

Fig. 9.3: Relation between point prevalence and incidence.

*Uses:*
- Mortality data is useful for prioritization of government action and resource allocation
- It helps in making comparison of deaths between two communities, or same community at different time interval
- Research purposes.

### Mortality Indicators

**Crude death rate (CDR):** It is number of deaths in a given time (usually a year) per 1,000 mid-year population.

**Case fatality rate:** It indicates severity of diseases. It measures number of deaths from a particular disease per 100 cases of same disease.

**Specific death rate:** Crude death rate does not reflect the true measure of death experience in community. Demographic composition of the community like age distribution, sex distribution, etc., has impact on CDR. Therefore, specific death rates like age specific death rate, sex specific rate, and cause specific death rate are epidemiologically more important and comparable.

$$\text{Crude death rate} = \frac{\text{Number of deaths in one year}}{\text{Midyear population}} \times 1{,}000$$

$$\text{Age specific death rate} = \frac{\text{Number of deaths in a particular age group in one year}}{\text{Midyear population of same age group}} \times 1{,}000$$

$$\text{Sex specific death rate} = \frac{\text{Number of deaths among a particular gender in one year}}{\text{Midyear population of that gender}} \times 1{,}000$$

$$\text{Disease specific death rate} = \frac{\text{Number of deaths from a specific disease in one year}}{\text{Midyear population}} \times 1{,}000$$

**Example: Calculation of crude and sex specific death rates**
In a subcenter area, total mid-year population is estimated to be 6,000, of them male was 3,200 and female was 2,800. Number of death in the year 2016 was 40, male 22 and female 18.

Crude death rate = $\frac{40}{6{,}000} \times 1{,}000 = 6.67/1{,}000$

Sex specific death rate for male = $\frac{22}{3{,}200} \times 1{,}000 = 6.87/1{,}000$

Sex specific death rate for female = $\frac{18}{2{,}800} \times 1{,}000 = 6.43/1{,}000$

**Proportional mortality rate:** Proportional mortality rate is useful when population data are not readily available to calculate specific death rates. It indicates the magnitude of mortality of a particular disease like cancer, or a group of diseases like cardiovascular diseases, communicable diseases, etc., or specific age group like above 50 years or under 5 years, in relation to total deaths in that population in a year. Proportional mortality rate gives an idea of major causes of death, but cannot reflect the risk of dying from a disease.

**Example: Calculation of proportional mortality rate**
In a community development block total yearly deaths were reported to be 720. Of them, 180 were CVA patients, 72 TB patients and 70 were under-fives.
Proportionate mortality from CVA

$\frac{\text{No. of deaths from CVA}}{\text{Total death from all causes}} \times 100 = \frac{180}{720} \times 100 = 25\%$

Under-5 proportionate mortality rate

$= \frac{\text{No. of under 5 deaths}}{\text{Total death from all causes}} \times 100 = \frac{70}{720} \times 100 = 9.7\%$

**Survival rate:** Though it is a mortality indicator, it is mostly used to measure prognosis of therapy particularly for cancer patients. 5 years survival rate is the measure of survival of cancer patients after diagnosis or initiation of therapy. If patient survives up to 5 years, it is usually considered prognostically good. Life table are computed from survival rates applying current survival rate to the population as of now. It is hypothetical data but gives us life expectancy at different age.

Five-year survival rate =

$\frac{\text{Number of patients alive five years after diagnosis or initiation of therapy}}{\text{Total number of patients diagnosed or treated}} \times 100$

**Example: Calculation of five-year survival rate**
In a cancer unit of a hospital, 40 cases of breast cancer were followed-up for 5 years after they were diagnosed and treated surgically. At the end of five years, 24 women were found to be alive.
Five-year survival rate = $24/40 \times 100 = 60\%$

### Adjusted or Standardized Rates

If we want to compare water content of 2 drums just by observing water level, these drums must be identical (**Fig. 9.4A**). If the diameter of one drum is larger than the other, even if the quantity of water of both drums is equal, water level of the larger one will be lower, and appears to have less quantity (**Fig. 9.4B**). In case of latter, comparability can be ensured by taking help of a third

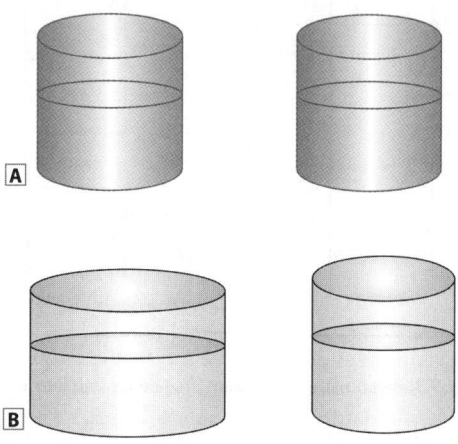

**Figs. 9.4A and B:** Difference of water level when capacity of jars is different.

jar (standard one). Water from the two jars can be poured into the standard one separately to see and mark water level, then conclusively we can say if water content is equal or one drum contains more or less quantity than the other.

It is true in case of crude death rate. CDR of 2 or more communities can be comparable, if they are identical with respect to composition by demographic characters like age, sex or other characteristics. But practically, they are not similar. Distorting effect of this dissimilar age or sex always modifies CDR. Specific death rates like age-specific, sex specific death rates are comparable, but it is cumbersome to use too many specific rates. This can be overcome by direct or indirect standardization for age, sex, socioeconomic status, etc. This is used mostly for death, but is equally useful for standardization of morbidity rates.

### Direct Standardization

When age-specific mortality rates for two or more populations are known, direct standardization method can be applied.

Calculate the age-specific mortality rates for each age group in each population A and population B **(Table 9.4)**. Then choose the standard (reference) population (*Note:* If the mortality rates of a specific community are compared to the national population, then the national population is considered as a "standard" population. Other example of standard population is the WHO world standard population, which is based on world overall average projected populations 2000-2025). Multiply the age-specific mortality rates of the population under study to the number of persons in each age group of the standard population. By this way, you will get the expected deaths for each age group of each population **(Table 9.5)**. Add the number of expected deaths from all age groups. Finally, to get the age-adjusted mortality rates, divide the total number of expected deaths by the standard population. Now you can conclude by comparing the age-standardized mortality rates of two populations.

**Table 9.4:** Crude and age specific death rate of community A and B.

| Age group (years) | Community A | | | Community B | | |
|---|---|---|---|---|---|---|
| | Population | Annual death | Age specific death rate per 1000 | Population | Annual death | Age specific death rate per 1000 |
| 0-24 | 18000 | 35 | 1.94 | 13000 | 30 | 2.31 |
| 25-49 | 11000 | 60 | 5.45 | 7000 | 50 | 7.14 |
| 50-74 | 9000 | 370 | 41.11 | 11000 | 400 | 36.36 |
| 75 and above | 3000 | 250 | 83.33 | 4000 | 380 | 95.00 |
| Total | 41000 | 715 | | 35000 | 860 | |
| | Crude death rate per 1000 = 17.44 | | | Crude death rate per 1000 = 24.57 | | |

As in given example from **Table 9.4**, seeing crude death rates, population B seems to have higher death rates than population A. But after age-standardization in **Table 9.5**, in fact the risk of death is higher in population A than in population B. It has clearly shown

**Table 9.5:** Calculation of expected deaths by applying direct standardization method (National population is taken as standard reference population).

| Age group (years) | Standard Population | Community A | | Community B | |
|---|---|---|---|---|---|
| | | Age specific death rate | Expected death | Age specific death rate | Expected death |
| 0-24 | 11000 | 1.94 | 21.34 | 2.31 | 25.41 |
| 25-49 | 17000 | 5.45 | 92.65 | 7.14 | 121.38 |
| 50-74 | 20000 | 41.11 | 822.20 | 36.36 | 727.20 |
| 75 and above | 3000 | 83.33 | 249.99 | 95.00 | 285.00 |
| Total | 51000 | | 1186.18 | | 1158.99 |
| Age adjusted mortality rate per 1000 (expected death/standard population) | | 23.3/1000 | | 22.7/1000 | |

that you may have misleading conclusion if you rely only on crude death rates.

- Standardization or adjustment eliminates distorting effect of population structure on CDR
- It is fictitious, only used for comparison
- Population of the block, district, state or national, from where study communities are drawn, may be used as standard population.

### Indirect Standardization (Standardized Mortality Ratio)

When age-specific mortality rates of the population (s) of interest are unknown, indirect standardization method is applied.

Choose a reference or standard population. Calculate the observed number of deaths in the population (s) of interest. For example—total observed deaths in population A is 120 and in population B is 30. Apply the age-specific mortality rates from the chosen reference population to the population(s) of interest. Multiply the number of people in each age group of the population(s) of interest by the age-specific mortality rate in the comparable age group of the reference population. Sum the total number of expected deaths for each population of interest. Divide the total number of observed deaths of the population(s) of interest by the expected deaths **(Table 9.6)**.

$$\text{Standardized mortality ratio (SMR)} = \frac{\text{Observed deaths}}{\text{Expected deaths}}$$

SMR for population A = 120/195.5 = 0.61
SMR for population B = 30/69.5 = 0.43

The risk of death is in fact higher in population A than population B after adjusting for differences by age. Common practice is to compare (SMR) in indirect method.

**(3) Nutritional status indicators:** Nutritional status is a positive health indicator. Three nutritional status indicators are considered important as indicators of health status: anthropometric measurements of preschool children, e.g., weight and height, mid-arm circumference; heights (and sometimes weights) of children at school entry; and prevalence of low birth weight (less than 2.5 kg).

**Table 9.6:** Calculation of expected deaths by applying indirect standardization method.

| Age group (years) | Age-specific death rate (per 1000) in standard population group | Community A | | Community B | |
|---|---|---|---|---|---|
| | | Population in each age group | Expected death | Population in each age group | Expected death |
| 0–24 | 4 | 2000 | 8.0 | 1000 | 4 |
| 25–49 | 7 | 2500 | 17.5 | 1500 | 10.5 |
| 50–74 | 10 | 3500 | 35.0 | 2500 | 25.0 |
| 75 and above | 30 | 4500 | 135.0 | 1000 | 30.0 |
| Total | | | 195.5 | | 69.5 |

**(4) Healthcare delivery indicators:** The frequently used indicators of healthcare delivery are:
a. Doctor-population ratio
b. Doctor-nurse ratio
c. Population-bed ratio
d. Population per health/subcenter and
e. Population per traditional birth attendant.

These indicators reflect the equity of distribution of health resources in different parts of the country, and of the provision of health care.

## TECHNIQUE OF COMMUNITY DIAGNOSIS

### Epidemiological Approaches in Community Diagnosis

***Know your Community:*** The essential prerequisite for community diagnosis is to know your community that means be familiar with your community. You have to identify which community you want to familiarize. Is it an urban slum or a village or a tribe or any occupational group? To know better you can have a transect walk through the area where the community lives and get various types of information like subgroup of population (ethnic or religious group), their customs and beliefs, health seeking behavior, healthcare resources with its location, sanitation and source of safe water. You can also draw a spot map **(Fig. 9.5)** with resource mapping like location of subcenter, primary healthcare center (PHC) or community health center (CHC), *anganwadi* center or availability of a Registered Medical Practitioner (RMP). This resource mapping can help you to assess the availability of healthcare services, transport or road condition or any barrier for accessing the health services. During implementation of health interventions, this will help you to overcome the obstacles.

***Which information you need:*** As a matter of fact, many factors combine together to affect the health of individuals and communities. In addition to genetics, factors such as demographic structure, literacy, environment and sanitation, access and transport, nutritional status, economic status and behavioral and sociocultural factors, all have considerable impacts on health.

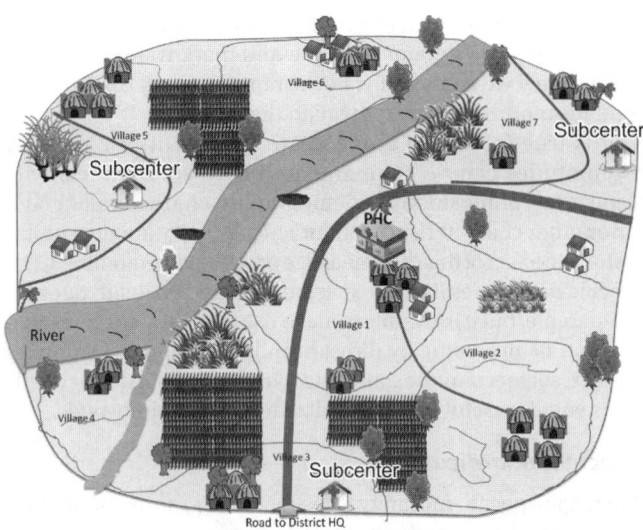

**Fig. 9.5:** Spot map.
(PHC: primary healthcare center; HQ: headquarters)

*Demographic characteristics*: Detailed information about the community is required for community diagnosis and identifying effective interventions. You need to know the community structure like total population, age and sex distribution of population, geographical locality with difficult terrains if any, education and occupation of them, people belonging to below poverty line (BPL) or any minority community, landholding pattern, caste structure, religious institutions, etc. You need to know the socioeconomic status of the community which is an important determinant of health.

*Opinion leaders*: In respect to get a better idea about the leadership in the community, you have to know the name of the influential persons in the locality, about the local self-government, opinion leaders, Mahila Mandals, nongovernment organizations (NGOs) and self-help groups. You need their help in community mobilization and successful implementation of any health intervention in that locality.

*Housing, sanitation and safe water supply*: You have to collect information about the source of safe drinking as well as household usable water, distance from the household, method of storage. How people dispose their garbage? Do the people use sanitary latrine? Is there any stagnation of water in the locality? Gather information about pets, mosquito or fly nuisance or menace rodents or pigs in the locality.

*Community nutrition*: Health status of the community directly depends on the availability, accessibility of food as well as food security measures. How many under-fives are under weight? What is the breastfeeding practices prevailing there? Is supplementary nutrition program available in *anganwadi* centers? Is there any misconception or cultural beliefs about food in the community? So, you have to know the staple diet in the community with its consumption pattern among population; cooking and food storage practices; provision of kitchen garden. You can proceed for diet survey at the household level with qualitative or quantitative estimation of the nutrients.

*Knowledge, attitude and practices*: People sometimes have poor or incorrect knowledge about the common health problems. Sometimes they have the knowledge but lack the practice. They know smoking inside rooms can cause repeated ARIs among children but still they practice it. People know about contraception, but lacks the attitude to adopt the method. You have to identify the gaps in the knowledge, attitude and practice of the people about the common health problems of the community. People know about the ideal age of marriage, but still the girls are being married below the age of 18. Some myths or wrong cultural practices might also prevail in the community. So your job is also to identify the key areas where the health promotion activities are to be strengthened.

*Health status of the community:* What are the health problems mostly prevailing in the community? Is undernutrition or anemia common in the community? If yes, in which age group? These types of questions you will encounter during data collection procedure. You can examine the members of the community to reach a tentative diagnosis (doctors' prescription if available, will help you) and can perform necessary investigations for confirmation. Otherwise, you can go through the available health records in the subcenter, *anganwadi* centers or with village health practitioners.

*Reproductive and child health:* Are the deliveries conducted at home or institution? Who conducts home deliveries in the locality? How many eligible couples are using contraception? Detailed information about the reproductive and child health is a prerequisite to arrive at a community diagnosis. You need to know the service coverage also like immunization status of the under-fives, birth and death registration and antenatal care coverage.

> **Relevant information**
> - Demographic characteristics, socioeconomic status
> - Housing, sanitation and safe water supply
> - Knowledge, attitude and practice
> - Health status of the community: Morbidity, mortality, nutritional status
> - Reproductive and child health
> - Healthcare seeking behavior
> - Available health resources.

*Healthcare seeking behavior of the community:* Knowledge about the healthcare seeking behavior of the community is of utmost importance for prioritizing the interventions and preventive care. Where do they go for delivery, hospital or nursing home? Which type of healthcare delivery they prefer for immunization or antenatal care? This will also help you to identify the gaps in judging the availability of adequate and quality healthcare to the community.

*Availability of health services*: What are the healthcare services available adjacent to the community? Is there any outreach session for immunization nearby? Does *anganwadi* worker perform growth monitoring or health check-up regularly? You know health status of the community also depend upon availability and accessibility of quality health services. You can encounter that antenatal mothers receive only iron and folic acid (IFA) and injection tetanus without any physical examination of mothers, thus neglecting early recognition of complications. It reflects that health services is available to the community, but may be inadequate or poor quality.

*Collection of information:* To obtain effective information about the community, you can utilize a variety of sources of information like existing health system records, active and passive surveillance, screening, survey results, or registration of vital events. Health Management Information System (HMIS) provides monthly data regarding different diseases or health problems as well as utilization status of various health services from the subcenters, PHCs and CHC. Few information can also be gathered from private practitioners, traditional healers and private and government laboratories.

Household survey data from National Family Health Survey (NFHS), District Level Household Survey (DLHS) or Sample Registration System (SRS) provide reliable information about various parameters related to demography, environment and Reproductive and Child Health (RCH) at district level. Similarly, data generated during surveillance or from Integrated Disease Surveillance Project (IDSP) also give you information about epidemic prone diseases.

Household level information can be collected by conducting survey through questionnaire or face to face interview or focus group discussion. Informal discussion with the stakeholders like ANM, AWW or ASHA; discussion with formal and informal leaders like Panchayat members, teachers, religious leaders or local club will help you to understand the health needs and bottlenecks of health services. Both quantitative and qualitative data can be compiled to have a basic understanding of the major issues in the community. Sometimes a dedicated team or working group is required, consisting of motivated individuals who will actively participate in data collection, analysis and adopting intervention.

Additional information is sometimes available from investigation of epidemic, testing the water for arsenic or coliform from Public Health Engineering department, health checkup or screening camps **(Table 9.7)**.

> **Methods of community diagnosis**
> - *Primary data collection technique:* Key informant interview, focus group discussion, observation, mapping, cross-sectional survey, longitudinal survey (to observe incident cases and time trend of diseases)
> - *Secondary data collection technique:* Census, hospital records, Health Management and Information System (HMIS), Sample Registration System (SRS), Integrated Disease Surveillance Project (IDSP), National Family Health Survey (NFHS), District Level Health Survey (DLHS), Laboratory Records, etc.

*Data analysis:* Collected data will be analyzed in terms of rate, ratio and proportions and can be utilized for comparison with other community. Graphical presentation is always better for easy understanding. Analysis of trends or projections will help in monitoring the disease for further planning.

*Felt need versus actual needs*: People may consider the availability of doctors and medicines are necessary for reduction of diarrhea in the community (felt needs), but the actual need

**Table 9.7:** Measurement of few indicators of sustainable development goals.

| Type of indicators | Indicators | Measurement strategy |
|---|---|---|
| Impact | Under-five mortality rate | • Registration of vital events<br>• Hospital data<br>• Household survey |
| | Malaria incidence rate | • Integrated Disease Surveillance Program (IDSP) data<br>• Active and passive surveillance report<br>• Longitudinal survey |
| Risk factors/ determinants | Proportion of the population using safely managed drinking water source | Household cross-sectional survey |
| Coverage | Proportion of births attended by skill health personnel | Health Management Information System data, cross-sectional household survey |
| System | Coverage of birth and death registration | Registration of vital events |

might be safe water and provision of sanitary latrine as revealed by the epidemiologist based on scientific evidence. When felt need and actual need will synchronize, health interventions will be successful.

> **Data analysis**
> - Rate, ratio and proportion like doctor-population ratio, mortality rate, morbidity rate
> - Graphical presentation like bar diagram, pie diagram, histogram, line diagram, etc.
> - Comparison with known indices or other community
> - Statistical test.

*Arriving at community diagnosis:* What has to be done? Based on the analysis of collected or available data, health status of the community, its determinants and potential intervention areas are identified. Then, health issues will be prioritized and suitable action plans for health intervention or prevention program can be formulated, viz. chlorination of drinking water, IFA supplementation and geriatric care services. But, these interventions should include not only treatment, but health promotion activities, legislation, environmental control, etc.

Sharing information to the community and the stakeholders will involve them in all health interventions. Community diagnosis is found to be ineffective without community participation in the health programs.

Your job will not end here. Follow-up of the community and evaluation through annual survey or HMIS data or rapid assessment survey will give you an estimate of the effectiveness of the interventions. Based on the information you can replan your services.

Thus, community diagnosis is a step by step scientific epidemiological method for identification of community health problems, with prioritization of the programs with team approach. This team will need intersectoral collaboration with Panchayat, health and ICDS *functionaries* **(Flowchart 9.1)**.

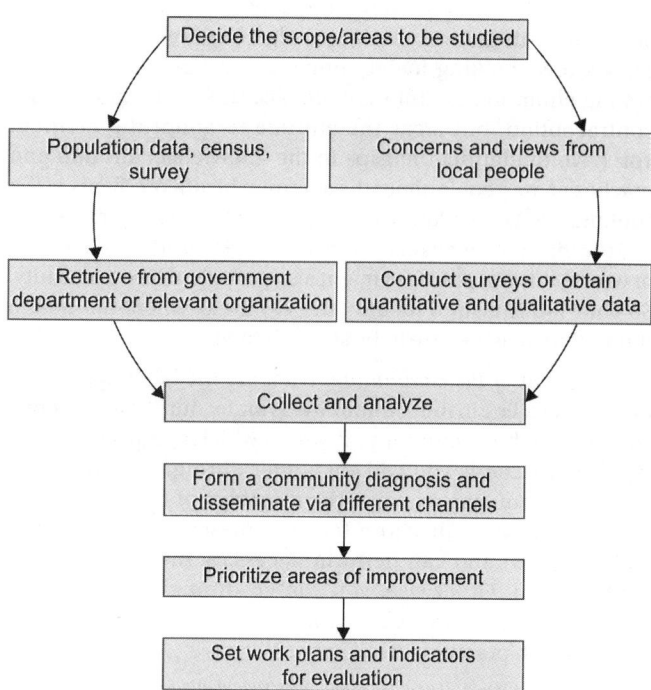

Flowchart 9.1: Community diagnosis process.

Community diagnosis is based on:
- Health problem of the community
- Determinants or risk factors in the community
- Areas for community interventions.

> **Points to Remember**
> **Community diagnosis**
> - Be familiar with the community you serve
> - Identify the factors that affect promotion of good health
> - Assess the current health problems and utilization of the existing health services
> - Adopt participatory approaches to assess community's health problem and understand any problem in accessibility and utilization of health services
> - Try to synchronize the "felt need" and "actual need" in order to make services successful
> - Empower the community; work with them by good rapport building to improve health services and health status.

## Epidemiological Studies (Conceptual Understanding)

An epidemiologist can approach to community diagnosis and solution of a particular problem, disease, death or disability by applying the principles of epidemiological studies. Under an observational study, one can observe the incidence or prevalence of disease or other health events without intervention. Descriptive and analytical studies come into the compartment of observational study.

Descriptive study simply describes the disease or health-related events as per time, place and person distribution. Simply by observing the data generated in IDSP, one can calculate the incidence of vector-borne diseases in a geographical area; can identify the seasonal pattern of malaria or dengue.

Under analytical epidemiology, you can find out the causes or risk factors behind the disease by case control or cohort study. You can find association between a sudden outbreak of vomiting and diarrhea among the students with the consumption of curd in the hostel feast last night by case control study. You can adopt a cohort study while following a group of low-birth-weight babies to find out the mortality or morbidity incidence among them compared to normal birth weight babies at the end of first year.

Intervention studies are undertaken to see the efficacy of a drug or a therapeutic procedure or a vaccine introduced as an intervention among the experimental and control group. In this manner comparison of home versus sanatorium treatment of tuberculosis was conducted by a Randomized Control Trial (RCT). One of the best examples of community trial is also the supply of iodized salt and reduction of prevalence of goiter in the community. Thus, one can undertake different types of epidemiological studies for community diagnosis of a particular disease or health problem with its associated risk factors.

**Epidemiological studies**
- Descriptive epidemiological studies describe place, person and time distribution diseases and health events
- Analytical epidemiological studies are used to determine risk factors or etiological agents
- Experimental epidemiological studies are applied to evaluate remedial or preventive measures.

# SUGGESTED READING

1. Bonita R, Beaglehole R, Kjellstrom T. Basic epidemiology, 2nd edition. Geneva: World Health Organization; 2006.
2. Census of India 2011. Houses, Household Amenities and Assets.
3. David L, Katz, Joann G, et al. Jekel's Epidemiology, biostatistics, Preventive Medicine, and Public Health, 4th edition. Philadelphia: Elsevier Saunders; 2013.
4. Department of Health. Basic principles of health cities: Community Diagnosis. [online] Available from https://www.chp.gov.hk/files/ pdf/hcp_community_diagnosis_en.pdf/.
5. Detels R, Gulliford M, Karim AQ. Oxford Textbook of Global Public Health, 6th edition. Oxford: Oxford University Press; 2015.
6. Government of India. Annual report of Department of Health and Family Welfare 2016-17. [online] Available from https:// mohfw.gov.in/sites/default/files/3201617.pdf
7. Graunt J. Natural and Political Observations Mentioned in a Following Index, and made upon the bills of Mortality. London. Reprinted. Baltimore: The John Hopkins Press; 1939. pp. 1662.
8. Greenood M. Epidemics and crowd diseases: an introduction to the study of epidemiology. Oxford: Oxford University Press; 1935.
9. International Institute for Population Sciences, Deonar, Mumbai. National Family Health Survey (NFHS-5) (2015-16), India. [online] Available from http://rchiips.org/nfhs/NFHS-5Reports/India.pdf/.
10. International Institute for Population Sciences, Deonar, Mumbai. National Family Health Survey (NFHS-5) (2019-21), India. [online] Available from http://rchiips.org/nfhs/NFHS-5Reports/India.pdf/.
11. Last JM (Ed). Dictionary of Epidemiology, 4th edition. New York: Oxford University Press; 2001.
12. Lilienfeld AM, Lilienfeld DE. Foundations of Epidemiology, 2nd edition. Oxford: Oxford University Press; 1980.
13. Lilienfeld DE. Celebration: William Farr (1807-1883): An appreciation on 200th anniversary of his birth. Int J Epidemiol. 2007;36(5):985-7.
14. Lilienfeld DE. Definitions of epidemiology. Am J Epidemiol. 1978;107(2): 67-90.
15. Loannidis JPA. Genetic and molecular epidemiology. J Epidemiol Community Health. 2007;61(9):757-8.
16. MacMahon B, Pugh TF. Epidemiology: principles and methods, 1st edition. Boston: Little, Brown; 1970.
17. Ministry of Health and Family Welfare, Government of India. Global Adult Tobacco Survey Fact sheet 2009-10.
18. Morris JN. Uses of epidemiology, 3rd edition. London: Churchill living stone; 1975.
19. National Tobacco Control Cell Ministry of Health and Family Welfare Government of India. (2012). Operational Guidelines National Tobacco Control Programme.
20. Porta M. A Dictionary of epidemiology, 5th edition. New York: Oxford University Press; 2008.
21. Roht LH, Selwyn BJ, Holguin AH, et al. Principal of epidemiology, a self-learning guide. Massachusetts: Academic press; 1982.
22. US Department of Health and Human Services/Centers for Disease Control and Prevention (CDC). Principles of Epidemiology in Public Health Practice, 3rd edition. Atlanta: CDC; 2012
23. Vaughan JP, Morrow RH. Manual of Epidemiology for District Health Management. Geneva: World Health Organization; 1989.

# CHAPTER 10

# Epidemiological and Research Studies

*Shikha Jain*

| | |
|---|---|
| CM7.5 | Enumerate, define, describe and discuss epidemiological study designs |
| CM7.8 | Describe the principles of association, causation and biases in epidemiological studies |

## INTRODUCTION

Epidemiology is not only important from public health aspect but also from clinical aspect as can be observed by looking to the history of epidemiology, most of the clinicians work in the field of epidemiology. Understanding of epidemiology is very important as it is the basic science of prevention and to make it simple, interesting and understandable is a herculean task.

## DEFINITION

John M Last in 1988 defined epidemiology as "the study of the distribution and determinants of health-related states or events in specified populations, and the application of this study to the control of health problems **(Table 10.1)**."

Epidemiology is not only the study of death, illness and disability but also positive health state and deals with health of human population and its subgroups. It is also used to describe the health situation of people. Information regarding disease burden in population is essential for stakeholders and policy implementers as limited resources would be utilized in best possible manner through identification of priority health programs for prevention and care.

## THE EPIDEMIOLOGIC APPROACH

To describe the health event, we need to answer six questions which is similar to what we are interested to know in case of any criminal incident. Questions are:
1. What health event it is?
2. How much is the magnitude of the health event?
3. Where did the event occur?
4. When did it happen?
5. Who all are affected?
6. Why did it occur?

The answers to the first five questions are given by **descriptive epidemiology** and the answer to the sixth question is given by **analytical epidemiology**. Thus, in descriptive epidemiology, hypothesis are generated and basic control measures are initiated; while in analytical epidemiology, the hypothesis that were generated are tested, underlying causes are established and scientifically sound health programs and intervention measures are suggested **(Table 10.2)**.

Both the type of studies complement each other. As the name suggests, observational studies allow nature to take its own

**Table 10.1:** Factors related to epidemiology of a disease.

| Term | Explanation |
|---|---|
| Study | Includes "surveillance, observation, hypothesis testing, analytical research and experiments" |
| Distribution | Refers to analysis of "time, place and population subgroups affected" |
| Determinants | Include factors that influence health, e.g. biological, chemical, physical, social, cultural, economic, genetic and behavioral |
| Health-related states and events | Refers to the diseases, causes of deaths, behavioral such as use of tobacco, positive health states, reactions to preventive regimens and provision of use of health services |
| Specified populations | Includes those with identifiable characteristics such as occupational groups |
| Application to prevention and control | The aim of public health to promote, protect and restore health |

**Table 10.2:** Classification of epidemiological studies.

| Epidemiological studies | |
|---|---|
| Study type | Unit of study |
| **1. Observational studies** | |
| i. Descriptive studies | |
| ii. Analytical studies | |
| Case-control study | Individuals |
| Cohort study | Individuals |
| Cross-sectional study | Individuals |
| Ecological study | Populations |
| **2. Experimental studies** | |
| Randomized controlled trials | Patients |
| Field trials | Healthy people |
| Community trials | Communities |

course; that is the investigator does not intervene. Descriptive type of observational studies is used to describe a health event in relation to time, place and person characteristics. While analytical studies are used to elucidate the etiology of and risk factors for human disease. Experimental or interventional studies involve an active attempt to change a disease determinant or the progress of a disease through treatment.

The essential requirement in all epidemiological studies is that the case should be defined clearly (i.e. whom to consider a case using operational case-definition using which the disease or condition can be identified and measured in the defined population with a degree of accuracy) and there should also be clear definition of an exposed person to interpret the data from an epidemiological study.

## DESCRIPTIVE STUDY

Describing the occurrence and distribution of disease by time, place and person and identifying those characteristics associated with the presence or absence of disease in individuals is critical for several reasons:
- Summarization of data using key demographic variables provides a comprehensive characterization of the disease-trends over time, its geographic distribution and the persons affected by the disease.
- From this characterization, population at risk can be identified.
- It provides idea about etiology, source and modes of transmission that can be tested (confirmed) using analytical epidemiological study.
- Descriptive epidemiology describes the where and whom of the disease, allowing to begin intervention and prevention measures.

### Time Distribution

The pattern of disease may be described by the time of its occurrence, i.e. by week, month, year, etc. This gives idea about whether the disease is seasonal, or whether the disease increases or decreases periodically or it follows a consistent time trend. During summer, diarrheal disease is most common, and in the winters, respiratory disease is most common. For diseases that occur seasonally, health officials can anticipate their occurrence and implement control and prevention measures, such as an influenza vaccination campaign or mosquito spraying. For diseases that occur sporadically, investigators can conduct studies to identify the causes and modes of spread, and then develop appropriately targeted actions to control or prevent further occurrence of the disease. Time series data are usually displayed in 2D graphs, in which X-axis contains time periods (days, weeks, months, years, etc.), and Y-axis contains number/rates of cases.

Three types of trends or fluctuations in disease occurrence are observed:
1. Short-term fluctuations
2. Periodic fluctuations
3. Long-term or secular trends.

### Short-term Fluctuations

An epidemic is the best example of short-term fluctuation. An epidemic is defined as "unusual increase in the number of cases of an illness or other health-related events in a defined geographic area and defined time period." But to decide whether the situation is of epidemic or not, one should have the idea of the usual level of cases of illness (endemicity). The type of curve can give an idea about the type of epidemic. There are different types of epidemic:
- **Common source epidemics**
  - Single exposure or point source epidemics
  - Continuous or multiple exposure epidemics
  - Interrupted exposure
- **Propagated epidemics**
  - Person to person
  - Arthropod borne
  - Animal reservoir
- **Slow epidemics.**

### Epidemic Curve

A special type of histogram is used to depict the time course of an epidemic. This graph is called an epidemic curve **(Fig. 10.1)**. It provides a simple visual display of the outbreak's magnitude and time trend. Epidemic curve is a basic investigative tool as it provides idea about:
- The magnitude of the epidemic over time as a simple, easily understood visual.
- The pattern of spread in the population (through the shape of the curve), e.g. point source versus intermittent source versus propagated.
- The course of epidemic (still on rise, on the down slope, or after the epidemic has ended).
- Are the intervention measures working?
- If the disease and its incubation period are known, the epidemic curve can be used to derive a probable time of exposure and that can be used to develop a questionnaire focused on that time period.
- Classical example is outbreaks of food poisoning, outbreaks of cholera, Bhopal gas tragedy in India (by industrial chemicals) and Minamata disease in Japan (due to consumption of fish containing high concentration of methyl mercury).

The example of time distribution curve of an epidemic is shown in **Figure 10.1**.

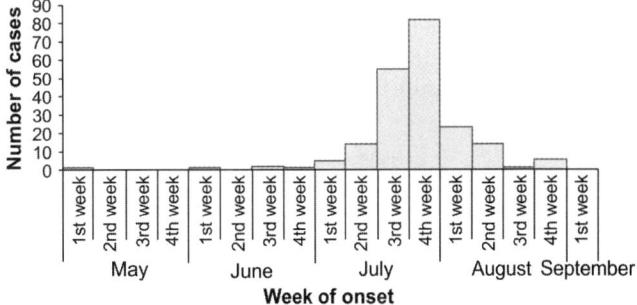

Fig. 10.1: Example of time distribution.

### Common Source (Vehicle) Epidemics

It occurs due to presence of an infectious or a chemical noxious agent in a common source or vehicle which acts as the mode of transmission, e.g. food, drink, air, pooled blood, etc. These are of three types depending upon the duration of presence of the

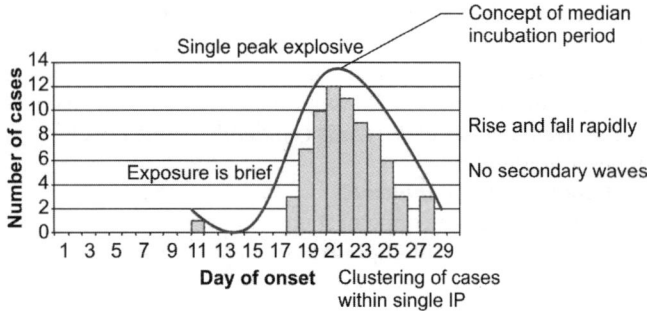

**Fig. 10.2:** Epidemic curve showing median incubation period (IP) during common source, single exposure epidemics.

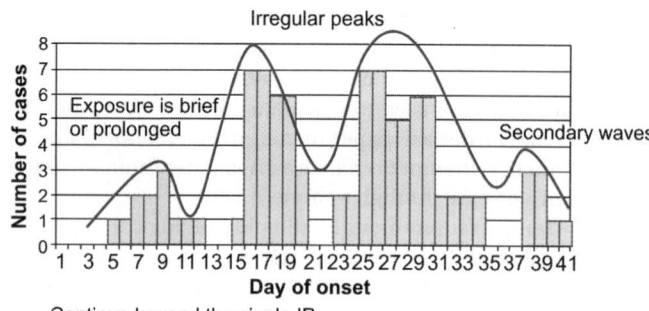

**Fig. 10.4:** Epidemic curve showing irregular peaks of single incubation period (IP) during common source, interrupted exposure.

infectious agent in the vehicle and the frequency of contact of the vehicle with the susceptible population.

a. **Common source, single exposure epidemics:** The infectious agent remains present in the vehicle for a short period of time; during this period all those who come in contact with the vehicle become exposed to the infection. The exposure is essentially simultaneous also. The epidemic of leukemia cases in Hiroshima following the atomic bomb blast and food poisoning among people who ate contaminated food at a restaurant are the examples of point source epidemic. The epidemic curve in common-source, single exposure epidemic shows **(Fig. 10.2)**:
   i. Sharp onset and fall with no secondary waves.
   ii. That all cases occur within one-incubation period of the disease.
   iii. The peak of the epidemic is sharp and coincides with median incubation period (median incubation period is the time required for half of the total cases to occur following exposure).

b. **Common source, continuous exposure:** In this type of epidemic, the infectious agent remains in the common vehicle for some time. The decline of the epidemic occurs either because the cause of contamination is removed or because of the reason that all possible "susceptible" have become infected. Example is the epidemic of infectious hepatitis or cholera due to contamination of surface/ground or piped water supplies with human excreta or food-borne typhoid fever due to carriers or contaminated tinned foods. The characteristic of epidemic curve in common source continuous exposure is **(Fig. 10.3)**:

   i. The epidemic curve rises slowly and also falls gradually.
   ii. The peak is not sharp but rather plateau-like.
   iii. The duration of epidemic is stretched out.

c. **Common source, interrupted exposure:** The source is common in such types of epidemic, but the source infects the vehicle only interruptedly. Example is an infected nurse posted in urological ward may be a carrier of *Pseudomonas aeruginosa* passing infection to the patients through the catheters on particular days of her duty. The characteristic of epidemic curve in common source, interrupted exposure is **Figure 10.4**:
   i. The curve will show an increase in frequency but the curve will be almost flat.
   ii. There will be occasional irregular waves coinciding with the periodic introduction of infection.

*Propagated Epidemics*

In this type of epidemics, the source itself multiplies. For example, a school child may be the index case of diphtheria and may pass on the droplet infection to other children. Those children may pass on the infection to other children and in this way the propagation of the epidemic will occur. The fall of the epidemic will occur when there will be sufficient herd immunity so that no more susceptible would be there. Other examples of such type of epidemics are seen in droplet infections like Measles, Mumps, vector-borne diseases like malaria, Japanese encephalitis, dengue, and in STDs and HIV epidemics. The characteristic of epidemic curve in propagated epidemic is **Figure 10.5**.

The curve rises slowly, in waves, reaches a flat plateau and then declines slowly.

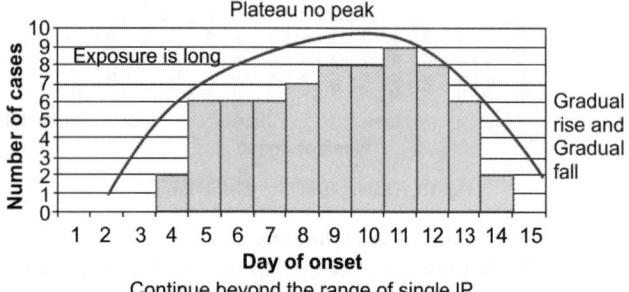

**Fig. 10.3:** Epidemic curve showing single incubation period (IP) during common source, continuous exposure.

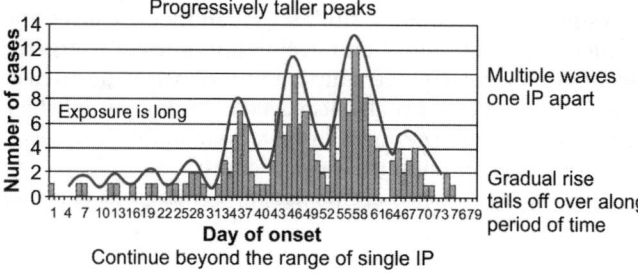

**Fig. 10.5:** Epidemic curve showing propagated epidemics.

*Periodic Fluctuations*

**Seasonal fluctuations:** Vector-borne diseases like malaria, dengue, chikungunya are common during monsoon and post-monsoon season due to favorable environmental factors such as increase in humidity and vector density. Upper respiratory tract infections are common in winters when overcrowding is there. Gastrointestinal infections are in summer season because of warm weather and increased vector density (flies). Sometimes noninfectious diseases also show seasonal fluctuations like asthma, heatstroke, snakebite, hay fever, etc. Seasonal fluctuations are presented graphically through line diagrams.

**Cyclical changes:** In this type, the disease occurs in a cyclical pattern spread over short periods of time which may be days, weeks, months or years. For example, measles in which the major peaks occur every 2–3 years because of accumulation of enough susceptible.

### Long-term Trends or Secular Trends

The changes in the occurrence (i.e. a progressive increase or decrease) of disease occur over a period of decades. A secular trend suggests a consistent tendency to change in a particular direction or a definite movement in one direction. For example, a progressive increase in lifestyle-related diseases such as coronary heart disease, lung cancer, diabetes, etc. and a decrease in infectious disease.

## Place Distribution

By knowing the distribution of diseases in different populations we get the idea about the differences in disease patterns not only between countries, but also within countries as many diseases have spatial relationships. The role of migration, genetic or environmental factors, diet or other etiological factors can be studied. Differences in the distribution of a disease according to place may be made according to political boundaries (e.g. international comparisons, regional comparisons within countries) or according to natural boundaries (e.g. rural urban differences, hilly or plain areas, etc.).

**International variations:** Pattern of disease is different in different regions. Although cases of cancer are reported from all over the world but there is a difference in the incidence of each cancer in different areas of the world. For example, oral cancer and cervical cancer is very common in India. Cancer of stomach is common in Japan.

Differences in the occurrence of diseases in different areas may be due to the role of environmental factors or genetic factors. This can be decided by carrying out studies in migrant population. Migrant studies can be carried out in two ways:
1. A group of people have migrated to a new country. Comparison of morbidity and mortality rates in these migrants with those of their relatives who are at their own country. This will be an example of genetically similar groups but living in different environmental conditions. If the morbidity and mortality rates of migrant population are similar to the population of the country where they have migrated, then it would be because of environmental factors.
2. If the morbidity and mortality rates of migrant population are different from the rates of population where they have migrated, then it would be because of genetic factors:

**Regional variations:** This means that occurrence of disease may be different in different areas of the country. For example, the distribution of lathyrism, fluorosis, endemic goiter, filariasis, malaria, Japanese encephalitis, etc.

**Rural-urban variations:** Certain diseases are more frequent in urban areas like accidents, cardiovascular diseases, drug dependence, mental illness, hypertension, etc. while certain diseases are more often seen in rural areas like soil-transmitted helminths, zoonotic diseases, skin diseases, etc. This may be due to differences in socioeconomic status, housing conditions, sanitation, education, accessibility to health care, etc.

**Local distribution:** Variations in the distribution of the disease within the area and outside the area can be best studied with the help of spot map. Spot map is a detailed layout map of the area showing the houses, water bodies and supply lines, sewage disposal system, vector breeding areas, etc. and other environmental factors which may be helpful in explaining the occurrence of disease in an area. In the same map, the cases of the disease can be plotted and if the numbers of cases are high in a particular area of the map then it can be correlated with the possible environmental factors. Spot map is very important tool in providing clue of the etiology of the disease and thus in formulating the hypothesis during epidemic investigation. John Snow's investigation on cholera epidemic in London and Maxcy's investigation on Typhus in USA are the examples of use of spot map in finding out the etiology of the disease.

Linking the distribution of the disease to a particular place may be proved strongly in case:
- The inhabitants of that place, by virtue of their genetic factors (higher rates of sickle cell anemia in tribes) or because of socio-environmental factors are different from those at other places.
- That particular geographic area may be playing an important role which can be demonstrated by higher rates of the disease in all the ethnic groups residing in that area as compared to similar ethnic groups residing in different area and also evidence of disease in animals residing in the same area.

In case of epidemic investigation, when more than one area is affected, the place distribution of the disease is very helpful in formulating the hypothesis regarding the source of outbreak.

***Example:*** **Figure 10.6** shows the three villages where the outbreak was reported including Mehragaon, Chauriagon and Dov. The yellow denotes the lowest incidence and the red the highest incidence. The blue elements on the slide represent the water supply system, including the springs, the reservoirs shown as blue rectangles and the pipelines shown as black arrows. Dov that had its own spring had the lowest incidence in yellow. Chauriagon that shared a spring with Mehragaon had an intermediate incidence in orange and Mehragaon that had almost only one source of water supply had the highest incidence in red. On the basis of the attack rate in villages, we generated the hypothesis that the spring that supplied both Mehragaon and Chauriagon was the source of the outbreak.

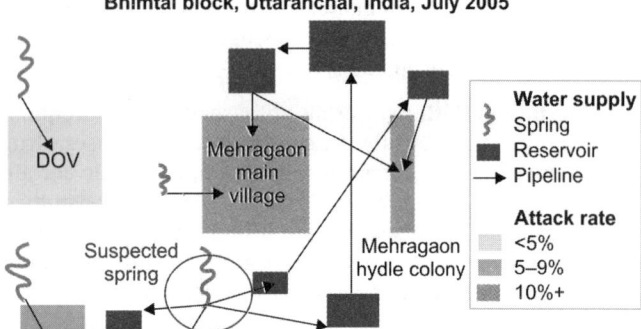

**Fig. 10.6:** Classic example of place distribution of a disease outbreak in India. *(For color version, see Plate 1)*

**Table 10.3:** Incidence of acute hepatitis by age and sex in 3 villages, Bhimtal block, Uttaranchal, India (July 2005) (CDC, Field Epidemiology Training Program Module, 2018).

| | | Population | Cases | Attack rate |
|---|---|---|---|---|
| Age (year) | 0–4 | 105 | 2 | 2% |
| | 5–9 | 110 | 4 | 4% |
| | 10–14 | 134 | 23 | 17% |
| | 15–44 | 729 | 139 | 19% |
| | 45+ | 261 | 37 | 14% |
| Sex | Male | 724 | 115 | 16% |
| | Female | 514 | 90 | 17% |
| Total | | 1238 | 205 | 16% |

## Person Distribution

Infinite variables can be used for describing person distribution of the disease which may be helpful in understanding the natural history of the disease, however the commonly studied person variables are:

- **Age:** It is strongly related to the disease. If we see the distribution of the disease, certain diseases are common in a particular age group. For example, vaccine preventable diseases are common in childhood; chronic diseases are commonly seen in the middle age (which may reflect a persistent and cumulative exposure to a risk factor), road traffic accidents in young/early middle age, etc. Some diseases also show bimodal distribution, i.e. incidence of the disease will be high in two different age groups, e.g. Hodgkin's lymphoma, which indicates that different sets of causal factors might be playing a role in the causation of the disease.
  
  To confirm that a particular disease is common in a particular age group, calculation of age-specific rates is very important. If the incidence rate is uniform in all the age groups, it suggests that all age groups are equally susceptible, and there was no previous immunity.

- **Sex:** Certain diseases are common in a particular sex, e.g. diseases of thyroid and gallbladder are common in females while lung cancer and CHD is more common among males. Sex-specific rates may be helpful in demonstrating the difference in the distribution of the disease in different sex. The difference in the distribution of the disease in a particular sex can be attributed to the biological differences between the sex, cultural and behavioral differences (smoking, use of automobiles, availing the health services, etc.)
  
  The example of person distribution is shown in **Table 10.3**. The attack rate was highest among persons 15–44 years of age (19%) followed by the 10–14 years of age (17%) and by those 45 years of age or older (14%). The lowest attack rate was found among children less than 9 years of age. Females were slightly more affected than males.

- **Ethnicity:** Ethnic group is a group of persons homogenous in respect of biologic inheritance and customs. The broad variables that are studied under ethnic group are: race, native place, religion and local social units (religious communities). Difference in the disease distribution between ethnic groups and other population may be because of genetic factors or because of customs, dietary factors, lifestyle or socioeconomic factors. Example is sickle cell anemia which is common in tribes or a particular community. High prevalence of Tay-Sachs disease is seen in Jews.

- **Social class:** Diseases are not distributed equally across the different social classes. Certain diseases are commonly seen in higher socioeconomic class, e.g. coronary heart disease, hypertension, diabetes, etc. while some diseases shows preponderance in lower socioeconomic class, e.g. respiratory illness, skin infections, tuberculosis, malnutrition, etc. which may be due to lack of personal hygiene, poor nutritional status, poor housing conditions, overcrowding, or not availing the health services. Limitation is there in comparison of studies in which social class is used as a variable as the social classification varies from country to country.

- **Occupation:** Occupation has an important bearing on the health status of an individual. It may affect the habit of the employee, e.g. sleep, consumption of alcohol, smoking, night shifts, etc. The high occurrence of a disease in a particular occupation may be because of exposure of the employee to various physical, chemical or biological agents or stress. Example of occupational diseases includes pneumoconiosis. Type of work also affects the health of the person, e.g. a person doing the sedentary type of work (mostly people in IT industry) may face the risk of heart disease. Sometimes, the investigator while conducting the study may come across the selection bias as people in certain occupation are selected on the basis of their physical and mental capabilities (army personnel, doctors).

- **Education:** As education is related to the increased knowledge (regarding the nutrition, vaccination, family planning, treatment seeking behavior, availing the health services, etc.) so it is likely to be associated with reduced risk of disease.

- **Marital status:** Studies have shown that mortality rates are lower for married people irrespective of sex. The reason could be that married people are more secure and feel protected. But, it can be a risk factor in certain diseases e.g. cervical cancer (because of multiple sexual contacts).

- **Behavior:** The chronic, noncommunicable diseases are also termed as lifestyle-related disease or behavior-related diseases as human behavior (smoking, consumption of alcohol, lack of physical activity, consumption of junk food, risky behavior such as involvement with multiple sex-partners, unprotective sex, drug addiction, non-use of helmets or seat belts while driving, etc.) may play a role of risk factor in such diseases. For example; coronary heart disease, diabetes, obesity, hypertension, cancers, etc.

- **Stress**: Patients response such as susceptibility to the disease, exacerbation of the symptoms, and compliance with medical regime may be related to the stress. Certain diseases are also related to the stress also known as psychosomatic disorders, e.g. peptic ulcer, hypertension, etc.

While interpreting the results of the descriptive studies based on the person distribution, it is very important to rule out the other explanations for the difference in the results, e.g. it may seem that the occurrence of STDs are less among affluent people but the actual reason may be that they may be going to the private practitioners for the treatment so the notification of those cases may not be there. Other example may be the higher morbidity in case of male child which may actually be due to girl child not being taken to the healthcare facility for the treatment.

### Uses of Descriptive Epidemiology

- We can get the idea about the magnitude of the problem (disease in terms of morbidity and mortality rates).
- It gives idea about the etiology of the disease and thus helps in formulation of the hypothesis regarding cause-effect relationship.
- As we can study the distribution of the disease in terms of time, place and person, we can identify the risk groups.
- It provides data which is helpful in planning, organizing and evaluating the health services.
- It is helpful in research.

### Steps of Designing a Descriptive Study

1. Write the research question and its background significance. (e.g. "To study the Epidemiological profile of the Dengue cases admitted in the year 2017 in a tertiary care hospital"). The study design may be cross-sectional or case-series.
2. Identify the variables to be studied.
   a. Main variables: Dengue cases
   b. Decide the other variables with which the main variable that is the Dengue cases will be associated, e.g. person related: age groups (may use standard age-groups), gender, socioeconomic status, etc. Time related: month wise cases. Place related: address (residence).
3. Any specific inclusion or exclusion criterion has to be stated.
4. Mention the methodology (study population, study period, study design, study area, sample size, etc.)
5. Collect the data. Take the informed consent from the subjects, maintain confidentiality.
6. Perform the data analysis. Prepare the tables, graphs and apply the appropriate statistical tests. In case of person analysis tables can be prepared. In case of time analysis, line diagram can be prepared to show the month wise cases and in case of place analysis map can be prepared.
7. Interpret the findings. Draw conclusion and make the recommendations.

In case of descriptive studies, there is no comparison group as only one group of subjects having the outcome of interest is studied. In such studies, no preformed hypothesis is there.

> **Points to Remember**
> - Descriptive epidemiological study describes the disease in relation to time, place and person.
> - There is no comparison in case of descriptive studies.
> - It is important for formulation of hypothesis regarding the cause of the disease which can be further tested by using analytical study.
> - Natural history of the disease can be studied by using descriptive epidemiological study.
> - Descriptive studies can be carried out in situations like:
>   - In a diabetic person what would be the course of H1N1 infection.
>   - How many cases of Dengue would occur in one year in a corporation area?
>   - How many anemic females are there in a field practice area?
>   - What is the proportion of road accident cases out of total hospital admissions in one year in a tertiary care hospital?

## ANALYTICAL STUDY

In analytical studies, hypothesis are specified in advance, new data are often collected, and differences between groups are measured to establish a cause-effect relationship.

### Ecological Studies (Correlational Studies)

To determine whether the association is there or not, the studies of group characteristics also known as ecologic studies can be conducted. **Figure 10.7** shows a study a study carried out in 20 developed countries to know the relationship between average dietary fat consumption and breast cancer incidence in each country. This diagram shows that higher the average dietary fat consumption for a country, the higher the breast cancer incidence for that country. So from this it can be concluded that high fat consumption could be a risk factor for development of breast cancer. But there is fallacy in drawing such conclusion from this type of study. The problem is that we do not know that dietary intake of fat was high or not in individuals in whom breast cancer developed. We only have the average values of dietary fat consumption for each country and the breast cancer incidence for each country. This is also known as "ecological fallacy" or "ecological bias". Ecological fallacy is described as that when the association observed between variables at group level does not necessarily represent the association at the individual level. This occurs because we have data for the groups and not for individual exposure and outcome.

### *Advantages of Ecological Studies*

- Such ecological studies are still helpful as they are easy to conduct and they can reflect light on cause-effect relationship and this could be further confirmed by conducting other types of analytical studies, like case-control or cohort studies.
- In such type of studies data can be used from populations with differing characteristics.
- Relationships may be studied between variables by comparing populations in different countries at same time or the same population in one country at different times.

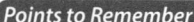

Fig. 10.7: Correlational between dietary fat intake and breast cancer by country.

> **Points to Remember**
> - Ecological studies are easy to carry out.
> - The unit of analysis in case of ecological studies is a group or a population.
> - But in case of ecological studies, the association between variables at the group level does not necessarily represent the association that exists at individual level.

*What type of study is required to explain the etiology of and risk factors for human disease? The answer to this is case-control and cohort studies.*

In the early 1940s, Alton Ochsner, a surgeon in New Orleans, observed that virtually all of the patients on whom he was operating for lung cancer gave a history of cigarette smoking. He hypothesized that cigarette smoking was linked to lung cancer. Again in 1940s, Sir Norman Gregg, an Australian ophthalmologist, observed a number of infants and young children in his ophthalmology practice presented with an unusual form of cataract. He noted that these children had been in-utero during the time of a rubella outbreak. He suggested that there was an association between prenatal rubella exposure and the development of the unusual cataract.

To determine the significance of such observations in a group of cases, a comparison or control group is needed. Comparison is an essential component of epidemiologic investigation.

## Case-control Study (Retrospective Study)

The distinctive feature of the case-control study is that it starts with people with the disease (cases) and compares them to people without the disease (controls). Three distinct features of the case-control study are:
- Both exposure and outcome (disease) have occurred before the start of the study.
- The study proceeds backward from effect (disease) to cause (exposure).
- It uses a control or comparison group to support or refute the inference.

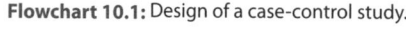

Flowchart 10.1: Design of a case-control study.

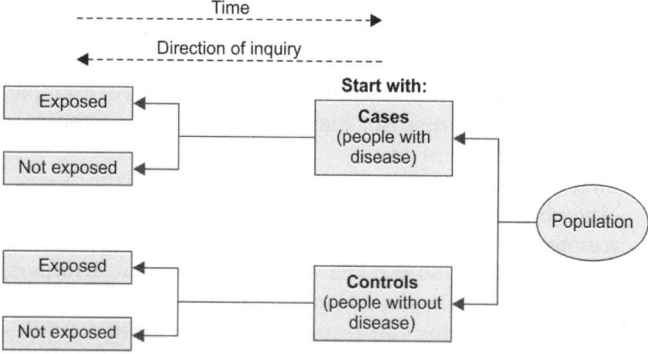

Table 10.4: Example of a case-control study.

| | First select | |
|---|---|---|
| Then measure past exposure | Cases (With disease) | Controls (Without disease) |
| Were exposed | a | b |
| Were not exposed | c | d |
| Total | a + c | b + d |
| Proportions exposed | a/a+c | b/b+d |

- In case-control studies, the unit is individual rather than the group.

Case-control studies are the choice of studies for the clinicians who have an easy access to the patients of a particular disease. The design of a case-control study is given in **Flowchart 10.1** and **Table 10.4**.

### Basic Steps in Conducting a Case-control Study

1. ***Specify the study population***: It is important as from this population, the cases have been selected and controls should also represent this population.
2. ***Specify the study variables***:
   - *Outcome variable*: The disease or outcome of interest
   - *Exposure variable*: Suspected cause that the investigator is studying
   - Potential confounding factors
3. ***Selection of cases***:
   - *Diagnostic criteria*: Mention clearly the diagnostic criteria for the disease
   - State the inclusion or exclusion criteria
   - *Source of cases*: Usually the cases are selected from hospitals. Cases can also be selected from OPDs of Private Practitioners or registries in case of cancer cases.
   - *Incident or prevalent cases*: It should be specified whether the incident cases will be selected or prevalent cases will be selected. It is preferable to use new cases of the disease in case-control studies of disease etiology to avoid the difficulty of disentangling factors related to causation and survival.
   - *Sampling*: Cases may be selected by simple random sampling method.
4. ***Selection of controls***:
   - *Selection of controls:* Control may also be selected from hospitals or population. Controls can also be selected from neighborhood or relatives. The important point is that the

controls should be representatives of the same population from which the cases come.
- *Inclusion/exclusion criteria*: Criteria for inclusion and exclusion of controls should be mentioned clearly.
- *Number of controls:* If the number of cases are less, then the ratio of cases to controls could be 1:2 or 1:4 and if the number of cases are 50 or more than the ratio of cases to controls could be 1:1.

5. *Matching*: It is a process of selecting the controls so that they are similar to the cases in certain characteristics, e.g. age, sex, socioeconomic status, occupation, etc. which can influence the outcome of the disease. There are two types: (1) group matching—selection of controls in such a manner that the proportion of controls with a certain characteristic is identical to the proportion of cases with the same characteristic, e.g. if 30% of the cases are from higher socioeconomic status then, 30% of the controls should also be from higher socioeconomic status. (2) Individual matching—in this, for each case selected for the study, a control is selected who is similar to the case in terms of specific variable, e.g. if the first case enrolled in a study is a 50-year-old male from urban area then the control should also be 50-year-old male residing in an urban area.

6. *Measurement of exposure:* Measurement of exposure should be done by obtaining information precisely the same manner for both cases and controls. This may be obtained by interviews, by questionnaires or by studying past records of cases such as hospital records, employment records, etc

### Bias in Case-control Study

One of the disadvantages of the case-control study is that it is susceptible to various forms of bias. There are different types of bias:

- **Selection bias:** Also known as Berksonian bias, selection of inappropriate controls, self-selection bias, incidence prevalence bias, selection of wrong control group.
  
  It is the difference in the characteristics of the people who are involved in the study and characteristics of the people who are not the part of the study population. Sometimes, the people themselves give their consent to be a part of the study. Studies carried out on children, many a times show selection bias, e.g. if a study is carried out for knowing the efficacy of a vaccine, then those parents who are educated, worried about their children's health may participate more and the results of the study could not be generalized. In case of studies carried out to know the effect of occupational exposure, one very important bias is there known as "healthy worker effect". This type of bias occurs when the workers who suffer from illness due to exposure to any chemical/dust, may leave the job or takes leave for rest and the investigator studies those occupational workers who are less affected and are on duty.

- **Memory or recall bias:** Since there is a collection of retrospective data, the recall of events would be better among the case than controls, because the cases are more likely to remember the past events better.

- **Interviewer's bias:** If the interviewer knows who is in the study group and who is in the control group there is a chance that interviewer may ask the questions thoroughly to the case then controls, like questions asked regarding history of exposure to suspected cases. This can be eliminated by applying blinding method in the study.

- **Measurement bias:** This type of bias occurs when the study does not measure correctly what it is supposed to measure. Measurement bias can occur if the basic technique of measurement is incorrect, due to defective instruments, etc. The basic measurement technique should be valid and reliable.
  - *Validity:* Study measures correctly what is supposed to be measured
  - *Reliability:* Study gives consistent results repeatedly.
  
  Measurement bias can also occur due to difference in data collection by two observers, e.g. reading of slides of peripheral smear for malarial parasite by two different observers may be different. Measurement bias can also occur because of variations in subjects on whom measurement is done, e.g. measurement of blood pressure in an individual during different time interval or after different activity will give different results.
  
  Measurement bias can also occur because of problems in the instrument being used for measurement if it is not calibrated. Recall bias faced during case-control studies is also an example of measurement bias.

- **Confounding bias**: A "confounding factor" is defined as one which is associated with both exposure and disease and is distributed unequally in study and control groups. It is independently a risk factor for the disease. Confounding variable should have the following properties:
  - It should be associated with the exposure of interest.
  - It should be known risk factor for outcome of interest.
  - It should not be an intermediary between exposure and the outcome (i.e. it must not lie on the causal pathway)

*Example of confounding variable:* A hypothesis that coffee drinkers have more heart disease than non-coffee drinkers may be influenced by another factor. Coffee drinkers may smoke more cigarettes than non-coffee drinkers, so smoking is a confounding variable in the study of the association between coffee drinking and heart disease. The increase in heart disease may be due to the smoking and not the coffee. More recent studies have shown coffee drinking to have substantial benefit in heart health and in the prevention of dementia. Confounding bias can be dealt with during study design by matching or during the stage of analysis by stratified analysis or regression (**Fig. 10.8**).

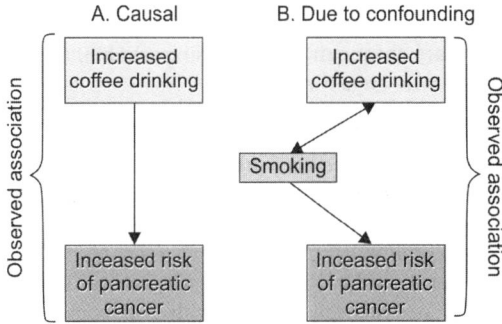

**Fig. 10.8:** Confounding variable.

7. **Analysis:** After conducting the entire study, the final step is to analyze for:
   - Calculation of exposure rates among cases and controls to suspected factor
   - Estimation of disease risk associated with exposure (odds ratio).

A study was carried out to find out the association between congenital malformation and maternal smoking **(Table 10.5)**.

**Table 10.5:** Association between congenital malformation and maternal smoking.*

| Maternal smoking | Congenital malformation | | |
| --- | --- | --- | --- |
| | Present (cases) | Absent (controls) | Total |
| Yes | 25 (a) | 45 (b) | 70 |
| No | 5 (c) | 25 (d) | 30 |
| Total | 30 | 70 | 100 |

*Exposure rates: Cases = 25/30 = 83.33%; Controls = 45/70 = 64.29% (P<0.01).

### Estimation of Risk

In case of a case-control study, we cannot calculate the incidence of the disease in the exposed and non-exposed population as we start the study with cases and controls and there is no appropriate denominator or population at risk to calculate the incidence rate. Hence, we calculate the odds ratio in case-control study as a measure of association.

**Odds ratio (cross-product ratio):** It is a measure of strength of association between risk factor and outcome. The formula for odds ratio is ad/bc.

*Interpretation of odds ratio:* If the odds ratio is 1 it indicates that the exposure is not related to the disease (null hypothesis). If the odds ratio is greater than 1 then it implies that the exposure is related to the disease (positive association) and if odds ratio is less than 1 then it means that there is negative association.

*Example:* Following is the data of a case-control study to study the association between use of seat belt and occurrence of a head injury during a car crash. Cases are persons who suffered a head injury in a car accident, while controls are persons who were in a car crash but did not have a head injury.

| | Cases (With head injury) | Controls (Without head injury) |
| --- | --- | --- |
| Did not use seat belt | 850 | 600 |
| Used seat belt | 150 | 400 |

Odds ratio: 850 × 400/600 × 150 = 3.78

The interpretation would be that the chances of head injury is 3.78 times more among drivers not using seat belt as compared to the drivers who are using seat belt.

### Examples of Case-control Study

- **Cigarette smoking and lung cancer:** In their landmark study, Doll and Hill (1950) evaluated the association between smoking and lung cancer. They included 709 patients of lung carcinoma (defined as cases). They also included 709 controls from general medical and surgical patients. The selected controls were similar to the cases with respect to age and sex. Thus, they included 649 males and 60 females in cases as well as controls.

They found that only 0.3% of males were non-smokers among cases. However, the proportion of non-smokers among controls was 4.2%; the different was statistically significant (P = 0.00000064). Similarly they found that about 31.7% of the female were non-smokers in cases compared with 53.3% in controls; this difference was also statistically significant (0.01< p <0.02).

- **Melanoma and tanning (Lazovic et al., 2010):** The authors conducted a case-control study to study the association between melanoma and tanning. The 1167 cases individuals with invasive cutaneous melanoma were selected from Minnesota Cancer Surveillance System. The 1101 controls were selected randomly from Minnesota State Driver's License list; they were matched for age (± 5 years) and sex.

The data were collected by self-administered questionnaires and telephone interviews. The investigators assessed the use of tanning devices (using photographs), number of years, and frequency of use of these devices. They also collected information on other variables (such as sun exposure; presence of freckles and moles; and color of skin, hair, among other exposures).

They found that melanoma was higher in individuals who used UVB enhances and primarily UVA-emitting devices. The risk of melanoma also increased in years of use, hours of use, and sessions.

- **Thalidomide study:** A classic example of a case control study was the discovery of the relation between thalidomide and unusual limb defects in babies born in the Federal Republic of Germany in 1959 and 1960; the study undertaken in 1961, compared affected children with normal children. Of 46 mothers whose babies had typical malformations, 41 had taken thalidomide during the fourth and ninth weeks of pregnancy for morning sickness, whereas none of the 300 control mothers, whose children were normal, had taken the drug at these stages. The term retrospective study is used for the case-control study. Some people have an erroneous impression that it is related to the calendar time but there are cohort studies (retrospective cohort) which also utilize data obtained in the past. The terminology retrospective is used as the investigator looks backward from the disease to a possible cause **(Table 10.6)**.

**Table 10.6:** Advantages and disadvantages of case-control study.

| Advantages | Disadvantages |
| --- | --- |
| It is easy to conduct | Problems of different types of bias are there (selection bias, recall bias, etc.) |
| Relatively inexpensive and less time consuming | Selection of control is difficult |
| Choice of study in case of rare diseases | Incidence cannot be estimated |
| Several etiological factors can be studied | Temporal association is not proven, only a matter of conjecture |
| Ethically there is no risk to the subjects | |
| Loss to follow-up is not there as these studies do not require the follow-up of the subjects | |
| It is also suited for diseases which have a long latent period (e.g. cancers) | |

> **Points to Remember**
> - Case-control studies are useful to study the cause of rare diseases.
> - Case-control studies include a comparison group.
> - The characteristic feature of case-control study is that it begins with cases and controls.
> - Several etiological factors can be studied.
> - One of the difficult tasks in conducting the case-control study is the selection of controls.

## Cohort Study (Synonym: Incidence Study, Follow-up Study, Longitudinal Study, Prospective Study)

Hallmark of the Cohort study: It begins with a group of people (cohort: a group of people who share a common characteristic or experience within a defined time period, e.g. age, occupation, etc.) free of disease, who are classified into subgroups according to exposure to a potential cause of disease or outcome **(Flowchart 10.2)**.

### Different types of cohort
- *Birth cohort:* Group of people born on the same day.
- *Exposure cohort:* People exposed to an infection, drug, etc.
- *Marriage cohort:* A group of males and females married on the same day or in the same period of time.

### Deciding when to Conduct a Cohort Study
- When there is evidence of an association between exposure and disease from clinical observations and supported by descriptive or case-control study.
- When the disease is common.
- When the follow-up is easy and the follow-up period is reasonably short.
- When the cohort is likely to continue the study.
- Funds are available.

### Basic Steps in Conducting a Cohort Study
1. State clearly the research question, objectives and background significance.
2. State the study population and cohort groups—exposed and unexposed.
3. State clearly the variables to be studied like exposure variable, outcome variable and possible confounding factors.
4. *Selection of study subjects:*
   a. *General population:* Subjects can be selected from the general population, so that the results can be generalized to the population sampled.
   b. *Special groups:*
      i. Special groups: Doctors, e.g. Doll's prospective study on smoking and lung cancer was carried out on British Doctors listed in the Medical Register of the UK in 1951.
      ii. Exposure groups: In case of rare exposure, such groups can be selected who are known to have the exposure, e.g. workers working in the industries, antenatal women having gestational diabetes for studying the outcome of pregnancy.
5. *Selection of comparison group*: It can be an inbuilt comparison group, e.g. all the antenatal women registered in antenatal clinic can be studied for the effect of Gestation diabetes on the outcome of pregnancy by dividing it into two groups: those having GDM and those not having GDM. Comparison with general population rates can also be done.
6. *Exclusion* of subjects having the disease or outcome of interest in both the exposed and unexposed groups
7. *Obtaining data on exposure*:
   a. Interview of study subjects
   b. Examination: Both exposed and unexposed group can be examined.
   c. Measurement of environment: Level of pollution at home, water pollution level, etc.
   d. Review of records: Medical records can be reviewed for obtaining data on exposure (dose of radiation, etc.)
8. *Follow-up and ascertainment of outcome of interest*: Frequency and time of follow-up and what to measure and how to measure to for detecting the outcome, should be decided prior to the start of the study. This can be done by reviewing the records, periodic examination of the subjects in the cohort, review of the death records, etc.

### Bias in Cohort Study
- **Measurement bias:** This type of bias can occur when there is a difference in determining the outcome of the disease because of disparity in the methods used by the observer.
- **Observer bias:** This type of bias occurs when the investigator knows about the exposure status of the subjects being studied. Blinding regarding the exposure status can avoid this type of bias.
- **Crossover bias:** Few subjects in the exposed group may shift to the non-exposed group and vice-versa (e.g. in the study of the effect of oral contraceptive pills on health, the women who were using OCPs may stop using it and adopt other method of contraception and vice-versa). This type of bias can be minimized by regular follow-up.
- **Loss to follow-up bias:** In spite of best efforts, a certain percentage of losses to follow-up are inevitable due to death, change of residence, migration, etc. However, it is recommended that 95% follow-up should be achieved if possible. Detailed address of the study subjects should be taken to avoid loss to follow-up.
- *Analysis*: As the cohort study is a follow-up study having a defined group of people, the incidence can be calculated. To measure the association between the exposure and the

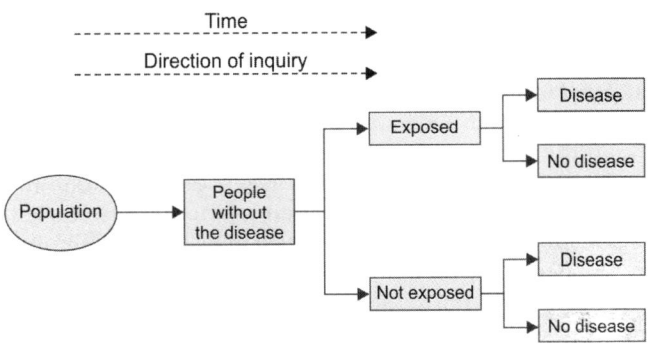
**Flowchart 10.2:** Design of a cohort study.

outcome in case of the cohort study, we calculate the relative risk (risk ratio).

### Estimation of Risk in a Cohort Study

**Relative risk:** It is defined as "The risk of disease in exposed individuals to the risk of disease in non-exposed individuals." RR is the measure of the strength of association and is a major consideration in deriving causal inferences.

$$\text{Relative risk} = \frac{\text{Disease risk in exposed}}{\text{Disease risk in non-exposed}}$$

*Interpretation of relative risk:* If relative risk is 1, then it indicates that there is no evidence of any increased risk in exposed individual or there is no association between the exposure and the outcome. If the relative risk is more than 1, it implies that the risk in exposed individuals is greater than the risk in non-exposed individuals. If RR is less than 1, it implies negative association, i.e. the risk in exposed persons is less than risk in non-exposed persons.

|  | Developed coronary heart disease | Did not develop coronary heart disease | Total |
|---|---|---|---|
| Intake of high fat diet | 90 | 1,710 | 1,800 |
| Intake of low fat diet | 45 | 1,755 | 1,800 |
| Total | 135 | 3,465 | 3,600 |

Incidence of disease among exposed = 90/1800 = 5 per 1,000
Incidence of disease among non-exposed = 45/1755 = 2.5 per 1,000

Relative risk = 5/2.5 = 2

Interpretation = The risk of developing coronary heart disease among those consuming high-fat diet is two times more than those consuming less-fat diet.

**Attributable risk (risk difference):** If the incidence of disease in exposed and unexposed groups were 0.5% and 0.1%, respectively, the relative risk would be 5.0. Similarly, if the incidence risks were 50% and 10%, the relative risk would also be 5.0. The major difference between these two situations is obvious: the actual amount of disease that is occurring is vastly different—in fact, in the second example it is 100 times greater. This vital public health information cannot be obtained from the relative risk. The approach to measuring the excess amount of disease occurring among those exposed to a potential risk factor is simple to calculate. We can calculate the extra amount of disease that is occurring in the exposed group by simply subtracting the incidence in the unexposed group from the incidence in the exposed group. This excess risk is known as attributable risk. [AR = IR (exposed) – IR (unexposed)]

In addition to the attributable risk, it may also be informative to consider the proportion of cases in the exposed group that would not have occurred in the absence of the exposure. This measure is often called the **attributable fraction or attributable risk percent.**

$$\text{Attributable risk percent} = \frac{\text{Incidence of disease among exposed} - \text{incidence of disease among unexposed}}{\text{Incidence of disease among exposed}}$$

*Importance of attributable risk:* If we are able to eliminate exposure to the agent in question, how much of the risk (incidence) of disease can we hope to prevent? It expresses the most that we can hope to achieve in reducing the risk of the disease if we completely eliminate the exposure, e.g. if relative risk of lung cancer among smokers is 10 times more than the risk among non-smokers, then attributable risk would be = 10 – 1/10 × 100 = 90%. If smoking is stopped, 90% of lung cancer cases could be reduced among the smokers.

Note that in the field of clinical epidemiology, what we have called the attributable risk is often called the **absolute risk reduction (ARR)** or **absolute risk increase (ARI)** depending on whether the event rate is reduced or increased in the treatment group.

**Population attributable risk (PAR):** It is the incidence of the disease (or death) in the total population minus the incidence of disease (or death) among those who were not exposed to the suspected causal factor. The concept of population attributable risk is useful in that it provides an estimate of the amount by which the disease could be reduced in that population if the suspected factor was eliminated or modified.

$$\text{PAR} = \frac{\text{Incidence of disease in total population} - \text{incidence of disease in nonexposed}}{\text{Incidence of disease in total population}}$$

For example, in a population of smokers, how much of the lung cancer that they experience is due to smoking and, consequently, how much of the lung cancer could be prevented if they did not smoke? However, to answer this question as to what effect the smoking cessation program will have on the city's population as a whole, we need to calculate the attributable risk for the total population:

Incidence of death among heavy smokers = 224
Incidence of death among non-smokers = 10
Incidence of death among total population = 74
Therefore, PAR# = 74 – 10/74 = 86%

86% of deaths from lung cancer could be avoided if the risk factor of cigarettes were eliminated.

Advantages and disadvantages of cohort study is described in **Table 10.7**.

### Examples of Cohort Studies

1. *Smoking and lung cancer by Doll and Hill:* In 1951, Doll and Hill sent a questionnaire about smoking habits to all the doctors resident in the UK through the British Medical Register. The responses were collected and long-term observation of their mortality was started. Follow-up of the cohort continued until 2001, and through the decades new questionnaires were sent to the study subjects (in 1957, 1966, 1971, 1978, 1991 and 2001) in

Table 10.7: Advantages and disadvantages of cohort study.

| Advantages | Disadvantages |
|---|---|
| • Temporal association can be proven as the study starts with the exposed and non-exposed groups and follows them till the outcome<br>• Stronger design as compared to case-control and cross-sectional study<br>• Several outcomes of a given exposure can be studied simultaneously<br>• Incidence can be calculated.<br>• No recall bias<br>• It is good for studying rare exposures<br>• It is a good design for studying rare exposure | • Not a good design for studying rare disease<br>• It is expensive and needs large number of subjects<br>• It takes long time to complete the study<br>• Problem of "loss to follow-up" is there<br>• Ethical issues are there<br>• Crossover can occur if some subjects from exposed group may leave the exposure and vice-versa |

order to gather information on changes in smoking habits and medical history. After the first 10 years of follow-up [3, 4], Doll and Hill reported 4597 deaths, and described an association between smoking and lung cancer, cancers of the upper respiratory and digestive tracts, chronic bronchitis, pulmonary tuberculosis, coronary disease without hypertension and peptic ulcer. A reduction of the death rate from lung cancer was seen in those who stopped smoking. The famous paper, published in 1976, on the 20-year follow-up and in 1999 on the 50-year follow up, clearly showed that smoking was an important cancer risk factor and co-factor for many other diseases.

2. *The Framingham Heart Study:* It is a long-term research project developed to identify risk factors of cardiovascular disease, including the effects of smoking, diet, and exercise. The study's findings further emphasized the need for preventing, detecting, and treating risk factors of cardiovascular disease in their earliest stages.

The Framingham Heart Study began in 1948 in the town of Framingham, Massachusetts. It was designed to track health information on men and women who initially did not show signs of heart disease. The original cohort (study group) included two-thirds of the adult population (more than 5,200 residents) of Framingham, with ages ranging from 30 to 62 years. Every two years people enrolled in the study submitted to medical tests and answered detailed questions about their lifestyle. Over the course of the study, researchers kept records of which individuals developed heart disease and which did not, and they studied the connections between disease and the data that had been collected.

In 1971 more than 5,120 new recruits, referred to as the Offspring Cohort, were added to the study. In 2001, a Third Generation Cohort, consisting of individuals who had at least one parent in the Offspring Cohort, was added.

This research has contributed very important discoveries related to the treatment of heart disease. Through the FHS, scientists have learned about the risk factors for heart disease, and they now know that many of those risks can be changed. It is why, in routine clinical examinations, doctors check for high blood pressure, high cholesterol, unhealthy eating patterns, smoking, physical inactivity or unhealthy weight. Researchers also know that these conditions can affect people differently depending on a patient's sex or race.

### Points to Remember

- The characteristic feature of the cohort study is that it starts with a group of people who are free of disease and followed over a period of time to study the outcome.
- Cohort studies provide measurement of risk of developing disease.
- This type of study can be used to study the multiple exposures.
- It is expensive and chances of loss to follow-up are there.

## Cross-sectional Studies (Synonym: Prevalence Study)

Hallmark of the cross-sectional study is that both the exposure and the effect (disease outcome) are determined simultaneously **(Flowchart 10.3)**.

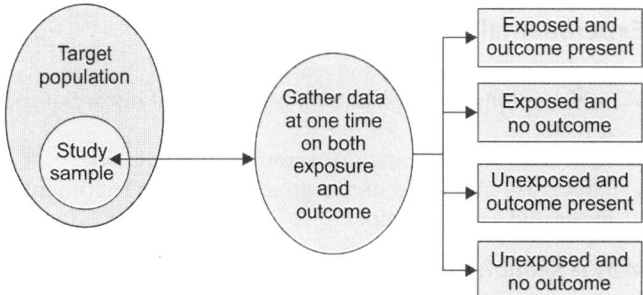

Flowchart 10.3: Design of a cross-sectional study.

Cross-sectional study is like viewing a photograph of the population at a certain point of time. They are known as cross-sectional study because it is like taking a cross-section of a sample of study population and determining both the exposure and the outcome at the same point of time. They are also known as prevalence study as the temporal relationship is not established between the exposure and the outcome.

### When to Conduct a Cross-sectional Study

1. It is useful to conduct cross-sectional study when the exposures are fixed characteristics of the individual, e.g. socioeconomic status, blood group, etc.
2. It is useful in knowing the utilization of health services by the population.
3. In such diseases which have wide clinical spectrum so that all cases are not reported in the hospital.

### Advantages of Cross-sectional Study

1. We can get the idea about the possible risk factor if the association between two continuously distributed variables is found.
2. It is helpful in assessing the health needs of the population.

### Steps of Conducting a Cross-sectional Study

1. Write the research question, hypothesis, objectives, and purpose of doing the study.
2. Clearly define the reference population and the study population.

3. Mention the study variables which are to be measured.
4. Calculate the sample size.
5. Describe the sampling method.
6. Collect the data.
7. Analyze the data.

> **Points to Remember**
> - In this type of study both exposure and disease outcome are determined simultaneously, e.g. in an individual there is history of smoking as well as family history of hypertension is also there and when we measure the blood pressure it comes out to be 140/100 mm Hg.
> - This is also known as prevalence study.
> - Cross-sectional studies are useful for investigation of exposures that are fixed characteristics of individuals, e.g. gender, blood group, etc.

# INTERVENTIONAL STUDIES (EXPERIMENTAL STUDIES)

## Experimental Epidemiology

- Also known as intervention epidemiology.
- Interventions are used to modify the natural history of the disease.
- It involves experimentation in groups or community.
- Effects are measured in two groups namely: experimental group and control group.

### Why is Reliable Evidence Important?

"Hormone replacement therapy for postmenopausal women provides an instructive example". Data from one of the observational studies showed that:

Giving hormone replacement therapy to postmenopausal women reduces cardiovascular risks.

## Types of Experimental Studies

1. **Clinical trial (therapeutic trial):** Drug trials, trials of surgical procedures etc. Unit of study is "patient" suffering from a given disease.
2. **Field trial (preventive trial):** Units of study are healthy individuals. The trial is undertaken in respect of a preventive procedure as a vaccine or personal protective measure, etc. Use of injectable polio vaccine is the biggest example of field trial.
3. **Community intervention trial:** Randomization done at the community level although assessment of outcome is done at the individual level. Such types of trials are good in knowing the effects of environmental variables or health educational measures, e.g. health education provided to people of one village regarding the hand hygiene practices and the other village the health education is not provided and study the outcome in terms of decreased episodes of illness.
4. **Health services evaluation trial:** The design is same as that of the community intervention trial, but one component of cost effectiveness is added. Example is: To reduce the incidence of diarrhea whether the ORS packets should be distributed or the health education regarding the hygienic practices should be provided to the mothers.
5. **Risk factor trial:** It is similar to preventive trial. A preventive step is introduced as an intervention, e.g. one of the risk factors of lifestyle-related diseases is the more consumption of junk food and less consumption of protective food like fruits and vegetables. One group may be asked to consume more of the vegetables and fruits in the diet while the other group is not.
6. **Cessation experiment:** A harmful factor is removed from the intervention group. A group of people who are leading sedentary lifestyle are divided into two groups and then one group is asked to perform daily physical exercise for at least 30 minutes while the other group is not and study the outcome (development of CHD in both the groups).

## Clinical (Therapeutic) Trials

Interventional clinical studies may be categorized into two large classifications: true experimental designs and quasi-experimental designs. The randomized, blinded clinical trial (RCT) is the prototypical example of a true experimental design.

### History of Clinical Trials

- Unintentional trial conducted by a surgeon Ambroise Pare (1510-1590) during the Renaissance. The standard treatment for war wounds was the application of boiling oil at that time as it solved the purpose of cauterization. Ambroise Pare was given the responsibility of treating the wounded after the war. After one war, when there were several people who were wounded, there was shortage of oil. So, he prepared a mixture by adding egg yolks, rose oil and turpentine. He was not able to sleep that night, as he was not sure of the role of this mixture on the wound. Surprisingly on next day he found that those people on whom the mixture was applied were feeling less pain as compared to those to whom boiled oil was applied.
- A planned trial by the Scottish surgeon, James Lind in 1747. He was interested in scurvy, as it leads to the death of thousands of British seamen each year. He took 12 patients in the scurvy on a ship to Salisbury. They were divided into six groups of two people each and given cider, elixir vitriol, vinegar, sea water, oranges and lemon in their diet. The best result was seen in people who received lemons and oranges. Scurvy essentially disappeared from the sailors as lime juice was included in the standard diet of the sailors.

### Randomized Control Trials (RCT)

In an RCT, patients are allocated to treatment arms in a prospective, random fashion in an attempt designed to ensure comparability between groups. The intervention and outcome are then administered and recorded, often with blinding of the interventionalist, the evaluator and the subject to reduce bias.

### Evidence from RCTs

An article published in "The New England Journal of Medicine" in August 2003 by Joann E Manson, et al. on "Estrogen plus Progestin and the risk of Coronary Heart Disease" concluded that:

Estrogen plus Progestin does not confer cardiac protection and may increase the risk of CHD among generally healthy postmenopausal women, especially during the first year after the initiation of hormone use. This treatment should not be prescribed for the prevention of cardiovascular disease.

### Uses of RCTs

- For evaluating new drugs and other treatments of disease
- For evaluating newer tests of medical care technology
- To assess new programs for screening and early detection
- For evaluation of effectiveness and efficiency of health services.

### Essential Requirements of a Clinical Trial

- Outcome benefits should be clinically important and measurable
- The intervention must be compatible with the health care needs of the patients in the trial
- There must be reasonable doubt regarding the efficacy of the intervention
- The intervention must be acceptable to both patient and provider
- There should be reasonable belief that the benefits will outweigh risks.

### When is an RCT not Appropriate?

- In knowing the etiology or natural history of disease
- Unethical to randomize
- Very rare outcomes (Cohort/case control)
- Outcomes may take a long time to develop (Cohort/case control)
- When the effect of an intervention is so powerful that a trial is not necessary.

### Steps of Conducting RCT (Flowchart 10.4)

1. ***Prepare a plan of study or protocol***
   a. Define clear objectives
   b. State the inclusion and exclusion criteria of case
   c. Determine the sample size, place and period of study
   d. Design of trial (single blind, double blind and triple blind method)
2. ***Define study population***: Most often the patients are chosen from hospital or from the community. For example, for a study for comparison of home and sanatorium treatment, open cases of tuberculosis may be chosen.
3. ***Selection of participants by defined criteria as per plan***: Selection of participants should be done with precision and should be precisely stated in writing so that it can be replicated by others. For example, out of open cases of tuberculosis those who fulfill criteria for inclusion may be selected (age groups, severity of disease and treatment taken or not, etc.)
4. ***Randomization of participants:*** Randomization is a statistical procedure by which the participants are allocated into groups usually called "study" and "control" groups, to receive or not to receive an experimental preventive or therapeutic procedure, maneuver or intervention. Randomization is an attempt to eliminate "bias" and allow for comparability.

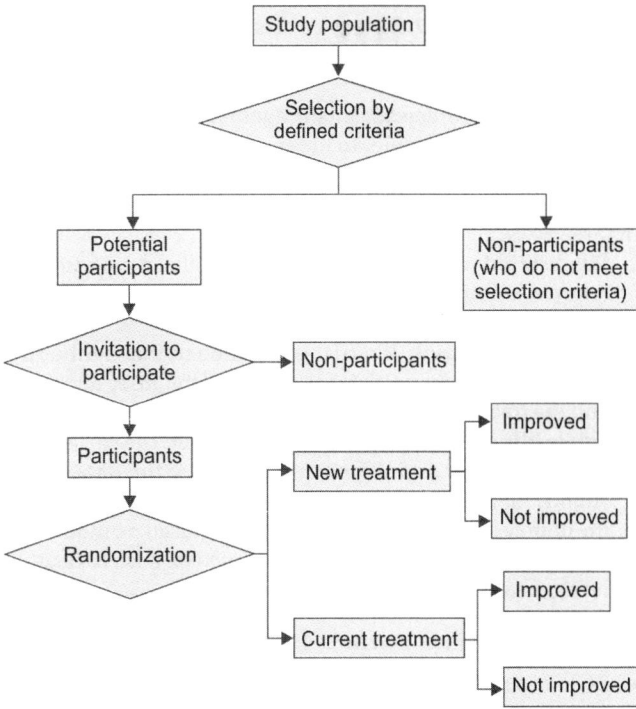

Flowchart 10.4: Design of randomized controlled trials.

Randomization is the "heart" of a control trial. It will give the greatest confidence that the groups are comparable so that "like can be compared with like". It ensures that the investigator has no control over allocation of participants to either study or control group, thus eliminating what is known as "selection bias". In other words, by random allocation, every individual gets an equal chance of being allocated into either group or any of the trial groups. Randomization is done only after the participant has entered the study, that is after having been qualified for the trial and has given his informed consent to participate in the study. It can be done by—token method, random number table, etc. The essential difference between a randomized controlled trial and an analytical study is that in the latter, there is no randomization because a differentiation into diseased and non-diseased (exposed or non-exposed) groups has already taken place. The only option left to ensure comparability in analytical studies is by matching.

5. ***Follow-up and analysis***: Final outcome in treatment and control group is observed with passage of time. Outcomes are determined as per laid down criteria under the plan of study. The final outcomes are compared between the treatment group and control group.

### Bias in RCT

- **Subject variation:** First, there may be bias on the part of the participants, who may subjectively feel better or report improvement if they knew they were receiving a new form of treatment.
- **Observer bias:** The investigator measuring the outcome of a therapeutic trial may be influenced if he knows beforehand

the particular procedure or therapy to which the patient has been subjected.
- **Evaluation bias:** There may be bias in evaluation - that is, the investigator may subconsciously give a favorable report of the outcome of the trial.

Randomization cannot guard against these sorts of bias, nor the size of the sample. In order to reduce these problems, a technique known as "blinding" is adopted, which will ensure that the outcome is assessed objectively. Blinding can be done in three ways:

1. **Single blind trial:** The trial is so planned that the participant is not aware whether he belongs to the study group or control group.
2. **Double blind trial:** The trial is so planned that neither the investigator nor the participant is aware of the group allocation and the treatment received.
3. **Triple blind trial:** This goes one step further. The participant, the investigator and the person analyzing the data are all "blind". Ideally, of course, triple blinding should be used; but the double blinding is the most frequently used method when a blind trial is conducted. When an outcome such as death is being measured, blinding is not so essential.

### Examples of RCTs (Flowchart 10.5)

- RCTs in tuberculosis: Comparison of home and sanatorium treatment—a study undertaken by tuberculosis chemotherapy center (Chennai) to study the emergence of relapse cases in these two groups. Study population: 163 newly diagnosed and previously untreated sputum positive patients of pulmonary tuberculosis from poor section of the community.
- TB attack rates among close family contacts—a study undertaken by tuberculosis chemotherapy center (Chennai) to determine the relative risks for contacts of patients treated at home and in the sanatorium. Study population: 256 close family contacts of patients treated in homes and 272 similar contacts of patients treated in sanatorium were followed-up by X-ray and bacteriological examination for 5 years.

> **Points to Remember**
> - In case of interventional studies, the investigator changes a variable.
> - In one or more groups of people, e.g. giving the micronutrient supplements to one group of children and placebo to the other group of children and then comparing the outcome in two groups by comparing their growth.
> - This type of study can be used to study any new preventive or therapeutic regime or any new procedure.
> - Randomization provides the best evidence of association because they can control both known and unknown confounding factors.

## Nonrandomized Interventional Study Designs (Quasi-Experimental Designs)

### 1. *Nonrandomly assigned control (or comparison) group studies*

In this type of studies, at least two separate groups are evaluated— one of which receives the intervention of interest and another that serves as a control or comparison group. Thus, the nonrandom control group is similar in design to a RCT, except that patients are assigned to treatment groups in a nonrandom fashion. Quasi-experimental designs differ from that of an observational trial in that the patients are allocated to treatment groups by research protocol, whereas in an observational study the natural history of treatments is studied (i.e., there is no allocation to any intervention).

### 2. *Time series analysis*

Time series analysis can provide a more concrete method for addressing the problem of secular trends in clinical care. Essentially, the investigator measures the outcome of interest several times before initiating the experiment to establish a baseline value and trend in the data and again after the intervention, the investigator will measure the outcome several times to establish the impact of the intervention. This design differs from a standard cohort design because the investigator manipulates patient care to estimate the effect of the intervention and from a pre/post design because it can identify trends in the outcome rate that existed before the intervention.

### 3. *Comprehensive cohort trials/patient preference trials*

As a result of the invasive nature of surgical interventions, patients may be reluctant to agree to random assignment. Consequently, the representativeness of surgical RCTs may be substantially compromised, thus making extrapolation of results to the general population concerning. In the comprehensive cohort study (CCS) or patient preference trial (PPT) designs, patients who decline to participate in the randomized portion of a trial continue to be followed in their chosen therapeutic arm. At the conclusion of the trial, comparisons are made for four groups of patients: patients randomized into intervention A, patients who selected intervention A, patients randomized into intervention B, and patients who selected intervention B.

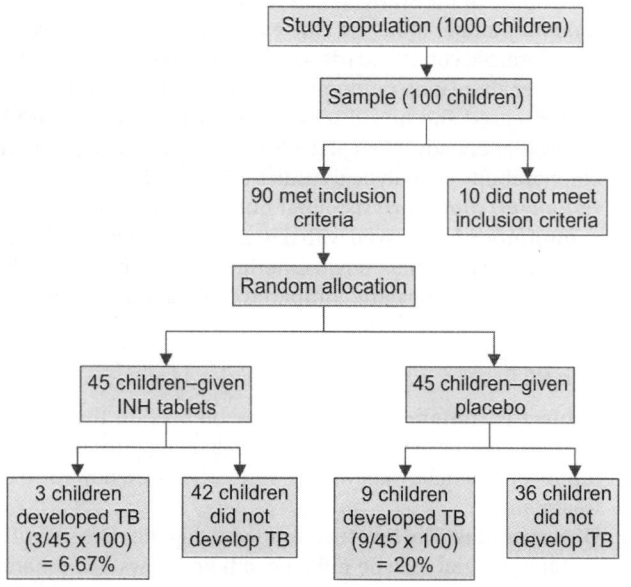

**Flowchart 10.5:** Example of RCT—whether it is worthwhile to give INH chemoprophylaxis to children who are close contacts of open cases of pulmonary TB? (RR = 1/3).

# ASSOCIATION AND CAUSATION

In previous topics, we discussed a variety of designs of epidemiologic studies that are used to determine whether an association exists between an exposure and a disease outcome. We then addressed different types of risk measurement that are used to quantitatively express an excess in risk. If we determine that an exposure is associated with a disease, the next question is whether the observed association reflects a causal relationship. Association is defined as occurrence of two variables together more often than would be expected by chance. Association doesn't always mean a causal relationship.

Conceptually, a two-step process is followed in carrying out studies and evaluating evidence.
1. We determine whether there is an association or correlation between an exposure or characteristic and the risk of a disease. To do so, we use:
   a. Studies of group characteristics: Ecologic studies
   b. Studies of individual characteristics: Cohort, case-control, and other types of studies.
2. If an association is demonstrated, we determine whether the observed association is likely to be a causal one.

## Types of Association

Association broadly grouped into:
1. Spurious association
2. Causal association—direct or indirect

### Spurious Association

- Observed association between disease and an agent may not be real.
  - Spurious associations are non-causal associations by chance, bias, confounding factor, etc. Association between a characteristic and a disease may be due to presence of a third factor (known or unknown) that is common to both characteristic and disease. This third factor is known as confounding factor. Bias due to confounding factor is explained in detail in description of case control studies.

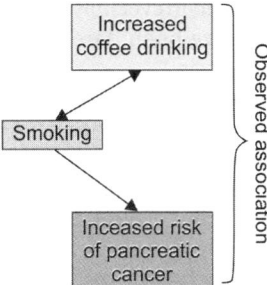

In this example, there seems to be a false association between coffee consumption and pancreatic cancer. This is because of the simultaneous presence of smoking in coffee drinkers, and smoking is responsible for causing pancreatic cancer.

### Causal Association

We have already looked at how we measure health (or disease) and how we look for associations between exposure and disease. Being able to identify a *relation* between a potential cause of disease and the disease itself is not enough, though. If our goal is to change practice or policy in order to improve health then we need to go one step further and decide whether the relation is causal because, if it is not, intervening will have no effect.

A causal pathway can be either *direct* or *indirect* **(Fig. 10.9)**. In *direct* causation a factor directly causes a disease without any intermediate step. In *indirect* causation a factor causes a disease but only through an intermediate step or steps. In human biology, intermediate steps are virtually always present in any causal process.

If a relationship is causal, four types of causal relationships are possible: (1) necessary and sufficient **(Fig. 10.10)**, (2) necessary but not sufficient **(Fig. 10.11)**, (3) sufficient but not necessary **(Fig. 10.12)**, and (4) neither sufficient nor necessary **(Fig. 10.13)**.

## What is the Importance of Knowing the Cause?

The knowledge of cause is not only important from the aspect of its prevention but also for the diagnosis and treatment of the disease.

### Cause and Criteria for Judging Causality (Bradford and Hills Criteria for Causality)

Cause is defined as an event, condition, characteristic or a combination of these factors which plays an important role in producing the disease.

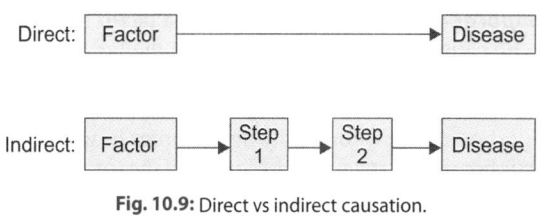

**Fig. 10.9:** Direct vs indirect causation.

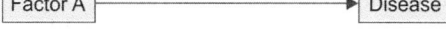

**Fig. 10.10:** Factor A is both necessary and sufficient.

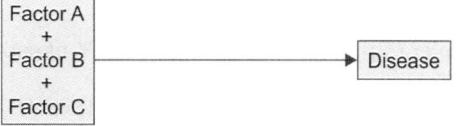

**Fig. 10.11:** Each factor A, B, C is necessary, but not sufficient in itself.

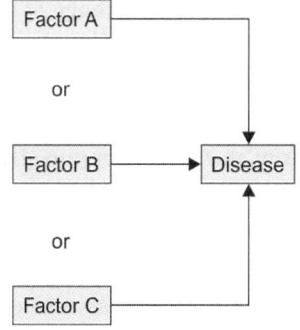

**Fig. 10.12:** Each factor A, B, C is sufficient, but not necessary in itself.

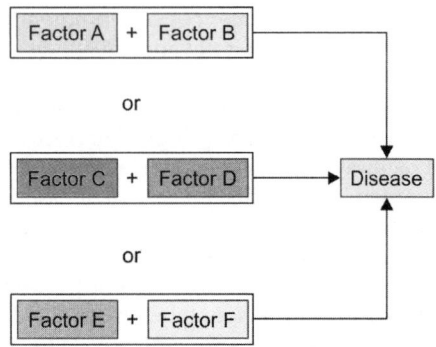

**Fig. 10.13:** Each of the factors is neither sufficient nor necessary.

Logically, the cause must precede the effect (disease). A cause is termed sufficient when it inevitably produces or initiates a disease and is termed necessary if a disease cannot develop in its absence. Each sufficient cause has a necessary cause as a component. For example, in case of tuberculosis several factors play role in the causation of the disease like, nutritional status, housing conditions, overcrowding, lower socioeconomic status but the bacteria *Mycobacterium tuberculosis* is necessary cause.

Causal inference is the process of determining whether the observed associations are likely to be causal. Guidelines for causation are prepared based on the concepts provided by the United States Surgeon General and Sir Bradford Hill.

1. ***Temporal relation:*** It is clear that if a factor is believed to be the cause of a disease, exposure to the factor must have occurred before the disease developed.

    The temporal relationship of exposure and disease is important not only for clarifying the order in which the two occur but also in regard to the length of the interval between exposure and disease.
    **Example:** About 11% of chronic gastritis patients will go on to have duodenal ulcers over 10 years period.
2. ***Strength of the association:*** The strength of the association is measured by the relative risk (or odds ratio). The stronger the association, the more likely it is that the relation is causal.
    **Example:** *H. pylori* is found in at least 90% of patients with duodenal ulcer.
3. ***Dose-response relationship:*** As the dose of exposure increases, the risk of disease also increases. If a dose-response relationship is present, it is strong evidence for a causal relationship. However, the absence of a dose-response relationship does not necessarily rule out a causal relationship. In some cases in which a threshold may exist, no disease may develop up to a certain level of exposure (a threshold); above this level, disease may develop
    **Example:** Density of *H. pylori* per mm of gastric mucosa is higher in patients with duodenal ulcer.
4. ***Replication of the findings:*** If the relationship is causal, we would expect to find it consistently in different studies and in different populations. Replication of findings is particularly important in epidemiology. If an association is observed, we would also expect to be seen consistently within subgroups of the population and in different populations, unless there is a clear reason to expect different results.
    **Example:** Many studies have demonstrated the role of *H. pylori* in duodenal ulcers.
5. ***Biologic plausibility:*** Biologic plausibility refers to coherence with the current body of biologic knowledge. Examples may be cited to demonstrate that epidemiologic observations have sometimes preceded biologic knowledge. The implication of high oxygen concentration in the causation of retrolental fibroplasia, a form of blindness that occurs in premature infants, preceded any biologic knowledge supporting such a relationship. Nevertheless, we seek consistency of the epidemiologic findings with existing biologic knowledge, and when this is not the case, interpreting the meaning of the observed association may be difficult. We may then be more demanding in our requirements about the size and significance of any differences observed and in having the study replicated by other investigators in other populations.
    **Example:** *H. pylori* induces mediators of inflammation, damages mucosa making it susceptible to damaging effects of acid.
6. ***Consideration of alternate explanations:*** We have discussed the problem in interpreting an observed association in regard to whether a relationship is causal or is the result of confounding. In judging whether a reported association is causal, the extent to which the investigators have taken other possible explanations into account and the extent to which they have ruled out such explanations are important considerations.
    **Example:** From the available data it has been observed that smoking can increase the risk of duodenal ulcer in *H. pylori*-infected patients but not in patients in whom *H. pylori* has been eradicated.
7. ***Cessation of exposure:*** If a factor is a cause of a disease, we would expect the risk of the disease to decline when exposure to the factor is reduced or eliminated. When cessation data are available, they provide helpful supporting evidence for a causal association. However, in certain cases, the pathogenic process may have been irreversibly initiated, and the disease occurrence may have been determined by the time the exposure is removed.
    **Example:** Long-term ulcer recurrence rates were zero after *H. pylori* was eradicated using antimicrobial therapy.
8. ***Consistency with other knowledge:*** If a relationship is causal, we would expect the findings to be consistent with other data.
    **Example:** The prevalence of ulcer disease peaked in later part of 19th century.
9. ***Specificity of the association:*** An association is specific when a certain exposure is associated with only one disease; this is the weakest of all the guidelines.
    When specificity of an association is found, it provides additional support for a causal inference. However, as with a dose-response relationship, absence of specificity in no way negates a causal relationship.
    **Example:** Prevalence of *H. pylori* in patients with duodenal ulcers is 90–100%.

## SUMMARY

- Epidemiology is not only the study of death, illness and disability but also positive health state and deals with health of human population and its subgroups. It is also used to describe the health situation of people. Information regarding disease burden in population is essential for stakeholders and policy implementers as limited resources would be utilized in best possible manner by identifying priority health programs for prevention and care.
- Epidemiological studies can be categorized into two types: observational and experimental. Observational studies are descriptive and analytical studies.
- To describe the health event we need to answer six questions: what, how much, where, when, who and why. The answers to first five questions are given by descriptive epidemiology and the answer to sixth question is given by analytical epidemiology.
- Descriptive studies describe any health-related event or disease in terms of time, place and person and are helpful in the formulation of the hypothesis. Analytical studies which may be cross-sectional, cohort or case-control studies are useful in testing the hypothesis.
- In describing the time distribution of a disease, epidemic curve is a very important tool in describing the short-term fluctuations.
- Case-control studies and cohort studies use the comparison group. In case of cohort study the temporal association can be proven.
- The strength of association in case of cohort study, is measured by calculating the relative risk and in case of case-control study it is measured by calculating the odds ratio.
- In cross-sectional studies the exposure and outcome are ascertained at the same time.
- Experimental or interventional studies where the participants are randomly allocated into exposed and non-exposed groups give strong evidence regarding the causal association.
- Different types of errors can occur while carrying out the epidemiological studies such as random error, systematic error, confounding, etc.

## SUGGESTED READING

1. Beaglehole R, Bonita R, Kjellstrom T. Basic Epidemiology. Hyderabad: Orient Longman/WHO; 1993.
2. CDC. Field Epidemiology Training Program Module. Atlanta: Centre for Disease Control and Prevention; 2018.
3. CDC. Principles of Epidemiology in Public Health Practice, 3rd edition. Atlanta: Center for Disease Control and Prevention; 2006.
4. Gordis L. Epidemiology, 3rd edition. Philadelphia: Elsevier Saunders; 2004.

# CHAPTER 11

# Research Methodology and Biostatistics

*Paragkumar Chavda, Mihir Rupani, Kalpita Shringarpure, Kedar Mehta*

**CM6.1** Formulate a research question for a study

**CM6.2** Describe and discuss the principles and demonstrate the methods of collection, classification, analysis, interpretation and presentation of statistical data

**CM6.3** Describe, discuss and demonstrate the application of elementary statistical methods including test of significance in various study designs

**CM6.4** Enumerate, discuss and demonstrate common sampling techniques, simple statistical methods, frequency distribution, measures of central tendency and dispersion

**CM7.3** Enumerate, describe and discuss the sources of epidemiological data

**CM7.9** Describe and demonstrate the application of computers in epidemiology

## INTRODUCTION TO HEALTH RESEARCH

> Dr Aavishkaar is a Medical Officer at the antiretroviral therapy (ART) center of a medical college hospital. He is concerned about patients presenting very late for treatment after human immunodeficiency virus (HIV) diagnosis. He discusses this with another senior colleague, Dr Vaigyanik. The two of them come to a conclusion that many patients who are diagnosed at primary health centers do not turn up for treatment initiation at the ART center. This problem makes Dr Aavishkaar wonder what should be done to motivate these patients for initiating treatment.
>
> He wishes to explore the possibility of giving reminders to such patients through phone calls. Since most of the patients now possess mobile phones, this idea should work. He discusses this plan with Dr Vaigyanik; who finds it interesting. Dr Aavishkaar plans to find out the percentage of newly diagnosed HIV patients from this district, being registered at ART center by the end of 1 month after diagnosis. Dr Vaigyanik suggests that he should also collect such data from another district; where such telephonic reminders will not be given to get a comparative picture.
>
> Dr Aavishkaar trains the counselors of intervention district for giving weekly phone reminders for registering at the ART center for treatment. After 6 months, Dr Aavishkaar collects the data from both the districts. He feels happy to find out that in the intervention district 90% of newly diagnosed HIV patients were registered at the ART center by the end of 1 month of diagnosis; whereas, in the comparison district, this proportion was 70%. Thus concluding that this intervention was found effective, the state acquired immune deficiency syndrome (AIDS) control society decides to take up mobile phone reminders as a routine service across all districts in the state.

As we read the story of Dr Aavishkaar we realize that doctors come across such situations in their life where they want to pursue a clinical problem to find a solution. What Dr Aavishkaar did differently was pursuing the problem using a sound scientific methodology. His suggested solution was found effective and it could become part of policy of HIV program. Thus, clinical problems in routine medical practice, if pursued methodologically, can bring about the desired changes. For this, we need to learn a bit about the scientific way of enquiry. This chapter explains methodological aspect of scientific medical research.

While reading the history of medical science in this book, you would have come across the fact that in ancient times the physicians tested a variety of treatments by trial and error method. Some of them worked, while others did not. This was known as empirical practice. As medical science evolved, physicians started following experience-based practice; that which worked well for the patients became a practice. Lately, medical science has moved to a more rationalist approach, the evidence-based medical practice. This evidence comes from research studies which are scientifically robust. So the journey of medical practice has passed through three "Es"—*empirical, experience, and evidence-based practice.*

Doctors, while treating patients, come across newer methods/modalities of treatment for diseases. A surgeon discovers a new technique of performing a surgery and feels that it is a better method compared to the standard way of performing that surgery. How does this surgeon convert his experience into evidence? It can be done only if the new method is tested and proven to be better using a scientifically planned and methodologically detailed research study.

In simple terms, research in medical science is nothing but a *scientific enquiry. Enquiry* means an investigation to find out the facts. The word "*scientific*" means that our investigation is carried using some scientific method.

In this chapter, we will go through the steps of this scientific process. But before that, let us understand broad domains of medical or health research. The scope of research is increasing in multiple fields related to medical science. **Table 11.1** outlines a simple grid to understand classification of health research.

Depending on the object of analysis, the research might be focused on the existing health problems or healthcare responses to such health problems. Depending on the level of analysis the research might be focused on analyzing information from individuals or from populations. Thus, the research that focuses

**Table 11.1:** Domains of health research.

| | | Object of analysis | |
| --- | --- | --- | --- |
| | | Health problems | Healthcare responses |
| Level of analysis | Individual or subindividual | Biomedical research:<br>• Biological processes<br>• Body structure and function<br>• Pathological mechanisms | Clinical research:<br>• Natural history of diseases<br>• Efficacy of preventive, diagnostic or therapeutic interventions |
| | Population—community health | Epidemiological research:<br>Frequency, distribution, and causes of diseases | Health systems research:<br>• Policy research<br>• Operational research |

on the description of health problem or disease in individuals falls under the domain of biomedical research.

When research focuses on the description of diseases at population level, it falls under the domain of epidemiological research. A research trying to find out the prevalence of goiter in a district would fall under this category. While a research testing the efficacy of new drug or therapy on individuals falls in the domain of clinical research. When the research focuses on studying the organized response to health problems at population level it falls under domain of health systems research. An example of research in this domain would be; trying to find out whether active case finding through home visits is more economical than passive case finding through clinics for detection of tuberculosis cases in a district under National Tuberculosis Control Program. You will learn more about the health systems research in a separate chapter in this book.

Whatever be the domain of research, it has a potential to change *policy* or *practice*. For example, a new research providing evidence that a new medication helps to reduce blood pressure among hypertensive patients may influence the practice of the doctors as they start prescribing this new medication. Similarly, under National Tuberculosis Control Programme research evidence showed that two sputum smear examinations were nearly as good compared to three sputum smears. This evidence changed the national policy from conducting three sputum smears to two sputum smears for diagnosis of tuberculosis.

> **Note**
> Research outcome: Change in health policy or medical practice.

### Where will I Use it in My Professional Life?

> **Note**
> A medical professional is always a consumer of research and can also become a contributor to research.

We consider medicine as a science, which can progress when new knowledge is added on a continuous basis. A doctor's work is termed as medical practice, since each encounter with a patient teaches the doctor a new thing. The robust process of research helps in converting all such learnings to meaningful evidence. Such evidence will be used by other doctors as well. In this sense every medical practitioner is a potential researcher. This is one of the reasons why research work in the form of a dissertation is mandatory in all postgraduate medical courses. A dissertation is the first exposure to research in the life of a medical specialist practitioner. Realizing the increasing importance of research, its training has become an integral part of undergraduate medical students curriculum. By now, most of you would have heard of the Indian Council of Medical Research (ICMR) Short Term Research Studentships given to undergraduate students for carrying out research. A medical professional is expected to contribute continuously to the field of medicine by engaging in research throughout their professional life.

Another encounter is when doctors become consumers of medical research. We as doctors depend on research-based evidence for our day-to-day clinical decisions; be it choosing a correct diagnostic test or choosing a preferred therapy for a patient. As consumers of research evidence we should not accept whatever is presented to us as scientific information at face value. One of the objectives of this chapter is to train students to critically evaluate any research evidence they read in form of research reports or publications.

Thus, going through this chapter, you will be better equipped to deal with your role as *contributor* as well as *consumer* of research.

## QUANTITATIVE AND QUALITATIVE APPROACHES TO RESEARCH

> **Dr Curious goes on a research expedition!**
>
> Dr Curious, a resident doctor in pulmonary medicine department of a medical college, observed many patients with drug-resistant tuberculosis coming to his outpatient department (OPD). The increasing proportion of drug-resistant cases intrigued him. When he shared his concern with his professor, she suggested that part of the problem lies in discontinuation of treatment of tuberculosis by patients—a phenomenon termed as "loss to follow-up".
>
> Interested in this problem, the resident doctor decided to find out the proportion of the lost to follow-up tuberculosis patients treated at primary health centers of his district. He collected the information of primary health centers of his district, as well as information regarding patients who were initiated on tuberculosis treatment in last 6 months and the number of those who discontinued treatment. He gathered data of 200 patients and found out that 40 of them had discontinued the treatment. Thus, around 20% patients were lost to follow-up.
>
> Alarmed by such high proportion of patients lost to follow-up on treatment (expected proportion <5%), he was curious to know why these patients had defaulted. He visited the homes of the patients who were lost to follow-up on treatment and interviewed them in detail for the reasons for discontinuing treatment. As he wanted to find out all possible reasons, he continued interviewing patients till the time he could not get a newer reason for default. In total, he interviewed 18 such patients. He audio recorded the interviews and wrote the scripts of the interview. He read and reread the interview scripts to understand in depth the context that lead to default. At the end of this process, he identified the following reasons: patients felt no further need for treatment once symptoms subsided, they were not able to tolerate the side-effects, traveling long distance for taking treatment was not feasible for them, their work timings and health center timings collided and they could not afford to lose work!
>
> Now Dr Curious had a reasonable idea of the magnitude of the problem and possible reasons.

As you read the story of Dr Curious, you must have observed that in the first scenario he was interested in answering the question "*What* is the proportion of patients lost to follow-up on treatment?" In the next scenario he was trying to find out the answers to the question, "*Why* do patients discontinue the treatment?" In the first instance Dr Curious has used a quantitative approach to research, while in the second scenario, he has used a qualitative approach to research. Let us briefly go through the salient features of both the approaches.

| | Quantitative research | Qualitative research |
|---|---|---|
| The purpose | Here the purpose is often to "estimate" a number (e.g., prevalence of patients defaulting on treatment) | Here the purpose is often to "explore" the different perspectives of the problem (e.g., to explore the reasons for default) |
| Basic process | We use numbers to quantify the problem. We have collection of numbers and data, e.g., we quantified the problem treatment default | We use words to understand the problem in detail. We have narrative descriptions which are collection of words, e.g., we have the patient's story of why he or she defaulted from treatment |
| Primary information unit | The information collected is in form of numbers | The collected information is in form of words |
| Viewpoint | While deciding in whose perspective data is to be collected, the researcher's viewpoint (etic perspective) is given priority | While deciding in whose perspective data is to be collected, the respondent's viewpoint (emic perspective) is given priority |
| Design of research | The research design is very structured. The epidemiological study designs that you learned in previous chapter are used here | The research design is not fixed but it is flexible. The design evolves as the researcher collects data |
| Sample | This approach often involves collecting small amount of data from large number of people | This approach involves collecting large amount of data but from a small sample |
| Methods of data collection | The methods of data collection include surveys, interviews, and experiments | The methods of data collection include observation and interviews. Experiments are usually not used here |
| Analysis | Since we are dealing with large amount of data we often make use of statistical software to analyze the data | We deal with narratives and hence software has limited role in analysis of such qualitative data. Much of the processing of such data happens within researcher's mind |
| Chronology of data management | Data analysis is possible only after the data is collected from all study participants | Data collection and analysis goes hand in hand, e.g., researcher starts analyzing the reasons for default in her mind right from the time she takes interview of the first patient |
| Training required | The researcher is required to be trained in intricacies of research design and statistical analysis | The researcher is required to be trained in the art of qualitative data collection and analysis |
| To whom can the findings be applied | The findings of research are often generalizable to other populations too | The findings are specific to the individuals studied and often not generalizable to other populations |

Let us take few more examples of questions and see which approach would be better suited to obtain their answers.
1. Does intestinal anastomosis using stapler result in better treatment outcome compared to hand-sewn intestinal anastomosis?
2. Which is a better predictor of obesity, sugar consumption or fat consumption?
3. What is the prevalence of dental caries in school going children aged 5–10 years?
4. Does mobile phone reminder reduce the loss to follow-up rate among people on ART?
5. What are the reasons for patients discontinuing tuberculosis treatment?
6. Why do parents in tribal areas not prefer to vaccinate their children?
7. Why do adolescents in a particular geographic area use addictive drugs?
8. What coping mechanism do medical students use to relieve exam-related stress?

Answers to questions 1 to 4 are better obtained through quantitative approach while those for questions 5 to 8 are better sought for through qualitative approach.

Irrespective of the approach chosen, it is important to understand that for both the approaches the primary intention is to uncover the truth. Thus, now you would understand that each approach has its own strength and hence no approach is superior to the other. Both have their own utility. Depending on the type of truth you want to uncover you would differ in your chosen approach.

Researchers over the time have realized that both the approaches are complementary to each other. Hence, recently there is a new approach which makes use of both these approaches together. Such approach is known as mixed methods approach. The research by Dr Curious described above is an example of mix-method approach.

We had the conceptual understanding of the quantitative and qualitative approaches to research in this section. From the next section onwards we will describe the quantitative approach to research in detail. The detailed discussion on qualitative research is beyond scope of this book.

## INTRODUCTION TO QUANTITATIVE RESEARCH

Quantitative research is a *systematic* process of collecting, analyzing, and interpreting data to answer a question or to solve a problem. Systematic means that research process is not a haphazard chain of activities, but an organized process to get meaningful answers and solutions to health problems. To ensure being systematic we make use of the concepts and methods of epidemiology. Epidemiologic study designs form the core of research design in quantitative research—differentiated into descriptive, analytical, and experimental types of studies.

We would like to visit the hierarchy of evidence that you have covered earlier. We understand that hierarchy starts at the base with descriptive studies such as case reports and case series and goes till meta-analysis. Meta-analysis is at the top of this hierarchy, thus being the strongest form of evidence. Let us understand this using real-life examples, viz. the issue of feeding an infant up to 6 months of age. There would be studies conducted across the world on breastfeeding and bottle feeding, in fact some studies also comparing both these approaches. Once sufficient numbers of such studies are available in published literature, an interested group of researchers might take up the task to conduct a systematic review of all such published studies. If the systematic review concludes that breastfeeding is better compared to bottle feeding for first 6 months of life, the ministry of health for a country can use such evidence to promote breastfeeding for the first 6 months of life in the general population. It may also enact a law to offer a period of maternity leave for all employees, so that working mothers have an opportunity to breastfeed their child. An individual practicing doctor or pediatrician will use this evidence to advice all the postnatal mothers for breastfeeding. Thus, this evidence may be used by practicing doctors, policy makers as well as general public at large.

What is the source of information for whatever we read in medical textbooks? You guessed it right! Most of the information and facts that you read from medical textbooks are based on the evidence generated by systematic reviews. The authors of medical textbooks prefer to use systematic reviews as the basis of scientific facts while describing the risk factors of a disease, identifying the preferred methods of diagnosing or treating a disease.

## Generic Steps in Conducting Research

We will now take you through the generic steps followed while conducting any quantitative research study. With small modifications, many of these steps are also applicable while conducting qualitative or mixed methods research. We will discuss each of these steps in detail in the subsequent sections of this chapter.

### *Selecting a Topic for Research*

It is important to understand at this stage how our general curiosity about a topic is different from scientific curiosity. As part of our general curiosity, we may be interested in many aspects of a particular topic, but to convert it to scientific curiosity, we need to narrow our focus on a single aspect. Quantitative research, being a systematic detailed process, does not allow us to study multiple aspects of a topic simultaneously. If we attempt to do that, we will end up studying multiple problems superficially and may not be confident about the findings of our research. This is the reason why quantitative research expects the researchers to study only one aspect of a health problem with scientific rigor so that the findings and evidence generated is usable.

### *Searching for Existing Knowledge on the Topic*

When we narrow down to a specific issue for research, we need to search if other people have worked in this area. It is possible that the topic that was interesting for us might have interested others also who might have already done research on this topic. So the first step is to search for existing literature to know the current status of evidence in a particular issue of our interest (termed as review of literature). Earlier, researchers spent hours in libraries sifting through the library catalogues to find out related research. Fortunately, there are databases available in electronic format nowadays that make this Herculean task of finding the "relevant" literature an easy one. Google scholar (https://scholar.google.co.in/) and PubMed (https://www.ncbi.nlm.nih.gov/pubmed/) are two of the commonly used tools for literature search.

### *Refining Research Question*

Once we are done with reviewing the existing literature on the topic of our interest, we would be able to find out the gaps in the existing body of knowledge. It is prudent to refine our topic of inquiry towards the direction of this gap. While refining the research question, we will clarify what exactly we want to study and on whom.

### *Defining Study Variables and Study Population*

Having a systematic approach expects us to be accurate in our measurements. So defining what we want to measure in our study (input and output variables) is important. It is also important to select the group of people from whom we will gather our data.

### *Planning for Data Management*

Many novice researchers skip this step unknowingly. For being systematic in our approach, we not only have to be specific about what information is to be collected, but also how we are going to collect such information. We have to plan in advance on what would be the sources of data, as well as methods and tools that will be used for data collection.

This step also involves preparing a plan for analysis. This is the advantage of quantitative research.

### *Preparing a Proposal and Ethics Review*

Having completed all the earlier steps we are ready with most of the ingredients for writing a proposal. A *study protocol* is a formal document containing the "plan for research". A "protocol" to a researcher is similar to that of a "blue print" to an architect. All scientific research involving human participants needs to process the study protocol through an ethics review committee before starting data collection.

> **Contents of a Study Protocol**
> - Project title
> - Project summary
> - Project description:
>   - Background explaining need for study
>   - Study objectives
>   - Study methodology
>   - Data management and analysis plan
> - Ethical issues
> - References

For the undergraduate or postgraduate students (as part of dissertation) conducting research, the protocol may have to be processed through departmental or college level scientific and ethical review committee. Sometimes this protocol is referred to as *synopsis*.

For research that requires financial support, the proposal would need to be sent to the funding agency. This *research proposal* usually includes a study protocol, budget plan, and curriculum vitae of the study investigators and sanction letter from the ethics committee.

For clinical trials, the researcher team has to register the study protocol with the Clinical Trial Registry-India (http://ctri.nic.in/Clinicaltrials/login.php). The registry now encourages the researchers to register observational studies also.

### Collecting Data from the Study Sample

Having completed all the above steps, the researcher is now set to collect the data. If the data collection is done on paper, the collected data will have to be entered in a database later on.

### Analyzing Data

In quantitative research, we take help of the methods of statistics to analyze the data. Fortunately powerful statistical software are now available and is commonly used by researchers for statistical analyzes.

You will learn about statistics, an elaborate science in itself, in detail in this chapter. Sometimes we get caught up in the complexities of statistics. It is fine if you are not able to memorize the detailed steps of the statistical calculations. What is more important is to know the correct interpretation of those calculations. If something goes wrong in calculation, it can be corrected by the computer but if things go wrong in interpretation no computer or statistical program can correct it.

### Making Interpretation of the Results

Making interpretation of the findings is one of the most crucial steps in the research process. The preceding step of statistical analysis takes care of chance errors in interpretation of results. Taking care of the systematic errors (bias) is also equally important. It is here that the researcher applies wisdom to examine the results in its entirety and not in isolation. The thought process which goes in this step often finds a place in the discussion section of the research report or published article.

### Disseminating the Results to Stakeholders

The research process does not end at writing a research report. The findings of the study are commonly shared by researchers in form of a peer reviewed publication or presentation at a scientific conference. If the project involves receiving funding from an agency, a research report also needs to be shared with such an agency. When the research involves immediate policy implications, it should be shared with the policy makers. The research findings should also be shared with the study participants and public at large, since they are the beneficiaries of research.

With this background information on the steps to conduct research we are now ready to learn how to frame a research question.

## FIRST STEP: FRAMING A GOOD RESEARCH QUESTION

(*Garbage in = Garbage out—Anonymous*)
The impact of good research goes to improving clinical practice and health of the community. Hence, it is vital that the first step of research is done correctly.

### Converting a Research Topic into Answerable Research Question

A research question is the starting point of the entire research project. It provides a roadmap for implementing the study. Generally, the *study protocol* is written only after the investigator finalizes the research question.

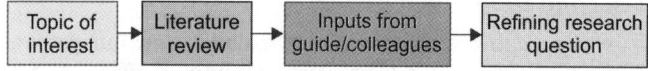

Any research usually starts with an idea or a topic of interest of the investigator. These ideas originate from clinical practice, teaching experience, meetings, journal articles, newspapers, talks with colleagues, and new technologies. The initial idea or topic is generally broad to start with. For example, the investigator is interested in addressing the issue of rising trend of heart disease in India. Heart disease is a very broad topic for research and the investigator, based on her interest, needs to choose a domain—screening, treatment or prognosis of heart diseases—in order to make the topic more specific.

Next step would be to search the existing literature for what is already known on the topic. Research usually being a team work; at the third step, the inputs from a guide or a colleague are valuable in making our scientific curiosity focused and relevant.

## Elements of a Research Question

There are two primary elements in a research question: the variable of interest and the population under study. In case of analytical research designs, there are two variables of interest: a predictor and an outcome variable.

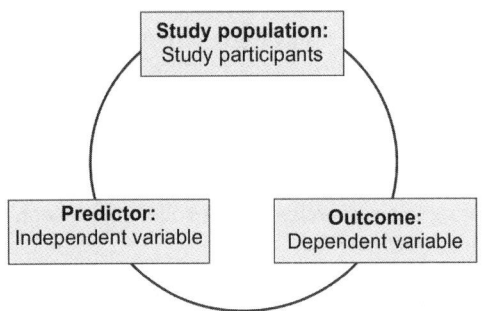

Predictor variable is the risk factor (in observational studies) or the intervention (in experimental studies), which has its effect on the outcome variable. In a clinical trial, it is the drug that is administered or the procedure that is performed.

The outcome variable is the effect (disease) caused by the predictor (risk factor) or the consequence of the intervention. In analytical studies, it is the disease caused by the risk factor, while in clinical trials, it is the effect of the drug administered or the result of the performed procedure.

The study population comprises of the research participants. It is the population to which the investigator wants to generalize the study findings to. Depending on the research topic, this can be children of a certain age, adults of a specific gender or a geriatric population with specific disease.

For analytical studies, putting together these three elements into a question form, a research question can be framed as: "Does the *predictor* cause the *outcome*, among the *study population*?" A research question should be phrased as a question; should be brief, clear, and focused. A few examples of analytical research questions are as follows:

- Does *brisk walking for at least 1 hour daily* reduce *fasting blood sugar level* among *adult type 2 diabetes mellitus patients*?
- Does *labetalol* decrease *blood pressure* as compared with *methyldopa* among *pregnant women with hypertension*? (*Note*: In clinical trials, it is prudent to add a comparator)
- Is *prenatal depression* associated with *infant mortality* among *pregnant women belonging to the low-income population*?
- Is *high-fat diet* associated with *development of dementia* among *adults older than 65 years*?

For descriptive studies measuring the prevalence of predictor variables (risk factors) or prevalence of outcome variables (disease), the research question would be slightly different in order to include two of the three elements described above. A few examples of descriptive research questions are as follows:

- What is the prevalence of high blood pressure [defined as systolic blood pressure (SBP) >120 or diastolic blood pressure >90 mm Hg] among adults above the age of 30 years residing in an urban slum?
- What is the prevalence of anemia [defined as hemoglobin (Hb) <12 g/dL] among adolescents between 10 years and 19 years of age residing in a village?

## Criteria for a Good Research Question

- Feasible
- Interesting
- Novel
- Ethical
- Relevant

For a research question to be useful, there are a few criteria defined in the form of an acronym: FINER. The FINER criteria stand for feasible, interesting, novel, ethical, and relevant.

**Feasible:** For all researchers, the research question selected should be manageable within their scope, time, expertise, and funds available.

**Interesting:** The research question should be interesting to colleagues and experts working in the research area as well as to the funding agency.

**Novel:** A key characteristic of any research is that it brings out findings that were otherwise not known.

**Ethical:** A research study is ethical when the risk of research is acceptable in relation to the likely benefits.

**Relevant:** It is important to do research on a topic that is relevant to the current times. This ensures that the findings will be useful.

## Framing Objectives of the Research

> **Note**
> Descriptive studies: "Estimate"
> Analytical studies: "Determine"

The objective/s of any research is/are translated from the research question itself. The difference is that the objectives are framed in scientific/epidemiologic terms making use of no more than one verb for each objective. Usually, the objectives are divided into primary (main) objective and secondary objectives (when applicable). The objectives differ according to the type of research questions: descriptive or analytical, and accordingly, the verb used will differ. In descriptive research questions, the prevalence of a risk factor or a disease is estimated. Therefore, the correct verb to be used is "estimate". In analytical studies, the association between a predictor and an outcome is to be determined. Therefore, the correct verb to be used is "determine". The objectives of the research should be SMART (specific, measurable, achievable, relevant, and time-bound).

For some of the research questions described above, the primary objectives can be framed as:

- To *determine* the effect of brisk walking for at least 1 hour daily on fasting blood sugar level of patients with adult type 2 diabetes mellitus.
- To *determine* the effect of labetalol on blood pressure of pregnant women with hypertension compared with methyldopa.
- To *determine* the effect of a high-fat diet on the development of dementia among adults older than 65 years.

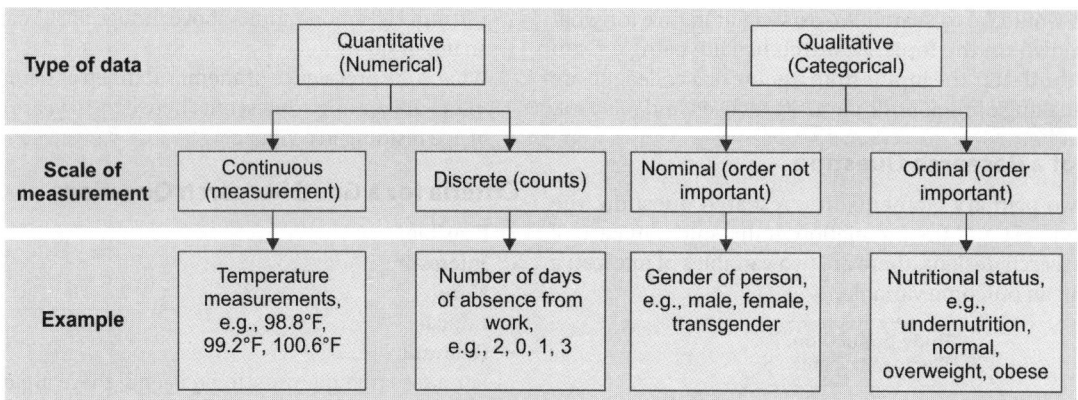

**Fig. 11.1:** Types of data and measurement scales.

- To *estimate* the prevalence of high blood pressure (defined as SBP >120 or diastolic blood pressure >90 mm Hg) among adults above the age of 30 years residing in an urban slum.
- To *estimate* the prevalence of anemia (defined as Hb <12 g/dL) among adolescents between 10 years and 19 years of age residing in a village.
- To *estimate* the prevalence of obesity [defined as body mass index (BMI) >25 kg/m$^2$] among patients who have had an episode of acute myocardial infarction in the last 1 year.

> **Note**
> **Applied aspect**
> A good research question passes the "FINER" criteria test and contains all the necessary elements of a research question.

## DEFINING STUDY VARIABLES

Variable of interest is one of the two primary elements in a research question.

| Concept | Example |
| --- | --- |
| Variable | Systolic blood pressure |
| Observational unit | The person whose blood pressure is measured |
| Observation | The value of measurement (e.g., 122 mm Hg) |

*Variable* is that attribute which varies. If we take Systolic Blood Pressure (SBP) as example, its value varies from person-to-person. The person on whom blood pressure is measured is an *observational unit*. The value of SBP measurement on a person is known as *observation*. Thus, we might have several observational units in our study each one of whom would give us an observation on our variable of interest. SBP is a variable whose value varies not only from person-to-person, but also from time-to-time within the same person. When we measure blood pressure of a person twice in a day we have two observations coming from the same observational unit. Such types of observations are called "paired observations". Later in this chapter we will explore the concept of paired observations in detail.

If there are 50 patients who participate in a research, each patient's weight would be different. Hence, patient's weight is a variable. Thus, we have information on weight of 50 patients participating in a research study. A collection of such values in kilogram is known as "data".

The data of a variable of interest is commonly collected in one of the two forms; quantitative and qualitative **(Fig. 11.1)**. (This is different from the quantitative and qualitative approaches for research that we discussed earlier in this chapter.)

### Qualitative (Categorical) Data

Gender of the patient (data collected from those participating in research) is qualitative data. Unlike quantitative data, gender cannot be measured on a numbered range. But, it is expressed as different categories such as males, females, transgender, etc. Thus, rather than numbers, qualitative data segregates people into different categories. The categorical data can be measured using two scales of measurement; nominal and ordinal. Data is said to be measured on an ordinal scale when the categories can be arranged in a meaningful order. For example, a patient's weight may be classified as normal, overweight or obese. Here order matters and hence it is said to be measured on an ordinal scale. Let us assume that we collect the data of patient's area of residence in categories such as urban, rural, and tribal. Here when the order is not important it is said to be measured on nominal scale. Thus, variables measured on nominal scale have no hierarchy. The choice of a statistical test to be applied will depend on whether the data is measured on nominal or ordinal scale. Qualitative data is summarized using proportions of people belonging to different categories.

### Quantitative (Numerical) Data

Systolic blood pressure of patients measured in mm Hg is an example of quantitative data. Here, blood pressure can take any value across a range of numbers such as 80–200 mm Hg. Depending on whether the quantitative data is measurements or counts; they are put on a continuous or discrete scale. Later, we will see that quantitative data is summarized using mean or median.

In certain situations, we may want to convert the quantitative data into qualitative data for ease of understanding. For example, data on SBP which is otherwise measured on a continuous scale (numerical data) may be converted to categories such as normal, high normal, and hypertension which is ordinal scale (categorical data). Such conversion makes it easy for us to understand the data.

## CHOOSING STUDY POPULATION

In real-life situations, the researcher does not have access to the whole population of interest. Thus the researcher ends up conducting study with only a small group of people. In this regards, let us understand three concepts: (1) reference population, (2) accessible population, and (3) study sample. Let us take the following research question: Does brisk walking for at least 1 hour daily reduce fasting blood sugar level among patients with adult type 2 diabetes mellitus? Here type 2 diabetes mellitus patients of the whole world could be our reference population. This means that if this research proves that walking exercise reduces blood sugar, this evidence would be possibly useful for all the type 2 diabetics of the world. However, in real life we do not have access to all type 2 diabetics of the world. (Spoiler alert: We will discover in the subsequent section that neither is it necessary to study all of them!). The researcher might have access to only those diabetic patients coming to her clinic. Such patients form what is known as a set of accessible population. Further, not entire accessible population would participate in research. For example, some of them might not be willing to start a walking exercise. Thus, only those patients actually enrolled in the study would form the study sample.

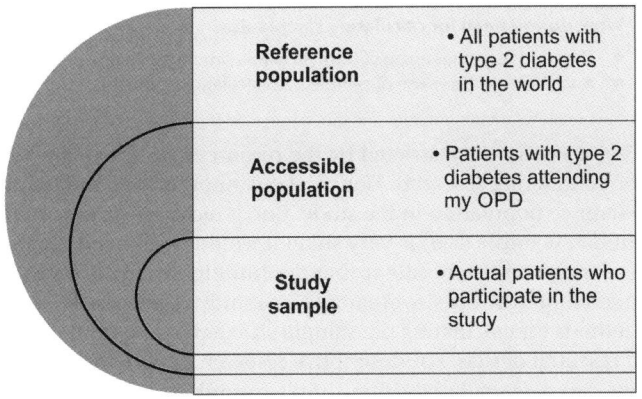

For each of following research questions identify which is the reference population.
- What is the prevalence of anemia among adolescents of a district X?
- What percentage of secondary schools are routinely procuring iron and folic acid supplements for their students in district X?
- What proportions of households in city Z are consuming green leafy vegetables at least thrice a week?

As you have observed in the first research question, all adolescents of the district are the reference population. In the second question, the secondary schools are reference population, while in the third question the households form a reference population. The population can consist of not only human beings but also hospitals, schools, or household, and many more such entities depending on the research question.

## Sampling

> **Note**
> **Key message**
> Probability sampling methods helps to ensure the sample is representative of the reference population.

To gain an idea of the next concept that we are going to cover let us visit a grocery shop. From your past experience of visiting a grocery shop, you would realize that the shopkeeper keeps a sample of different qualities of grains for our inspection. We make the buying decision based on our assessment of quality of the sample of grains. Imagine if the shopkeeper cheats and mixes half amount of poor quality grains to the lot you purchase from this shop. This means that the sample you were shown was not representative of the lot you received. For quantitative research, there are many reasons that makes the study sample not representative of the reference population. For the research question, estimating the prevalence of anemia among adolescents residing in a village, what if adolescents coming to our OPD are enrolled for the sake of convenience? In such scenario, our estimate of anemia prevalence might be falsely high since adolescents coming to OPD are more likely to be anemic. Thus, we will falsely overestimate the anemia prevalence.

When the sample is representative of the reference population, the researchers would be confident that the findings also apply to whole reference population. Fortunately there are methods available to ensure that the sample we choose is representative of the reference population. Such methods are known as probability sampling methods.

### Probability Sampling Methods

In probability sampling methods, every unit of the accessible population has a known probability of being selected. We briefly describe different probability sampling methods below.

### Simple Random Sampling

Theoretically, this is the simplest method. The logic behind all type of random sampling methods is to eliminate the human

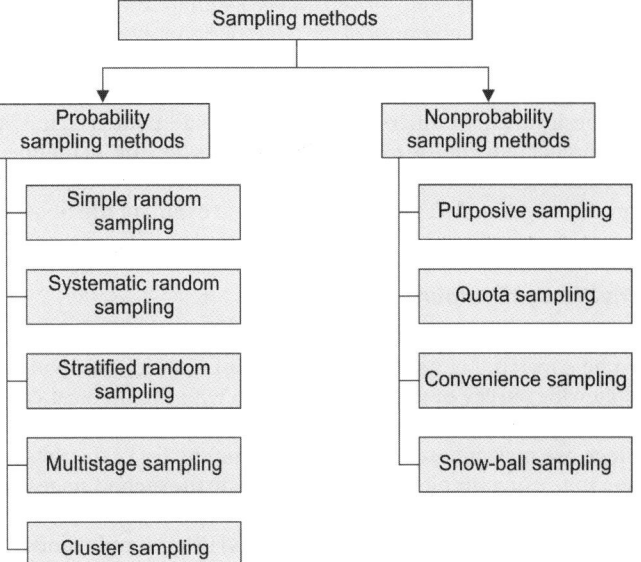

choice from selecting study participants. If human choice is allowed, there are chances that some bias would make the study sample non-representative of the population. In simple random sampling, we eliminate this human selection by making use of a computer program or random number tables to select which numbers from the list get selected in sample. A prerequisite for using this method is that a complete enumeration list of all members of the set of accessible population should be available. This is sometimes difficult. Imagine conducting the study of effect of walking on fasting blood sugar among diabetics. If accessible population patients coming to our OPD we may not be sure who will come for OPD visit on a particular day. Thus, it becomes difficult to implement this method when we do not have a list of entire accessible population.

### Systematic Random Sampling

In this method, the name-wise enumeration of all the people of accessible population is not needed; a count of the accessible population is sufficient. Suppose we denote the required number of people in our study sample as "n". If we divide the number of people in accessible population by n, what we get is a sampling interval commonly denoted as "k". Suppose for our study on prevalence of hypertension among adults above 30 years of age in an urban slum, we estimate that there are 100 households in the slum. Let us assume that the number of households required to be enrolled as study sample is 20. The calculation would be as follows: size of accessible population/size of study sample = k. Substituting the numbers, we get: 100/20 = 5. We take every kth (every 5th in this example) household in our study sample. We select the first unit in our study sample by generating a random number between 1 and k. In this case, if that random number comes out to be 4, the first unit in our sample will be house no. 4 and then every fifth house will be taken in study sample till we reach the last (20th) unit of study sample which will be 99th house in this slum. Advantage of this method is that it uniformly covers all parts of accessible population.

### Stratified Random Sampling

At times, we may want to separately estimate the variable of interest in some subgroups of the reference population. If we are conducting a research on estimating the prevalence of obesity among patients having acute myocardial infarction, prevalence of obesity might be different in male and female patients. Thus, a researcher may choose to stratify the patients into the two gender groups and then select the study sample from each of these two groups separately. This will enable us to estimate the obesity prevalence separately among the patients of both the genders.

### Multistage Sampling

This method is useful in situations where a large population is to be covered. Let us take an example of research involving a statewide survey of patient satisfaction with the medical care received from government primary health centers. For the first stage, we may choose some districts from the list of districts in the state using simple random sampling. In the second stage, we choose primary health centers from the list of all primary health centers (for each of the selected districts) using simple random sampling. This method adds convenience, since field visits for taking patient interviews need to be conducted in selected districts only.

### Cluster Sampling

This is another popular method used in field research, when reference population is aggregated in naturally occurring clusters such as villages. In simple cluster sampling, 30 clusters are selected using simple random sampling from the list of all clusters. For example, if a district X has 300 villages 30 villages will be selected using simple random sampling. In the next stage, the study sample will be selected from each of these clusters. The advantage of cluster sampling is that the list of accessible population is not needed, but the list of only the clusters is enough. Less travel is required since fixed (e.g., 30) number of clusters are to be visited. This method is commonly used to study the immunization coverage of particular area.

## Nonprobability Sampling Methods

There are other methods which are known as nonprobability samples. Here, the probability of being selected is not known for the members of accessible population. These methods are used more frequently in qualitative research as we will discuss in later part of this chapter.

## Adequacy of the Study Sample: Sample Size

> **Note**
> **What do you need for calculating sample size?**
> - Descriptive studies—use of formula with a simple calculator
> - Analytical studies—use of sample size calculation software.

The researcher is restricted by the resources and time she has for conducting research. Hence, she cannot include the entire reference population in the study. But, if the number of people studied (sample size) is very small it would be difficult for the researcher to be confident that the findings are true. So how much should be the size of sample for a study? There are different methods for calculating the sample size depending on the type of research design. For descriptive research design, the sample size can be calculated using simple formula with a paper and pen. For analytical research designs the formula for calculating the sample size are a little complex and hence we use computer programs to calculate the sample size for such analytical studies. We discuss here both the methods one by one.

### Sample Size for Descriptive Studies

The first task in calculating sample size for descriptive studies is to determine if the variable of interest is measured on quantitative or qualitative scale.

*Calculating sample size when variable is qualitative:*

$$n = \frac{Z^2 pq}{L^2}$$

Here,
- n = sample size
- Z = confidence level
- p = proportion of variable of interest (%)

- q = compliment of p, [1-p] (%)
- L = allowable error on either side of the estimated 'p'.

| Confidence level | Z score |
|---|---|
| 80% | 1.28 |
| 90% | 1.64 |
| 95% | 1.96 |
| 98% | 2.32 |
| 99% | 2.57 |

Let us take an example. In an earlier research, the researcher wanted to estimate prevalence of anemia among the adolescent boys residing in a district. Based on literature review, suppose the prevalence of anemia is reported to be around 30% among adolescent boys (p = 30). We decide that we want to detect anemia prevalence in this district with precision of 5% on either side of the expected prevalence (L = 5). As researchers we want to be 95% confident about our results so we keep the confidence level at 95%.

The corresponding Z value is 1.96 (Z = 1.96). We will learn more about Z later in this chapter. Now replacing the numbers in formula we get the following result.

$$n = \frac{Z^2 pq}{L^2} = \frac{(1.96)^2 \times (30) \times (70)}{5^2} = \frac{3.84 \times 2100}{25} = 322.5 = 323$$

Thus, we need to enroll 323 adolescent boys from the district to be able to estimate the anemia prevalence with 95% confidence level and 5% precision on either side of the estimated prevalence. Here, we assume that the sample will be chosen using simple random sampling.

What does allowable error at 5% on either side of p actually mean? It means that if the prevalence of anemia among adolescent boys in this study comes at 32% then the true prevalence of anemia among adolescent boys in this district is likely to be in the range of 32 ± 5, i.e., anywhere between 27% and 37%. 95% confidence level means that if this study were to be repeated 100 times, for 95 of such studies the sample mean would be in the range of 27 to 37%. Now, let us try calculating sample size while changing the allowable error.

$$n = \frac{Z^2 pq}{L^2} = \frac{(1.96)^2 \times (30) \times (70)}{3^2} = \frac{3.84 \times 2100}{9} = 896$$

$$n = \frac{Z^2 pq}{L^2} = \frac{(1.96)^2 \times (30) \times (70)}{7^2} = \frac{3.84 \times 2100}{49} = 164.6 \approx 165$$

$$n = \frac{Z^2 pq}{L^2} = \frac{(1.96)^2 \times (30) \times (70)}{20^2} = \frac{3.84 \times 2100}{400} = 20.1 \approx 20$$

You will observe that as we try to become more precise in our estimate (keeping L small) the required sample size increases. Inversely, if we relax our allowable error, the required sample size would decrease. We saw in this last example that by increasing allowable error we can complete the research by studying a sample as small as 20 participants. But the drawback of such a choice would be that the estimate of true prevalence will be very wide, i.e., if prevalence of anemia in the study sample is 30%, the true prevalence in the district could be anywhere from 10% to 50%. Such a wide range of the estimated prevalence of anemia for the district is practically unusable for any policymaker. The allowable error chosen for a study has to be small enough to give a reasonably precise estimate and large enough that it is feasible for the researcher to collect data within the limited resources.

**Sample size when variable is quantitative**

$$n = \frac{Z^2 \sigma^2}{L^2}$$

Here,
- n = sample size
- Z = confidence level
- σ = standard deviation (SD)
- L = allowable error on either side of the estimated mean

Let us take a hypothetical study which aims to estimate the SBP of adults in an urban slum. At 95% confidence level, Z = 1.96. We can find out the estimated mean and SD of SBP among adults from previous similar published studies or through a small pilot study. Suppose, a previous study from another city reports the mean SBP among adults at 120 mm Hg with a SD of 15 mm Hg. Let us keep the allowable error at 2 points on either side of the estimated mean. What do these 2 points on either side of the mean signify? It means that, if at the end of our study the mean SBP in our study sample came out to be 124 mm Hg, the true mean SBP of the adults of urban slums of this city would be anywhere from 122 to 126 mm Hg.

We have Z = 1.96, σ = 15, and L = 2.

$$n = \frac{Z^2 \sigma^2}{L^2} = \frac{(1.96)^2 \times (15)^2}{2^2} = \frac{3.84 \times 225}{4} = 216$$

With a SD of 15 mm Hg and keeping an allowable error of 2 points on either side of mean, the calculated sample size for estimating the mean SBP of adults of urban slums of this city comes at 216 at 95% level of confidence. As we tried altering the allowable error for qualitative variable, here also we can alter the allowable error.

### Choosing Sample Size for Analytical Studies

> **Note**
> Keep the following handy before using softwares for sample size for analytical studies:
> - Scale of measurement for the variable of interest
> - Magnitude of difference in variable
> - Acceptable level of α and β errors

Since the formulae for calculation of sample size for analytical studies are complex ones, we make use of computer programs. OpenEpi is one such free to use online tool that helps in calculating the sample size. Demonstration of sample size calculation with use of software is beyond the scope of this book. However, a list of broad parameters to keep handy to feed in the sample size calculating software is provided in the box here.

## DATA COLLECTION: SOURCES, METHODS, AND TOOLS

Once the study variables and study population are defined, the researcher has to plan how the collected data will be managed. This has to be decided before the actual data collection starts. The following are the steps in management of collected data:

- Defining the source of data
- Defining data collection method
- Developing data collection tool
- Developing data documentation sheet
- Developing dummy tables for analysis
- Data collection process
- Data entry
- Data analysis

## Sources of Data

The source of data for a research study can be primary or secondary. **Primary data** is when the researcher collects the data afresh for the specific purpose of the research study. **Secondary data** is one which is already collected for some other purpose which the researcher uses for her study. Commonly, researchers can use the data available from the census, national sample surveys such as National Family Health Survey (NFHS), data from the national health program records, hospital records, etc. The advantage with primary data is that it is more reliable since the researcher clearly defines the variables under study and data collection method. In our country, there are ample amount of clinical records generated by the hospitals. There lies a great opportunity in making use of this data to generate meaningful evidence. As we have already started moving towards digitization (electronic health records) in India, it will also be a very good source of data for research purpose in the days to come.

## Data Collection Methods

### Interviews

Interviews are nothing but a one-to-one verbal dialog with the respondent for collecting data required for the study. Interviews can be face-to-face or telephonic. An interview guide is a document containing instructions for the interviewer and a list of questions with space for recording answers. The questions and answers are made available in the language that the respondent understands.

### Questionnaires

A questionnaire is an especially designed set of questions which the respondent herself/himself is expected to answer. Traditionally, questionnaires were made available to the respondent on paper. Nowadays electronic questionnaires are becoming popular. Researchers can use the generic survey tools such as Google forms (www.forms.google.com) and Survey Monkey (www.surveymonkey.com) or especially designed tools such as EpiCollect (www.five.epicollect.net). Questionnaire has a limitation that it can be used only when the respondents are able to read/write.

### Observation/Examination/Investigations

Health research often involves collecting data on biological variables through patient examination by doctors or healthcare professionals. Sometimes, the variable under study may require laboratory investigations or radiological investigations. Whenever such measurements are used it would be important to pay attention to the accuracy of measurement.

## Data Collection Tool

Whatever be the method of data collection, a researcher will always need a data collection tool. This is nothing but a set of variables on which the data will need to be collected. A questionnaire is a commonly used data collection tool.

### Anatomy of a Questionnaire

A questionnaire is the heart of the research study. It commonly contains the following elements.

- **Title** of the study and name and contact details of the investigator.
- A paragraph on **background information:** This will include the purpose of the study, an indication of what kind of information is being sought, and approximate duration it will take to complete the questionnaire.
- **Directions for answering:** Directions can be of two types. General directions for answering can be put at the start of the questionnaire. Directions for specific questions can be put at the start of that particular set of questions.

---

**A sample Questionnaire on tobacco usage survey among adults attending OPD**

**XYZ Hospital**

Principal investigator of study: Dr ABC, Contact No XXXXX XXXXX Dear respondent,

We have planned this survey to gather information about the usage of tobacco among the people attending the OPD of this hospital. The purpose of this survey is to devise plans to help the tobacco users. The survey will take 2 minutes of your time.

Directions: Please fill the answers with a pen. Where applicable put a tick (√) mark within the available box to indicate the choice of your response.
1. Your age in years
2. Your gender is
    a. Male ☐
    b. Female ☐
    c. Other ☐
3. You are educated up to
    a. Primary schooling ☐
    b. Secondary/higher secondary schooling ☐
    c. Graduation/Postgraduation completed ☐
    d. Beyond postgraduation ☐
4. Did you smoke tobacco in any form in last 30 days?
    a. Yes ☐
    b. No ☐           [Go to question 7]
    c. Do not want to answer ☐           [Go to question 7]
5. Number of beedi or cigarettes smoked per day
6. Since how many years are you smoking
7. Would you or any of your known people like to use services of a tobacco cessation clinic if we start one?
    a. Yes ☐
    b. No ☐
    c. Do not want to answer ☐

Thank you for completing the survey!

---

- **Set of questions:** This is the list of questions with space for recording answers organized in a logical order. This set of questions would be primarily covering information related to predictor, outcome, and confounding variables as well as some background information of the study participants. Two type of questions commonly used in questionnaires are:

Table 11.2: Sample data documentation sheet for a tobacco usage survey among adults.

| Sl. No. | Question | Measurement scale<br>• Nominal<br>• Ordinal<br>• Numerical | Possible answers/answer range (including assigned codes if any) | Comments (skip/jumps) | Plan for summarization<br>• Mean + SD<br>• Median + IQR<br>• Percent |
|---|---|---|---|---|---|
| 1. | Age | Numerical | 18–99 | | Mean + SD |
| 2. | Gender | Nominal | • Male<br>• Female | | Proportion |
| 3. | Education of respondent | Ordinal | • Primary schooling<br>• Secondary/higher secondary schooling<br>• Graduation/Postgraduation completed<br>• Beyond postgraduation | | Proportion |
| 4. | Did you smoke tobacco in any form in last 30 days? | Nominal | • No<br>• Yes<br>• No answer | If Yes go to Q. No. 5; otherwise go to Q. No. 7 | Proportion |
| 5. | Beedi/cigarette smoked per day | Numerical | 1–50 | | Mean + SD/median + IQR |
| 6. | Since how many years smoking | Numerical | 0–99 | | Mean + SD/median + IQR |
| 7. | Would you like to use services of a tobacco cessation clinic if we start one? | Nominal | • No<br>• Yes<br>• Cannot say | | Proportion |

(IQR: interquartile range; SD: standard deviation)

- **Open-ended questions:** These are questions where the scope of answering is kept open for the respondent to decide. Here the respondent is given freedom of length to provide an answer. Take example of this question:
  ♦ "What causes your psoriasis skin rashes to flare up?"
  _____
  _____
  _____

- **Close-ended questions:** Here options available for the respondent when answering this question are limited. The example we used for open-ended question can be converted to a close-ended question like this:
  ♦ "From the list of following options please choose what causes your psoriasis skin rashes to flare up. [Tick all that apply]
    i. Winter ☐
    ii. Stress ☐
    iii. Alcohol ☐
    iv. Smoking ☐
    v. Drugs ☐
    vi. Pregnancy ☐
    vii. Others ☐
  In quantitative research questionnaires, most questions are close ended questions.

- **Ending note:** A questionnaire should not end abruptly. A thank you note to the respondent is a good way of ending a questionnaire.

## Data Documentation Sheet

The purpose of the study tool is to collect the required data on the variables under the study. To make our questionnaire focused and analysis-ready we need to prepare a plan for data management. This plan is referred to as data documentation sheet. We present here a sample data documentation sheet for a tobacco usage survey among adult OPD attendees of a primary health center **(Table 11.2)**.

We observe in this sample sheet that for each of the variable, it is important to define the measurement scale. The sheet also helps in deciding in advance the *possible answers* and the proposed methods for summarizing or analysis. While using paper-based forms with large samples, it is advisable to use codes for each possible answers (*codes* are the numbers you see against the option categories in **Table 11.2**). This makes the job of data entry easier and more efficient.

Once the data documentation sheet is ready it would be possible to prepare *dummy tables* for analysis. Dummy tables are nothing but a framework of how the analyzed data will be summarized, what statistical tests will be applied, and how they will be presented. Preparing dummy tables is a good practice in quantitative research. Once this is done, the researcher is ready to *collect data* for the study.

### Data Entry Tools

When data is collected on paper-based questionnaire it will have to be entered in a database file on the computer. When data is collected through the electronic means the data entry step is skipped since the data is directly available in a database. The data capture features of tools such as EpiInfo™, Microsoft Access or EpiData Manager provide a range of options to add checks on what can be entered in a field for a particular question. This helps in minimizing the data entry errors.

> **Note**
> **Commonly used data entry tools**
> • Microsoft Excel spreadsheet
> • EpiInfo™
> • Microsoft Access
> • EpiData Manager

### Data Analysis and Interpretation

Summarizing and analyzing the data using statistical tools is the step of data analysis. These will be discussed in detail in subsequent sections of this chapter. However, the process of data analysis is not limited to statistical processing through software. When we summarize the data and make use of relevant statistical tests, we convert the data into usable information. But this information is not sufficient. When we use the technical knowledge of the relevant field of research topic and apply clinical wisdom to make meaningful inference out of this information, it is known as intelligence. In the chapter on epidemiologic methods, you learned about the difference between association and causation; that all associations that we observe when we plot data in a 2 × 2 table may not necessarily be causation. Multiple errors can possibly influence our data. You also learned about these errors in the section that dealt with bias (systematic error). When we apply our wisdom to identify such possible errors and interpret the results in this context, we convert the information into intelligence or evidence.

It is very difficult to understand such raw data. So, if the same values are presented in a simple tabular form as given below it becomes easy to understand.

| Hemoglobin (g/dL) | No. of patients |
|---|---|
| 9–9.9 | 3 |
| 10–10.9 | 4 |
| 11–11.9 | 4 |
| 12–12.9 | 5 |
| 13–13.9 | 2 |
| 14–14.9 | 1 |
| 15–15.9 | 1 |
| Total | 20 |

### Methods of Data Presentation

Data can be presented in three different forms as described in **Flowchart 11.1**.

### Text

It is not always necessary to have a table or diagram to represent the data. Sometimes, even a simple sentence in the text is sufficient to present essence of the data. For example, the temperature in ice-lined refrigerator for five primary health centers is as given in table below:

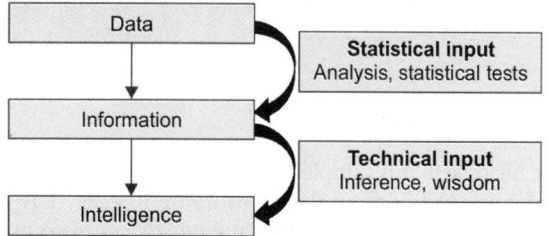

## PRESENTATION OF DATA

### Importance of Data Presentation

It is important to summarize the data to give clear message from the results of the research study. So, data should be presented in a simple form to make it easy for the readers to understand. It should be concise without losing the important information and need few words to explain. Overcomplicated presentation is often ignored by the readers.

For example, Hb measurements (g/dL) of 20 patients of a research study are as below:

9.0, 11.3, 10.6, 11.8, 13.2, 9.2, 11.6, 10.8, 12.4, 14.7, 12.2, 11.5, 12.1, 12.4, 10.7, 13.1, 15.0, 12.4, 10.5, 9.6.

| Primary health center (PHC) | Temperature in ice-lined refrigerator (°C) |
|---|---|
| PHC 1 | 4 |
| PHC 2 | 5 |
| PHC 3 | 3 |
| PHC 4 | 5 |
| PHC 5 | 4 |

This data can be presented in simple text, "the temperature in the ice-lined refrigerator of all five primary health centers was in the range from 3 to 5°C". It is not necessary to have a separate table for such study findings.

**Flowchart 11.1:** Methods of data presentation.

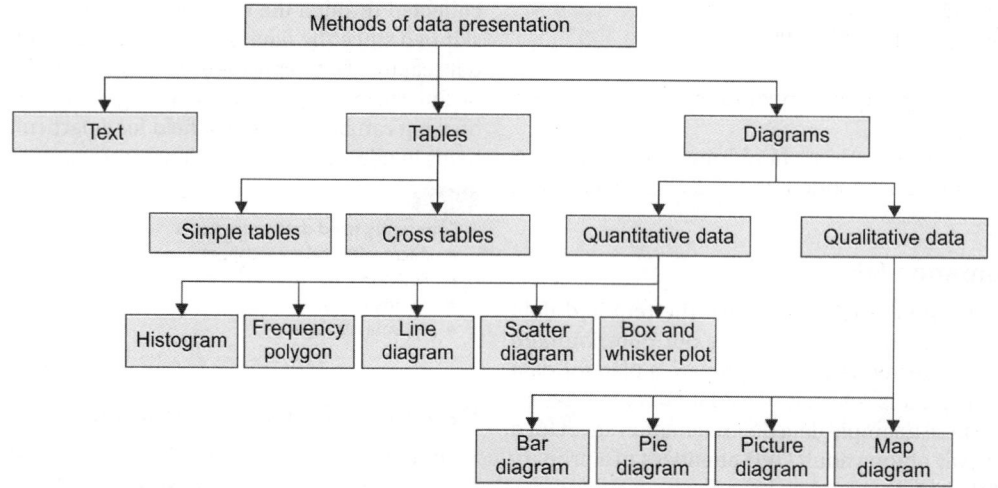

## Table

It is a basic form of data presentation. A table should have following components to be able to give a complete picture: table title, column titles, table body (data), and footnotes. For instance, hypothetical example of a table on clinical profile of dengue patients is given below:

Clinical profile of dengue patients admitted in a hospital, 2017 (N = 50) → Table title

| Clinical variables | Frequency | Percentage |
|---|---|---|
| Fever | 45 | 90 |
| Rash | 20 | 40 |
| Vomiting | 10 | 20 |
| Headache | 8 | 16 |
| Bleeding tendency* | 4 | 8 |

*Bleeding from nose or ear or hematemesis or melena → Footnote

Column title → (Frequency, Percentage); Table body → (data rows)

Table title should be clear and stand-alone. It should mention time, place, and person details of the data it contains. Every column of the table should have a title. Table body includes data or text. Short forms should be avoided in a table. Conventionally, data is usually presented to the precision of only one digit after decimal, unless more precise information is needed in a specific table. As shown in the example, when arranging the categories in order, try to follow descending or ascending order of frequency of the data to highlight the common findings of the study. Footnotes are used to give that additional information related to data which is difficult to incorporate in the table body.

Depending on the complexity involved, the tables can be simple table or cross table.

***Simple table:*** This is also known as frequency table. A simple table can be used to present qualitative as well as quantitative data.

**Simple table presenting qualitative data:** The above mentioned example of clinical profile of dengue patients is an example of such table. The clinical profile is presented in the form of categories of symptoms. In such tables usually the first column lists the categories. The second column gives frequency against each category.

**Simple table presenting quantitative data:** The example at the start of this section providing the Hb values of 20 patients in a tabular form is an example of such a table. Here the range of possible Hb values is divided into different categories in the first column. The second column gives frequency against each category.

While preparing such a table, it is advised to keep the number of categories in the range of four to eight. More than eight categories make it complex for the reader to understand data.

We observe here that each category covers a range of 1 g%. This is known as class interval. To decide the class interval, we find out the maximum and minimum values in our data set. In this given data set maximum Hb is 15 g% while minimum is 9 g%. We calculate the range using formula: maximum value – minimum value. Thus, here 15 – 9 = 6. The range divided by desired number of classes gives the class interval. In this case, 6/6 = 1. This is how we decided that each class will cover 1 g%. The first class chosen is one which covers the minimum value.

**Table 11.3:** Relationship between obesity and depression among adolescent boys of XYZ school.

| | Depression | No depression | Total |
|---|---|---|---|
| Obese | 5 | 25 | 30 |
| Non-obese | 10 | 60 | 70 |
| Total | 15 | 85 | 100 |

If we take example of the first class the value 9 is known as lower limit of the class and 9.9 as upper limit of the class.

**Tips while preparing table:**

- Avoid overlapping classes: In the example of the table on Hb values, if the first class was defined as 9–10 and second class as 10–11, there would be confusion about where to put a person whose Hb value is exactly at 10 g%. Hence, we prefer to keep first class as 9–9.9 and second class as 10–10.9.
- Last class can be kept open ended: Suppose we are presenting the data of age of persons segregated in 5 years class intervals. Now, it is likely that there are very few people in the age categories beyond 70 years of age. In such case, we can club all 5-year categories beyond 70 years age and label the last class as ">70". Such class is known as an open-ended class.

***Cross table:*** A cross table is used when we want to compare two or more different groups or want to see association between two variables. The simplest form of a cross table is a 2 × 2 table. The following 2 × 2 table contains first variable (obesity) split into two categories occupying two rows and second variable (depression) split into two categories occupying two columns **(Table 11.3)**.

## Diagram/Graph

It is a visual form of data presentation. The advantage is that it gives a quick picture of the data. Similar to table construction, diagram should also have components such as title, X-axis, label to X-axis, Y-axis, label to Y-axis, key to symbols, and footnotes.

For example, the immunization coverage of different states in India, 2017 (as per NFHS-4 survey) is given below.

**Immunization coverage* of different states in Western India, 2017**

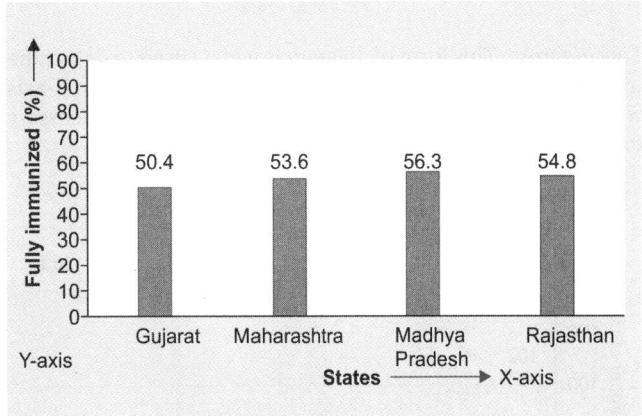

*Source*: National Family Health Survey-4 Data.

Diagrams can be prepared easily in a computer using Microsoft Excel program. Choice of type of diagram depends on the type of data as shown below.

## Quantitative

*Histogram:* Frequency distribution of continuous variables like age, height, weight, and Hb can be presented using a histogram. Variable is represented on X-axis while frequency is plotted on Y-axis. The frequency of each group/range will construct a column graph without the spaces between columns. It is also known as an area diagram since the area of the column varies with the frequency.

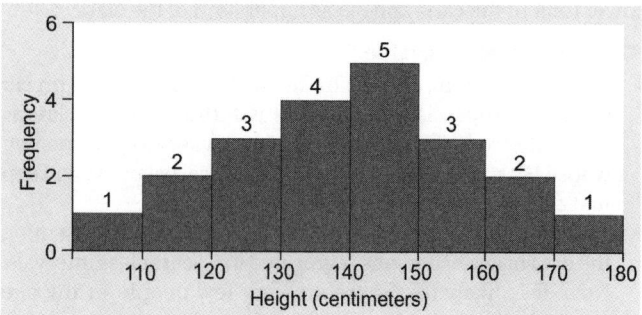

*Frequency polygon:* Frequency polygons are analogous to line graphs, and just as line graphs make continuous data visually easy to interpret. They can be used to graph large data sets with data points that repeat. The literal meaning of polygon is figure with many (poly) angles (gon). It is developed over histogram. When the midpoints of the class interval of the variables are joined together at the height of their frequencies by straight lines, a frequency polygon is developed.

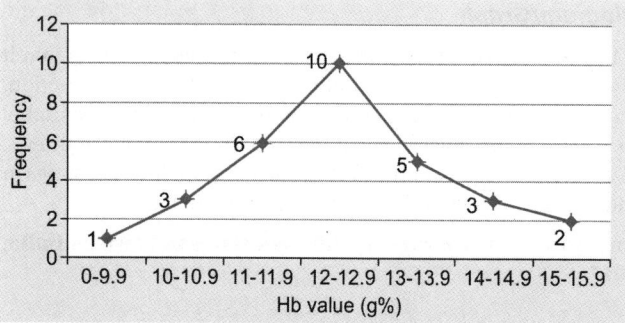

*Line diagram:* This form of diagram is widely used to depict the trend of an event over a period of time. Time is shown on X-axis while frequency of variable is shown on Y-axis. It is not necessary to start with zero on the Y-axis.

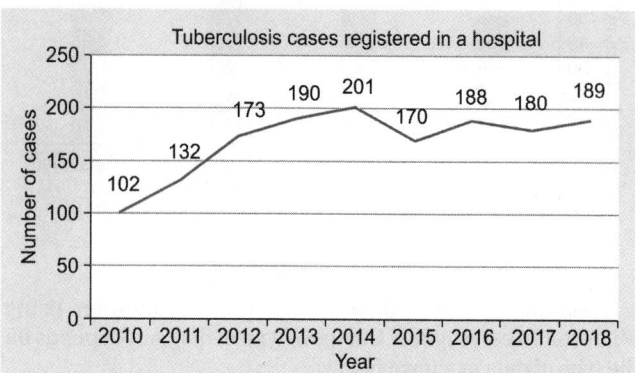

*Scatter/dot diagram:* This type of figure is used when we want to show the relationship between two quantitative variables. It is used to show the correlation between two variables like age and weight, so it is also known as correlation diagram. Perpendicular lines are drawn for relationship between two variables and the point at which those lines would meet is represented by a dot. The different frequencies of the variables would give many such dots, which is a scatter. Finally, a line is drawn to show the type of correlation at one glance.

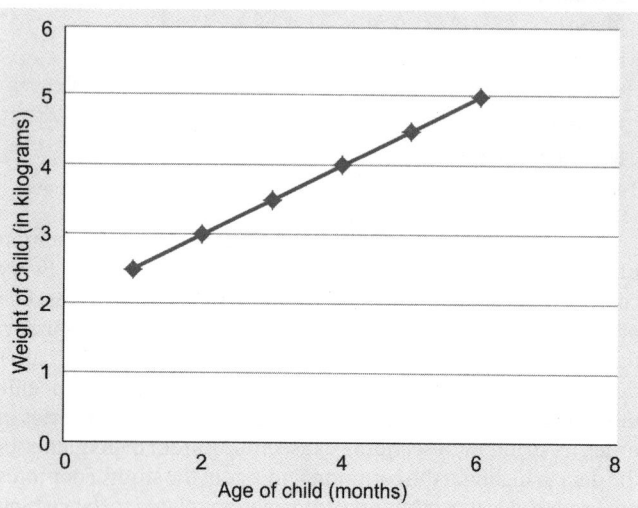

*Box and whisker diagram:* When numerical data is to be compared between two groups, a box and whisker chart is preferred over a histogram. The middle line inside the box is median, the ends of box are 1st and 3rd quartiles, and ends of whiskers are minimum and maximum values in data range. Sometimes, data not included between the whiskers is plotted as an outlier with dots.

For example, the box and whisker diagram below shows the distribution of BMI among male and female patients.

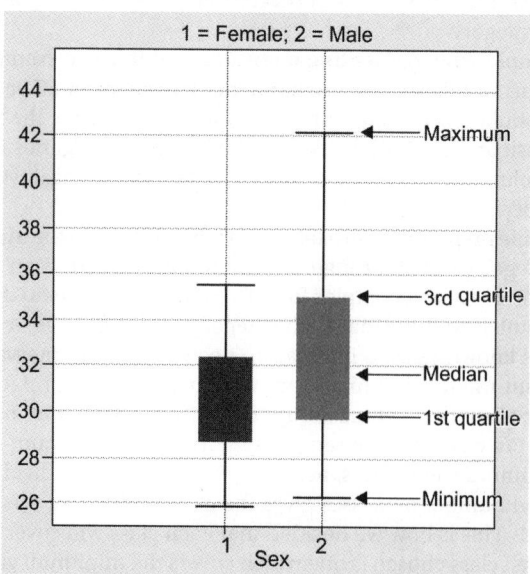

## Qualitative

*Bar diagram:* Bars can be drawn horizontal or vertical. Length of bar is proportional to the frequency of the variable. Width of each bar is same. Distance between two bars is at least half the width of the bar. There are three types of bar diagrams: simple, multiple, and component bar diagram.

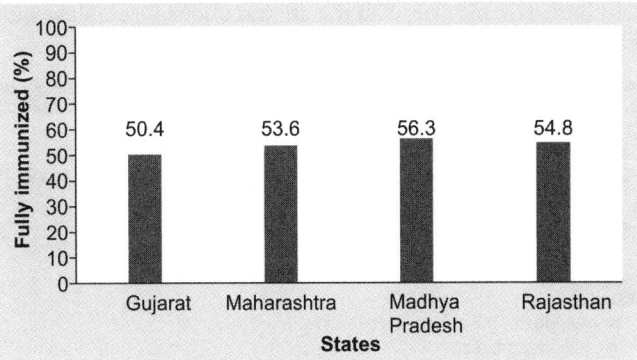

1. *Simple bar diagram:* As shown above, coverage of children fully immunized in different states of India is compared according to NFHS-4 data.
2. *Multiple bar diagram:* Multiple bars can be drawn within the same category. For example, comparison of coverage of fully immunized children as per NFHS-3 and NFHS-4 for selected states of India is shown in the multiple bar diagram.

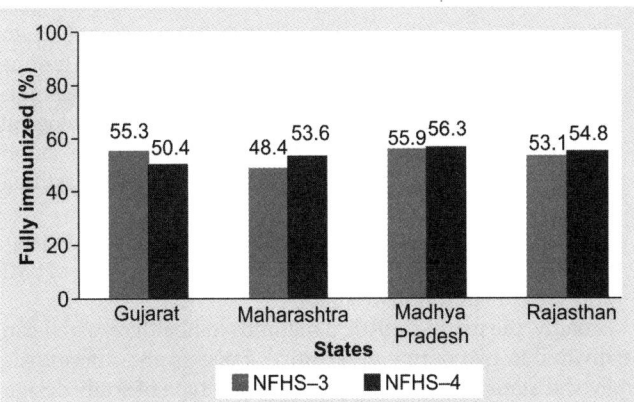

3. *Component bar diagram:* It is also known as proportional bar diagram. Total height of bar indicates the frequency of the category. Subcategories within these categories can be shown by splitting the height of the bar into different colored components. This bar diagram is used when we want to focus on the relative proportion of subcategories out of the total frequency.

For example, average number of patients per day in various OPDs of the hospital is shown in component bar diagram above.

First bar indicates on an average 100 patients per day attends medicine OPD, out of which the proportion of males and females is 60 and 40, respectively.

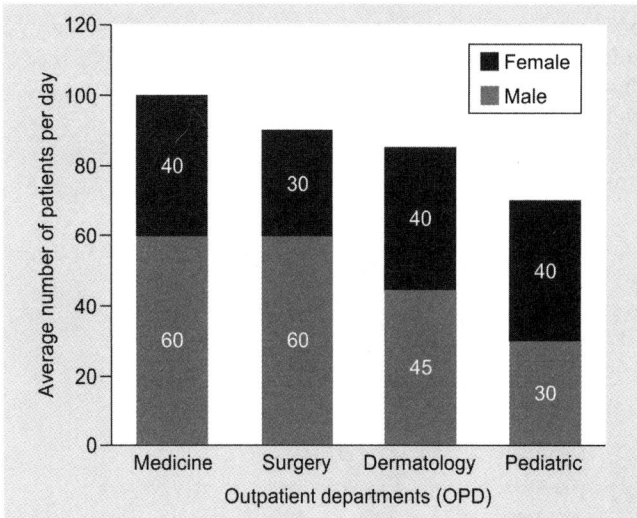

*Pie diagram:* Qualitative data can also be presented by pie chart. It is commonly used to present causes of morbidity or mortality in a population. The frequency of each group is shown in a circle, depicted by the degrees of the angle. The group with more frequency will have more degrees of angle. Each angle size is calculated by dividing the class frequency with total observations and then multiplying with 360°. It can be easily prepared in the Microsoft Excel worksheet without manual calculations of such degrees for angle size.

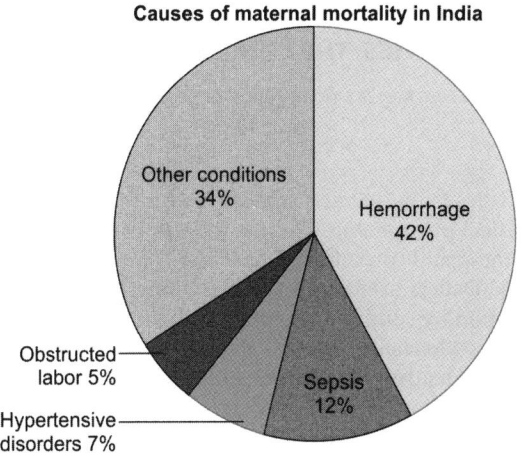

*Map diagram:* Such diagram is prepared to show geographical distribution of frequencies of some characteristic. Some symbols or colors in the map denote the frequency of the characteristic. For example, state-wise estimation of new HIV infections in India during 2015 is shown in the map below using different colors.

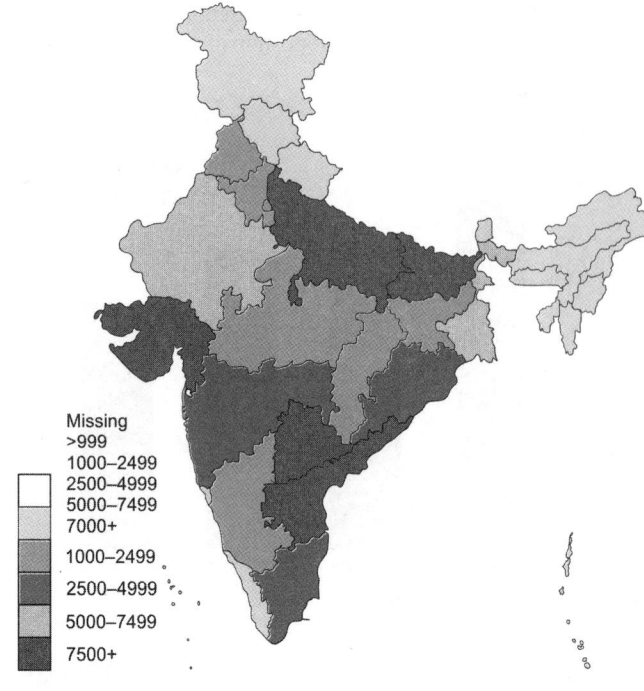

**Note**

**Some practical tips to consider while preparing a table/figure:**
- Anatomy—include all parts of the table/figure
- Keep it as simple as possible
- Easy to understand
- Keep axis units and intervals appropriate
- Avoid using dark colors
- Avoid making 3-dimensional figures

## BIOSTATISTICS: THE CONCEPT

*"It is the mark of a truly intelligent person to be moved by statistics"*

—GB Shaw

Biostatistics is the science of dealing with numbers related to biomedical phenomena. These numbers, when put into a set of columns and rows, form a "dataset" or simply referred to as "data". Data is useful only when it is inferred in the form of information by counting, dividing, and comparing (CDC) the numbers, which helps in decision making.

Usage of statistical methods and their interpretation have guided important health policies worldwide **(Box 11.1)**. A health professional also deals with numbers in daily practice. A large part of this chapter deals with the usage of biostatistics in health research. Apart from health research, biostatistics is also useful on day-to-day basis for management of medical practice as well as community health programs. Both the medical practice and community health programs generate a lot of data on routine basis. Health professionals are expected to analyze and interpret these data to make a meaning and data-informed decisions periodically. For example, a health professional in charge of a large hospital would be interested in knowing the average bed-occupancy rate of different departments or average length of stay for different diseases in his hospital. A doctor running a clinic would be interested in monitoring the stock of medicines in pharmacy or finding out the average waiting period for patients in OPD. In community health programs, one would be interested to monitor the monthly blood examination rate for malaria program or monitor the quarterly treatment outcome for tuberculosis. Thus, every doctor/healthcare professional need to familiarize themselves with the art and science of dealing with data.

**Box 11.1: History of achievements due to biostatistics.**
- Safety and efficacy of life-saving vaccines
- Statistics on use of seat belts led to Motor Vehicle Safety Act
- Framingham heart study: Well-designed statistical study established major risk factors for heart diseases
- Statistical evidence led to tobacco control laws

**Note**

Knowledge of biostatistics is useful in:
- Medical practice
- Community health practice
- Research

## Application of Biostatistics in Health Research

The science of biostatistics has manifold applications in health research, as below:

- To *describe* the biological characteristics/health outcomes (e.g., proportion of patients of a hospital suffering from hypertension)
- To find the *significance of differences* in values of biological characteristics/health outcomes between two groups (e.g., to compare the mean number of hours of exercise in two groups of patients with normal cholesterol and elevated cholesterol)
- To know the *association/relationship* between two biological characteristics/health outcomes (e.g., to know the association between family history of allergy and development of asthma among children)
- To *predict* the biological characteristics/health outcomes (e.g., to predict the value of blood pressure for a given value of BMI and salt consumption in a day).

Broadly, the use of statistical methods in health research can be divided in two parts—descriptive statistics and inferential/analytical statistics. It also depends on the type of study design that is covered under the epidemiological study designs. For most of descriptive studies only descriptive statistics is used, wherein, the variable of interest is summarized as measured among the study participants. In case of analytical studies, descriptive statistics is used to describe the background of the study participants, whereas inferential statistics is used to find out if the difference in variable of interest among groups is statistically significant. In this inferential statistics, we make use of various statistical tests.

**Note**

Use of statistics in health research:
- Descriptive statistics
- Inferential statistics

# DESCRIPTIVE STATISTICS: MEASURES OF CENTRAL TENDENCY AND VARIATION

## Concept of Central Tendency and Dispersion

When we collect a large amount of data, it is always a good practice to concise it and express it in a manner which will be easily understood by the statistician, clinician as well as a lay person. A good method to express data is through tables and figures.

However, if we are dealing with a very large amount of quantitative data, viz. Hb levels of all the adolescent girls in a district, the average Hb level of adolescent girls in a district would be more useful information rather than presenting all the individual values. This summarized single information is called the central tendency. It is also useful to know how much the individual data varies from the single summary measure. This measure is called the measure of dispersion.

## Measures of Central Tendency

Measures of central tendency give an idea about the value around which the observations are concentrated. Mean, median, and mode are measures of central tendency.

### Mean

This is a measure of central tendency used for normally distributed data.

It is the sum of all observations divided by the number of observations. Mean for a sample is denoted as $\bar{x}$, while that for a population is denoted by $\mu$.

Mean ($\bar{x}$) = Sum of all observations ÷ number of observations
$= \dfrac{\Sigma x}{n}$

Though mean is the simplest measure of central tendency, it is affected by extremes of observations; so sometimes it may not give the central value correctly.

*Example:* Calculation of mean

Hemoglobin levels (g%) of 10 boys was found to be 10.8, 12, 11.8, 13, 13.2, 14, 13.4, 13, 12.6, and 14.2. Calculate the mean Hb.

The above data is quantitative. Mean is sum of observations divided by the number of observations viz. 10
$x = (10.8 + 12 + 11.8 + 13 + 13.2 + 14 + 13.4 + 13 + 12.6 + 14.2)/10$
$= 128/10 = 12.8\ g\%$

*Example:* Calculation of mean from grouped data
In order to calculate the mean from grouped data:
- Find the midpoint of the class interval (denoted by x)—add the upper and the lower limit of the class interval and divide by 2 for the midpoint.
- Multiply the class frequency with the midpoint.
- Find the sum of all these multiplied values.
- Divide it by the number of observations.

The serum cholesterol levels (mg/dL) of 10 patients were found to be as follows: 192, 242, 203, 212, 175, 284, 256, 218, 182, and 228.

This can be converted into grouped data by preparing a frequency table with class intervals as shown below:

| Serum cholesterol level (mg/dL) | Midpoint (x) | Frequency (f) | x*f = fx |
|---|---|---|---|
| 175–199 | (175 + 199)/2 = 187 | 3 | 561 |
| 200–224 | 212 | 3 | 636 |
| 225–249 | 237 | 2 | 474 |
| 250–274 | 262 | 1 | 262 |
| 275–299 | 287 | 1 | 287 |
| Total | | 10 = Σf | 2,220 = Σfx |

Mean is calculated as = 2,220/10 = 222 mg/dL

### Median

Median is that value which divides the complete data set into two equal parts; when the data is arranged in ascending or descending order. It is the middle most value of the data when arranged in ascending or descending order. When total observations are an odd number, there is single middle value. When total observations are an even number, there are two middle values. The median is then calculated by taking mean of these two middle observations.

Median = (n + 1)/2 when the number of observations (n) is odd
= mean of n/2th and [(n/2) + 1]th observation when the observations (n) is even

Continuing with example of serum cholesterol levels, the ascending order of these observations is 175, 182, 192, 203, 212, 218, 228, 242, 256, and 284.

The median = mean of the 5th and 6th value = (212 + 218)/2 = 215

Advantages of median are as follows:
- Median is not affected by extreme high- and low-values.
- Median is often used for non-normal distributions wherein, it helps to convey the middlemost value.

*Example:*
Calculate the mean for the given observations: 4, 5, 6, and 7
Mean = 22/4 = 5.5
Median = Mean of 5 and 6 = 5.5

However, in the above example, if we have an additional observation viz. 20
Mean = 42/5 = 8.4
Median = 6

From the above example, it is apparent that the extreme value 20 affects the mean, however, it does not affect the median as much.

### Mode

The most commonly occurring value or the most often repeated value is mode. In case two values repeat themselves same number of times, the distribution may be bimodal or multimodal. Mode is a less commonly used measure in health research.

### Relation between Mean, Median, and Mode

- For a symmetric curve (normal curve): Mean = Median = Mode
- For positively skewed curve: Mean > Median > Mode
- For negatively skewed curve: Mean < Median < Mode

- For skewed data, median and mode are better indicators of central value as compared to the mean.

## Measures of Dispersion/Variability

Variability is an inherent biological phenomenon. As we saw in previous examples if we measure Hb of 10 boys, each of the boy's Hb value would be different. We can calculate the mean Hb level but each boy's Hb would be a little different than this central value. Thus, when we have a data of observations on a biological variable (e.g., Hb) not all observations fall on a certain point, but they are spread across a range. This spread is called variability or dispersion of data. As there are measures to calculate the central tendency in single value, there are measures to calculate this variation in data into a single measure. Following is a list of such possible measures of variability within the data in a sample and variability across samples.

| Measures of variability of individual observations within a sample | Measures of variability of samples (will be discussed in the next section) |
|---|---|
| 1. Range<br>2. Interquartile range<br>3. Mean deviation (MD)<br>4. Standard deviation<br>5. Coefficient of variation | 1. Standard error of mean<br>2. Standard error of difference between means<br>3. Standard error of proportion<br>4. Standard error of difference between proportions |

### Measures of Variability of Individual Observations within a Sample

***Range:*** Range is a simplest measure of variation. Range can be calculated as difference between the maximum and the minimum value of observations in a sample (range = maximum value–minimum value). In the previous example of serum cholesterol levels of 10 patients, the range = 284–175 = 109 mg/dL. Thus, it uses only extreme values.

***Interquartile range:*** Centiles are levels which divide the entire dataset into equal parts. Percentiles divide the data set into 100 equal parts. Similarly, quartiles divide the data set into four equal parts. There are three quartiles, viz. Q1, Q2, and Q3. Q1 divides the data set into 25:75 (25% observations are below and 75% observations are above it) observations, while Q3 divides it into 75:25 observations when observations are arranged in ascending order. The interquartile range (IQR) gives observations which are between Q1 and Q3. Thus, it gives the range of middle 50% observations. It is estimated by Q3 – Q1. Interquartile range is often used along with median in order to express the data which is non-normally distributed. Thus, they are not affected by the extremes of values.

***Mean deviation:*** For calculation of MD, for each observation, we measure how far away it is from mean. Thus we calculate deviation of each observation from mean. So, we have a parallel dataset of deviations of observations. If we take a mean of these deviations, it is known as MD.

$$MD = \frac{\Sigma[X - \bar{X}]}{n}$$

Mean deviation is not much used in statistical analysis, but its improved version SD is frequently used.

***Standard deviation:*** While calculating MD, we took a modulus to ignore the negative signs for the observations lying on the left side of mean in a distribution. Another mathematical process for overcoming this negative sign is to take a square of the deviations. But when we take square of deviation, the unit of deviation also gets squared (e.g., if the observations are height of individuals in cm then such deviation would be in cm$^2$). So to bring back the deviation in original units (e.g., cm) we take a square root of the entire calculation. In the denominator we place (n – 1) instead of n in formula for SD.

Thus, formula for SD is:

$$SD = \sqrt{Var} = \sqrt{\frac{\Sigma(X - \bar{X})^2}{n}} = \sqrt{\frac{\Sigma X^2 - \frac{(\Sigma X)^2}{n}}{n-1}}$$

Steps for calculation of SD are as follows:
- Find mean
- Find difference of each observation from the mean (deviation)
- Square this difference (deviation$^2$)
- Add up all these squared values (sum of squares of deviation)
- Divide this by the number of observations minus one (gives the variance)
- Find out the square root of this variance (gives SD).

Hence, SD is root mean squared variance. Small SD means that the observations are spread closely around the mean, while a wider SD means they are spread farther from the mean.

Uses of SD are as follows:
- It gives the dispersion of observations around the mean in a single unit.
- It helps to decide whether this dispersion from mean is real or by chance (using statistical tests).
- It helps to find out the standard error (SE); whether two samples are different from each other.
- It helps to calculate the sample size for a study when variable is measured on a quantitative scale.

***Example***: Let us carry forward the previous example of serum cholesterol level (mg/dL) of 10 patients to calculate the SD of this dataset. The serum cholesterol values were 192, 242, 203, 212, 175, 284, 256, 218, 182, and 228.

From the above example we know that mean = 222 mg/dL. We can calculate the SD as follows:

| Observations (x) | Deviations (x - x̄) | Squared deviations [(x - x̄)$^2$] |
|---|---|---|
| 192 | –30 | 900 |
| 242 | 20 | 400 |
| 203 | –19 | 361 |
| 212 | –10 | 100 |
| 175 | –47 | 2,209 |
| 284 | 62 | 3,844 |
| 256 | 34 | 1,156 |
| 218 | –4 | 16 |
| 182 | 60 | 3,600 |
| 228 | 6 | 36 |
| | | Σ(x - x̄)$^2$ = 12,622 |

$$SD = \sqrt{\frac{\Sigma(x-\bar{x})}{n-1}} = \sqrt{\frac{12622}{10-1}} = \sqrt{\frac{12622}{9}} = \sqrt{\frac{12622}{10-1}}$$

$$= \sqrt{1402.4} = 37.4 \text{ mg/dL}$$

**Coefficient of variation:** Coefficient of variation (CV) is used when variations in two different datasets have to be compared. For example, to know whether variation is more in the height or weight of individuals. CV converts the variation in a single value, which can then be compared. CV is in fact SD expressed as percentage of the mean.

$$CV = \frac{SD}{Mean} \times 100$$

*Example:* Mean height of adults is 160 cm and the SD is 10 cm. Mean height of 3 months old children is 60 cm and SD is 5 cm. Which group shows greater variation?

Here, CV of adult is $(10/160) \times 100 = 6.25\%$

Coefficient of variation of 3 months old children is $(5/60) \times 100 = 8.33\%$

Coefficient of variation of children is more than that of adults. Thus, the height of children shows greater variability than that of adults.

## Concept of Standard Error and Confidence Intervals

Imagine that a specific population comprises of 10,000 people. If you can measure the height of all 10,000 and then calculate the mean of all 10,000 you get the population mean. Now, measuring height of 10,000 people is a huge task. So, in real life, it is acceptable to take only a small sample of people and measure their height. We understand that when we take only a small sample, the mean height as derived from this sample will not be exactly same as population mean but it might be a little different. We would be interested in knowing how different it would be from population mean. The concept of SE helps us determine how different this value of sample mean would be from population mean.

Suppose you are going to take sample of 100 people from a population of 10,000. You can take many such samples of 100 people with replacement from this population of 10,000. Each of these sample would have its own mean and SD.

Imagine you have taken many samples and so, now you have many sample means. You might be surprised to note that if the values of these sample means are plotted to form a frequency distribution curve, the curve would be similar to normal distribution curve. It is expected that the mean of all the sample means (if you have considered all possible samples) will be equal to the population mean. Of course, now you would like to know the dispersion of sample means from the population mean and this measure is called standard error of mean (SEM) (denoted by "s") and is calculated by following formula. (Here, n is sample size)

$$SEM = \frac{Standard\ deviation}{\sqrt{n}}$$

### Concept of Confidence Interval

As discussed earlier, it is not always possible to study the entire population to understand its characteristics or estimate its central tendency or variability. Hence, based on sampling techniques, the investigator studies a sample and tries to estimates the population mean (µ) or population proportion (P) based on the sample mean (x) or sample proportion (p).

When we try to estimate population parameter based on the sample statistic, we may not get the exact value, some error is bound to occur. Hence, we try to estimate a range within which the population parameter is expected to lie. This interval range is known as confidence limits or CI.

Standard deviations describe the spread of individual observations around sample mean. Similarly, SE describes the spread of sample means around population mean. We have seen that, when individual observations in a sample follow normal distribution mean ±1SD covers around 68% observations and mean ±2SD covers around 95% observations. Similarly, we discussed that the distribution of sample means also follow normal distribution. Hence, sample mean +1SE covers 68% of such sample means and sample mean ±2SE covers around 95% of such sample means.

Imagine we take 100 samples each having 100 individuals from the original population of 10,000. All samples combined together, the total number of people studied is possibly 10,000. Thus, with 100 such samples, we are close to studying the entire population. If we had the resources, we could actually do such a study taking 100 samples. The average (mean) of these sample means would be the actual population mean. In real life, we usually do not have resources to take 100 such samples. However, the statistical measure of SE can help us know the range within which 95% of such sample means would possibly lie. In real life, most scientists are satisfied with 95% cutoff level. Thus, to know the population mean in real life, we do not have to study the entire population. We only study a sample and using the SD within sample and the sample size (n) we can estimate the range (2SE on either side of sample mean) within which 95% of such sample means would lie. We can say that we are 95% certain that the population mean would lie in this range.

This range calculated using 2SE is known as 95% confidence limit or 95% confidence interval (CI). As SE is dependent on sample size (recall: $SE = SD/\sqrt{n}$) we understand that larger the sample size, smaller will be SE and hence more precise will be the confidence limit.

Let us take an example to understand how 95% CI is used in real life in descriptive research studies.

A researcher wanted to estimate the average salt consumption per person per day among adults in a tribal village. She found that the mean salt consumption was 14 g with SD of 3 g from her study among 30 adults. How do we interpret findings?

Here, we want to calculate the 95% CI.

$$SE = SD/\sqrt{n} = 3/\sqrt{30} = 0.54 \text{ hence, } 2SE = 1.08$$

95% CI for population mean = sample mean + 2SE = (14 − 1.08) to (14 + 1.08) = 12.92 to 15.08 g.

We are 95% certain that the mean salt consumption among adults per day in this village lies within range of 12.92–15.08 g.

We understood how to calculate the SE of mean. What do we do when the variable is measured on a qualitative scale? Suppose we conduct a survey in a tribal district to know the prevalence of sickle cell trait among children. We carry out a survey among 400 children and find out that 80 of them have sickle cell trait. This converts to a prevalence of 20%. What would be the population prevalence of sickle cell trait?

As we took help of SE of mean in case of quantitative data we can take help of SE of proportion when we have measured our variable on qualitative scale.

The formula for SE of proportion (SEP) is as follows:
$$SEP = \sqrt{pq/ns}$$

Replacing the values of our survey we get SEP =
$$SEP = \sqrt{20 \times 80 / 400} = \sqrt{4}s = 2\%. \text{ So, } 2 \text{ SEP} = 4\%.$$

95% CI for population proportion = sample proportion + 2 SEP = (20 – 4) to (20 + 4) = 16 to 24.

We are 95% certain that the proportion of sickle cell trait among children population in this district would be within the range of 16–24%.

Let us read a story on utility of CIs in real-life situation.

> Mr Visionary was the District Development Officer of a district. He was very much interested in the health and education of children. He aimed to vaccinate all children so that no child suffers from a vaccine preventable illness. They were able to achieve vaccination coverage of 90% of the children last year. This year efforts were intensified and special vaccination drives were held. The survey conducted this year showed the vaccination coverage to be 91%. Mr Visionary was shocked to see the results. In spite of so much of efforts, there was only 1% improvement in the coverage. He called a meeting with the Chief Health Officer of the district, Dr Professional.
>
> *Mr Visionary:* I am shocked to see vaccine coverage reports! In spite of all our efforts the situation is not improving. What could be the reason, Dr Professional?
>
> *Dr Professional:* I sympathize with your feelings Mr Visionary! Let me go into a bit of technicalities of the way we interpret the coverage report. In the survey, we go to only few selected households that form part of our sample so we get only an estimate and not the exact data of the vaccination coverage. This year's report mentions that the vaccination coverage was 91% with a range of 85–97%.
>
> *Mr Visionary:* So you mean the actual coverage could be 97%?
>
> *Dr Professional:* It means that the actual coverage could be as high as 97% or as low as 85%, i.e., anywhere in the range of 85–97%.
>
> *Mr Visionary:* You mean the coverage could have decreased as well?
>
> *Dr Professional:* Well, we are saying so because we believe the last year's coverage was 90%, whereas actually we should interpret it with the range that was given by last year's survey.
>
> *Mr Visionary:* So what is the solution now? How do we get to know the precise answers?
>
> *Dr Professional:* One of the solutions would be to increase the number of households studied. This measure will give us a bit more precise measurement. But resources we have to conduct such survey are limited. Even with large sample we will only reduce the range of estimated coverage, but we will still not be able to tell the exact number.
>
> *Mr Visionary:* I now understand the limits of the survey report, Dr Professional. Thank you for providing this explanation.

## NORMAL DISTRIBUTION

We learnt about the use of frequency polygon to present numerical data collected on a variable of interest. When large number of observations of a quantitative variable are divided into small class

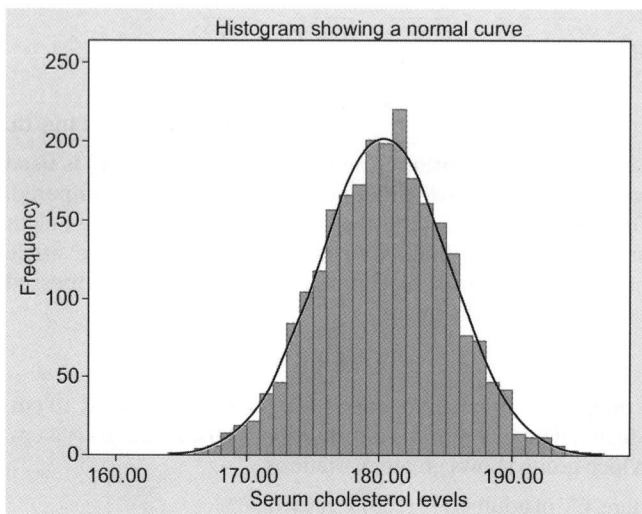

**Fig. 11.2:** A normal curve drawn over a histogram.

intervals and presented as a frequency polygon; and if it is seen that:
- The highest frequency is around the mean, lowest is at the extremities, and frequency is decreasing on either side of the mean, and
- Half of the observations lie on the right of mean and a half on left, i.e., observations symmetrically distributed on either side of mean. Then, in such a situation, we get a curve which is called a normal curve and the distribution is called as a normal distribution. It is also known as "Gaussian distribution" in honor of the scientist Carl Friedrich Gauss who first described it. **Figure 11.2** shows the normal distribution as a frequency polygon drawn on a histogram (as a curve) for a simulated data of serum cholesterol levels of 2,500 people with a mean of 180 and SD of 5. It can be seen that that the above mentioned bullet points holds true for the curve shown in **Figure 11.2**.

**Figure 11.3** shows the normal curve without the histogram.

The ***characteristics of a normal curve*** are as follows:
- It is bell-shaped
- It is symmetric around the mean: Two halves of the curve are the same size (mirror images)
- Mean, median, and mode are at the same value
- Since histogram represents all the values in the dataset, the area under curve (AUC) is 100%. The proportional area enclosed between mean and multiples of SD is constant and is as described below and shown in **Figure 11.3**:
  – Mean $\pm$ 1SD = 68.26% of the total area
  – Mean $\pm$ 2SD = 95.44% of the total area
  – Mean $\pm$ 3SD = 99.74% of the total area.

It is interesting to note that most of the biological variables that we deal with in medical science follow a distribution called as the normal distribution. In earlier section, we observed that dataset of sample means also follow normal distribution.

### Standard Normal Distribution

We use multiple units of measurement for variables measured on quantitative scale. For example, height can be measured in

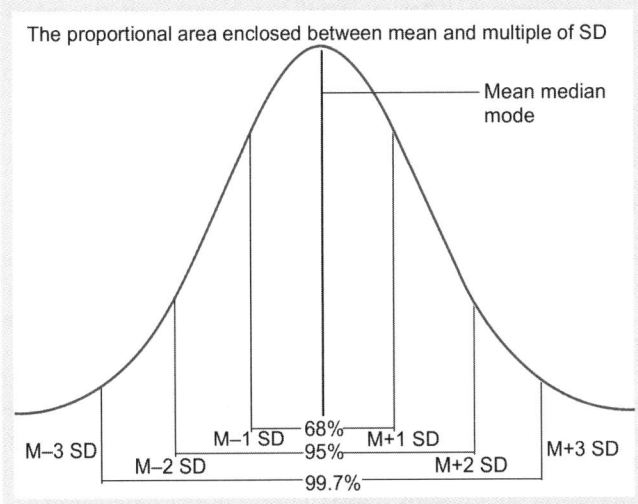

**Fig. 11.3:** A normal curve showing proportional area enclosed between mean and multiples of standard deviation.

centimeters or inches. To avoid discrepancy due to choice of units, we can take help of characteristics of normal distribution to express data in a unit free form (data can be "normalized"). This normalized value is called z-score or standard normal deviate.

$$\text{Standard normal deviate (z)} = \frac{\text{X-mean}}{\text{SD}}$$

z-score indicates how many SDs away from the mean an observation lies. Thus, instead of describing value of an observation in the original units, we can describe it in terms of z-score. z-score is used at many places in real life. The variable "weight of child" follows normal distribution. World Health Organization (WHO) has come up with growth charts with values of weight at 2 and 3SD around mean, for different age groups. Thus, in place of describing the weight of a male child at age of 1 year as 7 kg we can also mention that it is at 2SD point on left side of mean on the curve. Pediatricians define a child to be undernourished when weight is less than 2SD. Thus, when we convert the weight of child from original units (kg) to z-score, it helps in classifying the child as normal weight or underweight.

## INFERENTIAL STATISTICS: STATISTICAL TESTS USED IN HEALTH RESEARCH

*"Good statistical inference never strays very far from the data"*
—**Brian S Yandell**

We differentiated between descriptive and analytical research studies earlier in this chapter. We used means and proportions and CIs for descriptive studies. The analytical studies are different in that they try to find out association between two variables or compare the variable of interest between two groups. In any case, there is a comparison involved in analytical studies. In this situation, a hypothesis comes into picture. It is a statement describing the intent of the researcher to prove a specific finding from the study. A research hypothesis is stated when a research question has terms like: *compared with, greater than, less than, associated with, correlated with, leads to, causes,* etc. The research hypothesis should be focused on the primary objective of the study. A few examples of testable research hypothesis from analytical studies are described below:

- Fasting blood sugar level of type 2 diabetes patients who do brisk walking for at least 1 hour daily is *lower as compared with* those who do not.
- Reduction in blood pressure of pregnant women by labetalol is *greater than* that by methyldopa.
- Prenatal depression is *associated with* infant mortality among pregnant women belonging to the low-income population.
- Mobile phone usage of 6 hours daily for over 30 years causes cancer of the central nervous system.

We take help of statistical significance tests to check whether the researcher's hypothesis is true or not. A number of statistical tests are available for use while analyzing the health research data **(Table 11.4)**. The choice of a statistical test depends on the measurement scale for the variable of interest, the sample size, number of groups in the study, and whether the observations are paired or coming from independent samples.

### Null and Alternate Hypothesis in Statistical Significance Testing

In medical research, there are two type of hypothesis. Suppose a researcher is comparing the height of boys and girls. A null hypothesis in this example would be that the height of boys and girls are similar, any difference observed between the heights is just by chance. An alternative hypothesis (which usually the researcher is interested in) would be the height of boys is higher than the height of girls, so the observed difference between heights is real. Thus, the null hypothesis (denoted by $H_0$) is the hypothesis of no difference and the alternate hypothesis (denoted by $H_1$) is the hypothesis of difference.

**Table 11.4:** A simplified guide to choose a statistical test.

| Goal | Quantitative data (numerical) | Qualitative data (categorical) |
|---|---|---|
| Compare two different groups | Unpaired t-test of difference of two means (if n < 30 in any group); Z-test of difference of two means (if n >30 in both groups) | Chi-square test of proportion (if n < 30 in any group); Z-test of difference of two proportions (if n >30 in both groups) |
| Compare two paired measurements (before and after any intervention) | Paired t-test for difference of means of same sample | McNemar chi-square test *(out of the scope of this book)* |
| Determine association between two variables | Correlation coefficient | Chi-square test of association |
| Compare two or more different groups | One-way ANOVA (analysis of variance) | Chi-square test of proportion/ association |
| Predict value of outcome variable (disease) for a given value of exposure variable (risk factor) | Simple linear regression | Simple logistic regression |

*Note:* The calculations for one-way ANOVA, McNemar chi-square, correlation coefficient, and regression coefficients are out of the scope of this book, hence, only the concepts are explained.

## Errors in Medical Research

In any medical research, there are possibilities of committing two types of statistical errors while conducting the study. For explaining these errors, let us take an example of raising an alarm in case of a fire:

| There was a fire or not | You raised an alarm | You did not raise an alarm |
|---|---|---|
| Yes, there was a fire | Correct decision | Wrong decision |
| No, there was no fire | Wrong decision | Correct decision |

As given in the table above, there are two correct decisions and two wrong decisions.

In terms of null and alternate hypothesis, the above example can be explained as: null hypothesis ($H_0$)—there was no fire and alternate hypothesis ($H_1$)—there was a fire.

How does this relate to analytical studies? The fire in the above example is analogous to a real-life difference in values between two groups (e.g., suppose the height of boys were more than that of girls in reality). The alarm is analogous to researcher finding a difference in study sample (e.g., researcher finds that mean height is more among boys than girls in study sample).

| In reality | In study sample you find | |
|---|---|---|
| | Height of boys is more than girls (reject $H_0$) | Height of boys and girls is similar (do not reject $H_0$) |
| Height of boys is more than girls ($H_0$ not true) | Correct decision Power (1-β) | Wrong decision (type 2 error-β) |
| Height of boys and girls are same ($H_0$ true) | Wrong decision (type 1 error-α) | Correct decision Level of confidence (1-α) |

Suppose in real life, there is a difference in height between boys and girls then there are two possibilities; the probability of researcher finding a difference in his study sample is known as power of study (1-β) and probability of researcher not finding a difference is known as type 2 error (β).

Thus, ideally if there is a real difference the researcher would wish to detect this difference in his sample and so would like the power to be 1 and β to be 0, but practically most scientists are satisfied if we keep the power at 0.8 and β at 0.2.

Suppose in real life there is no difference in height between boys and girls then there are two possibilities; the probability of researcher finding a difference in his study sample is known as type 1 error (α) and probability of researcher not finding a difference is known as level of confidence (1-α).

Thus, ideally if there is no difference in real life then the researcher would wish his study sample does not show a difference and so would like the level of confidence to be 1 and α to be 0, but practically most scientists are satisfied if we keep the level of confidence at 0.95 and α at 0.05.

Thus, the two correct and two wrong decisions can be written as:
- **Level of confidence (1-α):** Accepting null hypothesis when it is true—you find no difference, when actually there is no difference.
- **Type I error (α):** Rejecting null hypothesis when it is true—you find a difference, when actually there is no difference.
- **Power (1-β):** Rejecting null hypothesis when it is false—you find a difference, when actually there is a difference.
- **Type II (β):** Accepting null hypothesis when it is false—you find no difference, when actually there is a difference.

## Probability (p-value)

Much of the statistical significance testing revolves around this type 1 error. Type 1 error occurs when the study finds a difference when in reality there is no difference. Why would a study find a difference? We studied the concept of variability earlier. When variability is at play, certain amount of variation in data is bound to occur by chance alone. So the difference in our study sample might be observed just by chance. How much of a difference should be attributed to chance? We have to make use of statistical tests to find out the limit of this chance. Further, a statistical test cannot tell with certainty that the difference is not by chance. It will tell us what the probability of this difference occurring by chance is. This probability of difference being by chance is known as p-value. Most scientists are satisfied if this probability is kept less than 5% (in fraction: <0.05). This cutoff mark of 0.05 is also called as level of significance. Although traditionally, it is kept at 0.05 we can also keep it at 0.01 if we want to be more stringent.

If α is predecided at 5% and the p-value in a research study is obtained as 0.20. It implies that the probability of this difference being by chance is 20% which is more than the cutoff level of 5%. Thus, there is high probability that this difference is observed just by chance and hence we call it statistically insignificant.

If α is predecided at 5% and the p-value in a research study is obtained as 0.03. It implies that the probability of this difference being by chance is 3% (and the probability of the difference being real is 97%). The probability of difference being by chance is less than the predecided cutoff level of 5%. Thus, the probability of this difference being just by chance is very small and hence this difference is likely to be real. Hence, we call it statistically significant.

> $p < 0.05$: Statistically significant
> $p > 0.05$: Statistically insignificant

## Elements of Statistical Inference Procedure (Hypothesis Testing)

For the purpose of statistical analysis, a logical flow of steps has to be followed. For the purpose of explanation, a research study comparing the mean serum triglyceride levels among cardiovascular disease (CVD) patients and normal individuals is taken. The steps of hypothesis testing and their explanation for this example are as follows:

### Step 1: Stating the null and alternate hypothesis.
For our example, the null hypothesis is "there is no difference in mean serum triglyceride levels among CVD patients and normal individuals. Whatever difference is found in study is by chance". The alternate hypothesis is "the difference between mean serum

triglyceride levels among CVD patients and normal individuals is real".

***Step 2: Calculate the summary measures of the data.***
Next, depending on the measurement scale of variable of interest, we calculate the summary measures such as mean and SD for quantitative variable and proportions for qualitative variable. In our example, we will calculate the mean and SD for serum triglyceride levels in both groups.

***Step 3: Choose a statistical test.***
Depending on the number of groups in the study, the sample size in each group and measurement scale for variable of interest, appropriate statistical test is chosen by referring to **Table 11.4**. In this example, variable (serum triglyceride levels) is measured on quantitative scale and compared between two different groups. Let us assume that one of the two groups sample size is less than 30 and since the difference of means is to be compared, the unpaired t-test will be applied.

***Step 4: Set cutoff value for type 1 error ($\alpha$).***
Alpha is commonly set at 0.05. (i.e., 95% confidence level).

***Step 5: Calculation of test statistic (as applicable along with formula).***
This is detailed in the subsequent section.

***Step 6: Comparison of test statistic with table value.***
At a particular significance level, table values for test statistics are the maximum points till which the difference is considered by chance. If test statistic is more than this table value it is less likely to be by chance, more likely to be true.

Thus, if we are checking the table values at 0.05 level of significance and calculated value of test statistic is more than allowable table value of test statistics, the obtained *p*-value is less than 0.05 meaning thereby the probability of difference being by chance is less than 5% and hence difference is likely to be real (accept alternate hypothesis).

Alternately, while checking the table values at 0.05 level of significance, if the calculated value of test statistic comes less than the allowable table value of test statistic, the obtained *p*-value is more than 0.05 meaning thereby the probability of difference being by chance is more than 5% and hence the difference is likely to be by chance and not real one (accept null hypothesis).

***Step 7: State the statistical inference.***
If *p*-value is less than 0.05, we can conclude that at 95% confidence level the difference in mean serum triglyceride levels among CVD patients and normal individuals is found to be real and not by chance.

If *p*-value is more than 0.05, we can conclude that at 95% confidence level the difference found in mean serum triglyceride levels among CVD patients and normal individuals is likely to be by chance and so it is not a real difference.

***Step 8: State the conclusion.***
If *p*-value is more than 0.05, conclusion would be, "mean serum triglyceride levels are *significantly higher* (p <0.05) among CVD patients compared to normal individuals.

If *p*-value if more than 0.05, conclusion would be, we would conclude, "the study failed to detect any significant difference in mean serum triglyceride levels among the CVD patients and normal individuals".

## Applied Aspect

When we obtain a *p*-value less than 0.05 and we conclude that the difference observed in study is statistically significant. This statistical significance means that researchers could reasonably eliminate the possibility of chance error in their study findings. However, researchers have to check if other types of errors (bias and confounding) are there in study findings. Further, it is important to understand that a difference which is found statistically significant may not always be clinically or epidemiologically relevant. Researchers have to apply their mind to decide the utility of study findings.

## Tests of Significance: Significance of Difference in Means and Proportions

We will now describe how different statistical tests are applied in some sample study situations. The steps of statistical inference procedure as described earlier are to be followed in these calculations also.

## Concept of Degrees of Freedom

Degrees of freedom are the "space" available for observations to vary. For example, there are three numbers x, y, and z which add up to a total of 100. The first two numbers x and y can be freely chosen, but the third number z will be restricted to z = 100 – x – y. Thus, three observations have only two free "spaces" to vary. Similarly, n observations have n – 1 degrees of freedom.

As described previously in the steps of statistical inference, the calculated test statistic is to be compared with the table value. For deciding the table value, the t-distribution and chi-square distribution tables (given in the Annexures 1 and 2) have to be looked at. The tables have degrees of freedom in the first column and table values in subsequent columns according to the level of significance. For instance, in t-distribution table, for degrees of freedom of 5, the corresponding table value for t is 2.571. Similarly, in chi-square distribution table, for degrees of freedom of 1, the corresponding table value for chi-square is 3.84.

For a one-sample t-test of mean and for a paired t-test, the formula for degrees of freedom is n – 1. For unpaired t-test, the formula for degrees of freedom is $n_1 + n_2 - 2$. For chi-square test, the formula for degrees of freedom is the number of rows –1 multiplied by the number of columns –1 = (r – 1 × c – 1).

## Concept of One-tailed and Two-tailed Hypothesis

The first two rows in t-distribution table are that for a one-tailed and two-tailed test and the values of t-distribution differ accordingly. Deciding on which row to look at depends on the type of hypothesis in research study.

When the investigator does not know whether mean of any one group will be higher or lower than the other, then it is said to be a two-tailed hypothesis. Many times based on clinical experience or biological plausibility the investigator would know if mean of one group will be higher than the other. In this situation, it will be a one-tailed hypothesis. Thus, the direction of hypothesis, whether it is two-tailed or one-tailed, is to be decided by the researcher before the study starts.

For z-tests, the table value for two-tailed tests is 1.96 while the table value for one-tailed tests is 1.64. The degrees of freedom concept does not apply to z-tests.

## Significance of Difference of Means of Two Different Groups when n < 30 (Unpaired t-test)

The unpaired t-test is applied to compare means of two different groups. Before applying the unpaired t-test, the data needs to meet a few requirements and assumptions as follows:
- Variable is being compared between two different groups in the hypothesis
- Variable is measured on quantitative scale
- Variable follows normal distribution
- *Equality of variance*: Data in both groups have the same variance
- Sample size (n) in either of the two groups is less than 30.

Please note that while applying t-test, the assumption of normal distribution stands true even when it is an approximately normal data because it is quite robust to deviations from normality.

The formula for applying unpaired t-test is as follows: $t = \dfrac{\bar{x}_1 - \bar{x}_2}{SE}$

Where, $\bar{x}_1$ is mean of the first group, $\bar{x}_2$ is mean of the second group, and SE is standard error of difference between two means.

Standard error (SE) = $Sp \sqrt{\dfrac{1}{n_1} + \dfrac{1}{n_2}}$, where $Sp = \sqrt{\dfrac{SD_1^2(n_1-1) + SD_2^2(n_2-1)}{(n_1 + n_2 - 2)}}$

The unpaired t-test is explained with the following example:

"A group of 69 CVDs patients had a mean serum triglyceride levels of 230 mg/dL with an SD of 4.9 and another group of 29 normal individuals had a mean serum triglyceride levels of 180 mg/dL with an SD of 8.4. Apply appropriate statistical test to test the hypothesis that the mean serum triglyceride levels among CVD patients are different than normal individuals. (*Note*: Two-tailed table value of t at degrees of freedom of 96 is 1.985.)"

On doing the calculations, standard error (SE) = 1.36.

Therefore, $t = \dfrac{230 - 180}{1.36} = 36.85$

Degrees of freedom for unpaired t-test = $n_1 + n_2 - 2 = 69 + 29 - 2 = 96$; table t-value = 1.985.

At degree of freedom of 96, since the calculated t-value (36.85) is more than the table value of 1.985, null hypothesis is rejected and alternate hypothesis is accepted. Hence, the difference in mean serum triglyceride levels among CVD patients and normal individuals is statistically significant ($p < 0.05$). The study found that mean serum triglyceride levels is significantly higher among CVD patients compared to normal individuals ($p < 0.05$).

## Significance of Difference of Means of the Same Group (Paired Data)—Paired t-test

The paired t-test is applied to compare means of the same sample before and after any intervention/procedure. Before applying the paired t-test, the data needs to meet a few requirements and assumptions as follows:
- Data comes from paired observations from only one group (before-after)
- Data to be compared should be quantitative
- Variable follows normal distribution.

The sample size for calculation of paired t-test can be any number as far as the above assumptions stand true.

The formula for applying paired t-test is,

$$t = \dfrac{\text{Mean of difference}}{\dfrac{\text{SD of differences}}{\sqrt{n}}}$$

The paired t-test is explained with the following example:

"A new drug for weight loss was being tested and the reduction in weight among 10 patients is given below:

| Weight in kilograms before taking the drug | Weight in kilograms after taking the drug | Difference |
|---|---|---|
| 52 | 51 | 1 |
| 109 | 105 | 4 |
| 112 | 113 | −1 |
| 98 | 95 | 3 |
| 87 | 80 | 7 |
| 128 | 120 | 8 |
| 115 | 114 | 1 |
| 69 | 65 | 4 |
| 80 | 82 | −2 |
| 85 | 80 | 5 |

Apply appropriate statistical test to find out whether the drug is significantly reducing the weight among the 10 individuals. (*Note*: Table value of t at degrees of freedom of 9 is 2.26)."

On doing the calculations, $\dfrac{\text{Mean of differenes}}{\dfrac{\text{SD of differences}}{\sqrt{n}}} = \dfrac{3}{\dfrac{3.26}{\sqrt{10}}} = 2.9$

Degrees of freedom = n − 1 = 9. At degrees of freedom of 9, since the calculated t-value (2.9) is more than the table value of 2.26, the null hypothesis is rejected and alternate hypothesis is accepted. Hence, the difference in mean weight before and after taking the drug is statistically significant. The new drug significantly reduces weight among the study participants ($p < 0.05$).

## Analysis of Variance

In previous example, we compared means between two groups. ANOVA test is applied to compare means of more than two different groups. If the ANOVA test is statistically significant ($p < 0.05$), it implies that the mean is significantly different in at least one of the n different groups being tested. In order to find out exactly which group is significantly different, a post-hoc test is applied. The calculations of ANOVA test and post-hoc tests are beyond the scope of this book.

## Chi-square Test

Chi-square test is a nonparametric test mainly used to test the difference between two proportions or for testing associations between two categorical variables. There are three types of chi-square tests:
1. Chi-square test of association
2. Chi-square test of proportion
3. Chi-square test of goodness of fit.

### Chi-square Test of Association

Chi-square test of association is applied to test the association between two categorical variables. Before applying the chi-square test, the data needs to meet a few requirements and assumptions as follows:
- Both the variables between which association is to be tested should be categorical
- At least 80% of expected cell values should be more than 5
- None of the expected cell values should be less than 1.

The calculation of expected cell values is explained below. The minimum sample size required for applying chi-square test of association can be any number as far as the above assumptions stand true. Also, as chi-square is a nonparametric test, the assumption of normal distribution does not apply here.

Classically, for a chi-square test, a 2 × 2 contingency table between an exposure and a disease as given below is to be constructed.

| Exposure | Disease present | Disease absent | Total |
|---|---|---|---|
| Present | a | b | a + b |
| Absent | c | d | c + d |
| Total | a + c | b + d | a + b + c + d |

The cells a, b, c, and d are observed values or values from findings of the study. The first step in calculating a chi-square test is to calculate expected values for each of the observed values.

In the above table, expected value for cell "a" =

$$\frac{(\text{row total}) \times (\text{column total})}{\text{table total}} = \frac{(a+b) \times (a+c)}{a+b+c+d}$$

Similarly, the expected value for "b" = $\frac{(b+d) \times (a+b)}{a+b+c+d}$ and so on for "c" and "d".

For a 2 × 2 contingency table, the observed values are denoted by $O_1$, $O_2$, $O_3$, and $O_4$ and the expected values are denoted by $E_1$, $E_2$, $E_3$, and $E_4$. While the formula for calculation of chi-square ($\chi^2$) is

$\chi^2 = \chi_1^2 + \chi_2^2 + \chi_3^2 + \chi_4^2$ where $\chi_1^2 = \frac{(O_1 - E_1)^2}{E_1}$, $\chi_2^2 = \frac{(O_2 - E_2)^2}{E_2}$ and so on.

The chi-square test is explained with the following example:

"A study was conducted to find out the association between parity and development of breast cancer. A group of 450 women with less than 3 parity and another group of 400 women with more than or equal to 3 parity were followed up for the development of breast cancer. Out of 450 women with less than 3 parity, 26 developed breast cancer and out of 400 women with more than or equal to 3 parity, 10 developed breast cancer. Apply appropriate statistical test to check whether parity less than 3 is associated with the development of breast cancer. (*Note*: Table value for $\chi^2$ at degrees of freedom of 1 at 0.05 level of significance is 3.84.)"

The 2 × 2 contingency table prepared from the provided data is as below:

| Parity groups | Developed breast cancer | Did not develop breast cancer | Total |
|---|---|---|---|
| <3 parity | 26 | 424 | 450 |
| ≥3 parity | 10 | 390 | 400 |
| Total | 36 | 814 | 850 |

On doing the calculations, $\chi^2 = \chi_1^2 + \chi_2^2 + \chi_3^2 + \chi_4^2 = 2.6 + 0.11 + 2.9 + 0.13 = 5.74$

At degree of freedom of 1, the calculated $\chi^2$ value (5.74) is more than the table value (3.84). Hence, the null hypothesis is rejected and alternate hypothesis is accepted. Thus, at 95% confidence level, parity less than 3 is associated with the development of breast cancer ($p < 0.05$). Women with parity less than 3 are at higher risk of developing breast cancer than women with more than or equal to 3 parity ($p < 0.05$).

### Chi-square Test of Proportion

Chi-square test of proportion is applied to compare the difference between two proportions. Before applying the chi-square test of proportion, the data needs to meet a few requirements and assumptions as follows:
- There should be two different groups in the hypothesis
- Data to be compared between the two groups should be qualitative (categorical, i.e., either nominal or ordinal)
- Sample size (n) in either of the two groups is less than 30
- At least 80% of expected cell values should be more than 5
- None of the expected cell values should be less than 1.

As chi-square test is a nonparametric test, the assumption of normal distribution does not apply here. The formula for applying chi-square test of proportion is same as described for chi-square test of association above.

The calculation of chi-square test of proportion is explained with the following example:

"Out of 20 hypertensive adolescent patients in a hospital, 10 had obesity and out of 45 normotensive adolescent patients in the hospital, 10 had obesity. Apply appropriate statistical test to compare whether the proportion of adolescent obesity is different among hypertensive and normotensive patients. (*Note*: Table value for $\chi^2$ at degrees of freedom of 1 at 0.05 level of significance is 3.84.)"

The 2 × 2 contingency table prepared from the provided data is as below:

| Obesity | Hypertensive patients | Normotensive patients | Total |
|---|---|---|---|
| Present | 10 | 10 | 20 |
| Absent | 10 | 35 | 45 |
| Total | 20 | 45 | 65 |

Looking at the table, we can see that among hypertensives 50% are obese while among normotensives 22.2% are obese. Let us apply test to see if this difference is statistically significant.

On doing the calculations, = 2.41 + 1.07 + 1.07 + 0.48 = 5.03 At degree of freedom of 1, the calculated $\chi^2$ value (5.03) is more than the table value (3.84). Hence, the null hypothesis is rejected and alternate hypothesis is accepted. Thus, at 95% confidence level, the difference in proportion of obese among hypertensive and normotensive patients is statistically significant ($p < 0.05$). Obesity is significantly higher among hypertensive patients than normotensive patients ($p < 0.05$).

### Chi-square Test of Goodness of Fit (2 × 1 Chi-square)

Chi-square test of goodness of fit is used to compare the difference between two proportions of the same sample. Before applying the chi-square test, the data needs to meet a few requirements and assumptions as follows:
- There should be only one variable, which should be categorical (i.e., nominal or ordinal)
- At least 80% of the expected cell values should be more than 5
- None of the expected cell values should be less than 1.

The minimum sample size required for applying chi-square test of goodness of fit can be any number as far as the above assumptions stand true. In this test, the observed values are compared with the "normally" expected values for that variable.

The calculation of chi-square test of goodness of fit is explained with the following example:

"In a random sample of 100 people in a city, it was found that 70 persons were male and 30 were female. Apply an appropriate statistical test to find out whether the proportion of males is higher than the proportion of females in this sample. (*Note*: Table value for $\chi^2$ at degrees of freedom of 1 at 0.05 level of significance is 3.84.)"

Number of males ($O_1$) = 70, number of females ($O_2$) = 30. It is "normally" expected that in a sample of 100 people, there should be 50 males and 50 females. Therefore, expected values $E_1$ = 50 and $E_2$ = 50.

On doing the calculations, $\chi^2 = \chi_1^2 + \chi_2^2 = 8 + 8 = 16$

At degrees of freedom of 1, the calculated $\chi^2$ value (16) is more than the table value (3.84). Hence, the null hypothesis is rejected and alternate hypothesis is accepted. Thus, at 95% confidence level, the difference in proportion of males versus females in the sample is statistically significant ($p < 0.05$). Proportion of males is significantly higher than that of females in the sample ($p < 0.05$).

**Annexure 1:** t-distribution table.

| One-tail | 0.1 | 0.05 | 0.025 | 0.01 | 0.005 |
|---|---|---|---|---|---|
| Two-tails | 0.2 | 0.1 | 0.05 | 0.02 | 0.01 |
| df | | | | | |
| 1 | 3.08 | 6.31 | 12.71 | 31.82 | 63.66 |
| 2 | 1.89 | 2.92 | 4.30 | 6.96 | 9.92 |
| 3 | 1.64 | 2.35 | 3.18 | 4.54 | 5.84 |
| One-tail | 0.1 | 0.05 | 0.025 | 0.01 | 0.005 |
| 4 | 1.53 | 2.13 | 2.78 | 3.75 | 4.60 |
| 5 | 1.48 | 2.02 | 2.57 | 3.36 | 4.03 |
| 6 | 1.44 | 1.94 | 2.45 | 3.14 | 3.71 |
| 7 | 1.41 | 1.89 | 2.36 | 3.00 | 3.50 |
| 8 | 1.40 | 1.86 | 2.31 | 2.90 | 3.36 |
| 9 | 1.38 | 1.83 | 2.26 | 2.82 | 3.25 |
| 10 | 1.37 | 1.81 | 2.23 | 2.76 | 3.17 |
| 11 | 1.36 | 1.80 | 2.20 | 2.72 | 3.11 |
| 12 | 1.36 | 1.78 | 2.18 | 2.68 | 3.05 |
| 13 | 1.35 | 1.77 | 2.16 | 2.65 | 3.01 |
| 14 | 1.35 | 1.76 | 2.14 | 2.62 | 2.98 |
| 15 | 1.34 | 1.75 | 2.13 | 2.60 | 2.95 |
| 16 | 1.34 | 1.75 | 2.12 | 2.58 | 2.92 |
| 17 | 1.33 | 1.74 | 2.11 | 2.57 | 2.90 |
| 18 | 1.33 | 1.73 | 2.10 | 2.55 | 2.88 |
| 19 | 1.33 | 1.73 | 2.09 | 2.54 | 2.86 |
| 20 | 1.33 | 1.72 | 2.09 | 2.53 | 2.85 |
| 21 | 1.32 | 1.72 | 2.08 | 2.52 | 2.83 |
| 22 | 1.32 | 1.72 | 2.07 | 2.51 | 2.82 |
| 23 | 1.32 | 1.71 | 2.07 | 2.50 | 2.81 |
| 24 | 1.32 | 1.71 | 2.06 | 2.49 | 2.80 |
| 25 | 1.32 | 1.71 | 2.06 | 2.49 | 2.79 |
| 26 | 1.31 | 1.71 | 2.06 | 2.48 | 2.78 |
| 27 | 1.31 | 1.70 | 2.05 | 2.47 | 2.77 |
| 28 | 1.31 | 1.70 | 2.05 | 2.47 | 2.76 |
| 29 | 1.31 | 1.70 | 2.05 | 2.46 | 2.76 |
| 30 | 1.31 | 1.70 | 2.04 | 2.46 | 2.75 |
| 40 | 1.30 | 1.68 | 2.02 | 2.42 | 2.70 |
| 50 | 1.30 | 1.68 | 2.01 | 2.40 | 2.68 |
| 60 | 1.30 | 1.67 | 2.00 | 2.39 | 2.66 |
| 100 | 1.29 | 1.66 | 1.98 | 2.36 | 2.63 |
| 120 | 1.29 | 1.66 | 1.98 | 2.36 | 2.62 |

## CORRELATION AND REGRESSION

### Correlation

Scatter diagram is a visual method of checking if there is a relationship between two quantitatively measured variables. If a relationship exists between the two variables; with changes in value of one variable the other variable will also change.

**Annexure 2:** Chi-square distribution table.

| df | $\chi^2$ at 0.1 | $\chi^2$ at 0.05 | $\chi^2$ at 0.025 | $\chi^2$ at 0.01 | $\chi^2$ at 0.005 |
|---|---|---|---|---|---|
| 1 | 2.71 | 3.84 | 5.02 | 6.64 | 7.88 |
| 2 | 4.61 | 5.99 | 7.38 | 9.21 | 10.60 |

| df | χ² at 0.1 | χ² at 0.05 | χ² at 0.025 | χ² at 0.01 | χ² at 0.005 |
|---|---|---|---|---|---|
| 3 | 6.25 | 7.82 | 9.35 | 11.35 | 12.84 |
| 4 | 7.78 | 9.49 | 11.14 | 13.28 | 14.86 |
| 5 | 9.24 | 11.07 | 12.83 | 15.09 | 16.75 |
| 6 | 10.65 | 12.59 | 14.45 | 16.81 | 18.55 |
| 7 | 12.02 | 14.07 | 16.01 | 18.48 | 20.28 |
| 8 | 13.36 | 15.51 | 17.54 | 20.09 | 21.96 |
| 9 | 14.68 | 16.92 | 19.02 | 21.67 | 23.59 |
| 10 | 15.99 | 18.31 | 20.48 | 23.21 | 25.19 |
| 11 | 17.28 | 19.68 | 21.92 | 24.73 | 26.76 |
| 12 | 18.55 | 21.03 | 23.34 | 26.22 | 28.30 |
| 13 | 19.81 | 22.36 | 24.74 | 27.69 | 29.82 |
| 14 | 21.06 | 23.69 | 26.12 | 29.14 | 31.32 |
| 15 | 22.31 | 25.00 | 27.49 | 30.58 | 32.80 |
| 16 | 23.54 | 26.30 | 28.85 | 32.00 | 34.27 |
| 17 | 24.77 | 27.59 | 30.19 | 33.41 | 35.72 |
| 18 | 25.99 | 28.87 | 31.53 | 34.81 | 37.16 |
| 19 | 27.20 | 30.14 | 32.85 | 36.19 | 38.58 |
| 20 | 28.41 | 31.41 | 34.17 | 37.57 | 40.00 |
| 21 | 29.62 | 32.67 | 35.48 | 38.93 | 41.40 |
| 22 | 30.81 | 33.92 | 36.78 | 40.29 | 42.80 |
| 23 | 32.01 | 35.17 | 38.08 | 41.64 | 44.18 |
| 24 | 33.20 | 36.42 | 39.36 | 42.98 | 45.56 |

| df | χ² at 0.1 | χ² at 0.05 | χ² at 0.025 | χ² at 0.01 | χ² at 0.005 |
|---|---|---|---|---|---|
| 25 | 34.38 | 37.65 | 40.65 | 44.31 | 46.93 |
| 26 | 35.56 | 38.89 | 41.92 | 45.64 | 48.29 |
| 27 | 36.74 | 40.11 | 43.20 | 46.96 | 49.65 |
| 28 | 37.92 | 41.34 | 44.46 | 48.28 | 50.99 |
| 29 | 39.09 | 42.56 | 45.72 | 49.59 | 52.34 |
| 30 | 40.26 | 43.77 | 46.98 | 50.89 | 53.67 |
| 40 | 51.81 | 55.76 | 59.34 | 63.69 | 66.77 |
| 50 | 63.17 | 67.51 | 71.42 | 76.15 | 79.49 |
| 60 | 74.40 | 79.08 | 83.30 | 88.38 | 91.95 |
| 70 | 85.53 | 90.53 | 95.02 | 100.43 | 104.22 |
| 80 | 96.58 | 101.88 | 106.63 | 112.33 | 116.32 |
| 90 | 107.57 | 113.15 | 118.14 | 124.12 | 128.30 |
| 100 | 118.50 | 124.34 | 129.56 | 135.81 | 140.17 |

## Types of Correlation

In the figure, chart A shows *no correlation* between two variables. Chart B shows a *positive correlation*. Which means that with increase in value of variable put on X-axis the value of variable on Y-axis also increases. Chart C shows *negative correlation*, where with increase in one variable the value of other variable decreases. Chart D shows a *perfect positive correlation* where there is a linear relationship between the two variables. Chart E shows such *perfect negative correlation*.

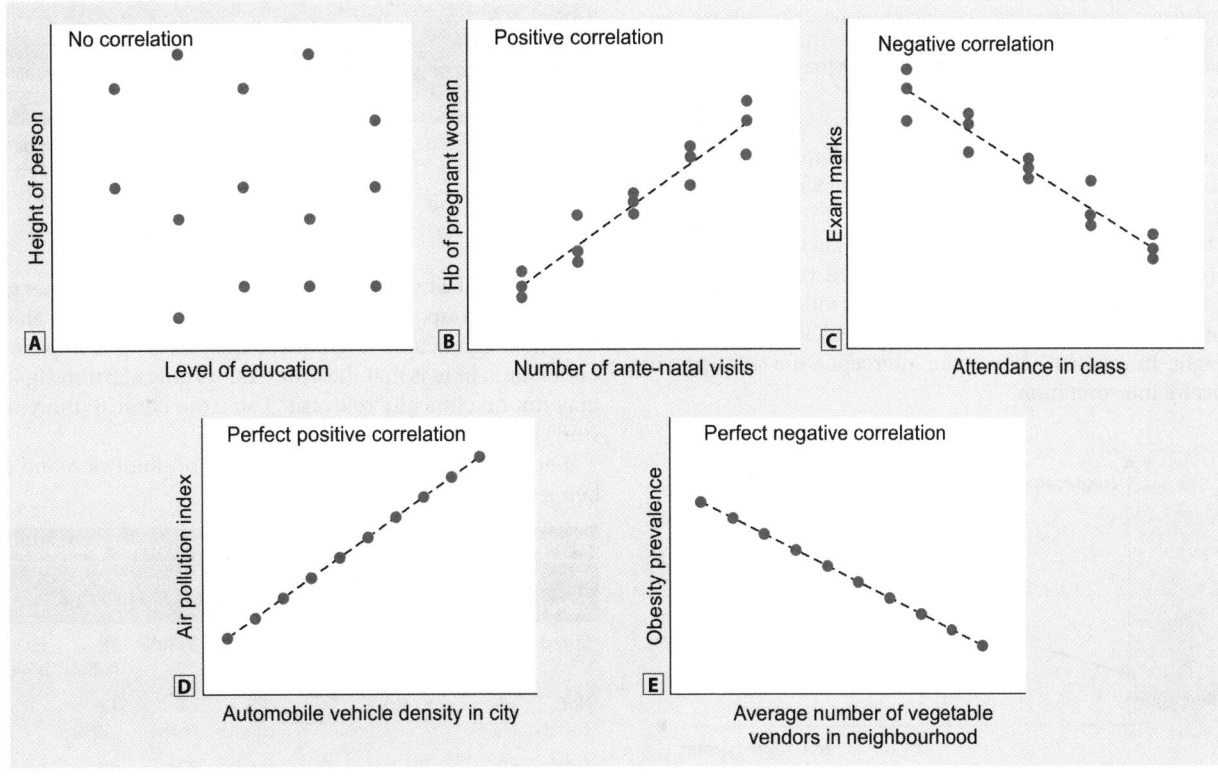

## Correlation Coefficient (r)

The degree of relationship between the two variables is measured by correlation coefficient (denoted by "r"). The value of "r" ranges from –1 for a perfect negative correlation (chart E) to +1 for a perfect positive correlation (chart D). Value of "r" at 0 indicates that there is no relationship between the two quantitative variables (chart A). There are two methods for calculation of correlation coefficient. When the variables follow normal distribution the formula of Karl Pearson's product-moment correlation coefficient is used and when they do not follow normal distribution formula of Spearman correlation coefficient is used. Irrespective of the formula used for calculation of "r", its interpretation is same which is as follows.

| Value of "r" | Interpretation |
|---|---|
| 0–0.3 | Negligible correlation |
| 0.3–0.5 | Low positive correlation |
| 0.5–0.7 | Moderate positive correlation |
| 0.7–0.9 | High positive correlation |
| 0.9–1 | Very high positive correlation |

Same way interpretation of negative correlation goes from 0 to –1.

## Regression

While correlation is used to know the strength of association between two quantitative variables, regression goes a step further. Regression is used to predict the value of one variable (dependent variable) with each unit change in another variable (independent variable).

> **Note**
> **Key message**
> *Correlation* gives degree and direction of relationship between two variables
> *Regression* predicts the values of one variable on the basis of the other variable.

The regression equation is $y = a + bx$ where; y is dependent variable, "a" is intercept, "x" is independent variable, and "b" is the regression coefficient.

If the regression equation for height (cm) as independent variable (x) and weight (kg) as dependent variable (y) is y = –133.1 + 1.16 x; then its interpretation is as follows:

For each 1 cm increase in height there will be 1.16 kg increase in weight. In medical science the intercept a does not provide any useful interpretation.

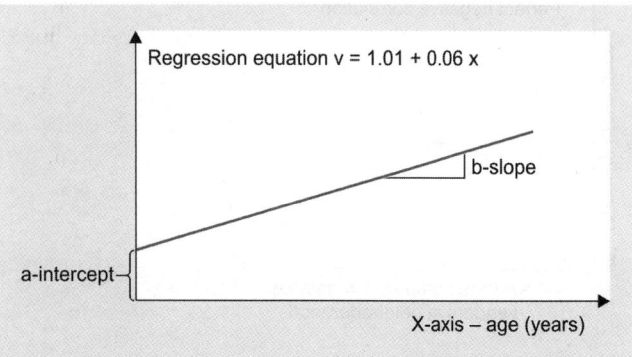

## Multivariate Regression Analysis

Earlier we saw how change in one independent variable can predict the change in a dependent variable. In real life many of the outcome variables are dependent on more than one independent variables. In such situations, if we look at the equation we will have one y and more than one x.

$$Y = a + \beta_1 x_1 + \beta_2 x_2 + \beta_3 x_3 + \beta_4 x_4$$

For example, SBP might be dependent on age ($x_1$), gender ($x_2$), waist circumference ($x_3$), and height ($x_4$).

## Types of Multivariate Regression

The type of multivariate regression depends on the nature of dependent variable.
- Multiple linear regression is used when the dependent variable is measured on quantitative scale (e.g., serum cholesterol level).
- Multiple logistic regression is used when the dependent variable is measured on binary categorical scale (e.g., treatment outcome measured in two categories success or failure).
- Cox regression model is used when dependent variable is survival data.

## INTERPRETING THE STUDY FINDINGS

*Are all statistically significant results also clinically significant?* The following table shows findings from a study comparing the antihypertensive effect of drugs A and B on SBP. Observe the result of statistical significance testing when sample size is increased from 100 per group to 300 per group.

| Situation 1: With original sample size | | | Situation 2: Using very high sample size | | |
|---|---|---|---|---|---|
| Groups | Mean ± SD of SBP | Statistical test | Groups | Mean ± SD of SBP | Statistical test |
| Group A (n = 100) | 140 ± 10 mm Hg | Unpaired t-test p = 0.15 | Group A (n = 300) | 140 ± 10 mm Hg | Unpaired t-test, p = 0.01 |
| Group B (n = 100) | 138 ± 10 mm Hg | | Group B (n = 300) | 138 ± 10 mm Hg | |

We see that when sample size is increased from 100 per group to 300 per group, the result of statistical significance changes from non-significant to significant difference. More important to understand here is that the difference is only of 2 mm Hg which may not be clinically relevant. Thus, the clinical utility of the study results should also be examined.

Let us take another example where antibiotics A and B are being compared.

| With small sample | | | | With a small increase in sample size | | | |
|---|---|---|---|---|---|---|---|
| Status | Group A | Group B | | Status | Group A | Group B | |
| Cured | 6 (30%) | 12 (60%) | $\chi^2$ = 3.6 p = 0.056 | Cured | 9 (30%) | 18 (60%) | $\chi^2$ = 5.4 p = 0.019 |
| Not cured | 14 (70%) | 8 (40%) | | Not cured | 21 (70%) | 12 (40%) | |
| Total | 20 | 20 | | Total | 30 | 30 | |

With a sample size of 20 patients in each group, there is a large difference found in the study where only 30% patients in group A are cured versus 60% in group B. In spite of the large difference the statistical significance testing through chi-square test shows a nonsignificant difference ($p > 0.05$). Looking at the large difference when the researcher increases the sample size to 30 in each group now, the difference is statistically significant ($p < 0.05$).

Thus, going through these two examples we understand that at times a small difference may come statistically significant and large difference may come statistically nonsignificant because of the sample size involved, hence checking whether the findings are clinically meaningful or not is also important to check while interpreting study results.

## Interpreting Study Findings

### Descriptive Studies

Descriptive studies are done to estimate the average value of variable of interest in given reference population. It is important to make use of CIs rather than only stating point estimates.

### Analytical Studies

The analytical studies could be a risk factor study that tries to find association between exposure and outcome variable or an intervention study trying to find out the difference in outcome variable between two groups. Below is an example of findings from an analytical study trying to see if owning a mobile phone among school students is associated with low physical activity. Commonly the results of such study are presented as below.

| | Low physical activity | Moderate physical activity | Total | Relative risk (95% CI of RR) | p-value |
|---|---|---|---|---|---|
| Owns mobile phone | 40 (80%) | 10 (20%) | 50 | 2 (1.5–2.6) | $p = 0.000003$ Chi-square test |
| Does not own mobile phone | 40 (40%) | 60 (60%) | 100 | | |

Ask these questions while interpreting analytical studies
1. What is the value of measure of strength of association?
2. What is the range of confidence interval?
3. What is the likelihood of chance error (p-value)?
4. What is the likelihood of systematic error?
5. Utility of results:
   a. Is association causative?
   b. Intervention's safety, acceptability, and cost.

In this table, the relative risk indicates the strength of association. With help of computer applications, we can also easily calculate the 95% CI of relative risk. This CI in this example means that students possessing mobile phones are 1.5 to 2.6 times more likely to have low physical activity level. In other words, CI indicates how precise our estimate of the relative risk is. Larger the sample size more precise would be this estimate. Results of chi-square test here show that the association is statistically significant. The low or high p-value does not indicate anything about the strength of association, it only tells that the probability of chance error in our results. In this case since p is very small researchers have reasonably eliminated the chance error in study results. Apart from chance errors the systematic errors (selection and measurement bias and confounders) are also important. So in this example also the researchers should discuss how the findings of this table are free from these systematic errors. Finally, not all associations are causations. So, applying the criteria for determining causation (described in epidemiology) is necessary to check if this apparent association is really causative.

If the research study is an intervention study assessing the efficacy of one intervention with the other on the outcome variable, the steps of interpretation would be largely the same. Here also, for assessing efficacy we would interpret the relative risk reduction, its 95% CI, chance error (p-value), and systematic error. In last step, the researchers should also discuss the acceptability (tolerability) of the intervention by the patients, its safety, and costs associated with such investigational new intervention.

## CONCEPT OF ETHICS IN HUMAN RESEARCH

### What is Medical Ethics?

Ethics refers to "a set of moral principles or values which determines the code of conduct in medical profession so as to serve in the best interest of individual and society".

### Why Ethics in Research?

Similar to the expectation of ethical conduct by a health professional in medical practice, it is also expected while performing health research. Ethics is about safeguarding the dignity, rights, safety, and well-being of the human research participants.

### History

In past, medical research witnessed few cruel forms of exploitation of human beings for research purpose.

During World War II, medical experiments were performed on camp prisoners without their consent leading to death and permanent disability. The *Nuremberg trial* considered it as violation of human rights. In *Tuskegee Syphilis study* which was planned to understand the natural progression of syphilis disease, around 600 male participants were enrolled but they were never told they had syphilis. Researchers became aware of penicillin for treatment in 1947, but knowingly did not treat patients and prevented them for taking treatment. Thus many men, their wives, and children suffered from dreaded consequences of syphilis. A series of brutal medical experiments with freezing temperatures, high altitude, head injury, sea water submersion, and mustard gas were performed during World War II.

After these series of unethical conduct in medical research, a series of meetings and guidance reports were generated. The

Belmont Report (1979) drafted by the National Commission for the Protection of Human Participants of Biomedical and Behavioral Research in United States is widely used as a guiding document on ethical conduct of health research. It focused on three important principles of ethics.

> **Note**
> **Three important principles of ethics:**
> 1. Respect for persons
> 2. Beneficence and nonmaleficence
> 3. Justice

1. ***Respect for persons:*** This principle tells that each person should be treated as autonomous individual capable of taking decisions for him/herself. Hence each human being participating in research should be given an opportunity to choose what would or would not happen to them. This opportunity is given in form of informed consent process explained below. This underscores that participation in research study should be voluntary and not forced. This principle also mentions that special protections be provided to those individuals who have reduced capacity to take decisions for themselves such as children or vulnerable people such as prisoners when they participate in research.
2. ***Beneficence and non-maleficence:*** It means that research should maximize the possible benefits to the subjects and minimize the possible harm.
3. ***Justice:*** This principle means that there should not be exploitation of some vulnerable population group or community for research purpose. The community that runs the risk by participating in research should also get the benefits of the research outcome.

## Informed Consent

The word "informed" in this term means informing the research participants of the risks and benefits of participating in research. Consent means human beings are not forced to participate in research, but they participate in it voluntarily after knowing the risks and possible benefits. The recent guidelines suggest audiovisual recording of this entire consent process in case of clinical trials involving human participants. It includes two main components: (1) participant information sheet (PIS) and (2) informed consent form.

1. ***Participant information sheet:*** This is a document containing all relevant information of the study that a possible participant needs to know. This document should include answers to a list of questions provided in the box in simple language which can be easily understood by the study participants. A copy of the PIS is to be provided to all the study participants preferably in the local vernacular language.
2. ***Informed consent form:*** It is the statement of declaration by the study participants and the researcher as shown in the sample form in the box below. This written informed consent form has to be signed or thumb impressed by the study participant for literate or illiterate participants, respectively. It has to be signed by the participant in presence of the third party witness, who is neither related to the study participant nor to the researcher. It has to be preserved by the researcher.

> **A participant information sheet answers the following questions:**
> - What is this study about?
> - Why are you being invited to participate?
> - What will you be asked to do?
> - Will there be any benefits to you?
> - Will there be any risks to you?
> - Will there be recordings or photos?
> - Who will get the results?
> - Where can you get the results?
> - Are there any costs?
> - Any questions?
> - Who to contact if there are questions later?

## Why there is a Need for an Ethics Committee?

If the opinion on ethical aspects of a proposed research study is left to the individual researcher, there is a risk of running a biased decision. Researchers might feel that their study is ethical and there is no harm to their study participants. Having understood the dark history and recommendations for ethical research, we now appreciate the need to have an unbiased opinion from a third eye on proposed research.

Most countries have established rules for an ethics committee. Committee performs an objective and unbiased review on ethical aspects of the project proposals received by it. Thus, it attempts to safeguard the interest of research participants. It has different names in different countries like institutional review board (IRB)/Institutional Ethics Committee (IEC). This committee is composed of people with interest and experience of ethical issues including persons from basic medical science, clinicians, legal expert like lawyer or judge, social scientist, philosopher, and a layperson from the community. It should be independent of researchers and sponsors.

> **SAMPLE CONSENT FORM**
> **Declaration by participant**
> By signing below, I…. agree to take part in a research study entitled "(Title of the study)"
> **I declare that:**
> - I have read this information and consent form and understand the contents
> - I have had a chance to ask questions and all my questions have been adequately answered
> - I understand that taking part in this study is voluntary and I have not been pressurized to take part
> - I may choose to leave the study at any time and will not be penalized or prejudiced in anyway
> 
> Signed at (place) ……………………..………………….. on (date) ……….……….
> 
> ……………………. Signature of participant or mark X if cannot sign and name
> 
> **Declaration by researcher**
> I, Dr XYZ (name of the researcher), declare that:
> - I explained the information in this document to ……………………….
> - I encouraged him/her to ask questions and took adequate time to answer them.
> - I am satisfied that he/she adequately understands all aspects of the research, as discussed above
> 
> Signed at (place) ……………………..………………….. on (date) ……….……….

*Source*: Union SORT-IT course module.

Most of the academic institutions have their local IEC. Researchers are required to submit the detailed study protocol to IEC in the prescribed format. Member secretary of IEC screens the received proposals and depending on the possible risk involved, the type of review will be decided as: (1) *exemption from review* (proposals with less than minimal risk like educational surveys), (2) *expedited review* (proposals with minimal risk like review of secondary records or minor deviations from previously approved proposals) or (3) *full review* (proposals with more than minimal risk like blood collection, investigations or intervention trials). Meetings of IEC are held at regular intervals and full reviews of the proposals are conducted. Based on the discussion during the meetings, the study proposal is either approved in the same state or approved with some major/minor suggestions or disapproved. Approval from IEC is mandatory before conducting any research study.

# DISSEMINATION OF RESEARCH FINDINGS: WRITING A RESEARCH REPORT

## Importance of Writing a Research Report

Dissemination of the research findings is an important responsibility of the researcher. Without dissemination of the research findings, the research process is incomplete.

## Format of Writing a Research Report

The most commonly used format is known by the acronym "IMRAD".

> **Note**
>
> | | |
> |---|---|
> | I—Introduction | Why did you study? |
> | M—Methodology | How did you study? |
> | R—Results [A—and] | What did you find |
> | D—Discussion | What does it mean anyway? |

### *Introduction*

In this section, the background of the study is mentioned. We answer three questions in this section. (1) Why this topic or problem is important to study? What is already known about this topic or problem through existing evidence? (2) What are the gaps in existing knowledge or what is still not known about this topic or problem? (3) How this study plans to answer this unanswered question or fill the gap in knowledge? This section usually ends with specific objectives of the study.

### *Methodology*

Also described as "materials and methods", this section explains "how the study was done?" Dictum is that it should be sufficiently detailed to enable other interested researcher to conduct a similar study in her setting by reading this section of the research project.

> **Components of methodology section:**
> Study design
> Study setting
> Study duration
> Study population
> Sample size
> Inclusion criteria
> Exclusion criteria
> Study procedure
> Data collection
> Outcome measures
> Data entry and analysis
> Quality assurance
> Ethical considerations

The following are common headings for describing methodology:

- ***Study design:*** Mention the type of study design used like cross-sectional or case-control or cohort.
- ***Study setting/site:*** Where was the study conducted? Hospital or community-based study?
- ***Study duration:*** When was the study conducted? Mention the period of data collection.
- ***Study population:*** Among whom was the study conducted? Whether among patients or healthy population or pregnant women or children or adolescents? Sampling method is also mentioned here.
- ***Inclusion and exclusion criteria:*** What criteria were used to enroll the study participants? For instance, adult patients above age of 18 years only were enrolled in the study and severely ill patients were excluded.
- ***Sample size:*** How many study participants were enrolled? How was sample size calculated and whether calculated sample size was achieved?
- ***Study procedure:*** We mention the flow of activities for this study here. It is usually starting from participant enrolment till the completion of all possible follow-up with the study participant.
- ***Data collection:*** How was the data collected from the study participants? Whether any validated tool or study questionnaire or any equipment was used? Here, we also mention about various variables in study questionnaire. Who collected the data? When and where was the data collected? Any challenges faced during data collection?
- ***Outcome measures:*** The main outcome variable including its scale of measurement and operational definition is explained.
- ***Data entry and analysis:*** Which software was used for data entry and analysis? How were data entry errors handled? How was data analyzed? Which statistical tests were applied? What was the level of significance accepted?
- ***Quality assurance:*** What were the quality assurance measures taken during this study? For instance, conducting double data entry with validation to minimize data entry errors; use of standard validated tool for data collection; blinding/random

allocation of participants in randomized control trial (RCT) are examples of quality assurance measures.
- **Ethical considerations:** Whether the study was approved by the IEC? Whether written informed consent was obtained from the study participants? How privacy and confidentiality were maintained?

### Results
This section presents the findings of the research study. Findings are presented in text, tables, and figures. The statistical tests with *p*-value will be found in this section. We should try to avoid the repetition of all the result findings mentioned in the tables and figures.

### Discussion
Discussion is meant to write the interpretation of the study findings and their implications. Here, we summarize the important findings of the study and explain possible reasons for such study findings. We compare our findings with other research studies. We need to discuss similarities and contradictions with other studies by appropriate logical reasoning. We also state the strengths and limitations of the study. We can also mention the directions for future research. Lastly, it ends with conclusion summarizing the most important study findings. Conclusion should always be aligned with the objectives of the research study. This section gives the researchers a liberty to write in a story telling fashion to maintain the flow of reading.

### References
It is the list of all resources, books or reports or previous research article used as reference in the research study. Reference list is placed at the end after the discussion section in appropriate format such as the Vancouver style.

## USES OF COMPUTER IN HEALTH RESEARCH
Computer applications are helpful in different stages of health research starting from protocol writing till the dissemination of research findings. Following is a brief on uses of computer at different stages.

### During Protocol Writing
Literature search includes finding of reports, health statistics, and existing evidence in the topic of research. Google scholar (http://scholar.google.com) is a generic search engine while PubMed (https://www.ncbi.nlm.nih.gov/pubmed/) is specific for field of medicine. Softwares for sample size calculation, such as Epi Info™ (https://www.cdc.gov/epiinfo/index.html) as well as Statulator (http://statulator.com/SampleSize/ss1P.html) and (http://powerandsamplesize.com) are also available. Epi Info™ also helps to create a structured questionnaire.

### During Research Project Implementation
EpiCollect (https://five.epicollect.net/) is a free electronic data collection tool especially designed for health research. Microsoft Excel can be used for generating random numbers in simple random sampling or for randomized clinical trials.

### For Data Management
Although Microsoft Excel is used for data entry by many researchers, EpiData (http://www.epidata.dk) is a more appropriate tool since it provides facility of more stringent quality checks and double data entry and validation. Basic and some descriptive statistics, e.g., mean, SD and proportion, and t-test can be easily calculated in Microsoft Excel. For other statistical tests EpiData, EpiInfo, and OpenEpi (https://www.openepi.com) are the freely available packages while SPSS, Stata are available to only licensed users. For presentation of data, tables and charts can be easily prepared in Microsoft Excel.

### For Dissemination of Research Findings
Nowadays, the entire process of processing of a research manuscript for publication in a scientific journal is online through the journal's online manuscript submission system. PowerPoint is commonly used for presenting the research findings in conferences meetings for oral or poster presentation.

## SUMMARY
- Purpose of research is to add to the scientific knowledge, change policy or medical practice.
- The quantitative approach of research is done to estimate a problem using numbers, while the qualitative approach is used to explore the different perspectives of the health problem.
- Variable of interest and study population are two important components to define while conducting research. Type of variable and scale of measurement decide how data will be collected and analyzed.
- Probability sampling methods allow the study sample to be representative of reference population.
- Sample size calculation helps us to keep study sample big enough for our study to be scientifically robust while being small enough to be feasible.
- Defining the data collection tool, and analysis plan at the start of the study makes it scientifically robust.
- Methods of data presentation help the researchers communicate research findings in clear and concise manner.
- The tools of biostatistics are useful as descriptive statistics to describe the data in concise form and as inferential statistics to find the chance errors in analytical study findings.
- Interpretation of the research results is as important as applying correct statistical tool. Ensuring ethical conduct in research is important.
- Research report should be sufficiently detailed to allow a scientific critique by another researchers and possible users of the results.

## SUGGESTED READING
1. Bewick V, Cheek L, Ball J. Statistics review 8: Qualitative data—tests of association. Crit Care. 2004;8(1):46-53.
2. Brereton RG. The normal distribution. J Chemom. 2014;28(11): 789-92.
3. CDC. (2017). Epi InfoTM. [online] Available from https://www.cdc.gov/epiinfo/index.html.
4. CDC. (2017). Top 10 Great Public Health Achievements in the 20th Century. [online] Available from http://www.cdc.gov/about/history/tengpha.htm.
5. Cummings S, Browner W, Hulley S. Conceiving the research question and developing the study plan. In: Hulley S, Cummings S, Browner W, Grady D, Newman T (Eds). Designing clinical research: an epidemiologic approach, 4th edition. Philadelphia: Lippincott Williams & Wilkins; 2013. pp. 17-9.

6. Daniel WW, Cross CL. Biostatistics: A foundation for analysis in health sciences, 10th edition. Wiley, New Jersey: John Wiley & Sons; 2013. pp. 614-6.
7. David B. Medical Statistics from Scratch: An Introduction for Health Professionals, 2nd edition. West Sussex: John Wiley & Sons Ltd; 2008.
8. Efficient, Quality-assured Data Capture and Analysis using EpiData. Course Manual. International Union against Tuberculosis and Lung Disease, South East Asia Office, New Delhi.
9. EpiData. (2013). EpiData software. [online] Available from http:// www.epidata.dk.
10. Fathalla MF, Fathalla MMF. A Practical Guide for Health Researchers. Cairo: World Health Organization Regional Office for the Eastern Mediterranean; 2004.
11. Gauss CF. Theoria Motus Corporum Coelestium in Sectionibus Conicis Solem Ambientium, 1st edition. Crawley, United Kingdom: ABC Books, Lowfield Heath; 1809. pp. 1-266.
12. Gupta P, Singh N. How to write the thesis and thesis Protocol: a primer for medical, dental and nursing courses. 1st edition. New Delhi: Jaypee Brothers Medical Publishers (P) Ltd; 2014.
13. Hulley S, Cummings S, Browner W, et al. Designing clinical research: an epidemiologic approach. 4th edition. Philadelphia: Lippincott Williams & Wilkins; 2013.
14. ICMR. (2018). Short Term Studentship. [online] Available from http://14.139.60.56:84/Homepage.aspx.
15. Julio Frenk. The new public health. Annu Rev Publ Health. 1993;14: 469-90.
16. NACO. National Strategic Plan for HIV/AIDS and STI 2017-2024.
17. National Ethical Guidelines for Biomedical and Health Research Involving Human Participants. New Delhi: Indian Council of Medical Research; 2017.
18. OpenEpi. (2013). Open Source Epidemiologic Statistics for Public Health. [online] Available from https://www.openepi.com/Menu/OE_Menu.htm.
19. Structured Operational Research Course material. South-East Asia Office, New Delhi: International Union against Tuberculosis and Lung Disease.

# CHAPTER 12

# Population Science

*Chandresh Pandya, Paragkumar Chavda, Vikas Doshi*

| CM1.8 | Describe the demographic profile of India and discuss its impact on health |
| CM9.1 | Define and describe the principles of demography, demographic cycle, vital statistics |
| CM9.2 | Define, calculate and interpret demographic indices including birth rate, death rate, fertility rates |
| CM9.3 | Enumerate and describe the causes of declining sex ratio and its social and health implications |
| CM9.4 | Enumerate and describe the causes and consequences of population explosion and population dynamics of India |
| CM9.7 | Enumerate the sources of vital statistics including census, SRS, NFHS, NSSO, etc. |

## DEMOGRAPHY—CONCEPT AND DEFINITION

Demography word is derived from the Greek words (***Demo:*** population and ***Graphy:*** measurement or study).

### Definition

*"Demography deals with population size, composition, and geographic distribution and growth in a given geographical area. It also deals with their relationship with social, economic, and behavioral factors."*

Let us understand:
- ***Size*** refers total number of persons residing in the country. It can be enumerated by census. It refers to quantity of the population.
- ***Composition*** deals with the age, sex, literacy level, occupation, income, marital status, languages spoken, and religion. It refers to quality aspect of population.
- ***Population growth*** refers to growth of the population over a period of decades (it may be positive or zero or negative growth. The difference between birth rate and death rate is expressed as a number, which is called as "demographic gap"). It depends upon fertility, mortality pattern, and migration of population.
- ***Distribution:*** Geographic distribution of population in a given country or given area.

> **Note**
> *Main sources for demographic data:*
> - Census (conducted at every 10-year interval)
> - Vital events registration (births, deaths, and marriages)
> - Population surveys
> - Sample registration system (SRS)
> - National Family Health Survey (NFHS)

## Importance of Demography in Public Health

Demographic factors play important role in understanding of health and disease etiology, e.g. age, sex, family size, number of births and deaths, mortality rates, contraception acceptance, literacy level, and marital status.

It is essential to have the knowledge about population with respect to its size, structure, change in its size, and their developments. The application of knowledge of demography is helpful to public health fields for different purposes:
- Mortality rates by age-sex and its geographical distribution with respect to various diseases are helpful to identify the public health importance diseases with respect to age-sex-location, for planning prevention and control measures for the diseases, for determining leading causes of mortality, and for planning manpower and logistics (like medicines, equipment, etc.).
- Population distribution according to age-sex-location is helpful to understand health and healthcare needs of various age groups by sex and location.
- Demographic data are useful for effective planning, designing, evaluation, and execution of health and healthcare needs for the whole population for current and future needs.
- To know the success or failure of health programs.
- To identify the leading causes of mortality and morbidity.

## CURRENT POPULATION TREND AT GLOBAL AND NATIONAL LEVEL

### Global Population Trend

Around 2000 years ago, at the beginning of Christian era, population of world was around 250 million. World population

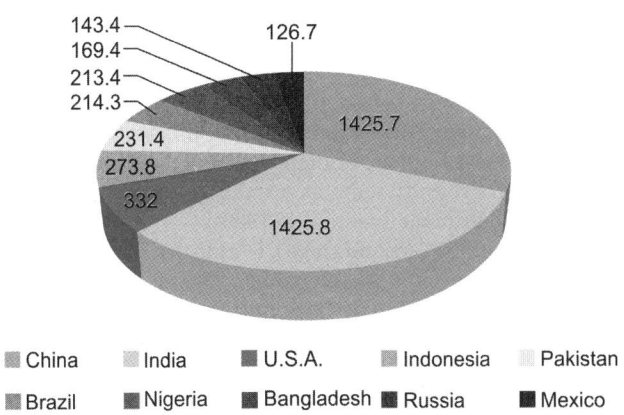

Fig. 12.1: Ten most populous countries of the world (2023) (Population in million).
Source: Worlddata.info

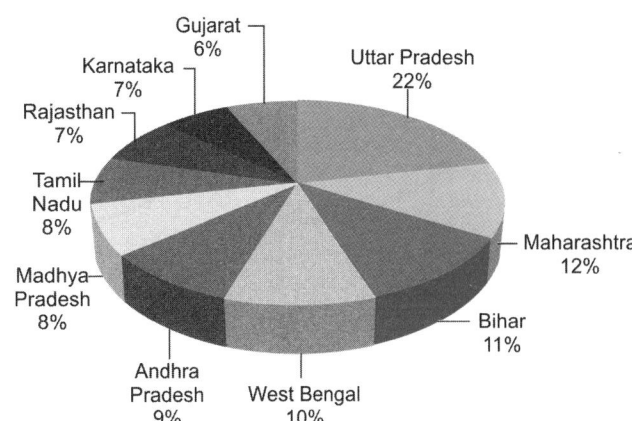

Fig. 12.3: Ten most populous states of India (Census 2011). (*Note:* Percentage shows proportion of each state's population out of total population of these 10 states).

grown slowly for thousands of years to reach 1 billion, thereafter it took almost 200 years to reach 7 billion in 2011 and currently as per United Nations, world's total population has reached 8 billion in November 2022. Current Crude Birth rate of 17 per 1000 population and Crude Death rate of 9 per 1000 population (2021) (data.Worldbank.org).

This growth is due to improvement in living standards and better healthcare services. These have reduced childhood and maternal mortality rates and fertility levels have declined but not at the same rate as mortality rates. Life expectancy is increased over the years, which has added total population.

The top 10 countries of the world according to their population (in million) are shown in **Figure 12.1**. Presently, India is world's most populous country followed by China. Amongst South-East Asia Region (SEAR), three countries—(1) India, (2) Indonesia, and (3) Bangladesh are among the top 10 most populous countries of the world. According to United Nations (UN) projections India's population will reach 1.53 billion by the year 2050.

## India's Situation

Census is main source of information for the population trend in the country. **Figure 12.2** shows trend in census population in

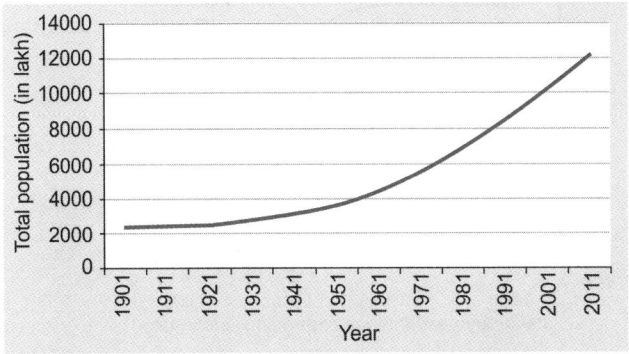

Fig. 12.2: Trend of census population in India (1901–2011).
Source: Office of the Registrar General and Census Commissioner.

India from 1901 to 2011. India's population stood at 121 crore comprising of 62.3 crore (51.5%) males and 58.7 crore (48.5%) females on 1st March, 2011 and this contributes to world's 17.5% population. About 83.4 crore (68.9%) population live in rural areas while 37.7 crore (31.1%) live in urban areas. India has overtaken China with 1425.8 million population in 2023.

India's population was 238 million in 1901, approximately doubled in 60 years to 439 million (1961); doubled again in only 30 years to reach 846 million by 1991. It has crossed 1 billion in 2000, and is projected to reach 1.53 billion by the year 2050.

**Figure 12.2** shows increasing trend of the total population in India during 1901–2011. Only exception is the year 1921 known as "year of great divide" because absolute number of people added to the population during each decade since 1921.

**Figure 12.3** shows the 10 most populous states in India. Uttar Pradesh comes first with about 199.581 million people, Maharashtra comes second with 112.372 million people, and Bihar comes third with 103.804 million people. These 10 states account for about 71% of the total population of India.

## BIRTH RATE AND DEATH RATE

Crude Birth Rate is defined as total number of live births in a given area per 1,000 mid-year population while crude death rate is defined as a total number of deaths in a given area per 1,000 mid-year population.

The pattern of crude birth rate (CBR) and crude death rate (CDR) of India is shown below. According to SRS Bulletin 2022, CBR and CDR of India (for the year 2020) are 19.5 and 6.0 (per 1,000 mid-year population), respectively.

**Figure 12.4** shows declining trend of birth and death rates in India. However, decline in death rate is obvious due to improvement in sanitation, hygiene, and successful implementation of various maternal and child health programs (vaccination, diarrheal diseases, etc.) and better diagnostic facilities and control or treatment of the infectious diseases. Birth rate is also showing declining trend but it is not as per the expected.

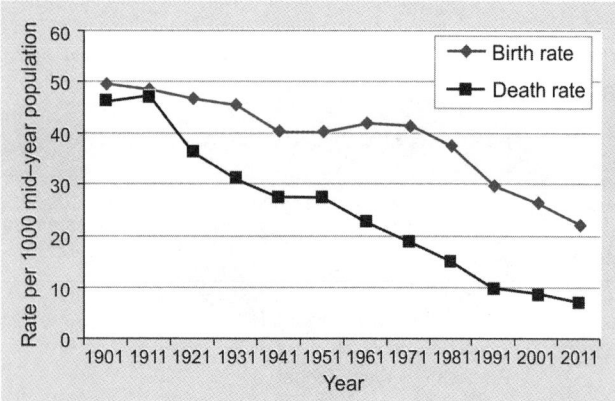

**Fig. 12.4:** Trend of crude birth rate in India (1901–2011).
Source: GOI, Office of the Registrar General and Census Commissioner.

# POPULATION TRANSITION AND DEMOGRAPHIC CYCLE

Demographic composition of the country is changing due to changes in births, deaths, and migration. Demographic indicators are showing population size, population growth rate, geographic distribution, and gender composition, changes in the components like mortality, fertility, mortality, and morbidity.

Demographic indicators are divided into two components—(1) population and (2) vital statistics.

> **Note**
> "Population statistics shows trend of population size and growth, sex ratio, and population density"
> "Vital statistics shows trend of birth rate, death rate, life expectancy at birth, natural growth rate, and mortality and fertility rates."

## Demographic Cycle

It is divided in five demographic stages. Each country passes through these stages over a period of time **(Fig. 12.5)**.

1. **High stationary (first stage):** During this stage, *birth rate and death rate both are at high level* results in no change in population size and it remains at stationary level. Our country had passed through this stage in 1920.
2. **Early expanding (second stage):** During this stage, *death rate starts declining but birth rate remains high or unchanged* and due to this, population of the country may increase. Decline in death rate may be due to improved health conditions and better cure.
3. **Late expanding (third stage):** During this stage, *birth rate starts declining while death rate starts declining more*. Population of country is increasing due to more number of births then deaths. India has entered in this phase. India's current birth rate and death rate are showing declining trend but still birth rate exceeds death rate.
4. **Low stationary (fourth stage):** During this stage, *birth rate and death rate both are at low level* and resulting into stationary population. However, certain countries have achieved zero growth rate also. Most of the developed countries have passed through the stage of low stationary population. UK, Australia, Denmark, and Sweden were in this stage during 1980s.
5. **Declining (fifth stage):** During this stage, *birth rate is lower than death rate and population showing declining trend*. This stage is known as "declining stage". Germany and Hungary are in this stage.

## India's Population Trajectory

**Figure 12.6** shows population trajectory from 1950 to 2023 and projections of United Nations through the year 2100. Current line is of the year 2023. As shown in the image, annual growth

| Stage | Stage name | BR | DR | Examples |
|---|---|---|---|---|
| Stage 1 | High stationary | ↑↑ | ↑↑ | India was in this stage till 1920 |
| Stage 2 | Early expanding | ± | ↓ | South Asia and Africa |
| Stage 3 | Late expanding | ↓ | ↓↓ | India, China, Singapore |
| Stage 4 | Low stationary | ↓ | ↓ | UK, Denmark, Sweden, Belgium |
| Stage 5 | Declining | ↓↓ | ↓ | Germany and Hungary |

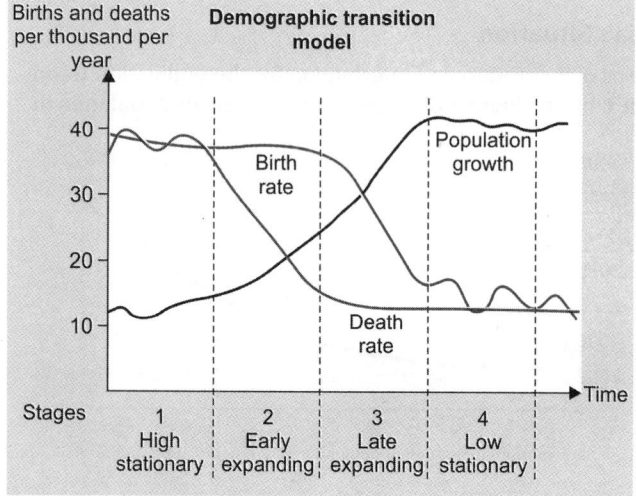

**Fig. 12.5:** Demographic transition model.

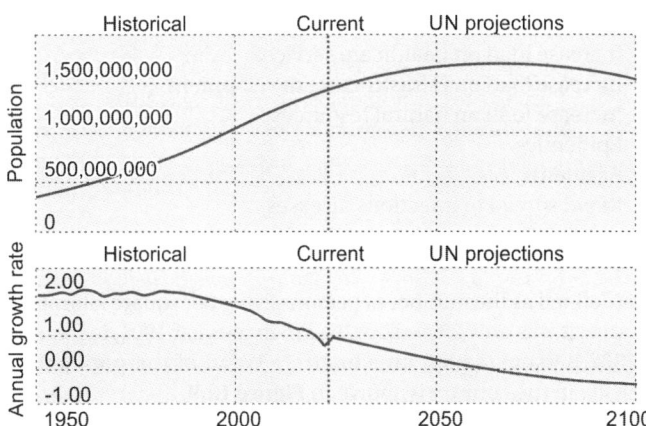

**Fig. 12.6:** India population trajectory 1950-2100.
(*Source:* <ahref='https://www.macrotrends.net/countries/IND/india/population-growth-rate'>India Population Growth Rate 1950-2023</a>.www.macrotrends.net. Retrieved 2023-11-27.)

rate is now in decreasing trends and similarly population will stabilize and eventually a phase will come where annual growth rate will fall below zero and population will have declining trend covering all phases of demographic cycles.

## AGE AND SEX COMPOSITION AND POPULATION PYRAMID

### Age and Sex Composition

The composition of the population age and sex at any particular time-period shows the population trends of fertility, mortality, and migration in recent past and it has impact on current birth and death rates and also future population growth.

Age-sex composition is important consideration for planning of economic development, social and health services, and human resources management in the country. However, age and sex composition of our country has not changed to a large extent but the proportion of 0-6 years age group has declined indicating fall in fertility.

Age composition by age groups for the year 2020 of India is shown in **Table 12.1**. It is observed that for most of the age groups, male-female differences are noticeable in the some age-groups. In the age-group 0-14, male population is about 0.9% more than female, whereas in the age-group 65+, percentage of females is 0.5% point more than males. The proportion of population in the age group 0-14 is higher in rural areas (26.5%) than in urban areas (21.6%) both for male and female.

**Table 12.1:** Percentage distribution of estimated population by age and sex, India (SRS 2020).

| Age group (years) | Population (%) | | |
|---|---|---|---|
| | Total | Male | Female |
| 0-4 | 7.5 | 7.7 | 7.4 |
| 5-9 | 8.3 | 8.4 | 8.1 |
| 10-14 | 9.0 | 9.2 | 8.9 |
| 15-64 | 70.0 | 69.8 | 70.3 |
| 65+ | 5.2 | 4.9 | 5.4 |
| **Total** | **100.0** | **100.0** | **100.0** |

### Population Pyramid

*Population pyramid shows age and sex composition of the population in a graphical way.*

India's age pyramid has broad base and steeply sloping sides, which indicates a large proportion of children and young when we compare the age pyramid of developed countries like Japan, it is in rectangular shape with bulge in the middle and sloping at the younger and older ages. This reflects a less number of children and a higher number of the adults and elderly population. Population pyramid graph of India and Japan for the year of 2020 and 2017 respectively is shown in **Figures 12.7 and 12.8**.

> **Note**
> **Basic differences in population pyramid are:**
> - *Developing country like India:*
>   - Broad base due to high birth rate and more number of younger populations
>   - Concave border and acute apex suggesting less number of elderly population.
> - *Developed country like Japan:*
>   - Narrow base due to low birth rate
>   - Convex border facing outwards
>   - Apex is obtuse due to more number of elderly population.

### Population Explosion

It is defined as massive increase in the population of a country in a very short span of time. As per current estimate India has

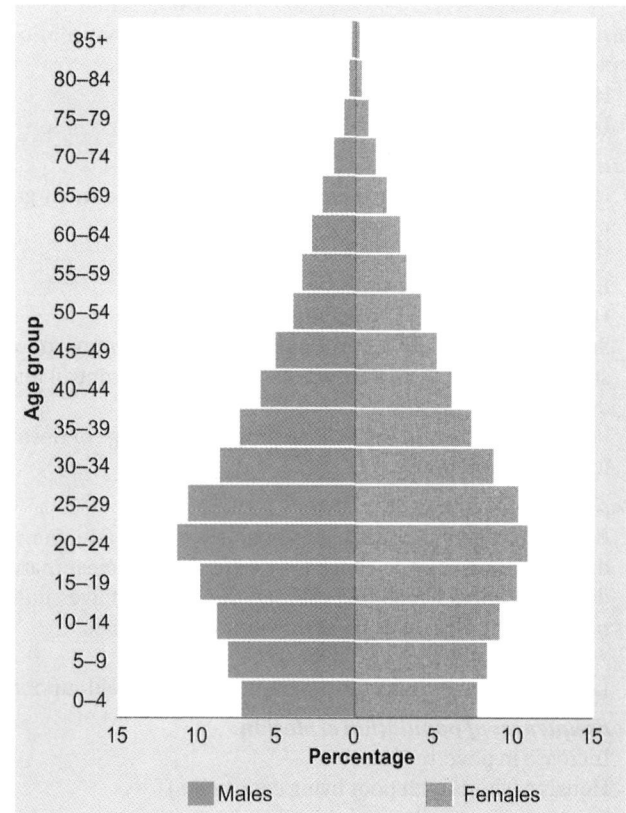

**Fig. 12.7:** Population pyramid of India (2020).
*Source:* SRS Statistical Report 2020.

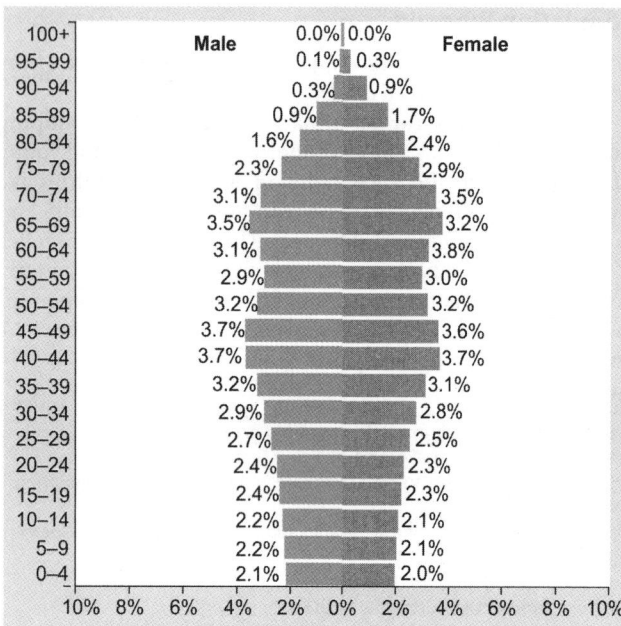

**Fig. 12.8:** Population pyramid of developed country.
*Source:* United Nations. World Population Prospects: The 2019 Revision.

recently overtaken China and now has the highest population (1.43 billion) among all the countries of world. The rampant population growth is the greatest obstacle to the social and economic development of the country.

*Causes:* Mainly two reasons are responsible for population explosion:
1. High birth rate
2. Low death rate

*Causes of high birth rate:*
- Universality of marriage which means everyone must get marry and prove their fertility
- Early onset of puberty
- Early age at marriage
- High proportion of young adults
- Social and cultural factors like poverty, illiteracy, poor standard of living, religious factors against birth control and desire of having a son
- Poor access low availability or no proper knowledge or desire for contraception use

*Causes of low birth rate:*
- Better medical facilities: Medical science made many discoveries because of which they were able to defeat many diseases, illness which had claimed thousands of lives until now were cured because of the invention of vaccines.
- Availability of healthcare facility is also improved
- Launching of various health programs and foreign aid support

*Consequences of population explosion:*
- Increase in poverty
- Housing (slums with poor living conditions)
- Environmental pollution (air, soil and water, etc.)
- Vector problems
- Unemployment
- Increase load on healthcare services
- Increase load on infrastructure development
- Increase load on natural resources
- Epidemics
- Accidents
- Rapid spread of infectious diseases

## Population Density

It is defined as the number of persons living per square kilometer of area. It was only 77 persons/sq.km in the year 1901, increased to 382 persons/sq.km area in 2011. Trend of the population density in the country is shown in **Figure 12.9**.

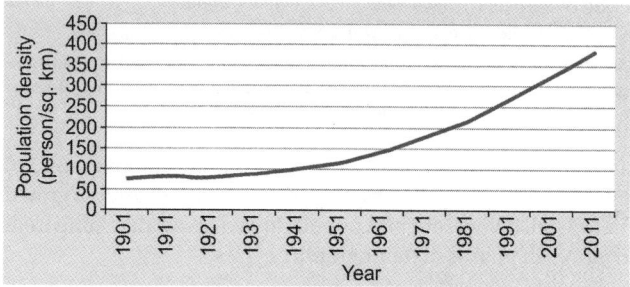

**Fig. 12.9:** Population density of India (1901–2011).
*Source:* Registrar General of India.

# SEX RATIO

*Sex ratio is defined as "the total number of females per 1,000 males".* In an ideal situation there should be equal number of males and females but in reality it is mostly in favor of males.

***Trends in the sex ratio (Census 2011):*** The sex ratio in India has been historically negative or in other words, unfavorable to females. A look at the **Figure 12.10** reveals that in the pre-independence period, the sex ratio declined consistently up to 1951 when it rose marginally. In the post-independence period, the trend continued and the sex ratio slipped down for two consecutive decades after 1951 to reach 930 in 1971. After 1971 Census, trends were not consistent, showing increase in one decade and decline in the next. However, it was hovering around 930, and has shown increasing trend in last two decades.

The patterns in sex ratio among the States and Union Territories are distinct. The top three States recording the highest value of overall sex ratio are neighbors located in the southern part of India namely Kerala (1084), Tamil Nadu (995), and Andhra Pradesh (992). Among the Union Territories (UTs), the top two are Puducherry (1038) and Lakshadweep (946).

The lowest sex ratio among the States has been recorded in Haryana (877), Jammu and Kashmir (883) and Sikkim (889). Among the UTs the lowest sex ratio has been returned in Daman and Diu (618), Dadra and Nagar Haveli (775) and Chandigarh (818).

## Child Sex Ratio (0–6 Years)

Child sex ratio is defined as "The total number of girl children (0–6 years) per 1,000 boys (0–6 years)". Child sex ratio at birth

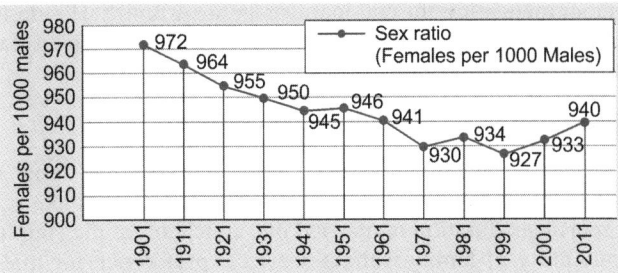

Fig. 12.10: Trend of sex ratio in India (1901–2011).
Source: Census 2011.

is better indicator as it shows pre-birth and post birth situation of girl child in the country. While the overall sex ratio presents encouraging trends across the country encompassing 29 States and Union Territories, the same is not true in the case of the girl child in the age group 0-6 years. **Figure 12.10** clearly brings out the fact that after 1991 there has been consistent rise in overall sex ratio. On the other hand, there is consistent fall in child sex ratio since 1961. As per the population totals of Census 2011, it has declined to reach an all-time low of 914.

The top three States recording the highest value of child sex ratio in the age group 0-6 years are Mizoram (971), Meghalaya (970) and Chhattisgarh (964). Among the UTs, the top three positions are held by Andaman and Nicobar Islands (966), Puducherry (965), and Dadra and Nagar Haveli (924).

The lowest child sex ratio (0-6 years) among the States have been observed in the States of Haryana (830), Punjab (846) and Jammu and Kashmir (859) while among the UTs, Delhi (866), Chandigarh (867) and Lakshadweep (908) occupy the bottom position.

**Adverse sex ratio due to various social and medical reasons:**
- Preference for the male child
- Poor care of girl child—leading to higher mortality of girl child during early age
- Female feticide (sex specific)
- Female child infanticide
- High maternal mortality
- Low social status of female in some parts

*Catalyst factors:*
- Easy access for sex determination testing
- Availability of services for medical termination of pregnancy (MTP)

### Social and Health Implications of Declining Sex Ratio

According to a Youth in India report brought out by the ministry of statistics and program implementation, the sex ratio is declining steadily. It is projected to fall to 898 by 2031. This could have serious repercussions.
- There is a sharp rise in violence against women.
- Likely increase in crimes like trafficking and forced marriages.
- A number of illegal abortions/medical termination of pregnancies (MTP) are conducted leading to poor health of women.
- Male dominated society will lead to reinforcement of patriarchy.
- The economic consequences are grave for this means that a huge proportion of the productive population is missing
- Lower political representation of women will ultimately make it difficult to address their concerns.

Detection of genetic abnormalities and techniques for sex determination are available in the country since 1975 but these utilities were misused for the sex determination and if female fetus is found termination of pregnancy often occurs due to social reasons. Government of India is promoting for the "Save daughters, educate daughters" scheme. This is known as "Beti Bachao, Beti Padhao" scheme. Government has started strict implementation of PC and PNDT (Pre-Conception and Pre-Natal Diagnostic Techniques) Act. Sukanya Samriddhi Account, meant to help families' save for their daughters, Poshan Abhiyan to address the challenges of malnutrition in children, adolescent girls, pregnant women and lactating women and various other schemes like Pradhan Mantri Matru Vandana Yoana, JSSK, JSY, Sakhi and Shakti Sadan are also implemented for upliftment of women in our country.

## DEPENDENCY RATIO

It reflects the economic dependency in any population and it is subdivided into dependency ratio for young age (0–14 years age) and dependency ratio for old age (>65 years of age).

The proportion of persons above 65 years of age and children below 15 years of age are considered to be dependent on the economically productive age group (15–64 years).

It measures number of dependents per 100 (working population) and computed based on three broad age groups, below 15 years, 15–64 years, and 65 years and above.

Total dependency ratio =

$$\frac{\text{Children (0–14 years)} + \text{Population} > 65 \text{ years}}{\text{Population of 15–64 years}} \times 100$$

However, dependency ratio is relatively crude, since it does not take into consideration elderly or young persons who are employed or working age persons who are unemployed. Old age dependency ratio has increased from 7.7% (2001) to 8.1% in the year 2011 due to increase in life expectancy.

It is useful to study dependency burden of population. As fertility declines and life expectancy increases, there is a shift from child dependency to old-age dependency. The rapid decline in dependency ratios, especially the child dependency ratio, has been identified to be a key factor underlying rapid economic development. The term **"demographic bonus"** is called as the period when the dependency ratio in a population declines due to decline in fertility, until it starts to rise again because of increasing longevity. If the switch to small families is fast, the demographic bonus can give a considerable thrust to development. If during this period, investment in healthcare and education are made, maximum advantage can be taken of the demographic transition with high economic growth rates.

The term **"demographic burden"** is called when total dependency ratio is increased due to increase in old age dependency ratio.

## LITERACY RATE

For the purpose of Census, a person aged 7 and above, who can both read and write with understanding in any language, is treated as literate. Ability to read and not to write is not literacy. 'Everyone has a Right to Education' was stated by the Declaration of Human Rights 1948. Education plays a crucial role in economic and social development. Without education, development can neither be broad based nor persistent. Literacy is generally affected by urbanization and industrialization. It plays an important role in the overall development of individuals, which leads to their social, political, and cultural environment better. Higher levels of literacy lead to a greater awareness and also add the improvement to economic conditions which leads to betterment and improvement in their social, political, and cultural environment. Higher levels of literacy also lead to a greater awareness and improved economic conditions.

The literacy rate taking into account the total population in the denominator has now been termed as 'crude literacy rate', while the literacy rate calculated taking into account the age 7 and above population in the denominator is called the 'effective literacy rate'. Effective literacy rate and literacy rate have been used interchangeably in this chapter.

Crude literacy rate =

$$\frac{\text{number of literate persons aged 7 and above}}{\text{total population}} \times 100$$

Effective literacy rate =

$$\frac{\text{number of literate persons aged 7 and above}}{\text{population aged 7 and above}} \times 100$$

Literacy rate of India in different census year is shown in **Figure 12.11**.

Effective literacy rate is defined as the national percentage of literates in the population aged 7 years and above. It is about 74.04 with literate males about 82.14% and females 65.46% in 2011. Also literacy rate varies from states to states. Highest literacy rate is of Kerala (93.91%) followed by Lakshadweep (92.28%), Mizoram (91.58%), Goa (88.70%), and Tripura (87.22%). The literacy rate of Bihar and Arunachal Pradesh is only 63.82 and 66.9%, respectively. The states which have literacy rates below the national average are Arunachal Pradesh, Andhra Pradesh, Bihar, Jharkhand, Jammu and Kashmir, Uttar Pradesh, Rajasthan and Odisha, etc.

## FAMILY SIZE

It means the "total number of children" a woman has borne at a given point of time. This depends upon the factors like age at marriage, duration of married life, education of the couple, availability of family welfare services, preference for male children, etc. The country's family size was 3.9 in 1990 and declined to 3.1 by 2000 year, and 2.5 in 2015 year. It is 4.7 in Nepal, 2 in USA, 1.8 in China, and 1.4 in Japan. If the couples adopt "small family norm", it can further be reduced.

## LIFE EXPECTANCY (EXPECTATION OF LIFE)

It is the average number of years a person is expected to live, according to the mortality pattern existing in that country. This is considered as one of the best indicators of health of the country. Unless otherwise specified, it always refers to $LE_0$ (life expectancy at birth). This includes the risk of infant mortality. The life expectancy at age 1, is the average number of years, an 1-year-old child is expected to live. This excludes the risk of infant mortality. During independence, the combined $LE_0$ for both the sexes in India was 46 years and it reached up to 63–64 years in 2011. It indicates the country's development. $LE_0$ is highest in Japan—80 years for male and 86 years for female.

## FERTILITY AND FERTILITY INDICATORS

Fertility usually refers to actual child bearing. High fertility in India is attributed due to several factors **(Table 12.2)**.

**Table 12.2:** Fertility Indicators of India (SRS Report 2020) (per 1,000 population).

| | Age Groups | Total | Rural | Urban |
|---|---|---|---|---|
| Age-specific fertility rate | 15–19 | 11.3 | 13.2 | 6.6 |
| | 20–24 | 113.6 | 128.1 | 81.8 |
| | 25–29 | 139.6 | 152.5 | 115.2 |
| | 30–34 | 84.4 | 89.4 | 75.5 |
| | 35–39 | 35.6 | 38.9 | 29.5 |
| | 40–44 | 11.7 | 13.5 | 8.5 |
| | 45–49 | 4.7 | 5.2 | 3.9 |
| Age-specific marital fertility indicators | 15–19 | 353.0 | 361.2 | 318.2 |
| | 20–24 | 339.1 | 350.0 | 306.5 |
| | 25–29 | 199.3 | 206.2 | 183.9 |
| | 30–34 | 95.1 | 98.4 | 88.8 |
| | 35–39 | 38.1 | 41.2 | 32.1 |
| | 40–44 | 12.6 | 14.5 | 9.2 |
| | 45–49 | 5.2 | 5.6 | 4.4 |
| Crude birth rate | | 19.5 | 21.1 | 16.1 |
| General fertility rate | | 67.0 | 73.7 | 53.7 |
| Total fertility rate | | 2.0 | 2.2 | 1.6 |
| Gross reproduction rate | | 0.9 | 1.0 | 0.8 |
| Total marital fertility rate | | 5.2 | 5.4 | 4.7 |

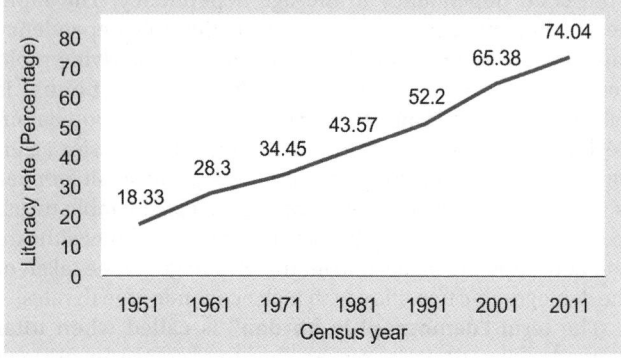

**Fig. 12.11:** Literacy rate (percentage) of India during different census years.

> **Reasons for high fertility in our country:**
> - Universality of marriage
> - Age at marriage (early marriage practices)
> - Early child-bearing
> - Less spacing between children
> - Duration of married life
> - Educational status particularly women
> - Poor socioeconomic status
> - Poor acceptance of family planning and unmet need for family planning
> - Caste and religion their customs and beliefs
> - Nutritional status of women
> - Social status of women.

Some of the factors, which have drawn attention of demographers since long are discussed below:

- *Age at marriage*: Earlier the marriage, more will be the number of children. The Child Marriage Restraint Act, 1978, Hindu Marriage Act, 1925 has governed the age of marriage. The minimum age approved for marriage in India is 18 years for girls and 21 years for boys. If the marriages are postponed for 4–5 years, number of births would decrease by about 20–30%.
- *Duration of married life*: Longer the duration of married life, more will be the fertility. Family planning efforts should be concentrated in the first few years of married life.
- *Spacing of children*: Studies have shown that when all births are delayed by 1 year, in each age group, there was a decrease in total fertility. It means spacing of children may have a significant influence on the general reduction in the fertility rates.
- *Education*: The fertility and educational status are associated inversely. Education provides knowledge; increased exposure to information, and media; forms skill for gainful employment; and increases female involvement in family decision making.
- *Economic status*: Research studies show that economic status has an inverse relationship with fertility. The total number of children born decreases with an increase in per capita expenditure of the household. The World Population Conference at Bucharest stressed that economic development is the best contraceptive and brings about reduction in fertility.
- *Caste and religion*: Muslims have a higher fertility than Hindus. Among this, the lower castes have a higher fertility rate as compared to the higher castes.
- *Nutrition*: Virtually, all well-nourished societies have low fertility as compared to poorly-nourished societies. The effect of nutrition on fertility is mostly indirect.
- *Family planning*: It is another important factor in fertility reduction. In a number of developing countries, family planning has been a key factor in declining fertility. Family planning programs can be initiated rapidly and require only limited resources, as compared to other factors.
- *Other factors*: Fertility is affected by a number of factors such as place of women in society, value of children in society, widow remarriage, breastfeeding, customs and beliefs, industrialization and urbanization, better health conditions, housing, and opportunities for women.

## Fertility Indicators

Fertility can be measured by a number of indicators. Some of the important indicators are described here.

### Crude Birth Rate

*"It is defined as total number of live births in a given area per 1,000 midyear population."*

$$\text{CBR} = \frac{\text{Total number of live births during the year}}{\text{Mid-year population}} \times 100$$

Crude birth rate is simplest measure of fertility and crucial determinants of population growth. However, it is not taking into consideration of child-bearing age group so it does not give true picture of fertility. The CBR of India had declined from 36.9 in 1971 to 19.5 in 2020 over four decades (SRS 2020 Report, published in Oct 2022). However there is a difference in CBR of rural area 21.1 and urban area 16.1 during the year 2020.

In 2020, highest birth rate was in Bihar (25.5) while Andaman and Nicobar had lowest birth rate of 10.8.

### General Fertility Rate

*"It is a refined measure of fertility and defined as the number of live births per thousand women in the reproductive age-group 15–49 (15–44) years."*

$$\text{GFR} = \frac{\text{Number of live births in one year}}{\text{Mid-year female population in the age group 15–44 years (15–49 years)}} \times 1000$$

General fertility rate (GFR) considers the women of reproductive age so it is better indicator over CBR. Though, all the women in the age group of 15–49 years are not bearing child birth.

### General Marital Fertility Rate (GMFR)

*"It is defined as the number of live births per thousand married women in the reproductive age-group 15–44/49 years. This takes into account of only the married women."*

$$\text{GMFR} = \frac{\text{Number of live births in one year}}{\text{Mid-year married female population in the age group 15–44 year (15–49 years)}} \times 1000$$

### Age Specific Fertility Rate (ASFR)

*"It is defined as the number of live births in a year per 1000 women in any specified age group."*

$$\text{ASFR} = \frac{\text{Number of live births in a particular age group}}{\text{Mid-year female population of same age group}} \times 1000$$

It shows fertility in specific age group and in turn reflects effective use of contraception.

### Age Specific Marital Fertility Rate

*"It is defined as the number of live births to married women per 1,000 women in the same age group."*

$$\text{ASMFR} = \frac{\text{Number of live births in a particular age group}}{\text{Mid-year married female population of same age group}} \times 1000$$

### Total Fertility Rate

*"It is the average number of children a woman would have if she passes through the current fertility rates during her reproductive age"* (*Source*: Health and Family Welfare Statistics in India 2017). Total fertility rate (TFR) is one of the most useful indicators reflecting completed family size. It is calculated by summation of all the age specific fertility rates (ASFRs) of all the age groups (If 5-year age group is used).

$$\text{TFR} = 5 \times \frac{\sum_{15-19}^{45-49} \text{ASFR}}{1000}$$

### Total Marital Fertility Rate

Average number of children a married woman would have if she experiences the current fertility pattern throughout her reproductive span.

$$\text{TMFR} = 5 \times \frac{\sum_{15-19}^{45-49} \text{ASMFR}}{1000}$$

### Gross Reproduction Rate

Average number of girls that woman would have if she experiences the current fertility pattern throughout her reproductive span (15–44 or 49 years), assuming no mortality.

$$\text{GRR} = 5 \times \frac{\sum_{15-19}^{45-49} \text{ASMFR for female live births}}{1000}$$

### Net Reproduction Rate

*"It is defined as the average number of daughters a newborn girl will bear during her lifetime assuming fixed age-specific fertility and mortality rates."*

Net reproduction rate (NRR) of 1 is reflects achieving the two children norm. However, for achieving this, 60% of the eligible couples must be covered by any of the approved contraceptive method.

### Couple Protection Rate

*"It is defined as percentage of eligible couples using or protected by one or other approved method of family planning and protected against childbirth."* Current approach is to attain couple protection rate (CPR) more than 60% to achieve goal of NRR = 1. *(This concept is further explained in Chapter 24: Reproductive Health and Family Welfare).*

### Child-Woman Ratio

It is the number of children between the age group of 0–4 years per 1,000 reproductive age group (15–44 or 49 years) women during a given year. It is useful in those areas where birth registration is poor. This data is acquired from census report.

$$\text{Child-woman ratio} = \frac{\text{Number of children between 0 – 4 years}}{\text{Number of women of reproductive age groups}} \times 1,000$$

### Pregnancy Rate

It is the ratio of number of pregnancies in a year to married women of reproductive age group (15–44/49 years) irrespective of outcome, i.e. as live births, stillbirths, or abortions.

### Abortion Rate

The number of all types of abortions, usually per 1,000 reproductive age group (15–44/49 years) women.

### Abortion Ratio

This is calculated by dividing the number of abortions during a particular time period by the number of live births over the same period.

## SOURCES OF VITAL STATISTICS

### Census

Census is one of most important activity of each country for getting information related to population. Census is carried out national wide every 10 years to enumerate total population. India had conducted its first census in the year 1881. Since then census is uninterrupted in the country every 10 yearly.

It is usually carried out in the months of January–March of the first year of every decade. Trained teams visit each and every household for collecting sociodemographic and economic information. National population register was prepared during last census of 2011.

It requires many trained manpower and other recourses. This activity also requires preparation for planning, organizing, training, and actual collection of information from the citizens of country. In India, "de-facto" method is used to collect data. The persons are enumerated according to their exact location at the time of enumeration and under the overall responsibility of Census Commissioner of India.

> **Note**
> **Key points of last census of 2011**
> - Total Population–121 crore (As on 1st March, 2011) comprising of 62.3 crore (51.5%) males and 58.7 crore (48.5%) females
> - Second highest country in total population (17.5%) in the world next to China (19.4%) with only 2.4% of world land
> - 83.4 crore (68.9%) population live in rural areas and 37.7 crore (31.1%) live in urban areas
> - Annual growth rate: 1.8%
> - Population density: 384/km²
> - Overall literacy rate: 74% (males: 82%, females: 65%)

> **Uses of census**
> - It provides demographic information regarding population composition—age and sex-wise composition
> - Social and economic characteristics of people
> - Useful in calculating vital statistical rates and demographic indicators
> - This data is useful for planning, action, and research.

## Civil Registration System

The Registration of Birth and Death Act, 1969
- This is an important act passed by the Government of India for compulsory registration of births and deaths in any part of the country. It includes compulsory Marriage registration also
- After 21 days till 30 days with late fee
- After 30 days till 1 year: Late fee + District registrar written permission (affidavit)
- After 1 year: Late fee + order of Executive Magistrate
- Registration of Name of child: Within 12 months; No charge
- After 12 months of birth till 15 years with charges

## The Sample Registration System (SRS)

This is a large-scale demographic survey conducted by the Office of the Registrar General, India for providing reliable annual estimates of Infant mortality rate, birth rate, death rate and other fertility and mortality indicators at the national and sub-national levels at regular intervals on a dual recording system.

## National Family Health Survey (NFHS)

This is a large-scale, multi-round survey conducted in a representative sample of households throughout India on a periodical basis. The survey provides national and state information on fertility, infant and child mortality, the practice of family planning, maternal and child health, reproductive health, nutrition, anemia, utilization and quality of health and family planning services. International Institute for Population Sciences (IIPS), Mumbai, as the nodal agency, responsible for providing coordination and technical guidance for the survey. NFHS-1 (1992–93), NFHS-2 (1998–99), NFHS-3 (2005–06), NFHS-4 (2015–16) and NFHS-5 (2019–20) are completed.

*Further reading for these is given in Chapter 48: Monitoring and Evaluation System in India.*

## CURRENT APPROACHES IN HEALTHCARE SERVICES

## Program and Policies Related to Population Sciences

You will learn more detail in some other sections on reproductive health but few salient features are narrated.

### National Family Welfare Program

National Program for Family Planning was launched in the year 1952 by Government of India and became the first country to launch Family Planning Program. After implementation of this program, it gained some success but not as per the desired level in fertility control. Effective use and access to contraceptives are essential to achieve goals and these will have impact on maternal, infant, and child mortality. Subsequently shift from family planning to the reproductive child health approach toward community needs assessment approach.

### National Population Policy (NPP)

Government of India launched NPP in the year 2000 to accelerate fertility reduction by target free approach and population norms.

### Pre-conception and Pre-natal Diagnostic Techniques (Prohibition of Sex Selection) Act, 1994 (PC and PNDT Act)

This act was implemented in the country from January 1996 and also amended in the Year 2003 and renamed as "Pre-Conception and Pre-Natal Diagnostic Techniques (Prohibition of Sex Selection) Act, 1994" (PC&PNDT Act)". This act is very much helpful in prevention of sex determination with the use of technology.

*Note: The programs are explained further in detail in Chapter 47: Health Policies and Programs in India. PC and PNDT Act is explained in detail in Chapter 49: Health Legislations in India.*

## SUGGESTED READING

1. Govt. of India, Central Bureau of Health intelligence, Ministry of Health and Family Welfare, New Delhi. (2018). National Health Profile of India-2018.
2. Govt. of India, Ministry of Health and Family Welfare, New Delhi. (2017). Health and Family Welfare Statistics in India 2017, Statistics Division.
3. Govt. of India, Ministry of Health and Family Welfare, New Delhi. (2018). Annual Report of Health and Family welfare 2017-18.
4. Govt. of India, Office of the Registrar General & Census Commissioner, India, Ministry of Home Affairs.
5. National Family Health Survey, India, International Institute for Population Sciences (IIPS) Mumbai.
6. Population pyramid. Population Pyramids of the World from 1950 to 2100.

# CHAPTER 13

# Social Medicine

*Late Shobha Mishra, Shalini Sundaram, Kalpita Shringarpure, Niyati Parmar*

**CM2.5** Describe social security measures and its relationship to health and disease

## SOCIAL MEDICINE: INTRODUCTION

It is an interdisciplinary field of medicine that focuses on interplay between socioeconomic and individual health outcomes. It seeks to understand how specific social, economical, and environmental conditions directly impact health, diseases and the delivery of medical care, and to promote conditions and interventions that address these determinants, aiming for a healthier and more equitable society.

Historical development of social medicine can be traced back to the early 19th century after the advent of the Industrial Revolution which resulted in an increase in poverty and disease among workers and raised concerns about the effect of social processes on the health of the poor and marginalized.

The term "social medicine" was coined by Rudolf Virchow (1821-1902), a German physician and politician who urged physicians to go beyond individual explanations of diseases and instead consider the social factors that may play role in the health and illness of their patients. Now he is remembered as "the founder of Social Medicine". The British Public Health specialist Thomas McKeown in his published thesis "The role of medicine: Dream, mirage or nemesis?" argued that decline in mortality due to infectious diseases was primarily due to better nutrition and better hygiene and marginally due to interventions such as Antibiotics. Though criticized at his times for his ideas, his work is equally significant in present understanding of Social Medicine.

Some of the aims of social medicine are:
- To understand and address the complex relationships between social, economic, cultural and environmental factors on individual health as well as that of the community.
- To promote health equity, prevent diseases, improve health systems and foster collaboration between different stakeholders and disciplines.

## Objectives of Social Medicine

Objectives are measurable and specific targets through which the discipline sets to achieve its aims. Some notable objectives of social medicine are:
- To investigate how factors like income, education, employment, race, gender, caste, class, housing and social support impact health outcomes.
- To study disparities in health outcomes in different groups based on racial, economic gender, caste, class or other demographic factors and create strategies to promote equal health opportunities for all.
- To examine psychological factors such as attitudes, beliefs, emotions, behaviors and its effect on health outcomes.
- To apply epidemiological methods to study the distribution and determinants of diseases in population.
- To evaluate how different health policies and programs, health care systems and structures impact health outcomes.
- To develop strategies to improve the health status of people through prevention, promotion, interventions or management.

Since then, social medicine has evolved into a vast and diverse field that covers a wide range of topics concerning the intersection of health and society. Community Medicine is extension of the same. Important topics in this regard include:
- ***Social determinants:*** Social determinants of health are the factors that influence health outcomes. They represent the conditions in which people are born, grow, work, live and age. They also include the wider set of forces and systems that shape people's daily life. e.g. income, education, employment, race, gender, housing and social support's impact on health outcomes.
- ***Health equity and disparity:*** Studying disparities in health outcomes among different groups based on racial, economic, gender, caste or other sociodemographic factors and creating strategies to promote equal health for all.
- ***Health systems and policies:*** Evaluating how different healthcare systems, structures and policies impact health outcomes.
- ***Social epidemiology:*** Applying epidemiological methods to study the distribution and determinants of diseases in populations.

- ***Social psychology:*** Examining how social-psychological factors such as attitude, beliefs, emotions, behaviors and interactions influence health behavior and outcomes.
- ***Health economics:*** Analyzing the costs and benefits of health interventions from a societal perspective.

## SOCIAL DIAGNOSIS

Clinical diagnosis needs to be supplemented by social diagnosis by exploring the social dimensions associated with the medical issue. Drawing parallels with "clinical medicine", it can be called as a "social pathology". These factors may be related, e.g., to the place of work, to various social institutions, to social customs, or to the working of government. Research and methods to find out these factors can be conducted in various ways, some of which are given below:

### Social Surveys

Social surveys play an important part in development of public health. They disclose social pathology. The foundation of the General Board of Health in 1848 in Great Britain was laid by a survey conducted by Chadwick. There is a strong kinship between epidemiological survey and social survey. When the objective of the research is to study the role of social factors in the etiology of disease, the two merge into "social epidemiology". Socio-epidemiological studies have investigated the relationship of the social factors leading to heart disease, cancer and arthritis.

### Case Studies and in-depth Interviews

A case study explores and analyzes the life of a social unit—a person, a family, an institution, culture group or even an entire community. Case study determines the factor that accounts for the complex behavior patterns of the unit and the relationship of the units to its surrounding milieu. The case study attempts to collect a large amount of information from a small number of units. It is a complete workup of the patient that will involve information gathering from the records, from their family members, and if necessary, conduct certain investigations to complete the picture. Thus, it yields valuable data about the cases. A combination of case study and survey can provide more information about a population of interest then either method could do alone. However, case study has its limitations, i.e. a single instant may or may not be representative of a larger population. In-depth interviews (IDI) of key informant individuals are like case studies, but they are not extensive follow-ups or study of the associated records, but the case studies may extend beyond one session or months depending upon objective, research question and purpose.

### Focus Group Discussion

Focus group discussion (FGD) is *"A group interview centered on a specific topic which seeks to generate primarily qualitative data, by capitalizing on the interaction that occurs within the group setting"*. It consists of around eight participants excluding the moderator and the recorder for the discussion. A typical FGD lasts for about 45 minutes. The participants in a group should be such that they belong to the same group so that they can share and discuss their issues. There should be no administrative or social hierarchy among the participants which can lead to lack of information sharing. A sociogram should be drawn by the recorder to ensure that all participants are interacting equally among themselves in the FGD **(Fig. 13.1)**. The venue selected for a FGD should be a neutral venue, acceptable to all. A series of FGDs is required to arrive at saturation, when no new information is further available **(Fig. 13.2)**.

### Field Study

Surveys are concerned with the breadth of knowledge (systematic collection of data from populations or samples of populations

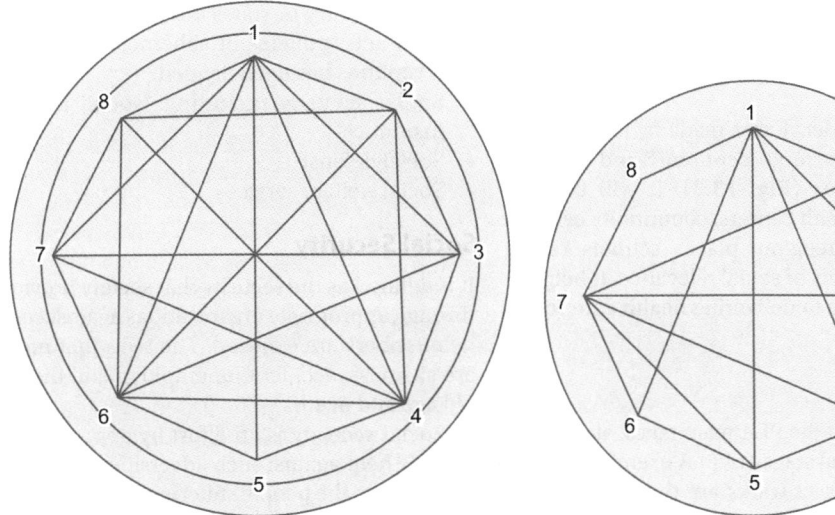

Sociogram representing good FDG     Sociogram representing limited participation

**Fig. 13.1:** A sociogram.

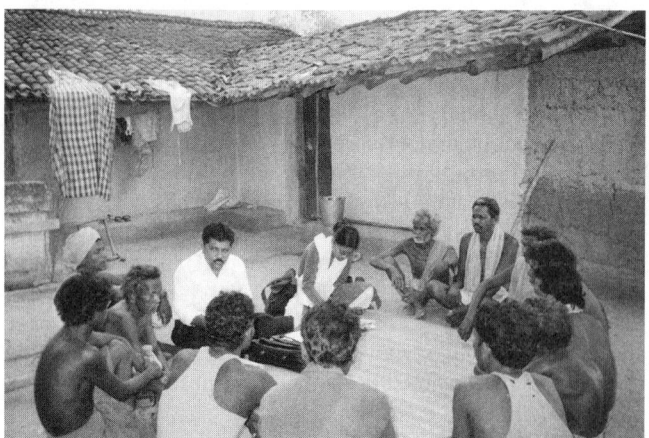

**Fig. 13.2:** Focus group discussion (FGD) setting.

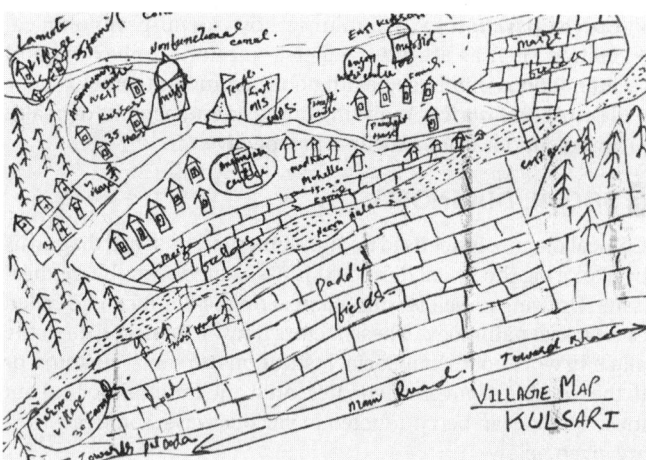

**Fig. 13.3:** Social map.

through personal interviews or other data gathering devises). Field studies, however, are concerned with depth of knowledge; they involve observation of people in situ.

## Participatory Rural Appraisal/Participatory Learning Action/Participatory Action Research (PRA/PLA/PAR)

In the mid-80s people's participation in rural development was realized, that led to Rapid Rural Appraisals (RRA). RRA since 1990s is known as PRA/PLA/PAR, i.e., participatory rural appraisal/learning action/action research.

Community-based knowledge is *first hand*, elicits and uses local and comprehensive information. Hence, community participation in problem analysis and solution planning (decentralized planning) can bring community ownership and sustainability of proposed managerial and operational solutions.

It empowers people by increasing their problem analysis, identification and solving capacities. This is effective for quick managerial and operational solutions, required for fixing the problems. For those program managers who aim to develop programs/strategies "with" than "for" people, it is an important tool in the field. Social mapping and transect walk are useful methods of PRA/PLA.

## Social Mapping

It is a visual representation of local area made by local people to explain sociocultural, behavioral, economic and political dimensions of the study area (**Fig. 13.3**). It will capture information such as roads, health centers, community centers, water drinking points, lakes, religious places, schools, refuse collection sites, and other points of social relevance. It helps in better planning with reference to delivering health care to the community.

## Transect Walk

These are purposive walks that the PLA team takes, along with community people in the initial stages of PLA exercise, usually after mapping exercise. Transect walks are therefore spatial data gathering tools. Transect walks help PLA team observe the people, surroundings and resources and understand their issues, problems and opportunities for interventions. This is done by marking different areas on the social map that you aim to observe with a line and reason/plan, make an observation guide, talk to local people in the marked area during the walk to assess situation, come back, make a diagram and notes, debrief and make final notes.

## SOCIAL THERAPEUTICS/SOCIAL INTERVENTIONS

Most of the diseases require that social factors are addressed along with the medical treatment to effectively tackle the public health problem. For example, for health promotion and better health outcomes nutritional supplements or supports are provided to vulnerable section of the society and group. For protecting people from ill-environmental conditions support for acquiring decent housing to the people living in slums is provided. Communities with better social support system build healthier community. This social support system is formed traditionally by communities as an informal community behavior, culture or custom or formal social system build by society. Country or states are providing social support through various acts, policies or schemes. Social support in form of interventions has been divided:

- Social security including "social assistance and social insurance"
- Social defense
- Social welfare services

## Social Security

It is defined as the security that society provides to its members through appropriate organizations against certain risks to which its members are exposed. The risks that most countries cover are sickness, accident, unemployment, disabilities, maternity, old age and death.

Social security is an effort by appropriate organizations to provide help against such adversities. It is important to provide such help to the people suffering from adversity in life because if they are not secured timely, then their number in the community will increase which may in turn lead to social pathology affecting the development of the entire community and country. Thus, social security is a safety net, providing income and support to such individuals facing life's challenges and aims for a society where everyone feels secured and empowered to reach their full potential.

Social security has two faces: 1. Social Assistance and 2. Social Insurance.

**Difference between the two are as follows:**

| Social Assistance | Social Insurance |
|---|---|
| Beneficiaries are unemployed widows, orphans, handicapped, old-age people who cannot contribute money. | Beneficiaries are industrial workers, employees of central and state government who can contribute money. |
| Noncontributory | Contribution by beneficiary and the employer |
| Involves feeling of charity or sympathy | Remittances are received as matter of right |
| Not backed by legislation | There are several legislations |
| Motive is maintenance of minimum level of living | Motive is planning for future |
| Benefits may be in form of cash or in kinds of food aid | Benefits are in proportion to the contributions made by the individual |
| Designed to supplement income of the vulnerable group | Designed to supplement income of the individual as a part of future planning |
| Members may become permanently dependent on the scheme | Members may not become permanently dependent on the scheme |
| Examples: Pension for old age, widow maternity benefit schemes, PM-JAY | Examples: Private Insurance, contributory pension scheme, provident fund |

In India, social security policies aim to deliver cash and quasi-cash payments to individuals and families. Generally, India's social security schemes cover the following types of social insurances: (1) Pension, (2) Health Insurance and Medical Benefit, (3) Disability Benefit, (4) Maternity Benefit, and (5) Gratuity.

Legislations act as the backbone to ensure such securities reaches to the workers, women, children and disenfranchised people safeguarding their rights and well-being throughout their employment journey. These laws also serve a multitude of purposes, ranging from establishing minimum living standards to promoting fairness and fostering responsible work environments.

### Some Key Social Security Acts for Workers in India

1. Employees' State Insurance Act, 1948: Provides healthcare benefits to employees and their dependents.
2. Employees' Provident Funds and Miscellaneous Provisions Act, 1952: Mandates contributions to a provident fund for retirement benefits.
3. Payment of Gratuity Act, 1972: Entitles employees to gratuity payments upon retirement or leaving the company.
4. Maternity Benefit Act, 1961: Provides paid maternity leave and other benefits to pregnant and lactating women.
5. Employees' Compensation Act, 1923 (Amendment 2017): Compensates workers for injury, disability, or death arising from work-related accidents.
6. Mines Act, 1952: Regulates working conditions and safety standards in the mining industry.
7. Building and Other Construction Workers (Regulation of Employment and Conditions of Service) Act, 1996: Ensures welfare and safety of construction workers.
8. The Unorganized Workers' Social Security Act, 2008: Aims to provide social security benefits to unorganized sector workers
9. The Code on Social Security, 2020: Subsumes nine central labor legislations, simplifying and streamlining social security provisions.
10. Employment Exchange Act, 1972: This act sets up machinery for the registration of unemployed persons and for notifying vacancies to them by employment exchanges. It also provides for vocational guidance and training to the unemployed.
11. National Food Security Act 2013, also known as Right to Food Act, is an Indian Act of Parliament which aims to provide subsidized food grains to approximately two thirds of the country's people.

Some of the key social security schemes in India are shown in **Table 13.1**.

### Social Defense

A new concept has come into vogue in recent times—the concept of social defense. Social defense is a system developed to defend the society against criminality not merely by treating and defending the offended, but also by creating such conditions and taking remedial steps in the community which are conducive for health and wholesome growth of human life. Included in this are measures related to the prevention and control of juvenile delinquency, eradication of beggary, social and moral hygiene program, welfare services in prisons, prison reforms, elimination of prostitution and control of alcoholism and drug addiction. Many States in India have enacted the "Children Act for the Prevention and Control of Juvenile Delinquency". Under the services of the "Immoral Traffic Act in Women and Girls Act", services are provided for the elimination of prostitution in society.

### Social Welfare

Despite economic progress, India faces persistent poverty, inequality, and vulnerabilities. While social security schemes are aimed to provide cash and cash-like payments to individuals and families, social welfare system delivers assistance in the form of services.

Under Social Welfare, various services and benefits are provided by government and non-governmental organizations which are crucial to bridge the gaps of social inequality and ensure that marginalized vulnerable groups have a chance to thrive. Reservation in education and occupation is conventions social welfare approaches. Scholarship, boarding schools for tribal are some of the other examples for addressing social determinant like education.

There are many social welfare schemes run by Government of India for different sections of the society. Some of the targeted vulnerable groups are:

**Table 13.1:** Social security schemes.

| Scheme | Beneficiaries | Support and Eligibility Criteria | Launch Date | Implementing Agency |
|---|---|---|---|---|
| **Pensions** | | | | |
| Atal Pension Yojana (APY) | All citizens aged 18-40 | Regular contributions starting from ₹42/month | May 2015 | Ministry of Finance (MoF) |
| National Pension Scheme (NPS) | All citizens | Flexible contributions and investment choices | January 2004 | Ministry of Finance and Pension Fund Regulatory and Development Authority (PFRDA) |
| Old Age Pension Scheme (OAP) | Varies by state (e.g., senior citizens) | State-specific eligibility criteria and benefits | Varies by state (1960s-2000s) | Department of Social Welfare (DSW) within state governments |
| National Social Assistance Programme (NSAP) | Disadvantaged groups (e.g., widows, disabled, transgender) | Financial assistance under NOAPS (National Old Age Pension Scheme), NFBS (National Family Benefit Scheme), IGNWPS (Indira Gandhi National Widow Pension Scheme), IGNDPS (Indira Gandhi National Disability Pension Scheme) | April 1995; IGNWPS and IGNDPS added in 2009 | Ministry of Social Justice and Empowerment |
| **Elderly and Maternity** | | | | |
| Pradhan Mantri Vaya Vandana Yojana (PMVVY) | Senior citizens | Assured returns & pension benefits for 10 years | April 2017 | Ministry of Social Justice and Empowerment) |
| Maternity Benefit Scheme | Pregnant & lactating mothers from low-income families | Financial assistance | Varies by state (1990s-2010s) | Department of Women and Child Development |
| **Health Insurance** | | | | |
| Pradhan Mantri Jan Arogya Yojana (AB-PMJAY) | Eligible beneficiaries (e.g., below poverty line) | Cashless treatment for various illnesses and hospitalization | September 2018 | Ministry of Health and Family Welfare |
| Rashtriya Swasthya Bima Yojana (RSBY) | Families below poverty line | Health insurance coverage of ₹30,000 per family per annum. | October 2003 | Ministry of Labor and Employment |
| **Life and Accidental Insurance** | | | | |
| Ayushman Bharat Pradhan Mantri Jeevan Jyoti Bima Yojana (PMJJBY) | Saving bank account holders in 18-50 years age group. | Life cover of ₹2 lakh for ₹436/year premium | March 2015 | Ministry of Finance and Department of Financial Services |
| Pradhan Mantri Suraksha Bima Yojana (PMSBY) | All citizens | Accidental death cover of ₹2 lakh for accidental death or permanent disability and ₹1 lakh for partial disability for ₹12/year | May 2015 | Ministry of Finance and Department of Financial Services |
| Aam Aadmi Bima Yojana (AABY) | All individuals aged 18-70 | Accidental death cover of ₹2 lakh and disability cover of ₹1 lakh for ₹20/year | May 2015 | Ministry of Finance Department of Financial Services |
| **Other Schemes** | | | | |
| National Safai Karamcharis Finance and Development Corporation (NSKFDC) | Sanitation workers and their dependents | Financial assistance and skill development programs | January 1997 | Ministry of Social Justice and Empowerment |
| Pradhan Mantri Shram Yogi Maan-dhan (PM-SYM) | Unorganized sector workers aged 18-40 years age, monthly income ₹15000 or less. | Monthly pension of ₹3,000 after attaining age 60 for regular contributions | March 2019 | Ministry of Labor and Employment |

- Scheduled tribes/scheduled caste/backward caste welfare
- Women and child development
- Unorganized sector
- Differentially-abled welfare
- Senior citizen welfare, and
- Urban rural poverty alleviation.

Some of the key social welfare schemes in India are shown in **Table 13.2**.

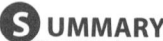

## UMMARY

Illness is not only a medical problem, but also a social problem. Person and/or community suffer from disease or could not enjoy good health are due to underlying social factors, like income, education, nutrition, inequality, etc. Understanding of biological science is alone is not sufficient for health and diseases outcomes. Knowledge and application of social medicine are also require for holistic management of health and disease for an individual and community. Formal and informal social support mechanisms are the most important measures under social medicine.

**Table 13.2:** Social welfare schemes.

| Scheme | Beneficiaries | Eligibility Criteria and Support | Launch Date | Ministry |
|---|---|---|---|---|
| **Poverty Alleviation and Financial Inclusion** | | | | |
| Mahatma Gandhi National Rural Employment Guarantee Act (MNREGA) | Adult members of rural households, who demand and volunteer to do unskilled manual labor | Guranteed 100 days of minimum wage employment per year. Otherwise unemployment allowance is given. | Feb 2006 | Ministry of Rural Development |
| Pradhan Mantri Jan Dhan Yojana (PMJDY) | All households in India | No income or banking history required. | August 2014 | Ministry of Finance |
| Pradhan Mantri Ujjwala Yojana (PMUY) | Primarily rural women living below the poverty line | BPL card holders. LPG connections are provided. | May 2016 | Ministry of Petroleum and Natural Gas |
| Pradhan Mantri Gramin Awaas Yojana (PMGAY) | Rural households below the poverty line | BPL card holders. | April 2016 | Ministry of Rural Development |
| **Rural and Village Development** | | | | |
| Pradhan Mantri Sahaj Bijli Har Ghar Yojana (SAUBHAGYA) | All households in the country | BPL card holders. | September 2017 | Ministry of Power |
| Pradhan Mantri Adarsh Gram Yojana (PMAGY) | Rural villages with more than 50% SC population | Set performance indicators for integrated development into model villages | October 2014 | Ministry of Social Justice and Empowerment |
| **Skill Development and Livelihood Generation** | | | | |
| Pradhan Mantri Kaushal Vikas Yojana (PMKVY) | Unemployed youth aged 18-35 | Aadhaar card and educational qualification (varies by course) | July 2015 | Ministry of Skill Development and Entrepreneurship |
| **Healthcare and Women's Empowerment** | | | | |
| Pradhan Mantri Matru Vandana Yojana (PMMVY) | Pregnant and lactating women for their first living child | Bank account and Aadhaar card | January 2017 | Ministry of Women and Child Development |
| Pradhan Mantri Surakshit Matritva Yojana (PMSMVY) | Pregnant and lactating mothers for first child | ANC care especially during 2nd and 3rd trimester, on 9th of every month | Jan 2017 | Ministry of Women and Child Development |
| Janani Shishu Suraksha Karyakram (JSSK) | Pregnant and lactating women and children under 5 years | Free delivery and essential child healthcare services | June 2011 | Ministry of Health and Family Welfare |
| Mission Shakti | Women (focus on marginalized and vulnerable) | Aims for safety, security, and empowerment of women through legal, economic, and social initiatives | 2021-22 | Ministry of Women and Child Development |
| **Early Childhood Development** | | | | |
| Integrated Child Development Services (ICDS) | Children aged 0-6 years, pregnant and lactating mothers | No specific criteria, focuses on underserved communities | October 1975 | Ministry of Women and Child Development |
| Mid-day meal scheme (POSHAN abhiyan) | School going children up to 8th standard. | Meal is provided | August 1995 | Ministry of Education |
| Beti Bachao Beti Padhao (BBBP) | All girls and women | Promotes gender equality, girl child education, and women's empowerment | Jan 2015 | Ministry of Women and Child Development |
| Mission Vatsalya | Children in difficult circumstances (juveniles, orphans, abandoned, street children) | Ensures holistic care and protection for children in need | April 2022 | Ministry of Women and Child Development |

# SUGGESTED READING

1. Health & Family Welfare | National Portal of India [Internet]; 2022. Available from: https://www.india.gov.in/topics/health-family-welfare.
2. Marmot M, Wilkinson R. Social determinants of health, 2nd edn. Oxford: Oxford University Press; 2005.
3. Nettleton S. The sociology of health and illness, 4th edn. John Wiley & Sons; 2020.
4. Schemes | National Portal of India [Internet]. 2022. Available from: https://www.india.gov.in/my-government/schemes.
5. Social policy and inclusion [Internet]. www.unicef.org. Available from: https://www.unicef.org/india/what-we-do/social-policy-inclusion.

# CHAPTER 14

# Health Communication

*Tulika Goswami, Tushar Manohar Rane, Abu Hasan Sarkar, Veena Kumari, Manjit Boruah*

| | |
|---|---|
| **CM 1.6** | Describe and discuss the concepts, the principles of health promotion and education, IEC and Behavioral change communication (BCC) |
| **CM 4.1** | Describe various methods of health education with their advantages and limitations |
| **CM 4.2** | Describe the methods of organizing health promotion and education and counselling activities at individual family and community |

## DEFINITION AND CONCEPTS

Communication can be defined as the process of transmitting information and common understanding from one person to another (Keyton, 2011). The word communication is derived from the Latin word, communis, which means common.

The definition underscores the fact that unless a *common understanding* results from the exchange of information, there is no communication. **Figure 14.1** reflects the definition and identifies the important elements of the communication process (Cheney, 2011).

## NEED FOR COMMUNICATION IN HEALTH

### Clinical

A fruitful doctor-patient communication is the most important clinical function required in building a therapeutic doctor-patient relationship. This is important as this can lead to the delivery of better healthcare. Many a time, patient dissatisfaction and complaints are due to the breakdown in doctor-patient communication.

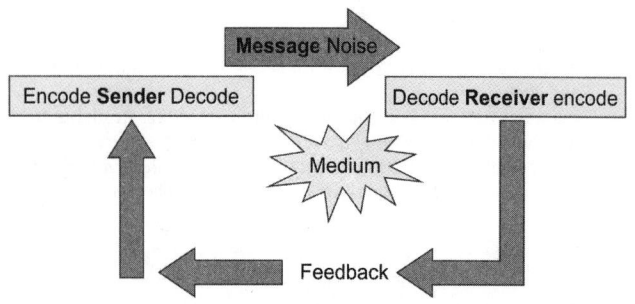

Fig. 14.1: The communication process.

The three main goals of current doctor-patient communication are: (1) creating a good interpersonal relationship, (2) facilitating exchange of information, and (3) including patients in informed decision making. Effective doctor-patient communication is determined to a large extent by the doctors' "bedside manner," which patients judge as a major indicator of their doctors' general competence. Patients reporting good communication with their doctor are more likely to be satisfied with their care, follow advice, and adhere to the prescribed treatment. Patients' agreement with the doctor about the nature of the treatment and need for follow-up is strongly associated with the treatment outcome.

### Public Health

Many of the threats to global public health (through diseases and environmental calamities) are rooted in human behavior. As public health practitioners, you ask tough questions, meticulously analyze data, craft policies, and work on behalf of entire populations of people. Those activities alone are challenging, but they are not finished until they are understood by the community.

Mostly, public health programs are based on two specific pillars—(1) supply of services and (2) its utilization and demand by community members. Behavior and practice of community members are essential and primary drivers of good health, e.g., breastfeeding practices. Therefore, it is critical to acknowledge the participation and ownership of communities in making any health program successful. Communication is needed in healthcare to harness community participation and ownership, which are critical to success of any health program.

Public health communications attempt to bring a change either in behavior or belief. While influencing public opinion or actions, consistent messaging and tone help to position the communicator as stable and dependable. The cohesiveness of materials will help the public build-confidence and accept change with less resistance. Public health communication draws from numerous disciplines, including mass and speech communication, health education, marketing, journalism, public relations, psychology, informatics, and epidemiology. Although, it is transdisciplinary in nature, the core principles of public health communication are firmly anchored in the central tenets of public health.

# COMMUNICATION PROCESS

The key elements in communication process (refer **Fig. 14.1**):
- **Communicator (the originator of the message)**: A communicator must know clearly about the objectives, target audience (their type, interest, and abilities), the accurate message (content and usefulness), and the available channels of communication.
- **Message (it is the information the communicator wishes to give)**: A good message will get good results so it should be carefully chosen, clearly understandable, specific to the needs, timely, appropriate, appealing, and fit to the audience customs, beliefs, and attitudes. It should not hurt the sentiments of the audience as that may lead to a negative impact.
- **Audience (they are the consumers of the message)**: They may be a total population or a specific group in the population, i.e. target audience.
- **Channels of communication (i.e. medium of communication)**: The selected medium should be cost-effective, easily available. A two-way communication is the most effective medium of communication. This should be adjusted to the local cultural pattern of the people. It should create interest among the people.
- **Feedback**: It is the most important component of communication loop. It signifies the importance of establishing the accurate transmission of information from sender by checking with the receiver, if the intended message has been received by him/her. It also reflects that communication is effective only if it is two-way.

# TYPES OF HEALTH COMMUNICATION

## One-way Communication (Didactic Method) and Two-way Communication (Socratic Method)

- **One-way communication**: The flow of communication is "one-way" from the communicator to the audience. The familiar example is the lecture method in classrooms. The drawbacks of the didactic method are:
  - Knowledge is imposed
  - Learning is authoritative
  - Little audience participation
  - No feedback
  - Does not influence human behavior.
- **Two-way communication**: The Socratic method is a two-way method of communication in which both the communicator and the audience take part. The audience may raise questions, and add their own information, ideas, and opinions to the subject. The process of learning is active and "democratic". It is more likely to influence behavior than one-way communication.

## Verbal Communication and Nonverbal Communication

- **Verbal communication**: The traditional way of communication has been by word of mouth. The advent of written and printed matter is of comparatively recent origin. Direct verbal communication by word of mouth may be loaded with hidden meanings. It is persuasive. Nondirect or written communication may not be as persuasive as the spoken word.
- **Nonverbal communication**: Communication can occur even without words. It includes a whole range of bodily movements, postures, gestures, and facial expressions (e.g. smile, raised eyebrows, frown, staring, gazing, etc.). Silence is nonverbal communication. It may at times speak louder than words.

## Formal and Informal Communication

Communication has been classified into formal (follows lines of authority) and informal (grape-vine) communication. Informal network (e.g. gossip circles) exists in all organizations. The informal channels may be more active, if the formal channels do not cater to the information needs.

## Visual Communication

The visual forms of communication comprise—charts and graphs, pictograms, tables, maps, posters, etc.

## Telecommunication and Internet

Telecommunication is the process of communicating over distance using electromagnetic instruments designed for the purpose. Radio, television (TV) and internet, etc. are mass communication media, while telephone and telegraph are known as point-to-point telecommunication systems. The point-to-point systems are closer to interpersonal communication (IPC). With the launching of satellites, a big explosion of electronic communication has taken place all over the world.

# METHODS IN HEALTH COMMUNICATION

Communication methods may be grouped into individual communication, group level, and community level.

## Individual and Family Level

Detail information can be given about the illness such as causation, mode of transmission, complications, treatment, prevention, sanitation, hygiene, etc. to individual and family. Here, the role of the doctor is very high and responsibility is very great because the patient and the family members constitute "captive audience". Health education at family level is best given by health workers and health assistants. The biggest advantage is that the educator may persuade the individual to change his/her behavior. Population covered is small in this type of communication method.

## Group Level

### Lecture

It is a presentation of the facts on a particular topic in an organized way by a qualified person.
- *Merits:* It is simple, accepted, and one-way method. It can be made more effective by using aids like chalk and writing legibly on the blackboard. This method can be made much more impressive and effective by using audiovisual aids. However, "chalk and talk" is traditional method of teaching.

- *Demerits:* Audience may get bored and lose the interest in-between. Learning is passive. It may fail to influence the health behavior of the people.

### Demonstration

In this method, procedure is performed and shown to the participants, e.g. preparation of oral rehydration salt (ORS) solution, accurate method to use condom. The participants repeat that skill by doing. Since this method involves active participation of the participants so they develop interest, understand it better, and then they change or improve in their behavior. This method involves the participants in discussion.

### Discussion Methods

- **Group discussion:**
  - The group usually comprises of 6–12 persons, with common interest and almost of the same educational level. They all seat in a circular fashion facing each other. Group "leader", initiates the subject and manages the discussion by preventing tangential conversation, motivates everyone to participate and finally summarizes the entire discussion. A "recorder" prepares a sociogram and a report on the discussion and on the decision taken.
  - Group discussion is effective as it permits free exchange of thoughts and ideas and also the decision taken by the group, tends to be adopted more readily. The demerits are that those who are shy, do not take active part in discussion and some may dominate in the discussion or there may be irrelevant discussion.
- **Panel discussion:** A group of 4–6 experts in a particular topic get around the table in the presence of audience. One among them is the Chairman who opens the meeting, welcomes the audience, introduces the panel of speakers to the group of audience and then introduces the topic briefly, and initiates discussion. The panel members discuss among themselves about the particular topic. Audience does not participate. However, if there is an arrangement for the audience to throw questions toward the end, then it is called "panel discussion forum". *Advantages:* Exploration of a problem in different angles; change of speakers maintains attention and interest among the audience. *Disadvantages:* Panel may not cover all aspects of the topic and audience remains passive listener throughout.
- **Symposium:** It is also a lecture form but the difference is that different speakers (experts) give lecture on different topics (aspects) of the same subject. The Chairman, who is also an expert, opens the symposium with a brief introduction, introduces the speakers and calls upon them one after the other to speak. At the end of each speech and before the next person begins, the Chairman makes some transitional remarks to serve as a link between what has been presented and what is to be followed and also to give his own views if any. For example, symposium on sexually transmitted disease (STD) will be as follows:
  - Anatomy expert—talks on anatomy of reproductive system.
  - Physiology expert—talks on physiology of reproduction and sexuality.
  - Pathologist—talks on pathological changes in the reproductive organs in STD.
  - Pharmacologist—talks on the list of treatment to cure STD.
  - Physician—talks on the clinical features and complications of STD.
  - Specialist in community medicine—talks on epidemiology, prevention, and control of STD.

  There is no discussion among the experts unlike in panel discussion. Symposium is of particular application to a mature group who has the listening attitude and the capacity to appreciate.
- **Seminar:** In this method of health education, one expert will speak about the different components of the same subject, to a group, having a common interest or discipline. These are usually conducted in academic or research institutions to have a high-level academic discussions, which will help for research purposes. There is a coordinator for the seminar. Preliminary planning is essential for seminar.
- **Workshop:** It consists of group of members, who are subdivided into small groups, each of about 4-6, each group having a chairman and recorder, discussing a part of the problem and leave the workshop finally with a plan of action, decided by the group. The guidance is given by the experts, who act as resource persons. Since, the participants share the knowledge, learning takes place in a friendly and happy atmosphere.
- **Conference:** It is a get together of experts or learned people being held usually once in a year, wherein the recent advances or the research work taken up will be presented before the audience, thereby gives an opportunity not only to meet their colleagues but also to learn recent advances. It is almost a continuing education usually held at State or National level.
- **Role playing (sociodrama):** In this method, education is given by a group in the form of a drama, to make the communication more impressive and effective, especially to school children, illiterate villagers, and such others. Role playing is followed by a discussion of the problem.
- **Brainstorming:** In this method, a problem is solved by group discussion. A group of 5–20 people participate, collecting, and recording the ideas or suggestions of each of the member and finally the decision is made. Brainstorming is done in four stages. In the first stage, the problem for which solutions are required is defined, so that the members are clear about their suggestions. In the second stage, the group leader invites suggestions and records them irrespective of whether it is right or wrong. No discussion is permitted among them. In the third stage, each suggestion is reviewed, so that it is made clear to everyone what the suggestion is and whether the suggestion to be included or excluded for further discussion. In the last and fourth stage, all suggestions are discussed to decide which one to be accepted and to develop the ideas further.
- **Tutorial:** A small group of learners are guided by a teacher to help clear the doubts, and confusions, improve understanding of the subject.
- **Colloquy:**
  - In this method of group discussion, the members from the audience initiate discussion by asking questions to

the experts on the stage, who will answer on the various aspects.
- Colloquy is especially useful when there are specific problems to be discussed for solution. One of the experts acts as a moderator who conducts the discussion. The effectiveness of the colloquy depends upon the efficiency of the moderator. The advantage is that there is a direct participation of the audience. It provides opportunities to extract information from experts. The experts will try to solve the controversial problems also if any.
- **Debate**: In this type of discussion method, two sets of speakers talk on "For" and "Against" a particular resolution or a statement and give their opinion.

## Community Level (Approach)

It consists of educating the whole community (mass approach). It is not possible by one or two persons. It usually employs "*mass media communication*". There are various ways to achieve community level communication. They are as follows:
- **Television**: It is the most potent of all the media because it appeals to both eyes and ears. It can mold the attitude and behavior of the people effectively. It is cost-effective.
- **Radio**: This appeal only to the ears. It is the cheapest mass media communication and quite potent also. Radio talk should not exceed more than 10–15 minutes.
- **Press materials**: These cater only to the eyes. The most widely disseminated form and most powerful press material is the newspaper. Other materials are posters, pamphlets, books, internet so on. Only demerit is that illiterate persons are not educated through press materials. They can be educated only through first-two methods.
- **Folk medias**: These are the indigenous methods such as kirtan, harikatha, folk dance, folk songs, dramas, puppet shows, qawwali, ghazals, etc.
- **Role play (sociodrama)**: Acting out a situation by a team of members, simulating a real-life situation, thereby the audience understand and appreciate the situation and implement in their daily life. Thus, it helps in changing (improving) their knowledge, attitude, and behavior of the people. Even though the community approach is "one-way" communication, it is effective in reaching millions of people.
- **Health magazines**: Good health magazines are also important channels of communication, e.g. Swash Hind (from Delhi), Herald of Health (from Pune), etc.

## LEVELS OF IMPACT OF COMMUNICATION

Health communication may be attempted at a number of different levels, and following levels of impact have been identified by the Centre for Disease Control and Prevention:
- **The individual:** The individual is the most fundamental target for health-related change, since it is individual behaviors that affect health status. Communication can affect the individual's awareness, knowledge, attitudes, self-efficacy, and skills for behavior change. Activity at all other levels ultimately aims to affect and support individual change.
- **The social network:** An individual's relationships and the groups to which an individual belongs can have a significant impact on his or her health. Health communication programs can work to shape the information a group receives and may attempt to change communication patterns or content. Opinion leaders within a network are often a point of entry for health programs.
- **The organization:** Organizations include formal groups with a defined structure, such as associations, clubs, and civic groups; worksites; schools; primary healthcare settings; and retailers. Organizations can carry health messages to their membership, provide support for individual efforts, and make policy changes that enable individual change.
- **The community:** The collective well-being of communities can be fostered by creating structures and policies that support healthy lifestyles and by reducing or eliminating hazards in social and physical environments. Community-level initiatives are planned and led by organizations and institutions that can influence health—schools, worksites, healthcare settings, community groups, and government agencies.
- **The society:** Society as a whole has many influences on individual behavior, including norms and values, attitudes and opinions, laws and policies, and the physical, economic, cultural, and information environments. Health communication alone, however, cannot change systemic problems related to health, such as poverty, environmental degradation, or lack of access to healthcare, but comprehensive health communication programs should include a systematic exploration of all the factors that contribute to health and the strategies that could be used to influence these factors. Well-designed health communication activities can help individuals better understand their own and their communities' needs so that they can take appropriate actions to maximize health.

## BARRIERS TO COMMUNICATION

Communication is not adequate if the message the sender wishes to convey is not identical to what is actually understood by the receiver.
- **Physical barriers:** Faulty equipment, surrounding noise, closed doors, poor lighting, etc. can act as physical barriers.
  - *Physiological*—difficulties in hearing, expression, and delivery of speech
  - *Psychological*—emotional disturbances, neurosis, levels of intelligence, language, or comprehension difficulties
- **Linguistic barriers:** India is a land of many languages and dialects. Differences in knowledge and understanding of these between the sender and the receiver of the message can act as a barrier.
- **Cultural barriers:** Ethnic, religious and social differences can act as another barrier. How one greets another person on meeting is mostly a cultural phenomenon specific to the culture. For example, a handshake between a man and a woman may be alright in some cultural contexts but may be considered highly offensive in another.
- **Semantic barrier:** This occurs due to the difference in interpretation of meanings of words in messages. There are various contributors to semantic barriers, viz. use of multi-meaning words, misleading translation, use of long and complex sentences, use of too many jargons, etc.

Even when health services are readily available, the social and cultural barriers can present serious problems to the achievement of health behavior change. These barriers should be identified and removed.

## APPLICATION OF HEALTH COMMUNICATION

- **IEC**—stands for information, education, and communication. It aims to generate specific awareness to target audiences. IEC is usually done for all health programs in three stages, viz. (1) planning, (2) implementation and (3) evaluation.
- **BCC**—behavioral change communication attempts to generate awareness among targeted recipients with an ultimate aim to change their behavior. BCC may be positive for health promoting habits and attitude or negative for harmful attitudes and habits.
- **SBCC**—social BCC (SBCC) is an interactive, researched, planned, and strategic process with the aim to change social conditions and individual behaviors. *The "C-planning" communication planning model* is strongly related to socioecological model where first step of C-planning is drawn from the socioecological model. It emphasizes on identification of *barriers and facilitators of change* as well as their indirect and underlying causes in terms of "understanding the situation".
- **Interpersonal communication**—one-to-one dialogue-based communication.
- **Group communication**—group discussions and street plays.
- **Mass media**—TV, radio, and newspapers.
- **New information technologies**—social media platforms using mobile phones.

## SUCCESS STORY: "COMMUNICATION" THE GAME CHANGER IN SUCCESS OF POLIO

India achieved one of the biggest achievements in global health—it was certified as polio-free by the World Health Organization (WHO) after 3 years without an endemic case of polio. After almost 20 years of fighting the disease, the Government of India (GOI), with the support of the World Bank, the United Nations International Children's Emergency Fund (UNICEF), WHO, Rotary International, civil society organizations, and millions of volunteers, finally graduated from being one of the four last countries in the world where the polio virus remains endemic.

The social mobilization strategy of SBCC was the game changer in this movement against Polio in India. UNICEF had led the social mobilization and communications side of efforts. Experience of professionals involved in this initiative tells that the focus was on creating demand for the vaccination and raising awareness about its benefits in public. The India model of community support was also used in Nigeria in efforts toward polio eradication.

The social mobilization strategy for polio-free India had the objective of establishing credibility for immunization in public. For building credibility for immunization, much of the focus was laid on bringing in influential leaders, like religious and local political leaders and doctors to participate in local functions to build sense of trust in public regarding immunization.

Another important communication technique that was used in the polio program in India is branding. Pink and yellow colors were used to symbolize the polio campaign and public or communities associated the colors with immunization and knew that there was a campaign on seeing such visuals. Use of celebrities as spokes people for the campaign across variety of media such as TV, radio (mass media), posters, banners, newspapers (print), in group communications in remote areas, and text messages played a critical role in making the program successful.

The success in India came down to creating a universal understanding and agreement among local and national government and among faith leaders that immunization was important. All relevant stakeholders took ownership of the program within their particular responsibility.

## SKILLS FOR GOOD INTERPERSONAL COMMUNICATION

Interpersonal communication is face-to-face verbal or nonverbal exchange of information, ideas, and feelings between two or more people. Each time, a doctor or health service provider has contact with a client or patient, communication is taking place.

Improved doctor-patient communication tends to increase patient involvement and adherence to recommended therapy; influence patient satisfaction, adherence, and healthcare utilization; and improve quality of care and health outcomes.

The key elements of effective IPC—there are three main types of communication interactions that occur within a provider-client relationship. They are:

1. **Caring**: The goal is to establish and maintain a positive rapport with the patient.
2. **Problem solving**: The goal is for the patient and provider to share all necessary information for accurate diagnoses and appropriate treatment.
3. **Counseling**: The goal is for the patients to understand their condition and adhere to their treatment.

While they occur throughout an interaction, these types of communication often happen sequentially, with caring communication to establish a positive tone, then problem solving to diagnose, and finally counseling to provide relevant health education. To communicate effectively through these different interactions, it can help to keep in mind some key elements of effective IPC.

The following techniques help providers improve client-patient interactions:
- **Effective questioning** helps to obtain useful information from the client. Questioning is a way to determine what service the patient wants. It is also a way to determine whether the patient has understood well. Open-ended questions like "how are you feeling?" encourage the patient to offer information. Close-ended questions like "Do you have any allergies?" help to obtain specific information.
- **Active listening** helps in getting the information needed to assist the patient with problems. Active listening means paying attention to what is being said, observing nonverbal communication of the patient, and using actions such as having eye contact and nodding.

- **Reflection or echoing** occurs when a provider observes a client's emotions and reflects them back to him/her. This helps the provider check whether the emotions he/she has observed are correct. It also helps to show that the provider has empathy and respect for the client's feelings.
- **Summarizing and paraphrasing** means repeating back to the client what you heard him/her say in a short form. It helps to ensure that you have understood correctly and provide an opportunity for clarification.
- **Praise and encouragement** build a patient's sense of confidence and reinforce positive behaviors. This occurs when providers use words and gestures that motivate and ensure a patient of their approval.
- **Giving information** clearly and simply with visual aids helps equip clients with accurate and relevant health information that is based on what the client already knows.

**Good interpersonal skills** can be attained by receiving training on communication skills and emotional intelligence. Understanding the concept of emotional intelligence enhances the doctor-patient relationship by a large extent. Further discussion on emotional intelligence is beyond the scope of this chapter.

# HEALTH EDUCATION

The ultimate aim of health communication is to understand the dynamics of health education. Health education is the way of transferring current scientific knowledge in a simple way to adapt or abandon certain health behaviors and or health concepts. Health education has been defined in various ways. According to John M Last health education is "the process by which individuals and groups of people learn to behave in a manner conducive to the promotion, maintenance, or restoration of health".

**The Declaration of Alma-Ata (1978)** defines health education as "a process aimed at encouraging people to want to be healthy, to know how to stay healthy, to do what they can individually and collectively to maintain health, and to seek help when needed".

## Approaches to Health Education

1. **Regulatory approach**—any direct or indirect intervention taken by the government to bring change in the existing behavior. Example of Cigarettes and Other Tobacco Products Act (COTPA), 2003 may be considered here. It prohibits the use of cigarettes in public places to prevent passive smoking.
2. **Service approach**—services may be delivered to people at their home irrespective of their acceptance or denial. This approach was tried by the government earlier; however, it failed to bring in the desired change.
3. **Health education approach**—people usually do not belief in something which they are not aware of. Providing health education to people results in change of understanding and change of perception. It helps in creating demand of the services by the people.
4. **Primary healthcare approach**—this is based on the concept of primary healthcare where people participate, think, and decide for themselves with the help of government, e.g., role of Anganwadi workers in ICDS.

## Principles of Health Education

Health education cannot be "given" to one person by another. It involves, among other things, the teaching, learning and inculcation of habits concerned with the objective of healthful living. There are certain principles of learning which can be used in health education.

- **Credibility:** It is the degree to which the message to be communicated is perceived as trustworthy by the receiver.
- **Interest:** It is a psychological principle that people are unlikely to listen to those things which are not to their interest. It is salutary to remind ourselves that health teaching should relate to the interests of the people.
- **Participation.**
- **Motivation.**
- **Comprehension:** In health education we must know the level of understanding, education and literacy of people to whom the teaching is directed.
- **Reinforcement:** Few people can learn all that is new in a single period. Repetition at intervals is necessary. If there is no reinforcement, there is every possibility of the individual going back to the preawareness stage.
- **Feedback.**
- **Learning by doing.**
- **Setting an example.**
- **Good human relations.**

# HEALTH PROMOTION

Health promotion is the process of enabling people to increase control over their health and its determinants, and thereby improving their health.

The first International Conference on Health Promotion was held in Ottawa in 1986 and was primarily a response to growing expectations for a new public health movement around the world. The basic strategies for health promotion identified in the Ottawa Charter (Fig. 14.2) were: *advocate* (to boost the factors which encourage health), *enable* (allowing all people to achieve health equity) and *mediate* (through collaboration across all sectors). Since then, the WHO Global Health

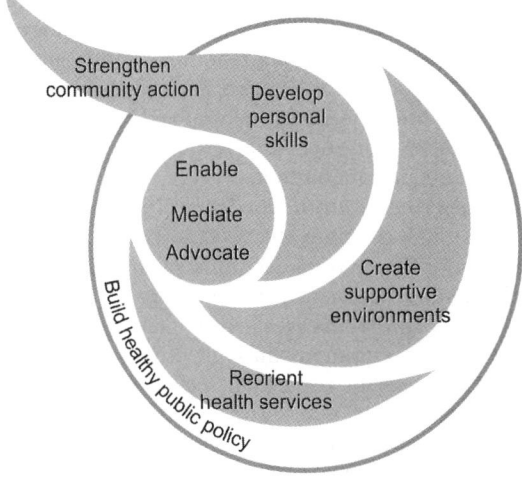

**Fig. 14.2:** Ottawa Charters Health Promotion Emblem.

**Table 14.1:** Methods of organizing health promotion, education and counseling activities at different levels in community.

| Level for health education | Example | Methods | Advantages | Limitations | Suggested Aids |
|---|---|---|---|---|---|
| Single person | • HIV/STD Counseling | • Counseling<br>• Personal/key person interview | • Complete attention<br>• Confidentiality<br>• Two-way process | • Requires long time<br>• Trained counselors required | • Pen and paper<br>• Photographs<br>• Models<br>• Charts |
| Family or group | • HIV/STD Counseling<br>• Training of trainers for different health programs | • Focus group discussions<br>• Practical<br>• Demonstration<br>• Workshops<br>• Counseling | • Attention level is high<br>• Understanding is good<br>• Good for training purposes<br>• Nearly two-way process | • Require well train educators who can make group people concentrate throughout the time<br>• Homogenous or common interest group is required<br>• People may start discussion among themselves | • Overhead projection system<br>• Charts<br>• Models<br>• Chalk and board<br>• Videos |
| Large group | • Education of students<br>• Training of large population groups (ASHA, Anganwadi workers, etc.) | • Lecture<br>• Panel discussion<br>• Symposium<br>• Role playing | • Education reach to large number of persons<br>• Collective questions can be attended<br>• Understanding is good | • Mostly one-way communication<br>• Managing target audience will become difficult sometimes<br>• No individual attention so requirement of individual understanding level is high | • Chalk and board<br>• Miking and announcement system<br>• Overhead projector system |
| Communities | Health education starting from village level and can be up to country level | • Exhibition<br>• Pamphlet distribution<br>• Posters/Banners<br>• Mass medias (Television, News Papers, Radio, Internet, Social Media) | • Message is conveyed very quickly and will reach to very large number of population living even in far areas<br>• Cost effective | • Target audience attention might be less<br>• Only general messages in simple language can only be provided | - |

Promotion Conferences have established and developed the global principles and action areas for health promotion.

These strategies are supported by five priority action areas:

1. ***Build healthy public policy:*** Health promotion puts health on the agenda of policy makers in all sectors and at all levels, combines diverse but complementary approaches including legislation, fiscal measures, taxation and organizational change and contributes to ensuring safer and healthier goods and services, healthier public services, and cleaner, more enjoyable environments.
2. ***Create supportive environments for health:*** Systematic assessment of the health impact of a rapidly changing environment—particularly in areas of technology, work, energy production and urbanization, is essential and must be followed by action to ensure positive benefit to the health of the public. The protection of the natural and built environments and the conservation of natural resources must be addressed in any health promotion strategy.
3. ***Strengthen community action for health:*** Health promotion works through concrete and effective community action in setting priorities, making decisions, planning strategies and implementing them to achieve better health.
4. ***Develop personal skills:*** Health promotion supports personal and social development through providing information, education for health, and enhancing life skills. This has to be facilitated in school, home, work and community settings.
5. ***Re-orient health services:*** The responsibility for health promotion in health services is shared among individuals, community groups, health professionals, health service institutions and governments. Reorienting health services also requires stronger attention to health research as well as changes in professional education and training. This must lead to a change of attitude and organization of health services which refocuses on the total needs of the individual as a whole person.

Methods of organizing health promotion, education and counselling activities at different levels in community is shown in **Table 14.1**.

## SUMMARY

Health communication has become an accepted tool for promoting community health. Health communication principles are often used today for various disease prevention and control strategies including advocacy for health issues, marketing health plans and products, educating patients about medical care or treatment choices, and educating consumers about healthcare quality issues. At the same time, the availability of new technologies and computer-based media is expanding access to health information and raising questions about equality of access, accuracy of information, and effective use of these new tools. The many roles that health communication can play have been highlighted by the Centers for Disease Control and Prevention. These roles include:
❖ Increase knowledge and awareness of a health issue, problem, or solution
❖ Influence perceptions, beliefs, attitudes, and social norms
❖ Prompt action
❖ Demonstrate or illustrate skills
❖ Show the benefit of behavior change
❖ Increase demand for health services
❖ Reinforce knowledge, attitudes, and behavior
❖ Refute myths and misconceptions
❖ Help coalesce organizational relationships
❖ Advocate for a health issue or a population group.

## SUGGESTED READING

1. Bernhardt JM. Communication at the core of effective public health. Am J Public Health. 2004;94(12):2051-3.
2. Brédart A, Bouleuc C, Dolbeault S. Doctor-patient communication and satisfaction with care in oncology. Curr Opin Oncol. 2005;17:351-4.
3. Dahama OP, Bhatnagar OP. Education and Communication for Development, 2nd edition. New Delhi: Oxford and IBH; 1987.
4. Effective Interpersonal Communication: A Handbook for Health Care Providers [Internet]. 2008. Available from: https://ccp.jhu.edu/documents/EffectiveInterpersonalCommunication_HandbookforProviders_0.pdf.
5. FAO. Communication for Rural Development. Guidelines for Planning and Project Formulation (2014).
6. Garland JV. Discussion Methods, New York: MH Wilson; 1951.
7. HIPS. Effective interpersonal communication: A handbook for health care providers. John Hopkins University; 2008.
8. Hubley J. Communicating Health: An Action Guide to Health Education and Health Promotion, 1st edition. London: The Macmillan Press Ltd; 2004.
9. IGNOU. Information, Education and Communication.PGD, MCH-1, Preventive MCH. New delhi: IGNOU.
10. Last JM. A Dictionary of Public Health. London:Oxford University Press; 2006.
11. Lilbert JJ. Educational Handbook for Health Personnel. Geneva: WHO; 1977.
12. Malik A. International Business Communication. National Programme on Technology Enhanced Learning (Phase II). Ministry of Human Resource Development. Govt of India.
13. Sarkar AH, Senapati J. Emotional Intelligence in Medical Practice. RHiME. 2016;3:31-6.
14. Thomas RK. Health communication. USA: Springer Publications; 2006.
15. University of Twente. Health Belief Model; 2017.
16. WHO. Vector Control in Primary Health Care. Tech Report Series; 755.

# SECTION 3
# Community Health Problems and Vulnerable Groups

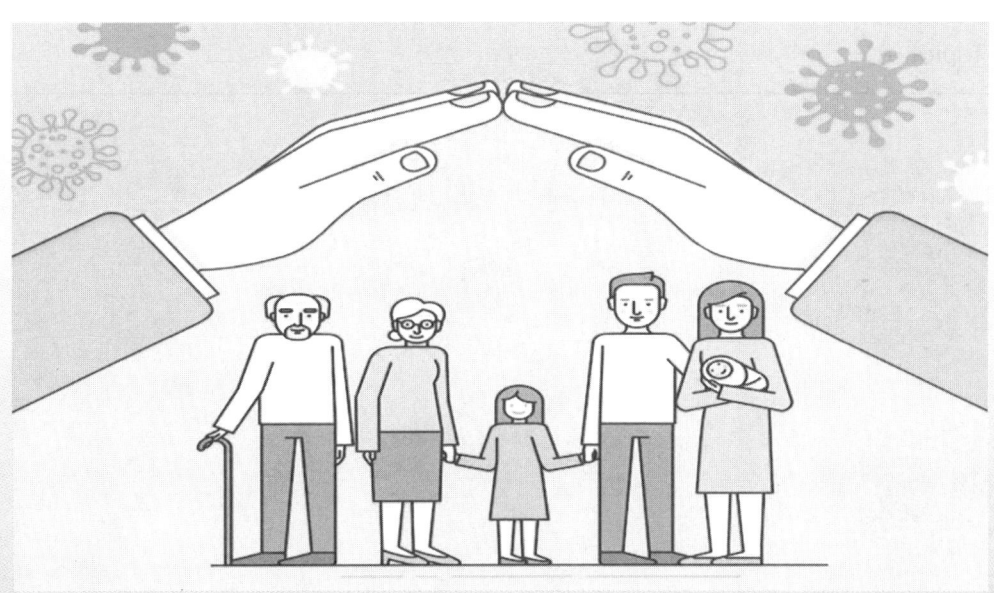

*'Few' affects 'Many' and 'Few' are affected by 'Many'. Master the art of 'Few' and 'More' to make community healthy.*

# SECTION OUTLINE

15. History and Important Events in Community Health
16. General Epidemiology of Infectious Diseases and its Prevention and Control
17. Specific Epidemiology of Infectious Diseases
18. General Epidemiology of Noncommunicable Diseases and its Prevention and Control
19. Specific Epidemiology of Noncommunicable Diseases
20. Primary Health Care Approach to Noncommunicable Diseases
21. Screening for Noncommunicable Diseases
22. Noncommunicable Disease Surveillance
23. Epidemiology of Nutrition and Food-related Diseases and its Prevention and Control
24. Reproductive Health and Family Welfare
25. Maternal Health
26. Child Health
27. Adolescent Health
28. Geriatric Health
29. Occupational Health
30. Mental Health
31. Urban Health, Rural Health and Tribal Health
32. Traveler's Health
33. Genetics and Health
34. Special Topics

# CHAPTER 15

# History and Important Events in Community Health

*Devraj R, Bishan S Garg*

*We are not makers of History. We are made by History*
—*Martin Luther King Jr*

## INTRODUCTION

The history of public health dates back to antiquity (before 500 AD), and was substantially revived during the medieval period that was marked by plague epidemics in Europe. The Renaissance witnessed the rise of eminent scholars like Paracelsus. The age of liberalism started in 1790, which included a wide range of philosophical, political, economic, and religious ideas which marked the revival of public health. During the 18th and 19th centuries, breakthroughs occurred in the development of smallpox vaccination and the formulation of epidemiologic methods such as spot mapping. The period from the beginning of the 20th century to the present has seen a rapid growth in public health; two of the landmark achievements of this period being the eradication of smallpox and identification of smoking as a cause of cancer.

The historical events in community health are dealt under two sections:
1. Emergence of public health issues—key milestones
2. Public health interventions.

## EMERGENCE OF PUBLIC HEALTH ISSUES— KEY MILESTONES

### Plague—The Black Death (1347)

The Black Death stands out as the most dramatic life changing event during the middle ages. From 1347 AD when the first signs of Plague were seen in Europe, the next three years witnessed the Black Death killing almost one-third of all the people in Europe. This drastic demographic change in the late middle ages caused great transitions in European culture and lifestyle.

Though the origins of Plague could be traced back to the Gobi Desert of Mongolia in the 1320s, the exact cause of this sudden eruption still remains unknown. From the Gobi Desert, the spread out was in all directions but the most important one was the eastward spread to China, resulting in an emergence of bubonic plague during the early 1330 AD. As the trade routes with China were strengthened during this period, European traders, particularly Italians, travelled to China regularly.

One such group of traders from Genoa who arrived in Sicily in the October of 1347, fresh from a Voyage to China, is believed to have carried the plague bacteria to Europe, along with the Chinese goods on board. The ship rats and even some sailors contributed to this most likely introduction of the plague to European lands. In the last decade of the last millennium, India too witnessed a plague epidemic. A total of 693 cases of bubonic and pneumonic plague cases, seropositive to *Y. pestis* were reported in 1994 from five Indian States with Maharashtra and Gujarat accounting for nearly eighty percentage of those cases. Also 56 deaths were reported due to plague during that period. This epidemic was an alarm, which alerted to us, the necessity for a national database for surveillance of seemingly isolated cases and also the rodents (**Fig. 15.1**). (CDC, International Notes Update: Human Plague-India, 1994).

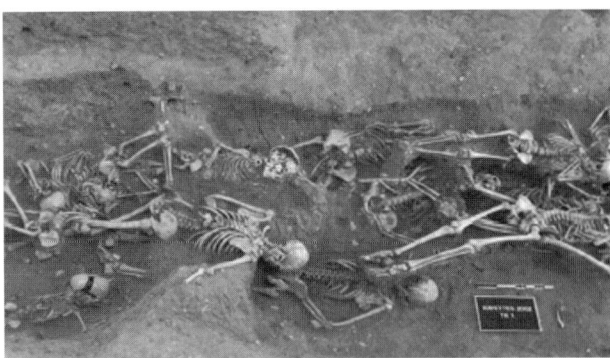

**Fig. 15.1:** Skeletons in a mass grave from 1720–21 in Martigues, France, yielded molecular evidence of the orientalis strain of *Yersinia pestis*, the organism responsible for bubonic plague.

### Global Cholera Epidemic (1826)

There were six cholera pandemics which struck parts of Asia, Europe, North Africa, and the Americas in the 19th century. The first cholera pandemic of 19th century originated in India in 1817, spread into the Caucasus of central Asia and reached its climax in 1823. However, the 'Asiatic cholera' reappeared in Russia in 1829 and during the next summer of 1830, in Astrakhan province, it took more than 20,000 lives and it even spread to Poland, Hungary, and later much of Europe. Subsequently, Cholera claimed thousands of lives, unleashing a nightmare in larger cities such as Paris and London. This epidemic peaked in 1831–32, and then it was observed that the social problems connected with industrialization and urbanization such as pervasive overcrowding and poor sanitation of Europe's blossoming cities contributed to high death rates. (WHO, Global Epidemics and Impact of Cholera).

### Pandemic Influenza (1919)

In 1918, when the world was recovering from the great war, a flu like illness was erupting in some pockets. In the next 2 years, twenty percent of the world population was affected. Also known by the names of Spanish Flu and La Grippe, this pandemic killed 50–100 million people globally. An estimated 675,000 Americans died of influenza during the pandemic, ten times as many as in the World War. (Katz DL et al., Elsevier Health Sciences, 2013)

One hypothesis is that the influenza virus could have had some interactions with respiratory bacteria, and bacterial pneumonias might have led to many deaths. The numbers of death were so high that cemeteries were packed with dead bodies pending burial. Supplies of coffins fell short drastically and the morticians were seldom available to perform the rites. To tackle this huge influx of patients, special field hospitals were set up. This epidemic also showed a different pattern by affecting people aged 20–40, unusual for influenza which was usually a killer of the elderly and children.

Towards the end of first decade of this millennium, there was a global scare due to a new strain of human H1N1 influenza virus, identified in Mexico in 2009. The 2009 swine flu pandemic lasted about 19 months, from January 2009 to August 2010. The number of lab-confirmed deaths reported to the WHO was 18,449 by August 2010 (WHO Pandemic H1N1 2009—update 112), though the 2009 H1N1 flu pandemic is estimated to have actually caused about 2,84,000 (range from 150,000 to 575,000) deaths (Mortality Estimates of H1N1 2009 Pandemic by CDC Led Collaboration in 2012).

### Great Smog of London (1952)

In December 1952, a mixture of smoke and cold fog, called Smog, drifted over the London City, which resulted in the deaths of nearly 12,000 people. Infants, and elders suffered from respiratory illnesses like bronchial asthma and pneumonia. Widespread asphyxiation of cattle was reported from Smithfield Market and surrounding areas. Though thick fogs often descended on the London city in late autumn, this was a consequence of severe air pollution, and not an atmospheric effect (**Fig. 15.2**). (Encyclopedia Britannica, The Great Smog of London: Environmental Disaster, England, 1952).

### PUBLIC HEALTH INTERVENTIONS

Just as we have mentioned some historical public health-related problems, there have also been great interventions to improve community health in the world. Here we present some of them.

In 1662, John Graunt published 'Natural and Political Observations made upon the Bills of Mortality' by observing the deaths in London. He is known as the first compiler of vital statistics.

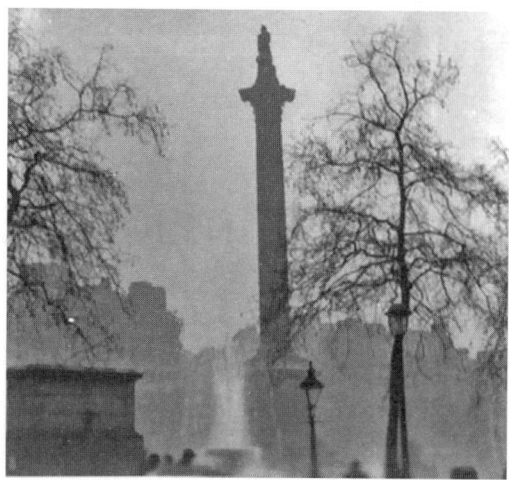

**Fig. 15.2:** Nelson's Column during the Great Smog of 1952, Central London.

The 17th and 18th centuries witnessed various exciting discoveries. Harvey's discovery of blood circulation, Leeuwenhoek's discovery of microscope, and Jenner's vaccination against smallpox changed the face of modern medicine.

### James Lind and Scurvy

James Lind was the son of an Edinburgh merchant and became a medical apprentice in the city before joining the Royal Navy as a surgeon's mate in the late 1730s. In 1747, on board HMS Salisbury, carried out one of the first controlled clinical trials recorded in medical science. He took 12 men suffering from similar symptoms of scurvy, divided them into six pairs and treated them with remedies suggested by previous writers— cider, sea-water, vinegar, oranges and lemon, elixir of vitriol, a white paste with garlic plus barley water. Though the group on oranges and lemon could be treated for only 5 days as they ran out of stock, both of the sailors had almost recovered by that time. Though Dr Lind's 'Treatise of the Scurvy' got published in 1753, it took 42 years for the administration at that time to issue an order for the distribution of lemon juice to sailors (**Fig. 15.3**). (The James Lind Library. James Lind and scurvy: 1747 to 1795).

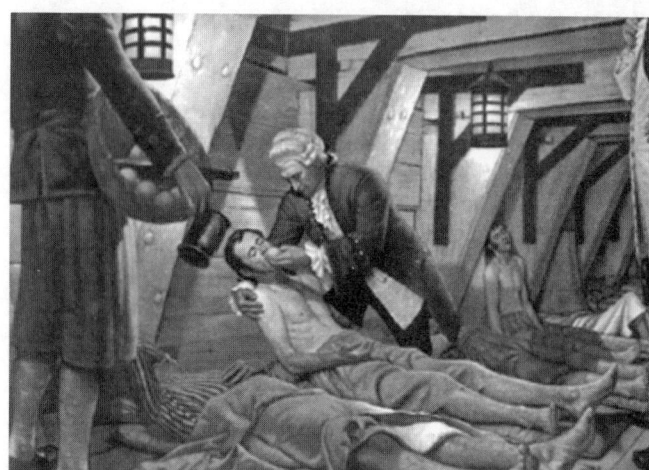

**Fig. 15.3:** James Lind's experiment with citrus fruit was one of the first reported clinical trials in medicine.

## Edward Jenner and Smallpox

Edward Jenner (1749-1823) was an English doctor who introduced the vaccine for smallpox. Folklore existed that milkmaids never caught smallpox. Jenner speculated that getting infected with cowpox provided immunity against smallpox. He also happened to meet locals who claimed to have acquired immunity against smallpox by deliberately infecting themselves with cowpox. In 1796, to prove his theory, he inoculated a local boy named James Phipps with pus collected from Sarah Names, a milkmaid with cowpox. Jenner exposed the boy to smallpox some days later and as speculated he was found to be immune.

As the Latin word for cow was 'vacca', Jenner called this method vaccination. He submitted a paper to the Royal Society though he had no explanation for why this method worked. As he was asked further proof, he proceeded to vaccinate several other children, including his own son and monitored them. In 1798, he published the full results of his study and it was opposed and even ridiculed by many. But 30 years after Jenner's death, in 1853, smallpox vaccination was made compulsory in England and Wales.

Because of a highly effective surveillance and vaccination program that was intensified during the late 1960s, the ancient menace of Smallpox, that had wreaked havoc for more than, 3000 years, was eradicated. The last known naturally acquired case was reported in Somalia in 1977.

## Handwashing and Semmelweis

Ignaz Semmelweis (1818-1865 CE) was a Hungarian physician who proposed to the medical community that simply by washing their hands, they could bring down the mortality rates.

In 1846, there were two obstetrical clinics in University of Vienna Allgemeine Krankenhaus, now known as General Hospital in Vienna, 'the first and the second'. Pregnant women were admitted for delivery alternatively to the first clinic or to the second clinic rotating every 24 hours. The first clinic was managed by physicians and medical students and the second by midwives. Semmelweis took care of the First Obstetrical Clinic in July 1846. In the first clinic, every day, physicians and medical students had to perform autopsies on women who had died from childbed fever before providing clinical care for pregnant women whereas the midwives in the second clinic did not have to perform any autopsies.

Semmelweis made an observation that the mortality rate in the first clinic was 16% whereas the second clinic was a mere 7%. He proposed that multiple examinations of the pregnant women by the physicians and medical students, traumatized the tissues of the vagina and cervix and that their hands which carried disease-causing particles from the cadavers, unknowingly transferred those particles to the pregnant women while performing these examinations. Semmelweis's suspicion was strengthened in 1847 by the death of his colleague Jakob Kolletschka following an injury by a medical student's knife while performing an autopsy and Jakob's autopsy revealed similar pathology to childbed fever.

Hence, Semmelweis reached the conclusion that physicians and medical students were in fact responsible for the high mortality rates from childbed fever in the first clinic as they carried the infection from the autopsy room to the pregnant women in the first clinic. To tackle this, Semmelweis devised a policy in the first clinic-physicians and medical students should wash their hands and brush under their finger nails after they finish the autopsies and before they come in contact with any of the patients. This simple step witnessed the death rate in first clinic drop tremendously. Semmelweis's findings and recommendations though initially ridiculed and criticized, eventually had worldwide effects on the practice of medicine. Awe inspiring, his observations and suggested interventions were before the actual discovery of microbes.

## Edwin Chadwick's Report and the Sanitary Awakening

The industrial revolution in the 18th century led to various problems affecting the life of the people, such as overcrowding and slums, accumulation of filth in cities and towns, infectious diseases like tuberculosis, and high rates of sickness and death. The mean age at death in London varied from 22 years for the working class and 44 for the elite. Edwin Chadwick studied the health of inhabitants of large towns in London and submitted a report on 'The Sanitary Conditions of the Laboring Population in Great Britain'. Chadwick's report can be considered as the first ever lifestyle modifying public health document as it paved the way to anti-filth crusade and the great sanitary awakening, which eventually led to the first ever legislation in public health—The Public Health Act of 1848 in England. Later, it was Sir John Simon, the first medical officer of Health of London, who is credited with building a Public Health System.

## John Snow and Cholera

*John Snow (1813-1858),* Father of Modern Epidemiology/field epidemiology, was an English anesthetist who developed many modern epidemiologic methods like spot map that remain valid even today.

London's water supply system during 1850s included a series of shallow public wells where people could use hand pumps to draw their own water to carry home. In September 1854, there was a cholera outbreak in England which was centered in the Soho district. John Snow made a map of 13 public wells and marked all the known cholera deaths around Soho in that same map. He noted the clustering of cholera cases around one particular water pump on the southwest corner of the intersection between Broadwick Street and Lexington Street **(Fig. 15.4)**. He also did examine water samples from different wells under a microscope and could confirm the presence of an unknown bacterium (*Vibrio cholerae* was not yet discovered) in the Broadwick Street samples. In spite of considerable skepticism from the authorities, John Snow had the pump handle removed from the Broadwick Street pump, which is considered as a landmark event in public health.

## Louis Pasteur and Germ Theory

Swan neck flask experiment conducted by Louis Pasteur changed the age old belief of spontaneous generation, that life can essentially arise from anything. This experiment by Pasteur confirmed one of the basic tenets of biology that 'life begets life'.

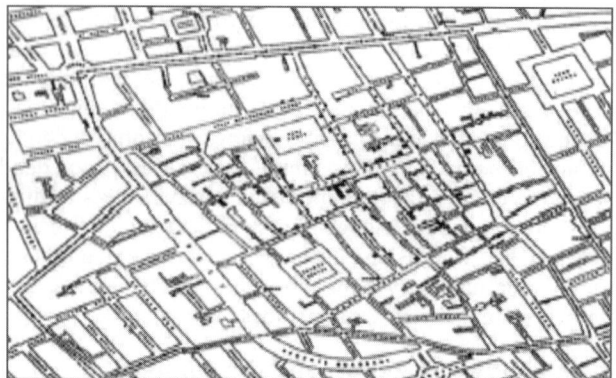

**Fig. 15.4:** Original map made by John Snow in 1854. Cholera cases are highlighted in black.

Pasteur used a swan necked flask for the experiment which contained heat sterilized nutrient broth in it. Though the mouth was open, all the dust and microorganisms were trapped in the neck itself owing to its shape. The broth did not show any growth of microbes. When microbes were directly introduced to the broth, their rapid multiplication was seen again. This proved the fact that there was no spontaneous generation of microbes in the broth but was introduced from outside. This led Pasteur, along with his contemporary Robert Koch to study various diseases closely and to conclude that specific microbes caused specific diseases. This established the germ theory of disease which led to the successful identification and treatment of many infectious diseases. This was in fact the base on which modern medicine flourished in tackling the infectious diseases and saved millions of lives.

## Robert Koch and his Postulates

Robert Koch summarized in his four postulates how to ascertain diseases to specific causative organisms.
1. The organism must be observed in every case of the disease
2. It must be isolated and grown in pure culture
3. The pure culture must, when inoculated into a susceptible animal, reproduce the disease
4. The organism must be observed in, and recovered from, the experimental animal.

Koch's postulates were criticized on certain grounds, but till date it remains the backbone of the 'causation theory' of communicable diseases. For non-communicable diseases, Framingham Heart Study provided the much needed breakthrough.

## Framingham Heart Study

Until 1940s, very little was known about the general causes of heart disease and stroke, though the death rates for cardiovascular diseases (CVD) were seen to be going up as much that America was said to be witnessing a new kind of non-communicable epidemic. The National Heart Institute [now National Heart, Lung, and Blood Institute (NHLBI)] took up this challenge in 1948, and rolled out the Framingham Heart Study.

The first generation group had 5,209 men and women recruited, between the ages of 30 and 62 years from the town of Framingham, Massachusetts who were followed up extensively every two years. A second-generation group which included 5,124 of the original participants' adult children and their spouses were recruited in 1971. A third generation of 4095 participants, the grandchildren of the original cohort were recruited in April 2002.

Framingham Study populations over the years have helped us to determine the major risk factors of CVD—high blood pressure, high blood cholesterol, smoking, obesity, diabetes, and physical inactivity. Much light was also thrown on the other related factors such as blood triglyceride, HDL cholesterol, age, gender, and psychosocial issues. The importance of this study is so huge that the concept of CVD risk factors is now an integral part of the modern medical curriculum and effective preventive strategies are much sought after in clinical practice as well.

Framingham investigators have collaborations with other leading researchers from around the world on research projects in stroke, dementia, osteoporosis, arthritis, nutrition, diabetes, eye diseases, hearing disorders, lung diseases, and genetic patterns of common diseases which are expected to reveal newer valuable information in future.

## Doll and Hill Study

Sir Richard Doll and Sir Austin Bradford Hill started the world's first large prospective study in October 1951 to explore the link between smoking and mortality. They sent a questionnaire on smoking habits to all registered British doctors and hence this study came to be known as 'The British Doctors Study' They mailed 59,600 questionnaires and received 41,024 replies, of which 40,701 complete ones (34,494 males and 6,207 females) were included in the follow-up. Changes in smoking habits were assessed by follow-up questionnaires sent in 1957, 1966, 1971, 1978, 1991, 1998, and 2001. Women were excluded owing to their lesser numbers and lesser exposure to tobacco and hence the study focused on men. The study demonstrated the risk of death among smokers due to lung cancer (1954) myocardial infarction and chronic obstructive pulmonary disease (1956). The questionnaire sent out in 1978 sought information on alcohol consumption and self-reported body mass index and also invited the doctors to be part of a randomized controlled trial for determining the prophylactic role of daily aspirin to prevent death from cardiovascular causes.

## Typhoid Fever Epidemic in Sangli, Maharashtra, India (1975)

In December 1975, India witnessed probably the world's largest single source typhoid outbreak in Sangli town of Maharashtra. From a population of about 1,35,000, more than 9,000 cases were reported during the next three months. The epidemiological investigation that followed to identify the cause revealed that fecal contamination of municipal water supply was the culprit. Chlorine treatment was found to be inadequate. This highlighted the importance of safe water supply and proper excreta disposal systems.

These were some glimpses of certain important historical events and actions in community health. These have changed the paradigm of preventive and public health globally. We continue to benefit from them and look forward to not only utilize this knowledge to the fullest but also to generate further community health related evidence in future for bettering tomorrow's history. (WHO, A Study of Typhoid Fever in Five Asian Countries, 2018).

> **Note**
> **Some Great Scientists of Public Health**
> - *Father of Medicine*: Hippocrates
> - *First Man of Modern Science*: Andreas Vesalius
> - *Father of Modern Surgery*: Joseph Lister
> - *First Compiler of Vital Statistics*: John Graunt
> - *Founder of Occupational Medicine*: Bernardino Ramazzini
> - Father of Public Health: Cholera
> - *Father of Modern Epidemiology*: John Snow

## ACKNOWLEDGMENT

Dr Dhanya R, Assistant Professor, Public Health Dentistry, Government Dental College, Thiruvananthapuram, Kerala, India.

## SUGGESTED READING

1. British Doctors Study—Oxford Clinical Trial Service Unit & Epidemiological Studies Unit (CTSU). [online] Available from https://www.ctsu.ox.ac.uk/research/british-doctors-study.
2. CDC, International Notes Update: Human Plague-India, 1994.
3. Detels R, Beaglehole R. Oxford textbook of public health, 5th edition. Oxford, New York: Oxford University Press; 2011. p. 1922.
4. Encyclopedia Britannica, The Great Smog of London: Environmental Disaster, England, 1952.
5. Friis et al., Jones and Bartlett Publishers, 2010.
6. Henry E. Sigerist: medical historian and social visionary. Am J Public Health. 2003;93(1):60.
7. History Today: Black Death: The Greatest Catastrophe Ever.
8. Katz DL, Elmore JG, Wild D, et al. Jekel's Epidemiology, Biostatistics and Preventive Medicine. Elsevier Health Sciences; 2013. p. 423.
9. Katz DL et al., Elsevier Health Sciences, 2013.
10. Mortality Estimates of H1N1 2009 Pandemic by CDC Led Collaboration in 2012.
11. NHLBI, Framingham Heart Study.
12. Robert Koch and the "golden age" of bacteriology. Int J Infect Dis. 2010;14(9):e744-51.
13. Strick J. Pasteur's Swan-necked flasks: the invention of an experimentum crucis. ResearchGate. 2016.
14. The James Lind Library. James Lind and scurvy: 1747–1795.
15. WHO, A Study of Typhoid Fever in Five Asian Countries, 2018.
16. WHO, Global Epidemics and Impact of Cholera.
17. WHO, Health Principles of Housing, 2009.
18. WHO, Historical Perspective on Hand Hygiene and Health Care, 2009.
19. WHO Pandemic H1N1 2009 - update 112.
20. World Health Organization. (2009). Historical perspective on hand hygiene in health care.
21. World Health Organization. Health Principles of Housing; 1989.

# CHAPTER 16

# General Epidemiology of Infectious Diseases and its Prevention and Control

*Pankaj Bhardwaj, Akhil Dhanesh Goel*

## CAUSATION OF DISEASES

| | |
|---|---|
| CM7.2 | Enumerate, describe and discuss the mode of transmission and measures for prevention and control |
| CM8.1 | Describe and discuss the epidemiological and control measures at the primary care level for communicable diseases |

## HISTORICAL PERSPECTIVE: GERM THEORY

Before 1789, the Hippocrates, Galen, and humoral medicine along with the astrology dominated the conceptual framework of disease causation. The epidemic was explained with the doctrine of miasma that is the poisoning of the air or malaria. In 1860, very well referred to as the year with the remarkable development in the golden era of microbiology that the concept of germ theory of disease emerged. This theory completely changed the concept of the causation of diseases. The French Bacteriologist, Louis Pasteur (1822-1895) conducted formal experiment to establish the relationship between germ and disease, and thus rejecting the theory of "Spontaneous Generation". The concept of germ theory emerged from his experiments on fermentation. Pasteur was a chemist as well as a biologist. He began his work on the fermentation of wine and beer, in particular their spoilage. He confirmed that living microorganisms causes fermentation and it is not a chemical process. These microorganisms were later identified as bacteria in the microscope. The concept of "Germ Theory of Disease" was confirmed by another scientist, Robert Koch. Koch with the help of different experiments established that the causes of Anthrax is a bacterium *Bacillus anthracis*. After these experiments by Pasteur and Koch, different microbes were isolated and their role in the disease causation could be established. This led to the development of modern medicine. It would not be wrong to say that it was only after the isolation of these pathogens, the work on the vaccines could be started along with the introduction of antiseptics during the surgery. The germ theory of disease established the concept of "One to one" relationship between the causal agent and the disease.

Causal agent → Man → Disease

For years together the causation of diseases was explained with the help of concept of germ theory of disease. But later on epidemiologists studied the causation of diseases with greater depth and started looking at the germ theory of disease with limitations. The questions were quite clear. Why all of the hosts who are exposed to the causal agent do not get the disease? Why only few of the hosts manifest diseases? It was the era when epidemiologists started their discussion on the concept of "Epidemiological Triad".

## EPIDEMIOLOGICAL TRIAD

The epidemiologic triad explains the interaction between the causal agent, host as well as environment **(Fig. 16.1)**.

The presence of an agent is must for the causation of disease. In an infectious disease, the microorganism (bacteria, virus, etc.) is described as the "agent" and in noninfectious diseases, the term "agent" may also include chemical and physical components.

"Host" refers to that specific entity that shall contract the disease once it is lodged with the disease agent. The different characteristics of host which includes the intrinsic factors like the genetic makeup, immunity status, the overall general condition of the host, exposure level, etc., determine whether the host will contract the disease or not.

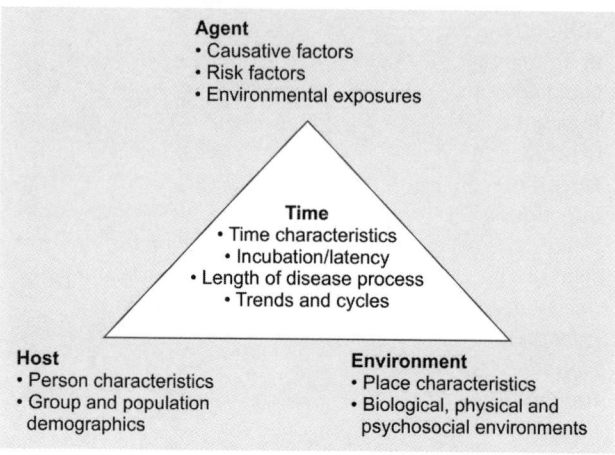

**Fig. 16.1:** The "Epidemiological Triad".
*Source:* Miller, R. (2002). Epidemiology for Health Promotion and Disease Prevention Professionals. New York: Routledge. pp. 63.

In the epidemiological triad, usually "environment" which is external to the host. This includes physical environment like the climatic conditions, biological environment like the changing vector bionomics, or even the socioeconomic factors. The "internal environment" is to describe the factors within the host like psycho-social environment which determines the causation of disease.

For a normal state of health, the interaction between the agent, host, and environment determines the state of health of an individual. A person remains healthy until the equilibrium is maintained.

## COMPONENT CAUSES AND CAUSAL PIES

It was quite evident to the epidemiologists working for the causation of diseases that all diseases whether infectious or noninfectious cannot be explained by one model alone. The diseases are multifactorial in nature and the search for different models to explain causalities continued. The "Causal Pies" model proposed by Rothman consists of the concept of "Component Cause" "Sufficient Cause," and "Necessary Cause" as discussed below:

### Piece of Pie

A piece of pie is an individual factor that contributes to the cause of disease. The disease is said to occur when all the pieces of the pie (representing the various possible causal or risk factors) fall into place and the pie is complete.

*Component causes:* These are the individual factors in the pie.

*Sufficient cause:* A complete pie can be considered as a causal pathway and is called as the sufficient cause. There is a possibility that certain diseases may have multiple pies, i.e., more than one sufficient cause. The various component causes in each pie of sufficient cause may or may not overlap.

*Necessary cause:* This is that component that will appear in every pie. If this component is missing, disease does not occur. **Figure 16.2** shows that component cause A appears in every pie and hence is a necessary cause.

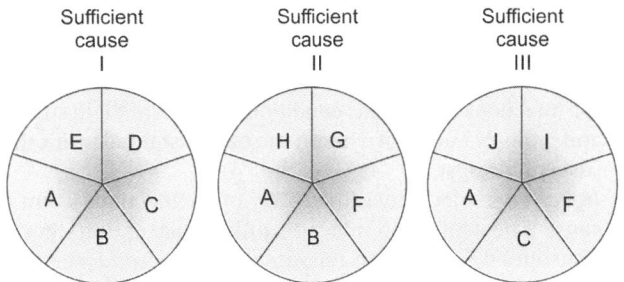

**Fig. 16.2:** Rothman causal pies.
*Source:* Rothman KJ. Causes. Am J Epidemiol. 1976;104(6):587-92.

## SUGGESTED READING

1. Merril RM, Timmereck TC. Introduction to Epidemiology, 4th edition. United States: Jones and Bartlett Publishers; 2006. pp. 1-352.
2. Rothman KJ. Causes. 1976. Am J Epidemiol. 1995;141(2):90-5.
3. US Department of Health and Human Services. Principles of epidemiology in public health practice, 3rd edition. An introduction to applied epidemiology and biostatistics. Atlanta: CDC; 2012. pp. 1-511.

# DYNAMICS OF DISEASE TRANSMISSION

## DEFINITIONS

- *Infectious disease (or communicable disease):* Illness caused by a specific infectious agent or its toxic product that results from transmission of that agent or its products from an infected person, animal, or reservoir to a susceptible host, either directly or indirectly through an intermediate plant or animal host, vector or inanimate environment. Some are contagious and some non-contagious.
- *Infectious agent:* Microorganisms or macroorganisms capable of producing an infection or an infectious disease.
- *Infection:* Entry and development or multiplication of an infectious agent in a human or animal body, whether or not it develops into a disease. The state in which there are no signs of a recognized disease is called *inapparent/subclinical infection*.
- *Infective dose:* Number of units of the infectious agent required to produce the disease.
- *Incubation period:* Interval between the effective exposure of the susceptible host to an infectious agent and the appearance of signs and clinical symptoms of the disease in that host. In noninfectious diseases the period is known as Latent period or induction period.
- *Infectivity:* Infectivity is the ability of an infectious agent to cause a new infection in a susceptible host, and in directly transmitted diseases it is measured by the Secondary Attack Rate, which is the proportion of susceptible individuals that develop the infection after exposure to a primary case.
- *Endemic:* The continuous occurrence at an expected frequency over a certain period of time and in a certain geographical location.
- *Holoendemic:* When a high level of infection is registered beginning at a young age and predominantly affecting the young population.
- *Hyperendemic:* When the infection equally affects all age groups.
- *Epidemic:* The occurrence of a disease that is definitely greater than that expected in a certain geographical region.
- *Pandemic:* When the epidemic is generalized and involves different countries and a large population.
- *Outbreak:* When the epidemic is restricted to a small geographical area or population.
- *Epizootic:* When the epidemic occurs in animal population.
- *Host:* a person or animal that affords lodgment of an infectious agent.
- *Definitive host:* The host that harbors an agent in a mature stage or in a sexually active phase.

- **Intermediate host:** Host that harbors the agent in a larvae stage or asexual developmental stage.
- **Vector:** The transmission of an agent is intermediated by an arthropod, which is called as vector. The vector may be simply mechanical—that is, it may merely carry the agent that accidentally contaminated it, or it may be biological when the infectious agent obligatorily requires the vector to pass from one phase to another in its development.
- **Vectorial capacity:** A property of the vector, measured by means of parameters such as abundance, survival, and house infestation rates, and has a direct influence on the capacity of transmission of an infectious agent.
- **Reservoir of infection:** Primary source of infection in which the infectious agent finds conditions that permit it to survive and multiply and from where it can be transmitted to another susceptible host.
- **Infectivity:** Infectivity is the ability of an infectious agent to cause a new infection in a susceptible host, and in directly transmitted diseases it is measured by the *Secondary Attack Rate*, which is the proportion of susceptible individuals that develop the infection after exposure to a primary case.
- **Latent infection:** Condition when infectious agents may remain silent in the host for long periods of time without any sign of their presence but may eventually cause disease.
- **Virulence:** The capacity of an infectious agent to provoke disease after having infected the host is called virulence, numerically expressed as the ratio of the number of cases of the disease in relation to the total number of individuals infected.
- **Case fatality rate:** Proportion of deaths in relation to the number of cases of a disease within a specified time.

There are three pre-requisites for the transmission of a disease namely:
- The reservoir and source of infection
- The susceptible person and
- Different routes of transmission from the reservoir to the susceptible persons.

## RESERVOIR

The causative organism lives, multiplies and depends primarily for its survival (i.e., the natural habitat of the organism) in **reservoir.** Such a reservoir may be human being, animal, arthropod or soil. A homologous reservoir state is the one, in which both the reservoir and the susceptible person belong to the same species. For example, chickenpox, measles (Human-Human being). A heterologous reservoir state is the one, in which both the reservoir and the susceptible belong to the different species. For example, salmonellosis (Cattle-human being), Rabies (Dogs-human being), etc.

**Source of infection** is a person, animal, arthropod, soil or the substance from which the organism is disseminated directly to the host.

The terms reservoir and source are not synonymous always. "Source" means immediate source of infection and may or may not be a part of reservoir.

There are three types of reservoir:

### Human Reservoir

A human reservoir can either be a case or carrier.

**Case:** A case is an infected person having clinical features of the disease. Such a case may be mild, moderate or a severe case. Mild cases are more dangerous than the severe cases because they are ambulatory and keep on spreading the disease. Severe cases are usually bedridden. The subclinical cases are variously referred to as inapparent, covert, missed or abortive cases are equally important in the silent spread of the disease because the disease agent may multiply in the host but does not manifest itself by signs and symptoms.

Cases act as source only during the 'period of communicability', which varies from disease to disease. For example, in typhoid from 1st day of fever until two stool samples (24 hours apart) are negative the cases can transmit the disease. In measles, communicability is from 1st day of fever to 4th day of onset of rash.

In epidemiological studies, 'Primary case' refers to the first person developing the disease in an outbreak, in the defined population. 'Index-case' is the first case which comes to the attention of the investigator. 'Secondary cases' are those who get the disease by contact from the primary case.

**Carrier:** A carrier is an infected person but not having the clinical features of the disease (thus harboring the organisms) and serves as a source of infection to others in the community. Such carriers can be seen in typhoid, diphtheria, gonorrhea, AIDS, hepatitis B, meningitis, salmonellosis and amoebiasis, etc. They can be detected only by doing laboratory investigations. The carriers constitute the submerged portion of ice in iceberg phenomenon.

***Carrier can be classified as below on different basis:***
A. *According to the stage in the disease cycle:*
  1. *Incubatory carrier:* The disease spread occurs during the incubation period. Such a state occurs in diseases like measles, mumps, diphtheria, poliomyelitis, pertussis, influenza and hepatitis A and B. After the incubation period, that individual develops the clinical features and become a case.
  2. *Convalescent carrier:* Is a carrier during the period of convalescence (recovery) from an illness during which clinical cure is observed but not bacteriological cure. This may be due to incomplete course of treatment. Such a state occurs in conditions like diphtheria, typhoid fever, amoebiasis.
  3. *Healthy or contact carrier:* Sub-clinical cases which act as a source of infection to others. The nursing staff, the patient's attendants or the family members who are in close association with the cases often become healthy carriers. They never suffer from the disease, e.g., diphtheria and cholera.

B. *According to the duration of the carrier state:*
  1. *Temporary carriers:* Spread of the disease for a short period of time (for several days). All incubatory, convalescent and healthy carriers are temporary carriers.

2. *Chronic carriers:* Transmission of the disease for a long period of time, several weeks to several months. This is due to the persistence of the organisms in the organs like gallbladder in typhoid fever, tonsils in diphtheria, liver in hepatitis B, etc.

C. *According to the route of exit of the organism:*
   1. Urinary carriers, where the focus of organisms is the kidney as in typhoid
   2. Intestinal carriers, where the focus of organisms is the intestine, as in typhoid, amoebiasis
   3. Biliary carriers, where the focus of organisms is the gallbladder as in typhoid
   4. Cutaneous carriers as in staphylococci
   5. Nasal carriers as in nasal diphtheria
   6. Genital carriers as in gonorrhea, AIDS.

Thus, from epidemiological point of view, the carriers are more dangerous than the cases because they are not recognized and are ambulatory. Among the carriers, chronic carriers are more dangerous than temporary carriers. Longer the duration of carriers, greater the risk to the community. Such carriers may shed the organisms intermittently or continuously. They are called as intermittent and continuous carriers respectively. Carriers are responsible for the endemicity of the disease in the community. They may spread the disease to those areas also, which are otherwise free of infection. They correspond to the 'submerged' portion of ice in iceberg phenomenon. Therefore, their detection and treatment are essential to limit the spread of the disease in the community and that is a challenge to the modern technique of community medicine.

## Animal Reservoir

There are many animals, which act as reservoir and transmit the diseases to human beings. These diseases are called zoonotic diseases (anthropozoonoses).

| Animal reservoir | Disease transmitted |
|---|---|
| Cattle | Bovine tuberculosis, salmonellosis, tetanus, brucellosis, Q-fever, Taenia saginata |
| Horse | Tetanus |
| Dog | Rabies, hydatid disease |
| Monkey | Yellow fever, dengue fever, Kyasanur forest disease |
| Sheep | Anthrax, liver fluke (Fasciola hepatica) |
| Pig | Japanese encephalitis, tenia solium |
| Rodent | Plague, leptospirosis, endemic typhus |
| Birds | Psittacosis, histoplasmosis, ornithosis |

For most of the zoonotic diseases, there is no treatment. Prevention is the only intervention. These animal diseases occur among human beings, because of our close association with them.

## Soil Reservoir

Soil acts not only as a reservoir but also as source of infection and transmit diseases like tetanus, gas-gangrene, ankylostomiasis, anthrax, malignant edema, aspergillosis, coccidioidomycosis, mycetoma (Soil borne diseases).

## MODE OF TRANSMISSION OF DISEASES

There are different ways of classifying the mode of transmission of a disease. One such classification as mentioned in CDC is:
1. Direct transmission:
   a. Direct contact
   b. Droplet spread
   c. Inoculation into skin or mucosa
   d. Contact with soil
   e. Transplacental
2. Indirect transmission:
   a. Airborne
   b. Vehicle-borne
   c. Vector-borne (biologic or mechanical)
   d. Fomite-borne
   e. Unclean hands and fingers

### Direct Transmission

Transfer of an infectious agent from a reservoir to a host directly, without any inanimate objects (vehicles) or animate intermediaries (vectors).
a. **Direct contact:** The transmission occurs through
   - skin-to-skin contact
   - intimate contacts including sexual intercourse
   - contact with the soil or vegetation fostering the infectious organisms
b. **Droplet spread:** Here the mode of transmission is through contact of host with the comparatively large aerosols generated by sneezing, coughing, or even talking. Droplets are those infectious particles which are more than five microns in size. They travel from the respiratory tract of the infected host directly to the susceptible host usually over short distances of at least 1 m. Droplet distribution depends on the force of expulsion and is limited by gravity. However, droplets are also known to be transmitted indirectly to mucosal surfaces (e.g. via hands). Examples of such transmission are influenza virus and *Meningococcus*.
c. **Inoculation into skin or mucosa:** The disease causing pathogen can enter the skin or mucosa directly by animal bites, contaminated needles or syringes or can get inoculated through skin eruptions or open wounds, e.g. hepatitis B virus through contaminated needles and rabies virus by dog bite.
d. **Contact with soil:** The disease agent may be acquired by direct exposure of susceptible tissue to the pathogen in soil or decaying vegetable matter, e.g. tetanus spores in soil and dust, hookworm larvae, etc.
e. **Transplacental or vertical transmission:** The disease agent can be transmitted from mother to the child through placenta directly, e.g. TORCH agents (*Toxoplasma gondii*, rubella, cytomegalovirus and herpes virus), varicella virus, syphilis, hepatitis B, AIDS, etc.

### Indirect Transmission

In indirect transmission infectious agents are carried from a reservoir to a host through the medium of suspended air particles, inanimate objects (vehicles), or animate intermediaries (vectors).

a. **Airborne transmission:** The infectious agents get transferred by dust or droplet nuclei suspended in air. Dust particles are either the materials settled on surfaces which become re-suspended by air currents or they may be infectious particles blown from the soil by the wind. Droplet nuclei are dried residue measuring less than five microns. While the larger droplets can travel up to few feet only, in contrast, droplet nuclei have the potential to remain suspended in the air for long periods of time and can get blown over great distances. There are mention of cases of measles occurring in a group of children who contracted the disease when they entered in the pediatrician chamber who recently examined a measles afflicted child and the air of the clinic still have the droplet nuclei of the infection. To prevent this mode of transmission in hospital settings, wet mopping is recommended over dry mopping.
b. **Vehicle-borne:** Vehicles, for example, food, water, biologic products (blood), and fomites (inanimate objects such as handkerchiefs, bedding, or surgical scalpels) carry an infectious agent from the infective person to the susceptible host. The vehicle may also help in providing the suitable environment where agent may grow, multiply, or may produce toxin.
c. **Vector-borne:** These are the animate bodies like mosquitoes, fleas, and ticks. The vectors transmit the diseases in the following ways:
    – *Mechanical transmission:* Carrying the pathogens from the filthy substances to food substances by soiling the legs, e.g., house-fly transmitting typhoid, trachoma, etc.
    – Biting and inoculating the pathogens percutaneously, e.g. mosquitoes, fleas, ticks, etc.
    – *Defecation:* Scratching in of the infected feces, into the abrasions of the skin, e.g., epidemic typhus, trench fever transmitted through the feces of infected louse.
    – Contamination of the abraded skin of the host by the body fluid of the infected arthropod when it is crushed, e.g., transmission of relapsing fever, when infected louse is crushed in the scalp.
    – *Biological transmission:* The pathogen undergoes multiplication or development from one stage to another stage or both multiplication and development, inside the body of the vector and then the transmission observed. Thus, biological mode of transmission is of three types:
        1. *Propagative type:* The pathogen undergoes only multiplication inside the vector, e.g., plague bacilli in the body of the rat-flea; yellow fever virus in the body of female Aedes mosquito; KFD virus in the body of hard tick.
        2. *Cyclopropagative type:* The pathogen undergoes not only multiplication but also a phase of development in its life cycle, e.g., plasmodium (malarial) parasites in the body of the female anopheline mosquito (Zygote → Ookinite → Ocyst → Sporozoites).
        3. *Cyclodevelopmental type:* The pathogen undergoes only a phase of the development but not multiplication, e.g., microfilariae developing into larval stage in the body of female culex mosquito; Guinea worm embryos developing into larva in the body of Cyclops.
d. **Fomite-borne:** Fomites are inanimate objects or substances (other than food or water) contaminated by infectious discharges from a patient harboring it to a healthy person. Fomites include soiled clothes, linen, towels, cups, plates, door handles, taps and surgical instruments and dressings. Diseases transmitted are hepatitis A, typhoid fever, eye and skin infections.
e. **Unclean hands and fingers:** The transmission of pathogenic agents takes place both directly (hand-to-mouth) from skin, nose, bowel, etc. and indirectly, e.g. dysentery, intestinal parasites, hepatitis A, staphylococcal and streptococcal infections.

## SUSCEPTIBLE HOST

A susceptible person is the one who is likely/prone to develop the disease. For a disease to occur in an individual, there must be a portal of entry, a site of election and poor defense mechanism.
- Portal of entry may be respiratory route, alimentary route, per cutaneous route or genital route. There may be even more than one route of entry, e.g. AIDS, Hepatitis B, etc.
- A site of election means, a site (an organ) where the pathogen finds optimum favorable condition for its growth, development, multiplication and survival. It is called 'Target Organ'.
- Defense mechanism is at three levels—anatomical protection by healthy and intact skin, chemical protection by gastric acidity, and biological protection by immunity.

For successful parasitism, there must be a portal of entry, a site of election, a portal of exit (similar to portal of entry) and must survive in the external environment for a sufficient period till it finds a new host, to propagate its species. If there is a portal of entry, site of election and no portal of exit, it is called 'Dead-end' infections. That means they are infectious diseases but not communicable from person to person, e.g., hydatid disease, rabies in man (Hydrophobia), Japanese encephalitis, tetanus, Kyasanur forest disease, Bubonic plague, trichinosis. The disease agent dies in human being.

A successful disease agent is the one which has a portal of entry, a site of election, a portal of exit, survives in the external environment, enters a new host, propagates its species and does not cause the death but produces only a low grade of immunity, so that the host is vulnerable again and again to the same infection. For example, common cold virus.

### Incubation Period

***Definition:*** It is defined as a 'period between the successful entry of a pathogen and the appearance of the first clinical sign or symptom of the disease', in an individual. It is also called 'intrinsic incubation period'.

After entering the body the pathogen circulates and reaches the target organ, where it lodges, gets adopted, multiplies and reaches an optimum number, overcomes the body's defense mechanism, disturbs the structure and function of that organ, produces changes in the body fluid and body tissues, disturbs the health equilibrium and ultimately results in the manifestations of clinical signs and symptoms of the disease.

Certain factors that influence the incubation period: These are virulence of the pathogens, infective dose and the susceptibility of the individual.

Every infectious disease has an incubation period. It varies from disease to disease and in the same disease it varies from person to person, depending upon the below factors.

| Very short incubation period (few hours to few days) | Food-poisoning, bacillary dysentery, gonorrhea, meningococcal meningitis, cholera, etc. |
|---|---|
| Incubation period varying from few days to few weeks (1 to 3 weeks) | Chickenpox, common cold, chancroid, measles, mumps, malaria, diphtheria, tetanus, pertussis, typhoid, poliomyelitis, yellow fever, etc. |
| Incubation period varying from few weeks to few months | Amoebiasis, hepatitis A and B, kala-azar, rabies, etc. |
| Incubation period varying from few months to few years | Tuberculosis, leprosy, filariasis, AIDS, etc. |

**Extrinsic incubation period:** It is the period between the entrance of the pathogen inside the body of the arthropod till the arthropod (vector) becomes infective. For example, 10 to 14 days in malaria, filariasis and yellow fever.

**Serial interval:** It is a period between the onset of the primary case and the secondary case. From a series of such secondary cases, the range of the incubation period of a particular disease can be guessed. Since the exact time of entry of the organism in the body cannot be known in practice, serial interval is used.

**Generation time:** It is a period between the onset of the infection and the maximum infectivity of the host. This period may be shorter than the incubation period as in mumps or longer than the incubation period as in measles.

**Latent period:** It is similar to incubation period but with reference to noncommunicable diseases such as diabetes, hypertension, cancer, etc. It is a period between the initiation of the disease and the detection of the disease.

**Minimum and maximum incubation period:** Since the incubation period always varies, every infectious disease has a minimum and a maximum incubation period.

**Median incubation period:** It is the time required for 50 percent of the cases to occur following exposure.

**Communicable period:** It is a period during which the reservoir is infectious to others. This can be reduced by making an early diagnosis and correct treatment. The communicability of a disease can be measured by an indicator 'Secondary attack rate', i.e. percentage of the exposed persons or susceptible contacts developing the disease, following exposure to primary case (The rate at which the disease is spreading in the community).

## Uses of Incubation Period

1. **Helps in making diagnosis:** Short incubation period helps in making the diagnosis, as in food poisoning, gonorrhea, donovanosis, etc.
2. **Helps to trace the contacts or the source of infection:** As in diseases having short incubation period (mentioned above). This is not possible if the incubation period is long. Tracing the source of infection or contacts helps to implement the control measures.
3. **For quarantine purposes:** Quarantine means limiting the movement of the healthy persons, who are suspected to have been exposed to a communicable disease, for such a period equal to the longest incubation period of the disease. This was adopted to prevent the international spread of the diseases like smallpox, cholera, plague and yellow fever by quarantining those who were not producing the valid International Certificate of Vaccination, in the international airports and seaports.
4. **For immunization purposes:** The at-risk person can be protected by immunizing after exposure to the disease by making use of the long incubation period as in rabies, tetanus, etc.
5. **Helps to assess the prognosis:** Shorter the incubation period, worse is the prognosis, as in tetanus.

## Host Defense Mechanisms (Immune Responses)

The immune response is how body recognizes and defends itself against bacteria, viruses, and substances that appear foreign and harmful. Broadly, there are two types of immune responses—innate and acquired (**Flowchart 16.1**)

**Flowchart 16.1:** Types of immunity.

```
                    Types of immunity
                    /              \
              Acquired            Innate
              /       \
      Active immunity   Passive immunity
      /       \           /         \
  Natural   Acquired   Natural    Acquired
  
  Antibodies  Antibodies  Maternal    Antibodies
  develop     develop     antibodies  developed in
  after       after       transferred an infected
  infection   vaccination to baby     host or in vitro
                          transplacentally are given to
                          or through  index host
                          breast milk
```

The first line of defense against pathogens is the innate, or non-specific immune response or natural immunity. The innate immune response consists of physical, chemical and cellular barriers against pathogens. The main purpose of the innate immune response is to immediately prevent the spread and movement of foreign pathogens throughout the body. Examples of innate immunity include:
- Cough reflex
- Enzymes in tears and skin oils
- Mucus, which traps bacteria and small particles
- Skin
- Stomach acid
- Innate immunity also comes in a protein chemical form, called innate humoral immunity. Examples include the body's complement system and substances called interferon and interleukin-1 (which causes fever).

The second line of defense against pathogens is called adaptive immune response. Adaptive immunity is also referred to as acquired immunity or specific immunity. It comes into play once microorganisms have breached local defense mechanisms. By virtue of these acquired immunity, the host is able to recognize, destroy and eliminate antigenic material (e.g., bacteria, viruses, proteins, etc.) foreign to his own. A person is said to be immune when he possesses "specific protective antibodies or cellular immunity as a result of previous infection or immunization, or from maternal antibodies so as to respond adequately to prevent infection and/or clinical illness following exposure to a specific infectious agent".

Active immunity is acquired after natural exposure to an antigen which actually stimulates an adaptive response (natural active immunity), or after administration of vaccines (acquired active immunity). In passive immunity, IgG antibodies are administered to protect against acute infection. It gives immediate, but shorter protection lasting from several weeks to 3 or 4 months. Passive immunity can also be classified as natural or acquired. The transplacental transfer of maternal measles antibody (mainly IgG) provides "natural passive immunity" for the newborn baby for several weeks/months. "Acquired passive immunity" can be developed in an individual by administrating the immunoglobulin fraction which is usually obtained from the serum of those individuals (humans or equine, etc.) who are immune to this infection.

## MATHEMATICAL MODELS APPLIED TO INFECTIOUS DISEASES

The efforts to discern the infectious diseases dynamics has been made by the epidemiologists for years together. These models use equation systems to understand dynamics of infectious diseases in depth with the application of mathematics.

One such model is known as *SIR model of Infectious Diseases*, where the population is described under three categories: Susceptibles (S) are those who are capable of acquiring an infection; Infectives (I) are those who are capable of transmitting infection to susceptible; and Removals (R) are those who become immune or die after an infection. In a virgin host population, all the hosts will be susceptible to a newly introduced infectious agent. Thus, at first contact of host and agent S = 1 and I and R = 0. As the infection propagates, S decreases and I increases.

R0: Basic Reproductive number. Expected number of secondary cases of a disease produced directly by an average infectious individual entering an entirely susceptible population.

$R_0 > 1$: Epidemic occurs    $R_0 < 1$: No epidemic occurs

## APPROACHES FOR PREVENTION AND CONTROL

If we have to control a disease, the chain of transmission needs to be broken. This chain of transmission has multiple links and as a public health specialist, one has to identify the weakest link and to attack on this link. The three major targets are needed to be identified:
1. Reservoir or source of infection
2. Route(s) of infection
3. Susceptible host(s)

### Controlling the Reservoir or Source of Infection

The chain of transmission of a disease starts from the source or reservoir. If the source or reservoir is an animal, one can try to eliminate the same to break the chain of transmission like in case of brucellosis. But, where the source or reservoir is a human than different steps are to be taken to attack on this link. The different steps comprises of:

### Early Diagnosis and Prompt Treatment

This is a very crucial step in controlling the source or reservoir. In any disease outbreak, for example, in swine flu, SARS, etc. the team of specialists comprising of a clinician, epidemiologist and a laboratory personnel need to develop an algorithm to diagnose an infection in a quick way and provide a prompt treatment of the cases to halt the communicability of disease to others.

### Notification

Once an infectious disease is suspected, the same should be mandatorily notified to the local health authorities or the global health authorities depending upon the regulatory mechanisms as well as the type of disease. Notification of disease provides a good data set for the epidemiological information needed for the preparedness plan for the control of infection or disease.

The International Health Regulations (IHR) have mandated notification of four infectious diseases irrespective of when or where they occur. Other diseases also become notifiable when they represent an unusual risk or situation.

**Always Notifiable:**
1. Smallpox.
2. Poliomyelitis due to wild-type poliovirus.
3. Human influenza caused by a new subtype.
4. Severe acute respiratory syndrome (SARS).

**Other Potentially Notifiable Events:**
1. This may be diseases due to pneumonic plague, cholera, yellow fever, viral hemorrhagic fevers, and West Nile fever or any others that meet the IHR criteria.
2. Other biological, radiological, or chemical events that meet IHR criteria.

After the revised IHR 2005, WHO has declared four **Public Health Emergencies of International Concerns (PHEICs):**
1. H1N1 influenza (2009).
2. Polio (2014).
3. Ebola (2014).
4. Zika virus (2016).

### Isolation

When a case of a disease is the most important source of infection in comparison to a carrier, one of the important step for control activity is isolating the case from the susceptible population. Isolation is defined as the separation for the period of communicability, of infected persons or animals from others so as to protect from direct or indirect transmission of disease from the infected ones to the susceptible. The best way of isolating a case is to put him/her under strict surveillance in a hospital. In some cases, the home isolation is also recommended, though difficult to achieve but carry meaning during outbreaks of infections like H1N1 and Covid-19 active cases where suspected cases are recommended home isolation though with few precautions.

## Quarantine

This refers to the restriction of movement of those persons or animals who are well but are potentially susceptible to contract the disease due to being exposed to the infected case. The period of quarantine is approximately equal to the longest incubation period of that disease. The quarantine measures are also applied by the health authorities at the portal of entry or exit like ship, aircraft, and train, etc. The quarantine may be of three types:
1. Complete quarantine.
2. *Modified quarantine:* In case of infectious diseases in children, the restriction of movement of children is just by their limitation of going to school and mixing with other children.
3. *Segregation:* Removal of susceptible children to the homes of immune persons.

Currently, quarantine is replaced by better methods of control of infection-largely by active surveillance.

## Interruption of Transmission

The most important step of the control of a communicable disease is to break the chain of transmission. The chain of transmission can be broken based on the type of diseases.
- For the vector-borne diseases, e.g., malaria, dengue, etc. the chain of transmission can be broken by source reduction, i.e., removal of water bodies where the vector breeding can take place.
- In case of food-borne diseases hand hygiene and ensuring safe drinking water break the chain of transmission.
- For zoonotic diseases like rabies, the chain of transmission can be broken by vaccinating the canine population.

### Disinfection as a Method to Interrupt the Transmission of Disease

*Disinfectants* are antimicrobial agents applied to the surface of non-living objects. In comparison to sterilization, disinfection is not that powerful. Disinfectants are frequently used in healthcare settings both medical surgical dental wards, and even in household use like in kitchens and bathrooms. Unlike sterilization, it does not affect all types of life.

*Disinfection:* Use of physical procedures or chemical agents to destroy most microbial forms; however, bacterial spores and relatively resistant organisms may remain viable.
- **Precurrent (prophylactic) disinfection:** Disinfection of water by chlorine, pasteurization of milk and handwashing may be cited as examples of precurrent disinfection.
- **Concurrent disinfection:** Disinfection is done as soon as possible after the discharge of infectious material from the body of an infected person, or after the soiling of articles with such infectious discharges. This way further spread of the agent is stopped. Concurrent disinfection consists of usually disinfection of urine, feces, vomit, contaminated linen, clothes, hands, dressings, aprons, gloves, etc. throughout the course of an illness.
- **Terminal disinfection:** Disinfection is done after the patient has been removed by death or to a hospital or has ceased to be a source of infection or after other hospital isolation practices have been discontinued.

*Sterilization:* Use of physical procedures or chemical agents to destroy all microbial forms including bacterial spores, mycobacteria, nonenveloped viruses and fungi. Sterilizer is the apparatus used to sterilize medical devices, equipment or supplies by direct exposure to the sterilizing agent.

*Antiseptic:* Substance that prevents or arrests the growth or action of microorganisms by inhibiting their activity or by destroying them. The term is used especially for preparations applied topically to living tissue.

*Sanitizer:* Agent that reduces the number of bacterial contaminants to safe levels as judged by public health requirements. Commonly used with substances applied to inanimate objects.

*Detergent:* Surface cleaning agent that makes no antimicrobial claims on the label. They comprise a hydrophilic component and a lipophilic component. It acts by lowering surface tension, e.g., soap which removes bacteria along with dirt.

Disinfectants are used to rapidly kill bacteria. They kill off the bacteria by damaging the proteins and outer layers of the bacteria resulting in subsequent leakage of DNA material **(Table 16.1 and Fig. 16.3)**.

**Table 16.1:** Levels of resistance to disinfectants.

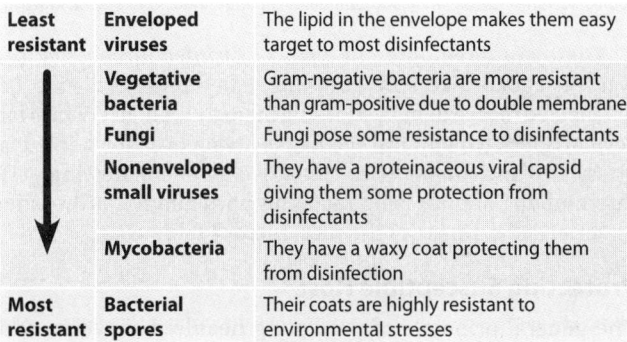

| | | |
|---|---|---|
| Least resistant | Enveloped viruses | The lipid in the envelope makes them easy target to most disinfectants |
| | Vegetative bacteria | Gram-negative bacteria are more resistant than gram-positive due to double membrane |
| | Fungi | Fungi pose some resistance to disinfectants |
| | Nonenveloped small viruses | They have a proteinaceous viral capsid giving them some protection from disinfectants |
| | Mycobacteria | They have a waxy coat protecting them from disinfection |
| Most resistant | Bacterial spores | Their coats are highly resistant to environmental stresses |

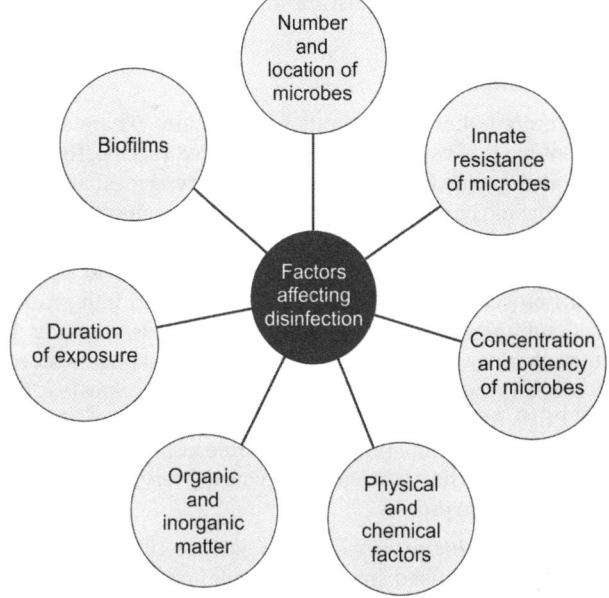

**Fig. 16.3:** Factors affecting efficacy of disinfection and sterilization.
*Source:* CDC, Guideline for Disinfection and Sterilization in Healthcare Facilities, 2008.

**Table 16.2:** Commonly used chemical disinfectants.

| Disinfectant | Activity | Advantages | Disadvantages | Recommendation |
|---|---|---|---|---|
| Glutaraldehyde | Broad-spectrum microbicidal and sporicidal | Good compatibility | Requires activation produces irritant fumes | For fibroscope and respiratory equipment |
| Orthophthaldehyde | Broad-spectrum microbicidal and sporicidal | No activation required No fumes | Costly Stains equipment | For scopes Alternative to glutaraldehyde |
| Iodine compounds | Microbicidal spares *M. tuberculosis* and spores | Rapid action | Corrosive to metals, plastic and rubber stains items | As an antiseptic |
| Alcohols | Wide microbicidal activity Non-sporicidal | Non-staining | Flammable | Hand disinfection for endoscopes |
| Phenols | Wide microbicidal activity Non-sporicidal | Easily available low cost | Irritant to skin | As surface disinfectant |
| Quaternary Ammonium compounds | Microbicidal spares *M. tuberculosis*, not sporicidal, not virucidal | Less irritant Good detergent property | Occupational asthma | As surface disinfectant for non-critical items |
| Peracetic acid | Broad-spectrum microbicidal and sporicidal | No activation required Wide compatibility | Expensive Irritant to eye and skin | For fibroscopes |
| Chlorines | Wide microbicidal activity Non-sporicidal | Low cost fast acting | Corrosive to metals | Surface disinfectant To clean blood and body fluid spills |
| Hydrogen peroxide | Broad-spectrum microbicidal and sporicidal | No activation required | Serious eye damage incompatible with some metals | Fogging of operating room for endoscopes |
| Formaldehyde | High level disinfectant | Non-corrosive | Pungent odor and irritant fumes carcinogenic | Withdrawn from use |

*Source:* Juwarkar CS. Cleaning and sterilisation of anaesthetic equipment. Indian J Anaesth. 2013;57:541-50.

There are three different types of disinfection agents: (a) Natural agents like sunlight—linen, beddings etc., can be disinfected to an extent by exposing them to sunlight UV rays for several hours, (b) Physical agents like hot air oven for sterilizing glasswares and similar items; autoclave for linen, dressings, OT instruments; and ionizing radiation particularly for dressing material and sutures, (c) chemical agents **(Table 16.2)**.

## Protecting Susceptible Host

The general principle of promoting healthy behaviors, and the specific protection by active or passive immunization or chemoprophylaxis to the host are important measures to protect the susceptible host.

### Active Immunization

It is acquired after administration of vaccines. There are four different types of vaccines (a) Live attenuated vaccine, (b) Killed inactivated vaccine, (c) Toxoid, and (d) Subunit vaccines (containing only antigenic part of the microbe) (Refer **Flowchart 16.2**). The subunit vaccines can be those produced by recombinant DNA technology or those obtained through the usual bacteriological growth processes. They can be further classified into protein-based subunit vaccines (e.g. acellular pertussis, hepatitis B), polysaccharide vaccines (e.g. meningococcal and pneumococcal polysaccharide vaccines) and conjugate subunit vaccines (e.g. HiB, MCV, PCV). All vaccines contain additional excipients which may function as an adjuvant (improves immune response), stabilizers, preservatives, carriers (vehicle for vaccine delivery) or are residual of the production process.

*Immunization history:* Evidence as early as 1000 CE suggests that the Chinese used smallpox inoculation (or variolation). Edward Jenner in 1796 successfully used material from cowpox infected cows to develop immunity against smallpox in susceptible humans. His methods over the next 200 years eventually lead to eradication of smallpox in 1979. The term vaccination is derived after the virus affecting cows (latin: *vacca* "cow"). Next to make an impact was rabies vaccine by Louis Pasteur in 1885.

India launched its Expanded Program of Immunization (EPI) in 1978 immediately after the country was declared smallpox free in 1977. In 1985, the program was renamed to Universal Immunization Program where measles (first dose) was added and a major focus was shifted to establishing quality of service, improving cold chain system along with district-wise monitoring and evaluation system and in towards self-sufficiency in manufacturing of vaccines and cold-chain equipment.

A well thought immunization schedule should be epidemiologically relevant, immunologically effective, operationally feasible and socially acceptable.

### National Immunization Schedule
*This topic has been covered in detail in Chapter 47: Health Policies and Programs in India.*

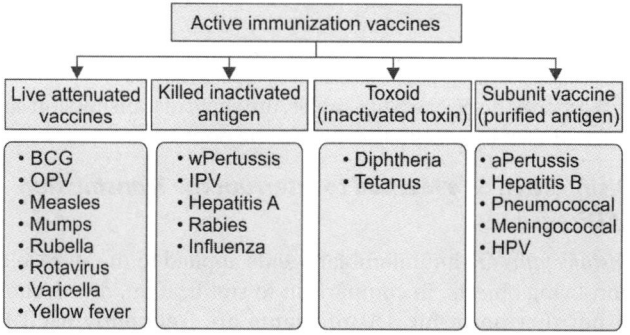

**Flowchart 16.2:** Active immunization agents.

## Recommended Vaccines for Adult Immunization:

| Vaccine | Indication | Previously immunized | Not immunized | Type of vaccine | Dose and route of administration | Brand |
|---|---|---|---|---|---|---|
| Diphtheria, Pertussis and Tetanus* | Universally accepted to all (Except any contraindications) | **1 dose** Tdap, then Td or Tdap booster every 10 years up to 64 years; Td booster every 10 years for ≥65 years | **3 doses** of Td or Tdap vaccine: 2 doses to be administered 4 Weeks apart 3rd dose to be given 6-12 months after the 2nd dose | Combination Vaccine | 0.5 mL; IM | Td- Tenivac, Tdvax; Tdap-Boostrix, Adacel |
| MMR | Recommended in adults up to 59 years (Contraindicated in pregnancy and immunosuppressed states) | Not indicated | **Single dose** | Live Vaccine | 0.5 mL; SC | Tresivac |
| Influenza | Recommended in all especially if some risk factor is present (e.g. based on medical, occupational or other indication) | **Single dose** once every year | **Single dose** once every year | Inactivated | 0.5 mL; IM | Fluvac |
| Pneumococcal Polysaccharide Vaccine (PPSV 23) | • Recommended for all above 65 years; • <65 years- only those at risk [Age 19-64 years with chronic medical conditions (chronic heart, lung, or liver disease, diabetes), alcoholism, or cigarette smoking] | If administered prior to age 65 years, administer **1 dose** at least 5 years after previous dose | **Single dose** at the age of 65 years | Polysaccharide | 0.5 mL; IM | Pneumovax 23 |
| Pneumococcal Conjugate Vaccine (PCV 13) | Recommended vaccination for adults age 19 years or older with immunocompromising conditions, chronic renal failure, nephrotic syndrome, leukemia, lymphoma, Hodgkin disease, generalized malignancy, iatrogenic immunosuppression, solid organ transplant, or anatomical or functional asplenia | | • 1 dose PCV13 followed by 1 dose PPSV23 at least 8 weeks later, then another dose PPSV23 at least 5 years after previous PPSV23; • At age 65 years or older, administer 1 dose PPSV23 at least 5 years after most recent PPSV23 (note: only 1 dose PPSV23 recommended at age 65 years or older) | Conjugate | 0.5 mL; IM | Prevnar 13 |
| Varicella | For all who are not immune or who did not have chickenpox | Not required if titres are adequate | **2 doses**; 4–8 weeks apart | Attenuated live VZV (Oka strain) | 0.5 mL; IM | Varilrix, Okavax, Varivax |
| Human Papillomavirus | • Recommended for young adults aged 19–26 years • 27–45 years, based on shared clinical decision-making | Not required | 9–14 years- **2 doses** are given 6 months apart 15–26 years- **3 doses** at 0,1 and 6 months | Recombinant | 0.5 mL; IM | Gardasil (Quadrivalent, HPV types 6,11,16 and 18) Cervarix (Bivalent HPV types 16 and 18) |
| Zoster | Recommended for >60 years age | **Single dose** | | Live attenuated | 0.65 mL; SC | Zostavax |
| | Recommended for >50 years age | **2-dose**; 2–6 months apart | | Recombinant | 0.5 mL; IM | Shingrix |
| Hepatitis A | At risk for infection due to chronic liver disease, HIV infection, healthcare workers in close contact with patients; infection during pregnancy; travel to endemic countries | **Single dose** if high-risk | • **2 doses**; 6 months apart • **3 doses**: 0, 1 and 6 months (for combination vaccine) | Inactivated; Combination | 0.5 mL; Parenteral | HAV antigen- Biovac-A, Harvix Combination Vaccine (HAV+HAB)- Twinrix |
| Hepatitis B | At risk for infection due to chronic liver disease, HIV infection, healthcare workers in close contact with patients, sexual exposure, percutaneous exposure, injectable drug use; infection during pregnancy; travel to endemic countries | Not indicated | **3 doses**: 0, 1 and 6 months | Recombinant; Combination | 1 mL; Parenteral | Shanvac-B, Engerix-B; Twinrix |

*Contd...*

*Contd...*

| Vaccine | Indication | Previously immunized | Not immunized | Type of vaccine | Dose and route of administration | Brand |
|---|---|---|---|---|---|---|
| Meningococcal@ | High-risk individuals – <br>• Anatomical or functional asplenia, HIV infection, persistent complement deficiency: **2 doses** at least 8 weeks apart and revaccinate every 5 years if risk remains <br>• Travel to countries with hyperendemic or epidemic of disease: **1 dose** and revaccinate every 5 years if risk remains | | | Conjugate; Polysaccharide | 0.5 mL; SC | Quadrivalent MenAWCY- Menactra, Menveo |
| HiB@ | At risk individuals like <br>• Anatomical or functional asplenia: **1 dose** if previously did not receive Hib; if elective splenectomy, 1 dose, preferably at least 14 days before splenectomy <br>• Hematopoietic stem cell transplant: **3-doses;** 4 weeks apart starting 6–12 months' after successful transplant, regardless of Hib vaccination history | | | Conjugate; Combination | 0.5 mL; IM | GSK |
| Rabies | Recommended in high-risk groups such as veterinary personnel, medical doctors, dog catchers, postmen, wild life wardens | Pre-exposure prophylaxis: 0, 7 and 28 days <br>Post-exposure prophylaxis: 0, 3, 7 and 28 days with Rig | | Human Diploid Cell Culture Vaccine | 1 mL; IM <br>0.1 mL; ID over deltoid | Abhayrig, Abhayrag, Berirab-P, Rabipur |
| Typhoid | To individuals during outbreak and high-risk travelers | Booster dose every 3 years | **Single dose**, than every 3 years | Polysaccharide (conjugated with tetanus toxoid) | 0.5 mL; SC/IM | Typbar TCV Vi-TT |
| Cholera | High-risk groups (children, pregnant women, and the elderly) | Booster dose within 2 years | **2 doses**, 1-6 weeks apart for those aged over 6 years | Inactivated | Oral | Dukoral ShanChol |
| Japanese encephalitis | Not recommended for routine use in adults | **Single dose** followed by booster dose at 1 year | | Live attenuated; Inactivated | 0.5 mL; SC <br>0.5 mL; IM | SA 14-14-2; Jenvac |
| Polio | Individuals travelling to endemic countries | **Single dose** of IPV | **3 doses** of IPV/ OPV spaced by 1 month | Live attenuated; Inactivated | 2 drops; oral <br>0.5 mL; IM | Polio Saven, Poliovac, Imovax Polio |

*DTaP: 6 weeks through 6 years; Td: 7 years of age and older; Tdap: 11 years of age and older
(Upper case "T" means there is about the same amount of tetanus in DTaP, Tdap and Td. Upper case "D" and "P" means there is more diphtheria and pertussis in DTaP than in Tdap and Td; lower case letters ("d""p") means there is less.)
@ Dose depends upon vaccine and indication.
*Sources:* Muruganathan A, Mathai D, Sharma SK, editors. Adult immunization. J Assoc Physicians India. 2014:1–270.
Guidelines for vaccination in normal adults in India. Indian J Nephrol. 2016.

## Vaccines to be given to travelers

| Category | Vaccine |
|---|---|
| Routine | • Diphtheria/tetanus/pertussis (DTaP) <br>• Hepatitis B virus (HBV) <br>• Measles, mumps, rubella (MMR) <br>• Inactivated poliomyelitis (IPV) |
| Recommended | • Influenza <br>• Hepatitis A virus (HAV) <br>• Japanese encephalitis <br>• Meningococcal meningitis <br>• Pneumococcal disease <br>• Rabies <br>• Tick-borne encephalitis <br>• Typhoid fever <br>• Yellow fever (for individual protection) <br>• Cholera |
| Required (mandatory) | • Yellow fever (for protection of vulnerable countries) <br>• Meningococcal meningitis (for Hajj, Umrah) |

## Passive Immunization

It involves standard serum immunoglobulin and specific targeted immunoglobulin (Refer **Flowchart 16.3**).

## Herd Immunity

"Herd immunity" is a concept where vaccination protects more than just the vaccinated person. It refers to protecting the whole community from a communicable disease by immunizing a critical mass of its population. In a community, those who are vaccinated have not only protected themselves from disease but also protect other members of the community who are not vaccinated. This is achieved by preventing the chain of disease and limiting potential outbreaks. Every vaccinated person thus adds to the effectiveness of community-level protection **(Table 16.3)**.

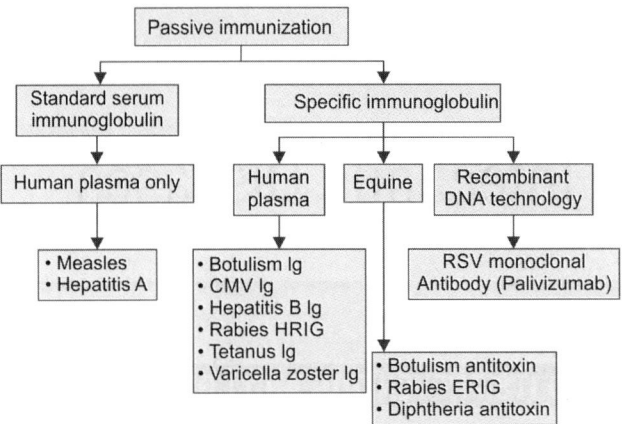

**Flowchart 16.3:** Passive immunization agents.

(ERIG: equine rabies immunoglobulin; CMV: cytomegalovirus; HRIG: human rabies immunoglobulin; RSV: respiratory syncytial virus)

**Table 16.3:** Herd immunity levels (Crude) for common vaccine preventable diseases.

| Disease | $R_0$ | Herd immunity threshold |
|---|---|---|
| Measles | 12–18 | 83–94% |
| Pertussis | 12–17 | 92–94% |
| Rubella | 6–7 | 83–85% |
| Diphtheria | 6–7 | 85% |
| Smallpox | 5–7 | 80–85% |
| Polio | 5–7 | 80–86% |
| Mumps | 4–7 | 75–86% |

Herd immunity is possible by mass immunization against directly transmitted infections from person-to-person like measles, pertussis, influenza and polio. On the other hand, herd immunity is not possible in those infections that are not generally transmitted from person-to-person or humans are not an important reservoir of infection (e.g. tetanus, rabies).

Herd immunity is based on a critical vaccine coverage which depends on following factors:
- *Infectiousness:* This has been described by Basic Reproduction Number ($R_0$) which is defined as "the average number of other individuals each infected individual will infect in a population that has no immunity to the disease".
- *Vaccine effectiveness:* Lesser the effectiveness, higher will be the critical vaccine coverage that will be required for heard immunity.
- *Waning immunity:* Pertussis and measles immunity may wane over time which may open up transmission pathways and dent the herd immunity.
- *Population heterogeneity:* A highly interconnected population will favor transmission dynamics and higher $R_0$.

## Chemoprophylaxis

Chemoprevention (also chemoprophylaxis) refers to the administration of a medication for the purpose of preventing disease or infection. Antibiotics, for example, may be administered to patients with disorders of immune system function to prevent bacterial infections (particularly opportunistic infection). Antibiotics may also be administered to healthy individuals to limit the spread of an epidemic, or to patients who have repeated infections (such as urinary tract infections) to prevent recurrence. It may also refer to the administration of heparin to prevent deep venous thrombosis in hospitalized patients.

## SUGGESTED READING

1. Bailey NJ. The Mathematical Theory of Infectious Diseases and its Applications. 2nd edition. [ISBN 0852642318] Charles Griffin; 1975. p. 413.
2. Barreto ML, Teixeira MG, Carmo EH. Infectious diseases epidemiology. J Epidemiol Community Health. 2006;60(3):192-5.
3. CDC. Global Health – International Health Regulations.
4. Fine PEM. Herd Immunity: History, Theory, Practice. Epidemiol Rev [Internet]. Oxford University Press; 1993.
5. Lahariya C. A brief history of vaccines and vaccination in India. Indian J Med Res [Internet]. 2014 [cited 2018 Jul 29];139(4):491–511. Available from: http://medind.nic.in/iby/t14/i4/ibyt14i4p491.pdf.
6. Last JM. A dictionary of epidemiology, 4th edition. New York: Oxford University Press; 1988. pp. 1-372.
7. Remington PL, Hall WN, Davis IH, et al. Airborne transmission of measles in a physician's office. JAMA. 1985;253(11):1574-7.
8. Siegel JD, Rhinehart E, Jackson M, et al. Guideline for isolation precautions: preventing transmission of infectious agents in healthcare settings. Atlanta: United States Centers for Disease Control and Prevention (CDC); 2007. p. 17.
9. WHO. Case definitions for the four diseases requiring notification in all circumstances under the International Health Regulations (2005).

# CHAPTER 17

# Specific Epidemiology of Infectious Diseases

## A. EPIDEMIOLOGY OF AIRBORNE DISEASES AND ITS PREVENTION AND CONTROL

### GENERAL EPIDEMIOLOGY OF AIRBORNE DISEASES AND GENERAL PRINCIPLES OF PREVENTION AND CONTROL

*Malatesh Undi, Vidya R*

| | |
|---|---|
| **CM7.2** | Enumerate, describe and discuss the mode of transmission and measures for prevention and control of airborne diseases |
| **CM8.1** | Describe and discuss the epidemiological and control measures applicable in airborne diseases |

> *Case Scenario*
>
> In May 1994, a lady traveled from Chicago to Honolulu by flight and the journey lasted about 8 hours 45 minutes. She died a few months later and was diagnosed to have Multi-Drug Resistant Tuberculosis (MDR-TB). Following this, the other people who had traveled on the same flight were tested. Among all the people in that flight, 15 passengers were found to be infected with Tuberculosis. Of these, six passengers did not have any other risk factors to develop Tuberculosis. It was also observed that they had sat on the same section of the plane as the lady.
> - So, how did the transmission happen even though they did not come in physical contact with that lady?
> - What factors could have led to the high number of secondary cases in this scenario?

## INTRODUCTION

The respiratory system is an open system. The air breathed out and the droplets released into the air during sneezing and coughing get easily transported in the air as there are no barriers to filter them. These contaminants can be transported through the air to great distances and hence anyone in the vicinity is prone for exposure.

Respiration is a vital activity. It is a constant activity. A person cannot stop breathing for longer than a few minutes without serious effects on the brain and other vital organs. During normal respiration, a person breathes in about 500 mL of air. Based on this, the volume of air that a person breathes in and out in a day is about 14,400 liters.

The quality of air that is present around a person depends on various factors which include the locality (urban, rural, and industrial), presence of contaminants due to industries or infected people, release of poisonous gases from the exhaust of vehicles and other such factors. This quality can play an important role in the health of the community because a whole of the same air is inhaled by all the people in the community. This can act as a health threat and a public health problem. *Airborne diseases* are defined as "the diseases caused by pathogenic organisms that remain suspended in the air (on dust particles, respiratory and water droplets) and transmitted from person-to-person via coughing, sneezing, talking, laughing and close personal contact or aerosolization of the pathogenic microbes" **(Box 17A.1)**.

> **Box 17A.1: How does one get infected by airborne diseases?**
> - One may be exposed to airborne diseases if he/she has spent time near someone with airborne disease of the lungs or throat.
> - One can get infected by breathing in the microorganisms that an infected person coughs/sneezes into the air.

## CHARACTERISTIC OF AIRBORNE DISEASES

- *Transmission of airborne diseases* can occur by two means of *aerosolization*:
  - Airborne transmission
  - Droplet transmission
- *Airborne transmission* is defined as "the transmission of infection by expelled particles that are comparatively smaller in size and thus can remain suspended in air for long periods of time".
- *Droplet transmission* is defined as "the transmission of diseases by expelled particles that are likely to settle to a surface quickly, typically within three feet of the source". A susceptible individual must be close enough to the source of the infection in order for the droplet (containing the infectious microorganism) to make contact with the susceptible individual's respiratory tract, eyes, mouth, nasal passages, and so forth.

- *Droplet and airborne transmission are not mutually exclusive.* Independent of its origin, particles carrying infectious microorganisms do not exclusively disperse by airborne or droplet transmission, but by both methods simultaneously.
- Airborne particles are particularly worrisome because they can *remain suspended in the air for extended periods of time.*
- Airborne diseases have potential to *spread across large geographical areas in short span of time* to cause *epidemics and pandemics.*
- Many airborne diseases are vaccine preventable diseases, e.g. measles, rubella, etc.
- One of the airborne diseases, smallpox has been successfully eradicated from the world **(Box 17A.2).**

### Box 17A.2: Common airborne diseases.
1. Acute respiratory infections (Pneumonia)
2. Chickenpox
3. Measles (Rubeola)
4. Mumps
5. Rubella
6. Influenza (Seasonal/Swine/Avian flu, SARS)
7. Tuberculosis
8. Diphtheria
9. Whooping cough (Pertussis)
10. Meningococcal meningitis
11. Covid-19 (Novel Coronavirus Induced Disease)

## EPIDEMIOLOGY OF AIRBORNE DISEASES (FIG. 17A.1)

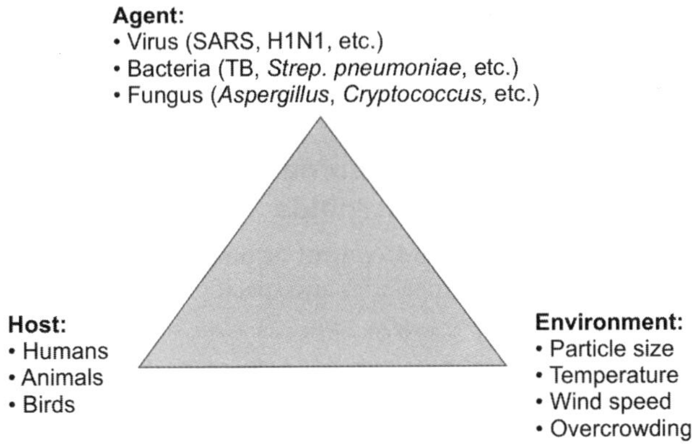

**Agent:**
- Virus (SARS, H1N1, etc.)
- Bacteria (TB, *Strep. pneumoniae*, etc.)
- Fungus (*Aspergillus, Cryptococcus*, etc.)

**Host:**
- Humans
- Animals
- Birds

**Environment:**
- Particle size
- Temperature
- Wind speed
- Overcrowding

**Fig. 17A.1:** Epidemiological triad depicting interrelationship between agent, host, and environmental factors responsible for airborne diseases.

## Host Factors

Most of the humans are susceptible to airborne diseases like seasonal flu, avian flu, swine flu, common cold, etc. Susceptibility of humans to airborne diseases depends on the following factors:

- *Vaccination status:* Many airborne diseases are vaccine preventable. For example, measles, rubella, diphtheria, pertussis, *H. influenzae*, etc. Unimmunized individuals remain susceptible for these airborne diseases.
- *Immunity:* Immunocompromised individuals are more susceptible for airborne diseases like tuberculosis, measles, etc. They also have a higher risk of developing complications.
- *Age group:* Airborne diseases like diphtheria, pertussis, measles, mumps, and rubella occur in children, more commonly in those less than 5 years. Some of the airborne diseases cause complications among elderly, e.g. avian flu, swine flu, etc.
- *Comorbidities/chronic illness:* Individuals with co-morbidities/chronic illness like diabetes, sickle cell disease, asplenia (no spleen), HIV infection, antibody and complement deficiency syndromes, cancer, bone marrow stem cell transplant, etc. has an increased risk of contracting airborne diseases and its complications, e.g. H1N1, *H. influenzae*, etc.
- *Occupation:* The individual's occupation may make him/her susceptible for airborne diseases. For example, individuals with silicosis are susceptible for tuberculosis infection, healthcare professionals treating infectious patients (H1N1, SARS, etc.) suffering from airborne diseases are themselves at risk of contracting the airborne diseases.
- *Travel:* Travelers especially frequent travelers are at increased risk of contracting airborne diseases from infected co-travelers. Air travel enables individual coming into contact with pathogenic organisms existing in far off places too.
- *Personal habits:* Habits like smoking makes them more susceptible to airborne disease like pulmonary tuberculosis infection and active tuberculosis.
- *Sex:* Most airborne diseases do not have a predilection to sex and ethnicity.

## Agent Factors

The virulence and pathogenicity of agent factors influence the infectivity and severity of disease **(Table 17A.1).**

**Table 17A.1:** Causative agent of various airborne diseases.

| Airborne disease | Causative agent |
| --- | --- |
| Common cold | Rhinovirus (common) and many other viruses |
| Pneumonia | Streptococcus pneumonia, Haemophilus influenzae (also causes meningitis) |
| Chickenpox | Varicella zoster virus |
| Measles (Rubeola) | Measles virus |
| Mumps | Mumps virus |
| Rubella | Rubella virus |
| Influenza (seasonal) | Influenza virus (Types A, B, C) |
| Avian flu | Influenza A virus: More virulent: H5N1, H5N6, H7N9, H10N8 Less virulent: H6N1, H7N4, H9N2 |
| Swine flu | Influenza A virus—H1N1 |
| SARS (Severe acute respiratory syndrome) | SARS-coronavirus (SARS-CoV) |
| MERS (Middle East respiratory syndrome) | Middle east respiratory syndrome coronavirus (MERS-CoV) |
| Tuberculosis | Mycobacterium tuberculosis |
| Diphtheria | Corynebacterium diphtheriae |
| Whooping cough (Pertussis) | Bordetella pertussis |
| Meningococcal meningitis | Neisseria meningitides (A, B, C, W, X and Y) |
| Hantavirus pulmonary syndrome (HPS) | Hantavirus |
| Smallpox (eradicated) | Variola virus (smallpox virus) |

(SARS: severe acute respiratory syndrome; MERS: middle east respiratory syndrome)

## Environmental Factors

Transmission of airborne diseases depends on several factors:

### Physical

- ***Particle size (i.e. the diameter of the particle):*** A particle with diameter of ≤5 mm (airborne) is capable of reaching the lower respiratory tract of humans and particle with diameter >5 mm (droplet) remains suspended in air and aids transmission of airborne diseases.

  Particle size is an important variable in airborne and droplet disease transmission because the ability of an infectious disease to cause an infection depends on the concentration of the microorganism, the human infectious dose, and the virulence of the organism.

- ***Level of infectious particles and the extent of desiccation:*** Humans can acquire devastating infectious diseases through exposure to very low levels of infectious particles. For example, infectious dose of influenza A for humans is very low. Similarly only a few cells of *Mycobacterium tuberculosis* are required to overcome normal lung clearance and inactivation of defence mechanisms. A single sneeze can generate around 40,000 large droplet particles; most will desiccate immediately into small, infectious droplet nuclei, with 80% of the particles being smaller than 100 microns.

- ***The frequency of the initiating activity:*** A single sneeze may produce more total infectious particles than a cough.

- ***Temperature:*** An important factor which influences survival of virus/bacteria. For example, low temperatures are ideal for airborne influenza virus survival and there is a less chance of survival at higher temperatures. However, bacteria are more resistant to temperature variations than viruses.

- ***Relative humidity:*** Relative humidity has an inconsistent relation with survival of airborne bacteria, e.g. *S. pneumoniae* survives poorly at intermediate relative humidity and *Pseudomonas* survives at high relative humidity.

- ***Ventilation:*** Poor ventilation favors increased density of infectious particles and transmission of airborne diseases.

### Social

- ***Overcrowding*** can lead to close exposure to droplets, concentration of the atmosphere with droplets, and infectious material.
- ***Close proximity*** to one another increases the risk of transmission of airborne diseases. *Close contact* includes kissing/hugging/talking to someone within three feet, sharing eating or drinking utensils and touching someone *directly.*
- ***Poverty:*** People living in poverty tend to live in poorly ventilated houses, have poor respiratory hygiene and personal hygiene, poor immunity and inadequate access to health service, all of which may favor transmission of airborne diseases and its complications.
- ***Urbanization:*** Increased density of population both at home and workplace increases the risk of transmission of airborne diseases.
- ***Travel:*** Frequent travelers, air travelers, travelers in crowded transport vehicles are at increased risk of contracting the airborne diseases as well as transmitting the diseases if they are infectious **(Table 17A.2)**.

**Table 17A.2:** Dynamics of airborne diseases transmission.

| Source of infection | Portal of exit | Mode of transmission |
|---|---|---|
| • Infectious humans<br>• Air/dust/fomites containing infectious material<br>• Air-conditioning systems<br>• Nonhuman sources—molds and its toxins, pollen, pet dander, and pest droppings<br>**Reservoir of infection**<br>• Infected humans<br>• Infected rodents<br>• Infected animals<br>**Infective material**<br>• Air with infected particles<br>  ➤ Droplets<br>  ➤ Aerosols<br>  ➤ Droplet nuclei<br>• Lesions (skin and mucosa)<br>• Fomites | Oral cavity and nasal cavity of infected persons<br>**Portal of entry**<br>Nasal cavity and oral cavity of susceptible persons | • Aerosolization of the pathogenic microbes<br>• Coughing<br>• Sneezing<br>• Talking<br>• Laughing<br>• Close personal contact<br>• Vomiting<br>• Flushing the toilet (aerosolization of toilet water) |

## PREVENTION AND CONTROL MEASURES OF AIRBORNE DISEASES

Prevention and control of airborne diseases can be achieved by *focusing on exposure to* droplet nuclei and dust/fomites containing infectious material:

### Strategies to Prevent Airborne Disease Transmission in Community and Households

Strategies to prevent and control airborne diseases can be classified into general measures and specific measures:

#### General Measures

These include all measures to prevent and control any infectious disease.

- ***Personal hygiene:*** This can get rid of any infectious material that is present on the skin surface following exposure.
  - *Hand washing and hygiene:* This is the single most important preventive measure against spread of airborne infections. Measures include washing of hands with soap and water before and after eating food and after using the toilet.
  - *Hand drying:* Use of disposable paper towels or air dry. Avoid cotton/linen towels or hot-air driers.
  - *Hand disinfection:* Alcohol and other disinfectants supplied in spray bottles that can be manipulated by users' elbow.
  - *Sanitation and cleanliness:* Avoiding open air defecation, open air urination, and spitting in public places can prevent transmission of several diseases including airborne diseases. Maintaining a clean living environment,

free from dust and any contamination can reduce the possibility of exposure to infectious material.

### Specific Measures

This includes measures that focus on prevention and control of airborne diseases.

- **Adequate ventilation:** Ventilation plays a major role in the prevention of airborne diseases. Adequate ventilation and cross-ventilation can reduce the concentration of the infectious microorganisms in the atmosphere and hence reduce the exposure. It is advised that the window area in a living area should occupy at least one-fifth space of the floor. There should also be cross-ventilation available. In work areas where there cannot be open windows, mechanical ventilation should be provided. In large factories and industries, it is advisable to install devices which can create negative airflow ventilation. It is advised that there should be a minimum of six air changes every hour.
- **Avoiding overcrowding:** Overcrowding is a major factor for airborne disease outbreaks in developing countries. Overcrowding can lead to close exposure to droplets, concentration of the atmosphere with droplets and infectious material. A minimum floor area of 6 meter squares should be available for each person in the living area. Overcrowding can be calculated based on two parameters—number of persons per room and square feet area per person. When sleeping or in hospital wards, there is a minimum distance that is recommended between two beds and this is usually 2 meters.
- **Immunization:** Many airborne diseases can be prevented by timely vaccination among susceptible humans, e.g. measles, mumps, rubella, diphtheria, pertussis, *H. influenzae*, etc.
- **Personal protective measures:**
  - *Cough etiquette/Good respiratory hygiene*: Covering the mouth and nose when coughing or sneezing, using tissues and disposing them correctly.
  - *Isolation*: Early self-isolation of those feeling unwell, feverish and having other symptoms of airborne diseases.
  - *Avoiding close contact* with sick people.
  - *Avoiding touching* one's eyes, nose or mouth.
  - *Regular hand washing* and proper drying of hands.

## Strategies to Prevent Airborne Disease Transmission in Healthcare Settings

Guidelines of WHO, CDC, and International Union of Tuberculosis and Lung Disease, focuses on healthcare facilities for the prevention and control of airborne diseases in developing and developed nations.

- **Administrative control:** Reduces the chances of exposure of non-infected individuals to infected patients. The measures include:
  - Training and education of healthcare staff
    - Infection control measures to be taken.
    - Standard operating procedures for different cadres of healthcare staff.
    - Proper handling of infectious waste.
  - Measures to be taken in the outpatient department
    - Well-ventilated rooms for patients with respiratory symptoms.
    - Separate room for waiting area and consultation room for those with respiratory complaints.
    - Health education to the patients regarding cough etiquette.
  - Measures to be taken in the inpatient department
    - Provision of separate wards for respiratory diseases.
    - Proper disposal of sputum.
    - Early diagnosis and prompt treatment.
    - Educating the patients and family members regarding cough hygiene.
- **Environmental control:** Reduces the density of infectious microorganisms in the air in healthcare settings. Measures include:
  - *Patient segregation and adequate spacing between the beds (at least 2 m)* to prevent close transmission.
  - *Adequate ventilation* to provide proper circulation of air.
  - *Special focus should be given to high-risk areas* like ART centers, bronchoscopy procedure rooms, respiratory wards, especially MDR-TB wards.
  - *Strategies for environmental control* are natural and mechanical ventilation, air replacement every hour, and UV light.
  - *Quarantine and isolation*: This shall be followed for airborne diseases based on their potential of causing outbreaks and known period of communicability.
- **Personal respiratory protection:** Measures to be taken *by the patients* to prevent transmission of infectious disease. These include:
  - *Wearing masks*: Patients with respiratory symptoms can wear masks (surgical/respirators) to prevent dispersion of droplets into the atmosphere. When used by the patient, it prevents the infectious material from getting dispersed into the atmosphere in the form of droplets following an episode of sneezing or coughing.
  - *Respiratory hygiene*: Cough etiquette, if followed properly, can reduce the dispersion of droplets.
  - *Personal hygiene*: Maintaining personal hygiene can help prevent the transmission through contact.
  - *Proper disposal of sputum*: Avoiding spitting of saliva or sputum in open areas and usage of sputum cup can help reduce the transmission **(Box 17A.3)**.

---

**Box 17A.3: Personal protective measures for health care workers (HCW).**

- **Respiratory protection devices:** These include surgical masks and specific respirators (N95). These should be used by healthcare workers at high-risk of frequent exposure to airborne diseased patients. These act as a barrier, preventing exposure of healthcare worker to the droplets.
- **Plastic aprons/impermeable aprons:** Prevents exposure of HCWs body to droplets. These should be used while doing aerosolization procedures and in isolation wards.
- **Gloves:** HCWs should wear gloves while collecting/handling infectious specimens (e.g. throat swab) of airborne disease patients and direct handling of the patients.
- **Eye protection with goggles/face shield:** These shall be worn by HCWs during aerosolization procedures, collection of specimen and in isolation wards.
- **Hand hygiene:** HCWs must regularly wash hands and dry them properly after handling every patient and/or specimens/equipment.

## CURRENT APPROACHES IN HEALTH

### Regulations for Prevention and Control of Airborne Diseases

International and National regulations exist for prevention and control of various airborne diseases especially for the ones which have potential to cause epidemics and pandemics.

#### International Health Regulations (IHR), 2005

As per IHR, 2005, Public Health Emergency of International Concern (PHEIC) is defined as "an extraordinary event which is determined, as provided in these regulations:

As an international treaty, the IHR are legally binding; all countries must report events of international public health importance **(Box 17A.4)**.

> **Box 17A.4: When does WHO declare an airborne disease as PHEIC?**
> Under IHR, a Public Health Emergency of International Concern is declared by the World Health Organization if the situation meets two of four criteria:
> 1. Is the public health impact of the event serious?
> 2. Is the event unusual or unexpected?
> 3. Is there a significant risk of international spread?
> 4. Is there a significant risk of international travel or trade restrictions?

#### Notification of Airborne Diseases

Some of the airborne diseases are notifiable both internationally and nationally **(Table 17A.3)**.

**Table 17A.3:** Notifiable airborne diseases.

| Notifiable under IHR, 2005 | Notifiable under GOI (Govt. of India) |
|---|---|
| • Human influenza caused by a new subtype<br>• Severe acute respiratory syndrome (SARS)<br>• Smallpox | • Tuberculosis*<br>• Human influenza-H1N1<br>• SARS<br>• Smallpox |

*Healthcare providers shall notify every TB case to local authorities (DHO/CMO/MHO)

## SUGGESTED READING

1. Blachere FM, Lindsley WG, Pearce TA, et al. Measurement of airborne influenza virus in a hospital emergency department. Clin Infect Dis. 2009;48(4):438-40.
2. Central Bureau of Health Intelligence. National Health Profile 2018. New Delhi: Directorate General of Health Services Ministry of Health and Family Welfare; 2018.
3. Centre for Disease Control and Prevention. Global Health Security: International Health Regulations (IHR), Division of Global Health Protection, Global Health. [Online] Available from: https://www.cdc.gov/globalhealth/healthprotection/ghs/ihr/index.html.
4. Cole EC, Cook CE. Characterization of infectious aerosols in health care facilities: An aid to effective engineering controls and preventive strategies. Am J Infect Control. 1998;26(4):453-64.
5. DHHS Maine. Airborne and Direct Contact Diseases—Infectious Disease Epidemiology Program—MeCDC. [Online] Available from https://www.maine.gov/dhhs/mecdc/infectious-disease/epi/airborne/.
6. Fernstrom A, Goldblatt M. Aerobiology and its role in the transmission of infectious diseases. J Pathog. 2013;2013:493960.
7. Garner JS. Guideline for isolation precautions in hospitals. The Hospital Infection Control Practices Advisory Committee. Infect Control Hosp Epidemiol. 1996;17(1):53-80.
8. Gralton J, Tovey E, McLaws ML, et al. The role of particle size in aerosolised pathogen transmission: A review. J Infect. 2011;62(1):1-13.
9. Plotkin B. Human rights and other provisions in the revised International Health Regulations (2005). Public Health. 2007;121(11):840-5.
10. Practical Guidelines for Infection Control in Health Care Facilities. Vol. 41. Manila, Philippines, New Delhi: World Health Organization, WPRO Regional Publication; 2005. pp. 1-103.
11. Shrivastava SR, Shrivastava PS, Ramasamy J. Airborne infection control in healthcare settings. Infect Ecol Epidemio. 2013;3.
12. TB India. 2019—RNTCP Annual Status Report. New Delhi: Central TB Division, DGHS, Ministry of Health and Family Welfare; 2019.
13. Wells WF. On air-borne infection. Study II. Droplets and droplet nuclei. Am J Epidemiol. 1934;20(3):611-8.
14. World Health Organisation. (2005). Case definitions for the four diseases requiring notification in all circumstances under the International Health Regulations (2005). [Online] Available from http://www.who.int/ihr/Case_Definitions.pdf?ua=1.
15. World Health Organization. (2018). IHR Procedures concerning public health emergencies of international concern (PHEIC). [Online] Available from: http://www.who.int/ihr/procedures/pheic/en/.

# EPIDEMIOLOGY OF ACUTE RESPIRATORY INFECTIONS AND ITS PREVENTION AND CONTROL

*Rajesh Kumar Konduru, Anil J Purty, Preetam Mahajan, Amit Kumar Mishra, Kalaiselvi*

| | |
|---|---|
| **CM7.2** | Enumerate, describe and discuss the mode of transmission and measures for prevention and control of Acute Respiratory infections |
| **CM8.1** | Describe and discuss the epidemiological and control measures applicable in Acute respiratory infections |

> *Case Scenario*
>
> ❑ Master X, a 4-year-old male child was brought by his parents to Rural Health Training Center OPD with a chief complaint of fever of moderate to high-grade since four days, cough for seven days, and difficulty in breathing for two days. It was informed that the child was apparently normal one week back after which he developed cough which was initially dry in nature and later, on 3rd day, became productive in nature. He developed fever for past four days, high grade fever, intermittent, associated with chills. The fever subsided on medication.
>
> He developed dyspnea with stridor and was associated with chest in-drawing since last two days. The child had similar history in the past at 2½ years of age for which he was hospitalized and diagnosed to have pneumonia and treated for the same.
>
> ❑ His mother informed that history of the child during antenatal period was uneventful and he was born through normal delivery. His birth weight was 2.65 kg and breastfeeding was initiated within 45 minutes after birth. His growth has been satisfactory and there were no delays in the development of milestones. The child is immunized for age as per National Immunization Schedule.
>
> ❑ Environmental history revealed that they were residing in a pucca house with adequate ventilation with overcrowding, and the kind of fuel used for cooking was LPG.
>
> ❑ On General examination, the child is lethargic and inactive, Cyanosis was present (generalized and mild), with Heart rate—88/min, Respiratory rate—45/min, and Temperature—102°F.

> - On systemic examination, it was found that chest in-drawing was present while inspiration, impaired note on right side (on percussion), and crepitations were present along with bronchial breath sounds on right side (on auscultation).
> - Provisional diagnosis: Master X, a 4-year-old male child is suffering from very severe pneumonia and requires hospital admission for further investigations and treatment.

# INTRODUCTION

The acute infections occurring in various parts of respiratory tract starting from nostrils to the alveoli of the lungs are considered as Acute Respiratory Infections (ARIs) and these infections contribute significantly in both adults and children in terms of morbidity and mortality. Due to low immune status, children, especially those aged under five years, would be the most vulnerable group experiencing the wrath of the severity of these infections. Acute respiratory infections can be classified against the anatomical backdrop. Those ARIs occurring from the nostrils to the vocal cords in the larynx including the Para Nasal sinuses and middle ear are considered as upper Respiratory tract infections (URTIs). Those acute infections occurring in the airways from trachea, bronchi (right and left bronchus), bronchiole, and alveoli are considered as lower respiratory tract infections (LRTIs). The different acute respiratory tract infections vary from common cold, being the simplest condition to pneumonia being the most serious condition. Other conditions include acute pharyngitis, otitis media, sinusitis, laryngitis, epiglottitis, tonsillo-epiglottitis, bronchitis, and bronchiolitis.

# BURDEN OF ARI

Acute respiratory infection (ARI) is consistently ranked among the top causes of morbidity and mortality worldwide. It has been referred to as a "forgotten pandemic", which kills more than 4 million people each year globally. The burden of pneumonia as the primary cause of mortality among children under 5 years of age is well established. Worldwide, ARIs are the third most common cause of mortality in all ages, particularly in lower income settings (WHO-EMRO 2016).

Studies have shown that despite dramatic advancement in the diagnostic and curative fields of medicine, there are still many communities in the world where 30% of the children die before their 5th birthday due to ARIs. Evidence from several studies has proven that the acute lower respiratory tract infections (ALRIs) are the major contributor to morbidity and mortality in under-five children and human respiratory syncytial virus (RSV), a common viral pathogen has been identified to be most commonly associated with ALRI though there are other viral and bacterial pathogens responsible for ALRIs and they would be explained later. Data shows that in 2016, 3% of neonatal and 13% of post neonatal deaths were due to pneumonia. This high case fatality rate due to ARI is due to a diversified clinical picture (signs and symptoms), difficulty in diagnosis (pack of a standardized diagnostic criteria), and the delay in the need to bring the children to healthcare facilities by the parents due to the lack of awareness on warning signals, thereby leading to delay in initiating the treatment or not being taken to health facilities on time (GHO data, Causes of Child Mortality, 2016).

As of 2019, 17.2 billion upper respiratory infections accounted for 42.8% of all-cause illnesses globally (Jin X, et al. Global burden of upper respiratory infections in 204 countries and territories, from 1990 to 2019.) National Health and Family Survey 5 (NFHS-5) data shows that in India 2.7% of under five children (2.3% in urban and 3.0% in rural area) had symptoms of ARIs at the time of survey or two weeks preceding the survey and among those who had symptoms of ARI, 69% of the victims had to be taken to a health facility.

To tackle the ARIs, emphasis was given to home based care (including the identification of warning signs) by UNICEF and this was the concept that lead to the birth of Integrated Management of Neonatal and Childhood Illness (IMNCI) which would be explained in the later part of the chapter. The presence of certain medical and social conditions, comorbidities like use of certain medications (e.g. steroids), malnutrition (common in under developed countries including India), poor living conditions, and physiochemical changes in non-specific host defense system such as cilia and mucus of the respiratory tract, will increase the overall morbidity and mortality rates due to ARI.

# EPIDEMIOLOGY OF ARI

The human respiratory tract is exposed to many pathogens through the smoke and dust that is inhaled along with air. To overcome these pathogens, the respiratory system is enabled with physiological defense mechanisms—the anatomy of the respiratory tract (mucus and cilia lining the respiratory tract), the normal microorganisms (commensals) residing in the respiratory tract, and the host's immune response. The inhaled microorganisms (pathogens) manifest clinical signs and symptoms and end up in illness when—the host's immune system fails (due to certain reasons like malnutrition, certain drugs, aging, certain medical conditions, etc.), when the virulence of the pathogens is high, high dosage of pathogens entering the host or a combination of above. There are many causes for the occurrence and spread of ARIs and these can be explained under the following headings:

## Agent Factors

Acute respiratory infections are caused by a wide range of bacterial and viral agents. Most of the acute upper respiratory tract infections (AURIs) are caused by viruses but the role of bacterial agents should not be neglected. Acute lower respiratory tract infections (ALRIs) are mostly attributed to bacterial agents but recent evidence shows that the role of viral agents has increased. Among the viral infections, the most important and foremost contender is influenza virus followed by respiratory syncytial virus (RSV). The other viral agents responsible for AURIs are parainfluenza virus, adenovirus, human metapneumovirus, and corona virus. Among bacterial infections, the most common pathogen responsible is *Streptococcus pneumoniae* (accounts to almost 50% of bacterial infections), and this is followed by *Haemophilus influenzae, Mycoplasma pneumoniae, Staphylococcus aureus*, and Gram-negative rods like *E. coli* and *Klebsiella pneumoniae* **(Table 17A.4)**.

A brief overview of agents causing various acute respiratory infectious conditions:

Table 17A.4: Causes of pneumonia with respect to specific pathogens responsible for different age groups.

| Age range | Most common causative organism |
|---|---|
| Neonates (from birth to 30 days after birth) | Streptococcus pyogens, Staphylococcus aureus and E. coli |
| Infants (from three weeks to four months) | Streptococcus pneumoniae |
| Infants older than four months to preschool age | Respiratory viruses and S. pneumoniae |
| Children in developing countries | S. aureus, Haemophilus influenzae |
| Adults-outpatient | S. pneumoniae, Mycoplasma pneumoniae, H. influenzae, Chlamydophila pneumoniae and respiratory viruses |
| Adults-inpatient | S. pneumoniae, Mycoplasma pneumoniae, H. influenzae, Chlamydophila pneumoniae, respiratory viruses, Legionella pneumophila and aspiration |
| Adults-intensive care unit | S. pneumoniae, H. influenzae, Chlamydophila pneumoniae, respiratory viruses, Legionella pneumophila, Gram-negative bacilli and aspiration |

## Acute Coryza (Common Cold)

Common cold is a conglomerate of symptoms like nasal congestion, sneezing, rhinorrhea, pharyngitis, and sometimes cough. Rhinovirus is the most common etiological agent but there are over 200 different viral agents including respiratory syncytial virus, corona viruses, influenza, and parainfluenza viruses known to cause coryza and common cold. Incubation period is generally 48–72 hours.

## Acute Pharyngitis

A wide range of bacterial and viral pathogens is present which can cause acute pharyngitis. Acute pharyngitis can occur not only due to any individual combination of viral and bacterial agents, it can also occur as a part of common cold. Among the bacterial agents, beta-hemolytic streptococci and *Chlamydia pneumoniae* are the most common agents. Among the viral agents, respiratory syncytial virus is the most common etiological agent followed by influenza and parainfluenza virus, corona virus, etc.

## Acute Sinusitis

A variety of microorganisms has been found to cause acute sinusitis including viruses. However, acute sinusitis is very rare in children under five years of age. In adults, *Haemophilus influenzae, Streptococcus pneumoniae,* and *Moraxella catarrhalis* account to majority of acute sinusitis cases.

## Acute Epiglottitis

Acute epiglottitis resulting in swelling and inflammation of epiglottis can be life-threatening situation (air way occlusion and asphyxiation) especially in children aged 2–3 years. The most common microorganism responsible for acute epiglottitis is *Haemophilus influenzae* type-B.

## Acute Otitis Media (AOM)

This condition may arise due to direct infection of the middle ear by viral and bacterial agents and as a sequelae to acute pharyngitis (due to blockage of eustachian tube). Study has shown that human respiratory virus has been isolated from the middle ear fluids in AOM cases. To conclude acute otitis media can be viral, bacterial, or combination of both.

## Acute Bronchitis

Acute bronchitis is the inflammation of large conducting airways. Clinically, it will present similar to a case of pneumonia except for the absence of signs of consolidation on chest examination and chest X-ray. Corona virus and respiratory syncytial viruses appear to be the most common contenders.

## Pneumonia

Previously, it was thought that pneumonia is caused predominantly by bacterial agents. But recent evidence shows that the role of viral agents in causing pneumonia has increased. Among the viral agents, the most common pathogen responsible for pneumonia is influenza virus followed by RSV. Among bacterial agents, the most pathogen responsible is *Streptococcus pneumoniae* followed by *Haemophilus influenzae*.

## Host Factors

### Age

Although ARI can occur in all age groups, evidence shows high morbidity and mortality among children is probably due to low immunity.

### Sex

Both males and females are equally affected.

### Maternal Education/Literacy of Mother

The burden of ARI is highest in children whose mothers had low literacy. This was probably due to low level of awareness regarding the identification warning signs and prevention and control/measures.

### Birth Weight

Studies show that the prevalence of ARI was higher among children whose birth weight was <2.5 kg.

### Nutritional Status

The Nutritional status of the child plays a vital role in the incidence of ARI. The burden of ARI is high among malnourished children.

### Immunization Status

Immunization plays an important role in incidence as well as prevention of ARIs. DPT vaccine is a proven example for the reduction of pharyngitis cases due to *Corynebacterium diphtheriae*. Vaccines against influenza and parainfluenza virus and respiratory syncytial virus would reduce the morbidity (since most of the viral infections are self-limiting) and vaccines against *Streptococcus pneumonia* and *Haemophilus influenzae* would prevent the mortality.

### Number of Children in the Household

There is a direct relationship between the total number of children and the incidence of ARIs. This is probably due to the increased spread of pathogens through direct and indirect modes resulting from increased contact between the siblings.

### Under-immunization Status

Even the measles vaccine gives protection (indirectly) against ARI, as pneumonia is a complication of measles. Thus, we can conclude that the MR campaign taken up by the Government of India, primarily is targeted against Measles and Rubella, but it will also help in the reduction of pneumonia (acute respiratory tract infection).

### Environmental Factors

The incidence and prevalence of ARI exhibit seasonal variation. Acute respiratory infections (both URTI and LRTI) are more common during monsoon and winter months. The other environmental factors linked to epidemiology of ARI are overcrowding, any family member suffering from cough and cold either currently or in the recent past, exposure to air pollution, including indoor air pollution (smoking chulas, indoor tobacco smoking), poor ventilation, use of fuels other than LPG for cooking, type of flooring and frequency of floor cleaning, etc.

### Mode of Transmission

Acute respiratory infections spread mainly by droplet infection (air borne). Droplet spread can be either direct or indirect. During the droplet spread by direct transmission, there is projection of droplets (with the infective pathogens) of saliva and secretions of nasopharynx, during coughing, sneezing, spitting, talking into the surrounding atmosphere, and thereby enters the nasopharynx of susceptible host. In direct transmission, the droplet spread is limited to a distance of 30–60 cm between the infected individual and susceptible host. In the indirect transmission, the "droplet nuclei" are responsible for the spread of infection from the infected individual to the susceptible host. Droplet nuclei are the dried residue of the droplets. The droplet nuclei may become airborne due to the wind current and can travel to long distances (due to the wind velocity). These droplet nuclei after getting inhaled, can reach and settle in different parts of respiratory tract (including the alveoli) and initiate the disease process.

## CLASSIFICATION OF PNEUMONIA

There are many classifications and most commonly used ones are:
1. Anatomical classification.
2. Classification of pneumonia based on setting (Community acquired pneumonia and hospital acquired pneumonia).
3. WHO classification.

### Anatomical Classification

- ***Lobar pneumonia:*** The consolidation involves all or part of the lobe
- ***Bronchopneumonia:*** The consolidation involves scattered lobules
- ***Interstitial pneumonia:*** Mostly inflammatory, involves mainly interstitial tissue between the alveoli.

### Classification of Pneumonia based on Setting

***Community-acquired pneumonia:*** Mainly caused by *Streptococcus pneumoniae, Haemophilus influenzae, Mycoplasma pneumoniae,* Viral, *Legionella pneumophila.*

***Hospital-acquired pneumonia:*** Mainly caused by gram-negative bacteria, *Staphylococcus aureus, Streptococcus pneumoniae,* anaerobes and fungi.

### WHO Classification

The original WHO guidelines classified the respiratory symptoms of children 2 to 59 months of age into four categories. Children with cough and cold who did not have signs of pneumonia were classified as "no pneumonia", and their caregivers were advised on appropriate home care. Children with fast breathing were classified as "pneumonia" and were given an oral antibiotic (at that time oral cotrimoxazole) to take at home for five days. Children who had chest indrawing with or without fast breathing were classified as "severe pneumonia" and were referred to the closest health facility for treatment with injectable penicillin. Children who had any general danger signs were classified as "severe pneumonia or very severe disease". These children received a first dose of oral antibiotic and were then urgently referred to a health facility for further evaluation and treatment with parenteral antibiotics.

However, the revisions in 2014 included changing the recommendation for the first-line antibiotic and re-defining the classification of pneumonia severity. The new WHO classification is therefore simplified to include only **two categories of pneumonia**; "**pneumonia**" with fast breathing and/or chest indrawing, which requires home therapy with oral amoxicillin, and "**severe pneumonia**", pneumonia with any general danger sign, which requires referral and injectable therapy **(Table 17A.5)**.

**Table 17A.5:** Classification of pneumonia in a child aged two months to five years.

| | Child age 2–59 months with cough and/or difficult breathing | | |
|---|---|---|---|
| | No pneumonia | Pneumonia | Severe pneumonia / Very severe pneumonia |
| Signs | • Cough<br>• Cold | • Fast breathing and/or<br>• Chest in-drawing | • General danger signs (Not able to drink, persistent vomiting, convulsions, lethargic or unconscious, stridor in a calm child or severe malnutrition) |
| Treatment | • Home care advice<br>• Advice mother to look for danger signs | • Oral amoxicillin<br>• Home care advice | • Give first dose of antibiotics<br>• Refer urgently to hospital |

### Classification of Pneumonia in a Young Infant

Young infants aged less than two months, are special category since they have *only non-specific* signs such as poor feeding, fever or low body temperature and are much less likely to cough with pneumonia. They can progress towards more severe sickness very easily and die very quickly if not diagnosed properly in the early stage and treated promptly. Further, in young infants, mild chest in-drawing is normal due to weak chest wall. A slight doubt regarding the clinical condition of a young infant should prompt towards referral to a higher center for further management.

> **Note**
> During the reassessment of the child with pneumonia (i.e. two days after the initiation of the antibiotics) if: (a) the condition is same, then change the antibiotic; (b) the condition improves, then continue the antibiotic therapy for five days and complete the course; (c) the condition has become worse (child stopped feeding, lethargic, etc.), refer urgently to higher center.

## HOW TO APPROACH CHILDREN PRESENTING WITH ACUTE RESPIRATORY INFECTIONS?

Acute respiratory infections are very common among children and it is expected that on an average a child may have at least 6–12 episodes in a year very early in life. Acute respiratory infection as mentioned earlier in the text includes wide range of conditions like common cold, sinusitis, tonsillitis, pharyngitis, laryngitis, tracheitis, bronchiolitis, bronchitis, pneumonia, etc. The last one can prove life threatening at times and need special strategy for early detection and appropriate management.

Children with ARI may present with features either singly or in combination depending upon underlying problem. These have been outlined in **Box 17A.5**.

| Box 17A.5: Common presentations in children with ARI. |
|---|
| • Nasal congestion (Rhinitis) |
| • Rhinorrhea |
| • Sore throat |
| • Cough |
| • Wheezing/Stridor |
| • Breathlessness/Dyspnea |
| • Fever |
| • Earache/Headache |

Nasal congestion usually progresses to rhinorrhea, common cold (viral rhinosinusitis) being the most common cause and has an acute presentation. It usually lasts for 7–10 days. Allergic rhinitis has a longer course and is a common cause of chronic rhinitis. In a fraction of cases (<15%) of common cold, symptoms might persist beyond 10 days and evolve into acute bacterial sinusitis (ABS), that would usually last for less than 30 days. Allergic rhinitis might contribute to poorly controlled asthma.

Fever is not an essential feature to diagnose common cold. Sneezing, pharyngitis, cough, postnasal discharge, and throat clearing are some of the other features that may be present. In sinusitis, headache and facial pain, with or without periorbital swelling may be present. Chronic cases are best referred to specialists to rule out other conditions like immunodeficiency, cystic fibrosis, ciliary dyskinesias, etc.

Most uncomplicated episodes of viral rhinosinusitis resolve within a week. One may consider use of analgesics, mechanical nasal clearance, and saline nasal drops in small children, and decongestants in older children (>6 years). Acute bacterial sinusitis is often caused by *Streptococcus pneumoniae*, *H. influenzae*, and *Moraxella catarrhalis*. Amoxicillin is used to treat ABS as a first-line agent. Azithromycin may be considered for children with allergy to penicillin.

Acute pharyngitis is among the most common conditions that bring children to health facility. We need to differentiate viral etiology from bacterial. Pharyngitis of viral origin manifest with cough, rhinorrhea, nasal congestion, red eyes, mouth ulcers, hoarseness of voice, and among age less than 3 years. While bacterial pharyngitis (seen more commonly among children >3 years of age) present with absence of URI symptoms, abrupt onset of fever, headache, throat pain, exudative pharyngitis, abdominal pain with or without vomiting, tender anterior cervical lymph nodes, scarlet fever rash, etc. This may lead to peritonsillar abscess, retropharyngeal abscess, etc. Group *A Streptococcus* (GAS) is a clinically important cause of pharyngitis and needs to be identified and treated accordingly to prevent acute rheumatic fever. Clinical judgment is often not reliable and laboratory diagnosis is important to confirm GAS. Cultures are more accurate as compared to Rapid Antigen Detection Tests, but reports are only available after three days. This can often delay or result in unnecessary treatment with antibiotics. Diphtheria also presents with pharyngitis and has been covered elsewhere. Penicillin continues to be first choice for GAS treatment due to its narrow spectrum and affordability. However, it has to be taken for 10 days. Suitable alternative could be amoxicillin and in allergic patients azithromycin may be considered.

A patient that progresses with severe pharyngitis and does not respond to oral antibiotics should be possibly evaluated for presence of peritonsillar abscess, retro- or lateral pharyngeal abscess. Some of the suggestive signs could be worsening of voice, unilateral tonsillar enlargement trismus, uvular deviation, unilateral neck pain, decreased neck movement, etc. These are indications for prompt referral to ENT department for possible incision and drainage procedure and IV antibiotic therapy.

Sometimes patient with severe pharyngitis may also present with stridor. In general, stridor should be evaluated for intrathoracic (expiratory stridor) or extra thoracic (inspiratory stridor) airway obstruction. Croup characterized by sudden onset barky cough, breathlessness and inspiratory stridor is very common in children presenting with stridor below three years of age. It is usually viral in origin (parainfluenza types 1 and 3, RSV, influenza virus and adeno virus) and in unimmunized children may be caused by laryngeal diphtheria and measles. Sometimes epiglottitis may cause inspiratory stridor, which is usually caused by Hib infections. Noninfectious causes like angioedema, foreign body aspirations may also contribute to inspiratory stridor and should be ruled out first as these can prove life threatening.

Early corticosteroid (CS) treatment can be beneficial in mild to moderate viral croup. So, any child presenting with mild stridor with anticipated delay to access higher centers should be observed for at least three hours after treatment with racemic epinephrine and CS, before deciding to return the child home. Failure to respond to CS/epinephrine or moderate to severe stridor at presentation is a case for prompt referral after initial first aid (steroid and antibiotic treatment) to allow airway visualization in a controlled environment.

Wheeze is yet another complaint that often finds children finding their way to health facilities. These children can be evaluated either based on the quality of wheeze or its chronicity and recurrence

Wheeze is an expiratory noise and is either monophonic (i.e. same sound across the chest) or polyphonic (heterogenous sound throughout the chest). Monophonic sounds arise due to obstruction of large central airways whereas polyphonic sounds are due to small airway obstructions. Since, it is not always easy to appreciate the quality of wheeze, it is easier to approach the child based on whether the onset is acute or chronic/recurrent. Cases with acute wheeze should be evaluated for foreign body aspiration. History is often suggestive and child may need X-ray and/or bronchoscopy which is only possible in an appropriate health facility.

In absence of foreign body, age less than 2 years, and symptoms of URTI, bronchiolitis should be strongly considered. In an older child and/or absence of URTI, trial with a dose of inhaled beta-agonist should be carried out. If the child responds and there is no reason to suspect any chronic cause, diagnosis of asthma can be made. Or else one should look for any compression/mass, etc. In an older child with symptoms of URTI, pneumonia should be ruled out.

Most of these symptoms are present in combination and one of these is predominating. Algorithmic approach is often helpful in systematically arriving at diagnosis.

The clinical picture of bronchiolitis and pneumonia is similar except that in bronchiolitis there would not be fever.

Bronchiolitis is a clinical condition characterized by wheezing, chest retractions, and tachypnea. Here, bronchioles or small airways are involved. RSV causes inflammation that results in necrosis, exudation, edema, and bronchospasm. Finally, there is air trapping, atelectasis, and ventilation perfusion mismatch. Respiratory rate helps to classify patients according to severity. Pulse oximetry if available to identify children that would need supplemental oxygen (with saturation below 90%). Chest X-ray (CXR) may be required in severe cases to rule out pneumonia. In bronchiolitis, CXR will show hyper-expansion of lungs with flattened diaphragm, peribronchial thickening, and patchy atelectasis with or without perihilar infiltrates.

Pneumonia typically presents with fast breathing, fever, and cough. Clinically, it is possible to differentiate between viral and bacterial etiology.

## Physical Examination

### Appearance of the Child

The appearance of the child—whether the child is normal, irritable or lethargic or unconscious at the time of examination gives an insight to the stage of pneumonia. Child is usually irritable in not severe pneumonia and lethargic or unconscious in severe pneumonia and very severe disease.

### Ability to Feed

Child will not be able to feed normally in severe pneumonia and very severe disease.

### Respiratory Rate

There would be increased respiratory rate in severe stages of pneumonia and this would be sometimes accompanied by chest in-drawing. So while examining the respiratory system to assess the respiratory rate, the child's chest and abdomen should be exposed and the respiration cycles are to be counted for one full minute and simultaneously intercostal spaces are to be examined carefully for chest in-drawing. As children get older, their respiratory rate comes down. So the criteria (cut-off point) to establish the fast breathing (increased respiratory rate) is as follows:
- In a young infant (child aged less than two months)—60 breaths per minute or more
- In a child aged 2–12 months—50 breaths per minute or more
- In a child aged 1–5 years—40 breaths per minute or more

> **Note**
> In young infants, occasionally the respiration may be erratic (They stop breathing for few seconds and then breathe rapidly) and this is normal.

### Chest in-drawing

A treating physician should look for chest in-drawing during inspiration (when the child breathes in); during inspiration the lower chest wall goes in and this is a positive test for chest in-drawing. The chest in-drawing is seen when greater effort is needed to pull the air into the lungs than normal.

### Noisy Breathing

A child may have noisy breathing called "Stridor" or "Wheeze", caused either due to obstruction or narrowing in larynx, trachea, pharynx, or in the air passages inside the lungs. Stridor is due to narrowing or obstruction in pharynx, larynx, or trachea and this can be elicited during inspiration. Wheeze is soft whistling noise produced during expiration (also expiration takes longer time than normal) and this is due to narrowing of air passages inside the lungs.

### Cyanosis

Cyanosis is the bluish discoloration of the body (in peripheral cyanosis only hands and legs are involved and in central cyanosis whole body including chest and abdomen is involved) and this is to be examined in good light (preferably in natural light). Cyanosis is the sign of hypoxia.

### Fever

Raised body temperature (hyperthermia) is common clinical feature of ARIs. In infants (especially young infants), there might be low body temperature during the acute infections.

### Malnutrition

Malnutrition should be ruled out among children with ARIs (especially with those signs and symptoms of pneumonia) as it is a major risk factor contributing to high case fatality. The children with malnutrition should be referred to higher centers as they need extra care during management.

## MANAGEMENT OF ARIs

In all ARIs (ARTIs and LRTIs), adequate bed rest, good nutrition, and proper hydration are very important. If the infection is suspected to be of viral origin, there is no role of antibiotics and only symptomatic treatment is advised. Regular monitoring is required to identify the progress of the condition (in some viral infections the clinical condition may deteriorate), secondary infections (Bacterial), and comorbidities, so that the course of the treatment can be changed as per the condition of the child. At most care (diagnosis and treatment) is needed for bacterial infections, especially pneumonia since the case fatality rate is high in children. In cases of bacterial pneumonia, choices of antibiotics would depend upon their spectrum and expected organisms for a given age of the presenting child. Higher fevers (>39°C), cough with sputum, and respiratory distress is suggestive of bacterial pneumonias. Chest X-ray showing lobar infiltrates/pleural effusions, or WBC > 15,000, or increased CRP, or Band neutrophils >1,000 further increase the chances of bacterial cause. Besides these, young infants, individuals with chronic illness, malnutrition, sickle cell anemia, and immunocompromised states increase risk in favor of bacterial pneumonias. On auscultation wheeze is suggestive of viral etiology, whereas crackles are in favor of bacterial cause.

If $O_2$ saturation drops below 90%, supplemental oxygen needs to be given. Therapy of bacterial pneumonia is based on age at presentation and severity of illness. Infants below four months should be admitted for IV antibiotics. Beyond this age, oral antibiotics can be prescribed in noncomplicated cases.

IV Ampicillin (100–200 mg/kg/24 h in 4–6 divided doses up to 8–12 g/24 h) and IV cefotaxime (100–200 mg/kg/24 hours in 3–4 divided doses up to 12 g/24 hrs) combination is recommended for children below three weeks and either of the two for children aged more than three weeks up to four months.

### Between 4 Months and 4 Years

High dose Amoxicillin (75–90 mg/kg/24 h divided every 12 hours, maximum 2–3 g/24 h), or

Amoxicillin + Clavulanic acid (*for a child of <40 kg*—80–90 mg of amoxicillin component/kg/24 h; *for a child of >40 kg*—250–500 mg every 8 hour or 875 mg every 12 h; maximum 2 g/24 5 h), or

Cefuroxime (30 mg/kg/24 h in two divided doses; maximum 1 g/24 h), or

Macrolides (Azithromycin—12 mg/kg/24 h once daily; maximum 500 mg/24 h) are indicated.

## PREVENTION AND CONTROL OF ARI

The burden of ARIs is high among the under developed and developing countries when compared to the developed world. This is mainly due to the environmental conditions like housing standards, water standards, garbage disposal, cooking fuels, poor standard of living, etc. and certain human factors like malnutrition and lack of awareness regarding the spread of the respiratory infections, etc. The prevention and control measures of ARI can be broadly explained under the following headings:

- Health promotion
- Specific protection

### Health Promotion

The bulk of the morbidity and mortality due to ARIs (especially pneumonia) occurs in poor and marginalized populations where in the problem like poor housing conditions, overcrowding, poor sanitary conditions, malnutrition prevail. Steps should be taken to address these predisposing factors of ARI and overall standard of living and nutritional status should be improved. It is clear that no amount government aid can solve these problems without the community participation. The importance of community participation is proven beyond doubt from the role of ASHA'S (selected from the community) in treating uncomplicated cases of ARI's and identification and prompt referral of complicated cases to higher centers for adequate management.

IEC activities to improve the level of awareness among general public about the warning signs of pneumonia and severe pneumonia (to reduce delayed and inappropriate management), role of nutrition, immunization, etc. should be taken up.

### Specific Protection

Vaccines play a very vital role in saving the lives of millions of children from pneumonia.

Measles vaccine, HIB vaccine and pneumococcal vaccine hold promise in reducing the morbidity and mortality due to ARI.

#### Measles Vaccine

Measles is a very contagious disease caused by an RNA Paramyxovirus. One of the most common and notorious complications of measles infection is pneumonia. Though measles vaccine primarily is targeted as a specific protection against measles, its role in the prevention and control of pneumonia cannot be overlooked since one of the common complications of measles is pneumonia. In India, measles vaccine is given as two doses (first dose at nine months of age and second dose between 18 months and 24 months of age). With a view to combat various vaccine preventable diseases in a comprehensive way and also to achieve a maximum immunization coverage of more than 95% of children, Government of India introduced two initiatives namely:

- Pentavalent vaccine
- Measles rubella vaccine campaign the burden of pneumonia due to *Haemophilus influenza* type b can be reduced by Pentavalent vaccine (DPT+ Hep B + HiB) which was introduced in India in phased manner. Pentavalent vaccine is given as a deep intramuscular injection in the anterolateral aspect of the thigh at 6, 10, and 14 weeks after birth. It should be stored between +2°C to + 8°C and are to be kept in the basket of ice lined refrigerator (ILR). Care should be taken to prevent the pentavalent vaccine vials from freezing.

In order to combat multiple vaccine preventable diseases in a comprehensive manner, the trend of introducing "single vaccine against multiple vaccine preventable diseases" has developed. With this viewpoint, National Technical Advisory Group for Immunization (NTAGI) has recommended measles-rubella vaccine (MR Vaccine) in 2014. The introduction of Rubella vaccine along with measles vaccine will not reduce the efficacy of measles vaccine and thereby will not downplay the prevention and control of pneumonia. Just like measles vaccine, MR vaccine is also given as two doses—first dose between 9 months and 12 months of age and second dose between 18 months and 24 months of age through subcutaneous route.

### Pneumococcal Vaccine

Center for Disease Control recommends pneumococcal vaccine for all children less than two years of age and all adults aged 65 years and above. In certain situations like splenectomy, pneumococcal vaccines are recommended for all age groups. Due to cost factor, these vaccines have not been incorporated in the routine immunization schedule in many countries including India. There are primarily two types of pneumococcal vaccines:
- Pneumococcal conjugate vaccines (PCV 10 and PCV 13)
- Pneumococcal polysaccharide vaccine (PPV 23)

***Pneumococcal conjugate vaccines:*** These are given primarily in children. Both PCV 10 and PCV 13 are preservative free and the appropriate temperature to store the vaccines is +2°C to +8°C (should not be frozen). These vaccines are contraindicated in children who had a past history of severe allergic reaction to any vaccine containing diphtheria toxoid, a dose of this similar vaccine. In cases of mild illness (common cold which is not severe), vaccine can be administered but in such cases where the illness is severe, then the vaccination schedule has to be postponed until the patient recovers.

WHO recommends two types of schedules for the vaccination of Pneumococcal Conjugate vaccines—three primary doses (3P + 0) or as an alternative, two primary plus one booster dose (2P + 1). In 3P + 0 schedule, the first dose can be given as early as six weeks of age. The time interval between the doses should be 4–8 weeks. Conveniently, the 3P + 0 schedule of PCV can be given at 6, 10, and 14 weeks after birth. In 2P + 1 schedule, the first dose can be given as early as six weeks. The time interval between the first primary and second primary doses can be eight weeks and the booster dose can be given between 9-15 months of age. Mild reactions like erythema, pain at the injection site, fever are common. In preterm babies and HIV babies, 2P + 1 schedule is more beneficial as booster dose during their second year gives better protection. However, if 3P + 0 was followed (where three primary doses are given before the first birthday), a booster dose to these vulnerable group during their second year gives better protection against pneumococcal infections.

***Pneumococcal polysaccharide vaccines:*** These vaccines are given primarily in adults. However in certain medical conditions like HIV, nephrotic syndrome, immune compromising conditions like sickle cell disease, chronic heart, lung and kidney diseases, these vaccines can be administered in children less than two years of age. Similar to pneumococcal conjugate vaccines, PPV23 is contraindicated in those who had serious life threatening allergic reactions with previous dose. A dose of 0.5 mL is injected intramuscularly and most preferred site for administration is deltoid muscle. Minor adverse reactions like pain at the site of injection, redness, fever are seen in 30–50% of those vaccinated.

A single dose of vaccination gives considerable protection for 5–8 years.

> **Note**
> 1. Whether PCV or PPV, in either case, the vaccine should not be mixed or loaded in the same syringe used to administer other vaccines, e.g. influenza vaccine, etc. But pneumococcal vaccines can be administered simultaneously with other vaccines at other site.
> 2. When primary immunization is initiated with either of these vaccines (either PPV or PCV), it is recommended that the remaining doses are administered with the same product.

## INTEGRATED MANAGEMENT OF NEONATAL AND CHILDHOOD ILLNESS

Various studies have shown that children who are most likely to die of ARIs (especially pneumonia) are mostly malnourished and belong to under privileged populations (low socioeconomic status) and low income countries. Quality of care in these settings is another issue. Surveys have shown that many sick children are not assessed properly and treated adequately by health care professionals and also parents are poorly advised. Most of the parents are clueless regarding the warning signals and when the child has to be taken to a higher center for better management. To overcome these challenges, in mid 1980s, the WHO initiated an integrated control program for the management of ARIs by the health workers, rendering services at the grassroots level in the health care delivery system. This strategy was adopted by the Government of India and was expanded to include all the neonates and so, it was renamed as "Integrated Management of Neonatal and Childhood Illness (IMNCI)". IMNCI utilizes a color coded triage system to classify the child's illness based on signs and symptoms and their nutritional status. The color codes used are green for home management, yellow for out-patient health facility based treatment, and pink for urgent referral for management on admission basis in a higher center. ***Further details regarding IMNCI would be discussed in Chapter 47: Health Policies and Programs in India.***

## SUMMARY

- The acute infections occurring in various parts of respiratory tract starting from nostrils to the alveoli of the lungs are considered as acute respiratory infections and these infections contribute significantly in both adults and children in terms of morbidity and mortality.
- The different ARIs vary from common cold, being the simplest condition to pneumonia being the most serious condition.
- The most common viral agent responsible for ARIs in children is respiratory syncytial virus (RSV) and the most common bacterial agent is *Streptococcus pneumoniae*.
- Acute respiratory infections spread mainly by droplet infection (air borne). Droplet spread can be either direct or indirect.
- Among the various ARIs, pneumonia is the most dreadful one due to its high case fatality rates if not treated adequately and promptly in children.
- Pneumonia can be classified as very severe disease, severe pneumonia, pneumonia, and no pneumonia. Very severe disease and severe pneumonia need referral to hospital for further management. *(Signs and symptoms of various stages of pneumonia are very important from exam point of view).*

- In all ARIs (ARTIs and LRTIs), adequate bed rest, good nutrition, and proper hydration are very important. If the infection is suspected to be of viral origin, there is no role of antibiotics, and only symptomatic treatment is advised.
- The prevention and control measures of ARI comprises of "Health Promotion" and "Specific Protection". As a part of specific protection, measles vaccine, HIB vaccine and pneumococcal vaccine hold promise in reducing the morbidity and mortality due to ARI.
- The strategy adopted by the Government of India to tackle the ARIs in children aged less than five years is IMNCI. IMNCI utilizes a color coded triage system to classify the child's illness based on signs and symptoms and their nutritional status. *(Please read IMNCI in detail).*

## SUGGESTED READING

1. Bajaj L, Berman S, Berman S. Berman's Pediatric Decision Making, 5th edition. Philadelphia: Elsevier/Mosby; 2011. pp. 1-788.
2. Center for Disease Control and Prevention. Pneumococcal Vaccination: What Everyone Should Know. Vaccines and Preventable Diseases. [online] Available from www.cdc.gov/vaccines/vpd/pneumo/public/index.html.
3. Detels R, Gulliford M, Karim QA, et al. Oxford Textbook of Global Public Health, Vol 3, 6th edition. Oxford: Oxford University Press; 2015. pp. 1083.
4. Food and Drug Administration. PNEUMOVAX® 23 (pneumococcal vaccine polyvalent) Sterile, Liquid Vaccine for Intramuscular or Subcutaneous Injection Initial U.S. Approval: 198.
5. Global Health Observatory (GHO) data. Causes of child mortality, 2016. [online] Available from: www.who.int/gho/child_mortality/causes/en/.
6. India—Key Indicators, National Family Health Survey-4 (2015-16), Ministry of Health and Family Welfare, Government of India.
7. Introduction of Measles-Rubella Vaccine (Campaign and Routine Immunization), National Operational Guidelines 2017, Ministry of Health and Family Welfare, Government of India.
8. Madhi SA, Levine OS, Hajjeh R, et al. Vaccines to prevent pneumonia and improve child survival. Bull World Health Organ. 2008;86(5): 365-72.
9. Mulholland K. Global burden of acute respiratory infections in children: Implications for interventions. Pediatr Pulmonol. 2003;36(6): 469-74.
10. Rogan M. Respiratory infections, Acute. In: Quah SR (Ed). The International Encyclopedia of Public Health, 2nd edition. London: Oliver Walter Publishing; 2017. pp. 332-6.
11. Shi T, McAllister DA, O'Brien KL, et al. Global, regional, and national disease burden estimates of acute lower respiratory infections due to respiratory syncytial virus in young children in 2015: A systematic review and modelling study. Lancet. 2017;390(10098):946-58.
12. Temani K, Mayenger A, Bairwa AL. Assessment of prevalence of acute respiratory tract infection and risk factors in under five children in Anganwadi of Kota city. Indian J Child Health. 2016;3(3):234-7.
13. Wallace RB (Ed). Maxy-Rosenau-Last Public Health and Preventive Medicine, 15th edition. New York: McGraw Hill; 2007. pp. 201-7.

---

# EPIDEMIOLOGY OF CHICKENPOX AND ITS PREVENTION AND CONTROL

*Shalini Pradeep*

| | |
|---|---|
| **CM7.2** | Enumerate, describe and discuss the mode of transmission and measures for prevention and control of Chickenpox |
| **CM8.1** | Describe and discuss the epidemiological and control measures applicable in Chickenpox |

*Case Scenario*

*A 7-year-girl presented with 4-day history of vesicular rash, initially at the feet but then spread up to the thighs bilaterally, abdomen and trunk. She presented to pediatrician with fever. On examination she was irritable but alert. She had fever for the first two days of the rash but since then has not had fever. She had diffuse vesiculopustular lesions over her entire body, with some areas showing older, crusted lesions. The liver and spleen were not enlarged. Her pediatrician examined her and confirmed a diagnosis of chickenpox.*

## INTRODUCTION

Chickenpox or Varicella is a communicable and a highly infectious disease acute in onset with 80-90% of susceptible individuals being infected after exposure. The etiological agent is varicella-zoster virus. This infectious agent is responsible for both chickenpox and herpes zoster (shingles). Based on the host response, it can manifest as either chickenpox or shingles. Clinical features due to zoster and that of chickenpox are similar. Herpes zoster can present locally either before or after chickenpox. The vesicles in herpes zoster are along the sensory nerves or a single dorsal ganglion or a group of ganglia. Shingles is more common in adults as compared to chickenpox in children.

## CHARACTERISTIC OF DISEASE

The disease starts as an itchy rash. Later blisters are formed which culminate into scabs. The rash is symmetrical. It first appears on the trunk where it is abundant, and then comes on the face, arms and legs, where it is less abundant. The mucosal surfaces of mouth, eyes, and genital area are involved. Rashes may be seen in Axilla, but palms and soles are unaffected. Once the blisters are formed, they change into scabs in a weeks' time.

## PROBLEM STATEMENT

### Global Burden

In the pre-vaccination era (1990-1994), the overall case fatality rate was 2-3/10,000 cases in high-income developed countries. Incidence in children was approximately 1/100,000 and 20-25 adults/100,000 cases. Most of these data are from community and that too in 4-5 developed countries only.

In Nigeria (1979-80), 65% who were admitted were more than 15 years. In South Africa (1985-96), measles accounted for 53% admissions and varicella, 23%. In India (1970), 155 cases were reported with 80% deaths in adults. This amounts to 52/100,000 cases, 20 times higher than high-income developed countries.

The majority of population-based data about the burden of varicella are from high-income countries, according to a World Health Organization (WHO) position paper. Approximately, 140 million cases of varicella are reported each year worldwide. There are also 4.2 million severe complications and 4200 deaths associated with varicella (WHO 2014).

## Burden in India

Total number of cases and deaths due to chickenpox were 66,963 and 50, respectively in 2018 (National Health Profile, 2019). Majority of outbreaks reported in 2017 were of acute diarrheal disease (21%), food poisoning (15%), followed by chickenpox and measles (13% each).

The burden of varicella is unevenly distributed in the country. The maximum number of cases was observed in states with the majority of the population living in low and lower-middle socioeconomic status states. States reporting high cases also ranked low in Sustainable Development Goals (SDG) ranking by NITI Aayog. There has been no fixed trend in the number of cases year-wise but the sudden rise of cases and deaths in 2016 can be noted. It decreased in 2020 which may be attributed to COVID 19 restrictions and non/under-reporting. (SDG India index 2020-2021 report, NITI Aayog of India).

## EPIDEMIOLOGY

### Host Factors

***Age:*** It can affect anyone but children <10 years are susceptible. Few persons escape infection until adulthood. The disease is very severe in adulthood.

***Sex:*** Both sexes are equally affected.

***Immunity:*** One episode of infection will give life-long immunity; second attacks are rare. The IgG antibodies persist for life and it is known to protect against Varicella-Zoster. The cell mediated immunity is known to be associated with prevention of reactivation of latent V-Z virus, and thus Varicella zoster infection. Maternal antibodies are known to protect the newborn for few months.

***Pregnancy:*** Infection during pregnancy may increase the risk for the fetus, resulting in congenital varicella syndrome.

> **Host Factors**
> - Commonly affects children less than 10 years.
> - Single episode will provide lifelong immunity.
> - Secondary attack rate in close household contacts is 90%.
> - Transplacental spread will result in congenital varicella syndrome.

### Agent Factors

***Types:*** The causative agent is human (alpha) herpes virus 3. This virus causes the primary infection.

***Infectivity:*** The period of communicability of patients with varicella is estimated to range from 1 to 2 days before appearance of rash, and 4 to 5 days thereafter.

***Recovery and Reactivation:*** After recovery from primary infection, the virus remains dormant for several years in cranial nerves, sensory ganglia and spinal dorsal root ganglia and may get reactivated. When the cell mediated immunity wanes with age, this dormant virus may reactivate, resulting in herpes zoster in 10-30% of cases.

***Viability:*** In vivo, it cannot survive for more than 48 hours. It can be readily killed by detergents and solvents.

> **Agent Factors**
> - Causative agent is Varicella Zoster virus, also called as Human (alpha) herpes virus 3.
> - The period of communicability of patients with varicella is estimated to range from 1 to 2 days before appearance of rash, and 4 to 5 days thereafter.
> - Dormant virus in sensory ganglia and spinal dorsal root ganglia, when get reactivated in adulthood, leads to herpes zoster.

### Environmental Factors

***Physical:*** VZV is heat labile. High temperature and humidity prevents transmission of the virus.

***Seasons:*** Chickenpox shows a seasonal trend in India. It occurs mostly during the first half of the year. However, In temperate climates, however there is no seasonal trend.

***Overcrowding:*** Overcrowding favors its transmission.

> **Environmental Factors**
> - Chicken pox shows seasonal trend, with peak incidence during winter and spring.
> - VZV is heat labile.

### Source

It is a patient with chickenpox lesions. The virus can be isolated in vesicular lesions during the first 3 days of illness. Herpes zoster may rarely be the source. It is observed that there are no subclinical cases, carriers, and animal reservoirs.

### Reservoir

Human are the only reservoir of infection. It can be in the respiratory tract even before the onset of symptoms, vesicular fluid, and in the nervous system after the rash resolves.

### Infective Material

Oropharyngeal secretions, skin, and mucosal lesions.

### Portal of Entry and Exit

The portal of exit is upper respiratory tract by droplet nuclei. The portals of entry is the upper respiratory tract or the conjunctiva and though close personal contact. The virus is also found to cross placental barrier and infect the fetus.

### Mode of Transmission

This occurs when an infected person sneezes, the tiny droplets which are released are inhaled by a non-immune person. Hence it is highly contagious. The risk of transmission is very high. There are 90% chances that children within the family can get chickenpox when one of siblings has the lesions.

### Incubation Period

The time period from the entry of the virus into the human body and clinical manifestations is 14–16 days. The range may vary from 10 to 21 days. For most people, getting chickenpox once provides immunity for life. Still, it is not uncommon for a person to get chickenpox for the second time in his life. It is reinfection which is mild without viremia.

## Period of Communicability

Begins 1–2 days before rashes are seen; terminates with formation of crusts. The time period may be 4–7 days after the appearance of the rash.

> **Chain of infection**
> - Humans are the only reservoir for chicken pox.
> - The respiratory system is the portal of entry and exit.
> - The incubation period of pertussis is commonly 14–16 days.
> - Period of communicability begins 1–2 days before rashes are seen; terminates with formation of crusts. The time period may be 4–7 days after the appearance of the rash.

## CLINICAL FEATURES

Prodromal symptoms include sudden onset of mild to moderate fever, back pain, chills, feeling tired, lack of desire to eat food, malaise and headache and this stage may last for 24 hours. All stages of rash seen together at a time are called "pleomorphism" which is unique for chickenpox. Lesions can occur in the mouth, cornea, tympanic membrane, and vagina. The rash is throughout the body and associated with scratching. The rash advances from macule to become a papule. Later, it changes to a fluid-filled vesicle. Finally, the lesion becomes crusted. The rash first appears on the trunk and then spreads to face, arms and legs **(Figs. 17A.2 and 17A.3)**. More number of lesions are seen on the chest and back. In children with good immunity, the disease is mild with prodromal symptoms of fever for 2–3 days and rash with itching. If it attacks infants, adults, and immunocompromised people, the disease is more severe with likelihood of complication **(Box 17A.6)**.

In 3% perinatal transmission, it can cause congenital varicella syndrome. The syndrome consists of low-birth weight, ophthalmic problems such as cataract, chorioretinitis, and micro-ophthalmia. There may be associated hypotrophic hypotonic limbs and zoster-like skin lesions. If the mother is infected in the last trimester, the fetus will have mild rashes. If the infection is in the last 5 days of pregnancy or 2 days of delivery, the neonate will have severe form of rashes.

Complications can occur in 5% of the cases. They are sepsis, pneumonia, encephalitis, and Reye's syndrome.

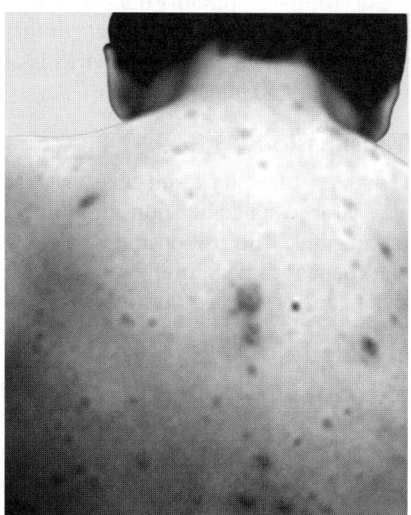

**Fig. 17A.2:** Chickenpox in an unvaccinated child.

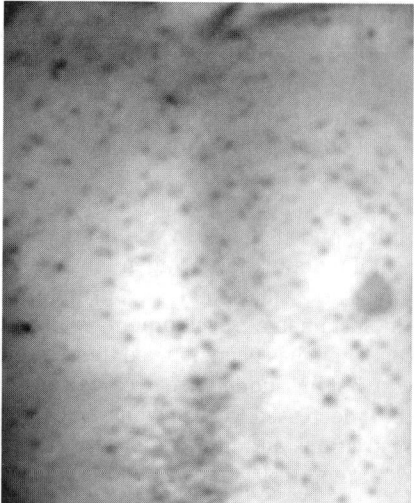

**Fig. 17A.3:** Chickenpox in an unvaccinated adult.

> **Box 17A.6: Breakthrough varicella.**
> - Can occur after 42 days of taking the vaccine
> - Milder, duration of illness shorter
> - Fever ±, fewer lesions, rashes may be maculopapular
> - Only 25–30% have classical chickenpox
> - Laboratory testing is very important due to diagnostic dilemma
> - Limited information about efficacy of two doses over single vaccine.

## DIAGNOSIS

It is indicated to—(1) corroborate the clinical findings, and (2) to identify antigenic strain of virus. For acute cases, PCR is preferred. The samples tested are vesicular fluid, scabs or scrapings from maculopapular lesions. Serological tests can be done where history of varicella is negative or uncertain. Viral genotyping is done when differentiation of wild strain from vaccine strain needs to be done.

Virus of chickenpox dies rapidly in crusts and hence it is not possible to infect susceptible children, but in the early phase of the illness the virus can waft and infect another patient at a distance.

## PREVENTION AND CONTROL MEASURES

### Controlling Source

Follow standard precautions as for any other communicable disease till the crusts fall off.

### Interrupting Transmission

Isolation is recommended. Persons with doubtful immunity should not be allowed entry into such a room. Period of isolation is from 10th day to 21st day postexposure or until 28th day if exposed individual receives varicella zoster immune globulin (VZIG).

## Protection of Susceptible Host

Acyclovir can be given orally or intravenously. This drug is most effective within 24 hours of rash onset. Oral therapy is indicated for children above 12 years of age. Intravenous acyclovir is indicated for complicated varicella, immune compromised, and those with recurrent zoster.

## Vaccine against Varicella in Healthy Subjects

Vaccine is safe and effective but expensive. It has not yet been introduced into the National Immunization Program. A single dose (0.5 mL SC) can be given from the age 1–12 years. Above the age of 12 years, two doses can be given 6–10 weeks apart.

## Special Situations

Children and adolescents with CD4 count of 15–24% and adults with CD4 count more than 200 cells/µL should receive two doses. During outbreaks, those who have received only one dose should take the second one.

## Postexposure Vaccination

One dose within 72 hours of exposure will prevent varicella to the extent of 98%. After 5 days, it is effective to the extent of 70%. Vaccination can be given after 72 hours because it can modify the disease or provide protection against future exposures.

Immunoglobulin is effective in reducing the severity when given 96 hours after exposure.

Decision is based on—(1) whether susceptible; (2) exposure is likely to result in infection; and (3) risk of complications is more than the general population.

*Dose*: 125 U/10 kg body weight up to 625 U/person.

Finally, studies have not been done to know whether giving vaccine will postpone the increased incidence to adulthood, make it more severe and prevent herpes Zoster in later life.

## PREVENTION

- Avoid healthy children and adults coming in contact with a case of chickenpox.
- Infected child should not attend school for a week.
- Wearing a surgical mask would reduce the spread to others.
- Trimming the nails would prevent spread of the virus.
- Disinfecting hands, clothes, and household surroundings also helps.
- Do not put finger in mouth or rub eyes after touching an infected person.

## SUMMARY

Chickenpox or Varicella is a highly infectious communicable disease, caused by varicella-zoster virus. which is responsible for both chickenpox and herpes zoster. The vesicles in herpes zoster are along the sensory nerves or a single dorsal ganglia or a group of ganglia.

**Epidemiology:** Commonly affects children less than 10 years. Single episode will provide lifelong immunity.

Transplacental spread will result in congenital varicella syndrome. The period of communicability of patients with varicella is estimated to range from 1 to 2 days before appearance of rash, and 4 to 5 days thereafter. Dormant virus in sensory ganglia and spinal dorsal root ganglia, when get reactivated in adulthood, leads to herpes zoster. Chickenpox shows seasonal trend, with peak incidence during winter and spring.

**Clinical features:** Prodromal symptoms with "pleomorphic rash is unique for chickenpox. The rash first appears on the trunk and then spreads to face, arms and legs. More number of lesions are seen on the chest and back.

In 3% perinatal transmission, it can cause congenital varicella syndrome. The syndrome consists of low-birth weight, ophthalmic problems such as cataract, chorioretinitis, and microphthalmia.

Complications can occur in 5% of the cases. They are sepsis, pneumonia, encephalitis, and Reye's syndrome.

**Diagnosis:** It is indicated to—(1) corroborate the clinical findings, and (2) to identify antigenic strain of virus.

**Prevention and control measures:** Isolation is recommended for the cases. Persons with doubtful immunity should not be allowed entry into such a room. Period of isolation is from 10th day to 21st day postexposure or until 28th day if exposed individual receives varicella zoster immune globulin (VZIG).

**Vaccination:** Vaccine is safe and effective but expensive. A single dose (0.5 mL SC) can be given from the age 1–12 years. Above the age of 12 years, two doses can be given 6–10 weeks apart.

Immunoglobulin is effective in reducing the severity when given 96 hours after exposure.

## SUGGESTED READING

1. Guriji D, Marin M, Seward JF. Varicella herpes zoster in diseases primarily controlled by vaccination. In: Vallace RB (Ed). Public Health and Preventive Medicine, 15th edition. New York: McGraw-Hill Professional Publishing; 2000. pp. 129-32.
2. Hobson W. Spread and control of airborne infections. The Theory and Practice of public Health, 5th edition. 1979. p. 236.
3. Integrated Disease Surveillance Programme (IDSP), Annual Report, GOI; 2017.
4. National Health Profile 13th issue, p.130-1.
5. Shrivastava SR, Shrivastava PS, Ramasamy J. Epidemiological investigation of a case of chickenpox in a medical college in Kancheepuram, India. Germs. 2013;3(1):18-20.

# EPIDEMIOLOGY OF MEASLES AND ITS PREVENTION AND CONTROL

*Rachana AR, Prince Alex Abraham*

*Measles will always show you if someone isn't doing a good job on vaccinations. Kids will start dying of measles.*
—Bill Gates

**CM7.2** Enumerate, describe and discuss the mode of transmission and measures for prevention and control of Measles

**CM8.1** Describe and discuss the epidemiological and control measures applicable in Measles

### Case Scenario

A 2-year-old female child was brought to primary health center by her mother, who complains that the child had fever associated with cough and cold since six days. The mother also complains that the child had developed rash over the body since two days, rash first appeared on the face and spread to all over the body. She also complains that baby is not eating well since one week. On probing mother also revealed that there is a child in neighboring house suffered with similar illness 15 days back. This was the 5th case of fever with rash (similar illness) reported since three days to the PHC. After looking into the records it revealed that all cases were from the same locality. A team of health workers including medical officer-in- charge of PHC visited the locality and did a survey. Survey revealed a total of 17 cases with similar illness in the age group of six months to three years in that locality. None of the cases had immunization card and most of the parents of the children were migrant construction workers. As a medical officer in-charge of PHC how will you handle the situation?

## INTRODUCTION

Measles is a viral disease which is highly contagious caused by the measles virus, an enveloped RNA virus which is single-stranded, and negative-sense RNA virus of the genus *Morbillivirus* within the family Paramyxoviridae. Though there is availability of safe and effective vaccine globally, it is an important cause of death among young children. Measles is also known as *rubeola* or *morbilli*.

Measles has been a menace for centuries; it affected millions of people. During 3rd century, physicians in North Africa and Asia identified and diagnosed measles as a highly contagious disease, which was similar to smallpox, which characterized with rashes and sores.

Chinese alchemist Ko Hung described the difference between smallpox and measles in 340 AD; around 300 years later a Christian priest, Ahrun, did the same in Egypt. In the year 910 AD, the Persian physician called Rhazes published a book on smallpox and measles. Rhazes described the early diagnoses of both the diseases, measles and smallpox, in his book.

## CHARACTERISTIC OF DISEASE

Measles is highly contagious, transmitted through respiratory droplets of the infected persons. 10–12 days after the infection initial symptoms appear which are high-grade fever, rhinitis, red eyes (conjunctivitis), and small white spots on the buccal mucosa (Koplik's spots). Several days later, a characteristic rash develops, starts on the face just behind the ear and upper part of the neck and later gradually spreading downwards.

## PROBLEM STATEMENT

### Before the Introduction of Measles Vaccine (1963)

Major epidemics occurred every 2–3 years and it is estimated that 30 million cases of measles and ≥2 million deaths occurred globally each year.

By the age of 15 years, more than 95% of individuals had been infected with measles virus. The disease was the one of the leading causes of death among young children globally (**Table 17A.6**).

**Table 17A.6:** Problem statement.

| World (Total number of deaths) | |
|---|---|
| 2000 | 550,100 |
| 2018 | 1,42,000 |
| India (Total number of deaths) (NHP, 2019) | |
| 2000 | 100,000 |
| 2019 | 34 |

### After the Introduction of Measles Vaccine

- In recent years, deaths due to measles have decreased by 84% worldwide—from 550,100 deaths in 2000 to 1,42,000 in 2018 (WHO, Fact Sheets: Measles, 2018).
- In many developing countries, measles is still common cause of death among children, particularly in Africa and Asia.
- Measles vaccination averted 56 million deaths being between 2000 and 2021.
- Even though a safe and cost-effective vaccine is available, in 2021, there were an estimated 128,000 measles deaths globally, mostly among unvaccinated or under vaccinated children under the age of 5 years.
- In 2021, about 81% of the world's children received one dose of measles vaccine by their first birthday through routine health services—the lowest since 2008.
- In India, the number of cases fell from one lakh to around fifty thousand after the vaccination. India have reported 20,895 measles cases in 2018 (NHP-2019).

### Measles and Rubella Surveillance Data by WHO: 2020

- According to World Health Organization (WHO), 277,846 suspected cases and 146,744 confirmed cases of measles reported from the six WHO regions in the year 2017.
- The share from South-East Asian region is 97,374 suspected cases and 75,362 confirmed cases of measles in the same year.
- India has topped the list among the top 10 countries by reporting 9,515 cases (**Fig. 17A.4** and **Table 17A.7**).

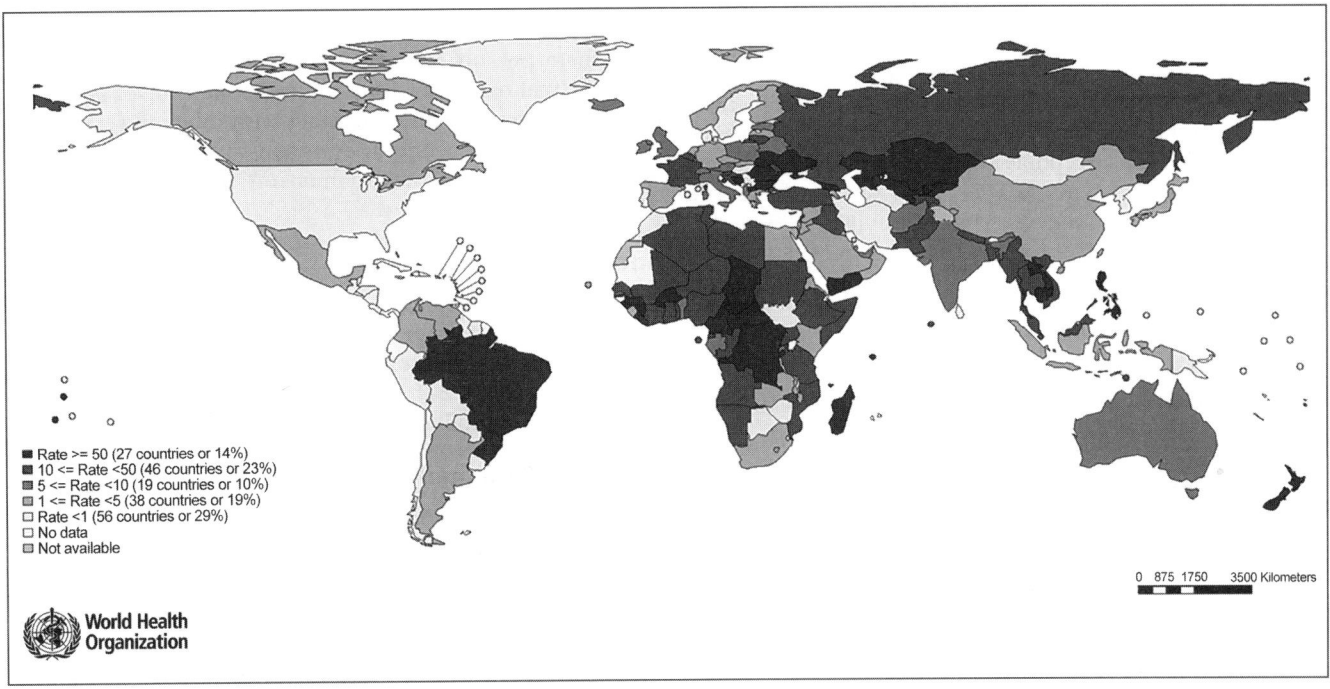

**Fig. 17A.4:** Measles incidence rate per million—12 months period (covering the period 06–2019 to 05–2020).
*Source:* Measles and Rubella Surveillance Data [Internet], World Health Organization. 2020.

**Table 17A.7:** Measles incidence rate per million population (covering the period 06-2019 to 05-2020).

| Top 10 Countries | | |
|---|---|---|
| Country | Cases | Rate |
| Brazil | 29,497 | 138.88 |
| DR Congo | 26,241 | 302.57 |
| Philippines | 10,916 | 100.97 |
| Nigeria | 9,572 | 47.63 |
| India | 9,515 | 6.95 |
| Kazakhstan | 7,467 | 401.6 |
| Ukraine | 6,750 | 154.13 |
| Bangladesh | 6,615 | 39.36 |
| Madagascar | 5,495 | 203.75 |
| Uzbekistan | 5,323 | 162.25 |

*Source:* Measles and Rubella Surveillance Data. World Health Organization 2020.

**Provisional data based on monthly reports to WHO (Geneva) as of August 2019.**

Measles outbreaks continue to spread rapidly around the world, in the first six months of 2019, reported measles cases are the highest they have been in any year since 2006. There have been almost three times as many cases reported to date in 2019 as there were at this same time last year.

Major outbreaks are ongoing in Angola, Cameroon, Chad, Kazakhstan, Nigeria, Philippines, South Sudan, Sudan and Thailand. The United States has reported its highest measles case count in 25 years.

For the period of January 1 through July 31, 2019, 182 countries reported 364,808 measles cases to WHO. For this same period last year, 129,239 measles cases were reported from 181 countries. For the current 2019 period, the WHO African Region has recorded a 900% (i.e. a 10-fold increase), the European Region 120% (more than two-fold increase), the Eastern Mediterranean Region 50% (1.5 fold increase), the Western Pacific Region 230% (a three-fold increase); the South-East Asia Region and the Region of the Americas—15% decrease in reported cases.

No country is exempt from measles, and areas with low immunization encourage the virus to circulate, increasing the likelihood of outbreaks and putting all unvaccinated children at risk.

India is the capital of the recent outbreak of measles in the world. There were 172 confirmed measles outbreaks from October 2021 to September 2022, with a total no. of cases of 12,589. As per the NFHS-5 (2019–2021) data, 87.9% of children aged 12–23 months received the first dose of the measles-containing vaccine, whereas only 31.9% of children aged 24–35 months received the second dose of the measles-containing vaccine. The recent COVID-19 outbreak severely dented the vaccination coverage that has been achieved over the past few years.

## EPIDEMIOLOGY (TABLE 17A.8)

### Host Factors

***Age:*** Measles is usually considered a childhood disease, but it can affect any age group. In low-income countries, with low population immunity, high birth rates and high population density will lead to increased transmission in younger age groups including infants and pre-school children. When there is increase in vaccination coverage, the age affected of measles infection can shift to adolescents and young adults because the older groups remain susceptible as they had not been vaccinated or exposed to wild-type measles virus due to decreased transmission among younger vaccinated groups.

*Sex:* Incidence is equal in both the sex.

*Immunity:* No age is immune, usually one attack of measles confers life-long immunity.

*Nutrition:* Measles tends to be very severe in malnourished, carrying mortality up to 400 times higher than in well-nourished child.

### Agent Factors

*Strain:* Measles is caused by the measles virus; it is a single-stranded, negative-sense, and enveloped RNA virus of the genus *Morbillivirus* belonging to the family Paramyxoviridae.

*Type:* Measles virus has only one serotype.

*Viability:* Virus can be stored in sub-zero temperature. It does not survive outside the human body for long time. Measles virus is readily inactivated by heat, ultraviolet rays, ether, and formaldehyde.

### Environmental Factors

*Physical:* In tropical zones, measles occur during dry season. In temperate climates, measles is a winter disease. Epidemics are seen both in winters and early spring.

*Overcrowding:* Like other respiratory infection overcrowding favors the spread of the disease.

**Table 17A.8:** Epidemiological triad of measles.

| Agent | Host | Environment |
|---|---|---|
| • Enveloped RNA virus<br>• Genus *Morbillivirus*<br>• Family Paramyxoviridae<br>• Virus has only one serotype | • Measles can affect any age group<br>• In low-income countries with lesser immunization coverage—younger age groups are affected<br>• In developed countries with better immunization coverage among younger age group—measles affects young adults and adolescents | • Overcrowding<br>• Ill ventilation favors the spread of the virus |

### Source/Reservoir of Infection

Humans are the only natural hosts, even though measles virus can infect susceptible monkeys, but there are no animal reservoirs.

**Infective material:** Secretions of the nose, throat and respiratory tract of a case of a measles during prodromal stage and the early stages of the rash.

### Portal of Exit, Transmission and Entry

Person-to-person transmission is mainly by respiratory droplets that disperse within minutes, and transmission can also occur through direct contact with infected secretions. Transmission from immune persons exposed to infection and asymptomatic person has not been demonstrated **(Table 17A.9)**.

### Incubation Period

The incubation period for measles usually lasts 10–14 days (range, 7–23 days) from exposure to onset of first symptoms, which generally consist of cough, fever, malaise, conjunctivitis, and coryza. After 2–4 days of onset of the prodrome the characteristic morbilliform rash appears.

### Period of Communicability

Patients are usually contagious from four days before eruption of the rash until four days after eruption, which is during the period when the load of measles virus in the respiratory tract is highest.

**Table 17A.9:** Dynamics of disease transmission of measles.

| Mode of transmission | Incubation period | Period of communicability |
|---|---|---|
| • Person-to-person transmission is mainly by respiratory droplets<br>• Rarely through direct contact | Usually 10–14 days (range, 7–23) from exposure to onset of first symptoms | Four days before the eruption of rash and until four days after eruption |

## CLINICAL FEATURES

Disease has two stages: (1) Pre-eruptive or initial stage, and (2) eruptive stage or rash stage **(Fig. 17A.5)**.

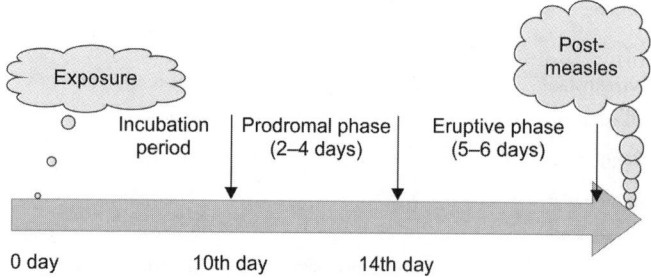

**Fig. 17A.5:** Schematic representation prepathogenic and pathogenic phase of measles.

### Pre-eruptive or Initial Stage

This stage starts after 10 days of infection and lasts for 14 days. The prodromal stage starts with fever of high grade (up to 104°F), lasts for 4–7 days, malaise, sneezing, rhinitis or coryza, congestion, conjunctivitis, and cough (3 Cs, classical triad of measles). Koplik's spots appear on the buccal mucosa, opposite the lower molars, which are pathognomonic feature of measles. Other associated symptoms may include photophobia, myalgia, and periorbital edema.

| Classical triad of measles (3 Cs) | Cough |
| --- | --- |
| | Coryza |
| | Conjunctivitis |

### Eruptive Stage or Rash Stage

The rash usually appears 1–2 days after the appearance of Koplik's spots; mild itching may be associated. The maculopapular rash develops about 14 days after exposure, which appears on the face (behind the ears) and upper neck first and then spreads to the extremities. Rash may not develop in immunocompromised patients. Early in the course the rash blanches on pressure. The rash fades in the order of appearance during the next 3–4 days and assumes a nonblanching appearance. The rash is more prominent than rubella and unlike rubella, often coalesces.

In uncomplicated measles, patient's improvement is seen by the third day after the onset of rash, and patients fully recover by 7–10 days after the onset of disease. The severity of measles varies widely, which depends on various host and environmental factors. The risk factors include children aged <5 years, overcrowding, malnutrition especially with vitamin A deficiency, and individuals with immunological disorders including AIDS.

## COMPLICATIONS

Complications occur in around 30% of reported cases depending on the age and predisposing conditions. Most common complications include otitis media, laryngotracheobronchitis (croup), diarrhea, and pneumonia. Among the children living in developed countries, 7–9% of cases may develop otitis media, diarrhea in 8% of cases, and pneumonia in 1–6%. Post-infectious measles encephalitis occurs in about 1–4 per 1,000–2,000 cases, and subacute sclerosing panencephalitis (SSPE) develops several years after the infection in about 1 per 10,000–100,000 cases. Immunocompromised individuals may develop severe complications of measles which include a characteristic giant cell pneumonia and acute progressive encephalitis (measles inclusion-body encephalitis).

Infants in developing countries may develop persistent diarrhea with protein-losing enteropathy. In these countries, secondary bacterial infection may develop among children with malnutrition, particularly vitamin A deficiency, and exposure to other infectious diseases are common.

The *case-fatality rate* of measles is 3–6%, but can be as high as 30%, particularly among displaced immunocompromised individuals. Case-fatality rate due to measles is rare in developed countries and it is usually as low as 0.01–0.1%. The greatest risk of death is in children younger than one year and in adults older than 30 years. In HIV-infected children, the case-fatality rate has been reported to be as high as 50%.

Recovery is delayed in children with Vitamin A deficiency, and post-measles complications are high among them. In addition, measles infection may precipitate acute vitamin A deficiency and xerophthalmia. Measles is one of the important causes of preventable childhood blindness.

## DIAGNOSIS ACCORDING TO WHO

*Suspected case of measles* is a case with fever and maculopapular (non-vesicular) rash or a case where a health-care worker suspects measles. Definitive diagnosis is by laboratory testing. Laboratory confirmation of measles is based on detection of anti-measles IgM antibodies by enzyme-linked immunosorbent assay (ELISA), or the detection of measles virus RNA by reverse transcriptase polymerase chain reaction (RT-PCR) from throat swabs, oral fluid, or nasopharyngeal secretions or urine.

## TREATMENT

There is no specific treatment for measles, only supportive care, and care should be taken to prevent post-measles complications including secondary infection. Patient isolation is an important intervention to prevent further spread. However, increasing population immunity through vaccination is the most effective way to prevent outbreaks. Supportive treatment should be given, including relieving common symptoms such as fever, cough, cold, conjunctivitis, and sore mouth.

Nutritional support is very important step to prevent malnutrition due to diarrhea, vomiting, and poor appetite associated with measles. Breastfeeding should be encouraged.

### Home-based Care for Measles

There is no specific treatment for measles. If there are no complications, most of the cases can be managed at home. Mothers should be encouraged to follow below instructions:

- Fever can lead to dehydration which can be aggravated by diarrhea; child should be encouraged to take plenty of fluids. Paracetamol can be given for fever. Aspirin should be avoided.
- *Nutrition:* Measles is severe in malnourished children. Malnutrition is an important cause of death in measles. Appetite is lost during any febrile illness. More calories are needed during the illness. Adequate nutrition ensures speedy recovery.
- *Diarrhea:* As diarrhea in measles is due to viral infection, antibiotics are not going to be useful. Oral rehydration is the mainstay of treatment.
- A child who is in the contagious stage should stay away from school and avoid close contact with others, especially those who are not immunized or have never had measles.
- *Prevention:* People who have already had measles are normally immune and they are unlikely to get it again. People who are not immune should consider the measles vaccine.
- Children develop vitamin A deficiency following measles. Hence supplementation with vitamin A will be helpful.

*Child should be brought to hospital if child develops following symptoms:*

- Unable to take feeds or fluids
- Rapid, difficult or noisy breathing (stridor)
- Increased respiratory rate, chest in-drawing
- Diarrhea, vomiting or blood in stools and dehydration
- Mouth ulcers, sore and discharge from ears and eyes, and white spots on eyes
- Corneal clouding or ulcers, or if vision is affected

- Mastoiditis—pain and swelling behind the ear
- Convulsions, lethargic or loss of consciousness

### Vitamin A Supplementation

All acute cases should be administered vitamin A. Vitamin A oral dosage should be given immediately on diagnosis and repeated the next day, irrespective of the previous doses; for infants aged more than 6 months 50,000 IU should be given, 100,000 IU to infants aged 6–11 months and 200,000 IU to children aged more than or equal to 12 months. In case of child who presents with ophthalmic signs of vitamin A deficiency such as Bitot's spots, a third dose should be given 4–6 weeks later.

### Postexposure Prophylaxis (PEP)

In unimmunized or insufficiently immunized individuals, measles vaccine may be administered within 72 hours of exposure to measles virus to protect against disease. For MCV is contraindicated in individuals like pregnant women, infants aged less than 6 months, and individuals with impaired immune systems, human immune globulin may be given after measles virus exposure, within 6 days of exposure. Passive immunization can prevent illness or reduce its severity **(Box 17A.7)**.

---

**Box 17A.7: Diagnosis and management of measles.**

- Suspected case of measles is case with fever and maculopapular rash.
- Definitive diagnosis is by demonstration of anti-measles IgM antibodies by (ELISA), or the detection of measles virus RNA by RT-PCR.
- There is no specific treatment for measles, only symptomatic management.
- All acute cases should receive Vitamin A, irrespective of the previous doses of vitamin A.
- Passive immunization can prevent illness or reduce its severity; it is given to the individuals with low immunity and pregnant mothers.

---

(ELISA: enzyme-linked immunosorbent assay; RNA: ribonucleic acid; RT-PCR: reverse transcriptase polymerase chain reaction)

## PREVENTION AND CONTROL MEASURES (BOX 17A.8)

Since human beings are the only hosts for the measles virus, measles can be eliminated by attaining and maintaining high population immunity (>95%). This can only be achieved by reaching 95% coverage with a measles-containing vaccine (MCV) in a country or a region. Hence, the primary method of measles prevention is by active immunization and in special circumstances, passive immunization is opted. General preventive and sanitary measures also have a preventive role in the spread of measles.

Once the polio cases reduced globally, i.e. after 2000 WHO has shifted its focus towards measles elimination and has been taking adequate measures to decrease measles-related morbidity and mortality.

---

**Box 17A.8: Prevention and control of measles.**

- Passive immunization is recommended among individuals where vaccine is contraindicated.
- Following general measures like isolation of the case, following cough etiquettes, disinfection of contaminated objects goes long way in prevention of the spread of measles.

---

(MCV: measles-containing vaccine)

### Controlling the Source and Interruption of Transmission

Once a measles outbreak occurs, it must be reported to the local health officials. The child can be excluded from school activities for a week from appearance of rash to prevent contact with susceptible children. In the hospital, strict isolation measures must be followed. The objects that are contaminated by secretions or fluids from the vesicles are incinerated.

### Protection of Susceptible Host

#### Vaccination

Active immunization is the best method to prevent measles.

Vaccines for measles are available either as single antigen vaccines or in combination with other antigens. The combination vaccines are measles with rubella (MR) or mumps and rubella (MMR) vaccines and with mumps, rubella, and varicella (MMRV) vaccine. When these above-mentioned combination vaccines are used, the protective immune response to each of the components remains unchanged.

The most commonly used strain is the Edmonston B strain with the propagation medium being chicken embryo cell culture. The vaccine is a live attenuated vaccine. The vaccine is presented as a freeze-dried product. Before use, the lyophilized vaccine is reconstituted with sterile diluent (double distilled water). As the vaccine is sensitive to both heat and light, once reconstituted vaccine should be stored in the dark at 2–8°C and used within four hours. Measles vaccine may contain sorbitol and hydrolyzed gelatin as stabilizers plus a small amount of neomycin, without thiomersal.

The vaccine should be stored in a refrigerator with a temperature of 2–8°C. The vaccine is administered through sub-cutaneous route. The second dose may be given as early as one month after the first dose. But under Universal Immunization Program second dose of measles (MCV2) is given at 16–24 months. Vaccine effectiveness of one dose of measles vaccine at nine months of age is around 85%. Vaccine effectiveness goes up to 95% and above when given at >12 months of age.

### Adverse Reactions to Measles Vaccine

Generally mild and transient adverse reactions following vaccination are seen and can be as follows:

- Within 24 hours of injection slight pain and tenderness at the site of injection may occur, which may be followed by mild fever; about 7–12 days after vaccination up to 5% of measles vaccine recipients may experience fever. In 2% of vaccinated children the fever may occasionally (1/3,000) induce febrile seizures; a transient rash may appear in few children.
- Approximately one in 30,000 vaccinated individuals, thrombocytopenic purpura may occur.
- One of the serious but extremely rare adverse effects due to measles vaccine is anaphylaxis. The risk is as low as to one in one million children vaccinated.

There is no evidence of an increased risk of encephalitis, permanent neurological sequelae or Guillain–Barré syndrome following vaccination.

## Contraindications to Vaccine

Measles vaccine should be avoided during high fever (>102°F/ 38-39°C) or serious illness and in pregnancy. Persons with a history of an allergic reaction to neomycin, gelatin or other components of the vaccine should not be vaccinated; severely immunocompromised individuals including HIV infection (full blown AIDS).

## Passive Immunization

Passive immunization involves subcutaneous administration of normal human immunoglobulin at a dosage of 0.25 mL/kg body weight within six days of exposure; indicated for children with low immunity status and pregnant women.

## Global Approach

In 2020, WHO and global stakeholders endorsed the Immunization Agenda 2021-2030. The agenda aims to achieve the regional targets as a core indicator of impact, positioning measles as a tracer of a health system's ability to deliver essential childhood vaccines. Based on current trends of measles vaccination coverage and incidence, the WHO Strategic Advisory Group of Experts on Immunization (SAGE) concluded that measles elimination is under threat, as the disease resurged in numerous countries that achieved, or were close to achieving, elimination. WHO continues to strengthen the Global Measles and Rubella Laboratory Network (GMRLN) to ensure timely diagnosis of measles and track the virus' spread to assist countries in coordinating targeted vaccination activities and reduce deaths from this vaccine-preventable disease. The Immunization Agenda (IA) 2030 Measles & Rubella Partnership (M&RP) is a partnership led by the American Red Cross, United Nations Foundation, Centers for Disease Control and Prevention (CDC), Gavi, the Vaccines Alliance, the Bill and Melinda French Gates Foundation, UNICEF and WHO, to achieve the IA 2030 measles and rubella specific targets.

The strategies for measles elimination include:
- To attain and maintain 95% immunization coverage throughout the country with two doses of the measles vaccine
- To build a patient-based surveillance system and monitor the vaccination coverage
- To improve the management of complications and supplement Vitamin A for a quick recovery **(Table 17A.10)**.

Table 17A.10: Dosage of vitamin A for measles case management.

| Age (in months) | Dose administered at diagnosis | Dose administered next day |
|---|---|---|
| 0–6 months | 50,000 IU | 50,000 IU |
| 6–11 months | 100,000 IU | 100,000 IU |
| >12 months | 200,000 IU | 200,000 IU |

## National Level

As per the Universal Immunization Program, measles vaccine was given subcutaneously. The first dose was given between 9 and 12 months, and the second dose is given between 16 and 24 months of age.

### MR Campaign

India launched one of the world's largest vaccination campaigns on 5th February 2017, against measles, which is a major childhood killer disease and congenital rubella syndrome (CRS) responsible for irreversible birth defects. The MR campaign aimed to vaccinate more than 35 million children in the age group of 9 months to 15 years.

Since the launch in 2017, the MR Vaccine campaign has covered nearly 20 crore children in 30 states and Union Territories. Further, to improve on this, the National Technical Advisory Group on Immunization (NTAGI) recommended the introduction of the Measles Rubella Vaccine in the routine immunization program. Both the doses of measles vaccine given subcutaneously at 9-12 months and 16-24 months, has been replaced by MR vaccine under routine immunization.

### Roadmap to Measles and Rubella Elimination in India by 2023

The roadmap is for charging and enabling each district to set goals towards achieving at least 95% MRCV2 coverage by age 2 years, or at the latest age 5 years and achieving and maintaining sensitive fever and rash surveillance.

### SDG Goals and Targets

Elimination of measles will contribute to achieving Sustainable Development Goal's target 3.2 which aims to end preventable deaths of newborns and children under five years of age by 2030.

### Mission Indradhanush

Although not measles-centric, the Government of India's initiative "Mission Indradhanush" launched on December 25, 2014, has concentrated on providing infant immunization in districts with poor vaccination coverage. Vaccination was given against eight vaccine preventable diseases nationally, i.e. Diphtheria, Pertussis, Tetanus, Polio, Measles, severe form of Childhood Tuberculosis and Hepatitis B and *Haemophilus influenza* type B. To further intensify the immunization program, Government of India launched the Intensified Mission Indradhanush (IMI) on October 8, 2017. **Further details of MI and IMI are discussed in Chapter 47: Health Policies and Programs in India**.

## SUMMARY

Measles is caused by a ss RNA, Paramyxovirus. It is one of the most important causes of death among under-fives globally. It is highly contagious. In countries with low vaccination coverage it affects infants and children. Incubation period is 10–14 days. Patients are contagious from four days before eruption of the rash to four days after eruption. Measles have two stages:
1. Preeruptive or initial stage
2. Eruptive or rash stage.

Common complications—otitis media, laryngotracheobronchitis (croup), diarrhea, and pneumonia.

**Diagnosis:** Laboratory confirmation of measles is based on detection of anti-measles IgM antibodies by ELISA, or detection of measles virus RNA by RT-PCR from throat swabs, oral fluid or nasopharyngeal secretions or urine.

**Treatment:** Symptomatic treatment is given. Patients should be isolated for preventing further spread. Vaccination is the most effective way to prevent outbreaks. All acute cases should be administered vitamin A, irrespective of the previous doses of vitamin A. In unimmunized or insufficiently immunized individuals, measles vaccine should be given within 72 hours of exposure.

**Prevention and control measures:** Measles can be eliminated by attaining and maintaining high immunity (>95%) in the population by reaching 95% coverage with a measles-containing vaccine. General preventive and sanitary measures are also important to control the spread of measles.

**Vaccination:** Measles vaccine is available as a single antigen or in combination.

**Global Approach:** The Immunization Agenda 2030 Measles & Rubella Partnership (M&RP) is the global approach for measles elimination.

**National approach:** The MR campaign aims to vaccinate more than 35 million children in the age group of 9 months to 15 years. The concept behind the MR vaccine campaign is to improve the herd immunity of the population

## SUGGESTED READING

1. Campbell H, Andrews N, Brown KE, et al. Review of the effect of measles vaccination on the epidemiology of SSPE. Int J Epidemiol. 2007;36(6):1334-48.
2. CDC. Measles Prevention: Recommendations of the Immunization Practices Advisory Committee (ACIP). [online] Available from: https://www.cdc.gov/mmwr/preview/mmwrhtml/00041753.htm.
3. Holzmann H, Hengel H, Tenbusch M, et al. Eradication of measles: Remaining challenges. Med Microbiol Immunol. 2016;205(3):201-8.
4. Measles and Rubella Surveillance bulletin, WHO Country Office for India for Ministry of Health and Family Welfare. 2022.
5. Ministry of Health and Family Welfare. Universal Immunization Programme. 2018.
6. Mission Indradhanush. National Health Portal of India [Internet]. Nhp.gov. in. 2019.
7. Palumbo P, Hoyt L, Demasio K, et al. Population-based study of measles and measles immunization in human immunodeficiency virus-infected children. Pediatr Infect Dis J. 1992;11(12):1008-14.
8. Perry RT, Halsey NA. The clinical significance of measles: a review. J Infect Dis. 2004;189(Suppl 1):S4-16.
9. Roadmap to Measles and Rubella Elimination in India by 2023 available from https://cms.pib.gov.in/WriteReadData/userfiles/PIB%20Mumbai/Roadmap%20towards%20Measles%20and%20Rubella%20Elimination%20in%20India%20by%202023%20.pdf
10. South-East Asia Regional Office. (2018). India's measles-rubella vaccination campaign a big step towards reducing childhood mortality, addressing birth defects. [online] Available from: http://www.searo.who.int/mediacentre/ features/2017/india-measles-rubella-vaccination-campaign/en.
11. WHO. Fact Sheet Measles. [online] Available from http://www.who.int/news-room/fact-sheets/detail/measles.
12. WHO. Global Measles and Rubella Update—February 2018. [online] Available from: http://www.who.int/immunization/monitoring_surveillance/burden/vpd/surveillance_type/active/Global_MR_Update_February_2018.pdf.
13. WHO: Measles fact sheets (31 May 2023 ) available from https://www.who.int/news-room/fact-sheets/detail/measles?gclid=CjwKCAjwtuOlBHBREiwA7agf1gq5N1w9wrh7T_pWFl4GI9vquFyzeL0mODmHwlt38HRX5P2RNiFYbxoCrPYQAvD_BwE
14. WHO provisional data based on monthly reports to WHO (Geneva) as of August 2019, World Health Organization, [Online]. 2019. [cited 2019 December 12]; [online]Available from: URL: https://www.who.int/ immunization/newsroom/new-measles-data-august-2019/en/
15. Wolfson LJ, Grais RF, Luquero FJ, et al. Estimates of measles case fatality ratios: a comprehensive review of community-based studies. Int J Epidemiol. 2009;38(1):192-205.
16. World Health Organization. (2018) Measles. [online] Available from: http:// www.who.int/immunization/diseases/measles/en.

## EPIDEMIOLOGY OF MUMPS AND ITS PREVENTION AND CONTROL

*Deepthi N Shanbhag*

*"Puffy cheeks and swollen jaw"*
—think of mumps

| | |
|---|---|
| CM7.2 | Enumerate, describe and discuss the mode of transmission and measures for prevention and control of Mumps |
| CM8.1 | Describe and discuss the epidemiological and control measures applicable in Mumps |

### Case Scenario

Mrs Lakshmi JHA(F) from Rampur PHC, on one of her routine visits to the Mogallur village, learns from the Anganwadi Worker that many of the children have not been attending due to fever and swollen jaw. Mrs Lakshmi then visits a few of the children in the village who have been sick and on examination of these children, she finds that they have fever with tender swelling just under ear mostly on one side. The children also found it painful to open their mouth. She immediately reports this to the Rampur PHC Medical Officer Dr Sheela for immediate future action.

**Questions for discussion:**
1. What may be the probable diagnosis in these children? What is the treatment?
2. How can an outbreak be confirmed?
3. What may be the steps taken to control the outbreak?
4. How could this have been prevented?

## INTRODUCTION

Mumps is an acute contagious viral illness of childhood which spreads through the respiratory tract. The name "mumps" is taken from an English verb meaning "grimace", reflecting the outcome of parotitis on facial expression. Historically in 5th century BC Hippocrates actually described "mumps" as a mild illness nonsuppurative swelling near the ears (parotitis) with occasional swelling of one or both testicles (orchitis). In the pre-vaccine era mumps used to be the cause of outbreaks among army personnel and one of important causes of aseptic meningitis and sensorineural deafness in childhood.

## PROBLEM STATEMENT

From 1999–2019, on average, about 500,000 mumps cases were reported to the World Health Organization annually; however, global mumps incidence is challenging to estimate as mumps is not a notifiable disease in many countries. As of 2021, mumps vaccine is routinely used in 123 of 194 (63%) countries. Since the introduction of the measles-mumps rubella (MMR) vaccine in 1968 there has been a significant decrease in the incidence of the infection globally. Recently, a global resurgence of mumps and recent outbreaks have mainly affected adolescents and young adults was observed. The resurgence of mumps began in 2004 and the confirmed cases occurred in the college going age group of 15–24 years. These age group individuals inadvertently are also more susceptible to the virus including its complications like orchitis. The incidence of orchitis in males with post pubertal mumps can be as high as 40%. This is very alarming as sporadic outbreaks of mumps orchitis are now being reported more often in many countries all over the world.

According to the WHO, the case-fatality rate of mumps encephalitis is low and overall mortality is 1/10,000 cases. The permanent sequelae followed by mumps infection occur in about 25% of encephalitis cases. Mumps is a leading cause of acquired sensorineural deafness among children, affecting approximately 5/100,000 mumps patients. Additionally, mumps infection during the first 12 weeks of pregnancy is associated with a 25% incidence of spontaneous abortion

In India, mumps, despite being a widely prevalent disease all over the country, is not considered as of public health importance mainly because of poor documentation, lack of surveillance of clinical cases and lack of published case studies. Even though outbreaks have been reported there is no national data on incidence of the disease from all the states of the country. However, individual research studies in limited geographic areas show that mumps meningoencephalitis was responsible for 2.3–14.6% of all hospitalized viral encephalitis or acute encephalitis syndrome cases. Three of such studies also studied the serological status of young children and adolescents against mumps, and found that the susceptibility rates vary from 32% to 80%. There is regular reporting of both sporadic cases and cyclic outbreaks from all the regions of the country (Vashishtha VM et al., Indian Pediatr, 2015).

## EPIDEMIOLOGY

### Host Factors

a. *Age:* In prevaccine era, mumps most commonly affected children aged 5–7 years and was characterized by interepidemic periods every 4–5 years. In the current era it has become more common among children in the age group of 5–15 years. However, in the unimmunized, it has the propensity to affect any age group. It tends to be more intense in adults as compared to children.
b. *Gender:* The incidence is equal in both males and females but the complication of orchitis in males is much more common as compared to oophoritis in females.
c. *Immunity:* One attack of mumps will give life-long immunity. Most of the infants below the age of 6 months are protected by maternal antibodies.

### Agent Factors

Mumps caused by an enveloped single-stranded RNA virus which is a paramyxovirus belonging to the genus *Rubulavirus* and the family Paramyxoviridae virus in the same group as parainfluenza and Newcastle disease virus. There are 12 mumps virus genotypes named from A to L. The geographic distribution of the genotypes varies—in the western hemisphere genotypes C, D, E, G, and H and in Asian countries, genotypes B, F, and I. The virus can be isolated or propagated in cultures of various human and monkey tissues and in embryonated eggs. It has been recovered from the saliva, cerebrospinal fluid, urine, blood, breastmilk, and infected tissues of patients with mumps. The lipid membrane renders the virus susceptible to ether and alcoholic disinfectants. Mumps virus is rapidly inactivated by formalin, ether, chloroform, heat, and ultraviolet light.

### Environmental Factors

Mumps is largely an endemic disease and cases are present throughout the year. The incidence predominantly peaks in late winter and spring. Epidemics are associated with overcrowding, poverty and rapid urbanization.

### Source/Reservoir

Mumps affects only the human beings predominantly. There are no known carrier states although persons with asymptomatic or atypical infection can transmit the virus.

### Mode of Transmission

The virus spreads by airborne transmission or can spread by direct contact with infected droplet nuclei or saliva. The virus lodges in the nasopharynx and regional lymph nodes and replicates. Viremia occurs after 12–25 days which lasts from 3 to 5 days. Through the viremia the mumps virus spreads to multiple tissues like the glands such as the salivary, pancreas, testes, and ovaries and including the meninges.

### Incubation Period

The incubation period of mumps is 12–25 days. The parotitis usually develops 16–18 days after exposure to mumps virus.

### Period of Communicability

Although mumps virus has been isolated from 7 days before and 11–14 days after the onset of parotitis onset, the optimum percentage of positive isolations and virus loads occur closest to the onset of parotitis and rapidly decreases thereafter. Mumps is therefore most infectious 4–6 days before and 7 days after the onset of parotitis. Transmission also likely occurs from persons with subclinical infections and from persons with only prodromal symptoms. The secondary attack rate is estimated to be as high as 86%.

## CLINICAL FEATURES

Mumps is a generalized viral infection. In 30–40% of cases, it is clinically nonapparent. The prodromal symptoms are mostly nonspecific like any other viral fever and includes generalized constitutional symptoms like myalgia, anorexia, malaise, headache, and low-grade fever. However in severe cases, there may be fever and headache. Parotitis is the most common symptoms of mumps. The proportion of those with mumps among those affected with classical parotitis in all age groups usually range from 31% to 65% although in specific age groups it can be as low as 9% or as high as 94%. This again depends on the age and immunity of the group. Parotitis may be unilateral or bilateral, and any combination of single or multiple salivary glands may be affected. Parotitis usually occurs within the first 2 days of infection and may initially show as earache and tenderness at angle of the jaw. The symptoms gradually decrease after 1 week and usually resolve within 10–14 days **(Table 17A.11)**.

**Table 17A.11:** Clinical presentations of mumps infection.

| Manifestations | Cases (%) |
|---|---|
| Clinical symptoms | 60–70% of infections |
| Parotitis | 95% of the patients with clinical symptoms |
| Epididymo-orchitis | 15–30% of adult men with infection |
| Bilateral orchitis | 15–30% of epididymo-orchitis |
| Oophoritis | 5% of adult women with infection |
| Meningitis | 1–10% of infections |
| Encephalitis | 0.1% of infections |
| Death | 1.5% of encephalitis cases |
| Permanent unilateral deafness | 0.005% of infections |
| Spontaneous abortion | 27% of the 1st trimester pregnancies |
| Pancreatitis | 4% of infections |

*Source:* Hviid A, Rubin S, Mühlemann K. Mumps Seminar. Lancet. 2008;371:932-44.

## CASE DEFINITION FOR CASE CLASSIFICATION

### Suspect

- "Parotitis, acute salivary gland swelling, orchitis, or oophoritis unexplained by another more likely diagnosis", or
- "A positive laboratory result with no mumps clinical symptoms (with or without epidemiological linkage to a confirmed or probable case)".

### Probable

- "Acute parotitis or other salivary gland swelling lasting at least 2 days, or orchitis or oophoritis unexplained by another more likely diagnosis, in a person with a positive test for serum anti-mumps immunoglobulin M (IgM) antibody", or
- "A person with epidemiologic linkage to another probable or confirmed case or linkage to a group/community defined by public health during an outbreak of mumps".

### Confirmed

"A positive mumps laboratory confirmation for mumps virus with RT-PCR or culture in a patient with an acute illness characterized by any of the following: acute parotitis or other salivary gland swelling, lasting at least 2 days with aseptic meningitis or encephalitis or hearing loss or orchitis or oophoritis or mastitis or pancreatitis".

## COMPLICATIONS

The most common complication is orchitis (testicular inflammation) especially among the post pubertal males. It has been observed that orchitis commonly occurs after an episode of parotitis, but it can occasionally precede it or in rarer instances begin simultaneously or even occur alone. This type of orchitis is usually associated with sudden onset of testicular swelling, tenderness, nausea, vomiting, and fever. The pain and swelling may subside within a week, but tenderness may last for longer extending to several weeks. Sterility from mumps orchitis, even if it is bilateral orchitis, is not common. In contrary, the rate of oophoritis among post pubertal females with mumps was less than 1% and moreover this was seen only during an outbreak of mumps. However, this did not have any relationship with infertility. Pancreatitis has also been reported in 3.5% of persons infected with mumps in some studies.

## DIAGNOSIS

The presumptive diagnosis of mumps is usually based more on clinical manifestations especially the presence of parotitis and other preceding prodromal symptoms. A patient meeting the clinical case definition should be reported as a suspect mumps in the absence of any other diagnosis.

Serology is the simplest method for confirming mumps virus infection and enzyme-linked immunosorbent assay (ELISA) is the most commonly used test. During the acute phase there is a presence of serum IgM along with a significant rise in serum IgG antibody titer which is present in both acute and convalescent phase. Sera should be collected as soon as possible after the onset of symptoms for IgM testing. IgM antibodies among the unvaccinated persons usually become detectable during the first 5 days of onset of illness and reach a peak about a week thereafter. It can remain elevated for several weeks or months.

In case of false positive results mumps virus can be isolated directly from the parotid duct, other affected salivary gland ducts, the throat, from urine, and from cerebrospinal fluid (CSF). The preferred sample for viral isolation is a swab from the parotid duct, or the duct of another affected salivary gland. It is preferable to obtain clinical specimens ideally within 3 days and not more than 8 days after onset of parotitis. Mumps virus can also be detected by real-time reverse transcriptase polymerase chain reaction (rRT-PCR).

## TREATMENT

Mumps infection does not have any specific therapy and the infection is usually self-limiting. The immediate treatment consists more of supportive and symptomatic measures such as analgesics and anti-inflammatory medicines, oral hygiene, plenty of fluids and soft diet and isolation of the patient. Treatment with intramuscular (IM) mumps immunoglobulin might be of use only in the early stages and only in certain cases, but shows no benefit whatsoever in an epidemic like situation. Treatment of mumps orchitis is also supportive which includes anti-inflammatory for pyrexia and analgesia for pain, bed rest and a good scrotal support. Local measures can include heat or cold packs. Symptoms resolve within 4–10 days. Only in cases of suspected secondary bacterial infection, broad-spectrum antibiotics can be used.

## PREVENTION AND CONTROL MEASURES

### Global Strategy

The main aim of global health security is to make whole world safe from infectious disease threats. This emphasizes need of global preparedness and response to emerging infectious diseases. Control of the international spread of infectious diseases is the primary and historical responsibility of WHO. The WHO's International health regulations, provides the legal instrument for consistent, proactive, coordinated and multilateral collaborative efforts to address any potential global health security threat that may spread beyond borders. The national governments should share the responsibility of serving those most in need.

- The group of paramyxoviruses is listed among the group of emerging and re-emerging infectious agents which have the potential to cause epidemics, and they need to be dealt with seriously by ensuring sustainable surveillance systems.
- WHO recommends integrating strategies to control mumps with existing high priority goals of measles and rubella control or elimination. Once the decision has been made to include mumps vaccine, the use of combined MMR vaccine is strongly encouraged.

### Indian Strategy

- The **Integrated Disease Surveillance Programme (IDSP)** of India has been recording outbreaks of diseases including mumps. The epidemiological methods employed in this instance involved collecting the number of outbreaks and diagnosing cases based on clinical signs and symptoms. The WHO-recommended clinical case definition is: 'acute onset of unilateral or bilateral tender, self-limited swelling of the parotid or other salivary gland, lasting two or more days and without other apparent cause'. The IDSP aims to strengthen and maintain decentralized laboratory-based disease surveillance systems for epidemic-prone diseases to monitor disease trends and to detect and respond to outbreaks promptly through trained Rapid Response Teams (RRTs)
- ***Controlling source/reservoir***: It is a little difficult due to the long and variable incubation period and the occurrence of subclinical cases. The disease is infective even before it is symptomatic and hence it becomes difficult to detect cases. Contacts can be kept under surveillance.
- ***Interrupting the transmission***: Most of the airborne transmission is likely to occur before and within 5 days of onset of parotitis. Transmission can occur even during the prodromal phase and among those who have subclinical infections. The updated guidelines by CDC (2007–2008) recommend a 5-day period of isolation of cases after onset of parotitis both in community and healthcare settings. It also suggests the usage of standard precautions and droplet precautions during this period of isolation.
    - Patients diagnosed with mumps should stay away with others for at least 5 days from the onset of symptoms.
    - Encourage the patient for good hand washing practices.
    - Encourage the patient to cover mouth and nose during coughing and sneezing with tissue, (put used tissue in the trash can) and if tissue is not available cover with upper sleeve or elbow, not the hands.
    - Drinks and eating utensils of patient should not be shared by others.
    - Frequently touched surfaces, such as toys, doorknobs, tables, counters should be kept clean.
- **Protection of susceptible host:** The Indian Government proposes that mumps is not a significant enough public health problem to warrant routine immunization despite being a widely prevalent disease in the Country. This may be mainly due to poor documentation of clinical cases and a lack of published studies. Hence, at present, the National Immunization Schedule does not include mumps.
- **Mumps vaccine:** The currently used strain of Jeryl Lynn constituting the live-attenuated mumps virus vaccine was licensed in December 1967. Mumps vaccine is also available as combination with measles and rubella vaccines (as MMR), or even as combined with measles, rubella, and varicella vaccine as MMRV in many countries. Mumps vaccine has been prepared in chick embryo fibroblast tissue culture. MMR and MMRV are supplied as a lyophilized (freeze-dried) powder which is then reconstituted with sterile water. The first dose (MMR) is given for children in the age group of 12–18 months old and second dose (MMR) is given at 4–6 years of age. Mumps vaccine produces an inapparent, or a mild infection which is noncommunicable. Approximately 94% (89–97%) of recipients of a single dose of vaccine has been observed to develop measurable mumps antibody titers. Seroconversion rates are found to be similar for single antigen mumps vaccine, MMR and MMRV. Adverse reactions following vaccination include allergic reactions, rash, pruritus and purpura. But these have been transient and generally mild. There are rare reported cases of fever, parotitis, orchitis, central nervous system (CNS) dysfunction, including deafness within 2 months of mumps vaccination **(Table 17A.12)**.

**Table 17A.12:** Characteristics of mumps vaccine.

| Characteristics | |
|---|---|
| Type of vaccine | Live-attenuated mumps virus |
| | Primarily administered as MMR combination |
| Common strains | Jeryl Lynn, RIT, 4385, Urabe Am9, Rubini, Leningrad-Zagreb and Leningrad—3 |
| Efficacy (prelicensure) | 95% (Jeryl Lynn strain in original randomized clinical trials in the USA) |
| Effectiveness (postlicensure) | 80% (the Rubini strain is associated with low effectiveness) |
| Safety | Local reactions, fever, rashes and parotitis. Aseptic meningitis for the Urabe and the Leningrad strains) |
| Schedule | First dose at age of 12–15 months, possibly a second dose from age 13 months to 13 years |

*Source*: Hviid A, Rubin S, Mühlemann K. Mumps Seminar. Lancet. 2008;371:932-44.

## SUMMARY

- Mumps is caused by an enveloped RNA virus belonging to the genus *Rubulavirus* and family Paramyxoviridae.
- Mumps has an incubation period of 12–25 days with period of communicability between 4–6 days before and 7 days after the onset of parotitis.
- Confirmed case of mumps includes laboratory confirmation with RT-PCR or culture in a patient with an acute illness characterized by acute parotitis or other salivary gland swelling, lasting at least 2 days.
- Mumps infection does not have any specific antiviral therapy since the infection is usually self-limiting. The immediate treatment consists more of supportive and symptomatic measures.
- The most common complication is orchitis (testicular inflammation) especially among the postpubertal males.
- As a preventive measure two doses of MMR is given, first dose at 12–18 months of age and second dose at 4–6 years of age.

## SUGGESTED READING

1. Clemmons N, Hickman C, Lee A, et al. Chapter 9: Mumps VPD Surveillance Manual. [online] Available from www.cdc.gov/vaccines/pubs/surv-manual/ chpt09-mumps.pdf.
2. Hviid A, Rubin S, Mühlemann K. Mumps Seminar. Lancet. 2008;371: 932-44.
3. Kadri SM, Rehman S, Rehana K, Brady AH, Chattu VK. Should Mumps Be Higher Up on the Public Health Agenda in India? A Concern for Global Health Security. Med. Sci. 2018;6(62):1-8
4. Kutty PK, Kyaw MH, Dayan GH, et al. Guidance for isolation precautions for mumps in the United States: a review of the scientific basis for policy change. Clin Infect Dis. 2010;50(12):1619-28.
5. Prevention of mumps. National Institute of Health and Family Welfare (NIHFW), by the Ministry of Health and Family Welfare (MoHFW), Government of India. Available from: https//www.nhp.gov.in/disease/ communicable-disease/mumps).
6. Smith KF et al., JR Soc Interface, 2014; WHO, Global and Regional Immunization Profile.
7. Vashishtha VM, Yadav S, Dabas A, et al. IAP Position Paper on Burden of Mumps in India and Vaccination Strategies. Indian Pediatr. 2015;52: 505-14.
8. WHO Position Paper, Mumps Virus Vaccines, Wkly Epidemiol Rec., 2007; Galazka et al., Bull WHO, 1999.
9. World Health Organization. Global and Regional Immunization Profile; South-East Asia Region. [online] Available from: http://www.who.int/immunization/monitoring _surveillance/data/gs_ seaprofile.pdf.
10. World Health Organization. Position paper. Mumps virus vaccines. Wkly Epidemiol Rec. 2007;7:51-60.

# EPIDEMIOLOGY OF RUBELLA AND ITS PREVENTION AND CONTROL

*Ravish HS, Nitu Kumari, Ramya MP*

| | |
|---|---|
| CM7.2 | Enumerate, describe and discuss the mode of transmission and measures for prevention and control of Rubella |
| CM8.1 | Describe and discuss the epidemiological and control measures applicable in Rubella |

## INTRODUCTION

Rubella is a viral disease caused by togavirus of the genus *Rubivirus*, characterized by mild, maculopapular rash affecting both children as well as adults in both the sexes. It is also called "German measles" or "3-day measles". The rash occurs in 50–80% of infected persons and sometimes misdiagnosed as measles or scarlet fever. When rubella infection occurs during pregnancy, especially during the first trimester, consequences such as miscarriages, fetal deaths/stillbirths and a constellation of severe birth defects known as congenital rubella syndrome (CRS) may occur.

## HISTORY

The name rubella is taken from Latin word "rubellus" meaning "little red". It was first described as a separate disease in German medical literature in 1814, hence the common name "German measles". In 1914, Hess postulated a viral etiology and in 1938, Hiro and Tosaka confirmed it by passing the disease to children using filtered nasal washings from infected persons. In 1941, Norman Gregg, an Australian ophthalmologist, reported the occurrence of congenital cataracts among 78 infants born following maternal rubella infection in early pregnancy. This was the first published CRS. Rubella virus was first isolated by Parkman and Weller in 1962.

## PROBLEM STATEMENT

### Global

Rubella has a worldwide distribution and circulates widely in Africa, Middle East and South-East Asia. Globally greater than 10,000 infants are born each year with CRS; greater than 80% of those are born in Africa and South-East Asia. In many developed and some developing countries, widespread rubella vaccination during the past decades has markedly reduced rubella and CRS.

## India

In India, rubella transmission was highly prevalent across the country, which affected susceptible pregnant mothers and had led to CRS in children. India has vaccinated over 348 million children between 2017 and March 2023 through nationwide measles-rubella vaccination campaign. Rubella cases decreased by 48%, from 2.3 to 1.2 cases per million population between 2017 and 2021.

## EPIDEMIOLOGY

### Host Factors

In the pre-vaccine era, the peak age of incidence was in the 5–9 years. After introduction of rubella vaccines in National Immunization Schedule, the frequency of rubella has marginally increased in the older age groups.

Infants of immune mothers are protected for 4 – 6 months. In India, 40% of women in child-bearing age are susceptible to rubella. One attack confers life-long immunity.

### Agent Factors

It is a single-stranded RNA virus, the only member of *Rubivirus* genus within the family Togaviridae. The virus is heat-liable and can be inactivated after 30 minutes at 56°C.

It is also susceptible to disinfectants and is inactivated by 1% sodium hypochlorite, 70% ethanol and formaldehyde.

### Environment Factors

The disease exhibits a seasonal pattern. Seasonal peaks are seen in late winter and spring, although infection remains endemic throughout the year.

### Mode of Transmission

Rubella is transmitted through direct contact/droplet infection from nasopharyngeal secretions.

### Incubation Period

The average incubation period is 17 days (range: 12–23 days). Persons with rubella are most infectious when rash is erupting and they can shed virus from 7 days before to 7 days after the onset of rash. Infants with CRS may shed large quantities of virus from bodily secretions, particularly from the throat and in the urine, up to 1 year.

## PATHOGENESIS

Rubella spreads when an infected person coughs or sneezes. The virus implants and multiplies in the nasopharynx; followed by spread to regional lymph nodes. Subsequently, viremia occurs and in pregnant women, it often results in infection of the placenta. Placental virus replication may lead to infection of the fetal organs and lead to CRS.

### Immunity

Antibodies appear in serum as rash fades and antibody titers rise rapidly in 1–3 weeks. Rash in association with detection of IgM indicates recent infection. IgG antibodies persist for life.

## CASE DEFINITION FOR CLASSIFICATION OF RUBELLA

### Suspected

Illness of acute onset and generalized rash that does not meet the criteria for probable or confirmed rubella or any other illness.

### Probable

The illness characterized by all of the following:
- Acute onset of generalized maculopapular rash
- Temperature greater than 99.0°F/37.2°C
- Arthralgia, arthritis, lymphadenopathy and/or conjunctivitis
- Lack of epidemiologic linkage to laboratory-confirmed case of rubella
- No serologic/virologic testing.

### Confirmed

A case with or without symptoms, but has laboratory evidence of rubella infection confirmed by one/more of the following:
- Isolation of rubella virus
- Detection of rubella-virus specific nucleic acid by reverse transcription polymerase chain reaction (RT-PCR)
- Significant rise between acute and convalescent phase titers in serum rubella immunoglobulin G (IgG) antibody level by any standard serologic assay
- Positive serologic test for immunoglobulin M (IgM) antibody [not explained by measles, mumps, and rubella (MMR) vaccination in the previous 6–45 days].

An illness characterized by all of the following:
- Acute onset of generalized maculopapular rash
- Temperature greater than 99.0°F/37.2°C
- Arthralgia, arthritis, lymphadenopathy or conjunctivitis
- Epidemiologic linkage to a laboratory-confirmed case of rubella.

## CLINICAL FEATURES

**Acquired rubella:** The clinical features are often mild and up to 50% of infection may be subclinical/in apparent. In children, rash is the first manifestation and a prodromal stage is rare. In older children and adults, there is often a 1–5 day prodrome with low-grade fever, malaise, lymphadenopathy and upper respiratory symptoms preceding the rash. The rash is maculopapular and occurs 14–17 days after the exposure; usually occurs initially on face and then progresses from head to foot. It lasts about 3 days and is occasionally pruritic and is often more prominent after a hot shower or bath. The rash is fainter than measles rash and does not coalesce.

Lymphadenopathy may begin a week before the rash and last for several weeks after the infection. Postauricular, posterior cervical and suboccipital nodes are commonly involved.

## COMPLICATIONS

Complications of rubella are not common, but they generally occur more in adult than in children. Arthralgia or arthritis may occur in 70% of adult women who contract rubella, but rare in children and adult males. Fingers, wrist and knees are often affected. Encephalitis occurs in 1 in 6,000 cases, more frequently in adult females.

Hemorrhagic manifestations occur in approximately 1/3,000 cases, more often in children than in adults. These manifestations may be secondary to low platelets and vascular damage, with thrombocytopenic purpura being the most common manifestation. Gastrointestinal, cerebral or intrarenal hemorrhage may occur. Additional complications include orchitis, neuritis and a rare late syndrome of progressive panencephalitis.

### Congenital Rubella Syndrome

Rubella infection during the first trimester of pregnancy leads to serious consequences, which include miscarriages, fetal deaths/stillbirths and a constellation of severe birth defects known as CRS that can affect all organ systems.

Deafness is most common and often the sole manifestation of congenital rubella infection, especially after the 4th month of gestation. Eye defects including cataracts, glaucoma, retinopathy and microphthalmia may occur. Cardiac defects such as patent ductus arteriosus, ventricular septal defect, pulmonic stenosis and coarctation of the aorta are possible. Neurologic abnormalities including microcephaly, mental retardation, and other abnormalities. Others include bone lesions, splenomegaly, hepatitis and thrombocytopenia with purpura.

Sometimes, manifestation of CRS may be delayed from 2 to 4 years. Diabetes mellitus appearing in later childhood occurs frequently in children with CRS. In addition, progressive encephalopathy resembling subacute sclerosing panencephalitis has been observed in few of the older children with CRS. Children with CRS have a higher incidence of autism.

## LABORATORY DIAGNOSIS

The suspected cases must be laboratory confirmed. Virus detection and serologic testing can be done to confirm acute or recent rubella infection. Demonstration of specific rubella IgM antibodies or significant increase in rubella IgG titer in acute and convalescent phase specimen is gold-standard. RT-PCR can also be used to detect virus infection; viral culture is also acceptable.

The optimum time for collection of serum is 5 days after the onset of symptoms (fever and rash) when greater than 90% of cases will be IgM positive. Enzyme-linked immunosorbent assay (ELISA) is sensitive, widely available and relatively easy to perform.

Rubella virus can be isolated from nasal, blood, throat, urine and cerebrospinal fluid specimens from infected patients; the best results are achieved with throat swabs. Virus may be isolated from the pharynx 1 week before and 2 weeks after the onset of rash.

## PREVENTION AND CONTROL

### Vaccine

Rubella is the leading vaccine-preventable cause of birth defects. The most effective method of preventing rubella and CRS is by vaccination. WHO recommends that all countries include two doses of rubella-containing vaccine (RCV) in their immunization program. Immunity is considered long-term and is probably life-long. Women of child-bearing age should avoid getting pregnant

Table 17A.13: Available rubella-containing vaccines (RCVs) in India.

| Vaccine | Brand name | Manufacturer | Price (₹) |
|---|---|---|---|
| MMR | Tresivac | SII | 96.25 |
| | Morupar | Sanofi Aventis | 75 |
| | Trimovax | Aventis Pasteur | 72 |
| MR | MR-Vac | SII | 90.47 |
| Rubella | R-Vac | SII | 86.60 |

for at least 4 weeks after receiving RCV and pregnant women should not get the RCV.

The rubella vaccine was developed by Maurice Hilleman and licensed in 1969. Later, in 1979, an improved live rubella vaccine RA27/3 was developed by Stanley A Plotkin, which replaced the previous one and is currently being used. Currently, majority of RCVs used worldwide; combines measles and rubella or MMR. A tetravalent measles, mumps, rubella, and varicella (MMRV) vaccine is also available, but is not widely used.

In India, the measles-rubella vaccine used in immunization program is live-attenuated lyophilized vaccine which requires to be reconstituted with diluents and each vaccine dose of 0.5 mL to be administered subcutaneously in the right upper arm. The vaccine induces both humoral and cellular immune responses, conferring long-term immunity for both measles and rubella.

In measles and rubella campaigns, nationwide supplementary immunization activity (SIA) with measles-rubella vaccine will be given for all children aged 9 months to 14 years, irrespective of previous immunization status or history of measles/rubella disease.

In the routine program, measles-rubella vaccine is administered in two doses; first dose is given to children between 9 months and 12 months of age and a second dose is given at 16–24 months of age. Vaccine potency is dependent on the vial being stored at the recommended temperature; following reconstitution, the vaccine must be stored at +2°C to +8°C and used within 4 hours. The presently available RCVs in India are shown in **Table 17A.13**.

### Treatment

There is not specific treatment for rubella; symptoms are mild and have to be managed with bed rest and symptomatic treatment such as paracetamol/acetaminophen for fever and other medicines as per the symptoms.

## CURRENT APPROACHES

### Global

**In 2020, WHO and global stakeholders endorsed the Immunization Agenda 2021–2030.**

The Immunization Agenda 2030 Measles & Rubella Partnership (M&RP) is a partnership led by the American Red Cross, United Nations Foundation, Centers for Disease Control and Prevention (CDC), Gavi, the Vaccines Alliance, the Bill and Melinda French Gates Foundation, UNICEF and WHO, to achieve the IA 2030 measles and rubella specific targets.

### India

#### MR Campaign

India launched one of the world's largest vaccination campaigns on 5th February 2017, against measles, which is a major childhood killer disease and congenital rubella syndrome (CRS) responsible for irreversible birth defects. Currently, the MR vaccine is provided in the national immunization program.

### Roadmap to Measles and Rubella Elimination in India by 2023

The roadmap is for charging and enabling each district to set goals towards achieving at least 95% MRCV2 coverage by age 2 years, or at the latest age 5 years and achieving and maintaining sensitive fever and rash surveillance.

***Rubella and CRS control:*** A 95% reduction of rubella and CRS as compared with the 2008 baseline nationally.

***Rubella elimination:*** The absence of endemic rubella virus transmission in a defined geographical area/country for greater than 12 months, as well as the absence of CRS cases associated with endemic transmission in the presence of a well-performing surveillance system.

### Mission Indradhanush

Although not rubella-centric, the Government of India's initiative "Mission Indradhanush" launched on December 25, 2014, has concentrated on providing infant immunization in districts with poor vaccination coverage. Vaccination was given against eight vaccine preventable diseases nationally, i.e. Diphtheria, Pertussis, Tetanus, Polio, Measles, severe form of Childhood Tuberculosis and Hepatitis B and Haemophilus influenza type B. To further intensify the immunization program, Government of India launched the Intensified Mission Indradhanush (IMI) on October 8, 2017. ***Further details of MI and IMI are discussed in Chapter 47: Health Policies and Programs in India.***

## SUMMARY

> Rubella is not only a vaccine preventable disease but also a leading cause of vaccine preventable birth defects. Usually a mild infection in adults, it can however cause congenital defects in the fetus if the pregnant women is infected especially so in the first trimester. One attack is known to confer life-long immunity. Currently, MR and MMR are the vaccines against rubella. MR is the vaccine is included in the National immunization schedule of the country. The vaccine strain is RA 27/3.

## SUGGESTED READING

1. Centers for Disease Control and Prevention. (2017). Facts about measles and rubella. [online] Available from https://www.cdc.gov/global health/rubella/facts.htm.
2. Introduction of measles-rubella vaccine (campaign and routine immunization). National Operational Guidelines 2017. Ministry of Health and Family Welfare, Government of India; 2017.
3. National Centre for Disease Control. (2019). Rubella. Available from https://ncdc.gov.in/index/rubella.
4. WHO-SEARO. (2019). India's measles-rubella vaccination campaign a big step towards reducing childhood mortality, addressing birth defects. [online] Available from http://www.searo.who.int/2017/india-measles-rubella-vaccination-campaign/en.
5. World Health Organization. (2019). Rubella. [online] Available from https://www.who.int/news-room/fact-sheets/detail/rubella.

# EPIDEMIOLOGY OF INFLUENZA AND ITS PREVENTION AND CONTROL

*Rajesh Kumar Konduru, Anil J Purty, Preetam Mahajan, Amit Kumar Mishra, Kalaiselvi*

| | |
|---|---|
| **CM7.2** | Enumerate, describe and discuss the mode of transmission and measures for prevention and control of Influenza |
| **CM8.1** | Describe and discuss the epidemiological and control measures applicable in Influenza |

> **Spanish Flu 1918: The Greatest Medical Holocaust in History**
> The H1N1 strain of influenza A emerged in 1918 to cause a disaster "Spanish flu pandemic" which was remembered for its high mortality during the pandemic. As per the estimation in 2002, around 50–100 million lives were lost during this pandemic period in 1918–1920. Though the actual data was not available, but it was believed that this pandemic had affected half of the population of the world that time. This pandemic not only affected the health status of the people but affected the economic status of the countries also. This pandemic taught a lesson regarding the need of public health measures which indirectly led to development of vaccines for flu and public health planning.

## INTRODUCTION

Avian influenza and pandemic influenza are the epidemic and pandemic diseases, respectively among human beings, caused by a RNA influenza virus of Orthomyxoviridae family. Avian influenza virus, a zoonotic disease virus does not normally infect humans. Sometimes, because of genetic reassortment, the novel strain developed in animals can infect people who are in close contact with the animals and leads to epidemics. Pandemic influenza virus, which is developed through genetic reassortment of animal, avian, and human strains can cause pandemics as there is no pre-existing immunity among human beings.

## CHARACTERISTIC OF DISEASE

There are four different types of influenza viruses—A, B, C and D. Influenza A virus infects human beings and many different animals. The development of a novel virus, which is different from the parent viruses, which has the ability to infect human beings and have sustained person to person transmission, can be responsible for pandemics. Influenza B virus usually circulates among humans and is responsible for seasonal epidemics. Influenza C virus can infect humans as well as animals such as pigs, but these infections are generally mild. Influenza D virus primarily infects animals such as cattle. Human cases of influenza D are not reported till date. Influenza causes respiratory disease. Once the virus enters the respiratory tract epithelium with the help of H antigen (tracheal, bronchial mucosa), it gets multiplied in the epithelial cells and the N antigen helps to release the new viral elements from the infected cells to invade new cells.

The process will continue and this cause inflammation and necrosis of the superficial epithelium. Later there is secondary bacterial infection of the dead tissue of the respiratory epithelium.

## PROBLEM STATEMENT

### Global Burden of Avian and Pandemic Influenza

In 1997, human infections with the Highly Pathogenic Avian Influenza (HPAI) A (H5N1 strain) were reported during an outbreak in poultry in Hong Kong SAR, China. Since 2003, this strain had spread from Asia to Europe and Africa, and to the Americas in 2021, and has become endemic in poultry populations in many countries. Other Avian strains causing human infections reported were A (H7N9), A (H7N7), and A (H9N2). In 2013, human infections with A(H7N9) viruses were reported for the first time in China. During the last 16 years (January 2003 to 21 November 2019), 861 human cases of Avian influenza were reported from 17 countries with 455 deaths. The maximum number of avian influenza cases was reported from Egypt, Indonesia, and Vietnam **(Table 17A.14)**.

**Table 17A.14:** Global burden of pandemic influenza.

| Pandemic | Virus strain | Year | Estimated deaths |
|---|---|---|---|
| Spanish flu | H1N1 | 1918–1920 | 40–50 million |
| Asian flu | H2N2 | 1957–1958 | 1–2 million |
| Hong Kong flu | H3N2 | 1968–1970 | 500,000–2 million |
| Swine flu | H1N1 | 2009–2010 | Up to 575,000 |

Very rarely a novel virus will arise by genetic reassortment, called antigenic shift, from two different influenza virus strains co-infecting the host. As there is no immunity for the novel virus among the population, this novel virus can infect humans and has pandemic potential. In the last hundred years, many pandemics such as Spanish flu, Asian flu, Hong Kong flu, and Swine flu had resulted due to the emergence of a new viral strain by genetic reassortment. On 25th April 2009, the Director-General of the World Health Organization (WHO) announced a Public Health Emergency of International Concern (PHEIC) and on 11 June of the same year, WHO declared it as an Influenza Pandemic. By 1 August 2010, worldwide laboratory-confirmed cases of pandemic influenza (H1N1) including over 18,449 deaths were reported from more than 214 countries (CDC, Disease Burden of Influenza). On September 2011 WHO had adopted a new nomenclature for 2009 pandemic influenza as influenza A (H1N1) pdm09.

### Burden of Avian and Pandemic Influenza in India

Till date in India not a single case of human avian influenza has been reported but as the virus is circulating in animals and birds and these viruses can easily go for antigenic shift, the population close to these animals and birds are at risk for Avian Influenza. After the influenza pandemic (H1N1) in 2009, the virus spread all over the globe and is responsible for epidemics afterwards in different countries including India confirmed Influenza cases and deaths in India are listed in **Tables 17A.15 and 17 A.16** (NCDC, Seasonal Influenza H1N1, 2023).

**Table 17A.15:** Lab confirmed cases and deaths of Influenza A H1N1 year-wise in India.

| Year | Confirmed cases | Deaths |
|---|---|---|
| 2009 | 27,236 | 981 |
| 2010 | 20,604 | 1,763 |
| 2011 | 603 | 75 |
| 2012 | 5,044 | 405 |
| 2013 | 5,253 | 699 |
| 2014 | 937 | 218 |
| 2015 | 42,592 | 2,990 |
| 2016 | 1,786 | 265 |
| 2017 | 38,811 | 2,266 |
| 2018 | 15,266 | 1,128 |
| 2019 | 28,798 | 1,218 |
| 2020 | 2,752 | 44 |
| 2021 | 778 | 12 |
| 2022 | 13,202 | 410 |
| 2023 | 1,995 | 26 |

*Source:* India. Seasonal Influenza H1N1. National Centre for Disease Control (NCDC) 2023.
Reports received from States/UTs to central surveillance units, IDSP, NCDC, Delhi

**Table 17A.16:** Differences between seasonal influenza and pandemic/avian influenza.

| Characteristics | Seasonal influenza | Pandemic/avian influenza |
|---|---|---|
| Antigenic reassortment | Antigenic drift | Antigenic shift |
| Public health problem | Endemic disease | Pandemic/Epidemic disease |
| Immunity | Active immunity develops due to previous infections | No immunity as the viral strain is new for human beings |
| People at risk | People without immunity are at risk for infection | All are at risk as there is no pre-existing immunity |

## EPIDEMIOLOGY

### Agent Factors

*Types:* The influenza virus is a RNA virus. There are four different types of influenza viruses—A, B, C and D.

**Genome:** The genome consists of eight segments, which can break easily in the invaded cell and combine with the genome segment of any other type of virus if invaded the same cell to give rise to a novel genome. Pigs play a great role in genetic reassortment of the influenza viruses. Pandemic influenza virus is the result of genetic reassortment of different human, avian, and swine strains of influenza viruses in the body of pig. The virus with the novel genome has new characteristics as it has different type of genome than its parents. Infection with this novel recombinant virus which has new characteristics from the parent genome can cause epidemics at its first contact to human population as this virus is new to human population with no pre-existing immunity **(Fig. 17A.6)**. Refer to seasonal flu section for more details.

# Chapter 17: Specific Epidemiology of Infectious Diseases

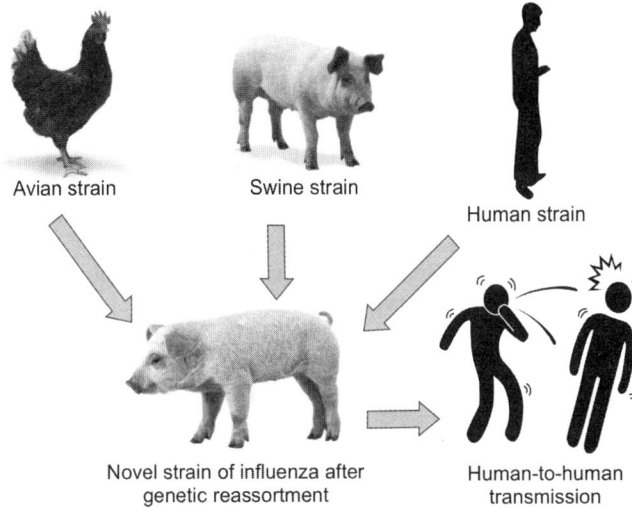

**Fig. 17A.6:** Genetic reassortment of pandemic influenza virus.

### Avian Influenza/Bird Flu

Avian influenza is a disease among birds which has outbreak potential (Epornithic disease). Due to its high pathogenic nature, the outbreak is always associated with high mortality among the birds. Rarely, it transmits to human beings. Till date human to human transmission is not reported. The transmission of virus can be possible to farmers through droplets because of their close contact with poultry.

### Pandemic Influenza (Swine Flu)

When there is genetic reassortment among human, avian, and swine viral strains (antigenic shift), the result is pandemic influenza strain, a novel strain with different characteristics than its parents. The human-to-human transmission of the novel viral strain depends on the nucleic acid segment received from parent human influenza strain; if it is sufficient then the virus can easily transmit from person to person and can cause pandemics.

## Host Factors

***Age:*** All people irrespective of age are susceptible to influenza infection. But severity of disease and case fatality is high among children, elderly and people with chronic diseases such as diabetes, chronic kidney disease, chronic heart disease and respiratory diseases.

***Sex:*** Both the gender are susceptible to influenza infection.

***Immunity:*** Immunity against influenza plays a great role in prevention of initiation of infection in seasonal influenza and influenza epidemic. Local secretory antibodies can help in prevention of infection. As the avian influenza and pandemic influenza viral strains (product of genetic reassortment) are mostly new to human population, there is no inbuilt immunity among the population. People vaccinated with inactivated influenza vaccine are protected from viral infection because of systemic immunity but can shed the virus through the nasal secretion as they do not have local immunity. Local immunity plays a great role to break the chain of transmission of infection (**Box 17A.9**).

> **Box 17A.9: High-risk groups for avian influenza.**
> - Children playing with infected poultry, particularly asymptomatic infected ducks
> - Poultry handlers in live animal markets/wet markets
> - Cullers without proper PPE
> - Those handling fighting cocks
> - Persons plucking and preparing of diseased birds in wet markets/backyard poultry/kitchens
> - Consumption of undercooked poultry products
> - Consumption of chicken or duck blood
> - Hospital functionaries managing human cases of AI without proper PPE.

***Occupation:*** The Avian influenza spread to the farmers who are in close contact with the poultry.

### Environmental Factors

***Seasons:*** The epidemics of influenza depend on country and seasons, it occurs in winter in temperate zones and in rainy seasons in tropical zones.

***Overcrowding:*** Overcrowding helps to spread the virus fast.

### Reservoir

Different strains of influenza viruses are isolated from many birds and animals such as wild birds, migratory waterfowl, pigs, swine, horses, etc. The novel strain of pandemic influenza develops by genetic reassortment of human, animal and bird influenza viruses in the body of pig. Migratory waterfowl is the natural reservoir of Avian influenza. It is interesting to note that the migratory waterfowl can get infection with all the H and N subtypes of Avian influenza virus.

### Source of Infection

A subclinical or clinical case of influenza being the source of infection. The viral load of the respiratory secretions is high in initial few days of infections. In epidemics, asymptomatic and mild symptomatic cases are primarily the source of infection. In cases of avian influenza, the influenza virus spreads through feco-orally among birds, farmers handing the infected birds/poultry can get the infection from the infected birds through direct or indirect methods.

### Portal of Exit, Transmission and Entry

Transmission can occur by both direct and indirect methods. Infected birds with avian influenza shed the virus in their feces. Farmers handling them can get the infection through direct or indirect modes. Human-to-human transmission for Avian influenza has not been reported till date. Pandemic influenza transmits through droplets and droplet nuclei. Indirect mode of transmission for pandemic influenza is also possible. Person-to-person transmission in pandemic influenza depends on the human component of the new influenza viral strain.

### Incubation Period

The incubation period is 2–5 days.

## Period of Communicability

The communicability period of influenza depends on the persistence of symptoms. Usually, it is one to two days before and one to two days after the onset of symptoms.

## CLINICAL FEATURES

### Avian Influenza

High-grade fever, cough, shortness of breath, and diarrhea are symptoms predominantly of lower respiratory tract infection. Later, the infection will cause bilateral pneumonia and then respiratory failure. Chest X-ray of the patient shows widespread collapse, consolidation, and interstitial shadowing.

### Pandemic Influenza (H1N1)

Fever, sore throat, runny nose, cough, headache, and myalgia. The pandemic influenza virus can cause rapidly progressive pneumonia by involving the lower respiratory tract of lungs in children and young-middle-aged adults. Complications such as otitis media, pneumonia, sinusitis, bronchiolitis myositis, and myocarditis may occur.

## LABORATORY CONFIRMATION

In the time of epidemics to confirm the diagnosis or to know more about the new viral strain the laboratory tests are required.

### Specimen

The clinical specimen required for the laboratory confirmation of diagnosis are the oropharyngeal or nasopharyngeal swab. In the case of avian influenza, the preferred specimen is endotracheal aspirate if available, than the oropharyngeal and nasopharyngeal specimens.

### Sample Collection

Only health care providers with universal precautions, i.e. with all Personal Protective Equipment (PPE) such as apron, goggles, head cover, N95 mask, and gloves should collect the specimen. Persons handling the samples should wash their hands before and after handling the specimens.

### Transportation of Samples

The samples after collections need to be packed properly (Triple Packaging System, WHO) in viral transport media and send to the reference laboratory maintaining the cold chain with the case history of the patient and sample ID.

### Laboratory Test

Following tests can be done in the laboratory for confirmation of diagnosis or for isolation of the virus. The viral antigen can be detected using rapid diagnostic kits. The nucleic acid of the virus can be identified by real time-polymerase chain reaction (RT-PCR). The virus can be isolated and identified by culture, which is the gold standard test in diagnosis of influenza.

## MANAGEMENT

### Case Definitions and Case Discharge Policy (Table 17A.17)

WHO with several partners has developed standardized case definitions for Avian influenza (H5N1) to facilitate:

- Reporting and classification of human cases of H5N1 infection by national and international health authorities.
- Standardization of language for communication purposes.
- Comparability of data across time and geographical areas.

### Medical Treatment

#### Concurrent Disinfection

It is the immediate disinfection of infectious materials of the patients (body fluids), infected articles used by them, and the materials soiled by them during their course of disease. This is to prevent transmission of the infectious agent to others close to the patient.

#### Supportive Treatment

Patients need oxygen therapy because of associated hypoxia. Severely-ill patients may require mechanical ventilation for respiratory failure. Some patients may need steroid for shock and antibiotics for associated bacterial infection.

#### Antiviral Drugs

*M2 inhibitors (Amantadin, Rimantadin):* Mechanism—it blocks the viral entry to the epithelial cells and prevents its multiplication.

*Neuraminidase inhibitors (Oseltamivir, Zanamivir, and Ribavirin):* Mechanism—it inhibits the neuraminidase (N) enzyme of virus and thus prevents the release of virus from infected host cell.

## CONTROL AND PREVENTIVE MEASURES

### Control Measures for Avian Flu

Whenever there is an epidemic of avain influenza among poultry, all the poultry birds of the infected farm should be culled. The farmer suspecting the influenza epidemic and the personnel handling the outbreak should use proper PPE.

### Control Measures for Pandemic Flu

The following measures can help to control and prevent transmission of influenza in pandemics:

- Proper hand washing practices
- Avoid public gathering/crowded places, if going to public gathering or crowded places then use N95 mask
- Cover nose and mouth with a cloth during sneezing and coughing
- Drink plenty of water
- Persons developing respiratory symptoms or fever, must stay at home and contact a local health care provider.

Table 17A.17: Case definitions of avian influenza (H5N1) and pandemic (H1N1).

| Case | Avian influenza (H5N1) | Pandemic influenza |
|---|---|---|
| Person under investigation | A person whom public health authorities have decided to investigate for possible H5N1 infection | |
| Suspected case | A person presenting with unexplained acute lower respiratory tract illness with fever (>38°C) and cough, shortness of breath or difficulty breathing<br>AND<br>One or more of the following exposures in the 7 days prior to symptom onset:<br>• Close contact with a person who is a suspected, probable, or confirmed H5N1 case;<br>• Exposure to poultry or wild birds or their remains or to environments contaminated by their feces in an area where H5N1 infections in animals or humans have been suspected or confirmed in the last month;<br>• Consumption of raw or undercooked poultry products in an area where H5N1 infections in animals or humans have been suspected or confirmed in the last month;<br>• Close contact with a confirmed H5N1 infected animal other than poultry or wild birds (e.g. cat or pig);<br>• Handling samples (animal or human) suspected of containing H5N1 virus in a laboratory or other setting | A person with acute febrile respiratory illness (fever ≥38°C) with onset:<br>Within 7 days of close contact with a person who is a confirmed case of pandemic influenza A (H1N1) virus infection, or<br>Within 7 days of travel to community where there are one or more confirmed pandemic influenza A (H1N1) cases, or<br>Resides in a community where there are one or more confirmed pandemic influenza cases |
| Probable case | *Probable definition 1:*<br>A suspected case AND<br>One of the following additional criteria:<br>• Infiltrates or evidence of an acute pneumonia on chest radiograph plus evidence of respiratory failure (hypoxemia, severe tachypnea)<br>• Positive laboratory confirmation of an influenza A infection but insufficient laboratory evidence for H5N1 infection.<br>*Probable definition 2:*<br>A person dying of an unexplained acute respiratory illness who is considered to be epidemiologically linked by time, place, and exposure to a probable or confirmed H5N1 case | A person with an acute febrile respiratory illness who:<br>• Is positive for influenza A, but unsubtypable for H1 and H3 by influenza RT-PCR or reagents used to detect seasonal influenza virus infection, or<br>• Is positive for influenza A by an influenza rapid test or an influenza immunofluorescence assay (IFA) plus meets criteria for a suspected case<br>• Individual with a clinically compatible illness who died of an unexplained acute respiratory illness who is considered to be epidemiologically linked to a probable or confirmed case. |
| Confirmed cases | A suspected or probable case AND<br>One of the following positive results conducted in a national, regional or international influenza laboratory whose H5N1 test results are accepted by WHO as confirmatory:<br>• Isolation of an H5N1 virus;<br>• Positive H5 PCR results from tests using two different PCR targets, e.g. primers specific for influenza A and H5 HA;<br>• A four-fold or greater rise in neutralization antibody titer for H5N1 based on testing of an acute serum specimen (collected 7 days or less after symptom onset) and a convalescent serum specimen. The convalescent neutralizing antibody titer must also be 1:80 or higher;<br>• A microneutralization antibody titre for H5N1 of 1:80 or<br>• Greater in a single serum specimen collected at day 14 or later after symptom onset and a positive result using a different serological assay, for example, a horse red blood cell hemagglutination inhibition titre of 1:160 or greater or an H5-specific western blot positive result | A person with an acute febrile respiratory illness with laboratory confirmed pandemic influenza A (H1N1) virus infection at WHO approved laboratories by one or more of the following tests:<br>• Real time PCR<br>• Viral culture<br>• Four-fold rise in pandemic influenza A (H1N1) virus specific neutralizing antibodies |
| Discharge policy | • Adult patients can be discharged 7 days after resolution of fever<br>• Children can be discharged 21 days after onset of illness | • Patients who responded to treatment after two to three days and became totally asymptomatic should be discharged after 5 days of treatment. There is no need for a repeat test<br>• Patients who continue to have symptoms of fever, sore throat, etc. even on the 5th day should continue treatment for 5 more days. If the patient becomes asymptomatic during the course of treatment there is no need to test further<br>• For patients who continue to be symptomatic even after 10 days of treatment or those cases with respiratory distress and in whom secondary infection is taken care of, and if patient continues to shed virus, then resistance of the patients to antiviral would be tested. The dose of antiviral may be adjusted on case to case basis |

## Hospital Infection Control

The following precautionary measures have to be followed by the hospitals and health care professionals to control the spread of infection in hospital:
- Proper hand washing practices
- Use of Personal Protective Equipment (PPE)
- Isolation of influenza case
- Cohorting of influenza cases in hospital
- Disinfection of patient's room
- Concurrent disinfection of patient's belonging.

## Chemoprophylaxis

The M2 inhibitors can be used for chemoprophylaxis for high-risk individuals such as children, elderly and debilitated persons. They have to take the drug till the epidemic is over. Oseltamivir can be used for chemoprophylaxis for avian influenza and should be taken within 2 days of exposure to cases of avian influenza.

## Vaccine (Pandemic Flu, H1N1)

Difference between intranasal and injectable vaccine (H1N1) has been listed in **Table 17A.18**.

## SURVEILLANCE

Influenza caused by H1N1 virus has been declared as one of the diseases under Public Health Emergency of International Concern (PHEIC) by WHO. The H1N1 and H5N1 cases should be reported with other diseases under Integrated Disease Surveillance Project (IDSP) in India for further reporting to WHO. The community spread of the disease (H1N1) is defined as "If there are 25 or more epidemiologically linked suspect cases of pandemic influenza A H1N1, of which at least 1 or more are laboratory confirmed, in 2 or more cities, over a period of 2 weeks, then the particular state would be considered to be having community spread."

## Influenza Surveillance Lab Network

The human health component of the avian influenza surveillance activity under india's IDSP aimed to minimize the threat posed to human population by these avian influenza viral infection and other zoonoses. This human health component also prepares for prevention, control, and response to an influenza pandemic in humans. This human component of surveillance system also supports the networking and strengthening of reference laboratories for prompt case confirmation and re-establishing seasonal influenza surveillance system for India (**Fig. 17A.7**).

## FluNet

It is a web-based platform for influenza virological surveillance. The data available or captured, e.g. number of influenza viral strain detected by subtypes in FluNet can help to track the movement of the virus in the world and for epidemiological interpretation. The data are updated every week in the web and publicly available.

## Global Influenza Surveillance and Response System

Known formerly as Global Influenza Surveillance Network (GISN), GISRS has been conducting global influenza virological surveillance for over half a century. GISRS (WHO) monitors the evolution of influenza viral strains and provides recommendations in different areas such as laboratory diagnostics, antiviral susceptibility, risk assessment, and vaccines. It serves as a global alert system for the emergence of influenza viral strains with pandemic potential.

The World Health Organization (WHO) global influenza surveillance standards define the surveillance case definitions for influenza-like illness (ILI) and severe acute respiratory infections (SARI) (**Table 17A.19**).

Points to be noted when using the case definitions:
- Influenza infection causes a clinical syndrome not easily distinguished from other respiratory infections.
- The case definitions for ILI and SARI are not necessarily intended to capture all cases but to describe trends over time.
- Using one common case definition globally will allow national health authorities to interpret their data in an international context.

Table 17A.18: Differences between intranasal and injectable vaccine (H1N1).

| Characteristics | Intranasal vaccine | Injectable vaccine* |
|---|---|---|
| Type | Live attenuated | Inactivated/killed |
| Dose | Single | 2 doses |
| Age | >2 years | >6 months |
| Local immunity | Yes | No |
| Systemic immunity | No | Yes |
| Route | Intranasal | Intramuscular/Subcutaneous |
| Contraindication(s) | Immunocompromised individuals, family members, and health care providers close to immunosuppressed persons | Allergy to chicken egg, anaphylactic reactions to any of the vaccine component, history of severe reaction to previous vaccine, moderate to severe illness with fever and Guillain-Barre syndrome within 6 weeks of last vaccination. |
| Spreading the disease | The vaccine receiver does not spread the disease as there is local immunity | The vaccine receiver is protected from the disease but spreads the virus in initial period as there is no local immunity |

*The serum antibody response to inactivated H1N1 influenza vaccine depends on age of the receiver and pre-existing antibody levels of the receiver. Pregnant women develop protective levels of influenza antibodies after the vaccination (inactivated vaccine) and the extra benefit of vaccinating pregnant women with inactivated influenza vaccine is providing passive transfer of anti-influenza antibodies to the neonates.

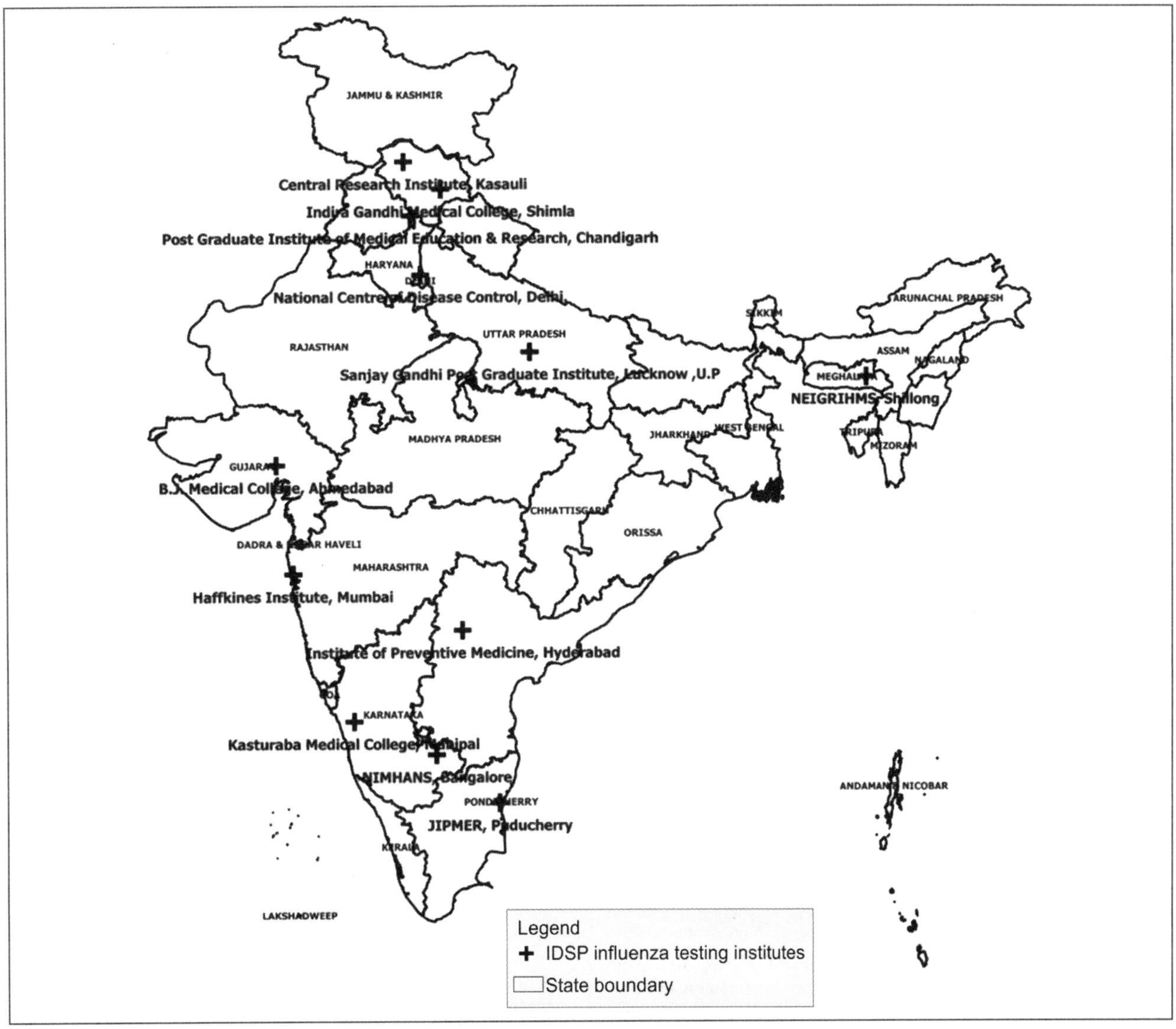

**Fig. 17A.7:** IDSP influenza network.
*Source:* IDSP, NCDC, Government of India.

Table 17A.19: Case definitions for influenza surveillance, World Health Organization.

| Illness | Case definition |
|---|---|
| Influenza-like illness | An acute respiratory infection with:<br>• Measured fever of ≥38°C<br>• Cough<br>• With onset within the last 10 days |
| Severe acute respiratory illness | An acute respiratory infection with:<br>• History of fever or measured fever of ≥38°C<br>• Cough<br>• With onset within the last 10 days<br>• Requires hospitalization |

## WHO'S 6 PHASES OF PANDEMIC ALERT FOR INFLUENZA PANDEMIC

Phases 1–3 of Pandemic influenza correlate with preparedness, including capacity development and response planning activities, and phases 4–6 clearly signal the need for response and mitigation efforts. The current phase for pdm09 Influenza pandemic is "the post-pandemic period" **(Fig. 17A.8)**.

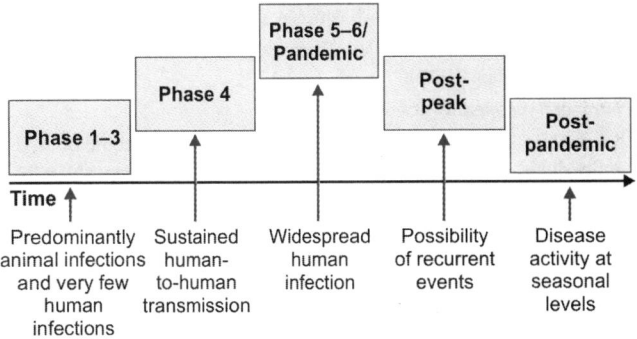

**Fig. 17A.8:** WHO's 6 phases of influenza pandemic (2009).
*Source:* Emergencies preparedness, response, WHO.

## IS IT POSSIBLE TO ERADICATE OR ELIMINATE INFLUENZA?

For many reasons, it cannot be possible to eradicate or eliminate influenza disease. First, it is known that avian species including certain other animal species such as swine, are the natural host of all known influenza A viruses. The swine helps some influenza A virus subtypes in circulation and provides the platform for genetic reassortment and development of novel viral strains. It is not possible to eliminate or eradicate the circulating influenza A viruses among all animal hosts. Second, the formation of novel strain viruses because of antigenic drift and antigenic shift restricts the use of vaccines as vaccines are to be updated based on the new strain of influenza virus.

## SUMMARY

*Pandemic flu:* Pandemic influenza can cause both epidemic and pandemic diseases, caused by a RNA influenza virus of Orthomyxoviridae family.

*Epidemiology:* All people irrespective of age are susceptible to influenza infection. A subclinical or clinical case of influenza being the source of infection. The incubation period is 2–5 days.

*Clinical features:* Fever, sore throat, runny nose, cough, headache, and myalgia. The pandemic influenza virus can cause rapidly progressive pneumonia by involving the lower respiratory tract of lungs in children and young-middle-aged adults. Complications such as otitis media, pneumonia, sinusitis, bronchiolitis myositis, and myocarditis may occur.

*Diagnosis:* The viral antigen can be detected on nasopharyngeal and throat swab using rapid diagnostic kits. The nucleic acid of the virus can be identified by real time-polymerase chain reaction (RT-PCR). The virus can be isolated and identified by culture, which is the gold standard test in diagnosis of influenza.

*Treatment: M2 inhibitors (Amantadin, Rimantadin):* Mechanism—it blocks the viral entry to the epithelial cells and prevents its multiplication.

*Neuraminidase inhibitors (Oseltamivir, Zanamivir, and Ribavirin):* Mechanism—it inhibits the neuraminidase (N) enzyme of virus and thus prevents the release of virus from infected host cell.

*Prevention and control measures:* The following measures can help to control and prevent transmission of influenza in pandemics:
- Proper hand washing practices
- Avoid public gathering/crowded places, if going to public gathering or crowded places then use N95 mask
- Cover nose and mouth with a cloth during sneezing and coughing
- Drink plenty of water
- Persons developing respiratory symptoms or fever, must stay at home and contact a local health care provider.

*Vaccination (Pandemic Flu, H1N1):* There are two vaccines, intranasal and injectable vaccine (H1N1).

*Intranasal vaccine:* Live attenuated

Single dose, given for >2 years. Contraindicated in immunocompromised individuals, family members, and healthcare providers close to immunosuppressed persons.

*Injectable vaccine:* Inactivated/killed given in 2 doses for those who are >6 months. This vaccine is given intramuscular/subcutaneous.

*Avaian influenza:* Avian influenza virus, a zoonotic disease virus does not normally infect humans. Sometimes, because of genetic reassortment, the novel strain developed in animals can infect people who are in close contact with the animals and leads to epidemics.

Avian influenza is a disease among birds which has outbreak potential (Epornithic disease). Rarely, it transmits to human beings. High-risk groups include Children playing with infected poultry, particularly asymptomatic infected ducks, Poultry handlers in live animal markets/wet markets, Cullers without proper PPE.

*Clinical features:* High-grade fever, cough, shortness of breath, and diarrhea are symptoms predominantly of lower respiratory tract infection. Later, the infection will cause bilateral pneumonia and then respiratory failure. Chest X-ray of the patient shows widespread collapse, consolidation, and interstitial shadowing.

*Diagnosis:* The viral antigen can be detected on nasopharyngeal and throat swab using rapid diagnostic kits. The nucleic acid of the virus can be identified by real time-polymerase chain reaction (RT-PCR). The virus can be isolated and identified by culture, which is the gold standard test in diagnosis of influenza.

*Prevention and control measures:* Whenever there is an epidemic of avain influenza among poultry, all the poultry birds of the infected farm should be culled. The farmer suspecting the influenza epidemic and the personnel handling the outbreak should use proper PPE.

*Chemoprophylaxis:* The M2 inhibitors can be used for chemoprophylaxis for high-risk individuals such as children, elderly and debilitated persons. They have to take the drug till the epidemic is over. Oseltamivir can be used for chemoprophylaxis for avian influenza and should be taken within 2 days of exposure to cases of avian influenza.

## SUGGESTED READING

1. DGHS, Ministry of Health and Family Welfare, Government of India. Pandemic Influenza A H1N1. Clinical management Protocol and Infection Control Guidelines. [online] Available from https://mohfw. gov.in/sites/default/files/2366426352.pdf.
2. Lab Confirmed Cases and Deaths of Influenza A H1N1 (Swine Flu). National Health Profile 2019.
3. National Centre for Disease Control, Govt. of India. (2018). Influenza Surveillance Lab Network. IDSP.
4. Plotkin S, Orenstein W, Offit P. Inactivated Influenza Vaccines. Vaccines, 6th edition. China: Elsevier Inc.; 2012. pp. 1-1570.
5. WHO. (1997). FluNet. Influenza. [online] Available from: http://www.who.int/influenza/gisrs_laboratory/flunet/en.
6. WHO. (2006). WHO case definitions for human infections with influenza A (H5N1) virus, Influenza.
7. WHO. (2009). Current WHO phase of pandemic alert for Pandemic (H1N1).
8. WHO. (2018). The pathogen, Influenza (Avian and other zoonotic). [online] Available from http://www.who.int/en/news-room/fact-sheets/detail/influenza-(avian-and-other-zoonotic).
9. WHO. Case definitions for influenza surveillance. WHO surveillance case definitions for ILI and SARI. [Online] Available from: https://www.who.int/influenza/surveillance_monitoring/ili_sari_ surveillance_case_definition/en/
10. WHO. Interim Guidelines for Avian Influenza Case Management. [online] Available from http://apps.searo.who.int/PDS_DOCS/B0634.pdf.
11. World Health Organization. Weekly Update Pandemic (H1N1) 2009. Geneva: WHO; 2010.

# SEASONAL INFLUENZA

**CM7.2** Enumerate, describe and discuss the mode of transmission and measures for prevention and control of seasonal influenza

**CM8.1** Describe and discuss the epidemiological and control measures applicable in seasonal influenza

> *Case Scenario*
>
> *Mithun 26-year-old adult male makes a visit to the emergency department in the evening. He says he is having fever, cough and coryza for the past 4 days also he complaints of having throat pain. When the doctor explored the history, Mithun told he is living in a hostel which has dormitory arrangements. One of his friends also suffered from similar complaints two days before. Mithun has informed the doctor that several times in a year he used to have similar kind of illness which is mild in nature. During those episodes, he did not consult any healthcare provider and he managed it with drugs from over the counters. But, this time he has severe breathlessness and cough which necessitated him to make a visit to emergency department.*
>
> *Following which many adults from the same hostel had made a visit to outpatient Medicine department with similar complaints. One of the senior citizens staying in that hostel also had similar complaints and because of the severe breathlessness and decreased $SpO_2$ level he was shifted to intensive care unit.*

## INTRODUCTION

Influenza viruses are one of the major causes of atypical pneumonia where the patient does not respond to the routine course of antibiotics. Though in many it is self-limited, annually it contributes to thousands of mortality. It can also cause millions of deaths in an epidemic scenario. Seasonal influenza illnesses contribute to the majority of school and industrial absenteeism. Hence, influenza is considered as one of the public health emergencies.

### Problem Burden

Influenza has a wide spectrum of illness from subclinical infection to fatal respiratory failure. Since only clinical cases are reported routinely, the actual number of influenza reported does not represent the true burden.

As per the recent estimates, there are around a billion cases of seasonal influenza annually, including 3–5 million cases of severe illness. It causes 290,000 to 650,000 respiratory deaths annually. Flu-like illnesses alone contribute to 14 to 16% of the febrile acute respiratory tract infections managed in OPD settings (WHO, Seasonal Influenza Factsheet, 2023).

In tropical countries, influenza has been associated with 5% of ARI. In temperate countries, the outbreak of influenza typically occurs during late autumn and winter months. However, in tropical countries the pattern of outbreak highly varied. In some of the countries (India and Thailand) there is a perennial sporadic outbreak and large outbreak during June, July and November-January. Several countries had shown consistent flu outbreak during winter (South Africa, Brazil) and some during the rainy season (Taiwan, Nigeria).

Annually, around 40,000 flu cases are reported throughout India under the Integrated Disease Surveillance Project. In recent years, the maximum number of Flu cases is reported from the state of Andhra Pradesh and Telangana, Maharashtra, Gujarat, Uttar Pradesh, Delhi, and Rajasthan. Case fatality rate was more in the state of Madhya Pradesh, Chhattisgarh, Jammu and Kashmir, and Kerela (MOH&FW, Seasonal Influenza-State/Ut, 2011-2018).

## EPIDEMIOLOGY

### Agent Factors

***Type:*** Seasonal flu is caused by influenza viruses. Influenza virus belongs to *orthomyxoviridae* family. It is a segmented spherical shaped RNA type of virus. Based on the nucleoprotein and capsid protein influenza virus has been divided into four major types namely type A, type B, type C and type D.

***Genetic mutation:*** The segmental nature of RNA facilitates the occurrence of mutation to happen in faster rate compared to other viruses. Also, this segmental nature allows exchange of genetic materials among various species. Avian influenza and H1N1 are examples for those genetic reassortments of human and mammals.

***Structure:*** The envelope or outer layer of influenza type A has two structural glycoproteins namely hemagglutinins which help the virus to bind with the host cell membrane and neuraminidase which penetrates and helps the virus to get released from the host cell. There are 17 hemagglutinin and 10 neuraminidase identified to date. Of the three influenza viruses, combinations of H and N results in more than 16 influenza type A viruses such as H1N1, H1N2, H2N2, H3N1, H3N2. Influenza H1N1 and H3N2 and influenza type B are recently circulating strains.

Since type A virus has the capacity to infect multiple species, there is a chance for genetic changes to occur in various degrees. Segmented genomic property of influenza viruses gives the tremendous opportunity for gene exchange to happen across various segments.

Based on whether antigenic changes occur within the genome or there is mix up of various genomes to result in complete gene reassortment these changes are named as antigenic drift and shift respectively. If there is a minimal genetic change occurs in the existing strain due to mutation that phenomenon is called antigenic drift. Since there is no cross-immunity between serotypes, based on the antigenic drift pattern of emerging strain in that particular year there may be a need for changing the vaccine type. The sequence of this antigenic drift mechanism is illustrated in **Figure 17A.9**.

Influenza is one of the epizootic diseases. The Avian (bird) flu strain can pass to intermediate host such as pigs without any change in the antigen structure of influenza. Similarly, human strain also can be passed to the intermediate host. *When there*

| | |
|---|---|
| Person gets immunized with influenza vaccine which has two A strains and one influenza B strains | 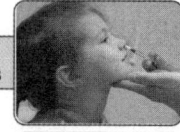 |
| Antibody is produced in the body against three influenza strains contained in the vaccine | 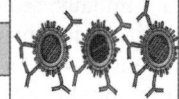 |
| When the person is exposed to influenza during the season these specific antibodies bind with hemagglutinin antigens. Hence the penetration of virus into the host cell is prevented | 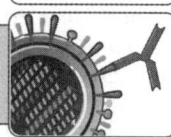 |
| Since influenza viruses are RNA viruses they are more prone for mutation compared to DNA viruses | 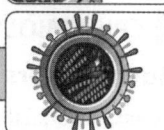 |
| Due to mutation the HA gene changes during the next season thereby the HA antigen also changes its shape | 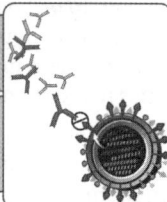 |
| Previously available antibodies in the body now cannot bind with HA antigen of newer influenza strain which in turn facilitates the virus to bind with the host cells and infect it | |

**Fig. 17A.9:** The sequence of antigenic drift process.

Though in a majority of the people it acts as a self-limiting illness certain following high-risk groups are prone for severe illness and influenza-related mortality:
- Age more than 50 years
- Chronic conditions related to pulmonary and cardiovascular system
- Residents or health care providers of nursing homes or who have potential direct contact with the patient
- Chronic metabolic conditions such as diabetes, renal failure, and immune suppressive state
- Pregnant women in second or third trimester
- Caretakers involved in residential care in groups

## Environmental Factors

***Physical environment:*** High temperature and humidity prevalent in the tropical countries expected to decrease the aerosol spread of infection. However, impoverished living conditions, poor access, and affordability to health care in tropical countries lead to the disproportionate amount of morbidity and mortality.

In developed countries, the majority of epidemic happened from January to April whereas in India all H1N1 and Avian Flu outbreaks had happened during September–December.

***Seasons:*** Rainy season is the usual influenza seasonal period for large parts of India. In north, north-west and Central India, the surge in cases usually occurs during winter months (January–March).

***Over-crowding:*** Living in overcrowded settings can increase the risk of acquiring the infection. That is the reason why there is clustering of cases often reported in institutional settings such as hostels, schools, etc.

***Socio-economic status:*** Moreover, low socio-economic status could co-exist with undernutrition and tuberculosis which also can independently increase the risk of infection.

## Source/Reservoir of Infection

Children and immune compromised hosts can shed the virus for a longer duration.

## Mode of Transmission

The primary mode of spread is person to person aerosol droplet. Due to the nature of droplet spread, shedding of virus from subclinical cases and narrow incubation period (24–72 hours) within a short span of time it can transmit the infection to many susceptible individuals. Direct contact with secretions through fomites also acts as a good source of infection.

### Incubation Period

Usually it is 2–3 days.

The detail of the natural history of disease is explained in **Figure 17A.11**.

During influenza season, around 20% of people can be affected by influenza. Among semiclosed groups such as schools and nursing home, the infection rate (secondary attack rate) can even go up to 70%.

The transmissibility of influenza virus is reported to be around 2 which means every new case of influenza can generate two secondary influenza cases within the serial interval of 2–3 days. Hence, in the case of a pandemic where the population is naïve to the current strain, it can lead to an explosive outbreak.

is a concomitant infection from two different species there is a chance of gene-reassortment within the intermediate host. These new strains can spread the infection from intermediate species to human beings. Since these strains are never exposed in the past among human species there is a threat of pandemic occurrence in this scenario. A schematic framework which explains the mechanism of antigenic shift is shown in **Figure 17A.10**.

Parainfluenza viruses (PIVs) are the second most common cause of respiratory infections next to rhinovirus among children. PIVs also are the second most common cause for lower respiratory tract infections and cause for hospitalization among children next to RSV. Unlike influenza viruses, PIVs do not have any animal reservoirs. By age 8, the majority of children will show seropositivity against PIVs.

It has been predicted that recent influenza the H1N1/pdm09 which caused major pandemic can continue to circulate as seasonal influenza virus for several years.

## Host Factors

***Age:*** Affects mainly old age people. And Children are the significant source of disease transmission in the community.

***Sex:*** Affects both the sex equally.

Influenza type A affects multiple species like human, swine, avian, equine, etc. Influenza type B and type C mainly affect human beings. Occasionally, type C affects pigs. Birds, pigs, equine acts as a reservoir of infection. Type D affects mainly cattle and there is no evidence of human transmission that has been reported.

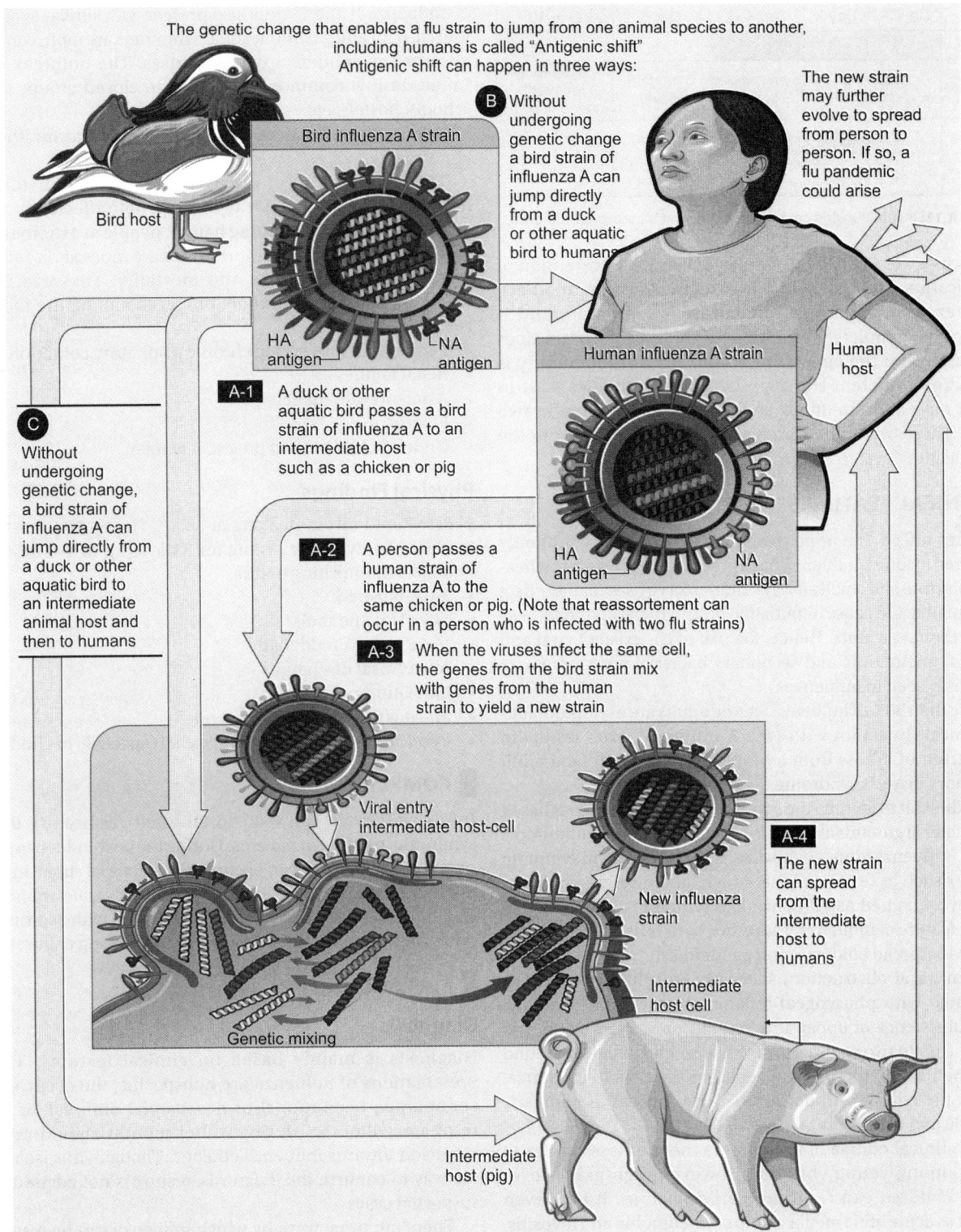

Fig. 17A.10: The framework on antigenic shift.

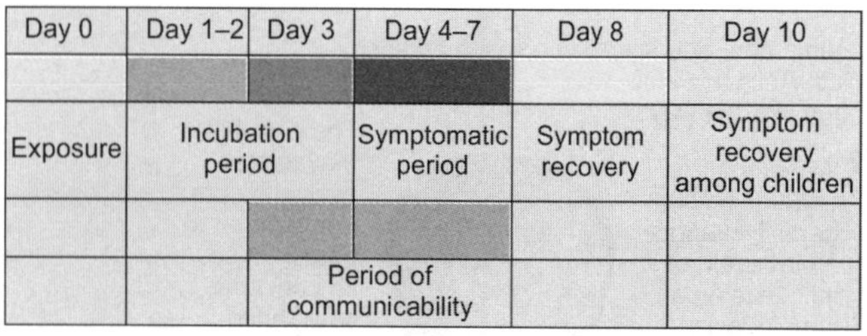

| Day 0 | Day 1–2 | Day 3 | Day 4–7 | Day 8 | Day 10 |
|---|---|---|---|---|---|
| Exposure | Incubation period | Symptomatic period | Symptom period | Symptom recovery | Symptom recovery among children |
| | | Period of communicability | | | |

**Fig. 17A.11:** Incubation and communicable period for seasonal influenza.

Vaccines are reported to be effective against prevention of complications, mortality and disease transmission to others. However, vaccine-induced immunity is temporary and it may not be completely protective, if the vaccine strain does not match with the circulating strain. No cross-immunity is seen across different sub-types/strains. Antibodies start to appear days after an attack and reach the maximum in two weeks. These antibodies gradually wean off and drop to the pre- infection level in 8–12 months.

## CLINICAL FEATURES

Influenza affects the upper respiratory tract more commonly compared to lungs. Influenza has a predilection towards trachea-bronchial tree and small airways. Influenza viruses mainly affect cilia function and cause denudation of superficial epithelial cells of the respiratory tract. Hence, the risk of co- existent viral and bacterial pneumonia and secondary bacterial pneumonia are commonly seen in influenza.

More than 50% of influenza among adults are asymptomatic/subclinical. Infection with type A influenza virus results in a spectrum of illness from asymptomatic stage to fatal adult respiratory distress syndrome.

It is difficult to identify the specific type of viral illnesses based on the clinical grounds alone. Basically, all types of pneumotropic viruses (influenza virus, adenovirus, RSV, etc.) result in symptom complex such as fever, malaise, cough, and myalgia which are collectively named as influenza-like symptoms. Probably, the unique feature of influenza from other virus is its predilection to cause widespread epidemic and pandemics.

Often nasal obstruction, sneezing, and rhinorrhea occur associated with pharyngeal inflammation without exudate. After subsistence of upper airway symptoms, a dry cough can continue up to two weeks. However, fever and cough are found to be the best predictors in diagnosing the case of influenza. Among the elderly without fever, it can present as anorexia, lassitude and confusion.

The clinical course of influenza is more or less similar to adults among young children. However, high-grade fever among children can result in febrile seizures. It may even present as acute otitis media, croup or pneumonia and myositis. Influenza A virus infection can also lead to exacerbation of bronchial asthma episodes. High proportions of elderly can present with pneumonia compared to children and young adults. There are two specific CNS involvements observed during influenza A virus infection influenza encephalopathy and post-influenza encephalitis.

Influenza B and C virus also present with similar symptoms. Muscle pain and gastrointestinal symptoms are more commonly observed in influenza type B viruses. The outbreak due to Influenza B is commonly observed in closed groups such as schools, hostels, etc.

Respiratory examination and radiography may not show any abnormality.

The presentation of disease differs from individuals to individuals. While a majority of the people affected by this flu gets cured by its self-limiting nature, people at extremes of age group and underlying comorbidities are more at risk of severe respiratory dysfunctions and mortality. The severity and mortality is more commonly observed among the following risk groups:

- People with underlying chronic respiratory conditions
- Renal failure
- A person with diabetes
- Elderly
- Under-5 children and pregnant women.

### Physical Findings

***Fever:*** Rapid onset, peaking at 38.4°C (up to 41°C, especially in children), typically lasting for 3 days (up to 4–8 days), and gradually diminishing nature.
- *Face*: Flushed
- *Skin*: Hot and moist
- *Eyes*: Watery, reddened
- *Nose*: Nasal discharge
- *Ear*: Otitis
- *Mucous membranes*: Hyperemic
- *Cervical lymph nodes enlargement* (especially in children).

## COMPLICATIONS

Influenza illness can lead to an adult respiratory distress syndrome in subset of patients. During the post-influenza period, pneumonia outbreak can occur due to bacterial super-infection mainly caused by *Staph. aureus, Streptococcus pneumoniae* and *H. influenzae*. If flu-like symptoms is treated with aspirin/other salicylates it can lead to Reye's syndrome among children.

## MANAGEMENT

### Diagnosis

Diagnosis is mainly based on clinical features. Though presentations of influenza are nonspecific, the occurrence of community, institutional or nosocomial outbreak of febrile respiratory illnesses during winter months should raise the suspicion towards influenza etiology. Though virus isolation is the way to confirm the diagnosis, testing is not advised for all suspected cases.

There are three ways by which influenza can be tested and confirmed:
1. Virus isolation from a swab taken from the respiratory tract
2. Paired serology of elevated IgG titre more than fourfold
3. Real time polymerase chain reaction (RT-PCR).

Influenza virus can be successively isolated from nasopharyngeal region up to five days of symptom onset.

Swabs from nasal and nasopharyngeal region have better isolation rates compared to throat swab when the specimen is collected within three days of onset. However, posterior pharyngeal swabs are suggested by the WHO to diagnose pandemic flu.

## Treatment

Since these seasonal flu strains are predisposed to create pandemic threat every health care provider should be aware of how to identify the cases and assess its severity. When a new viral strain is reported there could be panic among the public which may lead to patient overload at tertiary care hospital. Hence, following the standard case definition and treatment guidelines from the peripheral health institutes is mandatory to manage the public health emergency efficiently.

The following case definitions are used in the country to assess the severity. The management has to be planned accordingly as per the following:

| Category | Definition | Investigations | Management |
|---|---|---|---|
| Category A | Patients with mild fever with cough/sore throat associated with or without the following symptoms: body ache, headache, diarrhea and vomiting | No testing for influenza is required | • Symptomatic management for fever and cough<br>• Paracetamol 500 mg thrice daily. Avoid taking aspirin<br>• Drink plenty of water<br>• Eat nutritious food<br>• Take rest up to 24 hours after the fever has subsided<br>• Reassess after 24 hours<br>• The patient should restrict their stay at home.<br>• They should avoid contact people at crowded places and they should stay away from their family members and visitors who are at risk such as infants, elderly and pregnant women<br>• At least an arm level distance should be maintained from the susceptible contacts |
| Category B | Symptoms mentioned under category A<br>With high-grade fever (more than 102°F) and sore throat<br>(Or)<br>Symptoms mentioned under category A has been seen in one of the following high-risk groups:<br>Children with mild illness but with predisposing risk factors.<br>Pregnant women;<br>Persons aged 65 years or older;<br>Patients with lung diseases, heart disease, liver disease kidney disease, blood disorders, diabetes, neurological disorders, cancer and HIV/AIDS;<br>Patients on long-term cortisone therapy | No testing for influenza | • Oseltamivir 75 mg daily twice for 5 days<br>• Broad-spectrum antibiotics as per CAP guidelines<br>• The patient should restrict their stay at home<br>• They should avoid contact people at crowded places and they should stay away from their family members who are at risk such as infants, elderly and pregnant women |
| Category C | • Symptoms mentioned under category A and B<br>• Presenting with any one of the following critical signs<br>• Breathlessness, chest pain, drowsiness, fall in blood pressure, sputum mixed with blood, bluish discoloration of nails<br>• In case of children, if they show any one of the following danger signs:<br>&gt; Somnolence, high and persistent fever, inability to feed well, convulsions, shortness of breath, difficulty in breathing<br>&gt; Worsening of underlying chronic conditions | Testing for influenza specific strains through nasal/throat swab | Immediate hospitalization and treatment under inpatient/intensive care settings |

***Chemoprophylaxis:** Individuals belong to high-risk group and not vaccinated with current circulating strains of Influenza can be protected from disease transmission through Oseltamivir chemoprophylaxis. The schedule for Oseltamivir prophylaxis can be as follow: wt <15 kg: 30 mg OD; 15–23 kg: 45 mg OD; 24–39 kg: 60 mg OD; >40 kg: 75 mg OD. For infants <3 months: Not recommended; 3–5 months: 20 mg OD; 6–11 months: 25 mg OD.

## PREVENTION AND CONTROL (FIG. 17A.12)

Since the major mode of transmission is through droplets following certain personal hygiene measures and adherence to personal protective equipment (PPE) among healthcare providers can reduce the transmission to the larger extent. Though the vaccine is effective against the reduction of hospitalization and mortality in resource-poor settings it is impossible to include influenza vaccine under the universal immunization program. In developing countries, influenza vaccine is recommended for healthcare providers and people at risk.

Personal protective device such as masks play a major role to contain the aerosol transmission of influenza. There are two types of masks provided under the programmatic settings: (1) triple layer surgical and (2) N95 respirator. Healthcare provider collecting respiratory samples and who directly involved in aerosol generation activities such as intubation, suction and nebulization should use N95 respirators. Other types of healthcare providers such as a person working in community

## Section 3: Community Health Problems and Vulnerable Groups

### Protect yourself and others

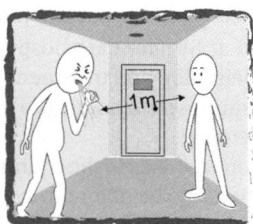 Avoid close contact with sick people

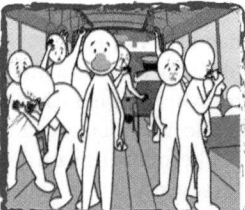 Wear a face mask in crowded places

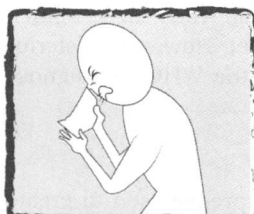 Cover your nose and mouth with a tissue when you cough or sneeze

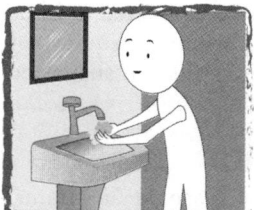 Wash your hands regularly with soap and water

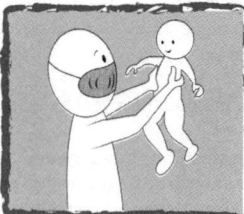 People at high-risk and those around them with influenza-like symptoms should take extra precautions

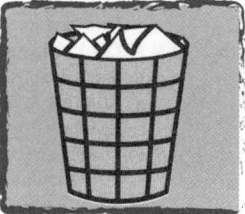 Throw away used tissues or disposable items used by sick people in a rubbish bin

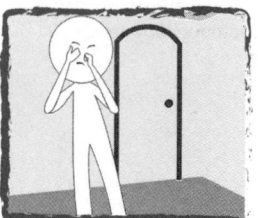 Avoid touching eyes, nose or mouth with unwashed hands

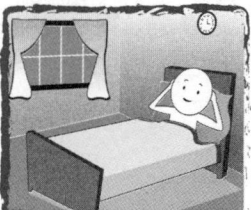 Try and stay home for at least 24 hours after your fever has gone

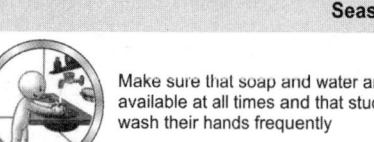

### How to protect students at schools and nurseries

#### Seasonal influenza

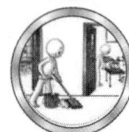 Make sure that soap and water are available at all times and that students wash their hands frequently

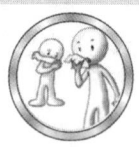 Educate students on the importance of covering their mouth and nose with their upper sleeve, a disposable tissue or a clean handkerchief when they sneeze or cough

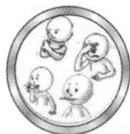 Bathrooms, floors and surfaces, including of tables, chairs, toys and door and window handles, should be regularly cleaned with disinfectants

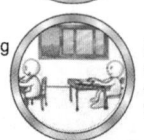 Keep windows of classrooms open, or at least during break times, even during cold weather, to ensure good ventilation

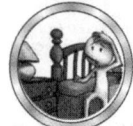 Watch out for the main influenza symptoms: high temperature (above 38°C), runny nose, cough, headache, muscle and joint pain

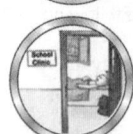 If a student suddenly develops influenza symptoms, separate him/her from classmates and inform parents as soon as possible

 Make sure that students and staff with influenza symptoms stay away from school

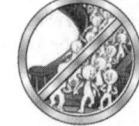 Plan student's entry and exit to and from classrooms as much as possible to minimize unnecessary crowding

Encourage students and staff not to hug or kiss when greeting during the influenza season, especially if the students have influenza symptoms

 Educate students to avoid sharing drinking cups, towels, etc. and to avoid touching their eyes, nose or mouth with unwashed hands

The vast majority of people infected with seasonal influenza get better with no medical intervention

**Fig. 17A.12:** Prevention of seasonal influenza in schools and nurseries.

surveillance, screening, ambulance and security are advised to use a triple layer surgical mask.

There is no supportive evidence to encourage the use of triple layer surgical mask among public except the susceptible/probable case and their household contacts and caretakers. Inappropriate use of surgical mask like wearing for more than six hours, reuse of mask, can actually increase the rate of transmission.

### Infection Control Practices

| Do's | Don'ts |
|---|---|
| • Use of triple layer mask<br>• Following principles of respiratory etiquettes<br>• Covering the nose and mouth with a piece of cloth whenever a cough or sneeze occurs<br>• Collection of sputum or nasal secretions in a covered container to reduce the aerosol generation | • Spit/blow nose here and there<br>• Consumption of Aspirin for a head, body ache and other flu like symptoms from nearby pharmacies as self-medication<br>• Close contact with other family members<br>• Using utensils of an affected person without washing* |

*Since, many respiratory pathogens are transmitted through fomites hand washing with soap and water after touching potentially contaminated items such as bathroom tap, door knobs, etc. should be encouraged.*

### Chemoprophylaxis

Prophylactic use of anti-viral drugs among unvaccinated individuals namely oseltamivir, zanamivir, amantadine and rimantadine can prevent the transmission of infection up to 70%.

Anti-viral drugs like amantadine and rimantadine is used prophylactically and therapeutically against influenza type A virus. When these drugs were used prophylactically during H3N2 epidemic it reduced the infection by 90%. However, amantadine is not commonly used due to the fear of CNS side effects and renal dysfunction among the elderly. Rimantadine is reported to have a better safety profile compared to amantadine.

Neuraminidase (NA) inhibitors such as oseltamivir and zanamivir also found to be 96% effective against viral shedding and 85% against infections. Also, the therapeutic use of oseltamivir has significantly reduced the duration of illness. However, NA inhibitors use among children less than one year is not encouraged.

Among individuals who were unable to receive flu vaccination before the season, vaccinated with non-circulating strains, contraindications to vaccines but likely to have contact with flu patients (healthcare providers, closed group) can be given prophylactic dose (half of the therapeutic dose) of anti-viral drugs such as oseltamivir or zanamivir to curtail the transmission.

### Vaccines

There are three types of inactivated Influenza vaccines available for use: (1) intact whole cell vaccine, (2) split vaccines, (2) sub-unit vaccines. Currently, split viruses are encouraged and it became mandatory to use only split virus vaccine among children less than 12 years.

The trivalent inactivated influenza vaccine (TIV) gives protection against infection in the range of 70-90% provided the vaccine strain matches with the circulating strain. However, the protection against hospitalization and mortality is found to be 25-39%, 39-75% respectively. US government suggests people more than 55 years, cardiopulmonary diseases, renal dysfunctions, diabetes, residents of health care facilities and health care workers to get vaccinated against influenza annually. This vaccine has to be administered at least four weeks before the expected season of an epidemic. Currently, CDC encourages shifting towards universal immunization for flu rather than targeting to the high-risk groups.

Live attenuated intranasal vaccines are effective and safe to be administered among healthy adults 2–49 years. Though these intranasal vaccines are safe, tolerable and easy to administer. This type of vaccine is not recommended among high-risk groups such as elderly, a person with comorbidities and immune suppressive state.

Irrespective of the vaccine type (inactivated/live attenuated) all children less than 9 years need two doses of inactivated vaccine over one-month interval to attain optimal response and vaccine effectiveness. These inactivated vaccines do not interfere with the efficacy of other co-administered vaccines. Adults who exposed to natural infection or previous influenza vaccination need one annual dose of influenza vaccine. Among children who are first time to get the flu vaccine are recommended to have live attenuated vaccine whereas in adults any type of vaccine gives an equal amount of protection. Continuous emergence of new antigenic variants and waning of immunity a year after the vaccination necessitates the need for annual administration of influenza vaccine.

> As per the recent guidelines by the Ministry of Health and Family Welfare (MoHFW), India **seasonal influenza vaccine is recommended for following high-risk people:**
> 1. Healthcare workers, working in hospital/institutional settings (doctors, nurses, paramedics) with the likelihood of exposure to Influenza virus such as emergency department, ICU, isolation wards, screening centers, laboratory technicians, rapid response team members, ambulance drivers should be vaccinated.
> 2. The vaccine is recommended for pregnant women, irrespective of the duration of pregnancy.
> 3. Persons with chronic illnesses such as chronic obstructive pulmonary disease, bronchial asthma, heart disease, liver disease, kidney disease, blood disorders, diabetes, cancer and for those who are immune compromised.
> 4. For children having chronic diseases like asthma; neuro-developmental condition like cerebral palsy, epilepsy, stroke, mentally challenged, etc. Heart disease like congenital heart diseases, congestive heart failures; blood disorders like Sickle cell disease; diabetes, metabolic disorder, all immune-compromised children, malignancy receiving immunosuppressive therapy, kidney disorder and liver disorder.
> Vaccine among elderly and children 6 months to 8 years is considered as desirable.

In line with WHO advisory group, the ICMR has recommended on the following seasonal influenza vaccine composition, for the period 2017-2018. The recommended trivalent vaccine should have:
1. an A/Michigan/45/2015 (H1N1)pdm09-like virus.
2. an A/Hong Kong/4801/2014 (H3N2)-like virus.
3. a B/Brisbane/60/2008-like virus.

The vaccine should be administered at least one month before the commencement of the predicted season. If any high-risk individual did not get vaccinated before, in the meanwhile chemoprophylaxis can be followed to prevent transmission.

## PUBLIC HEALTH MEASURES

As influenza is prone to cause epidemic and pandemic, global measures towards pandemic preparedness and risk assessment are coordinated by the earnest efforts of the WHO.

### Global Measures

As periodically, illnesses caused by influenza viruses caused major death toll in the form of epidemic and pandemics globally strict surveillance mechanism has been set up. Currently, the WHO GISRS (Global Influenza Surveillance and response systems) is a system of National Influenza centres and WHO collaborating centres around the world continuously monitor the influenza viruses circulating in the humans and updates the composition of influenza vaccines twice a year. Based on the currently circulating strains, the technical advisory group on vaccinations and immunizations informs the decision on the type of the vaccine to be administered for that particular year.

WHO convenes a meeting twice a year during the month of February (Northern hemisphere) and September (Southern hemisphere) to decide the influenza strain to be included in the vaccine during the next seasonal flu.

As of now, three countries namely United States of America, Japan and Canada have recommended and implementing annual vaccine against seasonal flu.

### Public Health Measures Initiated by Government of India

Rapid response teams were made and trained by all the states.

Capacity building workshops are conducted related to early identification of outbreak/epidemic.

### Early Identification of Outbreak

All levels of healthcare providers are trained under Integrated Disease Surveillance Project (IDSP) on standard case definitions to diagnose seasonal influenza. As per IDSP, age and gender disaggregated ARI episodes treated in the specific health facilities are reported on weekly basis. Based on the comparison of number of episodes treated in the previous month and number of cases treated in the last year of similar month epidemic warning signals are generated. Based on this, epidemic warning signals rapid response team is deployed from the routine health system for detailed investigations and disease control measures.

- The MoHFW is ensuring the availability of adequate stocks related to personal protective equipment, N95 masks, and supply of anti-viral drug oseltamivir.
- Technical guidelines have been shared with all the state governments regarding vaccination against flu for healthcare workers, testing and treatment guidelines, quality assurance for testing kits.
- Reference laboratories including regional ICMR institutes are set up to monitor quality assurance and supply of testing kits.
- Enhanced surveillance for influenza-like illnesses and severe acute respiratory infections through IDSP network is being implemented.
- 24 × 7 outbreak monitoring cell is functioning under the National Center for Disease Control (NCDC).
- Regular update of a burden on influenza through collaborative efforts with media.
- Periodic capacity building workshops are conducted on influenza surveillance and data management.
- Biomedical waste management guidelines have been circulated to all state health departments for strict adherence.
- Rapid points of care tests are made available to improve the surveillance during the emergency.
- Integration with animal husbandry is made under the one health strategy.

## SUGGESTED READING

1. Control C for D. Disease burden of Influenza [Internet]. Available from: https://www.cdc.gov/flu/about/disease/burden.htm.
2. WHO: influenza (seasonal ), factsheet. 12 Jan 2023
3. Guerrant RL, Walker D, Weller PF. Viral infections. 3rd edition. Tropical infectious diseases: principles, pathogens and practice. China: Saunders Elsevier; 2011. pp. 378-98.
4. Madeley JS. PCR. section 6: Viral Infections. Manson's Tropical Disease. Twenty Fir. London: Saunders; 2003. pp. 831-40.
5. Ministry of Health and Family Welfare G of I. Clinical Management for Seasonal Influenza [Internet]. Available from: https://mohfw. gov.in/sites/default/files/49049173711477913766.pdf
6. Ministry of Health and Family Welfare G of I. Guidelines on categorization of Seasonal Influenza cases during screening for home isolation, testing, treatment and hospitalization [Internet]. 2016. Available from: https://mohfw.gov.in/sites/default/files/394697031477913837_3.pdf
7. Ministry of Health and Family Welfare G of I. Guidelines on use of masks for health care workers, patients and members of public [Internet]. 2016.
8. Ministry of Health and Family Welfare G of I. Virology of Influenza [Internet]. 2016. Available from: https://mohfw.gov.in/sites/default/files/78665981141424950643.pdf
9. Nair H, Brooks WA, Katz M, et al. Global burden of respiratory infections due to seasonal influenza in young children: a systematic review and meta-analysis. Lancet. 2011;378(9807):1917–30. Available from: http://linkinghub.elsevier.com/retrieve/pii/S0140673611610519.
10. Neuzil PFWKM. RNA Viruses. Infectious Diseases. third. Philadelphia: Lippincot Williams & Wilkins; 2004. pp. 1987–2015.
11. Part II: Viral infections. Hunter's Tropical Medicine and Emerging Infectious Diseases. 8th edition. Philadelphia: Saunders; 2000. pp. 1071–104.
12. Targonski PV, Poland GA. Volume 4. The International Encyclopedia of Public Health. 2nd edition. Canada: Elsevier; 2017. pp. (4) 238-58.
13. Voulme 1. In: Oxford Textbook of Global Public Health. sixth. New York: Oxford University Press; 2015.
14. World Health Organisation. Vaccines against influenza WHo position paper. Wkly Epidemiol Rec. 2012;87:461–76.

## SEVERE ACUTE RESPIRATORY SYNDROME

**CM7.2** Enumerate, describe and discuss the mode of transmission and measures for prevention and control of Severe Acute Respiratory Syndrome

**CM8.1** Describe and discuss the epidemiological and control measures applicable in Severe Acute Respiratory Syndrome

## INTRODUCTION

During February 2003, worldwide panic was created due to the outbreak of severe acute respiratory syndrome (SARS). SARS is the first severe communicable new disease to emerge in the 21st century. By March 2005, SARS was declared eradicated by the WHO. Next to smallpox, SARS is the illness which received the label of eradication.

## EPIDEMIOLOGY

SARS is caused by the novel coronavirus (SARS-CoV). This virus is suspected to have a zoonotic origin. Initially, the disease was originated in Hong Kong as a hospital outbreak followed by it rapidly spread to other continents including North America and Europe. Almost 8,400 people were affected from 29 countries within a short span of time with a case fatality rate of 11%. China, Canada, Singapore and Vietnam are the countries which are heavily affected due to SARS.

*Risk factors:* Healthcare workers involved in procedures which generate aerosol such as nebulization procedure are estimated to have 21% of total SARS transmission. Close household contacts, air travel to countries with local transmission of SARS, increasing age, respiratory comorbidities are other factors which predispose to the condition of SARS. Children are affected rarely by SARS.

## CLINICAL FEATURES

SARS-CoV mainly transmitted through droplet origin. Fomites also frequently act as a source of infection. Among patients who have diarrhea, fecal contamination becomes the significant modes of spread. The mean incubation period is 6 days. Fevers with chills (100%), unproductive cough (50–100%), dyspnea (78%) are common manifestations of SARS illness. Unlike other coronaviruses, upper respiratory tract symptoms are unusual in SARS. The characteristic features which differentiate from other respiratory viral illnesses are rapidly progressive bilateral pneumonia, pulmonary thromboembolic manifestations and rapid response to immune-modulating agents such as steroids. Imaging techniques such as chest X-ray, CT thorax can help to identify the pneumo-mediastinum and pneumo-thorax and to assess the people who need intensive care and positive pressure ventilator support.

## DIAGNOSIS

SARS is diagnosed by the presence of clinical features such as fever >38°C, respiratory symptoms, radiographic evidence of pneumonia and the presence of virological markers either in the form of virus isolation, raising antibody titre or positive RT-PCR. The prerequisite to suspect SARS is history of contact with a SARS patient or history of visit to the hospital with a SARS outbreak in the precedent 10 days symptom onset.

Initially, the patient may present with normal blood counts. However, by day 3 or 4 many will develop thrombocytopenia and lymphopenia. Liver enzymes, creatinine phosphokinase and prothrombin can be elevated in certain patients.

> The following case definitions are used globally for surveillance of SARS including exit screening at airports at the time of emergency.
>
> **Suspect case**
> A person presenting after 1 February 2003 with a history of high fever (>38 °C)
>
> AND
>
> One or more respiratory symptoms including a cough, shortness of breath, difficulty breathing
>
> AND
>
> One or more of the following:
> close contact, within 10 days of onset of symptoms, with a person diagnosed with SARS;
> history of travel, within 10 days of onset of symptoms, to SARS-affected areas
>
> **Probable case**
> A suspect case with chest X-ray findings of pneumonia or respiratory distress syndrome
>
> OR
>
> A suspect case with an unexplained respiratory illness resulting in death, with an autopsy examination demonstrating the pathology of respiratory distress syndrome without an identifiable cause.

## TREATMENT

There is no randomized clinical trial evidence available to support any specific drug in the management of SARS. Supportive treatment under intensive care unit plays a major role in reducing the mortality. Empirical antibiotic therapy, ribavirin, ritonavir/lopinavir, steroids and use of other immune modulating agents have been tried in many hospital settings. However, these treatments are prone to result in side effects such as deranged liver functions, cerebrovascular accidents due to ischemic stroke, ventilator-associated pneumonia and sepsis.

Prognosis is poor among people with other comorbid conditions such as diabetes, COPD, elderly, coexisting other viral illnesses like hepatitis B.

## PREVENTION

Suspected patients should be isolated and managed in an isolation ward. The treating physician and allied health professionals should follow strict aseptic precautions and use the personal protective equipment. Wearing of N95 masks should be mandatory among health professions. Isolation wards should have at least 12 times per hour air exchange. Surface contaminated with any patient secretion should be disinfected with diluted bleach immediately. Nebulization therapy should be prescribed carefully for the patient with SARS to prevent

**306** | **Section 3:** Community Health Problems and Vulnerable Groups

SARS transmission to others. Research laboratories dealing with live coronavirus isolated from SARS patient should adhere to level 3 biosafety containment procedures.

## SUMMARY

SARS is caused by the novel coronavirus (SARS-CoV). This virus is suspected to have a zoonotic origin. Initially, the disease was originated in Hong Kong as a hospital outbreak followed by it rapidly spread to other continents including North America and Europe. Almost 8,400 people were affected from 29 countries within a short span of time with a case fatality rate of 11%. China, Canada, Singapore and Vietnam are the countries which are heavily affected due to SARS.

*Risk factors:* Healthcare workers involved in procedures which generate aerosol such as nebulization procedure are estimated to have 21% of total SARS transmission. Close household contacts, air travel to countries with local transmission of SARS, increasing age, respiratory comorbidities are other factors which predispose to the condition of SARS. Children are affected rarely by SARS. Prognosis is poor among people with other comorbid conditions such as diabetes, COPD, elderly, coexisting other viral illnesses like hepatitis B.

The mean incubation period is 6 days.

*Clinical Features*
Fevers with chills, unproductive cough, dyspnea are common manifestations of SARS illness. Unlike other coronaviruses, upper respiratory tract symptoms are unusual in SARS. The characteristic features which differentiate from other respiratory viral illnesses are rapidly progressive bilateral pneumonia, pulmonary thromboembolic manifestations and rapid response to immune-modulating agents such as steroids

*Diagnosis*
SARS is diagnosed by the presence of clinical features such as fever >38°C, respiratory symptoms, radiographic evidence of pneumonia and the presence of virological markers either in the form of virus isolation, raising antibody titer or positive RT-PCR.

*Treatment*
Empirical antibiotic therapy, ribavirin, ritonavir/lopinavir, steroids and use of other immune modulating agents have been tried in many hospital settings.

*Prevention*
Suspected patients should be isolated and managed in an isolation ward. The treating physician and allied health professionals should follow strict aseptic precautions and use the personal protective equipment. Wearing of N95 masks should be mandatory among health professions.

## SUGGESTED READING

1. Consensus document on the epidemiology of severe acute respiratory syndrome (SARS). 2003.
2. Peiris JSM, Guan Y, Yuen KY. Severe acute respiratory syndrome. Nat Med [Internet]. 2004;10(12s):S88–97. Available from: http://www.nature.com/doifinder/10.1038/nm1143.
3. Severe Acute Respiratory Syndrome. Weekly epidemiological record Relevé épidémiologique hebdomadaire. 2003;(14):97-120.
4. World Health Organization. WHO guidelines for the global surveillance of severe acute respiratory syndrome (SARS). Epidemic Alert and Response [Internet]. 2004;(October). Available from: http://www.who.int/csr/resources/publications/WHO_CDS_CSR_ARO_2004_1.pdf.

---

## EPIDEMIOLOGY OF TUBERCULOSIS AND ITS PREVENTION AND CONTROL

*Ritesh Singh*

*"TB Anywhere Is TB Everywhere"*

*End TB; to ensure no one is left behind. It's time for action! It's time to End TB - Mar 24, 2020*

| | |
|---|---|
| **CM7.2** | Enumerate, describe and discuss the mode of transmission and measures for prevention and control of Tuberculosis |
| **CM8.1** | Describe and discuss the epidemiological and control measures applicable in Tuberculosis |

*Case Scenario*

*A 60-year-old male who presented to hospital emergency after having 3 weeks cough, profuse nocturnal sweating, loss of appetite, unintended weight loss, nausea, shortness of breath, and a productive cough. His chest X-ray revealed extensive bilateral cavitary disease. His sputum specimens were collected for and were positive Acid Fast Bacilli (AFB). Further culture and sensitivity of the sample established it to be drug sensitive TB. Finally, he was diagnosed with bacteriologically confirmed case of active pulmonary tuberculosis.*

## HISTORY AND IMPORTANCE OF TUBERCULOSIS

Tuberculosis (TB) is an old disease. According to genetic studies, it has been presumed that the TB has been present in humans for at least 15,000 years. Mummies as old as of 3400 BCE have evidence of TB in their spines. The earliest written mentions of TB were in India about 3,300 years ago. In the *Rigveda*, it is mentioned as *Yaksma*. The *Sushruta Samhita*, written around 600 BCE, recommends that the disease be treated with breast milk, various meats, alcohol, and rest. The *Yajurveda* advises sufferers to move to higher altitudes. Hippocrates named the disease "*phithis*" or consumption, because of the significant weight loss associated with it. In the 1700s, TB was called "*the white plague*" due to the paleness of the patients. In the early 1800s, there were "*vampire panics*" throughout New England. When a TB outbreak occurred in a town, it was suspected that the first family member to die of TB came back as a vampire to infect the rest of the family. To stop the vampires, people used to dig up the suspected 'vampire' grave and perform a ritual. Johann Schonlein coined the term "tuberculosis" in the year 1834. On March 24, 1882, Dr Robert Koch, a German Scientist announced the discovery of *Mycobacterium tuberculosis* (MTB). Until the discovery of antibiotics, treatment for TB was limited to warmth, rest, and good food. In 1943, Selman Waksman, Elizabeth Bugie, and Albert Schatz developed streptomycin, a breakthrough in the treatment of TB.

Lives of many famous personalities have been cut short by TB. Emily Jane Brontë, the author of the classic English novel "*Wuthering Heights*" died at an early age of 30 due to TB. The famous romantic poet John Keats died at 25 years after suffering from TB. Louis Braille died at the age of 43 in 1852 of TB. Advancement in medical sciences has led to better treatment options for those suffering from TB, thus greatly bringing down the mortality rate. Despite this, unfortunate celebrity deaths from TB have happened even in last century. American actress Vivien Leigh, British writer George Orwel, Founder of Pakistan, Muhammad Ali Jinnah, all died due to TB in last century. Srinivasa Ramanujan, the famous mathematician was diagnosed with TB and put in a sanatorium. He died in 1920 at 32 years of age probably of TB. Mrs Kamala Nehru, wife of the first prime minister of India, died due to TB in Lausanne, Switzerland in 1936. While serving his 27-year prison term, Nelson Mandela was diagnosed with TB in 1988. Amitabh Bachchan is a TB survivor!

# INTRODUCTION

Tuberculosis is a contagious disease caused by the *Mycobacterium tuberculosis*. It can affect any part of the body, though lungs are most affected organs. Among all the forms of TB, pulmonary TB is most important, as diagnosing it early and treating it appropriately will prevent the spread of disease.

# CHARACTERISTIC OF DISEASE

The classic symptoms of active TB are chronic cough with sputum, fever and sweats usually at night, and weight loss. Symptoms also depend upon the body part affected. Once diagnosed, the cases should be promptly put on effective antibiotic treatment. More than one type of antibiotic is required to be given to patients for a longer duration to cure the patient. Cases of antibiotic resistant TB are on rise due to rampant use of inappropriate TB regimens over the years. TB can be prevented, if proper screening methods are applied to the vulnerable population.

TB bacteria reside in the lungs causing no symptom at all in about 90% of those infected. They are cases of latent TB infections (LTBI). There is a 10% risk that this latent infection will progress to post primary or reactivated tuberculosis disease in an individual throughout his lifetime. In those suffering from HIV or acquired immune deficiency syndrome (AIDS), the risk of developing TB increases to nearly 10% every year.

Due to high concentration of air, TB bacilli settle in either the upper part of the lower lobe or the lower part of the upper lobe of the lung leading to plenary TB. Any part of the body except hair, nail and teeth can be affected by the disease. Very few cases of TB of heart, skeletal muscles, pancreas, or thyroid are reported. The TB bacteria can enter the blood stream. Then, it can go to any part of the body and makes home a specific site or set up many foci. These tiny and white tubercles in the tissues dispersed throughout the body are known as miliary TB. Mostly children and HIV-positive individuals have this form of severe TB. Disseminated TB has a high fatality rate (about 30%) even with anti-TB treatment.

# PROBLEM STATEMENT

## Global

Tuberculosis is an important public health issue globally, present in all countries and age groups. But TB is curable and preventable. Tuberculosis is one amongst the top 10 causes of death worldwide. It is the leading killer of people with HIV. A total of 1.3 million people died from TB in 2022 (including 167,000 people with HIV). Worldwide, TB is the 13th leading cause of death and the second leading infectious killer after COVID-19 (above HIV and AIDS). In 2022, an estimated 10.6 million people fell ill with tuberculosis (TB) worldwide, including 5.8 million men, 3.5 million women and 1.3 million children **(Table 17A.20** and **Fig. 17A.13)**.

**Table 17A.20:** Estimates of TB Burden in India and worldwide, 2022.

| Indicator | Global (per lakh population) | India (per lakh population) |
|---|---|---|
| Incidence of TB (including HIV) | 10,600,000 (134) | 2,590,000 (188) |
| Mortality due to TB (HIV Negative) | 1,380,000 (17) | 49,300 (37) |
| Incidence of MDR-TB/RR | 450,000 (5.9) | 49,679 (9.6) |
| Incidence of HIV-TB | 703,000 (8.9) | 53,000 ((3.8) |
| Mortality due to TB (HIV Positive) | 187,000 (2.4 | 11,000 (0.78) |

(HIV: human immunodeficiency virus; MDR: multi-drug resistant; TB: tuberculosis; RR: rifampicin resistance)

*Source:* INDIA TB REPORT 2022 Coming Together to End TB Altogether Ministry of Health and Family Welfare Government of India

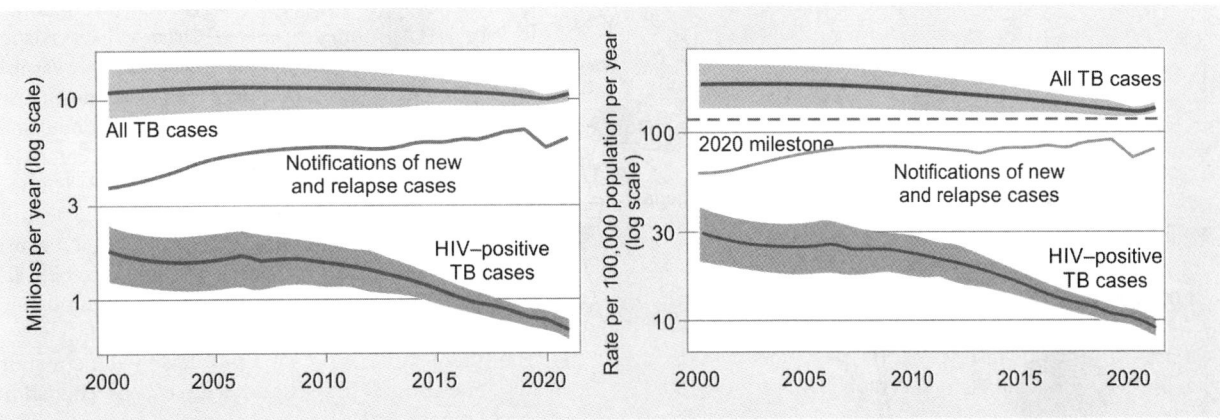

**Fig. 17A.13:** Global trends in the estimated number of incident TB cases (left) and the incidence rate (right) 2000–2021.
The horizontal dashed line shows the first milestone of the End TB Strategy, which was a 20% reduction in the TB incidence rate between 2015 and 2020. Shaded areas represent 95% uncertainty intervals.

Multidrug-resistant TB (MDR-TB) remains a public health crisis and a health security threat. Only about 2 in 5 people with drug resistant TB accessed treatment in 2022. Global efforts to combat TB have saved an estimated 75 million lives since the year 2000. US$ 13 billion is needed annually for TB prevention, diagnosis, treatment and care to achieve the global target agreed at the 2018 UN high level-meeting on TB. (WHO Factsheet, 2023)

The COVID-19 pandemic continues to have a damaging impact on access to TB diagnosis and treatment and the burden of TB disease. Progress made in the years up to 2019 has slowed, stalled or reversed, and global TB targets are off track. Intensified efforts backed by increased funding are urgently required to mitigate and reverse the negative impacts of the pandemic on TB. The need for action has become even more pressing in the context of war in Ukraine, ongoing conflicts in other parts of the world, a global energy crisis and associated impacts on food security, which are likely to further worsen some of the broader determinants of TB.

### Newly Diagnosed with TB (Fig. 17A.14)

The most obvious and immediate impact was a large global drop in the reported number of people newly diagnosed with TB. Reductions suggest that the number of people with undiagnosed and untreated TB has grown, resulting first in an increased number of TB deaths and more transmission of infection and then, with some lag-time, increased numbers of people developing TB. This is due to consequences of reduced access to TB diagnosis and treatment.

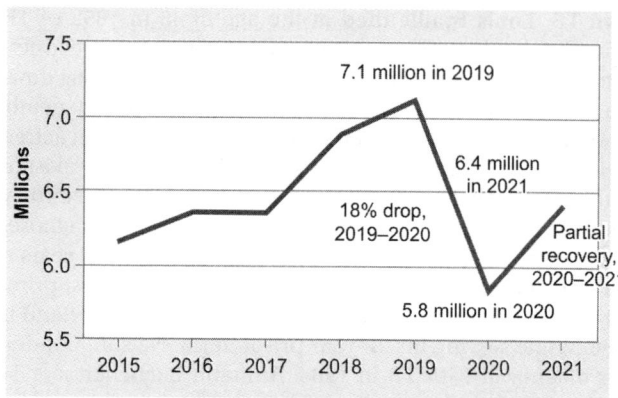

**Fig. 17A.14:** Number of people newly diagnosed with TB.

Estimated TB incidence in 2021, for countries with at least 100 000 incident cases. The countries that rank first to eighth in terms of numbers of cases, and that accounted for about two thirds of global cases in 2021, are labelled.

From a peak of 7.1 million in 2019, this fell to 5.8 million in 2020 (–18%), back to the level last seen in 2012. In 2021, there was a partial recovery, to 6.4 million (the level of 2016–2017). The three countries that accounted for most of the reduction in 2020 were India, Indonesia and the Philippines (67% of the global total) **(Fig. 17A.15)**. They made partial recoveries in 2021, but still accounted for 60% of the global reduction compared with 2019. Other high TB burden countries with large relative year-to-year reductions (>20%) included Bangladesh (2020), Lesotho (2020 and 2021), Myanmar (2020 and 2021), Mongolia (2021) and Viet Nam (2021) **(Fig. 17A.16)**.

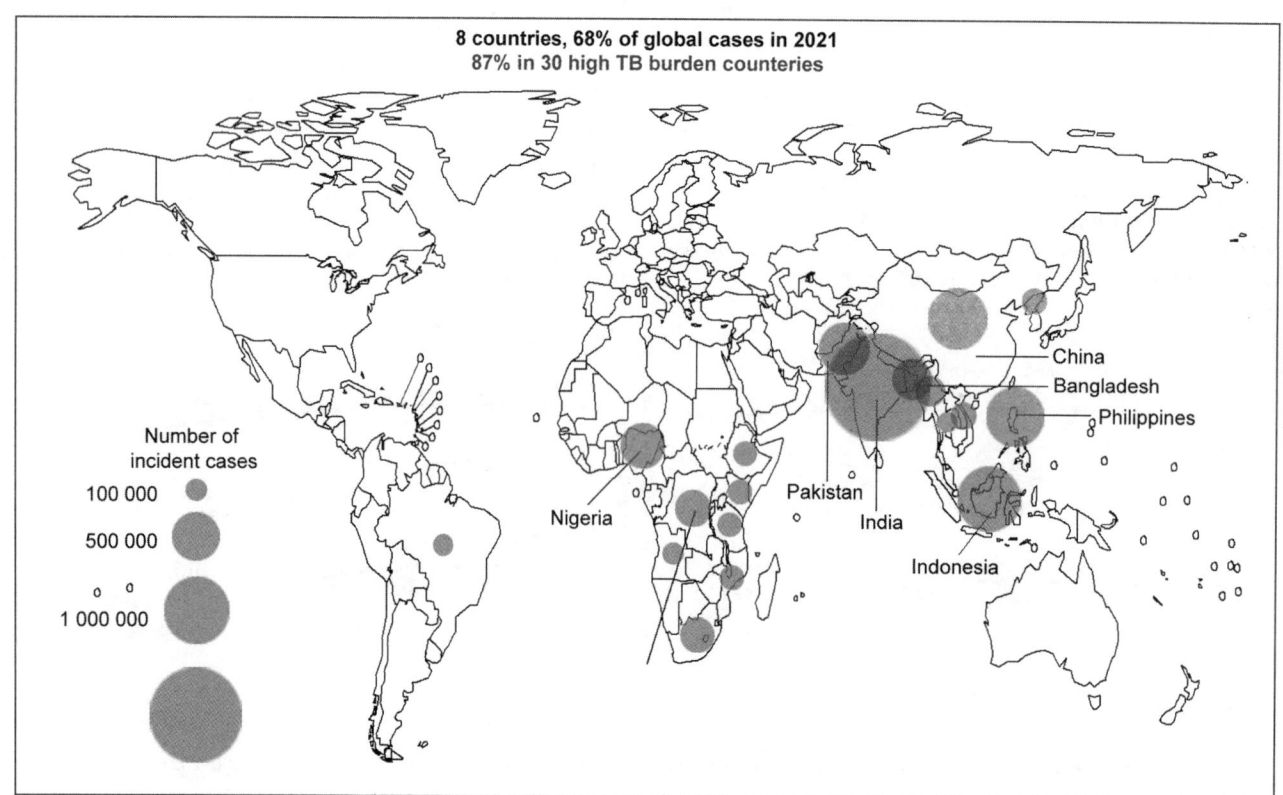

**Fig. 17A.15:** Number of incident cases of TB globally in 2021.

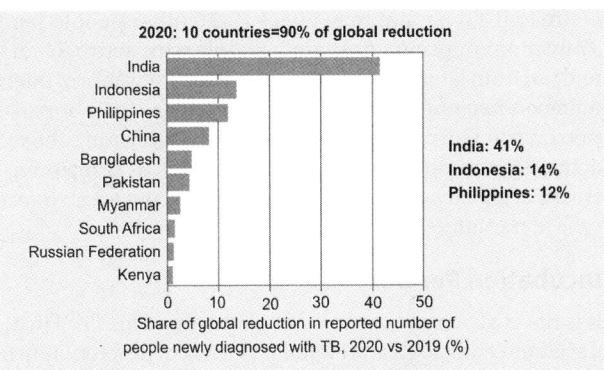
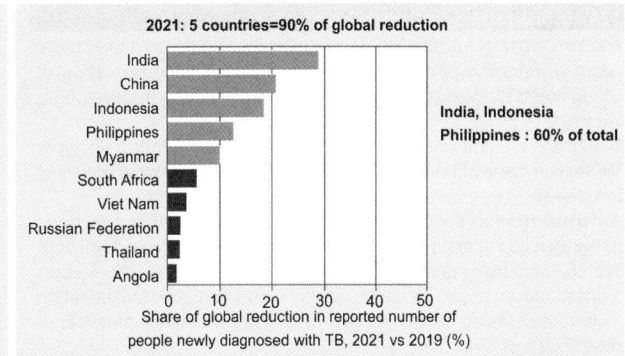

Fig. 17A.16: The top 10 countries that accounted for ≥90% of the global reduction in case notifications of people newly diagnosed with TB in 2020 and 2021, compared with 2019.
Countries that accounted for 90% of the reduction are shown in red.

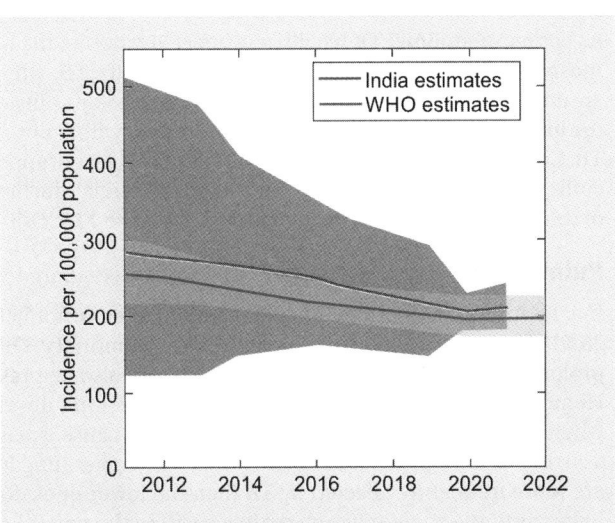
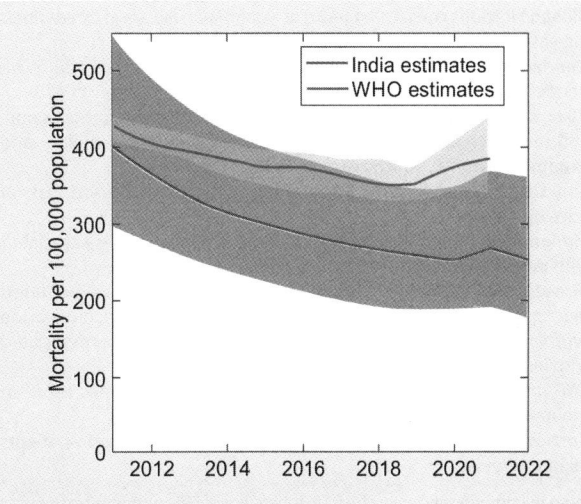

Fig. 17A.17: Comparison of estimates from Global TB Report 2022 for India (interim) and the in-country model (India) 2015-2022.
*Source:* India Tuberculosis Report 2023.

## India (India TB Report 2018, 2019 and 2020)

Tuberculosis continues to pose threat to the health of people in the country and become lethal with concurrent HIV infection. Despite the brief decline TB notifications in India in 2020-21, a record high notification of 24.2 lakh cases was seen in 2022; an increase of over 13% as compared to 2021. This translates to a case notification rate of 172 case per lakh population. The treatment initiation rate among the notified cases for 2022 was 95.5%. The highest case notification rate among States was seen in Delhi (546 per lakh population) and the lowest among States was seen in Kerala (67 per lakh population). The private TB case notification also saw highest notifications around 7.3 lakhs **(Fig. 17A.17)**.

The estimated incidence of MDR/RR-TB (as per the Global TB Report 2022) in 2021 for the country was 119,000 (93,000-145,000). The year 2022, an increase of 32% in the number of MDR/RR-TB cases detected under NTEP as compared to 2021. The presumptive TB examination rate (PTBER) for country rose to 1282 per lakh population (68% increase) from 763 in 2021. The task of TB prevention treatment (TPT) scale up reported 722 (94%) districts of India have expanded TPT.

## EPIDEMIOLOGY

### Host Factors

Though not everyone exposed to MTB becomes infected with TB bacilli, nearly one-third of the global population is infected with MTB. The probability of transmission of MTB from an infected person to an uninfected one depends on—infectiousness of the case, type of environment, and length of exposure to the case. Nearly 10% of infected persons will go on developing TB disease at some time in their lives. The major risk factors for development of TB disease in those infected with MTB are mentioned in the **Box 17A.10**.

### Agent Factors

*Mycobacterium tuberculosis* (MTB) is a small, acid-fast, aerobic, nonmotile, non-capsulated, and non-sporing bacillus. They are either straight or slightly curved rod of about 3 μm × 0.3 μm size. They occur either in pairs or small clumps. It has very high lipid content. Compared to other bacteria, it divides at an extremely slow rate of every 16–20 h. The bacteria are resistant to weak disinfectants and can survive in a dry state for weeks.

> **Box 17A.10: Risk factors for tuberculosis.**
> - ***HIV:*** The most important risk factor globally, five to six times more risk of developing primary progressive disease and reactivation of tuberculosis; TB most common opportunistic infection in developing country
> - ***Diabetes:*** Three-times increased risk of tuberculosis than nondiabetic; type I DM (insulin-dependent diabetes mellitus) more at risk, higher mortality from the TB
> - ***Undernutrition and vitamin deficiencies:*** Undernutrition, low body mass index, and vitamin D deficiency associated with increased risk of TB
> - ***Overcrowded living conditions:*** Increased exposure to infectious cases in closed spaces; prisons, homeless shelters, brick kilns, and rehabilitation centers where living conditions are not so good are vulnerable areas of transmission of TB bacilli
> - ***Smoking:*** Current smoking associated with two times increased risk of TB infection
> - ***Indoor air pollution:*** About two-times increased risk of active TB disease in individuals who are constantly exposed to indoor air pollution
> - ***Silicosis:*** Three-times greater risk of developing TB disease
> - ***Alcohol:*** Persons consuming >40 g of alcohol per day are at three-times increased risk of developing active TB disease
> - ***Gender:*** Incident TB disease in men: women about 2:1 in adults, no gender separation in children
> - ***Age:*** Risks of acquisition, form of disease, disease progression, and mortality risk depend on age; children have more miliary and extrapulmonary TB, which are more fatal
> - ***End-stage renal failure:*** More than 10-times increased risk of development of TB
> - ***Malignancy:*** Hematological and solid organ malignancies associated with increased risk of development of TB diseases
> - ***Genetic susceptibility:*** Genes for natural resistance-associated macrophage protein 1, interferon γ, mannan binding lectin, nitric oxide synthase 2A, vitamin D receptor, and some Toll-like receptors associated with increased susceptibility to TB.
> - ***TNF antagonist therapy:*** TB about one and a half times more in rheumatology patients taking TNF antibodies
> - ***Corticosteroid therapy:*** TB risk increases about two times in patients taking steroids.

(HIV: human immunodeficiency virus; TB: tuberculosis; TNF: tumor necrosis factor)

As MTB retains certain stains even after treatment with acidic solution, it is called an acid-fast bacillus. The most common acid-fast staining technique is the Ziehl–Nielsen stain. Auramine–rhodamine staining followed by fluorescence microscopy is a more sensitive tests and can diagnose TB even if less bacteria are present in the sputum.

The MTB complex (MTBC) includes four other TB-causing mycobacteria, *M. bovis*, *M. africanum*, *M. canetti*, and *M. microti*. *M. bovis* was once a common cause of TB, before pasteurization of milk became a routine phenomenon. *M. avium* and *M. kansasii* are classified as nontuberculous mycobacteria (NTM). They should be suspected, if the patent tests positive for acid-fast bacilli (AFB) repeatedly despite getting anti-TB drugs (ATDs).

## Transmission

The mode of transmission of TB is inhaling air contaminated with *Mycobacterium tuberculosis*. Infected persons with active TB release the bacteria in air when they cough, sneeze, speak, or spit, they expel infectious aerosol droplets of size 0.5–5.0 μm in diameter in air. A single sneeze can release up to 40,000 infectious droplets; as low as 10 bacteria may cause infection. Those who remain in prolonged, frequent, or close contact with TB cases are at particularly high-risk of becoming infected.

Untreated TB patient may infect 10–15 other people per year. Transmission occurs from only people with active TB disease and not from latent infectious cases. After 3–4 weeks of infection, a person becomes infectious to others. The chain of person to person transmission can be broken by segregating those with active TB and putting them on an effective ATD regimen. Two weeks of effective treatment are enough to convert an infectious case to noninfectious one.

## Incubation Period

It is not easy to predict the incubation period for TB. The risk of developing the disease is lifelong. The risk of development of the disease is age-dependent and depends on various risk factors described in **Box 17A.10**.

# CLINICAL FEATURES

As earlier mentioned TB bacilli may infect any part of the body, most common site being lungs. Extrapulmonary TB, which is around 15% of all TB cases, occurs when TB develops outside of the lungs. Extrapulmonary TB may also co-exist with pulmonary TB. Common signs and symptoms of TB are fever, loss of appetite, chills, weight loss, night sweats, and fatiguability. Natural history of tuberculosis of TB has been depicted in **Figure 17A.18**).

## Pulmonary

If a TB infection does become active, it most commonly (80–85%) affects the lungs. Main symptom of pulmonary TB is a prolonged cough with sputum. Chest pain may also be present. Hemoptysis can occur, and rarely massive bleeding develops when the pulmonary artery is involved. TB may cause extensive scarring in the upper lobes of the lungs. The upper lung lobes are more frequently affected by TB than the lower ones due to better airflow and poor lymph drainage within the upper lungs.

## Extrapulmonary

In 15–20% of TB cases, the infection spreads from the lungs to other sites, causing TB of that site. These are collectively known as "extrapulmonary TB". They occur more commonly in people with weak immune system and children. Common extrapulmonary infection sites include the pleura (tuberculous pleurisy), lymph nodes (tubercular lymphadenitis), central nervous system (CNS) (tuberculous meningitis), genitourinary system (urogenital TB), and the bones and joints (Pott's disease of the spine). Disseminated TB occurs when the disease spread to various organs of the body.

# DIAGNOSIS

## Active Tuberculosis

Though TB can be diagnosed clinically by classic symptoms of cough, night sweats, chest pain, hemoptysis, and fever, all efforts should be made for the microbiological diagnosis of the disease. According to the latest guidelines of NTEP, a chest X-ray and sputum examination for AFB are must for all presumptive TB cases. A definitive microbiological diagnosis of TB is made when AFB is either detected in microscopy, molecular test or grown in culture from a clinical sample. The clinical sample

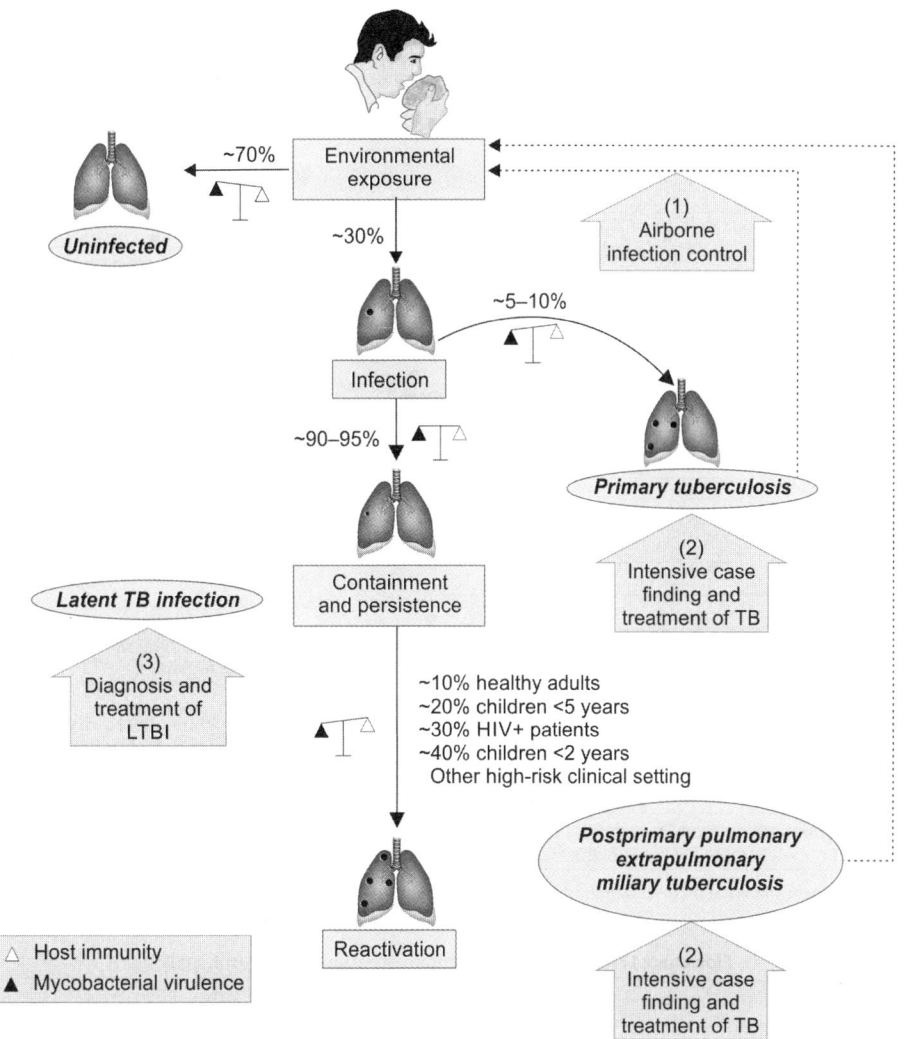

**Fig. 17A.18:** Natural history of tuberculosis (number in parentheses means ways to detect and manage cases of TB in community).

will depend on the organ affected. It may be sputum, pus, or a tissue biopsy. Culture of the organism takes time, as AFB is slow growing. Nucleic acid amplification test (NAAT) allows rapid diagnosis of TB. The cartridge based NAAT is emerging as the point of care test of choice for diagnosing drug resistant TB **(Fig. 17A.19)**. Blood tests to detect antibodies are not specific or sensitive. The diagnostic algorithm currently followed under NTEP is shown in **Flowchart 17A.1** for pulmonary TB and **Flowchart 17A.2** for extrapulmonary TB. Tests used to diagnose TB are mentioned in the **Box 17A.11**.

## Sputum Microscopy

Sputum smear microscopy remains the primary diagnostic technique used in many high TB burden countries. In patients with extrapulmonary TB, and in children, collection of samples for microscopy is often challenging. Children usually have paucibacillary disease. Therefore, a negative test result does not exclude TB in children. The diagnosis of TB in children is made based upon a careful history of exposure, clinical examination,

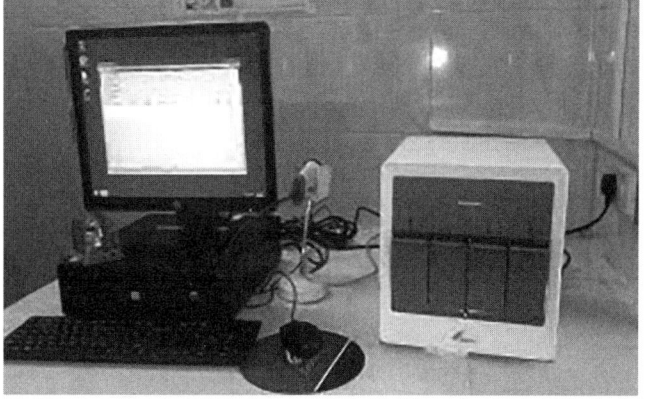

**Fig. 17A.19:** CBNAAT machine with computer.
(CBNAAT: cartridge-based nucleic acid amplification test)

and relevant investigations. At least two sputum specimens should be collected within a day or two consecutive days. One

## Section 3: Community Health Problems and Vulnerable Groups

**Flowchart 17A.1:** Diagnostic algorithm of pulmonary tuberculosis.

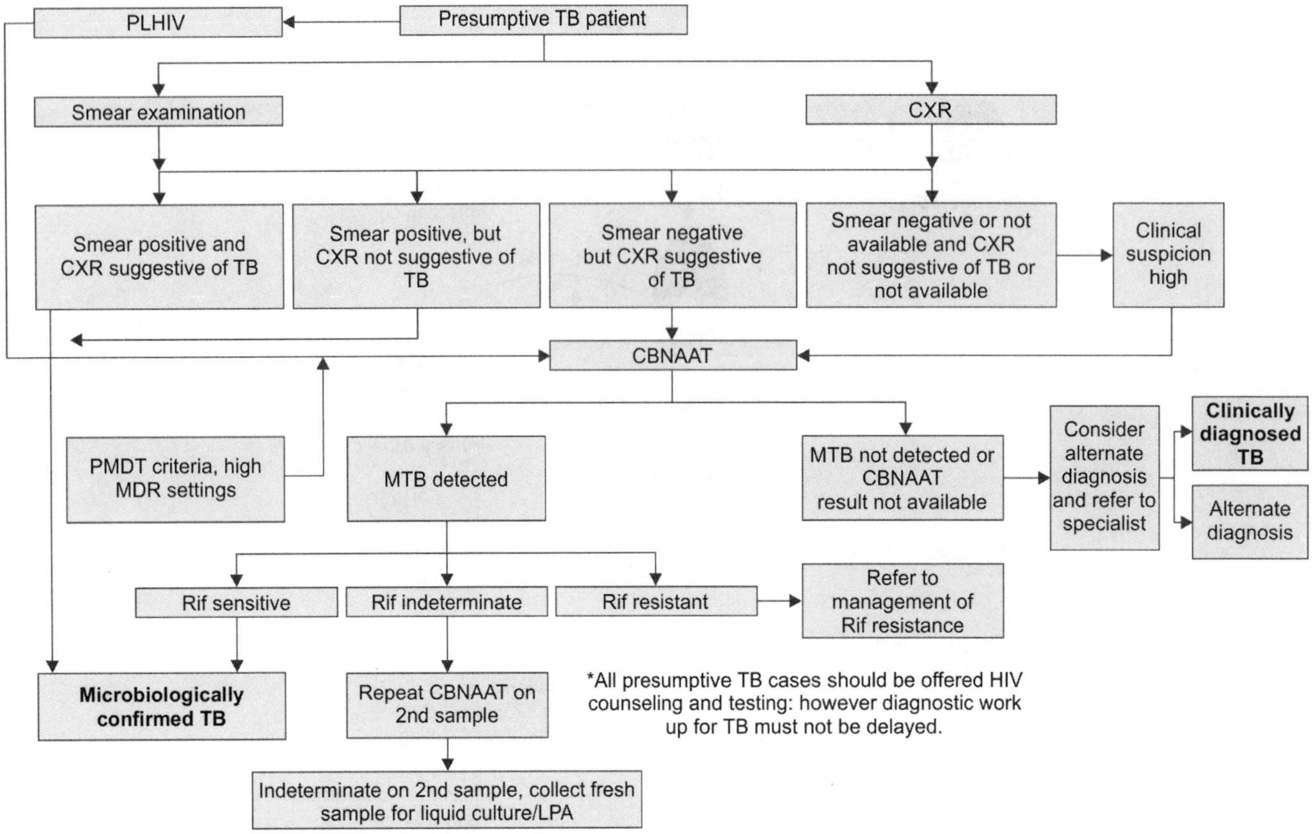

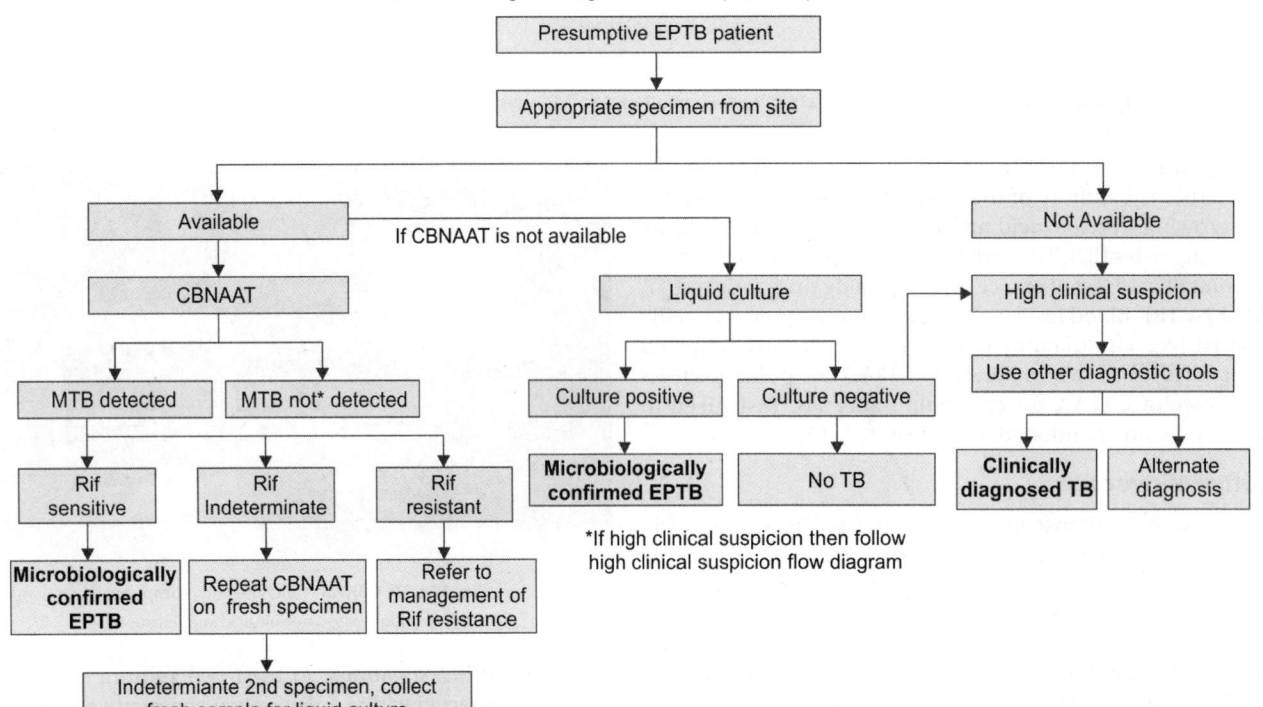

(CBNAAT: cartridge-based nucleic acid amplification test; CXR: chest X-ray; MTB: *Mycobacterium tuberculosis*; LPA: line probe assay; PLHIV: people living with HIV/AIDS; TB: tuberculosis)

**Flowchart 17A.2:** Diagnostic algorithm of extrapulmonary tuberculosis.

(CBNAAT: cartridge-based nucleic acid amplification test; EPTB: extrapulmonary tuberculosis; MTB: *Mycobacterium tuberculosis*)

## Chapter 17: Specific Epidemiology of Infectious Diseases | 313

**Box 17A.11: Commonly used tests for microbiological confirmation of TB.**
- Sputum smear microscopy (for AFB):
  - Ziehl–Nielsen staining
  - Fluorescence staining
- Culture:
  - Solid (Lowenstein Jensen) media
  - Automated liquid culture systems
- Drug sensitivity testing:
  - Modified DST for MGIT 960 system (for both first and second-line drugs)
- Rapid molecular diagnostic testing:
  - Line probe assay for MTB complex and detection of RIF and INH resistance
  - Nucleic Acid Amplification Test (NAAT): Xpert MTB/RIF testing using the Gene Xpert system

(AFB: acid-fast bacilli; DST: drug-susceptibility testing; MGIT: mycobacteria growth indicator tube; MTB: *Mycobacterium tuberculosis*)

**Table 17A.21:** Grading of slides under sputum microscopy.

| If the slide has | No. of fields to be examined | Grading | Result |
|---|---|---|---|
| No AFB in 100 oil immersion fields | 100 | 0 | Negative |
| 1–9 AFB per 100 oil immersion fields | 100 | Scanty* | Positive |
| 10–99 AFB per 100 oil immersion fields | 100 | 1+ | Positive |
| 1–10 AFB per oil immersion field | 50 | 2+ | Positive |
| >10 AFB per oil immersion field | 20 | 3+ | Positive |

*Record actual number of bacilli seen in 100 fields, e.g. "Scanty 4".

(AFB: acid fast bacilli)

sample is collected on the spot under supervision and the other is collected early in the morning. One specimen positive out of the two is enough to declare a patient as microbiologically confirmed TB. In designated microscopy centers sputum sample is stained with Ziehl–Nielsen stain. The slides are graded according to NTEP guidelines **(Table 17A.21)**. In places where the load of slide is high, Auramine–Rhodamine staining technique is used and the slides are examined under fluorescence light-emitting diode (LED) microscope. It is more sensitive for paucibacillary specimens, since it allows examination of more fields in less time. There is a robust system of external quality assessment (EQA) in place in all NTEP-designated microscopy centers.

### Chest X-ray

Chest X-ray as a diagnostic tool for TB is more sensitive but less specific with higher inter- and intra-reader variation. Abnormal chest X-ray, by itself, cannot confirm the diagnosis of TB, but can be used with other diagnostic indicators. Chest X-ray is useful for diagnosing extra pulmonary TB like pleural effusion, pericardial effusion, mediastinal adenopathy, and miliary TB. There are several limitations of chest X-ray as the sole method for TB diagnosis **(Box 17A.12)**.

**Box 17A.12: Limitations of chest X-ray as a diagnostic tool for tuberculosis.**
- High inter- and intra-reader variation
- No shadow is characteristic of TB
- 10–15% culture-positive cases remain undiagnosed (under reading)
- About 40% patients diagnosed as having TB by X-ray alone may not have TB disease (over reading)

### Rapid Diagnostics (Xpert MTB/RIF PCR-based Testing or Ultra Assays)

The Cartridge-based Nucleic Acid Amplification Test or CBNAAT is now the test of choice for diagnosing TB case. A completely closed automated system using real-time polymerase chain reaction (PCR), CBNAAT has a sensitivity of 70–90% even for smear negative cases. It has the added advantage of detecting Rifampicin Resistance (RR). The other advantages are that this highly automated system requires only a minimally trained staff to generate drug sensitivity and testing results, results are free of cross-contamination risk and are internally quality-assured. The result is available within 2 hours.

### Latent Tuberculosis

When a person has TB bacilli without the clinical manifestation of disease, the person is said to have LTBI. Due to persistent immune response by the bacilli, the person usually tests positive by tuberculin skin testing (TST) or an interferon- gamma (IFN-γ) release assay (IGRA).

### Mantoux Tuberculin Skin Test

Tuberculin skin test, commonly known as Mantoux test, is widely used for the diagnosis of LTBI. The test detects delayed hypersensitivity toward antigens of MTB and some related mycobacteria. Test specificity is affected by exposure to BCG vaccines. Test sensitivity decreases with age and impaired cellular immunity. Result of test should be interpreted cautiously depending upon the epidemiological situation, age, and general health of the individual.

About 0.1 mL of 5-TU of purified protein derivative (PPD) solution is injected intradermally using a 27-gauge needle. It produces a wheal of 6–10 mm in diameter. The induration, not erythema, is measured horizontally within 48–72 hours.

### Interpretation of TST Result

- About 5–10 mm of induration is considered positive in:
  - Organ transplant recipients who are on cytotoxic immunosuppressive drug
  - Persons who have chest X-ray findings consistent with prior healed TB
  - Close contacts of an infectious TB case
  - Human immunodeficiency virus-infected persons
  - Persons who are immunosuppressed [e.g. those taking the equivalent of ≥15 mg/d of prednisone for 1 month or those taking tumor necrosis factor-α (TNF-α) antagonists].
- About 10–15 mm of induration is positive in:
  - Recent immigrants (within last 5 years) from a high-prevalence country
  - Residents or employees of high-risk congregate settings
  - Persons with other high-risk medical conditions
  - Mycobacteriology laboratory personnel
  - Children less than 4 years of age
  - Injection drug users.
- More than or equal to 15 mm induration is positive in:
  - Persons with no known risk factors for TB.

### Interferon-gamma Release Assays

T cells, which are primed for MTB antigens, will respond to restimulation by releasing IFN-γ. IGRA uses this principle for diagnosis of LTBI. This advanced test has higher specificity and less cross-reactivity with the BCG vaccine than TST, thus generating fewer false-positive results. It must be borne in mind that neither IGRA nor TST accurately predicts the risk of developing active TB or diagnose a case of tuberculosis. IGRA can be conducted on persons found positive on TST.

## CASE DEFINITIONS (BOX 17A.13)

- *Presumptive pulmonary TB:* A person with any of the symptoms and signs suggestive of TB including cough more than 2 weeks, fever more than 2 weeks, significant weight loss, hemoptysis, and any abnormality in chest radiograph.
- *Presumptive extrapulmonary TB:* Presence of organ specific symptoms and signs like swelling of lymph node, pain and swelling in joints, neck stiffness, disorientation, and/or constitutional symptoms like significant weight loss, persistent fever for more than 2 weeks, night sweats.
- *Presumptive drug resistant TB:* Those TB patients who have failed treatment with first-line drugs, pediatric TB non-responders, TB patients who are contacts of DR-TB, previously treated TB cases, TB patients with HIV coinfection, and TB patients who are found positive on any follow-up sputum smear examination during treatment with first-line drugs.
- *Microbiologically confirmed TB:* Presumptive TB patients with biological specimen positive for AFB, positive for MTB on culture, or positive for TB through quality-assured rapid diagnostic molecular test.
- *Clinically diagnosed TB:* A patient who does not fulfil the criteria for bacteriologically confirmed TB but has been diagnosed with active TB by a clinician and who has decided to give the patient a full course of TB treatment. It includes cases diagnosed based on X-ray abnormalities or suggestive histology and extrapulmonary cases without laboratory confirmation.
- *Pulmonary TB:* Any bacteriologically confirmed or clinically diagnosed case of TB involving the lung parenchyma or the tracheobronchial tree. Miliary TB is classified as pulmonary TB because there are lesions in the lungs. Tuberculous intrathoracic lymphadenopathy (mediastinal and/or hilar) or tuberculous pleural effusion, without radiographic abnormalities in the lungs, constitute a case of extrapulmonary TB. A patient with both pulmonary and extrapulmonary TB should be classified as a case of pulmonary TB.
- *Extrapulmonary TB:* Any bacteriologically confirmed or clinically diagnosed case of TB involving organs other than the lungs, e.g. abdomen, genitourinary tract, joints and bones, lymph nodes, meninges, pleura, and skin.
- *New case of TB:* A patient, who has never been treated for TB or has taken anti-tubercular drugs (ATDs) for less than 1 month.
- *Retreatment case of TB:* A patient who has been treated for 1 month or more with ATDs in the past. Retreatment cases are further classified by the outcome of their most recent course of treatment into four categories:
    1. *Recurrent:* TB patient previously declared as successfully treated and is subsequently found to be microbiologically confirmed TB case.
    2. *Treatment after failure:* Previously been treated for TB and whose treatment failed at the end of their most recent course of treatment.
    3. *Treatment after loss to follow-up:* TB patient previously treated and was declared lost to follow-up in their most recent course of treatment and subsequently found microbiologically confirmed TB case.
    4. *Other previously treated patients:* Those who have previously been treated for TB, but whose outcome after their most recent course of treatment is unknown or undocumented.
- *Classification based on HIV status:*
    - **HIV-positive TB** patient refers to any bacteriologically confirmed or clinically diagnosed case of TB who has a positive result from HIV testing conducted at the time of TB diagnosis or other documented evidence of enrolment in HIV care, such as enrolment in the antiretroviral therapy (ART) register.
    - **HIV-negative TB** patient refers to any bacteriologically confirmed or clinically diagnosed case of TB who has a negative result from HIV testing conducted at the time of TB diagnosis. Any HIV-negative TB patient subsequently found to be HIV-positive should be reclassified accordingly.
    - **HIV status unknown TB** patient refers to any bacteriologically confirmed or clinically diagnosed case of TB who has no result of HIV testing and no other documented evidence of enrolment in HIV care. If the patient's HIV status is subsequently determined, he or she should be reclassified accordingly.
- *Classification based on drug resistance:*
    - **Monoresistance (MR)**: Resistance to one first line ATD only (except rifampicin).
    - **Polydrug resistance (PDR)**: Resistance to more than one first line ATD (other than both isoniazid and rifampicin).
    - **Multidrug resistance (MDR)**: Resistance to at least both isoniazid and rifampicin.
    - **Extensively drug resistance (XDR)**: Resistance to any fluoroquinolone and to at least one of three second-line injectable drugs (capreomycin, kanamycin, and amikacin), in addition to MDR.

---

**Box 17A.13: Active case finding of tuberculosis.**

Active case finding (ACF) or intensive case finding activity (ICF) is a provider-initiated activity with the primary objective of detecting TB cases early by active case searching in targeted groups and to initiate treatment promptly. For better yield ACF activity is focused on clinically, socially, and occupationally vulnerable populations. Screening is a dynamic process and the prioritization of vulnerable groups; choice of screening approach and screening interval should be regularly assessed. Decisions on when and how to screen for TB, which vulnerable groups to prioritize and which screening tool to use, depend on the vulnerable group, the capacity of the health system, and the availability of resources. As an added advantage, this creates mass awareness about the signs and symptoms of TB in general population.

- **Rifampicin resistance (RR)**: Resistance to rifampicin detected using phenotypic or genotypic methods, with or without resistance to other ATDs. It includes any resistance to rifampicin, whether monoresistance, MDR, polydrug resistance, or XDR.

## MANAGEMENT

Morphology and characteristics of MTB makes the treatment of TB disease a difficult one. A combination of antibiotics is required to successfully treat a case of TB. Inappropriate selection of drugs, less duration of treatment, and improper monitoring of long course of antibiotics are the main causes of treatment failure and emergence of drug resistant TB in community. In some developed countries, people with LTBI are treated to prevent them from progressing to active TB disease. Directly observed therapy (DOT) where a healthcare provider watches the person taking their medications, is recommended by the WHO to increase the compliance to anti-TB therapy. The drugs used for treatment of TB are shown in **Table 17A.22**.

**Table 17A.22:** Grouping of first line and second line drugs for tuberculosis as classified by WHO.

| | |
|---|---|
| Group 1: First-line oral anti-TB agents | Isoniazid (H); Rifampicin (R); Ethambutol (E); Pyrazinamide (Z); and Rifabutin (Rfb) |
| Group 2: Injectable anti-TB agents | Streptomycin (S); Kanamycin (Km); Amikacin (Am); Capreomycin (Cm); and Viomycin (Vm) |
| Group 3: Fluoroquinolones | Ciprofloxacin (Cfx); Ofloxacin (Ofx); Levofloxacin (Lvx); Moxifloxacin (Mfx); and Gatifloxacin (Gfx) |
| Group 4: Oral second-line anti-TB agents | Ethionamide (Eto); Prothionamide (Pto); Cycloserine (Cs); Terizidone (Trd); and Para-aminosalicylic acid (PAS) |
| Group 5: Agents with unclear efficacy | Clofazimine (Cfz); Linezolid (Lzd); Amoxicillin/clavulanate (Amx/Clv); Thioacetazone (Thz); Imipenem and cilastatin (Ipm/Cln); Meropenem clavulanate (Mpm); High dose isoniazid (High dose H); Bedaquiline (BDQ); Delamanid (Dlm); and Clarithromycin (Clr) |

### Treatment of Drug-sensitive TB (Tables 17A.23 to 17A. 26)

**Table 17A.23:** Treatment regimen for drug sensitive TB case.

| Type of TB case | (Months) Treatment regimen in IP | (Months) Treatment regimen in CP |
|---|---|---|
| New | (2) HRZE | (4) HRE |
| Previously treated | (2) HRZE | (4) HRE |

### Treatment Regimen for New TB Cases

The recommended treatment of new-onset pulmonary TB, according to the NTEP is 6 months of a combination of antibiotics daily in fixed dose combinations tablets divided in two phases:
1. **Intensive phase (IP):** 8 weeks of isoniazid, rifampicin, pyrazinamide, and ethambutol in daily dosages. There is no need for extension of IP.
2. **Continuation phase (CP):** 16 weeks of isoniazid, rifampicin, and ethambutol in daily dosages. CP may be extended by 12-24 weeks in certain forms of TB like CNS TB, skeletal TB, disseminated TB, etc.

### Treatment Regimen for Previously Treated TB Cases

In December 2018, it was decided in India that all previously treated patients should receive a standard six month first line treatment similar to new TB cases, if no resistance was detected to either rifampicin or isoniazid. It is however very important to ensure that drug susceptibility testing is carried out to ensure that the previously treated patient does not have any drug resistance. If any drug resistance is found, then treatment would be in the line of drug resistant TB discussed later.

**Table 17A.24:** Fixed-dose combinations (FDC) drugs for adult drug sensitive TB.

| | Number of tablets (FDC) per day | |
|---|---|---|
| | Intensive phase | Continuation phase |
| | 4FDC (HRZE) | 3FDC (HRE) |
| Weight category | 75/150/400/275 | 75/150/275 |
| 25–34 kg | 2 | 2 |
| 35–49kg | 3 | 3 |
| 50–64 kg | 4 | 4 |
| 65–75 kg | 5 | 5 |
| >75 kg* | 6 | 6 |

*Patients of weight more than 75 kg may be given 5 tablets/day if they do not tolerate this dose.

**Table 17A.25:** Drug dosages for adult drug sensitive TB.

| Type of TB case | Doses in IP | Doses in CP |
|---|---|---|
| New | 56 doses (7 days × 8 weeks) | 112 doses (7 days × 16 weeks) |
| Previously treated | 56 doses (7 days × 8 weeks) | 112 doses (7 days × 16 weeks) |

**Table 17A.26:** Side effects of first line anti-TB drugs used in NTEP and possible actions.

| Symptom | Drug | Action to be taken |
|---|---|---|
| Gastrointestinal upset | Any oral ATD | • Reassure patient<br>• Give drugs with less water<br>• Give drugs over a longer period of time (e.g. 20 min)<br>• Do not give drugs on empty stomach, if the above fails, give antiemetic if appropriate |
| Itching | Isoniazid (H) (other drugs also) | • Reassure patient<br>• If severe, stop all drugs and refer |
| Burning in the hands and feet | Isoniazid (H) | Give pyridoxine 100 mg/day until symptoms subside |
| Joint pains | Pyrazinamide (Z) | If severe, refer patient for evaluation |
| Impaired vision | Ethambutol (E) | Stop ethambutol, refer patient for evaluation |
| Ringing in the ears | Streptomycin (S) | Stop streptomycin, refer for evaluation |
| Loss of hearing | Streptomycin (S) | Stop streptomycin, refer for evaluation |
| Dizziness and loss of balance | Streptomycin (S) | Stop streptomycin, refer patient for evaluation |
| Jaundice | Isoniazid (H) Rifampicin (R) Pyrazinamide (Z) | Stop all drugs, refer patient for evaluation |

**Table 17A.27:** Classes of anti-TB drugs used for DR-TB patients.

| Group | Class | Drugs |
|---|---|---|
| A | Fluoroquinolone | Levofloxacin (Lfx), Gatifloxacin (Gfx) and Moxifloxacin (Mfx) |
| B | Second-line injectable agents | Amikacin (Am), Capreomycin (Cm), Kanamycin (Km), and Streptomycin (S) |
| C | Other second-line agents | Ethionamide (Eto)/Prothionamide (Pto), Cycloserine (Cs)/Terizidone (Trd), Linezolid (Lzd), and Clofazimine (Cfz) |
| D1 | (Add-on agents, not part of the core MDR regimen) | Pyrazinamide, Ethambutol, and High-dose Isoniazid |
| D2 | | Bedaquiline (BDQ) and Delamanid (Dlm) |
| D3 | | P-aminosalicylic acid (PAS), Imipenem Cilastatin, Meropenem, and Amoxicillin–Clavulanate (Thioacetazone) |

(DR-TB: drug resistant tuberculosis; MDR: multidrug resistant)

## Treatment of Drug-resistant Tuberculosis

Drug resistant TB may either be primary where the person becomes infected with a resistant strain of TB or secondary (acquired) where the initial susceptible TB bacilli develop resistance during therapy because of inadequate treatment, not taking the prescribed regimen appropriately or using low-quality medication. DR-TB is a serious community health problem in many developing countries. The treatment is longer and requires more expensive drugs, which many countries cannot afford to give to its patients. Totally DR-TB is resistant to all currently used drugs. Totally drug-resistant, TDR-TB was first observed in 2003 in Italy, but not widely reported until 2012, when some cases appeared in Mumbai, India. **Table 17A.27** shows the classes and drugs used for the treatment of DR-TB patients. **Table 17A.28** shows the current treatment regimen of DR-TB patients according to Programmatic Management of Drug resistant Tuberculosis (PMDT) 2019 guidelines.

## Definitions of Treatment Outcomes

The new treatment outcome definitions make a clear distinction between four types of patients **(Tables 17A.29)**:
1. Patients treated for drug-susceptible TB
2. Patients treated for all oral H mono/poly DR TB patients
3. Patients treated for RR/MDR-TB by shorter regimen
4. Patients treated for RR/MDR-TB by all oral longer regimen

## Adherence to ATDs

There are barriers to adherence to the ATDs. Despite much progress in society, TB still is a disease associated with stigma. Long duration of treatment, adverse reactions to medications, and lack of knowledge about TB and its treatment prevent many patients to complete the treatment. The onus of completing treatment is on the healthcare provider. Adherence can be increased by counseling the patient appropriately before commencing the treatment, DOT, managing adverse events, and by providing incentives. DOT is the best way to ensure adherence. As majority of the drugs are taken in presence of healthcare provider, it ensures compliance, reduces relapse and acquired DR-TB. The DOT-provider can be anybody who is accessible and acceptable to the patient, and accountable to the health system. NTEP now allows even family members to become DOT providers. Now under 99-DOTS patients are instructed to give a missed call to the number displayed on the medicine strip once they take out the tablet from the strip.

**Table 17A.28:** All oral MDR-TB regimen guidelines for PMDT in India 2019.

| Regimen class | Intensive phase (IP) | Continuation phase (CP) |
|---|---|---|
| **H mono/poly DR-TB (R resistance not detected and H resistance)** | | |
| All oral H mono-poly DR TB regimen | (6) Lfx R E Z | |
| **MDR/RR TB** | | |
| Shorter MDR-TB regimen | (4–6) High dose Mfxh Km/Am* Eto Cfz Z High dose H E | (5) High dose Mfxh Cfz Z E |
| All oral longer MDR-TB regimen | (18–20) Bdq (6) Lfx Lzd# Cfz Cs | |

*If the intensive phase is prolonged, the injectable agent is only given three times a week in the extended intensive phase.

#Reduce Lzd to 300 mg/day after 6 to 8 months.

Pyridoxine to be given to all DR TB patients as per weight band.

All oral H mono/poly DR TB regimen is of 6 months with no separate IP/CP. Shorter MDR-TB regimen is of 9-11 months with 4-6 months of IP containing injectables and 5 months of CP. If the IP is prolonged, the injectable is only given three times a week in the extended intensive phase. All oral longer MDR TB regimen is of 18-20 months with no separate IP/CP. New drugs like Bdq and Dlm would be given for 6 months duration while the dose of Lzd will be tapered to 300 mg after the initial 6-8 months of treatment. This regimen will also be used for treatment of XDR-TB patients with 20 months duration.

## PREVENTION OF TUBERCULOSIS

### BCG Vaccine

The most widely used vaccine worldwide, BCG, is the only available vaccine against TB. In children, it decreases the risk of getting the infection and the risk of infection turning into active disease by 20% and 60% respectively. BCG vaccine has a documented protective effect against meningitis and disseminated TB in children. It does not prevent primary infection in adults and, more importantly, does not prevent reactivation of latent pulmonary infection in adults, the principal source of bacillary spread in the community. The impact of BCG vaccination on transmission of MTB is therefore limited.

The BCG is a live attenuated vaccine derived from *M. bovis* that was originally isolated in 1902 from a tuberculous cow. The isolate was cultured for 13 years, during which time it lost its virulence. Since the 1920s, the original BCG strain has been passaged under different conditions in different laboratories worldwide, which has resulted in more than 10 manufacturing strains. To introduce standardization of BCG vaccines, a lyophilized seed lot system was introduced by the WHO in 1956.

**Table 17A.29:** Treatment outcomes in treated TB patients.

| Treatment outcome | Patients treated for drug-susceptible TB | Patients treated for all oral H mono/poly DR TB patients | Patients treated for RR/MDR-TB by shorter regimen | Patients treated for RR/MDR-TB by all oral longer regimen |
|---|---|---|---|---|
| Cured | A pulmonary TB patient with bacteriologically confirmed TB at the beginning of treatment who was smear or culture-negative in the last month of treatment and on at least one previous occasion | A microbiologically confirmed patient at the beginning of treatment who was smear negative at the end of the complete treatment and on at least one previous occasion | A microbiologically confirmed MDR/RR TB patient who has completed treatment without evidence of failure and was culture negative at end of treatment and on at least one previous occasion | A microbiologically confirmed MDR/RR TB patient who has completed treatment without evidence of failure and three or more consecutive cultures taken at least 1 month apart from 8 months onwards are negative including culture at the end of treatment |
| Treatment completed | A TB patient who completed treatment without evidence of failure but with no record to show that sputum smear or culture results in the last month of treatment and on at least one previous occasion were negative, either because tests were not done or because results are unavailable | A patient who has completed treatment according to guidelines but does not meet the definition for cure or treatment failure due to lack of microbiological results | | |
| Treatment failed | A TB patient whose biological specimen is positive by smear or culture at end of treatment | A patient whose biological specimen is positive by smear at 5 months or later | Treatment terminated or need for permanent regimen change of any anti-TB drugs in CP because of lack of microbiological conversion by the end of extended IP or microbiological reversion in CP after conversion to negative or evidence of additional acquired resistance for drugs in regimen or adverse drug reactions (ADR) | Treatment terminated or need for permanent regimen change of at least two or more anti-TB drugs from 8th months onwards because of lack of microbiological conversion by the end of the 8th month of treatment or microbiological reversion in the 8th month or later after conversion to negative or evidence of additional acquired resistance for drugs in regimen |
| Regimen changed | | A need for permanent discontinuation of existing regimen and initiation of new regimen with change of at least one or more anti-TB drugs prior to being declared as failed | | |
| Died | A TB patient who died from any cause during treatment | | | |
| Lost to follow-up | A TB patient whose treatment was interrupted for 1 consecutive month or more | | | |
| Not evaluated | A TB patient for whom no treatment outcome is assigned | | | |
| Treatment success | The sum of cured and treatment completed | | | |

(CP: continuation phase; DR: drug resistant; MDR: multidrug resistant; TB: tuberculosis; XDR: extensively drug resistant)

- ***Dosage, site of administration, and reactions:*** BCG vaccine is usually administered by intradermal injection. Correct vaccine administration technique by a trained health worker is important to ensure correct dosage, efficacy, and safety. BCG vaccination in majority of the cases causes a scar at the site of injection due to local inflammatory processes in about 6 weeks. However, scar formation is not a marker for protection and approximately 10% of vaccine recipients do not develop a scar, and it should not be repeated in those cases. The standard dose of reconstituted vaccine is 0.05 mL for infants aged less than 1 month and 0.1 mL for infants aged more than 1 month. The vaccine should not be exposed to direct sunlight or heat and should be stored at temperatures between 2°C and 8°C. Currently, BCG is administered to infants of age up to 1 year in India.
- ***Effectiveness:*** Evidence from trials and observational studies has shown that the effectiveness of BCG vaccination against TB differs considerably up to 80%. In some population, protection after primary infant BCG vaccination last for up to 15 years. Protection declines with time. BCG revaccination in adolescents and adults after primary BCG vaccination in infancy does not give protection against MTB infection or TB disease.
- ***Adverse events:*** Adverse events with BCG depend on several factors. Important ones are, strain used in the vaccine, number of viable bacilli, and injection technique. If vaccine is administered subdermally chances of local reactions like injection site abscess, severe ulceration, or suppurative lymphadenitis increase many folds. These cases can either be managed conservatively or by aspiration of the pus. Disseminated BCG disease may occur in about 1.56–4.29 cases per million doses and has a high case fatality rate. It occurs in high proportion of HIV-infected children. BCG immune reconstitution inflammatory syndrome (IRIS) occurs in association with HIV infection. Other events associated with BCG vaccination are skin reaction, erythema, rash, pyrexia, pain, hypotonic hyporesponsive episode, decreased appetite,

irritability, herpetic meningoencephalitis, Kawasaki disease, and osteomyelitis.
- **Pregnant and lactating women:** Though, BCG administered to pregnant women does not harm fetus, it should be avoided. Lactating women can be administered BCG vaccine.
- **HIV-infected infants:** BCG administration can cause severe adverse event following immunization (AEFI) in HIV-infected infants as described above. Children born HIV-positive and vaccinated with BCG at birth, and later developed AIDS, are at increased risk of developing disseminated BCG disease. BCG IRIS can be prevented, if anti-retroviral therapy is started promptly.
- **Preterm infants and low birth weight infants:** BCG vaccination at birth in healthy preterm infants born after 32 weeks of gestation is safe and effective. Evidence regarding BCG vaccination of very preterm and extremely preterm infants is limited.

## TB Preventive Treatment (TPT)

The following TPT treatment options are recommended under NTEP once active TB has been ruled-out:
a. Expanded eligible group which includes children >5 years, adolescents and adult House Hold Contact (HHC) of pulmonary TB patients notified in Nikshay from public and private sector and regimen of choice for contacts of drug sensitive (DS) TB patients.

| Target population | Treatment option |
|---|---|
| • People living with HIV (+ ART)<br>• Adults and children >12 months<br>• Infants <12 months in contact with active TB<br>• HHC below 5 years of pulmonary TB patients | • 6-month daily isoniazid (6H)<br>• 3-month weekly Isoniazid and Rifapentine (3HP) in persons older than 2 years |
| HHC 5 years and above of pulmonary TB patients | • 3-month weekly Isoniazid and Rifapentine (3HP)<br>• 6-month daily isoniazid (6H) |

b. Other risk groups

| Target population | Treatment option |
|---|---|
| Children/adult on immunosuppressive therapy, silicosis, anti-TNF treatment, dialysis, transplantation | • 3-month weekly Isoniazid and Rifapentine (3HP)<br>• 6-month daily isoniazid (6H) |

### Contraindications of TB Preventive Treatment (TPT)

- Active TB disease (absolute)
- Acute or chronic hepatitis
- Concurrent use of other hepatotoxic medications (such as nevirapine)
- Regular and heavy alcohol consumption
- Signs and symptoms of peripheral neuropathy like persistent tingling, numbness and burning sensation in the limbs
Allergy or known hypersensitivity to any drugs being considered for TPT

## TB-HIV

Tuberculosis and HIV duo forms the deadly combination. There are problems aplenty for a person coinfected with HIV and TB. Diagnosis is difficult, and treatment has many challenges. HIV infection increases the risk of progression of LTBI to TB disease. TB is the most common opportunistic infection and cause of death among people living with HIV (PLHIV). HIV-TB coinfected patients more often will have unfavorable outcomes.

### TB-HIV Collaborative Activities

The TB-HIV collaboration by RNTCP and National AIDS Control Programme (NACP) was started in the year 2001. Since then, TB- HIV activities have evolved over time in line with updated scientific evidences. National framework for joint TB-HIV collaborative activities was developed under which National and State TB/HIV coordinating mechanism were put in place. Service delivery level coordination bodies were established at district level. Components such as dedicated human resources, integration of surveillance, joint training, standard recording and reporting, joint monitoring and evaluation, and operational research were strategically implemented, and nationwide coverage was achieved in July 2012.

India adopted all recommendations suggested by the WHO recommended TB/HIV collaborative activities. HIV testing of TB patients is now routine through provider-initiated testing and counseling (PITC) scheme. Cotrimoxazole preventive therapy (CPT) is given to all HIV-infected TB patients. Intensified TB case finding has been implemented nationwide at all HIV care centers at Integrated Counselling and Testing Centres (ICTCs) and ART centers. Isoniazid preventive therapy is given to HIV positive-TB negative cases **(Flowchart 17A.3)**.

Interventions to reduce the burden of TB among PLHIV include the early provision of ART for PLHIV in line with WHO guidelines and the three I's for HIV/TB:
1. Intensified TB case-finding followed by high quality anti-TB treatment,
2. Isoniazid preventive therapy (IPT) and
3. Infection control in HIV care setting.

### Infection Control for Tuberculosis

The HIV patients are more at risk of getting TB infection while visiting the health centers for treatment. Since the HIV care is being decentralized and more and more people living with HIV/AIDS (PLWHA) are accessing antiretroviral drugs from the primary healthcare (PHCs) and DOTS center, there is high chance of intermingling of TB and HIV patients in the health centers under same roof. TB infection control practices should be in place in all settings, which includes personal, administrative, and environmental controls as well as health worker surveillance. Various ways to control TB transmission under different controls is shown below:
- **Administrative control:**
  - A triage system to identify presumptive TB cases
  - Separate patients with suspected or confirmed TB
  - Cough etiquette or respiratory hygiene
  - Rapid diagnostics with Xpert™ MTB/RIF test
- **Environmental control:**
  - Ventilation (mechanical)
  - Ventilation (natural)
  - Upper room ultraviolet germicidal irradiation.
- **Healthcare workers control:**
  - Surveillance and information
  - Package of care for HIV positive workers (ART and IPT)

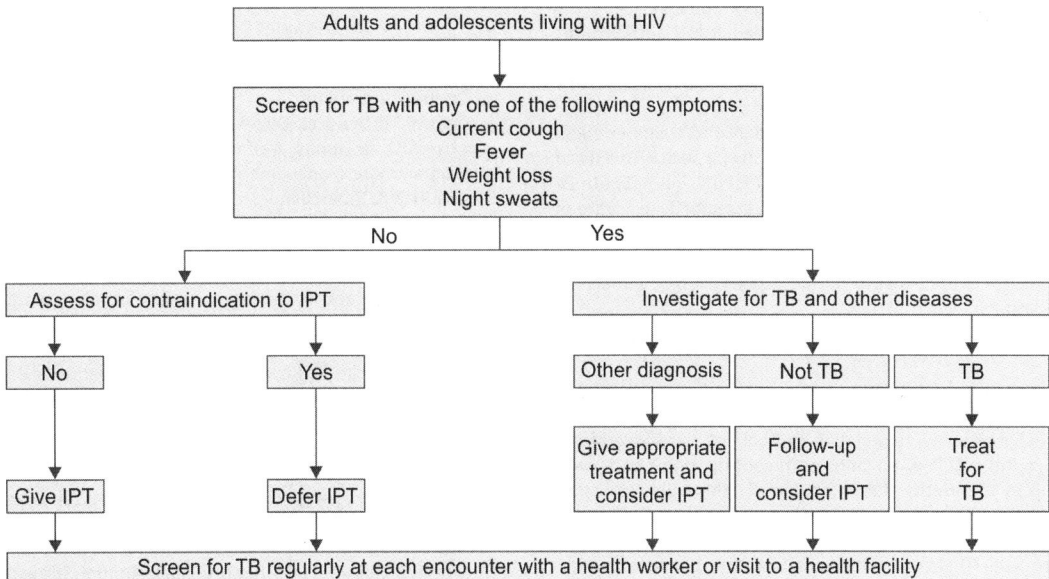

Flowchart 17A.3: Intensive case finding and INH preventive therapy in HIV patients.

(HIV: human immunodeficiency virus; IPT: isoniazid preventive therapy; TB: tuberculosis)

- Protective equipment (particulate respirator masks, which meet or exceed N95 standards)
- Relocation for healthcare worker living with HIV to lower risk area.
- **Personal control:**
  - Spend as much time as possible outside
  - Cough etiquette
  - Sleep alone while smear positive
  - Avoid congregate settings and public transport while smear positive.

## TUBERCULOSIS AND DIABETES

Though scientist knew the association between the diabetes and TB for more than thousand years now, recently with the increasing MDR-TB and DM cases in the world, the relationship is reemerging as a significant community health concern. Worldwide, 70% of diabetics live in TB endemic countries. The link of DM and TB is more prominent in developing countries where TB is endemic, and the prevalence of DM is rising.

### TB in Persons with Diabetes

Persons with diabetes are at increased risk of developing TB disease. Depressed cellular immunity, low levels of IFN-γ, dysfunction of alveolar macrophages, pulmonary microangiopathy, and micronutrient deficiency common in DM may be predisposing factors for the activation of LTBI. The risk of TB is higher among patients who are using insulin. There is an increased risk of MDR-TB among diabetics. The risk ranges from 2.1 to 8.8 times more in DM patients. Control of hyperglycemia is more difficult, and many patients need to switch to insulin for control of hyperglycemia. DM may have a negative impact on the outcome of TB treatment. Higher failure rates, higher rates of all-cause mortality, and death specifically related to TB has been reported in persons with diabetes and TB.

### Diabetes in TB

Isoniazid and rifampin have hyperglycemic effects. Also, pyrazinamide may result in difficult control of DM. Rifampin induces metabolism and decreases blood level of sulfonylureas, leading to hyperglycemia.

Following steps can be undertaken to prevent the occurrence of TB and DM in the same individual:
- Providing regular screening for the two diseases
- Administering quality-assured treatment to patients suffering from both diseases.

People with diabetes should be screened for symptoms of TB at the time of their diagnosis with diabetes. They should be regularly screened for TB throughout their life.

## CONTROL OF TB—GLOBAL AND INDIAN MEASURES

*The global and Indian efforts to control TB—End TB strategy, National TB Elimination Programme in India are discussed in Chapter 47: Health Policies and Programs in India.*

## RESEARCH

There is an urgent need to develop new drugs for appropriate treatment of TB. New diagnostics, drugs, and vaccines are necessary to achieve a TB free world. Currently, 23 drugs for the treatment of drug-susceptible TB, multidrug-resistant TB (MDR-TB) or latent TB infection are in Phase I, II or III trials. These drugs comprise 13 new compounds, three other drugs (bedaquiline, delamanid and pretomanid) that have already received regulatory approval, and seven repurposed drugs. Fourteen vaccine candidates are in clinical trials: three in Phase I, eight in Phase II and three in Phase III. They include candidates to prevent the development of latent TB infection and TB disease, and candidates to help improve the outcomes of treatment for TB disease.

**Box 17A.14: Success stories in TB control.**

**West Bengal: Regulating Sale of Antituberculosis Medicines**
As per a 2015 Government of India notification (schedule H1), anti-TB drugs can be sold in retail only on prescription by a registered medical practitioner and details of the prescriber as well as the patient are to be recorded in a register by the chemists or pharmacists. With increasing collaboration with the private sector, RNTCP is aiming to provide diagnostic, treatment, and patient support services even to patients in the private sector. To extend public sector services to all such patients, the district officials of South 24 Parganas in West Bengal contacted the Assistant Director, Directorate of Drug Control to strengthen this implementation and to share details of all listed patients with the TB department. A notice has also been issued to ensure implementation of Schedule H1 and submission of a quarterly report in this regard.

**West Bengal: Encouraging Adherence to Treatment through Peer Support**
Aminur Islam, a 20 years old orphan, was diagnosed with MDR-TB at the age of 17 years. He was started on MDR-TB regimen. Follow-up cultures in intensive phase were negative and patient was shifted from IP to CP after 6 months. Follow-up cultures in continuation phase were also negative up to 12 months. But unfortunately, there was reversion in subsequent follow-up cultures in continuation phase. Resistance was detected to second-line DST of his samples, and then he was diagnosed as an XDR-TB patient. After receiving the recommendation from DOT Plus site, he was initiated on Category V treatment (earlier regimen, not practiced now). At the time of counseling by DTO and other concerned medical officers of Dakshin Dinajpur District Hospital DR-TB committee, he never got frustrated and assured that he would continue his full course of treatment. He has now completed treatment, and all the sample results were negative and his weight also increased. He is playing an important role in MDR-TB patient provider meetings. He is an inspiration to many and encourages his peer group to continue their treatment course without missing a single dose. He cites his own journey and hardships and boosts the morale of his friends who may be going through difficulties in adhering to treatment.

(DOT: directly observed therapy; MDR: multidrug resistant; RNTCP: Revised National Tuberculosis Control Programme; TB: tuberculosis)

## SUGGESTED READING

1. Active TB Case Finding. Guidance Document. Central TB Division. Directorate General of Health Services. Ministry of Health & Family Welfare. Govt of India, June 2017.
2. Baghaei P, Marjani M, Javanmard P, et al. Diabetes mellitus and tuberculosis facts and controversies. J Diabetes Metab Disord. 2013;12:58.
3. Central TB Division, Directorate General of Health Services, Ministry of Health with Family Welfare. (2017). National Strategic Plan for Tuberculosis Elimination 2017–2025. Revised National Tuberculosis Control Programme.
4. Central TB Division. Directorate General of Health Services. Ministry of Health & Family Welfare. Govt. of India. (2017). Guidelines on Programmatic Management of Drug-Resistant Tuberculosis in India.
5. Chadha VK. Tuberculin Test. Indian J Pediatrics. 2001;68(1):53-58.
6. Dheda K, Gumbo T, Gandhi NR, et al. Global control of tuberculosis: from extensively drug-resistant to untreatable tuberculosis. Lancet Respir Med. 2014;S2213-2600(14)70031-1.
7. Dobler CC, Flack JR, Barrington G. Risk of tuberculosis among people with diabetes mellitus: an Australian nationwide cohort study. BMJ Open. 2012;2:e000666.
8. Dunn JJ, Starke JR, Revell PA. Laboratory diagnosis of Mycobacterium tuberculosis infection and disease in children. J Clin Microbiol. 2016;54:1434-41.
9. Global Alliance for TB Drug Development, USA. Handbook of Anti-Tuberculosis Agents. Tuberculosis. 2008;88(2):85-170.
10. Kaufmann SH, Lange C, Rao M, et al. Progress in tuberculosis vaccine development and host-directed therapies—a state of the art review. Lancet Respir Med. 2014;2(4):301-20.
11. MoHFW, GoI. India TB Report 2020. Annual Status Report. Revised National Tuberculosis Control Programme.
12. MoHFW, GoI. Technical and Operational guidelines for Tuberculosis Control in India 2016. Revised National Tuberculosis Control Programme.
13. Reuben Granich, Nancy J. Binkin, William R. Jarvis AND Patricia M. Simone. Guidelines for the prevention of Tuberculosis in health care facilities in resource-limited settings. Geneva; World Health Organization; 1999.
14. Vynnycky E et al., Am J epidemiology, 2000.
15. Weekly epidemiological record. World Health Organization. 2018;93(8);73-96.
16. WHO India. Report of the first national anti-tuberculosis drug resistant survey 2014-16. Revised National Tuberculosis Control Programme. MoHFW, GoI. [online] Available from: https://tbcindia.gov.in/showfile.php?lid=3315.
17. World Health Organization. (2009). WHO policy on TB infection control in health-care facilities, congregate settings and households.
18. World Health Organization. Global Tuberculosis Report 2019. [online] Available from: https://www.who.int/tb/publications/global_report/en.
19. Zumla AI, Gillespie SH, Hoelscher M, et al. New antituberculosis drugs, regimens, and adjunct therapies: needs, advances, and future prospects. Lancet Infect Dis. 2014;14:327-40.

## EPIDEMIOLOGY OF DIPHTHERIA AND ITS PREVENTION AND CONTROL

*Ayesha Siddiqua Nawaz, Ashwin Kumar*

| CM7.2 | Enumerate, describe and discuss the mode of transmission and measures for prevention and control of Diphtheria |
|---|---|
| CM8.1 | Describe and discuss the epidemiological and control measures applicable in Diphtheria |

*Case Scenario*

*A 13-year-old boy comes to your PHC with history of fever and cough since two weeks. On examination of the throat you find a thick gray membrane over the tonsils which bleeds when you try to remove it. Further examination reveals enlarged neck nodes. The boy is weak and has toxic appearance. He is not able to recall his immunization status and says few of his friends in the hostel too have the same symptoms. What is your diagnosis? How will you manage this situation?*

## INTRODUCTION

Diphtheria is an acute infectious disease caused by the toxin produced by the bacterium *Corynebacterium diphtheriae* and was one of the leading causes of mortality among children in pre-vaccination era. The disease mainly affects the throat and upper airways and the toxin leads to systemic manifestation. The earliest description of diphtheria like illness was given 2,500 years ago by Hippocrates in his work Epidemics III. The disease is known by different names around the world, such as *Syrian ulcer, membranous angina, malignant croup, and Boulogne sore throat*. In 1821 during an epidemic in Southern France, *Pierre Bretonneau*, a Physician described the clinical characteristics of diphtheria, its communicability and named it *Diphtérite*, a Greek word for leather, after the leathery texture of the pseudomembrane which is a classical feature of the disease. He was also the pioneer to practice tracheostomy successfully as a method of treatment for the disease.

The causative organism was first described in 1883 by Klebs in the stained preparations of diphtheritic membranes and successfully cultured a year later by Loeffler. Hence, this is also known as Kleb-Loefflers bacilli.

## CHARACTERISTICS OF THE DISEASE

Infection with the organism can cause respiratory diphtheria or less commonly cutaneous diphtheria. Respiratory diphtheria is more common and can be pharyngeal, laryngeal, or tracheal based on the anatomical location. Pharyngeal diphtheria is the most common form of disease seen in unimmunized population followed by laryngeal diphtheria which accounts for 25% of cases; isolated nasal diphtheria is seen less often. The infection can also cause cutaneous diphtheria especially in regions with warm climate and in rare cases cause systemic diphtheria. Respiratory diphtheria has a gradual onset with an incubation period of 2-5 days. The disease is spread by droplet nuclei and direct physical contact. Symptoms include mild fever (does not exceed 38.5°C), sore throat, diminished activity and irritability. A day after the onset of disease, small exudative patches appear in the pharynx, which over the next few days confluence to form a grayish, thick membrane covering the entire pharynx. Any effort to dislodge the membrane results in bleeding as the membrane is firmly adherent to the underlying mucosa. The patient has a toxic appearance.

## PROBLEM STATEMENT

### Global Burden

Diphtheria has been the most feared diseases since historical times, which gave rise to fatal epidemics mainly affecting children in both developed and developing countries. Several major outbreaks of diphtheria have been recorded during 1921-2018, in almost all global regions including the United States, Europe, Asia, the Newly Independent States of the former Soviet Union (NIS), Haiti, Venezuela and Yemen. The incidence declined in the developed world, owing to large scale use of diphtheria toxoid vaccine during the late 1940s, while in low and middle income countries where the vaccines were not easily accessible, diphtheria continued to cause an estimated one million cases including 50,000-60,000 deaths each year. With the launch of the Expanded Program on Immunization (EPI) in 1974, the cases reported worldwide also reduced dramatically thereafter. South-East Asia Region contributed 55-99% of all the cases reported during 2011-2015 with India contributing highest cases (18,350), followed by Indonesia (3,203) and Madagascar (1,633). However, significant under-reporting of cases especially from the African and Eastern Mediterranean regions, shadows the true burden of disease. In 2018, the WHO recorded 16,611 reported cases. Generally, diphtheria is under-reported from many regions, including Asian, African and Eastern Mediterranean countries.

### Disease Burden in India

In India 11,720 cases and 180 deaths were reported from Diphtheria in 2018 (NHP-2019). The coverage for DTP3 has improved in India from 78.4% (NFHS-4) to 86.7% (NFHS-5). India recorded 93% DPT3 coverage in 2022, surpassing pre-pandemic all time high of 91% in 2019, and a rapid increase from 85% recorded in 2021.

Diphtheria still persists in states like Delhi, West Bengal, and Rajasthan, while there have been outbreaks of diphtheria in states like Kerala, Karnataka, and Telangana where the cases and deaths due to the disease previously were very low. This resurgence is often due to fall in immunization coverage and population mobility as observed in Soviet Union during 1998 or due to resistance to immunization. A shift in the incidence of the disease has been observed from under five children to older children and adolescents in the outbreaks of the disease reported from North Kerala and Karnataka, suggesting waning immunity and reduced coverage with booster dose **(Box 17A.15)**.

> **Box 17A.15: Resurgence of diphtheria in recent times (WHO, Diphtheria Outbreak Response Update).**
>
> An outbreak of diphtheria occurred among the displaced Rohingya population living in makeshift camps at Cox Bazar, Bangladesh. With the first case reported in November 2017 by December 2017 there were about 1,841 suspected cases and 22 deaths reported as a result of this outbreak. Most of the affected were children above five-year age and adolescents. Co-existing malnutrition, low routine immunization coverage, and poor sanitation facilities facilitated the outbreak. Such outbreaks highlight the need to strengthen immunization coverage among the displaced and vulnerable population.

## EPIDEMIOLOGICAL DETERMINANTS

### Host Factors

#### Age

Diphtheria is mainly a disease of children of 1-5 years of age. Following the introduction of vaccines in population where the disease is endemic, the shift in age group was observed in two epidemiological stages. In the first stage, the shift in the incidence of the disease occurred from preschool age to school age, while in second stage, the cases were seen mainly in adolescents and young adults in greater proportion. Diphtheria is rare in infants younger than 6 months of age because of the presence of maternal antibody, and rare among adults, especially those living in urban areas, as a result of acquired immunity.

#### Sex

Both sexes are equally affected. But the recent outbreaks in Kerala showed a preponderance of cases among male preschool and school children, while among adults, cases were seen more in females.

### Agent Factors

*Corynebacterium diphtheriae* is a non-motile, non-sporing, and non-capsulated Gram-positive bacillus. It is a club-shaped facultative anaerobic species that exists in four biotypes (gravis, mitis, belfanti, and intermedius). These biotypes differ slightly in their colonial morphology and biochemical parameters, but do not differ much in severity of disease.

Exotoxin produced by the bacilli is the most important determinant of virulence, the production of which is dependent on β-coryne-bacteriophage. The toxin has two fragments A and B; fragment A consists of the enzymatic activity of toxin and B helps in binding of toxin to the cells. The cell-wall components such as the O and K antigens are also important in the pathogenesis of the disease. The toxin can result in both local as well as systemic effects.

### Resistance

When compared to other sporulating bacilli, more resistant to light and freezing. It is destroyed by heating at 58°C for 10 minute, at 100°C for 1 minute, by antiseptics. It is sensitive to antibiotics like penicillin and erythromycin.

### Environmental Factors

In temperate countries, diphtheria can occur throughout the year but most of the cases tend to occur in winter and in tropical countries diphtheria is more common and unrelated to season.

### Source of Infection

Humans are the only reservoir of infection. A case or a carrier can be the source of infection. A case can be a subclinical or a frank case. The carrier can be temporary or a chronic carrier, where the carrier state can last for a month or up to a year respectively. Transmission from person-to-person occurs predominantly by respiratory droplets or by direct contact with the respiratory secretions and discharges from skin lesions, the latter one commonly occurring under conditions of poor hygiene and overcrowding. The infective material is the nasopharyngeal secretions in respiratory diphtheria and discharge from skin lesions in cutaneous diphtheria. The most common portal of entry is respiratory tract and also occurs through non respiratory routes like skin sometimes if cuts, wounds and ulcers are not taken care of properly and under conditions of poor hygiene.

---

**Epidemiological Triad**

*Agent*
It is a non-motile, non-sporing, non-capsulated facultative anaerobic Gram-positive bacillus. The species consists of four biotypes (gravis, mitis, belfanti, and intermedius).
Virulence is determined by the exotoxin produced by the bacilli, which in turn is dependent on β-corynebacteriophage.
Easily destroyed by antiseptics and is sensitive to antibiotics like penicillin and erythromycin.

*Host*
Diphtheria is mainly a disease of children of 1–5 years of age, however showing a shift to the older age group among immunized population. Both the sexes are equally affected.

*Environment*
In tropical countries, diphtheria is more common and unrelated to season. The source of infection can be a case or a carrier. Transmission from person to person occurs predominantly by respiratory droplets or by direct contact with the respiratory secretions and skin lesions causing either respiratory or cutaneous diphtheria based on portal of entry.

---

## CLINICAL FEATURES

The incubation period of the disease is 2–5 days; the symptoms are gradual in onset and depend on the portal of entry of organism, manifesting either as respiratory or cutaneous forms.

The grayish white leathery membrane is pathognomonic of the disease.

### Respiratory Diphtheria

Based on the anatomical location of membrane it can be classified as anterior nasal, pharyngeal and laryngeal or tracheobronchial diphtheria, the pharyngeal diphtheria being the most common form.

### Anterior Nasal Diphtheria

It is commonly seen in infants. The symptoms are usually mild unless it occurs in combination with pharyngeal diphtheria. It is characterized by nasal discharge which is thin in the beginning and later becomes purulent and bloody and associated with excoriations of the nostril.

### Pharyngeal Diphtheria

Pharyngeal diphtheria is the most common form of diphtheria. It is gradual in onset and characterized by mild fever, malaise, sore throat, and painful swallowing. One or multiple patches of gray yellow adherent membrane surrounded by a red inflamed area might be seen over the tonsils, often making it appear as tonsillitis. Over a period of 2–3 days the disease progresses and the exudative patches organize to form a pseudomembrane that gradually extends into uvula, soft palate, oropharynx, nasopharynx or larynx. As it is firmly attached to the underlying tissue, any attempts to remove it results in bleeding. The pseudomembrane can result in obstruction of the airways if it extends into the nasal cavity and the larynx, which is a medical emergency, often requiring tracheotomy. The anterior cervical lymph nodes become enlarged and painful, and neck might be swollen due to inflammation and edema of surrounding tissues causing "bull-neck" appearance, which is associated with greater morbidity and mortality.

### Laryngeal or Tracheobronchial Diphtheria

It is the second most common variety of diphtheria characterized by fever, unproductive cough, dyspnea, and hoarseness of voice. It is life-threatening as any further expansion or detachment of the membrane and the associated edema can result in acute respiratory obstruction. The child is agitated, quiet, and cyanosed, and can suffocate and die if tracheostomy is not done on time.

### Cutaneous Diphtheria

Cutaneous diphtheria is more common in areas where the disease is less endemic. This is often seen among people living in overcrowded, unhygienic conditions and is characterized by a chronic nonhealing ulcer covered by a dirty gray membrane. Toxic manifestations are less likely and if occur can present as neuritis. Less common variants, include aural and vaginal diphtheria.

## COMPLICATIONS

***Due to obstructive effects of pseudomembrane:*** Life-threatening obstruction of the airways and pneumonia can result due to the pseudomembrane covering the larynx, Otitis media and sinusitis can result secondary to edema of the upper respiratory tract.

***Systemic effects of the absorbed toxin on the organs:*** The effects can damage the heart muscle (myocarditis), nerve damage (polyneuropathy), post-diphtheritic paralysis especially of the palate and ciliary muscles during 3rd or 4th week of disease, lung infection, and acute circulatory failure. Even with treatment, about 1 of 10 patients succumb to the illness but in the absence of treatment, 1 out of 2 patients can die due to the illness. Palatine and ciliary paralysis recover spontaneously without any specific treatment.

## DIAGNOSIS

Clinical diagnosis is based on the presence of sore throat with visible pseudomembrane. As laryngeal diphtheria often presents with pharyngeal involvement, any membranous pharyngitis with concomitant stridor should be considered as diphtheria unless proved otherwise. In about one-fourth of all the cases of laryngeal diphtheria, pharyngeal membrane might not be present often missing the diagnosis. Though laboratory confirmation of suspected cases is recommended, the treatment should be started immediately without waiting for the laboratory results to avoid unnecessary delay which can prove fatal.

## LABORATORY INVESTIGATIONS

***Culture:*** The investigation of choice is taking a throat swab and culture in appropriate media. The swabs are collected from the edges of the mucosal lesions and placed in appropriate *transport media (Amies or Stuart media)*. The swabs are then inoculated onto *Loeffler's serum slope, blood agar, and tellurite containing media*; the inoculation on blood agar is to rule out Streptococcal or Staphylococcal pharyngitis.
- The growth on Loffler's serum slope is seen in 4–6 hours, but if negative can be incubated for 24 hours while smears after inoculation on tellurite medium need incubation for at least 2 days before declaring as negative.
- Tellurite media are important for detecting growth among convalescents and carriers.
- On staining the smears with Albert's stain, the characteristic arrangement of bacilli in pairs at angles resembling letters V or L can be seen clearly.

***Elek immunoprecipitation test:*** It is used to test the suspected colonies for toxin production which takes about 24–48 hours. A positive culture with toxin-producing *C. diphtheria* confirms the diagnosis. Polymerase chain reaction (PCR) can be used to detect the diphtheria toxin gene (tox) from *C. diphtheriae* isolates.

## DIFFERENTIAL DIAGNOSIS

Differential diagnosis includes severe streptococcal sore throat, Vincent's angina, epiglottitis caused by *Haemophilus influenzae* type b (Hib), spasmodic croup, foreign body, and laryngotracheobronchitis.

## PREVENTION AND CONTROL MEASURES

### Prevention

a. ***Primary prevention:*** It consists of maintaining high level of immunity in population through vaccination.

   Diphtheria toxoid combined with tetanus and pertussis vaccines (DTP) has been part of the WHO Expanded Programme on Immunization (EPI) since its inception in 1974. Diphtheria toxoid is one of the safest vaccines available. Individuals with an anti-diphtheria toxin antibody level of more than 0.1 IU/mL are considered fully protected from disease.

   The **pentavalent vaccine** currently being used in the Universal Immunization Program (UIP) is a liquid pentavalent vaccine with five antigens in one formulation. Three primary doses of pentavalent vaccine (Diphtheria, Pertussis, Tetanus, Hep-B, Hib) are given at 6 weeks, 10 weeks, and 14 weeks. Booster doses of DPT are given at 16–24 months and at 5–6 years. It is available as a multi-dose vial (10 doses). The storage temperature is 2–8°C. 0.5 mL of the vaccine is given intramuscularly in the anterolateral aspect of the thigh.

   *Contraindications:* Contraindications are severe allergic reactions to any of the component of the vaccine in previous immunization and individuals with moderate to severe acute illness.

   In order to boost the waning immunity and prevent the outbreaks of Diphtheria, Td (Tetanus & Diphtheria) vaccine is included in UIP instead of TT (Tetanus Toxoid) vaccine at 10 and 16 years. It is a combination of Tetanus and Diphtheria with lower concentration of Diphtheria antigen. 0.5 ml of the vaccine should be given intramuscularly in the arm.

b. ***Secondary prevention:*** This includes interrupting the spread of the disease by identifying the close contacts of patients and their proper treatment. In case of exposed, unimmunized, and asymptomatic persons, the throat swab is taken for culture; immunization is given with diphtheria toxoid based on the age of the contact, and antibiotic prophylaxis with erythromycin or penicillin is given for seven days.

c. ***Tertiary prevention:*** Prevention of complications and death by early diagnosis and prompt management of cases.

### Treatment

***Diphtheria Antitoxin (DAT):*** DAT (polyclonal IgG antibody) is highly effective and continues to be the gold standard in the treatment of diphtheria. If administered as soon as possible following the disease onset, it can reduce complications and prevent deaths. It can be given either by intramuscular or intravenous route; the latter preferred in severe cases. Based on severity the amount of antitoxin recommended varies between 20,000 units – 100,000 units. The dose is the same for children and adults **(Table 17A.30)**.

**Table 17A.30:** Dosage of Diphtheria anti-toxin.

| Diphtheria | Onset | Dose of antitoxin |
|---|---|---|
| Pharyngeal and cutaneous diphtheria | < 24 hrs | 20,000–40,000 units |
| Pharyngeal and laryngeal diphtheria | >24 hrs | 40,000–80,000 units |
| Malignant diphtheria | – | 80,000–1,00,000 units |

Adverse events such as anaphylaxis may occur. However, the use of antitoxin for controlling outbreaks has no proven benefit as it is the asymptomatic carrier and not symptomatic cases who are the major source of transmission.

***Antibiotics:*** Antibiotics of choice are penicillin or erythromycin. The disease is usually not contagious 48 hours after antibiotics are started. The antibiotic penicillin G is given at a dose of 50,000 units/kg in four divided doses a day intramuscularly or erythromycin given at a dose of 5 mg/kg four times a day either orally or in parenteral form as an alternative in patients with penicillin allergy. The antibiotics are given for 2 weeks. Erythromycin is useful in eliminating the carrier state also. Airway management is crucial in dealing with patients with life-endangering respiratory obstruction due to pseudomembrane. Access to procedures like tracheotomy or mechanical removal of tracheobronchial pseudomembranes, intubation and ventilator support are vital to prevent the risk of sudden asphyxia.

## CURRENT APPROACHES IN HEALTH

### Surveillance

Case based surveillance with lab confirmation, contact tracing are to be carried out. All the outbreaks should be immediately reported from peripheral units to intermediate or central units. During outbreaks, the probable and suspected cases should be reported daily within 24 hours. Routine reporting is carried out at weekly intervals even if there are zero cases.

Routine immunization against Diphtheria is carried out under **Universal Immunization Program which is further explained in detail in Chapter 47: Health Policies and Programs in India.**

## SUMMARY

- Diphtheria is an acute infectious disease caused by the toxin produced by *Corynebacterium diphtheriae*.
- The disease mainly affects the throat and upper airways, and the toxin leads to systemic manifestation.
- A tough leathery pseudomembrane is the hallmark of the disease. (Hence named after the Greek word for leather Diphtherite).
- The incidence declined in the developed world, following the large scale use of diphtheria toxoid vaccine during the late 1940s.
- Incidence reduced further worldwide following launch of EPI in 1974.
- A major proportion of cases is from South-East Asian Region specially India, Indonesia, and Madagascar.
- The incidence of the disease has shifted from under five children to older children and adolescents among immunized population.
- Poor immunization coverage has resulted in disease re-emergence in several parts of India.
- Clinical features of the disease are based on the anatomical location of the membrane.
- Respiratory diphtheria can be pharyngeal, laryngeal or nasal. Pharyngeal is the most common form and laryngeal diphtheria often causes life-threatening obstruction of airway requiring tracheostomy.
- Cutaneous diphtheria is more common among population with poor standard of living.
- Diagnosis is based on clinical symptoms and presence of membrane, laboratory confirmation by culture is recommended. Elek immunoprecipitation test is used to detect toxin production.
- Primary prevention is by vaccination and secondary treatment involves early detection and prompt treatment of cases and carriers.
- Diphtheria antitoxin is the gold standard for treatment. Penicillin and erythromycin are the antibiotics of choice.

## SUGGESTED READING

1. 2017 Assessment Report of the Global Vaccine Action Plan Strategic Advisory Group of Experts on Immunization. Geneva: World Health Organization; 2017.
2. Ananthanarayan R, Paniker CK. Ananthanarayan and Paniker's Textbook of Microbiology, 7th edition. Hyderabad: Orient Longman Private Limited; 2005. pp. 1-658.
3. Center for Disease Prevention and Control. Diphtheria. Photos of the Disease and Images of People Affected by the Disease. [online] Available from: https://www.cdc.gov/diphtheria/about/photos.html.
4. Central Bureau of Health Intelligence (CBHI). Director General of Health Services, MOHFW.GOI. National Health Profile 2017. GOI. [online] Available from: http://www.indiaenvironmentportal.org.in/files/file/NHP_2017-1.pdf.
5. Etymologia. Diphtheria. Emerging Infectious Diseases. 2013;19(11):1838. [online] Available from: https://wwwnc.cdc.gov/eid/article/19/11/pdfs/et- 1911.pdf.
6. Hien TT, White NJ. Diphtheria. In: Farrar J, Hotez PJ, Junghanss T, Kang G, Lalloo D, White N (Eds). Manson's Tropical Diseases, 23rd edition. China: Elsevier Saunders; 2014. p. 342.
7. Indian Institute of Population Sciences. MOHFW. National Family Health Survey-4 2015-2016. Mumbai. IIPS. [online] Available from: http://www.rchiips.org/nfhs.
8. Ministry of Health and Family Welfare, GOI. Tetanus and adult Diphtheria (Td) Operational Guidelines.
9. Parande MV, Parande AM, Lakkannavar SL, et al. Diphtheria outbreak in rural North Karnataka, India. JMM Case Rep. 2014;1(3). [online] Available from: www.microbiologyresearch.org.
10. Sangal L, Joshi S, Anandan S, et al. Resurgence of Diphtheria in North Kerala, India, 2016: Laboratory supported case based survival outcomes. Front Public Health. 2017; 5:218. [online] Available from: www.frontiersin.org.
11. Tiwari TS, Wharton M. Diphtheria toxoid. In: Plotkin SA, Orenstein WA, Offit PA, Edwards KM (Eds). Plotkin's Vaccines, 7th edition. Philadelphia, PA: Elsevier; 2018. pp. xxi, 1691.
12. WHO, Diphtheria Vaccine: Position Paper, 2017; Clarke KEN, Review of Epidemiology of Diphtheria 2010–2016.
13. WHO. (2018). The Department of Immunization, Vaccines and Biologicals. WHO-recommended standards for surveillance of selected vaccine preventable diseases. WHO. [online] Available from: www.who.int/vaccines- documents/.
14. WHO Reported estimates of DTP-3 coverage and Diphtheria reported cases in 2018.
15. WHO South-East Asia Region lauds countries for routine immunization coverage scale-up, says accelerated efforts must continue. 18 July 2023. News release, New Delhi.
16. World Health Organization. Diphtheria vaccine: WHO position paper — August 2017. Wkly Epidemiol. Rec. 92, 417–435 (2017)
17. World Health Organization. Immunization, Vaccines and Biologicals. Diphtheria 2018. WHO. [online] Available from: http://www.who.int/immunization/diseases/diphtheria/en/.

# EPIDEMIOLOGY OF WHOOPING COUGH AND ITS PREVENTION AND CONTROL

*Swetha Rajeshwari, Ravikumar*

*"If you've had a cough that lasted for weeks, a cough that just doesn't seem to go away, chances are it was pertussis"*
—**Paul A Offit**

| | |
|---|---|
| **CM7.2** | Enumerate, describe and discuss the mode of transmission and measures for prevention and control of Whooping Cough |
| **CM8.1** | Describe and discuss the epidemiological and control measures applicable in Whooping Cough |

> *Case Scenario*
>
> Over the past one week, 13 children under the age of three years were referred to a tertiary care hospital from a nearby PHC with complaints of 1-week history of severe coughing and post-tussive vomiting. Coughing episodes were followed by central cyanosis associated with lethargy and respiratory distress. After getting a detailed clinical history, examination, and laboratory investigation, it was confirmed that it was an outbreak of Whooping cough. All the cases were treated accordingly with a 5-day course of azithromycin. On epidemiological investigation, it was found that the cases came from a tribal village where most of the children's immunization coverage was very low. The organism was also isolated from adults and adolescents in the community.
> All the cases with similar complaints were identified in the community and treated appropriately. Accordingly isolation and immunization activities were carried out thereafter.

## INTRODUCTION

Pertussis, also called as whooping cough (*Synonym*: Whooping cough, 100-day cough) is an acute infectious disease caused by fastidious Gram-negative bacteria "Bordetella Pertussis". The disease is typically manifested by exhaustive paroxysms of cough lasting over several weeks and often associated with inspiratory whooping and post-tussive vomiting. The coughing episode may last up to 100 days giving it another name "100-day cough". The word pertussis was coined by English physician Thomas Syndenhamin 1670—the word "per" means "thoroughly" and "tussis" means "cough".

The disease was first seen in the 16th century and the organism was first described by Jules Bordet and Octave Gengou in 1906 at Paris. Jules Bordet along with Octave Gengou saw ovoid bacterium in the sputum of 5-year-old child which was similar to *Haemophilus influenzae* but had distinct morphological features.

A separate Bordet and Gengou (BG) medium were prepared which consisted of glycerin extract of potato, agar, salt solution, and human blood. Interestingly the BG medium showed growth of colonies from the first day and isolated the bacterium very easily.

More than 2,00,000 cases of pertussis were reported annually in pre-vaccination era (Broder KR et al., MMWR Recomm Rep, 2006), its incidence has decreased by more than 80% currently with vaccination in place. Globally, there has been 151,074 reported cases according to WHO data in 2018. However, a publication modeling pertussis cases and deaths with data from 2014 estimates that there were 24.1 million pertussis cases and 160,700 deaths in children younger than 5 years worldwide.

In India, after launch of immunization against pertussis there has been a remarkable decline in the new cases. In 2018, 18,006 cases and 8 deaths from Whooping cough were reported in India (NHP-2019).

> **Pertussis**
> - It is an acute infectious diseases caused by Gram-negative bacteria *"Bordetella pertussis"*.
> - It is also known as whooping cough because it is characterized by "fits of intensive coughing".
> - The organism was first described by Jules Bordet and Octave Gengou in 1906 at Paris.

## EPIDEMIOLOGICAL DETERMINANTS

### Host Factors

***Age:*** Although case fatality has remained fairly constant, an increase in the number of deaths has been reported among neonates and very young infants. Adults play an important role in passing infection to young infants and sometimes with fatal consequences.

***Sex:*** Female children are most commonly affected when compared to male child.

***Immunity:*** Infants are susceptible from birth and maternal antibody does not give protection against the disease. Immunity following pertussis is not permanent. Secondary attack rate is found to be 80–90% in un-immunized children. The defense mechanism can be attained by production of antibody that prevents attachment of bacilli to the cilia of respiratory epithelium.

> **Host Factors**
> - Children below 5 years are most affected group and highest mortality is seen in infants below 6months
> - Secondary attack rate is found to be 90% in un-immunized children
> - Maternal antibody does not give protection against disease.

### Agent Factors

***Types:*** Pertussis is caused by two type of agents: *Bordetella pertussis* and *Bordetella parapertussis*.
*B. pertussis* occurs in more than 95% of the cases and no cross immunity with *B. parapertussis* is seen.

***Strains:*** A total of 11 suspected strains of *B. pertussis* have been isolated so far (Bp1-Bp11).

***Antigenicity:*** Multiple antigenic and biologically active products, including pertussis toxin (PT), filamentous hemagglutinin (FHA), agglutinogens, adenylate cyclase, pertactin, and tracheal cytotoxin exhibit its antigenicity.

***Viability:*** Pertussis bacilli do not survive outside the human body.

***Infectivity:*** The bacilli harbors enormously in nasal and bronchial secretions. The infection rate gradually increases during the catarrhal period and during the first two weeks after the cough onset.

> **Agent Factors**
> - Pertussis is caused by two types of agents: *Bordetella pertussis* and *Bordetella parapertussis*
> - Catarrhal stage is found to be most infective period.
> - The bacilli harbors enormously in nasal and bronchia lsecretions.

### Environmental Factors

Although cases are reported throughout the year, pertussis exhibits seasonal trend. More cases are seen in winter and spring months. Overcrowding and poverty increases the risk of acquiring the infection.

> **Environmental Factors**
> - Pertussis exhibits seasonal trend although cases have been reported throughout the year
> - Cases are more seen in winter and spring months.
> - The risk of getting the disease increases with overcrowding and also with poverty.

### Source/Reservoir of Infection

Pertussis is a human disease with no animal reservoirs. An important reservoir and source for infection for the infants are adolescents and adults **(Fig. 17A.23)**.

### Portal of Exit, Transmission and Entry

The bacteria exits the respiratory system of an infected person in the form of droplets when the patient coughs or sneezes. The bacilli get transmitted to the susceptible host mainly by contact with droplets through respiratory route, but can also occur by contact with the freshly contaminated articles.

### Incubation Period

Usually 7–10 days is the incubation period of pertussis. Rarely, it may be as long as 42 days.

### Period of Communicability

Pertussis infection is highly communicable. Secondary attack rate is as high as 80% among the susceptible household contacts.

> **Chain of Infection**
> - Adolescents and adults are an important reservoir for *B. pertussis*
> - The respiratory system is the portal of entry and exit
> - The incubation period of pertussis is commonly 7–10 days.
> - The infection rate increases during the catarrhal period.

## CLINICAL FEATURES

Pertussis is essentially a toxin-mediated disease. The bacterium gets attached to the cilia of the respiratory epithelial cells and produces toxins that paralyze the cilia and cause inflammation of the respiratory tract thereby impairing the mechanism of clearing the pulmonary secretions.

The clinical course of the illness can be explained in three stages.

Firstly, catarrhal stage, is characterized by the insidious onset of coryza (runny nose), sneezing, low-grade fever, and a mild, occasional cough, which is indistinguishable from viral upper respiratory tract infections.

In about 1–2 weeks, gradually the cough becomes more severe, typically, the patient presents with bursts or paroxysms of bouts of hacking cough, apparently due to difficulty in expelling thick mucus from the tracheobronchial tree. Typically, after a long inspiration follows a high-pitched whoop at the end of the paroxysmal attack. During such an attack, the patient may become cyanotic (turn blue); the paroxysmal episode is usually followed by vomiting and exhaustion causing more distress among children and young infants. The person does not appear to be ill between attacks. This stage usually lasts for about 1–6 weeks but may sometimes be prolonged for up to 10 weeks. Infants younger than six months of age have only paroxysms of coughing. The diagnosis of pertussis is suspected during this paroxysmal stage.

In the convalescent stage, recovery is gradual, as the cough becomes gradually less paroxysmal and disappears in about 2–3 weeks. However, chances of recurrence of paroxysms may occur following any respiratory infections for many months after the onset of pertussis. Fever is generally minimal throughout the course of illness **(Fig. 17A.24)**.

Partially immunized adolescents, adults, and children usually present with a milder form of the disease.

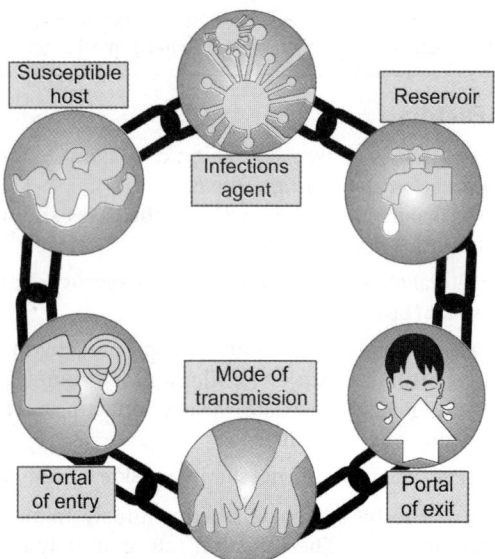

**Fig. 17A.23:** Chain of infection of pertussis.

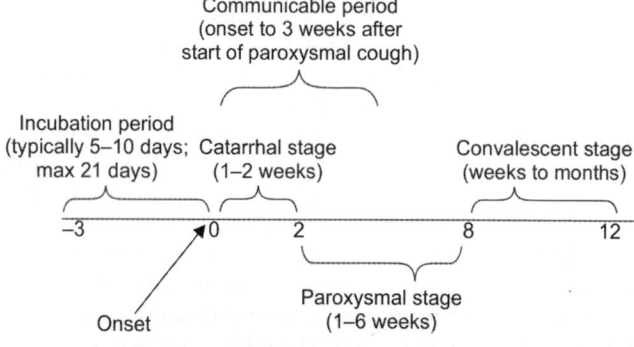

**Fig. 17A.24:** Clinical course of pertussis.

## COMPLICATIONS

Pertussis related mortality is most commonly due to secondary bacterial pneumonia.

As a result of hypoxia caused because of cough or probably from the toxin, neurologic complications such as seizures and encephalopathy may occur. These neurological complications are more common among infants. Otitis media, anorexia, and dehydration are few of the less serious complications of pertussis. Pneumothorax, epistaxis, subdural hematomas, hernias and rectal prolapse are few other complications noted mainly due to pressure effects **(Fig. 17A.25)**.

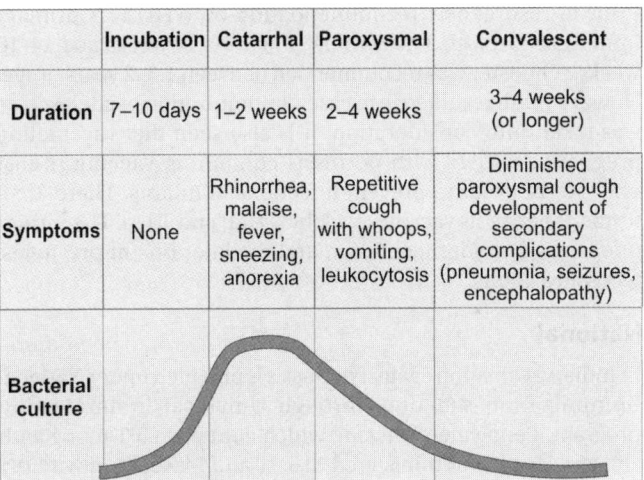

**Fig. 17A.25:** Three stages of pertussis diseases.

**Pertussis Complications in Children**
- Secondary bacterial pneumonia—most common
- Neurologic complications—seizures, encephalopathy more common among infants
- Anorexia, dehydration, epistaxis, pneumothorax, hernias, subdural hematomas, rectal prolapse

**Pertussis Complications in Adolescents and Adults**
- Difficulty in sleeping, urinary incontinence, pneumonia, rib fracture.

## DIAGNOSIS

The diagnosis of pertussis depends on atypical history, i.e. cough for more than two weeks with whoop, paroxysms, or post-tussive vomiting and also on laboratory tests, i.e. culture, polymerase chain reaction (PCR) and serology **(Fig. 17A.26)**. Culture is said to be the gold standard test and is the most specific of all the tests for pertussis. However, fastidious growth hampers the culture. The yield of culture can be increased by appropriate technique of specimen collection, transportation and isolation techniques. An appropriate method of collecting the specimen is shown in **Figure 17A.27**.

Specimens should be obtained from the posterior nasopharynx, using either Dacron or calcium alginate swabs. Cultural growth rate increases during first two weeks of disease.

A raised white blood cell count with a lymphocytosis is classical presentation in infants. The absolute lymphocyte count frequently reaches 20,000 or higher. But sometimes, there may not be lymphocytosis in infants and children or in persons with mild cases of pertussis.

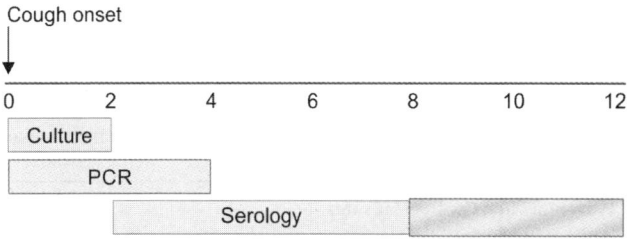

**Fig. 17A.26:** Optimal timing of pertussis diagnostic test.

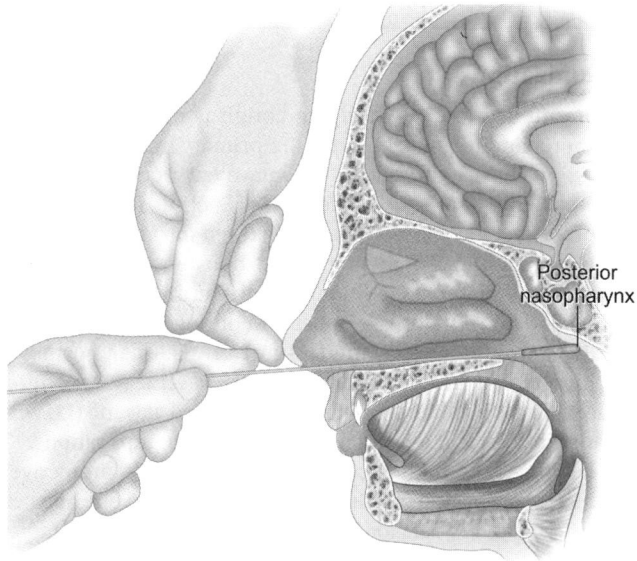

**Fig. 17A.27:** Proper technique of obtaining nasopharyngeal specimen.

**Pertussis Laboratory Diagnosis**
- Culture—gold standard
- Polymerase chain reaction (PCR) can confirm pertussis in an outbreak
- Serology can confirm illness late in the course of infection
- Direct fluorescent antibody test has low sensitivity and unpredictable specificity. Therefore, should not be used as a confirmatory test.

## PREVENTION AND CONTROL MEASURES

### Controlling Source/Reservoir

Since the major source/reservoir of infection includes adults and adolescents, care should be taken to avoid their exposure to other healthy individuals.

### Interrupting the Transmission

Patients must be advised to cover their mouth while coughing and if they have coughed into the object or tissue, ensure that the object does not come in contact with others.

Bacterial filters must be used to clean the room if the infected person is staying in same room.

### Protection of Susceptible Host

Important control measures are early diagnosis, isolation, and treatment.

Early diagnosis is made by examination of the nasopharyngeal secretions for bacteria.

***Contacts:*** Prophylactic antibiotic must be administered to all the contacts either with erythromycin or ampicillin for period of 10 days. Infants and young children must be isolated from cases.

> **Prevention and Control Measures**
> - To limit adults and adolescents exposure to other healthy individuals
> - Bacterial filters must be used to clean the room if the infected person is staying in same room
> - Cough hygiene must be maintained by all the patients

### Immunization

The immunization of whooping cough is given along with diphtheria and tetanus. In India, the primary immunization of pertussis is given as three doses of pentavalent vaccine at 6weeks, 10 weeks and 14 weeks, respectively. Each dose containing 0.5 mL of vaccine should be administered intramuscularly in anterolateral side of mid-thigh. First booster dose of DPT is given at anterolateral side of mid-thigh during 16–24 months and second booster dose on upper arm during 5–6 years.

Either whole cell vaccine (DTwP) or acellular pertussis vaccine (DTaP) is given. Acellular pertussis vaccine (DTaP) must be used for older children instead of whole cell vaccine (DTwP) because it is associated with less neurological complications.

The efficacy of both vaccines is said to be 85% protective. Duration of protection with three primary doses and one booster dose is up to 6–12 years for both types of vaccines. In principle, the same type of vaccine must be given throughout the primary course of vaccination.

Some adverse reactions following immunization are mild fever, irritability and in rare cases persistent screaming and collapse. Vaccine is contraindicated in febrile patients, anaphylactic reaction, encephalopathy, and epilepsy.

The role of passive immunization is not yet determined as efficacy of immunoglobulin is not yet established.

> **Immunization**
> - The primary immunization of pertussis is scheduled as 3 doses of pentavalent vaccine at 6 weeks, 10 weeks and 14 weeks respectively.
> - A booster Dose-1 of DPT is given at antero-lateral side of mid-thigh during 16–24 months and booster Dose-2 on upper arm during 5–6 years.

### TREATMENT

Antibiotics have little role in the management of pertussis and is mainly supportive. Antibiotics usually recommended are erythromycin, azithromycin, and clarithromycin. Sometimes, Trimethoprim-sulfamethoxazole (co-trimoxazole) can also be used.

An effective antibiotic must be administered to all the close contacts with pertussis cases, regardless of their age and immunization status.

> **Treatment of Pertussis**
> - The medical treatment of pertussis cases is basically supportive, with little role of antibiotics
> - Drug of choice is erythromycin
> - Dose is 40 mg/kg for 10 days
> - *Protection of susceptible host cases*: Erythromycin is drug of choice and it is administered 30–50 mg/kg of body weight in 4 divided doses for 10 days

### CURRENT APPROACHES IN HEALTH

#### Global

Prior to resurgence, recommendation by WHO was primary immunization with 3 doses of DPT at 6, 10–14 weeks and 14–18 weeks. A booster was recommended between 1.5–2 years of age. However, with resurgence in cases, immunization of adolescents was taken into consideration. It is also seen that vaccinating pregnant mothers with pertussis containing vaccine is cost effective in order to prevent infections in infants. There are 2 forms of pertussis vaccine available DTaP and Tdap. The former one is used in young children and the later one in pre-teens, teens and adults.

#### National

In India, vaccination against pertussis is provided under National Immunization schedule through Universal immunization program. Pentavalent vaccine which contains DPT along with HiB and Hep B is administered at 6, 10 and 14 weeks with a DPT booster—1st booster—16–24 months, 2nd booster—5–6 years of age. Vaccination along with continued active surveillance activities are the essential programs in the prevention and control of Pertusis.

### SUGGESTED READING

1. American Academy of Pediatrics. Pertussis. In: PickeringL, Baker CJ, Kimberlin D, et al. (Eds). Red Book: 2009 Report of the Committee on Infectious Diseases, 28th edition. Elk Grove Village, IL:American Academy of Pediatrics; 2009, pp.504-19.
2. ATrain Education. Pertussis (Whooping Cough)—retired. [online] Available from: https://www.atrainceu.com/course- module/1472862-zzz_015_pertussis-whooping- cough- module-1.
3. Broder KR, Cortese MM, Iskander JK, et al. Advisory Committee on Immunization Practices (ACIP). Preventing tetanus, diphtheria, and pertussis among adolescents: Use of tetanus toxoid, reduced diphtheria toxoid and acellular pertussis vaccine recommendations of the Advisory Committee on Immunization Practices (ACIP). MMWR Recomm Rep. 2006;55(RR-3):1-34.
4. Center for Disease Prevention and Control Pertussis. Photos of the Disease and Images of People Affected by the Disease. Available fromhttps://www.cdc.gov/pertussis/about/photos.html.
5. Centers for Disease Control and Prevention (CDC). Vaccine preventable deaths and the Global Immunization Vision and Strategy, 2006-2015. MMWR Morb Mortal Wkly Rep. 2006;55(18): 511-5.
6. Cherry JD. The epidemiology of pertussis: A comparison of the epidemiology of the disease pertussis with the epidemiology of Bordetella pertussis infection. Pediatrics. 2005;115(5): 1422-7.
7. Forsyth KD, Wirsingvon Konig CH, Tan T, et al. Prevention of pertussis: Recommendations derived from the second Global Pertussis Initiative round table meeting. Vaccine. 2007;25(14):2634-42.

8. Greenberg DP. Pertussis in adolescents: Increasing incidence brings attention to the need for booster immunization of adolescents. Pediatr Infect Dis J. 2005;24(8):721-8.
9. Immunization Action Coalition. Pertussis Photos.[online]Available from http://www.immunize.org/photos/diphtheria-photos.asp.
10. Kosuwon P, Warachit B, Hutagalung Y, et al. Reactogenicity and immunogenicity of reduced antigen content diphtheria-tetanus- acellular pertussis vaccine (dTpa) administered as a booster to 4-6 year-old children primed with four doses of whole-cell pertussis vaccine. Vaccine. 2003;21(27-30):4194-200.
11. Kretsinger K, Broder KR, Cortese MM, et al. Centers for Disease Control and Prevention; Advisory Committee on Immunization Practices; Healthcare Infection Control Practices Advisory Committee. Preventing tetanus, diphtheria, and pertussis among adults: Use of tetanus toxoid, reduced diphtheria toxoid and acellular pertussis vaccine recommendations of the Advisory Committee on Immunization Practices(ACIP) and recommendation of ACIP, supported by the Healthcare Infection Control Practices Advisory Committee (HICPAC), for use of Tdap among health-care personnel. MMWR Recomm Rep. 2006;55(RR-17):1-37.
12. Patrick BM, Rosenthal KS. Medical Microbiology, 7th edition. Philadelphia: Elsevier Sanduers; 2013.
13. Pertussis vaccination: Use of acellular pertussis vaccines among infants and young children. Recommendations of the Advisory Committee on Immunization Practices (ACIP). MMWR Recomm Rep.1997;46(RR-7):1-25.
14. Recommended antimicrobial agents for the treatment and postexposure prophylaxis of pertussis: 2005 CDC Guidelines. MMWR Recomm Rep. 2005;54(RR-14):1-16.
15. Summary of the Pertussis Vaccines: WHO position paper-September 2015 https://www.who.int/immunization/documents/pertussis_pp_2015_summary.pdf?ua=1
16. Von König CH, Halperin S, Riffelmanna M, et al. Pertussis of adults and infants. Lancet Infect Dis. 2002;2(12):744-50.
17. Ward JI, Cherry JD, Chang SJ, et al. Efficacy of an acellular pertussis vaccine among adolescents and adults. N Engl J Med. 2005;353(15):1555-63.

# EPIDEMIOLOGY OF MENINGOCOCCAL MENINGITIS AND ITS PREVENTION AND CONTROL

*Jayanthi Srikanth*

*Meningitis – It was a word you had to bite on to say it. It had a fright and a Hiss in it – Seamus Deane*
*"While the disease can only last a couple of days, the lasting impact can remain for lifetime" – World Meningitis Day 2016*

| | |
|---|---|
| **CM7.2** | Enumerate, describe and discuss the mode of transmission and measures for prevention and control of Meningococcal meningitis |
| **CM8.1** | Describe and discuss the epidemiological and control measures applicable in Meningococcal meningitis |

> A 18-year-old college student reported having sore throat for a week. A day prior to admission, he experienced nausea and vomiting. On the day of admission he noticed "spots" on his arms, legs, trunk, and abdomen. Shortly before his presentation to the emergency department, he developed fatigue, headache, neck pain, and photophobia. The patient did not have any history of abdominal pain, tick bites, sick contacts, sexually transmitted diseases, or recent travel.
> On examination following findings noticed: temperature -36.8°C; heart rate - 114 beats per minute; respiratory rate -24 per minute; blood pressure-88/54 mm Hg. Pertinent physical examination findings included tachycardia, hypotension, and purpuric lesions on his arms, legs, trunk, and genitals. He was acutely ill, well oriented and neurologic examination revealed nuchal rigidity (positive Brudzynski and Kernig signs).

## INTRODUCTION

Meningococcal meningitis is an acute infectious disease and serious infection of the meninges caused by bacteria *Neisseria meningitidis*. When untreated it can cause severe brain damage and is associated with high fatality rate of up to 50%. Around 1 in 6 people who get meningitis die and 1 in 5 have severe complications. This devastating disease has significant long-term sequelae in survivors (more than 10% of infections), remains a major global public-health challenge. Early antibiotic treatment is a very important measure to save lives and reduce complications (WHO, Fact Sheets: Meningococcal Meningitis, 2023).

**Characteristic of disease:** Meningococcal meningitis presents in the following clinical forms.

1. **Meningococcal meningitis** (meningococcal disease): The most common entity especially during epidemics, outcome is good if treated appropriately.
2. **Meningococcal sepsis** (bloodstream infection or meningo-coccemia): Less common form and is highly fatal even when actively treated.
3. Less common presentations of meningococcal infection pneumonia include (5 to 15% of cases), arthritis (2%), otitis media (1%), and epiglottitis (less than 1%). This group may be asymptomatic carriers and accounts for spread and occurrence of disease in sporadic form. Ratio of carriers to cases has been reported as high as 10000:1. Meningococcal disease can occurs as endemic or epidemic disease, both forms causes substantial illness and death as well as persistent neurological defects, particularly deafness.

## PROBLEM STATEMENT

### Global

Meningococcal meningitis clusters occur sporadically and also in the form of epidemics in all parts of the world. An enormous public health burden of Meningitis epidemics occur in the African meningitis belt in Sub-Saharan African countries stretching from Senegal in the west to Ethiopia in the east (26 countries) with a population of >400 million.

Historically, epidemics in this belt were mainly due to serogroup A meningococci. Since 2010 with the introduction of a serogroup A conjugate vaccine, epidemics due to this serogroup have disappeared, while those due to other meningococcal serogroups continue.

The Global Burden of Diseases, Injuries, and Risk Factors Study (GBD) 2016 reported an estimated 21% decrease in meningitis deaths between 2000 and 2016, whereas incident cases increased from 2.50 million in 2000 to 2.82 million during this period.

A new hyper-invasive strain of meningococcal meningitis serogroup C is circulating now represents the major risk of meningitis outbreaks in this region. While January to June 2018 cases due to meningitis serogroup C decreased, still 5000 suspected cases were reported in Niger and Nigeria alone. In 2017 the meningitis serogroup C strain had caused 18,000 cases in Nigeria and Niger.

## India

Cases of meningococcal meningitis are reported sporadically or in small clusters. In India, the predominant serogroup was meningococcal serogroup A.

*N. meningitidis* is the third most common cause of acute bacterial meningitis (ABM) in children <5 years, and accounts for an estimated 1.9% of all ABM cases regardless of age in India. The disease remains endemic in India, with major outbreaks reported in Delhi (2005-08), Meghalaya (2008-09), and Tripura (2009) over the last 25 years. During 2018, 3382 cases of meningococcal meningitis were reported with about 152 deaths (NHP-2019).

## EPIDEMIOLOGY

### Host Factors

**Age and Sex:** Primarily a disease of children and young adults of both sexes, however, no age is exempt. Incidence rates are highest between 6 months to 2 years and highest attack rates in infants aged 3-12 months.

**Immunity:** Younger age groups are more susceptible as their antibodies are lower. Infants get protection through maternal antibodies till the age of six months. Acquired immunity is developed by subclinical infection mostly, clinical disease or vaccination. Certain genetic factors and functional or anatomic asplenia also increase the risk of meningococcemia.

### Agent Factors

Meningococcus or *Neisseria meningitidis* is a gram negative, kidney shaped diplococci, occur in pairs with adjacent side flattened.

**Strain:** There are 13 serogroups based on the structure of the polysaccharide capsule of which majority of meningococcal disease worldwide is caused 6 serogroups namely by serogroup A, B, C, W135, X and Y. (5)

**Viability in different environmental conditions:** *N. meningitidis* is a delicate organism; it dies rapidly on exposure to heat, desiccation, disinfectants and alterations in pH. It can survive on glass and plastic for up to 72 hours.

### Environmental Factors

Outbreaks occurs more frequently in the form of seasonal epidemics during the dry and cold months of the year from December to June, during this season dust winds, cold nights and antecedent viral infections combine to damage the nasopharyngeal mucosa thereby increasing the risk of disease.

> **Risk factors for meningococcal meningitis are:**
> a. Overcrowding as occurs in schools, barracks, refugee camps
> b. Low socio-economic groups living under poor housing conditions, and
> c. Inadequate ventilation
> d. Smoking both active and passive
> e. Antecedent upper respiratory infection
> f. Asplenia
> g. Underlying chronic illnesses, and
> h. Travel to endemic areas
> i. Occupational (microbiologists)

### Source/Reservoir of Infection

Humans are the only **natural reservoirs**. As many as 10% of adolescents and adults are asymptomatic transient carriers of *N. meningitidis*, most strains of which are not pathogenic. The organism is found in the nasopharynx of cases and carriers. Spread of infection from clinical cases is negligible.

In majority of individuals the infection is trivial with atypical symptoms of nasopharyngitis, these individuals act as carriers and account for major source of spread of infection. During the epidemics the carrier rate may rise to 70-80 percent and the temporary carrier stage may last for a mean period of 10 months.

### Infective Material

Respiratory or throat secretions.

### Portal of Exit

Respiratory droplets produced through nose and mouth within a distance of one meter. Close contact like kissing can also spread the infection.

### Mode of Transmission

The bacteria are transmitted from person-to-person through droplets of respiratory or throat secretions from carriers and direct contact.

### Portal of Entry

Is the nasopharynx.

### Incubation Period

3 to 4 days but may range from 2 to 10 days.

### Period of Communicability

Generally limited, i.e., until meningococci are no longer present in the discharges of nose and throat. Cases rapidly lose their infectiousness within 24 hours of specific treatment.

## CLINICAL FEATURES

The disease presents in 3 clinical variants,
1. **Cerebrospinal meningitis** which is the most common form and is characterized by involvement of the meninges. Symptoms include headache, temperature of 37.3 to 38.9°C, slow pulse, vomiting, cervical rigidity, Kernig's sign and in young children opisthotonus. Even when disease is diagnosed early and adequate treatment is started, 8 to 15% of patients die, often within 24 to 48 hours after the onset of symptoms. If untreated, meningococcal meningitis is fatal in 50 percent of the cases and may result in brain damage, hearing loss or disability in 10 to 20 percent of survivors.
2. **Meningococcemia** alone, is uncommon which is characterized by acute septicemia, petechial rash and sometimes joint involvement. About 10 to 20 percent of such patients develop the "**Waterhouse Friderichsen syndrome**" resulting in vasomotor collapse and death.
3. **Nasopharyngitis** alone which is common and accounts for spread and occurrence of disease in sporadic form.

# DIAGNOSIS

Initial diagnosis can be made by clinical examination, rapid diagnosis testing, followed by a lumbar puncture showing purulent spinal fluid. Demonstration of typical organism in gram stained smear of spinal fluid. Culture of organism from blood and CSF. Demonstration of group specific meningococcal polysaccharide in spinal fluid by agglutination tests, by polymerase chain reaction or whole genome sequencing.

# TREATMENT

Meningococcal disease is a medical emergency as it is a potentially fatal disease. Admission of the patient to hospital is essential but isolation is not necessary. Antibiotic treatment should be started as soon as possible. The drug of choice is Penicillin. Ceftriaxone or any other third generation cephalosporin should be substituted if intolerance to penicillin is observed.

Treatment of carrier state is difficult and needs use of powerful antibiotic like rifampicin to eradicate the carrier state. Chemoprophylaxis is the preferred means of prevention of disease among close contacts of sporadic cases. In adults ciprofloxacin 500 mg single oral dose or rifampicin 600 mg twice a day for 2 days are options. In closed communities and communities who can be kept under surveillance, mass chemoprophylaxis is recommended. This brings about an immediate drop in the incidence rate of meningitis and in the proportion of carriers.

# PREVENTION AND CONTROL MEASURES

## Controlling Source and Reservoir

By early diagnosis and prompt treatment can reduce the morbidity and mortality due to meningitis. Isolation of cases has limited value as carriers outnumber cases and are primarily responsible for spread of disease. Treatment of cases and chemoprophylaxis is a preferred means for prevention of disease among close contacts and can interrupt the transmission of disease. The susceptible host can be protected by meningococcal vaccines which are serogroup specific and confer varying degrees of duration of protection. Vaccines available:

- Polysaccharide vaccines are used during a response to outbreaks, mainly in Africa. They are either bivalent (serogroup A and C), trivalent (A, C, and W 135), or tetravalent (A, C, Y and W135). This is administered as a single dose to persons above the age of 2 years. Route of administration is subcutaneous. Adverse reactions are mild; most frequent reaction is pain and redness at the site of injection which lasts for a day or two.
- Conjugate vaccines are used in prevention and outbreak response. They confer longer lasting immunity (5 years are more), prevent carrier state and induce herd immunity and can be used in young children (less than one year). Available vaccines are—Monovalent C, Monovalent A and Tetravalent (serogroups A, C, Y, W135). Monovalent A vaccine is given as a single dose to individuals 1–29 years of age. Children aged 2–11 months require 2 doses at an interval of 2 months followed by booster dose after a year.

## Vaccine is Recommended for Use in

- Controlling outbreaks of meningococcal disease targeting population at risk.
- Travellers (Hajj/Umra travellers)
- Subjects living in or visiting epidemic and highly endemic areas.
- Subjects living in closed communities (armed forces unit, training camps or boarding schools)
- Persons who are immunocompromised such as asplenia and inherited immunological immunodeficiencies.
- Subjects found to be in close contact with patients with disease caused by Meningococcus.

# CURRENT APPROACHES IN HEALTH CARE SERVICES

## Global Approach

WHO recommends strategies for epidemic preparedness, prevention and outbreak control. In countries with high and medium endemic rates of invasive meningococcal meningitis and frequent epidemics, WHO advices the introduction of appropriate large scale meningococcal vaccination programs.

The Global Meningococcal Initiative (GMI) was formed in 2009 and is led by a multidisciplinary group, whose mission is to effect change in MD through education, research, and international cooperation.

GMI Recommendations for Reducing the Global Burden of Meningococcal meningitis are:
a. Country-specific approaches to vaccine prevention are needed because of geographic and temporal variations in disease epidemiology.
b. Country-specific meningococcal vaccination policy should be based on local epidemiology and economic considerations.
c. Continued funding of the introduction of Men AfriVacTM is an important global and regional public health priority.
d. The Meningitis Vaccine Project (MVP) model should be considered when developing other products with markets that are primarily or exclusively in developing countries.
e. Travelers to high-risk areas should be vaccinated against MD.
f. Vaccines against all clinically relevant MD serogroups (A, B, C, W-135, X, and Y) should be developed.
g. Conjugate vaccines should replace polysaccharide vaccines whenever cost, availability, licensing, and immunization policy allow.
However, polysaccharide vaccines are still recommended where conjugate vaccines are not available.
h. Laboratory-based surveillance for MD should be strengthened (or initiated) to determine the true burden of disease.

Since the GBD 2016 report the WHO Defeating Meningitis 2030 Roadmap has set visionary goals to eliminate meningitis epidemics, reduce cases of and deaths from vaccine-preventable meningitis, reduce disability, and improve quality of life among survivors. The roadmap sets a comprehensive vision "Towards a world free of meningitis" and has 3 visionary goals:
1. Elimination of bacterial meningitis epidemics;
2. Reduction of cases of vaccine-preventable bacterial meningitis by 50% and deaths by 70%; and

**Section 3:** Community Health Problems and Vulnerable Groups

3. Reduction of disability and improvement of quality of life after meningitis due to any cause.

WHO is working on the intersectoral global action plan on epilepsy and other neurological disorders in consultation with Member States to address many challenges and gaps in providing care and services for people with epilepsy and other neurological disorders that exist worldwide.

### National Level Approach in India

In India, disease surveillance is not enforced, as there is no public health infrastructure within the central Ministry of Health. According to statute, meningococcal disease is a notifiable disease in India, but reporting is not enforced (passive surveillance). There is no national policy on routine meningococcal vaccination to control disease. Whenever there is an outbreak, immediate action needs to be taken by the government.

The measures used to prevent and contain meningococcal disease outbreaks in India are:
• Active case surveillance • Early diagnosis and prompt treatment • Chemoprophylaxis of close contacts (household members, healthcare professionals) • Fostering disease awareness within the community, including the need to seek medical help and to avoid crowded places • Respiratory isolation of patients for 72 h • Reactive vaccination of high-risk groups.

The National Centre for Disease Control (NCDC) launched the Integrated Disease Surveillance Project (IDSP) in 2004, so that outbreaks can be detected early in their course and appropriate and timely public health responses can be taken. Under the IDSP, state and district level surveillance units are coordinated by a central facility in Delhi. Currently, the IDSP receives weekly epidemiological reports from 85% of the country's districts.

### SUMMARY

1. Meningococcal meningitis is caused by *Niesseria meningitides*. It is predominantly a disease of children and young adults of both sexes.
2. There are 3 clinical variants of this disease namely nasopharyngitis, meningococcemia and cerebrospinal meningitis.
3. Overcrowding, poor living conditions and underlying chronic diseases predisposes the individual to high-risk of developing meningitis. Carriers are the most important source of infection. Infection is spread through respiratory droplets.
4. Treatment with antibiotics like penicillin or third generation cephalosporin should be started as early as possible. In untreated cases fatality can be as high as 50%. Carrier state to be treated with rifampicin.
5. Vaccination of susceptible population is advised; vaccines available are serogroup specific and confer adequate protection.

### Key Points
- Meningococcal disease is a medical emergency as it is a potentially fatal disease.
- Case fatality rate for meningococcal disease is 50% when untreated.
- Period of communicability lasts for 24 hours with specific treatment.

### SUGGESTED READING

1. Ananthanarayanan & Panikers Textbook of Microbiology, 9th edition.
2. DEFEATING_MENINGITIS_BY_2030. Available on https://www.who.int/immunization/sage/meetings/2019/april/2_DEFEATING_MENINGITIS_BY_2030_baseline_situation_analysis.pdf?ua=1)
3. Ghia CJ, Rambhad GS. Meningococcal Disease Burden in India: A Systematic Review and Meta-Analysis. Microbiology Insights. 2021 Nov;14:11786361211053344.
4. Jawetz, Melnick & Adelberg's, (2015), Medical Microbiology, 28th edition., A lange medical book.
5. John TJ, Gupta S, Chitkara AJ, Dutta AK, Borrow R. An overview of meningococcal disease in India: knowledge gaps and potential solutions. Vaccine. 2013;31(25):2731-7.
6. Kwambana-Adams B. Global burden of meningitis and implications for strategy. The Lancet Neurology. 2023 Aug 1;22(8):646-8.
7. National health profile, India 2018. Central Bureau of health Intelligence. (www.cbhidghs.nic.in) (ref: Vaccine preventable disease surveillance standards. Geneva: World Health Organization; 2018 (available from: http://www.who.int/immunization/monitoring_surveillance/burden/vpd/standards/en/).)
8. Pink Book: Immunology and Vaccine-Preventable Diseases—Meningitis. Available on https://www.cdc.gov/vaccines/pubs/pinkbook/downloads/mening.pdf)
9. Weekly epidemiological record, 31 March 2017, vol. 92,13 (PP.145-164)
10. WHO: Meningitis (April 2023 available from https://www.who.int/news-room/fact-sheets/detail/meningitis)
11. WHO: Meningococcal meningitis – factsheet (feb 2018): available on https://www.who.int/news-room/fact-sheets/detail/meningococcal-meningitis.

---

## OTHER AIRBORNE DISEASES OF COMMUNITY HEALTH IMPORTANCE

*Shubha Davalagi, Sanjana SN*

### INHALATIONAL ANTHRAX (WOOLSORTER'S DISEASE)

| | |
|---|---|
| CM7.2 | Enumerate, describe and discuss the mode of transmission and measures for prevention and control of Inhalational anthrax |
| CM8.1 | Describe and discuss the epidemiological and control measures applicable in Inhalational anthrax |

### BACKGROUND

Anthrax is primarily the disease of the herbivore animals; based on the occupational exposure humans contract either non-industrial (cutaneous) anthrax or industrial (inhalational) anthrax. Anthrax gained popularity in the early 1900s as the deadliest biological weapon of mass destruction for people, livestock or crops.

Indians have never been able to contain the disease for lack of adequate vaccination among animals. The situation is worsened due to lack of awareness particularly among people who handle the hide and/or consume the meat. Whereas, the pulmonary anthrax carries the risk of nearly 100% mortality, the presence of characteristic Gram-positive rods found abundantly in the smear of the cerebrospinal fluid, blood etc. make for confirmatory diagnosis in most of the cases. A major barrier in successful control of the disease is resistance to penicillin, which is the drug of choice for anthrax.

# INTRODUCTION

On October 2, 2001, an old man presented with fever, nausea, myalgia and malaise to the casualty department of Florida Medical Center (United States of America). Soon after admission, he had a seizure and in spite of aggressive medical treatment, the patient died.

It was found, the man was a photo editor and his duties involved reviewing photographs submitted by mail or the internet to the newspaper. His co-workers reported that he had closely examined a letter which contained suspicious granular powder, roughly eight days prior to the onset of his illness. Extensive samples taken from his work environment confirmed the presence of *Anthrax endospores*.

Above is the case report of the index case of Inhalational Anthrax which took place in United States in 2001. Over the course of several weeks beginning on 18th September 2001, letters containing anthrax spores were mailed to several media offices and two US senators as an attack of bioterrorism. As a consequence of this, 22 people were confirmed to have anthrax infection and 5 of them lost their lives to inhalational anthrax after 25 years of not a single case of anthrax being reported in the United States.

Anthrax, a zoonotic disease, is caused by the bacteria *Bacillus anthracis* which can transmit from animals to humans. Anthrax manifests in three forms—cutaneous, gastrointestinal, and inhalational. This section we will be discussing predominantly about inhalational anthrax.

# HISTORY

Anthrax first originated in Egypt and Mesopotamia, today's Iraq, and parts of Iran, Syria, and Turkey.

It is said that in Moses' time, during the 10 plagues of Egypt, anthrax may have caused the fifth plague, affecting animals primarily horses, cattle, sheep, camels and oxen.

# PROBLEM STATEMENT

## Global

Anthrax is a zoonotic disease, through control of disease in their livestock like cattle, goat, pig, sheep, etc. developed countries have been able to successfully control the disease incidence among humans.

The disease has never been fully contained in developing countries particularly in Asian, African and Central American countries, as the livestock in these countries are only marginally subjected to vaccination and the environmental conditions here favor disease transmission.

## India

India is an endemic region for animal anthrax because of unprotected livestock population. It is this which gives rise to emergence of human anthrax from time to time in some parts of the country, especially in southern India.

All the cases including three outbreaks of anthrax have been reported from southern states of India. The disease seems to be endemic particularly in tri-junction of southern Indian states of Andhra Pradesh, Karnataka and Tamil Nadu, and in Union Territory of Puducherry (National Health Portal, Anthrax: Disease/Condition Information). 6 outbreak of Anthrax were reported in India in 2019 (NHP-2019).

# EPIDEMIOLOGY

## Agent Factors

Anthrax is a zoonotic disease caused by *Bacillus anthracis*. Mostly anthrax is cutaneous (95%); to some extent inhalational (5%) and gastrointestinal (<1%). Anthrax caused by inhalation is usually fatal and bioterrorism is suspected in inhalational anthrax.

## Host Factors

Humans acquire inhalational anthrax after occupational exposure to infected or contaminated animal products. The incidence depends on the level of exposure of humans to affected animals.

Age- or sex-related bias is not seen in humans, though males generally have higher risk rates.

Reported animal-human case ratios reflect the economic conditions, quality of surveillance, social traditions, dietary behavior, etc. in that country or region.

People working in wool mills/slaughterhouses/tanneries are most vulnerable to anthrax spores.

## Environmental Factors

Environmental factors affecting sporulation and/or germination, like pH, temperature, water activity, and cation levels; and seasonal factors like land available for grazing of herbivorous animals, the health of the host, insect populations and human activities.

## Mode of Transmission

Inhalational anthrax is acquired from breathing in airborne anthrax spores while handling carcasses, hides, bones, etc. from animals that died of the disease. Thus, people particularly involved in occupations like processing of bones, hides, wool and other animal products are more exposed to spore laden dust **(Fig. 17A.28)**.

## Incubation Period

Infection usually develops within a week (1–5 days) after exposure, but it can take up to two months.

Inhalational anthrax can be mistaken for influenza like illness, particularly during winter season.

# CLINICAL FEATURES

It has a biphasic clinical presentation. The initial stage begins with the onset of myalgia, fatigue, cough (nonproductive), and fever. Some patients recover after the first few days.

The second stage develops suddenly with the onset of acute respiratory distress, hypoxemia, hypothermia, and shock. A

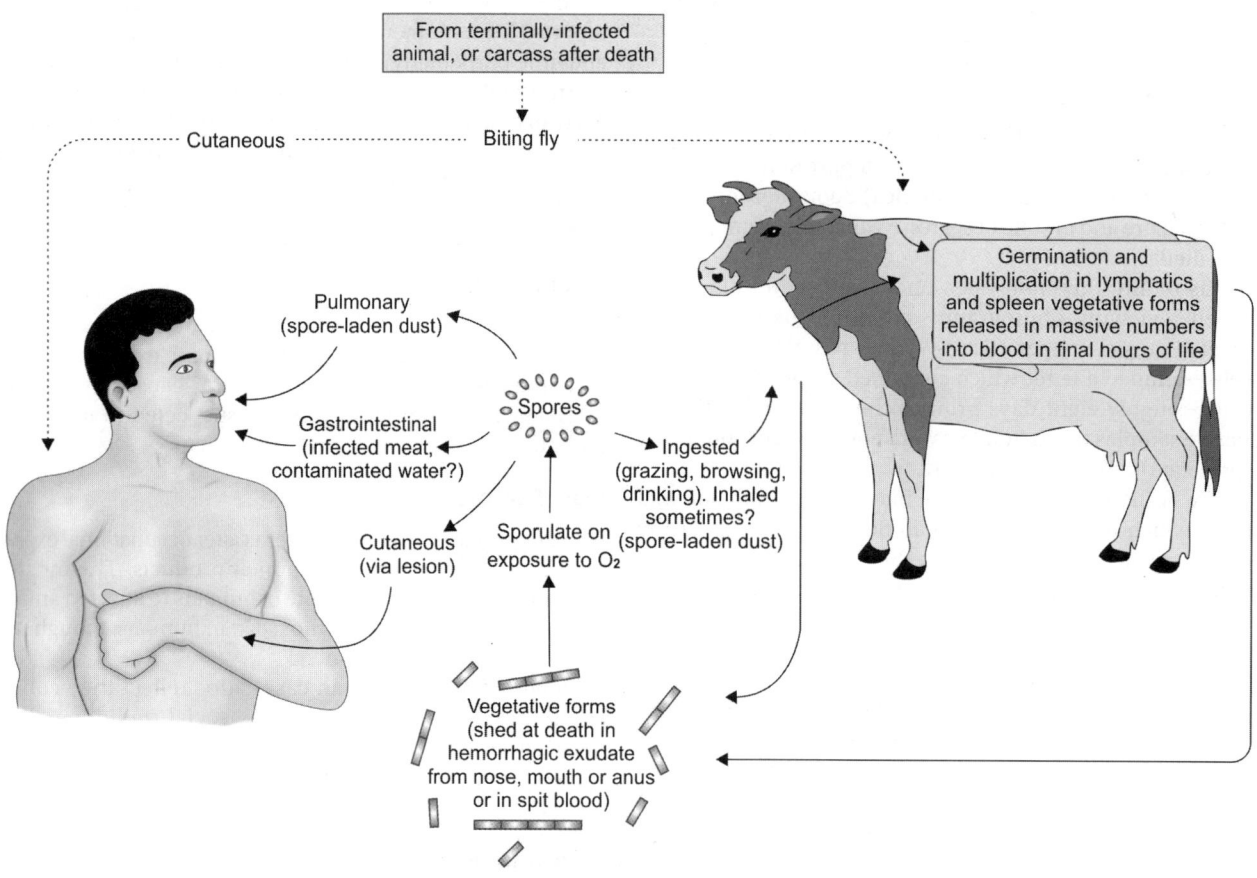

**Fig. 17A.28:** Mode of transmission in anthrax.
*Source:* WHO. Anthrax in humans and animals, 4th edition. Geneva: WHO; 2008. pp. 9-18.

characteristic radiographic finding is symmetric mediastinal widening with or without pleural effusion. Up to half of patients develop anthrax meningitis. Shock and death typically follow in less than 24 hours. The initial phase of the disease is very difficult to diagnose in the absence of a known outbreak. Presence of a widened mediastinum with normal chest X-ray findings suggest of an advanced inhalational anthrax. Inhalation anthrax must be distinguished from pneumonic plague.

Unlike patients with influenza or other viral respiratory illness, patients with inhalational anthrax are not contagious; they will have shortness of breath and vomiting; and they do not have sore throat or rhinorrhea.

## DIAGNOSIS

Clinical specimens taken before antibiotic therapy is started will grow *B. anthracis* in culture.

Severe cases of anthrax, especially the inhalation form, may have bacteremia, but by the time blood cultures become positive many patients will have died.

Laboratory confirmation can also be made by demonstration of *B. anthracis* in the clinical specimens by direct fluorescent antibody staining.

Serological tests are helpful in making a diagnosis, especially when prior antibiotics have eradicated the bacteria before cultures or smears were obtained.

However, patients with severe disease, especially inhalation anthrax, die so quickly that these tests may not be helpful to the clinician.

Useful tests include an enzyme-linked immunosorbent assay (ELISA), which detects antibodies to the capsular antigen and/or protective antigen (PA), and an electrophoretic immunotransblot test (Western blot), which detects antibodies. These tests are only available at national reference laboratories.

### Laboratory Diagnosis

- Serum—for testing anthrax lethal factor (LF) toxin
- Plasma—for testing LF toxin (Plasma preferred specimen for LF detection)
- Blood—before initiation of antimicrobial therapy for culture and real-time polymerase chain reaction (PCR)
- Pleural fluid—for culture, real-time PCR and LF toxin detection
- CSF—for culture and real-time PCR (especially in patients with severe headache, seizures, meningeal signs and altered sensorium

- Biopsy—pleural or bronchial biopsy for immunohistochemistry
- Autopsy tissues—for histopathology and immunohistochemistry

## TREATMENT

Most strains of *B. anthracis* are susceptible to penicillin, which should be started as soon as possible. In inhalation anthrax, intravenous penicillin G, 4 million units 4-hourly, should be administered.

Other drugs are intravenous ciprofloxacin (800 mg/day) or intravenous doxycycline (200 mg/day).

Most of the patients require intensive supportive care including vigilant monitoring and correction of electrolyte and acid–base disturbance, mechanical ventilation, and vasopressor administration.

## PROGNOSIS

Almost all cases of inhalation anthrax are fatal.

## PREVENTION AND CONTROL

Control of anthrax in animals is essential to control of the disease in humans. Routine immunization of animals is mandatory in areas with continuing cases of animal anthrax. All cases of animal or human anthrax should be reported to the appropriate authorities.

During an outbreak, suspected animals should be quarantined and infected herds sacrificed.

Carcasses of animals that have succumbed to anthrax are buried intact or cremated to avoid sporulation and further contamination of the environment.

Anthrax vaccines should be given to those at risk of acquiring the disease such as agricultural workers or veterinarians who have contact with potentially infected animals, laboratory workers who work with *B. anthracis*, and workers involved in the industrial processing of animal products.

The incidence of industrial anthrax has been further decreased by educating workers about how anthrax is transmitted, improvement in industrial hygiene, better manufacturing equipment and environmental control, as well as the decline in using fibers of animal origin as raw material.

Current anthrax vaccines for human use include cell-free preparations consisting of alum-precipitated and aluminum hydroxide-adsorbed extracellular components (primarily Protective Antigen component of anthrax toxin) of uncapsulated *B. anthracis*, available in the United Kingdom and the United States, respectively.

A live attenuated anthrax spore vaccine is available in countries of the former Soviet Union, but is not used elsewhere because of safety concerns.

The current cell-free vaccines are manufactured from an undefined crude culture supernatant. They must be given several times to ensure protection and local reactions have been reported. These drawbacks and the potential use of *B. anthracis* as a biological weapon have stimulated efforts to develop improved vaccines. A minimally reactogenic, recombinant PA vaccine has been investigated.

Other approaches, made possible by modern molecular biology technology, include cloning the PA gene into other bacteria or viruses and development of mutant avirulent strains of *B. anthracis*.

## SUGGESTED READING

1. Anthrax. National Center for Emerging and Zoonotic Infectious Diseases (NCEZID). Centers for Disease Control and Prevention. [online] Available from: https://www.cdc.gov/anthrax/index.html.
2. Anthrax in humans and animals. 4th edition. WHO Library. [online] Available from: http://apps.who.int/iris/bitstream/handle/10665/97503/9789241547536_eng.pdf.
3. Dutta TK, Sujatha S, Sahoo RK. Anthrax—Update on diagnosis and management. J Assoc Physicians India. 2011;59:573-8.
4. Kasper DL, Hauser SL, Jameson JL, et al. (Eds). Harrison's Principles of Internal Medicine. 19th edition. New York: McGraw Hill, Health Professions Division; 2015. pp. 1931-3.

# PNEUMONIC PLAGUE

| | |
|---|---|
| CM 7.2 | Enumerate, describe and discuss the mode of transmission and measures for prevention and control of Pneumonic plague |
| CM 8.1 | Describe and discuss the epidemiological and control measures applicable in pneumonic plague |
| CM 8.4 | Describe the principles and enumerate the measures to control a pneumonic plague epidemic |

## INTRODUCTION

"Ring around the rosy, a pocket full of posies, Ashes …Ashes, we all fall down".

A harmless nursery rhyme which children have recited for generations ironically takes its origin from one of the most devastating diseases in human history—Plague.

The simplistic words used in the nursery rhyme capture the essence of the plague's horror.

Dark-ringed red spots on the skin from infected flea bites or "ring around the rosy" would eventually turn black, producing putrid smelling lesions. People carried with them "pocket full of posies" (a fragrant herb) and held it to their faces to avoid the horrid odor associated with the plague. Many of the corpses were cremated—"ashes …ashes" and finally death would come to all and "we all fall down".

## HISTORY

Plague also known as "Black death" was first recorded in China in 224 BCE. It has been a dreaded killer from times immemorial. The first plague also called the Justinian plague took place in the sixth century and claimed nearly a hundred million victims. The second plague also called as "Black death" took place in the fourteenth century in Europe. It caused 50 million deaths wiping out nearly a quarter of Europe's population. The third pandemic began in Hong Kong in 1894. Within 10 years this pandemic had spread to all the continents. It resulted in 13 million deaths in India alone.

## PROBLEM STATEMENT

Between 1st January 2010 and 31st December 2015, 3,248 cases of plague in humans were reported, resulting in 584 deaths (WHO, Fact Sheets: Plague, 2017). Africa, Asia, and South America have been most affected by plague in the past; but since the 1990s, most human cases have predominantly occurred in Africa. The endemic countries for plague are Madagascar, The Democratic Republic of the Congo, and Peru. Presence of natural foci of plague, viz. the bacteria, animal reservoir, and vector co-existing with human populations always poses a threat for an outbreak of plague. The outbreak of pneumonic plague in September, 2017, in Antananarivo, the capital city of Madagascar was observed for 2 months till November 2017 with only 32 laboratory confirmed plague, with eight of these leading to death.

India (1994, 2002), Algeria (2003), and Indonesia (1997) are examples of countries who have reported outbreaks of plague after a lull of nearly 30–50 years.

India reported an outbreak of 16 cases of pneumonic plague including four deaths in February 2002. The last reported case had a date of onset of 8 February 2002 (WHO, Impact of Plague: a short history of recent outbreak, 2005).

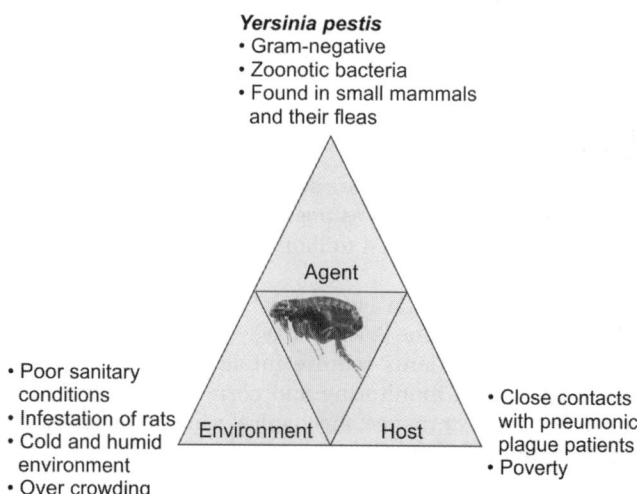

Fig. 17A.29: Epidemiology of pneumonic plague.

## EPIDEMIOLOGY

Plague is an infectious disease caused by the bacteria *Yersinia pestis*. Plague manifests in three different forms (**Flowchart 17A.4**).

**Flowchart 17A.4:** Manifestation of plague.

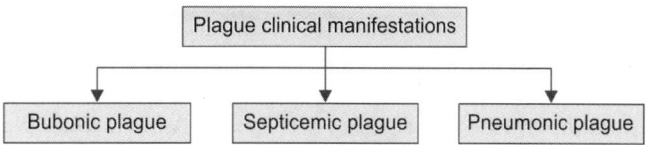

The bubonic and septicemia plague have been dealt with in detail in **Chapter 17D: Epidemiology of Zoonotic Diseases and its Prevention and Control**. This section will highlight particularly on pneumonic plague.

### Pneumonic Plague

It is the only form of plague to spread from person to person. There are two types of pneumonic plague.

#### Primary Pneumonic Plague

Disease results from direct infection of the airways and also could result from intentional release of aerosolized *Yersinia pestis*.

#### Secondary Pneumonic Plague

In a patient suffering from bubonic plague (never spreads from person to person) the bacteria may reach the lungs through hematogenous spread; these people develop secondary pneumonic plague.

It occurs in <5% of patients who are treated with bubonic plague (**Fig. 17A.29**).

## CLINICAL FEATURES

Incubation period: 2–4 day (Range 1–6 day).

### Initial Symptoms

Sudden onset of increased headache, chills, dyspnea, malaise, increased heart rate, and respiratory rate. Steady rise in body temperature.

### After 24 Hours

Cough develops which is initially dry and then progressively becomes productive and blood stained and/or purulent.

In secondary pneumonic plague, sputum production is scant and more likely to appear tenacious and inspissated.

### Final Stages (One to Several Hours before Death)

Patient produces copious amounts of bright red sputum with enormous amounts of plague bacilli in almost pure culture.

Pneumonic forms of plague have a case fatality ratio of 30–100% if left untreated.

## INVESTIGATIONS AND DIAGNOSIS

- Typical sudden onset and very rapid progression of symptoms should raise the suspicion of pneumonic plague.
- Radiology is helpful for early detection of pneumonia. Alveolar infiltrates usually bilateral are seen in the lower lobes, sometimes preceded by nodular or patchy lesions.
- Hilar lymphadenopathy is sometimes seen.
- Confirmation of plague requires identification of *Y. pestis* from a sample of pus from bubo, blood or sputum.
- Rapid dipstick test which detects a specific *Y. pestis* antigen F1 is used in endemic countries for identifying plague patients.

## TREATMENT

Antibiotic treatment is effective for plague. So, early diagnosis and treatment is the key.

Along with supportive care streptomycin, tetracycline, doxycycline, and levofloxacin are licensed by the US Food and Drug Administration for the treatment of plague. Tetracycline chloramphenicol and sulfonamides are preferred drugs for chemoprophylaxis.

Due to the high case fatality and contagious nature of pneumonic plague case notification and quarantine of patients is mandatory.

## PREVENTION

WHO recommends vaccination only for high-risk groups who are constantly exposed to the risk of contamination and health care workers.

When a zoonotic plague exists in the environment creating awareness about safe handling of animal carcasses and protection against flea bites goes a long way in preventing an outbreak.

## MANAGING PLAGUE OUTBREAKS

Avoid direct contact with infected body fluids and tissues. Follow standard precautions while handling potentially infected patients and collecting specimens **(Table 17A.31)**.

Table 17A.31: Management of plague outbreak.

| | |
|---|---|
| Find and stop the source of infection | • Look for clustered areas with deaths of small animals in large numbers<br>• Institute vector control before rodent control in order to avoid the fleas from jumping to new hosts |
| Protect health workers | • Health workers should wear PPE<br>• Health workers should recieve chemoprophylaxis for seven days or as long as they are exposed to infected patients |
| Ensure correct treatment | • Appropriate antibiotics should be given<br>• Ensure that supply of medicines is adequate |
| Isolate | • Patients should be isolated to curb spread via air droplets<br>• Provide masks for the pneumonic plague patients |
| Surveillance | • Monitor close contacts of patients of both pneumonic and bubonic plague<br>• These close contacts should be started on chemoprophylaxis |
| Specimen collection | Use appropriate infection prevention and control practices while collecting and transporting specimens for testing |
| Disinfection | • Routine hand washing with soap and water<br>• 10% of diluted household bleach can be used for larger area disinfection |
| Safe burial practices | Face or chest area should be covered with disinfectant soaked cloth or absorbent material |

## SUGGESTED READING

1. InfoPlease. Epidemics of the Past: Bubonic Plague. [online] Available from https://www.infoplease.com/science/health-and-body/epidemics-past-bubonic-plague/.
2. Kasper DL, Hauser SL, Jameson JL, et al. Harrison's Principles of Internal Medicine, 19th edition. New York: McGraw Hill, Health Professions Division; 2015.
3. Kool JL. Risk of person-to-person transmission of pneumonic plague. Clin Infect Dis. 2006;40(8):1166-72.
4. Mead P. Epidemics of plague past, present, and future. The Lancet Infectious Diseases. 2019;19(5):459-60.
5. WHO. (2005). Impact of plague: a short history of recent outbreaks. Available from http://www.who.int/csr/disease/plague/impact/en/.
6. WHO. (2017). Plague. [online] Available from: http://www.who.int/news-room/fact-sheets/detail/plague.

# B. EPIDEMIOLOGY OF INTESTINAL (WATERBORNE AND FOODBORNE) DISEASES AND ITS PREVENTION AND CONTROL

## GENERAL EPIDEMIOLOGY OF WATERBORNE DISEASES AND GENERAL PRINCIPLES OF ITS PREVENTION AND CONTROL

*Bhavani Kenche, Jyothi Lakshmi Naga Vemuri, Arundhathi B, Bhavana Laxmi Surity*

*"Sanitation is more important than Independence."*
—Mahatma Gandhi

**SDG Goal 6**—*Clean Water and Sanitation—the focus is on Universal Access to Clean Water, Sanitation and Hygiene (WASH)*

**World Water Day**—*22nd March every year*

| | |
|---|---|
| CM7.2 | Enumerate, describe and discuss the mode of transmission and measures for prevention and control of waterborne diseases |
| CM8.1 | Describe and discuss the epidemiological and control measures applicable in waterborne diseases |
| CM8.5 | Describe and discuss the principles of planning, implementing and evaluating control measures for disease at community level bearing in mind the public importance of waterborne diseases |

### Case Scenario

*In 1998, Nagasaki, Japan, there was a large outbreak of Shigella sonnei infection, with 470 confirmed cases and 821 epidemiological linked cases. The outbreak investigation started when six students were reported ill (five of whom were hospitalized); all of who had eaten lunch at the University cafeteria. Active case finding and a cohort study of University users (students, staff and visitors) was undertaken. This found that 25% of regular University users had symptoms that met the case definition.*

*Patient interviews provided no evidence of a common food, but consuming water on campus was suspected to be associated with illness. The campus was supplied from two shallow wells, with no water treatment other than chlorination. Disinfection, however, was thought to be inadequate with samples showing no evidence of residual chlorine. Additionally, microbial tests were positive for Shigella sonnei. The source of the contamination was traced to a leakage of raw sewage from a nearby sewerage pipeline (identified using a sodium chloride tracer). DNA fingerprinting, using pulse field gel electrophoresis revealed that the isolates of Shigella sonnei were identical from both clinical and water samples. The outbreak was halted by issuing instructions not to drink the campus water and then switching from the well source to a municipal supply.*

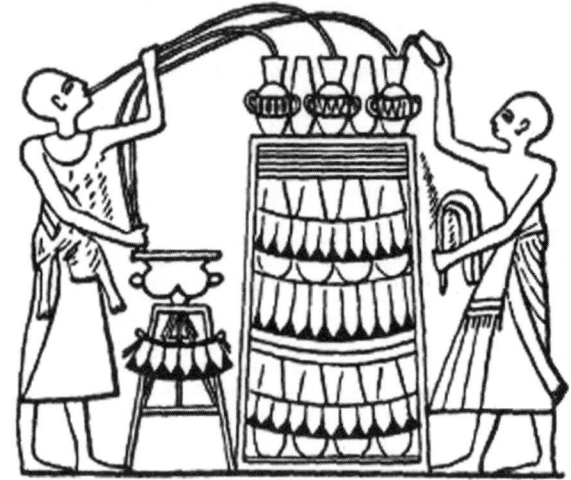

**Fig. 17B.1:** Egyptian clarifying device pictured in the tomb of Amenophis II at Thebes, 1450 BC (Baker, 1948).

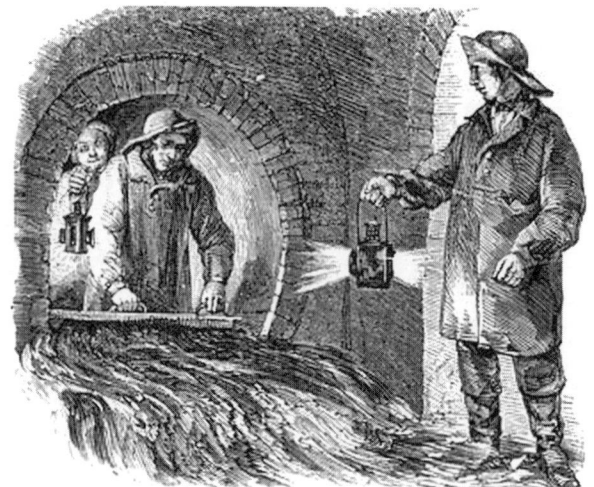

**Fig. 17B.2:** Flushing a London sewer (Mayhew, 1861).

## INTRODUCTION

Waterborne diseases are defined as the infections as a result of exposure to contaminated water in the form of ingestion of contaminated water either directly or through food; by the use of contaminated water for the purpose of personal hygiene and recreation.

### HISTORICAL PERSPECTIVE OF WATERBORNE DISEASES (FIGS. 17B.1 AND 17B.2)

**1677:** Leeuwenhoek's described protists and bacteria living in a range of environments including water.

**1800s:** The cause for cholera was attributed to miasmas, or poisonous air. William Farr supported the miasmatic theory.
**1817:** Cholera from India traveled across Russia into Europe and the US via trade routes, giving rise to the first pandemic.

*1842:* The sanitary movement started in London.
*1854:* John Snow proved that cholera is due to contaminated water by drawing spot maps of water supply to the households.
*Early 1900s:* The importance of water treatment and disinfection was realized.
*Early 2000s:* Early water treatment methods to improve the quality of drinking water were seen. Treatment to correct the color, taste and odor of drinking water was focused on.

# CLASSIFICATION

The classification of water-related diseases and categorization of waterborne disease agents is given in **Tables 17B.1 and 17B.2**.

# PROBLEM STATEMENT

Half of the world's population still does not have adequate access to safe drinking water, sanitation and hygiene (WASH) which could have prevented at least 1.4 million deaths and 74 million disability-adjusted life years in 2019, according to the latest report by the World Health Organization (WHO) and an accompanying article published in The Lancet.

# GENERAL EPIDEMIOLOGY OF WATERBORNE DISEASES

## Reservoirs

**Animals:** For example, *Campylobacter jejuni, Cryptosporidium, E. coli, Francisella tularensis, Giardia, Leptospira, Schistosoma, Salmonella* species.

These wild or domestic animal reservoirs can contaminate recreational water with feces, although contamination from animal carcasses can also occur. Some of these organisms, e.g., *E. coli, Cryptosporidium,* and *Giardia,* can also contaminate water through shedding from infected humans.

**Humans:** For example, *Shigella,* hepatitis A virus, *Salmonella typhi* (typhoid), *Vibrio cholerae* (cholera), norovirus, rotavirus and poliovirus.

**Environment:** For example, *Legionella, Vibrio parahaemolyticus, Mycobacterium, Schistosoma,* and free-living ameba. These are maintained in the soil or water.

## Modes of Transmission

Waterborne disease agents are transmitted through contaminated water, food cooked in unclean water, water source where animals are washed or animal carcass in water, or feco-oral contamination.

## Route of Entry

The most common route of entry of organism is by drinking or direct contact. Exposure can also occur through inhalation of aerosolized water (e.g. *Legionella*) or volatilized chemicals. Further intranasal exposure (e.g. *Naegleria fowleri*) also leads to disease.

Water gets contaminated under poor hygienic and insanitary conditions. Contamination can occur at the source of water supply, while passing through water pipes, which are broken,

**Table 17B.1:** Classification of water–related diseases (after Bradley, 1974).

| Category | Inclusion |
|---|---|
| Waterborne diseases | Caused by the ingestion of contaminated water with feces and urine, e.g., cholera, typhoid, viral, amebic and bacillary dysentery and other diarrheal diseases |
| Water-washed diseases | Caused by poor personal hygiene, e.g., scabies, trachoma, flea, lice and tickborne diseases |
| Water-based diseases | Caused by parasites having intermediate hosts living in water, e.g., dracunculiasis, schistosomiasis and some other helminths |
| Water-related diseases/vector-borne diseases | Transmitted by insect vectors which breed in water, e.g., dengue, filariasis, malaria onchocerciasis, trypanosomiasis and yellow fever |

*Source:* A public health perspective for establishing water-related guidelines and standards-WHO; available at www.who.int>dwq>iwachap11.

**Table 17B.2:** Categorization of waterborne disease agents.

| Category | Examples of waterborne disease agents |
|---|---|
| Virus | • Hepatitis A<br>• Hepatitis E<br>• Poliomyelitis<br>• Rotavirus |
| Bacterium | • Typhoid fever and Paratyphoid fever (*S. typhi* and other than typhoid causing *Salmonella* species)<br>• *E. coli*<br>• Bacillary dysentery (*Shigella*)<br>• Cholera<br>• *Campylobacter* species<br>• *Vibrio cholera* |
| Other bacterium | • *Francisella tularensis*<br>• *Legionella* species<br>• *Leptospira* species<br>• *Mycobacterium* species<br>• *Pseudomonas* species<br>• Non-cholerae *Vibrio* species that cause wound infections |
| Protozoa and trematodes | • Free-living ameba:<br>  ➤ *Naeglaria fowleri* (causes meningoencephalitis)<br>  ➤ *Balamuthia mandrillaris*<br>  ➤ *Acanthamoeba* species (causes granulomatous amebic encephalitis or disseminated or cutaneous infections)<br>• Parasitic protozoa:<br>  ➤ *Cryptosporidium* species<br>  ➤ *Giardia* species<br>  ➤ *Cyclospora cayetanensis*<br>• Helminthic: Roundworm<br>  ➤ Threadworm<br>  ➤ Hydatid disease.<br>  ➤ Leptospiral: Weil's disease |
| Schistosoma flatworms | • Cause of cercarial dermatitis, or swimmer's itch, local site<br>• Cause of schistosomiasis in tropical countries |
| Noninfectious | Toxins produced by some algae, e.g., cyanobacteriae heavy metals like copper, mercury, cadmium, etc. |

*Source:* A public health perspective for establishing water-related guidelines and standards-WHO; available at www.who.int>dwq>iwachap11.

or in the homes when water is not stored properly. The number of people affected will depend on the place of contamination.

> **The incidence of waterborne diseases is more in areas with:**
> ❖ Inadequate supply of water
> ❖ Poor quality of water and sewage pipelines
> ❖ Poor sanitary conditions
> ❖ Step wells and uncovered wells
> ❖ Defecation in the open especially near water sources
> ❖ Poor system of disposal of human waste
> ❖ Contaminated water is used for washing utensils
> ❖ Eating raw fruits and vegetables
> ❖ Ice prepared with water from unreliable sources

## OUTBREAK OF A WATERBORNE DISEASE

A waterborne disease outbreak is the occurrence in which both of the following criteria are met:
- Two or more persons experience a similar illness after exposure to the same water source; and
- There is evidence that the water is the likely source of the illness.

### Classification of Confirmed Case

*Confirmed case*: Any outbreak of an infectious disease, chemical poisoning or toxin-mediated illness where water is indicated as the source by an epidemiological investigation [Center for Disease Control and Prevention (CDC)].

### Investigation of a Waterborne Outbreak

- To collect information from cases to characterize the outbreak
- To confirm the existence of an outbreak
- To formulate a hypothesis about the agent and arrange for appropriate clinical laboratory testing, if necessary
- To develop a case definition including person, place, and time
- To carry out an environmental field investigation based on the data collected
- Implementation of immediate control measures based on the suspected agent and the source
- Testing hypotheses with an epidemiologic study (e.g. case-control or cohort)
- Implementation and evaluation of further control measures.

### Preventing Waterborne Diseases

- Ensuring safe water for drinking: The drinking water to be supplied regularly can be rendered safe by ensuring residual chlorine of 0.5–1 PPM with zero bacterial count.
- Prevention of open air defecation
- Enforcement of food hygiene
- Effective garbage removal
- Desilting of drains
- Health education/IEC activity
- Distribution of chlorine tablets
- Monitoring and surveillance.

Surveillance of drinking-water quality is the "continuous close assessment and review of the safety and acceptability of drinking-water supplies". — **WHO, 1976**

WHO recommends the household water treatment and safe storage (HWTS) in places where water supplies do not deliver safe water, or where water is subjected to recontamination.

Water purification methods—small scale and large scale (will be dealt in environment).

To prevent and control waterborne diseases in community, an integrated effort from health and other departments and agencies providing civic amenities is required. Health department can only tell about the distribution of disease in the community and can find the cause and remedy of the disease. On the other hand, other departments such as water supply department, sewerage department, enforcement department, sanitation wing and drainage department plays a vital role. With this coordinated effort waterborne diseases can be put under control.

## SURVEILLANCE SYSTEMS (FLOWCHART 17B.1 AND FIGS. 17B.3 AND 17B.4)

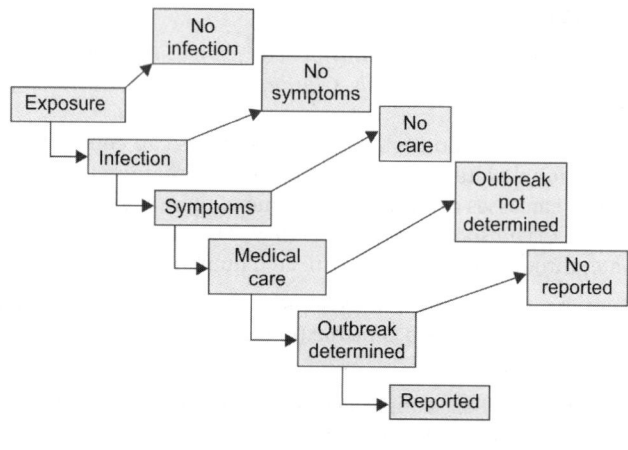

**Flowchart 17B.1:** Disease surveillance: Pathway from disease exposure to reporting as outbreak.

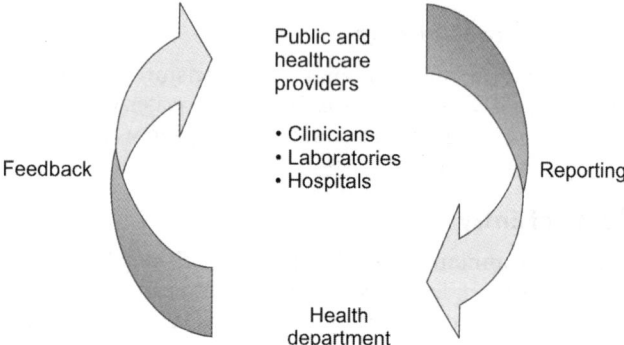

**Fig. 17B.3:** Surveillance cycle.

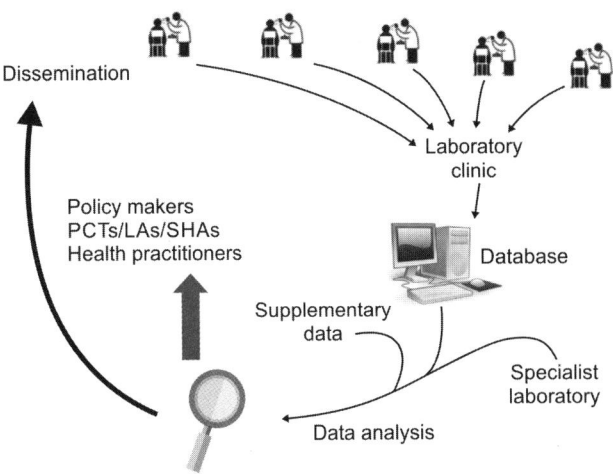

**Fig. 17B.4:** Surveillance systems.
(PCT: primary care trust; LA: local authority; SHA: strategic health authority)

## PROGRAMS FOR SAFE WATER AND SANITATION

- ***Swacch Bharat Abhiyaan (SBA):*** To stop open defecation and promote sanitation.
- ***National Rural Drinking Water Programme:*** Vision—safe and adequate drinking for all, at all times.
- ***Total Sanitation Campaign (TSC):*** This includes the construction and usage of toilets.
- ***Mission Bhageeratha in Telangana:*** To provide safe drinking water to each and every household.

*(Further details of SBA and TSC are described in Chapter 47: Health Policies and Programs in India.)*

## SUMMARY

- Waterborne diseases remain as leading causes of human morbidity and mortality worldwide.
- Over 95% of these are preventable.
- Ensuring universal access to water and sanitation is the major preventive action for preventing these diseases. It is one of the United Nation's Sustainable Development Goals for 2030.

## SUGGESTED READING

1. Center for Disease Control and Prevention. (2018). Waterborne Disease Prevention Branch (DFWED -NCEZID –CDC) files. [online] Available from https://www.cdc.gov/ncezid/dfwed/waterborne/index.html.
2. Eisenberg JNS, Bartram J, Hunter PR. (2001). A public health perspective for establishing water-related guidelines and standards.
3. Global Health Observatory (GHO) data: Mortality and burden of disease from water and sanitation. Available on https://www.who.int/gho/phe/water_sanitation/burden_text/en/
4. Health Department, New Delhi Municipal Corporation. (2017). Prevention and Control of Waterborne diseases, Action Plan-2017. [online] Available from https://www.ndmc.gov.in/departments/ Departments/Health/Vector_Borne_Action_plan-2017.pdf.
5. Improving access to water, sanitation and hygiene can save 1.4 million lives per year, says new WHO report. 28 June 2023 https://www.who.int/news/item/28-06-2023-improving-access-to-water--sanitation-and-hygiene-can-save-1.4-million-lives-per-year--says-new-who-report
6. National Institute of Environmental Health Sciences. (2017). Waterborne Diseases-files. [online] Available from https://www. niehs.nih.gov/research/ programs/geh/climate change/health_ impacts/waterborne_ diseases/ index.cfm.
7. Pine R, Marsee M, NMED Drinking Water Bureau. (2000). Waterborne Disease Outbreaks. [online] Available from https://www.env.nm.gov/dwb/whats_new/documents/ WaterborneDiseaseCaseStudies_3.29.12. pdf.
8. WHO. (2016). The situation of water-related infectious diseases in the pan- European region. [online] Available from http://www. euro.who.int/en/publications/abstracts/situation-of-water-related-infectious-diseases-in- the-pan-european-region-the-2016.
9. World Health Organization. Preventing waterborne disease-Ensuring safe drinking-water-WHO.

## GENERAL EPIDEMIOLOGY OF INTESTINAL (FOODBORNE) DISEASES AND GENERAL PRINCIPLES OF ITS PREVENTION AND CONTROL

*Abhishek Singh*

*"Let food be your medicine and medicine be your food."*
**—Hippocrates**
*World Health Day Theme—Food Safety - From Farm to Plate, Make Food Safe*

| | |
|---|---|
| **CM5.7** | Describe food hygiene |
| **CM7.2** | Enumerate, describe and discuss the mode of transmission and measures for prevention and control of foodborne diseases |
| **CM8.1** | Describe and discuss the epidemiological and control measures applicable in foodborne diseases |
| **CM8.4** | Describe the principles and enumerate the measures to control a foodborne diseases epidemic |

---

*Case Scenario*

*An outbreak of food poisoning occurred among recruits in a training establishment. Investigation of outbreak was undertaken, a total of 402 recruits reported with symptoms of gastroenteritis in a span of 3 days.*

*Of those affected, only 6 were admitted and rest recovered with treatment on OPD basis. No deaths were reported. It was a classical point source, single exposure gastroenteritis outbreak. When food histories and sickness histories were analyzed, revealed that risk of transmission of disease was associated with ingestion of the "Flavored milk," which was an outsourced item. From the clinico-epidemiological profile, it was ascertained that symptomatology (diarrhea predominantly with fever and without dysentery) was matching that of Salmonella species and hence a tentative diagnosis of Salmonella food poisoning was made.*

*Epidemiological investigation incriminated the dinner of previous day as the meal responsible for the outbreak with flavored milk as the most attributable food item which was an outsourced item. On investigation it was found that overall hygienic conditions of trainee's cookhouse and dining hall were satisfactory.*

> *All the food handlers were clinically found to be free from infection, and their monthly medical chart maintained in the cookhouse. The hygienic condition of the wet canteen was satisfactory. There was no rat nuisance or infestation found in the cook house and wet canteen. Water distribution and sewage disposal system were satisfactory and no cross-contamination found anywhere. The hygienic condition of butchery was satisfactory.*
>
> *On inspection of the civil factory, which manufactures flavored milk for recruits, hygiene conditions were found to be unsatisfactory. The cold chain system of the flavored milk from the place of manufacturing through the middle agent before reaching the consumer end was also found to be highly unsatisfactory (the storage facility was also found to be grossly inadequate).*
>
> *The laboratory findings of the samples collected from milk confirmed the presence of Salmonella food poisoning.*

## INTRODUCTION

Foodborne diseases encompass a wide spectrum of illnesses and are a growing public health problem worldwide. According to WHO, **"Foodborne diseases are defined as the infections which were the result of exposure to contaminated food."** Foodborne illnesses include foodborne intoxications and foodborne infections. It includes all the illnesses due to ingestion of contaminated food **(Table 17B.3)**. Commonly termed as "food poisoning". The contamination of food may occur at any stage in the process from food production to consumption ("farm to fork") and can result from environmental contamination, including pollution of water, soil or air.

**Table 17B.3:** Difference between foodborne infections and intoxications.

| Factors | Foodborne infections | Foodborne intoxications |
|---|---|---|
| Cause | Bacteria/viruses/parasites | Preformed toxins rather than organisms directly |
| Mechanism of action | Invade the lining of intestine | No invasion/multiplication of the gut epithelium |
| Incubation period | Hours to days | Minutes to hours |
| Symptoms | Diarrhea followed by nausea, vomiting, abdominal cramps, fever may or may not be present | Vomiting followed by nausea, diarrhea, double vision, weakness, numbness, paresthesia |
| Transmission | Feco-oral transmission | Not communicable |
| Related factors | Inadequate cooking of food, poor personal hygiene, direct hand contact, cross-contamination of food | Inadequate cooking, improper holding temperatures |

However, in this chapter, we shall discuss only food borne infections. All other food related diseases and disorders are discussed in **Chapter 23: Epidemiology of Nutrition and Food-related Diseases and its Prevention and Control.**

## PROBLEM STATEMENT

Worldwide, foodborne diseases carry a high burden of incidence and prevalence.

Every year, nearly one in 10 people around the world fall ill after eating contaminated food, leading to over 420,000 deaths. Children are disproportionately affected, with 125,000 deaths every year in people under 5 years of age. The majority of these cases are caused by diarrhoeal diseases. Other serious consequences of foodborne diseases include kidney and liver failure, brain and neural disorders, reactive arthritis, cancer, and death.

## EPIDEMIOLOGY OF FOODBORNE DISEASES

Foodborne diseases are closely linked to poverty in low- and middle-income countries but are a growing public health issue around the world. Increasing international trade and longer, more complex food chains increase the risk of food contamination and transport of infected food products across national borders. Growing cities, climate change, migration and growing international travel compound these issues and expose people to new hazards.

Increased consumption of street food, food from non-registered food establishments and lack of proper hygienic practices in food handlers, in addition to food adulteration are the frequent causes of foodborne illnesses in India.

### Bacterial Contamination of Food (Table 17B.4)

**Table 17B.4:** Types of diarrhea due to bacterial contamination of food.

| Cause | Site of action | Type of disease | Feces examination | Examples |
|---|---|---|---|---|
| Toxin mediated | Small intestine—proximal part | Watery diarrhea | No fecal leukocytes | *Vibrio cholerae*, ETEC, EAEC, viruses, *Giardia lamblia* |
| Invading | Small intestine—distal part | Bloody diarrhea/Inflammatory diarrhea | Fecal leukocytes | *Salmonella, C. jejuni*, EHEC, enterocolitica, *Vibrio para haemolyticus, E. histolytica* |
| Penetrating | Small intestine—distal part | Enteric fever | Fecal leukocytes | *Salmonella typhi* |

(EAEC: enteroaggregative *Escherichia coli*; EHEC: enterohemorrhagic *Escherichia coli*; ETEC: enterotoxigenic *Escherichia coli*)

### Bacterial Causes of Food Poisoning (Table 17B.5)

**Table 17B.5:** Bacterial causes of food poisoning.

| Incubation period | Probable cause | Presenting symptoms | Ingested foods |
|---|---|---|---|
| 1–6 hours | *Staphylococcus aureus* | Nausea, vomiting, diarrhea | Milk products, creams |
| | *Bacillus cereus* | Nausea, vomiting, diarrhea | Rice items |
| 8–16 hours | *C. perfringens B. cereus* | Pain abdomen, diarrhea (vomiting rare) | Vegetables, legumes, poultry items |

**Other causes:** Viruses—Norovirus, Hepatitis A virus, fungi; parasites—tapeworms like *Echinococcus spp* or *Taenia solium*; helminthes—*Ascaris, Cryptosporidium, Entamoeba histolytica* or *Giardia*.

### Transmission of Foodborne Diseases

*During production and processing of food*: Inadequate washing of vegetables, irrigating the vegetable growing area with sewage, and improper precautions during slaughtering of animals.

*During the preparation and handling of food*: Infected persons handling the equipment or food items, e.g., Typhoid Mary, cross-contamination from one food to another food if using same equipment for cooking both inadequate cooking temperature and inadequate pasteurization.

*Improper storage of food*: At temperatures favoring multiplication of pathogens, contamination by rodents and flies.

In 2015, World Health Day was celebrated under the theme slogan "From farm to plate, make food safe" highlighting the challenges associated with food safety. It emphasizes the need of safe food for every one that is "free from microbes, viruses, and chemicals". Food safety can be achieved if one can prevent contamination anywhere along the farm-to-plate continuum, viz. at production, procurement, processing, transport, cooking, storage, distribution, and finally serving and consumption of food as shown in **Figure17B.5**.

## Factors that Significantly Affect Food Safety

Foodborne illnesses have also been identified with demographic changes, increased meat demand (production and consumption), increased urbanization, environmental hazards, increased opportunities for travel, technological progress, and behavioral and other factors.

### Population Growth

Food production has to be increased to meet demand of increasing population. This means use of more and more agricultural chemicals. These provide greater chances for contamination, growth, multiplication, and survival of pathogenic organisms. Even more prone to food borne diseases and suffering are the geriatric population whose proportion in the population is increasing, and they have a weak immune system.

### Increased Meat Demand (Production and Consumption)

Meat consumption is on surge, demanding more production, particularly in developing countries. This demand can only be met by large-scale animal farming, which can result in rising animal populations having subclinical infections with foodborne pathogens. This may result in successive contamination of food obtained from such animals.

### Increased Urbanization

More and more people are flocking to the cities and towns to look for work and earn their livelihood. This has led to mushrooming of slum areas without proper health-related setup, like water supply and sanitation. Food contamination is common in such setups. Public health services are generally poor in such areas. Overcrowding increases, the opportunities for transmission of variety of infections.

### Environment

Environmental factors may also influence the occurrence of food borne illnesses. Spores persist in the environment for long periods depending on favorable and unfavorable conditions. Factors favoring the growth of fungi and the production of mycotoxins are climatic factors such as heat and humidity.

### Increased Opportunities for Travel

The world has become a global village. People travel more often, at far places, and more quickly than ever before because international travel is turning easier, more affordable, and widely available. Such movements ease the transfer of parasites and pathogens from one country to the other, thus blocking the measures for disease prevention and control.

### Food Processing Technologies (Table 17B.6)

Food processing is a necessary evil. Food processing technologies downgrade the dietary risks in two ways. One set of technologies destroys microorganisms by heat treatment, radiation, and newer technologies like hydrostatic pressure and pulsed light. Another set of technologies limits the contaminants within acceptable limits. Basically, these include preservation by chemicals (i.e. fermentation, use of bacteriostatic, and pH control), dehydration, and freezing and refrigeration.

Table 17B.6: Examples of commonly used food processing techniques.

| Pickling | Carbonation of cold drinks | Canning (juices, fruits, and fish) |
|---|---|---|
| Cooking, frying, and grilling of foods | Brewing (tea) | Pureeing (vegetables and fruits) |
| Baking of bread, cake, etc. | Making sprouts (pulses) | Pasteurization of milk |
| Jam and jelly (fruit, vegetables) | Hydrogenation of fats (ghee) | Sauce and ketchups (tomato) |

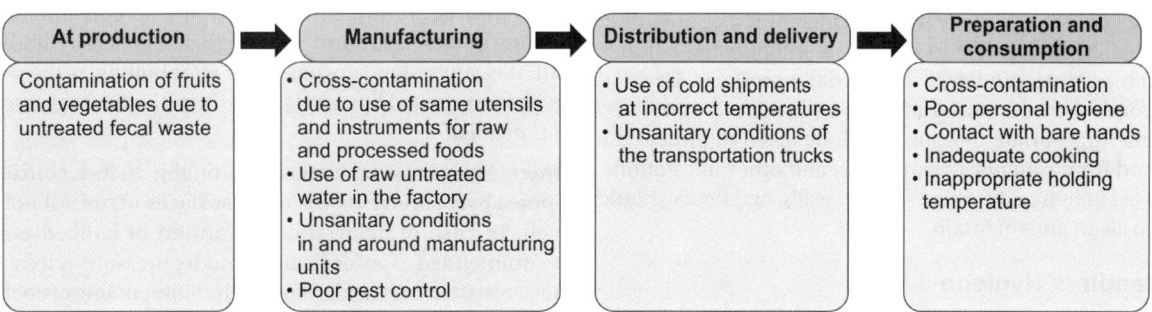

Fig. 17B.5: Points of food contamination and important factors related to it.

Effective application of these technologies in combination, works like a system. If one fails to apply any of discussed technologies at any stage, later technology may increase the risk of microbial growth. If during processing, oxygen is excluded from the faulty packaging (canning, foil, an oil layer), free production of toxins by anaerobic pathogens, such as *Clostridium botulinum* will occur, which may lead to botulism.

### Behavioral Factors

Human behavior directly affects food safety. Improper and unsafe behaviors anywhere along the farm-to-plate continuum, e.g., food procurement and storage practices, food handlers' hygiene practices, kitchen hygiene and sanitation practices, cooking practices, and eating and serving habits, may cause various foodborne illnesses. Handwashing, an easily overlooked habit, is a simple yet very effective technique to reduce cross-contamination and the transmission of foodborne pathogens.

### Other Risk Factors

Apart from factors already described, a few other factors also increase the opportunities for transmission of variety of foodborne infections. They are group gatherings, social events, contact with animals, food handling, suffering from a chronic infectious illness, etc.

## PREVENTION AND CONTROL OF FOODBORNE INFECTIONS

The prevention and control of foodborne infections starts right from the very early stages like production of food grain and continues till consumption of food by the consumer. These measures also include intermediary stages like procurement, processing, transport, cooking, storing, and serving of the food products.

### Procurement and Storage

Food should always be procured from an authorized dealer following and maintaining the hygiene standards. One needs to observe the facilities for cold and chilled storage of food items, facilities for segregating and handling of raw and cooked food items, apart from cleanliness of site and equipment. Raw meat, fish, milk, and cream should preferably be procured every day. It is not advisable to use refrigerated meat and fish beyond 72 hours. Vegetables should preferably be purchased fresh daily in quantities sufficient for everyday use. A lot of vegetables can be refrigerated otherwise these must be kept in a moisture controlled cool storage away from direct sunlight or any other heat source. It is advisable to refrigerate the perishable foods items such as meat, poultry, fish, and dairy products. Dry and canned foods are best stored in a dry and properly ventilated storeroom. Appropriate measures shall be taken to protect the stored food from rodents, cockroaches, and other infestations. Surfaces of kitchen and storage shelves, walls, and floors should be easy to clean and maintain.

### Food Handlers' Hygiene

Pathogens can be easily passed to the food by infected hands of cooks and food handlers. Therefore, practice of proper and appropriate personal hygiene by the workers is the cornerstone in the prevention of foodborne infections. Food handlers should be subjected to vigorous training and education as regards to personal hygiene and ways of handling food and utensils. Maintenance of hygiene from head to toe is essential and includes covering of the head, avoiding coughing or sneezing near the food items, trimming of nails, thorough washing and scrubbing of hands with soap and water before handling food and following each visit to the toilet, avoiding touching food with bare hands, or licking the fingers and wearing of clean clothes, etc. should be made obligatory.

Adequate amenities for hand washing with soap should be available for cooks. They should be provided with their special clothing to wear and mops to use while cooking. All the cooks and kitchen staff must take bath thoroughly before starting work every day.

The workers shall be periodically examined and may be sent for medical checkup if pointers like diarrhea, wound, boils, or other signs of any infectious disease that can be transmitted via food, are discovered. If any such sign is present, they must be kept away from the kitchen duties immediately and treated appropriately.

### Kitchen Hygiene and Sanitation

Besides personal hygiene, kitchen hygiene and sanitation must be given due attention. Cooking surface and also the other working surfaces must be thoroughly cleaned before and after cooking. Cooking utensils, tools, equipment, and mops, etc. should also be regularly cleaned.

### Sanitation of Specific Foods

Sanitation of some commonly used food items like vegetables/salad, fruits, milk, eggs, meat, and poultry are described here.

***Vegetables and fruits:*** Foods that are eaten raw may pose a problem in food sanitation. Areas where sewage is applied for irrigating agricultural fields, spread of pathogenic organisms, protozoa, and helminths are a serious menace. Vegetables and fruits may harbor pathogenic organisms, protozoans, and helminths on their surfaces. Vegetables, salad, and fruits, which cannot be peeled (e.g. spinach, cabbage, grapes, etc.) should be scrubbed and washed thoroughly, preferably in water with bleaching agent like hypochlorite. Vegetables that are cooked are free from this danger.

***Milk and eggs:*** Raw milk should not be consumed without boiling or pasteurization. Fresh eggs are generally sterile inside still it is advised to consume eggs after boiling as the shells can get contaminated by excreta of the hen. Cracked egg may harbor *Salmonella*.

***Meat:*** Meat must be cooked thoroughly before consumption. Spores may survive on the outer surfaces of meat if not cooked well. In case of delayed consumption of cooked meat, it is recommended to go for steaming under pressure as it can destroy heat-resistant organisms effectively. Slow cooling of cooked food and storage at atmospheric temperature should be discouraged as it favors quick multiplication of bacteria.

***Poultry:*** Poultry may carry pathogenic bacteria and virus not only on the skin but also inside the carcasses. Handling surfaces and utensils must be thoroughly cleaned following using them. Hands must be thoroughly washed once raw material is handled.

Use of clothes is not advised to wipe carcasses. Poultry must be thawed well before cooking.

# MILK HYGIENE

Milk hygiene is a study of all the methods necessary to ensure the production, handling, and final delivery to the consumer of clean, wholesome, unadulterated milk, or milk products—cream, butter, buttermilk, ice cream, etc.

Milk may act as a very good vehicle for a large number of disease agents compared to any other food item if it is not handled hygienically. Milk is a good medium for the organisms to grow thus, it may become a good nidus for many organisms. A great variety of diseases conveyed through milk are tabulated in **Table 17B.7**.

Prevention of milk-borne infections is done by procuring clean and safe milk through hygienic dairy, pasteurization, and sterilization.

**Table 17B.7:** Milk-borne infections.

| Infections | Organisms | Reservoir/Source |
|---|---|---|
| **Bacterial infections** | | |
| Tuberculosis | Mycobacterium tuberculosis (bovine) | Cattle |
| Brucellosis | Brucella abortus/Brucella melitensis | Cattle, goat |
| Q-fever | Coxiella burnetii | Cattle |
| Listeria | Listeria monocytogenes | Milk |
| Septic sore throat | Streptococcus pyogenes | Cattle, milk handlers |
| Food poisoning | Staphylococcus aureus | Cattle, milk handlers |
| Diarrhea and dysenteries | Shigella, Entamoeba histolytica | Milk handlers |
| Cholera | Vibrio cholerae | Water, milk |
| Enteric fever | Salmonella species | Milk |
| Diphtheria | Corynebacterium diphtheriae | Milk |
| **Viral infections** | | |
| Viral hepatitis | Hepatitis A, E viruses | Milk |
| Polio | Polio viruses | Milk |
| **Fungal infections** | | |
| Nocardiasis | Nocardia asteroides/Nocardia brasiliensis | Milk |
| Candidiasis | Candida tropicalis/Candida krusei | Milk |
| **Parasitic infections** | | |
| Taeniasis | Taenia spp. | Milk |
| Toxoplasmosis | Toxoplasma gondii | Milk |

## Sanitation of Dairy Farms

Dairy farms must ensure supply of pure and clean milk. To fulfill this, the process of milk hygiene must begin at the dairy farm, the source of production. The dairy contains milk receiving, pooling, cooling, and blending rooms. Essential components of any modern dairy are a milk depot, the pasteurization plant, bottling or packing plant, and a disposal yard for manure.

Hygiene of cattle, dairy workers, equipment, pasteurization process, as well as sanitary bottling or packing, and delivery all are extremely important to prevent occurrence of milk-borne infection. Examination of cattle by veterinary doctors, inspection of premises and equipment, periodical medical examination of dairy workers, and tests for process of pasteurization should be done on regular basis.

### Care of Cattle

Milk yield from the cattle in terms of both quality as well as quantity depends on a lot of factors like the breed of cattle, care, comfort, feeding, and cleanliness around the cattle. Therefore, a clean, well-ventilated shed with proper space is important. There should not be scarcity of water for drinking, bathing the cattle as well as to wash the cattle sheds. Ample amount of food for cattle (bran, fodder, oilcake, cottonseed, and coarsely crushed mixture of grains) should be available. These food storage places should be safe. Veterinary doctors should do examination or checkup of cattle regularly preferably on monthly basis. Animals found sick must be immediately isolated. Contact with sick cattle should be minimized and such cattle should be segregated.

### Cattle Sheds

The walls of cattle shed should be *pucca* (preferably be made of concrete) and white washed inside. It should have adequate cross-ventilation. A minimum of 6 m² floor area should be reserved for each cattle head. Drainage of the shed should be built a little high as compared to the surrounding level. The floor should preferably be made of impervious concrete. Cleanliness should be maintained. The cattle sheds should preferably be washed every day and cleaned on an alternate day. Insecticidal spray should be done on regular intervals.

### Disposal of Cattle Dung and Sullage

Cattle dung act as an important source of fly breeding. Thus, anti-fly measures should be in place. Those structures meant for carrying the sullage must always be built *pucca* (preferably of concrete). Similar arrangements should be made for carrying liquid cattle dung. Cattle dung should be transported to a depot situated minimum 200 m away from the cattle sheds. The walls of cattle dung depot should be made *pucca*.

### Health of Workers

Medical examination of all the dairy workers and dairy employees should be carried out on regular intervals. Illnesses among dairy workers must receive due attention especially the cases of diarrhea, dysentery, enteric fever, boils, or showing signs of active bacterial or viral infections. Carriers of communicable diseases should be excluded. Dairy workers should be immunized against enteric group of fevers. Sanitary as well as bathing facilities should also be provided to the dairy workers.

### Pasteurization

Milk constituents are heat-labile. Boiling destroys the microorganisms but it undesirably may affect the color, smell, taste, flavor, and composition of milk. Pasteurization is a process of preservation of milk, wherein the milk is heated to such temperature and time period so as to kill all the pathogenic organisms present in the milk and at the same time preserving the nutritive value of milk without changing the color, smell, taste, flavor, and composition. The nutritive value of milk does not change much following pasteurization. Fat and protein content of the milk remain same. Its calcium, phosphorus, as well as vitamin A and D contents also remain unaffected. A 10% loss of vitamin B and 20% loss of vitamin C are noted.

In the process of pasteurization, milk is rapidly heated to less than the boiling point; kept at that temperature for a specific period of time and then rapidly cooled. This process of rapid heating and followed by rapid cooling of the milk prevents the growth and development of any residual microbes. It may not sterilize the milk but it destroys most of the pathogenic microbes keeping its integral qualities like taste and flavor. Spores and thermoduric bacteria are not killed in the pasteurization process. Pasteurization also improves the keeping quality of the milk and it can safely be preserved upto 12 hours at 18°C. Pasteurization of milk is an example of *precurrent disinfection*. Sterilization is done by heating milk to 100°C or 212°F for 20–30 minutes. This process is capable of destroying 100% of pathogens as well as spores but on the other hand, this is not a popular method because it reduces the nutritive value of the milk. The comparison between sterilization and pasteurization is summarized here in **Table 17B.8**.

**Table 17B.8:** Comparison between sterilization and pasteurization processes.

|  | Sterilization | Pasteurization |
|---|---|---|
| Method/process | Boiling the milk to 100°C for 20–30 minutes | Three methods are:<br>1. Holder process (65°C for 30 minutes)<br>2. HTST process (72°C for 15 minutes)<br>3. UHT process (88°C for few seconds then at 125°C for few seconds) |
| Killing power | 100% of pathogens are killed including spores | Does not destroy all the pathogenic microorganisms |
| Survival | Nil | Spores are not destroyed |
| Physical changes | Some changes in the color, composition, taste, smell, and flavor | No changes in the color, composition, taste, smell, and flavor |
| *Nutritive value and chemical changes* | | |
| Carbohydrate | Lactose is completely charred or caramelized | Lactose is not charred or caramelized |
| Fat | Scum (cream) is formed so calcium and phosphorus are taken up | No scum is formed so calcium and phosphorus are not taken up |
| Protein | 100% lactalbumin is lost | Only 5% lactalbumin is lost |
| Vitamin | Vitamin C is lost | Vitamin C is reduced |
| Minerals | Ca and Mg salts are precipitated | Proportion of insoluble Ca salts is increased by 6%. Other salts are not affected |

(HTST: high-temperature short-time; UHT: ultra-high temperature)

### Methods of Pasteurization

There are several methods of pasteurizing milk. A few commonly used methods are as follows:

- ***Holder (Vat) method:*** In Holder method, temperature of the milk is raised to 65°C and maintained at this temperature for a period of 30 minutes before cooling it rapidly to 5°C. Pathogenic bacteria present in milk are killed with certainty. Rapid cooling prevents the growth of microorganisms. Milk flows toward the cooler and subsequently to the packing and bottling machine in a closed system from the holding tanks. It is a British method, recommended for small and rural communities. It is not recommended for large towns.
- ***Continuous flow method:*** This method is slight modification of the Holder (Vat) method. The temperature of the milk is raised to 63°C or more and then subjected to a series of heated metal coils. This keeps and maintains the milk at desired temperature in the coil for a period of 30 minutes.
- ***High-temperature short-time (HTST) (flash process) method:*** It is an American method. In HTST method, milk is quickly heated to 72°C for not less than 15 seconds and then quickly cooled to 4°C. This is now the most widely used method, recommended for urban areas as it can pasteurize large quantities of milk in short span of time.
- ***Ultra-high temperature (UHT) method:*** In this method, temperature of the milk is raised in two stages. In the first stage, heating is done under normal pressure to 88°C for few seconds, then in the second stage milk is heated to 125°C under pressure for a few seconds only. Milk is then quickly cooled and packed and bottled rapidly.

### Pasteurization in Bottles

There exists a risk of contamination even after pasteurization. The filled bottles can also be pasteurized. Pasteurization of filled bottles will eliminate any such risk. It is done by heating the sealed bottles under shower of hot water or steam. Sealed bottles are placed in water bath brought to 63°C for 30 minutes and then chilled.

After bottling, the milk should be kept at low temperature till consumer receives it as subsequent rise in temperature may favor bacterial growth.

### Supervision of Pasteurization Process

An efficient process of pasteurization demands supervision of various factors that may hamper the process at various points: (1) Raw milk being subjected for pasteurization process should be clean and free from any extraneous material; (2) Pasteurization chart should be maintained showing the details like temperature parameters and duration as per the method applied; (3) Milk contamination may occur especially at the stages of cooling, bottling, and packing. Therefore, protected coolers are desirable; (4) Excessive and disproportionate foaming of milk should be avoided because the temperature drops due to foam to such levels not sufficient to kill the pathogens. This favors the growth of thermophilic bacteria; (5) The apparatus should be thoroughly cleaned and sterilized every day after the process; and (6) The process of pasteurization should be checked regularly by tests of pasteurized milk.

***Tests for milk:*** Broadly, these can be grouped in two categories namely tests for adulteration and pasteurization.

1. **Tests for adulteration:**
   - *Gerber's test*: The Gerber's test is a chemical test applied for estimation of content of milk and other substances. Dr Niklaus Gerber developed this method in year 1891. Low fat content points toward removal of fat or addition of water in the milk.

     In this test, sulfuric acid is added to milk in order to separate milk fat from proteins. Amyl alcohol and centrifugation facilitates the process of separation of milk fat and proteins. Specially designed and calibrated butyrometer is used to measure the fat content of the milk.
   - *Specific gravity*: Normally specific gravity of milk ranges between 1.028 and 1.033 but the specific gravity of milk diluted with water can be easily reinstated to the normal values merely by adding sugar or cornflour. Specific gravity is recorded by using lactometer.
   - *Iodine test*: To perform this test, a few drops of iodine are added to 5 mL of milk. Development of blue color indicates addition of starch.
   - *Cane sugar*: To find out any addition of sugar in the milk, a few drops of hydrochloric acid and few grains of resorcin are added to test sample and then heated. Development of red color indicates addition of sugar.

2. **Tests for milk pasteurization:**
   - *Phosphatase test*: Phosphatase test is carried out to ascertain the efficiency of pasteurization process. The basis of phosphatase test is that the enzyme phosphatase is destroyed when the milk is heated as in the process of pasteurization. A buffer disodium phenyl phosphate is added and incubated. If the enzyme is present, it acts upon the buffer and liberates phenol, which is indicated by adding Folin's reagent, which turns the milk blue. Thus, if blue color appears, it indicates the enzyme is present. The color can be matched and comparison can be done against the standard colors provided in Lovibond colorimeter. Pasteurized milk should not have more than 2.3 Lovibond units.

     Positive test indicates that either milk is not pasteurized properly or raw milk is added.

     This test has ability to detect up to 0.25% of raw milk added in the pasteurized milk as that very small amount of raw milk still holds detectable amount of enzyme.
   - *Methylene blue test*: It is carried out to evaluate the microbiological quality of raw as well as pasteurized milk. This test is based on the principle that the blue color of methylene blue dye added to the milk gets decolorized when microbial activity exhausts the oxygen present in the milk. The rate and extent of reduction acts as an indicator of the extent of microbial contamination. The bacteriological quality of milk is presumed to be inferior, if decolorization occurs soon. In other words, the best quality milk is the one, which remains blue for longer period of time. Methylene blue test is generally performed at those places (reception of dairy, milk processing units, and milk chilling centers) where result of this test is used as criteria to accept or reject the raw and processed milk.
   - *Standard plate count*: This test is carried out to assess the bacteriological quality of pasteurized milk. Permissible limit is 30,000 bacteria/mL of pasteurized milk.
   - *Coliform count*: Pasteurization completely destroys the coliform organisms present in the milk. Any 1 mL of sample of pasteurized milk should have nil coliform count. Presence of coliform organisms in pasteurized milk suggests either inefficient pasteurization or possible contamination after the pasteurization.

## MEAT HYGIENE

Term "meat" includes all flesh foods like poultry, mutton, pork, beef, goat meat, veal (calves meat), etc. Meat hygiene may be defined as skilled supervision of all meat products for the purpose of providing wholesome meat for human use and preventing hazards to public health.

Nutritive value of meat is high but at the same time, it deteriorates fast. Thus, if meat hygiene gets compromised at any stage, it may become source of several types of bacterial infections as well as food poisoning. Meat hygiene is, thus, very essential at various stages of food processing.

### Diseases Transmitted through Meat

- ***Parasitic infestations:***
  - *Taeniasis, caused by the tapeworm species*:
    - *Taenia saginata* (beef tapeworm)
    - *Taenia solium* (pork tapeworm)
    - *Taenia asiatica* (asian tapeworm).
  - *Trichinella spiralis* through pork
  - Liver flukes (*Fasciola hepatica*) through mutton of sheep
  - Toxoplasmosis
  - Giardiasis.
- ***Bacterial infections:***
  - Anthrax
  - Tuberculosis
  - Actinomycosis
  - Listeriosis
  - Food poisoning (botulism).
- ***Viral diseases:***
  - Prion diseases
  - Norovirus.

### Inspection of Animals (Antemortem Examination)

Antemortem inspection identifies down, disabled, diseased, or dead [known as four-dimensional (4D) animals]. These 4D animals are considered unfit for human consumption. Antemortem examination should preferably be performed within a day of slaughter. Such examination should be repeated in case slaughter is postponed over a day. This must be performed at a place having sufficient lighting and where the animals can be inspected during at rest as well as motion. The general behavior, nourishment, cleanliness, presence of any disease, and any visible abnormality of animals should be noted down.

If any animal is found with clinical signs of disease, it must be detained for veterinary checkup and opinion. Such animals usually have dull eyes, nostrils covered with frothy excretions, tongue furred and hanging out of the mouth, rapid breathing, and febrile conditions. They should be segregated from other healthy animals.

Antemortem inspection is basically carried out to:
- Screen all the animals intended to slaughter
- Fetch clinical information, to make disease diagnosis and decision to slaughter
- Confirm that injured or suffering animals receive emergency slaughter
- Confirm proper cleaning and disinfection of vehicles transporting livestock.

Common causes of rejection of animals are emaciation, pregnancy, diseases like sheeppox, foot and mouth disease, anthrax, tuberculosis, brucellosis, rabies, etc.

### Inspection of Meat (Postmortem Examination)

The purpose of postmortem inspection is to ensure that any carcasses or parts that are unwholesome and unfit for human food do not enter food chain. Common causes of rejection of meat are various infections and infestations like cysticercus.

Human beings may get infected with these tapeworms by consuming raw or undercooked beef (*Taenia saginata*) or pork (*Taenia solium* and *Taenia asiatica*).

*Fasciola hepatica*, parasitic infections of lungs, nodular infections of liver, hydatidosis, abscesses, tuberculosis, etc.

Meat deteriorates rapidly when conditions favor. Pale pink or purple tint meat is not considered as good meat. Good meat is firm and elastic to touch, should have little or no odor, should not shrink on cooking, and should have marble appearance and water holding capacity.

The common signs of deterioration of meat, fish, and poultry are as follows:
- **Fresh meat:**
  - **Smell:** One should smell the outside of the carcass. Foul smell indicates that decomposition of meat has set in. Such meat is unfit for human consumption.
  - **Consistency:** Fresh meat is firm and elastic to touch. Meat becomes soft and slimy when decomposition sets in losing the firm and elastic consistency.
  - **Appearance and color:** Fresh meat has uniform pattern of color. Discolored patches emerge with passage of time. Pale pink or purple tint meat is not considered as good meat. Muscle appears dark brown to black on decomposition.
  - **Skewer thrust test:** It is a simple test of soundness of meat in which a skewer is pushed into the flesh and then smelt. If meat smells unpleasant, it is recommended not to consume such meat.
- **Fresh fish:**
  - **Smell:** It is most practical and simple test of assessing freshness of fish. If fish smells unpleasant, it is recommended not to consume such fish and should be rejected.
  - **Appearance:** Gills of fresh fish are bright pink. They turn darker with passage of time. If someone stores fish for longer period of time, pink gills will turn darker. Fish with pale or muddy gills should be discarded.
  - **Consistency:** Flesh of fresh fish is firm and stiff to touch. Soft pulpiness of flesh points toward decomposition. Put little pressure on flesh, if it pits readily, it should not be consumed.
  - **Color:** It should be uniform. Discolored patches on the skin of fish are sign of staleness. These appear first along the line of the backbone.
  - **Eyes:** These should be prominent, clear, and bright. Sunken eyes, collapsed eyes, or dull eyes point toward staleness of fish.
  - **Floatation test:** A sound fresh fish sinks in water whereas a decomposed and stale fish floats in water. Consumption of stale fish is not recommended.

> **Characteristics of Fresh Fish**
> ❖ Firm and stiff to touch
> ❖ Clear, bright, bulging, and prominent eyes
> ❖ Bright red gills
> ❖ Scales not easily detachable
> ❖ Tail should not drop when held flat on the hand
> ❖ A sound fresh fish sinks (decomposed one floats in water).

Diphyllobothriasis infection can occur when a person consumes raw or undercooked fish contaminated with fish tapeworm (*Diphyllobothrium latum*). Stale fish may carry pathogens causing salmonellosis, botulism, food poisoning, etc.

- **Tinned meat and fish:** Hermetically sealed cans remain sound for long period of time. Internal part of the tin and its contents receive heat treatment inhibiting the growth of remaining live organisms and spores **(Table 17B.9)**. One must look for the "date of packaging" and "best before or last date for usage" while purchasing tinned products **(Box 17B.1)**.

**Table 17B.9:** Examination of tins.

| On inspection | • Should look fresh and new<br>• Should not bulge<br>• Should be free from rust and indentations. |
|---|---|
| On palpation | • Should not give springy feeling—indicates loss of vacuum through hole<br>• Should not give sense of resistance—indicates internal pressure due to gas formation. |
| On shaking | Should not have loose sloppy sound—indicates decomposition |
| On opening | Should not be blown out—indicates formation of gas |

> **Box 17B.1: Tins/cans to be looked with suspicion.**
> • Damaged, leaking, bulging, dented, or rusted tins
> • Excessively convex tins
> • "Blown" tin (gas formation due to decomposition of contents)
> • Foul smelling, altered or bad taste of its contents.

- **Fresh poultry:** Bright prominent eyes are signs of fresh poultry where as dull and collapsed eyes point towards staleness. The feet of fresh poultry are limp and pliable, on contrary stiff and dry feet suggest staleness. Moderately firm flesh and pale skin indicate freshness; on the other hand, soft, flabby flesh, and greenish discoloration around the crop indicate staleness. Consumption of stale poultry is not recommended.

# SLAUGHTERHOUSE (ABATTOIR) SANITATION

A slaughter house or abattoir is a dedicated place where animals are slaughtered in sanitary conditions to ensure its safety and wholesomeness for human consumption as food products. Large volume of blood production along with shedding of urine and fecal matter in the nearby areas along with large collection of offal undergoing putrefaction may pose nuisance and serious threat to public health. Fly breeding and contamination of meat are serious concerns. Slaughtering activities must be performed in licensed public slaughterhouses adhering to sanitation and hygiene rules. A good slaughter house should have the following standards:

- **Design:** Building should be designed to have adequate ventilation. It should be fly proof. Necessary arrangements and machinery must be in place to treat blood, offal, and any kind of waste generated in this process. Facility must be fitted with scaffolding with chrome-plated hooks for the purpose of animals dressing.
- **Building:** Proper fencing should be raised all around the slaughter house area in order to check unauthorized entry of any individual or stray animals. The slaughterhouse should be built with *pucca* structures preferably of concrete. It should be well protected against animal nuisance especially dogs. Adequate amenities for toilet and hand washing with soap and water should be available.
- **Floor and walls:** All structures should be made of *pucca* structures. Cleanliness of floor should be paid due attention especially places where the carcasses are dressed. The interior walls should be lime washed regularly.
- **Waste disposal:**
    - **Separation of blood:** Sometimes, materials generated by coagulation of blood from slaughtered animals block drains of slaughterhouse. It is, thus, suggested that the blood may be collected and recycled for stock feed production or fertilizers, if it is permitted on religious and cultural grounds. It should be treated before disposal.
    - **Screening of solids:** Solid substance is generated due to trimming of skin, pieces of bones, bunch of hairs and hooves, etc. that may cause blockage of drains thus, should be screened. Vertical sieves placed at drains provide the solution.
    - **Trapping of grease:** Grease-like material is generally produced because effluent from slaughter house usually holds varying amounts of fat (melted fat or tiny sections of fat) often blockading the drains. Grease traps placed at drains solve the problem. Fat particles solidify and rise on the surface. Such matter should be removed on regular basis.
      The final disposal of the effluent depends as per legislation.
- **Drains:** Concrete channels should drain the waste within covered drains. Drains should be cleaned regularly. The manholes should also be inspected on regular basis.
- **Equipment:** The key concept is that the equipment like hooks, tables, and machines should be easy to dismantle or disconnect to facilitate their cleaning. Possibilities for cleaning and disinfection of equipment must be considered.
- **Employees:** The employees must not be suffering from any kind of communicable diseases. They should be subjected to periodical medical examination. They should also receive appropriate vaccines.

# HAZARD ANALYSIS AND CRITICAL CONTROL POINTS

The Hazard Analysis and Critical Control Points (HACCP) is an internationally recognized management system to identify and control critical points along the food production and entire distribution chain that may cause food hazard. It also helps in establishing prevention and control systems focusing on food safety from harvest to consumption.

The concept of HACCP is not new. During 1960s, three agencies: (1) National Aeronautics and Space Administration (NASA), (2) the US Army Laboratories, and (3) the Pillsbury Company collaborated to deliver safest and quality food possible for astronauts for the space program. The Codex Alimentarius and few others have recognized HACCP as one of the best process control management system available.

It acts as a process control system that recognizes possibilities of occurrence of hazards in the process of food production, distribution, and places strict actions to avoid them. Possibilities of occurrence of hazards are minimized by constant monitoring and strictly controlling every step of the process. HACCP is essential as it prioritizes and keeps robust check on probable threats in food production. Consumers are assured that its products are safe by eliminating main food risks like microbiological hazards, chemical and physical contaminants.

## Seven Principles of a Hazard Analysis and Critical Control Points Plan

1. **Conduct hazard analysis:** Hazards related to food hygiene can be biological in the form of microbes, chemical in the form of toxins, or physical in the form of ground glass or metal fragments. These probable threats can trigger injury or illness if not controlled.
2. **Identify critical control points (CCPs):** A CCP is a stage where control strategy can be applied. It is necessary to control such hazard or atleast minimize it. Examples include cooking, chilling, packaging, and metal detection.
3. **Establish critical limits:** A critical limit may be defined as maximum and/or minimum value to which various parameters (biological, chemical or physical) may be controlled at a CCP to down grade it to an acceptable level of a food safety hazard, e.g., setting up the temperature and time needed to confirm the killing of microbes while cooking.
4. **Establish monitoring procedures:** These are planned strategic sequence of observations to evaluate whether a CCP is in control or not and to determine if any deviation occurs at a CCP. Personnel accountable for such monitoring are frequently associated with production, quality control, or maintenance personnel.

5. **Establish corrective actions:** Corrective actions are necessary if any deviation is detected from established critical limits.
6. **Establish verification procedures:** Its purpose is to make sure that the entire management system is functioning as per the plan.
7. **Establish record keeping and documentation procedures:** This principle embraces identified hazards, their control approaches, and corrective actions taken for any deviation detected.

## INVESTIGATION OF A FOODBORNE DISEASE OUTBREAK

An epidemiologist investigating the matter of foodborne disease or infections frequently uses two similar looking terms: (1) Outbreak and (2) Epidemic. Many people may interchange them while using but actually they are not same. With reference to foodborne disease, "outbreak" denotes development of two or more cases developing from intake of a common food. The term "epidemic" is used when it involves greater number of individuals over a wide geographical region.

A detailed investigation of a foodborne disease outbreak regardless of the scale of the outbreak usually includes epidemiological investigations; environmental and food investigations, and laboratory investigations. These investigations are conducted in parallel. Different situations may demand change in chronological order of these steps. List of steps to be followed while investigating a foodborne disease outbreak in practical scenario are discussed here.

### Preliminary Assessment of the Situation

Sole purpose of this step is either to accept or negate the occurrence of food borne disease outbreak. This will assist us to get a better picture of the clinical scenario and epidemiological variables of the group under investigation.

- To assess if the cases presenting with the same kind of illness (or varied presentations of the same illness)
- To assess occurrence of outbreak by assessing the background activity of disease at that time.
- Arrange interviews with cases reporting in early phase. Following details are captured:
  - Demographic characteristics, details of occupation
  - Relevant clinical details, like onset, duration, presenting complaints, severity of symptoms, and visits to any health center or doctor
  - Reports of laboratory test
  - Whether respondent knows about affected persons with similar kind of illness
  - History of any contact with persons having same kind of illness
  - Details about food intake
  - Date of contact with suspected food items
  - Respondent's view on factors or reasons behind their illness
  - Listing the common exposures among affected persons with similar kind of illness.
- Collection of fecal and vomitus samples from affected persons
- Identification of common features or factors to all cases
- Carry out site investigation wherever possible
- Collection of food samples
- Formulation of preliminary hypotheses
- Introduce the suitable control measures
- Decide upon the need for additional exploration.

### Communication

- Establish communication route with patients, public, and all those who must know
- Accuracy and timeliness are important
- Prefer mass media.

### Descriptive Epidemiology

- Define the case definitions (confirmed, and probable cases)
- Try to include maximum cases
- ***Capture data on a standardized questionnaire:*** The difference between investigation taken up during preliminary phase and here is that in preliminary phase questions are mostly open-ended and wide ranging allowing us to generate hypothesis.
- ***Identifying information:*** To inform subjects about their laboratory results, opportunity to ask additional questions, and inform them about results of the investigation.
- ***Demographic information:*** Population at risk can be defined based on this information.
- ***Clinical information:*** To recognize cases, fulfillment of case definitions, presentation of disease, and to find out possible etiologies:
  - Presenting complaints
  - Appearance of first signs and symptoms
  - Description of presentation at an early and later phases
  - Severity of presenting and associated symptoms
  - Duration of presenting and associated symptoms
  - Visits to healthcare centers
  - Treatment received.
- ***Risk factor information:*** Normally, the questionnaire should include both food-related as well as personal risk factors.
  - *Food-related risk factors*:
    - Elaborated food history including food consumption outside home
    - Information about source of food and water supply
    - Details of food-handling practices.
  - *Personal risk factors*:
    - Details of contact with an implicated food item (if known)
    - History of any contact with persons having same kind of illness
    - History of recent travel (within or outside the country)
    - Particulars of group gatherings and social events in recent past
    - Employed as a food handler anywhere
    - History of any chronic illness, immunosuppression, and allergies
    - History of perceived recent changes in clinical presentation
    - Details of medication history, if any.

- Categorize subjects by time, place, and person characteristics. Spot map and epidemic curve should be drawn wherever needed.
- Develop the hypotheses.
- Match the hypotheses with the gathered details.
- Make a decision over need of analytical epidemiological study to test the developed hypothesis.

## Environmental (Sanitary) and Food Investigations

### Investigation of Food Establishments

While investigating a food firm or establishment, following things need to be done:
- Conducting interview of managers
- Conducting interviews of employees who were involved in preparation of suspected foods
- Try to find out if any employee was ill during the period of interest in the investigation
- Food and environmental sampling
- Assess the food worker's health status and hygiene, collect specimens if needed
- Conduct an appraisal of the water supply in food establishment
- Take the measurements of critical limits of equipment [temperatures, water activity (aw), and pH].

### Investigation of a Suspect Food

While investigating a suspect food, one needs to review overall processing and preparation history. It may include details about source, procurement of food article and ingredients used, particular equipment used, probable contaminants, and critical limits like time, temperature in which food was prepared. Investigation must cover work practices, cleaning methods adopted, overall hygiene, and sanitary practices including food handler's hygiene. Food-handling practices should not be missed.

### Interviewing Food Handlers

While conducting the interview of food handler, following details should be captured—movement of the suspect food among handlers, details of condition of food by individual handler while he received it, details of food preparation, and any unusual event during the period of interest noted by them. Details of recent sickness or illness of all food handlers working there must be noted keeping period of outbreak in mind. Specimens should be collected from those who are ill and sent to microbiology laboratory for further analysis.

### Food Sampling

Appropriate and adequate food samples should be taken and sent to the laboratory for further testing if such facilities are available. This step includes sampling of:
- Epidemiologically implicated food items in the menu
- Ingredients used in preparation of implicated foods
- Remaining and leftover food articles from a suspect meal
- Food items linked with the suspected pathogen, if any
- Food items likely to be affected by the environment favoring the growth of microbes.

### Environmental Sampling

It is known that if source of any food item is contaminated, it may lead to foodborne disease outbreak later on. Thus, environmental sampling is carried out to trace the sources of contamination, and assess the magnitude of contamination that may have resulted in the form of outbreak. Swabs are usually taken from equipment surfaces coming in contact of food, kitchen surfaces, utensils, containers, and refrigerator, etc. It is advised to take samples of water also.

### Food Handlers

Analysis of samples and swabs taken from food handler's assist in identification of potential carriers of diseases and probable sources of contamination. Such swabs include nasal, nasopharyngeal, rectal swabs, and from skin lesions (pimples, boils, infected cuts, etc.). Blood and stool samples are also taken. If illness of food handler is proved, then he has to be excluded from work till their symptoms resolve.

### Laboratory Investigations

The clinical and food laboratories must work together to supplement and support the epidemiological and environmental investigation teams in identifying, characterizing, and detecting the suspect pathogens, toxins, or chemicals in the suspected food item. They must work together to understand the occurrence of the outbreak.

Usually our setting seldom has necessary infrastructure and facilities, especially in terms of laboratory support, to follow all the steps but the best should be tried to do so.

## WORLD HEALTH ORGANIZATIONS' FIVE KEYS TO SAFER FOOD

1. ***Keep hygiene:***
   » Wash raw fruits and vegetables with running tap water.
   » Keep clean hands and cooking equipment all the time.
2. ***Separation of uncooked and cooked food:*** The separation of animal and plant products before cooking and during cooking is important.
3. ***Cooking food thoroughly:*** Meat, poultry foods need thorough cooking before consumption.
4. ***Safe temperatures for storing foods:***
   » Refrigerate cooked food within 2 hours of preparation.
   » Never defrost food. Defrost frozen food in the refrigerator, cold water or in the microwave.
5. ***Use safe water:*** Use safe drinking water for food preparation.

## SUMMARY

- Over 200 diseases are caused by eating food contaminated with bacteria, viruses, parasites or chemical substances such as heavy metals.
- These diseases contribute significantly to the global burden of disease and mortality.
- Foodborne diseases encompass a wide range of illnesses from diarrhea to cancers.
- Diseases causing diarrhea are a major problem in all countries of the world, though the burden is carried disproportionately by low- and middle-income countries and by children under 5 years of age.
- Prevention and control of foodborne diseases can be achieved by following World Health Organizations' five keys strategy to safe food.

## SUGGESTED READING

1. CD Alert—Monthly Newsletter of National Centre for Disease Control, Directorate General of Health Services, Government of India. Food-Borne Diseases. 2009;13(4).
2. WHO. (1997). Hazard Analysis and Critical Control Point, World Health Organization, 1997 [online] Available from http://apps.who. int/iris/handle/10665/63610.
3. WHO. (2008). Food borne disease outbreaks-guidelines for investigation and control, WHO–2008. [online] Available from apps. who.int/iris/handle/10665/43771.
4. WHO. Foodborne diseases; Impact 2023 available from https://www.who.int/health-topics/foodborne-diseases#tab=tab_2
5. WHO: Food safety. Available from https://www.who.int/en/news-room/fact-sheets/detail/food-safety.

# EPIDEMIOLOGY OF POLIOMYELITIS AND ITS PREVENTION AND CONTROL

*Bhavani Kenche, Jyothi Lakshmi Naga Vemuri, Arundhathi B, Bhavana Laxmi Surity*

*If you want to save your child from polio, you can pray or you can inoculate. ... Choose science.*
—**Carl Sagan**

**CM7.2** Enumerate, describe and discuss the mode of transmission and measures for prevention and control of poliomyelitis

**CM8.1** Describe and discuss the epidemiological and control measures applicable in poliomyelitis

---

*Case Scenario*

A 4-month-old boy presented to a hospital casualty with weakness of his left leg. On examination the child was afebrile and did not have difficulty in breathing. His left leg appears flaccid and no deep tendon reflexes or Babinski could be elicited whereas sensation was intact. The tone, movement, sensation, and reflexes of his other limbs were normal. Respiratory, cardiovascular and abdominal examinations were normal. On further investigation his parents revealed that he had a cough and fever of 38.3°C that resolved one week prior to presentation. His mother gave normal birth history, appropriate well baby checkups and up to date immunization, i.e. second doses of HiB, DTaP, OPV. Investigations of the child revealed normal complete blood count and serum immunoglobulin levels. CSF demonstrated raised protein with normal glucose levels. Radiographs of spine and left lower limb were unremarkable. Electromyography and nerve conduction studies illustrated absent motor responses to stimulation of her right tibial nerve. Fecal samples were sent to the CDC where the poliovirus was identified as a vaccine strain of poliovirus (not the "wild-type" strain).

---

## INTRODUCTION

Polio is an acute viral infectious disease contracted predominantly by children that can lead to acute flaccid paralysis and can ultimately cause death by paralyzing the respiratory muscles.

Poliomyelitis epidemic was unknown until 20th century; polio would paralyze or kill over half of million people worldwide every year. *Sir Walter Scott's* was the first recorded poliomyelitis case. Major epidemics occurred in Norway and Sweden which claimed many lives. With the advent of polio vaccine, the poliomyelitis cases were reduced.

### History

- In 1789, *British physician Michael Underwood* provided *first clinical description of polio disease.*
- In 1840, *Jacob Heine* described the *clinical features of disease as well as involvement of spinal cord.*
- In 1908, *Karl Landsteiner and Erwin Popper* identified virus as cause of polio by transmitting disease to monkey.
- In 1930, two strains of polio virus were discovered.
- In 1953, *Salk* and his associates developed a potentially safe *inactivated (killed) IPV vaccine* for polio.
- In 1957–1959 mass clinical trials of Albert Sabin live attenuated vaccine in Russia.
- In 1962 Sabin OPV vaccine replaced Salk IPV for easier administration and less expense.
- Till 18th century polio was a silent endemic, claimed many lives and left many disabled.
- In 1988, WHO started the Global Polio Eradication Initiative. Since then, the incidence of polio worldwide has been reduced by 99%, and the world stands on the threshold of eradicating a human disease globally for only the second time in history, after smallpox in 1980.

**Figures 17B.6 and 17B.7** give information regarding polio cases trends globally and certification of polio free zones (WHO July 2023).

- In 2020, Africa became the fifth region to be certified wild poliovirus-free
- South eastern Asian region certified as polio free in the year 2014
- Europe certified as polio free in the year 2002
- Western Pacific Region certified as polio free in the year 2000
- America certified as polio free in 1994.

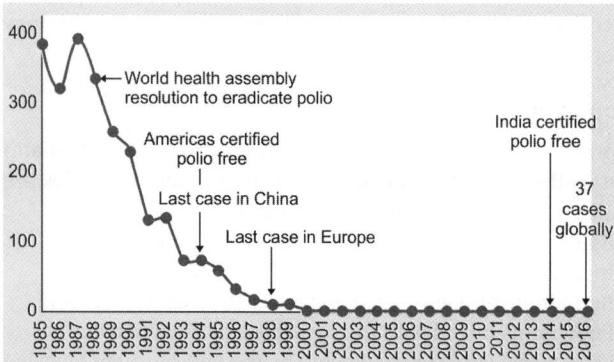

**Fig. 17B.6:** Polio trends globally.

## Chapter 17: Specific Epidemiology of Infectious Diseases

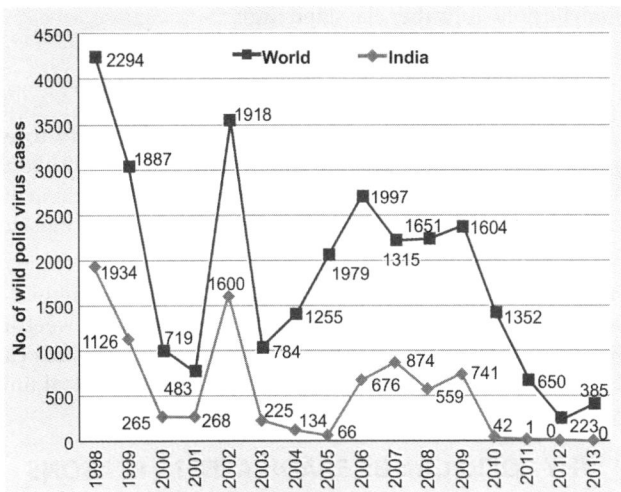

**Fig. 17B.7:** Worldwide trend of wild polio cases compared with India.
*Source:* Mane Abhay B. India Defeats Polio: Historical Health Milestone for Global Polio Eradication. Primary Health Care: 2014;4:e107.

### PROBLEM STATEMENT

Wild poliovirus cases have decreased by over 99% since 1988, from an estimated 350,000 cases in more than 125 endemic countries then 6 reported cases in 2021. Only 2 countries continue to report indigenous polio transmission—they are *Pakistan* and *Afghanistan*.

India successfully stopped polio transmission from January 2011. No natural case was reported since 13th January 2011 and was declared polio free in January 2014. No cases were reported due to type 2 and type 3 strains since 1999 and 2012, respectively. Vaccine derived polio virus (VDPV) type 2 was found in sewage sample collected in Hyderabad and Rangareddy districts of Telangana state during May-June 2016. Since detection of isolates, outbreak response campaigns have been implemented consisting of door to door immunization activities. Active surveillance for cases of acute flaccid paralysis was done and no children were found to be affected **(Figs. 17B.8A and B)**.

India's journey from the world's epicenter of a highly infectious viral disease to turning polio-free was like walking on eggshells: Every step we took mattered.

On 13 January 2023, India completes 12 polio-free years—a remarkable achievement that was made as a result of consistent, determined efforts and genuine commitment at all levels.

### EPIDEMIOLOGY

#### Host Factors

*Age:* Children are more susceptible than adult; children <15 years are at high risk.

*Sex:* Males are more prone than female in the ratio of 3:1.

*Risk factors:* Unvaccinated children, immunodeficiency, malnutrition, traveling to endemic areas.

*Immunity:* Maternal antibodies are protective until six months of age; this protection gradually disappears.

#### Agent Factors

Poliomyelitis is caused by polio virus belonging to human *Enterovirus* of *Picornaviridae* family. It is non-enveloped RNA type of virus. It consists of intranuclear Cowdry B inclusion bodies.

It cannot survive in external environment for more than 48 hours; it becomes inactivated by pasteurization and other physical and chemical methods of sterilization.

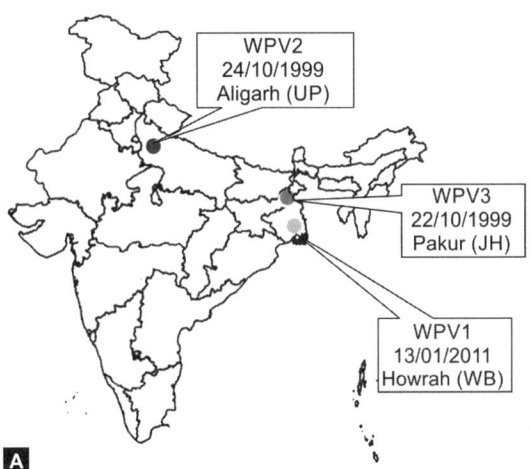
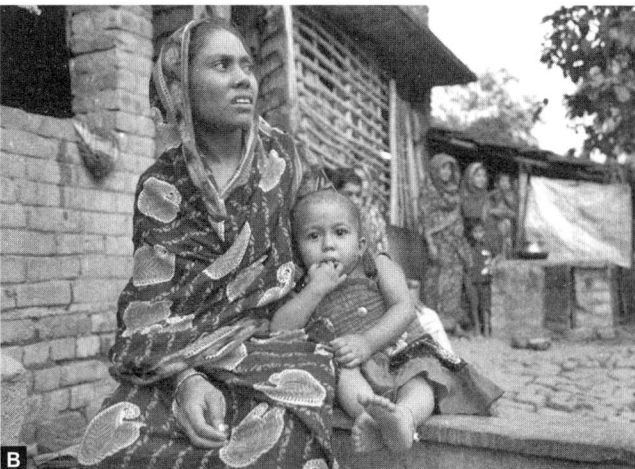

**Figs. 17B.8A and B:** Last cases of wild poliovirus in India: (A) Map showing last cases of polio; (B) Rukhsar Khatoon, last case of WPV in India (Jan 2011) with her mother (Shahpur village, West Bengal).

It is of three serotypes. They differ in capsid protein:
1. Type 1 is the most common wild type responsible of causing epidemics.
2. Type 2 is the most antigenic and cause endemic infection.
3. Type 3 is the most common cause for VAPP, and mostly associated with Sabin OPV.

Immunity to one serotype does not confer immunity to other two serotypes.

## Environmental Factors

Polio cases are more predominant in rainy season, appropriately 60% cases occur from the month of June to September. Contaminated water, food, and flies; poor sanitary conditions and overcrowding are favorable conditions for exposure of infection.

## Reservoir

Man (subclinical cases). There is no chronic carrier state. It is estimated that for one polio case there will be 1,000 subclinical cases in children and 75 in adults.

## Infective Material

Stools and oropharyngeal secretions of infected human being.

## Period of Communicability

Period of Communicability 7–10 days before and after onset of paralysis.

## Mode of Transmission

It is transmitted from person to person through feco-oral route. The virus is excreted in faeces for more than two months after infection with maximum occurring just before paralysis and during the first two weeks after the onset of paralysis.

*Clinical:* Subclinical ratio is one clinical case can cause 1,000 subclinical cases in children and 75 in adults.

*Clinical features:* Nonparalytic poliomyelitis presents with stiffness and pain in the neck and back it last for 2–20 days.

*Paralytic poliomyelitis:* Fever at the time paralysis suggestive of polio, malaise, anorexia, nausea, vomiting, sore throat, headache, constipation, stiffness in the neck and back muscles.

*Site:* Anterior horn cells of spinal cord.

*Earliest change in neuron:* Nissl body degeneration.

## CLINICAL TYPES

- 91–96% constitute in apparent infections,
- 4–8% cause abortive infection, and
- <1% cause paralytic cases.

Paralytic polio is further classified into:
- Spinal (80%)
- Bulbospinal (20%)
- Bulbar paralysis (2%)

In nonparalytic infections, the manifestations are fever, headache, nausea, diarrhea, and vomiting. In paralytic infections, these manifestations are accompanied by asymmetric acute flaccid paralysis of descending type, involving proximal muscles more than distal muscles.

*Diagnosis:* Virus can be isolated from blood sample within 3–5 days after manifestation of fever and in stools from first week till eight weeks of infection but ideally within two weeks. Virus can also be isolated from throat swab and CSF samples. Real time PCR is used for identification of the organism.

## WHY POLIO CAN BE ERADICATED? – REASONS

- Potent vaccine
- Only reservoir of infection is man
- Virus cannot survive in environment for >48 hours
- Availability of Rapid Response Team.

In 1988, World Health Assembly resoluted to eradicate Polio by end of the year 2000. India launched National Polio Eradication Program in the year 1995.

## Program includes

1. *Routine immunization:* To achieve and maintain high level of coverage for OPV about 85% and above.
2. *Pulse polio immunization (PPI):* Pulse polio immunization program was launched in India in the year 1995. Mass administration of OPV on a single day to children less than three years of age irrespective of the previous immunization status, first round of vaccine was administered on 9th December 1995 and 20th January 1996. Later, WHO recommended the age group 0–5 years under pulse polio immunization. The success of PPI was seen as a reduction in cases from 35,000 annually in 1995 to nil case in India.
3. *AFP surveillance:* To identify and report all cases of acute flaccid paralysis (AFP).
4. *Mopping up round:* Mass supplementary immunization activities (SIA) are organized to immunize all children aged 0–5 years.
5. *Protection of high-risk population:* Children belonging to migrant population, slums, construction sites, and brick-kilns.

## POLIO VACCINE

*Storage:* OPV is stored at –20°C and IPV at 2–8°C in cold chain.

*VAPP (Vaccine-associated paralytic poliomyelitis):* These polio cases are due to Sabin OPV vaccine. They occur in OPV recipients and their close contacts due to feco-oral transmission. They do not cause outbreak. About one case per 2.5 million doses of OPV and most commonly occur with 1st dose of OPV **(Table 17B.10)**.

**Table 17B.10:** Differences between Sabin and Salk vaccine.

| Vaccine characteristics | |
|---|---|
| **Salk (killed vaccine)** | **Sabin (live attenuated vaccine)** |
| Injectable form/IM | Oral form/oral drops |
| Composition = 80 units Type 1: 40 units; type 2: 8 units; type 3: 32 units | Composition Type 1: 3 lakhs; type 2: 1 lakh; type 3: 3 lakhs |
| 4 doses, first 3 doses with 1–2 months gap followed by booster dose at 6–12 months gap | 5 doses with one zero dose at birth followed by booster dose at 6–24 months |
| 80–90% efficient | 90–100% efficient |
| Slow immune response | Fast immune response |
| Short duration of protection | Long lasting |
| No herd immunity | Herd immunity present |
| Can precipitate paralysis | Can be used safely |

(IM: intramuscular)

# SWITCH

## Introduction

World Health Assembly in 2012 declared the completion of poliovirus eradication to be a "programmatic emergency for global public health". Polio End Game Strategy (2013–2018) was approved by WHO executive body in 2013, for removal of oral polio vaccine in phased manner to prevent vaccine derived paralytic poliomyelitis. WHO recommended introduction of at least one dose of IPV into all OPV using countries into their routine immunization scheduled.

As per latest WHO report over 90% of cVDPV cases and approximately 40% of VAPP cases are due to the type 2 component of tOPV.

The long-term strategy of endgame strategy is complete removal of OPVs and replacement of it by IPVs which is initiated with a switch from tOPV to bOPV to mOPV followed by complete replacement of OPVs by IPVs.

## Definition

Replacement of trivalent tOPV with bOPV, by removing type 2 strain from the trivalent oral polio vaccine, and with the introduction of one dose of IPV before withdrawal of type 2 strain from tOPV is called switch.

Primary objectives of the switch:
- Successfully recall tOPV and introduce bOPV in April 2016
- Successful disposal of the tOPV.
- All children should be vaccinated before switch
- Validate that country is free of tOPV.

All OPV using countries and territories should switch within a two weeks of window period, i.e. from 18 April to 1 May.

Globally synchronizing the switch reduces the re-emergence of polio cases due to type 2cVDPV.

Key dates for switch is described in **Table 17B.11**.

**Table 17B.11:** Key dates for switch.

| May 2015 | World Health Assembly endorsement of the process and tentative timelines |
|---|---|
| September 2015 | Finalization of national switch plan |
| October 2015 | Strategic advisory group of experts (SAGE) were assigned to assess the epidemiology of persistence of the type 2cVDPVs and confirm the switch date |
| December 2015 | Introduction of at least one dose of IPV into the routine immunization in all countries |
| April 2016 | SWITCH: Replace tOPV with bOPV globally and tOPV should not be used RIs and SIA in any country |
| May 2016 | Disposal of tOPV and validation of switch day by each country within two weeks of switch |

(SAGE: strategic advisory group of experts; IPV: inactivated polio vaccine; OPV: oral polio vaccines; SIA: supplementary immunization activities; RI: routine immunization)

## National Validation Day

Two weeks after switch day all countries will schedule a validation day.
- All tOPV must be fully disposed of as soon as possible after the switch day **(Fig. 17B.9)**.

# AFP SURVEILLANCE

Acute flaccid paralysis (AFP) is defined as sudden onset of weakness and floppiness in any part of body in a child <15 years of age or paralysis in a person of any age in whom polio is suspected. All cases of AFP among children <15 years of age should be reported and tested for wild polio virus or VDPV within 48 hours of onset. Active surveillance is done to detect circulation of polio virus by reporting all cases of AFP and investigating these cases for polio to ensure rapid response in the locality to interrupt the transmission. In India, AFP surveillance for polio started in the year 1997 by establishing National Polio Surveillance Project (NPSP) in collaboration with WHO and GOI.

## Objectives

- The primary objective is to recognize and report AFP cases at the earliest and to ensure prompt outbreak immunization response with OPV.
- The second objective is to confirm the cases of wild polio virus through isolation of virus in the stool samples.

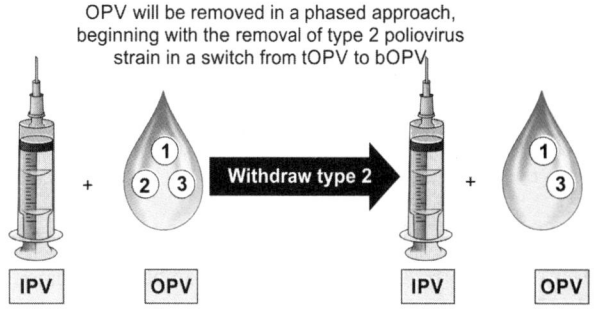

**Fig. 17B.9:** Switching of tOPV to bOPV.

- The third objective is to measure the impact of routine immunization and PPI in India.

All the districts in India should report AFP cases. AFP rates of at least one case per 1,00,000 population of children below 15 years of age per year should be achieved by each district. This measures the quality and adequacy of AFP surveillance.

### Steps for AFP Surveillance

The steps for AFP surveillance are shown in **Flowchart 17B.2**.

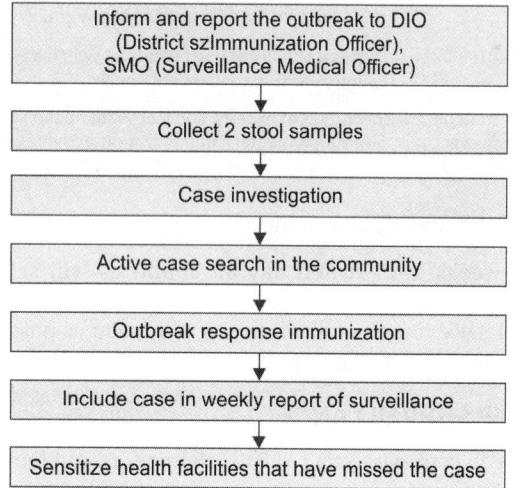

**Flowchart 17B.2:** Steps for AFP surveillance.

#### Stool Sample Collection

Two stool samples are collected at least 24 hours apart from suspected AFP case. The results are good when samples are collected within two weeks of onset of paralysis up to two months. The specimen should be of eight grams or thumb size in amount in a sterile container. Samples should be transported by maintaining reverse cold chain to the laboratory.

## PREVENTION

### Pulse Polio Immunization

Simultaneous and mass administration of OPV in a single day to all children of less than 5 years irrespective of their previous OPV coverage. These are considered as extra doses and does not replace the doses of national immunization schedule.

### Travel Advice

WHO's International Travel and Health recommends that all travelers to polio affected areas be fully vaccinated against polio and for residents (visitors more than four weeks) from infected areas should receive an additional dose of OPV or IPV within 4 weeks to 12 months of travel.

## END GAME STRATEGIC PLAN (2013–2018)

The strategies under end game strategic plan has been listed in **Table 17B.12**.

**Table 17B.12:** End game strategic plan (2013–2018).

| Goal | Strategies |
|---|---|
| Mass immunization at risk groups | • Routine immunization systems strengthening<br>• National and subnational immunization days<br>• IPV introduction<br>• Community engagement and social mobilization |
| Surveillance | • Outbreak response and mop-ups<br>• Stockpiles for emergency response<br>• Acute flaccid paralysis surveillance<br>• Environmental surveillance<br>• New diagnostics and special studies |
| Withdrawal of polio strain 2 | Cessation type 2 polio |
| Polio free certification | Bio-containment of residual polioviruses |
| | Certification of eradication and containment |

(IPV: inactivated polio vaccine)

### Objectives of End Game Strategic Plan

- Detection and interruption of all poliovirus transmission.
- Strengthen immunization systems, introduce IPV and withdraw oral polio OPV.
- Containment and certification.
- Plan polio legacy:
  - Polio detection and interruption
    - To stop all wild polio virus transmission by end of 2014
    - Strengthen global surveillance.
  - Strengthening immunization system
    - Maintain appropriate SIA schedule
    - Enhance OPV campaign quality
    - Enhance safety of OPV operations
    - Prevent and respond to polio outbreak.

  **December 2015:** Introduction of IPV into routine immunization program.
  **April 2016:** All nations should *switch from tOPV to bOPV* in two weeks' duration by observing National Switch Day in this period.
  **May 2016:** All tOPV disposed.
  **2019:** Administering IPV only, complete withdrawal of OPV.

  - Implementing containment of polio viruses and to certify world as polio free

  The primary requirements for certifying a WHO region as free of WPV are:
    - Absence of any WPV for a minimum of three years in all countries of the region
    - Presence of certification-standard surveillance in all countries during that three-year period
    - Completion of phase I biocontainment activities for all facility-based WPV stocks.
  - *Legacy planning:* The infrastructure, funds, manpower, knowledge, and experience acquired through polio program will be utilized for other health programs.

## Rehabilitation

Surgeries, calipers, physiotherapy.

Rehabilitation center for polio patients was started in 1992 at Kodaikanal situated in south India, polio home and orthotic workshop.

Calipers like *polio leg braces*.

## POLIO END GAME STRATEGY (2019–2023)

| Continue | Improve | Innovate |
|---|---|---|
| **GOAL 1:** Eradication | | |
| • Immunization campaign<br>• Stockpile management<br>• AFP and environmental surveillance | • Community engagement<br>• Accountability and supportive management, surge capacity<br>• Environmental surveillance network<br>• Communication for eradication | • Regional support to endemic countries.<br>• Expanded age groups for supplementary immunization activities<br>• Rapid respond team for outbreak<br>• Invest in antivirals and new IPV |
| **GOAL 2:** Integration | | |
| Delivery of bOPV and IPV as a part of National immunization schedules | • Integration of polio surveillance with VPD surveillance<br>• Engagement with CSOs for better reach in the communities<br>• Joint delivery and enhanced coordination between polio and other VPDs and SIAs. | • MoU formulation between WHO emergency programme and GPEI to harmonize outbreak and emergency response.<br>• Systematic collaboration between GAVI and immunization partners for joint accountability.<br>• Strengthening of immunization system in all outbreak responses.<br>• Harmonized data systems: POLIS and WIISE |
| **GOAL 3:** Certification and Containment | | |
| • Certification processes.<br>• Polio virus essential facility certification process<br>• National containment surveys and inventories. | • Containment guidance<br>• Communication (including VDPV plans).<br>• Data quality metrics | Introduction of genetically stable vaccine strains to eliminate the need to use and retain live poliovirus. |

(CSOs: Civil Society Organizations; VDP: vaccine preventable diseases; POLIS: polio information system; VPDV: vaccine derived polio virus; WIISE: WHO Immunization information system; MoU: memorandum of understanding; GAVI: Global Alliance for Vaccines and Immunization)

## POLIO ERADICATION STRATEGY 2022–2026: DELIVERING ON A PROMISE (FIG. 17B.10)

Before the emergence of COVID-19, polio was considered to be one of the most challenging infectious diseases of international concern, despite the consistent efforts of the Global Polio Eradication Initiative (GPEI) program to vaccinate every child in the endemic countries, Pakistan and Afghanistan. In June 2021, the GPEI launched a revised and strengthened plan 'Polio Eradication Strategy 2022–2026: Delivering on a Promise', replacing the previous plan from 2019 to 2023, to overcome the continuing challenges in polio eradication.

While polio cases have fallen 99.9% since 1988, polio remains a Public Health Emergency of International Concern (PHEIC) and persistent barriers to reaching every child with polio vaccines and the pandemic have contributed to an increase in polio cases. In 2020, 1226 cases of all forms of polio were recorded compared to 138 in 2018.

In 2020, the GPEI paused polio door-to-door campaigns for four months to protect communities from the spread of COVID-19 and contributed up to 30,000 program staff and over $100 million in polio resources to support pandemic response in almost 50 countries.

Leaders from the two countries yet to interrupt wild polio transmission—Pakistan and Afghanistan—called for renewed global solidarity and the continued resources necessary to eradicate this vaccine-preventable disease. They committed to strengthening their partnership with GPEI to improve vaccination campaigns and engagement with communities at high risk of polio.

The GPEI is committed to an integrated approach to program implementation that enables countries to fully leverage existing polio program assets and serve the health needs of vulnerable communities.

## SUMMARY

❖ Poliomyelitis (polio) is an acute communicable disease of humans caused by poliovirus of serotypes 1, 2 or 3.
❖ Mode of transmission of disease is fecal-oral and/or oral-oral mode of transmission, depending on standard of sanitation.
❖ Globally, the last case of poliomyelitis caused by naturally circulating WPV type 2 (WPV2) occurred in India in 1999. Global eradication of WPV2 was certified in 2015.
❖ No case due to WPV type 3 (WPV3) has been detected since 10 November 2012.
❖ No specific anti-viral drugs are available for poliomyelitis.
❖ For primary prevention, two types of poliovirus vaccines are available: live attenuated oral poliovirus vaccine and inactivated poliovirus vaccine.
❖ WHO no longer recommends an OPV-only vaccination schedule. For all countries currently using OPV only, at least 1 dose of IPV should be added to the schedule.
❖ Travelers to infected areas should be vaccinated according to their national schedules.
❖ All healthcare workers worldwide should have completed a full course of primary vaccination against poliomyelitis.

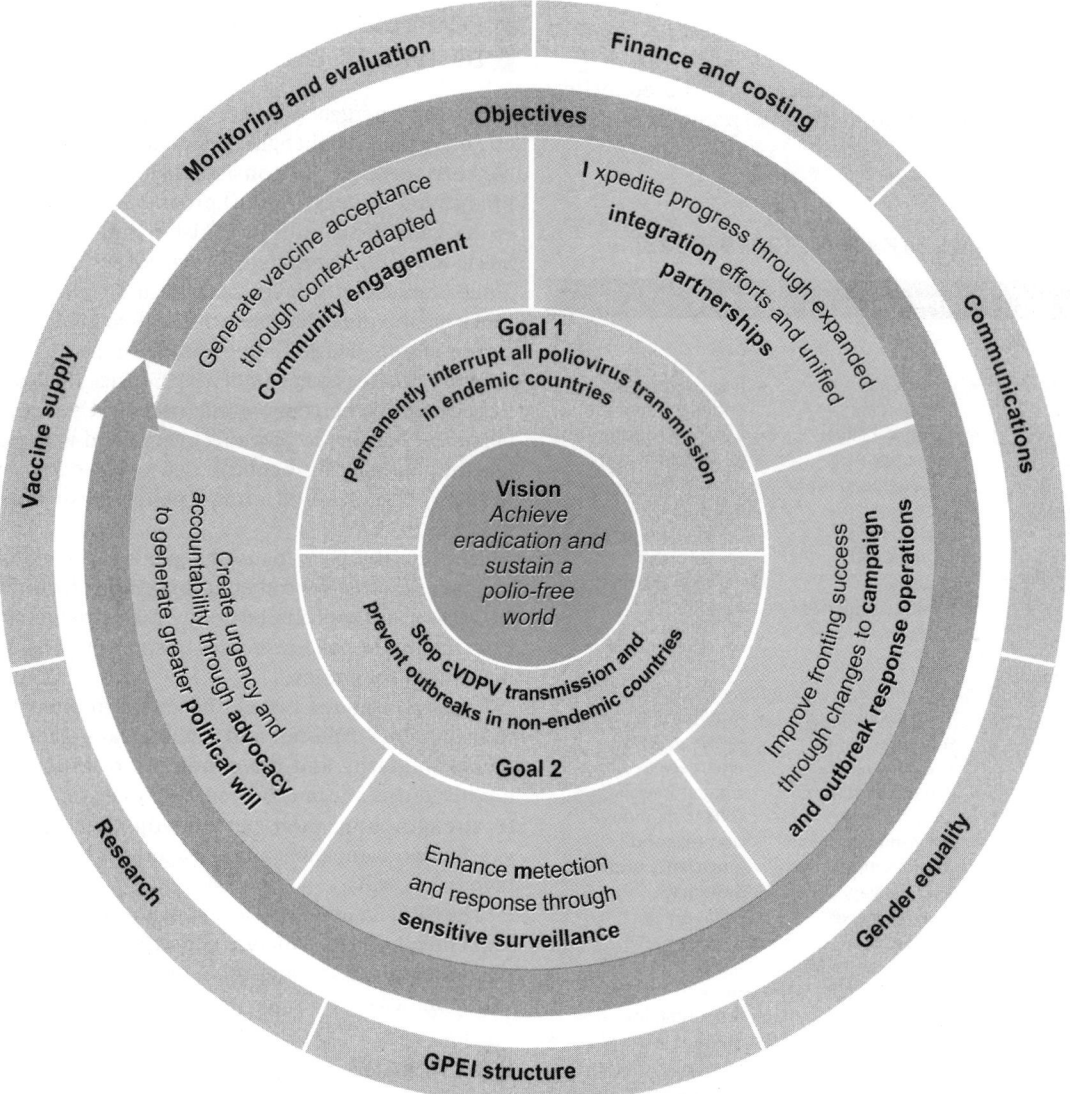

Fig. 17B.10: Polio Eradication Strategy 2022–2026 strategic framework.

## SUGGESTED READING

1. Cliff A, Smallman-Raynor M. Oxford Textbook of Infectious Disease Control. Oxford: Oxford University Press; 2009.
2. Global polio eradication initiative. Polio-free India: It seemed impossible until it was done available from https://polioeradication.org/news-post/polio-free-india-it-seemed-impossible-until-it-was-done/#:~:text=On%2013%20January%202023%2C%20India,genuine%20commitment%20at%20all%20levels.
3. Polio Eradication Strategy 2022-2026: Delivering on a promise) Published by the World Health Organization (WHO) on behalf of the Global Polio Eradication Initiative (GPEI).
4. UNICEF Polio Transition and Post-Certification Management Plan. New York; 2015.
5. WHO, Fact Sheets: Poliomyelitis July 22; Polioeradication. org, Endemic Countries.
6. WHO. Countries reaffirm commitment to ending polio at launch of new eradication strategy, June 2021.
7. WHO. Report on polio transition planning surveillance of AFP. Geneva: WHO; 2012. World health assembly (WHA) Global polio eradication initiative; 1988 report.

## EPIDEMIOLOGY OF CHOLERA AND ITS PREVENTION AND CONTROL

*Bhavani Kenche, Jyothi Lakshmi Naga Vemuri, Arundhathi B, Bhavana Laxmi Surity*

*There is Strength in Unity. Let us Help One Another Fight Against Cholera!*
—CDC

| CM7.2 | Enumerate, describe and discuss the mode of transmission and measures for prevention and control of cholera |
|---|---|
| CM8.1 | Describe and discuss the epidemiological and control measures applicable in cholera |
| CM8.4 | Describe the principles and enumerate the measures to control a cholera epidemic |

*Case Scenario*

On 14 November 2003, a primary health center in Dhenkanal district, Orissa, Eastern India, reported a cluster of acute, severe diarrhea with dehydration among adults in the village of Parbatia to the district public-health authorities. The population of the village in 2003 was 946. Cholera was suspected in the diagnosis. On 15 November 2003, an epidemiologist was assigned to the state of Orissa initiated an investigation and arrived in the village in the morning to investigate the outbreak. Forty cases were identified among the 946 residents of the village. There were no deaths. Of the 40 case-patients, 29% had vomiting, 47% had abdominal pain, and 32% had dehydration. None had blood in stools or fever. 64% of the cases could be reasonably attributed to the contaminated well as cases were clustered around an unprotected well located close to the residence of the index case, and for the remaining case-patients, we did not have any specific explanation. However, a certain amount of person-to-person transmission may have occurred towards the second part of the outbreak. Rectal swabs grew V. cholerae El Tor O1, serotype Ogawa confirming the epidemic as cholera.

*Source:* Amitav D, et al. J Health Popul Nutr. 2009;27(5):646–51.

## INTRODUCTION

Cholera is an acute bacterial infection of small intestine caused by *Vibrio cholerae (V. cholerae)* which manifest as profuse, painless, watery diarrhea. It has high potential of rapid spread leading to public health problem. Cholera has re-emerged as a major disease in recent past with a global increase in its incidence. It accounts for 5% of total diarrheal diseases in India.

In 1781, the disease entered Calcutta and there was high mortality and nearly a thousand people died within a short span. Those who witnessed these outbreaks regarded them as evidence of divine anger. The cholera epidemic of 1817 originated in district of Jessore in August of that year and shortly spread to an alarming extent in Calcutta and western and central districts of Bengal.

For centuries, cholera has been one of the most feared diseases. Even today, it remains a global threat to public health and one of the key indicators of social development. It remains a challenge in those countries where access to safe water and adequate sanitation cannot be guaranteed for all.

## PROBLEM STATEMENT

It is estimated that each year there are 1.3 million to 4.0 million cases of cholera, and 21,000 to 143,000 deaths worldwide due to cholera. Worldwide spread of cholera began in the year 1817, and by 1823 the first pandemic of cholera had spread from the Ganges river delta to much of Asia and Africa. Five periods of pandemic spread occurred before 1990 that is 1817–1823; 1826–1837; 1846–1862; 1864–1875; and 1887–1896. All these pandemics were due to *V. cholerae* classic strain and the case fatality rate was about 50%. Sixth pandemic occurred in 1902–1923 in Asia and seventh pandemic occurred during 1961–1980. These are due to *V. cholerae el tor* strain (WHO, Fact Sheets: March 2022: Cholera) **(Fig. 17B.11)**.

Description of cholera epidemics in India from late 18th century suggests that Bengal region of India and Bangladesh has been a continuous endemic region for cholera. The Indian subcontinent reported 23% of all cases notified from Asia, with India notifying a total of 2,635 cases and 3 deaths. According to National Health Profile 2019, India had 651 cases and 6 deaths from Cholera in 2018.

There were 565 reported outbreaks between 2011 and 2020 that led to 45,759 cases and 263 deaths. Outbreaks occurred throughout the year; however, they exploded with monsoons (June through September). In Tamil Nadu, a typical peak of cholera outbreaks was observed from December to January. Seventy-two percent of outbreak-related cases were reported in five states, namely Maharashtra, West Bengal, Punjab, Karnataka, and Madhya Pradesh.

National Institute of Cholera and other Enteric Diseases (NICED) located at Kolkata performs research and develop strategies for treatment, prevention and control of enteric infections.

## EPIDEMIOLOGY

### Host Factors

***Age:*** Cholera can affect all age groups of individuals.

***Sex:*** Both male and female sex is equally affected.

***Immunity:*** Individuals with lower immunity such as malnourished children or people living with AIDS are at greater risk of death if infected by cholera.

The incidence of cholera is high in low socioeconomic families due to poor hygiene practices.

### Agent Factors

Cholera is caused by bacteria *V. cholerae*. Koch first isolated vibrio from stools of patient with cholera in 1883. It is small curved (comma shaped) actively motile aerobic Gram-negative

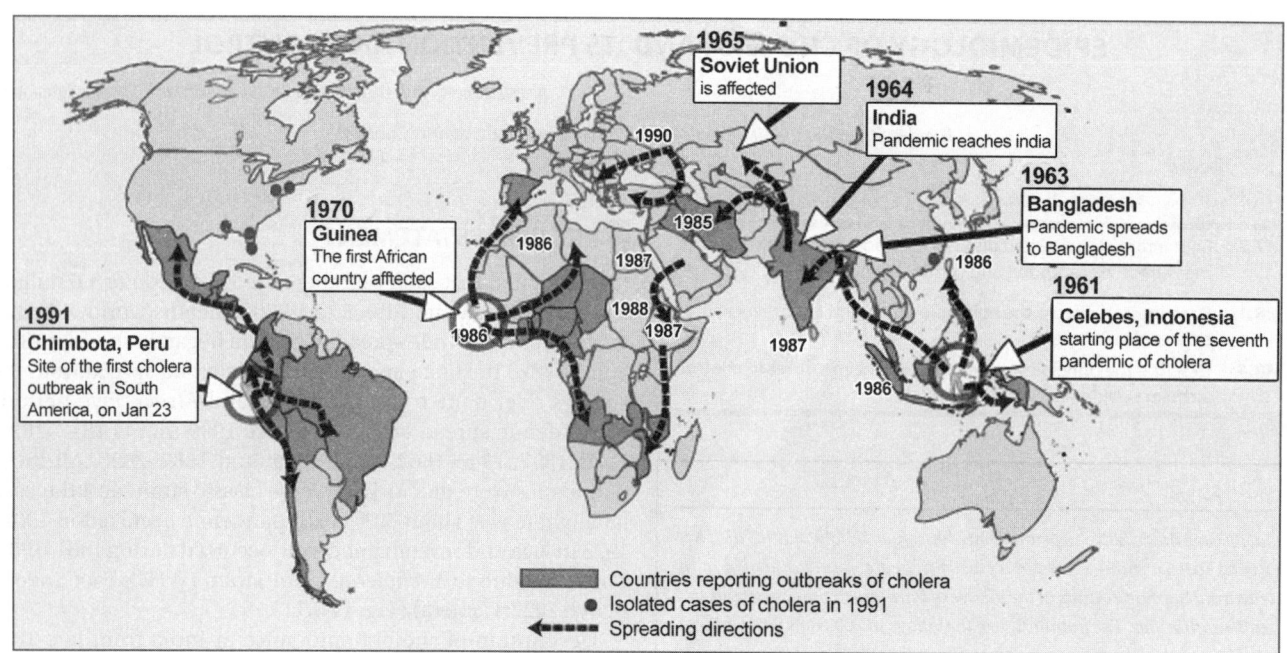

**Fig. 17B.11:** Worldwide distribution of cholera cases.

bacilli and non-sporing organism. It produces enterotoxin that disrupts the ion transport by intestinal epithelial cells.

***Serotypes:*** Three serotypes have been identified namely *V. cholerae* classic, *V. cholera el tor* and *V. cholerae* O139. After cholera outbreak in 1970 by classic *V. cholerae* hardly any classical strain has been isolated in India after 1980. *V. cholera el tor* has replaced old *V. cholerae* classic strain. El tor serotype is further classified into three sub-types namely Inaba, Ogawa and Hikojima. *V. cholerae* O139 Bengal emerged as a new strain of cholera in Madras in 1992.

Cholera due to El tor biotype differs from classical cholera **(Table 17B.13)**.

**Table 17B.13:** Differences between classic strain and el tor strain.

| Classic V. cholerae | V. cholerae el tor |
| --- | --- |
| Low incidence of mild and asymptomatic cases | High incidence of mild and asymptomatic cases |
| More secondary cases | Few secondary cases |
| Chronic carrier state is less | Occurrence of chronic carriers are more |
| Less resistant | More resistant and survive for longer duration in environment |
| Shorter duration of epidemics | Epidemics last longer |

### Environmental Factors

***Seasons:*** Incidence of cholera cases are seen more during monsoon seasons when the contamination of food and water with fecal matter is more common.

***Rain:*** Breeding of house flies is more during rainy season and spread of cholera from one person to other person increases as they act as vehicles for transmitting the infective material.

***Social factors:*** Cholera and poverty follow same distribution. Other social factors like urbanization, migration, overcrowding where there are low standards of personal hygiene and poor quality of life also play a key role in causing the disease.

***Safe drinking water:*** Spread of cholera is inherently linked with safe water supply. Consumption of water contaminated with *V. cholerae* will cause the disease.

***Sanitation:*** Risk of cholera incidence is more in places where the sanitation conditions are poor due to shedding back of bacteria into the environment which is a source of further potential infection.

***Physical:*** The *V. cholerae* is sensitive to acidity and drying, and commercially prepared acidic (pH 4.5 or less) or dried foods are therefore without risk.

***Temperature:*** Low temperatures limit proliferation of the organism and thus may prevent the level of contamination from reaching an infective dose. Gamma irradiation and temperatures above 70°C also destroy the vibrio.

### Reservoir of Infection

Man is the only reservoir for cholera. Both cases and carriers act as source of infection. The ratio of severe cases to mild or in apparent infections has been shown to be about 1:5 for classical cholera and 1:25 to 1:100 for El tor cholera.

***Carrier state:*** Carriers in cholera are of four types, viz. incubatory carriers, convalescent carriers, healthy carriers, and contact carriers. Person who has recovered from cholera infection may continue to excrete bacteria in stools for 2–3 weeks. In patients who are not effectively treated with antibiotics may also act as carrier. Majority of *V. cholerae* El tor and *V. cholerae* O139 are asymptomatic. They are responsible for carrier state.

***Infective material:*** Stools and vomitus of cases and carriers.

## Mode of Transmission

In 1853, John Snow described transmission of cholera was due to contaminated water with fecal matter in London. Transmission occurs from man to man through feco-oral route. Portal of entry is oral and portal of exit is fecal matter.

Ingestion of contaminated food and water with fecal matter causes cholera. It also occurs due to direct contact with contaminated fingers while handling excreta and vomitus of patients.

## Incubation Period

Cholera has short incubation period that is 12 hours to 5 days for development of symptoms. According to international health regulatory (IHR) 5 days of quarantine period has to be followed to prevent infection.

## Period of Communicability

Bacteria are present in their feces for 1–10 days after infection and are shed back into the environment, potentially infecting other people.

## PATHOPHYSIOLOGY

Produces protein enterotoxin which acts on mucosal epithelial cells of intestine. The toxin combines with substances in the epithelial cell membrane called gangliosides and this binds the vibrio to the cell wall irreversibly. This increases the activity of adenylate cyclase in the intestinal mucosa resulting in increased CAMP levels which inhibit NaCl absorption by villus cells and secretion of chloride and bicarbonate by secretory cells in the crypts of Liberkhun **(Fig. 17B.12)**.

## CLINICAL FEATURES

The severity of cholera is determined by duration of fluid loss. A typical case of cholera shows three stages.

### Stage of Evacuation

The onset is abrupt with profuse, painless, watery diarrhea followed by vomiting. The patient may pass as many as 40 stools in a day. Patient passes clear fluid with flakes of mucus called rice watery stools. They are non-offensive, sometimes fishy odor.

### Stage of Collapse

Signs and symptoms are due to loss of large volume of isotonic fluid. The classical signs are sunken eyes, hollow cheeks, scaphoid abdomen, sub-normal temperature, Washerman's hands and feet, absent pulse, unrecordable blood pressure, loss of skin elasticity, and shallow and quick respiration. The urinary output decreases and may ultimately cease. The patient becomes restless, and complains of intense thirst and cramps in legs and abdomen. Death may occur at this stage, due to dehydration and acidosis resulting from diarrhea.

### Stage of Recovery

The patient begins to show signs of clinical improvement. The blood pressure begins to rise, the temperature returns to normal and urine output is re-established. If anuria persists, the patient may die of renal failure.

Symptoms subside spontaneously within 2–7 days.

## DIAGNOSIS

Clinical features are obvious and suggest of cholera. Lab diagnosis is made to confirm diagnosis by detecting vibrio in stool samples. However, treatment should not be delayed till laboratory results.

### Stool Sample Collection

Fresh stool sample (cotton-tipped rectal swab soaked in liquid stool, placed in a sterile plastic bag) is collected from suspected patient before giving antibiotics and transported in media like Venkatraman-Ramakrishnan (VR) media, alkaline peptone water, Cary-Blair medium that allow better conservation of samples and are used to transport to laboratory. Rectal swabs can also be used for diagnosis.

Recently developed dipstick method for the rapid detection of *Vibrio cholerae* serotype O139 from rectal swabs has been successfully used to diagnose cholera. This is likely to improve surveillance for cholera, especially in remote settings and during epidemic outbreaks **(Table 17B.14 and Fig. 17B.13)**.

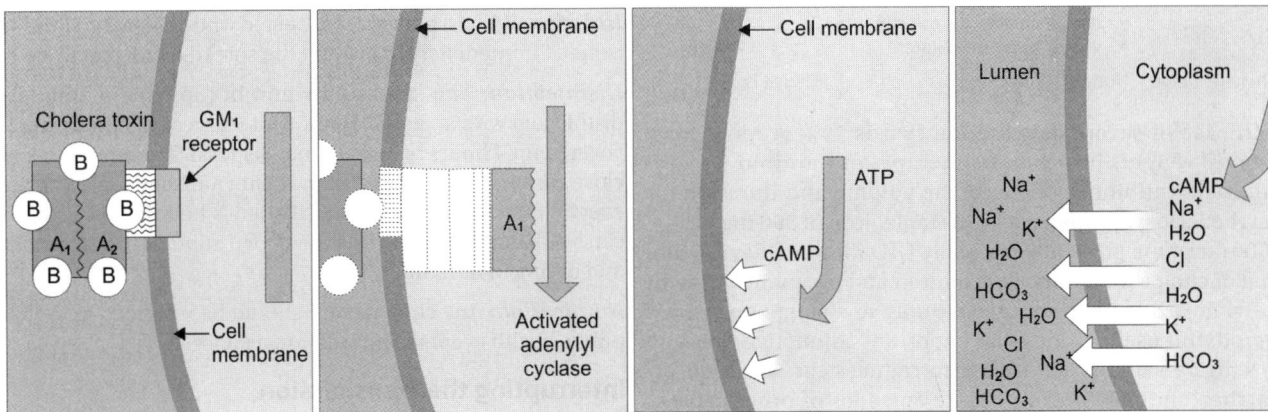

**Fig. 17B.12:** Mechanism of action of cholera toxin.

**Table 17B.14:** Types of culture media.

| Media | Name |
|---|---|
| Transport media | Venkatraman-Ramakrishna media<br>Alkaline peptone water<br>Cary-Blair media |
| Enrichment media | Tellurite media |
| Selective media | Thiosulfate Citrate Bile Salt Sucrose agar (TCBS) |

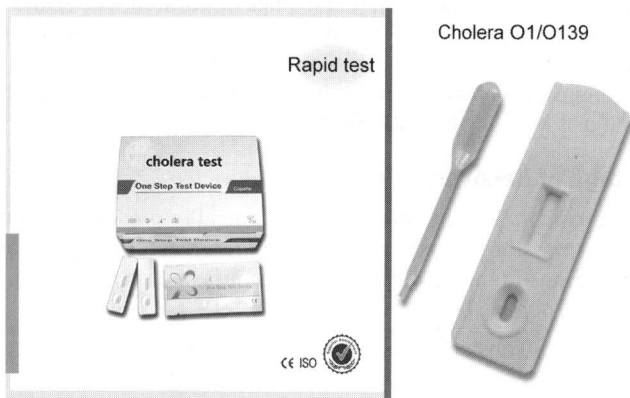

**Fig. 17B.13:** Rapid test for cholera.

## TREATMENT

Replacement and restoration of fluids and electrolytes is the main treatment. WHO recommends that use of oral rehydration solution (ORS) is the most suitable solution and nearly 80% of patients can be adequately treated **(Table 17B.15)**.

**Table 17B.15:** Classification and management of cholera.

| Dehydration stage | Signs | Treatment |
|---|---|---|
| Severe | • Lethargic, unconscious, floppy<br>• Very sunken eyes<br>• Drinks poorly, unable to drink<br>• Mouth, very dry<br>• Skin pinch goes back very slowly<br>• No tears (only for children) | IV therapy + antibiotics + ORS |
| Mild | • Restless and irritable<br>• Sunken eyes<br>• Dry mouth<br>• Thirsty, drinks eagerly<br>• Skin pinch goes back slowly<br>• No tears (only for children) | ORS + surveillance |
| No dehydration | None of the above signs | ORS at home |

In case of severe dehydration that is 10% or more loss of body weight, intravenous therapy and antibiotics are required. Antibiotics decrease the volume and duration of diarrhea. Doxycycline given in a single dose of 300 mg orally or Tetracycline given 500 mg orally QID for three days is the drug of choice for adults. For children and pregnant women, Co-trimoxazole 30 mg/kg given orally in a single dose, has been found useful. Zinc is an important adjunctive therapy for children under 5, which also reduces the duration of diarrhea and may prevent future episodes of other causes on acute watery diarrhea. If the child is breastfeeding, then it should be continued. Chemoprophylaxis (one dose of doxycycline) may be useful for members of a household who share food and shelter with a cholera patient.

## INVESTIGATION OF CHOLERA EPIDEMIC

Investigation of an epidemic is conducted if any increase in cases over the baseline in endemic areas or any single case reported in non-endemic areas.

*A case of cholera should be suspected when:*
- In an area where the disease is not known to be present, a patient aged 5 years or more develops severe dehydration or dies from acute watery diarrhea
- In an area where there is a cholera epidemic, a patient aged 5 years or more develops acute watery diarrhea, with or without vomiting.

*A case of cholera is confirmed when* V. cholerae O1 or O139 is isolated from any patient with diarrhea.

When an outbreak is suspected, an outbreak response team (ORT) or multidisciplinary team is convened to conduct the investigation in the field in order to confirm the outbreak and to take the first measures for controlling the spread of the disease.

A cholera emergency plan should list the essential elements of outbreak preparedness and response and should implement the control measures by providing safe water and ensuring safe disposal of excreta, and for education campaigns. Treatment of the source may be the best way to prevent the spread of cholera in the community. In emergencies, a free residual chlorine of about 0.5 mg/L is advisable.

Safe oral cholera vaccines should be used in conjunction with improvements in water and sanitation to control cholera outbreaks and for prevention in areas known to be high risk for cholera.

## PREVENTION AND CONTROL MEASURES

- Quick access to treatment, such as oral rehydration solution (ORS), which is used to successfully treat most cases, and intravenous fluids and antibiotics for severe cases.
- Enhanced epidemiological and laboratory surveillance to identify endemic areas and detect, confirm, and quickly respond to outbreaks.
- Community engagement for behavioral changes and improved hygiene practices.

### Controlling Source/Reservoir

*Isolation:* When a person is suspected with cholera he should be isolated immediately to prevent the spread of infection.

*Disinfection:* The stool and vomit of the patient should be disinfected with an equal quantity of 5% cresol solution and left covered for 4 hours before its final disposal. The attendants and close contacts should wash hands with antiseptic solution after every contact with the patient. Patient's bedding and clothing can be disinfected by stirring them for 5 minutes in boiling water and drying in the sun.

*Notification:* Any cholera case should be informed to WHO of public health events of international concern.

### Interrupting the Transmission

Provision of safe water and sanitation is critical to control the transmission of cholera and other waterborne diseases.

## Safety of Food and Water

Control of food and water from contamination is the most important method of control of an outbreak.
- All food must be protected against flies. It is necessary to ensure that food is prepared, cooked, stored and served under clean conditions.
- Uncooked vegetables and fruits should always be washed and then soaked in disinfectant solution before peeling.
- Drinking water should be super chlorinated. Washing and bathing water should be chlorinated.

## Improvement of Environmental Sanitation

There is no end to cholera without basic water sanitation and hygienic practices. Improvement in water supply and sanitation can reduce cholera morbidity by 80-100%. Main aspects of environmental sanitation are adequate chlorination and protected water supply, proper disposal of night soil/sewage. Health education is important for improvement of personal hygiene that is hand washing practice after defecation and before eating, and elimination of open defecation will significantly reduce the incidence of diarrheal diseases. WASH (water, sanitation and hygiene) are the key interventions to reduce the burden of disease associated with outbreaks and are commonly implemented in emergency response.

## Protection of Susceptible Host

### Immunization

- **Whole cell killed vaccine:** Given parenterally, provides protection for five months, efficacy is only 50% and has significant side effects.
- **B-subunit whole cell killed vaccine:** Given orally in two doses at an interval of 1-6 weeks and has an efficacy of 50-60%. It provides herd immunity in endemic setting. Oral cholera vaccines (OCVs) are now being considered as complements to traditional preventive measures.

### Oral Cholera Vaccine

In 2013, WHO established the Global Oral Cholera Vaccine stockpile and received long-term support from GAVI, the Vaccine Alliance for use of OCV in epidemic and endemic settings. To date (May 2018) over 25M doses have been administered through mass vaccination campaigns in 19 countries since the stockpile was created in 2013. Cholera vaccine provides up to 65% protection for about five years in cholera endemic areas. The use of OCV is an additional tool to the classic cholera control measures. Administration of vaccine is recommended in endemic countries as well as during outbreaks and emergencies **(Table 17B.16 and Fig. 17B.14)**.

**Table 17B.16:** Prevention and control measures.

| 1. Controlling source/reservoir | Isolation |
| --- | --- |
| | Disinfection |
| | Notification |
| 2. Interrupting the transmission | Safety of food and water |
| | Improvement of environmental sanitation |
| 3. Protection of susceptible host | Immunization |

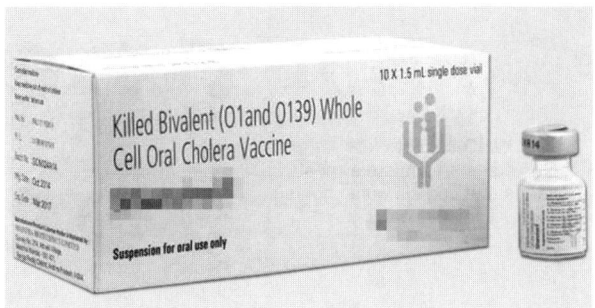

**Fig. 17B.14:** Oral cholera vaccine.

## CURRENT APPROACHES IN HEALTH CARE SERVICES

### Global Approach

- In 2016, WHO introduced the cholera kits which replaced the interagency diarrhea disease kit (IDDK). These cholera kits are used for preparedness and outbreak response. Each treatment kit provides enough material to treat 100 patients **(Fig. 17B.15)**.
- Cholera vaccination drive started during May-June 2018 with target of covering 2 million people across five African nations.
- WHO strategy "**Ending Cholera: A Global Roadmap to 2030**" was launched in 2017 with target to reduce cholera deaths by 90% and to eliminate cholera in as many as 20 countries by 2030 with the support of the global task force on cholera control (GTFCC). The Global Roadmap focuses on three strategic axes:
  1. Early detection and quick response to contain outbreaks: The strategy focuses on containing outbreaks—wherever they may occur—through early detection and rapid multisectoral response including community, engagement, strengthening surveillance and laboratory capacity, health systems and supply readiness, and supporting rapid response teams.
  2. A targeted multisectoral approach to prevent cholera recurrence: The strategy calls on countries and partners to focus on cholera "hotspots", the relatively small areas most heavily affected by cholera. Cholera transmission can be stopped in these areas through measures including improved WASH and through use of OCV.
  3. An effective mechanism of coordination for technical support, advocacy, resource mobilization, and partnership at local and global levels: The GTFCC provides a strong framework to support countries to intensify efforts to control cholera, building upon country-led cross-sectoral cholera control programs and supporting them with human, technical, and financial resources.
- A targeted multisectoral approach to prevent cholera recurrence with an effective mechanism of coordination for technical support, advocacy, resource mobilization, and partnership at local and global levels **(Fig. 17B.16)**.

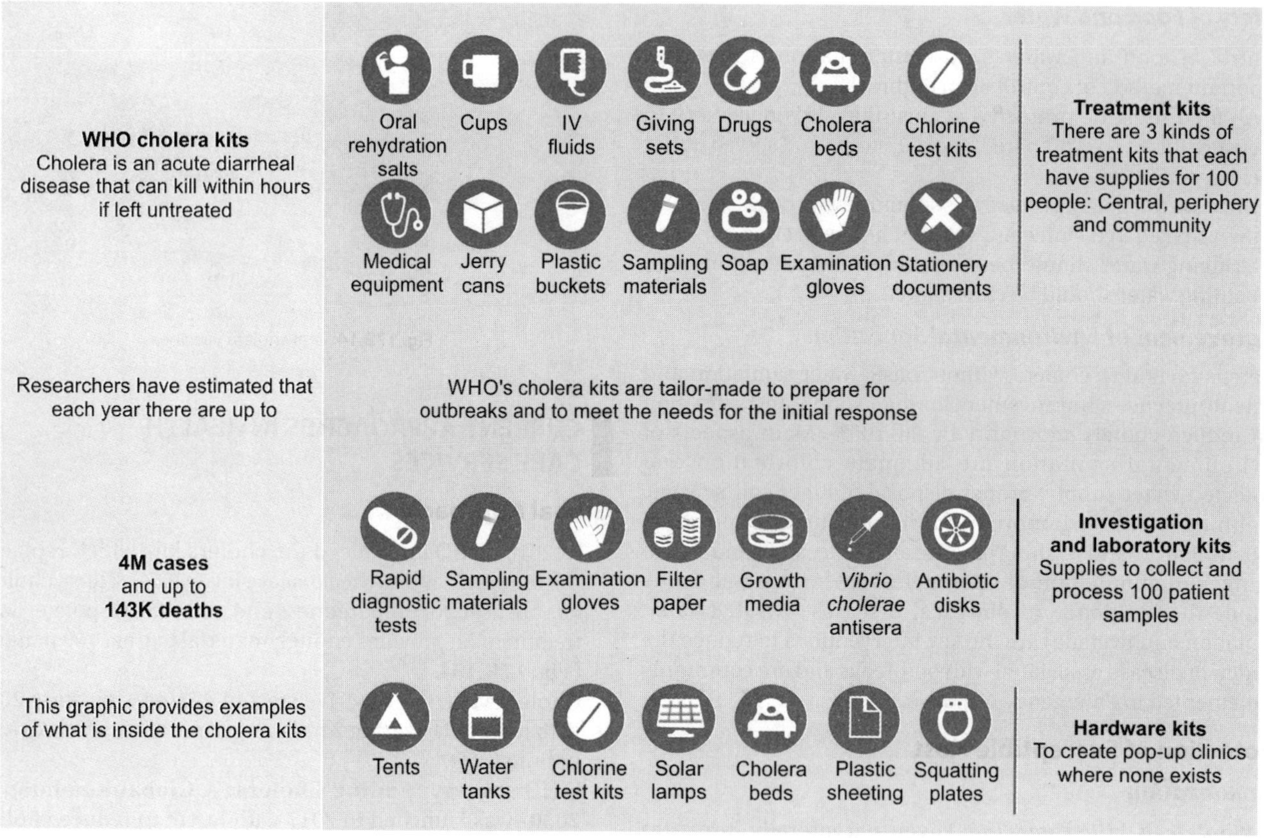

**Section 3:** Community Health Problems and Vulnerable Groups

**WHO cholera kits**
Cholera is an acute diarrheal disease that can kill within hours if left untreated

**Treatment kits**
There are 3 kinds of treatment kits that each have supplies for 100 people: Central, periphery and community

WHO's cholera kits are tailor-made to prepare for outbreaks and to meet the needs for the initial response

Researchers have estimated that each year there are up to

**4M cases** and up to **143K deaths**

**Investigation and laboratory kits**
Supplies to collect and process 100 patient samples

This graphic provides examples of what is inside the cholera kits

**Hardware kits**
To create pop-up clinics where none exists

Fig. 17B.15: Contents of cholera kit.

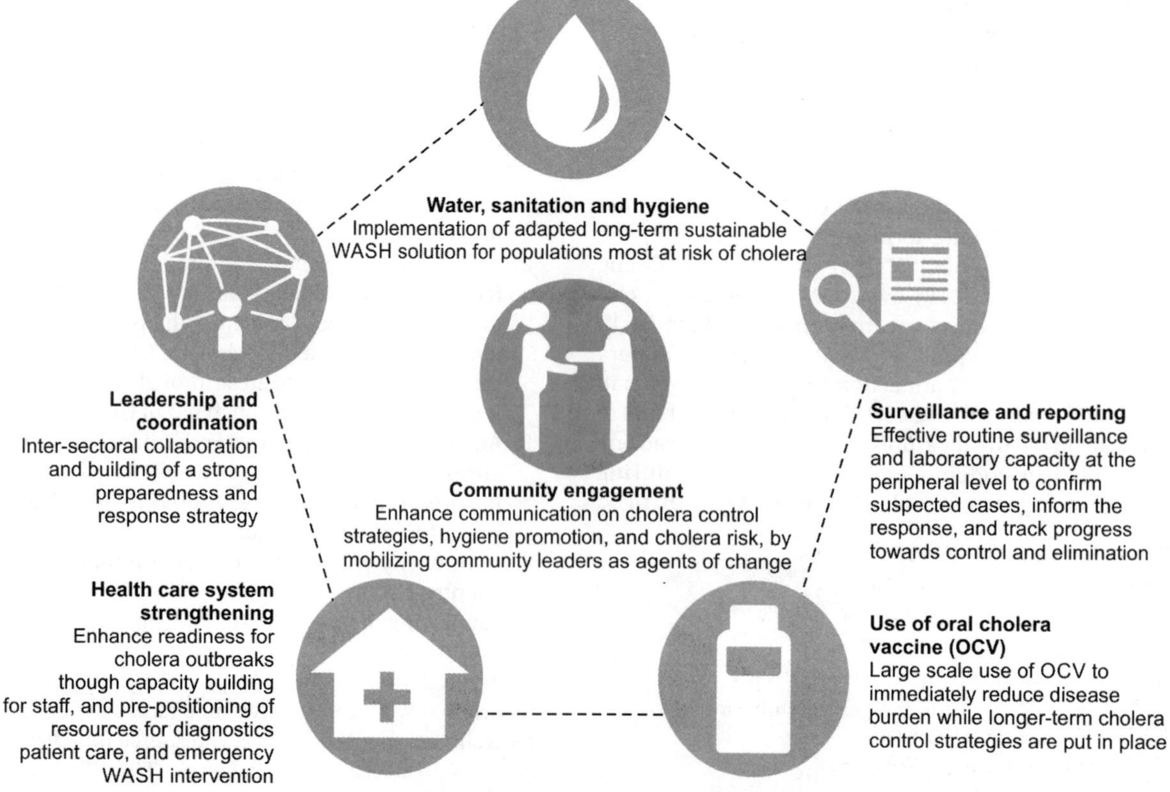

**Water, sanitation and hygiene**
Implementation of adapted long-term sustainable WASH solution for populations most at risk of cholera

**Leadership and coordination**
Inter-sectoral collaboration and building of a strong preparedness and response strategy

**Community engagement**
Enhance communication on cholera control strategies, hygiene promotion, and cholera risk, by mobilizing community leaders as agents of change

**Surveillance and reporting**
Effective routine surveillance and laboratory capacity at the peripheral level to confirm suspected cases, inform the response, and track progress towards control and elimination

**Health care system strengthening**
Enhance readiness for cholera outbreaks though capacity building for staff, and pre-positioning of resources for diagnostics patient care, and emergency WASH intervention

**Use of oral cholera vaccine (OCV)**
Large scale use of OCV to immediately reduce disease burden while longer-term cholera control strategies are put in place

Fig. 17B.16: Multisectoral interventions to end cholera.

## SUMMARY

- Cholera remains a major public health problem in developing countries.
- Cholera is caused by *V. cholerae* bacteria having 3 serotypes: *V. Cholera* classic, *V. Cholera El tor* and *V. Cholera* O139.
- Disease spreads from person-to-person by faeco-oral route through contaminated food and water and unhygienic environmental conditions.
- It manifests as profuse, painless, and watery diarrhea (rice watery stools). In severe stages, patient may collapse due to loss of large volume of isotonic fluids from body.
- Treatment constitutes replacement and restoration of fluids and electrolytes with ORS and IV fluids.
- WASH (water, sanitation, and hygiene) are the key interventions to reduce the burden of disease.
- Adequate chlorination and protected water supply and proper disposal of sewage can reduce the morbidity by 80–100%.
- In 2017, WHO launched "Ending Cholera: A Global Roadmap to 2030" with target to reduce cholera deaths by 90% and to eliminate cholera by 2030.

## SUGGESTED READING

1. Ali M, Lopez AL, You YA, et al. The global burden of cholera. Bull World Health Organ. 2012;90(3):209-18A.
2. Bengal Judicial Letter 114 129. (1817). Board's Collections, F/4/610, Asia Africa and Pacific Collections (APAC), British Library (BL).
3. Cholera prevention, control and elimination. A policy brief by the initiative against diarrheal and enteric diseases in Asia. Available from: http://www. idea-asia.info/index.php/component/search/?searchword=policy+brief&o rdering=&searchphrase= all.
4. Moore SM, Azman AS, Zaitchik BF, et al. El Niño and the shifting geography of cholera in Africa. Proc Natl Acad Sci. 2017;114(17): 4436-41.
5. Muzembo BA, Kitahara K, Debnath A, Ohno A, Okamoto K, Miyoshi SI. Cholera outbreaks in India, 2011–2020: A systematic review. International journal of environmental research and public health. 2022;19(9):5738.
6. Talavera A, Pérez EM. Is cholera disease associated with poverty? J Infect Dev Ctries. 2009;3(6):408-11.
7. World Health Organization. (2015). Cholera Kit 2015/Information Note. Available from: http://origin.who.int/cholera/kit/cholera-kit- information-note.pdf.
8. World Health Organization. Oral cholera vaccine stockpile. Available from: http://www.who.int/cholera/vaccines/ocv_stockpile_2013/ en/.
9. World Health Organization. The global task force on cholera control. Available from: http://www.who.int/cholera/task_force/en/.
10. WHO, Fact Sheets March 2022: Cholera. Available from: https://www. who. int/news-room/fact-sheets/detail/cholera

# EPIDEMIOLOGY OF ACUTE DIARRHEAL DISEASES AND ITS PREVENTION AND CONTROL

*Bhavani Kenche, Jyothi Lakshmi Naga Vemuri, Arundhathi B, Bhavana Laxmi Surity*

*"We shall not defeat any of the infectious diseases that plague the developing world until we have also won the battle for safe drinking water, sanitation, and basic health care".*

—Kofi Annan

| | |
|---|---|
| CM3.3 | Describe the etiology and basis of diarrheal diseases |
| CM7.2 | Enumerate, describe and discuss the mode of transmission and measures for prevention and control of acute diarrheal diseases |
| CM8.1 | Describe and discuss the epidemiological and control measures applicable in acute diarrheal diseases |
| CM8.4 | Describe the principles and enumerate the measures to control an acute diarrheal diseases epidemic |

### Case Scenario

*A 5-month-old girl presented to hospital with a 2-day history of watery diarrhea and fever developed in the 12 hours before admission. The infant was reported to have had 10 watery stools over the previous 24 hours, during which she was crying excessively and drinking half her usual amount of liquids. There was no history of vomiting. On the day of presentation, physical examination revealed an alert but irritable and ill-appearing infant with a temperature of 39.9°C, heart rate -180 beats/min, respiratory rate - 64 breaths/min, blood pressure of 102/55 mmHg, and oxygen saturation of 100%. The child's weight at admission was 4 kg, and noticed that she lost 10% of the previous reported weight. The skin was pale, tenting skin turgor, dry lips and dry buccal mucosa, normal looking eyes but reduced tears, soft fontanel, and capillary refill time of 3 seconds. The urine output was also decreased. Systemic examinations were normal. Abdominal and thorax radiographs were normal. There were no signs of meningeal irritation.*

*Routine stool specimen tested positive for rotavirus antigen, while results for blood and urine culture were negative. Serum electrolytes were significant for a sodium concentration of 146 mEq/L and a bicarbonate level of 8 mEq/L. Blood urea nitrogen was 61 mg/dL. The patient was admitted to the hospital and intravenous fluid therapy was promptly initiated and correction of electrolyte imbalance was done.*

## INTRODUCTION

Diarrhea is defined as the passage of three or more loose stools per day (or more frequent passage than is normal for the individual). Frequent passing of formed stools is not diarrhea, nor is the passing of loose and "pasty" stools by breastfed babies. It is usually the symptom of gastrointestinal infection, which can be caused by a variety of viral, parasitic and bacteria organisms.

Three clinical types of diarrhea:
1. **Acute watery diarrhea**—lasts several hours or days, e.g., cholera
2. **Acute bloody diarrhea**—also called dysentery, e.g., *Shigella*
3. **Persistent diarrhea**—lasts 14 days or longer.

## PROBLEM STATEMENT

Diarrhea is a leading killer of children, accounting for approximately 9% of all deaths among children under age five worldwide in 2019. This translates to over 1,300 young children dying each day, or about 484,000 children a year, despite the availability of a simple treatment solution. Deaths caused by diarrhea among children under-five are highest in south Asia and sub-Saharan Africa.

It is a leading cause of malnutrition in children under five years old. In the past, for most people, severe dehydration and fluid loss were the main causes of diarrhea deaths. Now, other causes such as septic bacterial infections are likely to account for an increasing proportion of all diarrhea-associated deaths. Children who are malnourished or have impaired immunity as well as people living with HIV are most at risk of life-threatening diarrhea. In developed countries diarrhea is a rare occurrence for most people where sanitation is widely available, access to safe water is high and personal and domestic hygiene is relatively good. Worldwide, 780 million individuals lack access to improved drinking-water and 2.5 billion lack improved sanitation. Diarrhea due to infection is widespread throughout developing countries. In low-income countries, children under three years old experience on average three episodes of diarrhea every year.

Globally, four billion episodes of diarrhea were estimated to occur each year, with >90% occurring in developing countries. Diarrheal disease is an important public health problem among under-five children in developing countries. Total diarrheal deaths in India among children aged 0-6 years were estimated to be 158,209 and proportionate mortality due to diarrhea in this age-group was 9.1%. Average estimated incidence of diarrhea in children aged 0-6 years was 1.71 and 1.09 episodes/person/year in rural and urban areas. According to National Family Health Survey-5 (NFHS-5) report, 7.3% of all under-five children were reported to be suffering from diarrhea in last 2 weeks of study data collection. Studies have shown that the incidence of acute diarrheal diseases was as low as 1 episode/child/year in some urban areas. During 2018, 330 acute diarrheal diseases outbreak were reported in India (NHP-2019).

Diarrhea is both preventable and treatable. Diarrheal disease is preventable through safe drinking-water, adequate sanitation, and hygiene. Inadequate access to proper nutrition, essential health services, safe water and sanitation facilities, and above all, having deficient knowledge and awareness about effective interventions like oral rehydration fluids are the most vulnerable and thus frequently suffer from and succumb to these diseases. Breastfeeding practices, complementary feeding, expanded immunization coverage, hand washing practices, improved water quality at the point of use and community sanitation practices, and zinc supplements have been identified as the important preventive strategies.

## EPIDEMIOLOGY

### Host Factors

Diarrhea is most common in young children specially among 6 months to 2 years of age with highest incidence between 6 months to 11 months. It suggests combined effects of decreasing maternal immunity, lack of innate immunity of infant and complimentary feeding of child with high risk of contamination. Diarrhea is also common among less than 6 months of age if the child is on infant feeding formulas or cow's milk. Most infectious causes of diarrhea are not sex-specific. Young age, low socioeconomic status, poor maternal literacy, presence of under-five sibling in the family, birth weight, inadequate breastfeeding, malnutrition, poor sanitation, low literacy level and hygiene practices of the mother are associated with a higher incidence of diarrheal diseases in young children. The leading cause of malnutrition in children under 5 years old is diarrhea.

### Agent Factors

Universally diarrhea in developing countries is infectious in origin. Following are some of the causes of diarrhea **(Table 17B.17)**.

**Bacteria:** *Campylobacter jejuni, Escherichia (E. coli), Shigella, Salmonella, Vibrio, Bacillus cereus, Staph. aureus, Clostridia, Aeromonas, Yersinia, Chlamydia, Neisseria.*

**Viruses:** Rotavirus, adenovirus, astrovirus, Norwalk virus, calicivirus, coronavirus, cytomegalovirus and enterovirus.

**Parasites:** *Giardia intestinalis, Giardia, Trichuriasis, Cryptosporidium,* intestinal worms, *Cyclospora.*

**Others:** Travelers' diarrhea, medication induced, food allergy or intolerance, food additives, digestive disorders.

**Table 17B.17:** Common etiological agents of persistent and bloody diarrhea.

| Persistent diarrhea | Bloody diarrhea |
| --- | --- |
| Enteropathogenic *Escherichia coli* | *Shigella* |
| Enteroaggregative *E. coli* | Nontyphoidal *Salmonella* |
| Nontyphoidal *Salmonella* | Campylobacter |
| Cryptosporidium | Enteroaggregative *E. coli* |
| Microsporidia | Enteroinvasive *E. coli* |
| *Giardia lamblia* | Shiga toxin-producing *E. coli* |
| *Ascaris lumbricoides* | *Entamoeba histolytica* |
| Cytomegalovirus | |
| Other viruses | |

*Source:* American Academy of Pediatrics (2009).

### Environmental Factors

Distinct seasonal patterns of diarrhea will occur as per the countries climatic conditions. Bacterial diarrhea is common during summer seasons whereas viral like rotavirus diarrhea is common during winter in temperate climates. Others factors like type of water source, presence of sanitation facilities, solid waste disposal system and floor type in the kitchen, poor knowledge on diarrheal cases and improved latrine, poor personal hygiene and no hand washing practices are found to be crucial contributors for the high prevalence of diarrheal diseases. Particularly, diarrhea occurrence is more associated with unsafe/unprotected water sources, e.g., ponds, wells, rivers, lakes. Drinking water storage and handling is also an important risk factor. Fish and seafood from water polluted by various causes may also contribute to the disease.

### Reservoir of Infection

It is not uniform for all the causative agents of diarrhea. For some of the pathogens human being is principal reservoir and transmission is mostly seen in humans, e.g., *E. coli, Shigella* species, *V. cholerae, Giardia, E. histolytica*. For others animals being reservoirs and transmission among both humans and animals observed, e.g., *Campylobacter jejuni, Salmonella* species and *Y. enterocolitica*.

## Mode of Transmission

Primarily eco-oral route through contaminated water of food or direct transmission via fingers or fomites or dirt which may be ingested by children.

## CLINICAL FEATURES

Acute diarrhea starts suddenly and is characterized by the passage of loose watery motions. Patients of diarrhea recover within 3–7 days. Persistent diarrhea may present with weight loss. Persistent diarrhea, which is recurrent or long lasting, due to non-infectious causes such as sensitivity to gluten or inherited metabolic disorders **(Table 17B.18 and Fig. 17B.17)**.

The threat posed by diarrhea is dehydration. During a diarrheal episode, water and electrolyte (sodium, chloride, potassium, and bicarbonate) losses occur. Dehydration occurs when these losses are not replaced.

The degree of dehydration is rated as:
- **Severe dehydration (at least two of the following signs):**
  Fluid deficit >10% body weight
  - Lethargy/unconsciousness
  - Sunken eyes
  - Unable to drink or drink poorly
  - Skin pinch goes back very slowly (≥2 seconds)

- **Some dehydration (two or more of the following signs):**
  Fluid deficit 5–10% body weight
  - Restlessness, irritability
  - Sunken eyes
  - Drinks eagerly, thirsty
- **No dehydration (not enough signs to classify as some or severe dehydration):** Fluid deficit <5% body weight.

Factors to be considered while investigating diarrhea and laboratory work up of diarrhea are shown in **Box 17B.2** and **17B.3**.

**Box 17B.2: Factors to be considered while investigating diarrhea.**
- Stool characteristics—consistency, color, volume, frequency
- Presence of associated enteric symptoms—nausea, vomiting, fever, abdominal pain
- Use of child daycare (rotavirus, astrovirus)
- Food ingestion history
- Travel history
- Water exposure (swimming pools, marine environment)
- Animal exposure (dogs/cats—campylobacter, turtle—*Salmonella* species)
- Predisposing conditions—hospitalization, antibiotic use, immunocompromised state

**Box 17B.3: Laboratory workup of diarrheal diseases.**
**Fecal laboratory studies:**
- Examination for ova and parasites
- Leukocyte count
- *pH level*: A pH level of 5.5 or less or the presence of reducing substances indicates carbohydrate intolerance, usually secondary to viral illness.
- Examination of exudates for presence/absence of leukocytes.
- Stool cultures
- Enzyme immunoassay for rotavirus or adenovirus antigens
- Latex agglutination assay for rotavirus

**Other laboratory studies:**
- Serum albumin levels—low in protein-losing enteropathies from enteroinvasive intestinal infections
- Fecal alpha1-antitrypsin levels—high in enteroinvasive intestinal infections
- Anion gap to determine the nature of diarrhea (i.e. osmolar vs. secretory)
- Intestinal biopsy—indicated in the presence of chronic or protracted diarrhea.

**Table 17B.18:** Differences between osmotic and secretory diarrhea.

| Osmotic diarrhea | Secretory diarrhea |
|---|---|
| This form of diarrhea involves the retention of water in the bowel, which results from the accumulation of non-absorbable substances. For instance, sugar substitutes like sorbitol and mannitol can slow down absorption while causing rapid motility of the small intestine | When electrolyte absorption is affected, the body releases water into the small intestine, causing loose bowel movements. This type of diarrhea is often a result of infection or the intake of certain drugs |

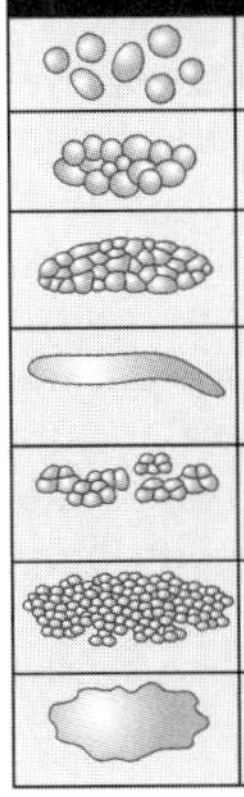

| Bristol stool chart | | |
|---|---|---|
| Type 1 | Separate hard lumps | Severe constipation |
| Type 2 | Lumpy and sausge like | Mild constipation |
| Type 3 | A sausage shape with cracks in the surface | Normal |
| Type 4 | Like a smooth, soft sausage or snake | Normal |
| Type 5 | Soft blobs with clear-cut edges | Lacking fiber |
| Type 6 | Mushy consistency with ragged edges | Mild diarrhea |
| Type 7 | Liquid consistency with no solid pieces | Severe diarrhea |

**Fig. 17B.17:** Bristol stool chart.

## PREVENTION AND CONTROL OF DIARRHEAL DISEASES

The Diarrhoeal Disease Control Programme launched by WHO in 1978 with the aim to reduce mortality and malnutrition due to diarrhea by making available oral rehydration salts and training in the treatment and prevention of diarrheal diaseses. It advocated following strategies.

### Strategies to Combat Diarrhea

The strategy comprised five major elements:
1. Appropriate case management
2. Preventive interventions
3. Community mobilization and empowerment
4. Surveillance, research, monitoring, and evaluation
5. Mobilizing national and international response.

## Appropriate Case Management

**Rehydration:** From epidemiological point of view all the diarrheal diseases are considered together due to common symptom, diarrhea, though the causes are diverse in nature. It is now established that regardless of causative agent and other determinants, oral rehydration forms the first line of treatment advocated by WHO/UNICEF.

**Aim:** To prevent dehydration and reduce mortality.
- *Basis of treatment:* Glucose given orally enhances the intestinal absorption of salt and water, and corrects the fluid-electrolyte balance.
- For the first time, the ORS prepared by WHO was sodium bicarbonate based.
- Inclusion of tri-sodium citrate in place of sodium bicarbonate has the following benefits:
  - Makes product more stable
  - Reduced stool output
  - Focused on reducing osmolarity of the solution to reduce the adverse effects of hypertonicity.

### Reduced Osmolarity ORS (Table 17B.19)

WHO and UNICEF updated the guidelines for managing diarrheal disease in all children in 2004 (WHO/UNICEF, 2004) and WHO updated the guidelines for integrated management of childhood illness in 2005 (WHO, 2005). The current recommendations for assessing and treating diarrhea involve evaluating dehydration, appropriate fluid replacement, continued feeding or increased breastfeeding, zinc supplementation, antibiotic regimens when indicated and appropriate referral, and follow-up.

Table 17B.19: Reduced osmolarity ORS-composition.

| Ingredients | Gram/L |
|---|---|
| Glucose, anhydrous | 13.5 |
| Sodium chloride | 2.6 |
| Potassium chloride | 1.5 |
| Trisodium citrate, dehydrate | 2.9 |
| Total weight | 20.5 |

*Source:* WHO/UNICEF Joint statement—Clinical Management of Acute Diarrhea.

Having assessed the degree of dehydration of the child, one of the following treatment plans should be followed:
- **Treatment Plan A:** To treat diarrhea at home—with homemade fluids to avoid dehydration
- **Treatment Plan B:** To treat some dehydration—with WHO recommended ORS
- **Treatment Plan C:** To treat severe dehydration—with IV infusion.

All children with diarrhea will be treated with Plan A, including both children who have not developed signs of dehydration and children who have already been treated for dehydration and have improved **(Fig. 17B.18)**.

### ORT Corner

It is the place in the primary health center or sub-center where mothers are taught of ORS preparation and assessment of child's dehydration.
- **Zinc supplements:** Zinc supplements reduce the duration of the episode.
- **Vitamin A supplementation.**
- **Exclusive breastfeeding** for first 6 months and proper weaning practices after 6 months.
- **Chemotherapy:** Unnecessary use of antibiotics is to be avoided in treatment of diarrhea. It should be considered when there is clear identification of causative agent like shigella, cholera or typhoid.

### Preventive Interventions

- Exclusive breastfeeding for the first 6 months followed by appropriate nutrient-dense, complementary feeding coupled with continued breastfeeding for 12–24 months.
- Good personal and food hygiene; Best practices on food handling, preparation, and storage prior to consumption.
- Promotion of behavior change in the community promoted through strong behavioral change communications (BCC) and information, education, and communication (IEC) efforts.
- Adequate access to safe drinking-water;
- Health education about how infections spread;
- Fly control measures to be adopted and
- Vaccines against diarrhea.

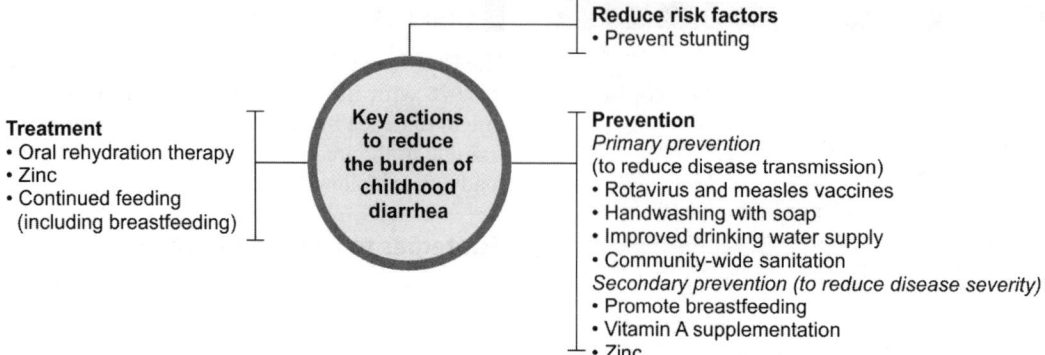

Fig. 17B.18: Nutrition, health and environmental factors all play a role in preventing and treating childhood diarrhea.
*Source:* The Child Health Epidemiology Reference Group, 2009.
*Diarrhea:* Why children are still dying and what can be done-WHO, Available at whqlibdoc.who.int>9789241598415_eng.

*Rotavirus vaccine:* Two new vaccines are live, attenuated—monovalent human rotavirus (Rotarix) and pentavalent bovine-human, reassortant vaccine (Rotateq).

Rotarix vaccine should be administered orally in a two-dose schedule at the time of the first and second doses of DTP and with an interval of 4 weeks between the doses. RotaTeq requires an oral three-dose schedule administered with DTP1, DTP2, and DTP3 and with an interval of 4-10 weeks between doses. WHO recommends that the first dose of rotavirus vaccine be administered as soon as possible after 6 weeks of age, along with diphtheria-tetanus-pertussis (DTP) vaccination.

Because most severe cases of rotavirus gastroenteritis occur earlier in life, vaccination of children older than 24 months is not encouraged.

Rotavirus vaccine was introduced in routine immunization schedule in India since 2016 in a phased manner, in selected states/districts: Andhra Pradesh, Assam, Haryana, Himachal Pradesh, Jharkhand, Madhya Pradesh, Odisha, Rajasthan, Tamil Nadu, Tripura and Uttar Pradesh.

*Typhoid vaccines:* Two types.
1. *Live vaccine:* Marketed as Typhoral. Three capsules—one capsule on alternate day for all above three years of age.
2. *Cellular extract vaccine*: Marketed as Typhim-Vi; it contains capsular, polysaccharide-Vi antigen of *Salmonella typhi*.

*Oral cholera vaccine:* Three oral cholera vaccines have been approved by the World Health Organization (WHO): Dukoral, ShanChol, and Euvichol-Plus.

This is given for above two years, intramuscularly or subcutaneously.

1. *Hepatitis B vaccine*.
2. *Parenteral cholera vaccine* and *shigella vaccine* are under trials.

## Community Mobilization and Empowerment

Improvement in care-seeking and child-rearing practices; health education and promotion; social accountability; and advocacy have been identified as the core components of the community mobilization strategy of the program.
- Increasing community sanitation
- Stopping open air defecation
- Avoiding outside street foods
- Taking adequate medication and preventing carrier state (e.g. in case of typhoid)
- Proper hand washing practices.

## Surveillance, Research, Monitoring and Evaluation

- Monitoring of disease occurrence, trends, outbreaks, and follow-up actions in the communities
- Periodic evaluations of the program outcomes and the impact on disease burden
- Surveillance of antibiotic use in the community and emergence of antimicrobial resistance.

## Mobilizing National and International Response

*Global approach:* WHO works with Member States and other partners to:
- Promote national policies and investments that support case management of diarrhoea and its complications as well as

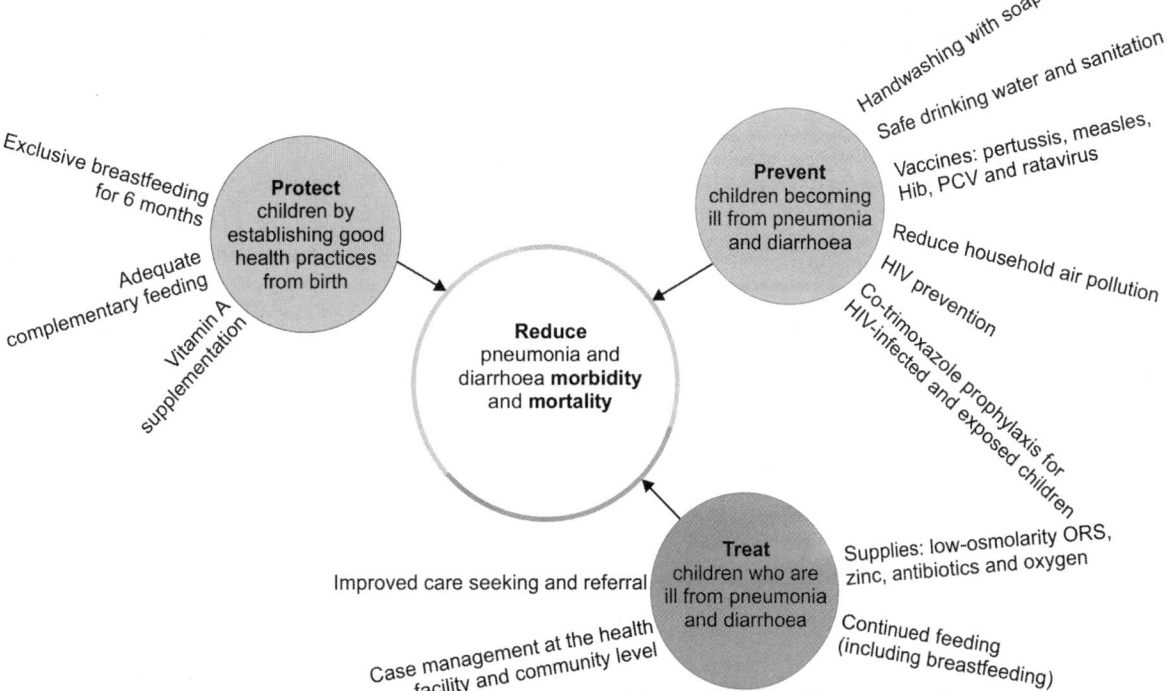

**Fig. 17B.19:** Integrated Global Action Plan for the Prevention and Control of Pneumonia and Diarrhoea (GAPPD).
*Source:* Global Action Plan for the Prevention and Control of Pneumonia and Diarrhoea (GAPPD).

increasing access to safe drinking-water and sanitation in developing countries;
- Conduct research to develop and test new diarrhoea prevention and control strategies in this area;
- Build capacity in implementing preventive interventions, including sanitation, source water improvements, and household water treatment and safe storage;
- Develop new health interventions, such as the rotavirus immunization; and
- Help to train health workers, especially at community level.
  - A program for the coordinated approach to prevention and control of acute diarrhea and respiratory infections—called the Coordinated Approach to Prevention and Control of Acute Diarrhea and Respiratory infections (CDR).
  - *The Integrated Global Action Plan for the Prevention and Control of Pneumonia and Diarrhea (GAPPD) by WHO/ UNICEF:* The goal is to see a drop in deaths from pneumonia to fewer than three children in 1,000 live births, and from diarrhea to less than one in 1,000 by 2025.

**Protect, Prevent and Treat Framework:** The Integrated Global Action Plan for the Prevention and Control of Pneumonia and Diarrhoea (GAPPD) sets forth an integrated framework of key interventions proven to effectively protect children's health, prevent disease and appropriately treat children who do fall ill with diarrhea and pneumonia **(Fig. 17B.19)**.
- Protective interventions provide the foundations for keeping children healthy and free of disease
- Preventative interventions help stop disease transmission and prevent children from becoming ill
- Treatment interventions – when timely and appropriate can cure children from diarrhea and ensure survival.

## SUGGESTED READING

1. Barr W, Smith A. Acute diarrhea in adults. Lawrence, Massachusetts: Family Medicine Residency; 2016.
2. Diarrhoea. UNICEF Data: Monitoring the situation of mother and child December 2022. Available from https://data.unicef.org/topic/child-health/diarrhoeal-disease/#:~:text=Diarrhoea%20is%20a%20leading%20killer,of%20a%20simple%20treatment%20solution.
3. Health Promotion and Communication Team—Waterborne Disease Prevention Branch—NCEZID—CDC_files.
4. Integrated Management of Childhood Illness (IMCI), Departments of Child and Adolescent Health and Development (CAH). WHO recommendations on the management of diarrhoea and pneumonia in HIV-infected infants and children. Geneva: WHO.
5. Integrated management of childhood illnesses. Department of child and adolescent health and development: WHO/UNICEF.
6. Intensified Diarrhoea Control Fortnight, Operational Guidelines—MOHFW, GOI10. Manual of Gastroenterology: Diagnosis and Therapy, 2008. Curr Gastroenterol Rep. 1999;1(5):389-97.
7. Malik A, Haldar P, Ray A, et al. Introducing rotavirus vaccine in the Universal Immunization Programme in India: From evidence to policy to implementation. Vaccine. 2019;37(39):5817-24.
8. UNICEF: Diarrheal disease October 2019. Available from https://data.unicef.org/topic/child-health/diarrhoeal-disease/
9. WHO. Diarrhea: Nutrition—why children are still dying and what can be done—prevention and treatment measures. Geneva: WHO/ UNICEF; 2016.
10. WHO. Strategy for coordinated approach to prevention and control of acute diarrhoea and respiratory infection in the South-East Asia Region. Geneva; 2016.
11. World Health Organization. The management and prevention of diarrhoea. Practical Guidelines, 3rd edition. Geneva: World Health Organization; 1993. pp. 1-50.

# EPIDEMIOLOGY OF SALMONELLOSIS AND TYPHOID FEVER AND ITS PREVENTION AND CONTROL

*Abhishek Singh*

**CM7.2** Enumerate, describe and discuss the mode of transmission and measures for prevention and control of salmonellosis and typhoid fever

**CM8.1** Describe and discuss the epidemiological and control measures applicable in salmonellosis and typhoid fever

---

*Case Scenario*

*A 37-year-old female was admitted to district hospital with high fever, headache, and abdominal symptoms for last 10 days. She gave a history of abdominal discomfort with diarrhea. She visited a local doctor 5 days back and received chloroquine for malaria, but her condition did not improve. The clinician suspects her to be suffering from typhoid fever.*
- *Describe the agent and host factors for typhoid fever.*
- *Describe the laboratory tests for diagnosis of typhoid fever.*
- *What are the vaccines available against the typhoid fever?*
- *Discuss about prevention of salmonellosis.*

---

**Typhoid Mary**

*Mary Mallon (1869–1938) was an Irish-American cook. She used to do household work in the homes of rich families before she settled down as a cook. New York-based banker Mr Warren hired Marry Mallon to be their cook for the summer of 1906. Within a week, six out of 11 members of Warren's family got infected with typhoid fever. Warren wanted to know how his family became infected with typhoid fever. For this purpose, Warren hired George Sober, a person having experience with typhoid fever outbreaks. Initially Sober thought soft clams as the reason but it was not so as not everyone got the disease had used them. But finally Sober cracked the case and became the first person to explain "healthy carrier" of Salmonella typhi in the US. In the same year, nearly 3,000 residents of New York city got infected with typhoid fever and perhaps Mary, a healthy carrier of Salmonella typhi, played a major role behind this outbreak. She became popular as "Typhoid Mary". She continued spreading the typhoid as she always denied out her illness. She was subjected to quarantine at different times on North Brother Island for a total period of 26 years and she expired there.*

# Chapter 17: Specific Epidemiology of Infectious Diseases

## INTRODUCTION

"Enteric fever" is a group of clinically similar, but immunologically distinct fever, caused by *Salmonella* spp. The characteristic features of the disease are continuous fever for 3–4 weeks, associated with relative bradycardia and lymphoid tissue involvement besides the constitutional symptoms. The disease varies in severity, and a spectrum of illness may present. The term "enteric fever" is a clinical term and covers both typhoid and paratyphoid fever, to differentiate the two requires laboratory support.

## MILESTONES

- *1829:* Louis distinguished typhoid from typhus fever.
- *1839:* Schonlein demonstrated that the lesions in the Payer's patches and mesenteric lymph nodes were specific for typhoid fever and not for typhus fever.
- *1856:* Budd specified that disease transmits through the excreta of patients.
- *1880:* Eberth demonstrated organisms in the lymphoid tissues.
- *1884:* Gaffky successfully grew the organisms in pure culture.
- *1890:* Pfeiffer, Wright, and Kolle carried out vaccination experiments independently.
- *1975:* Germanier and Fürer developed vaccine against typhoid.

## CHARACTERISTIC OF DISEASE

Typhoid fever is an infectious disease of the small intestine which is acute in onset, caused by *Salmonella typhi*, transmitted via food and water contaminated with fecal matter. *Salmonella typhi* and *Salmonella paratyphi* infections are prevalent in our country and are confined to human beings, whereas other *Salmonella* species are primarily infective to animals and humans are secondarily infected. Presence of typhoid is the barometer of the sanitation of the community. The *Salmonella* species predominantly cause three types of clinical syndromes, viz. (1) enteric fever, (2) septicemia, and (3) gastroenteritis.

## PROBLEM STATEMENT

### Global

Enteric (typhoid) fever is globally distributed everywhere. As of 2019, an estimated 9 million people get sick from typhoid and 110,000 people die from it every year.

### India

In developing countries also, it is a major health concern, where it constitutes 60–80% of the total foodborne diseases. The estimated incidence of typhoid fever from hospital surveillance ranged from 12 to 1622 cases per 100,000 child-years among children between the ages of 6 months and 14 years and from 108 to 970 cases per 100,000 person-years among those who were 15 years of age or older (2017-2020). In 2018, 2.3 million cases and 399 deaths were reported in India. It also has a huge socioeconomic impact on our society as typhoid patients may require several months to recover and resume work (NHP-2019).

> **Sangli Outbreak of Typhoid, 1975–1976**
>
> A common source epidemic of typhoid, perhaps the world's largest, was reported from Sangli (Maharashtra) during 1975–1976. More than 9,000 people were affected out of a total population of 135,000. The water supply to this region was from two wells on the banks of a nearby river. After filtration, water was subjected to chlorination inadequately many a times. An underground sewerage was existent but not operational so, most of the sewage drained by surface gutters, entered into a stream that opened into the main river near one of the wells. A dam was made on the sewage stream to prevent direct contamination of well. Accumulated sewage was fed down a ditch to enter the river further downstream. Some of contaminated water was allowed to enter rice fields. The problem occurred when due to prolonged monsoons the sewage overflowed onto the well area. This overflow choked the filtration beds of sand filters. As a result, raw water entered the water supply. Inadequate chlorination of water supply by the municipality added upon with heavy contamination by fecal matter, led to this explosive epidemic.

## EPIDEMIOLOGICAL DETERMINANTS

### Agent Factors

*Salmonella* is a large group of bacterium with many serotypes, which can infect humans. They can be broadly classified into three types according to host preference:

*Types:*
1. *Those affecting only human*: Salmonella typhi, Salmonella paratyphi A and C.
2. *Those that can affect humans as well as animals and no preference*: Salmonella typhimurium, Salmonella enteritidis.
3. *Those that affect animals primarily*: Salmonella cholerasuis, Salmonella abortus, and Salmonella gallinarum.

*Salmonella typhi* is a gram-negative bacillus, capsulated, flagellated, non-lactose fermenting, and actively motile organism. *Salmonella typhi* has three main antigens—(1) Somatic or "O" antigen (specific for the group), (2) Flagellar or "H" antigen (specific for the type), and (3) A surface/capsular or "Vi" antigen (related to the virulence of the organism). They are sensitive to heat and chemicals. The organism can be killed by heating at 60°C for 15 minutes and also by routine disinfectants like formalin, chlorine, and bleaching powder.

Natural habitat of *Salmonella typhi* is the human intestine. They also survive intracellularly in the tissues of various organs like spleen and kidney. On autolysis of bacilli, endotoxin is released. This endotoxin has a key role in the disease process. *Salmonella typhi* can survive in the environment for 15–20 days.

> **Vi Antigen**
> - Antibody disappears early in convalescence. If it persists, it denotes the development of carrier state
> - Complete absence of Vi antibody in confirmed case of typhoid fever denotes poor prognosis
> - Demonstration of the Vi antibody is not helpful in diagnosing the typhoid; thus, Vi antigen is not tested in Widal test.

### Infective Dose

The infective dose of *Salmonella typhi* is $10^2$–$10^5$ bacilli, i.e. a minimum dose of $10^5$ *Salmonella typhi* cells is required to develop typhoid fever in 50 individuals of total 100 volunteers.

## Host Factors

**Age:** It can affect humans at any age; however, children are affected more than adults and the common age group is 5–20 years.

**Sex:** Males have a higher disease proportion as compared to females but carrier rate is more in females.

**Immunity:** Individuals of all age groups are susceptible to get infection. Infection or immunization may stimulate the antibody production. There is an acquired, cell-mediated, and partial immunity following a clinical illness. Antibody to the somatic antigen (O) is generally in the higher range in diseased individuals, i.e. cases of typhoid. Antibody to the flagellar antigen (H) is frequently found in higher range in the immunized persons. Antibody to the capsular antigen (Vi) is usually higher among carriers. *Salmonella typhi* is an intracellular organism therefore, cell-mediated immunity has a critical role in the disease process. Gastric juice and local intestinal immunity confer resistance to *Salmonella typhi* infection in the host.

**Predisposing factors:** Typhoid is a social disease with clinical manifestations. Many social factors are implicated in dynamics of the disease, e.g., poverty, illiteracy, lack of sanitation, poor standard of living, lack of personal hygiene, lack of protected water supply, open air defecation, etc.

## Environmental Factors

*Salmonella* is distributed in the environment in animals, birds, insects, mammals, sewage, soil, vegetables, water, manure, etc. They can grow in warm environment and at high temperatures as in subtropical countries. The highest incidence is seen during rains as conditions favor breeding of houseflies, the medium of transmission being water, food, ice, milk, vegetables, and soil.

## Reservoir of Infection

The reservoirs of infection, viz. cases and carriers, are humans only. Cases or carriers are infectious till, they shed bacilli in stool or urine. (1) *Cases:* A case may be an active clinical case or a subclinical case. For every clinical case, there are about 10 subclinical cases and (2) *Carriers:* All types of carrier stages are seen in typhoid. Carriers constitute the submerged portion of ice in the iceberg phenomena. They maintain the endemicity of disease in the community. A carrier may be, according to the type, an incubatory, convalescent, or a contact carrier and depending upon the duration may be temporary or chronic and depending upon the portal of exit, may be intestinal, urinary, or biliary carrier. The bacilli are excreted in convalescent carriers for 6–8 weeks. Chronic carrier's term is used if the bacilli are excreted for a period of more than 12 months after initial illness and may last as long as 50 years. Most of subclinical cases and 2–5% of cases become carriers. "Typhoid Mary", a worker in food establishment, is an excellent example of chronic carrier who solely, was responsible for more than 1,300 cases of typhoid in her lifetime.

> **Points to Remember**
> - Convalescent carriers: Patients excreting typhoid bacilli in feces for 3 weeks–3 months after declaring clinically cured
> - Temporary carriers: Patients shedding bacilli for >3 months but <1 year
> - Chronic carriers: Patients excreting bacilli for >1 year.

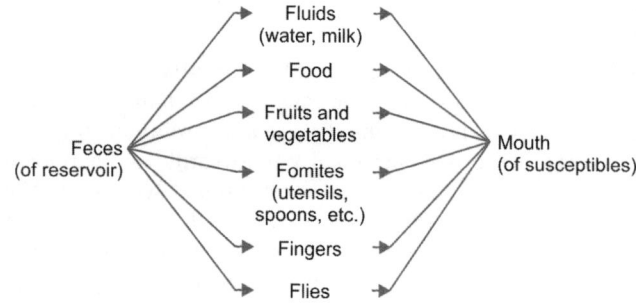

**Fig. 17B.20:** Feco-oral route of transmission.

## Sources of Infection

Chief sources of infection are excreta of cases and carriers.

## Modes of Transmission

Enteric fever is spread primarily through fecal (sewage) contamination of water, food, milk, and vegetables, i.e. through feco-oral route. The pathogen is transmitted from one "F", through six "Fs" to a susceptible person as shown in **Figure 17B.20**. Flies constitute an important subsidiary vehicle of transmission. A small fraction of cases may result because of direct transmission of infection from an actual case/carrier via contaminated hands, while handling patients or their excreta.

## Incubation Period

It is usually 10–14 days for *Salmonella typhi* and 4–5 days for *Salmonella paratyphi*. The period of communicability persists till the case excretes the bacilli in the excreta, in the convalescent carriers it is for 6–8 weeks, whereas in chronic carriers it is for years.

# CLINICAL FEATURES

The clinical features vary according to the syndrome.

## Typhoid (Enteric) Fever

Clinical symptoms start appearing towards the end of incubation period and may vary from mild pyrexia to a fatal fulminating disease. The symptoms are gradual in appearance in form of dull frontal headache, anorexia, malaise, lethargy, myalgia, and congestion of mucous membranes. In early part of the disease, many patients present with *constipation or pea soup diarrhea*, along with marked abdominal distention. In the 2nd week, the signs could be hepatosplenomegaly, *stepladder pattern* of persistent fever with *relative bradycardia* and leukopenia. *The rash (rose spots)*, are pink papules 2–3 mm in diameter fading on pressure, are found principally on the trunk which frequently appear during the 2nd week of disease and disappears by 3–4 days. The organisms may appear in stool in 2nd–3rd weeks and in urine in 3rd–4th weeks. The Peyer's patches in the ileum may develop necrosis, which may lead to intestinal hemorrhage and perforation and are dreaded complications.

## Septicemia

The common serotypes associated with this are *Salmonella cholerasuis*, *Salmonella paratyphi* C. The infection occurs through the oral route; however, the invasion of the bloodstream occurs early, leading to local suppuration in different organs. The local signs may vary according to the organ system involved. The suppuration may be a cause of osteomyelitis, pneumonia, pulmonary abscess, meningitis, or endocarditis.

## Gastroenteritis

It is a common foodborne illness caused by *Salmonella* species, resulting from ingestion of food harboring the bacilli. The incubation period ranges from 12 hours to 24 hours but can be upto 36 hours. Fever, vomiting, pain in abdomen, and diarrhea are the characteristic symptoms. The poisoning is of infective type in which the organism grows in intestine. It is generally not associated with bacteremia. The illness is self-limiting with symptoms disappearing within a few days with little or no complications.

## Carrier State

These are the subjects who had infection in the past and have the organism harbored in gallbladder. They continue to shed the organism in stool sometimes continuously and sometimes intermittently. They act as a source for disease to affect the healthy individuals.

## DIAGNOSIS

Clinically, diagnosed enteric fever is classified as salmonellosis, typhoid fever, or paratyphoid by the laboratory support. In laboratory, the diagnosis is made by isolating the bacilli or by demonstration of organism-specific antibodies or circulating antigens. **Figure 17B.21** depicts the culture and serologic diagnosis of typhoid fever.

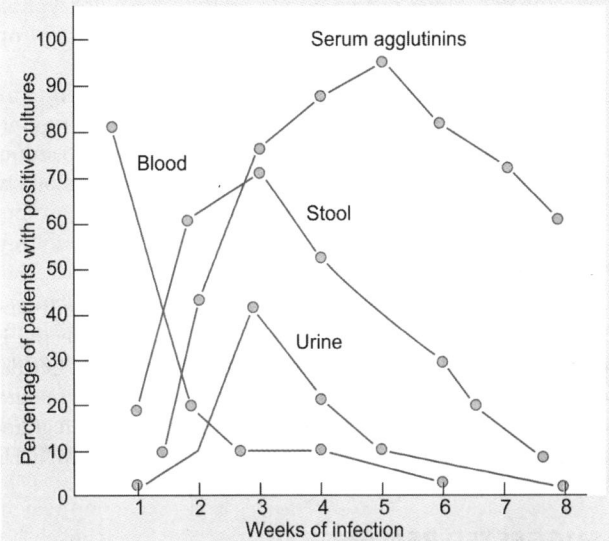

**Fig. 17B.21:** Culture and serologic diagnosis of typhoid fever.
*Source:* Winn WC. Koneman's Color Atlas and Textbook of Diagnostic Microbiology. Philadelphia: Lippincott Williams and Wilkins; 2006.

**Table 17B.20** depicts the percentage positivity and the specimen to be used according to the duration of the disease. The diagnosis of the carriers is done by the detection of the organism in their stool or urine. In some cases, specimen from bile or duodenal drainage may be required. The serological tests are Felix-Widal test (having moderate sensitivity and specificity), other tests using antibody detection are Typhidot-M, IDL Tubex test, and dipstick test **(Table 17B.21)**.

**Table 17B.20:** Clinical investigation for diagnosis at different duration of illness.

| Test of diagnosis (percentage positivity) | Time of diagnosis | Remarks |
|---|---|---|
| Blood culture (90%) | 1st week | Mainstay of diagnosis |
| Antibodies (Widal test) (low titer) | 2nd week | Moderate sensitivity and specificity |
| Stool culture (80%) | 3rd week | – |
| Urine test | 4th week | – |

**Table 17B.21:** Newer modalities of diagnosis of typhoid fever.

| IDL tubex test | Detects IgM antibodies |
|---|---|
| Typhidot | Detects IgM and IgG antibodies |
| Typhidot-M | Detects IgM antibodies |
| Dipstick test | Detects IgM antibodies |

(IgG: immunoglobulin G; IgM: immunoglobulin M)

## STRATEGIES FOR TREATMENT, PREVENTION AND CONTROL MEASURES

### Treatment

Treatment of the cases is by fluoroquinolones or cephalosporins. The alternative drugs are chloramphenicol, amoxicillin, and cotrimoxazole. Fluoroquinolone such as ciprofloxacin 750 mg orally twice daily or levofloxacin 500 mg orally once daily, 5–7 days for uncomplicated enteric fever and 10–14 days for severe infection, is the treatment of choice.

> **Chloramphenicol-resistant *Salmonella typhi***
>
> In our country, Kerala is the first state to report the epidemics of multidrug-resistant *Salmonella typhi*. First such incident occurred in Calicutin 1972. The situation was endemic and was confined to boundaries of Kerala till 1978. Other states started reporting of such resistant strains later on. These strains were having resistance to streptomycin, sulfadiazine, and tetracycline. Reason behind this was a plasmid having transmissible property, carried resistance to the antibiotics. In early phase, these strains were not resistant to ampicillin, amoxicillin, co-trimoxazole, and furazolidone. Resistance began to emerge from many regions of India to many drugs in late 1980s.

### Carriers of Typhoid

Carriers are detected during follow-up of cases by culture of duodenal drainage or serological examination (Vi antibodies). Most successful treatment approach for carriers is cholecystectomy coupled with an intensive therapy using ampicillin/amoxicillin and probenecid for 6 weeks (up to 80% cure rate). The carriers should be kept under surveillance and must not be allowed to handle food, milk, or water for others.

Disinfection of the stool and urine of the cases by 5% cresol with a contact period of 2 hours is important.

## Prevention

The prevention of salmonellosis is three-pronged.
- **Controlling source/reservoir:** As cases or carriers are primarily the source of typhoid, the cases are to be diagnosed early and prompt treatment must be instituted. There is a role of isolation, until three stool or urine samples on different days are negative for the bacterium.
- **Breaking the chain of transmission (interruption of transmission):** Feco-oral route of transmission is interrupted effectively by creating the "sanitation barrier" in its way **(Fig. 17B.22)**. It consists of construction and use of sanitary latrine, which prevents access of the pathogens from feces to six Fs.

  This interruption can be made more effective by supplementing following measures:
  - Chlorination of drinking water.
  - Pasteurization of milk.
  - Disinfection of vegetables and fruits with potassium permanganate ($KMnO_4$) before consumption.
  - Practicing personal hygienic measures.
- **Sanitation:** Provision of safe water supply and basic sanitation along with health education plays an important role in reducing the morbidity because of *Salmonella*.
- **Immunization:** Though not 100%, immunization confers specific protection, it lowers incidence and severity of the infection. It is recommended for the populations living in the endemic areas, the household contacts of the cases or carriers, children, healthcare staff, and travelers to the endemic areas.
  - *Typhoral (live oral Ty21a) vaccine:*
    - Contains more than $10^9$ viable organisms of attenuated *Salmonella typhi*
    - The lyophilized vaccine is available in two formulations: (1) as enteric-coated capsules or (2) a liquid suspension. The liquid formulation consists of the vaccine in one sachet and a buffer in another, which are combined with water before oral administration. The capsules are licensed for use in individuals aged more than or equal to 5 years whereas liquid vaccine can be administered from the age of 2 years.
    - *Schedule:* A three-dose regimen, one capsule each on days 1, 3, and 5 (booster of three doses, once every 3 years).
    - Protective immunity is achieved a week after the last dose with the three-dose regimen.
    - *Duration of protection:* 3 years
    - *Salmonella typhi* Ty21a strain is a stable mutant lacking the enzyme UDP-galactose-4-epimerase. On ingestion, the strain begins infection, but after four or five cell divisions causes self-destruction. Thus, it cannot cause illness. The vaccine appears to stimulate both serum and intestinal antibodies and cell-mediated immune responses but mechanism remains unknown.
  - *Typhim Vi vaccine:*
    - Vi polysaccharide containing vaccine is given as a single dose via intramuscular (IM) or subcutaneous (SC) route in 0.5 mL dose
    - Not given in age less than 2 years.
  - *TAB vaccine:* It confers immunity against *Salmonella typhi*, *Salmonella paratyphi* A, and *Salmonella paratyphi* B.

## Global Approach

- In October 2017, the Strategic Advisory Group of Experts on Immunization (SAGE), which advises WHO on vaccine use, issued a recommendation for the typhoid conjugate vaccine to be added to routine childhood immunization programs in typhoid endemic countries. SAGE also called for the introduction of typhoid conjugate vaccine to be prioritized for countries with the highest burden of typhoid disease or high levels of antibiotic resistance to *Salmonella typhi*.
- Starting in 2019, Gavi, the Vaccine Alliance has provided funding to support typhoid conjugate vaccine use in eligible countries.
- As at March 2023, WHO has prequalified two conjugate vaccines for the prevention of typhoid. Typhoid conjugate vaccine has longer-lasting immunity than the older typhoid vaccines and can be given as a single dose to children from the age of 6 months.
- In addition to decreasing the disease burden in endemic countries and saving lives, widespread use of the typhoid conjugate vaccine in affected countries is expected to reduce the need for antibiotics for typhoid treatment and slow the increase in antibiotic resistance in *Salmonella typhi*.

## Indian Approach

The national immunization schedule in places like Delhi and Chandigarh have incorporated Vi polysaccharide vaccine in their schedule. The basic sanitation and hand hygiene, besides provision of drinking water which is safe, is one of the integral components of village health and nutrition days, the Integrated Child Development Services (ICDS) Program, and RMNCHA Program under National Health Mission.

## SUGGESTED READING

1. Braunwald EB, Fauci AS, Kasper DL, et al. Harrison's Principles of Internal Medicine, 15th edition. New York: Tata McGraw Hill; 2001.

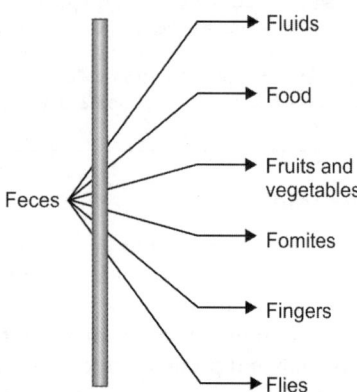

**Fig. 17B.22:** Sanitation barrier.

2. Connor BA, Schwartz E. Typhoid and paratyphoid fever in travellers. Lancet Infect Dis. 2005;5:623-8.
3. Eddleston M, Davidson R, Wilkinson R, et al. Oxford Handbook of Tropical Medicine, 2nd edition. New Delhi: Oxford University Press; 2005.
4. Farrar J, Hotez PJ, Junghanss T, et al. Manson's Tropical Diseases. New York: Elsevier Health Sciences; 2013.
5. Gordan CC, Alimuddin Z. Manson's Tropical Diseases, 21st edition. London: Saunders; 2003.
6. Kaufmann SH, Raupach B, Finlay BB. Introduction: microbiology and immunology: lessons learned from Salmonella. Microbes Infect. 2001;3:1177-81.
7. John J, Bavdekar A, Rongsen-Chandola T, et al. Burden of typhoid and paratyphoid fever in India. New England Journal of Medicine. 2023;388(16):1491-500.
8. John ML, Robert BW. Maxey-Rosenau—Last Public Health and Preventive Medicine, 15th edition. New York: McGraw-Hill Companies Inc.; 2008.
9. Kimberlin DW, Brady MT, Jackson MA, et al. Red Book (R) 2015: Report of the Committee on Infectious Diseases, 30th edition. United States: American Academy of Pediatrics; 2015.
10. Kliegman RM, Behrman RE, Jenson HB, et al. Nelson Textbook of Pediatrics. New York: Elsevier Health Sciences; 2007.
11. Levine MM. Typhoid fever vaccines. In: Plotkin S, Orenstein W, Offit P, Edwards KM (Eds). Plotkin's Vaccines, 7th edition. New York: Elsevier; 2018. pp. 1114-44.
12. Parija SC. Textbook of Microbiology and Immunology. New York: Elsevier Health Sciences; 2014.
13. Winn WC. Koneman's Color Atlas and Textbook of Diagnostic Microbiology. Philadelphia: Lippincott Williams & Wilkins; 2006.

# EPIDEMIOLOGY OF SHIGELLOSIS AND ITS PREVENTION AND CONTROL

*Abhishek Singh*

**CM7.2** Enumerate, describe and discuss the mode of transmission and measures for prevention and control of shigellosis

**CM8.1** Describe and discuss the epidemiological and control measures applicable in shigellosis

## INTRODUCTION

Shigellosis is ubiquitous. It causes approximately 165 million cases of severe dysentery. A great number of such cases are reported from developing countries and the age group involved is under 5 years of children. *Shigella* is closely related to *Escherichia coli*; however, it is not a part of normal gastrointestinal flora. The organism *Shigella* causes enteric bacillary dysentery. It has four species identified by serology and each species has many serotypes. It is one of the important causes of dysentery in our country.

## PROBLEM STATEMENT

### Global

Each year slightly more than a million cases die from *Shigella* infection. Nearly 99% cases are reported from the developing countries. Approximately, 580,000 cases of shigellosis are reported among travelers from developed countries. Nearly 1.1 million people die from *Shigella* infection every year (Kotloff KL et al., Bull World Health Organ, 1999; Peirano G et al., Mam Inst Oswaldo Cruz, 2006). Since 1969, *Shigella dysenteriae* has been implicated for many outbreaks in many countries such as in Central America in 1969-1972; in Zaire, Rwanda, and Burundi in 1979-1982; in India in 1984; in Burma in 1985; in Bangladesh in 1988; and in Zimbabwe and Zambia in 1992-1994. The strains held responsible behind these outbreaks were found to be resistant to antimicrobials used in normal circumstances.

The World Health Organization (WHO) was notified on 4 February 2022 of an unusually high number of cases of extensively drug-resistant (XDR) *Shigella sonnei* which have been reported in the United Kingdom of Great Britain and Northern Ireland and several other countries in the WHO European Region since late 2021. Although most infections with *S. sonnei* result in a short duration of disease and low case fatality, multi-drug resistant (MDR) and XDR shigellosis is a public health concern since treatment options are very limited for moderate to severe cases.

### India

The accurate estimates of morbidity and mortality due to shigellosis are lacking, though it is endemic in India. In India, the outbreak reported in year 1984 was due to multiresistant strain of *Shigella dysenteriae* type 1 and the worst hit state was West Bengal. After that, many states have reported such outbreaks.

*Shigella sonnei* causes shigellosis in industrialized countries in 77% of cases (compared to 15% in developing countries). *Shigella flexneri* is commonly found in developing countries (60%). *Shigella dysenteriae* (Sd1) causes epidemic dysentery and has potential to cause outbreaks particularly in confined populations, like refugee camps.

## EPIDEMIOLOGICAL DETERMINANTS

### Host Factors

**Age:** Severity of illness is higher at the extremes of age, affecting children aged less than 1 year and subjects aged 50 years and above. The other risk groups are: children who are not breastfed, children who are malnourished, or who are recovering from illnesses like measles. Mortality is higher among them.

### Agent Factors

The genus *Shigella* consists of four species that are biochemically similar and are serologically classified as:
1. *Shigella dysenteriae (group A)*: Most virulent type
2. *Shigella flexneri (group B)*: Antigenically most complex
3. *Shigella boydii (group C)*
4. *Shigella sonnei (group D)*: Causes mildest dysentery (most common in developed countries).

These are non-motile and non-lactose fermenting organisms. They are responsible for sporadic cases as well as epidemics of dysentery.

**Viability:** The organisms can be killed by physical and chemical agents such as disinfectants, high concentration of acids and bile. All *Shigellae* produce endotoxins on autolysis which is responsible for irritating effect on intestine and causes diarrhea and intestinal ulcers. Group A produces exotoxin as well as neurotoxin.

**Resistance:** The disease is highly communicable, a dose as low as 10–100 bacilli may be sufficient to initiate a disease in a healthy adult, as it can survive in gastric acid.

### Environmental Factors

It occurs in developing countries due to overcrowding and poor sanitation. It affects young children in daycare centers and people living in crowded and inadequate housing conditions.

### Reservoir

The only known reservoirs of *Shigella* are human beings.

### Modes of Transmission

The transmission may occur by direct contact with an infected person, by feco-oral route with carriers as the source. Flies, fingers, and food or water contaminated by infected persons, and inanimate objects also act as modes of transmission.

## CLINICAL FEATURES

The clinical features vary from asymptomatic to severe form of disease. In the initial stages of disease there may be fever which is high grade, associated with chills, abdominal pain may be present in form of cramps or tenesmus which typically occurs 24–48 hours after ingestion of organisms. The organisms multiply in small intestine and then move toward colon and can be isolated from there, 1–3 days after development of infection. Symptoms last for 3–7 days in most people. Initially, there may be watery diarrhea which may be followed by the bloody stool, containing mucus and leukocytes due to invasion of intestinal mucosa and inflammatory reaction. In young children, rectal prolapse may result from excessive straining. Severe cases of shigellosis may develop obstruction of intestines, toxic megacolon, and bacteremia due to dissemination of organism after invasion of intestinal mucosa. Complications include seizures, polyneuritis, coma, meningism, and hemolytic uremic syndrome (HUS).

## MANAGEMENT

Isolation of organisms from stool samples confirms the diagnosis. Stool microscopy reveals polymorphonuclear cells on methylene blue stain; however, culture differentiates *Shigella* from colitis. Uncomplicated shigellosis is self-limiting illness, dehydration has to be corrected promptly in infants and young children.

### Controlling Source/Reservoir

As the primary sources are cases or carriers, they need to be diagnosed early and prompt treatment to be instituted. Antibiotic treatment is reserved for serious cases. There is no evidence if antibiotic therapy hastens recovery or prevents carrier state.

### Prevention and Control Measures

The personal hygiene plays a vital role in prevention of shigellosis. Public health measures like provision of safe water supply and basic sanitation plays a key role in reducing the burden of shigellosis. The basic sanitation and hand hygiene besides safe drinking water are essential for prevention of disease transmission.

## SUGGESTED READING

1. Bhalwar R, Vaidya R. Textbook of Public Health and Community Medicine. Pune: Armed Forces Medical College; 2009.
2. Niyogi SK. Shigellosis. J Microbiol. 2005;43:133-43.
3. Pazhani GP, Sarkar B, Ramamurthy T, et al. Clonal multidrug-resistant Shigella dysenteriae type 1 strains associated with epidemic and sporadic dysenteries in eastern India. Antimicrob Agents Chemother. 2004;48:681-4.
4. Peirano G, Souza FS, Rodrigues DP, et al. Frequency of serovars and antimicrobial resistance in Shigella spp. from Brazil. Mem Inst Oswaldo Cruz. 2006;101:245-50.

---

# EPIDEMIOLOGY OF VIRAL HEPATITIS (A AND E) AND ITS PREVENTION AND CONTROL

*Abhishek Singh*

| | |
|---|---|
| CM3.3 | Describe the etiology and basis of waterborne jaundice/hepatitis |
| CM7.2 | Enumerate, describe and discuss the mode of transmission and measures for prevention and control of hepatitis (A and E) |
| CM8.1 | Describe and discuss the epidemiological and control measures applicable in hepatitis (A and E) |

## INTRODUCTION

The term "Jaundice" is derived from old French word "Jaunice" or "Yalnice". "Icterus" means yellow in a Greek. Hepatitis (hepat, the Greek word for liver) is a term used for inflammatory condition of the liver caused by one of the heterogeneous group of "hepatotropic viruses". It can be caused due to viral infection or when liver is exposed to harmful or toxic substances, autoimmune diseases, and some infections.

Hepatitis is termed "acute" or "chronic" according to the duration which is considered as less than or more than 6 months, respectively. The hepatitis A and E viruses primarily transmit through the feco-oral route, resulting in an acute self-limited infection. The hepatitis B, C, and D viruses are transmitted by the parenteral route or sexual route and may result in both acute and chronic types of infection.

# HEPATITIS A (ACUTE INFECTIOUS HEPATITIS, EPIDEMIC JAUNDICE, BOTKIN'S DISEASE, AND AUSTRALIA ANTIGEN NEGATIVE HEPATITIS)

## Introduction

The hepatitis A virus (HAV) causes this infection and is a common form of viral hepatitis occurring globally. It is an acute, inflammatory disease of liver. It can be easily transmitted from one person to other. Specific protection against this disease is conferred by a vaccine. The route of entry of the organism is feco-oral and is due to consumption of food or water contaminated by fecal matter. Hepatitis A resolves on its own and usually does not progress to chronicity. The case fatality rate is extremely low, less than 0.2%.

## Problem Statement

### Global

Hepatitis A is estimated to cause over 100 million cases and around 15,000–30,000 deaths per year worldwide. It occurs intermittently and is known to cause outbreaks, with a trend of cyclic recurrences. Globally, food contaminated with HAV accounts for 2–7% of all HAV. According to global estimates, approximately 600 million cases of foodborne illness related to 31 pathogens are reported annually, of which 14 million cases are due to HAV infection with 1,353,767 Disability-Adjusted Life-Years (DALYs), which reflects the ability of the virus to persist in the environment and withstand food-production processes. Food handlers play a major role in preparation of safe food, and they may transmit HAV to susceptible individuals, if infected themselves.

### India

Hepatitis A is an endemic disease in all the developing countries, because of insanitary conditions and poor hygiene. In India, very little epidemiological data is available on HAV. HAV infection was hyperendemic in India with high infection rates in initial years of life and most people acquired antibodies to HAV by 10 years of age. In India, lack of knowledge and awareness of preventing foodborne diseases and practice of proper hygiene among food handlers is a major concern as it may lead to a significant disease burden due to foodborne infections such as hepatitis.

Seroprevalence of anti-HAV was in lower range (54.5%) in the higher socioeconomic group as compared to the lower socio-economic group (85%). As per recent reports, seroprevalence of anti-HAV differ in different areas of country. Certain areas are showing a gradual shift with rise of infection in adult population (Batra Y et al., Bull World Health Organ, 2002; Jindal M et al., Indian J Med Res, 2002; Das K et al., Eur J Epidemiol, 2000).

## Epidemiological Determinants

### Host Factors

Susceptibility for HAV is universal. In countries with suboptimal sanitary conditions and poor hygienic practices, infection with the HAV occurs within 10 years of age in 90% of children. Severity of infection increases with age, i.e. infection tends to be mild among children and severe among adults.

### Agent Factors

*Type:* Hepatitis A is a non-enveloped virus. The genetic material is single-stranded RNA. It belongs to Picornaviridae family of viruses. The virus is shed in feces in late incubation and early illness period.

*Viability:* It can stay unaffected in the environment and can withstand the routinely used processes of food production. It can withstand heat at 60°C for 1 hour but at 100°C, it gets destroyed shortly. Virus survives more than 10 weeks in well water. Formalin and 0.5% sodium hypochlorite are effective disinfectants. Virus survives in routine chlorination process but inactivated beyond 1 ppm. Exposure to ultraviolet (UV) radiations or autoclaving or by boiling for 5 minutes can inactivate the virus.

### Environmental Factors

Poor standard of living with poor sanitation, poor personal hygiene (such as dirty hands), unsafe water, and overcrowding greatly influence the spread of the disease.

### Modes of Transmission

Many routes of HAV transmission are known; however, most common is via fecal-oral route or by direct contact with an infectious person. In some cases, the infection status of the member involved in preparing or processing food is responsible, through his hands which may be dirty or unclean. Rarely few water borne outbreaks, are also seen, they occur due to contamination of drinking water by sewage or inadequately treated water.

### Reservoir of Infection

The only known reservoir of infection is man. Such a human reservoir may be an active clinical case or a subclinical case or a carrier of the disease. Subclinical cases or carriers maintain endemicity of disease in community.

### Infective Material

It is mainly the feces of the case or the carrier. Blood is infective during the period of viremia. Once the jaundice sets in, virus is no longer found in the blood but only in feces for about 2–4 weeks.

### Period of Infectivity and Incubation Period

The patient is highly infectious during the last 2 weeks of the incubation period and for about 1 week after the onset of the disease. Infectivity reduces after development of jaundice. The incubation period of hepatitis A is usually 14–28 days.

## Clinical Features

The symptoms are non-specific and ranging from mild to severe. The common presentation includes fever, malaise, and loss of appetite associated with diarrhea, nausea, and abdominal pain. Patient may report passing of pale or clay-colored stool, dark-colored urine, and jaundice. All symptoms may not be present in those infected with HAV. Patients with HAV infection are similar in presentation to other types of acute viral hepatitis. Relapses are reported to occur in HAV. Those who recover from hepatitis A develop lifelong immunity. Rarely, hepatitis A could lead to death from fulminant hepatitis.

### Diagnosis

Isolation of HAV or demonstration of specific antigens in the feces, bile, and blood is required for diagnosis. HAV can be detected in the stool of the patient, about 2 weeks before the onset of jaundice and up to 2 weeks after the onset of jaundice. Serologic detection of immunoglobulin M (IgM) in single acute-phase serum sample can be done. IgM anti-HAV is usually detectable from 5 days before to the appearance of symptoms and then reduces to levels which cannot be detected, 6 months after infection. Antibody (IgG anti-HAV) is used to detect previous infection as it usually persists for lifelong after infection (Fig. 17B.23).

### Treatment

Specific treatment is not available for hepatitis A. Treatment mainly includes of symptomatic management with bed rest and low protein diet. The guidelines do not recommend use of paracetamol or anti-emetics.

### Prevention

As main mode of transmission of HAV infections is by feco-oral route thus, improvement in the sanitation, better personal hygiene maintenance, and provision of high quality standards for drinking water, food safety, management of sanitary waste, and immunization are the basis of prevention and control of infective hepatitis.

#### Immunization

*Active immunization:* Availability of two types of HAV vaccines, namely (1) inactivated vaccine and (2) live attenuated vaccine are there but none is recommended to be used in children younger than 1 year of age.

- **Inactivated vaccine:** It is cell-culture liquid vaccine using HM-175 strain of HAV. Each 1 mL contains not less than 720 Elisa units of viral antigens. Adults and children are given 1 mL and 0.5 mL dose, respectively. It should be given as IM injection in deltoid region. Primary course consists of two doses with 4–6 weeks' interval. A booster dose is required after 6–12 months. Immunity lasts for about 15–20 years. Storage temperature is 2–8°C. It is marketed as "Havrix". Schedule of combined vaccine is 0 month, 1 month, and 6 months.
- **Live vaccine:** A live, attenuated freeze-dried vaccine containing H2 strain of HAV cultured on human diploid cells, has been developed. The diluent is sterile distilled water. Single SC dose of 0.5 mL is injected in the deltoid region. Immunity lasts for 15 years. No booster dose is required. Storage temperature is 2–8°C. Hepatitis A freeze-dried vaccine is recommended for both pre-exposure prophylaxis of high-risk individuals traveling to endemic areas and postexposure prophylaxis to young close contacts because of long incubation period (15–50 days). It is marketed as "Biovac-A".

*Passive immunization:* Passive immunization with human immunoglobin that contain anti-HAV are more than 85% effective in preventing symptomatic HAV infection if given before, or within 2 weeks of exposure. With the availability of hepatitis A vaccines, immunoglobin is primarily recommended for postexposure prophylaxis for unvaccinated persons who are exposed to HAV. A single IM dose of immunoglobin (0.02 mL/kg) is recommended for young close contacts and to travelers going to endemic areas.

## HEPATITIS E [ENTERICALLY TRANSMITTED NON-A, NON-B HEPATITIS (HNANB)]

### Introduction

Hepatitis E virus (HEV) was discovered in 1990. It is commonly found in developing countries where environmental sanitation is poor. It is essentially water borne disease transmitted through water or food supplies contaminated by feces. Mostly, it presents as a mild and self-limiting infection.

### Problem Statement

#### Global

Every year, around 20 million HEV infections reported worldwide leading to an estimated 3.3 million symptomatic cases of hepatitis E. WHO estimates that hepatitis E caused approximately 44,000 deaths in 2015 (accounting for 3.3% of the mortality due to viral hepatitis). Fulminant form of HEV is common (up to 20% cases) during pregnancy with high case fatality rate, up to 80% (Teshale EH et al., World J Hepatol, 2011).

#### India

HEV infection and disease are highly endemic in India, with nearly 60% of blood donors having circulating anti-HEV IgG antibodies, indicating prior exposure to the virus. The

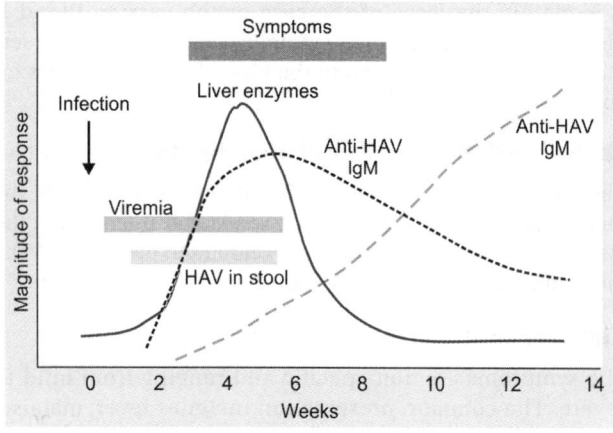

**Fig. 17B.23:** The appearance of symptoms and protective antibodies with duration of illness.
(HAV: hepatitis A virus; IgG: immunoglobulin G; IgM: immunoglobulin M)

*Source:* Murray PR, Rosenthal KS, Pfaller MA. Medical Microbiology. New York: Elsevier Health Sciences, 2015.

seroprevalence rates vary by age, being higher in the elderly. Overall, hepatitis E accounts for nearly 50% of acute hepatitis cases and for a similar proportion of acute liver failure (ALF) cases.

The epidemiology of hepatitis E in India has not changed much over time. The outbreaks occur periodically, during the years 2011 to 2013, 291 outbreaks of hepatitis were reported to the country's Integrated Disease Surveillance Programme of the 163 outbreaks with a known cause, 78 were related to hepatitis E.

The first retrospectively (serologically) confirmed outbreak of hepatitis E was reported from New Delhi during 1955-1956. Out of total 1.6 million people, approximately 29,300 jaundice cases were reported, with about 67,700 non-icteric cases (Cainelli F, World J Hepatol, 2012). Another epidemic of hepatitis E was from Kanpur in year 1991 affected over 79,000 cases of jaundice (Labrique Ab et al., Epidemiol Rev, 1999).

A few special reported large outbreaks of hepatitis E are described in **Table 17B.22** (Geng Y et al., Springer, 2016).

Table 17B.22: Selected reported large outbreaks of hepatitis E.

| Location | Year | Cases | Transmission |
|---|---|---|---|
| India | 1955–1968 | 29,300 | Waterborne |
| India | 1991 | 79,000 | Contaminated river water |
| China | 1991 | 119,000 | Waterborne |
| Pakistan | 1993–1994 | 3,827 | Contaminated plant water |
| Sudan | 2004 | >2,600 | Safe water insufficient |
| Uganda | 2008 | >10,000 | Person-to-person |
| Sudan | 2014–2015 | >1,117 | Safe water insufficient |

## Epidemiological Determinants

### Host Factors

*Age:* It occurs predominantly in young to middle-aged adults aged 15-40 years. HEV is most common cause of sporadic hepatitis in adults. Interestingly, young children are often spared in most hepatitis E epidemics. HEV among children results only in mild illness, i.e. anicteric hepatitis. It does not lead to chronic disease or carrier state. The virus is excreted from few days prior to clinical disease onset till 3-4 weeks after the onset of disease.

Hepatitis E virus infection occurs predominantly in young to middle-aged adults aged 15-40 years; however, among children it results in mild illness only.

### Agent Factors

*Types:* Hepatitis E virus is RNA virus, which belongs to family *Calciviridae*, a nonenveloped virus. It has four different genotypes of which types 1 and 2 are known to affect humans, the types 3 and 4 are found primarily in animals and occasionally affect humans.

### Environmental Factors

The risk factor for hepatitis E is poor sanitation, which permits the virus excreted in the feces of infected people to reach drinking water source; however, two patterns are observed:

1. Resource-limited areas with frequent water contamination, and
2. Areas with safe drinking water supplies.

### Source

The source of hepatitis virus is man and some animals. The most common route by which HEV transmitted is through the feco-oral route contaminating drinking water. This route accounts for a majority of cases.

### Modes of Transmission

Other routes of transmission include:
- Ingestion of inadequately cooked meat or meat products derived from infected animals
- Transfusion of infected blood products
- Vertical transmission from a pregnant woman to fetus.

### Incubation Period

The incubation period ranges from 2 weeks to 10 weeks, average 5-6 weeks.

## Clinical Features

Clinically, HEV infection is characterized by the same features as those of viral hepatitis A, followed by recovery on its own, in most of the cases. Patients usually present with mild fever, anorexia, nausea, and vomiting, in some cases abdominal pain, itching (without skin lesions), skin rash, and tender hepatomegaly. Jaundice with dark urine and pale stool are common. Disease severity is higher among pregnant women resulting in fetal loss and high mortality. Around 20-25% of them develop fulminant hepatitis (acute liver failure), the disease is severe and carries a risk of fatality in the 2nd or 3rd trimester.

## Diagnosis

Diagnosis may be strongly suspected clinically in disease endemic area, on exclusion of hepatitis A. Diagnosis of HEV is made by detection of anti-HEV antibodies in blood. The gold standard for diagnosis is detection of HEV-RNA by reverse transcriptase-polymerase chain reaction (RT-PCR).

## Treatment

Hepatitis E resolves on its own by 2-6 weeks. Recovery is almost complete. Treatment is required in fulminant cases only.

## Prevention

Most effective approach for prevention is by sanitation barrier. Maintenance of personal hygiene, adhering to safe water and food practices protects the individuals. Vulnerable subjects like pregnant mothers and those having cirrhosis need special attention to protect against HEV infection.

The "Global Health Sector Strategy on Viral Hepatitis, 2016-2021" aims to reduce new infections by 90% and deaths due to viral hepatitis by 65% by year 2030. Achievement of these targets requires the following actions to be taken by countries: Generating awareness, partnership promotion, and resource mobilization; devising evidence-based policy and making use of data for action; prevention of transmission; and treatment services.

## SUGGESTED READING

1. Aggarwal R, Goel A. Hepatitis E: Current Status in India. Clin Liver Dis (Hoboken). 2021;18(3):168-172.
2. Braude AI. International Textbook of Medicine. In: Braude AI (Ed). Medical Microbiology and Infectious Diseases. Philadelphia: Saunders Company; 1981.
3. Kar P. Is there a change in seroepidemiology of hepatitis A infection in India? Indian J Med Res. 2006;123:727-9.
4. Khuroo MS, Kamali S, Jameel S. Vertical transmission of hepatitis E virus. Lancet. 1995;345:1025-6.
5. Pinto MA, de Oliveira JM, González J. Hepatitis A and E in South America: new challenges toward prevention and control. In: de Oliveira JM, González J (Eds). Human Virology in Latin America. Cham: Springer; 2017. pp. 119-38.
6. Shenoy B, Andani A, Kolhapure S, Agrawal A, Mazumdar J. Endemicity change of hepatitis A infection necessitates vaccination in food handlers: An Indian perspective. Hum Vaccin Immunother. 2022;18(1):1868820.
7. Who. Hepatitis E ; Fact sheet. 2023.
8. Wu X, Chen P, Lin H, et al. Hepatitis E virus: Current epidemiology and vaccine. Hum Vaccin Immunother. 2016;12:2603-10.

# EPIDEMIOLOGY OF CAMPYLOBACTERIOSIS AND ITS PREVENTION AND CONTROL

*Abhishek Singh*

| CM7.2 | Enumerate, describe and discuss the mode of transmission and measures for prevention and control of campylobacteriosis |
| --- | --- |
| CM8.1 | Describe and discuss the epidemiological and control measures applicable in campylobacteriosis |

## INTRODUCTION

*Campylobacter jejuni* is an important cause of bacterial gastroenteritis, globally. It is a zoonotic disease. In developing countries, diarrhea caused by *Campylobacter* species constitutes an important cause of child morbidity, in healthcare and community settings. Campylobacter infections are generally mild, but can be fatal among very young children, elderly, and immunosuppressed individuals.

## PROBLEM STATEMENT

### Global

*Campylobacter* is 1 of 4 key global causes of diarrheal diseases. It is considered to be the most common bacterial cause of human gastroenteritis in the world. It Incidence of campylobacteriosis is on rise. The high incidence of *Campylobacter* diarrhea, as well as its duration and possible complications, makes it highly important from a socio-economic perspective. In developing countries, *Campylobacter* infections in children under the age of 2 years are especially frequent, sometimes resulting in death (WHO 2023).

It is estimated that *Campylobacter* species are responsible for over 172 million episodes of diarrhea annually worldwide and account for over 75,000 deaths due to diarrhea as per the Global Burden of Disease Study 2016.

In developing countries, it is estimated that *Campylobacter* isolation rates for foodborne illness are between 5% and 20%.

Endemicity of this infection has been reported from certain areas of North America, Europe, and Australia. As per the estimates from developed world, an average incidence of *Campylobacter* bacteremia is estimated to be 1.5/1,000 patients with enteritis (Kaakoush NO et al., Clin Microbiol Rev, 2015).

### India

In developing nations, where *Campylobacter* is endemic, infection mostly affects children.

Recent data from Kolkata reported that, during 2008-2010, 7.0% of admitted patients with gastroenteritis proved to be culture positive for *Campylobacter* species. *Campylobacter jejuni* was isolated in 70% of these cases (Palmer SR et al., Lancet, 1983). *Campylobacter jejuni* is regularly isolated from stool of healthy under five children. Isolation rates in children fall between 8% and 45%. Annual incidence is estimated to be 2.1 episodes of *Campylobacter*-associated diarrhea per child (Mukherjee P et al., Emerg Infect Dis, 2013).

## EPIDEMIOLOGICAL DETERMINANTS

### Host Factors

*Age:* In children below 2 years of age, this infection is hyperendemic. The infection may remain asymptomatic in children as well as in adults. It rarely causes outbreaks.

### Agent Factors

*Type:* Term *Campylobacter* comes from the Greek word Kampylos, which means curved rod. *Campylobacter* is a spiral, "S"-shaped, or curved gram-negative bacilli. *Campylobacter* and *Vibrio* are similar in context of motility by polar flagella, shape curved gram-negative bacilli, and oxidase positive activity. They differ in certain aspects, as *Campylobacter* are microaerophilic, do not ferment carbohydrates, and have lower guanosine and cytosine content of DNA.

*Strain:* *Campylobacter jejuni* (subspecies *jejuni*) and *Campylobacter coli* are the most common species infecting humans. Other species such as *Campylobacter laridis* and *Campylobacter upsaliensis* are reported less frequently.

*Viability:* Outside the gut, *Campylobacter jejuni* does not replicate and its survival is poor. It grows nicely in environment with less oxygen and in a temperature range of 37-42°C. The organism has high sensitivity to harsh conditions such as freezing, drying, acidic conditions (pH < 5.0), and salinity.

### Environmental Factors

It follows a seasonal trend in occurrence in developed countries; however, in India no seasonality is seen.

### Reservoir/Source of Infection

Infected animals act as the main reservoir of the infection. Dogs, cats, and other pets act as reservoir. Organisms are found in the intestines of the reservoirs. Food products of infected animal act as the source of infection.

### Modes of Transmission

*Campylobacter* species are commonly found in animal-derived foods such as poultry, cattle, pigs, and sheep. Consumption of improperly cooked meat and meat products, and contaminated milk are implicated for transmission. At the time of sacrifice of animals, their meat or carcasses may become contaminated with feces. Upto 50–70% of the *Campylobacter* infection can be attributed to infected chickens. Other modes of transmission are feco-oral route, through sexual contact. Of all the earlier sources, consumption of undercooked meat is considered as a chief source.

*Campylobacter enteritis* is quite common in under five children in developing countries. In contrast, *Campylobacter bacteremia* occurs in patients more than 65 years.

## CLINICAL FEATURES

*Campylobacter* infections are generally mild and self-limiting. Usually within 2–5 days, symptoms of illness develop in most cases, this can delay up to 7 days after exposure in some cases. The illness usually lasts 7 days after onset. Infection with *Campylobacter jejuni* usually presents as enteritis, which is manifested by abdominal pain, vomiting, diarrhea, fever, and malaise. Watery diarrhea is very important manifestation and seen in approximately 10% of children. Severity of diarrhea can vary from loose stool in mild cases, progressing to bloody stool in severe cases, or sometimes pus in stool. Chronic sequelae in the form of Guillain-Barré syndrome, Reiter's syndrome, and relapses are known to occur.

## DIAGNOSIS AND TREATMENT

Isolation of organisms from diarrheal stool samples confirms the diagnosis. The culture or fecal smear by Gram staining and dark-field microscopy is used to visualize the bacteria. Treatment is generally not needed, except electrolyte replacement and rehydration, which are the principal therapies for most patients. Antibiotic cover is advocated in severe cases (when bacterial invasion of intestinal mucosa cells and tissue damage ensues) or to prevent formation of carrier state (the condition where asymptomatic subjects keep shedding the bacteria).

## PREVENTION AND CONTROL MEASURES

To prevent disease, hygienic practices need to be reinforced at every step of food chain from production level till consumer level. Wide occurrence of *Campylobacter* acts as a barrier in devising the control strategies along the food chain. Heating and thorough cooking of food are effective in killing *Campylobacter* species.

Multiple strategies used for prevention of campylobacteriosis are:

- Prevention revolves around control measures implementation at every stage of the food chain, from production level on a farm, during processing in industry, till consumption of food.
- Feces and items soiled with feces must be disinfected before disposal, in countries where adequate sewage disposal systems do not exist.
- To reduce the contamination of carcasses by feces, hygienic slaughtering practices need to be followed. Training of abattoir workers and raw meat producers about handling of food hygienically are crucial to reduce contamination.
- Chlorination of drinking water for chickens and chemical rinses to inhibit bacterial flora on poultry carcasses are other options.

Heating or irradiation is an effective bactericidal method to eliminate organism from contaminated food.

## SUGGESTED READING

1. Borkakoty B, Jakharia A, Sarmah MD, Hazarika R, Baruah PJ, Bora CJ, et al. Prevalence of campylobacter enteritis in children under 5 years hospitalised for diarrhoea in two cities of Northeast India. Indian J Med Microbiol. 2020;38:32-6.
2. Kliegman RM, Behrman RE, Jenson HB, et al. Nelson Textbook of Pediatrics. New York: Elsevier Health Sciences; 2007.
3. Nachamkin I, Szymanski CM, Blaser MJ. Campylobacter. United States: ASM Press; 2008.
4. WHO. Campylobacter; Fact sheet. 2020.

# EPIDEMIOLOGY OF ESCHERICHIA COLI INFECTION AND ITS PREVENTION AND CONTROL

*Abhishek Singh*

**CM7.2** Enumerate, describe and discuss the mode of transmission and measures for prevention and control of *Escherichia coli*

**CM8.1** Describe and discuss the epidemiological and control measures applicable in *Escherichia coli*

---

*Case Scenario*

Dr X got news about outbreak of diarrhea among infants in a nursery of hospital Y. On probing, it was found that the illness was associated with low-grade fever, malaise, and vomiting. On gross examination of stool, Dr X observed that the stool contained large amounts of mucus but gross blood was absent.
- Which could be the organism responsible? (a) EPEC, (b) ETEC, (c) EIEC, and (d) EHEC serotype O157:H7.
- Describe laboratory investigations need to be carried out to confirm the diagnosis.
- Suggest measures to prevent such outbreaks in the future.

---

## INTRODUCTION

Bacteria *Escherichia coli* (*E. coli*) is commonly seen in the lower intestine of human beings and warm-blooded animals. It has been recognized as harmless commensal and also as a versatile pathogen. These strains can be commensal, existing in a symbiotic state providing resistance against pathogenic organisms, or be pathogenic and cause diseases of intestinal and extraintestinal sites. Some strains can cause diarrhea and infection occurs through contact with contaminated food or water while other strains can cause respiratory illness, urinary tract, meningeal (particularly in the newborn), and wound infections. *E. coli* is also implicated for many diarrheal illnesses.

*Note*

*E. coli* ferment lactose (i.e. they are Lac+) in contrast to the major intestinal pathogens. *Salmonella* and *Shigella* cannot ferment lactose (i.e. they are Lac–).

Five major types of *E. coli* which cause diarrheal illnesses based on distinct epidemiology, O:H serotypes, and clinical features are as follows:
1. Enteropathogenic *E. coli* (EPEC)
2. Enterotoxigenic *E. coli* (ETEC)
3. Enteroinvasive *E. coli* (EIEC)
4. Enterohemorrhagic *E. coli* (EHEC) serotype O157:H7
5. Enteroaggregative *E. coli* (EAEC).

## PROBLEM STATEMENT

### Global

Diarrhea is a second leading killer of children, accounting for the deaths of 370,000 children in 2019 (WHO). EHEC is contributing largely to burden of foodborne disease in northern United States and Canada. These regions have reported outbreaks of HUS among children causing mortality in them.

### India

In India, 13% of deaths in the same age-group are because of diarrhea, leading to 300,000 deaths among children every year; though the actual incidence may be manifold. EPEC and EAEC are frequently reported to cause infections in developing countries. ETEC is an important cause of infantile diarrhea especially in poor and developing nations (Okeke IN et al., Lancet Infect Dis, 2001).

*Key Points*

Typing strains is based on differences in three structural antigens: (1) O, (2) H, and (3) K.

**O antigens (somatic or cell wall antigens):**
- Found on the *polysaccharide portion* of the lipopolysaccharide
- Heat stable
- Commonly used to *serologically type* many of the enteric Gram-negative rods.

**H antigens:**
- Are associated with flagella
- Only flagellated (motile) Enterobacteriaceae such as *E. coli* have H antigen.

**K antigens:**
- Located within the *polysaccharide capsules*.

## ENTEROPATHOGENIC ESCHERICHIA COLI

Enteropathogenic *E. coli* is very important cause of infant diarrhea in tropical countries. EPEC strains are associated with infantile diarrhea and such outbreaks have occurred in hospital nurseries. Disease is uncommon among older children and adults. Infection results when EPEC adheres to epithelial cells of the small intestine and then destroys the microvillus. Low-grade fever, malaise, vomiting, and diarrhea are characteristic features of the illness. The stool contains large amounts of mucus but gross blood is usually absent. In children aged less than 1 year, severe diarrhea infection with EPEC must be suspected.

*Key Points*

**Enteropathogenic *E. coli***
- An important cause of diarrhea in infants.
- *Characteristic lesions in the small lintestine*:
  » Attaching and effacing lesions (A/E)
  » Destruction of the microvilli
  » Caused by way of a type III secretion system (T3SS).
- Being noninvasive EPEC does not cause bloody diarrhea.

## ENTEROTOXIGENIC ESCHERICHIA COLI

Diarrhea caused by ETEC is still endemic in the developing countries. It is prevalent in all age groups of the population. ETEC strains causes diarrhea in infants, when it occurs in adults, it is sometimes referred as "traveler's diarrhea". ETEC infection occurs frequently by consumption of contaminated water or food. The major determinants of disease transmission are poor hygiene, unsafe drinking water, and improper sanitation.

> **Key Points**
>
> **Enterotoxigenic E. coli**
>
> - A common cause of traveler's diarrhea
> - Colonize the small intestine
> - Enterotoxins cause prolonged hypersecretion of chloride ions and water by the intestinal mucosal cells and inhibit the reabsorption of sodium.
> - *Heat-stable toxin*: Works by causing an elevation in cellular cyclic guanosine monophosphate (cGMP) levels
> - *Heat-labile toxin*: Causes elevated cyclic adenosine monophosphate (cAMP) and is essentially identical to choleratoxin.

Enterotoxigenic *E. coli* strains release one or both the toxins into the small intestine, a heat-labile toxin (LT) and a heat stable toxin (ST). Two fragments (A and B) make up the LT; the B fragment binds on the receptor site present on intestinal mucosa. This binding facilitates entry of A fragment, which then acts on adenylyl cyclase, activating the conversion of ATP to cAMP. The accumulation of cAMP in the intestinal mucosa initiates the hypersecretion of electrolytes and fluid in the lumen. These accumulated luminal secretions result in a watery diarrhea. The ST stimulates guanylate cyclase, leading to an increased production of cGMP and subsequent hypersecretion.

Enterotoxigenic *E. coli* strains usually causes low-grade fever, nausea, and non-bloody watery diarrhea often associated with abdominal cramps. The illness may last from 1 day to 5 days. Characteristic clinical features and isolation of lactose-fermenting organisms on differential media form the basis of diagnosis.

## ENTEROINVASIVE ESCHERICHIA COLI

Enteroinvasive strains are named so as they cause dysentery associated with invasion and destruction of the intestinal mucosa. The illness resembles that produced by shigellae. Transmission is directly from person-to-person via the fecal-oral route. Fever, abdominal cramps, malaise, and watery diarrhea accompanied by toxemia are the characteristic features of the illness. Scanty stool containing pus, mucus, and blood follows the watery diarrhea. EIEC strains do not ferment lactose and do not decarboxylate lysine. Newly developed technique for screening the stool samples involves DNA probes.

> **Key Points**
>
> **Enteroinvasive E. coli**
>
> - Cause a dysentery-like syndrome with fever and bloody stool
> - Plasmid-encoded virulence factors are nearly identical to those of *Shigella* species
> - These virulence factors allow the invasion of epithelial cells (Ipa)
> - In addition, EIEC strains produce a hemolysin (HlyA).

## ENTEROHEMORRHAGIC ESCHERICHIA COLI SEROTYPE O157:H7

The serotype O157:H7 is probably the most important public health Shiga toxin-producing *Escherichia coli* (STEC) serotype of *E. coli*. STEC may cause severe foodborne disease. It can survive for up to 6 months in mud. STEC is heat-sensitive. Incubation period is 3–8 days. Cattle is the main reservoir of this pathogen. Vehicles of transmission include raw milk, undercooked meat, raw apple juice, and fecal contamination of vegetables. Person-to-person (oral-fecal route) is an important mode of transmission. An asymptomatic carrier state may also be present. STEC may be excreted up to less than 1 week in adults but for longer period in children.

> **Key Points**
>
> **Enterohemorrhagic E. coli**
>
> - Produce one of two exotoxins (Shiga-like toxins 1 or 2)
> - *Result in a severe form of copious, bloody diarrhea* (hemorrhagic colitis) in the absence of mucosal invasion or inflammation
> - Associated with outbreaks of *acute renal failure (hemolytic uremic syndrome, or HUS)*
> - Detected on Mac Conkey sorbitol agar
> - Primary reservoir of EHEC is cattle
> - Possibility of infection can be greatly *decreased by thoroughly cooking ground beef and pasteurizing milk.*

The toxin produced by STEC is known as Shiga toxins because of its similarity to the toxins produced by *Shigella dysenteriae*. STEC grows at 7–50°C, with an optimum temperature of 37°C. Some STEC can grow in acidic foods, at a pH of 4.4, and in foods with a minimum aW of 0.95.

> **Note**
>
> Enterohemorrhagic *E. coli* infection should be suspected in all patients with acute bloody diarrhea, particularly if associated with abdominal tenderness and absence of fever.

Watery diarrhea and severe crampy abdominal pain are the characteristic presentation. Fever is typically absent in most of the cases. Symptoms usually last for 5–10 days. In most cases, the illness is self-limiting, but it may lead to a life-threatening disease including hemolytic uremic syndrome (HUS), especially in young children and the elderly. Up to 10% of patients harboring O157 develops HUS, this usually occurs about a week after the onset of diarrhea and has an associated case-fatality rate of 3–5%. HUS is characterized by thrombocytopenia, renal failure, and central nervous system (CNS) involvement. In young children, HUS is the most common cause of acute renal failure. Definitive diagnosis can be made by stool culture. The stool contains no leukocyte which differentiates it from shigellae-induced dysentery. Antibiotics are not recommended in treatment of patients with STEC disease as they may increase the risk of subsequent HUS.

## ENTEROAGGREGATIVE ESCHERICHIA COLI

Enteroaggregative *Escherichia coli* (EAEC) strains are so called because they show a typical "stacked brick" arrangement on Hep-2 cells or glass due to their autoagglutination. EAEC causes increased secretion of mucus. This forms a layer of biofilm on the epithelium of the small intestine, trapping the organisms in the epithelium of the small intestine. Adherence to the intestinal mucosa is the reason for EAEC strains to cause diarrhea. These strains adhere to Hep-2 cells on and between the cells. These organisms produce symptoms such as watery diarrhea, vomiting, and occasionally, abdominal pain. Symptoms may persist for more than 2 weeks.

> **Key Points**
>
> **Enteroaggregative *E. coli***
> - Also cause traveler's diarrhea and persistent diarrhea in young children
> - Adherence to the small intestine is mediated by *aggregative adherence fimbriae*
> - The adherent rods resemble *stacked bricks*
> - Result in *shortening* of microvilli
> - Produce a *heat-stable toxin* that is plasmid encoded.

**Table 17B.23** summarizes the major characteristics of the five major types of diarrheagenic *E. coli*.

**Table 17B.23:** Summary of the five major types of diarrheagenic *E. coli*.

| Groups | Mechanism of infection | Symptoms | Infectious dose | Source of infection |
|---|---|---|---|---|
| ETEC | LT and ST toxin | Traveler's diarrhea, watery diarrhea, abdominal cramps, nausea, and no mucus or blood | $10^8$ bacteria | Food and water |
| EAEC | Adherence to intestinal mucosa, toxin, or inflammation-induced damage | Watery diarrhea, occasional bloody stools, and vomiting | $10^{10}$ bacteria | Nosocomial and community acquired |
| EPEC | Attachment and effacement | Watery, non-bloody diarrhea with mucus, without fecal leukocytes, fever, and vomiting | 10 bacteria | Formula, food contaminated with fecal material (fecal-oral) |
| EIEC | Invasion of colon epithelium | Either watery diarrhea or dysentery (bloody, watery stool with mucus), fecal leukocytes, and fever | $10^6$ bacteria | Food and water |
| EHEC | Shiga toxins | Range from watery diarrhea to hemorrhagic colitis (bloody diarrhea with abdominal pain) | $<10^2$ bacteria | Food and water |

(EAEC: Enteroaggregative *E. coli*; EHEC: Enterohemorrhagic *E. coli*; EIEC: Enteroinvasive *E. coli*; EPEC: Enteropathogenic *E. coli*; ETEC: Enterotoxigenic *E. coli*)

**Remember:** Gastroenteritis caused by *Escherichia coli*.

| Diseases | Site and mechanism of action (MOA) | Group of *E. coli* |
|---|---|---|
| Infant diarrhea | Acts on small intestine, adhesion | EPEC, EAEC |
| Dysentery | Acts on large intestine, invasion and destruction of epithelial cells | EIEC |
| Traveler's diarrhea | Acts on small intestine, heat-stable/heat-labile toxin | ETEC |
| Hemorrhagic colitis | Shiga toxin | EHEC |
| Chronic diarrheal disease | Acts on small intestine | EAEC |

## PREVENTION AND CONTROL MEASURES

In general, the prevention of infection from *E. coli* requires institution of measures at all levels of the food chain, from the farm in agricultural production, to the processing, manufacturing, and preparation of foods at domestic and commercial level. At home while preparing the food, one should follow the basic food hygiene practices.

"Five keys to safer food" can effectively prevent the foodborne diseases. These are: (1) Keep clean, (2) Separate raw and cooked, (3) Cook thoroughly, (4) Keep food at safe temperatures, and (5) Use safe water and raw materials. Regular hand washing, particularly before food preparation or consumption and after toilet contact, is highly recommended to reduce the incidence of diarrhea illnesses.

## SUGGESTED READING

1. Chin J. Control of Communicable Diseases Manual. United States: American Public Health Association; 1917.
2. Donnenberg MS. Escherichia coli: Virulence Mechanisms of a Versatile Pathogen. New York: Elsevier; 2002.
3. Meng J, Doyle MP. Emerging and evolving microbial foodborne pathogens. Bull Instit Past. 1998;96:151-63.
4. Nguyen TV, Le Van P, Le Huy C, et al. Detection and characterization of diarrheagenic Escherichia coli from young children in Hanoi, Vietnam. J Clin Microbiol. 2005;43:755-60.
5. Scheiring J, Andreoli SP, Zimmerhackl LB. Treatment and outcome of Shiga-toxin-associated hemolytic uremic syndrome (HUS). Pediatr Nephrol. 2008;23:1749-60.
6. Thapar N, Sanderson IR. Diarrhoea in children: an interface between developing and developed countries. Lancet. 2004;363:641-53.
7. Who. Diarrhea Factsheet. 2019 available from https://www.who.int/health-topics/diarrhoea#tab=tab_1
8. Woodward DL, Clark CG, Caldeira RA, et al. Verotoxigenic Escherichia coli (VTEC): a major public health threat in Canada. Can J Infect Dis. 2002;13:321-30.

## C. EPIDEMIOLOGY OF SOIL HELMINTHS AND ITS PREVENTION AND CONTROL

*Manoj Bansal, Dhiraj Kumar Srivastava, Ashok Mishra, Roopa M*

## EPIDEMIOLOGY OF DRACUNCULIASIS AND ITS PREVENTION AND CONTROL

*"Zero transmission in 2015 – Historic Opportunity, New Challenges, Steadfast resolve"*
—**WHO slogan towards eradication of Dracunculiasis**

| | |
|---|---|
| CM7.2 | Enumerate, describe and discuss the mode of transmission and measures for prevention and control of Dracunculiasis |
| CM8.1 | Describe and discuss the epidemiological and control measures applicable in Dracunculiasis |

*Case Scenario*

*A 25-year-old man from rural area of Jodhpur district in Rajasthan, presented with the history of pain in left leg and ulcer on left shin of 15 days duration and these symptoms were recurring since last 4 years. Treatment with antibiotics at primary care level used to heal the ulcer but it used recur after few days. On examination a 3 × 3 cm ulcer was noticed with a healed ulcer below the present one. Sensation was intact. There were no thickened nerves or lymphadenopathy. His general and systemic examination and laboratory investigations were within normal limits. Biopsy of the ulcer by the treating doctor showed only chronic inflammatory infiltrate. X-ray did not report any evidence of osteomyelitis of underlying bone however; it revealed a linear calcification ending in the ulcer. He was also given anti-tubercular therapy and then multidrug therapy (MDT) for leprosy but the ulcer recurred. A provisional diagnosis of Guinea worm disease (GWD) was made and decided to surgically remove the worm. A long linear calcified worm was found which was removed from the subcutaneous plain. Skin was sutured in layers. Wound healed completely and there was no recurrence thereafter.*

## INTRODUCTION

Dracunculiasis is a parasitic disease caused by thread-like nematode *Dracunculus medinensis*. The disease is commonly known as *Guinea worm disease* because of the existence of parasite on the Guinea coast of West Africa. Other names given to the parasite are *dragon worm, medina worm, serpent worm*. Human get the disease when they swallow cyclops-containing larvae in drinking water.

## PROBLEM STATEMENT

The global burden of dracunculiasis has fallen significantly since the launch of eradication efforts in the 1980s when 20 countries were endemic for the disease. **Dracunculiasis is a crippling parasitic disease on the verge of eradication**. During the mid-1980, worldwide estimated cases were 3.5 million. Over the past eight years, human cases have stayed at double digits (54 in 2019 and 27 human cases in 2020). These human cases were reported from countries: Angola (1), Chad (12), Ethiopia (11), Mali (1), South Sudan (1) and Cameroon (1) – likely imported from Chad.

During 1984, almost two-thirds cases were reported from Rajasthan, Madhya Pradesh, Karnataka, Andhra Pradesh, Maharashtra and Gujarat. Last case of GWD was reported in Jodhpur, Rajasthan in year 1996. In 2000, WHO declared India as free of GWD (National Health Portal: Dracunculiasis, 2015).

Certification of India as a Guinea Worm disease free country by the World Health Organization in February 2000 is a major milestone in the history of disease eradication in India. Guinea worm is the second communicable disease after smallpox, which has been eradicated from the country, by the efforts of NICD and the concerned states.

## EPIDEMIOLOGY

### Host Factors

Humans are universal hosts. In general, about the same number of men and women get infected. GWD occurs in all age groups but it is most common among young adults 15–45 years old, may be due to type of work done. Humans are definitive host while cyclops acts as an intermediate host.

### Agent Factors

*Dracunculus medinensis* (Guinea worm) is the largest of the tissue parasite affecting humans. The adult female, which carries about 3 million embryos, can measure 60–100 cm in length and 2 mm in diameter. The male worm is short about 2–3 cm and it dies after mating. The parasite migrates through the victim's subcutaneous tissues causing severe pain especially when it occurs in the joints. The worm eventually emerges (from the feet in most of the cases), causing an intensely painful edema, a blister and an ulcer accompanied by fever, nausea and vomiting about 10–14 months after the infection. Transmission of disease begins from water source where fertilized adult female worm discharges thousands of larvae in the water source and these larvae are then ingested by cyclops. Larvae developed in its infective stage in about 2 weeks. When people consume water containing infected cyclops, the larvae are liberated into stomach and migrates to small intestine then penetrate the mucosa of gut **(Fig. 17C.1)**.

### Environmental Factors

GWD is common in rural or remote areas where safe drinking water is not available instead major source of drinking water is natural or artificial ponds or step wells. The transmission of Guinea worm has a seasonal pattern. In dry regions, people generally get infected during the rainy season, when stagnant surface water is available. In wet regions, people generally get infected during the dry season, when surface water is drying up and becoming stagnant.

### Reservoir of Infection

An infected person harboring gravid female worm.

### Mode of Transmission

The disease is transmitted entirely through the consumption of stagnant water containing cyclops harboring the infective stages of the parasite.

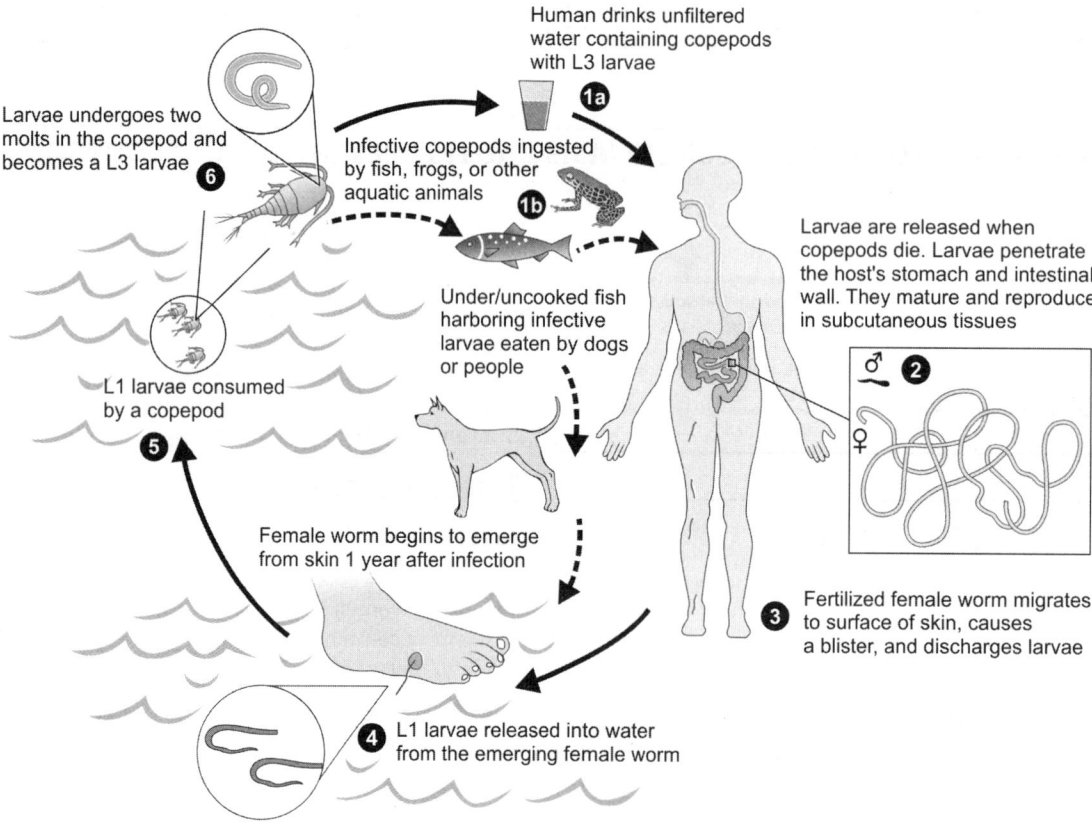

Fig. 17C.1: Life cycle of *Dracunculus medinensis*.
(L1: first developmental stage of larvae; L3: third developmental stage of larvae)
Source: CDC. Parasites—Guinea worm. [online] Available from https://www.cdc.gov/parasites/guineaworm/biology.html.

### Incubation Period

It takes between 10 and 14 months for the transmission cycle to complete until a mature worm emerges from the body.

### CLINICAL FEATURES

- Infected persons usually do not present any symptom for about 12 months
- Urticaria and pruritis
- Nausea and vomiting
- Fever with burning pain and swelling or blister can be seen at the site where adult worm comes out
- Secondary bacterial infection can also occur at this site
- Crippling disability.

### TREATMENT

No drug is available to prevent or heal this parasitic disease as it is exclusively associated with drinking contaminated water.
- Slow removal of adult worm from wound by slowly twisting it on the stick, try to avoid breakage otherwise may cause cellulitis and/or secondary bacterial infection
- Antibiotics—to prevent secondary bacterial infection
- Analgesics
- Antihelminthics are ineffective.

### PREVENTION

Dracunculiasis is relatively easy to eliminate and eventually eradicate. Strategy to achieve eradication are:
- Effective strengthening of surveillance activities.
- Containment of cases by early detection within 24 hours.
- Provision of safe drinking water and converting unsafe sources to safe ones.
- The construction of copings around well heads or the installation of boreholes with handpumps.
- Regular and systematic filtering of drinking water derived from ponds and shallow unprotected wells or from surface water. Finely-meshed cloth or better still, a filter made from a 0.15 mm nylon mesh, is all that is needed to filter out the cyclops from the drinking water.
- Treatment of unsafe water sources with temephos to kill the cyclops.
- Cleaning, treatment, and bandaging the wound to facilitate the expulsion of worm and to prevent secondary bacterial infection.
- Health education should be given to infected persons and to volunteers of the community in endemic area and social mobilization to encourage affected communities to adopt healthy drinking water behavior.
- No vaccine or drug is available for Guinea worm prevention.

## SUMMARY

- Dracunculiasis is caused by the large female of the nematode *Dracunculus medinensis*, which emerges painfully and slowly from the skin, usually on the lower limbs.
- The disease can infect animals, and sustainable animal cycles occur in North America and Central Asia but do not act as reservoirs of human infection.
- The disease is endemic across the Sahel belt of Africa from Mauritania to Ethiopia, having been eliminated from Asia and some African countries.
- Temporary disability due to disease has a significant socioeconomic impact.
- Dracunculiasis is exclusively caught from drinking water, usually from ponds.
- A campaign to eradicate the disease was launched in the 1980s and has made significant progress.
- The strategy of the campaign is discussed, including water supply, health education, case management, and vector control. Current issues including the integration of the campaign into primary health care and the mapping of cases by using geographic information systems are also considered.

**Key Points**

There is no immunity for Guinea worm. Person infected once may get infected many times.

## SUGGESTED READING

1. Dracunculiasis (guinea-worm disease). [online] Available from https://www.nhp.gov.in/disease/communicable disease/dracunculiasis-guinea-worm-disease.
2. Guinea Worm Disease Frequently Asked Questions (FAQs). [online] Available from https://www.cdc.gov/parasites/guineaworm/gen_info/faqs.html.
3. National centre for disease control. Guinea Worm Eradication Programme (GWEP). https://www.ncdc.gov.in/index1.php?lang=1&level=1&sublinkid=142&lid=73#:~:text=Guinea%20Worm%20disease%20(Dracunculiasis)%20was,two%20hosts%20%E2%80%93%20Man%20and%20Cyclops.
4. Sharma R, Singla LD, Singh BB. Zoonoses: parasitic and mycotic diseases, Volume 3. Guru Angad Dev Veterinary and Animal Sciences University; Ludhiana. pp. 86-94.
5. WHO factsheet - Dracunculiasis, Latest situation as of 16 March 2020 available on https://www.who.int/en/news-room/fact-sheets/detail/dracunculiasis-(guinea-worm-disease).

# EPIDEMIOLOGY OF AMOEBIASIS AND ITS PREVENTION AND CONTROL

*Dhiraj Kumar Srivastava*

*Strong people cannot bend for emotions but he can bend for dysentery.*

**CM7.2** Enumerate, describe and discuss the mode of transmission and measures for prevention and control of Amoebiasis

**CM8.1** Describe and discuss the epidemiological and control measures applicable in Amoebiasis

*Case Scenario*

*A 60-year-old, 50 kg woman was admitted to emergency department with a 14-day history of diarrhea with blood and mucus, recent urge incontinence, cramping abdominal pain and three episodes of vomiting. Further patient was lethargic with poor appetite. On examination vitals, general physical and systemic examination found to be in normal limits except for abdominal tenderness. Stool samples for culture were negative for Salmonella, Campylobacter, Shigella, Clostridium difficile toxin. Stool microscopy was negative for helminth ova and amebic cysts. However, Entamoeba histolytica trophozoites were seen in fresh stool samples and PCR was positive for E. histolytica DNA. The patient was diagnosed with amebic dysentery.*

## INTRODUCTION

Amoebiasis, or commonly known as amebic dysentery, is a protozoal disease caused by *Entamoeba* group. It is a third deadliest parasitic disease in the world. The disease spectrum ranges from asymptomatic infections for years to fumigant colitis as well as variety of extraintestinal infections. The disease occurs throughout the world but it is more endemic in countries with poor sanitation system. Epidemic of amoebiasis occurs when there is mixing of sewage water with drinking water. In developed countries, majority of the infections occurs due to food exposure when food handlers shed or food grown in soil contaminated with feces contains the cysts of *Escherichia coli*.

## CHARACTERISTICS OF DISEASE

Nearly 90% of the diseases present as an asymptomatic infection and the remaining 10% of the infections present as an invasive disease along with extraintestinal disease. Immunological studies has shown that majority of the asymptomatic individuals who shed cysts in their feces are infected with noninvasive species of *Entamoeba* group like *E. dispar* or *E. moshkovskii* whereas invasive and extraintestinal infection are caused by *E. hystolytica*. Among *E. histolytica*, out of 18 zymodemes recognized till now (on the basis of electrophoretic mobility of one or more enzymes), seven are found to be potentially pathogenic in nature.

## PROBLEM STATEMENT

Amoebiasis is the third deadliest parasitic disease in the world. Around 10% of the world's population is thought to be infected by parasitic amebae. Amoebiasis is a leading cause of diarrhea globally and is one among the top 15 causes of diarrhea in the first 2 years of life in children living in the developing world, where diarrhea remains the third leading cause of death, accounting for 9% of all deaths in children under the age of 5 years. The disease is responsible for 40,000 to 100,000 deaths each year, mainly in poorest regions of South-East Asia, South-Eastern and Western Africa, and Central and South America, where the hygiene conditions and the lack of effective sewage treatment plants encourage the spread of amebae. In some regions of India, Mexico, Bangladesh, and South Africa, up to 20% of the population can be infected. In developed countries the disease is rarer, with sporadic cases in travelers returning from endemic areas. The prevalence rate ranges from 2 to 60% from the countries with well-developed sanitation system to countries with poor sanitation system, respectively. It is responsible for about 40,000–100,000 deaths annually. The disease is prevalent throughout the world (Pasteur.fr: Disease Sheets: Amoebiasis 2023).

The disease is found in endemic proportion in South East Asia, South Eastern and Western Africa, and Central and South America. In India, the disease is found throughout the country. Approximately 15% of the population are infected by the amoebiasis (National Health Portal: Amoebiasis, 2015).

## EPIDEMIOLOGY

### Host Factors

All the ages and both the sexes are equally affected by amoebiasis. However, the disease is more invasive in males then in females. High-risk group includes persons on immunotherapy, malnourished, prisoners, migrant workers, etc. Cell-mediated immunity seems to have some protective effects and prevent from reinfection. Although the patients with AIDS do not have an increased risk of infection, patients who are MSM (men who have sex with men) are seen to have high risk.

### Agent Factors

Initially, the disease was thought to be caused by *Entamoeba histolytica*, but now it is proven that the disease is caused by other members of *Entamoeba* group like *E. dispar*, *E. moshkovskii*, etc.

The agent exist in three different phases in the human beings, namely trophozoite phase, precystic phase, and cystic phase. Trophozoite and precystic predominantly resides in the mucosa of the large intestine. During the encystment, the parasite become rounded surrounded by a highly refractile membrane to become cyst. These cysts are then shed in the feces to transmit the infections. They are quite resistant and can survive for days to months in moist damp environment at low temperature. They are not destroyed by the chlorine in the amount used for water purification. However, they are destroyed by the heat at temperature above 55°C or on freezing. In contract to cyst, trophozoites are readily destroyed outside the body.

On ingestion of the cyst, the trophozoites are released from it through the process of excystation in the alimentary canal which again move ahead to large intestine and colonize there to complete the life cycle **(Fig. 17C.2)**.

### Environmental Factors

Amoebiasis is closely associated with poor sanitation and low socioeconomic conditions. Overcrowding also increases the risk of infection in noninfected persons. Higher prevalence of amoebiasis has been noted in the communities where human night soil is used for agriculture purposes. In the countries where there is a marked variation between wet and dry seasons, higher transmission is noted during the wet seasons.

### Reservoir of Infection

Man is the only known reservoir of the infection. An infected man can discharge up to $1.5 \times 10^7$ cyst per day. However, experimentally the disease has been produced in cats, monkeys, and dogs.

*Infective material:* Food or water contaminated with entamoeba cysts.

### Modes of Transmission

- The fecal–oral route, either directly by person-to-person contact or indirectly by eating or drinking fecally contaminated food or water, and direct hand to mouth transmission.
- Sexual transmission, through rectal-oral contact especially among male homosexuals.
- **Vectors:** Flies, cockroaches and rodents are capable of carrying these parasites contaminating food and water.

### Period of Communicability

The person is infective as long as the cyst is shed in the feces which may range up to years in noninvasive cases where the diseases are not recognized and not treated.

### Incubation Period

Incubation period ranges from 2 to 4 weeks or longer.

## CLINICAL FEATURES

Nearly 90% of the infections are asymptomatic for years and the infected person can shed the cyst in their feces.

Symptomatic colitis develops after 2–6 weeks of ingestion. These patients present themselves as a slow onset of lower abdominal pain and mild diarrhea which is followed by malaise and weight loss. Patients with full blown colitis may present with dysentery with 10–12 stool per day which mostly consist of little fecal material and a mix of blood and mucus. These patients have typical flask-shaped ulcers in their large intestinal mucosa. On invasion of blood vessels, the disease spreads to liver where it presents as amebic liver abscess. These patients may present as a right upper quadrant pain associated with fever and jaundice. The disease may also spread to other parts of the body like spleen, brain, and genitourinary tract.

## DIAGNOSIS

Stool examination, serological examination, and noninvasive technique are the main stay of the diagnosis. Stool examination can show trophozoites or cysts along with heme. Definitive diagnosis of amoebiasis can be made by demonstration of hematophagous trophozoites of *E. histolytica*. Because the trophozoites are readily destroyed in the external environment, three fresh stool samples should be examined before giving negative reports.

Serological test like ELISA (enzyme-linked immunosorbent assay) can be positive in nearly 90% of the patients of colitis or extraintestinal amoebiasis.

Noninvasive techniques like ultrasonography, CT scan or MRI play an important role in the diagnosis of extraintestinal amoebiasis like amebic liver diseases.

## TREATMENT

Metronidazole is the drug of choice for the management of amoebiasis. It is given as 30 mg/kg body weight either orally or intravenously (IV) three times a day for 5–10 days. Other antiamebic drugs like tinidazole, paromomycin, diloxanide furoate or

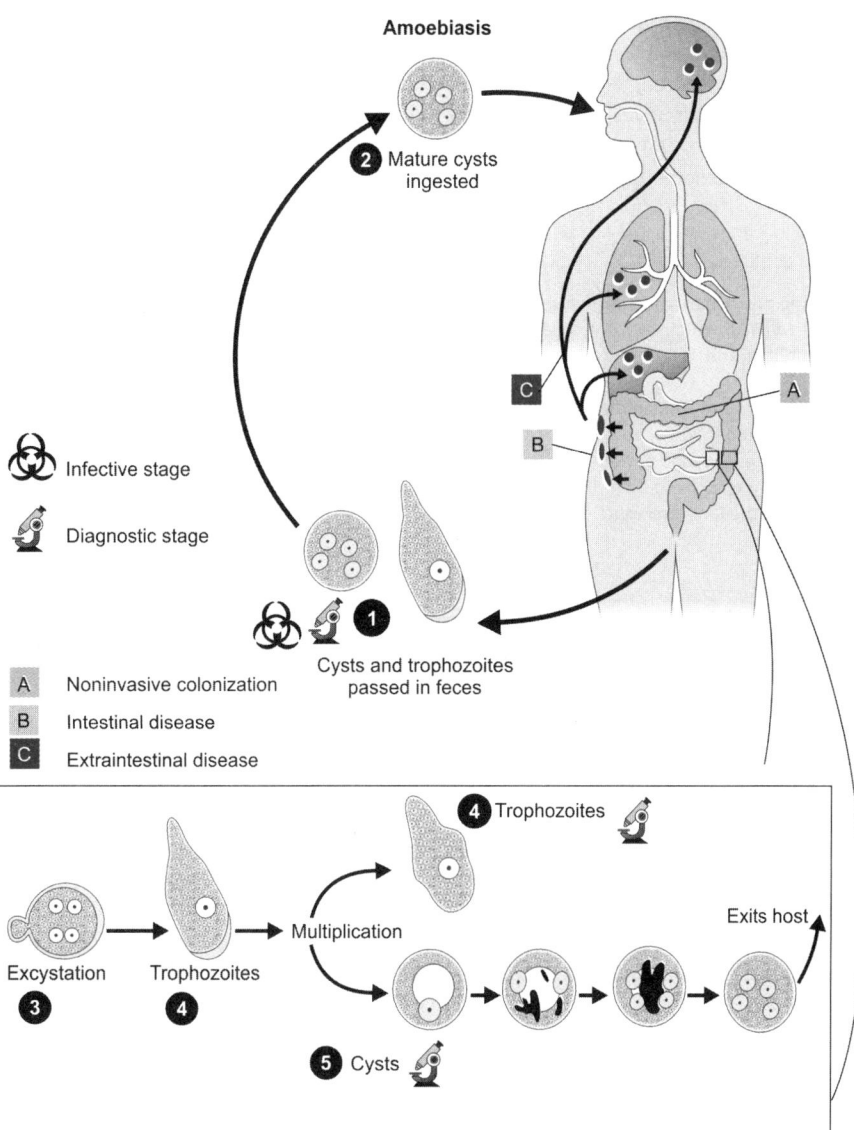

**Fig. 17C.2:** Life cycle of amoebiasis.
*Source:* CDC. Parasites amoebiasis—*Entamoeba histolytica* infection. [online] Available from https://www.cdc.gov/parasites/amoebiasis/pathogen.html.

iodoquinol can be used either as an alternative or as an adjunctive to one of the ongoing treatment.

Asymptomatic cases are generally not treated as there is a chance of reinfection in the endemic area, however, they should be treated if they are food handlers. They should be treated with oral diloxanide furoate 500 mg three times a day for 10 days or with diiodohydroxyquin 650 mg three times a day for 20 days.

At present no vaccine is available for the prevention of amoebiasis. Also there are no guidelines suggesting use of chemoprophylaxis for endemic area.

# PREVENTION AND CONTROL

Prevention and control of amoebiasis primarily centers around adopting proper sanitation practices and preventing contamination of food and water with human feces.

- ***Sanitation:*** Adoption of proper sanitation practices like washing hand after defecation or before cooking or eating is important in the prevention of amoebiasis. Cysts remaining under the nail bed are important source of autoinfection. Building of sanitary latrines and proper disposal of human feces are also important in the control of amoebiasis. Building of the sanitary latrines requires local body or central or state government support whereas maintenance of it requires community participation.
- ***Water supply:*** Drinking water sources should be well protected from contamination by human fecal matter. Sand filters are quite effective in removing the cyst of *Entamoeba* group, therefore water filtration at a large scale using sand filters and boiling water at a small scale are the most effective way for prevention of amoebiasis.

- **Health education:** People should be motivated to practice food hygiene like washing fruit and vegetables with an aqueous solution of acetic acid (5–10%) or full strength of vinegar. Even through washing in running water removes a large amount of the cyst from the raw fruits and vegetables. Food handlers should be motivated for the regular screening of amoebic cyst in their stool samples.

## SUMMARY

- Amoebiasis is an anaerobic protozoan infection caused by the protozoal organism *E. histolytica*, which can give rise both to intestinal disease (e.g., colitis) and to various extraintestinal manifestations.
- Several species of amebae are found in mammals, but the only known pathogen is *Entamoeba histolytica*.
- Humans become infected by ingesting food or water contaminated with feces containing infective cysts.
- Transmission usually occurs via the fecal-oral route when traveling in an endemic region.
- Stool examination, serological examination, and noninvasive technique are used to diagnose depending on type of infection.
- Treatment and prevention are the main mode of control of amoebiasis.

## SUGGESTED READING

1. Chatterjee KD. Parasitology, 25th edition. Kolkata: Chatterjee Medical Publisher; 1995. pp. 14-33.
2. Harrison's Principle of Internal Medicine, 17th Edition. New York: MCGraw Hills Medicine; 2009. pp. 1275-80.
3. Melnick and Adelberg's Medical Microbiology, 25th Edition. New York: A Lange Publication; 2010. pp. 1450-2.
4. National Health Portal. Amoebiasis. [online] Available from https://www.nhp.gov.in/disease/digestive/amoebiasis.
5. Sargeaunt PG, Jackson TF, Simjee A. Biochemical homogeneity of Entamoeba histolytica isolates, especially those from liver abscess. Lancet. 1982;1(8286):1386-8.
6. WHO. International travel and health—Amoebiasis. [online] Available from http://www.who.int/ith/diseases/amoebiasis/en/.
7. WHO. Technical Report Series. World Health Organization, Geneva, 1969. p. 421.

# EPIDEMIOLOGY OF GIARDIASIS AND ITS PREVENTION AND CONTROL

*My handbag turned into diaper bag for the chronically ill.*
—**Tracey Burkowitz**

| CM7.2 | Enumerate, describe and discuss the mode of transmission and measures for prevention and control of Giardiasis |
|---|---|
| CM8.1 | Describe and discuss the epidemiological and control measures applicable in Giardiasis |

### Case Scenario

*A 35-year-old male presented with an attack of diarrhea followed by intense pain in epigastric region on day one then it was intermittent and dull in nature. Patient also complained of constant headache, nausea and dizziness, fatigability. Blood picture showed leukocytosis with highest normal limit of eosinophils. Stool examination revealed the presence of cysts of giardia of varying dimensions. The diagnosis of Giardiasis was made.*

## INTRODUCTION

Giardiasis is a diarrheal disease which may be of acute or chronic in nature and caused by a protozoa *Giardia intestinalis*. It is a cosmopolitan protozoan which inhabits small intestine of human or other mammals. From epidemiological perspective this disease is similar to amoebiasis as far as mode of transmission or preventive and control measures are concerned.

## CHARACTERISTICS

The disease is characterized by a biflagellate trophozoite which mostly resides in the lumen of proximal part of small intestine and does not have hematogenous spread. It is more common in children than in adults. Other groups which are at risk are homosexuals and immune deficient persons.

## PROBLEM STATEMENT

Giardiasis has been reported throughout the world. It is present both in temperate as well as tropical countries. The prevalence rate of giardiasis ranges between 4 and 43% in different parts of the world and 1–7% in low and high income countries respectively with less prevalence in developed countries with better sanitation facilities and higher prevalence in undeveloped or developing countries where sanitation facilities are poor. The prevalence rate among children less than 10 years of age ranges between 15 and 20% and it is a major cause of malnutrition amongst children (Caccio SM et al., Trends Parasitol, 2005).

In India, prevalence of giardiasis ranges from 0.4 to 70% in different studies and asymptomatic passage of cyst was reported to be as high as 50% in one study in rural south India (Laishram S et al., Indian J Gastroenterol 2012).

## EPIDEMIOLOGY

### Host Factors

#### Age and Sex

Giardiasis is primarily a disease of human beings. All the ages and both the sexes are susceptible to the infection. However, children under the age of 5 years have higher rate of infection than adults.

#### High-risk Group

Patients having immunodeficiency like AIDS can present with prolonged and serious illness. Also, persons involved water-related recreational activities also have a higher risk of giardiasis infection.

## Agent Factor

*Giardia intestinalis* is a biflagellate protozoan. Ingestion of as low as 10 cyst is sufficient to cause an infection. The cyst undergoes excystation in the proximal part of small intestine to release two trophozoites which further multiplies by binary fission. These trophozoites remain free either in lumen of proximal part of small intestine or attached to the mucosa by the ventral sucking disk. The process of encystations occurs in colon from where cysts are released out of body along with the feces to infect others.

The number of cyst production may vary and it may reach up to $10^7$ cyst/g of the stool. The cysts are resistant to the routine chlorination and are killed by boiling or filtration. Heating water is a time-proven method of killing contaminants. While giardia cysts die at temperature below boiling (130–145°F), to be safe you should maintain a rolling boil for several minutes-longer at high altitudes.

Cysts are resistant forms and are responsible for transmission of *giardiasis*. Both cysts and trophozoites can be found in the feces. The cysts are hard and can survive several months in cold water. In cold temperature (around 4°C/39.2°F), giardia can survive for approximately 7 weeks (49 days). At room temperature (around 25°C/77°F), giardia can survive for approximately 1 week (7 days).

## Environmental Factor

Giardiasis is primarily a disease of poor sanitation condition. Person-to-person transmission occurs in condition where fecal hygiene is poor. Foodborne transmission mostly occurs when person infected with giardiasis cooks food in the absence of proper sanitation practices. Waterborne transmission occurs when the large water bodies are contaminated with fecal material or there is a contamination of the water supply by the sewage water **(Fig. 17C.3)**.

## Reservoir of Infection

Giardiasis do infect other animals, however their importance as reservoir is still not established.

## Modes of Transmission

Infection occurs by the process of ingestion of cyst contaminated food and water or by hand through fecal-oral route.

## Period of Communicability

Duration of cyst excretion is variable but can range from weeks to months. Giardiasis is communicable for as long as the infected person excretes cysts.

## Incubation Period

Usually 3–25 days or longer; median 7–10 days.

## CLINICAL FEATURES

The spectrum of clinical manifestations of giardiasis ranges from asymptomatic infections to fulminant diarrhea and malnutrition. Acute symptomatic cases mostly present with diarrhea associated with abdominal symptoms like abdominal pain, belching, bloating, nausea, and vomiting. Chronic cases may present with increase severity of abdominal symptoms

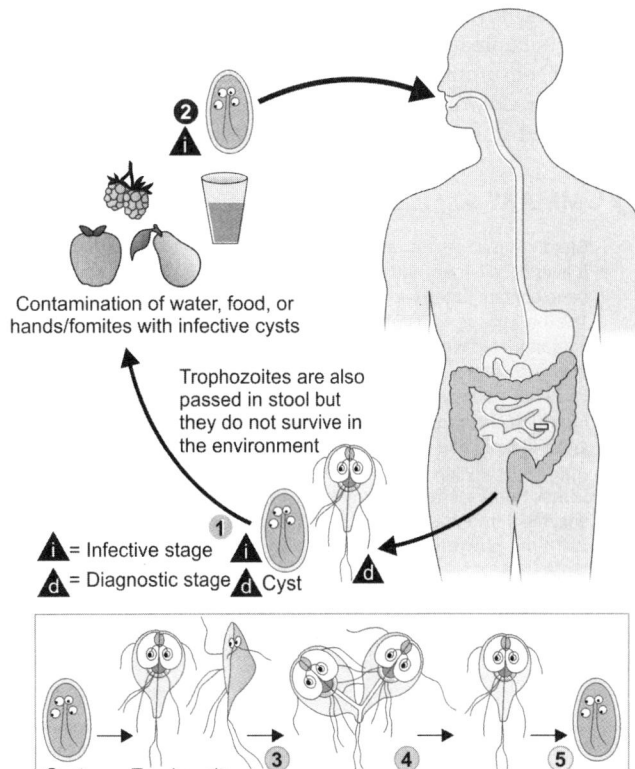

**Fig. 17C.3:** Life cycle of giardiasis.
*Source:* CDC. Parasites—Giardia. [online] Available from https://www.cdc.gov/parasites/giardia/pathogen.html.

which is not associated with diarrhea. Asymptomatic cases are mostly malnourished and have weight loss. Giardiasis in children mostly present with profound malnutrition associated with steatorrhea.

## DIAGNOSIS

Diagnosis is made by the demonstration of cyst or trophozoites in the fresh or properly preserve stool using concentration methods. Sometimes repeated stool examination is required for the demonstration of cyst or trophozoites. Antigen detection test on stool sample can also be used for the diagnosis.

## TREATMENT

Metronidazole is the drug of choice for the treatment of giardiasis. It is given in a dose of 250 mg thrice daily for 5 days. Other drug like tinidazole 2 g single dose can also be used for the treatment of giardiasis. In pregnant women paromomycin can be used for the treatment of giardiasis.

## PREVENTION AND CONTROL

Prevention and control of giardiasis can be done by adoption of proper sanitation practices.
- **Sanitation:** Proper disposal of human feces is pivotal in the control of giardiasis. Open field defecation near water bodies should be stopped by construction of sanitary latrines.

- **Water supply:** Drinking water supply should be protected from contamination by human feces. Water filtration or boiling before consumption can prevent the infection by giardiasis. However, chlorination is of limited use, as the cyst are not destroyed at the normal chlorination doses.

## SUMMARY

- Giardiasis is an illness caused by a parasite called *Giardia intestinalis*. It lives in soil, food, and water. It may also be on surfaces that have been contaminated with waste.
- The parasite is transmitted by the fecal-oral route, ingestion of contaminated water and food or person-to-person transmission.
- Risk factors for infection include children in day-care settings, child-care workers, institutionalized individuals, travelers in endemic areas, ingestion of contaminated or recreational water, immunodeficiency, cystic fibrosis, and oral-anal sex.
- Approximately 50–75% of infected children are asymptomatic.
- Direct fluorescent antibody tests that detect intact organisms, enzyme immunoassays that detect soluble antigens, and multiplex real-time polymerase chain reaction assays that detect specific genes of the parasite in stool samples have improved sensitivity and specificity compared with microscopic examination of stool specimens for the detection of giardia trophozoites or cysts.
- The best way to prevent giardia infection is to practice good hygiene, including frequent hand washing.

## SUGGESTED READING

1. Cacciò SM, Thompson RC, McLauchlin J, et al. Unravelling Cryptosporidium and Giardia epidemiology. Trends Parasitol. 2005;21(9):430-7.
2. CDC. Parasite Giardiasis. [online] Available from https://www.cdc.gov/parasites/giardia/general-info.html [Last assessed January 2019].
3. Chatterjee KD. Parasitology, 25th edition. Kolkata: Chatterjee Medical Publisher; 995. pp. 36-8.
4. Harrison's Principle of Internal Medicine, 17th Edition. New York: MCGraw Hills Medicine; 2009. pp. 1311-3.
5. Waldram A, Vivancos R, Hartley C et al. Prevalence of Giardia infection in households of Giardia cases and risk factors for household transmission. BMC Infect Dis. 2017;17:486.

# EPIDEMIOLOGY OF ASCARIASIS AND ITS PREVENTION AND CONTROL

*10 August 2018: National deworming day; a step towards building a healthy nation.*

**CM7.2** Enumerate, describe and discuss the mode of transmission and measures for prevention and control of Ascariasis

**CM8.1** Describe and discuss the epidemiological and control measures applicable in Ascariasis

### Case Scenario

*A 5-year-old male child coming from village presented to pediatric OPD with abdominal pain, nausea, and decreased appetite since last 6 months. On examination the child found to have growth stunting and cognitive delays. The mother also gave the history of passage of large worms in the stool suggesting ascariasis infestation. Microscopic examination of stool specimens demonstrate the characteristic ascaris eggs.*

## INTRODUCTION

Ascariasis, most common helminthic infection caused by *Ascaris lumbricoides, also known as roundworm*. World Health Organization has included it under the list of "Neglected Tropical Diseases". It is prevalent throughout the world with higher prevalence in low socioeconomic communities where limited access to clean water, poor personal hygiene, and sanitary facilities are widespread. Majority of the infections are asymptomatic especially in adults. However, children may present with symptoms of malnutrition, pneumonitis, etc.

## PROBLEM STATEMENT

It is estimated that approximately 25% of the world population are infected with ascariasis with approximately 60,000 annually (Bethony J et al., Lancet, 2006). In India, the prevalence of ascariasis is highest amongt all nematodes. Its prevalence ranges from 6 to 69% in different studies. In 2020, 6 deaths have been reported in India. Highest transmission has been reported during rainy season (Kumar H et al., Med J Armed Forces India, 2017).

## EPIDEMIOLOGY

### Host Factors

Ascariasis is primarily a disease of human beings. All the ages and both the sexes are susceptible to the infection. However, children have higher rate of infection.

### Agent Factor

The adult worm resembles like an earthworm. When fresh from intestine, it is pink or light brown in color, however as the time passes it becomes white in color. Its shape is rounded with tapering at both the ends. Females are longer and wider in size than their male counterpart. Average female is 25–40 cm in length and 5 mm in width whereas male is about 15–25 cm in length and 3–4 mm in width. The tail end of the male is more curved ventrally.

A mature female worm lay approximately about 150,000–200,000 unembryonated eggs daily. These eggs have a rough mammillated coating and are discharged into the intestinal lumen to be passed out through feces. Their population is regulated by temperature, moisture, oxygen pressure or ultraviolet rays. Cold temperature inhibits the development of these eggs. Once deposited in the soil they become embryonated and infectious and remain viable for years despite extreme temperature and moisture. Once ingested, these eggs reach the small intestine and get converted into rhabditiform larvae. These larvae penetrate the intestinal mucosa to reach the portal vein and from there to liver and then subsequently to lung. In the lung, they penetrate through the alveoli and move into the bronchioles and are coughed up and swallowed and again return to small intestine where they develop into adult worm.

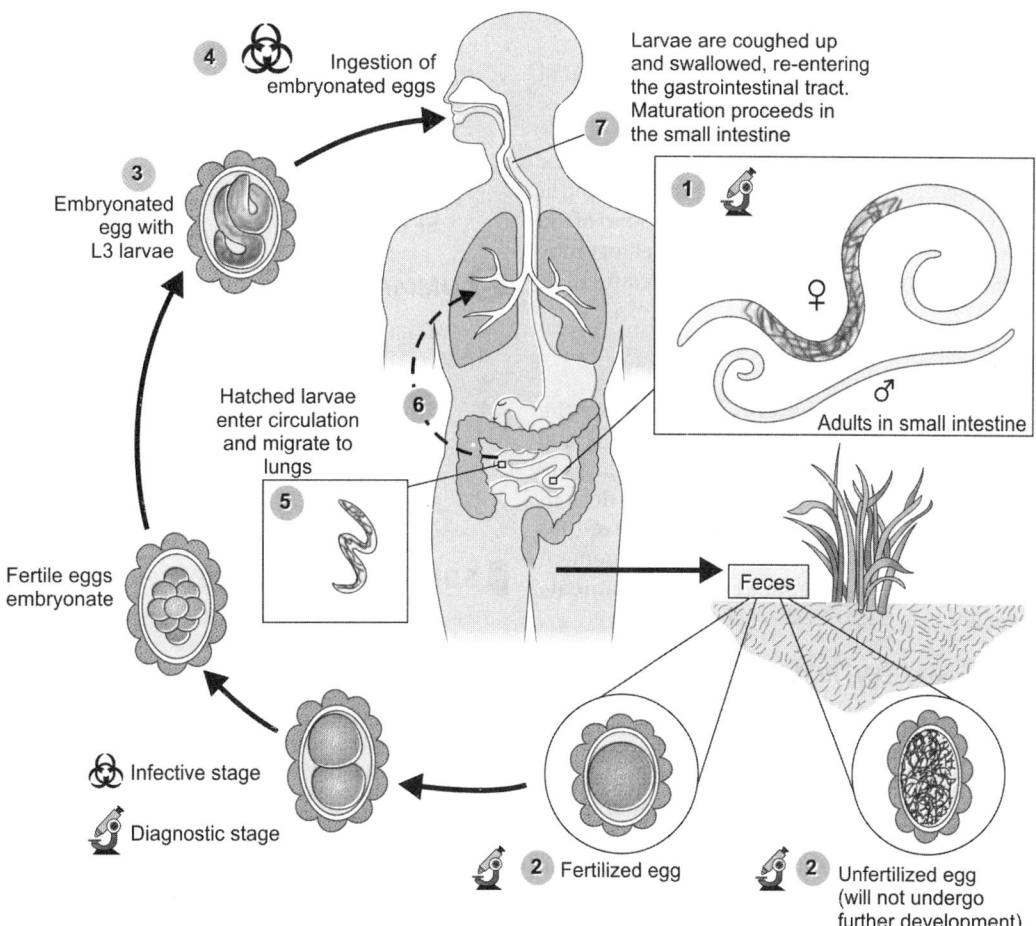

Fig. 17C.4: Life cycle of *Ascaris lumbricoides*.
(L3: third developmental stage of larvae)
Source: CDC. Parasites ascariasis. [online] Available from https://www.cdc.gov/parasites/ascariasis/biology.html.

## Environmental Factors

The disease is cosmopolitan in nature and has been reported throughout the world. It is primarily a disease of lower socioeconomic group associated with poor sanitation. Higher transmission rates have been reported in warmer climate regions and during rainy seasons (Fig. 17C.4).

## Reservoir of Infection

Man is the only known reservoir of the infection. It has no intermediate host.

## Modes of Transmission

Primarily fecal-oral route; ingestion of water or food contaminated with Ascaris eggs. To little extent duct may also disseminate ascaris in arid areas.

## Period of Communicability

The time period between the ingestion of eggs and its appearance in the stool is approximately 2 months.

## Incubation Period

Its incubation period is about 18 days to several weeks.

## CLINICAL MANIFESTATION

Majority of the infections in adult are asymptomatic. However, symptoms are related to the number of worm harbored. According to WHO heavy infection are said to happen when there are more than 50,000 eggs/g of feces. During the migration through the lungs they may produce the symptoms of pneumonitis associated with transient eosinophilia. In intestine, they may produce the symptoms like diarrhea, abdominal pain, and malaise along with generalized signs of malnutrition.

In children, migrating larvae may produce symptoms of allergic manifestation, fever, urticaria, etc. Pulmonary manifestation may resemble like Loffler's syndrome associated with eosinophilia. Adult worm in children may cause volvulus, intestinal obstruction or intussusception. Sometime wandering worms may cause symptoms of severe pancreatic or hepatobiliary diseases.

## DIAGNOSIS

Diagnosis of ascariasis can be established by demonstration of characteristics eggs in the feces of infected persons. Sometimes, the larvae can be demonstrated in the sputum or the gastric aspirate in the early stages of the disease. During the pulmonary movement of the larvae, there can be marked eosinophilia seen in the blood picture. Occasionally, X-ray of chest, ultrasound of the abdomen or endoscopic retrograde cholangiopancreatography (ERCP) can be used for the diagnosis as well as treatment of ascariasis.

## TREATMENT

Albendazole or mebendazole is the drug of choice for the treatment of ascariasis. Albendazole can be used as 400 mg single dose in adult or 200 mg single dose in children. Mebendazole can be used in a dose of 500 mg single dose in adult. Sometime, ivermectin can also be used in a dose of 150–200 µg per body weight in a single dose in the management of ascariasis. However, during pregnancy pyrantel pamoate 10 mg/kg body weight in a single dose is used.

## PREVENTION AND CONTROL

Prevention of ascariasis is primarily based on sanitary disposal of human waste and provision of safe drinking water.

- **Sanitation:** Construction of sanitary latrine for the proper disposal of human feces is the main element in the interruption of the chain of transmission of ascariasis. Proper disposal of human feces does not allow the embryonated eggs to come in contact with food and water to be used by human beings.
- **Safe drinking water:** Provision of safe water for drinking and personal use is also pivotal in the management of ascariasis.
- **Health education:** Communities should be motivated for—
  - Washing hands after defecation and before cooking food.
  - Constructing sanitary latrines for the dwellings and thus avoid open air defecation.
  - To take antihelminth drugs regularly when given during the mass chemotherapy campaigns.

## SUMMARY

- Ascariasis, most common helminthic infection of humans.
- Persons get infected through fecal-oral route.
- Majority of the infections in adult are asymptomatic.
- It is found in association with poor personal hygiene, poor sanitation, and in places where human feces are used as fertilizer.
- The best way to prevent people from getting ascariasis is through health education, hand washing practices, avoiding open air defecation, building up effective sewage disposal systems.

## SUGGESTED READING

1. Bethony J, Brooker S, Albonico M, et al. Soil-transmitted helminth infections: ascariasis, trichuriasis, and hookworm. Lancet. 2006;367(9521):1521-32.
2. Chatterjee KD. Parasitology, 25th Edition. Kolkata: Chatterjee Medical Publisher; 1995. pp. 182-8.
3. Harrison's Principle of Internal Medicine, 17th Editions. New York: McGraw Hills Medicine; 2009. pp. 1319-20.
4. Helbig S, Adja AM, Tayea A, et al. Soil Transmitted Helminths. Global Health Education Consortium and Collaborating Partner; 2012.
5. Wallace Public Health and Preventive Medicine, 15th Edition. New York: McGraw Hills Medicine; 2008. pp. 473-6.
6. WHO. Data; Mortality—Ascariasis.
7. WHO. Technical Report Series. World Health Organization: Geneva; 1981. p. 666.

---

# EPIDEMIOLOGY OF TRICHURIASIS AND ITS PREVENTION AND CONTROL

**CM7.2** Enumerate, describe and discuss the mode of transmission and measures for prevention and control of Trichuriasis

**CM8.1** Describe and discuss the epidemiological and control measures applicable in Trichuriasis

### Case Scenario

*A 62-year-old male was referred to the gastroenterology clinic with complaints of right lower abdominal pain, diarrhea and unintentional weight loss over the past couple of weeks. Laboratory and X-ray tests revealed no abnormalities. No ovum or parasite was found on repeated stool examinations. However, colonoscopic examination demonstrated the presence of a parasite on the edematous mucosa of cecum. The adult male whipworm (Trichuris trichiura) was then removed endoscopically. Her symptoms disappeared quickly, and also got treated with mebendazole for additional parasites followed by repeated stool examinations which failed to show any ova as this patient was infected by a single male whipworm.*

## INTRODUCTION

Trichuriasis also commonly known as whipworm infection is caused by *Trichuris trichiura* belonging to class nematode. It is called as whipworm because of it is typical whip like structure. It is a soil-transmitted helminthes and third most common roundworm infection of human being. It is prevalent throughout the world with highest prevalent in tropical and subtropical countries with poor sanitation conditions or where human feces are used as fertilizers. WHO has included it under the "Neglected Tropical Disease" list.

## CHARACTERISTICS OF DISEASE

The disease is mainly asymptomatic however when the disease load increases it may present with variety of gastrointestinal symptoms. The disease is found in tropical and subtropical countries with warm and humid climate. In temperate countries, it is more noted during the warmer seasons.

## PROBLEM STATEMENT

Globally, it is estimated that nearly 450 million to 1 billion active cases of trichuriasis with most diagnosed in children (CDC, Trichuriasis). In majority of the cases, the disease remains asymptomatic. It is only when the disease load increases, it may present as a *Trichuris* dysentery syndrome. Worldwide, almost half of the 5 billion people that live in developing countries are infected with at least one soil-transmitted helminth species, and 10% with two or more helminth species.

In 2014, the WHO estimated that by number, India has the highest burden of soil transmitted helminth (STH) infections in the world, with 223 million children aged 1–14 years at risk. Although the published studies indicate heterogenous burden of STH in the country, with prevalence ranging from 0.6% to 91% with A. lumbricoides as the predominant species. In India, the prevalence of trichuriasis is reported to range from 0.08 to 32% with majority of the transmission taking place in autumn.

## EPIDEMIOLOGY

### Host Factors

Trichuriasis is primarily a disease of human beings. Although all the ages and both the sexes are equally susceptible to trichuriasis but children of primary school age group are more commonly affected.

### Agent Factor

Trichuriasis is caused by *T. trichiura, T. vulpis, and T. suis* worldwide. The person became infected by the ingestion of embryonated egg from the environment. On reaching small intestine, the eggs are lodged in the crypts of small intestine up to 14 days before completing their maturation in large intestine especially cecum. The adult worm shed their eggs in the feces. These eggs later develop into rhabditiform larvae depending upon the climatic condition. In tropical countries, it takes around 3–4 weeks to develop whereas in temperate countries it takes around 6–12 months to develop. When man ingests these embryonated eggs, it completes their cycle **(Fig. 17C.5)**.

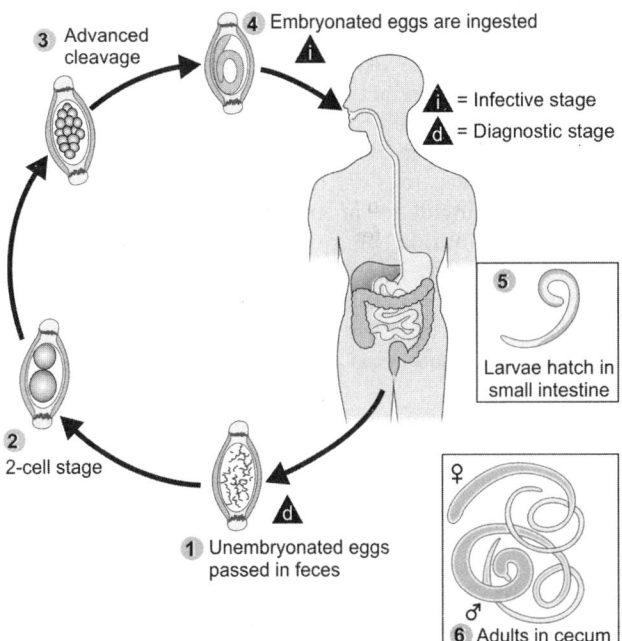

**Fig. 17C.5:** Life cycle of trichuriasis.
*Source:* CDC. Parasites—Trichuriasis. [online] Available at https://www.cdc.gov/parasites/whipworm/biology.html.

### Environmental Factors

The disease is primarily associated with poor sanitation condition and low socioeconomic status. The worm grows well in warm, moist, and densely shady places. Higher transmission rates are reported during rainy seasons.

### Reservoir of Infection

Man is the only known reservoir of the infection. It has no intermediate host.

### Modes of Transmission

Ingestion of infective eggs from contaminated soils, hands, food, or water (eggs require a minimum of 15–30 days in warm moist soil to become infective).

### Period of Communicability

The person is infective as long as the cysts are shed in the feces which may range up to years where the diseases are not recognized and not treated.

### Incubation Period

Generally around 60 days.

## CLINICAL FEATURES

Milder forms of infection are generally asymptomatic or have eosinophilia. Heavy infection can cause chronic diarrhea which may be bloody. This may be associated with abdominal pain and distention, nausea, vomiting, flatulence, headache, and weight loss along with the signs of malnutrition and anemia. Some cases may even present as appendicitis, colitis, and proctitis. Rarely, children may even present as a rectal prolapsed.

## DIAGNOSIS

Definitive diagnosis can be established by demonstration of characteristics egg by direct microscopical examination of a saline emulsion of the stool. Adult worms may occasionally be present in the stool. Severity of the infection can be established by Kato-Katz method of counting egg per gram of feces. Egg count above 30,000/g of feces may be considered as a sign of heavy infection. On doing colonoscopy classical signs of "Coconut Cake Rectum" can be seen.

## TREATMENT

Tablet albendazole 400 mg for 3 days or a single tablet mebendazole 500 mg can be used for the treatment of trichuriasis. Tablet ivermectin (200 µg/kg body weight) for 3 days can also be used for the treatment of trichuriasis.

## PREVENTION AND CONTROL

Like other soil-transmitted helminthes proper sanitation and prevention of contamination of food and water by human feces are the core element in the prevention of trichuriasis.

- **Sanitation:** Proper disposal of human feces has a pivotal role in the control of trichuriasis as the embryonated eggs are the main infective organism.

- **Health education:** Community members should be motivated to properly wash their raw fruits and vegetables before consuming them.

## SUMMARY

- The intestinal nematode *Trichuris trichiura* is among the most common causes of human infectious disease worldwide.
- The disease is primarily associated with poor sanitation condition and low socioeconomic status.
- The person is infective as long as the cysts are shed in the feces which may range up to years.
- Whipworm gets transmitted through ingestion of contaminated water, food and soil.
- All soil-transmitted helminthes infestation can be prevented by proper sanitation avoiding fecal contamination of food, water and soil.

## SUGGESTED READING

1. CDC. Trichuriasis. [online] Available from https://www.cdc.gov/parasites/whipworm/index.html.
2. Chatterjee KD. Parasitology, 25th Edition. Kolkata: Chatterjee Medical Publisher; 1995. pp. 164-7.
3. Ganguly S, Barkataki S, Sanga P, Boopathi K, Kanagasabai K, Devika S, et al. Epidemiology of Soil-Transmitted Helminth Infections among Primary School Children in the States of Chhattisgarh, Telangana, and Tripura, India, 2015-2016. Am J Trop Med Hyg. 2022;107(1): 122–9.
4. Harrison's Principle of Internal Medicine, 17th Edition. New York: MCGraw Hills Medicine; 2009. p. 1322.
5. Trichuriasis. Centre for food security and public health. [online] Available from http://www.cfsph.iastate.edu/Factsheets/pdfs/trichuriasis.pdf.
6. Viswanath A, Yarrarapu SNS, Williams M. Trichuris trichiura Infection. [Updated 2022 Aug 22]. In: StatPearls [Internet]. Treasure Island (FL): StatPearls Publishing; 2023 Jan-. Available from: https://www.ncbi.nlm.nih.gov/books/NBK507843/.

# EPIDEMIOLOGY OF ANCYLOSTOMIASIS AND ITS PREVENTION AND CONTROL

*The nation that destroys its soil destroys itself.*
—**Franklin D Roosevelt**

| CM7.2 | Enumerate, describe and discuss the mode of transmission and measures for prevention and control of Ancylostomiasis |
|---|---|
| CM8.1 | Describe and discuss the epidemiological and control measures applicable in Ancylostomiasis |

### Case Scenario

*A 10-year-old boy was hospitalized with a severe anemia in the pediatric department. The patient had fatigue, paleness, dizziness and weight loss since one month. As there were no hematologic factors associated with severe anemia; the stool examination was also performed. The stool microscopy of the patient revealed numerous ova of hookworm. General condition of the patient was improved with anti-parasitic and anti-anemia treatment suggesting the need for patients with iron deficiency anemia diagnosed in health centers should be also examined for the intestinal parasitic diseases.*

## INTRODUCTION

Hookworm is a soil-transmitted helminthic intestinal infection. Two species mainly associated with human infection are *Ancylostoma duodenale* and *Necator americanus*. These two hookworms, together with the roundworm, Ascaris lumbricoides, and the whipworm, Trichuris trichiura, are often referred to collectively as soil-transmitted helminths (STHs). Hookworm infection is commonly found in rural areas where night soil has been used as a soil fertilizer.

## PROBLEM STATEMENT

The geographic distributions of the hookworm *Ancylostoma duodenale* and *Necator americanus*, are worldwide in areas with warm, moist climates and are widely overlapping. Geographically hookworm infection is prevalent in Africa, Latin America, Mediterranean region, South East Asia, and the Western Pacific region. An estimated 576–740 million people in the world are infected with hookworm. The highest prevalence of hookworm occurs in sub-Saharan Africa and eastern Asia. It is estimated that more than 1.5 billion people worldwide are at risk for infection with *Ancylostoma* and other STH. Half of the infections occur in Asia and the Pacific where tropical climate, overcrowded population, poor hygiene, and poor sanitation are present. *Ancylostoma*, along with the other hookworms, cause more disability than mortality. Hookworm-associated malnutrition and anemia account for the loss of up to 4.1 million disability-adjusted life-years (DALY) annually. The highest at-risk population to contract Ancylostoma infections are the pre-school and school-aged children and travelers who returned from tropical countries. Additionally, people in close contact with dogs and cats are at risk to acquire zoonotic *Ancylostoma* infection. The incidence of *Ancylostoma* infection is tied to seasonal distribution where during the summer-autumn period, the incidence is more prevalent. Mixed infections with more than one *Ancylostoma* species are common in humans. High transmission occurs in other areas of rural poverty in the tropics, including southern China, the Indian subcontinent, and the Americas.

*Necator americanus* was widespread in the Southeastern United States until the early 20th century but improvements in living conditions have greatly reduced hookworm infections.

Hookworms infect approximately one-tenth of the population in the Indian subcontinent, mostly school-aged children and pregnant women. In India, the hookworm prevalence is estimated to be 71 million cases and *A. lumbricoides* contributes 140 million. In India, the maximum prevalence is seen in Karnataka (47%) followed by Andhra Pradesh (40%). The prevalence rate in Tamil Nadu is 3.2% whereas in Puducherry, it is 4.8% (Ananthakrishnan S et al., Natl Med J India 1997).

As the intensity of the infection determines the rate of prevalence and morbidity based on the egg count, the WHO proposed three classes of the intensity of STH—light, moderate, and heavy intensity infections. Few people harbor very high worm burden whereas most individual harbor less intense infections. These heavily infected people were the major source of environmental contamination and transmission of infection.

| Helminth involved | Light intensity | Moderate intensity | Heavy intensity |
|---|---|---|---|
| Ascaris | 1–4,999 epg | 5,000–49,999 epg | >50,000 epg |
| Trichuris | 1–999 epg | 1,000–9,999 epg | >10,000 epg |
| Hookworm | 1–1,999 epg | 2,000–3,999 epg | >4,000 epg |

(epg: eggs per gram of stool)

It has been observed that direct correlation exists between the initial worm burden before treatment and worm burden during reinfection. If high-intensity infections were present before treatment, then during reinfection, the individual is predisposed to have high-intensity infections. This pattern is seen in children affected with *A. lumbricoides*, *T. trichura*, and adults with hookworm (Parija SC et al., Trop Parasitol, 2017).

## EPIDEMIOLOGY

### Host Factors

Hookworm infection affects all age groups; however, children are affected at higher rate due to outdoor activities. Because of same reason males are more commonly affected than females, specially among barefoot walkers **(Fig. 17C.6)**.

### Agent

Intestinal hookworm disease in humans is caused by *Ancylostoma duodenale*, *A. ceylanicum*, and *Necator americanus*. Classically, there are two primary intestinal hookworm species worldwide *A. duodenale* and *N. americanus* but a parasite infecting animals, *A. ceylanicum*, is also an important emerging parasite infecting humans in some regions. Occasionally larvae of *A. caninum*, normally a parasite of canids, may partially develop in the human intestine and cause eosinophilic enteritis, but this species does not appear to reach reproductive maturity in humans.

Another group of hookworms infecting animals can penetrate the human skin causing cutaneous larva migrans (*A. braziliense*, *A. caninum*, *Uncinaria stenocephala*). Other than *A. caninum* noted above, these parasites do not develop further after their larvae penetrate human skin.

Hookworm eggs present in the soil hatch in the favorable conditions (warm and moist) and release rhabditiform larvae, which further grow and become infective filariform larvae.

Infective larvae penetrate bare skin and reach the lung through blood circulation. From there they ascend to throat, swallowed and migrate to small intestine.

### Environmental Factors

- Warm and moist environment
- Poor hygiene and sanitation
- Animal keeping practices.

### Reservoir of Infection

Humans are the definitive hosts for both *Necator americanus* and *Ancylostoma duodenale*. *Ancylostoma caninum* primarily

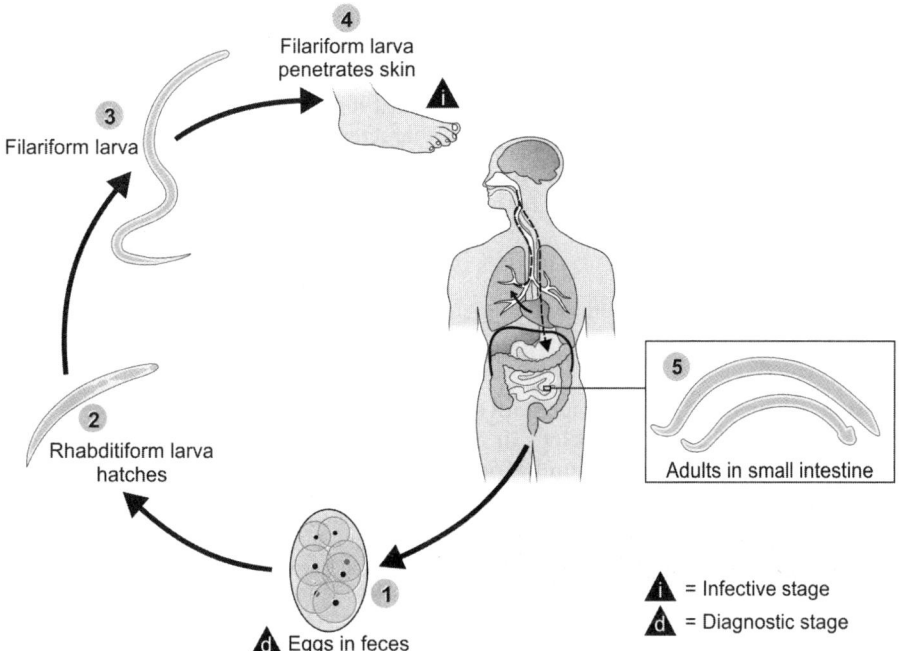

**Fig. 17C.6:** Life cycle of *Ancylostoma*.
*Source:* CDC. Parasites—Hookworm. [online] Available from https://www.cdc.gov/parasites/hookworm/biology.html.

infects dogs, but humans can be dead-end hosts that prevent the larvae from completing their life cycle.

## Mode of Transmission

*Necator* can only be transmitted through penetration of the skin whereas *Ancylostoma* can be transmitted percutaneously, orally, and probably transplacentally. When *A. duodenale* is transmitted orally, the early migrations of the larvae cause Wakana disease which is characterized by nausea, vomiting, pharyngeal irritation, cough, dyspnea, and hoarseness.

## Incubation Period

Total time taken from the entry of larvae through skin contact to appearance of eggs in the feces is around 6–8 weeks.

## Period of Communicability

As long as the person harbors the infective larvae.

## CLINICAL FEATURES

- Most of the infections are asymptomatic
- Pruritic maculopapular rash at the site of entry of larvae
- Fever
- Pale skin
- Reduced appetite
- Epigastric tenderness
- Constipation.

## COMPLICATIONS

- Iron deficiency anemia—*A. duodenale* causes greater blood loss than *N. americanus*
- Hypoproteinemia
- Other nutritional deficiencies due to poor absorption
- Ascites.

## DIAGNOSIS

Microscopic examination of stool for identification of eggs is the most common method of diagnosing hookworm.

Steps for microscopic examination are as follows:
- Collect a stool specimen
- Fix the specimen in 10% formalin
- Concentrate using the formalin–ethyl acetate sedimentation technique.
- Examine a wet mount of the sediment.

**Chandler's index:** It is used to identify the importance of hookworm infestation as a public health problem in a community. It is calculated based on average number of hookworm eggs/gram of stool.

| Average no. of hookworm eggs/g of stool | Significance of hookworm infestation |
|---|---|
| <200 | Not much significance |
| 200–250 | Potential danger |
| 250–300 | Minor public health problem |
| >300 | Major public health problem |

## TREATMENT

World Health Organization recommends antihelminthic drugs like albendazole 400 mg once orally, mebendazole 100 mg orally twice daily for 3 days, and pyrantel pamoate 11 mg/kg (maximum 1 g) orally for 3 days which are effective, inexpensive, and easy to administer by nonmedical person.

Iron supplements should be given in case of anemia. Nutritional supplements should also be given to prevent malnutrition.

## PREVENTION

- Best way to prevent hookworm infection is to avoid barefoot walking on the soil in areas where fecal contamination is common.
- Avoid open field defecation.
- Periodic deworming of at-risk groups especially children should be done with oral albendazole in endemic areas.
- Sewage disposal system should be adequate.
- Health education should be given to maintain proper hygiene and sanitation.
- Promotion of hand washing practices.

## GLOBAL TARGET

The global target is to eliminate morbidity due to soil-transmitted helminthiases in children by 2020. This will be achieved by providing regular treatment to at least 75% of the children in endemic areas (an estimated 836 million in 2016).

## CUTANEOUS LARVA MIGRANS ALSO KNOWN AS "CREEPING ERUPTIONS"

It is a zoonotic hookworm infection commonly caused by *A. braziliense* and *A. caninum*. Dogs and cats are definitive hosts for these hookworm species. These animals shed the eggs in their feces. Humans get infected by skin contact with soil contaminated with infective form of larvae. After 1–5 days of entry of larvae, typical serpiginous eruptions with intense itching can be seen. Characteristic skin lesions are usually helpful to diagnose the condition clinically. This is a self-limiting condition.

Oral albendazole 400 mg once daily for 3–7 days is the most effective drug. People must be made aware to avoid bare skin contact of soil or surface contaminated with animal feces.

Cutaneous larva migrans may be complicated by a self-limiting pulmonary reaction called Loffler syndrome (patchy pulmonary infiltrates and peripheral blood eosinophilia).

## SUMMARY

- Ancylostomiasis, also known as *hookworm infections*, is related to *necatoriasis* and *ascariasis*, and has symptoms including *anemia*, *abdominal pain* and *intestinal bleeding*.
- Ascariasis can be transmitted if the person walks barefoot on soil that contains the larvae, swallows soil particles, e.g., on unwashed salad leaves.
- Malnutrition and iron deficiency anemia is the most common complication.
- Periodic deworming of at-risk groups should be done.
- Best way to prevent hookworm infection is by avoiding barefoot walking and open air defecation.

## SUGGESTED READING

1. Aziz MH, Ramphul K. Ancylostoma. InStatPearls [Internet] 2022. StatPearls Publishing.
2. Nath TC, Eom KS, Choe S et al. Molecular evidence of hookworms in public environment of Bangladesh. Sci Rep. 2023;13:133.
3. CDC. Chapter 3: Infectious Diseases Related to Travel. Available from https:// wwwnc.cdc.gov/travel/yellowbook/2018/infectious-diseases-related-to- travel/cutaneous-larva-migrans.
4. CDC. Parasites—Hookworm. Available from https://www.cdc.gov/parasites/ hookworm/epi.html.
5. Chatterjee KD. Parasitology, 13th Edition. Kolkata: Chatterjee Medical Publisher; 2009. pp. 212-20.
6. Hotez PJ, Simon B, Jeffrey MB, et al. Current concepts: hookworm infection. The New England Journal of Medicine. 2004;351:799-807.
7. WHO. Prevention and control of intestinal parasitic infections: WHO Technical Report Series N° 749. [online] http://www.who.int/neglected_diseases/resources/who_trs_749/en/.

# D. EPIDEMIOLOGY OF ZOONOTIC DISEASES AND ITS PREVENTION AND CONTROL

*Mohua Moitra, Shailee Vyas*
**Rabies Part:** *Ashok Mishra, Sasmita Mungi, Manoj Bansal, Priyesh Marskole*

## GENERAL EPIDEMIOLOGY OF ZOONOTIC DISEASES AND GENERAL PRINCIPLES OF ITS PREVENTION AND CONTROL

**CM7.2** Enumerate, describe and discuss the mode of transmission and measures for prevention and control of zoonotic diseases

**CM8.1** Describe and discuss the epidemiological and control measures applicable in zoonotic diseases

### INTRODUCTION

Since the beginning of time, animals have been an integral part of human lives, may it be in the form of domestic and agricultural help or for the purpose of consuming them as food. In animals, humans have found some of the best companions apart from other utilities and animals have got the love and protection in turn. But inevitably, there also has been a definite transfer of disease causing agents between the two. Human health; therefore, remains at a constant threat from animals—wild or domestic.

This interaction and the resultant diseases impact public health and the social and economic well-being of the world population mightily. These diseases, transmissible from animals to humans, either through direct or indirect contact via the agencies of food, water, environment, etc. are referred to as "zoonoses".

The word "zoonoses" has been derived from the Greek words—"Zoo" means animals and "noses" meaning disease. Zoonotic diseases constitute a unique group of infectious diseases that affect man as well as animals.

The zoonoses have been defined by the World Health Organization (WHO) as, "those diseases and infections (the agents of which) are naturally transmitted between (other) vertebrate animals and man".

The ability of the pathogen to spread from one species to another is called "crossing or jumping the species gap", hence any pathogen, which may cross the species gap is considered to have this "zoonotic potential". Thus by definition of zoonosis, human beings is one such host between the two species involved. This makes it an important public health concern.

These have serious consequences on different aspects like livelihood, farming, animal husbandry and food scarcity. In modern times, the fast modes of human travel and emergent lifestyles affecting the natural equilibrium in the nature "eco-niche" are often the reasons for outbreaks of disease. Thus, proper education about the spread of infection and the actual risk of getting the disease is of utmost importance.

### IMPACT OF ZOONOSIS

- **Human health:** There have been evidences of serious illnesses and high case fatality rate following zoonotic infections. Many a times the diseases result in clinical complications and debilitating disorders. This result in limitations for the patient as well as the family, like less earning capacity, a vicious cycle of malnutrition and infection, turbulent family and social dynamics, etc.
- **Animal health:** The animal health is compromised when infected. This may lead to reduction in the production and availability of milk, meat, eggs and other dairy products, wool, as well as the working capacity of these animals.
- **Health services:** Zoonotic diseases create an additional burden on resources and hospital services, especially in diagnosis, treatment, prevention, and control measures. Sometimes the events like bird flu or Nipah virus scare create an emergency situation, due to which routine services get diverted from routine services.
- **Economic burden:** Zoonotic diseases have significant impact on the national economic development. Since, it affects both, animals and humans, it exhibits two-fold impact.
- **Bioterrorism:** Some zoonoses like anthrax and plague have the potential of being used as weapons of bioterrorism.

### CLASSIFICATION

Zoonoses can be classified in many ways, but the most reasonable, scientific, and consistent method would be as per:

- **Etiological agents:**
  - Bacterial—brucellosis, leptospirosis, and listeriosis
  - Viral—rabies and Japanese encephalitis
  - Rickettsial and chlamydial—Q-fever, scrub typhus, and ornithosis
  - Mycotic—dermatophytosis, cryptococcosis, and histoplasmosis
  - Parasitic—toxoplasmosis, visceral larva migrans, and hydatidosis.
- **Transmission cycle:** This classification is based on the type of lifecycle of the infective organism.
  - **Direct zoonoses:** These are the zoonoses that have been existing in the nature by a *single vertebrate animal species*. The infection gets transmitted through either direct contact (anthrax) or indirectly through food (teniasis), air (tuberculosis), etc. If at all a vector is involved in transmission, there is no development of the pathogen in the vector (i.e. just mechanical transmission happens), e.g. anthrax, rabies, tuberculosis, scabies, etc. **(Fig. 17D.1)**.
  - **Cyclozoonoses:** These zoonoses require two or more vertebrate animal species hosts to complete the transmission cycle of an infectious agent. They are further classified into:
    - ◆ *Obligatory cyclozoonoses:* In these diseases, man is a must to complete the life cycle of the infective agent,

i.e. a compulsory host. For example *Taenia solium* and *Taenia saginata* **(Fig. 17D.2)**.
- *Nonobligatory cyclozoonoses:* In these zoonoses, man is accidentally involved in transmission cycle. Many times, these zoonoses have a dead end in man, e.g. hydatidosis (*Echinococcus granulosus*) **(Fig. 17D.3)**.
- **Metazoonoses:** In this, both vertebrate and invertebrate species are involved in the transmission of the infective agent. In the invertebrate species, the infectious agent may multiply, develop, or remain dormant. These are further divided into four subtypes depending on the number of vertebrate and invertebrate hosts involved in maintaining the cycle.
  - *Metazoonosis type I*: One vertebrate and one invertebrate host (e.g. yellow fever, and plague) **(Fig. 17D.4)**
  - *Metazoonosis type II:* One vertebrate and two invertebrate hosts (e.g. paragonimiasis) **(Fig. 17D.5)**
  - *Metazoonosis type III*: Two vertebrate and one invertebrate host (e.g. clonorchiasis) **(Fig. 17D.6)**
  - *Metazoonosis type IV*: Transovarian transmission (e.g. tick-borne encephalitis) **(Fig. 17D.7)**.
- **Saprozoonoses:** These zoonotics require an inanimate substance for completion of lifecycle in addition to vertebrate or invertebrate host. The infective agent may multiply or develop or propagate in the inanimate site. The inanimate site may serve as a reservoir or source of infection. The inanimate site may be food, soil, clothing, water, and grass of plants. These are subdivided into three types:
  1. *Saproanthropozoonoses:* Transmitted via inanimate substances to humans, e.g. cutaneous larva migrans and ancylostomiasis **(Fig. 17D.8)**.
  2. *Saproamphixenoses*: Man and animals equally are involved in the nature but are transmitted through inanimate objects, e.g. histoplasmosis and fungal infection **(Fig. 17D.9)**.

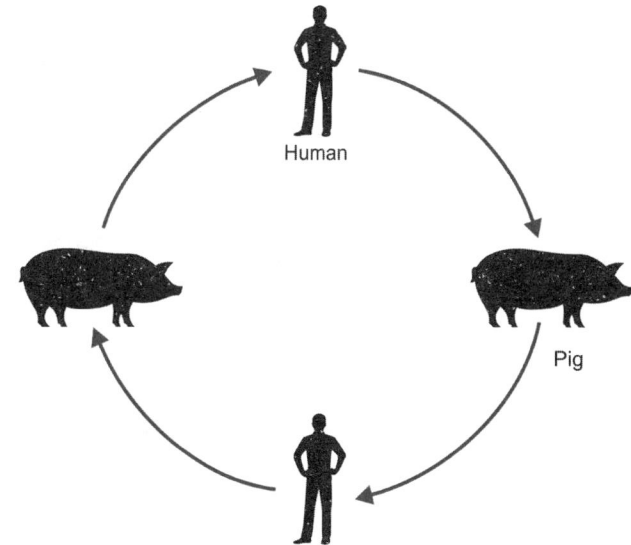

**Fig. 17D.2:** *Taenia solium.*

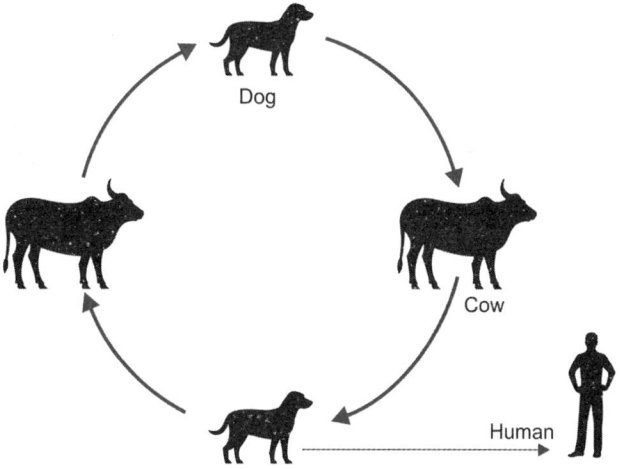

**Fig. 17D.3:** Hydatidosis.

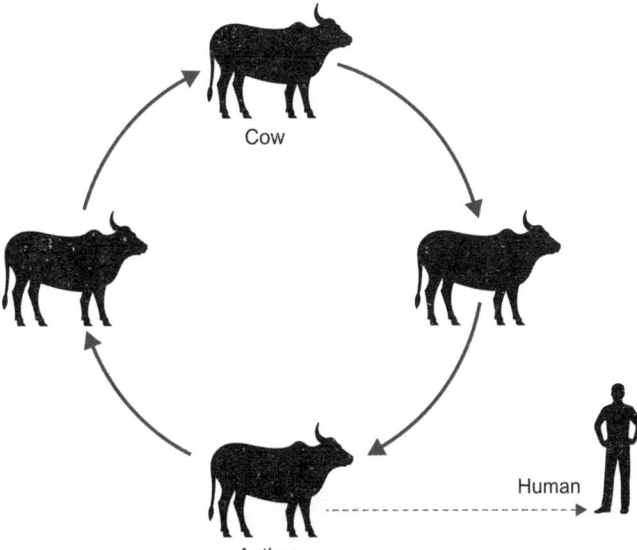

**Fig. 17D.1:** Solid line represents obligatory pathway, broken line represents alternate pathway.

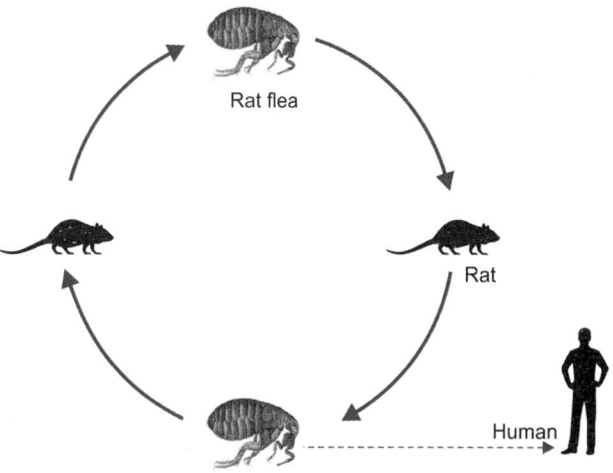

**Fig. 17D.4:** Plague.

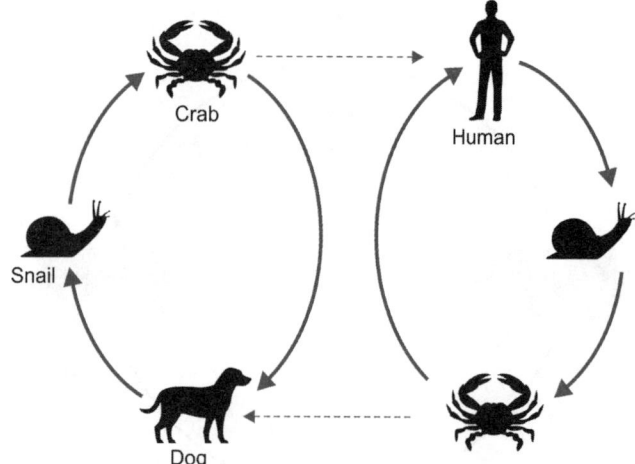

**Fig. 17D.5:** Paragonimiasis.

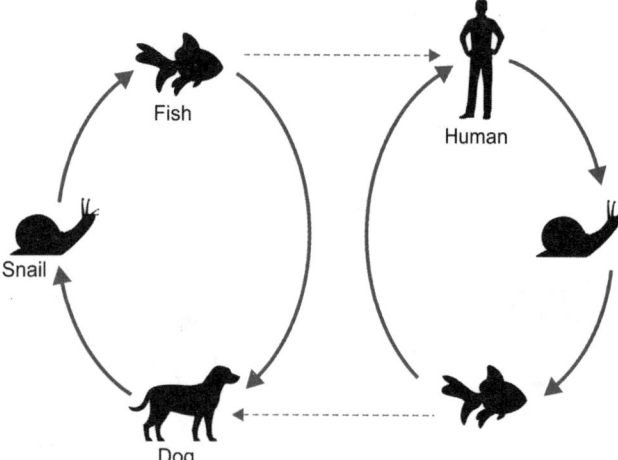

**Fig. 17D.6:** Clonorchiasis.

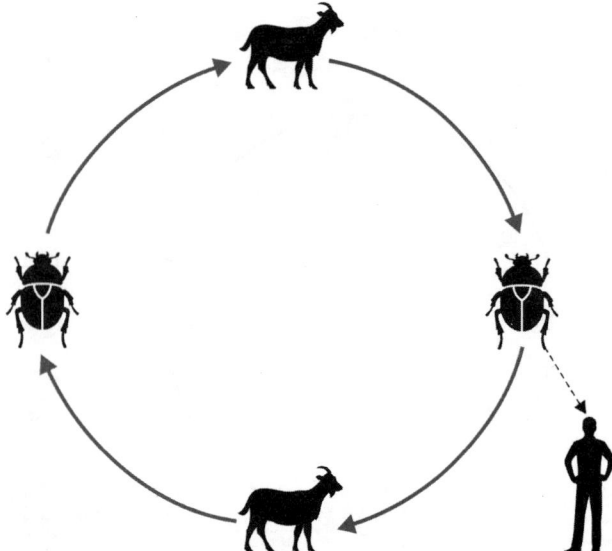

**Fig. 17D.7:** Tick-borne encephalitis.

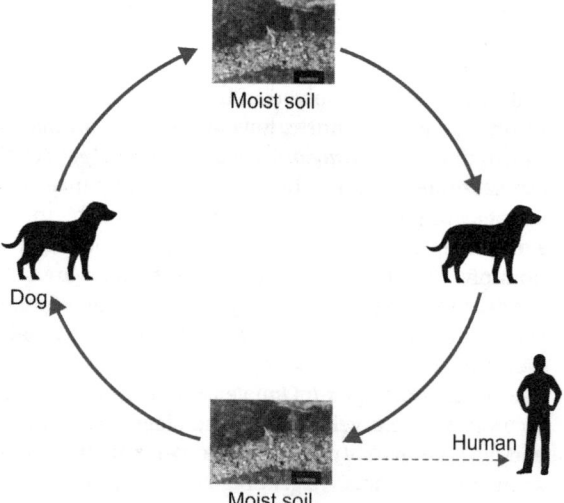

**Fig. 17D.8:** Cutaneous larva migrans.

3. *Saprometa-anthropozoonoses*: These diseases require an inanimate object, and vertebrate host and invertebrate host for completion of the transmission cycle, e.g. fascioliasis **(Fig. 17D.10)**.

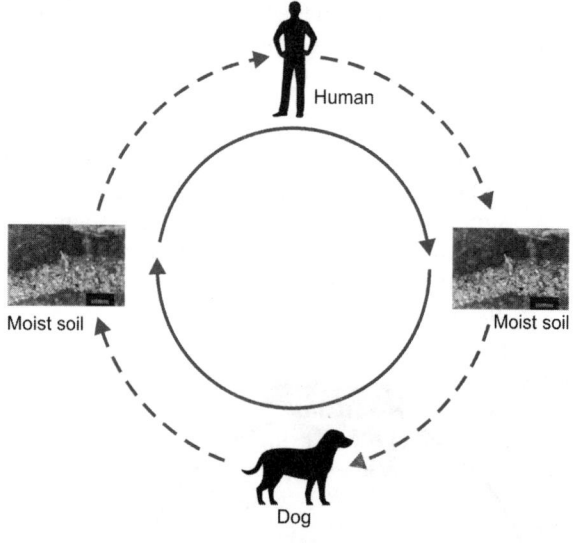

**Fig. 17D.9:** Histoplasmosis.

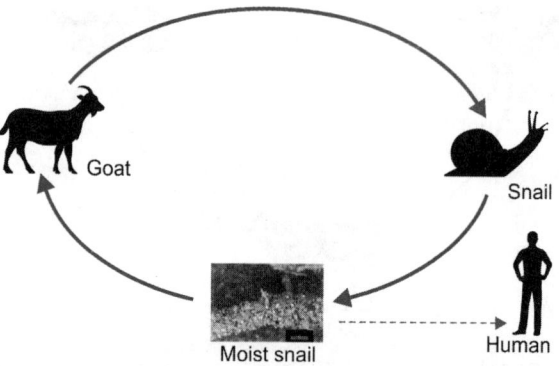

**Fig. 17D.10:** Fascioliasis.

- *Reservoir host:*
  - **Anthropozoonoses:** These are the diseases of domestic or wild animals, which occur in them independent of man. Humans get infected accidentally in specific circumstances like occupational exposure to the diseased animals or through food and the dead-end hosts, i.e. no further transmittion, e.g., leptospirosis, tularemia, rift valley fever, hydatidosis, and rabies
  - **Zooanthroponoses:** These are the zoonotics, which normally do pass from man to other vertebrate animals, e.g. tuberculosis (human type), amebiasis, and diphtheria (human type)
  - **Amphixenoses:** These are universal diseases, which can be transmitted from man to other vertebrates and vice versa. The humans as well as the other vertebrates can act as a host, e.g., streptococcosis, nonhost specific salmonellosis, and staphylococcosis

## TRANSMISSION OF ZOONOTIC DISEASES

Zoonoses may be transmitted from the source or reservoir of infection to the susceptible host through many ways:
- *Direct transmission:*
  - **By direct contact**—through direct contact between the source of infection and the susceptible host, e.g. leptospirosis, pox, and dermatophytosis.
  - **Droplet infection**—through direct projection of droplet sprays of either saliva or nasopharyngeal secretions on conjunctiva or mucous membrane of the susceptible host. This usually happens during sneezing, coughing, or even talking, e.g. tuberculosis, common cold, and diphtheria.
  - **Contact with soil**—through exposure of the susceptible host to the infective agent present either in soil or in decaying materials, e.g. tetanus and hookworm infection.
  - **Bite of an animal**—rabies
  - **Transplacental or vertical transmission**—toxoplasmosis and hepatitis B.
- *Indirect transmission:*
  - **Vector-borne transmission:** A vector is either an arthropod or any other living agent (e.g. snail), which can transmit an infectious agent to the susceptible host. This transmission can be mechanical or biological.
    - ♦ *Mechanical transmission*: The infectious agent is merely mechanically transmitted or inoculated into the susceptible host. There is neither development nor multiplication in the vector, e.g. amebiasis, cholera, and serum hepatitis.
    - ♦ *Biological transmission*: The infectious agent either multiplies or undergoes growth in the vector. This also needs some incubation period before it can actually transmit the disease. There are four types of biological transmission:
      1. *Propagative*: The agent undergoes multiplication in the vector without development into various stages, e.g. plague bacilli in rat fleas.
      2. *Cyclopropagative:* The agent undergoes both multiplication and grows and develops in the vector, e.g. malaria parasites in mosquitoes.
      3. *Cyclodevelopmental:* The agent only undergoes development, but does not multiply in the vector, e.g. microfilaria in mosquitoes.
      4. *Transovarian:* The agent gets transmitted from one generation to the next generation of the vector, e.g. tick-borne encephalitis.
  - **Vehicle-borne transmission:** The infectious agent gets transmitted through some media like water, food (milk, meat, fish, fruits, etc.), blood, serum, and other biological products like tissues, organs, etc. Further, the transmission may be mechanical or biological, e.g. hepatitis A through water, salmonellosis through infected meat, brucellosis and tuberculosis through milk, and hepatitis B through blood.
  - **Air-borne transmission:** The infectious agent gets transmitted through the agency of air. It can be of four types:
    1. *Droplet nuclei:* [already will be covered in general epidemiology] e.g. tuberculosis, Q-fever.
    2. *Droplet infection:* During act of coughing, talking, sneezing, etc. which settle down with dust particles and cause air-borne transmission, e.g. fungal infections.
    3. *Fomite-borne transmission*: Through soil, clothes, towels, utensils, e.g. diphtheria and typhoid.
    4. *Unclean hands and fingers*: Hands are the most common media through which the pathogens get transmitted by various ways such as food, skin, etc. e.g. staphylococcosis and salmonellosis.

## SUGGESTED READING

1. Joshi SK. Introduction to Zoonoses. In: Joshi SK, Singh MK. Textbook of Zoonotic Diseases; Delhi: Satish serial publishing house; pp. 1-8.
2. Sherikar AT, Bachhil VN, Thapliyal DC, for ICAR, Govt. of India. Introduction and general aspects of zoonosis; In: Sherikar AT, Bachhil VN, Thapliyal DC (Eds). Textbook of Elements of Veterinary Public Health; Fifth reprint. New Delhi: Indian Council of Agricultural Research; 2018. pp. 287-304.
3. Wallace R. Public health and preventive medicine, Fifteenth edition. USA; McGraw Hill Companies; 2007.
4. World Health Organization. Managing public health risk at the human-animal-environment interface. [online] Available from: http://www.who.int/zoonoses/en/.

## EPIDEMIOLOGY OF RABIES AND ITS PREVENTION AND CONTROL

| | |
|---|---|
| CM7.2 | Enumerate, describe and discuss the mode of transmission and measures for prevention and control of rabies |
| CM8.1 | Describe and discuss the epidemiological and control measures applicable in rabies |

## INTRODUCTION

Rabies is an acute fatal encephalomyelitis caused by a ribonucleic acid (RNA) virus under the genus *Lyssavirus* and family Rhabdoviridae. It is the most important viral zoonosis of warm-blooded animals like dogs, cats, jackals, etc. recognized worldwide because of its global distribution, incidence, veterinary and human health costs, and extremely high case fatality rate. Rabies occurs in more than 150 countries and territories. It causes tens of thousands of deaths every year, mainly in Asia and Africa, 40% of whom are children under 15 years of age.

Dogs are main source of human rabies deaths, contributing up to 99% of all rabies transmissions to humans. Rabies can be prevented through vaccination of dogs and prevention of dog bites (WHO: Rabies: Factsheet; Jan 2023). India is endemic for rabies, and accounts for 36% of the world's rabies deaths. True burden of rabies in India is not fully known; although as per available information, it causes 18,000–20,000 deaths every year. About 30–60% of reported rabies cases and deaths in India occur in children under the age of 15 years as bites that occur in children often go unrecognized and unreported.

## CHARACTERISTIC OF DISEASE

Rabies now features among the 17 identified neglected tropical diseases (NTDs) by the WHO. The acute viral infection is characterized by inflammation of the central nervous system (CNS). When the disease occurs in man, the most characteristic symptom is fear of water (hydrophobia) which develops due to painful spasms of the muscles of deglutition. Rabies is an extremely dangerous disease with a frequently long incubation period, highly distressing symptoms and as a rule, a lethal outcome. The violent symptoms associated with the illness and usual inevitability of death make it one of the most terrifying diseases.

## HISTORICAL PERSPECTIVE

Rabies or hydrophobia is probably the oldest recorded infection of mankind. Even today, it is as frightening a disease as it was in the past.

The famous Indian Physician Sushrut, observed this condition in dogs, foxes, etc. which manifests as a state of confusion, drooping of tail, and lower jaw and profuse salivation. He emphasized that this condition was fatal, once clinical symptoms became apparent.

Dr Louis Pasteur in 1885 developed the first antirabies vaccine (ARV), which was first administered on July 6, 1885 to Joseph Meister, the young boy who had been severely bitten 14 times by a rabid dog. After Jenner and his concept of protection against smallpox, rabies vaccine was the third vaccine developed in history, long before recognition of the nature of viruses (Fig. 17D.11).

## GLOBAL SCENARIO

September 28 is being observed as World Rabies Day. This viral disease, which is almost invariably fatal, kills 50,000–70,000 people per year. Around the world, rabies kills around 100 children every day because they cannot afford the vaccine. In Africa and Asia alone, the disease threatens 3.3 billion people—just under half the world's population (Liane Wimhurst, the Independent, Health News 2011).

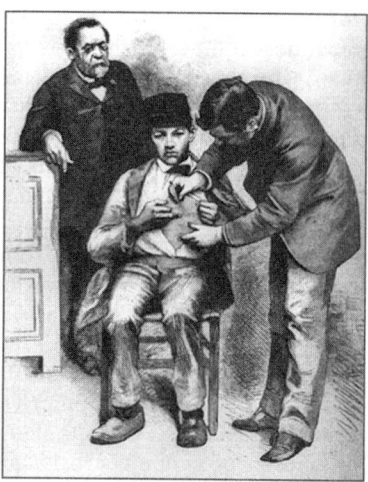

**Fig. 17D.11:** Dr Louis Pasteur in 1885 giving the first antirabies vaccine to Joseph Meister.

In Newark, New Jersey, four boys were bitten by a rabid dog. A fund raising effort arose to send the boys to France for treatment by Pasteur. Donors raised $1,000 which sent the boys overseas via ocean liner. The healthy boys returned home in January 1886 after treatment with the new rabies vaccine.

More than 99% of all human deaths from rabies occur in the developing world, and rabies still remains a neglected disease throughout most of Asia (Knobel DL et al., Bull World Health Organ, 2005). Asia accounts for 40–60% of all animal bites occurring in children under 14 years. Dog bites are the primary source of human infection in all rabies endemic countries in the region and account for 96% of human rabies cases (Meslin Fx et al., Vaccine, 2006). The annual incidence of suspect bites from rabid dogs is 6.5 per million humans in Asia (WHO, Vaccine Research, gvrf).

India, Bangladesh, and Myanmar are highly endemic countries among the South East Asian region. The estimated number of human rabies deaths in Asia is approximately 30,000–40,000 annually (20,000 in India, 2,000 in Bangladesh, remainder in the rest of Asia). (APCRI Journal, 2010).

## INDIAN SCENARIO

In India, about 15 million people are bitten by animals, mostly dogs every year and need postexposure prophylaxis (PEP). The incidence of animal's bites is 17.4 per 1,000 population. In India 2018, there were 110 Rabies cases and 110 deaths were reported (WHO). Cats are the second most common source of human rabies exposures in Asia and virus samples collected from Asian rabid cats and other domestic animals revealed only canine street virus strains.

Rabies occurs in more than 100 countries. Water seems to be the most effective natural barrier to this disease. Geographic boundaries play a very important role. Norway, Sweden, Finland, The Liberian Peninsula, Iceland, United Kingdom, Ireland, Cyprus, Australia, New Zealand, the Western Pacific Islands, Japan, Malta, and China (Taiwan) are rabies free countries. Some countries have achieved "rabies free" status by employing vigorous measures for elimination. In India, Andaman and

Nicobar Islands and Lakshadweep are free of the disease. A "rabies free" area is one in which no case of indigenously acquired rabies has occurred in man or other warm-blooded animals for 2 years.

# EPIDEMIOLOGY

## Agent Factors

***Type:*** The causative agent (*Lyssavirus* type 1) is a very small (size 120 × 80 nm), bullet shaped, i.e. round at one end and flat at another, and neurotropic RNA containing virus. The virus is present in the saliva of rabid animals, saliva of human rabies patients, and also in the urine in low titers. On biting, scratching or licking on broken skin and intact mucous membrane, the virus enters the body, multiplies locally in the tissues and muscles, and then travels to brain at the speed of 3-10 mm/h via neurotropic nerves. Here it affects the brainstem function, causing hydrophobia (fear of water), aerophobia (fear of breeze) and/or photophobia (fear of light), and finally resulting in respiratory paralysis and death.

***Viability:*** Virus is highly resistant against cold, dryness, and decay and can remain infectious for weeks in dead bodies. It is inactivated by formaldehyde, sunlight, lipid solvents, and various antiseptics.

***Structure:*** Rabies virus particles contain two distinct major antigens—(1) a glycoprotein antigen from the virus membrane, and (2) an internal nucleoprotein antigen. The glycoprotein seems to be the only antigen capable of inducing the formation of virus-neutralizing antibodies **(Fig. 17D.12)**.

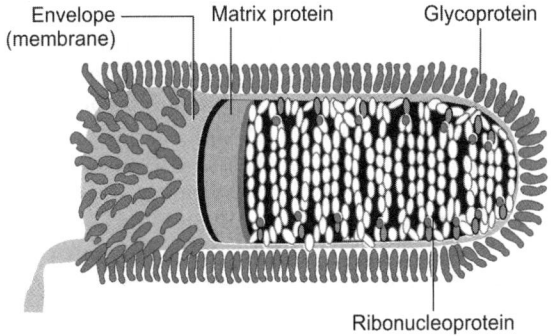

**Fig. 17D.12:** Rabies virus particles.

The virus recovered from naturally occurring cases of rabies is called "street virus". It is pathogenic for all mammals and shows a long variable incubation period (20-60 days in dogs). Serial brain-to-brain passage of the street virus in rabbits modifies the virus such that its incubation period is progressively reduced until it becomes constant between 4 and 6 days. Virus isolated at this stage is called a "fixed virus". A fixed strain of virus is one that has a short, fixed, and reproducible incubation period (4-6 days) when injected intracerebrally into suitable animals. It does not form Negri bodies. The fixed virus is used in the preparation of ARV.

## Host Factors

**Age:** Incidence of rabies is maximum in children less than 15 years of age.

**Susceptibility:** All warm-blooded animals including man are susceptible to rabies. Bites around head and neck are most dangerous.

**Occupation:** Animal handlers, forest staff, hunters, field naturalists, veterinarians, and laboratory workers dealing with rabies virus are much more vulnerable for exposure to rabies virus.

***Reservoirs of infection:*** Rabies exists in three epidemiological forms:

1. **Urban rabies:** The transfer of infection from wildlife to domestic dogs results in the creation of urban cycle, which is maintained by dog and is responsible for 99% of human cases in India. Cats can also be the source of human infection.
2. **Wild life rabies:** Wild life or sylvatic rabies is perpetuated by the jackal, fox, hyena, etc. In South Africa, the disease is enzootic in the mongoose. These animals maintain a cycle amongst themselves and transmit the infection to dogs and domestic animals. Man may contract rabies through intrusion into this wild lifecycle of rabies.
3. **Bat rabies:** In some Latin American countries like Brazil, Venezuela, Mexico, Trinidad, Tobago, and Parts of USA, the vampire bat is an important host and vector of rabies. They can transmit rabies to animals and humans. This form of rabies is responsible for killing hundreds of thousands of cattle annually. Human is affected while sleeping outdoors. Recently, rabid bats have been found in Germany, Denmark, and Holland but not reported in India. Rabies virus is probably transmitted between vampire bats by either bite or aerosol.

***Source of infection:*** The source of infection for man is the saliva of rabid animals. In dogs and cats, the virus may be present in the saliva for 3-4 days (occasionally 5-6 days) before the onset of clinical symptoms and during the course of illness till death. Only half of rabid animals have virus in saliva so the chances of getting rabies following the bite of a rabid animal are 50%.

**Carrier states:** In rare cases, carrier states have also been reported where the animal although apparently healthy, has transmitted the disease.

## Mode of Transmission

- ***Animal bites:*** In India, most of the human rabies cases occur due to bite of a rabid dog. Rabies can also be contracted through the bites of cats, monkey, horses, sheep, goat, etc. For transmission to occur the saliva of the biting animal must contain the virus at the time of bite.
- ***Licks:*** Licks on broken skin and mucosa can transmit the disease. Rarely the disease may be transmitted through bone splinter or other object contaminated with saliva of a rabid animal.
- ***Aerosols:*** Aerosol (respiratory) transmission can occur in two ways, laboratory workers can become infected due to aerosols

created during homogenization of infected animal brains or in caves where rabid vampire bats are present.
- ***Person-to-person:*** Man-to-man transmission although rare, is possible either through bite by a hydrophobia patient or through corneal or organ transplants.

### Incubation Period

The incubation period in man is highly variable, commonly 1–3 months following exposure, but it may vary from 4 days to many years. The incubation period depends on number of factors:
- Site of the bite
- Severity of the bite
- Number of wounds
- Amount of virus injected, i.e. virus inoculum
- Species of the animal
- Protection provided by clothing and
- Treatment provided.

Generally, incubation period is shorter in severe bites, bites by wild animals, and also bites on head and neck region and upper extremities. Rabies is one of the, communicable disease where the incubation period is variable and dependent on so many factors.

## PATHOGENESIS

The live virus multiplies on entering through the epidermis or mucous membrane and ascends centripetally up the peripheral nerves to the CNS resulting in generalized encephalomyelitis. Once it reaches the CNS, it multiplies exclusively in the gray matter and then travels centrifugally along autonomic nerves spreading to other tissues including salivary glands and also cornea **(Fig. 17D.13)**.

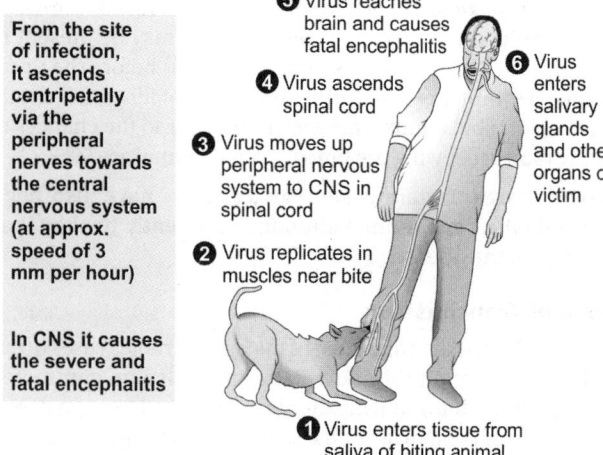

**Fig. 17D.13:** Pathogenesis of rabies.

The pathognomonic lesion of rabies is an intracytoplasmic eosinophilic inclusion body, which is commonly known as Negri body. These Negri bodies are seen only with infection of "Street virus" and not with "fixed virus".

So far, the virus has not been isolated from the blood of rabies patients and hence, the hematogenous route of spread is ruled out.

In rabies, initial viremia is absent and the virus is not accessible to the normal immune mechanism of the body. The viremia or the stimulation of the normal immune mechanism is only during the end-stages of the fatal disease therefore the role of naturally acquired infection is practically nonexistent.

## CLINICAL PRESENTATION

***Clinical features in man:*** Rabies in man is known as hydrophobia in general. The disease can be divided into different stages:
- **Prodromal stage:** The virus enters the CNS. Nonspecific symptoms and signs develop. The disease begins with symptoms like malaise, anorexia, fever, headache, chills, myalgia, sore throat, diarrhea and vomiting, and depression. There is pain and tingling or numbness at the site of bite in about 50% of cases. It is the most important complaint at this time and is due to the multiplication of virus at the local site. This stage may last for 2–10 days.
- **Acute neurologic stage:** This period is characterized by objective signs of developing CNS disease. The duration is 2–7 days. This stage is further divided into two substages:
  1. *Stage of acute encephalitis:* This stage is characterized by excessive motor activity and agitation. There are symptoms like confusion, hallucination, muscle spasms, and convulsions. There is increased intolerance to noise, bright light, touch, or currents of air. Aerophobia (fear of air) may also be present and considered to be pathognomonic of rabies.
  2. *Stage of brainstem dysfunction:* The characteristic symptom of hydrophobia appears which is pathognomonic of rabies and is absent in animals. This fear of water is due to painful, violent, involuntary contraction of diaphragm, respiratory, pharyngeal, and laryngeal muscles, initiated by swallowing of liquids. Progressively, even the sight, smell or sound of liquids can precipitate spasm of muscles of deglutition. More than 80% patients die during this stage. Death is due to respiratory arrest, convulsions or choking. Rest of the patients may progress to next stage.
- **Stage of coma:** Can occur at anytime during the course of illness, usually within 10 days. Now, the muscle spasms cease and paralytic symptoms appear. There is generalized flaccidity, apathy, stupor, and coma. Death occurs due to hypoxia or heart failure.

Occasionally, rabies may present as Guillain-Barre type of ascending paralysis. This may be seen with bite of a vampire bat or in patients who have received PEP against the disease.
- **Death:** Once the symptoms develop, the disease is fatal and the patient dies within 2 weeks.

There are no quarantine restrictions for a rabies patient. However, since the saliva, urine or tears, etc. may contain the virus, all the persons coming in contact should be immunized against rabies. Transmission from man to man, though uncommon is possible.

## DIAGNOSIS

The *clinical diagnosis* can be possible on the basis of classical signs and symptoms. Hydrophobia is pathognomonic of rabies. There is history of animal bite.

*Laboratory diagnosis:* The laboratory tests are not routinely done for the management of animal bite cases, as these are not cost effective for management purposes and have limited availability in specific centers of big cities.

Several biological samples like saliva, cerebral spinal fluid (CSF), skin biopsies containing hair follicles collected at the nape of neck, extracted hair follicles, tears, and urine can be used. Positive results of viral RNA in samples should be confirmed by sequencing to avoid false positives. Sensitivity of a single skin biopsy is about 98% but by collecting and testing 3 serial daily saliva samples per patient, it is possible to achieve maximal, i.e. 100% sensitivity. Fluorescent antibody test is a very reliable test and can establish the diagnosis within a few hours. If the brain biopsy is negative by this test a person need not be treated. Fluorescent antibody titers in clinical rabies are more than 1:10,000 which help to differentiate between rabies and vaccine reaction.

Fluorescent antibody test can be performed on corneal impressions. After 7–10 days of illness virus neutralizing antibodies appear in the serum and CSF, which can be measured by the Rapid Fluorescent Focus Inhibition Test (RFFIT) or enzyme-linked immunosorbent assay (ELISA). Histopathologically, the necrosed ganglia, demyelinized cord sheaths, glial proliferation, and Negri body inclusions are typical feature for a specific encephalomyelitis due to rabies.

*Rabies specific ELISA technique:* ELISA techniques for detection of rabies antigen or antirabies immunoglobulin G (IgG) are rapid, easy to use, and safe.

*Differential diagnosis:* Before the appearance of hydrophobia and in those cases where it does not manifest, rabies needs to be differentiated from other clinical conditions such as tetanus (lockjaw), encephalitis, hysteria, acute polyneuritis, poliomyelitis, and belladonna poisoning.

## RABIES IN DOGS

### Clinical Features in Dogs

Two clinical forms of manifestation are known in dogs:
1. **Furious rabies:** Dog behaves abnormally and becomes very restless and aggressive, and now tends to bite objects, animals and man indiscriminately and without provocation. There is profuse salivation due to paralysis of muscles of deglutition and tone of bark changes due to partial paralysis of vocal cords. In terminal stages of illness there are generalized convulsions followed by muscular incoordination and paralysis of muscles of trunk and limbs.
2. **Dumb rabies:** It is characterized by predominantly paralytic clinical features. The excitation phase, if at all present, tends to be very short. Paralysis is progressive beginning from head and neck region. Animal has difficulty in swallowing. The dog withdraws itself from being disturbed and lapses into a stage of sleepiness and dies in about 3 days.

Once the symptoms of rabies develop in an animal, it rarely survives more than a week.

*Observation of an animal for 10 days from the day of biting for signs of rabies* is applicable for dogs and cats only and not for other domestic or wild animals. The rationale for observation is that if these animals are having infective saliva with rabies virus, they will show signs of disease in the next 3–5 days and die subsequently in another 3–5 days.

## MANAGEMENT OF A CASE OF HUMAN RABIES (HYDROPHOBIA)

Although no specific treatment for rabies is available, a case has to be managed according to following procedure:
- The patient should be sedated and kept in a quiet room, with shades drawn on windows. No external stimuli like noise, bright light, etc. should be present as it may lead to convulsions. Patient should be treated symptomatically and proper hydration and diuresis should be maintained. Intensive respiratory and cardiac therapy is given.
- The nursing attendants and all persons coming in contact with the patient should be adequately protected, as these patients are potentially infectious.
- The intensive care and nursing support are a must for rabies patients and there are seven cases of human rabies on record who survived this dreaded disease.

## PREVENTION OF HUMAN RABIES

The prevention concerns the two main immunization strategies, namely vaccination for post-exposure prophylaxis (PEP) and vaccination for pre-exposure prophylaxis (PrEP). The following sections summarize the main points of the updated WHO position as endorsed by the Strategic Advisory Group of Experts on immunization (SAGE) at its meeting in October 2017.

### Postexposure Prophylaxis for Rabies

The following World Health Organization (WHO) classification is used for grading the exposure to rabies and guide to provide rabies prophylaxis **(Table 17D.1)**.

The PEP has broadly four components, i.e.
A. Wound management
B. Vaccination

**Table 17D.1:** Assessment of exposure—according to WHO.

| Category | Type of contact | Recommended postexposure prophylaxis |
|---|---|---|
| I | • Touching or feeding of animals<br>• Licks on intact skin<br>• Contact of intact skin with secretions or excretions of rabid animal or human case | None, if reliable case history is available |
| II | • Nibbling of uncovered skin<br>• Minor scratches or abrasions without bleeding | • Wound management<br>• Antirabies vaccine |
| III | • Single or multiple transdermal bites or scratches<br>• Licks on broken skin<br>• Contamination of mucous membrane with saliva (i.e. licks) and suspect contacts with bats | • Wound management<br>• Antirabies vaccine<br>• Rabies immunoglobulin |

*Source:* National Centre for Disease Control. National Guidelines on Rabies Prophylaxis, Govt. of India and WHO. Rabies Jan 2023.

C. RIG infiltration
D. Counseling

**A. Wound care and treatment:** Appropriate wound care is a very important step as it may bring down the risk of infection to the extent of 50–70%. This step is however often neglected. The objective is to reduce the virus deposited at the site of bite as much as possible. The wound treatment must be done immediately or as early as possible after the bite. The steps are as follows:

- Gentle washing of the wound using a detergent soap, preferably under running tap water for at least 10 minutes.
- Application of household antiseptics like povidone-iodine, 40–70% alcohol, or 0.01% aqueous solution of iodine can be done.
- In some extensive deep wounds, the exploration of wound followed by debridement, removal of dirt, and dead tissue may be required in a hospital setting and sometimes under anesthesia **(Table 17D.2)**.
- *Suturing must be generally avoided as a rule*, as it may lead to the risk of inoculation of virus deep into the wound defeating our purpose. However, if it cannot be avoided, it should be done as late as possible, from a few hours up to 1 or 2 days. The suturing should be loose and minimum possible stitches should be given. Before the suturing equine RIG (ERIG) or human RIG (HRIG) should be infiltrated into the wound.
- *Generally, animal bite wound should not be dressed or bandaged as the virus grows in anaerobic conditions* and if unavoidable, it should be loose and not occlusive.
- *Proper tetanus prophylaxis* (two doses of tetanus toxoid vaccine 0.5 mL IM 4 weeks apart) wherever necessary, systemic antibiotics to prevent wound sepsis should be given.
- The use of any local applicant or irritant like turmeric, neem, red chilli, lime, plant juices, coffee powder, coin, etc. should be discouraged and avoided, as these will further propel the virus deeper into the wound causing nerve infection, encephalitis, and death.

**B. Administration of modern ARV:**
i. **Intradermal rabies vaccination (IDRV)**
   - In the government institutions as a policy, only IDRV is provided free of cost to treat animal bite victims. The vaccine supplied shall be reconstituted only with the diluent provided with it. Disposable Insulin syringe with fixed needle or a suitable alternative 1 mL syringe provided shall be used for ID vaccination. The recommended regimen consists of injecting one dose of 0.1 mL of the reconstituted vaccine at two sites on days 0, 3,7 and 28 (2-2-2-0-2). This is known as the updated "Thai Red Cross (TRC)" regimen. The opened vials having reconstituted vaccine shall not be exposed to sunlight, used in 6–8 hours and any leftover vaccine shall be discarded at the end of the day. Day 0 is the day of first dose of vaccination and not necessarily the day of bite/exposure.
   - The commonly recommended site/s of ID vaccination is the deltoids. The alternate sites are suprascapular and rarely lateral thighs only if necessary and with the consent of the patient; in case of women strictly in the presence of a female attendant. A successful ID injection is evident by the appearance of a bleb (3–4 mm) and peau de orange (orange peel) effect. If ID injection fails (no appearance of a bleb) at one site, than at an adjacent area the ID dose shall be injected. The patient shall be informed not to rub or apply any applicant to the injection sites.
   - The common side effects of IDRV are soreness, redness, itching, occasionally slight pain, etc. and these are self limiting and no medication is ordinarily needed. Spirit swab shall not be used before ID vaccination.
   - The vaccination series may be discontinued if the biting dog or cat (not other animals) is alive after ten days of observation. In the process, if the patient has received at least two doses of rabies vaccine then he/she is considered to have received pre-exposure rabies vaccination/prophylaxis (PrEP) and in future in the event of a re-exposure to rabies than such patients require wound management, one dose (0.1 mL) of rabies vaccine at one site on day 0 and 3 and no RIG.

ii. **Intramuscular rabies vaccination**

In the private sector, PEP is provided for a fee by IM route. The currently available vaccines and regimen in India for IM administration are described below.

1. *Cell culture vaccines:* Human Diploid Cell Vaccine (HDCV), Liquid (Adsorbed), 1 mL: Produced locally in private sector. Purified Chick Embryo Cell Vaccine (PCECV), 1 mL: Produced locally in private sector, Purified Vero Cell Rabies Vaccine (PVRV), 0.5 mL and 1 mL: Imported and also produced locally in public and private sectors.
2. *Purified Duck Embryo Vaccine (PDEV), 1 mL:* Produced locally in private sector and is currently being exported.

**Regimen:** Essen regimen (1-1-1-1-1): Five dose intramuscular schedule – the course for post-exposure prophylaxis consists of intramuscular administration of five injections, one dose each given on days 0, 3, 7, 14 and 28. Day 0 indicates date of administration of first dose of vaccine.

**Site of injection:** The deltoid region is ideal for the administration of these vaccines. Gluteal region is not recommended because the fat present in this region retards the absorption of antigen and hence impairs the generation of optimal immune response. In case of infants and young children anterolateral part of the thigh is the preferred site.

**Table 17D.2:** Wound(s) management.

| Do's | | |
|---|---|---|
| Physical | Wash with running water | Mechanical removal of virus from the wound(s) |
| Chemical | • Wash the wound(s) with soap and water<br>• Apply disinfectant | Inactivation of the virus |
| Biological | Infiltrate immunoglobulin into the depth and around the wound(s) in category III exposures | Neutralization of the virus |
| **Don'ts** | | |
| Touch the wound(s) with bare hand | | |
| Apply irritants like soil, chilies, oil, lime, herbs, chalk, betel leaves, etc. | | |

### C. Administration of rabies immunoglobulin (RIG) for passive immunization

The RIGs or ARS (antirabies serum) are readymade antirabies antibodies providing passive immunity and immediate protection. Even the best of modern vaccines take 10–14 days to elicit the protective antibody titer of more than 0.5 IU/mL of serum and therefore RIGs cover this vulnerable period in category III exposure.

The combination of ARV and RIG is almost 100% effective "at prevention" of clinical symptoms and disease; however, attempts to use vaccine or RIG after the onset of symptoms have not been successful. Some salient points related with use of RIG should always be kept in mind. These are:
- The RIG should be administered in all individuals with category III exposure and in those with category II exposure who are immunodeficient.
- The RIG is administered only once and as soon as possible after the initiation of PEP. RIG is not indicated beyond the seventh day after the first ARV dose.
- The dose of Human Rabies Immunoglobulin (HRIG) is 20 IU/kg body weight and for Equine Rabies Immunoglobulin (ERIG), 40 IU/kg body weight.
- All of the RIG, or as much as anatomically possible, should be administered into or around the wound site(s).
- Remaining RIG, if any, should be injected IM at a site distant from the site of vaccine administration. RIG may be diluted to a volume sufficient for all wounds to be effectively and safely infiltrated. There are no scientific grounds for performing a skin sensitivity test prior to ERIG administration. So, it is not mandatory.

The RIG should be immediately given after exposure to inhibit viral spread because vaccination needs time to induce a humoral response. RIG can be diluted with normal saline whenever the calculated dose (20 IU/kg body weight for HRIG subject to a maximum of 1,500 IU and 40 IU/kg body weight for ERIG subject to a maximum of 3,000 IU) is inadequate to infiltrate all wounds without previous dilution. However, the overall dose of HRIG or ERIG should not be increased because it may interfere with vaccination and may lead to reduced rate of seroconversion.

Rabies human monoclonal antibodies: These are approved by DCGI in October 2016 and can be used as an alternative to RIGs. They induce rabies virus neutralizing activity, which is noninferior to HRIG regimen. They are safe, well tolerated and more cost effective. Dose is 3.33 IU/kg body weight, which is the same for children and adults. The monoclonal antibodies should be given along with first dose of ARV and not beyond seventh day of first dose of ARV just like RIG. It should be infiltrated in and around the wound and if dose remains, it is injected intramuscularly in mid-thigh.

### D. Counseling

Animal bite, more so when severe and in children is distressing. A word of advice and comforting the patient by the doctor, informing the patient to comply with the series of vaccination and not to default; no dietary restrictions; no alcohol and no strenuous physical exercises during the course of vaccination are to be given.

## Pre-exposure Prophylaxis

It is recommended for high-risk groups like laboratory staff handling the rabies virus and infected material, physicians and paramedics attending the hydrophobia cases, veterinarians, animal handlers and catchers, wild life wardens, pet owners, and travelers from rabies free to rabies endemic areas.

The PrEP should consist of three 1 mL IM or 0.1 mL ID (one dose of 0.1 mL ID on each shoulder) doses of CCV, one dose each given on day 0, 7, and 28 with one booster after 1 year. Persons in high-risk group should have their neutralizing antibody titers checked every 6 months. If it is less than 0.5 IU/mL a booster dose of vaccine should be given. If these persons after successful PrEP get exposed to rabies virus irrespective of time interval between previous vaccination and re-exposure, they require only two booster doses of CCV on day 0 and 3 without any RIG, whatever be the category of exposure or bite.

## Management of Re-exposure following Pre-exposure or Postexposure Prophylaxis with CCV

In case of re-exposure, if a person has previously received complete PrEP of three doses with one booster after 1 year or PEP of five doses with a potent CCV, he/she should be given only two booster doses, IM or ID on days 0 and 3 but no RIG is necessary in them.

## CONTROL OF RABIES

As the major source of infection is dog, the control of dog population along with their mass immunization in the shortest possible time remains the most logical approach for the control of this dreaded disease. A canine rabies control program has been launched by the ministry of agriculture. This type of program should incorporate three basic elements:
1. Epidemiological surveillance.
2. Control of dog population and animal birth control (ABC) programs.
3. Mass immunization of dogs by giving primary vaccination at 3 months of age and booster 1 year later and then every year. Nowadays, safe oral vaccines have become available and can be used for mass immunization. Oral immunization can cover 75% of dog population.

Oral vaccination of wild animals with attenuated as well as recombinant vaccines by using "oral vaccine baits" has successfully reduced and controlled wild life rabies in foxes in some countries of Europe like Germany, Switzerland, etc. and also in Canada.

*Health education:* Health education of public regarding prevention and control of rabies and management of animal bite is crucial to save lives. It is a real tragedy that this disease, which is 100% preventable, is still a major cause of mortality in developing countries.

## Indications for Doubling the First Dose of CCV

In some situations, it becomes necessary and appropriate to double the first dose of antirabies CCV, whatever route or schedule is used. These are patients with:
- Underlying chronic disease (e.g. liver cirrhosis)
- Severely malnourishment
- Treatment after a delay of 48 hours or more
- Congenital immunodeficient or suffering from acquired immunodeficiency syndrome
- Immunosuppressive drugs (including corticosteroids, antimalarials, and anticancer drugs)
- Very high degree of exposure or extensive wounds, i.e. on head, neck, face, hands and genitals, etc. following bites by suspect or proven rabid animals or by wild animals like fox, jackal, mongoose, etc.
- Where RIG is indicated but unavailable.

## Global and National Approach

Rabies is included in WHO's 2021–2030 Roadmap for the global control of neglected tropical diseases, which sets regional, progressive targets for the elimination of targeted diseases. Rabies is one of these. As a zoonotic disease, it requires close cross-sectoral coordination at the national, regional and global levels.

WHO, Food and Agriculture Organization (FAO) and World Organization for Animal Health (WOAH, founded as OIE) have launched the United Against Rabies Forum (UAR), a multi-stakeholder platform to advocate for action and investment in rabies control.

Rabies can significantly contribute to building of capacity of the One Health workforce.

WHO works with partners to guide and support countries as they develop and implement their national rabies elimination plans, but the data are weak. Strengthening disease surveillance, data reporting and monitoring rabies programs remains a priority focus.

WHO develops technical guidance on rabies and supports the capacity development in countries.

In 2019, Gavi, the Vaccine Alliance included human rabies vaccines in its Vaccine investment strategy 2021–2025, which would support scaling up rabies PEP in Gavi-eligible countries. Currently the roll out of this strategy is still on hold following the COVID-19 pandemic.

The key towards implementing effective rabies elimination programs is to engage with local communities, start small, catalyze long-term investment through stimulus packages, ensure the ownership of governments, demonstrate success and cost-effectiveness, and scale up quickly.

Rabies elimination is feasible and achievable if this goal is prioritized and adequately supported financially and politically.

### Key Points

- *Pregnancy and lactation:* There are no contraindications regarding the use of modern CCV for PEP during pregnancy and lactation.
- *Extremes of age:* The dose of CCV is not dependent on age and weight. The dose is exactly the same from pediatric to geriatric age group.
- If a dog is vaccinated against rabies, it cannot suffer from or transmit the disease. But in view of questionable maintenance of cold chain, it is very difficult to say that a vaccinated dog is immune against rabies unless it is confirmed by a serological test. However, a modern tissue culture vaccine of adequate potency, if given regularly to dog following strict schedule should prove to be sufficiently protective.
- According to WHO, rabies virus has not been isolated from the raw milk of rabid animal, therefore PEP is not indicated in case of consumption of such raw milk. But, it is always better to consume milk after boiling or pasteurization.
- The WHO document states that no human cases resulting from consumption of raw meat of rabid animal have been reported. However, consumption of raw meat of rabid animal is not advisable.
- If a person presents after a considerable delay of weeks to months with a history of animal bite, it is mandatory to give complete course of postexposure treatment including infiltration of wound site with RIG in view of the 100% mortality with this disease. It may be appropriate to double the first dose of vaccine. If there is no visible wound then give the RIG by IM route away from the site of ARV.
- The saliva of rabies patients contains rabies virus and is infective, hence in case of suspicion about contact with saliva of a rabies patient during kissing the contact requires rabies postexposure vaccination. If ulcers are present in the mouth then Ig should be advised by IM route.
- Rabies virus is present in the semen and to some extent in vaginal secretions. In some male patients, priapism and in both male and female patients increased libido may be observed. Hence, a complete course of postexposure vaccination should be given to the healthy contact. If abrasion on penis or vagina, RIG is to be given by IM route.
- There have been some instances of failure even after complete course of antirabies treatment. During discussions at WHO and other expert committee meetings, it was found that the efficacy and immunogenicity of modern CCV were never in doubt, but failures were either due to delay in getting vaccination or RIG was not used or there was already immunosuppression in patients.
- There is no contraindication of giving ARV along with Expanded Program on Immunization (EPI) or pediatric vaccines in case of postexposure vaccination, however, an interval of 3–4 weeks between the two types of vaccines is advisable in case of PrEP.
- Modern ARV can be safely given to children having chickenpox, measles, or any other eruptive fevers.
- If during antirabies vaccination any dose is missed then patient is counseled regarding strict adherence to schedule and schedule is completed as soon as possible.
- No dietary restrictions are required during vaccination but alcohol, tobacco, gutka, and smoking must be avoided.
- There is no single shot ARV till date and a full course of antirabies vaccination does not guarantee or provide life-long immunity against the disease.

## SUMMARY

Rabies is still a very dreadful as well as dreaded disease. Strict measures to control or eliminate the disease in domestic as well as wild animals must be taken if we are ever to achieve control of rabies.

Rabies is an acute fatal encephalomyelitis caused by a ribonucleic acid (RNA) virus under the genus *Lyssavirus* and family Rhabdoviridae. It is the most important viral zoonosis of warm-blooded animals like dogs, cats, jackals, etc. recognized today because of its global distribution, incidence, veterinary and human health costs, and extremely high case fatality rate.

Upon biting, scratching or licking on broken skin and intact mucous membrane, the virus enters the body, multiplies locally in the tissues and muscles, and then travels to brain at the speed of 3–10 mm/h via neurotropic nerves. There, it affects the brain stem function, causing hydrophobia (fear of water), aerophobia (fear of breeze) and/or photophobia (fear of light), and finally resulting in respiratory paralysis and death.

**Chapter 17:** Specific Epidemiology of Infectious Diseases | 411

The incubation period in man is highly variable, commonly 1–3 months following exposure but it may vary from 4 days to many years.

**Clinical features**
1. *Prodromal stage*
2. *Acute neurologic stage:* Further divided into two substages:
    a. Stage of acute encephalitis
    b. Stage of brainstem dysfunction
3. *Stage of coma*
4. *Death*

**Diagnosis:** Several biological samples like saliva, cerebral spinal fluid (CSF), skin biopsies containing hair follicles collected at the nape of neck, extracted hair follicles, tears, and urine can be used. Positive results of viral RNA in samples should be confirmed by sequencing.

**Prevention:** Care of the bite wound and postexposure prophylaxis for rabies with vaccine (IM/ID) and rabies Immunoglobulin (RIG) for passive immunization.

**Pre-exposure Prophylaxis**
It is recommended for high-risk groups like laboratory staff handling the rabies virus and infected material, physicians and paramedics attending the hydrophobia cases, veterinarians, animal handlers and catchers, wild life wardens, pet owners, and travelers from rabies free to rabies endemic areas.

Cases of human rabies would be extremely rare, if all patients knew whom to approach for treatment in case of bite, if ARV and Igs were readily available and if the postexposure treatment was strictly and diligently carried out following the guidelines.

# SUGGESTED READING

1. Batra RK, Kaul HL. Rabies—pathophysiology and current status of management. J Gen Med. 1994;6(4).
2. Both L, Banyard AC, van Dolleweerd C, et al. Passive immunity in the prevention of rabies. Lancet Infect Dis. 2012;12(5):397-407.
3. Dietzschold B, Rupperecht CE, Fu ZF, et al. Rhabdoviruses. In: Fields N, Knipe DM, Howley PM, Chanock RM, Melnick JL, Monath TP, Roizman B, Straus SE (Eds). Fields Virology, 3rd edition. Philadelphia: Lippincott-Raven Publishers; 1996. pp. 1137-59.
4. Gode GR. Treatment of Human rabies, problems and possibilities: In: Kaul HL (Ed). Advances in Anaesthesiology, proceeding of V Asian and Austral. New Delhi: Sagar Publishers; 1978. pp. 229-303.
5. Gogtay N, Munshi R, Ashwath Narayana DH, et al. Comparison of a Novel Human Rabies Monoclonal Antibody to Human Rabies Immunoglobulin for Postexposure Prophylaxis: A Phase 2/3, Randomized, Single-Blind, Noninferiority, Controlled Study. Clin Infect Dis. 2018;66(3):387-95.
6. Gompf SG. Rabies Clinical Presentation. Medscape; 2016.
7. Nandi S, Kumar M. Global perspective of rabies and rabies related viruses: a comprehensive review. Asian J Anim Vet Adv. 2011;6(2):101-16.
8. Perrin P, Lafon M, Sureau. Rabies vaccines from Pasteur's time up to experimental subunit vaccines today. In: Plotkin S (Ed). Viral vaccines, New York: Wiley-Lisss, Inc.; 1990. pp. 325-45.
9. Rabies Emerging Trends. Delhi: An IJCP Group Publication, IJCP Medinews; 1998.
10. Sehgal S, Bhatia R. Rabies: Current status and proposed control programmes in India Shamnath Marg, Delhi: NICD; 1985.
11. Shantavasinkul P, Wilde H. Postexposure prophylaxis for rabies in resource- limited/poor countries. Adv Virus Res. 2011;79:291-307.
12. Sudarshan MK. Rabies Prevention. India: Macmillan Medical Communications; 2010.
13. Sudarshan MK. Rabies Prophylaxis. India: Macmillan Medical Communications; 2012.
14. WHO, World Rabies Day Report, 2011.
15. WHO. Rabies in India. Accessed in July 2023 available from https://www.who.int/india/health-topics/rabies.
16. WHO. World Rabies Day 2011 Report.
17. WHO Position Paper: Rabies Vaccine, 2010; Sudarshan MK et al., APCRI J, 2004; NHP-2019.
18. WHO publication. Rabies vaccines: WHO position paper-recommendations. Vaccine. 2010;28:7140-2.
19. WHO Rabies: Factsheet. Jan 2023. Available from https://www.who.int/news-room/fact-sheets/detail/rabies#:~:text=Overview,both%20domestic%20and%20wild%20animals.
20. WHO Technical Report Series, 1012. (2018). WHO Expert Consultation on Rabies, third report. [online] Available from: http://apps.who.int/iris/bitstream/handle/10665/272364/9789241210218-eng.pdf.
21. Wilde H. Editorial Commentary: Rabies Postexposure Vaccination: Are Antibody Responses Adequate? Clin Infect Dis. 2012;55(12):206-8.

# EPIDEMIOLOGY OF PLAGUE AND ITS PREVENTION AND CONTROL

*"Black death", "Mad rat disease", "Mahamari" and "Pest".*

| CM7.2 | Enumerate, describe and discuss the mode of transmission and measures for prevention and control of plague |
|---|---|
| CM8.1 | Describe and discuss the epidemiological and control measures applicable in plague |

# INTRODUCTION

Plague is an infectious, zoonotic, bacterial disease caused by the bacteria *Yersinia pestis*, transmitted to humans by the infectious fleabite. Plague has always been able to generate panic whenever suspected. This is due to the fact that it can be a severe disease, especially in its septicemic and pneumonic forms, where the case-fatality ratio ranges from 30 to 100%, if left untreated (WHO, Plague, 2018).

Moreover, considering the recent threat of bioterrorism and inclusion of the causative organism, *Y. pestis*, as a bioterrorism agent, has added to the irrational response this disease gathers.

# HISTORICAL PERSPECTIVE

Three major pandemics of plague have been documented in the history dated as early as the sixth century. These involved many parts of Asia, Europe, etc. and accounted for mass casualties. These events gave birth to some of the most important public health measures like quarantine.

# PROBLEM STATEMENT

Being a zoonotic disease, plague is found in all the continents, except Oceania. There is a definite risk of human plague at all places where there is coexistence of the natural foci of plague (the bacteria, an animal reservoir, and a vector) and human population **(Fig. 17D.14)**.

The three countries that are on the top list for being endemic for plague are the Democratic Republic of Congo, Madagascar, and Peru. In Madagascar, cases of bubonic plague are reported nearly every year, during the epidemic season (between

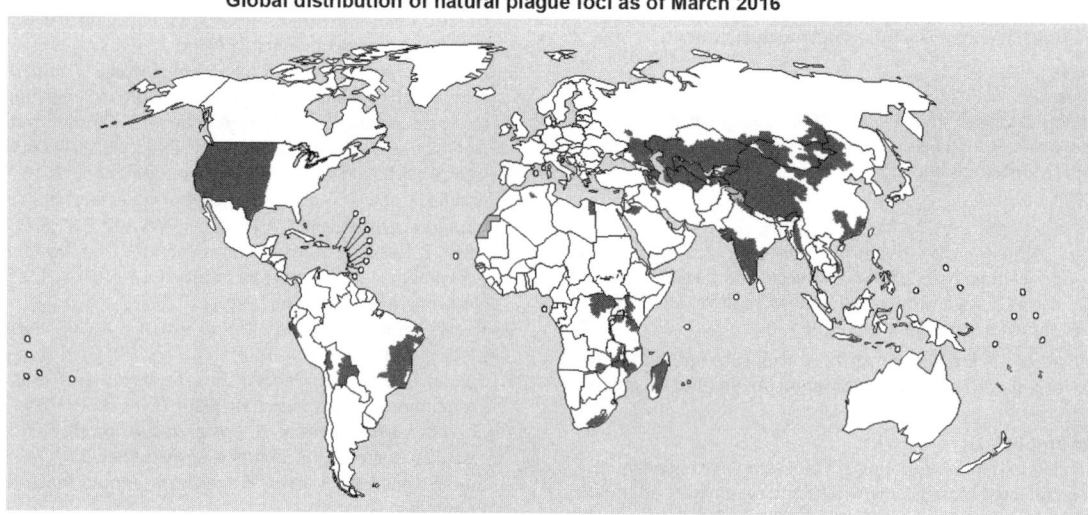

**Fig. 17D.14:** Distribution of plague across the world in 2016.
*First administrative level representation.*
Source: WHO/PED, as of 15 March 2016.

September and April). From 2010 to 2015 there were 3,248 cases reported worldwide, including 584 deaths. As of 15 September 2021, a total of 20 suspected and 22 confirmed cases of plague have been notified. (WHO, Fact Sheets: Plague 2022, Plague - Madagascar Oct 2021).

## EPIDEMIOLOGY

### Agent Factors

**Agent:** Plague is a bacterial disease caused by the bacteria *Y. pestis*.
**Strain:** They are gram negative, bipolar staining, nonsporulating, and nonmotile coccobacilli belonging to the Enterobacteriaceae family.

### Host Factors

Plague is primarily a disease of rodents in which humans become accidental host. It has been observed to be occurring in epizootic and enzootic forms.

### Environmental Factors

Epizootics are usually observed with involvement of these domestic rats and affects overcrowded areas. This kind of epizootics are most hazardous to humans since they occur in domestic environment (often where there is overcrowding) and the oriental flea are the most efficient vector that readily feeds on humans.

### Reservoir

The domestic rats (*Rattus rattus* and *Rattus norvegicus*) and its fleas have been known to be associated with plague since ages.

### Mode of Transmission

Fleas are the only arthropods known to transmit *Y. pestis* in nature. The efficiency of transmission varies by the flea species and also environmental conditions like temperature, humidity, etc. High vector flea density on the rodent hosts is associated with increased likelihood of transmitting the infection.

Among the different varieties of fleas, the oriental flea is the most efficient vector. When a flea takes an infected blood meal, the bacilli multiply in a huge number in it. This results in blocking of the foregut of the flea. The resultant starving flea seek new host. And on biting them, it regurgitates the *Y. pestis* from the blocked foregut into the bite wound. There can be partially blocked and completely blocked fleas. A partially blocked flea is more dangerous than a completely blocked one, since it lives longer, around a year.

## CLINICAL MANIFESTATIONS

After the incubation period of 1–7 days, those who are infected with plague, mostly develop initial acute febrile disease with other constitutional symptoms like, chills, head and body aches, weakness, vomiting, etc.

There are primarily three forms of plague, depending on the route of infection—bubonic, pnuemonic and septicemic.

- ***Bubonic plague:***
  - The most common form.
  - In this type, the bacilli enter the body at the site of fleabite and then entering into the lymphatic system, reaches to the nearest lymph node, where it undergoes replication.
  - This leads to inflammation of the lymph node, which becomes inflamed, tense, and painful. This is called a "bubo".

- As the disease progresses, the inflamed lymph nodes may turn into open sores, filled with pus.
- Human to human transmission of bubonic plague is rare.
- In advance cases, bubonic plague can spread to the lungs and attains a more severe form, called pneumonic plague.
- *Pneumonic plague (lungs affected):*
  - The most virulent form.
  - Incubation can be as short as 24 hours.
  - Any person with pneumonic plague may transmit the disease via droplets to other humans.
  - Untreated pneumonic plague, if not diagnosed and treated early, can be fatal.
  - However, recovery rates are high, if detected and treated in time (within 24 hours of onset of symptoms).

## DIAGNOSIS

To diagnose plague, a careful epidemiological history is must. This should be followed by prompt collection of diagnostic samples. And if the epidemiological and clinical evidence are adequate, initial specific treatment may be commenced without waiting for the laboratory results.

### Samples

- For bubonic plague, the best sample is aspirates from a bubo. If the aspirate is "dry", sterile saline can be injected into it and then aspiration can be reattempted.
- *Other samples:* Exudates, respiratory secretions, throat swab, sputum, and blood.

Samples may be cultured for isolation of the organism. The specimen for culture must be taken prior to the commencement of treatment.

The sample specimen may be used to prepare smear for identification of the bacilli. For the same Giemsa or Wayson's stain may be used.

Fluorescent antibody test may be used to demonstrate the F1 antigen of the bacilli. But this is a presumptive test and at times its results may be inconclusive.

Rapid test (dipstick test) is also available for detection of the same antigen.

Confirmatory diagnosis is provided by isolation of the bacteria and demonstration of its lysis by a specific bacteriophage and four-fold rise in the titer of the antibody in paired sera.

## TREATMENT

Antibiotic of choice for *Y. pestis* is streptomycin. Gentamicin, although not approved for this purpose is more widely available and an acceptable alternative. Other alternatives include, tetracyclines and chloramphenicol (agent of choice for plague meningitis, pleuritis, and endophthalmitis—due to its higher permeability). However, recently multidrug resistance had been observed in the *Y. pestis*. The penicillins, cephalosporins, and macrolides have not been observed to be effective against *Y. pestis*, and hence should not be used.

## PREVENTION AND CONTROL

Surveillance, education, and environmental management are the main pillars for prevention and control of plague.

- Active identification and monitoring of plague foci must be carried out by the health authorities. This should be coupled with a system for rapid identification and evaluation of any suspect human cases or epizootics of plague.
- People living in plague foci should protect themselves and their pets form the fleas.
- Living and working environment free of rodents should be maintained—for the same extensive and ongoing rodent control measures should be taken, like, rodent proofing of buildings, removal of any rodent food source such as garbage or animal feeds, removal of any potential harborage sites like wood piles, junk heaps, etc.
- In the situations of epizootics:
  - Killing the fleas with insecticides is the principal control measure. In addition to this, rodents' burrows, rodent runs, etc. where the rodents along with the fleas dwelling on them are found, should be dusted or sprayed with appropriate insecticides like dichlorodiphenyltrichloroethane (DDT) or benzene hexachloride (BHC).
  - Killing the rodents is entirely the decision of the health authorities. And this should be done only when adequate flea control measures have already been done.
  - Control of rodents without environmental sanitation may worsen the situation. This is likely to happen because, the void created by removal of the existing rodents will be quickly filled by immature and more susceptible population of rodents which will make the situation even worse.

## SURVEILLANCE

As per the IHR (International Health Regulations), all the countries and their health authorities are to notify to the WHO regarding all plague cases and presence of any plague bacilli foci in their territory.

The case definitions for plague according to WHO are:
- *Suspected plague:*
  - Compatible clinical and epidemiological features and
  - Suspicious organisms seen or isolated from clinical specimen.
- *Presumptive plague:*
  - *Y. pestis* F1 antigen detected in clinical materials by direct fluorescent antibody testing or by some other standardized antigen detection method, or
  - Isolate from a clinical specimen demonstrates biochemical reactions consistent with *Y. pestis* or polymerase chain reaction (PCR) positivity, or
  - A single serum specimen is found positive for diagnostic levels of antibodies to *Y. pestis* F1 antigen, not explainable on the basis of prior infection or immunization.

- *Confirmed plague:*
  - Isolate identified as *Y. pestis* by phage lysis of cultures, or
  - A significant (≥ four-fold) change in antibody titer to the F1 antigen in paired serum specimens.

## MANAGING PLAGUE OUTBREAKS

- *Identification and control of the source of infection:*
  - First of all, the source of infection needs to be rapidly identified. This includes looking for clustering of large numbers of small animal deaths.
  - For the same, appropriate infection, prevention and control measures need to be implemented with urgency, including vector control, then rodent control.
- *Protection of the health workers:*
  - Information and training of the health workers on infection prevention and control is of paramount importance.
  - Those in direct contact with pneumonic plague patients must wear standard precautions and also receive chemoprophylaxis with antibiotics for 7 days or as long as they are exposed to infected patients.
- *Ensuring correct treatment:*
  - Verify that patients are being given appropriate antibiotic treatment.
  - It should be made sure that in such a situation, local supplies of antibiotics are adequate and uninterrupted.
- *Isolating patients with pneumonic plague:*
  - Patients should be isolated at the earliest. This is mandatory to prevent infection to others via air droplets.
  - Simple measure like providing masks for pneumonic patients can significantly contribute in reduction of spread.
- *Surveillance:*
  - Identifying and monitoring close contacts of pneumonic plague patients and providing a 7-day chemoprophylaxis.
  - Chemoprophylaxis should also be given to household members of bubonic plague patients.
- *Obtaining specimens:* The specimen should be collected carefully with use of appropriate infection, prevention and control procedures, and sent to laboratories for testing.
- *Disinfection:*
  - Routine handwashing is recommended with soap and water or use of alcohol hand rub.
  - Larger areas can be disinfected using 10% of diluted household bleach (made fresh daily).
- *Ensuring safe burial practices:* Spraying of face or chest area of suspected pneumonic plague deaths should be discouraged. The area should be covered with a disinfectant-soaked cloth or absorbent material.

## TRAVEL AND TRADE

- Considering the current information and understanding, there is very low-risk of international transmission of plague.
- The WHO advises against any restriction on travel or trade on Madagascar based on the available information. However, the international travelers should be informed about the current plague scenario. The fact that plague is endemic in Madagascar, travelers should receive advice on prevention, postexposure chemoprophylaxis, and where to seek medical treatment should they develop plague-related symptoms.

## VACCINATION

The WHO does not recommend vaccination against plague, except for high-risk groups (such as laboratory personnel who are constantly exposed to the risk of contamination, and healthcare workers).

The plague vaccine is no longer commercially available. The original vaccine against plague, which was formalin inactivated, was providing partial protection against bubonic plague, and also had many side effects. Research is ongoing to develop a vaccine that will protect against both bubonic as well as pneumonic types with fewer side effects.

## CHEMOPROPHYLAXIS

Short-term prophylaxis with either tetracycline or trimethoprim–sulfamethoxazole can be considered for people who are either caring for the plague patients or have an unavoidable exposure to plague in epizootic or enzootic situations.

Some facts about plague are highlighted in **Figure 17D.15**.

## SUMMARY

Plague is an infectious, zoonotic, bacterial disease caused by the bacteria *Yersinia pestis*, transmitted to humans by the infectious fleabite.

The domestic rats (*Rattus rattus* and *Rattus norvegicus*) and its fleas have been known to be associated with plague since ages. Epizootics are usually observed with involvement of these domestic rats and affects overcrowded areas.

An incubation period is 1–7 days.

There are primarily three forms of plague, which depend on the route of infection—bubonic and pneumonic and septicemic

*Diagnosis:* Fluorescent antibody test may be used to demonstrate the F1 antigen of the bacilli.

Rapid test (dipstick test) is also available for detection of the same antigen.

*Treatment:* Antibiotic of choice for *Y. pestis* is streptomycin. Gentamicin, although not approved for this purpose is more widely available and an acceptable alternative. Other alternatives include, tetracyclines and chloramphenicol (agent of choice for plague meningitis, pleuritis, and endophthalmitis—due to its higher permeability).

**Prevention and Control**

Surveillance, education, and environmental management are the main pillars for prevention and control of plague.

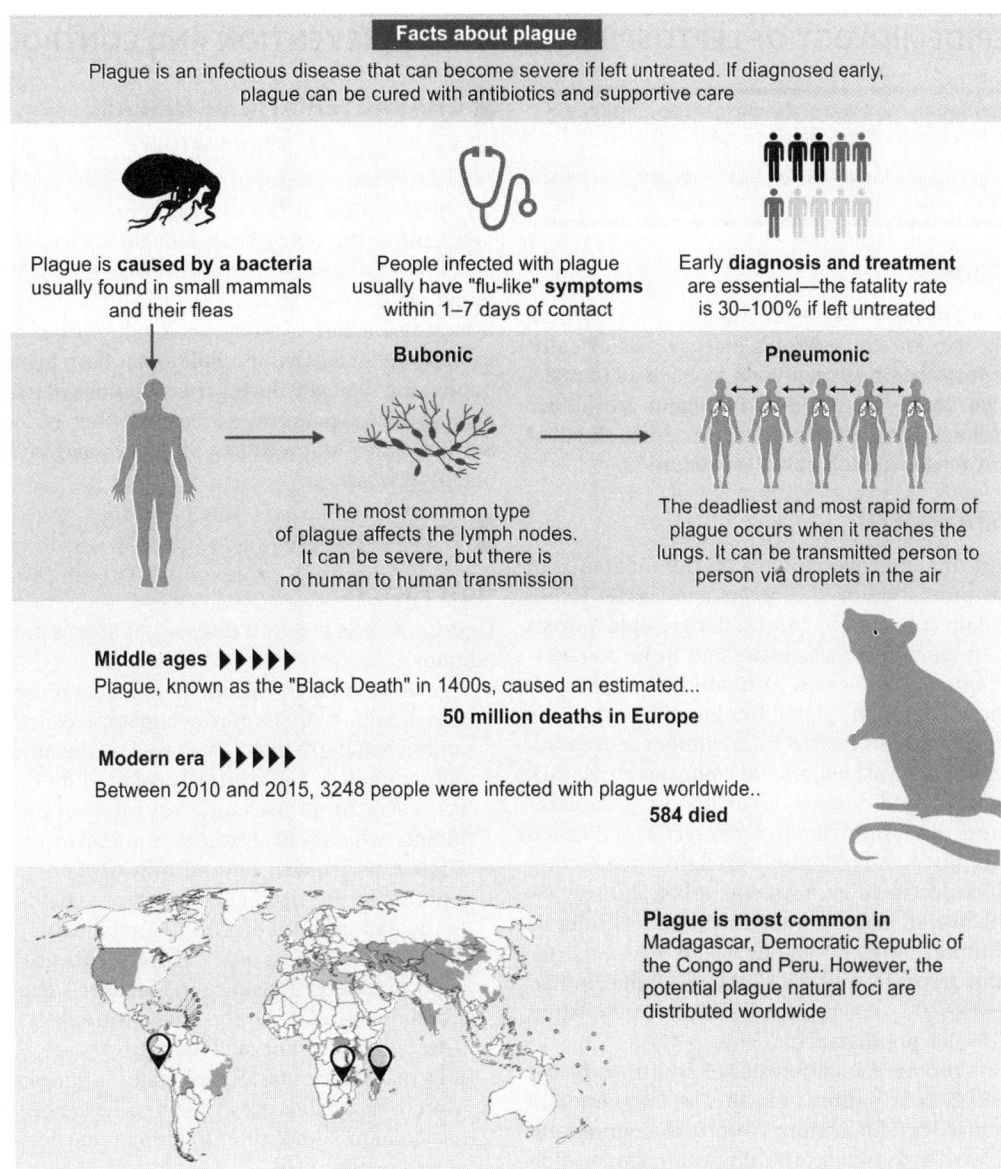

**Fig. 17D.15:** Some facts about plague.
*Source:* https://www.who.int/images/default-source/infographics/plague-february-2017-jpg.jpg?sfvrsn=af65c05c_0.

## SUGGESTED READING

1. Cavanaugh DC. Specific effect of temperature upon transmission of the plague bacillus by the oriental flea, Xenopsylla cheopis. Amer J Trop Med Hyg. 1971;20(2):264-73.
2. Cavanauh DC, Marshall JD Jr. The influence of climate on the seasonal prevalence of plague in the Republic of Vietnam. J Wildl Dis. 1972;8(1): 8-94.
3. Centers for Disease Control and Prevention. Plague. The Yellow Book: Health Information for International Travel, 2003–2004. Atlanta: US Department of Health and Human Services, Public Health Service; 2003.
4. Dennis DT, Campbell GL. Plague and other Yersinia infections. In: Kasper DL, Braunwald E, Fauci AS, Hauser S, Longo D, Jameson JL (Eds). Harrison's Principles of Internal Medicine, 16th edition. New York: McGraw–Hill; 2005. pp. 921-9.
5. Dennis DT, Gage KL, Gratz N, Poland JD, Tikhomirov E. Plague Manual: Epidemiology, Distribution, Surveillance and Control. Geneva: World Health Organization; 1999.
6. Galimand M, Guiyoule A, GerbaudG, et al. Multidrug resistance *in* Yersinia pestis mediated by transferable plasmid. N Engl J Med. 1997;337(10):677-80.
7. Hinnebusch BJ. Transmission factors: Yersinia pestis genes required to infect the flea vector of plague. Adv Exp Med Biol. 2003;529:55-62.
8. Hoogstraal H. The roles *of* fleas and ticks in epidemiology of human diseases. In: Traub R, Stracker H (Eds). Fleas Rotterdam: AA Balkema; 1980. pp. 241-4.
9. Perry RD, Fetherston JD. Yersinia pestis etiological agent of plague. Clinical Microbio Rev. 1997;10(1):35-66.
10. Programme for Prevention and Control of Leptospirosis, National Guidelines. Diagnosis, Case Management, Prevention and Control of Leptospirosis. India: National Centre for Disease Control; 2015.
11. Sehdev PS. The origin of quarantine. Clin Infect Dis. 2002;35(9):1071-2.
12. World health Organization. (2017). Plague. [online] Available from: http://www.who.int/en/news-room/fact-sheets/detail/plague.
13. World Health Organization. International Health Regulations (1969). Geneva: World Health Organization; 1983.

# EPIDEMIOLOGY OF LEPTOSPIROSIS AND ITS PREVENTION AND CONTROL

**CM7.2** Enumerate, describe and discuss the mode of transmission and measures for prevention and control of leptospirosis

**CM8.1** Describe and discuss the epidemiological and control measures applicable in leptospirosis

## INTRODUCTION

Leptospirosis is a zoonotic bacterial infection with global distribution. It is also known as Weil's disease. Historically, its severe icteric form has been reported as back as in 1886. Although it has worldwide distribution, the major prevalence is found in tropical and subtropical regions. Extreme rainfall or flooding invariably results in outbreak of leptospirosis.

## PROBLEM STATEMENT

An initial attempt to gather global data on the incidence of leptospirosis was published over 15 years ago (WHO 1999). Based on global data collected by International Leptospirosis Society surveys, the incidence was estimated to be 350,000–500,000 severe leptospirosis cases annually (Ahmed et al. 2012). Despite these efforts, the global burden of leptospirosis was felt to be largely underestimated for a number of reasons, including the fact that the vast majority of countries either lack a notification system or notification is not mandatory (Ahmed et al. 2012). To address these shortcomings, the WHO established the Leptospirosis Burden Epidemiology Reference Group (LERG). The LERG report included a systematic literature review that estimated the overall global annual incidence of endemic and epidemic human leptospirosis at 5 and 14 cases per 100,000 population, respectively (WHO 2011). Endemic human leptospirosis rates varied by region from 0.5/100,000 population in Europe to 95/100,000 population in Africa.

Leptospirosis is reported in a number of countries of the South-East Asia Region from time to time. The magnitude of the leptospirosis problem differs from country to country and depends on awareness and attitude of public healthcare decision makers. Most human cases have been reported from India, Indonesia, Thailand and Sri Lanka during the rainy season. Major outbreaks in South-East Asia were reported in the past in Jakarta (2003), Mumbai (2005) and Sri Lanka (2008). Seasonal outbreaks are reported in northern Thailand and in Gujarat, India following heavy rainfall and flooding. A few human cases have been reported from Maldives. According to currently available reports, incidences range from approximately 0.1–10 per 100,000 per year globally. During outbreaks and in high-exposure risk groups, disease incidence may reach over 50 per 100,000.

There are anecdotal reports of human and animal cases in Bangladesh, Myanmar, Nepal and Timor-Leste. However, no information is available about leptospirosis in Bhutan and Democratic People's Republic of Korea. (World Health Organization. Leptospirosis: Fact Sheet 2009).

## CHARACTERISTIC OF DISEASE

Leptospirosis can occur worldwide, but a few risk factors have been found to be associated with the disease, which influence the distribution of the disease. Leptospirosis is found most frequently in the slums with insufficient sewage disposal facilities and water treatment. It also occurs as an occupational disease in people who work outdoors or in close proximity of animals. It may also occur as a recreational hazard in those taking part in water-related activities. Epidemics have been observed to be happening typically during the situations like flooding, shifting environmental patterns, extreme weather, etc. In India, parts of South Gujarat, Maharashtra, etc. have relatively high proportion of leptospirosis.

## EPIDEMIOLOGY

### Host Factors

Leptospirosis is chiefly a disease of animals and seldom infects humans.

- *Age and sex distribution:* Males suffer more frequently than females due to their more occupation related exposure to the animals that are infected as well as the environment that is contaminated. Leptospirosis is found more often in the age bracket of 20–45 years and very rarely in young children and infants, which is likely due to minimal exposure.
- *High-risk groups:* Agricultural workers, especially those working in the rice fields, sugar cane fields, and pineapple fields, laborers involved in canal cleaning processes and livestock handlers are subjected to greater degrees of exposure. Other at risk occupations are—fishermen, cesspool workers, and all those persons who are likely to work in rodent infested environment. Truck drivers are also at risk since they may use contaminated water in washing their vehicles. Moreover, masons are at risk too. This is because they might use contaminated water to prepare the cement mixture and get exposed.

### Agent Factors

The causative agents are pathogenic spirochete of the genus *Leptospira*, especially *Leptospira interrogans* and *Leptospira biflexa*.

### Environmental Factors

- *Drainage, congestion, and water logging:* A lot of surplus water gets collected in events of heavy rainfall. Additionally, developmental activities like canal network, roads and railway lines, disrupt and hinder natural drainage of rain water, and leads to its accumulation for longer periods. And water logging, forces the rodent population to abandon their burrows, which ultimately leads to contamination of the stagnant water by their urine.

- **Soil salinization:** Water logging is closely related with soil salinity. The salinity of the soil and alkaline pH create an environment, which is conducive for the survival of *Leptospira*, for months.
- **Soil temperature:** In the endemic areas, the soil is found to have lesser base saturation. And the mean annual soil temperature at the depth of 50 cm, remains 22°C or more. Additionally, there is less than 5°C difference between the mean summer (June-August) and mean winter (December-February) temperature.

***Seasonal variation:*** Leptospirosis is typically a seasonal disease, which begins with the beginning of the rainy season and drops as the rains reduce. However, there may be occurrence of sporadic cases throughout the year. In India, it is frequently found during the postmonsoon period. The disease may acquire epidemic potential during the natural disasters like floods.

### Reservoir

A wide range of rodent and nonrodent animals are reservoirs as well as carriers of the disease. Reservoirs include rats, rabbits, etc. and carriers include domestic animals, like cattle, buffalo, pigs, sheep, and goats, who contain the microorganisms in their bodies.

There is excretion of the organism in huge amount by the rodents and cattle. This contaminates the soil and water bodies (small and large both).

### Mode of Transmission

When the abraded skin or mucus membrane comes in contact with water contaminated by urine of either rodents or carrier or diseased animals, infection takes place. There are very scarce chances of direct transmission of the disease.

### Incubation Period

Typically of 5–14 days, ranging from 2 to 30 days.

## CLINICAL PRESENTATION

- **Clinical types:** Leptospirosis has a very wide spectrum of clinical manifestations ranging from the mild anicteric presentation to severe leptospirosis, which involves severe jaundice and multiorgan involvement. Various clinical presentations of leptospirosis are as follows:
  - **Anicteric leptospirosis:** This is the milder variety of the disease. Patients present with:
    - *Fever:* There exists moderate to high grade, remittent fever with chills.
    - *Myalgia:* This is a very typical feature of leptospirosis, with predominant involvement of the muscles of calf, abdominal, and lumbosacral areas. This symptom helps in differentiating leptospirosis from other febrile illnesses. There is also associated rise in serum creatinine phosphokinase (CPK). This helps in differentiating leptospirosis from other illnesses.
    - *Conjunctival suffusion:* The reddish discoloration of conjunctive is a very peculiar sign of leptospirosis. It is generally bilateral and is most manifest on palpebral conjunctiva.
    - *Headache:* Generally, frontal headache, which is intense and throbbing, is often seen. And it does not get relieved by analgesics.
    - *Renal manifestations:* Some form of renal involvement consistently occurs in leptospirosis. This might range from asymptomatic urinary abnormality manifested as mild proteinuria with few casts and cells to severe renal involvement resulting in acute renal failure, (which occurs in icteric leptospirosis). The latter is rare, though.
    - *Pulmonary manifestations:* The primary manifestations are cough and chest pain. In a few cases, hemoptysis might occur. However, such involvement, which might lead to respiratory failure, does not occur in anicteric leptospirosis.
    - *Hemorrhage:* Some cases might exhibit hemorrhagic tendencies.
  - **Icteric leptospirosis:** This form of leptospirosis, which is more severe and is characterized by development of jaundice. Others features are:
    - *Fever:* Similar to the anicteric phase but more severe and prolonged.
    - *Myalgia:* Calf muscles exhibit more tenderness. It may be so severe, the patient may stop walking and hence may be mistaken for paraplegia. The myalgia may be result of myositis, myonecrosis, or bleeding into the muscles.
    - *Headache:* Most of the patients present with diffuse type of headache, which rarely becomes severe.
    - *Conjunctival suffusion:* Icterus, congested vessels and subconjunctival hemorrhage together give the reddish yellow discoloration to eyes of the patients.
    - Oliguria or anuria and/or proteinuria may occur due to acute renal failure.
    - Nausea, vomiting, diarrhea, and abdominal pain.
    - Hypotension and circulatory collapse.
  - **Severe leptospirosis:** The more severe form of disease with severe liver and kidney involvement is known as Weil's disease. Salient features of the organ involvements are described below:
    - *Hepatic:* Jaundice is the most important clinical feature, varying from mild to severe, which occurs 4–7 days after the development of cardinal symptoms. Hepatic failure resulting in hepatic encephalopathy or death is rare.
    - *Renal:* Leptospirosis invariably shows renal involvement, either as acute tubular necrosis (ATN) or as interstitial nephritis. Hematuria with complaints of Cola colored urine and red blood cell (RBC) casts in urine microscopy is common. In severe cases, renal involvement manifests as oliguria or even anuria, edema on face and feet, signs of uremia like breathlessness, convulsion, delirium, and altered level of consciousness. This usually occurs in very severe cases.

- *Pulmonary*: Mild illness usually presents with cough, chest pain, and blood tinged sputum. In severe cases, patients show cough, hemoptysis, rapidly increasing breathlessness culminating in respiratory failure and death. On examination, increased respiratory rate with crepitation in the basal region rapidly spreading upwards to middle and upper lobes. X-ray shows basal and mid zone opacity in severe cases. Pulmonary hemorrhage and severe respiratory distress may lead to death. Pulmonary pathology is the most frequent cause of death in leptospirosis. More than 90% of deaths in leptospirosis result due to pulmonary or renal causes.
- *Cardiovascular system involvement*: Patients might present with one or more of the following features:
  - *Shock*: Manifested as severe hypotension, cold clammy extremities, and tachycardia. This might be due to due to either dehydration or peripheral vasodilatation.
  - *Arrhythmias*: Manifested as palpitations, syncope, and irregular pulse. Supraventricular tachyarrhythmia and various degrees of atrioventricular (AV) blocks with segment depression and T-wave inversion in some cases.
  - *Central nervous system*: This frequently presents as meningitis. Most common manifestations are headache, irritability, restlessness, seizures, and coma. However, encephalitis, focal deficits, nystagmus, paralysis, spasticity, peripheral neuropathies, nerve palsies, and radiculitis also have been observed.
  - *Skin*: Macular and maculopapular erythematous skin eruptions with occasional purpura are observed on face, trunks, and/or extremities in many patients. These bleeding manifestations are not directly linked to the level of thrombocytopenia in leptospirosis. They resolve in 2–3 days without any specific intervention.
  - *Leptospirosis in pregnancy*: Leptospirosis during pregnancy is invariably associated with poor prognosis and high chances of fetal loss, especially during first trimester and near term.

It is imperative to refer all the patients with severe, multiple organ involvement, to a tertiary care center.

- *Differential diagnosis*:
  - Falciparum malaria
  - Dengue fever/hemorrhagic fever
  - Scrub typhus
  - Typhoid
  - Viral hepatitis closely resembles leptospirosis and is prevalent in areas reporting leptospirosis.
- *Recommended case definition*:
  - *Suspected*: Acute febrile illness with headache, myalgia, and prostration associated with a history of exposure to infected animals or an environment contaminated with animal urine with one or more of the following:
    - Calf muscle tenderness
    - Conjunctival suffusion
    - Anuria or oliguria and/or proteinuria
    - Jaundice
    - Hemorrhagic manifestations (intestines and lung)
    - Meningeal irritation
    - Nausea, vomiting, abdominal pain, and diarrhea.
  - *Probable*: Suspected case with positive presumptive laboratory diagnosis.
  - *Confirmed*: Suspect or probable case with confirmatory laboratory test.

*Note*: The classification of suspected, probable, and confirmed does not in any way explains the severity and that has to be assessed based on the severity and rapidity of organ involvement.

## LABORATORY DIAGNOSIS

- *Criteria for diagnosis:*
  - *Presumptive diagnosis*:
    - A positive result in IgM-based immune-assays, slide agglutination test or latex agglutination test, or immunochromatographic test.
    - A microscopic agglutination test (MAT) titer of 100/200/400 or above in single sample based on endemicity.
    - Demonstration of leptospires directly or by staining methods.
  - *Confirmatory diagnosis:*
    - Isolation of leptospira species from clinical specimen
    - Four-fold or greater rise in the MAT titer between acute and convalescent phase serum specimens run in parallel. Positive by any two different types of rapid test.
    - Seroconversion.
    - Polymerase chain reaction test.
- *Collection and transportation of samples:*
  - *Blood sample:* While collecting blood and separating serum proper procedures should be followed to avoid lysis or contamination. Store and transport at –80°C to 4°C in vaccine carriers or icebox. If transportation in the cold chain is not possible then use quickest mode of transportation.
  - *Cerebrospinal fluid sample:* CSF should be collected in a sterile container by lumbar puncture under aseptic conditions before the institution of antibiotics. CSF should be transported immediately to laboratory without delay.
  - *Urine sample:* Urine should be collected in sterile wide-mouth container, if delay is expected, specimen should be kept cool preferably at –80°C to 4°C (serology and molecular tests) and ambient temperature (culture) and sent to laboratory as early as possible.

## PREVENTION AND CONTROL MEASURES

- *Personal protection:*
  - Avoiding direct and indirect human contact with animal urine is recommended as preventive measures.
  - While working in situations like flooded fields, utmost precautions should be taken to prevent any direct contact with contaminated water or mud, which can be done

by using rubber shoes and gloves. In case of any cuts or abrasion on the lower extremities of the body, an antiseptic ointment, e.g. Betadine, must be applied prior to entering the field and after exit.

- **Health education:**
  - The primary modality for prevention of leptospirosis is by generating awareness about the disease and its prevention.
  - This can be achieved through intensive educational campaign, IEC through audiovisual, print, press, and maximizing the use of new and emerging electronic media.
- **Chemoprophylaxis:**
  - Chemoprophylaxis with doxycycline 200 mg, once a week, may be given to agricultural workers (e.g. paddy field workers and workers who clean canals/sewage) during the peak transmission season in the endemic areas.
  - This should be for 6 weeks and not to be extended beyond 8 weeks.
- **Rodent control:**
  - Four species of rodents *Rattus rattus* (House rat), *Rattus norvegicus* (Norway rat), *Bandicota bengalensis* (Lesser bandicoot), and *Bandicota indica* (Larger bandicoot) are found to be reservoirs for this bacterium in India.
  - The strategic planning should cover the following:
    - Identifying the reservoir species of affected area
    - Delineating areas for antirodent activities
    - Completion of activities in premonsoon months
    - Adopting appropriate technology for antirodent operations
    - Capacity building
    - Creating awareness in general community and community participation.

***Mapping of Water Bodies for Establishing a Proper Drainage System:*** Mapping of water bodies and human activities in water-logged areas will help in identifying the high-risk population. Education to the farmers regarding drainage of the cattle urine into a pit instead of letting it flow and contamination of water bodies would be helpful. The farmers can be educated to make a system by which the cattle's urine gets collected in a pit and does not flow in the main drainage system. This will prevent contamination of the water bodies and thus will reduce the chances of spread of the infection.

***Vaccination of Animals:*** Leptospiral vaccines provide immunity for a limited time period and need boosters every 1–2 years. Vaccination should be considered very conservatively in routine situations and only in endemic situations having high incidence of leptospirosis.

The vaccine must be the one containing the locally prevalent serovars. It must be kept in mind that vaccination has a role in only prevention of illness, and not in protecting from infection and renal shedding.

## SUMMARY

- Leptospirosis is a zoonotic bacterial infection with global distribution. It is also known as Weil's disease. Leptospirosis is found most frequently in the slums with insufficient sewage disposal facilities and water treatment. It also occurs as an occupational disease in people who work outdoors or in close proximity of animals.
  - The causative agents are pathogenic spirochete of the genus *Leptospira*, especially *Leptospira interrogans* and *Leptospira biflexa*.
  - *Reservoir and carrier hosts:* A wide range of rodent and nonrodent animals is reservoirs as well as carriers of the disease. Reservoirs include rats, rabbits, etc. and carriers include domestic animals, like cattle, buffalo, pigs, sheep, and goats, who contain the microorganisms in their bodies.
- ***Mode of transmission:*** When the abraded skin or mucus membrane comes in contact with water, which has been contaminated by urine of either rodents or carrier or diseased animals, infection takes place. There are very scanty chances of direct transmission of the disease.
- ***Incubation period:*** Typically of 5–14 days, ranging from 2 to 30 days.
- ***Case fatality rate:*** 0–15%
- ***Clinical types:***
  - Anicteric leptospirosis
  - Icteric leptospirosis
  - Severe leptospirosis
- ***Criteria for diagnosis:***
  - *Presumptive diagnosis:* A positive result in IgM-based immune-assays, slide agglutination test or latex agglutination test, or immunochromatographic test.
  - *Confirmatory diagnosis:* Isolation of leptospires from clinical specimen

Four-fold or greater rise in the MAT titer between acute and convalescent phase serum specimens run in parallel.

**Prevention**
- ***Personal protection:*** Avoiding direct and indirect human contact with animal urine is recommended as preventive measures.
- ***Health education:*** The primary modality for prevention of leptospirosis is by generating awareness about the disease and its prevention.
- ***Chemoprophylaxis:***
  - Chemoprophylaxis with doxycycline 200 mg, once a week, may be given to agricultural workers (e.g. paddy field workers and canal cleaning workers in endemic areas) during the peak transmission season in the endemic areas.
  - This should be for 6 weeks and not to be extended beyond 8 weeks.
- ***Rodent control***

## SUGGESTED READING

1. Haake DA, Levett PN. Leptospirosis in humans. Curr Top Microbiol Immunol. 2015;387:65-97.
2. World Health Organization. Leptospirosis. [online] Available from: https://www.who.int/zoonoses/diseases/leptospirosis/en/.
3. World Health Organization. Leptospirosis: Fact Sheet; 2009.
4. World Health Organization. Leptospirosis Burden epidemiology Reference Group. [online] Available from: http://www.who.int/zoonoses/diseases/lerg/en/index2.html.

## E. EPIDEMIOLOGY OF VECTOR-BORNE DISEASES AND ITS PREVENTION AND CONTROL

*Rashmi Sharma*

*Small bite, Big threat*
*World Health Day theme, 2014*

| | |
|---|---|
| CM7.2 | Enumerate, describe and discuss the mode of transmission and measures for prevention and control of vector-borne diseases |
| CM8.1 | Describe and discuss the epidemiological and control measures applicable in vector-borne diseases |

## INTRODUCTION

Occurrence of vector-borne rather vector transmitted diseases is largely influenced by climatic variability leading to unexpected weather (rain/draughts), affecting the density and survival and in turn the transmissibility of vectors. As reported by Liverpool University, IICT, Hyderabad and NIPER, an increase in temperature from 17 to 30°C can hike transmission rates by 3–4 times by increase in feeding of *Aedes aegypti* and decrease in extrinsic incubation period (EIP). Presence of Japanese encephalitis (JE) in North-East states of India, and recent invasion of Nipah virus in Kerala are the few examples. In addition to the toll, the premature deaths and disability can have significant impediment to economic development as a result of lost working hours, high cost of treatment and vector control. Malaria and dengue fever are among the most important vector-borne diseases in the tropic. Looking at the severity of this public health problem World Health Organization (WHO) in 2014 chose a theme for world health day (WHD) **"small bite big threat".**

### Vector

An invertebrate, arthropod or any living carrier (snail) or host, which allows (transmits) the development or multiplication of parasite, inside its own system and transmits the infective forms of parasites to another host.

### Vector Density

The critical density is important at which transmission takes place and is different for different species. But change in longevity of vector can alter the transmission even at low vector density. Vector density and gametocyte density have an inverse relationship, i.e., lower vector density and higher gametocytemia and vice versa can establish malaria transmission.

### Vector Longevity

Even small variations (mainly climatic), can seriously affect the probability of completion of the cycle and further affects the subsequent period of survival, which is necessary for successful transmission.

### Vector Feeding Habits

***Anthropophily:*** Preference of parasite in feeding humans over other animals (the frequency of feeding in most species depends on the temperature, typically in tropical conditions). Under optimal condition biting takes place in every 2–3 days.

### Vector Receptivity/Susceptibility

Within one species of mosquito there may be strains or types which are more susceptible to malaria parasite than others, it may also so happen that an Anopheline may be more susceptible to one species of *Plasmodium* than to another, the same species may be a vector of malaria in one area and not in another due to genetic difference.

### Receptivity of the Vector

Receptiveness to pathogenic organisms by a vector depends on following:
- Whether anthropophagic in nature
- Can survive up to 12–14 days
- Temperature of surrounding around 30°C
- About 60% relative humidity
- Closeness to reservoir of infection with presence of high density, and
- Efficient in biting species.

### Vector-Borne Diseases Primarily of Public Health Significance

- Malaria
- Dengue
- Lymphatic filariasis
- Yellow fever (not in India)
- Japanese encephalitis
- Chikungunya
- Leishmaniasis.

## EPIDEMIOLOGY OF MALARIA AND ITS PREVENTION AND CONTROL

| | |
|---|---|
| CM7.2 | Enumerate, describe and discuss the mode of transmission and measures for prevention and control of malaria |
| CM8.1 | Describe and discuss the epidemiological and control measures applicable in malaria |
| CM8.6 | Educate and train health workers in disease surveillance, control and treatment and health education regarding malaria |

*Case Study*

*Radha aged 24 years wife of an army officer posted in Nagaland. She is in the seventh month of her first pregnancy. She was taken to a Peripheral Health Unit as she became ill 5 days ago, with chills, profuse sweating and headaches. An antibiotic was prescribed and her condition seemed to improve, but yesterday she developed rigors and persistent vomiting. A blood film at the local clinic revealed presence of malaria parasites (Plasmodium falciparum) and oral quinine (600 mg every 8 hrs) was prescribed. She took two doses.*

*Today she has been referred to Military Hospital, at Dimapur, Nagaland because of restlessness and increasing mental confusion. Examination reveals altered sensorium, semi-consciousness and inability to talk. She withdraws her hand from a painful stimulus. There is no neck stiffness, jaundice, pallor or rash. Axillary temperature is 39°C, pulse 90 beats/minute, blood pressure 110/70 mm Hg. The uterine fundus is palpable (26–28 weeks) and the fetal heart can be heard.*

## INTRODUCTION

Malaria is the oldest disease in the history of tropical medicine. Survey report of 1935 conducted in India revealed that due to malaria annually about 10 million people suffered and 1 million died along with economic loss of 1,000 crore rupees. During the 2nd World War in India, more soldiers died from an attack of malaria than military operations. Out of all vector-borne diseases malaria is by far the most important in terms of the number of individuals it affects and of deaths it causes. It was essentially a rural disease due to the large number of breeding places. Dichlorodiphenyltrichloroethane (DDT) was a great land mark in malaria control and was used in India since 1946. It may be noted that various vector control measures focused on malaria are also relevant to a large extent in prevention and control of other vector-borne diseases such as plague, kala-azar, etc.

## DEFINITION

Malaria literally means bad air. A characteristic odor was prevalent in the marshy and water-logged areas which provided breeding ground for malaria transmitting vectors. High incidence of malaria cases in such areas resulted in this nomenclature of disease. Malaria is a mosquito-borne protozoal disease of human being resulting from infection of the parenchyma cells of the liver and erythrocytes by SPOROZOA belonging to the genus *Plasmodium* and a typical attack presents with three stages and clinical features varying from mild-to-severe and with/without complications.

## MILESTONES OF MALARIA

- **Hippocrates** described features of malaria first time
- **Charaka and Sushruta mentioned** description and bite of mosquito
- **Laveran** discovered *P. malariae* parasite in the blood of a soldier (1880–81)
- **Ronald Ross**, documented disease transmission by mosquitoes
- **Grassi and Feletti** discovered *P. vivax* parasite (1890)
- **Welch** discovered *P. falciparum* parasite (1897)
- **Stephenes** discovered *P. ovale* parasite
- **Romanowski** developed a method of staining the blood films
- **Manson** hypothesized that mosquito transmits the disease (1900)
- **Mesnil** established family Plasmodiae (1903)
- **Sacharov** discovered Leeches experiment for PF (1894)
- **Romanowsky** discovered staining of malaria parasite (1861–1921)
- **Paul Muller** discovered the insecticidal property of DDT.

### Interesting fact

Dr Ronald Ross, recipient of Nobel Prize in Medicine (1902) was born in 1857 in Almora, India. Based in Secunderbad, in 1895 got serious on his quest regarding malaria transmission. He reared 8 adult brown mosquitos and had them feed on a volunteer named Husein Khan who had malaria. The volunteer was paid 8 annas (1 anna per mosquito)! On dissecting these 8 mosquitoes on different days spanning 5 days in total, he found the parasites in different stages of development which proved to be a critical finding to show that parasite grows within mosquitoes and thus are the causes of spread. He got his findings published in the British Medical Journal on 18 December 1897.

## PROBLEM STATEMENT

### Global Scenario

Globally in 2022, there were an estimated 249 million malaria cases in 85 malaria endemic countries and areas, an increase of 5 million cases compared with 2021. The main countries contributing to the increase were Pakistan (+2.1 million), Ethiopia (+1.3 million), Nigeria (+1.3 million), Uganda (+597,000) and Papua New Guinea (+423,000). In 2015, the baseline year of the Global technical strategy for malaria 2016–2030 (GTS), there were an estimated 231 million malaria cases. Malaria case incidence declined from 81 per 1000 population at risk in 2000 to 58 in 2022. The WHO African Region, with an estimated 233 million cases in 2022, accounted for about 94% of cases globally. The WHO South-East Asia Region accounted for about 2% of malaria cases globally. Malaria cases in this region declined by 76%, from 23 million in 2000 to about 5 million in 2022 (WHO World Malaria Report, 2023).

Globally, malaria deaths declined steadily from 864,000 in 2000 to 608,000 in 2022, with a sharp dip in 2019 (576,000 deaths). The percentage of total malaria deaths in children aged under 5 years decreased from 87% in 2000 to 76% in 2015. Since then, there has been no change. Globally, the malaria mortality rate (i.e. deaths per 100,000 population at risk) halved from about 29 in 2000 to 15 in 2015. It then continued to decrease but at a slower rate, falling to 14.3 in 2022. Four countries accounted for just over half of all malaria deaths globally in 2022 – Nigeria (31%), the Democratic Republic of the Congo (12%), Niger (6%) and the United Republic of Tanzania (4%). In WHO African Region, the malaria mortality rate decreased by 60% between 2000 and 2022, from 143 to 56 deaths per 100,000 population at risk. In the WHO South-East Asia Region, malaria deaths decreased by 77%, from about 35000 in 2000 to 8000 in 2022. India and Indonesia accounted for about 94% of all malaria deaths in the WHO South-East Asia Region (WHO World Malaria Report, 2023).

### Indian Scenario

Problem of malaria was virtually eliminated from India in mid-sixties with nil deaths, but resurgence was seen in 1976 with 6.47 million cases. In 2022, India accounted for 66% of cases in the

WHO South-East Asia Region. Almost 46% of all cases in the region were due to *P. vivax*. India and Indonesia accounted for about 94% of all malaria deaths in the WHO South-East Asia Region. India achieved a reduction of 83.34% in malaria morbidity and 92% in malaria mortality between the year 2000 and 2019. The World Malaria Report (WMR) 2023 by WHO indicates that India has made considerable progress in reducing its malaria burden. WHO has initiated the High Burden to High Impact (HBHI) initiative in 11 high malaria burden countries, including India. Among the HBHI countries, India reported the highest relative reduction in cases among these countries (about 30%). In 2022, there were 176,522 cases and 83 deaths reported due to Malaria.

## EPIDEMIOLOGICAL TYPES OF MALARIA

*Tribal malaria:* 50% PF (Andhra Pradesh, Madhya Pradesh, Gujarat, Chhattisgarh, Bihar, Maharashtra, Jharkhand, Rajasthan, Odisha).

*Rural malaria:* Irrigated arid or semi-arid plains of Haryana, Punjab, Western UP, Rajasthan.

*Urban malaria:* 15 major cities including 4 meters (account for 80% of malaria cases).

*Malaria in project areas:* Under construction areas.

*Border malaria:* High transmission belts along international borders (mixing of population and poor administration due to remote location).

## EPIDEMIOLOGY

### Host Factors

- *Age:* All ages are susceptible or at risk to acquire the infection however newborn are resistant to PF due to presence of fetal hemoglobin (HbF).
- *Sex:* Outdoor activity or better clothing.
- *Race:* Sickle cell trait have mild illness with PF, Duffy negative RBCs resistant to PV.
- *Pregnancy:* Malaria during pregnancy especially of PF type has severe manifestations including intrauterine death, abortion, and premature labor.
- *Socio-economic development:* More in developing countries.
- *Immunity:* Acquired after repeated exposure. People staying in endemic area develop immunity gradually. It is species specific.
- *Housing:* Ill-ventilated or ill-lighted house (resting habit) and it also depends upon on type of construction, type of wall (vector control).
- *Population mobility:* Migration malaria
- *Occupation:* Agricultural practice
- *Human habits:* Sleeping outdoor

### Agent Factors

Disease is caused by mainly 4 species of protozoa called *Plasmodium*; species are *P. falciparum*, *P. vivax*, *P. malariae*, and *P. ovale*. As of now more than 60% cases are due PF, 1% due to *P. malariae*, 4–8% are due to mixed and rest are caused by PV. Genus *Plasmodium* belongs to order Coccidiadae, family Hemosporia, and family Plasmodiidae.

### Environmental Factors

- *Season:* Seasonal disease (July-November): Especially, the post-monsoon period which provides ample opportunities through water collections. Heavy rains wash away the breeding sites so light to moderate rainfall lasting for longer duration is more conducive for the vector breeding.
- *Temperature:* 20–30 (<16 and >30 lethal): Temperature within this range ensures survival long enough to facilitate the picking up of infection and its subsequent transmission to susceptible host (after undergoing extrinsic incubation period).
- *Humidity:* An environmental relative humidity of around 60% ensures long life span and active mosquitoes.
- *Rainfall and droughts:* Breeding places, humidity.
- *Altitude:* Anophelines are not found above 2,000 meters.
- *Man-made malaria:* Man-made activities like construction of buildings, canals, tanks, dams, garden pools, and other engineering projects provide water collections which support vector breeding.

### Source of Infection and Reservoir

Source of infection is infected female anopheles mosquito having sporozoites and reservoirs are clinical, subclinical, chronic cases of malaria. There is no animal reservoir except chimpanzees of tropical Africa. Children are likely to be gametocyte carrier from an adult and may act as a better reservoir than adult. In order to act as a reservoir of infection a person:
- Must harbor both the sexes of gametocytes.
- Gametocytes must be mature and viable. If patients receive antimalarial drugs, gametocytes lose the viability or infectivity to the mosquito.
- Must have gametocyte in sufficient quantity in blood at least 12/mm$^3$ of blood.

### Modes of Transmission

The critical density is important at which transmission take place and is different for different species. Method of biological transmission is cyclopropagative as the agent undergoes multiplication as well as development from one form to another. Most common mode of transmission is indirect (vector-borne) by the bite of female mosquito which carry sporozoites in salivary glands, followed by direct transmission through blood transfusion (parasites remain infective 14 days in blood stored at–4°C), vertical transmission from mother-to-newborn (congenital malaria) and Cryptic malaria (route of transmission cannot be established).

### Malaria Vector in India

Important species of vectors which play an important role in transmission are **(Table 17E.1)**:
- *Anopheles culicifacies:* Rural/peri-urban orzoophilic
- *Anopheles stephensi:* Malaria in urban or industrial
- *Anopheles fluviatilis:* Hilly areas or forest fringes
- *Anopheles minimus:* Foot hills of north eastern India
- *Anopheles dirus:* Forest vector in the north-east
- *Anopheles epiroticus:* Andaman and Nicobar Islands.

Table 17E.1: Breeding habits as per Anopheles species.

| Anopheles species | Breeding habits | Anopheles species | Breeding habits |
|---|---|---|---|
| An. culicifacies | Clean water, river margin, rice field, pits, pools | An. sundaicus | Brackish water, near cost, river mouth |
| An. stephensi | Urban domestic water container, construction sites, rural borrow pits, rice fields | An. minimus | Hills and foot hills |
| An. fluviatilis | Foot hills and hills | An. annularis | Clean water ground stagnant water |
| An. philippinensis | Tanks, pools, burrow pits with vegetation | An. dirus | Shaddy pools mainly in forest |

## Incubation Period

Time interval in days between bite of infective mosquito and the first appearance of clinical signs. It varies from species to species.
- *Plasmodium falciparum:* 12 days (9–14)
- *Plasmodium vivax:* 14 days (8–17)
- *Plasmodium ovale:* 17 days (6–18)
- *Plasmodium malariae:* 28 days (18–40)

## Extrinsic Incubation Period (in Mosquitoes)

Time taken in days by mosquito from entry of gametocyte to presence of sporozoites in its salivary glands to become infective and is usually 10 (10–20) days.

## Incubation Interval

Period between infectivity one person (case) to the infectivity of another person from whom the former case acquires the infection. Extrinsic plus intrinsic incubation period is called incubation interval.

## Period of Communicability

Malaria is communicable till gametocytes are present in the human blood. In *P. vivax* gametocyte appear 4–5 days after appearance of asexual parasites while in *P. falciparum* gametocyte appear 10–12 days after the appearance of asexual parasite. Gametocytes are more numerous in the early phase of clinical illness and usually it is 1,000/mm³ of blood.

## Life Cycle of Malaria Parasite

Though there are differences in the life cycle of various species, largely for human malaria parasite shares the common life cycle.

Life cycle is completed in intermediate and definitive host **(Fig. 17E.1)**.

The malaria parasite life cycle involves two hosts:
1. ***Exoerythrocytic and erythrocytic schizogony:*** Human is intermediate host.
2. ***Sporogony:*** Mosquito is definitive host.

During a blood meal, a malaria-infected female Anopheles mosquito inoculates sporozoites into the human host. Sporozoites infect liver cells and mature into schizonts. Schizonts are large, yellowish-brown, coalesced pigment, which rupture and release 12–24 merozoites. [In *P. vivax* and *P. ovale*, a dormant stage (hypnozoites) can persist in the liver (if untreated) and cause relapses by invading the bloodstream weeks, or even years later. There are no hypnozoites in *P. falciparum*, hence no relapse but recrudescence occurs as parasite may go into deeper tissue)].

After this initial replication in the liver (exo-erythrocytic schizogony), the parasites undergo asexual multiplication in the erythrocytes (erythrocytic schizogony). Merozoites infect red blood cells. Trophozoites show amoeboid cytoplasm, large chromatin dots, and have fine, yellowish-brown pigment. Schüffner's dots may appear more fine in comparison to those seen in *P. ovale*. The ring stage trophozoites mature into schizonts, which rupture releasing merozoites. Some parasites differentiate into sexual erythrocytic stages (gametocytes). Blood stage parasites are responsible for the clinical manifestations of the disease. The gametocytes, male (microgametocytes) and female (macrogametocytes), are ingested by an Anopheles mosquito during a blood meal. The parasites' multiplication in the mosquito is known as the sporogonic cycle. While in the mosquito's stomach, the microgametes penetrate the macrogametes generating zygotes. The zygotes in turn become motile and elongated (ookinetes) which invade the midgut wall of the mosquito where they develop into oocysts. The oocysts grow, rupture, and release sporozoites, which make their way to the mosquito's salivary glands. Inoculation of the sporozoites into a new human host perpetuates the malaria life cycle.

## CLINICAL FEATURES

*P. falciparum* is a major cause of death. Fever is cardinal symptom (with or without periodicity). Many cases have chills and rigors accompanied by anorexia or arthralgia or headache or myalgia or nausea or vomiting and can mimic viral or typhoid infection. Suspect malaria in endemic areas; investigate it in presence of running nose or cough or respiratory infection, diarrhea or dysentery or burning micturition, abscess or ear discharge or lymphadenopathy.

Rigors may be absent with prolongation of cold stage. Anemia and splenomegaly may not be well-marked.

Low mortality among deficits of G6PD, and Hbs, Hbc, HbE, HbF, thalassemia. Plasma becomes viscous, rise in bilirubin and vitamin K, A/G ratio reversed, total plasma level falls. One paroxysm may extend into the next.

### Complications of P. falciparum

It is an acute, diffuse encephalopathy clinically characterized by confusion, convulsion, and comma. It is a cause of mortality among young children especially with severe malnutrition. It also occurs in nonimmune individual, it is due to inflammatory responses which are due to release of kinins, loss of water to tissues, petechial hemorrhages, edema with hemorrhage, endothelial thickening, necrosis of vein wall, hyaline micro thrombosis and granuloma formation. Clinically, manifestations are cerebral malaria, peripheral neuritis, acute renal insufficiency, acute respiratory insufficiency, pulmonary edema, hyperparasitemia, hyperpyrexia. Generalized vascular collapse with shock and low BP is due to adrenal failure along with severe abdominal pain, diarrhea and vomiting, dysenteric, jaundice, dehydration, metabolic acidosis, bleeding disorders, and splenic

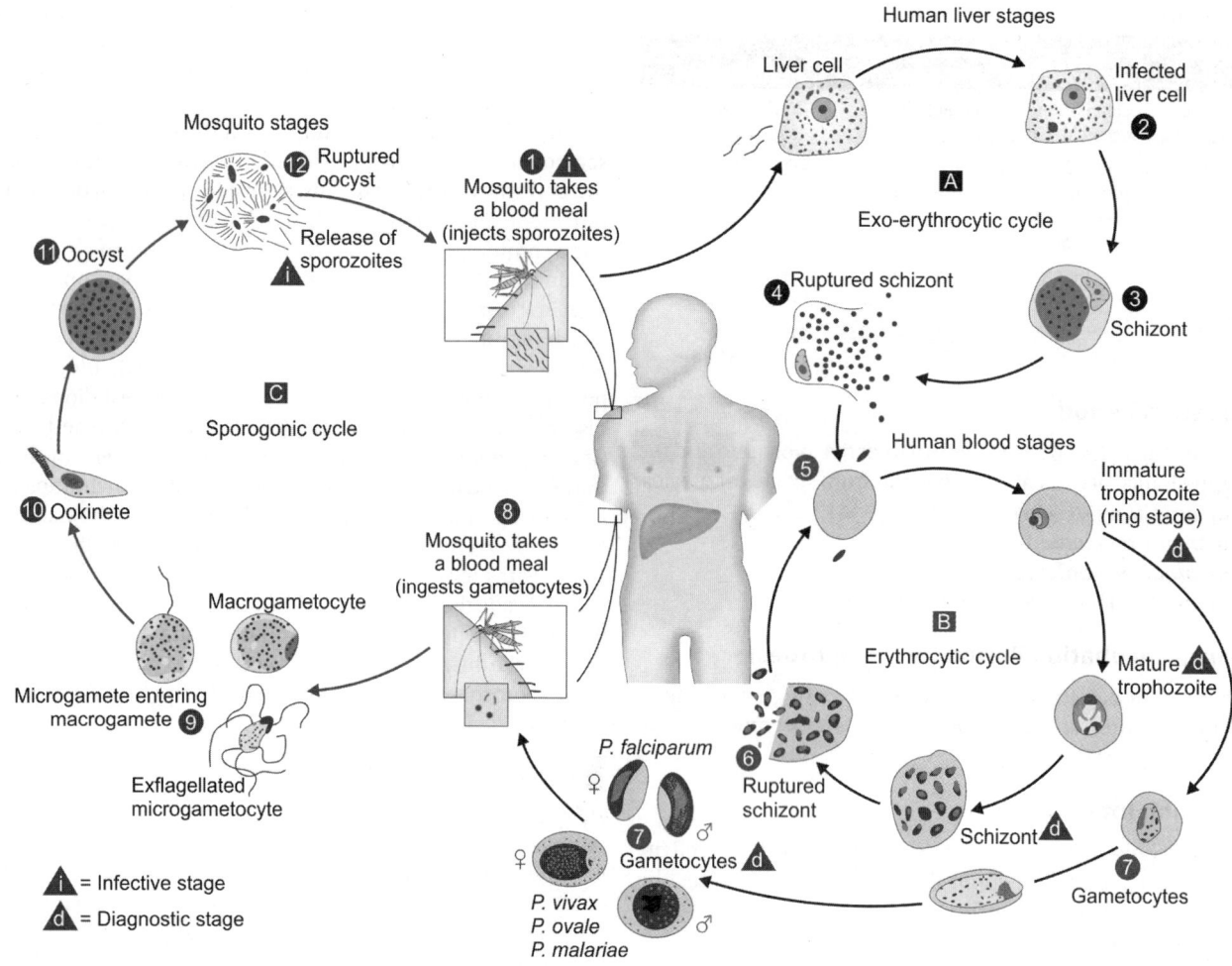

**Fig. 17E.1:** Life cycle of malaria parasite.

rupture. Cerebral malaria is unarguable coma not attributed to any other cause in a patient infected with PF (in Africa 10–40% of patients hospitalized). With cerebral malaria patient may die even when treatment is optimal.

### Pathogenesis and Pathology of Severe Malaria

- *P. vivax* predominately affects young RBCs whereas *P. falciparum* affects RBCs of all ages. Thus, the infective load and severity of infection are more in case of *P. falciparum*.
- *P. falciparum* infections causes release of malaria antigens, pigments and toxins which initiates cascade of pathological events like production of cytokines specially tumor necrosis factor (TNF). TNF and cachexin are the cause of malarial fever.
- Mechanical changes in infected RBCs causes cyto-adherence of *P. falciparum*-infected erythrocytes to endothelial cells.
- Sequestration of mature parasites in capillaries and venules causing blockage.
- Development of knobs (helps in sequestration) on membrane of infected RBCs.
- *Resetting:* Infected RBCs bind with uninfected erythrocytes causing narrowing of blood vessels and restricted blood flow. Causes higher micro-vascular obstruction responsible for cerebral malaria, encourages cyto-adherence to endothelium.

- **Black water fever** is characterized by marked intravascular hemolysis with hemoglobinuria. Patients with G6PD deficiency may develop it after therapy with primaquine.

### Pathological Changes in Placenta

Due to the high glucose in maternal blood in the intervillous spaces favoring the development of the parasite. Sinusoids packed with infected RBCs. Stickier parasitized cells tend to sludge in eddies of the slow moving placental stream and also favors fibrin deposition on the villi and hastens the degenerative process and by interfering with the nutrients of the fetus causing stillbirths. Malaria in pregnancy may be asymptomatic and is one of the important causes of premature labor pain.

### Differential Diagnosis of PF

Typhoid meningitis, enteritis, head stroke, hypoglycemia, malarial granuloma of brain.

## DIAGNOSIS OF MALARIA

### Microscopy

It holds as a gold standard. Blood cells fixed thus enables parasites to be seen in RBCs, parasitized cells oval/enlarged

**Table 17E.2:** Demonstration of parasites.

| Grading | Interpretation of result |
|---|---|
| + | 1–10 parasites/100 thick film fields |
| ++ | 11–100 parasites/100 thick film fields |
| +++ | 1–10 parasite/field |
| ++++ | >10 parasite/field |

or stippled are helpful in identification of mixed infection and monitoring treatment Stains used are Giemsa stain, JSB stain (developed by two scientists in the national program namely, Jaswant Singh and Bhattacharya and used extensively in the PHCs, etc.) and Leishman's stain.

### Demonstration of Parasites—Thick and Thin Smear

Staining by Giemsa or Leishman or Field stain (JSB) **(Table 17E.2)**.
- **Thick smear:** Advantages are it concentrates parasites by 20–40 times—high sensitivity and useful for detection of parasite.
- **Thin smear** is required to confirm the species, blood cells are fixed thus enabling parasites to be seen in RBCs, parasitized cells are oval or enlarged or stippled and helpful in identification of mixed infection. It helps in monitoring the treatment.

### Fluorescence Microscopy

**Quantitative buffy coat (QBC) method:** Advantages are rapid or easy to perform, number of parasites must be more than 100/μL, sensitivity and specificity is equal to thick smear, disadvantages are that it needs special training and expensive equipment supplies are required.

### Antigen Detection: Rapid Diagnostic Test Kits

Detects *P. falciparum* or *P. vivax* on the basis of circulating parasitic antigens ensure—kit kept at recommended temperature, within expiry period and user's manual adhered. Highly sensitive or rapid test takes 15–20 minutes, simple to perform (finger prick method) based on Histidine-rich protein (HRP-2) produced only by *P. falciparum* and based on parasite lactate dehydrogenase (PLDH) antigen which is produced by all 4 species both antigen are secreted in the blood by asexual stages of parasites. PLDH is also secreted by gametocytes, sensitivity and specificity are more than 90%, if parasite count is less than 60–100/μL.

## EPIDEMIOLOGICAL INDICES

### Pre-eradication Era

- **Spleen rate:** Percent of children (2–10 years) showing enlargement of spleen. It has a poor specificity.
- **Average enlarged spleen:** Average size of the enlarged spleen.
- **Parasite rate:** Children (2–10 years) showing malaria parasite in blood film.
- **Parasite density index:** Average degree of parasitemia in a sample where the denominator is all malaria positive slides.
- **Infant parasite rate:** Percent of infants showing malaria parasite in blood. It is a sensitive indicator of ongoing transmission and of new infection.
- **Proportional case rate:** Number of cases diagnosed as clinical malaria for every 100 patients.

### Eradication Era (Current Incidence Levels)

- **Annual parasite incidence (API):**
  API = Confirmed cases during 1 year/population under surveillance in the same year × 1,000. It can be either active surveillance or passive surveillance. Cases are confirmed by blood examination.
  API more than or equal to 2/1,000 high-risk area (vector control)

  $$API = \frac{\text{Total number of confirmed cases in a year}}{\text{Total population under surveillance in the same year}} \times 1,000$$

  Based on API as primary criteria, all the states and UTs are divided into four categories. Specific milestones and targets are set up for each of these categories and strategies will be implemented accordingly. For further read, refer the document on National Strategic Plan for Malaria Elimination (2017–2022) by NVBDCP.

- **Annual falciparum incidence (AFI):**

  $$AFI = \frac{\text{Total number of confirmed cases of PF in a year}}{\text{Total population under surveillance in the same year}} \times 1,000$$

- **Annual blood examination rate (ABER):** Number of slides examined/population under surveillance × 100. It has nothing to do with malaria situation and is an index of operational efficiency, depends upon annual blood collection and examination rate. The idea of ABER is that a sufficient no. of blood slides must be systematically obtained and examined before commenting up on the malaria situation. It must be 10% of the population presuming that around 10% people will develop fever in a year. However, during the transmission season, examination rate must be 1% per month.

  $$ABER = \frac{\text{Total number of sides examined}}{\text{Total population under surveillance in the same time period}} \times 100$$

- **Slide positivity rate (SPR):** Number of slides found positive for any one or more (mixed infection) malaria parasites/total number of slides examined. It shows trend of malaria transmission. It shows parasitic load on the population and helps in estimation of the transmission level to see the impact of control measures, built up of parasite reservoir and possibility of an epidemic build up and identify high-risk areas.

  $$SPR = \frac{\text{No. of slides positive for parasite}}{\text{Total number of slides examined}} \times 100$$

- **Proportion of P. falciparum cases:** To know the load of falciparum, out of total malaria cases how many are confirmed falciparum cases, as falciparum is more dangerous than PV it shows trend of shifting from PV to PF infection.

  $$\text{Proportion of } P.\text{ falciparum cases} = \frac{\text{No. of confirmed falciparum cases}}{\text{Total confirmed malaria cases}} \times 100$$

## Vector Indices

- *Human blood index:* Proportion of freshly fed female anopheline mosquitoes whose stomach contains human blood it shows **degree of anthrophilism** (preference to bite human subjects).
- *Sporozoite rate:* Percent of female anopheles with sporozoite in their salivary glands and indicate proportion of infective (capable to freshly infect) mosquitoes.
- *Mosquito density:* Number of mosquitoes per man hour catch.
- *Man biting rate (Biting density):* Average incidence of anopheline bites per day per person.
- *Inoculation rate:* The man biting rate multiplied by the infective sporozoite rate. For prevention and control of malaria, mosquitos' control has an important role and integrated approach is required.

## PREVENTION AND CONTROL OF MALARIA

### Vector Control Measures

Vector control measures should take advantage of the specific characteristics or survival pattern of the different vectors. The various control options are aimed at eliminating vector and/or its production, reducing adult vector populations, reducing the life span of adult females and preventing vector contact with humans. The recommended measures by WHO includes two types of interventions:
1. *Core interventions:* Use of ITN (Insecticide Treated Nets) and IRS (Indoor Residual Spray)
2. *Supplementary interventions:*
   - Source reduction measures to kill larval forms and prevent breeding sites
   - *Personal protective measures:* Use of repellants
   - *Other interventions:* Space spraying
   - Entomological surveillance

### Continuous Monitoring of Activities

*Active surveillance:* This is done by community level health workers like the ANM or MPHW by fornightly door to door visit. Those individuals with fever and chills in past 14 days are tested using rapid diagnostic test (RDT) kits. If the test turns positive, then the treatment is initiated.

*Passive surveillance:* This includes detection of malaria among those individuals who go to the health facility of their own accord for febrile illness. This indirectly also signifies health seeking behavior among the people in the community.

*Sentinel surveillance:* Sentinel sites are established in selected hospitals in high endemic districts. Functionaries include a SSMO (sentinel surveillance medical officer) and a lab technician. The SSMO is in-charge of activities undertaken at the sentinel sites regarding malaria.

### Integrated Vector Management

It includes usage of tools in combination and synergistically, i.e., using both chemical and nonchemical methods.

## Effective Treatment of Malaria under the Revised Drug Policy 2013

It is primarily aimed for early diagnosis and treatment for complete cure not only clinically but also parasitological to interrupt transmission (prevent new cases by gametocidal drugs), prevent relapse by giving radical treatment. The other objectives are prevention of progression of uncomplicated malaria to severe (prevent mortality) and judicious use of drugs to minimize occurrence or spread of drug resistance.

### Algorithm

Algorithm for diagnosis and treatment of malaria as per revised drug policy where microscopic result is available within 24 hours has been described in **Figure 17E.2**. Where microscopic result is not available within 24 hours, do RDT and follow the same algorithm as given.

### Treatment of Uncomplicated P. vivax Malaria (Table 17E.3)

*P. vivax* cases should be treated with chloroquine (CQ) for 3 days and primaquine for 14 days. Chloroquine is the drug of choice which is given 25 mg/kg divided over 3 days (10 + 10 + 5) and to prevent relapse due to hypnozoites. Primaquine is given as 0.25 mg/kg daily for 14 days, but contraindicated in pregnant, infants and G6PD deficiency. Follow-up and close monitoring of all cases are required and should be instructed to report back

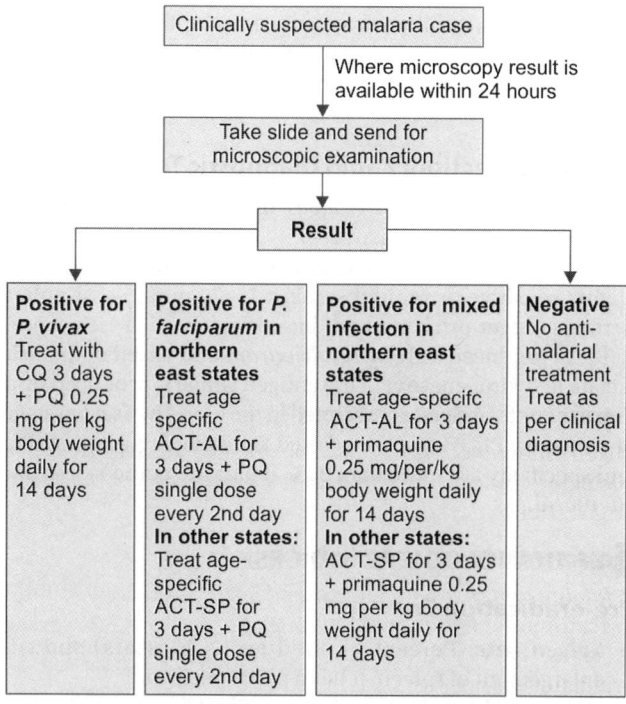

**Fig. 17E.2:** Drug schedule for treatment of malaria under NVBDCP. (ACT-AL: artemisinin-based combination therapy-artemether-lumefantrine; ACT-SP: artemisinin-based combination therapy-artesunate + sulfadoxine pyrimethamine; CQ: chloroquine; PQ: primaquine)

*Note:* If a patient has severe symptoms at any stage, then immediately refer to a nearest PHC or other health facility with indoor patient management or a registered medical doctor.

**Table 17E.3:** Doses (no of tablets) of antimalarial drugs as per age.

| Age | CHQ 150 mg | | | Primaquine (2.5 mg) |
|---|---|---|---|---|
| Years | Day 1 | Day 2 | Day 3 | Day 1 to 14 |
| <1 | 1/2 | 1/2 | 1/4 | Nil |
| 1–4 | 1 | 1 | 1/2 | 1 |
| 5–8 | 2 | 2 | 1 | 2 |
| 9–14 | 3 | 3 | 1/14 | 4 |
| >15 | 4 | 4 | 2 | 6 |
| Pregnancy | 4 | 4 | 2 | Nil |

**Table 17E.4:** Dosage chart for treatment of falciparum malaria with ACT-SP.

| Age group (years) | 1st day | | 2nd day | | 3rd day |
|---|---|---|---|---|---|
| | AS | SP | AS | PQ | AS |
| 0–1* (pink blister) | 1 (25 mg) | 1 (250 + 12.5 mg) | 1 (25 mg) | Nil | 1 (25 mg) |
| 1–4 (yellow blister) | 1 (50 mg) | 1 (500 + 25 mg) each | 1 (50 mg) | 1 (7.5 mg base) | 1 (50 mg) |
| 5–8 (green) | 1 (100 mg) | 1 (750 + 37.5 mg each) | 1 (100 mg) | 2 (7.5 mg base each) | 1 (100 mg) |
| 9–14 red blister | 1 (150 mg | 2 (500 + 25 mg each) | 1 (150 mg) | 4 (7.5 mg base each | 1 (150 mg |
| 15 and above white blister | 1 (200 mg) | 2 (750 + 37.5 mg each) | 1 (200 mg) | 6 (7.5 mg base each) | 1 (200 mg) |

*SP is not to be prescribed for children less than 5 months of age and should be treated with alternate ACT

* ACT-AL is not to be prescribed of children weighing less than 5 kg

in case of hematuria or high-colored urine or cyanosis or blue discoloration of lips, nausea, vomiting, or abdominal pain.

### Treatment of Uncomplicated P. falciparum Malaria

All cases should be confirmed by microscopy or RDT and be treated with artemisinin combination therapy (ACT)—Artesunate (4 mg/kg BW)/day for 3 days and SP (Sulfadoxine—25 mg/kg BW and Pyrimethamine 1.25 mg/kg BW) single dose—on first day and Primaquine single dose (0.75 mg/kg BW) on 2nd day. Oral artemisinin monotherapy is banned as it can lead to drug resistance **(Table 17E.4)**.

### Treatment of Mixed Infections

Mixed infections with *P. falciparum* should be treated as falciparum malaria. Anti-relapse treatment with primaquine to be given for 14 days.

### Treatment of Malaria in Pregnancy

*P. falciparum cases:* ACT in 2nd and 3rd trimesters and quinine in 1st trimester (if quinine NA, use ACT).
*P. vivax cases:* Chloroquine in all trimesters, however primaquine is not given.

### General Recommendations

- Avoid treatment on an empty stomach.
- First dose to be given under observation and repeat if vomiting occurs within 30 minutes.
- Ask to report back, if no improvement after 48 hours or situation deteriorates (Not responding to treatment). Also examine for concomitant illnesses.

## Chemoprophylaxis

Recommended only in selective groups for travelers to endemic areas, migrant laborers and military personnel exposed to highly endemic areas.

### Short-term Chemoprophylaxis (<6 Weeks)

*Doxycycline:* 100 mg daily in adults and 1.5 mg/kg body weight for children more than 8 years old, drug is started 2 days before travel and continued for 4 weeks after leaving the malarious area. Contraindicated in pregnant or lactating women and children less than 8 years, in whom personal protection is advised.

### Long-term Chemoprophylaxis (>6 Weeks)

*Mefloquine:* The drug of choice in doses of 5 mg/kg BW (up to 250 mg) weekly. To be taken 2 weeks before, and till 4 weeks after leaving the area. Contraindicated in cases with history of convulsions, neuropsychiatric and cardiac conditions.

### Treatment Failure or Drug Resistance

"Cure" if no fever or parasitemia till 28 days otherwise—treatment failure or drug resistance:

- *Early treatment failure (ETF):* Development of danger signs or severe malaria on Day 1, 2, or 3, in presence of parasitemia, or parasitemia on Day 2 higher than day 0, irrespective of axillary temperature, or parasitemia on day 3 with axillary temperature more than 37.5°C, or parasitemia on day 3 if more than 25% of count on day 0 irrespective of axillary temperature then early treatment failure should be suspected.
- *Late clinical failure (LCF):* Development of danger signs or severe malaria in the presence of parasitemia on any day between 4 and day 28 (42) or presence of parasitemia on any day between 4 and day 28 (42) with axillary temperature more than 37.5°C, provided it did not meet criteria of ETF.
- *Late parasitological failure (LPF):* Presence of parasitemia any day between 7 and 28 irrespective of axillary temperature, such cases should get alternative ACT or quinine with Doxycycline.

## CURRENT APPROACHES

*Global level:* WHO has put forth the **WHO Global technical strategy for malaria—2016-2030,** updated in 2021, which provides technical guidelines for malaria endemic countries.

It is intended to guide and support regional and country programmes as they work towards malaria control and elimination. The strategy sets ambitious but achievable global targets, including:

- Reduce the burden of malaria case by 90% by 2030
- Reduce deaths by malaria by 90% by 2030
- Eliminate malaria in at least 35 countries by 2030
- Prevent resurgence of malaria in the current malaria free countries.

Guided by this strategy, the Global Malaria Programme coordinates the WHO's global efforts to control and eliminate malaria by:

- Playing a leadership role in malaria, effectively supporting member states and rallying partners to reach Universal Health Coverage and achieve goals and targets of the Global Technical Strategy for Malaria;

- Shaping the research agenda and promoting the generation of evidence to support global guidance for new tools and strategies to achieve impact;
- Developing ethical and evidence based global guidance on malaria with effective dissemination to support adoption and implementation by national malaria programmes and other relevant stakeholders; and
- Monitoring and responding to global malaria trends and threats.

*National level:* In line with the **WHO strategy India has brought out a National Framework for Malaria Elimination in India (2016–2030)**, with the objective of:
- Eliminate malaria from 26 low and moderate transmission states/UT by 2022
- Reduce incidence of malaria to less than 1 per case per 1,000 population per year in all states and UTs and their districts by 2024
- Interrupt the indigenous transmission of malaria in the country including high transmission states and UTs by 2027
- Prevent the re-establishment of local transmission of malaria in areas where it has been eliminated and thus maintain the national malaria status by 2030 and beyond.

*National program:* National Vector Borne Disease Control Programme (NVBDCP). Malaria along with other vector borne disease is managed under this program which is further explained in *Chapter 47: Health Policies and Programs in India.*

> **Key Points**
> - The main clinical presentation is fever with chills; however, nausea and headache can also occur.
> - Diagnosis is confirmed by microscopic examination of a blood smear (gold standard) and rapid diagnostic tests
> - In India, the major vector for rural malaria is *Anopheles culicifacies*, and breeds in clean ground water collections
> - In urban areas, malaria is mainly transmitted by *Anopheles stephensi* which breeds in man-made water containers in domestic and peri-domestic situations such as tanks, wells, cisterns, which are more or less of permanent in nature and hence can maintain density for malaria transmission throughout the year.
> - It is also necessary to check whether the insecticide has been applied at the appropriate time in relation to the onset of transmission.

## SUMMARY

Malaria has shown an overall decline in terms of morbidity and mortality since fifties when it was a major health issue with medical and economic implications.

Clinical presentation of malaria cases have also undergone considerable change during the recent past due to change in host characteristics, environmental changes (extreme and unexpected weather conditions), demographic changes like migration, drug resistance and increased potential for epidemics and increase in proportion of falciparum cases.

All these factors have contributed to the increase in the complicated malaria thereby increasing mortality rate. Hence a proper referral system has to be strengthened further for an early access to proper treatment.

Early Diagnosis and Prompt Treatment (EDPT) is the key to prevent not only complications and death but also reduce the sickness duration and prevent community transmission. Apart from that environmental control to keep the vector density below the critical level is also crucial in this regard.

## SUGGESTED READING

1. Kumar A, Valecha N, Jain T, et al. Burden of Malaria in India: Retrospective and Prospective View. Defining and Defeating the Intolerable Burden of Malaria III: Progress and Perspectives. Am J Trop Med Hygien; 2007.
2. National drug policy on malaria, 2013, NVBDCP, MOHFW, Government of India.
3. WHO (2017). World malaria report 2017 [online]. Available from http://www.who.int/malaria/publications/world-malaria-report-2017/en/.
4. World Malaria Report 2022. Geneva: World Health Organization; 2022.

# EPIDEMIOLOGY OF DENGUE AND ITS PREVENTION AND CONTROL

| CM7.2 | Enumerate, describe and discuss the mode of transmission and measures for prevention and control of dengue |
|---|---|
| CM8.1 | Describe and discuss the epidemiological and control measures applicable in dengue |

> *Case Study*
>
> A 19-years-old male laborer residing in a slum was admitted to a hospital with a 3 days history of high-grade continuous fever with chills, frontal headache, vomiting and loose stools. He did not have systemic symptoms suggestive of dengue. He had no past history of dengue fever. Upon investigations, his test of nonstructural protein (NS1) for dengue virus was found positive. On day three post-admission, he developed tachycardia, mild abdominal pain, tenderness, and fall in blood pressure. He also had generalized weakness, and bleeding from nose. Platelet count dropped to 60,000 per mm³ (baseline 220,000/mm³) and hematocrit increased by 25% since the time of admission.
> - What is the important information from the point of view of public health and clinical management?

## INTRODUCTION

Dengue fever is the most important arboviral (viral infection transmitted by arthropod/vector) and a major international public health concern as it occurs as not only as endemic or epidemic but as pandemic too and characterized by classical dengue fever (DF). Dengue hemorrhagic fever (DHF) and DHF with shock (DSS) and transmitted by *Aedes* mosquito. Every year, thousands of individuals are affected and contribute to the burden of health care. It is a self-limiting disease found in tropical and subtropical regions around the world, predominantly in urban and semi-urban areas.

## PROBLEM STATEMENT

As per the revision of the International Health Regulation (IHR) dengue is considered as a public health emergency due to its peculiar tendency for rapid epidemic spread beyond national borders causing international concern for health security.

## Global Scenario

Dengue hemorrhagic fever has been showing a rising trend in the past few decades. Prior to 1970 only nine countries were affected but now it is endemic in more than 100 countries (mostly Asian countries) and is a leading cause of childhood deaths. First time, its complications were recognized in 1950s during the dengue epidemic (Philippines and Thailand).

About half of the world's population is now at risk of dengue with an estimated 100–400 million infections occurring each year. Dengue is found in tropical and sub-tropical climates worldwide, mostly in urban and semi-urban areas.

Globally, incidence has grown 30 times around the world in the last 50 years. The incidence of dengue has grown dramatically around the world in recent decades, with cases reported to WHO increased from 505,430 cases in 2000 to 5.2 million in 2019. A vast majority of cases are asymptomatic or mild and self-managed, and hence the actual numbers of dengue cases are under-reported. Many cases are also misdiagnosed as other febrile illnesses.

The disease is now endemic in more than 100 countries in the WHO Regions of Africa, Americas, Eastern Mediterranean, South-East Asia and Western Pacific. The Americas, South-East Asia and Western Pacific regions are the most seriously affected, with Asia representing around 70% of the global disease burden.

Dengue is spreading to new areas including Europe, and explosive outbreaks are occurring. Local transmission was reported for the first time in France and Croatia in 2010 and imported cases were detected in 3 other European countries.

The largest number of dengue cases ever reported globally was in 2019. All regions were affected, and dengue transmission was recorded in Afghanistan for the first time. (WHO, Fact Sheets: Dengue and Severe Dengue; March 2023).

## Indian Scenario

Though dengue outbreaks have continued since the 1950s, severity of disease has increased in the last two decade. In India, first major outbreak associated with hemorrhagic manifestation occurred in Calcutta in 1963 followed by a major outbreak in Delhi in 1996 and 2003. Since, the mid 1990 epidemics have spread to new regions due to rapid or unplanned urbanization, poor water storage or management, such as Orissa, Arunachal Pradesh, and Mizoram, where dengue was historically nonexistent. Trends in recent decades include larger and more frequent outbreaks; geographic expansion of endemic transmission; spread of the disease from urban to peri-urban or rural areas, an increasing proportion of severe cases leading to deaths and progression to hyperendemicity particularly in large urban areas (Chakravarti A et al., Trans R Soc Trop Med Hyg, 2012).

By 2012–13, the face of dengue incidence in India radically transformed. Dengue has become an annual epidemic in many parts of southeast Asia, and the disease is becoming more hazardous as the environment changes. According to the most recent data, 110,473 dengue cases were documented in India between January and October, 2022, which is similar to the number of cases reported in 2018 (101,192). Notably, there was a substantially higher number of dengue cases recorded in previous years: 188,401 in 2017; 157,315 in 2019; and 193,245 in 2021. When the COVID-19 wave began in India in 2020, dengue incidence reduced by 56–60% (44,585).

## EPIDEMIOLOGY

Determinants of dengue are those which determine high vector density like conductive environment and vulnerable population. Post-rainy season, collected water facilitates breeding, high humidity and temperature favors long survival of the mosquito.

### Host Factors

It affects people from all walks of society but the poor, living in water scarcity and in inadequate waste disposal infrastructure provides a more favorable environment for breeding of *Aedes aegypti*. All ages and both sexes are susceptible to infection. Vulnerable population mainly includes infants, young children (less able than adults to compensate for capillary leakage) and young adults (more exposed to day biter).

### Agent Factors

Causative agent belongs to group B arbovirus belonging to genus *Flavivirus* of family, Flaviviridae a single-stranded virus and serotypes include 1, 2, 3, and 4 (DEN-1, DEN-2, DEN-3, and DEN-4). Although all 4 serotypes are antigenically similar, the cross protection is only for a short time. However, infection with one serotype confers life-long immunity to that serotype. Also the second infection later by another serotype increases the likelihood of suffering from DHF. DEN-1 and DEN-2 serotypes are widespread in India.

### Environmental Factors

*Aedes aegypti* survives best between 16 and 30°C and a relative humidity of 60–80%. The outbreaks usually occur in post-monsoon period when vector density is pretty high. Urban areas, having high population density, poor sanitation and rural areas where the environment is also friendly for mosquito breeding like storage water for cattle feeding and drinking, etc. are places where the mosquito breeds.

Breeding areas are found in and around households, construction sites and factories; natural larval habitats are tree holes, leaf axils and coconut shells which are water receptacles. During hot and dry seasons, overhead tanks and ground water storage tanks are the usual breeding grounds. Some most common breeding sites are flower pots, coolers and unused tyres.

### Reservoir of Infection

Man and mosquito.

### Incubation Period

Ranges for 5–6 days but may vary from 3 to 10 days.

## CLINICAL MANIFESTATIONS AND SPECTRUM OF DISEASE (FIG. 17E.3)

Dengue is one disease entity with different clinical presentations and often with unpredictable clinical evolution and outcome.

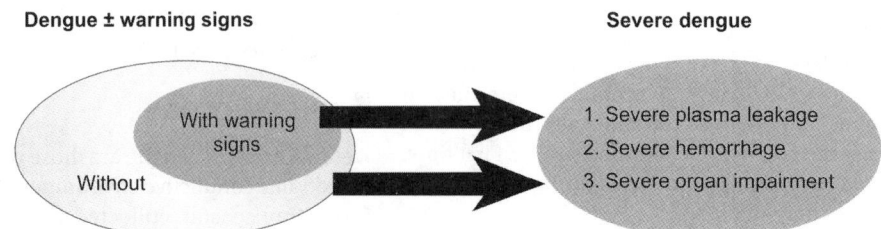

Fig. 17E.3: Manifestations of dengue virus infections.

It varies with age as infants and young children may have a nonspecific febrile illness with rash.

## Tourniquet Test

The test is part of the WHO algorithm for diagnosis of DF.

A blood pressure cuff is applied to the arm and inflated to register a pressure midpoint between the systolic and diastolic blood pressures and maintained for five minutes. The test is positive, if there are more than 10–20 petechiae per square inch in the antecubital fossa. Test may be positive in hemorrhagic conditions due to bleeding from nose, gums and gastrointestinal track.

- Thrombocytopenia (platelets <100,000/mm³), and
- Evidence of plasma leakage due to increased capillary permeability manifested by one or more of the following:
  – More than 20% rise in hematocrit for age and sex
  – More than 20% drop in hematocrit after therapy with fluids as compared to baseline
  – Signs of plasma leakage (pleural effusion, ascites or hypoproteinemia).

## LABORATORY DIAGNOSIS

- Direct diagnosis includes isolation of virus which is difficult
- For sero-diagnosis three criteria are required for definitive diagnosis
  – Detection of dengue virus RNA in acute phase serum or tissues
  – Detection of anti-dengue virus IgM or
  – Detection of anti-dengue IgG antibody titer, serum samples should be collected between 10 and 14 days, detection of IgM antibodies by IgM capture ELISA, detection of total immunoglobulin through hemagglutination inhibition and detection of IgG antibodies by ELISA.

## EPIDEMIOLOGICAL INDICES (TABLE 17E.5)

*Larval surveys:* The extent of prevalence of vectors in certain selected high-risk areas especially from where dengue cases are reported to plan vector control measures, environment management and improved water storage practices.

Table 17E.5: Epidemiological interpretation of various entomological indices.

| Entomological index | High-risk of transmission | Low-risk of transmission |
|---|---|---|
| Breteau index | >50 | <5 |
| House index | >10% | 1% |
| Larval house index | >10% | <1% |

*Note:* One more parameter for high-risk of transmission is landing/biting rate.

- *House index (HI):* Number of houses found positive for larvae of *Aedes aegypti* per 100 houses searched.
- *Container index (CI):* Number of water holding containers positive for *Aedes aegypti* larvae breeding per 100 wet containers. CI is mostly helpful in drawing vector control strategy.
- *Breteau index (BI):* Number of positive containers for *Aedes aegypti* per 100 houses inspected.
- *Aedes aegypti* **index** is the ratio expressed as percentage of the number of houses in a well-defined limited area in surrounding of which breeding places of *Aedes aegypti* has been identified to the total number of houses surveyed in that area.

*Pupae surveys:*
- **Pupa index (PI)**—number of pupae per 100 houses inspected.

*Adult surveys:* Estimating adult population density using ovi traps, sticky traps, human landing collections or any similar traps. Adult mosquito surveillance will help in finding out the susceptibility status of insecticides.

- **Adult landing or biting rate:** *Aedes* mosquito can be collected on human bait and landing rate on bait per hour is calculated. The mosquitoes thus collected can be used for virus isolation.

  Surveys will reflect any change in vector density and all indices needs to be monitored.

# PREVENTION AND CONTROL

## Vector Control Measures

- *Environmental modification:* By improving water supply, proofing of overhead tanks, cisterns or underground reservoirs against mosquitoes.
- *Personal protection:* Reducing man-mosquito contact by mosquito proofing the houses with screens on doors/windows, using repellants, wearing full sleeved clothing, etc.

## Continuous Monitoring of Activities–Surveillance

Surveillance is a prerequisite for monitoring the dengue situation in the areas and should be carried out regularly for impending outbreak and to initiate timely prevention and control measures. It includes epidemiological, laboratory, and entomological surveillance discussed below:

- **Fever surveillance:** Diagnosis is based on standard case definition.
  - Reporting of DF/DHF cases to state health authorities is the pre-requisite. If 5-10% of the sample collected from the clinically suspected or diagnosed cases is positive by laboratory then it suggests an outbreak. Apart from it peripheral health staff should have high index of suspicion and alertness for reporting, if increase of clustering of acute febrile illness compatible with case definition of DF/DHF and needs to be investigated along with vector density in the same area.
- **Laboratory surveillance:** Here the objective is to detect new strain or serotype of dengue virus to detect any unusual increase in dengue transmission. It will support and confirm the diagnosis to provide report to the public health authority within 24 hours mentioning the serotypes involved for early detection of epidemic. The location of cases in the area of the neighboring states should also be monitored, as this will be helpful to evaluate the impact of prevention or early preparedness of any epidemic.
- **Entomological surveillance:** Timely forecasting of vector-borne epidemics depends upon quality of in-depth integrated entomological and epidemiological surveillance conducted in the urban, semiurban as well as in rural areas. *Aedes aegypti* density is important in determining factors related to dengue transmission, in order to prioritize areas and seasons for vector control.
  - **Sample size:** A minimum of 50-100 houses should be searched for *Aedes* mosquitoes in a given locality and in case if 25 houses are continuously found negative for *Aedes* mosquitoes then a change of the locality (at least 100 meters) away from the previous one is required.

Intensified epidemiological and entomological surveillance along with reporting of fever cases needs to be monitored closely. Active surveillance for dengue by health workers in the community should take place on a regular basis.

## Integrated Vector Management

*Biological methods:* Using larvivorous fish/bacillus thuringiensis.

*Chemical methods:*
- Larvicide like Temephos
- Adulticides—
  - Pyrethrum: 0.1-0.2% concentration used in indoor space spray
  - Malathion fogging or Ultra Low Volume (ULV) fogging

*Legislative measures:* Building bye laws under the Building Construction Regulation Act, appropriate disposal of junk through Environmental Health Act, etc.

The above measures along with health education at the community combined with vector control measures form make up for an effective integrated management of the vector in Dengue.

## Treatment of Dengue Fever and Dengue Hemorrhagic Fever (Table 17E.6)

**Febrile phase:** Difficult to distinguish DF from DHF. Same treatment symptomatic and supportive. Requires antipyretics and sponging along with oral fluids and electrolytes.

**Table 17E.6:** DF/DHF Management charts for dengue fever as per guidelines given by WHO.

| Phase | Manifestations | Management |
|---|---|---|
| **Febrile phase** | | |
| Duration 2–7 days | • Temperature 39–40°C<br>• Headache<br>• Retro-orbital pain<br>• Muscle pain<br>• Joint/bone pain<br>• Flushed face<br>• Skin hemorrhage, bleeding from nose gums, positive tourniquet test<br>• Liver often enlarged<br>• Leukopenia<br>• Platelet and hematocrit normal | • At home bed rest<br>• Keep the body temperature below 39°C<br>• Paracetamol, yes<br>• Aspirin, no<br>• Brufen, no<br>• Oral fluids and electrolyte therapy<br>• Follow-up for any change-in plate late and hematocrit |
| **Afebrile phase (critical stage)** | | |
| Duration 2–3 days | • Same C/F as in febrile phase<br>• Improvement in general conditions, platelet and hematocrit normal<br>• Appetite rapidly regained | • Bed rest<br>• Check plate late hematocrit<br>• Oral fluids and electrolyte therapy |
| **Convalescent phase** | | |
| Duration 7–10 days after critical stage | Further improvement in general conditions and return of appetite, Bradycardia, confluent petechial rash with white central itching Weakness for 1–2 weeks | No special advice, no restrictions, normal diet |

*Note:* Paracetamol should be administered not more than 4 times in 24 hours period PCM (250 mg): <1 yr 1/4 tab, 1–4 years: 1/2 tab; 5 years and above—one tablet.

- Rest.
- Paracetamol (<4 times/day) as per age for fever above 39°C.
- Do not use Aspirin/Brufen. Aspirin can cause gastritis and/or bleeding.
- No use of antibiotics.
- ORS for patients with moderate dehydration (vomiting/high temperature.
- Food as per appetite.
- Parenteral fluid therapy.
- No satisfactory vaccine.
- Isolation under bed nets during first few days.

Main culprit in DHF is leakage of plasma in the pleural and abdominal cavities leading to hypovolemic shock usually these changes occur before the subsidence of fever and before the onset of shock and are correlated with the disease severity. Therefore, it requires continuous monitoring of hematocrit value and platelet count for early identifications of critical cases.

### Don'ts

- Do not give Aspirin/Brufen
- Avoid IV therapy before the evidence of hemorrhage and bleeding
- Avoid BT unless indicated (reduction in hematocrit/severe bleeding)
- Avoid steroids or antibiotics
- Do not change the speed of fluid rapidly
- Insertion of NG tube to determine concealed bleeding/stop bleeding (by cold lavage) not recommended.

### For DHF Grades I and II

Dengue with thrombocytopenia, high hem-concentration, epistaxis, black tarry stools, bleeding from gums, needs to be hospitalized. Shock usually develops between the transition from febrile to afebrile phase. This needs to be carefully monitored, it is usually around the 3rd day. A rise in hematocrit indicates plasma leakage and this has to be managed by IV fluid replacement along with continued fever management.

### For DHF Grades III and IV

Along with IV fluid replacement, blood transfusion becomes necessary.

## CURRENT APPROACHES

### Global Level

WHO supports countries in the development of dengue prevention and control strategies and adopting the Global Vector Control Response (2017–2030).

WHO had put forth the **Global dengue situation and strategy for prevention and control 2012–2020,** the specific objectives of which are the following:

- To reduce dengue deaths by at least 50% by 2020.
- To reduce dengue morbidity by at least 25% by 2020.
- To better ascertain the true burden of the disease by 2015, which provides technical guidelines for malaria endemic countries.

*National level:* A conceptual framework for dengue has been developed as a mid-term plan with OCTALOGUE in place that consists of the following:

- Surveillance
- Case management
- Vector management
- Outbreak response
- Capacity building
- Behavior change communication
- Inter-sectoral coordination
- Monitoring and supervision

*National program:* National Vector Borne Disease Control Programme (NVBDCP). Dengue along with other vector borne disease is managed under this program which is further discussed in *Chapter 47: Health Policies and Programs in India.*

### Key Points

- All patients of DF do not need hospitalization.
- ORS should be initiated on the first day of illness as it prevents DHF and decreases risk for hospitalization.
- Health care personnel need to be sensitized about the treatment protocol to avoid inappropriate referral to tertiary care hospital.
- The severity of disease in DHF/DSS depends on the quantum of plasma leakage, which is the major pathophysiological abnormality differentiating DF from DHF/DSS.
- Plasma leakage is due to generalized vasculopathy caused by dengue virus.
- Platelet count is not at all predictive of hemorrhage in DHF/DSS, the risk factors of severe hemorrhage and subsequently mortality are duration of shock and low normal hematocrit at the time of shock.

## SUMMARY

Out of all vector borne diseases, Dengue cases are increasing alarmingly all over India. Risk of dengue has increased considerably in last two decades due to rapid urbanization, life style changes and defective water management (improper water storage practices) due to water scarcity leading to potential to large scale outbreaks. There is no specific treatment for dengue fever. Dengue vaccine has a long way to go. One of the common and major problems in management of dengue is misinterpretation and incorrect evaluation of hemodynamic state to assess for judicious fluid replacement at several point of management. Deaths due to dengue are largely avoidable if crucial decision is made about the volume, rate and type of fluid infusion. Prevention of this disease through integrated vector management is still the mainstay and most cost effective intervention in the program.

## SUGGESTED READING

1. Arasada MR. Guidelines for prevention & control of Dengue. New Delhi: Zoonosis Division, National Institute of Communicable Disease.
2. Chaturvedi UC, Nagar R. Dengue and dengue hemorrhagic fever: Indian perspective. J Bio Sci. 2008;33:429-41.
3. Mayxay M, Phetsouvanh R, Moore CE, et al. Predictive diagnostic value of the tourniquet test for the diagnosis of dengue infection in adults. Trop Med Int Health. 2011;16(1):127-33.
4. Mondal N. The resurgence of dengue epidemic and climate change in India. The Lancet. 2023;401(10378):727-8.
5. WHO (2018). Dengue and severe dengue [online]. Available from http://www.who.int/news-room/fact-sheets/detail/dengue-and-severe-dengue.
6. WHO (2018). Vector surveillance [online]. Available from http://www.who.int/denguecontrol/monitoring/vector_surveillance/en/.
7. WHO, Fact Sheets: Dengue and Severe Dengue;2023.

# EPIDEMIOLOGY OF CHIKUNGUNYA AND ITS PREVENTION AND CONTROL

**CM7.2** Enumerate, describe and discuss the modes of transmission and measures for prevention and control of chikungunya

**CM8.1** Describe and discuss the epidemiological and control measures for chikungunya

---

*Case study*

*A 28-year-old teacher in government primary school in Ahmedabad experienced sudden onset of fever with chills accompanied with severe joint pain in wrists, ankles and neck for which he visited Urban Health Centre. Initially he was treated for malaria and his fever resolved after three days and IgM antibodies demonstrable by ELISA was negative. After recovery from acute illness, he was still experiencing joint pain and restricted range of motion in affected joints. He was referred to the corporation run Medical College. Two and a half months after his initial symptoms of persistent polyartheritis and minimal pain relief with the use of nonsteroidal anti-inflammatory drugs (NSAIDs). On physical examination all vital signs were normal with no enlargement of lymph nodes or liver or spleen or effusion of joints. No Significant pathogonomic hematological findings were observed but Erythrocyte Sedimentation Rate (ESR) was elevated. Rheumatoid (RH) factor and titre to chikungunya immunoglobulin G (IgG) antibodies was found elevated. He was diagnosed with chikungunya fever and was prescribed ibuprofen and physical therapy.*

❑ *Identify the important clinical and public health factors supporting the diagnosis in this case?*

---

## INTRODUCTION

Chikungunya, a relatively rare type of a mosquito-borne zoonotic disease in the world is caused by an arbovirus and transmitted by *Aedes aegypti* mosquito. The name Chikungunya is derived from the Makonde word, (language spoken by South-East Tanzania) other word *SWAHILI* meaning "that which bends up" in reference to the stooped posture developed as a result of the arthritic symptoms of the disease. It resembles dengue and is reported mainly from Africa, South-East Asia including India and Pakistan. It occurs principally during the rainy season. Chikungunya outbreaks typically result in large number of cases but deaths are rarely encountered.

## PROBLEM STATEMENT

### Global Scenario

Chikungunya virus (CHIKV) was first identified in the United Republic of Tanzania in 1952 and subsequently in other countries Africa and Asia. CHIKV was first isolated from a febrile patient and was first described by Robinson and Lumsden in 1953. Urban outbreaks were first recorded in Thailand in 1967 and in India in the 1970s (2). Since 2004, outbreaks of CHIKV have become more frequent and widespread, caused partly due to viral adaptations allowing the virus to be spread more easily by Aedes albopictus mosquitoes. CHIKV has now been identified in over 110 countries in Asia, Africa, Europe and the Americas. Epidemics shows secular trend with a gap of more than ten years and has been identified in nearly in 40 countries, Since 2003, there has been a resurgence of Chikungunya outbreaks in the islands of the Pacific Ocean, including Madagascar, the Comoros, Mauritius and Reunion Island.

### Indian Scenario

In India, the disease reemerged after 32 years in 2005. Earlier major epidemics were reported from Kolkata (1963), Pondicherry (1965), Tamil Nadu, Andhra Pradesh, Madhya Pradesh and Maharashtra (1973), thereafter, sporadic cases continued to be recorded in Maharashtra (1983 and 2000). There was a very large epidemic in Reunion Island (2006) followed quickly by the one in India. Resurgence of Chikungunya has been attributed to various factors including globalization, increase in the mosquito population, loss of herd immunity and the mutation. The number of cases reported are increasing, probably because of better reporting through IgM detection kits of National Institute of Virology as per 148587 suspected cases and 8067 confirmed cases were reported on 2022 due to Chikungunya (NVBDCP, Chikungunya fever, 2022).

## EPIDEMIOLOGY

### Host Factors

Man is the natural host. There is neither animal reservoir nor the carrier.

### Agent Factors

Chikungunya virus (CHIKV, buggy Creek Virus) is a member of the genus *Alphavirus* and family Togaviridae. Wild cycle of virus is similar to yellow fever involving jungle primates and mosquitoes (*A. africanus, A. furcifer/taylori*). This virion is 60–70 nm in size, enveloped, single-stranded, positive-sense RNA. Two genera in Togaviridae are Alpha virus and Rubivirus. Alpha viruses shows two disease patterns: Fever+/-Encephalitis and Fever + Arthritis.

### Environmental Factors

Mainly occurs in rainy season, rising cases coinciding with increase in vector population.

### Source/Reservoir of Infection

Mosquitoes become infected when they feed on a person infected with CHIKV. Infected *Aedes* is the source of infection. Hence, all types of cases, monkeys, and possibly other wild animals, may also serve as reservoirs of the virus **(Fig. 17E.4)**.

### Incubation Period

It ranges between 2 and 12 days, but is usually 3–7 days. "Silent" CHIKV infections (infections without illness) do occur.

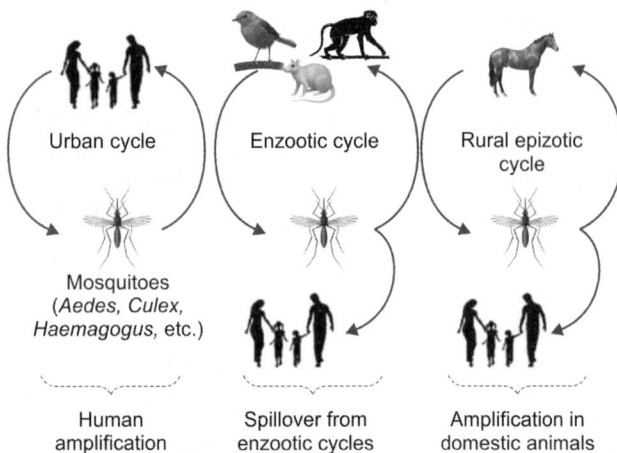

Fig. 17E.4: Life cycle of chikungunya.

## CLINICAL FEATURES

It is important to differentiate Chikungunya from Dengue as it is a disease of urban resembling dengue in terms of epidemiology, modalities of transmission with the important differences like shock due to hemorrhagic complications like petechiae, hypovolemic shock, thrombocytopenia and high hematocrit more seen in dengue than in Chikungunya. Whereas fever with abrupt onset accompanied by headache, fatigue, muscle pain without any serious complications (mostly cases recover fully) but arthralgia which lasts more than a month are more common in Chikungunya. Occasionally, some cases have reported eye, neurological complications but serious one occurs rarely. In case of older adults (≥65 years), newborns infected around the time of birth and people with medical conditions such as high blood pressure, diabetes, heart disease may have more severe form of disease which may lead to death.

Symptoms of infection generally last for 3–7 days. After an incubation period, there is a sudden onset of flu-like symptoms including fever, chills, headache, nausea, vomiting, severe joint pain (arthralgia) and rash. Rash may appear at the outset or several days into the illness; its development often coincides with defervescence, which takes place around day 2 or day 3 of the disease. The rash is most intense on trunk and limbs and may desquamate. Migratory polyarthritis usually affects the small joints. The joints of the extremities in particular become swollen and painful to touch. Although rare, the infection can result in meningoencephalitis, especially in new borns and those with pre-existing medical conditions. Pregnant women can pass the virus to their fetus. Residual arthritis, with morning stiffness, swelling and pain on movement may persist for weeks or months after recovery. A full blown disease is most common among adults, in whom the clinical picture maybe dramatic. Severe cases of Chikungunya can occur in the elderly, in the very young (newborns) and in those who are immune-compromised.

## LABORATORY DIAGNOSIS

- ***Isolation of virus from blood during viremia phase by cell-line:*** Diagnosis is confirmatory but difficult and time consuming.
- ***Serology:*** Diagnostic serological approach comparing acute and convalescent–phase sera. ELISA may confirm the presence of IgM and IgG antibodies to Chikungunya virus. IgM level are highest at 3–5 weeks after the onset of illness and persist for about 2 months.
- Indirect immunofluorescence, hemagglutination inhibition test and complement fixation test, but the limitations are that these tests are technically demanding and do not show positive results in early phase of illness.
- ***PCR diagnosis (RT-PCR):*** Blood sample need to be obtained in viremia phase (1–5 days), sensitive, specific and for early diagnosis, 427-bp fragment of *E2* gene, RTPCR and Nested PCR combination, amplification of 172-bp amplicon are helpful (few as 10 genomic strands can be detected).

## TREATMENT

No specific antiviral drug treatment is recommended it is primarily at relieving the symptoms using antipyretics for fever and pain of muscle and joint and plenty of fluids.

## PREVENTION AND CONTROL

### Vector Control Measures

This remains to be the mainstay of prevention of Chikungunya.

Measures are similar in lines with control as described for dengue (Refer Dengue prevention and control). They include (elimination of breeding places, filling and drainage operation for source reduction, piped water supply, proper covering of stored water) and also include "Observation of weekly dry day". Health education focusing on symptoms of disease and role of vector and breeding places elimination via media like TV, Radio, Cinema slides involving local leaders, faith healers, etc. and community ownership plays an important role in control of the disease.

There is no specific treatment against Chikungunya. It is mostly self-limiting and hence management is mainly symptomatic. Rest, supportive care and nutrition remain the mainstay of case management. Patients should be advised against self-medication particularly with antibiotics, steroids and other painkillers. Aspirin should be strictly avoided.

> **Key Points**
> - Principal vector, *Ae. aegypti* is same for Dengue and Chikungunya hence vector control measures are same.
> - Though chikungunya outbreaks typically result in large number of cases but rarely deaths occur.
> - Occasionally some cases have reported eye, neurological complications but serious one occurs rarely.
> - In case of older adults (≥65 years), newborns infected around the time of birth and people with medical conditions such as high blood pressure, diabetes, heart disease may have more severe form of disease that may contribute to death.
> - Man is the natural host and there is no animal reservoir and no carrier state.
> - It resembles dengue and shock due to hemorrhagic complications petechiae, hypovolemic shock, thrombocytopenia and high hematocrit are more seen in dengue than in chikungunya.

## SUMMARY

This emerging vector-borne disease is a public health problem in countries of South-East Asia Region including several outbreaks of chikungunya in recent years in India. Although not a killer disease, it has high morbidity and prolonged polyarthritis resulting into the prolonged disability and associated socioeconomic impact. There is no specific treatment or vaccine available for chikungunya fever. Patient is the reservoir of infection, hence public health measures to break the chain of transmission needs to be strengthened for prevention and control of this disease.

## SUGGESTED READING

1. Cecilia D. Current status of dengue and chikungunya in India. WHO South-East Asia J Public Health. 2014;3(1):22-7.
2. Chikungunya situation in India. National Centre for Vector borne disease control program. DGHS, MoHFW GOI, 2022.
3. Das S, Kohler RP, Mane BG, et al. Chikungunya epidemic: Global and Indian. J Comm Dis. 2007;39(1):37-43.
4. National Vector Borne Disease Control Program (2013). Chikungunya fever 2013. [online] Available from http://nvbdcp.gov. in/chikun-status.html.
5. Ravi V. Re-emergence of Chikungunya virus in India. Indian J Med Microbiol. 2006;24:83-8.
6. Ross RW. The Newala epidemic. III. The virus: Isolation, pathogenic properties and relationship to the epidemic. J Hyg. 1956;54:177-91.
7. WHO (2017). Other vector borne arbo-viral diseases [online]. Available from http://www.who.int/denguecontrol/arbo-viral/other_arboviral_chikungunya/en/.
8. WHO. Dengue and Severe Dengue: Key facts; 2022.
9. WHO. Regional office India. Investigation and Control of Outbreaks. Dengue Fever and Dengue Hemorrhagic Fever. National Institute of Communicable diseases. New Delhi: Directorate General of Health Services; 2001.

# EPIDEMIOLOGY OF YELLOW FEVER AND ITS PREVENTION AND CONTROL

**CM7.2** Enumerate, describe and discuss the mode of transmission and measures for prevention and control of yellow fever

**CM8.1** Describe and discuss the epidemiological and control measures applicable in yellow fever

### Case Study

A. Mr Gandhi a businessman from Mumbai, India is going to New York via Rio de Janeiro, Brazil. He took the yellow fever vaccine 15 days before commencing on the journey.

B. What if Mr Gandhi lands at New York airport without the vaccination?

**Question:**
1. Will Mr Gandhi require this vaccine if takes a direct flight from Mumbai to New York?
2. What should be the minimum gap in days between taking the vaccine and commencement of the journey?
3. What action will be taken by the airport authorities in the scenario B?

## INTRODUCTION

Yellow fever; historically known as "yellow plague (known so due to yellow pigmentation of skin because of hepatic involvement)", is an acute viral hemorrhagic disease. It is a first known zoonotic viral disease of man. It principally affects monkeys and other vertebrate animals and clinical features are similar to DHF. Severe cases have involvement of liver and/or kidneys. Case fatality rate (CFR) can be as high as 80% in severe cases and death can occur within 5-10 days.

## PROBLEM STATEMENT

### Global Scenario

It is one of the three internationally notifiable disease under the International Health Regulation; other two being cholera and plague. Yellow fever is endemic in 44 countries and 110 countries are at risk of disease transmission. The disease probably evolved in Africa and reached to South America from slave trade in the 17th century. There have been several regular and devastating epidemics in parts of Caribbean, Central and South Africa and South America (Ernest AG et al., Adv Virus Res, 2003). As of 2023, 34 countries in Africa and 13 countries in Central and South America are either endemic for, or have regions that are endemic for, yellow fever. A modeling study based on African data sources estimated the burden of yellow fever during 2013 was 84,000–170,000 severe cases and 29,000–60,000 deaths (WHO).

### Indian Scenario

#### Yellow Fever does not occur in India

However, India, with largest susceptible populations, presence of vector and suitable environmental conditions have skipped from this disease but does offer a very fertile ground for yellow fever. As a yellow fever receptive zone and with high volume of International travel, India needs to take preventive measures against this unwanted illness. Effective checking for valid yellow fever vaccination certificate at point of entry, regular entomological surveillance, expansion of yellow fever vaccination centers, generating public awareness and epidemic preparedness strategy are some of the steps against emergence of this fatal disease in India. Yellow fever has not entered into Indian Territory till date but no stone should be left unturned to stop this disease from entering into the country.

## EPIDEMIOLOGY

### Host Factors

- All ages and both sexes are susceptible to yellow fever
- All occupations related to forest (forest workers, tourists, veterinarians) are at higher risk of contracting the disease
- One infection provides life-long immunity
- Infants born to immune mothers have antibody till 6 months of life.

### Agent Factors

It belongs to the *Flavivirus fibricus*, a group B arbovirus from Toga virus family.

### Environmental Factors

Temperature more than or equal to 24°C is needed for the virus to survive along with a relative humidity more than 60%.

### Social Factors

Some social factors also play a role in causation of yellow fever such as:
- Urbanization
- Deforestation
- Migration
- Travel

### Vector Bionomics

The vectors of yellow fever in forest areas in Africa are Aedes africanus. In South America, the primary vector is the *Haemagogus* species.

In urban areas of both Africa and South America, the vector is *Aedes aegypti*.

The mosquitoes either breed around houses (domestic), in forests or jungles (wild), or in both habitats (semi-domestic).

### Reservoir

The natural host for the yellow fever virus in forest areas is non-human primates (usually monkeys and chimpanzees).

### Transmission of Infection (Fig. 17E.5)

There are three types of transmission cycles:
1. ***Sylvatic (or jungle) yellow fever:*** Here, monkeys, which are the primary reservoir of yellow fever in tropical rainforests, thus passing the virus to other monkeys. Humans working or traveling in these forest regions can get bitten by these infected mosquitoes and develop yellow fever.
2. ***Intermediate yellow fever:*** Here the semi-domestic mosquitoes (those mosquitoes that breed in the wild as well as around households) infect both monkeys and people. Thus an increased contact between people and infected mosquitoes leads to an increased transmission in humans. This can also lead to an outbreak of cases in adjacent dwellings and villages.
3. ***Urban yellow fever:*** Here infected mosquitoes in the urban areas transmit the virus from human to human thus affecting large number of people in heavily populated areas with high density of mosquito.

### Period of Communicability

Man is communicable in the first 3-4 days of illness while monkeys are communicable for several days, African monkeys do not die due to yellow fever.

### Extrinsic Incubation

It is 8-12 days. Mosquitoes are infective for life and show transovarian transmission similar to dengue.

### Incubation Period

It lasts for 3-6 days (6 days by IHR).

## CLINICAL FEATURES

The clinical disease varies from nonspecific, abortive illness to fatal hemorrhagic fever. Disease starts with abrupt onset of fever, chills, malaise, headache, lower back pain, generalized myalgia, nausea,

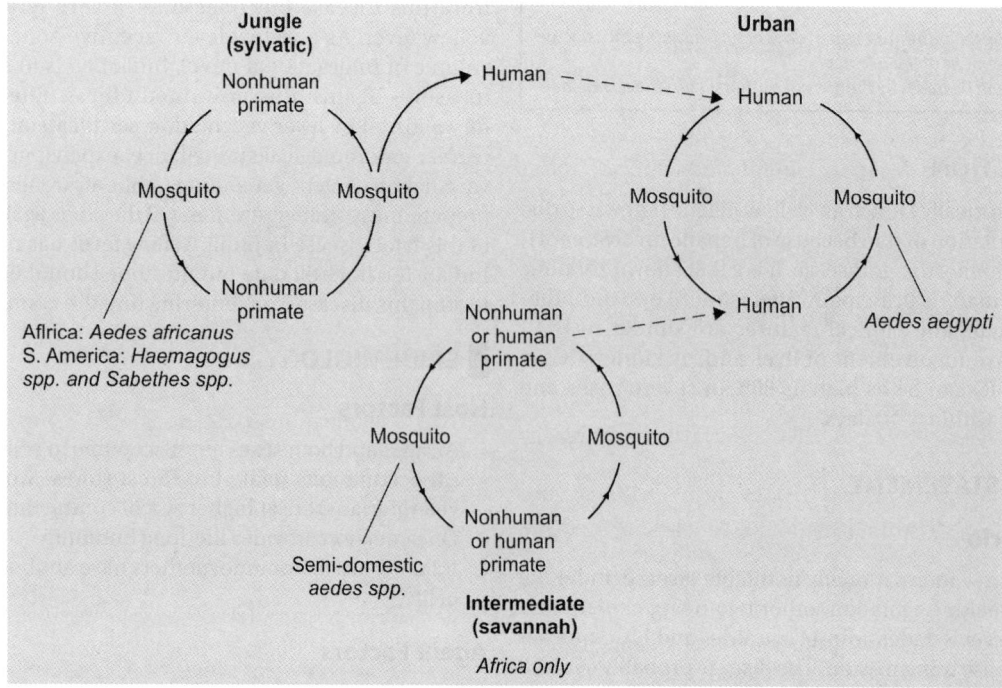

**Fig. 17E.5:** Transmission of yellow fever virus.
*Source:* CDC.

and dizziness. On examination, Fagets sign may be elicited, i.e relative bradycardia along with high fever. The conjunctiva may be congested. Young children may present with febrile convulsions. Laboratory findings may show leukopenia along with a relative neutropenia. Jaundice may develop between 48 and 72 hours after onset and there may be a rise in serum transaminase levels. This period may last for several days followed by remission.

In approximately 15–25% of people affected, the illness reappears in a more severe form with fever, vomiting, epigastric pain, jaundice, renal failure, and a hemorrhagic diathesis. Hemorrhagic manifestations like petechiae, ecchymoses, epistaxis, and oozing of blood from the gums and at needle puncture sites. Many of such individuals may show coffee-grounds hematemesis, melaena, or metrorrhagia. Laboratory abnormalities would reveal reduced platelet count, prolonged clotting and prothrombin times, reduced fibrinogen and factors II, V, VII, VIII, IX, and X, and the presence of fibrin split products suggesting consumption coagulopathy.

About 20–50% of patients with hepato-renal disease die, typically 7–10 days after onset.

True yellow fever viral encephalitis is rarely seen.

## TREATMENT

As it is viral disease, so as such no specific treatment is there, symptomatic measures need to be undertaken as a precautionary measure, case should be hospitalized for treatment of their symptoms and close observation for monitoring the symptoms. Certain medications like in dengue should be avoided, such as aspirin or other nonsteroidal anti-inflammatory drugs, because these may increase the risk of bleeding. The disease can be fatal.

## PREVENTION AND CONTROL OF YELLOW FEVER

Main thrust areas for prevention and control of yellow fever are vaccination and vector control coupled with surveillance.

### Vaccination

17D vaccine is a freeze dried, live attenuated which contains a nonvirulent 17D strain prepared from chick embryo and sensitive to heat. A single dose of 0.5 mL s/c at the insertion of deltoid is required. Vaccine being thermosensitive has to be stored between 2 and 8°C and cold physiological saline is used as a diluent. Once brought out, vaccine should be kept on ice, away from sun and used within half an hour. Immunity develops from 7th day and remains life-long,. From 11th July 2016, the certificate of vaccination is valid for the life of the person vaccinated according to WHO. Yellow fever vaccine is recommended for people aged nine months or older who are traveling (even during the transit) to or living in areas at risk for yellow fever virus transmission in South America and Africa. Proof of this vaccine is officially required under International Health Regulations for entry into some countries if the traveler is entering from a yellow fever endemic area.

Vaccine is to be avoided during pregnancy and infancy, if there is no risk of exposure. Mild post-vaccination reactions occur but anaphylaxis is rare. Cholera vaccine also required for international travel at the same time may interfere with seroconversion, hence two vaccines should be given 3 weeks apart.

### *International Certificate of Vaccination and India*

On arrival, every one including infants, coming from a yellow fever affected areas (even during transit) requires a valid certificate. **Validity of vaccination is from 10 days of vaccination to the life of the person vaccinated.**

In India, the vaccine is given at specified authorized centers for yellow fever vaccination by the DGHS and ministry of health and family welfare.

### Vector Control Measures

For yellow fever, a vector surveillance for *Aedes aegypti* and other *Aedes* species will helpful.

Personal protective measures for prevention of mosquito bites are useful.

Integrated approach of vector control that involves source reduction along with other measures are effective. Spraying aircrafts and ships with insecticides on arrival from endemic areas. *Aedes aegypti* index maintained below 1% in 400-meter surrounding airports and seaports.

### Surveillance

Clinical or serological or histopathological and entomological surveillance (discussed in dengue) are required. "*Aedes aegypti* index" should not be more than 1%.

## CURRENT APPROACHES

### Global Level

A Global Strategy to Eliminate Yellow Fever Epidemics (EYE) 2017–2026 had been developed jointly by WHO along with GAVI and UNICEF with three objectives:
1. Protect at-risk populations,
2. Prevent international spread and
3. Contain outbreaks rapidly

### National Level

The main purpose of the Point of Entries Health (POEs) Organizations is to prevent spread of disease (Public Health Emergencies of International Concern) from foreign countries to India and similarly any disease outbreak of international importance should not be transmitted from India to other foreign countries.

Other main purpose of the Point of Entries Health (POEs) Organizations is to ensure provision of safe healthy environment at point of entries for travelers and the staff working at the POEs. The safe healthy environment includes provision of safe food, safe drinking water, sanitation and Vector control at POEs.

In this regard:
- All international passengers of all International flights are screened by the immigration officials for history of travel to yellow fever endemic countries within last 6 days of arriving in India.
- They are checked for yellow fever vaccination certificate. If they do not possess a vaccination certificate then they are

quarantined and observed as per the Indian Aircraft (Public Health) Rules, 1955.
- As per rule, Airport up to the radius of 400 meters has to be mosquito free (container/house Index has to be zero) therefore vector control/surveillance activities primarily for *Aedes aegypt* mosquito, which is vector for many diseases including yellow fever disease, are performed by APHO in coordination with NVBDCP (National Vector Borne Disease Control Programme) and necessary measures taken.
- Aircraft disinfection measures are taken as per need.

### Key Points
- First known viral disease of man, zoonotic disease. It principally affects monkeys and other vertebrate animals and clinical features are similar to DH, Lassa fever, etc.
- It is one of the notifiable diseases under the IHR.
- Though, it does not occur in India, but because India has largest susceptible populations, presence of vector and suitable environmental conditions, it provides a fertile ground for yellow fever. As a yellow fever receptive zone and with high volume of International travel, India needs to take preventive measures against unwanted epidemics.
- Vaccination and mosquito control are only weapons to prevent yellow fever.

## SUMMARY

The containment of Yellow fever in the countries of South America and Central Africa is a triumph of preventive medicine. It is largely due to the international travel policy focusing mainly on a valid vaccination to any one visiting the endemic countries even during transit. Couple of other actions are also taken to ensure that the cases of yellow fever do not occur outside the endemic belt (including India), where the susceptible population and vector are present in abundance.

## SUGGESTED READING

1. Alan DT, Stephen H. Yellow fever: A disease that has yet to be conquered. Ann Rev. 2007;52:209-29.
2. Ernest AG, Xavier DL, Pablo MA, et al. Origins, evolution and vector/host co coadaptations within the genus *Flaviviruses*. Adv Virus Res. 2003;59:277-314.
3. Monath TP. Treatment of yellow fever. Antiviral Res. 2008;78(1):116-24.
4. Paul S, Sahoo J. India's Preparedness against Yellow Fever. Indian J Hygiene Pub Health. 2015;1(2):77.
5. World Health Organization (2017). Increased risk of urban yellow fever outbreaks in Africa. Global alert and response (GAR). [online] Available from http://www.who.int/csr/disease/yellowfev/urbanoutbreaks/en/.
6. WHO. Yellow fever: Keyfacts; 2023.

# EPIDEMIOLOGY OF FILARIASIS AND ITS PREVENTION AND CONTROL

**CM7.2** Enumerate, describe and discuss the mode of transmission and measures for prevention and control of Filariasis

**CM8.1** Describe and discuss the epidemiological and control measures applicable in Filariasis

### Case Study
During Mass Drug Administration (MDA) in 2005, in rural areas from an endemic district of Gujarat, 4 subjects developed fever, bodyache urticaria and wheezing. Symptoms persisted for 2 days and then subsided after this event, community became hostile and refused to participate in MDA.
- How do we handle such challenges?

## INTRODUCTION

Lymphatic filariasis (LF) also known as elephantiasis, is a chronic debilitating infection primarily caused by two thread-like, parasitic filarial worms namely, *Wuchereria bancrofti* and *Brugia malayi*. It has been a major public health problem in India mainly due to the grotesque swelling of the limbs and genitalia and has been a neglected tropical disease (NTD). Infection is transmitted from one person to other by bite of an infective mosquitoes (Culex/Mansonia and rarely anopheles) when the infective larvae penetrate the host skin and enters to the nearest lymphatic vessel. It is a highly disfiguring and debilitating disease causing enormous amount of stigma, shame, psychological problems and social and economic deprivation. Consequences are borne by the affected individuals as well as the family members in terms of effects due to acute and chronic sequalae and loss of employment opportunities.

## HISTORY

- Disease was known since 6th Century BC, when famous Indian physician, Sushruta in his book *Sushruta Samhita* reported it. In 7th century AD, Madhavakara described signs and symptoms in his treatise *Madhava Nidana*.
- Clarke (1709) called elephantoid legs in Cochin as Malabar legs. Lewis discovered microfilaria (MF) in peripheral blood in Kolkata (1872).
- Patrick Manson (1844–1922) called "Father of Tropical medicine" discovered that filarial worms are present in the blood of the patients during night and he also demonstrated the worms in the stomach of a mosquito which was fed up on a patient of filariasis.

## PROBLEM STATEMENT

### Global Scenario

In 2021, 882.5 million people in 44 countries were living in areas that require preventive chemotherapy to stop the spread of infection. It is the fourth most common cause of disability worldwide. The global baseline estimate of people affected by lymphatic filariasis was 25 million men with hydrocele and over 15 million people with lymphoedema. At least 36 million people remain with these chronic disease manifestations.

Lymphatic filariasis can be eliminated by stopping the spread of infection through preventive chemotherapy with safe medicine combinations repeated annually. More than 9 billion cumulative treatments have been delivered to stop the spread of infection since 2000.

As of 2018, 51 million people were infected—a 74% decline since the start of WHO's Global Programme to Eliminate Lymphatic Filariasis in 2000. Due to successful implementation of WHO strategies, 740 million people no longer require preventive chemotherapy (WHO 2023).

## Indian Scenario

The infection is endemic in more than 80 countries with more than 1.3 billion people at risk and 120 million already infected globally. Two-thirds of the endemic population reside in Southeast Asia, and one-thirds live in India with Andhra Pradesh, Bihar, Jharkhand and Madhya Pradesh among the worst-affected states in the country. 49 million Indian (20 million chronic forms and 29 million carriers) are affected either with *W. bancrofti or B. malayi*. Northern and Northwest states of India are spared (similar to leprosy) especially Jammu and Kashmir, Himachal Pradesh, Punjab, Haryana, Delhi and Rajasthan as well as northeastern states are not endemic while 20 states (250 districts) have indigenous transmission.

## EPIDEMIOLOGY

### Host Factors

Man is the natural host and all ages are susceptible to infection as in endemic areas infection was recorded even in infants aged 6 months, so it starts mostly in childhood and rise with age up to 20–30 years and not consistently thereafter, manifestations are seen, several years later in adulthood. Filarial disease appears in a small percentage of infected individual aged more than 10 years. Repeated infections provide some immunity.

### Agent Factors

Filariasis is caused by nematodes from the family Filarioidea. There are eight main species which infect humans; three of them are responsible for most of the morbidity due to Filariasis. *Wuchereria bancrofti* and *Brugia malayi* cause lymphatic filariasis while *Onchocerca volvulus* causes onchocerciasis (river blindness). The other five species are *Loa loa, Mansonella perstans, M. streptocerca, M. ozzardi*, and *brugiatimori*. *W. bancrofti* and *B. malayi* are the two species responsible for this disease. The former accounts for almost 99.4% of the disease burden in the tropical countries, while the latter is responsible for most of the remaining 0.6% of cases. Both of them exhibit nocturnal periodicity of microfilaremia. Infection is prevalent both in urban and rural areas. *Brugia malayi* is seen more in Kerala, Tamil Nadu, Andhra Pradesh, Odisha, Madhya Pradesh, Assam, and West Bengal. Adult worms live in the lymphatic system while the larvae (microfilaria) circulate in the blood.

### Social Factors

Migration due to industrialization and unplanned urbanization especially creation of slums with presence of open drainage-based excreta disposal and characteristic absence of any sanitary system is important social factor leading to extension of infection from endemic to nonendemic areas. At times migration is not a cause but the effect of disease where the victim due to the deformities and associated stigma are compelled to leave their native places and move to the newer areas.

### Environmental Factors

Climate is an important factor in the epidemiology of filariasis. It influences the breeding of vector mosquitoes, their longevity and determines the development of parasite in mosquitoes.

- **Temperature:** The maximum prevalence of *Culex quinquefasciatus* (formerly known as *Culex fatigans*) is observed when the temperature ranges between 22 and 38°C.
- **Humidity:** It influences the longevity of the mosquitoes and the longevity is optimum when the relative humidity is around 70%.
- **Drainage:** Filaria is associated with poor drainage as the vector breeds profusely in clogged and polluted water.

*Town planning:* Inadequate sewage disposal and lack of town planning aggravate the problem by providing more breeding sites nearer to human dwellings.

### Vector

Female mosquitoes of the species Culicine/*Aedes*/*Anopheles* depending upon their geographical prevalence are responsible for the spread. *Culex quinquefasciatus* is the most predominant one and it breeds in dirty and polluted water but can also breed in clear water in the absence of polluted water. *Brugia malayi* is mainly restricted to rural or coastal areas due to peculiar breeding habits of the primary vector (*Mansonia annulifera* and less commonly *M. uniformis*) requiring aquatic plants like *Pistia stratiotes* (floating vegetation). The breeding of these mosquitoes is just not possible in the absence of these plants.

### Mode of Infection

- Through the bite of certain culicine mosquitoes.
- **Infective forms:** Third stage larvae of developing microfilaria.
- **Portal of entry:** Skin.
- **Site of localization:** Lymphatic system of the host in superior or inferior extremities is according to the site of bite, most commonly of inguinoscrotal region.
- **Reservoir of infection:** Reservoir or source of infection is a person with circulating microfilaria in peripheral blood. Microfilaria carriers are usually without any recognizable symptoms of illness. Individuals with advanced disease often turn out to be negative for microfilaria.

## CLINICAL FEATURES

Spectrum of LF ranges from the initial phase of asymptomatic microfilaremia to the later stages of acute and chronic clinical manifestations. The disease manifestations caused by *Brugia malayi* differ from those of *Wuchereria bancrofti* in that, in the former the lymphedema involves only the legs below the knee and upper limbs below the elbow and there is no genital involvement.

Disease manifest mainly in two forms namely, lymphatic filariasis and occult filariasis in which MF are not seen in blood but are found in the affected tissues (mainly lungs but also found in liver and spleen). In lungs due to immunological reaction (raised eosinophilia) symptoms like dyspnea, cough (more at night), and wheeze are common and condition is known as tropical pulmonary eosinophilia (TPE).

## STAGES OF ACUTE FILARIASIS

- Asymptomatic amicrofilaremic stage
- Asymptomatic microfilaremic stage
- Stage of acute manifestation
- Stage of obstructive (chronic) lesions.

### Asymptomatic Amicrofilaremic Stage

In spite of exposure to infective larva, similar to those who become infected, a proportion of population does not show microfilaria or any symptom, including by means of laboratory technique.

### Asymptomatic Microfilaremia

In any endemic area for LF, among the infected individuals, the largest group consists of otherwise healthy young adults and children who have microfilaria in their peripheral blood without any overt clinical manifestation. Even at this stage, there are abnormalities of the lymph vessels like dilation which may be irreversible even after treatment. This is important because approximately 30% of children in certain endemic communities have been shown to acquire LF infection by the age of 4 years, as shown either by the presence of microfilaria or *Wuchereria bancrofti* antigen in blood.

### Acute Manifestations

During initial months and years, there are recurrent episodes of acute inflammation in the lymph vessel or node of the limb and scrotum that are related to bacterial and fungal superinfections and various manifestations are as follows:

### Filarial Fever—Acute Dermatolymphangioadenitis

In 97% of cases, symptoms are fever and chills. Even though acute dermatolymphangioadenitis (ADLA) occurs both in the early and late stages of the disease, it is more frequent in higher grades of lymphedema. The affected area is usually in the extremities or sometimes in the scrotum which is extremely painful, warm, red, swollen and tender. The draining lymph nodes in the groin or axilla become swollen and tender. Acute attacks recur several times a year in patients due to precipitating factors with filarial swelling. Acute episodes are due to secondary bacterial infections by streptococci. In higher grades of lymphedema, fungal infection tends to occur in the webs of the toes and becomes aggravated during rainy season or due to household work where the feet are soaked in water. In such situations, the ADLA are more frequent and are responsible for the persistence and progression of lymphedema leading on to elephantiasis which leads not only to stigma and discrimination but also affects earning capacity.

### Acute Epididymo-orchitis and Funiculitis

Inflammation of structures in the scrotal sac may result in acute epididymo-orchitis or funiculitis in bancroftian filariasis. This is characterized by severe pain, tenderness and swelling of scrotum, usually with fever and rigor. The testes, epididymis or the spermatic cord may become swollen and extremely tender. Like acute ADLA, these attacks are also precipitated by bacterial infections.

### Acute Filarial Lymphangitis

Usually seen when the adult worms are killed in the lymphatic either spontaneously or by DEC. Where adult worms die, small tender nodules are seen at the location, either in the scrotum or along the lymphatic, these episodes are not associated with fever, toxemia or evidence of secondary bacterial infection. At the site of dead adult worms rarely abscess formation may be seen.

### Chronic Manifestations

Most common chronic manifestation of LF is lymphedema of the extremities and Elephantiasis, which on progression leads on to elephantiasis. Even though lower limbs are the ones frequently affected, upper limbs and male genitalia may also be involved. In females, rarely the breasts may also be affected.

### Genitourinary Lesions

Hydrocele is a common chronic manifestation of bancroftian filariasis in the males. This is characterized by accumulation of fluid in the tunica vaginalis, the sac covering the testes. The swelling gradually increases over a period of time and in long standing cases the size of the scrotum may be enormous. Microfilaria may be detected in the peripheral blood or in the hydrocele fluid in some of these subjects. Occasionally, the Hydrocele may have an acute onset when the surrounding lymphatics are inflamed due to the death of adult worms. This is usually self-limiting and may disappear over a period of time. Lymphedema of the scrotum and penis may occur in bancroftian filariasis. In some subjects, the skin of the scrotum may be covered with vesicles distended with lymph known as "lymph scrotum". These patients are prone for acute ADLA attacks involving the skin of genitalia. The other genitourinary manifestations associated with LF are hematuria, chyluria and chylocele.

Lymphedema of the limbs is graded as below:
- *Grade 1 lymphedema:* Pitting edema (mostly) which is spontaneously reversible on elevation.
- *Grade 2 lymphedema:* Nonpitting edema (mostly) which is not spontaneously reversible on elevation.
- *Grade 3 lymphedema:* Also known as elephantiasis, more edema than grade two with dermatosclerosis and papillomatous lesions.

## DIAGNOSIS

It is based on history of mosquito bites in endemic areas, clinical findings and presence of microfilaria in blood samples collected at night. Identification of microfilaria by microscopic examination is the most practical diagnostic procedure. Laboratory confirmation of diagnosis is necessary to identify asymptomatic patients and those with nonspecific symptoms and to identify endemicity of the area and to document impact of mass drug administration (MDA). The decision on

Chapter 17: Specific Epidemiology of Infectious Diseases | 441

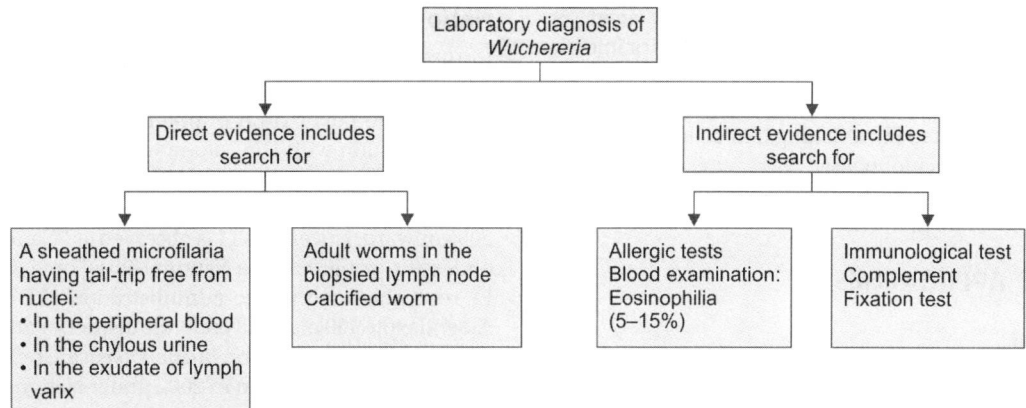

Fig. 17E.6: Diagnosis of *Wuchereriasis* (filariasis).

whether to continue annual rounds of MDA will depend on the laboratory results. The main diagnostic test is the examination of night blood smear collected from 8:30 pm to 12 midnight. Examination of blood samples will allow identification of microfilaria of *Wuchereria bancrofti*. It is important to time the blood collection with the known periodicity of the microfilaria. The blood sample can be a thick smear, stained with Giemsa or hematoxylin and eosin (JSB-I). For increased sensitivity, concentration techniques can be used. These include centrifugation of the blood sample lysed in 2% formalin (Knott's technique), or filtration through nucleo pore membrane **(Fig. 17E.6)**. ***Immunochromatographic (ICT) card test*** can also be done for circulating filarial antigen assay as it detects infection during day time with high sensitivity and specificity; it is simple, rapid and easy to perform.

## EPIDEMIOLOGICAL INDICES

### Parasitological Indices

Microfilaria rate (%) = $\dfrac{\text{No. of slides +ve for MF}}{\text{Total number of slides examined}} \times 100$

Average MF density (This is expressed as mean number of MF per 20 mL blood)

Average MF density = $\dfrac{\text{Total number of microfilariae}}{\text{No. of +ve blood smears}} \times 100$

Disease rate = $\dfrac{\text{No. of persons +ve for disease}}{\text{Total number of persons examined}} \times 100$

### Entomological Indices

From ten catching stations and spot check site using flash light and aspirator tube in the early morning between 6 and 10 am after collecting all *Culex quinque fasciatus* shall be dissected to find out the filarial infection. They are as follow:

### Ten Men Hour Vector Density

$\dfrac{\text{No. of male and female } C. \text{ Quenque fasciatus collected}}{\text{No. of man hours spent for mosquito collection}} \times 100$

If it is less than 50, it is considered to be low density.

Between 50 and 83 moderate density and more than 84 per 100 MHC is considered high or alarming level of vector density.

### Infection Rate (%)

$\dfrac{\text{No. of mosquitoes +ve for infection (L1/L2/L3)}}{\text{No. of female mosquitoes dissected}} \times 100$

### Vector Infectivity Rate (%)

$\dfrac{\text{No. of mosquitoes +ve for infection (L3)}}{\text{No. of female mosquitoes dissected}} \times 100$

If it is more than 1.5%, it indicates high transmission potential and between 0.2 and 1.5% indicates moderate transmission potential.

### Mean Number of L3/Infective Mosquito

$\dfrac{\text{No. of infective larvae found}}{\text{No. of mosquito}} \times 100$

## PREVENTION AND CONTROL OF FILARIASIS

It is interesting to note that wherever proper sewage disposal system and environment sanitation was in place filariasis is eliminated hence these nonhealth interventions play much more significant role apart from preventive chemotherapy.

**Vector control measures** alone or with MDA till now have successfully eliminated LF. There are some challenges of sustainability with MDA in long run as to how long microfilarial suppression is required compounded with factors like mobility of infected cases or their nonparticipation, with possibility of drug resistance in areas co-endemic with Loasis. Hence, integrated vector control measures are required (refer to entomology chapter) along with prevention of mosquito bite at night by using mosquito nets and between dusk and dawn avoid mosquito bite by wearing proper clothing (full sleeves/trousers) and using mosquito repellents.

### Case Management

This **foot care program** to prevent ADLA attacks consists of the following steps:
- Washing the affected area (webs of the toes/deep skin-folds) with soap and water twice a day or at least once before going to bed and wiping dry with a clean cloth.

- Clipping the nails at intervals and keeping them clean.
- Preventing or promptly treating any local injuries or infections using antibiotic ointments.
- Applying antifungal ointment in the webs of the toes, skin folds and sides of the feet to prevent fungal infections.
- Regular use of proper footwear.
- Keeping the affected limb raised at night, using bricks to elevate the foot end of the cot.

## CURRENT APPROACHES

### Global Level

**Global program for elimination of LF (GPELF)** was launched in 2000.

This program has two components:

1. **Interruption of transmission:** The first component of GPELF is to interrupt transmission of filarial infection in the entire "at risk" population of an endemic region by administration of single annual doses of a two-drug regimen which in India consists of administration of Diethylcarbamazine (DEC) at 6 mg/kg and Albendazole 400 mg for a period of 4–6 years. Children under 2 years of age, pregnant women and severely ill-patients are excluded from MDA. The principle behind this strategy is that the transmission of LF infection in a community depends on the MF load in the human carriers and density of vector mosquitoes. Vector control is ideal in theory, but is difficult to achieve due to the difficulties encountered and the cost involved. So, the next best thing is to reduce the load of MF in a given community to such low levels that the mosquitoes will be unable to effectively transmit the infection. The two-drug combination, in the doses mentioned above is shown to bring down the blood microfilaria levels drastically even after annual single dose administration which when repeated for up to 6 years would achieve the target of preventing transmission of LF infection. The estimated fecundity life of the adult parasite is 4–6 years which is the basis for continuing the program for the duration mentioned. It has been shown further that at least 80% of the "at risk" population should consume the drug once annually to achieve transmission control in the timeframe mentioned above. Otherwise the drug administration will have to be continued for many more years.

2. **Alleviation of the disability:** By caring for patient to reduce the suffering and improve the quality of life of the patient in those who already have the disease.

   In 2020, GPELF set the following goals for the new NTD Road Map (2021–2030):
   - 58 (80%) endemic countries have met the criteria for validation of elimination of lymphatic filariasis as a public health problem, with both sustained infection rates below target thresholds for at least 4 years after stopping MDA and providing the essential package of care in all areas with known patients;
   - 72 (100%) endemic countries implement post-MDA or post-validation surveillance; and
   - Reduction to 0 of the total population requiring MDA.

### National Level

In 1955, India launched National Filariasis Control Programme (NFCP) which was limited to urban population and was later extended to cover rural population also in 1994. Mass drug administration with DEC alone was launched (1996) as a pilot project in 13 districts of 7 states covering a population of 41 million. In 2004, districts targeted for MDA were 202 and since, 2006 onward, November 11 is observed as "National Filaria Day" and in the same year, the National Task Force on Elimination of LF recommended the co-administration of DEC 6 mg/kg and Albendazole 400 mg to all endemic districts. Later NFCP became a part of National Vector Borne Disease Control Programme (NVBDCP) in 2003. Then in 2002 under National Health Policy, India set an ambitious goal to elimination of transmission of disease due to lymphatic filariasis by the year 2015. The country has brought out a "Accelerated Plan for Elimination of Lymphatic Filariasis" in 2018 with a goal to eliminate lymphatic filariasis by 2020. It mainly aims to

- Accelerate support and commitment from all stakeholders in eliminating filariasis
- To increase awareness about the disease, symptoms, transmission, and benefits of MDA
- To ensure enhanced MDA in all districts
- To introduce evidence-based chemotherapy strategies for elimination
- To improve monitoring and supervision of the filarial control program.

### Need for Microfilaria Survey

It will give baseline data on MF, current prevalence and impact assessment of MDA. It is also required to facilitate for continuance of MDA and/or certification of elimination of LF.

> **Key Points**
> - Filariasis is not a cause of mortality but has morbidity and deformities with social and economic implications.
> - Globally including India 90% cases are caused by *W. bancrofti* and rest by *B. malayi* and others.
> - It is interesting to note that wherever proper sewage disposal system and environment sanitation has been put in place, filariasis is eliminated hence these public health interventions play significant role apart from preventive chemotherapy.
> - National average prevalence rate is 0.26%. Disease is most common among migrants mainly because of their deformities and social handicaps, patients have to leave their native place and move to other places.
> - Interestingly those having circulating microfilariae are outwardly healthy but transmit the infection to others through mosquitoes while those with chronic filarial swellings or with disabilities can no longer transmit the infection.
> - Vector for filariasis: *Culex quinquefasciatus* is the most predominant one and it breeds in dirty and polluted water but can also breed in clear water in the absence of polluted water. *Brugia malayai* is mainly restricted to rural areas due to peculiar breeding habits of the vector requiring floating vegetation.
> - Type of biological transmission is cyclodevelopmental and third stage larvae are infective to human.
> - Tropical pulmonary eosinophilia (TPE) characterized by symptoms like dyspnea, cough (more at night), and wheeze is an immunological reaction leading to raised eosinophilia.

Chapter 17: Specific Epidemiology of Infectious Diseases | 443

❖ To interrupt community transmission mass drug administration (MDA) by giving DEC 6 mg/kg and Albendazole 400 mg is required for a period of 5 years excluding pregnant women, children under two years and severely ill-patients.

## SUGGESTED READING

1. Addiss DG, Beach MJ, Streit TG, et al. Randomized placebo-controlled comparison of ivermectin and albendazole alone and in combination for Wuchereria bancrofti microfilaremia in Haitian children. Lancet. 1997;350(9076):480-4.
2. Amaral F, Dreyer G, Figueredo-Silva J, et al. Live adult worms detected by ultrasonography in human Bancroftian filariasis. Am J Trop Med Hyg. 1994;50(6):753-7.
3. Burri H, Loutan L, Kumaraswami V, et al. Skin changes in chronic lymphatic filariasis. Trans R Soc Trop Med Hyg. 1996;90(6):671-4.
4. Norões J, Addiss D. The silent burden of sexual disability associated with lymphatic filariasis. Acta Trop. 1997;63(1):57-60.
5. Seim AR, Dreyer G, Addiss DG. Controlling morbidity and interrupting transmission: twin pillars of lymphatic filariasis elimination. Rev Soc Bras Med Trop. 1999;32(3):325-8.
6. Shenoy RK, Kumaraswami V, Suma TK, et al. A double-blind placebo controlled study of the efficacy of oral penicillin, diethyl carbamazine or local treatment of the affected limb in preventing acute adenolymphangitis in lymphoedema caused by brugian filarial. Ann Trop Med Parasitol. 1999;93(4):367-77.
7. Suma TK. Indian scenario of elimination of lymphatic filariasis. Med Update; 2013.
8. Weekly Epidemiological Record. Global program to eliminate lymphatic filariasis. WER. WHO, Geneva. 2009;84(42):437-44.
9. World Health Organization. Bridging the Gaps. World Health Report; WHO, Geneva; 1995.
10. WHO. Lymphatic filariasis; Factsheet; 2023.
11. Kumar D, Kumar A, Vikas K, Kumar C, Sircar S. Coverage of mass drug administration (MDA) and operational issues in elimination of lymphatic filariasis in selected districts of Jharkhand, India. J Family Med Prim Care. 2023;12(1):111-116.

# EPIDEMIOLOGY OF JAPANESE ENCEPHALITIS AND ITS PREVENTION AND CONTROL

**CM7.2** Enumerate, describe and discuss the mode of transmission and measures for prevention and control of Japanese enchephalitis

**CM8.1** Describe and discuss the epidemiological and control measures applicable in Japanese enchephalitis

---

*Case Scenario*

*A 25-year-old man working in piggeries in Assam returned from job and had acute onset high grade fever, headache with stiff neck and was not able to speak, emotionally unstable and lost bladder and bowel control. Investigations findings in CSF showed mild increase in pressure with normal glucose and mildly elevated protein. Later on antibodies to JE virus was positive and antigenic detection by PCR was positive.*
❑ *What is the important information from the point of view of public health and clinical management?*

---

## INTRODUCTION

**Japanese encephalitis** is an arboviral (Arthropod born viral) mosquito-borne zoonotic disease. It has immense public health importance due to its potential of causing outbreaks and high mortality in severe cases. Young children particularly those in 3–6 years present with highest age-specific attack rates, where approximately one-thirds of patients die and half of the survivors are left with severe neuropsychiatric sequelae. Currently, there is no cure for JE virus (JEV) and treatment is mainly symptomatic and supportive in nature. No antiviral drug has shown a convincing improved outcome in cases of JEV. Patients are though not infectious should avoid further mosquito bites.

## HISTORY OF JAPANESE ENCEPHALITIS

- *1870's:* Japan "Summer encephalitis" epidemics.
- *1924:* Great epidemic in Japan with more than 6,000 cases and a high case fatality rate of 62%.
- *1935:* JE virus was first isolated from a fatal human case and in 1938 it was isolated from *Culex tritaeniorhynchus*.
- *1940–54:* Disease spread with epidemics in China (1940), Korea (1949), and India (1954).
- *1983:* Immunization for the first time in South Korea started at age of 3 years (in endemic areas at 1 year).

## ECONOMIC IMPLICATIONS

Economic implications are tremendous due to: (1) high mortality among piglets (rare in adult pigs), food industry is affected; (2) morbidity and mortality (CFR between 5 and 35%) involving high cost for immunization, treatment for serious neurologic sequel (seizures/paresis) which are as high as 50% among survivors leading to loss of productivity (wages) of patients; and (3) expenditure on vector control.

## PROBLEM STATEMENT

### Global Scenario

- JEV is the main cause of viral encephalitis in many countries of Asia with an estimated 68,000 clinical cases every year.
- Although symptomatic Japanese encephalitis (JE) is rare, the case-fatality rate among those with encephalitis can be as high as 30%. Permanent neurologic or psychiatric sequelae can occur in 30%–50% of those with encephalitis.
- 24 countries in the WHO South-East Asia and Western Pacific regions have endemic JEV transmission, exposing more than 3 billion people to risks of infection.

It was first time reported in Japan in 1924 and epidemics were reported from China, Korea, but from 1950s onwards disease is also reported from India. The first encephalitis outbreak attributed to JEV occurred in Japan in 1871. Thereafter, epidemics have been reported with regular frequency including one in 1924 where over 6,000 cases were reported in Japan. Now, it has spread to previously non-affected Asian regions (Kabilan L et al., India J Pediatr, 2004).

### Indian Scenario (Fig. 17E.7)

Epidemics of JE are reported from many parts of the country, first recorded in Vellore and Pondicherry in mid 1950s as in 1955 it was recognized by serological surveys in Tamil Nadu. Subsequent surveys carried out by the National Institute of Virology, Pune indicated that approximately half of the population in Southern India has neutralizing antibodies to the virus. Since 1955, major outbreaks in different parts of the country have been reported. A major outbreak resulting in a 42.6% fatality rate was reported in Bankura, West Bengal in 1973. Subsequently, the disease spread to other states and caused a series of outbreaks in different parts of the country. In 1978, cases were reported from 21 states and union territories. In Uttar Pradesh (UP) (1978), the first major JE epidemic (1,002 cases and 297 deaths) occurred in Gorakhpur and thereafter many were reported with varying intensity and magnitude. Since, 1978–2005, it has taken away more than 10,000 lives in the state.

JE is a leading cause of viral encephalitis in Southeast Asia. It is a serious public health issue in India, and cases have been emerging in newer areas of the country. Although vaccination efforts have already been initiated in the country since 2006 and later through the Universal Immunization Programme in 2011, still a significant reduction in the number of cases has to be achieved since an escalating trend of JE incidence has been reported in certain States such as Assam, Uttar Pradesh and West Bengal.

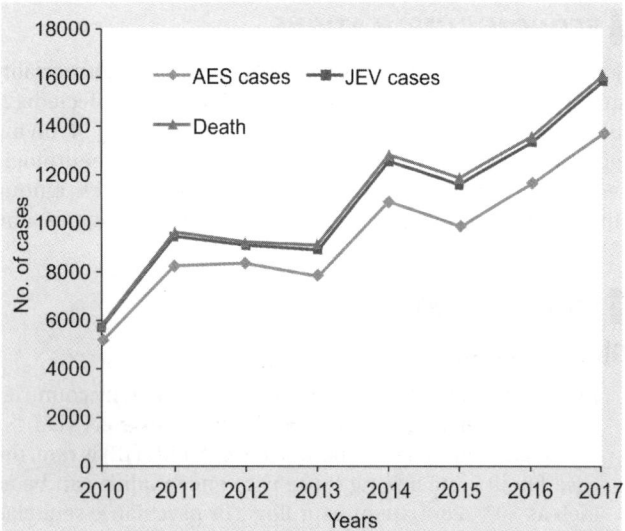

**Fig. 17E.7:** Trend of JE incidence in India (2010-2017).
*Source:* NVBDCP, India. (JE, Japanese encephalitis)

## EPIDEMIOLOGICAL DETERMINANTS

### Host Factors

Mostly affects children and young adults. Most cases (85%) do occur in children (<15 years) while in elderly (>60 years) it is about 10%. Rates of infection in the 3–15-year age group are five to ten times higher than in older individuals while the epidemics in non-endemic regions have affected all age groups with a bimodal age distribution (young children and elderly), indicating an increased risk in elderly people. In endemic areas, nearly all residents have sustained infection by young adulthood. Presence of one clinical case in the community suggest 300–1,000 infections. Various host factors apart from age which influence occurrence of infection are genetic make-up, general health, and pre-existing immunity.

- **Amplifying host:** Pig
- **Incidental host:** Infection in human is incidental.

### Pigs Act as Amplifiers While Cow or Buffalo Act as Brakes of Transmission

Pigs act as extra human reservoir and are the major vertebrate host and act as amplifying hosts in different parts of India 12–44% of pig population are found positive for JE antibodies in endemic areas. Human cases of JE are often preceded by several cycles in pig who develop only viremia and later when mosquitoes bite human (overflowing infection). Infection in man appears to be correlated with living in close proximity with animal reservoirs (pigs), providing a link to human through their proximity to housing or staying outdoor also facilitate transmission (more pigs in an area more JE cases). In absence of pigs, cycle is maintained by birds (less common), cow, etc. and when bitten develop antibodies and transmission stopped (brakes).

### Extra Human Reservoir

Natural cycle is maintained between vertebrates and mosquitoes mainly in Aquatic birds like egrets, pond herons, etc. Animal hosts mainly include pigs, while other animals such as cattle and horses have no significant role in disease transmission.

### Agent Factors

Causative organism is a flavivirus (Flavus in Latin means "yellow" refers to yellow fever virus which incidentally belongs to the same group) belongs to Flaviviridae. It is an enveloped, single-stranded RNA virus and has two serotypes namely Nakayama and Beijing. Nakayama strain (1935) was isolated from the brain of encephalitis patient. It belongs to flaviviruses as a group B arbovirus of family Togaviridae.

### Environmental Factors

Epidemics usually coincide with period (monsoons and post monsoons—referred as paddy season) when the vector density is high. It is primarily rural disease affecting communities engaged in agricultural practices as well as those residing at the outskirts of towns where people are engaged in agricultural practices.

### Mode of Transmission

It is transmitted indirectly through bite of an infected culicine mosquito. Transmission cycle is maintained in animals and birds.

### Vectors

Out of many species of *Culex* mosquitoes which can transmit JE in India, most important are group of *Culex vishnui*. It breeds in water bodies with vegetation like irrigated paddy fields, shallow ditches and pools. Mosquitoes are primarily zoophilic feeding on animals and wild birds.

## Incubation Period

About 6–8 days.

## PATHOGENESIS

After the bite of an infected mosquito, virus replicates in the skin and reaches to dendritic cells regional lymph nodes for viral replication, amplifies peripherally, causing a transient viremia before invading the central nervous system (CNS). The clinical manifestations of many infections are dependent on whether or not the virus gains access to susceptible cells within the CNS which leads to encephalitis, However, JEV crosses the blood-brain barrier is not known.

## DIAGNOSIS

Diagnosis is based on epidemiological and clinical features.

### Clinical Progression of Disease

Not all infected, develop disease as it follows iceberg phenomenon and around 1 out of 300–1,000 infected develop JE. Encephalitis cases are usually scattered, 1–2 per village. Human cases of JE may be suspected in persons visiting endemic areas and demonstrating neurological sign accompanied by a fever.

### Signs and Symptoms

As mentioned earlier, most cases are asymptomatic. It usually starts with a fever above 38°C, chills, myalgia, and meningitis-type headaches accompanied by vomiting. Most JEV infections are mild (fever and headache) or without apparent symptoms, but approximately 1 in 250 infections results in severe clinical illness. Severe disease is characterized by rapid onset of high fever, headache, neck stiffness, disorientation, coma, seizures, spastic paralysis and ultimately death. The case-fatality rate can be as high as 30% among those with disease symptoms. Of those who survive, 20–30% suffer permanent intellectual, behavioral, or neurological problems such as paralysis, recurrent seizures or the inability to speak.

### Usual Course of Disease has Three Stages

1. ***First stage (prodromal):*** There is an acute and abrupt onset of symptoms and characterized by fever, headache, lethargy, malaise and gastrointestinal disturbances abrupt onset of high fever accompanied by headache, with nonspecific symptoms including malaise, anorexia, nausea and vomiting.
2. ***Second stage (acute stage):*** Includes changes in the level of consciousness ranging from mild clouding to stupor, semi-coma, or coma. Generalized or focal convulsions are common, with neck stiffness and weakness of extremities. In this stage, fatal cases progress rapidly and die. The third is a late stage characterized by defervescence with improved neurologic sequelae in uncomplicated cases. The last stage is the sequelae phase, which includes complete recovery in mild cases, while severe cases also improve but are left with neurological deficits.
3. ***Third (late) stage:*** Recovery with signs of neurological loss persists or worsens while fever disappears.

### Clinical Signs (Severe)

They include signs of acute encephalitis like headache, high fever, stiff neck, stupor, severe encephalitis, paralysis, seizures, convulsions, coma and death. Neuropsychiatric sequelae occurs 30–50% of survivors. In utero, infection may lead to abortion of fetus.

## LABORATORY DIAGNOSIS

A tentative diagnosis of JE can be based on a four-fold rise in antibody titer using several methods such as hemagglutination inhibition (HI), immunofluorescent antibody titer (IFA), complement fixation (CF), or IgG enzyme-linked immunosorbent assay (ELISA). Caution should be used when interpreting these results since cross-reactivity can occur with other flaviviruses. Additionally, the antibody response may have already peaked by the time, the patient presented for care and therefore fail to demonstrate a rise in titer. Additionally, demonstration of JE specific IgM in serum or cerebrospinal fluid (CSF) may be useful in acute phases of the disease. Definitive diagnosis of JE is done by viral isolation. Samples of CSF can be used. Brain tissue can be used for virus isolation in postmortem situations. There is no specific treatment for JE and supportive care is recommended.

## PREVENTION AND CONTROL

- Field-based management
- Management of case
- Vector control
- Personal protective measures
- Vaccination-animal and humans
- Notification to authorities

### Field-based Management

#### Case Definitions

- ***Suspected case:*** Acute fever of 5–7 days with altered mental status with or without new seizures (except febrile).
- ***Probable case:*** A suspected case in geographical or temporal proximity of a confirmed case.
- ***Confirmed case:*** A suspected case with any one of the following: (1) presence of JE specific IgM in blood or CSF; (2) four-fold raised titer of IgG (paired sera); or (3) isolation of virus or antigen or nucleic acid.

#### Early Case Detection and Treatment

It helps in reducing case fatality by early case detection from community to various health facilities at PHCs/CHCs and District Hospital through strengthening of diagnostic and clinical management. To reduce JE-related morbidity, complications, and mortality in endemic areas estimation of actual disease burden for timely intervention is must. Suspected cases referred from field to referral hospital should be confirmed with two diagnostic tests, one for detection of JE reverse transcriptase–polymer chain reaction (RT-PCR) and one for detection of virus antigen or virus genome.

### Management of Case

- To be differentiated from non-JE
- Management is symptomatic and supportive, if any one develops Lethargy/Convulsions/Unconsciousness.

Refer to nearest FRU, and refer to higher treatment center (tertiary care) directly, if develops shock hypotension-feeble pulse, poor respiration (ventilators are required), unmanageable cyanosis even with oxygen therapy.

### Vector Control

Vector control is a serious challenge for JE simply due to exophilic and exophagic behavior of JE vectors as conventional method of vector control (e.g., indoor residual spray) may not be effective but may work in high-risk pockets where vector is endophilic like *Mansonia annulifera*.

### *Fogging*

Fogging is a very cost intensive vector control tool with limited effect and hence not recommended as a routine vector control measure. In case of containment of JE outbreak due to exophilic and zoophilic behavior of vector peri-domestic fogging could be resorted. Besides the impact on adult population fogging efforts are visible in the community.

### *Anti-larval Operations*

On regular basis for JE vector control it is neither cost effective nor operationally feasible. But environmental measures like reduction of breeding sources for larvae are more feasible and few of them are control of breeding places in paddy field by incorporating neem products as a fertilizer to enhance grain production as well as to suppress the breeding and a strategy of alternate drying and wetting water management system are more effective.

### *Larvivorous Fish*

Composite fish culture for mosquito control in rice fields and release of fish in large and small water bodies.

### *Biolarvicides*

Biocides like *Bacillus thuringiensis israelensis* and *Bacillus sphaericus* were promoted and anticipated to have great implications as biological larvicides against different mosquito species.

### Personal Protective Measures

While creating community awareness, use of long-lasting insecticide (pyrethroid) treated bed nets (LLITBN) and curtains mosquito repellants, proper clothing to cover exposed body parts to avoid biting hours should be encouraged. LLITBN is superior to earlier technology of repeated impregnation at 6–9 months and periodic assessment of insecticide resistance.

### Control of Pig

Pigs being amplifying host, require control measures such as immunization, slaughtering pig, and use of mosquito proof piggeries. Segregating pigs 4–5 km away from human habitations can be through legislative measures.

### Immunization of Animals

Effective as there is reduction in animal transmission. Inactivated or attenuated vaccines are available for swine but challenge is difficult to ensure complete coverage due to the requirement of repeated doses specially for rapidly breeding animals like pigs annually as period of vaccine effectiveness is limited.

### Vaccination in Human

Three types of vaccines are in use in endemic or epidemic areas.
1. Inactivated brain derived and purified type used in India
2. ***Cell-culture derived (CCD):*** Inactivated based on Beijing strain
3. CCD live attenuated used only in China.

### *Vaccination Schedule*

Apart from children, it is also recommended for at risk person like; laboratory staff and travelers who are visiting for more than 30 days.

### *Doses and Schedule*

0.5 mL (<3 years) or 1.0 mL (>3 years)—S/C—2 doses—1 month apart, booster at 1 year and subsequent boosters every 3rd year till 15 years of age. Protection comes in 1 month after 2nd dose, hence best given prior to transmission season. It is contraindicated in pregnancy and immunodeficiency.

### Vaccination under Universal Immunization Programme

Cell-culture derived (CCD) live attenuated has been introduced in Universal Immunization Programme (UIP) in 83 endemic districts of UP, Bihar, Assam, West Bengal only 1 dose given with a booster at 1 year to children up to 15 years of age. Not given below 6 months of age due to maternal antibodies interference. Oct 2013: JENVAC–CCD live attenuated vaccine with local strain "SA14-14-2" was indigenously developed by Bharat Biotech, Hyderabad, India.

## CURRENT APPROACH

### Global

WHO responds to JE by:
- Providing recommendations for control of JE, on use of vaccines.
- It recommends immunization against JE in regions where JE is detected.
- Provides support for implementation of immunization programs.
- Provides technical guidance on surveillance in JE.

### National

- Strengthening surveillance activities across the nation on JE and acute encephalitis syndrome.
- Having sentinel surveillance and laboratory facilities for detection.
- JE immunization is a part of routine immunization in areas endemic for JE.

### *Notification to Authorities*

If an outbreak of JE is suspected, it must be reported immediately to the District Health office by means of quickest mode of communication like telephone, e-mail sharing the details of outbreak including investigation and control measures initiated.

**National program:** National Program for Prevention and Control of Japanese Encephalitis/Acute Encephalitis Syndrome is a part of NVBDCP programme which is further discussed under *Chapter 47: Health Policies and Programs in India.*

### Key Points
- Mostly affects children and young adults
- Vector control is a serious challenge for JE simply due to exophilic and exophagic behavior of vectors as insecticidal indoor residual spray (IRS) may not be effective
- As pigs are the amplifying host, hence control methods have to extend to pig population including immunization, slaughtering pig, use of mosquito proof piggeries
- Diagnosis is based on epidemiological and clinical feature
- Definitive diagnosis of JE is done by viral isolation.

## 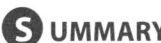 UMMARY

Japanese encephalitis has its natural cycle among vertebrates and mosquitoes and pigs are the main host and water birds have significant role in maintain the natural cycle whereas other animals such as cattle and horse do not play significant role in disease transmission and man is accidental and dead end host. Cases represent the tip of the iceberg of total infected ones. If outbreak is suspected, it must be reported immediately to the local health officials. In India, indigenously developed vaccine by Bharat Biotech, Hyderabad called "JENVAC" has been put to use recently.

## SUGGESTED READING

1. Burke DS, Monath TP. Flaviviruses. In: Knipe DM, Howkey PM (Eds). Fields Virolgy. 4th edition. Philadelphia, PA: Lippincott-Ravin Publishers; 2001. pp. 1043-125.
2. Dhillon GP, Raina VK. Epidemiology of Japanese encephalitis in context with Indian scenario. J Indian Med Assoc. 2008;106:660-3.
3. Diagana M, Preux PM, Dumas M. Japanese encephalitis revisited. J Neurol Sci. 2007;262:165-70.
4. Grossman RA, Edelman R, Chiewanich P, et al. Study of Japanese encephalitis virus in Chiangmai valley, Thailand. II. Human clinical infections. Am J Epidemiol. 1973;98:121-32.
5. Hoke Jr CH, Vaughn DW, Nisalak A, et al. Effect of high-dose dexamethasone on the outcome of acute encephalitis due to Japanese encephalitis virus. J Infect Dis. 1992;165:631-7.
6. Kabilan L, Rajendran R, Arunachalam N, et al. Japanese encephalitis in India: an overview. Indian J Pediatr. 2004;71:609-15.
7. Kabilan L. Control of Japanese encephalitis in India: a reality. Indian J Pediatr. 2004;71:707-12.
8. Miyake M. The pathology of Japanese encephalitis. A review. Bull World Health Organ. 1964;30:153-60.
9. Rajaiah P, Kumar A. Japanese encephalitis virus in India: An update on virus genotypes. Indian J Med Res. 2022;156(4&5):588-597.
10. Tsai TF. Factors in the changing epidemiology of Japanese encephalitis and West Nile fever. In: Saluzzo JF (Ed). Factors in the Emergence of Arboviral Diseases. Amsterdam: Elsevier; 1997. pp. 179-89.
11. WHO (2015). Japanese encephalitis [online]. Available from http://www.who.int/news-room/fact-sheets/detail/japanese-encephalitis.
12. WHO. Japanese Encephalitis; Factsheets. May 2019.
13. World Health Organization country office of India. Guidelines for Prevention and Control of Japanese Encephalitis. New Delhi: Zoonosis division, National Institute of Communicable diseases, Directorate General of Health services; 2019.

---

# EPIDEMIOLOGY OF KALA-AZAR AND ITS PREVENTION AND CONTROL

| | |
|---|---|
| CM7.2 | Enumerate, describe and discuss the mode of transmission and measures for prevention and control of Kala-azar |
| CM8.1 | Describe and discuss the epidemiological and control measures applicable in Kala-azar |

### Case Study

*30-year-old male, presented with prolonged intermittent fever, weight loss, generalized body ache for about 6 months along with yellow discoloration in the eye for 4-5 months. On a general examination he had significant pallor and jaundice. Systemic examination showed severe splenomegaly and hepatomegaly. Malaria test was negative. Bone marrow aspiration revealed LD bodies. He was diagnosed to have kala-azar.*

## INTRODUCTION

A deadliest parasitic disease labeled as NTD, caused by small *Leishmania* protozoan and transmitted by sandflies and is fatal, if remains untreated. Disease is characterized by irregular fever with double rise of temperature, progressive emaciation, anemia and enlargement of spleen and liver. It usually occurs in rural agricultural villages where houses are frequently constructed with mud walls and earthen floors, and cattle and other livestock are kept close to human dwellings.

## HISTORY

People of Assam and Garo hills (1869) called this as kala-azar literally meaning "Black Death". Dr Clarke (1889) published a report about it when whole of the Assam was affected. Sir William Leishman (1903,) discovered the parasite in the blood of the spleen puncture of a soldier who later died due to chronic fever. Donovan in the same year observed the same parasite in the splenic puncture of a patient from Madras and since then parasite is known as *Leishmania donovani* (LD) body.

## PROBLEM STATEMENT

### Global Scenario

The disease has a wide distribution in all continents except Australia. The parasites causing Leishmaniasis are found in 88 countries, mainly in South and Central America, Africa, Asia, and Southern Europe. The disease affects some of the world's poorest people and is associated with malnutrition, population displacement, poor housing, a weak immune system and lack of financial resources. An estimated 700,000 to 1 million new cases occur annually. Only a small fraction of those infected by parasites causing leishmaniasis will eventually develop the disease.

Leishmaniasis is caused by a protozoan parasite from over 20 Leishmania species. There are three main forms of the disease:

1. ***Visceral leishmaniasis (VL),*** also known as kala-azar is fatal, if left untreated in over 95% of cases. It is characterized by irregular bouts of fever, weight loss, enlargement of the spleen and liver and anemia. Most cases occur in Brazil, East Africa and in South-East Asia. An estimated 50,000–90,000 new cases of VL occur worldwide each year with only 25–45% reported to WHO. It has outbreak and mortality potential.
2. ***Cutaneous leishmaniasis (CL):*** Most common form of Leishmaniasis and causes skin lesions, mainly ulcers, on exposed parts of the body, leaving life-long scars and serious disability. It is estimated that 600,000 new cases occur worldwide annually but only around 200,000 are reported to WHO. About 95% of CL cases occur in the Americas, the Mediterranean basin, the Middle East and Central Asia. In 2015 over two-thirds of new CL cases occurred in 6 countries: Afghanistan, Algeria, Brazil, Colombia, Iran, and the Syria.
3. ***Mucocutaneous leishmaniasis (ML)*** leads to partial or total destruction of mucous membranes of the nose, mouth, and throat. Over 90% cases occur in Bolivia, Brazil, Ethiopia and Peru (WHO, Fact Sheets: Leishmaniasis, 2018).

### Indian Scenario

Kala-azar (visceral Leishmaniasis, VL) is a major public health problem affecting the poor sections of the society. In India, an estimated 130 million at risk population in 54 districts of four states where the disease is endemic: Bihar (33 districts, 458 blocks), Jharkhand (4 districts, 33 blocks), West Bengal (11 districts, 120 blocks) and Uttar Pradesh (6 districts, 22 blocks).

Elimination of visceral leishmaniasis as a public health problem in WHO's South-East Asia Region is defined as achieving an annual incidence of less than 1 case per 10,000 population at the district level in Nepal and at the subdistrict level in Bangladesh and India.

The disease was targeted for elimination by 2017. Actually National Health Policy, 2002 had set the goal of kala-azar elimination by the year 2010 which was revised to 2015. Since 1992, after years of accelerated program implementation, the number of kala-azar cases in India has dropped by 97%. Fatalities have fallen from 1419 in 1992 to 58 in 2018. In 2020, only 37 deaths, 4 were reported (July 2021).

## EPIDEMIOLOGY

### Host Factors

#### Socioeconomic Conditions

Poverty increases the risk for *Leishmaniasis*. Poor housing and domestic insanitary conditions (such as a lack of waste management or open sewerage) may increase fly breeding and resting sites, as well as their access to humans. Sandflies are attracted to crowded housing as these provide a good source of blood-meals. Human behavior, such as sleeping outside or on the ground, may increase risk.

#### Age and Gender

About 5–20 years of age are usually affected. Male are affected more than female.

#### Season

More prevalent in the winter and spring after rains.

#### Malnutrition

Diets lacking protein-energy, iron, vitamin and zinc increase the risk that an infection will progress to kala-azar.

#### Population Mobility

Epidemics of both cutaneous and visceral leishmaniasis are often associated with migration and the movement of non-immune people into areas with existing transmission cycles. Occupational exposures as well as widespread deforestation are other important factors.

### Agent Factors

*Leishmania donovani* belonging to family Trypanosomidaeisa minuteuni cellular organism, resides in the reticuloendothelial system (RES) of human body. They feed and multiply by binary fission inside the monocytes, polymorph and endothelial cells of the RES. When the number of parasites inside the cell reaches between 50 and 200, it bursts and liberates the parasite into blood, which again invades the new cell. The cycle continues and the number of parasites goes on increasing. The patient suffering from the disease always bears certain number of these parasites in their blood in *Leishmania* or amastigote form. LD is a ***digenetic parasite,*** i.e., it completes its life cycle in two hosts. The primary host is man whereas the secondary host is sandfly.

### Environmental Factors

The incidence of Leishmaniasis can be affected by changes in urbanization, and the human incursion into forested areas.

### Climate Change

Leishmaniasis is climate-sensitive and has effect on its epidemiology in multiple ways. Changes in temperature, rainfall, and humidity can have strong effects on vectors and reservoir hosts by altering their distribution and influencing their survival and population sizes; small fluctuations in temperature can have a profound effect on the developmental cycle of *Leishmania promastigotes* in sandflies, allowing transmission of the parasite in areas not previously endemic for the disease; drought, famine and flood can lead to massive displacement and migration of people to areas with transmission of *Leishmania,* and poor nutrition could compromise their immunity.

### Vector Bionomics

Over 90 sandflies are known to transmit *Leishmania* parasites. Sandflies are insects belonging to genus *Phlebotomus* and *Sergentomyia.* About 30 species of sandflies have been recorded in India. The important ones are *Phlebotomus argentipes,*

*P. sergenti* and *Sergentomyia punjabensis*. This troublesome nocturnal pest is smaller than mosquitoes of light or dark brown in color and is incapable of flying long distances. They are active during night. In day time they hide in holes and crevices in wall, dark store rooms, stables and dark dense vegetation. While male usually feed upon fruit and plant juices, females require blood meal before ovi position, hence the female alone are actual vector of the disease. They feed up on the blood of wide variety of vertebrates, which include both warm blooded forms, like man, domestic pets, cats, dogs, rodents, cattle, jackal, foxes, domestic birds and cold blooded forms like lizards, snakes, frogs, toads, etc. Among different genus, Sergentomyia frequently feed on avian and reptilian blood and *Phlebotomus* has a liking for human blood.

## Breeding Habits

Sandflies breed in the cracks and crevices in the soil, treeholes, caves, etc., where decaying organic substance are present. Their number is more in rural areas as compared to the urban ones because the conditions for breeding readily exist there. Sandflies generally, remain confined within 50 yards of their breeding place as they simply hop about from one place to another and cannot fly (contrary to the suggestion by their names). Suitable places of breeding are tree holes, rock holes; dark and damp places in the vicinity of cattle shed and poultry farm, etc.

## Mode of Infection

When a sandfly sucks the blood of kala-azar patient, the *Leishmania* or amastigote stage enters the gut of sandfly. Inside the gut, *Leishmania* changes into Leptomonad or promastigote form. Leptomonad form divide by longitudinal binary fission and within 6–9 days becomes ready to be transmitted to a new definitive host (human-beings). On the basis of the site of development of Leptomonad form in the gut of sandfly, three types of development may take place.

The sandfly which subsists on fruit or plant juice after the first blood meal shows a heavy flagellate infection. The buccal cavity of the fly gets completely blocked by the parasites. Bite of such blocked sandflies to human beings; almost invariably causes infection, as in order to take blood meal sandfly has to liberate the parasites into the wound caused by its proboscis. In this way, the infection of kala-azar reaches a man mainly through the bite of the infected sandflies. Transmission may also take place by contamination of the bite wound or by contact when the insect is crushed during the act of feeding.

## Mode of Transmission

It is transmitted to humans and other mammals by phlebotomine sandflies. When sandfly bites; it is crushed on the skin at the point of bite, by the host. Infant do not suffer as they cannot crush the vector during bite. Rarely non vector transmission can also occur by accidental laboratory infection, blood transfusion, or organ transplantation.

## Reservoir

Domestic dogs, rodents, sloths, and opossum.

## Incubation Period

6 weeks to 6 months.

## CLINICAL FEATURES

*Leishmania* species determines which of the main two forms of the Leishmaniasis (CL and VL) will result from infection. Progression, and severity of infection as well as treatment regimen and outcome is dependent on a range of other factors, including parasite strain, characteristics of sandfly saliva, parasite infection with *Leishmania* RNA virus, host genetics, and immunosuppression, particularly due to HIV coinfection. CL typically presents as cutaneous nodules or lesions at the site of the bite(localized cutaneous Leishmaniasis).In some cases, parasites disseminate through the skin and present as multiple nonulcerative nodules [Diffuse Cutaneous Leishmaniasis, (DCL)] or propagate through the lymphatic system resulting in naso-bronchial and buccal mucosal tissue destruction (ML). Localized CL may resolve spontaneously and usually responds well to treatment while VL generally affects the spleen, liver, or other lymphoid tissues, and, if left untreated, is fatal; a fraction of successfully treated VL cases may result in maculopapular or nodular rashes known as **post-kala-azar dermal leishmaniasis**.

## LABORATORY DIAGNOSIS

Diagnosis and treatment of kala-azar now include rapid tests; most widely used is rk39 rapid test which is easy to perform, quick (results in 10–20 minutes), and inexpensive. In VL form, diagnosis is made by combining clinical signs with parasitological or serological tests (such as RDTs). In CL and ML serological tests have limited value and clinical manifestation with parasitological tests confirms the diagnosis.

## PREVENTION AND CONTROL

It requires a combination of intervention strategies because transmission occurs in a complex biological system involving the human host, parasite, sandfly vector and in some causes an animal reservoir host. Key strategies for prevention are listed below.

### Vector Control

To reduce or interrupt transmission of disease by controlling sandflies.

### *Use of Insecticides*

The sandflies can be killed by the use of different types of insecticides. DDT is the first choice as the vector of kala-azar. Phlebotomus argentipes is highly susceptible to this pesticide. A single application of 1–2 $g/m^2$ of DDT or 0.25 $g/m^2$ of Lindane has been found effective in reducing the number of sandflies. DDT residue may remain effective for a period of one to two years while Lindane is effective only for a period of three months. Spraying should be done in cattle shed, around poultry farms and human dwellings. Control methods include insecticide spray, use of insecticide-treated nets, environmental management and personal protection. Effective disease surveillance is important to promptly monitor and take action during epidemics and situations with high case fatality rates under treatment.

Control of animal reservoir hosts is complex and should be tailored to the local situation. Social mobilization and strengthening partnerships–mobilization and education of the community with effective behavioral change interventions must always use locally tailored communication strategies. Partnership and collaboration with various stakeholders and other vector-borne disease control programs is critical.

### *Sanitation*

Mainly include removal of shrubs and vegetation within 50 yards of human dwellings, filling up cracks and crevices in walls and floor of houses. Cattle sheds and poultry houses should be constructed at a fair distance from human habitations.

### *Personal Prophylaxis*

Use of mosquito net or screen (22 meshes in a square inch), avoiding the ground floor for sleeping purposes and periodic fumigation of sleeping quarters.

No vaccines or drugs to prevent infection are available. The best way for travelers to prevent infection is to protect themselves from sandfly bites, follow these preventive measures:
- Avoid outdoor activities especially from dusk to dawn, when sandflies generally are the most active.
- Minimize the amount of exposed (uncovered) skin as per climate or insecticide-treated clothing.
- Apply insect repellent to exposed skin and under the ends of sleeves and pant legs. Follow the instructions on the label of the repellent. The most effective repellents generally are those that contain the chemical DEET (N, N-diethyl met-atoluamide).

### Early Diagnosis and Effective Treatment

It reduces the prevalence of the disease and prevents disabilities and death. It also helps to reduce transmission and to monitor the spread and burden of disease. Currently, there are highly effective and safe anti-Leishmania medicines particularly for visceral Leishmaniasis. Access to these medicines has significantly improved thanks to a WHO-negotiated price scheme and a medicine donation program through WHO. Leishmaniasis is a treatable and curable disease, but requires an immune competent system because medicines will not get rid of the parasite from the body, thus the risk of relapse is always there, if immune suppression occurs. The treatment depends on several factors such as type of disease, concomitant morbidities, parasite species, and geographic location. All patients diagnosed with visceral Leishmaniasis require prompt and complete treatment. Management of DCL and ML cases is more difficult and cases may take considerably longer to resolve. Single dose treatment using Liposomal Amphotericin B (Ambisome) is the main stay of treatment. Second treatment option is combination of paromomycin and miltefosine.

### Other Measures

#### *When Indoors*

Stay in well-screened or air-conditioned areas. Keep in mind that sand flies are much smaller than mosquitoes and therefore can get through smaller holes. The mosquito nets used to prevent mosquito bite may not effective here. Spray living or sleeping areas with an insecticide to kill insects. If you are not sleeping in a well-screened or air-conditioned area, use a bed net and tuck it under your mattress. If possible, use a bed net that has been soaked in or sprayed with a pyrethroid-containing insecticide. The same treatment can be applied to screens, curtains, sheets and clothing should be retreated after five washings.

## CURRENT APPROACHES

### Global

WHO supports nations technically and financially towards elimination of kala-azar. It ensures access to quality medicines for treatment of kala-azar and develops guidelines and evidence-based policies for prevention, control and monitoring of Leishmaniasis.

### National

According to National Health Policy-2002, kala-azar elimination was to be achieved by 2011, later prolonged to 2015. However, the country is still seeing cases of kala-azar at various sites.

India has signed a memorandum along with Bangladesh and Nepal towards elimination of kala-azar from SEAR region. In India, elimination for kala-azar is defined as reducing annual incidence of kala-azar to <1 case/10,000 population at the sub-district (block PHCs).

**National program:** After the resurgence of kala-azar in the 70's the government of India launched the Kala-azar Control Programme in 1990–91 in endemic states. Currently called kala-azar elimination program all activities are carried out through the existing NVBDCP program.

> **Key Points**
> - New tools for diagnosis and treatment of kala-azar include rapid tests and most widely used is the rk39 rapid test which is easy to perform, quick (results in 10–20 minutes), and cheap
> - Prevention and control requires combination of intervention strategies because transmission occurs in a complex biological system
> - DDT is the first choice as the vector of kala-azar Phlebotomus argentipes is highly susceptible to it
> - No vaccines or drugs to prevent infection are available
> - The best way for travelers to prevent infection is to protect themselves from sandfly bites
> - Single dose treatment using Liposomal amphotericin B (AmBisome) is the main stay of treatment.

## SUMMARY

Kala-azar is a slow progressing indigenous disease caused by a protozoan parasite of genus *Leishmania*, primarily infecting the reticuloendothelial system. Man gets affected by bite of sandflies and can present with various forms of Leishmaniasis. Sanitation plays an important role in prevention of the disease by reducing the vector population. Amphotericin B is the mainstay of treatment of an affected individual.

## SUGGESTED READING

1. Alvar J, Vélez ID, Bern C, et al. Leishmaniasis worldwide and global estimates of its incidence. PLoS One. 2012;7(5):e35671.

2. Directorate of National Vector Borne Disease Control Program (2014). National Road Map for Kala-azar Elimination [online]. Available from http:// nvbdcp.gov.in/Doc/Road-map-KA_2014.pdf.
3. WHO, Fact Sheets: Leishmaniasis, 2023.
4. Jongejan F, Uilenberg G. The global importance of ticks. Parasitol. 2004;129(Suppl 1):S3-14.
5. WHO. Visceral leishmaniasis elimination: India gears-up to overcome last-mile challenges. July 2021.
6. Mathers CD, Ezzati M, Lopez AD. Measuring the burden of neglected tropical diseases: the global burden of disease framework. PLoS Negl Trop Dis. 2007;1.
7. Ministry of Health and Family Welfare (2014). National Health Policy 2015 Draft [online]. Available from http://www.nhp.gov.in/sites/default/files/pdf/ draft_national_health_policy_2015.pdf.
8. Murray HW, Berman JD, Davies CR, et al. Advances in leishmaniasis. Lancet. 2005;366(9496):1561-77.
9. Pigott DM, Bhatt S, Golding N, et al. Global distribution maps of the leishmaniases. eLife. 2014;3:e02851.
10. WHO (2018). Leishmaniasis. [online]. Available from http://www. who.int/news-room/fact-sheets/detail/leishmaniasis.

## OTHER VECTOR-BORNE DISEASES

**CM7.2** Enumerate, describe and discuss the mode of transmission and measures for prevention and control of other vector borne diseases

**CM8.1** Describe and discuss the epidemiological and control measures applicable in other vector borne diseases

*Case Study*

*In the month of January, 2020, monkey deaths were reported at a district in Chikkamagaluru, Karnataka. The Viscera samples of the dead monkeys confirmed the presence of the KFD. The ticks samples from the same area showed presence of the KFD virus. Outbreak of KFD was confirmed and people within the vicinity of areas where infected ticks were found were vaccinated and awareness and other preventive measures undertaken.*

### INTRODUCTION

Other vector-borne diseases have less public health significance as some of them are restricted to some specific districts of specific states or few cases occurs but for surveillance and emerging and remerging phenomenon must be under watch. They are mainly louse and tick-borne diseases.
- Kyasanur Forest Disease (KFD)
- Zika Virus
- Crimean–Congo hemorrhagic fever (CCHF)
- Murine typhus or endemic typhus or flea-borne typhus
- Louse-borne epidemic typhus
- Trench fever
- Louse-borne relapsing fever
- Tick-borne relapsing fever
- Rocky Mountain spotted fever
- Rickettsial pox
- Indian tick typhus

Globally, ticks are the important arthropod vectors for transmission of numerous infectious agents and are responsible for causing human and animal diseases. Various wild and domestic animals are reservoir hosts for tick-borne pathogens live stock, pets and humans. Ticks are obligatory blood sucking ecto-parasites that infest mammals, birds, reptiles, and amphibians. Tick-borne diseases are prevalent only in specific risk areas where favorable environmental conditions exist for individual tick species. *Hyalomma anatolicum* and *Haemaphysalis spinigera* are the two important species of ticks present in India, which are responsible for causing the fatal tick-borne viral diseases of CCHF and KFD, respectively. The tick species are widely distributed in different parts of world, including India (**Tables 17E.7** and **17E.8**).

### KYASANUR FOREST DISEASE

#### Introduction

About 80% of the world's tick fauna are hard ticks and the remaining 20% are soft ticks. However, only 10% of the total hard and soft tick species are known to be involved in disease transmission to domestic animals and humans. Ticks suck host blood during their lengthy attachment period (7–14 days); this may extend, depending on the association of the tick species and host. KFD is a zoonotic disease and has so far been localized only in a southern part of India. The exact cause of its emergence in the mid 1950's is not known. It is a febrile arboviral hemorrhagic disease, transmitted by infective ticks. There is antigenic similarity with Russian hemorrhagic fever and role of Siberian migratory birds hence may be targeted as biological weapon for biological warfare. Monkeys and small mammals are common host for KFD hence locally known as "Monkey Fever Disease". Good surveillance system is required to monitor mortality in monkeys.

#### Problem Statement

It was first recognized as a febrile illness and first reported (1957) as fatal epizootic of monkeys in Kyasanur forest in the Shimoga district of Karnataka state of India.

**Table 17E.7:** Detail description of tick-borne diseases (KFDV and CCHFV) in India.

| Virus name | Family/Genus | Tick species | Natural vertebrate host | First isolation |
|---|---|---|---|---|
| CCHFV | Bunyaviridae/ Nairovirus | *Hyalomma marginatum* and *Ixodid* species | Hare | 2011: *Hyalomma anatolicum* pool of ticks collected from domestic animals, Gujarat |
| KFDV | Flaviviridae/ Flavivirus/ | *Haemaphysalis spinigera* and *Ixodid* species | Monkeys (*Semnopithecus entellus*, *Macaca radiata*), rodents, shrews, bats | 1957: Langur, monkey (*Semnopithecus entellus*) moribund adult organs and tissues, Kyasanur Forest Baragi village, Karnataka |

(CCHFV: Crimean-Congo hemorrhagic fever; KFDV: Kyasanur forest disease virus)

Table 17E.8: Clinical, diagnostic and hematologic description of tick-borne viral disease in India.

| Disease | Phase of illness | Post onset days | Diagnostic test | Disease signs and symptoms | Hematological changes | CFR (%) |
|---|---|---|---|---|---|---|
| KFD | Acute | 2–7 days | IgM ELISA, virus isolation (in vitro and in vivo), RT-PCR and real-time RT-PCR | Fever, cephalalgia, myalgia, diarrhea, cough, hepatomegaly, splenomegaly, epistaxis, bradycardia, oral and intestinal hemorrhage, menigoencephalitis | Leukopenia, thrombocytopenia, neutropenia, eosinopenia, elevated liver enzymes | 2–10% |
| | Convalescent phase | 8–12 day | IgM ELISA | | | |
| CCHF | Acute phase | 1–7 days | RT-PCR and real-time RT-PCR (1–10 days), IgM ELISA (4 days–4 months), virus isolation (in vitro): 1–7 days | Fever, myalgia, arthralgia, dizziness, malaise, mucosal hemorrhage, hemorrhagic rash, multi-organ failure, disseminated intravascular coagulopathy | Leukocytopenia, thrombocytopenia, increase clotting times, increased pro-inflammatory cytokines/chemokines, elevated-liver enzymes | 3–60% |
| | Convalescent phase | 7–12 days can extend up to 4 months | IgM ELISA, IgG ELISA (7 days onwards) | | | |

(ELISA: enzyme-linked immunosorbent assay; RT-PCR: reverse transcriptase polymerase chain reaction)

During 1957-2012, KFDV activity was limited to Shimoga, Chikmagalur, Uttara Kannada, Dakshina Kannada and Udupi districts of Karnataka State.

In 2012, KFD cases were reported in Nilgiris of Tamil Nadu.

During 2013-2015, confirmed cases were reported from Wayanad, Malappuram, Palakkad and Nilambur districts of Kerala State.

Some cases were reported from Sattari taluk of Goa during 2015.

During 2016, KFD cases were reported from Dodamarg and Sindhudurg districts of Maharashtra and Dharbandora taluk of Goa.

The number of cases increased in 2017 from Dodamarg, Sawantwadi, Sindhudurg districts of Maharashtra and Valpoi, Pernem, Dharbandora taluk of Goa state.

Cases from Karnataka were reported regularly during these years. Since the last seven decades, the virus activity was known only in Karnataka and for the past five years the cases have been reported from adjacent States of Karnataka such as Tamil Nadu, Kerala, Goa and Maharashtra. This is a cause of concern considering the similar ecology of the affected areas, which are all situated in the Western Ghats. It is not clear whether these areas are endemic or disease has spread due to movement of monkeys and small rodents (those harbour ticks), which act as reservoir for the virus. Rodents develop very low-level of asymptomatic viral load in their system, which is sufficient to transmit infection to vector tick during blood meals. Earlier sero-surveillance studies have reported positivity in Gujarat, West Bengal and Andaman Nicobar Islands.

## Epidemiology

### Host Factors

Age group commonly affected is between 20 and 40 years.

### Agent Factors

Group B Toga (flavi) virus. The causative agent, KFD virus (KFDV), is a highly pathogenic member in the family Flaviviridae, producing a hemorrhagic disease in infected human beings.

### Reservoir

Monkeys and small mammals are common host for KFD. Infection with KFDV may cause epizootic in high primate with high fatality. Rats, mice, squirrels, birds and bats are less important host. Larger animal like cattle, sheep, and goat may be infected but play limited role in disease transmission. Monkeys are amplifier, but ineffective as maintenance host as most of them die due to the infection.

### Environmental Factors

KFD, a tick-borne viral hemorrhagic fever that occurs as seasonal outbreaks during January–June.

### Modes of Transmission

Bites of tick's transmission to human occurs once the infected tick bites or contact animal, most commonly sick or dead monkey. No person-to-person infection occurs, human are dead end infection. Human cases occur in dried summer (November-June) in south west and south India. Local residents visiting-collect fire wood may acquire the infection through tick bite. People with recreational exposure to rural and outdoor setting (farmer, hunter, road making charcoal) in Karnataka State, South India are potentially at risk of infection. Man-man transmission does not occur.

### Vector

Hard or soft ticks (species *Haemaphysalis*). The hard tick *Haemaphysalis spinigera* is the reservoir and vector of KFD, once infected will pass the infection (KFDV) to their off-spring via eggs.

### Incubation Period

3–8 days.

## Clinical Features

Some of the initial phase symptoms include persistent headaches, fever, and muscle weakness. However, the neurological symptoms begin to appear only in the second phase of the viral attack. At this stage, viral encephalopathy, meningoencephalitis, or even meningitis could manifest and lead to vast deficits.

## Case Definition

There is variability in clinical illness associated with KFD infection and the lack of data available on clinical diagnosis of KFD, it is essential to emphasize the importance of laboratory confirmation of the disease.

"A patient of any age presenting with acute fever, headache and myalgia, and a history of exposure to ticks and/or a visit to a forest area and/or living in a KFD-endemic area particularly forest in Karnataka".

### Suspected Case

Patient, within a radius of 5 km surrounding the villages reporting recent monkey deaths or laboratory confirmed KFD cases, with sudden onset of high fever and one the following: headache or myalgia.

### Probable Case

A clinically compatible illness that does not meet the SOPs for a confirmed definition, but with one of the following: epidemiological link to a documented exposure to a KFD affected area (one or more of the following exposures within the 3 weeks before onset of symptoms). Positive result on testing of clinical serum specimens using the immunoglobulin M (IgM) ELISA.

### Confirmed Case

A case that fulfills the criteria for a probable KFD case and in addition it should cover any of the following:
- Exposure to secretions from a confirmed acute or convalescent case of viral hemorrhagic fever (VHF) within 10 days of onset of symptoms
- Isolation of KFDV in cell culture or in a mouse model, from blood or tissues.
- Detection of KFDV-specific genetic sequence by RT-PCR or real time RT-PCR from blood or tissues.

## Diagnosis

In the KFD-endemic area of Karnataka state, India, the differential diagnosis should include consideration of influenza, typhoid and rickettsial group of fevers, e.g. Q-fever and mite-borne typhus in mild cases, and malaria, leptospirosis in moderate to severe cases.

***Hospital laboratory testing:*** The following tests should be performed on blood samples from enrolled patients, according to standard hospital procedures:
- *Complete blood count (CBC):* Total leukocytic count (TLC) or differential leukocyte count (DLC), hemoglobin level and platelet counts
- *Liver function tests (LFT):* Aspartate aminotransferase (AST) or alanine aminotransferase (ALT), serum bilirubin, alkaline phosphatase
- Serum electrolytes, blood urea, serum creatinine
- Smear for malaria parasite or malaria RDT

## Prevention and Control of Tick-borne Diseases

***Vaccination:*** Vaccination with formalin-inactivated tissue-culture vaccine has been the primary strategy for controlling KFD. The formalin-inactivated KFDV vaccine produced in chick embryo fibroblasts is currently in use in the endemic areas in Karnataka state of India. The vaccine was found to be immunogenic, potent, stable and safe. The production of inactivated vaccines carries the inherent risk of utilizing large quantities of potentially highly pathogenic viruses and the possibility of incomplete inactivation of viruses. In addition, vaccines based on inactivated viruses as antigens have shown a certain level of adverse reactions, especially in children, and this has to be carefully balanced with their efficacy and durability. The strategy involves mass vaccination in areas reporting KFD activity [i.e. laboratory evidence of KFD virus (KFDV) in monkeys, humans, or ticks] and in villages within a 5-km radius of such areas. For population at risk killed or live attenuated KFD vaccine. Two vaccine doses are administered at least 1 month apart to persons 7–65 years of age. Vaccine-induced immunity is short-lived, so the first booster dose of vaccine is recommended within 6–9 months after primary vaccination; thereafter, annual booster doses are recommended for 5 years after the last confirmed case in the area.

***Control of vector (Ticks):*** Destruction of infected ticks would necessitate control of ticks throughout the entire forest area, but is not technically and economically feasible. This is the main reason why, once focus of this disease becomes established in any biotope, it cannot be eliminated easily. As association of human infections in the vicinity of dead monkeys has been shown, and the use of spray insecticides has been recommended in a 50-m radius around a dead monkey. However, although recommendations have been made for spraying of insecticides around the place of monkey death, it is technically difficult in certain inaccessible areas to transport the large volumes of water needed for the spray. Economic and logistical problems associated with regular insecticide spray in a large area makes implementation of a control program difficult. Under these circumstances, the prevention of tick bites by the use of repellents should be considered. Aircraft-mounted equipment to spray in hot spots-using Fenthion, Propoxur.

## Current Approaches–National

The strategies in place are:
- *Surveillance:* Human surveillance, Monkey surveillance and Tick surveillance
- Vaccination as required
- Routine IEC activities at hot spots
- Tick control measures
- *Inter-sectoral co-ordination between the various stakeholders:* Health department, Veterinary Public Health department, Forest and Wild life departments, Vector control division, District administration, Tribal welfare, Fire control departments, and many more are the key stake holders in its control.

> **Key Points**
> - Infected Ticks can cause arboviral hemorrhagic fever.
> - KFD is a tick borne (hard tick) diseases typically restricted to South India.
> - Enzootic cycle of KFD is maintained by many small rodents, shrews, insectivorous bats and birds.
> - The Ixodius hard tick are the reservoirs and vectors of thr disease.
> - Cattle are important to maintain the tick population.

## SUMMARY

KFD is a re-emerging zoonotic disease. An outbreak is preceded by monkey deaths. As of now, KFD is found only in India especially in South India. Man happens to be an incidental dead end host of the disease. The epidemic usually peaks between January and April. For diagnosis, human blood sample, monkey viscera and tick samples are required from suspected areas. There is no specific treatment available. Vaccine that is currently available is a formalin inactivated vaccine. Tick control in cattle and domestic animals will reduce density of tick population.

## CRIMEAN-CONGO HEMORRHAGIC FEVER

Crimean-Congo hemorrhagic fever is a disease caused by a tick-borne virus (*Nairovirus*), belonging to the Bunyaviridae family. The infection leads to intense viral hemorrhagic fever outbreaks. The case fatality rate as high as 10–40% (CDC, Control and Prevention: CCHF). The disease got its name from the place where it was first identified, i.e., Crimea, in the year 1944 and in Congo in the year 1969. Historically, epidemics of CCHF have occurred during World War II in the Crimea provided the first modern recognition. The causative agent of the disease was finally isolated in newborn mice in 1968.

### Problem Statement

Crimean-Congo hemorrhagic fever is frequently found in the Eastern part of Europe, predominantly in the previous Soviet Union, all over the Mediterranean, in Northwestern part of China, Central part of Asia, Southern part of Europe, Africa, the Middle East, and also in the Indian subcontinent.

### Epidemiology

#### Agent Factors

Crimean-Congo hemorrhagic fever is a prevalent disease, which is caused by a tick-borne virus (*Nairovirus*), belonging to the Bunyaviridae family.

#### Host Factors

***Risk groups:*** The CCHF virus gets transmitted through tick bites or contact with infected animal blood or tissues. This exposure happens typically in people involved in slaughter, dealing with livestock, agriculture workers and veterinarians. Those people and international travelers who come in contact with the livestock in endemic areas may be exposed as well.

#### Reservoir

Ixodid (hard) ticks, particularly those belonging to the genus, *Hyalomma*, act as a reservoir as well as a vector for the CCHF virus. Several wild as well as domestic animals, like, cattle, sheep, goats, and hares, function as amplifying hosts.

#### Mode of Transmission

It is transmitted to humans from animals by contact to infected ticks or animal blood. Human to human transmission may occur by contact with blood or body fluids. Inappropriate sterilization of medical equipment has also been shown to spread the infection.

### Incubation Period

- Its length primarily depends on how the infection is acquired.
- If the virus is acquired through a tick bite, typically the incubation period is 1–3 days, and a maximum of 9 days.
- If the route of infection is through infected blood or tissues, the incubation period is 5–6 days, and a maximum of 13 days, as per documented evidence.

### Clinical Features

- There is sudden onset of the following symptoms:
  - Fever
  - Myalgia
  - Dizziness
  - Neck pain, stiffness
  - Backache
  - Headache
  - Photophobia
  - There may also be other constitutional symptoms like, nausea, vomiting, diarrhea, pain in abdomen and sore throat, etc.
  - These initial symptoms precede the onset of acute mood swings and confusion.
- After 2–4 days, this initial agitational behavior would be replaced by contrast behavior like sleepiness, depression, and lethargy.
- Moreover, the generalized abdominal pain may get localized to the right upper quadrant, with detectable hepatomegaly.
- Other clinical signs include:
  - Tachycardia
  - Lymphadenopathy
  - Enlarged lymph nodes
  - Petechial rash on mucosal surfaces which may progress to ecchymoses, and
  - Other hemorrhagic manifestations.
- In the later course of the illness, with rise in the intensity there are evidences of multiorgan involvement with rapid kidney deterioration, acute liver failure, and pulmonary failure. These are observed mostly after the fifth day of illness. Around 30% mortality rate has been reported in CCHF in which death occurs in the second week of the illness.
- In those who demonstrate recovery, the improvement usually manifests from the ninth or tenth day after the onset of illness.
- In the reports of CCHF outbreaks, there is a wide range of fatality rates in the hospitalized patients, ranging from as low as 9% to as high as 50%. Since no studies have been conducted on long-term effects of CCHF infection in the survivors, it is difficult to determine, if any specific complications exist. However, recovery is slow.

### Diagnosis

- The diagnosis is essentially based on laboratory confirmation since the signs and symptoms are shared by many other viral hemorrhagic illnesses.
- Laboratory tests used are:
  - Antigen-capture ELISA
  - Real time-PCR (RT-PCR)
  - Virus isolation attempts
  - Detection of antibody by ELISA (IgG and IgM)

- Reverse transcriptase-PCR (RT-PCR) assay
- Virus isolation by cell culture.
- Laboratory diagnosis in patients in the initial period of illness with suspected CCHF through clinical history can be made by using the combination of detection of the viral antigen (ELISA antigen capture), viral RNA sequence (RT-PCR) in the blood or in tissues collected from a fatal case and virus isolation.
- Immunohistochemical staining can be used to demonstrate the viral antigen in formalin-fixed tissues.
- In the later phases of infection, in the survivors, antibodies can be found in the blood. But antigen, viral RNA and virus are absent and undetectable.
- Since the patient samples of CCHF used for laboratory tests pose significant biohazard, they must be handled with maximum caution. Nevertheless, if the samples are inactivated (e.g., using virucides, gamma rays, formaldehyde, heat, etc.), then they can be handled in a setting with basic biosafety.

### Treatment
- Treatment for CCHF is chiefly supportive.
- Care includes vigilant attention to fluid and electrolyte balance, oxygenation and hemodynamic support, and appropriate care for prevention and treatment of secondary infections.
- The virus has been found to be sensitive in vitro to the antiviral drug ribavirin, which has been used in the treatment of CCHF patients with some benefit.

### Prevention
- ***Control of CCHF in animals and ticks:***
  - It is quite challenging to prevent or control the infection of CCHF in animals and ticks. This is because the tick-animal-tick cycle commonly goes unnoticed and unapparent infections occur in domestic animals. And there is abundance of the tick vectors, which worsens the situation.
  - Thus, controlling the ticks with acaricides (chemicals used to kill ticks) is the choice for facilities with well-managed livestock production.
  - No vaccine is available for use in animals.
- ***Risk reduction for infection in people:***
  - Public health advice should be focused on the following aspects:
    - Risk reduction of tick-to-human transmission:
      - Using protective clothing like those with long sleeves, long trousers
      - Wearing light colored clothes which will aid in easy detection of ticks on the clothes
      - Using correct acaricides and repellant on skin and clothing
      - Regular examination of clothes and skin for ticks; and safe removal of the same if found
      - Elimination or control of tick infestations on the animals or in stables and barns
      - Avoiding places with plenty of ticks as well as seasons when they are the most active.
    - Risk reduction of transmission from animal to human:
      - Using gloves and other protective clothing at the time of handling animals or their materials, especially in the endemic areas. More so, notably during the process of slaughtering, butchering, and culling either in slaughterhouses or at home.
      - Quarantine of the animals before they enter slaughterhouses.
      - Treating the animals routinely with pesticides 2 weeks before slaughter.
    - Risk reduction of human-to-human transmission:
      - Avoiding any kind of close physical contact with people infected with CCHF.
      - Taking personal protective measures, like wearing gloves and using proper equipment while taking care of the sick.
      - Adequate washing hands after caring for or visiting ill people.
      - At present, there is no safe and efficacious vaccine available. Although an inactivated, mouse brain-derived vaccine that has been developed is being used on a small scale in Eastern Europe.
      - Hence, the primary mode of reducing the risk of acquiring the infection is by raising the awareness regarding the disease and enabling the people to take utmost preventive measures.
    - Control of the infection in healthcare facilities.
    - All the standard infection control measures should be strictly followed by all the healthcare providers who are involved in the care of either suspected or confirmed cases of CCHF.
    - These include:
      - Following basic hand hygiene
      - Using personal protective equipment
      - Following safe injection practices
      - Observing safe burial practices
      - Cautiously handling the samples taken from the patient, by the trained staff working in suitably equipped laboratories.

## SUMMARY

Crimean-Congo hemorrhagic fever is a prevalent disease, which is caused by a tick-borne virus (*Nairovirus*), belonging to the Bunyaviridae family. The infection leads to intense viral hemorrhagic fever outbreaks. This has case fatality rate as high as 10–40%.

**Transmission:** Human to human transmission may occur by contact with blood or body fluids. Inappropriate sterilization of medical equipment has also been shown to spread the infection.

Typically the incubation period is 1–3 days, which may be as long as 9 days.

**Clinical features:**
- Fever
- Myalgia
- Dizziness
- Neck pain, stiffness
- Backache
- Headache
- Photophobia
- There may also be other constitutional symptoms like, nausea, vomiting, diarrhea, pain in abdomen and sore throat, etc.

The diagnosis is essentially based on laboratory confirmation since the signs and symptoms are shared by many other viral hemorrhagic illnesses.
- Laboratory tests used are:
  - Antigen-capture ELISA
  - Real time-PCR (RT-PCR)
- *Treatment* for CCHF is chiefly supportive.

**Prevention:** Includes control of ticks and following standard precaution.

## SUGGESTED READING

1. Akram SM, Tyagi I. Rickettsia Akari (Rickettsial pox). Stat Pearls Publishing LLC; 2018.
2. CDC (2015). Tick-borne Relapsing Fever (TBRF) [online]. Available from https://www.cdc.gov/relapsing-fever/index.html.
3. CDC (2018). Rocky Mountain Spotted Fever (RMSF) [online]. Available from https://www.cdc.gov/rmsf/#whatis.
4. DHR-ICMR guidelines for diagnosis and management of rickettsial diseases in INDIA. Available from https://www.icmr.nic.in/sites/default/files/guidelines/DHR-ICMR%20Guidelines%20on%20Ricketesial%20Diseases.pdf.
5. ECDC (2019). Facts about louse-borne relapsing fever [online]. Available from https://ecdc.europa.eu/en/louse-borne-relapsing-fever/facts.
6. Geevarghese G, Mishra AC. Hemaphysalis ticks of India. 1st edition. United States: Elsevier; 2011.
7. Ghosh S, Azhahianambi P, Fuente J. Control of ticks of ruminants, with special emphasis on livestock farming systems in India: present and future possibilities for integrated control—a review. Experiment. Appl Acarol. 2006;40:49-66.
8. Kasabi GS, Murhekar MV, Sandhya VK, et al. Coverage and effectiveness of Kyasanur Forest disease (KFD) vaccine in Karnataka, South India, 2005–10. PLoS Negl Trop Dis. 2013;7:e2025.
9. Munivenkatappa A, Sahay RR, Yadav PD, Viswanathan R, Mourya DT. Clinical and epidemiological significance of Kyasanur forest disease. Indian J Med Res. 2018;148(2):145-150.
10. Parola P, Paddock CD, Raoult D. Tick-borne rickettsioses around the world: Emerging diseases challenging old concepts. Clin Microbiol Rev. 2005;18(4):719-56.
11. Parola P, Raoult D. Ticks and tick-borne bacterial diseases in humans: an emerging infectious threat. Clin Infect Dis. 2001;32:897-928.
12. Sharma A, Mishra B. Rickettsial disease existence in India: resurgence in outbreaks with the advent of 20th century. Indian J Health Sci Biomed Res. 2020;13:5-10.
13. WHO. (2018). HO South-East Asia Journal of Public Health [online]. Available from http://www.searo.who.int/publications/journals/seajph/seajphv3n1p8.pdf.
14. Yadav PD, Gurav YK, Mistry M, et al. Emergence of Crimean-Congo hemorrhagic fever in Amreli District of Gujarat State, India, Juneto July 2013. Int J Infect Dis. 2014;18:97-1000.

# RICKETTSIAL DISEASES

**CM7.2** Enumerate, describe and discuss the modes of transmission and measures for prevention and control of Rickettsial diseases

**CM8.1** Describe and discuss the epidemiological and control measures of Rickettsial diseases

## INTRODUCTION

It is the most important disease caused by *Rickettesia* as a public health problem so during the 1st and 2nd World War. In 1829, it was first time differentiated from typhoid fever by French physician Louis. Four principal diseases in the typhus group have been classified as per vector involved. The microorganism *Rickettesia* is the intermediate in character between virus and bacteria and they only grow in living tissue and do not grow in ordinary media.

## PROBLEM STATEMENT

### Global Scenario

Rickettsia are one of the most neglected tropical diseases. Data from countries with existing surveillance systems, i.e., South Korea, Japan, China, and Thailand have been reporting increase in incidence in scrub typhus. It is also widely distributed around Asia. If not treated Scrub typhus can lead to a median mortality of 6% and 1.4% in treated individuals. It has been noted that both scrub typhus and murine typhus cause a good proportion of pyrexia of unknown origin in many tropical countries.

### Indian Scenario

During 1960's and 1970's scrub typhus was endemic in many parts of India. There was a gap of another 20 years where it was thought that the disease ceased to exist when cases started getting reported in 1990 amongst the Indian soldiers at the Pakistan border. Since the year 2000 there have been many outbreaks reported across the country. Most of the reported cases are scrub typhus, murine typhus and the Indian tick typhus. Scrub typhus is the most common amongst the reported variety. The disease has been reported from various parts of the country, i.e., Himachal Pradesh, Jammu and Kashmir, Uttarakhand, Rajasthan, Assam, Maharashtra, West Bengal, Kerala, Tamil Nadu, Karnataka.

## EPIDEMIOLOGY

### Host Factors

All ages and both sexes are susceptible to infection. However, the incidence is more in men compared to women due to increased outdoor activity. The disease is also common amongst children.

### Agent Factors

There are various agents of rickettsia causing the different types of rickettsial disease in man **(Table 17E.9)**.

### Environmental Factors

*Seasonal trends:* Outbreaks are more common during climatic conditions that favor increase in vector density. More common between August to November. This is more so with mites the eggs hatch into larva during the post monsoon humidity.

### Mode of Spread

Louse becomes infected by sucking blood from its host after the organism gains entry into the stomach of louse where it multiplies rapidly and fills the surface cells of the intestinal tract and appears in the feces' in 3–5 days after a feed on infected person. The infected louse bites a person makes a small puncture in the skin and defecates at the site of bite and inoculates himself with infected feces.

## DIAGNOSIS

Typical signs and symptoms are sudden onset of fever with headache and eruptions appear on 4th day.

Table 17E.9: Epidemiological description of other vector borne diseases.

| Disease | Vector | Agent | Clinical features | Lab diagnosis | Treatment |
|---|---|---|---|---|---|
| Murine typhus Or Endemic tyhus Or Flea borne typhus | Flea- Xenopsylla cheopis | R. prowazekii | Abdominal pain, backache, rash and fever that may last up to 2 weeks, dry cough, headache, joint/muscle pain, nausea and vomiting | PCR and fluorescent antibody testing | Doxycycline |
| Louse-borne epidemic typhus | Louse—P. humanus corporis | Rickettsia prowazekii | Severe headache, high fever, cough, rash severe muscle pain, chills, falling blood pressure, stupor, sensitivity to light, delirium and death | IFA, ELISA or PCR positive after 10 days | Tetracycline, chloramphenicol doxycyclline |
| Trench fever | Louse (Pediculus humanus corporis) | Rochalimea quintana | Fever, rashes and splenomegaly | Blood culture | Macrolide/ doxycycline |
| Louse-borne relapsing fever | Louse (Pediculus humanus corporis) | Borrelia recurrentis | Fever chills, headaches, muscle or joint aches, and nausea | Direct identification in the stained (Giemsa) | Tetracycline, penicillin G, erythromycin or chloramphenicol |
| Tick-borne relapsing fever | Soft ticks Ornithodoros species | Bacterial spirochete species including Borrelia hermsii (most common) Borrelia parkeri, or Borrelia turicatae | High fever headache, muscle and joint aches | Sample of blood under microscope | Antibiotics |
| Rocky Mountain spotted fever | Tick: Dermacentor ticks | Rickettsia | Fever/nausea, emesis, headache muscle pain, lack of appetite | Low platelet count and blood sodium concentration elevated liver enzyme serology testing and skin biopsy are considered to be the best methods of diagnosis. Although immunofluorescent antibody assays | Tetracycline, chloramphenicol |
| Rickettsial pox | House mouse mite, Liponyssoides sanguineus | R. akari | Triad of fever, rash and eschar | 4-fold rise (convalescent titers) complement fixation or indirect fluorescent antibodies using spotted fever group as antigens | Doxycycline |
| Indian tick typhus | Brown dog tick, Rhipicephalus sanguineus | Rickettsia conori | Headache, fever, arthralgia maculopapular rash, eschar at the site of bite | Based on signs and symptoms and h/o of exposure | Tetracycline |

## Serological Test

**Weil-Felix reaction:** Serum from typhus patient will agglutinate suspension of proteus OX 19 and this test is positive after 1st week.

## PREVENTION AND CONTROL OF RICKETTSIAL DISEASES

- Notification of the first case to the nearest health facility.
- Isolation of the patients after diagnosis.
- All contacts should be kept under medical supervision for 2 weeks.
- Vaccination with Cox's vaccine–formalin killed *Rickettsia* developed in chick embryo.
- Delousing measures with 5 cc DDT powder or emulsion.

Avoid infestation with body lice as transmission of the body lice primarily occurs by direct contact with an infected person, also occurs through fomites, like clothes or bedding. Body lice infestations are linked to low socioeconomic status, overcrowding and improper personal hygiene (homeless and migrants). Lice multiply rapidly and a population can increase by 11% per day. They are found on clothing close to the human skin. Discarding infected clothes is an effective way to control the infestation. If this is not possible, steam disinfection of clothing along with sun drying or washing it at a temperature of 60°C or above.

### During Outbreaks

Dusting powder with an appropriate insecticide has been applied to obtain a rapid decrease of infested persons with some lasting benefits.

### Other Measures

About 10% DDT powder dusting of garments, anti-lice shampoo- permethrin 1%, fenitrothion, delamethrin.

### Key Points

- Epidemiological transition refers to gross changes in the diseases causing morbidity and mortality from communicable to noncommunicable in nature.
- The key identified factors for the epidemiological transition are tobacco use, physical inactivity, the harmful use of alcohol, and unhealthy diet.
- From point of view of prevention, these risk factors may be divided as modifiable or nonmodifiable.
- Web of causation refers to complex interactions between various risk factors, ultimately leading to development of disease in question.

### SUMMARY

Rickettsial diseases are the most coveted emerging and re-emerging infections. Human beings are accidental hosts. Spotted fever group and the typhus group are the most common. They are difficult to diagnose and adequate probing into history on exposure to vector along with understanding the epidemiology are important for early diagnosis. The disease, if manifests into a severe form can result in high morbidity, hence requires extensive workup for PUO (Pyrexia of Unknown Origin). Treatment for rickettsia is easily available and shows dramatic results. Control and prevention of man vector contact is of utmost importance.

# F. EPIDEMIOLOGY OF BLOOD-BORNE DISEASES AND ITS PREVENTION AND CONTROL

*Abhik Sinha, Palash Das, Sukamal Bisoi, Dibakar Haldar*

## INTRODUCTION

We know from the concept of dynamic transmission of disease that a communicable disease is transmitted from one person to other person or from an animal to a man or vice versa. The same principle is observed in blood-borne diseases.

The disease agent uses the blood or other body fluid as a good vehicle or medium for its survival, multiplication, and transmission from one person to another person. A blood-borne disease is spread through contamination by blood and also other body fluids infected with microorganisms. Microorganisms such as viruses or bacteria are blood-borne pathogens, they exist in blood and other body fluids and they are carried in blood from one person to other and can cause disease in these new infected people.

Exposures to blood and other body fluids occur through a wide variety of activities. Healthcare workers and their assistants, emergency response and public safety personnel, and other workers dealing with blood and blood products can be exposed to blood through needlestick and other sharps injuries, broken mucous membrane, and skin exposures.

The pathogens of primary concern are hepatitis B virus (HBV), hepatitis C virus (HCV), and the human immunodeficiency virus (HIV). ***HIV is dealt in next Sub-Chapter: Epidemiology of contact diseases***.

Healthcare workers and employers should take advantage of available engineering controls to prevent their possibility of infection. Universal precautionary measures in everyday work maintaining standard workplace precautions and their practices are desirable to prevent exposure to blood and other body fluids.

## EPIDEMIOLOGY OF HEPATITIS B AND ITS PREVENTION AND CONTROL

| | |
|---|---|
| CM7.2 | Enumerate, describe and discuss the mode of transmission and measures for prevention and control of Hepatitis B |
| CM8.1 | Describe and discuss the epidemiological and control measures applicable in Hepatitis B |

## INTRODUCTION

Hepatitis B is a viral infection that attacks the liver and can cause inflammation of liver resulting in both acute and chronic disease. The virus is transmitted through contact with the blood (transfusion transmission) or other body fluids (saliva, menstrual, vaginal, and seminal fluids, etc.) of an infected person. Hepatitis B is an important occupational hazard for healthcare workers. However, it can be prevented by safe and effective vaccine.

A vaccine against hepatitis B has been available for a quite longtime. The vaccine is highly (95%) effective in preventing infection and the development of chronic liver disease and liver cancer due to this hepatitis B.

## PROBLEM STATEMENT

Hepatitis B is an endemic disease and its existence poses a problem in most of the countries of the world.

### Global Situation

Approximately 2 billion people are affected by HBV worldwide. Chronic infection with hepatitis B may be defined as hepatitis B surface antigen (HBsAg) positive for at least 6 months.

WHO estimates that 296 million people were living with chronic hepatitis B infection in 2019 with 1.5 million new infections each year. In 2019, hepatitis B resulted in an estimated 820,000 deaths, mostly from cirrhosis and hepatocellular carcinoma (primary liver cancer).

Hepatitis B is a major global health problem. The burden of infection is highest in the WHO Western Pacific Region and the WHO African Region, where 116 million and 81 million people, respectively, are chronically infected. WHO South-East Asia Region reported 18 million cases.

About 1% of persons living with HBV infection (2.7 million people) are also infected with HIV. Conversely, the global prevalence of HBV infection in HIV-infected persons is 7.4%. Since 2015, WHO has recommended treatment for everyone diagnosed with HIV infection, regardless of the stage of disease.

According to latest WHO estimates, the proportion of children under-five years of age chronically infected with HBV dropped to just under 1% in 2019 down from around 5% in the pre-vaccine era ranging from the 1980s to the early 2000s (WHO; 2023).

An estimated 84% coverage by hepatitis B dose of vaccine was found and 97% of countries integrated hepatitis B vaccine in routine immunization (WHO, Fact Sheets: Hepatitis B, 2017).

The overall prevalence of hepatitis B infection varies from country to country. Depending upon the HBsAg positivity the world has been divided into three areas (Puri P et al., J Clin Exp Hepatol, 2014).

1. The disease may be found relatively rare and it is acquired primarily in adulthood with a prevalence of HBsAg positive less than 2% among population. The areas where prevalence rate is less than 2% are called *low endemicity areas*. North America, West Europe, and Australia including Nepal and Sri Lanka fall in this group.
2. In Asia and most of Africa, HBV infection is common and usually acquired perinatally or in childhood with a prevalence of HBsAg positive 2–7% (with an average of 4%) *in intermediate endemicity areas*. India, Bhutan, Indonesia, Maldives, Japan, and East Europe fall in this group.
3. Prevalence rate of HBsAg may be more than or equal to 8% up to 20% in some countries including Bangladesh, Myanmar, Thailand, Korea, Russia, China, part of Africa, etc. These countries may be called *high endemicity areas*.

### India

All subtypes of viral hepatitis have been reported by National Health Profile, 2018. The NHP has reported a total of 145,970 cases and about 451 acute hepatitis B related deaths. Of these 81,966 were males and 64,004 were females and the death rates among males and females was found to be 314 and 137 respectively.

Based on the prevalence of hepatitis B surface antigen, different areas of the world are classified as high (≥8%), intermediate (2–7%) or low HBV endemicity. India falls under the category of intermediate endemicity zone (average of 4%). Hepatitis B surface antigen (HBsAg) positivity in the general population ranges from 1.1% to 12.2%, with an average prevalence of 3–4%. Chronic HBV infection accounts for 40–50% of hepatocellular carcinoma (HCC) and 20–30% cases of cirrhosis.

The transmission of HBV in India is primarily through horizontal and to a lesser extent via perinatal transmission. The outcome of HBV infection depends upon the age of infection. In case of vertical transmission among newborns the risk of chronicity is higher (>90%), around 30% in children aged 2–5 years and this is very low (<5%) in adults. The blood related or body fluid-related transmission may be seen at any age through transfusion of infected blood or blood products, intravenous drug use, unsafe therapeutic injections, occupational injuries, or nosocomial transmission during healthcare-related procedures such as surgery, hemodialysis, and organ transplantation.

> **Key Points**
> - Hepatitis refers to an inflammation of liver caused by a viral agent—HBV
> - Approximately 2 billion people are affected by HBV worldwide
> - Depending upon the HBsAg positivity the world has been divided into three areas—high, intermediate and low endemicity areas. India belongs to intermediate endemicity area
> - The outcome of HBV infection depends upon the age of affection; the risk of chronicity is higher in case of vertical transmission.

## EPIDEMIOLOGY

### Host Factors

Human beings are the only natural host for HBV.
- *Age:* All ages are susceptible to HBV infection. HBVs are strictly species specific and they are hepatoautotrophic. Outcomes of HBV infection depend upon age of infection. The age of infection with HBV is inversely proportional to the adverse outcomes, higher the age at infection lesser is the risk of chronic infection. However, fulminant hepatitis is more common among adults which significantly contributes to mortality rates due to HBV infection in adults. Infection in adulthood leads to chronic hepatitis in less than 5% of cases. Conversely, fulminant infections are seen very low among infants, low in children and very high in adults. Mortality is high in fulminant HBV infection.
- *Sex:* Both sexes are susceptible, however, men are more often found to carry HBsAg infection in adults aged 35 years and above compared to the females.
- *Ethnicity:* The seroprevalence of chronic HBV infection is found high in migrant populations particularly among those from East Asia, sub-Saharan Africa, and Eastern Europe. More than 50% were found to be susceptible to HBV.
- *Immunity:* Newborns, children as well as immune-deficient patients usually hardly produce efficient immune reactions. Therefore, an asymptomatic infection with a high viral concentration can persist in the body for a long period of time in these people. Adult patients can develop immunity to protect self in a good number of HBV infections.
- *Behavior:* This is an important issue in HBV infection. Homosexuals, female sex workers, and intravenous (percutaneous) drug users are highly susceptible to the infection. Body fluids play its role here. Healthcare workers such as Doctors, nurses, laboratory technicians, blood collectors, ward attendants, and sweepers are at risk. Surgeons are more commonly affected with HBV infection compared to other medical professional specialties. Recipients of organ transplantation and blood transfusion are also at risk. Tattooing, acupuncture and beauty treatments, heterosexuals with multiple partners are the behavior in favor of HBV transmission.
- *Occupation:* The people who deal with blood, blood products, other body fluids, etc. are affected more. The doctors who deal with tissue, healthcare providers, dentists, phlebotomists, and people with sexually promiscuous behaviors are more prone to be infected by HBV.

### Agent Factors

The agent of *hepatitis B* belongs to the virus family Hepadnaviridae. The HBV has a complex coiled genomic structure. The core of the virus is surrounded by an envelope. Based on the replication cycles, the DNA virus is close to the Retroviridae. Therefore, they are also named deoxyribonucleic acid (DNA) retroviruses. The HBV genome is a complex virus particle; spherical double shelled structure with overlapping ends of the double-strand DNA (dsDNA).

- BS Blumberg first described the surface antigen of HBV in 1963 as a new serum protein. He named the new antigen (protein) the Australia antigen as it was found first in Australian Aboriginals. In 1968, the Australia antigen was renamed as HBsAg. The complete HBV virion (also called Dane particle) is 42 nm in diameter. HBsAg remains in the outer lipoprotein coat of HBV.
- About 27-nm nucleocapsid core of HBV has been designated as hepatitis B core antigen (HBcAg).
- A soluble protein, known as hepatitis B early antigen (HBeAg), can be detected in the serum of patients who are suffering from acute HBV infection and chronic HBV infection with high viral load.

Reverse transcriptase is used in HBV replication and due to its intermediate action, viruses have the potential for higher number of mutations. This nature of virus causes increased virulence, decreased host response to treatment.

- **Infectivity**: HBV dies at 90°C after 1 hour and after which infectivity of the virus is destroyed. Virus survives at surface of any object for 1 week or longer. This property gives it inoculation in human being by some inanimate objects. In serum, it can retain its infectivity for at least 1 month, if stored at room temperature or cooled environment.

- **Effects of disinfectants and heat**: Resistance level of the HBV is high in normal temperature or in body fluid but not extreme. The HBV is also susceptible to other disinfectants like 1% sodium hypochlorite and 2% alkalinized glutaraldehyde and formaldehyde. The virus is not stable at temperatures above 60°C; however, HBsAg is not destroyed by ultraviolet (UV) of blood products.

### Environmental Factors

**Temperature:** The infectivity of HBV serum at low temperature is relatively stable and infectivity is lost in a short period of time at high temperature. Virus at outside of body survives in dried blood for long periods (weeks), stable on environmental surfaces for at least 7 days at 25°C. Seasonal variation of the occurrence of hepatitis B is not conclusive though some favors to speak its peak in either spring or summer. Improved sanitation reduces the risk of HBV infection. Overcrowding, poverty, urbanization, and migration will increase the incidence of HBV infection. They indirectly play their role for increased incidence of this infection.

### Source or Reservoir of Infection

Human beings are the only reservoir of HBV. Blood and other body fluids are the source of infection from a case of hepatitis B patient or carrier of HBV. HBV reaches blood through infected blood or other body fluids, transported to the liver and then multiplies through replication, establishes infection in liver. It may be aborted (more in adult), may cause in-apparent disease or frank disease or chronic infection (more in child). Chronic carriers possess HBsAg in their blood for more than 6 months. They become a major source of infection. These patients may suffer from cirrhosis of the liver and hepatic carcinoma in later period of life.

### Infective Material

Blood, body fluids like serum, semen, saliva, blood products, cerebrospinal fluid, serum-derived fluids, vaginal fluids, breast milk, unfixed tissues, and organs are the materials where HBVs are present in ample amount.

### Portal of Exit

Portals of exit are multiple. Blood from accidental wound or some operational wound, cut injury, unsterile hypodermic needle injections, menstrual blood, sexual route (oral, anal, and vaginal), placenta, penile (semen), etc. play as portal of exit for HBV.

### Mode of Transmission

These include percutaneous or mucosal exposure to infectious body fluids, contact with contaminated specimens in the laboratory; contaminated needles, syringes and IV infusion set; channel devices, contamination of wounds or lacerations by blood splash or contaminated fomites; exposure of mucous membranes; and sexual contact (homo and hetero), household contact through wound, perinatal transmission from mother to infant (placenta and breast milk) nosocomial exposure (catheterization or injections).

Hepatitis B is most commonly spread from mother to child at birth (perinatal transmission), or through horizontal transmission (exposure to infected blood) during the first 5 years of life in highly endemic areas. The development of chronic infection is observed in infants infected from their mothers or before the age of 5 years.

### Portal of Entry

Percutaneous (skin wound or injections) or mucosal contact (oral, anal, and vaginal), dermatologic lesions or breaks, blood vessel (transfusion), umbilical cord, etc. are acting as the portals of entry of HBV.

### Incubation Period

The average incubation period is 2–3 months with a range of 1–6 months.

### Period of Communicability

Blood becomes infective weeks before the development of symptoms in patients; remains infective through clinical and chronic carrier states. Infectivity of chronic HbsAg carriers varies depending on the presence of HbeAg, the index of infectivity. Serum or other body fluids of infected individuals contain huge number of infectious virions per unit of fluid.

## CLINICAL FEATURES

During the acute infection phase, people may not experience any symptoms. Few people may experience the symptoms that last several weeks including yellowish discoloration of the skin and eyes (jaundice), dark urine, extreme fatigue, weakness, tiredness, nausea, vomiting, and abdominal pain.

A small group of suffering persons with acute hepatitis can develop acute failure of liver and this can lead to loss of life.
- In a fraction of affected people, HBV can cause a chronic liver infection, which can later lead to cirrhosis of the liver or carcinoma of liver.
- Most of the healthy adults (90%) who are infected with the HBV recover naturally within the first year.

---

*Case Scenario 1*

*25-year-old male, who is an injecting drug user, has presented with features of yellowish discoloration of eyes and dark urine. On examination he is also found to have an enlarged tender liver. What is the most likely diagnosis and why?*

**Suggested Solution**

*One of the most likely diagnosis is hepatitis B. The risk factor of being an injecting drug user means the most likely route of acquiring the infection is contaminated needles. The presence of jaundice and tender hepatomegaly also points toward this diagnosis. To confirm the diagnosis blood tests will have to be done, especially to differentiate from hepatitis caused by other viral agents.*

---

### Natural History of HBV Infection

The likelihood of development of chronic HBV infection depends upon the age at which a person becomes infected. The earlier the age of infection, the higher the likelihood of development of chronic HBV infection. Infants (80–90%) infected during the first year of life may develop chronic infections more frequently. Children (30–50%) infected before the age of 6 years may develop chronic infections in good number. In adults, it is low (5%) among otherwise healthy people.

Adults who are chronically infected will develop cirrhosis of liver and/or cancer of liver in 20-30% of affected people.

## DIAGNOSIS

Diagnosis of hepatitis B should be done by:
- At first level, complaints of the patients should be judged to get guidance or direction what system(s) may be involved. The patient will complain of yellowish discoloration of the skin and eyes (jaundice), dark urine, extreme fatigue, weakness, tiredness, nausea, vomiting, and abdominal pain. History of associated conditions can be elicited. History of injection, blood transfusion, organ donation, hospitalization, sexual contact with infected person, age of the affected persons, etc. will direct physicians toward the HBV infection.
- At the second level, clinical examination by doctors will augment the decision in favor or in disfavor to reveal the truth. The symptoms expressed here will guide the clinician that this is related to liver dysfunction. Clinically, the physician will find jaundice, yellowish discoloration of the skin and eyes, dark urine (jaundice), enlarged tender liver (hepatomegaly), etc. and these will guide the physician that the affected person is suffering from hepatitis. Now a question comes regarding identification of specific cause of the disease. On clinical grounds it is difficult to differentiate hepatitis B from hepatitis caused by other viral agents and even from non-viral agents.

Laboratory examination for hepatitis B infection is carried out by detection of the HBsAg.

Acute HBV infection is diagnosed based on the presence of HBsAg and antibody to the core antigen, anti-HBcAg [immunoglobulin M (IgM)]. It is evident from the **Figure 17F.1**

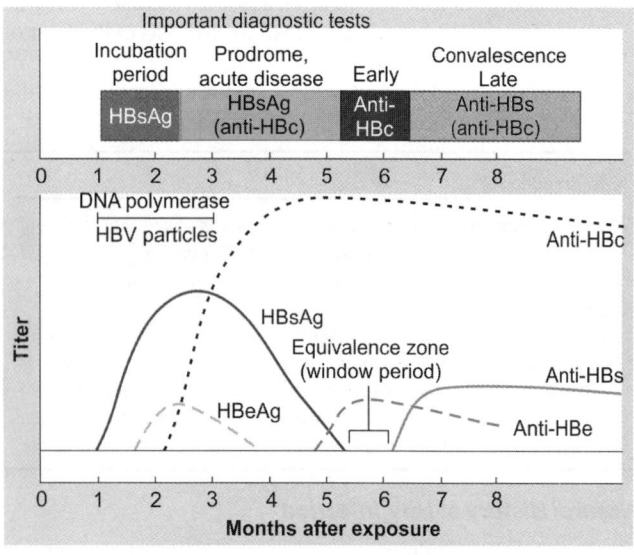

**Fig. 17F.1:** Diagnosis of hepatitis B.

*Sources:*
1. Tassopoulos NC, Papaevangelou GJ, Roumeliotou-Karayiannis A, et al. Serologic markers of hepatitis B virus (HBV) and hepatitis D virus infection in carriers of hepatitis B surface antigen who are frequently exposed to HBV. Hepatogastroenterology. 1986;33(4):151-4.
2. Kao JH. Diagnosis of hepatitis B virus infection through serological and virological markers. Expert Rev Gastroenterol Hepatol. 2008;2(4):553-62.

that at the initial phase of infection, patients are seropositive for HBeAg. This indicates high levels of replication of the virus. The presence of HBeAg provides information that the blood and body fluids of the affected individual are highly infectious.

Chronic HBV infection is diagnosed by the presence of HBsAg for more than or equal to 6 months irrespective of status of HBeAg. The presence of HBsAg for more than or equal to 6 months increases the risk of developing chronic liver disease and liver cancer (hepatocellular carcinoma) in later life.

## TREATMENT

No specific treatment for acute hepatitis B is available. Symptomatic treatment is aimed at providing and maintaining comfort to the patient.

Adequate nutritional balance, including replacement of fluids lost from vomiting and diarrhea should be taken care of. Drugs are offered to treat chronic HBV infection as oral antiviral agents. Treatment is given to slow the progression of cirrhosis and to reduce the transmission of HBV, to reduce incidence of liver cancer and to improve long-term survival.

Tenofovir or entecavir is the most potent drugs to suppress HBV. In comparison with other antiviral drugs, these two generally do not lead to resistance. They have few side effects. These drugs are given once a day which improves the patient compliance. Other drugs such as alpha-interferon, pegylated interferon, lamivudine, adefovir, etc. can be advocated to the patient but these are costlier and adverse effects are found high. These drugs suppress replication of HBVs, cause remission of liver disease. High pretreatment alanine aminotransferase (ALT) level is one of the predictors for response. About half of the patients become HBeAg negative in proper treatment. Most of the people who start hepatitis B treatment must continue for whole of the life.

In general, the outcome of HBV infection is poor. In low-income countries, most people die within months of diagnosis as it was late identification. In high-income countries, surgery and chemotherapy can be applied and it may prolong life up to years. Liver transplantation is sometimes considered and used in people with cirrhosis with variable success.

> **Key Points**
> - Behavior and occupation are 2 important host factors determining the risk of HBV infection
> - The HBV is a DNA virus with the surface antigen (HBsAg), core antigen (HBcAg) and the early antigen (HBeAg)
> - Some of the modes of transmission of infection include percutaneous or mucosal exposure to infectious body fluids, contaminated needles, contamination of wounds by blood splash or contaminated fomites; exposure of mucous membranes; and sexual contact, perinatal transmission and nosocomial exposure
> - Most of the healthy adults who are infected with the HBV recover naturally
> - Focus of laboratory examination for hepatitis B infection falls on the detection of the HBsAg
> - No specific treatment for acute hepatitis B is present up till now.

## PREVENTION AND CONTROL MEASURES

### Controlling Source or Reservoir

Reservoir of HBV is a patient (acute or chronic hepatitis) from whom the HBV spreads to a susceptible host. Source is the product of patient with which the virus is transmitted. Blood, blood-derived products, and other body fluids are the vehicles or medium through, which virus reaches to a susceptible host.

Controlling a reservoir with its products will be one of the strategies by which man can prevent or reduce the incidence of hepatitis B in the community. Few measures by which transmission of HBV can be prevented include:
- Screening of blood donors and blood.
- Preparation of plasma-derived products in a way that inactivates HBV virus.
- Implementation of infection control measures by following principles of universal precautions and injection safety.
- Administration of hepatitis B immune globulin following suspected exposure, especially for infants born to HBsAg-positive women,
- Rational disposal of biomedical waste, etc.

Patients who are known to be chronic carriers of HBsAg and are infective should be compliant to medication, follow appropriate disinfection and disposal of blood stained items like razors, towels and other inanimate objects.

## Interrupting the Transmission

- Newborns of pregnant women who carry HBV should receive both the passive and the active immunization. This interrupts infection from mother to child.
- Implementation of blood safety strategies (quality-assured screening of all donated blood and blood components used for transfusion) can prevent transmission of HBV.
- Safe injection practices, elimination of unnecessary and unsafe injections are effective strategies to protect against HBV transmission.
- Safer sex practices (minimizing the number of partners and use of barrier protective measures) protect against transmission of sexually transmitted diseases (STDs) including HBV.
- Treatment of acute or chronic cases reduces the viral load in blood or body fluid and thus possibility of viral transmission in some accidental way can be reduced.
- Blood transfusion should not be done before screening of blood for HBV.
- Soiled cotton, gauze, napkins, and other materials with blood or tissue fluid contact should be disposed in appropriate way.
- Disposable syringe should be used where available and needle should be cut at its hub. No attempt for recapping of needles should be followed and reuse of articles soiled with infected blood and body fluids should be discouraged.

Promote the use of simple, noninvasive diagnostic tests to assess the stage of liver disease and eligibility for treatment. Similarly, healthcare providers have to prioritize treatment for those with most advanced liver disease and at greatest risk of mortality and recommend the preferred use of tenofovir and entecavir, and entecavir in children aged 2-11 years for first-line and second-line treatment.

Lifelong treatment should be continued in cirrhosis of liver. Regular monitoring for disease progression, toxicity of drugs and early detection of liver cancer will be implemented. Awareness program should be launched for understanding of HBV infection in order to control and prevent HBV infection among population.

## Protection of Susceptible Host

The last and final link in the chain of infection is a susceptible host. Susceptibility of a host depends on genetic or constitutional factors, specific immunity, and other nonspecific factors. The genetic makeup of an individual may either increase or decrease susceptibility.

Specific immunity means development of protective antibodies directed against a specific antigen. Antibodies against HBsAg antigen may develop in response to infection, vaccine, or may be acquired by transplacental transfer from mother to fetus or by injection of immune globulin.

Nonspecific factors include the skin, mucous membranes, and nonspecific immune response. Factors that may increase susceptibility to infection by disrupting host defenses include malnutrition and or undernutrition, alcoholism, and disease or immunosuppressive therapy.

The hepatitis vaccine has an outstanding record of safety. This is really effective in preventing infection and its chronic consequences. More than 95% of infants, children, and adolescents (0-19 years) and more than 90% of healthy adults develop adequate antibody responses after three intramuscular doses. About 75% of immunized subjects develop protective antibody titers by 60 years of age.

Hepatitis B vaccine is available as monovalent formulations or in combination with diphtheria-tetanus-pertussis and *Hemophilus influenzae* type b. The number of normal adult dose is from two to four times or an increased number of doses may be required in hemodialysis patients or in other immunocompromised subjects to induce protective antibodies. A recombinant vaccine using alum and lipid A as adjuvant is available and may be considered for adult patients with renal insufficiency.

The primary hepatitis B vaccination consists of three doses; four doses may be administered for programmatic reasons according to the schedules of national routine immunization program. The use of routine booster doses does not appear necessary to maintain long-term protection in successfully vaccinated immunocompetent children.

### Primary Prevention

Advocacy and raising awareness for viral hepatitis infections will reduce transmission in the community. So, hepatitis education should be promoted in the general population. Safe and effective vaccines are widely available for the prevention of HBV infections. Vaccination program should be implemented in the countries. Other strategies include:
- Implementation of blood safety strategies
- Infection control precautions in health care and community settings
- Safe injection practices by healthcare providers
- Safer sex practices
- Harm reduction practices for injecting drug users
- Occupational safety measures

### Secondary and Tertiary Prevention

Early diagnosis and prompt treatment provide the best opportunities for effective medical support and prevention of further spread. Early diagnosis of chronic infection allows people to take precautions to protect the liver from additional damage, specifically by abstaining from alcohol and tobacco consumption and avoiding harmful drugs for liver. Counseling of blood donors who have reactive results detected during screening of donated blood provide unique opportunities for early diagnosis and medical support. Antiviral agents against HBV exist. Needs are required to ensure access to and availability of reliable and low-cost diagnostics and safe and simple treatment regimens, especially in resource constrained areas of the world.

> *Case Scenario 2*
>
> Ms Mary D' Souza is a 26-year-old nursing student has presented with history of needle stick injury for post exposure prophylaxis. She gives history of attempting to recap the needle due to which she sustained the injury. What level of prevention do you think has failed in this case and how would you rectify the same?
>
> **Suggested Solution**
> Primary prevention has which targets toward interrupting the transmission of hepatitis B has failed in this scenario.
>
> Promotion of safe injection practices by healthcare providers especially use of disposable syringes, avoidance of recapping, universal precautions and infection control precautions in health care are some of the corrective actions.

## CURRENT APPROACHES IN HEALTHCARE SERVICES

### Global Approach, Goals, and Targets

The World Health Assembly adopted the first "Global Health Sector Strategy on Viral Hepatitis, 2016–2021" in 2016. The strategy of Universal Health Coverage (UHC) has been aligned with those of the Sustainable Development Goals (SDGs). The vision to eliminate viral hepatitis as a public health threat by 2030 and included a roadmap towards elimination by implementing key prevention, diagnosis, treatment and community interventions strategies.

In May 2022, the 75th World Health Assembly noted a new set of integrated global health sector strategies on HIV, viral hepatitis and sexually transmitted infections for the period of 2022–2030. Based on the previous and now new strategies, a broad range of Member States have developed comprehensive national hepatitis programs and elimination strategies guided by the global health sector strategy.

To support countries in achieving the global hepatitis elimination targets under the Sustainable Development Agenda 2030, WHO is working to:
- Raise awareness, promote partnerships and mobilize resources
- Formulate evidence-based policy and data for action
- Increase health equities within the hepatitis response
- Prevent transmission
- Scale up screening, care and treatment services.

WHO organizes the annual World Hepatitis Day campaign (as 1 of its 9 flagship annual health campaigns) to increase awareness and understanding of viral hepatitis. For World Hepatitis Day 2022, WHO focuses on the theme "One life One liver" to highlight the importance of the liver for a healthy life and the need to scale up testing and treatment of viral hepatitis to prevent liver disease and achieve the 2030 elimination goals (WHO 2023).

### Health Programs and Schemes in India

World Health Organization (WHO) initiated program for elimination of public health problem due to HBV infection. Government of India launched National Programme for Prevention and Control of Viral Hepatitis during 12th Five-Year Plan period. On the occasion of the World Hepatitis Day, 28th July 2018, Ministry of Health and Family Welfare, Government of India has launched the National Viral Hepatitis Control Program (NVHCP). It is an integrated initiative to achieve SDG 3.3 which aims to "... Combat viral hepatitis". The Government of India is a signatory to the resolution 69.22 endorsed in the WHO Global Health Sector Strategy on Viral Hepatitis 2016-2021 at 69th WHA towards ending Viral hepatitis by 2030. National Viral Hepatitis Control Program is further explained in detail in **Chapter 47: Health Policies and Programs in India.**

### Applied Aspect

Hepatitis B vaccination is the mainstay for prevention. Hepatitis B vaccine was universalized nationwide in 2011. The UIP schedule recommends hepatitis B birth dose to all infants within 24 hours, followed by three doses at 6, 10 and 14 weeks to complete the schedule. National Immunization Schedule has been recommended by Government of India in infants and children.

- *Hepatitis B—birth dose* is offered at birth or as early as possible within 24 h of birth. Dose is 0.5 mL. Route of administration is deep intramuscular. Site of injection is anterolateral aspect of mid-thigh. This is highly immunogenic and seroconversion is seen in 95% cases. Seroconversion means the level of immunoglobulin at a good titer (≥10 mIU/mL) after 1–2 months of complete vaccination.
- *Pentavalent 1, 2, and 3:* Pentavalent vaccine includes 5 antigens for Diphtheria, Pertussis, Tetanus, *Haemophilus influenzae* type b, and HBV. Dose, site, and route are similar to hepatitis B birth dose vaccine. Time schedule for these vaccines is at 6 weeks, 10 weeks, and 14 weeks (can be given till one year of age).
- *No booster dose* are given to children. The immunocompromised children due to hereditary disease or drug or earned disease may be given after seeing the immunological assessment.

> **Key Points**
> - Prevention and control measures include controlling source/reservoir; interrupting the transmission and protection of susceptible host
> - Framework for Global Action in relation to Prevention and Control of Viral Hepatitis Infection has 4 distinct axes: (1) partnerships, resource mobilization, and communication axis; (2) data for policy and action axis; (3) prevention of virus transmission axis; and (4) screening, care, and treatment
> - Primary prevention include Advocacy and raising awareness; Implementation of blood safety strategies; Infection control precautions in health care and community settings; Safe injection practices; Safer sex practices; Harm reduction practices for injecting drug users; Occupational safety measures

- Early diagnosis and prompt treatment provide the best opportunity for effective medical support and prevention of further spread.
- Government of India has launched National Viral Hepatitis Control Programme
- Under the National Immunization Schedule; Hepatitis B vaccination is given as birth dose followed by Pentavalent 1, 2, and 3.

## SUGGESTED READING

1. Blumberg BS, Alter HJ, Visnich S. A "new" antigen in leukemia sera. JAMA. 1965;191:541-6.
2. Fares A. Seasonality of Hepatitis: A Review Update. J Family Med Prim Care. 2015;4(1):96-100.
3. Jin H, Zhao Y, Tan Z, et al. Immunization interventions to interrupt hepatitis B virus mother-to-child transmission: a meta-analysis of randomized controlled trials. BMC Pediatr. 2014;14:307.
4. Kao JH. Diagnosis of hepatitis B virus infection through serological and virological markers. Expert Rev Gastroenterol Hepatol. 2008;2(4):553-62.
5. Kobayashi H, Tsuzuki M, Koshimizu K, et al. Susceptibility of Hepatitis B Virus to Disinfectants or Heat. J Clin Microbiol. 1984;20(2):214-6.
6. Lozano R, Naghavi M, Foreman K, et al. Global and regional mortality from 235 causes of death for 20 age groups in 1990 and 2010: a systematic analysis for the Global Burden of Disease Study 2010. Lancet. 2012;380:2095-128.
7. National Action Plan Combating Viral Hepatitis in India. NHM, MoHFW; 2019.
8. Puri P. Tackling the Hepatitis B Disease Burden in India. J Clin Exp Hepatol. 2014;4(4):312-9.
9. Ray G. Current Scenario of Hepatitis B and its Treatment in India. J Clin Transl Hepatol. 2017;5(3):277-96.
10. Rossi C, Shrier I, Marshall L, et al. Seroprevalence of chronic hepatitis B virus infection and prior immunity in immigrants and refugees: a systematic review and meta-analysis. PLoS One. 2012;7(9):e44611.
11. Song XX, Ju LW, Wei GR, et al. Heat impact upon the infectivity of hepatitis B virus in serum. Zhonghua Yu Fang Yi Xue Za Zhi. 2011;45(8):723-6.
12. Tassopoulos NC, Papaevangelou GJ, Roumeliotou-Karayiannis A, et al. Serologic markers of hepatitis B virus (HBV) and hepatitis D virus infection in carriers of hepatitis B surface antigen who are frequently exposed to HBV. Hepatogastroenterology. 1986;33(4):151-4.
13. The Polaris Observatory Collaborators. Global prevalence, treatment, and prevention of hepatitis B virus infection in 2016: a modelling study. Lancet Gastroenterol Hepatol. 2018;3(6):383-403.
14. Vikaspedia. National Viral Hepatitis Surveillance Programme. [online] Available from: http://vikaspedia.in/health/nrhm/national-health-programmes-1/national-programme-on-prevention-and-control-of-viral-hepatitis.
15. Wallace RB. Maxcy-Rosenau-Last Public Health and Preventive Medicine, 15th dition. India; McGraw-Hill; 2007.
16. WHO. Hepatitis B; Factsheet July; 2023.
17. World Health Organization. (2012). Prevention & Control of Viral Hepatitis Infection: Framework for Global Action. [online] Available from: https://www.who.int/hiv/pub/hepatitis/Framework/en/.
18. World Health Organization. Global Hepatitis Programme. [online] Available from: https://www.who.int/hepatitis/about/global-hepatitis-programme/en/.
19. World Health Organization. Hepatitis B. [online] Available at http://www.who.int/news-room/fact-sheets/detail/hepatitis-b.

## EPIDEMIOLOGY OF HEPATITIS C AND ITS PREVENTION AND CONTROL

**CM7.2** Enumerate, describe and discuss the mode of transmission and measures for prevention and control of Hepatitis C

**CM8.1** Describe and discuss the epidemiological and control measures applicable in Hepatitis C

## INTRODUCTION

Hepatitis C is an infectious disease characterized by fever, dark yellow urine, abdominal pain, and yellow tinged skin, caused by the HCV, an enveloped RNA virus. The virus primarily affects the liver. Majority of the initially affected persons (75–85%) harbors the virus in the liver. Affected people have mild or no symptoms during the initial stage of the disease.

HCV leads to chronic liver disease like cirrhosis of liver after a long period of time (many years). In some cases, cirrhosis of liver will develop life-threatening complications such as liver failure, liver cancer or esophageal varices, and others.

In healthcare setting, HCV primarily spreads by blood-to-blood contact associated with poorly sterilized medical equipment, needle-stick injuries, intravenous use of drugs, and blood and blood products transfusions. It may spread vertically from an infected mother to her baby at perinatal period. Diagnosis is done by testing of blood for either viral RNA or antibodies to the HCV. Testing is recommended in all people who may complain of symptoms of hepatitis C or at risk.

There is no vaccine against hepatitis C. Prevention strategy is the preferred choice to tackle hepatitis C. It prescribes harm reduction efforts for the at-risk people.

In most of the cases, indication for liver transplantation is seen for long standing chronic HCV infection. Recurrence of HCV infection occurs in transplanted liver. Prevention modalities should be implemented to avoid all these health problems of HCV infection.

## CHARACTERISTIC OF HEPATITIS C

The spectrum of acute hepatitis C ranges from an asymptomatic infection to frank hepatitis. Fulminant hepatitis is rarely seen. Most of the newly affected persons (60–80%) are without any symptoms. Jaundice is seen among 15–20% of affected persons. Others may be present with nonspecific symptoms. Diagnosis of hepatitis C is only made after serologic screening and tests. Most of the affected persons (up to 85%) develop persistent infection among both the adult and the children. A good number of chronic HCV infections (58–81%) develop chronic hepatitis within 6 months of acute infection with elevated ALT. Some factors like alcohol use, older age at infection, males, immunodeficiency states are associated with higher risk of infection.

## PROBLEM STATEMENT

### Global

HCV infection is present worldwide and wide variation in distribution exists among countries.

Globally, an estimated 58 million people have chronic hepatitis C virus infection, with about 1.5 million new infections occurring per year. There are an estimated 3.2 million adolescents and children with chronic hepatitis C infection. WHO estimated that in 2019, approximately 290,000 people died from hepatitis C, mostly from cirrhosis and hepatocellular carcinoma (primary liver cancer). Direct-acting antiviral (DAAs) medicines can cure more than 95% of persons with hepatitis C infection, but access to diagnosis and treatment is low.

There is currently no effective vaccine against hepatitis C.

Acute HCV infections are usually asymptomatic and most do not lead to a life-threatening disease. Around 30% (15–45%) of infected persons spontaneously clear the virus within 6 months of infection without any treatment. The remaining 70% (55–85%) of persons will develop chronic HCV infection. Of those with chronic HCV infection, the risk of cirrhosis ranges from 15% to 30% within 20 years. Anti-Hepatitis C virus (HCV) antibody prevalence in the general population is estimated to be between 0.09–15%.

About 2.3 million people (6.2%) of the estimated 37.7 million living with HIV globally have serological evidence of past or present HCV infection. Chronic liver disease represents a major cause of morbidity and mortality among persons living with HIV globally.

- **Incidence:** Productive population was highly affected (2.8–3.1-fold increase, 2.2/lakh population). On the contrary population of extreme age (child and old) was least affected. Men exceed women in hepatitis incidence caused by HCV (1.1-fold).
- **Risk exposure or behavior:** Risky behaviors or contributors include injection drugs (68.2%); occupational exposure (1%), dialysis or kidney transplant (0.2%), surgery (12.2%), and accidental needle-stick or puncture (7.7%).
- **Deaths:** Mortality rate in males greater than that in females. 50% deaths were seen in older population. Two-third deaths were found due to cirrhosis of liver and one-third deaths were due to liver cancer in hepatitis C patients. Cirrhosis of liver and hepatocellular carcinoma cause most of the deaths each year from hepatitis C (Pal S, Infectious Disease, 2017).

## India

According to global estimates, the prevalence rate of HCV viremia in India in 2015 was 0.5%, affecting about 4.7 to 10.9 million people. Among the 36.7 million persons living with HIV in 2015 2.3 million had been infected with HCV. Liver diseases are a major cause of morbidity and mortality among those living with HIV and co-infected with viral hepatitis.

Since India has one-fifth of the world's population, it accounts for a large proportion of the worldwide HBV burden. India harbors 10-15% of the entire pool of HBV carriers of the world. It has been estimated that India has around 40 million HBV carriers. About 15–25% of HBsAg carriers are likely to suffer from cirrhosis and liver cancer and may die prematurely.

Anti-hepatitis C virus (HCV) antibody prevalence in the general population is estimated to be between 0.09 and 15%. Based on some regional level studies, it is estimated that there are 6–12 million people with hepatitis C in India. Chronic HBV infection accounts for 40–50% of hepatocellular carcinoma (HCC) and 20–30% cases of cirrhosis and chronic HCV infection accounts for 12–32% of HCC and 12–20% of cirrhosis in the country. (National Action Plan Combating Viral Hepatitis in India; 2019).

Genotype 3 is reported as the most common genotype in India (54–80%) (Verma V et al., Diagn Microbiol Infect Dis, 2008; Narahari S et al., Infect Genet Evol. 2009).

> **Key Points**
> - Hepatitis C is an infectious disease the primarily affects the liver caused by the HCV, an enveloped RNA virus
> - The HCV leads to chronic liver disease like cirrhosis of liver after a long period of time
> - HCV infection is a global problem with worldwide distribution
> - Productive population is affected with mortality rate in males greater than that in females
> - The estimated prevalence of HCV infection is about 1–1.9% in India with interstate variations.

## NATURAL HISTORY OF HEPATITIS C

Most of the hepatitis C infected persons (75–85%) may develop chronic HCV infection and rest 10–20% will develop cirrhosis over 20–30 years. Susceptible individuals for cirrhosis are male, more than or equal to 50 years, alcoholics, patient with nonalcoholic fatty liver disease, coinfected people with hepatitis B virus or HIV, recipient of immunosuppressive drugs, etc. With each passing year, among individuals infected with hepatitis C and with hepatitis C related cirrhosis, the annual risk of liver failure is 3–6% and the annual risk of liver cancer is about 1–5%.

## EPIDEMIOLOGY

### Host Factors

All individuals irrespective of age and sex have equal susceptibility to hepatitis C. People at increased risk of HCV infection are injectable drug users, intranasal drug users, recipients of infected blood or blood products, persons with invasive procedures in healthcare facilities, children born to infected mothers, persons with multiple sexual partners, people with HIV infection, prisoners, or previously incarcerated persons; people practicing tattooing, healthcare providers, scavengers, etc. Tribal people are more affected. Hemophiliacs, dialysis patients are especially highly prone to get infection.

- **Age:** HCV infection is seen more in extremes of age (<10 years, ≥ 60 years). No age is a bar of HCV infection.
- **Sex:** HCV infection disproportionately affects more men than women. Slower rate of disease progression is seen among women. HCV related complications occur more commonly in men.
- **Ethnicity:** The African American population in USA was found disproportionately affected by HCV and had lower response rates to current treatments. Internal racial and external factors (genetic, metabolic, social, economic, and cultural) in disease outcomes are well-known issues.
- **Immunity:** Immunological factors associated with progression to the persistent HCV infections and HCV-related chronic diseases are not evident. Antibodies developed against various viral epitopes are found to be high in persistent infection but these do not provide protection in reinfection. Both the innate and adaptive immune responses remain intact before the onset of advanced liver damage.
- **Behavior:** Sexual behavior may be considered as primary one to acquire the HCV infection. Unprotected anal sex, multiple sex partners, use of intranasal and intravenous narcotic drugs, vaginal sex during menstruation and in presence of

sexually transmitted infections (STIs), etc. are considered such behaviors which increase the likelihood of infection. Tattooing and piercing are other favorable behavior. Illicit drug injection practices including the shared use of syringe-needles; sharing a straw to snort drugs and drug preparation equipment, such as drug cookers, filtration cotton and rinse water has been shown to be associated with HCV transmission.

- **Occupation:** Body art by tattooists and piercers. They can be exposed to blood containing HCV during the set-up, procedure, break down, and clean-up stages. These exposures occur through needle-sticks, contact with dried blood on equipment or surfaces, or blood splashes in the eyes, nose, or mouth. Similarly, correctional healthcare workers, first responders or emergency response personnel, healthcare workers, and maintenance and waste workers are exposed to blood and or body fluids containing HCV.

### Agent Factors

**Types and strain:** The HCV belong to the genus *Hepacivirus*, a member of the Flaviviridae family. The HCV particle (60 nm) has a core of genetic material (ssRNA), covered by an icosahedral, protective protein shell, is encased in a lipid (fatty) envelope of cellular origin. Structural proteins made by the HCV include core protein, two envelope proteins E1 and E2, and other nonstructural proteins include protease, helicase, and polymerase.

The HCV replicates mainly in the hepatocytes of the liver. It is estimated that each HCV infected cell produces approximately 50 virions (virus particles) in a day.

**Effects of disinfectants:** Exposures to aldehyde (formaldehyde and glutaraldehyde) and ionic or nonionic detergents can destroy HCV infectivity effectively in the presence of cell culture medium or human serum. UVC light irradiation efficiently inactivates HCV within 2 min. Bleach at recommended concentration is efficient to decontaminate article. HCV survives 63 days in high volume syringe (high dead space).

### Environmental Factors

HCV infected patients with history of alcohol, tobacco, cannabis abuse were found to have accelerated liver fibrogenesis and steatosis.

- **Temperature:** Heat inactivates HCV in 8 and 4 min when incubated at 60°C and 65°C. At room temperature, HCV survives weeks after drying on inanimate surface.
- **Rain and seasons:** Definite and consistent seasonal pattern or association with rainfall has not been observed. Some evidence points toward spring and summer peak for peak transmission.
- **Humidity:** Lower the humidity higher are the chances of viral transmission.
- **Sanitation:** Sanitation directly does not play any role in transmission. Disposal of biomedical waste is relevant in HCV prevention and control.

### Social Factors

- **Overcrowding:** Overcrowded conditions promote shared supplies particularly drug use. In prison inmates, higher rates of infection with HCV is seen.
- **Poverty:** People living with hepatitis C are disproportionately affected by poverty. People in isolation, poverty and the erosion of culture are forced to engage in risky activities. These people suffer more with chronic HCV infection and its complication due to poor access to treatment.
- **Urbanization:** Social up liftment with proper education, healthy habits diminishes, any kind of infections including HCV. On the contrary, people conglomeration in poor living conditions promote the environment to abuse drugs including injectable. This will increase the risk of HCV infection.
- **Migration:** The incidence of new cases of HCV increases in the context of migration. Country with low prevalence suffers from high HCV infection due to migration from high prevalent countries. Screening of migrants is cost-effective. National programs will have to address the linguistic, cultural, social, and medical insurance barriers for the migrants with viral hepatitis.

---

*Case Scenario 3*

Mr Akash, A 36-year-old male long-distance trucker is found on screening laboratory testing to have mildly elevated liver enzymes; an enzyme immunoassay (EIA) shows that the patient tests positive for hepatitis C virus. He gives history of alcoholism in the past and injectable drug use and also has been a client for FSW in the past. Enumerate the risk behavior in the patient that might have resulted in him contracting the infection.

**Suggested solution**

Patient is a PWID, who also gives history of alcohol consumption. History of being a client of a Female Sex worker with the possibility of unprotected sexual intercourse may also be significant for him having contracted the infection.

---

### Source or Reservoir of Infection

HCV is a blood-borne virus and human blood or its product is the source of infection. In human, HCV enters, replicates at liver and reaches through its portal of exit to a susceptible person. Human being is the principal reservoir of HCV.

### Infective Material

Blood and blood products are the infective material which can cause HCV infection. Other body fluids may cause infection due to micro- or microtear exposing blood.

### Portal of Exit

Blood for transfusion, blood products for treatment, cut injury of skin or mucous membrane, ulcers in reproductive tract or penile surface, venepuncture, etc. may be considered as portal of exit of the virus from an infected person.

### Mode of Transmission

The most common mode of transmission is exposure to blood. This may happen through the transfusion of unscreened blood and blood products, injectable drug use through the sharing of injection equipment, unsafe healthcare injection practices, unsafe use (reuse or inadequate sterilization) of medical instruments (syringes and needles).

The HCV can be transmitted sexually. HCV can be passed from an infected mother to her baby vertically. These modes of transmission occur less commonly.

### Incubation Period

Incubation period of acute symptomatic hepatitis C is 6–7 weeks (2 weeks–6 months). Window period may extend up to 9 weeks.

### Period of Communicability

After development of viremia, most of the infected people will continue spreading the disease agent thoroughout life.

## CLINICAL FEATURES

Following initial HCV infection, approximately 80% of people do not exhibit any symptoms.
- HCV causes both acute and chronic infection. Acute HCV infection is usually asymptomatic, and is rarely (if ever) associated with life-threatening disease. About 15–45% of infected persons spontaneously clear the virus within 6 months of infection without any treatment. Acutely symptomatic patient of hepatitis C will complain of fever, fatigue, decreased appetite, nausea, vomiting, abdominal pain, dark urine, gray-colored feces, joint pain, and jaundice (yellowish skin, palm, sclera of the eyes, and under surface of tongue).
- The remaining 60–80% of persons will develop chronic HCV infection. Of those with chronic HCV infection, the risk of cirrhosis of the liver is between 15% and 30% within 20 years.

## SCREENING AND DIAGNOSIS

Nucleic-acid amplification test (NAT), antigens (NS3 and NS5), and antibodies (anti-HCV) are the important markers for screening and diagnosis of HCV infection.

World Health Organization suggests that screening should be done among the populations at increased risk of HCV infection regularly. People with positive history should go for diagnosis.

The antibodies are stable over 10–15 years after the hepatitis C infection and these antibodies can be detected. Screening by NAT and HCV antibodies can differentiate between an acute HCV infection (NAT positive and HCV antibody negative) and a chronic HCV disease (NAT positive and HCV antibody positive). The diagnostic window for HCV is long for antibody development and it is about 2 months. The current diagnostic window could be reduced between 6–8 days where the virus is in the replication process depending on different NAT methods. This is fact that acute HCV infection is usually asymptomatic and as a result, few people are diagnosed during the acute stage. In those people who develop chronic HCV infection, the infection remains undiagnosed because the infection does not produce symptoms until decades after infection. Symptoms develop after serious damage to the liver cells.

The HCV infection is diagnosed in two steps:
1. Screening for anti-HCV antibodies by a serological test. Tests remain positive for anti-HCV antibodies even in absence of infection in a good number of patients.
2. If the test is positive for anti-HCV antibodies, a nucleic acid test for RNA of HCV is done to confirm chronic infection. About 30% of people infected with HCV spontaneously clear the infection by a strong immune response without the need for treatment.

Patients of chronic hepatitis C infection require assessments to determine the degree of liver damage (fibrosis and cirrhosis of liver and hepatoma). Liver biopsy or a variety of noninvasive tests is advised.

Patients should have a laboratory test to identify the genotype of the HCV. Different genotypes respond differently to treatment. A person may be infected with more than one genotype. The degree of liver damage and virus genotype are used to guide management.

Status of liver should be assessed to support the person with HCV infection. In resource-limited settings, the aminotransferase or platelet ratio index (APRI) should be determined for the assessment of hepatic fibrosis.

## TREATMENT

In some of the HCV infections, immune response clears it. In some people with chronic infection, it is observed that liver damage is minimal. So, treatment may not be required. If the treatment is required by the patient than the goal will be to cure, which will depend on the strains of the virus and the type of treatment given.

WHO recommends therapy with pangenotypic direct-acting antivirals (DAAs) for all adults, adolescents and children down to 3 years of age with chronic hepatitis C infection. The short-course oral, curative DAA treatment regimens has few if any side-effects. DAAs can cure most persons with HCV infection, and treatment duration is short (usually 12 to 24 weeks), depending on the absence or presence of cirrhosis. In 2022, WHO included new recommendations for treatment of adolescents and children using the same pangenotypic treatments used for adults. The most widely used and low-cost pangenotypic DAA regimen is sofosbuvir and daclatasvir.

The availability of sofosbuvir, ledipasvir, and daclatasvir (direct acting antiviral agents—DAAs) created a paradigm shift in the management of chronic hepatitis C. Better response rates have been observed with the use of these drugs. These antiviral medicines (DDAs) cure more than 95% of hepatitis C infection and this reduces the risk of liver cancer, cirrhosis, and death. Diagnostic and treatment accessibility are still far behind our expectation. Sofosbuvir, daclatasvir, and the sofosbuvir or ledipasvir combination are part of the preferred regimens. These medicines are more effective, safer, and better-tolerated than the older medicines. Therapy with DAAs is shorter (usually 12 weeks). Pegylated interferon and ribavirin were used before the advent of these modern drugs and these drugs have very limited role.

An alcohol intake assessment has been recommended for all persons with HCV infection. Behavioral alcohol reduction intervention should be offered to persons with moderate-to-high alcohol intake.

> **Key Points**
> - Most of the hepatitis C infected persons develop chronic HCV infection and rest 10–20% will develop cirrhosis
> - HCV is a blood-borne virus and principally human blood or its product is the source of infection

- The HCV particle is a core of genetic material (ssRNA), covered by protein shell, and further encased in a lipid (fatty) envelope
- People at increased risk of HCV infection are drug users, recipients of infected blood or blood products, persons with invasive procedures in healthcare facilities, children born to infected mothers, persons with multiple sexual partners, people with HIV infection, prisoners, or previously incarcerated persons; people practicing tattooing, healthcare providers, scavengers, etc.
- Some of the contributory social factors include overcrowding, poverty, urbanization and migration
- Nucleic-acid amplification test (NAT), antigens (NS3 and NS5), and antibodies (anti-HCV) are the important markers
- Direct acting antiviral agents—DAAs have a major role in the management of chronic hepatitis C.

## PREVENTION AND CONTROL MEASURES

### Controlling Source or Reservoir

The reservoir is a person with HCV infection. These persons should be informed and motivated not to donate blood and organs. This will prevent direct transmission. Health education to increase awareness on the different issues. Reduction of or abstinence from alcohol consumption, avoidance of multiple sex partners, avoidance of intravenous drug use, no more piercing or tattooing, etc. in the day-to-day life.

### Interrupting the Transmission

The strategies include:
- Avoidance of reuse of syringe-needles, infusion sets, proper disposal of soiled articles in the healthcare settings (hospital ward, operation theaters, pathology, biochemistry, microbiology, vaccination unit, emergency block, etc.).
- Appropriate management of biomedical waste, etc.
- Injection safety (no recapping, hub cutting, disinfection using hypochlorite solution, etc.)

### Protection of Susceptible Host

There is no vaccine for HCV infection. Appropriate healthy behavior should be practiced by susceptible people. Susceptible population should not receive blood or blood products. The behaviors which will increase the risk of HCV infection should be avoided by these non-affected groups.

### *Primary Prevention*

As there is no vaccine, reduction of the risk of exposure to the virus in healthcare settings and in high-risk populations is primary activity.

Primary prevention interventions are:
- Hand hygiene—including surgical hand preparation, hand washing, and use of gloves
- Safe and appropriate use of healthcare injections
- Safe handling and disposal of sharps and waste
- Provision of comprehensive harm-reduction services to PWID including sterile injecting equipment
- Testing of donated blood for hepatitis C
- Training of health personnel; and
- Promotion of correct and consistent use of condoms.

### *Secondary and Tertiary Prevention*

Education and counseling on options for care and treatment, immunization with the hepatitis A and B vaccines to prevent coinfection from these hepatitis viruses and to protect their liver, early and appropriate medical management including antiviral therapy, if appropriate, and regular monitoring for early diagnosis of chronic liver disease are the issues in this level.

### Global Approach, Goals, and Targets

The World Health Assembly adopted the first **"Global Health Sector Strategy on Viral Hepatitis, 2016–2021"** in 2016. The strategy of Universal Health Coverage (UHC) has been aligned with those of the Sustainable Development Goals (SDGs). The vision is to eliminate viral hepatitis as a public health problem.

Targets were specified by reduction of new viral hepatitis infections by 90% and reduction of deaths due to viral hepatitis by 65% by 2030. Following actions were outlined in the strategy.

- In May 2022, the 75th World Health Assembly noted a new set of integrated global health sector strategies on HIV, viral hepatitis and sexually transmitted infections for the period of 2022–2030. Based on the previous and now new strategies, a broad range of Member States have developed comprehensive national hepatitis programmes and elimination strategies guided by the global health sector strategy.
- The WHO will support countries toward achieving the global hepatitis goals under the Sustainable Development Agenda by 2030 by (1) raising awareness, promoting partnerships and mobilizing resources; (2) formulating evidence-based policy and data for action; (3) preventing transmission; and (4) scaling up screening, care, and treatment services.

### Health Programs and Schemes, and Goals in India

#### *National Viral Hepatitis Control Program*

The Government of India launched the National Viral Hepatitis Control Program (NVHCP) in 2018 with the aim to prevent and treat viral hepatitis (A, B, C, and E) and provide screening, diagnosis, treatment, and counseling services free of cost to all. The NVHCP synergizes with other national programs, such as the National AIDS Control Program, to promote safe blood and blood products, preventive services for the high-risk population, and injection safety practices. Therefore, an integrated approach will lead to better utilization of resources, promote screening and early treatment, and prevent attrition. NVHCP is further explained in ***Chapter 47: Health Policies and Programs in India***.

In case of blood and organ donation, HCV is screened and if found positive, the blood or organ is rejected. Every blood bank is dedicated to screen blood for HCV with others. Public health approach for HCV control should consider the following aspects.

- ***Prevention issues*** should include (1) screening of all donated blood for HCV, (2) reduction of unnecessary injections, (3) implementation of infection control measures and (4) provision of clean needles and opiate substitution therapy.
- ***Screening*** may be done among the most affected populations, including those exposed to unsafe blood, key populations, and people living with HIV/AIDS. Standardized diagnostic algorithms should be developed.

- **Treatment** should consider use effective, well-tolerated, short-duration, and affordable regimens in national guidelines.

### Key Points

- Prevention and control measures include controlling source/reservoir; interrupting the transmission and protection of susceptible host
- Avoidance of high-risk behavior, appropriate management of biomedical waste and injection safety are strategies to interrupt transmission
- "Global Health Sector Strategy on Viral Hepatitis, 2016–2021" has been aligned with those of the Sustainable Development Goals
- National Viral Hepatitis Control Program (NVHCP) was launched in 2018 with the aim to prevent and treat viral hepatitis (A, B, C, and E) and provide screening, diagnosis, treatment, and counseling services free of cost to all.

## SUMMARY

1. Hepatitis refers to an inflammation of liver and may be caused by viral agents like HBV and HCV.
2. Many of the high-risk groups are shared by both the viral infections. These homosexuals, heterosexuals with multiple partners female sex workers, and intravenous (percutaneous) drug users, health care workers such as doctors, nurse, laboratory technicians; recipients of organ transplantation and blood transfusion; Tattooing, acupuncture and beauty treatments.
3. Prevention and control measures for both viral infections include controlling source/reservoir; interrupting the transmission and protection of susceptible host.
4. Some of the *Key Strategies of Blood Safety Program* include Assessing blood needs and requirements of the country; Increasing regular voluntary nonremunerated blood donation to meet the safe blood requirements of the country; Promoting component preparation and availability along with rational use of blood in healthcare facilities; Capacity building of healthcare providers; Enhancing blood access through a well networked centrally coordinated, efficient, and self-sufficient blood transfusion services; Establishing quality management systems to ensure safe blood and building implementation structures and referral linkages.
5. One of the key strategies to enhance blood safety is to focus on promoting voluntary blood donation by motivating nonremunerated blood donors.

## SUGGESTED READING

1. Baden R, Rockstroh JK, Buti M. Natural History and Management of Hepatitis C: Does Sex Play a Role? J Infect Dis. 2014;209(3):81-5.
2. Chakravarti A, Ashraf A, Malik S. A study of changing trends of prevalence and genotypic distribution of Hepatitis C virus among high risk groups in North India. Indian J Med Microbiol. 2013;31(4):354-9.
3. Chandra M, Khaja MN, Farees N. Prevalence, risk factors and genotype distribution of HCV and HBV infection in the tribal population: a community based study in south India. Trop Gastroenterol. 2003;24(4):193-5.
4. Hagan H. Agent, host, and environment: hepatitis C virus in people who inject drugs. J Infect Dis. 2011;204(12):1819-21.
5. Mallat A, Hezode C, Lotersztajn S. Environmental factors as disease accelerators during chronic hepatitis C. J Hepatol. 2008;48(4):657-65.
6. Paintsil E, Binka M, Patel A, et al. Hepatitis C virus maintains infectivity for weeks after drying on inanimate surfaces at room temperature: implications for risks of transmission. J Infect Dis. 2014;209(8):1205-11.
7. Puri P, Anand AC, Saraswat VA. Consensus statement of HCV task force of the Indian National Association for Study of the Liver (INASL). Part I. Status report of HCV infection in India. J Clin Exp Hepatol. 2014;4(2):106-16.
8. Simon TL, McCullough J, Snyder EL, et al. Rossi's Principles of Transfusion Medicine, 5th edition. Garsington Road, Oxford: John Wiley & Sons, Ltd.; 2016.
9. Song H, Li J, Shi S, et al. Thermal stability and inactivation of hepatitis C virus grown in cell culture. Virol J. 2010;7:40.
10. Terilli RR, Cox AL. Immunity and hepatitis C: a review. Curr HIV/AIDS Rep. 2013;10(1):51-8.
11. WHO. Hepatitis C: Factsheet; July 2023.
12. World Health Organization. Hepatitis C. [online] Available from: http://www.who.int/en/news-room/fact-sheets/detail/hepatitis-c.

# G. EPIDEMIOLOGY OF CONTACT DISEASES AND ITS PREVENTION AND CONTROL

## EPIDEMIOLOGY OF HIV AND ITS PREVENTION AND CONTROL

*Mausumi Basu, Abhik Sinha, Mohua Moitra, Sukumal Bisoi*

**World AIDS Day Theme 2019:** *"Ending the HIV/AIDS Epidemic: Community by Community".*

| | |
|---|---|
| **CM7.2** | Enumerate, describe and discuss the mode of transmission and measures for prevention and control of HIV |
| **CM8.1** | Describe and discuss the epidemiological and control measures applicable in HIV |

## INTRODUCTION

Human Immunodeficiency Virus (HIV) continues to be a major global public health problem. However, with increasing access to effective HIV prevention, diagnosis, treatment and care, including for opportunistic infections, HIV infection has become a manageable chronic health condition, enabling people living with HIV to lead long and healthy lives.

The human immunodeficiency virus targets the immune system and weakens people's defense systems against infections and some types of cancer. As the virus destroys and impairs the function of immune cells, infected individuals gradually become immune-deficient. Immune function is typically measured by CD4 cell count. Immunodeficiency results in increased susceptibility to a wide range of infections, cancers and other diseases that people with healthy immune systems can fight off. Unlike some other viruses, the human body cannot get rid of HIV completely, even with treatment. So once you get HIV, you have it for life.

Acquired immunodeficiency syndrome (AIDS) is the most advanced stage of HIV infection, which can take from 2 to 15 years to develop if not treated, depending on the individual. AIDS is defined by the development of certain cancers, infections or other severe clinical manifestations.

## HISTORY OF HIV/AIDS

In 1970s, the disease was confined to green monkeys of Africa; in 1981, a new syndrome reported by Centers for Disease Control and Prevention (CDC), Atlanta, USA—pneumonia, caused by *Pneumocystis carinii* pneumonia and Kaposi's sarcoma (in a homosexual man who died due to loss of immunity). In 1982, it was named AIDS. In 1983, French scientist Luc Montagnier, Pasteur Institute, Paris identified the virus named lymphadenopathy-associated virus (LAV). In 1984, it was confirmed LAV as causative agent of AIDS in USA. In 1985, the virus was renamed as "human T-cell lymphotropic virus (HTLV)". In 1986, International Expert Committee on Taxonomy called the virus by a new name "human immunodeficiency virus" type 1. In 1987, a new virus of same characteristics was identified in West Africa as HIV type 2. In 1988, WHO announced December, 1st of each year as "World AIDS Day". In 1991, red ribbon was launched as an international symbol of AIDS awareness. In 1992, combination drug therapy AZT (azidothymidine) + DDC (zalcitabine) became successful for the first time. In 1994, AZT was shown to reduce the risk of transplacental transmission by 60%. In 1996, combination antiretroviral therapy (ART) was first introduced. In 1998, first human trial of an AIDS vaccine was performed by AIDSVAX® company on 5,000 volunteers. In 1999, single-dose Nevirapine was found to be effective in prevention of mother-to-child transmission (MTCT) of HIV. In 2010, WHO revised treatment guidelines—earlier initiation of ART at CD4 less than 350/mm$^3$.

## PROBLEM STATEMENT

### Global

The global burden of the epidemic continues to vary considerably between countries and regions. The WHO African region remains most severely affected, with nearly 1 in every 25 adults (3.9%) living with HIV and accounting for more than two-thirds of the people living with HIV worldwide.

HIV remains a major global public health issue, having claimed 40.4 million [32.9-51.3 million] lives so far with ongoing transmission in all countries globally, with some countries reporting increasing trends in new infections when previously on the decline. There were an estimated 39.0 million [33.1-45.7 million] people living with HIV at the end of 2022, two thirds of whom (25.6 million) are in the WHO African Region.

In 2022, 630,000 [480,000–880,000] people died from HIV-related causes and 1.3 million [1.0–1.7 million] people acquired HIV.

By 2025, 95% of all people living with HIV (PLHIV) should have a diagnosis, 95% of those should be taking lifesaving antiretroviral treatment (ART) and 95% of PLHIV on treatment should achieve a suppressed viral load for the benefit of the person's health and for reducing onward HIV transmission. In 2022, these percentages were 86(%) [73–>98%], 89(%) 75–>98%] and 93(%) [79–>98%], respectively (WHO. HIV-AIDS; Factsheet July 2023.

Despite the fact that 51% of people living with HIV globally are female, higher treatment coverage and better adherence to treatment among women have driven more rapid declines in AIDS-related deaths among females. Deaths from AIDS-related illnesses were 27% lower among women and girls in 2016 than they were among men and boys. Nonetheless, AIDS-related illnesses remain the leading cause of death among women of reproductive age (15–49 years) globally, and they are the second leading cause of death for young women aged 15–24 years in Africa. Since 2010, the annual number of new HIV infections (all ages) has declined by 16% to 1.7 million. Differences in the number of new HIV infections between men and women are more pronounced at younger ages. In 2016, new infections among young women (aged 15–24 years) were 44% higher than those were among men in the same age group. Since 2010, new infections among young women globally (aged 15–24 years) have declined by 17% and new infections also declined among young men (aged 15–24 years) during that time, falling by 16% in 2016 (UNAIDS Report, 2017).

## India

HIV burden estimations are a periodic exercise under the robust surveillance and epidemiology system of NACP in India. NACO has designated the Indian Council of Medical Research, National Institute of Medical Statistics (ICMR-NIMS) in Delhi as the nodal institute to anchor the HIV burden **(Table 17G.1 and Fig. 17G.1)**.

**Table 17G.1:** National Summary of the HIV/AIDS Epidemic in 2021.

| Indicator | Category | Value |
|---|---|---|
| Adult (15–49 years) prevalence | Total | 021% [0.17–0.25] |
| | Male | 022% [0.18–0.28] |
| | Female | 019% [0.15–0.23] |
| Number of people living with HIV | Total | 24,01,284 [19,92,058–29,06,772] |
| | Adult (15+ years) | 23,31,476 [19,37,759–28,18,674] |
| | Women (15+ years) | 10,50,251 [8,72,579–12,68,579] |
| | Children (<15 years) | 69,808 [54,266–89,260] |
| | Young people (15–24) | 1,70,403 [1,30,096–2,26,182] |
| PLHIV per million population | Total | 1762 [1462–2133] |
| HIV incidence per 1,000 uninfected population | Total | 0.05 [0.03–0.08] |
| | Male | 0.05 [0.03–0.09] |
| | Female | 0.04 [0.02–0.07] |
| New HIV Infections | Total | 62,967 [30,715–1,04,058] |
| | Adults (15+ years) | 57,969 [33,488–96,528] |
| | Women (15+ years) | 24,550 [14,268–40,694] |
| | Young people (15–24) | 15,078 [8,597–25,172] |
| Change in new HIV infections since 2010 (%) | Total | –46.25 |
| | Adults (15+ years) | –44.48 |
| | Female (15+ years) | –43.75 |
| | Children (<15 years) | –60.82 |
| AIDS-related deaths | Total | 41,968 [26,499–67,451] |
| | Adults (15+ years) | 39,462 [25,141–63,261] |
| | Women (15+ years) | 11,258 [5,789–20,460] |
| | Children (<15 years) | 2506 [1125–4389] |
| | Young people (15–24) | 1118 [644–1954] |
| AIDS-related deaths per 100,000 population | Total | 3,08 [1.94–4.95] |
| | Male | 4.21 [2.77–3.41] |
| | Female | 1,88 [0.97–6.40] |
| Change in AIDS related deaths since 2010 (%) | Total | –76.54 |
| | Adults (15+ years) | –76.44 |
| | Female (15+ years) | –82.74 |
| | Children (<15 years) | –77.92 |
| PMTCT need | Total | –20,612 [16,379–26,359] |
| Final MTCT Rate of HIV (%) | Total | 24.25 [18.50–29.50] |

*Source:* Technical Report India HIV Estimates 2021; National AIDS Control Organisation & Indian Council of Medical Research – National Institute of Medical Statistics (ICMR-NIMS) Ministry of Health & Family Welfare, Government of India.

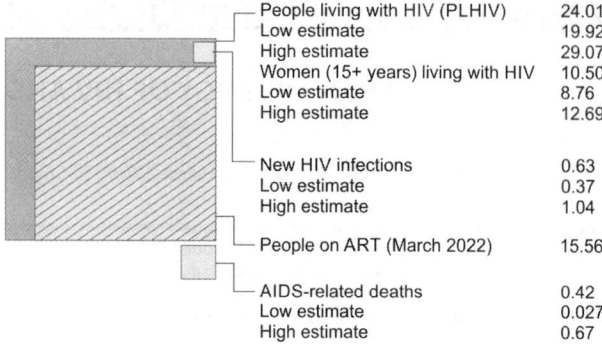

**Fig. 17G.1:** Overview of HIV/AIDS epidemic in India, 2021 (all figures in lakhs).
*Source:* Sankalak. Status of National AIDS Response 4th edition NACO, MoHFW, GOI, 2022

**Table 17G.2:** Categorization of states according to prevalence of people living with human immunodeficiency viruses (PLHIVs).

| Category of states | Criteria | States |
|---|---|---|
| High-prevalence states | ANC prevalence >1% HRGs prevalence >5% | Maharashtra, Tamil Nadu, Karnataka, Andhra Pradesh, Manipur, Nagaland |
| Moderate prevalence states | ANC <1% HRGs >5% | Gujarat, Goa, Puducherry |
| Low-prevalence states | ANC <1% HRGs <5% | Rest of the states |

(ANC: antenatal clinic; HRG: high-risk group)

The occurrence of HIV infections also varies across the state/UTs as well as the urban-rural divide **(Fig. 17G.2 and Table 17G.2)**. In addition, young women of childbearing age are also at a higher risk of infection and are a potential source of onward transmission to their infants, during birth, labor, and through breastfeeding.

There are various other determinants such as social, economic, access to health care, below par literacy level and awareness regarding HIV/AIDS, gender inequalities, and marginalization and discrimination; all of which account greater risks and vulnerabilities. In addition, many technological advances and liberal practices like premarital sex, travel and information technology (IT), mobile phones, and social media, all have consequences on exposure to risk and the capacity to protect oneself.

Nationally, annual new HIV infections in 2019 have decreased by 37% since 2010. There has also been a fall in the estimated number of AIDS-related deaths by 56%, largely due to increasing coverage of ART, and this, together with reductions in new HIV infections, has contributed to stabilizing the number of people living with HIV.

In addition to HIV, there are various co-infections and comorbidities including other sexually transmitted infections (STIs), reproductive tract infections (RTIs), tuberculosis (TB), hepatitis B and C, and cervical cancer, which need to be addressed.

A focus on consolidation of convergence with reproductive health, maternal and child health, and adolescent health departments will be fundamental in this regard.

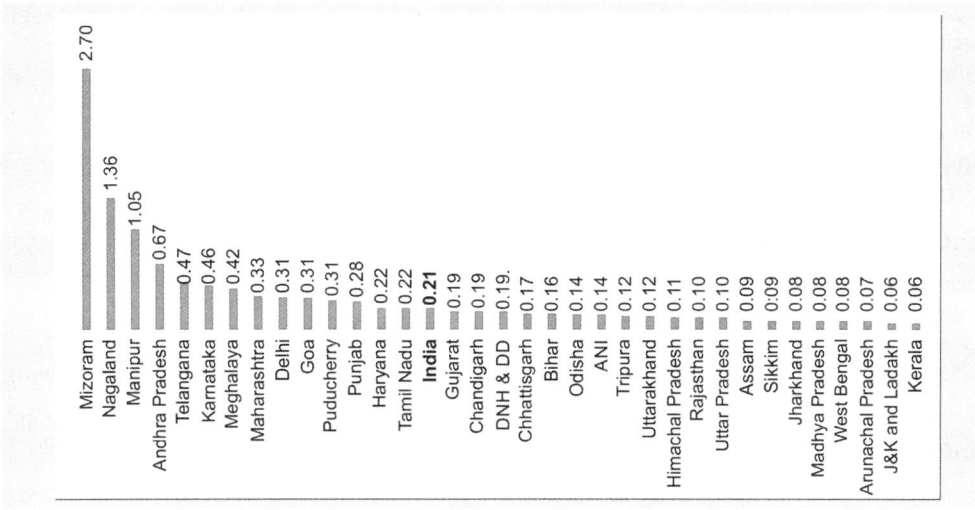

**Fig. 17G.2:** Adult prevalence (in %) in India by states.
*Source:* India HIV Estimate Factsheet 2021, NACO

# EPIDEMIOLOGY OF HIV/AIDS

## Host Factors

The period of infectivity is throughout life for an infected person. It is not an occupational disease, but surgeons, dentists, obstetricians, commercial sex worker (CSW), blood bank and laboratory workers are at risk. HIV is common among sexually active and productive age group of life (15–40 years, <3% among children). Sex incidence in India is M:F = 3:2. Incubation period varies from 5 to 10 years.

## Agent Factors

AIDS is caused by HIV. The virus has reverse transcriptase enzyme in it. The enzyme is used to generate complementary deoxyribonucleic acid (DNA) from a ribonucleic acid (RNA) template. The structure of the virus is depicted in **Figure 17G.3**.

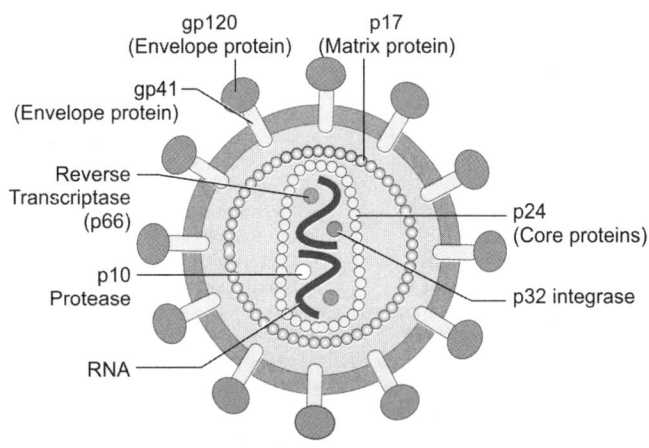

| Three types of antigens | Three enzymes |
|---|---|
| 1. Core antigens: GAG (p17), (p24), | 1. Reverse transcriptase (p66) |
| 2. Polymerase antigens: POL | 2. Integrase (p32) |
| 3. Envelope antigens ENV: gp120 and gp41 | 3. Protease (p10) |

**Fig. 17G.3:** Structure of the human immunodeficiency virus.

## Reservoir of Infection

The reservoirs of infection are only human case and carriers. Carrier state is found among 85% of infected persons. For every case of AIDS, there are about 8–10 subclinical cases, who act as carriers (tip of iceberg). Carriers are highly infectious during the "Window Period" (6–12 weeks).

## Source of Infection

Infective materials are blood, semen, vaginal secretion, and breast milk.

Saliva, cerebrospinal fluid (CSF), tears, urine, and joint fluid are usually not infective but become infective when contaminated with HIV-infected blood.

## Routes of Transmission

- **By direct physical sexual contact**, viz by having unprotected sex (without condom). The factors, which favor sexual transmission, are the type of sexual act, protection, if any, age and sex of the infected partner, presence of STI, stage of illness of infected partner, virulence of HIV strain, and period of menstruation. It is the most common route of transmission.
- **By blood transfusion**: HIV/AIDS can be spread, if the transfused blood is infected with HIV/AIDS. It is the most efficient route of transmission.
- **By percutaneous route**: By sharing needles/syringes or using unsterile needles, syringes or other surgical or dental instruments, contact between HIV-infected blood and broken skin.
- **By vertical transmission**: During pregnancy, during childbirth, or during breastfeeding.

## High-risk Groups

Some groups of population are at increased risk of developing HIV/AIDS. They are as follows:
- Male homosexuals (MSM)
- Transgender/transsexual/*Hijras*
- Men/women having multiple sexual partners

- Female sex workers
- Intravenous drug users
- Sexually transmitted infection patients
- Newborn of infected mothers.

Bridge population is the population, which forms a link between the general population and the high-risk population like long-distance truckers and migrants.

### Stages of Untreated HIV Infection

The stages of untreated HIV Infection are: *Acute retroviral syndrome* for 2–3 weeks followed by *seroconversion* by 2–20 weeks followed by *asymptomatic chronic HIV infection* by 8 years (average) and *symptomatic HIV infection/AIDS* by 1.3 years (average).

### Opportunistic Infections

The opportunistic infections that can occur in a patient with HIV/AIDS are as follows:
- **Bacteria:** Atypical mycobacteria, *Mycobacterium tuberculosis* (pulmonary tuberculosis), *Legionella*.
- **Viruses:** Cytomegalovirus (retinitis and blindness), Herpes virus, Epstein–Barr virus.
- **Protozoa:** *Pneumocystis carinii* (pneumonia), *Toxoplasma gondii* (toxoplasmosis and encephalitis), *Cryptosporidium* (cryptosporidiosis).
- **Fungi:** *Candida albicans* (esophageal candidiasis), *Cryptococcus* (meningitis), *Coccidioides* (coccidioidomycosis), *Histoplasma* (histoplasmosis).
- **Helminth:** *Strongyloides stercoralis* (strongyloidiasis)
- **Unusual cancers:** Kaposi's sarcoma and nonHodgkin's lymphoma.

## CLINICAL FEATURES OF AIDS (FIG. 17G.4)

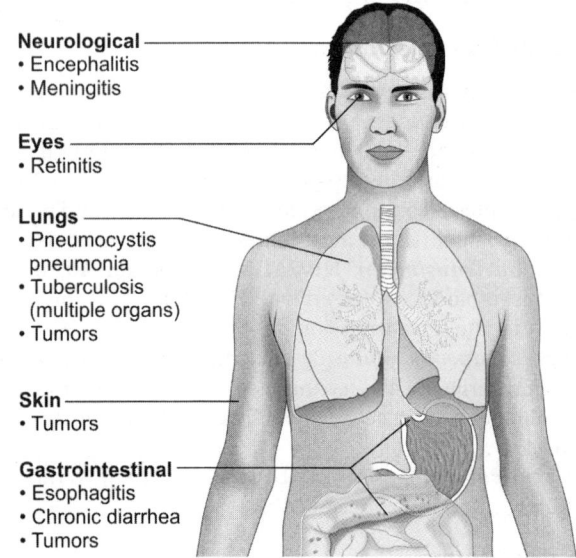

**Fig. 17G.4:** Main symptoms of AIDS.
(AIDS: acquired immunodeficiency syndrome)

### Acute HIV Syndrome

It is usually manifested as transient symptomatic illness and affects 40–90% of HIV-positive individuals. It ranges from mild and nonspecific illness to severe illness that can result in hospitalization.

### WHO Clinical Staging

#### WHO Clinical Staging 1
- Asymptomatic
- Persistent generalized lymphadenopathy (PGL):
  - Painless enlarged lymph nodes more than 1 cm
  - In two or more noncontiguous sites (excluding inguinal), in the absence of known cause
  - Persisting for 3 months

#### WHO Clinical Staging 2 for Adults and Children

The WHO clinical staging 2 for adult and children is discussed in **Table 17G.3**.

**Table 17G.3:** World Health Organization clinical staging 2.

| Adults | Children |
|---|---|
| • Moderate unexplained weight loss (<10% of presumed or measured body weight) <br>• Recurrent respiratory tract infections (sinusitis, tonsillitis, otitis media, pharyngitis) <br>• Herpes zoster <br>• Angular cheilitis <br>• Recurrent oral ulceration <br>• Popular pruritic eruption <br>• Fungal nail infections <br>• Seborrheic dermatitis | • Unexplained persistent hepatosplenomegaly <br>• Recurrent or chronic upper respiratory tract infections (otitis media, otorrhea, sinusitis, tonsillitis) <br>• Herpes zoster <br>• Lineal gingival erythema <br>• Recurrent oral ulceration <br>• Popular pruritic eruption <br>• Fungal nail infections <br>• Extensive wart virus infection <br>• Extensive molluscum contagiosum <br>• Unexplained persistent parotid enlargement |

#### WHO Clinical Staging 3 for Adults and Children

The WHO clinical staging 3 for adult and children is discussed in **Table 17G.4**.

**Table 17G.4:** World Health Organization clinical staging 3.

| Adults | Children |
|---|---|
| • Unexplained severe weight loss (>10% of presumed or measured body weight) <br>• Unexplained chronic diarrhea for longer than 1 month <br>• Unexplained persistent fever (intermittent or constant for longer than 1 month) <br>• Persistent oral candidiasis <br>• Oral hairy leukoplakia <br>• Pulmonary tuberculosis <br>• Severe bacterial infections (such as pneumonia, empyema, pyomyositis, bone or joint infection, meningitis, bacteremia) <br>• Acute necrotizing ulcerative stomatitis, gingivitis, or periodontitis <br>• Unexplained anemia (<8 g/dL), neutropenia (<0.5 × 10$^9$/L) and/or chronic thrombocytopenia (<50 × 10$^9$/L) | • Unexplained moderate malnutrition not adequately responding to standard therapy <br>• Unexplained persistent diarrhea (14 days or more) <br>• Unexplained persistent fever (above 37.5°C, intermittent or constant, for longer than 1 month) <br>• Persistent oral candidiasis (after first 6 weeks of life) <br>• Oral hairy leukoplakia <br>• Lymph node tuberculosis <br>• Pulmonary tuberculosis <br>• Severe recurrent bacterial pneumonia <br>• Acute necrotizing ulcerative gingivitis or periodontitis <br>• Unexplained anemia (<8 g/dL), neutropenia (<0.5 × 10$^9$/L) or chronic thrombocytopenia (<50 × 10$^9$/L) <br>• Symptomatic lymphoid interstitial pneumonitis <br>• Chronic HIV-associated lung disease including bronchiectasis |

## WHO Clinical Staging 4 for Adults and Children

The WHO clinical staging 4 for adult and children is discussed in **Table 17G.5**.

**Table 17G.5:** World Health Organization clinical staging 4.

| Adults | Children |
|---|---|
| • Kaposi sarcoma | • Kaposi sarcoma |
| • Cytomegalovirus infection (retinitis or infection of other organs) | • Cytomegalovirus infection (retinitis or infection of other organs with onset at age more than 1 month) |
| • Central nervous system toxoplasmosis | • Central nervous system toxoplasmosis (after the neonatal period) |
| • HIV encephalopathy | • HIV encephalopathy |
| • Extrapulmonary cryptococcosis, including meningitis | • Extrapulmonary cryptococcosis, including meningitis |
| • Disseminated nontuberculous mycobacterial infection | • Disseminated nontuberculous mycobacterial infection |
| • Progressive multifocal leukoencephalopathy | • Progressive multifocal leukoencephalopathy |
| • Chronic cryptosporidiosis | • Chronic cryptosporidiosis (with diarrhea); chronic isosporiasis |
| • Chronic isosporiasis | |
| • Disseminated mycosis (extrapulmonary histoplasmosis, coccidioidomycosis) | • Disseminated endemic mycosis (extrapulmonary histoplasmosis, coccidioidomycosis, penicilliosis) |
| • Lymphoma (cerebral or B-cell nonHodgkin) | • Cerebral or B-cell nonHodgkin lymphoma |
| • Symptomatic HIV-associated nephropathy or cardiomyopathy | • HIV-associated nephropathy or cardiomyopathy |
| • Recurrent septicemia (including nontyphoidal *Salmonella*) | |
| • Invasive cervical carcinoma | |
| • Atypical disseminated leishmaniasis | |

(HIV: human immunodeficiency virus)

## TESTS FOR DIAGNOSING HIV

- ***Screening tests:*** Antibody tests: Rapid tests and enzyme-linked immunosorbent assays (ELISA).
- ***Confirmatory/supplemental tests:*** Second and third rapid/ ELISA tests to confirm first HIV test and Western blot assay.
- Same blood sample is utilized for performing all the tests for identifying HIV antibodies.

Screening is done either by rapid test or ELISA. In order to call a person HIV positive, the blood must be tested at least three times with three different test kits on the same sample. The tests are available in the Integrated Counseling and Testing Centers (ICTC). At present, to ensure accuracy, for all HIV-positive cases, a confirmatory test, usually a Western blot, is a highly specific test. It is based on detecting viral core protein (p24) and envelops glycoprotein (gp41) **(Fig. 17G.5)**.

## Counseling in HIV/AIDS

Counseling in HIV/AIDS is very important **(Table 17G.6)**. It consists of the following points:
- Acceptance of serostatus
- Normalize HIV/AIDS
- Reference of social support
- Psychological support

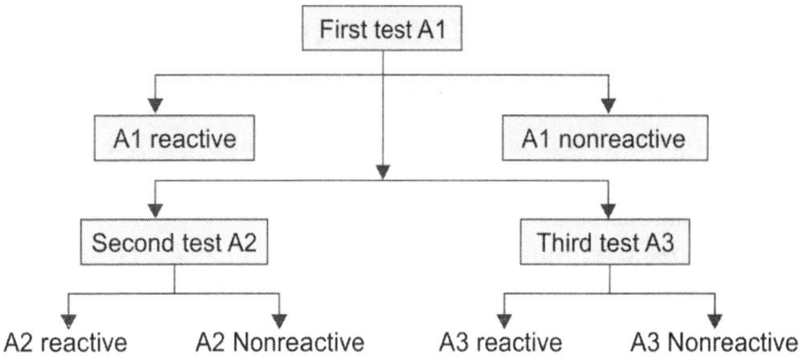

| Report | | |
|---|---|---|
| | A1+, A2+, A3+ | Reactive to HIV Ab |
| | A1– (or) A1+, A2–, A3– | Nonreactive to HIV Ab |
| | A1+, A2–, A3+ (or) A1+, A2+, A3– | Indeterminate |

**Fig. 17G.5:** Strategy for HIV testing.
(HIV: human immunodeficiency virus)

- Facilitates behavior change
- Reduces MTCT
- Early management of opportunistic infections
- Preventive therapy (TB) or contraceptive.

*If the test result is positive:*
The person is informed gently and allowed to react. It is not a death sentence. It only means that the person is educated about taking special care to prevent progression to AIDS in himself/herself by taking the treatment (ART) in right stage and adhering to it.

The person is also educated about not to infect others by the following measures:
- Not donating blood, blood products, or any organs
- Consistently using condoms while having sex
- Not to become pregnant
- Not to share needles.
- The person is encouraged to tell spouse about the HIV status.

***Advice to couple, if both are HIV positive:*** They should avoid getting children. They are permitted to adopt a child legally. They must explain about the need to practice safe sex, by using condoms.

**Table 17G.6:** Counseling in HIV/AIDS.

| Pretest counseling | Post-test counseling |
|---|---|
| • It prepares the client for undergoing test and changing his/ her behavior | • Prepare the client to understand the meaning of positive and negative test and benefits of changing the risk behavior |
| • Provides an opportunity for educating about the risk of transmission | • *If the result is negative:* The person is educated: |
| • To assess how the person may react, if HIV positive | ➤ About self-protection by reducing the high-risk behavior |
| | ➤ The negative result does not mean that the patient cannot get HIV infection |
| | ➤ That if he/she has had a recent exposure, stress the need to undergo test again after the window period |

(HIV: human immunodeficiency virus; AIDS: acquired immunodeficiency syndrome)

## PREVENTION AND CONTROL OF HIV/AIDS

### Prevention of Sexually Transmitted HIV Infection

- Having single sexual partner and being faithful to the partner
- *Having less risky sexual behavior*: Anal sex carries more risk than vaginal sex.
- *Condom use*: Main route of HIV transmission is through sexual route, so main mode of HIV prevention is by correct use of condom consistently.
  - **Male condom:** Since 1990s, condom promotion has gained a significant drive as an important intervention method and use of condom among high-risk populations have also shown growing trends.
    
    There are three types of male condoms available in India: (1) free supply condoms (named as Nirodh), (2) social marketing condoms (Deluxe Nirodh) (available at highly subsidized rate), and (3) commercial sales condoms. Among these, social marketing is the major force for increasing the condom use in India. It is recommended that every sex, which carries a risk of HIV transmission, should be protected by condom use.
    
    Freely distributed condoms in India are available via different Government service delivery outlets, like ICTC, ART centers, Suraksha/STI clinics, immunization centers, and postpartum units. They are usually meant for poor people who cannot afford but who are at risk. The problem of free supply condom is that as it does not bear any cost to the receiver, its value became low leading to more wastage. Moreover, there is a misconception that they are of inferior quality. But factually they are of the same quality like socially marketed condoms.
    
    Potential outlets of social marketed condoms are: Traditional drug stores, nontraditional paan shops, tea/coffee shops, beauty parlors, telephone booths, brothels, hotels/lodges, dhabas, petrol pumps, massage parlors, wine shops, liquor bars, dance parlors, night clubs, private clinics or quacks or dispensing doctors, cinema theaters, etc.
  - **Condom-vending machines (CVM)** were installed by National AIDS Control Organization (NACO) at public places to provide anytime access to quality condoms without embarrassment for shy population. There were three types of condom-vending outlets: low-traffic dispensing outlet (LTDO), medium-traffic dispensing outlet (MTDO), and high-traffic dispensing outlets (HTDO). However, this project was not so popular and nowadays almost not working.
  - **Female condom (FC)** is the only existing prophylactic method for females against STI, HIV, and unwanted pregnancy, and it is a symbol of women empowerment, especially for FSWs to protect herself in a nonnegotiable situation when their male partner denies for using condom. It is available at a heavily subsidized rate via social marketing. However, they are not so much acceptable in India by NACO and are being scaled up in India.
  - **MSM condom:** Thick, with additional lubricants, condoms are needed for anal sex by MSM.
  - **Efficacy of condoms:** Male condoms reduce 80% transmission of heterosexual route and 64% anal sex transmission in MSM and female condoms also have almost same prevention.
- *Voluntary medical male circumcision (VMMC)*: WHO recommended that VMMC can also be an important preventive strategy for 60% risk reduction of female-to-male heterosexual transmission.
- *Early detection and prompt treatment of STI/RTI*: Management of STI/RTI through syndromic approach is a very important part of HIV/AIDS control. For this, NACO has established STI/RTI clinics in medical colleges and district hospitals named as "*Suraksha Clinics*". Different *syndromic drug kits* with color coding are available there.

> Safer sex using condom correctly and consistently is the mainstay to prevent the sexually transmitted HIV infection.
> Other preventive measures to reduce transmission by this route are having single faithful sexual partner, and management of STIs/RTIs through syndromic management.

### Prevention of Parent-to-Child Transmission

The HIV infection can transmit from mother to child in antenatal period, intranatal period during birth, and postnatal period via breastfeeding. The chance of mother/parent-to-child transmission is ranged from 20 to 45% without any intervention. However with antiretroviral drug (ARV) prophylaxis, this can be reduced dramatically.

In India, Nevirapine tablet single dose to the mother during labor followed by Nevirapine syrup to the newborn was started in 2002 and scaled up till 2012, which significantly reduced the risk of transmission to less than 10%.

World Health Organization (WHO) recommended a multidrug ARV regimen in 2013, which could reduce the transmission risk to less than 5%, if stated early in pregnancy and continued during delivery and breastfeeding.

In line with WHO recommendations, Government of India (GOI) decided that from January 1st, 2014, all confirmed HIV-infected pregnant women including those appeared for first time in labor and even breastfeeding women presented for first time should be provided with a fixed dose combination (FDC) of lifelong triple antiretroviral therapy irrespective of WHO clinical staging and CD4 count. For this, *Tenofovir (TDF) (300 mg) + Lamivudine (3TC) (300 mg) + Efavirenz (EFV) (600 mg)*, once daily, is recommended as a FDC in a single tablet for first-line ART lifelong.

- Antiretroviral therapy should be initiated only at ART center.
- *Cotrimoxazole prophylaxis therapy (CPT)* should be initiated, if CD4 count is less than or equal to 250 cells/mm$^3$ and continue throughout antenatal, intranatal, and postnatal period as per national guidelines, to prevent opportunistic infections (OI) (Dose: Double strength tablet—1 tablet daily).
- *Intrapartum*: HIV-positive pregnant women should have normal delivery and cesarean sections to be performed for obstetric indications only.

- *Care of exposed child less than 18 months*: Package of services for the baby: free ARV prophylaxis, co-trimoxazole (CTX) prophylaxis, HIV DNA polymerase chain reaction (PCR) or antibody testing to know the HIV status of the infant/child depending on his/her age, follow-up, immunizations, appropriate infant feeding, and ART when indicated.

    Baby of the mother who is receiving ART must receive daily syrup Nevirapine at least for 6 weeks irrespective of exclusively breastfeeding (EBF) or exclusively replacement feeding (ERF) **(Table 17G.7)**, positive for HIV, a repeat sample is tested for HIV DNA PCR, and if HIV positivity is confirmed by two DNA PCR test, the baby is started on lifelong ART.

**Table 17G.7:** Schedule of daily nevirapine (NVP) prophylaxis for infants.

| Weight (at birth) | Once daily NVP (in mg) | Once daily NVP (in mL) | Duration |
|---|---|---|---|
| Infants who have birth weight less than 2 kg | 2 mg per kg of body weight | 0.2 mL per kg of body weight | For 6 weeks for all HIV-exposed infants, irrespective of exclusively breastfeeding or exclusively replacement fed. It may be extended to 12 weeks, and provided the mother has not received ART for at least 24 weeks |
| Birth weight 2–2.5 kg | 10 mg | 1 mL | |
| Birth weight >2.5 kg | 15 mg | 1.5 mL | |

*Note:* 10 mg Nevirapine in 1 mL suspension.
*Source:* WHO Guidelines.

- *Early infant diagnosis (EID)*: HIV-exposed infants and sick infants with sign and symptoms of HIV should be tested at 6 weeks, 6 months, and again at 12 months using dry blood spot (DBS) by DNA PCR test.

    Final infant diagnosis should be done at 18 months by three rapid antibody tests at ICTC. If the antibody is reactive in all the three tests then the baby is HIV infected and initiate lifelong ART.
- *Update on early infant diagnosis of HIV*: As per the recommendation by WHO in 2016, virological testing of HIV should be done for diagnosis of HIV among infants and children less than 18 months, ART must be started immediately, and all positive test results to be confirmed by collecting a second specimen at the same time or even before.

*Five things to be done at 6 weeks for HIV-exposed infants*:
1. Exclusive breastfeeding (EBF) should be reinforced up to first 6 months.
2. Early infant diagnosis testing
3. Immunization
4. Initiation of CPT and continue till the child is 18 months/continue, if tested positive
5. Stop NVP prophylaxis (extended up to 12 weeks, if mother started late ART).

*Infant feeding guidelines for HIV-exposed and HIV-infected infants less than 6 months (2011 National Guidelines)*:
- Exclusive breastfeeding up to 6 months
- In situations like maternal death, severe maternal illness where breastfeeding cannot be done, ERF can be considered as per *AFASS* criteria (Affordable, Feasible, Acceptable, Sustainable, Safe).

*Remember—no mixed feeding at any cost within first 6 months.*

- To prevent parent-to-child transmission, fixed dose combination of Tenofovir (TDF) (300 mg) + Lamivudine (3TC) (300 mg) + Efavirenz (EFV) (600 mg) is recommended once daily lifelong (irrespective of WHO clinical stage and CD4 count).
- Cesarean sections should be performed for obstetric indications only.
- Infants should receive at least 6 weeks of daily syrup nevirapine.
- Early infant diagnosis should be done at 6 weeks, 6 months, 12 months, and final infant diagnosis at 18 months.
- Exclusively breastfeeding (EBF) should be up to 6 months.

## Prevention of Blood-borne Route of HIV Transmission

Risk of HIV infection following transfusion of HIV-positive blood is 90% irrespective of age and gender of the recipient, type of component transfused, and reason for transfusion.

Annual requirement of blood for India is 12.8 million units as per WHO norm of 1% of the population. In 2002, GOI launched the National Blood Policy for access to good quality, adequate, and safe blood.

*Professional blood donors have been prohibited in India since January 1st, 1998.* So to meet the requirement of this huge amount of safe blood, voluntary blood donors should constitute the main source (WHO recommendation).

### Voluntary Blood Donation

*Voluntary nonremunerated blood donor* means a person who gives blood, plasma, or cellular components as per his/her own will but not get any incentive for this service, either in cash or kind.

The blood safety division is renamed as division of blood transfusion services. Blood Transfusion Councils have set up both at national and state levels, namely National Blood Transfusion Council (NBTC) and State Blood Transfusion Council (SBTC) respectively. Zonal blood testing centers (ZBTCs) are also established. Moreover, establishment of Blood Component Separation Unit (BCSU), model blood banks, modernization of some major blood banks, and procurement of equipment, kits, and reagents has also been done. Some major blood banks and district level blood banks are converted to BCSU, which acts mainly as access points for rural population. Blood transportation vans transfer blood under cold chain from linked mother blood bank to blood storage center (BSC) regularly and also during demand/emergency.

As per National Blood Safety Policy of India, it is mandatory to test every unit of donated blood for detecting HIV1 and HIV2, hepatitis B surface antigen (HBsAg), hepatitis C (HCV), malaria parasite (MP), and syphilis (VDRL).

High-risk group like FSW, MSM, injecting drug users (IDUs), and clients of sex workers should not donate blood, body organs, sperm, or other tissues.

All blood units should be collected from healthy, nonpaid, voluntary donors.

All blood units should be screened for HIV using highly sensitive, specific, and validated tests. Only nonreactive blood units should be used.

- For prevention of blood-borne HIV, professional blood donors have been prohibited in India since January 1st, 1998.
- Blood from voluntary blood donors is the main source of blood supply.
- Every unit of donated blood is tested for HIV, hepatitis B, hepatitis C, malaria parasite, and syphilis.

## Prevention of Infected Syringe/Needle Transmission of HIV

Injecting drug users play an effective route in HIV transmission in India, more than 5% prevalence consistently. The surveillance data for 2008–2009 showed that there is a decreasing trend of HIV among FSW but increasing trend was observed among IDUs and MSM in many states (NACO, 2010).

Blood-borne infections, namely HIV, hepatitis B, and hepatitis C are spreading among IDUs by double burden of risky behaviors due to contaminated needles/syringes and high-risk sexual behaviors under the influence of drugs, thus facilitating the transmission of HIV infection from IDU group to sex workers and ultimately to the general population.

### An Injecting Drug User

A person "who uses any psychoactive substance via injection without a medical purpose for at least once last 3 months" is considered as an IDU. However, *National AIDS Control Programme IV (NACP)* proposed to broaden the definition of IDU as a person who has injected at least once in the last 12 months.

Majority of the IDUs (98%) are dependent on opioids, due to which IDUs incur harms associated with opioid dependence as well.

*For reduction of getting HIV infection via injection route*:
- Stop injecting drugs
- Counseling and treatment for substance use disorder (SUD)
- Try to avoid injections unless they are absolutely necessary
- If injection is necessary, use disposable/auto-disable syringes/needles
- Never share needles
- Safe disposal of the used needles
- *Syringe service program (SSP)*: Some countries have SSP where free sterile syringes and needles are available
- Proper sterilization practices in hospitals, nursing homes, and private clinics.

*Following are some preventive components in the comprehensive package for IDUs (WHO)*:
- Needle and syringe program (NSP)
- Opioid substitution therapy (OST)
- HIV counseling, testing, and referral
- Antiretroviral therapy (ART)
- Prevention of sexually transmitted infections
- Condom programming
- Information, education, and communication (IEC)
- Hepatitis vaccination (for hepatitis A and B), hepatitis diagnosis, and treatment (for hepatitis A, B, and C)
- Tuberculosis diagnosis and treatment
- Behavioral interventions.

*Some recommendations of NACP IV harm reduction program*:
- Female injecting drug user (FIDU), an extra typology
- Definition of IDU expanded from 3 months up to 12 months
- Service should include hepatitis B and hepatitis C prevention
- Availability of naloxone in public healthcare settings
- Proper waste disposal system
- Provision of detoxification like support in detoxification centers, detoxification camps, and home-based detoxification.

*Agonist maintenance treatment with opioids (commonly referred to as OST in India)* has shown better outcomes and better retention rates than other existing treatment strategies, because it helps in retaining the patient in treatment, reducing the use of illicit opioids and other substances, and improving the individual's productivity and quality of life.

There is a difference between illicit opioids and the opioids used as medicines.

The opioids used as OST medicine have slower onset of action, longer duration, and absorbed through safer routes. The use of OST in India is going on since last three decades, with initial use of low-dose buprenorphine followed by higher strength *buprenorphine as well as buprenorphine-naloxone* combination. Other medications such as slow-release oral morphine, and recently, *methadone maintenance treatment (MMT)* have also been started.

**For prevention of infected syringe/needle transmission of HIV**
Harm reduction intervention—among many components, needle and syringe program (NSP) and opioid substitution therapy (OST) are most important.

## Health Education/IEC/BCC

Finally, HIV transmission from any route—be it sexual, blood-borne, infected syringe/needles/parent to child—can only be prevented by fruitful awareness generation via effective IEC to change unhealthy behavior to healthy behavior. In the absence of any vaccine and/or cure, HIV infection is entirely preventable through awareness raising—as awareness raising brings behavior change.

*Information, education and communication should be focused on*:
- To increase knowledge among general population about safer sex, e.g., avoid indiscriminate sex, having one sexual partner, use condoms, and avoid use of shared razors and toothbrushes
- To retain the behavior change among high-risk groups and bridge populations
- To generate demand for care, support, and treatment
- To improve the environment by strengthening changes in societal norms, which allow positive attitudes, beliefs, and practices
- To address discrimination and stigma.

*Targeted audience for IEC/BCC*: Youths, women, sex workers, migrants, others.

*Educational materials*: As Indian people come from different social, cultural, traditional, and religious backgrounds, the language, and content of those materials also vary.
- *Mass media campaigns (targets a mass)*: Doordarshan, public TV service, live music, music videos, private TV channel services via cable and satellite, radio, FM private radio networks, advertisements through movies—the messages

should target on consistent and correct use of condom, STI management services, voluntary blood donation (VBD), prevention of parent-to-child transmission (PPTCT) and stigma and discrimination reduction. The messages can be translated into different languages.

- *Mid media*: Folk drama, folk performance, street theater, puppet shows, IEC video vans, fairs and exhibitions—they use local cultural contexts of the audience. Stress should be given in *haats* and *bazaars* especially during state-specific major festivals where large gatherings are easily available.
- *Print media (is a part of mass media)*: Printed materials, posters, newspapers, newsletters, magazines, journals, books, brochures, posters, flyers, directories, direct mail, letters and postcards, leaflets, handbills, etc.
- *Broadcast media*: TV and radio news.
- *Mobile media*: Flyers, WhatsApp messages, mobile phone messages.
- *Outdoor advertising* like banners, billboards, hoardings, wall paintings, bus panels, kiosks, tabloids, railway stations and trains and metro rails.

For youth, there are two awareness programs:
1. *Adolescence education program (AEP)/school-based sexuality education*—means imparting sex education to school-going adolescents in India in a regular basis—implemented in all states in India through the Department of Education (DoE) and State AIDS Control Societies (SACS)—aim is to cover cent per cent senior schools from class IX to XI, so that they have accurate life-skill knowledge about HIV/AIDS.

    As per the draft of National Education Policy 2016, the schools should impart "sex education in schools for adolescent for safety measures".
2. *Red ribbon clubs*: Red Ribbon Club (RRC) was launched by GOI in the educational institutions, namely colleges to create awareness about HIV/AIDS by providing correct information through peer-to-peer message on safe lifestyles, to clarify their doubts and myths about HIV/AIDS, and to promote voluntary blood donation.

## Other Strategies

1. **Address stigma and discrimination**: Fear of stigma, discrimination, and violence discourages PLHIV to disclose their status. So to uncover the stigma, there should be services that use a human rights-based approach and making more comfortable environment for HIV-positive patients.
2. **Available, accessible, and acceptable HIV health services.**
3. **Community empowerment**-oriented approach.
4. **Violence from key populations against people** should be prevented by monitoring and timely reporting.

> The IEC/BCC use of mass media, mid media, outdoor advertisement should be advocated.
> For youth, there are two awareness programs:
> 1. Adolescence Education Program (AEP)/School-based sexuality education
> 2. Red Ribbon Club

## CARE, SUPPORT AND TREATMENT

### Antiretroviral Drugs

The HIV can be prevented and treated by *ARV* (antiretroviral) drugs.

#### Following are the uses of ARV drugs for HIV infection:
- To prevent parent-to-child transmission of HIV (PPTCT)
- To reduce HIV transmission in serodiscordant couples
- For postexposure prophylaxis (PEP), and
- For pre-exposure prophylaxis (PrEP).

### Antiretroviral Therapy

The ART is defined as lifelong use of combination of ARV drugs for treating HIV infection. There is suppression of HIV virus but these drugs cannot eliminate the virus from the body, thus they cannot cure HIV/AIDS.

*Goal of ART*:
- Viral load suppression
- Drug toxicity minimization
- Pill burden reduction
- Immunity reconstitution
- To increase treatment adherence.

*Benefits of antiretroviral therapy*:
- **Virological**: Maximally suppresses the HIV virus replication to undetectable level.
- **Immunological**: Restores the immune system both qualitative and quantitative.
- **Transmission**: Prevents onward transmission of HIV and thus halts the progression of HIV disease.
- **Therapeutic**: Huge reductions in mortality and morbidity.
- **Opportunistic infections**: Reduces chance of opportunistic infections.
- **Clinical**: Increases longevity, improves quality of life, and helps to lead more productive life with reduced stigma and discrimination.
- **Familial**: Expanded access to ART has an impact on orphanhood and preserve families.
- **TB-HIV**: Prevented resurgence of TB.
- **Others**: Delay the onset of AIDS, thus transformed the common perception of HIV from "virtual death sentence" to "a chronic manageable illness".

*Risks of antiretroviral therapy*:
- Adverse events, short, and long term—like cardiovascular and renal diseases
- Side effects
- Long-term drug toxicities
- Drug–drug interaction
- Immune reconstitution inflammatory syndrome (IRIS).

ART is accessible, and available to all who need it, at free of cost, in public health facilities.

*Milestones of ART global*:
- The first ARV drug AZT or Zidovudine was US FDA approved in 1987 (NRTI).
- In 1995, first PI, Saquinavir, was approved.

- In 1996, first nonnucleoside reverse transcriptase inhibitor (NNRTI), nevirapine, was approved.
- In 1997, first combination ARV tablet was approved (Combivir).
- In 2002, ten antiretroviral drugs were added to the list of "Essential Medicines" by WHO.
- In 2003, "3 by 5" initiative of WHO/UNAIDS—supply of free ART drugs to 3 million people by end of 2005 in developing countries.
- 2006 guidelines of WHO: ART to be started to those who have advanced clinical disease and/or CD4 cell count less than or equal to 200/mm$^3$.
- In 2007, first integrase inhibitor was approved
- In 2010, WHO recommended to start ART at CD4 count less than or equal to 350/mm$^3$
- In 2013, WHO guidelines set threshold to start ART at CD4 count less than or equal to 500/mm$^3$
- In 2015, pre-exposure prophylaxis for HIV was undertaken and implemented since 2016.
- In 2016, WHO recommended the treatment for all, at any CD4 cell count, WHO clinical staging, population, and age.

### Milestones of ART in India

The image of HIV disease was considered as a death sentence previously, and was completely changed due to access to ART in India. ART program of India has been identified as one of best national healthcare programs.

Though the so-called "AIDS cocktail therapy"/HAART or highly active ART, which is triple drug therapy or combination antiretroviral therapy (cART), was launched in 1996, it was unavailable and unaffordable as the costs were very high. Moreover, people had to take higher number of pills and scared due to adverse effects of drugs. PLHIV had to take 32 pills/day in 1998, with a price of nearly ₹ 30,000/month.
- Government of India announced free ART program on November 30th, 2003 and started it on April 1st, 2004 and scaled up in a phased manner.
- The CD4 testing was made free from 2006.
- Second-line ART was launched in January, 2008, which was expanded later on, EID with care of exposed infants was initiated in 2010.
- The ART plus was launched in October, 2010 to increase access to second-line ART.
- Starting of ART at CD4 count less than 350 was launched in 2011.
- Stavudine was stopped in 2012.

In 2014, the country adapted the new WHO guidelines for earlier initiation of ART at CD4 count less than 500, with simplified ARV regimen, third-line ART, etc. Finally in 2017, it was decided to "treat all PLHIV with ART" at any CD4 cell count, WHO clinical staging, age or population as per revised guideline.

India's ART program is world's second largest, only after South Africa, which has the world's biggest ART program.

### Generic ARVs from India:
The generic ARVs from India are listed in **Table 17G.8**.

**Table 17G.8:** The generic antiretrovirals (ARVs) from India.

| Nucleoside reverse transcriptase inhibitors (NRTIs) | Nonnucleoside reverse transcriptase inhibitors (NNRTIs) | Protease inhibitors (PIs) |
|---|---|---|
| • Zidovudine (AZT) <br> • Didanosine (ddI) <br> • Stavudine (d4T) <br> • Lamivudine (3TC) <br> • Abacavir (ABC) <br> • Emtricitabine (FTC) | • Nevirapine (NVP) <br> • Efavirenz (EFV) <br> • Rilpivirine (RLP) <br> • Etravirine (ETV) <br> *Nucleotide reverse transcriptase inhibitors (NtRTIs)* <br> • Tenofovir (TDF) <br> *Entry inhibitors* <br> • Maraviroc (CCR5) <br> • Enfuvirtide (ENF, T20) <br> *Integrase inhibitors:* <br> • Raltegravir (RAL) <br> • Elvitegravir (ELV), Bictegravir (BIC) <br> • Dolutegravir (DTG) | • Saquinavir (SQV) <br> • Indinavir (IDV) <br> • Ritonavir (RTV) <br> • Nelfinavir (NFV) <br> • Lopinavir/ritonavir (LPV/r) <br> • Atazanavir (ATV) <br> • Darunavir (DRV) <br> *Postattachment inhibitor* <br> • Ibalizumab |

### ART for advanced HIV:
Though mortality and morbidity associated with HIV have decreased due to access of increased ART, still around "*1 in 3 PLHIV has an advanced HIV*", who has a high death risk, even after ART initiation, which increases with reduction of CD4 cell count. The common causes of death among them are tuberculosis, severe bacterial infections, and cryptococcal meningitis. WHO new guidelines recommend that "*PLHIV with advanced HIV disease should be offered a package of care including screening, rapid ART initiation, prevention/treatment of major opportunistic infections, and intensified treatment adherence support*" to reduce morbidity and mortality.

**Following is the *definition of advanced HIV disease as per WHO*:**
- Adults, adolescents, and children more than or equal to 5-year old, advanced HIV disease is considered as a CD4 count less than 200/mm$^3$ or WHO clinical stage 3 or 4.
- All children younger than 5-year old with HIV infection should be considered as having advanced HIV disease.

### Timing for initiation of ART:
First consolidated guidelines about timing of initiation of antiretroviral (ARV) drugs in HIV was published in 2013 by WHO. Revised WHO consolidated guidelines published in 2016, which recommended that ART should be used for all PLHIV immediately on diagnosis irrespective of CD4 count.

Countries are now following these recommendations within their epidemiological settings. *Majority of the countries adopted and implemented this policy to "treat all"* **(Box 17G.1)**.

### Government of India guidelines:
As per the recommendations of technical resource group on ART and review of evidence of WHO 2016 ART guidelines, the guidelines for timing of initiation of ART under NACP has revised and it was clear cut that all PLHIV should be treated with ART irrespective of CD4 count and WHO clinical stage.

### What to Start: Antiretroviral Therapy Regimens

Fixed-dose combinations of ARVs are preferred because they are easy to prescribe and easy for patients to take, thereby facilitating

## Box 17G.1: Why initiate ART early?
- Longer life
- More effective and safe
- Convenient antiretroviral regimens are available
- Reduced chance of nonAIDS-related diseases in HIV-infected population (cancer, cardiovascular disease)
- Prevent serious AIDS-related diseases
- Less chance of neurocognitive decline
- Likelihood of CD4/CD8 ratio normalization is three times greater
- Lesser chance of immune reconstitution inflammatory syndrome
- Lesser risk of developing antiretroviral (ARV) resistance
- Lesser likelihood of toxicities
- Prevention of transmission to HIV uninfected partners
- More economic sense.

improved and desirable treatment adherence. This is essential for PLHIV as the treatment is life-long and we need to minimize the chances of developing drug resistant mutants in their body and the resultant treatment failure. Further, FDCs have distinct advantages in drug procurement and distribution, essentially the drug stock management itself. The national experience has shown that regimens with FDCs are more acceptable, well tolerated and adequately complied with.

### Antiretroviral regimens for prevention and treatment of HIV infection (2018):
- In 2017, WHO felt that optimization of antiretroviral drug regimens is a critical component to support country efforts to achieve the *Target-90-90-90*: which means that 90% of HIV-positive people should know their HIV status, among these diagnosed people, 90% should be on treatment, and 90% of those put on treatment should have fully viral load suppression.
- To achieve this target, new *WHO interim guidelines, 2018* recommend preferred first-line ARV drug schedules for adults, adolescents, and children, which include dolutegravir (DTG) and raltegravir (RAL): as per this guideline, DTG-based regimen might be considered as a preferred first-line regimen for PLHIV initiating ART in:
  - Adults and adolescents
  - Women and girls of childbearing potential
  - Infants and children with approved DTG dosing.
- An RAL-based regimen may be considered as an alternative first-line regimen for infants and children where approved DTG dosing is not available. Moreover, an RAL-based regimen may be considered as a preferred first-line regimen for neonates.
- *Rationale*: WHO has revealed that DTG-based regimens are better tolerated, less adverse events (AEs) compared with EFV600, more rapid viral suppression, higher genetic resistance barrier, effective against HIV-2 (which is resistant to NNRTIs), and 10–15% less expensive than current EFV formulations.
- Also, DTG in combination with an optimized NRTI backbone is a preferred second-line regimen among people for whom nonDTG-based regimens has failed.

**Table 17G.9** shows summary of options for first-line, second-line, and third-line ART regimens for adults in sequential order (including pregnant women and adolescents) and children (2018).

**Table 17G.9:** Summary of options for first-line, second-line, and third-line antiretroviral therapy (ART) regimens for adults in sequential order (including pregnant women and adolescents) and children (2018).

| Population | First-line regimens | Second-line regimens | Third-line regimens |
|---|---|---|---|
| Adults and adolescents (including women and adolescent girls who are of childbearing potential or are pregnant) | 2 NRTIs + DTG | 2 NRTIs + (ATV/r or lopinavir/ ritonavir (LPV/r) | Darunavir/ ritonavir (DRV/r) + DTG + 1–2 NRTIs (if possible, consider optimization using genotyping) |
|  | 2 NRTIs + EFV | 2 NRTIs + DTG |  |
| Children | 2 NRTIs + DTG | 2 NRTIs + (ATV/r or LPV/r) |  |
|  | Two NRTIs + LPV/r | Two NRTIs + DTG |  |
|  | Two NRTIs + NNRTI | Two NRTIs + DTG |  |

(NRTI: nucleoside reverse transcriptase inhibitor; DTG: dolutegravir)

### Three-tier Model of HIV Treatment Service
Three-tier model of HIV treatment service is depicted in **Figure 17G.6**.

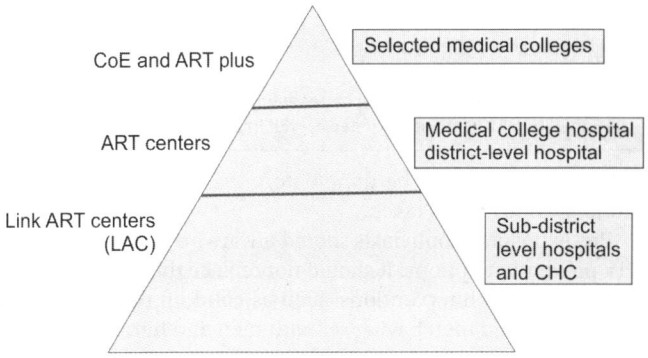

**Fig. 17G.6:** Three-tier model for ART services.
(ART: antiretroviral therapy; CoE: center of excellence; CHC: community health center)

**ARV drugs:**
Uses—PPTCT, reduce transmission of HIV in serodiscordant couples, post-PEP and pre-exposure prophylaxis (PrEP).
The ART should be used for all PLHIV immediately on diagnosis irrespective of CD4 count.
Tenofovir (TDF) + 3TC (or FTC) + EFV in a fixed dose combination is the preferred regimen.
The WHO Interim Guidelines, 2018 include DTG and RAL.

### Pre-exposure Prophylaxis for Prevention of Acquisition of HIV (WHO Recommendation)
Oral PrEP for HIV infection is the consumption of ARV drugs before potential exposure by people who are HIV-uninfected to occlude the acquisition of HIV. Daily PrEP decreases the risk of getting HIV through sexual route by more than 90% and among inject drug users (IDU) by more than 70%.

**Target group:** HIV uninfected people who are at substantial risk of getting HIV infection.

In 2012, WHO recommended PrEP among serodiscordant couples, MSM, and TG people.

In 2014, WHO developed consolidated HIV guidelines for KPs, which include MSM, IDU, sex workers, TGs, prisoners, and other closed settings, which replaced the earlier WHO recommendations on PrEP and *entitled the offer of PrEP for people who are at substantial risk of getting HIV infection, rather than limiting the recommendation to only specific population.*

This recommendation covered a *wider range of populations to be benefitted from this additional prevention option and allowed the offer of PrEP to be based on individual assessment, and not only limited to risk group.*

Thus, WHO has expanded the recommendation to include all population groups at substantial risk of HIV infection.

> **Definition of "substantial risk" of HIV infection:**
> Initially, it was defined as HIV incidence more than 3/100 person–years in the absence of PrEP, which was seen among some groups of MSM, transgender, and heterosexual men and women who had undiagnosed/untreated HIV-infected sexual partners.
>
> As per recommendation of International Antiviral Society, USA expert panel in 2014, HIV incidence more than 2/100 person–years is sufficient for offering oral PrEP.
>
> Thus, there are variable thresholds for offering PrEP depending on epidemiological patterns, resources available, costs, feasibility, demand, and other opportunities.
>
> In 2016, risk assessment tools for better definition of substantial risk were designed by WHO and incorporated in PrEP implementation guidance.

The HIV testing to be done before PrEP and then every 3 months while PrEP is taken.

Pre-exposure prophylaxis should always be given with other HIV prevention options. It should not replace the other existing HIV prevention interventions, such as condom promotion for sex workers and men having sex with men and harm reduction for people who inject drugs.

### Which drug should be given?
World Health Organization (2016) recommended that *countries can consider all of the following three drug regimens* for PrEP (including pregnancy and breastfeeding):
1. TDF alone,
2. TDF/FTC, and
3. TDF/3TC—depending on their populations at risk, availability of tenofovir-containing drugs and other considerations.

Pre-exposure prophylaxis either can be taken orally, using an antiretroviral drug (either tenofovir or tenofovir plus emtricitabine), or topically in the form of vaginal gel-containing tenofovir.

Pre-exposure prophylaxis is highly effective only when used:
- People who start PrEP may have side effects in the first few weeks like nausea, headache, abdominal cramp, etc. These are usually so mild and self-limiting that do not need discontinuation of PrEP.
- Pre-exposure prophylaxis is needed during risky periods, which start when there is a change in relationship status, leaving school, leaving home, alcohol and drug use, trauma, migration, or other events.
- PrEP may be stopped, if the person taking PrEP is no longer at risk.
- PrEP starts its full protection after 7 doses for anal sex and 20 doses for vaginal sex and injecting drug use.
- If people report exposure to HIV before full protection, they should be addressed for postexposure prophylaxis also.
- When they are on both PrEP and PEP, PrEP can be discontinued 28 days after the last potential exposure to HIV-infected fluids.
- PEP started after recent HIV exposure can be converted to PrEP after 28 days, if there is continuing substantial risk.

***India:*** In India, PrEP for HIV was launched at Sonagachi of West Bengal in December, 2015 by National AIDS Control Organization under Health Ministry with the financial support of Melinda Gates Foundation. In this project, some medicines (TDF/FTC) are given to HIV-negative sex workers who are engaged sexually with a HIV-positive person to prevent HIV/AIDS.

> The PrEP should be offered for people who are at substantial risk of getting HIV infection, along with other HIV preventive options like condom, etc., and should be continued as long as the person is at risk.
>
> World Health Organization recommends that countries can choose all three drug regimens for PrEP (including pregnancy and breastfeeding):
> 1. TDF alone
> 2. TDF/FTC
> 3. TDF/3TC

## Postexposure Prophylaxis (Table 17G.10)

***Definition:*** Postexposure prophylaxis for HIV is a method to prevent the chance of getting HIV after a recent potential exposure (either through occupational exposure or via sexual intercourse) using a short course (28 days course) of an antiretroviral treatment.

### When PEP should be initiated?
Postexposure prophylaxis (PEP) for HIV has its greatest effect if begun within 2 hours of exposure, it is essential to act immediately. There is little benefit if > 72 hours have lapsed but PEP can still be used if the health care worker presents after 72 hours of exposure. It is seen that, if PEP started early after exposure, it can reduce the risk of being infected by HIV by over 80%. However, it may not be possible for many individuals to access these PEP services within 72 hours. Thus, PEP providers

**Table 17G.10:** Recommended PEP regimens.

| Dosages of the drugs for PEP for adults | Recommendation for PEP | Duration |
|---|---|---|
| Tenofovir (TDF) 300 mg + Lamivudine (3TC) 300 mg One Tab (FDC) once daily (1–OD) | One tab immediately within 2 hours of accidental exposure, either at day time or at night time | Next day one tab once OD, continue for 4 weeks |
| Lopinavir (200 mg) + Ritonavir (50 mg) Two Tab (FDC) twice daily (2-BD) | Two Tab Immediately within 2 hours of accidental exposure, either at day time or at night time | Next day two-tab BD, continue for 4 weeks |
| If LPV/r is not available/can not be used, Tenofovir (300 mg) + Lamivudine (300 mg) + Efavirenz (600 mg), One Tab OD may be given for 4 weeks. | | |

should offer other essential interventions and referrals for those clients presenting after 72 hours.

*Duration:* 4 weeks (28 days)

*Complete a full course of PEP is important:* It is evidenced that only 57% of the people who initiated PEP have completed the full course.

Assessment of eligibility for PEP depends on *HIV status of the source (status code)*, background prevalence, and local epidemiological patterns.

*Following are the potential exposures warranting HIV PEP (exposure code):*
- *Body fluids:* Like blood, blood-stained saliva, vaginal secretions, semen, breast milk, cerebrospinal fluid, amniotic fluid, peritoneal fluid, synovial, pericardial fluid, pleural fluid
- Mucous membrane, i.e., sexual exposure; splashes to eye, nose, or oral cavity
- Parenteral exposures.

*Following exposures do not need HIV PEP:*
- Exposed individual is already HIV infected;
- Established source is HIV negative; and
- Exposures to body fluids, which do not have a significant risk, i.e., saliva, tears, urine, and sweat.

If PEP is not needed, the exposed person should be counseled for limiting future exposure and HIV testing can be provided, if the exposed person desires.

## MANAGE COMMON COINFECTIONS AND COMORBIDITIES

### Co-trimoxazole Prophylaxis

Co-trimoxazole is a fixed-dose combination of two antimicrobial drugs (sulfamethoxazole and trimethoprim); it treats and prevents a variety of bacterial, fungal, and protozoan infections. CTX prevention is a feasible, well-tolerated, and cost-effective intervention to prevent opportunistic infections (OI) and to reduce HIV-related mortality and morbidity in PLHIV.

The first WHO guidelines on CTX prophylaxis was published in 2006, it was reviewed and updated in 2014. Evidence is showing that with expanded access to ART, there is a wider benefit of CTX prophylaxis over and above the prevention of some AIDS-associated opportunistic infection. These benefits include prevention of malaria and/or severe bacterial infections (SBIs) in PLHI.

### Tuberculosis

The most common cause of death among hospitalized PLHIV is TB. Timely initiation of *ART* and implementing the *"three I's"* for HIV/TB (increased TB case-finding, *isoniazid preventive therapy/IPT,* and infection control) are important to prevent mortality from TB-HIV.

### Cryptococcal Disease
- *For induction phase:* Two-week combination antifungal regimens are recommended.
- *For consolidation phase:* 8-week antifungal regimen is recommended by fluconazole.
- *For maintenance treatment:* Treatment by oral fluconazole 200 mg once daily is recommended.
- *Timing of ART initiation:* ART initiation is not recommended immediately due to the high risk of life-threatening immune reconstitution inflammatory syndrome.
- ART initiation should be started after 4 weeks treatment with amphotericin B-containing regimens along with flucytosine or fluconazole, or after 4–6 weeks treatment with a high-dose oral fluconazole regimen.

### Hepatitis B Coinfection

The HIV-infected adults are at high risk of acquiring HBV. Therefore, screening of all PLHIV should be done for HBsAg and vaccination should be given, if needed.

### Hepatitis C Coinfection

It is advisable to clinically stabilize HIV using ART before initiating treatment for HCV, especially with advanced immunosuppression. The newer oral direct-acting antiviral HCV regimens (DAAs) are efficacious for HIV/HCV coinfection.

### Malaria

In high malaria prevalent areas, CTX should be started irrespective of CD4 cell count or WHO stage.

Patients having HIV/AIDS and uncomplicated *Plasmodium falciparum* malaria do not use artesunate + sulfadoxine-pyrimethamine, if they are treated with CTX.

### Sexually Transmitted Infections

Integration of STI services should be an important part of comprehensive HIV care.

### Cervical Cancer

The HIV-infected women have a greater chance of getting precancer and invasive cervical cancer. Therefore, screening of all women with HIV should be done for cervical cancer irrespective of age. Prompt treatment for precancerous and cancerous lesions should be provided. WHO recommendations cover HPV vaccination, prevention, screening, treatment, and palliative care of cervical cancer.

### Vaccines for PLHIV

The HIV-exposed infants, children, and adolescents with HIV should receive all recommended vaccines according to national immunization schedules. For adults, influenza, hepatitis B, pneumococcal, and tetanus vaccines are usually indicated.

### HIV-related Skin and Oral Conditions

Antiretroviral therapy is the treatment of choice for many skin conditions, which are associated with HIV like Kaposi sarcoma, eosinophilic folliculitis, molluscum contagiosum, etc.

## Assessment and Management of Cardiovascular Diseases (WHO Recommendation)

Strategies for prevention of cardiovascular diseases address modifiable risk factors like hypertension, tobacco, obesity, unhealthy diet, and lack of exercise to all PLHIV.

## Assessment and Management of Depression

As per WHO guidelines, assessment and management of depression can be included in the package of HIV care services.

### Palliative Care

Through all stages of HIV disease, PLHIV experience different types of pain and other discomfort. So, caregivers should identify the cause and should control the pain. WHO is now working to develop guidelines of palliative care.

> **Prevention of Opportunistic Infections**
>
> The CTX prevention is a feasible, well-tolerated, and inexpensive intervention to prevent OI and reduce HIV-related mortality and morbidity in PLHIV.
> - Timely initiation of ART and implementing the "three I's" for HIV/TB (increased TB case-finding, isoniazid preventive therapy/IPT and infection control) are important to prevent TB and mortality from HIV-associated TB.
> - Antifungal regimens are recommended for cryptococcal disease.
> - Assessment and management of cardiovascular disease in PLHIV are needed.
> - Assessment and management of depression in PLHIV should be addressed.
> - WHO is now working to develop guidelines of palliative care.

## GLOBAL HEALTH SECTOR STRATEGY ON HIV 2022–2030 TOWARDS ENDING AIDS

Global health sector strategies on HIV, viral hepatitis, and sexually transmitted infections for the period 2022–2030 (GHSSs) guide the health sector in implementing strategically focused responses to achieve the goals of ending AIDS, viral hepatitis B and C and sexually transmitted infections by 2030. This strategy outlines both what countries need to do and what WHO will do. If implemented, these fast-track actions by countries and by WHO will accelerate and intensify the HIV response in order for the "end of AIDS" to become a reality.

The strategy builds on the extraordinary public health achievements made in the global HIV response since WHO launched the Special Programme on AIDS in 1986. It continues the momentum generated by the Millennium Development Goals and the universal access commitments.

### India

To respond to the challenge, the Government of India established the National AIDS Committee in 1986, which led to the establishment of National AIDS Control Organization in 1992 to oversee the policies for prevention and control of the HIV infection. The first phase of the National AIDS Control Programme (NACP) started in 1992 and lasted until 1999. The first phase contained initial interventions focused on understanding modes of transmission and on prevention, blood safety and information, education and communication strategy to increase awareness. This was followed by NACP-II (2000–2005), NACP-III (2006–2011), NACP-IV (2012–2017), which was extended for a further four years till March 2021). In the meanwhile, a seven-year National Strategic Plan on HIV/AIDS and STIs (2017–2024) was initiated overlapping phases IV and V. In the NACP-IV, the focus was on consolidating the gains achieved in the previous phases, dealing with emerging vulnerabilities and balancing between prevention and growing need for treatment. NACP-IV aimed at improving integration and mainstreaming HIV care in the general health system. In the current phase of NACP- V (2021–2026), the focus is on ensuring PLHIV survive longer and lead productive lives. This will be achieved through improving retention in HIV care and adherence to ART. The program is transitioning towards a client-centric approach to providing care, support and treatment services through differentiated care service delivery models, community system strengthening and community-based service delivery. The current strategic plan aims to achieve zero new infections, zero AIDS-related deaths and zero discrimination for paving the way for an end of AIDS as a public health threat by 2030. NACP-V is further explained in *Chapter 47: Health Policies and Programs in India.*

## SUGGESTED READING

1. Ministry of Health and Family Welfare, NACO. (2016). NACP 4 Programme document. [online] Available from http://naco.gov.in/ strategy-document.
2. Ministry of Health and Family Welfare, NACO. (2017). ART treatment guidelines. http://www.naco.gov.in/om-revised-guidelines-art.
3. Ministry of Health and Family Welfare, NACO. Operational Guidelines for Condom promotion by State Aids Control Societies.
4. Ministry of Health and Family Welfare. (2015). National Health Portal of India. National Blood Policy (2003).
5. NACO. (2013). Prevention of Parent to Child Transmission(PPTCT). Available from http://naco.gov.in/prevention-parent-child- transmissionpptct.
6. NACO. HIV sentinel surveillance 2016-17 technical brief Dec 2017.
7. NACO. Department of AIDS Control, Ministry of Health and Family Welfare, Government of India. (2013). Updated Guidelines for Prevention of Parent to Child Transmission (PPTCT) of HIV using Multi Drug Anti-retroviral Regimen in India.
8. NACO; Ministry of Health and Family Welfare, Government of India. (2014). Journey of ART Programme in India. Story of a Decade. Care, Support and Treatment Division. Department of AIDS Control.
9. NACO; Ministry of Health and Family Welfare, Government of India. (2017). Revised Guideline for ART. [online] Available from http:// www.naco.gov.in/ om-revised-guidelines-art.
10. NACO; MoHFW, GOI. (2017). Red Ribbon Club. [online] IEC and Mainstreaming. Available from http://naco.gov.in/iec-mainstreaming-division.
11. National AIDS Control Organisation, Ministry of Health and Family Welfare, Government of India. (2017). National Strategic Plan for HIV/AIDS and STI, 2017–2024.
12. National AIDS Control Organisation. (2016). Injecting Drug Use Strategy Report for NACP IV.
13. National AIDS Control Organisation. (2017). STI/RTI Services. [online] Available from http://naco.gov.in/sti-rti-services.
14. Rao R. The journey of opioid substitution therapy in India: Achievements and challenges. Indian J Psychiatry. 2017;59(1):39- 45.
15. Sankalak. Status of National AIDS Response, 4th edition. NACO, MoHFW, GOI, 2022.
16. Smith DK, Herbst JH, Zhang X, et al. Condom effectiveness for HIV prevention by consistency of use among men who have sex with men in the United States. J Acquir Immune Defic Syndr. 2014;68(3):337-44.
17. Technical Report India HIV Estimates 2021 National AIDS Control Organisation & Indian Council of Medical Research – National Institute

of Medical Statistics (ICMR-NIMS) Ministry of Health & Family Welfare, Government of India.
18. U.S. Global Health Policy. (2012). The Global HIV/AIDS Epidemic, fact sheet, 2012.
19. UNAIDS. (2017). UNAIDS DATA BOOK 2017. [online] Available from: http://www.unaids.org/en/resources/documents/2017/2017_ data_book.
20. Weller SC, Davis-Beaty K. Condom effectiveness in reducing heterosexual HIV transmission. Cochrane Database Syst Rev. 2001;(3):CD003255.
21. WHO, Geneva. (2015). Guideline on when to start antiretroviral therapy and on pre-exposure prophylaxis for HIV. [online] Available from: http://www. who.int/hiv/pub/guidelines/earlyrelease-arv/en.
22. WHO, UNICEF and UNAIDS. (2013). Global update of HIV Treatment 2013, Results, Impact and Opportunities. [online] Available from: https://www.who.int/hiv/pub/progressreports/update2013/en/.
23. WHO. (2012). Voluntary medical male circumcision for HIV prevention. Fact sheet: 2012. [online] Available from: https://www. who.int/hiv/topics/ malecircumcision/fact_sheet/en/.
24. WHO. (2015). From MDGs (Millennium Development Goals) to SDGs (Sustainable Development Goals). [online] Available from: https:// www.who.int/gho/publications/mdgs-sdgs/en/.
25. WHO. (2016). Consolidated guidelines on the use of Antiretroviral Drugs for treating and preventing HIV infection, recommendation for a Public Health Approach, 2nd edition.
26. WHO. (2017). HIV Treatment. Policy Brief. Guidelines for managing advanced HIV disease and rapid initiation of antiretroviral therapy.
27. WHO. (2018). Dolutegravir (DTG) and the fixed dose combination (FDC) of tenofovir/lamivudine/dolutegravir (TLD).
28. WHO. Appropriate Medicines: Options for Pre-Exposure Prophylaxis. Geneva: World Health Organization; 2018.
29. WHO. Consolidated guidelines on the use of antiretroviral drugs for treating and preventing HIV infection-recommendations for a Public Health Approach. 2nd edition. Geneva: World Health Organization; 2016.
30. WHO. Global Health Sector Strategy on HIV 2016–2021 towards ending AIDS. June 2016.
31. WHO. Guidelines on post-exposure prophylaxis for HIV and the use of co-trimoxazole prophylaxis for HIV-related infections among adults, adolescents and children: recommendations for a public health approach—December 2014 supplement to the 2013 consolidated guidelines on the use of antiretroviral drugs for treating and preventing HIV infection. Geneva: World Health Organization; 2014.
32. WHO. HIV/AIDS;Factsheet July 2023
33. WHO. Policy Brief: Updated recommendations on first-line and second- line antiretroviral regimens and post-exposure prophylaxis and recommendations on early infant diagnosis of HIV: HIV treatment, interim guidance. Geneva: World Health Organization; 2018.
34. World Health Organization. Blood Transfusion Safety. Voluntary Non-remunerated Blood Donation. [online] Available from https:// www.who.int/bloodsafety/voluntary_donation/en/.

# EPIDEMIOLOGY OF SEXUALLY TRANSMITTED DISEASES AND ITS PREVENTION AND CONTROL

*Abhishek Mishra, Neeraj Agarwal*

| | |
|---|---|
| CM7.2 | Enumerate, describe and discuss the mode of transmission and measures for prevention and control of STD |
| CM8.1 | Describe and discuss the epidemiological and control measures applicable in STD |

*Case Scenario 1*

Dr Anirudh has joined a Community Health Center (CHC) recently which is close to International Border. Soon he has noticed that most of the Adults and Adolescents clients attending OPD have complained of unexplained Urethral discharge and genital ulcer without rash. After proper counselling at "Suraksha clinics", laboratory clinic results are found to be positive for one or more Sexually Transmitted Infections positive. Prepacked color coded drug packs are being given to patients and soon they got relieved from their symptoms. Health awareness generation camps through "Nukkad Nataks" and IEC Posters being displayed at prominent public places regarding safe sexual practices. After six months, Dr Anirudh has noticed a significant decline in patients complaining of similar complains in his CHC.

*Case Scenario 2*

A medical officer has noticed high rate of infertility and unwanted birth outcomes in a group of migrant population in her area. She has visited to that community and came to know that in most of the family the male members are working outside for a livelihood for most part of the year. She advised all female members of reproductive age group for clinical check-up and laboratory examination at the health center which is free of cost. Most of the results come out positive for one or more STIs for which color coded drug packs are being distributed. They are advised to bring their partners for counseling and check up at "Suraksha clinics" and drug is given to them too. After couple of month improved fertility rate and declined unwanted birth outcomes have noticed in that population.

## INTRODUCTION

These are a group of diseases usually transmitted by sexual contact and being caused by a wide range of bacteria, viruses, fungus, protozoal and ectoparasites. Some of these may also be spread through blood or blood products (nonsexual means). Moreover, few sexually transmitted diseases are transmitted from mother to child and thereby lead to poor pregnancy, neonatal, and child health outcomes.

From earlier periods these infections were called as "venereal diseases" (VD). The word veneral is derived from a word Venus meaning "Goddess of love" in Egypt. Keeping in view the high degree of social stigma attached with it, World Health Organization rephrased it to sexually transmitted diseases (STDs) since 1974. The current name sexually transmitted infections, 1999 onwards has gained momentum, as many times these are manifested as asymptomatic infections only.

Sexually transmitted infections have prominent sequelae—for example, roughly one-third of pregnant women infected with syphilis experience adverse birth outcomes including stillbirth, human papillomavirus (HPV) infection leads to an estimated 266,000 cervical cancer deaths annually, and some bacterial STIs cause pelvic inflammatory disease, female infertility, preterm delivery, and low birth weight. Other factors which aggravates these infections as a concern in modern times are:

- Under reporting of the infections and cases
- Associated stigma and shame
- Often not diagnosed properly at lower levels of health care delivery system
- Adverse effects on neonatal, fetal outcomes and female fertility
- Self-intake of medication and incomplete treatment
- Growing antimicrobial resistance in agents causing sexually transmitted infections.

Some researchers have established the fact that the presence of STIs increases the chance of getting HIV 6–10 times higher, in compared to that of noninfected persons.

## PROBLEM STATEMENT

### Global

More than 1 million sexually transmitted infections are acquired every day worldwide, the majority of which are asymptomatic. In 2020, WHO estimated 374 million new infections with 1 of 4 STIs: chlamydia (129 million), gonorrhea (82 million), syphilis (7.1 million) and trichomoniasis (156 million). More than 500 million people 15–49 years are estimated to have a genital infection with herpes simplex virus (HSV or herpes). Human papillomavirus infection is associated with over 311 000 cervical cancer deaths each year. Almost 1 million pregnant women were estimated to be infected with syphilis in 2016, resulting in over 350 000 adverse birth outcomes. (WHO. Sexually transmitted infections. Factsheet 10 July 2023) **(Fig. 17G.7)**.

### Indian Scenario

In India, the prevalence of four curable STI among general populations is in between 0 and 3.9 percent. and consistently this number is on rise. Some of the major STIs burden in India is given in **Table 17G.11** (Bhatta M et al.).

**Table 17G.11:** Number of major STI cases in India, 2018.

| STIs | No. of cases | Male | Female |
|---|---|---|---|
| Syphilis | 15,995 | 6,126 | 9,869 |
| Gonococcal infection | 55,470 | 15,836 | 39,634 |

*Source:* National Health Profile (NHP) of India-2019, Central Bureau of Health Intelligence, GOI.

## EPIDEMIOLOGY

### Host Factors

#### Age

Almost all STIs are common in 20–30 years of age group, followed by 15–19 years and more than 30 years.

#### Sex

The morbidity rate is high among men than women, however severity of the diseases are more in women than men.

#### Socioeconomic Status

Peoples from lower socioeconomic classes are having higher morbidity rate.

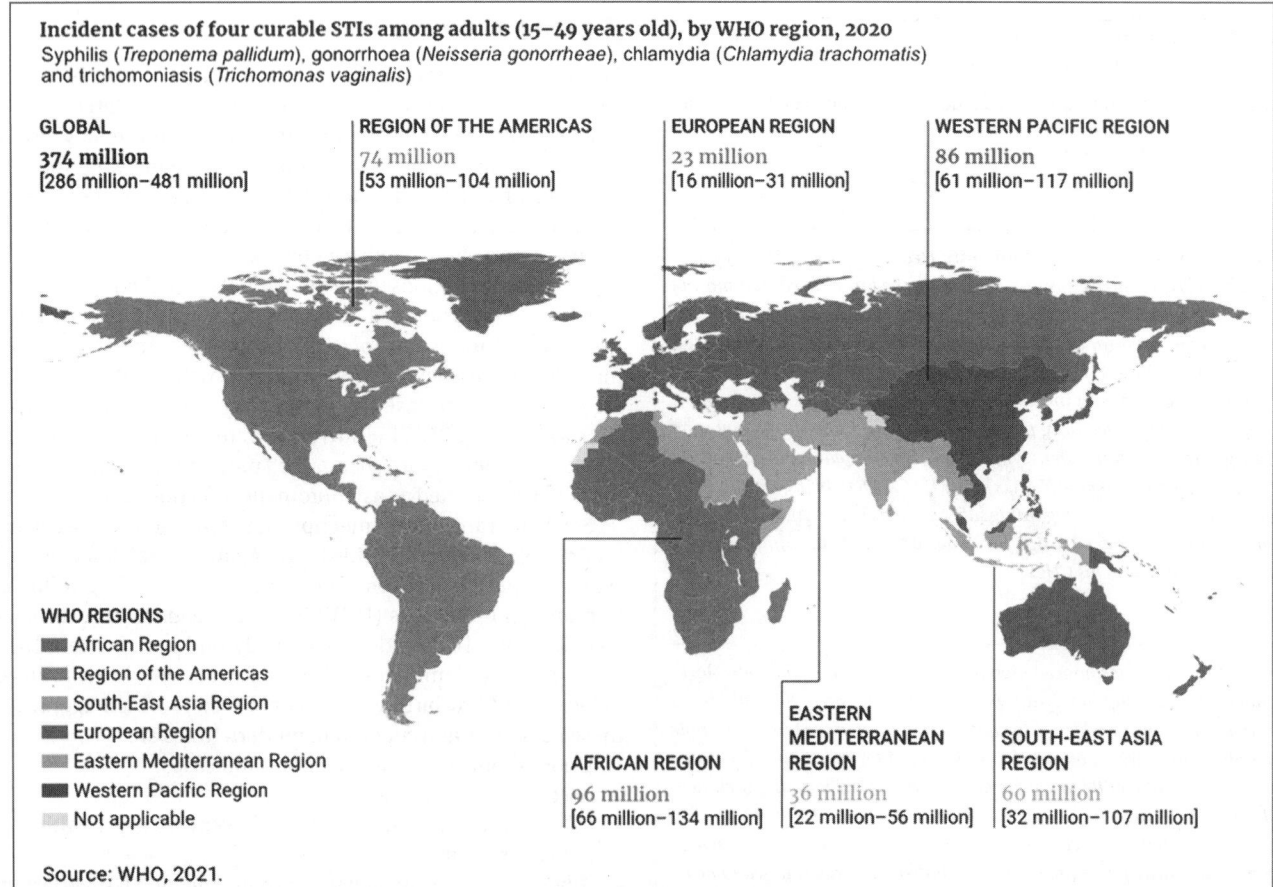

**Fig. 17G.7:** Incident cases of STI among adults, by WHO region, 202.
(WHO. Global Sexually Transmitted Infections Programme, Accessed in July 2023 and available from https://www.who.int/teams/global-hiv-hepatitis-and-stis-programmes/stis/overview.)

## Marital Status

The frequency of STIs are high among unmarried (singles), divorced and separated individuals than that of married couples.

## Vulnerable Groups for Sexually Transmitted Infections—High-risk Groups

In certain group of individual the incidence and prevalence of the STIs are generally more than normal population, they are called "Core Groups" from the point that of view of the transmission, prevention and control of STIs. They are (Fig. 17G.8):
- Commercial sex workers (CSWs)
- Injecting drug users (IDUs) and their sexual partners
- Prisoners, where juveniles stay with long stay inmates
- Street children (School drop outs and working in unorganized sectors)
- Group of individuals which are often clients of CSWs
    - Long distance truckers
    - Tourists/Travelers
    - Men having sex with men—homosexual and bisexual men.

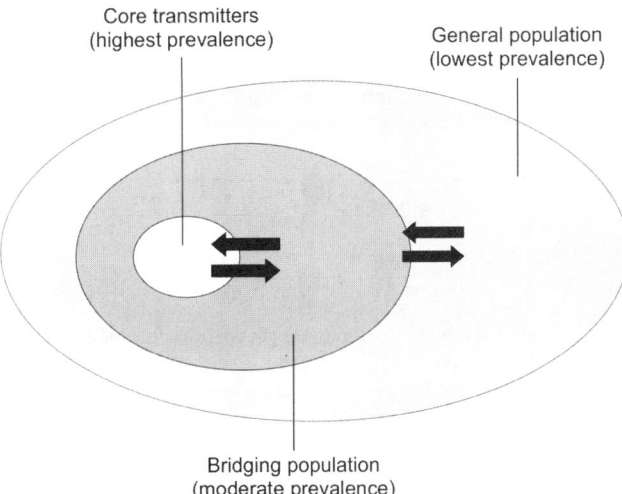

Fig. 17G.8: Core population, bridge population in relation to sexually transmitted infections.

## Agent Factor

There are about 30 different bacteria, viruses and parasites are known to be transmitted through unprotected sexual contact. Most of these require a breech in the skin or mucosal epithelium to enter to host body and such erosion can readily occur during sexual contact. The disease agents and the disease caused by them are given in **Table 17G.12**.

## Social Factors

Sexually transmitted infections are truly a social disease due to the following factors:

### Illiteracy

Illiterates are often victims of risk behavior and acquire STIs easily.

Table 17G.12: Major STIs and their causative agents.

| Agents | Disease |
|---|---|
| **Bacteria** (including spirochetes) | |
| *Treponema pallidum, Haemophilus ducreyi, Neisseria gonorrheae* | • Syphilis, Yaws, Pinta<br>• Chancroid (Soft sore)<br>• Gonorrhea, urethritis<br>• Cervicitis, Epididymitis, Salpingitis, PID, Ophthalmia neonatorum, |
| *Calymmatobacterium granulomatis* | Donovanosis (Granuloma inguinale) |
| *Chlamydia trachomatis* (L1, L2, L3) | Lymphogranuloma venereum (LGV) |
| *Chlamydia trachomatis* (D to K) | Nongonococcal urethritis (NGU) |
| | Cervicitis |
| *Mycoplasma hominis* | NGU |
| *Ureaplasma urealyticum* | NGU |
| *Shigella* spp. | Proctocolitis (due to anal sex) |
| *Campylobacter* spp. | Proctocolitis (due to anal sex) |
| Bacterial vaginosis-associated organisms<br>Group B streptococci | Bacterial vaginosis<br>Vaginitis, urethritis, cervicitis, balanitis, cystitis |
| **Viral agents** | |
| Human (alpha) herpesvirus 1 and 2 | Herpes genitalis |
| Human (beta) herpesvirus 5 | Cervicitis, NGU |
| Hepatitis B virus | Serum hepatitis |
| Human papillomavirus | Genital warts |
| Molluscum contagiosum virus | Genital molluscum contagiosum |
| Human immunodeficiency virus | AIDS |
| **Protozoal agents** | |
| *Entamoeba histolytica* | Amebiasis |
| *Giardia lamblia* | Giardiasis |
| *Trichomonas vaginalis* | Trichomoniasis (vaginitis) |
| **Fungal agents** | |
| *Candida albicans* | Vaginal candidiasis |
| **Ectoparasites** | |
| *Pthirus pubis* | Pubic pediculosis (it is not a disease but infestation) |
| *Sarcoptes scabiei* | Genial scabies |

(PID: pelvic inflammatory diseases; LGV: lymphogranuloma venereum; NGU: nongonococcal urethritis; HIV: human immunodeficiency virus; AIDS: acquired immune deficiency syndrome)

### Prostitution

These often act as core group (reservoir) and readily spread the infection.

### Polygamy/Polyandry Behavior

Polygamy (one male with many female partner) and polyandry (one woman having many male partner) are still practiced in many parts of the world, predisposes the contact and spread of STIs.

### Broken Homes

In families where there is death or divorce of the parents, the young individuals are likely to practice unsafe sexual behavior, predisposing to STIs.

### Social Disruption

War, famine, floods and other disasters favor the spread of the sexually transmitted infections.

### Social Stigma

The huge social stigma attached with the STIs make it difficult in screening and diagnosis.

### Demographic Factors

#### Migration

Selective movement of the individuals for education, employment and better life opportunities to different parts of the country and globe accelerates the spread of STIs.

#### Changing Life Style Pattern

Isolation from family, eccentric life style, lack of mental relaxation and addiction together precipitates the risky behavior of the individual for spread of STIs.

## COMPLICATIONS OF SEXUALLY TRANSMITTED INFECTIONS

STIs if left untreated can cause serious complications in both the genders and neonates. Millions of men, women, and children globally are affected by the long-term complications of STIs.
- ***Complications in male:*** Infertility, carcinoma of penis (HPV infection)
- ***Complications in female:***
  - Pelvic inflammatory diseases (PIDs) due to untreated Gonococcal and Chlamydial infections
  - Adverse outcomes of pregnancy like stillbirth, spontaneous abortions and low birth weight
  - Infertility
  - Ectopic pregnancy
  - Cervical cancer (HPV infection)
- ***Complications in neonates:***
  - Perinatal and neonatal infections like—congenital syphilis, conjunctivitis, herpes simplex virus 1-2, hepatitis B and HIV
  - Prematurity—STIs in pregnancy especially bacterial vaginosis and trichomoniasis may result in preterm delivery, which can lead to prematurity and associated complications in the neonate.
  - Low birth weight.

## PREVENTION AND CONTROL

The main components of STI control can be categorized into following heads:
A. Elimination of reservoirs (for core groups)
B. Breaking the channel of transmission (for bridge population)
C. Protection of the susceptible (for normal population)
D. Other measures.

### Elimination of the Reservoir

The main emphasis under this approach is the detection and control of infection in core group members either asymptomatic infections or symptomatic cases.

### Case Detection

Early detection of infection and cases are the backbone in controlling STIs.

### Screening

As STIs show the iceberg phenomena, selective screening for core group population and opportunistic screening for at risk population are very much relevant. Screening should be done for other groups like antenatal mothers and blood donors.

### Contact Tracing

Tracing the sexual partner (contacts) of diagnosed STI cases by rapid means to identify them before incubation period of the disease **(Fig. 17G.9)**.

After proper identification counselling regarding STI clinic visit, examination and treatment can be provided to the contacts.

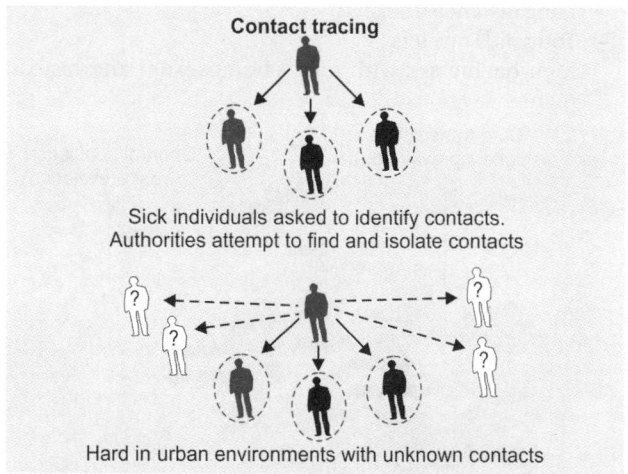

**Fig. 17G.9:** Contact tracing in relation to sexually transmitted infections.

### Cluster Testing

This is the identification of other HRGs or core group members who reside or move in to the same socio-sexual environment of any diagnosed STI cases. If proper confidentiality is maintained it is the most effective way of identification of CSWs, Homosexual communities.

### Case Holding and Treatment

After identification of the case by proper screening procedure complete, correct treatment is to be provided with confidentiality. Follow-up of cases is mandatory as incomplete treatment and drop out are the major concern resulting in antimicrobial resistance. Administration of full course of treatment to all the contacts or to recently exposed people before getting the investigation results is referred to as "epidemiological treatment" or "contact treatment". Sexually transmitted infections clinics and social workers play a pivotal role in controlling STIs. The treatment of most of the STIs is based on the identification of a group of symptoms and easy recognizable signs called "syndromic management", which is highly effective in resource poor countries like India.

## Breaking the Chain of Transmission

Abstinence from sex is the absolute but impractical method in controlling STIs. Safe sex practice (with barrier methods) to be advised and encouraged in the bridge population.

## Protection of the Susceptible

Safe sex to be practiced in the community
- Faithful to one sexual partner
- Using barrier methods (condoms), if having multiple sexual partner
- Condom use to be practiced correctly, consistently and continuously.

## Other Measures

### Health Education

It is an integral component of STIs control program. The chief objective of this education should aim at changing behavior of individual to minimize the disease acquisition and spread.

### Vaccination

At present hepatitis B vaccine is the only vaccine available for control of this STI.

### Sexually Transmitted Infections Clinics

These clinics have been popularly known as "Suraksha Clinics" which deliver sexual and reproductive health services. National AIDS Control Organization through its network of 1,160 designated STI/RTI clinics (situated at government health care facilities at district level and above) is providing free standardized STI/RTI services.

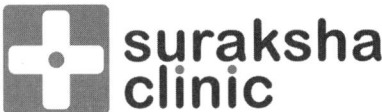

Standardized training to the health (medical and paramedical) personnel as per syndromic case management approach is being provided at these clinics. Rapid plasma reagin (RPR) test kits and color coded syndromic drug kits are being centrally procured and supplied to these clinics for rapid diagnosis and treatment of STI patients. Free counseling services to patient and their partners are amongst the foremost services being delivered by trained counselor at these designated sites.

### Legislative Measures

Implementation of legislative measures to restrict prostitutions, human trafficking and addictive substance abuse can minimize the load of STIs. Newer legislative approaches ensuring contact identification, early treatment and notification by general practitioner to be in place.

*The Immoral Traffic Prevention Act, 1986* (Surpassing the earlier Suppression of Immoral Traffic Prevention Act, 1956) covers all person (male and female), who are exploited sexually for commercial purposes. The offences are liable for stringent punishment.

The "*Ujjawala Scheme*" under Ministry of Women and Child Development, Government of India has been launched since 1st April 2016. This is a Comprehensive Scheme for Prevention of Trafficking, for Rescue, Rehabilitation and Re-Integration of Victims of Trafficking for Commercial Sexual Exploitation.

### Social Welfare Measures

Sexually transmitted infections can be labeled as social issues with medical aspects. Hence social welfare measures "Social therapy" should be in place such as:
- Rehabilitation of CSWs
- Proper recreation facilities in community
- Decent living conditions (home discipline)
- Marriage counseling
- Sex education in educational institutions
- Prohibition on selling and advertisement of pornographic materials, books and photographs.

### Elimination of Parent-to-Child Transmission of Syphilis (EPTCT)

Under this initiative NACO and maternal division of Government of India are aiming for early registration, early screening for both Syphilis and HIV and treat those found reactive. There is also promotion for institutional delivery and follow-up of the newborn up to 24 months of age.

### The STI/RTI Services Under National AIDS Control Programme

The STI/RTI control is an important component of NACP. The program aims to provide quality services to people in need especially the high risk groups and vulnerable population. It works through a convergence along with the National health mission and also involves private sector in service delivery. Colored kits are provided for syndromic management of STI.

## SYNDROMIC CASE MANAGEMENT OF STIs/RTIs

Syndromic case management of STIs/RTIs refers to the approach of treating STIs based upon a consistent group of symptoms and easily recognizable sign, the treatment protocol will deal with the organism most commonly responsible for producing such syndrome in that geographical area.

### Community-based Examples for "Syndromic Management" of STI/RTI

> Daily case load in a community health center serving a local "high-risk population" is very high often leading to long outpatient department (OPD) hours. The residents posted there have started managing patients by "flowchart approach" developed by NACO for symptoms and signs suggesting of STIs after proper history taking and clinical examination. The decision making by this approach have saved a lot of time and uniformity in drug dispensing as well.

The basic differences between "clinical diagnostic" approach and "syndromic" approach may be summarized as shown in **Table 17G.13**.

The third type of approach, i.e., "etiologic" approach involves laboratory tests and investigations has many challenges in

**Table 17G.13:** Advantages and disadvantages of sexually transmitted infections/reproductive tract infections (STIs/RTIs) diagnostic approaches.

| Diagnostic approach | Advantages | Disadvantages |
| --- | --- | --- |
| **Clinical** | | |
| Clinical experiences is being used to identify the apparent symptoms which are specific for a particular STI, then treat specifically | • Saves time of patient<br>• Reduces laboratory expenses | • Requires reasonable good clinical skills<br>• Mixed infections may be ignored<br>• Does not identify cases without symptoms (asymptomatic one) |
| **Syndromic** | | |
| Identifying clinical syndrome based upon sign and symptoms, providing treatment regime focusing toward all the known possible pathogens which might have caused the syndrome | • Complete STI treatment offered at very initial visit<br>• Rapid, simple, and cost-effective<br>• Treatment for all possible mixed options<br>• Reduces case load at hospitals<br>• Accessibility is high as can be given by health counselor and workers | • Risk of over treatment<br>• Require prior research for proper identification of syndromes<br>• Asymptomatic infections are missed |

developing countries like India. It requires huge manpower, sophisticated laboratory instruments, and a time consuming process.

Since 1990, WHO has recommended the "syndromic approach", a scientific valid approach which offers immediate treatment, easy accessibility, effective, and efficient management for STIs in countries like India.

**Common STI Syndromes**
- Genital ulcer
- Urethral discharge in men
- Inguinal bubo
- Vaginal discharge
- Lower abdominal pain
- Scrotal swelling
- Neonatal conjunctivitis
- Acquired immunodeficiency syndromes (AIDS)

## Steps Involved in Adopting Syndromic Approach (Fig. 17G.10 and 17G.11)

The diagnosis and treatment of STI under syndromic approach relies upon a proper history taking, physical examination, and fitment of collective signs and symptoms to an appropriate flowchart **(Table 17G.14)**. The steps may be summarized as:

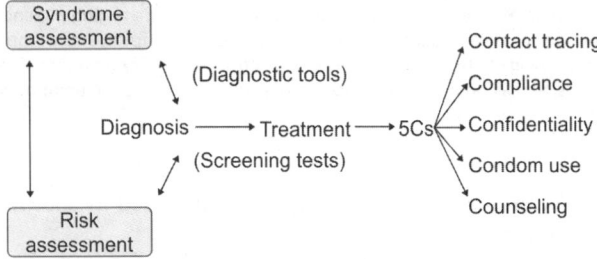

**Fig. 17G.10:** Steps involved in adopting syndromic approach.
(STI: sexually transmitted infection)

**Table 17G.14:** Specific histories to be elicited during STI management.

| Specific symptoms | Important history to be taken |
| --- | --- |
| Urethral discharge or burning sensation on urination in men | Onset, progression, the amount of discharge, and history of unprotected sex |
| Vaginal discharge | Change in color, amount and odor of discharge, STI in the partner or multiple sexual partners and change in sexual partner |
| Genital ulcer in men and women | The onset, history of recurrence, painful or painless, location, and single or multiple nature of the ulcer |
| Lower abdominal pain in women | About onset, nature of pain, severity, radiation, last menstrual period, presence of vaginal discharge, and certain systemic symptoms like fever, nausea, and vomiting |
| Scrotal swelling | Regarding onset, pain, history of trauma, and concomitant urethral discharge |
| Inguinal bubo | Presence of pain, ulceration, discharges, and the locations of the swelling |
| Neonatal conjunctivitis | Onset, presence of unilateral or bilateral eye involvement, sticky eyes, and swollen eyelids |

*Source:* Sexually transmitted infections, World Health Organization, 2017.

- Proper history taking and elaborate on chief complaint of the patient
- The demographic detail and gender of the patient to be kept in mind
- Gentle clinical examination
- Depending upon the symptoms and signs appropriate treatment flowchart to be taken
- If laboratory investigations are available then choose appropriate treatment flowchart
- Ensure confidentiality and privacy
- Encourage for the partner treatment
- Educate the patient regarding condom promotion.

## Steps in Examining the Male and Female Patient (Table 17G.15)

**Table 17G.15:** Specific examinations of suspected sexually transmitted infection (STI) male and female client.

| Male patient | Female patient* |
| --- | --- |
| Ask the patient gently to stand up and lower his pants up to knees | Ask the patient to remove her clothes below waist<br>Ask the patient to lie down in lithotomy position |
| Palpate for enlarged lymph nodes in the inguinal region | Palpate the inguinal region for enlarged lymph nodes |
| Palpate the scrotum | Palpate the lower abdomen for any pelvic mass/tenderness |
| Examine the penis for rashes and sores | Examine the vulva and look for discharge if any |
| Look at the urethral meatus and the glans after asking the patient to retract the foreskin | Speculum examination of vagina to differentiate between cervical and vaginal discharge |
| Look for any discharge after asking the patient to milk the urethra to express it | Digital bimanual per vaginum examination for adnexal or cervical motion and tenderness |
| Examine the oral and anal region | Examine the oral and anal region |
| Record all the observations | Record all the observations |

*Examine the female client always in the presence of female staff member.

## Chapter 17: Specific Epidemiology of Infectious Diseases

| Urethral discharge | Cervical discharge | Painful scrotal swelling | Vaginal discharge | Genital ulcer-non-herpetic | Genital ulcer-herpetic | Lower abdominal pain (LAP) | Inguinal bubo (IB) |
|---|---|---|---|---|---|---|---|
| • Urethral discharge (Pus or muco-purulent)<br>• Pain or burning while passing urine<br>• Increased frequency of urination<br>• Systemic symptoms like malaise, fever | • Nature and type of discharge (quantity, color and odor)<br>• Burning while passing urine, increased frequency<br>• Genital complaints by sexual partners<br>• Low backache (Take menstrual history to rule out pregnancy) | • Swelling in inguinal region which may be painful<br>• Preceding history of genital ulcer or discharge<br>• Systemic symptoms like malaise, fever<br>• History of urethral discharge | • Nature and type of discharge (quantity, color and odor)<br>• Burning while passing urine, increased frequency<br>• Genital complaints by sexual partners<br>• Low backache (Take menstrual history to rule out pregnancy) | • Genital ulcer, single or multiple, painful or painless<br>• Burning sensation in the genital area<br>• Enlarged lymph nodes | • Genital ulcer or vesicles, single or multiple, painful, recurrent<br>• Burning sensation in the genital area | • Lower abdominal pain<br>• Fever<br>• Vaginal discharge<br>• Menstrual irregularities like heavy, irregular vaginal bleeding<br>• Dysmenorrhea, dysparenunia, dysuria, tenesmus<br>• Lower backache<br>• Cervical motion tenderness | • Swelling in inguinal region which may be painful<br>• Preceding history of genital ulcer or discharge<br>• Systemic symptoms like malaise, fever, etc |
| Tab. Azithromycin 1 g OD stat + Tab. Cefixime 400 mg OD stat | Tab. Azithromycin 1 g OD stat + Tab. Cefixime 400 mg OD stat | Tab. Azithromycin 1 g OD stat + Tab. Cefixime 400 mg OD stat | Tab. Secnidazole 2 g OD stat + Cap. Fluconazole 150 mg OD stat | Inj. Benzathine penicilin (2.4 MU)-1vial Tab. Azithromycin (1 g)–single dose | Tab. Acyclovir 400 mg TDS for 7 days | Tab. Cefixime 400 mg OD stat + Tab. Metronidaole 400 mg BD X 14 days + Doxycycline 100 mg BD X 14 days | Tab. Azithromycin 1 g OD stat + Tab. Doxycycline 100 mg BD for 21 days |
| | | | | If allergic to Inj. Penicillin: Doxycycline 100 g (Bid for 15 days) Azithromycin 1 g (Single dose) | | | |
| KIT 1/Grey | KIT 1/Grey | KIT 1/Grey | KIT 2/Green | KIT 3/White | KIT 4/Blue | KIT 5/Red | KIT 6/Yellow | KIT 7/Black |
| Treat all recent partners | Treat partners when symptomatic | Treat all recent partners | Treat partners when symptomatic | Treat all sexual partners for past 3 months | No partner treatment | Treat male partners with kit 1 | Treat all sexual partners for past 3 weeks |

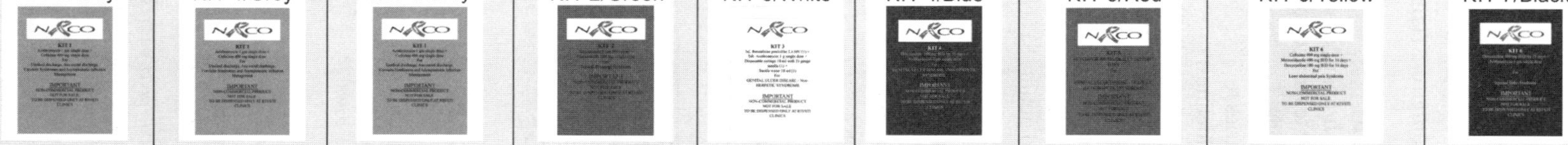

**Important Considerations for Management of All STI/RTI**
- Educate and counsel client and sexual partners regarding STI/RTI, safer sex practices and importance of taking complete treatment
- Treat partners
- Advise sexual abstinence or condom use during the course of treatment
- Provide condoms, educate about correct and consistent use
- Refer all patients to ICTC
- Follow-up after 7 days for all STI, 3rd, 7th, 14th day for LAP and 7th, 14th, and 21st day for IB
- If symptoms persist, assess whether it is due to re-infection and advise prompt referral
- Consider immunization against hepatitis B

Fig. 17G.11: Seven colored prepacked drug kits for sexually transmitted infection (STI) syndromic management.
(Tab.: tablet; Inj.: injection)

## GLOBAL AND NATIONAL APPROACH

**Global health sector strategy on HIV, Hepatitis and Sexually Transmitted Infections, 2022–2030.**

Within this framework, WHO:
- Develops global targets, norms and standards for STI prevention, testing and treatment;
- Supports the estimation and economic burden of STIs and the strengthening of STI surveillance;
- Globally monitors AMR to gonorrhea; and
- Leads the setting of the global research agenda on STIs, including the development of diagnostic tests, vaccines and additional drugs for gonorrhea and syphilis.

As part of its mission, WHO supports countries to:
- Develop national strategic plans and guidelines;
- Create an encouraging environment allowing individuals to discuss STIs, adopt safer sexual practices, and seek treatment;
- Scale-up primary prevention (condom availability and use, etc.);
- Increase integration of STI services within primary healthcare services;
- Increase accessibility of people-centered quality STI care;
- Facilitate adoption of point-of-care tests;
- Enhance and scale-up health intervention for impact, such as hepatitis B and HPV vaccination, syphilis screening in priority populations;
- Strengthen capacity to monitoring STIs trends; and
- Monitor and respond to AMR in gonorrhea.

The National goals and strategies to control STIs in India are covered under National AIDS Control Program, Phase V (2021-2026) which is *explained in further details in Chapter 47: Health Policies and Programs in India*.

## SUMMARY

STIs have a profound impact on health and lives of children, adolescents and adults all over the world. It has a major impact on sexual and reproductive health. It leads to varied complications like IUDs, neonatal deaths, cervical cancer, infertility, risk of HIV, etc. Along with this it also leads to physical, psychological and social consequences thus hampering the quality of life of an individual. Syndromic management of STIs have been found to be the most feasible approach to reach out to a larger affected individual also providing an opportunity to treat the partners as well.

## SUGGESTED READING

1. Bhatta M, Majumdar A, Ghosh U, Ghosh P, Banerji P, Aridoss S, et al. Sexually transmitted infections among key populations in India: A protocol for systematic review. PLoS ONE 18(3): e0279048.
2. Cohen MS, Hoffman IF, Royce RA, Kazembe P, Dyer JR, Daly CC, et al. Reduction of concentration of HIV-1 in semen after treatment of urethritis: Implications for prevention of sexual transmission of HIV-1. AIDSCAP Malawi Research Group. Lancet. 1997;349(9069):1868-73.
3. Low N, Broutet N, Turner R. A Collection on the prevention, diagnosis, and treatment of sexually transmitted infections: Call for research papers. PLoS Med. 2017;14(6):e1002333.
4. Low N, Broutet NJ. Sexually transmitted infections—Research priorities for new challenges. PLoS Med. 2017;14(12):e1002481.
5. NACO. (2007). National Guidelines on Prevention, Management and Control of Reproductive Tract Infections including Sexually Transmitted Infections.
6. NACO. (2012). Operational Guidelines for Programme Managers and Service Providers for Strengthening STI/RTI Services.
7. WHO. (2001). Management of Sexually Transmitted Infections. Report of an intercountry workshop Yangon. Myanmar.
8. WHO. (2004). Guidelines for management of sexually transmitted infections.
9. WHO. (2017). Sexually transmitted infections: implementing the global STI Strategy.
10. WHO. Global Sexually Transmitted Infections Programme, Accessed in July 2023 and available from https://www.who.int/teams/global-hiv-hepatitis-and-stis-programmes/stis/overview.
11. WHO. Sexually transmitted infections (STIs). Factsheet 10 July 2023
12. World Health Organization. Sexually transmitted infections factsheet. [Cited 2017 May 18].
13. Yin YP, Han Y, Dai XQ, et al. Susceptibility of Neisseria gonorrhoeae to azithromycin and ceftriaxone in China: A retrospective study of national surveillance data from 2013 to 2016. PLoS ONE. 2023;18(3):e0279048.

---

# EPIDEMIOLOGY OF LEPROSY AND ITS PREVENTION AND CONTROL

*Anku Moni Saikia, Kumaril Goswami*

*Eliminating leprosy is the only work I have not been able to complete in my lifetime.*
—**Mahatma Gandhi**

| | |
|---|---|
| CM7.2 | Enumerate, describe and discuss the mode of transmission and measures for prevention and control of leprosy |
| CM8.1 | Describe and discuss the epidemiological and control measures applicable in leprosy |

### Case Scenario

*Mr Mohan, a 35-year-old rickshaw puller noticed a pale patch on the skin of his forearm one year ago. Initially, he ignored it but later consulted an ASHA worker. He was assured by the ASHA worker that there was nothing to worry about for such a simple skin infection and he started applying turmeric paste on and off. Mohan had no time to visit the nearby PHC for this small issue. A few days later, he noticed another similar patch on his abdomen and found that the previous patch had become bigger. Further more, he noticed that he had developed some weakness in the same hand while pulling his rickshaw. He also did not feel any sensation when touching the patch. This time without consulting the ASHA, he went to the nearby medical officer of the PHC, where he was diagnosed as a case of leprosy.*

- ❏ What ASHA could have done when Mohan reported for the first time?
- ❏ What are the points in the narration that favor the diagnosis of leprosy?
- ❏ What are the gaps in the description that led to the late diagnosis of the disease?
- ❏ What are the likely complications Mohan might develop due to late diagnosis?
- ❏ How does the disease may affect the livelihood of Mohan?

## INTRODUCTION

Leprosy is a well-known disease since the days of Sushruta and Charkas. It mainly affects the skin and peripheral nerves.

But it can also affect the other sites like mucosa of the upper respiratory tract, eyes, testes, etc. It is one of the important causes of permanent physical disability. The impact of disability on the life of the affected person, family, and as a whole in the society, is tremendous.

Simultaneous to physical suffering, the disease is full of superstitions and social stigma. The social stigma has a great impact not only on the person affected with leprosy but also on the family and society as well.

Until the early part of 19th century, leprosy was believed to be terrible and highly contagious incurable disease and transmitted by inheritance. The person with leprosy was often isolated, rejected, not allowed to participate in different social activities, and displaced from work. They were kept or treated in asylum or sanatoria. The fight to remove the stigma associated with leprosy started long back by Mahatma Gandhi and he continued this throughout his life. Gandhiji met different persons suffering from leprosy several times. Their sufferings evoked a strong determination in his mind to fight against the disease, social stigma in particular. Removing the deeply rooted stigma from the minds of people has been a major challenge in controlling the disease over the decades.

During the Satyagraha in India, while Gandhiji was in the Yeravada prison in 1932, Parchure Shastri, a Sanskrit scholar was also in the same prison, but locked up in an isolated room as he was suffering from leprosy. Nobody was allowed to meet Shastri and Gandhiji had to correspond with him through letters only. The law of land at that time "The Leprosy Act, 1898" recommended strict segregation of leprosy patients. Years later, Shastri wrote a letter mentioning his willingness to stay at Gandhiji's Ashram at Sevagram. Initially, Gandhiji was in dilemma because of the nature of the disease and on the other side his vow to fight against it. Gandhiji could raise the empathy of the Ashramites and not only gave him accommodation but also nursed him personally until he recovered sufficiently. The image of Gandhiji nursing Shastri, the leprosy patient, during those days is an epic image and was depicted on the postage stamp as a bold message on social stigma and untouchability.

The term "Lepra" derived from a Latin word meaning "Scaly". The disease is also known as Hansen's disease as the causative organism *Mycobacterium leprae* was first identified by Dr Gerhard Armauer Hansen of Norway in 1873. In India, this disease is still known as "Kusht" meaning "Eating away".

Introduction of Sulphones (Dapsone) in the treatment of leprosy initiated a new era in leprosy control. Before Sulphones came, the mainstay of treatment in India was an oil derived from Chaulmoogra tree. However, the duration of Dapsone monotherapy was pretty long (5–10 years) which led to non-compliance with the treatment and eventually resulted in development of dapsone resistance. In 1982, World Health Organization after extensive trials recommended the use of multi-drug therapy (MDT) which included the addition of rifampicin and clofazimine to tackle Dapsone resistance. The spectacular results after use of MDT in terms of reducing the number of leprosy cases led to the realization that elimination of disease is possible in the community. In 1991, WHO passed the resolution of "Elimination of Leprosy" by the year 2000 and accordingly outlined the strategies.

## PROBLEM STATEMENT

Indicators for assessment of burden of leprosy are as follows:

### 1. Prevalence Rate

This is defined as the number of leprosy patients receiving MDT per 10,000 populations during a year. This rate is useful to compare the outcome of the program in the reduction of the disease load in the community in successive years.

### 2. Annual New Case Detection Rate

New cases detected during a year per 100,000 population is the annual new case detection rate (ANCDR). However, we need to understand that all new cases are not the actual new case (incident cases), some may be old cases reported/detected during that particular year.

### 3. Grade II Deformity Among Newly Detected Cases

Deformity is the end result of nerve damage. The cases, which are being undiagnosed and untreated for a long time may present with Grade II deformity. Inadequate community awareness along with lack of skills and commitment on the part of health functionaries influence the diagnosis of the disease. So, Grade II deformity among new cases clearly indicates a delay in diagnosis and treatment. Grade II deformity is always measured in absolute numbers and the global goal is to reduce the disability to less than one per million by 2020.

### 4. Proportion of Child (Less than 15 years) Cases

The occurrence of disease among children indicates the long duration exposure to an untreated case either in the household or among the close contacts. In spite of having effective medications and easy diagnostic approach, the presence of such cases and subsequent infection in children reflects the failure of the system in detecting the cases in time. The higher proportion of cases in children indicates active transmission in the community. The chance of developing deformities significantly increases if nerve damage occurs in this age group.

### Global Scenario

Leprosy was eliminated at the global level in the year 2000. *Criteria for elimination of leprosy as a public health problem is prevalence <1 case per 10,000 population.*

The current scenario is described using the epidemiological indicators.

### Prevalence

The overall burden of leprosy has declined over the last couple of years. In the year 2018, global prevalence was 0.2/10,000 population, which is much below the elimination criteria. But, regional disparities still exist. Some countries have not attained the elimination status and still reporting a good number of cases.

As per data of 2019, Brazil, India and Indonesia reported more than 10,000 new cases, while 13 other countries (Bangladesh, Democratic Republic of the Congo, Ethiopia, Madagascar, Mozambique, Myanmar, Nepal, Nigeria, Philippines, Somalia, South Sudan, Sri Lanka and the United Republic of Tanzania) each reported 1,000–10,000 new cases. Forty-five countries reported 0 cases and 99 reported fewer than 1,000 new cases. (WHO 2023)

Elimination at the global level has been possible due to the following reasons:
- Intensified case detection effort globally
- Effective antileprosy treatment, i.e., MDT
- Strong commitment at every level (national, international).

However, WHO has identified 22 "Global Priority Countries", having a higher burden of leprosy and together contributed more than 90% of cases in the last 10 years. These countries are prioritized for intensifying control activities.

### New Cases

The major burden of new cases was from *India, Brazil, and Indonesia* during the year 2016. According to recent statistics, a small reduction (3.4%) was reported during 2017 in comparison to 2016. This global reduction of new cases was mainly due to the reduction of cases reported from India (WHO, Weekly Epidemiological Report 2017).

### Grade II Deformity

Majority (92%) of Grade II deformity cases were reported from 22 priority countries. However, a declining trend has been observed over the last three years in the Global Priority Countries. Currently, leprosy with Grade II disability is reported as 1.6 per million population and the target is less than one case per million population by 2020 (WHO Weekly Epidemiological Record 2018).

### Proportion of Child Cases

As per WHO report in 2016, the proportion of child cases among the newly infected cases was 9%.

### India Scenario

India achieved the elimination status at national level in the year 2005 following intensification of case detection and treatment activity under the National Leprosy Eradication Programme. Although elimination is achieved at the national level, regional or state wise disparities still exist. India is still among the "Global Priority Countries".

### Prevalence Rate

Prevalence Rate (PR) at National level was 0.84 per 10,000 population in 2005-06 which has been reduced to 0.57 per 10,000 population in 2019-20. Due to COVID-19 pandemic, case detection was compromised, which led to sudden downward trend of Prevalence Rate to 0.40 and 0.45 per 10,000 population in 2020–21 and 2021–22 respectively. Despite COVID-19 disruption of health services during 2020-2021, 65,147 new cases of leprosy were identified, diagnosed and provided free treatment. Continuity of these essential healthcare services during the pandemic response ensures that in the year 2021-22 a total of 61,678, leprosy cases were under treatment. PR was 0.45/10,000 population as of 31st March 2021. 34 States/ UTs (out of 36 States/UTs) and 645 districts (88%) out of total, 733 districts achieved elimination by March 2022.

"India is making progress and new leprosy cases are declining year after year. With the whole of government, whole of society support, synergy and cooperation, we can achieve the target of Leprosy Mukt Bharat by 2027, three years ahead of the SDG".

### Grade II Disability

A total of 1,863 Grade 2 Disabilities detected amongst the new Leprosy cases during 2021–22, indicating the G2D Rate of 1.36/million population and 2.47% G2D among new cases.

### Proportion of Child Cases

Trends of cases among children at national level shows a steady decline over the decade from 16,112 (9.98%) in 2005-06 (13,331) to 4,107 (5.45%) in 2021–22.

> **Key Points**
> - Leprosy causes permanent physical disability if not treated at the earliest.
> - All untreated and active leprosy cases can be a source of infection.
> - Leprosy is curable with multi-drug therapy.
> - Leprosy has been eliminated globally as well as from India. However, regional disparities still exist.
> - It is said to be eliminated if the prevalence is <1 per 10,000 population.

## EPIDEMIOLOGY

The epidemiological determinants will be described in the context of the epidemiological triad.

### Host Factors

#### Age

The maximum incidence is found between 10 and 20 years of age. Higher prevalence among this age group has a profound impact on social and economic productivity. Because of the long incubation period, the occurrence of leprosy is low among the very young age group.

#### Gender

Males are found to be more affected than females. A higher opportunity of exposure in male could be one reason for this. Again, females may report less fearing stigma and discrimination in society. However, this is not seen in children.

#### Immunity

Cell-mediated immunity (CMI) is the protective immunity in leprosy. Although humoral antibodies are also produced, they do not have a protective effect against *M. leprae*. Immunity can be acquired through:
- Subclinical infection
- *BCG vaccination: Mycobacterium tuberculosis* shares common antigen with *M. leprae*. BCG can give some degree of protection.
- Infection with other mycobacteria.

### HIV and Leprosy

There is no substantial evidence to show increase HIV prevalence among leprosy cases and vice versa.

### Genetic Factors

Leprosy is not a genetic disease. Certain HLA and nonHLA antigens have been identified in both TT (Tuberculoid) and LL (Lepromatous) leprosy and they may increase the susceptibility to leprosy.

### Risk Groups

Leprosy is seen to be more among the slum dwellers, migrant population, and the population living in hard to reach areas, etc. Besides being inaccessible to the care provider, ignorance and illiteracy in these communities prevent them from seeking treatment.

Household contacts of MB leprosy are more prone to acquire the infection.

### Agent Factors

- *M. leprae* is an intracellular, obligate, acid-fast, gram-positive, nonmotile, and rod-shaped organism.
- Under the microscope, it usually occurs in clumps or bundles and stained red with Ziehl-Neelsen stain. Viable bacilli are seen as solid and uniformly stained rods. The bacilli which stain irregularly are considered to be dead.
- *M. leprae* cannot be cultivated in artificial media under laboratory condition. This is the reason why the research related to leprosy has not progressed as expected in spite of the fact that *M. leprae* was the first bacteria to be identified causing human disease.
- It has got a strong affinity for Schwann cells of peripheral nerves. So, clinical manifestations are mainly because of damage to peripheral nerves.
- Leprosy bacilli have an extremely slow doubling time of 12–14 days. Hence, the incubation period is very long and prolonged exposure is required to acquire the infection. The pathogenicity and virulence of leprosy bacilli are also low.
- Prefers to grow well at 33-degree centigrade. That is the reason why *M. leprae* is more found in cooler places like extremities and ear lobules, etc.
- *M. leprae* can survive and remain viable in the environment outside the human body (humid environment: 9–16 days; moist soil: 46 days). Transmission through fomites and soil has been suspected.
- There are other mycobacteria (*Mycobacterium tuberculosis*, environmental mycobacteria) sharing some common antigen. Hence, exposure to these mycobacteria may offer some level of protection against *M. leprae*.

### Environmental Factors

#### Climate

Leprosy cases are found more in tropical and subtropical climate.

#### Overcrowding and Lack of Ventilation

As leprosy is primarily transmitted by droplet route, the transmission is more in overcrowded and ill-ventilated house.

#### Socioeconomic Status

Leprosy occurs more in lower socioeconomic status due to the adverse physical environment as well as low education and awareness level.

### Source of Infection

Man is the only established source of infection. All untreated and active leprosy cases can be a source of infection. However, as the bacterial load is more in multibacillary (MB) cases; they are more infectious to the community. Infectivity decreases significantly with MDT and rifampicin itself can kill more than 99.9% of the organism in a single dose.

Among the animal sources, *M. leprae* is also found in armadillos, mangabey monkeys, and chimpanzees. But their role in human transmission is not found till now.

### Portal of Entry and Exit

- Upper respiratory tract mainly through the nasal mucosa
- *Skin:* Less commonly through broken skin.

### Modes of Transmission

#### Droplet Infection

This is the major mode of transmission considering the fact that nose is the portal of the exit of *M. leprae*. Multibacillary leprosy cases harbor millions of organism in the nasal mucosa and shed the organism through droplets during talking, coughing, sneezing, etc., into the environment. Persons living in the vicinity of such a patient may get the infection.

#### Direct Contact

The epidemiological significance of direct contact with an open and active lesion route is debated by the observations that bacillary load in the epidermis is insufficient to transmit infection.

Transmission through fomites, soil, breast milk, insect, and tattooing, etc., has been suspected. However, these routes are not significant in the transmission of leprosy.

### Incubation Period

Leprosy has a long and variable incubation from few weeks to 20 years with an average of 2–5 years.

## PATHOGENESIS AND CLASSIFICATION

### Pathogenesis

Leprosy has got diverse clinical spectrum based on CMI of the affected person. Following exposure to *M. leprae* infection, the majority (95%) possess the adequate protective antibody and they do not develop the clinical disease.

Flowchart 17G.1: Pathogenesis of leprosy.

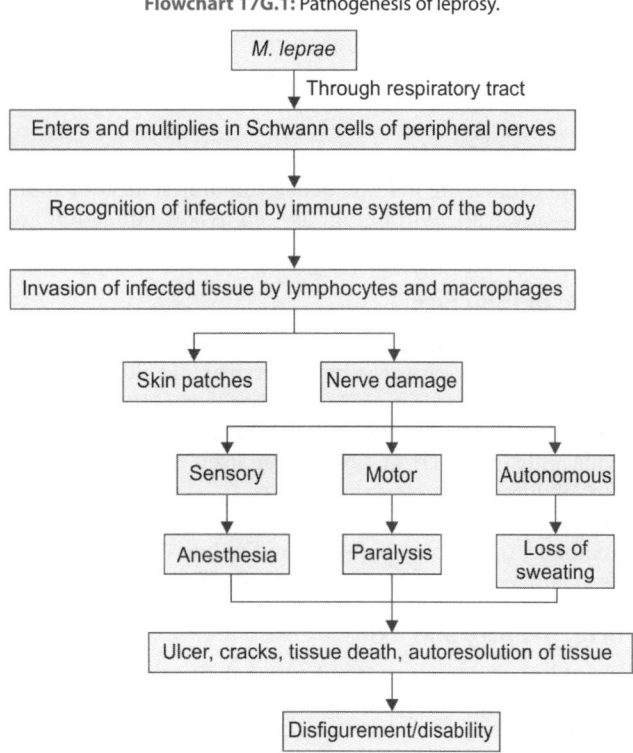

Only a small percentage (5%) develops the disease. The spectrum of severity depends on CMI which is shown in **Flowchart 17G.1**.

## Immunological Classification

The immunological basis of leprosy is depicted in **Flowchart 17G.2**.

In the middle of the spectrum, borderline leprosy exists which can go to either end of the extremes (TT/LL) depending on their change in immunity status.

Flowchart 17G.2: Immunological classification of leprosy.

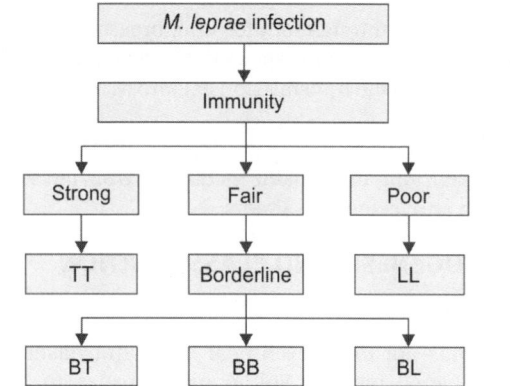

(TT: tuberculoid type, BT: borderline tuberculoid, BB: borderline-borderline, BL: borderline lepromatous, LL: lepromatous)

# CLINICAL CHARACTERISTICS

## Cardinal Features

a. Hypopigmented (pale) or erythematous skin patch with a definite sensory deficit.
b. Thickened, tender peripheral nerve(s) with sensory deficit.
c. Positive skin smears.

*Presence of one or more cardinal features is diagnostic of leprosy.*

### Hypopigmented (Pale) or Erythematous Skin Patch

Any person with hypopigmented or erythematous skin patches should be thoroughly examined under the good light. The most relevant point in the examination is testing for loss of sensation in the skin lesion(s). The lesion should be tested for touch sensation.

### Thickened, Tender Peripheral Nerve(s) with Sensory Deficit

Peripheral nerves should be examined for thickening and tenderness. Nerve functions (both sensory and motor function) are also to be assessed **(Fig. 17G.12)**.

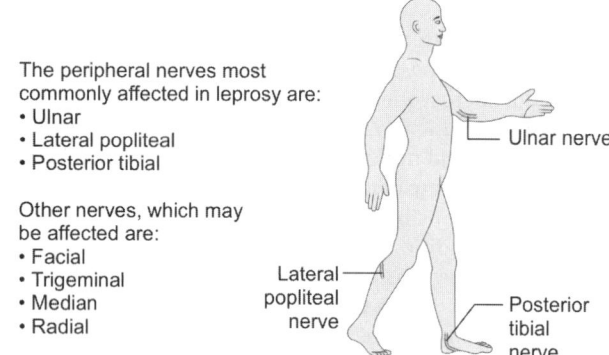

Fig. 17G.12: The commonly affected nerves and the sites of their examination.

In the advanced stage of disease, the patient may present with nodular infiltration of face and extremities and some deformities like claw hand, claw feet, and loss of limb or fingers. Lepromatous leprosy patients may exhibit characteristic "leonine facies" **(Fig. 17G.13A)** with thick earlobes **(Fig. 17G.13B)**, collapse nose, thickened skin of the forehead and lost eyebrows. Due to damage

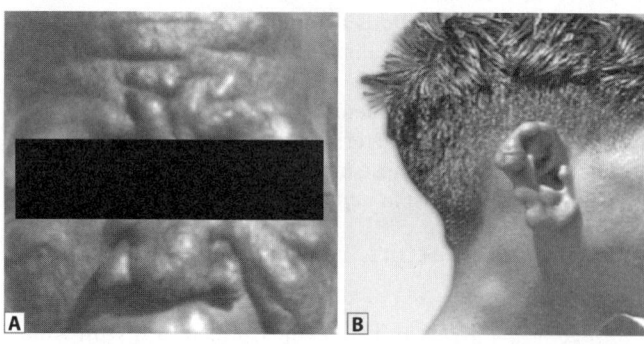

Figs. 17G.13A and B: (A) Leonine facies; (B) Nodular infiltration of ear.

of facial nerve, the patient becomes unable to close the eyes (lagophthalmos). This may cause exposure associated infection and later lead to blindness.

As the disease advances, a person affected with leprosy may present with various types of disabilities. WHO classifies disability based on its severity which is depicted in **Table 17G.16**.

Table 17G.16: WHO's grading of disability.

| Hands and feets | Grade 0 | No anesthesia over palm/sole no visible deformity or damage |
| --- | --- | --- |
| | Grade 1 | Anesthesia present over palm/sole but no visible deformity or damage |
| | Grade 2 | Visible deformity or damage present |
| Eyes | Grade 0 | No eye problem due to leprosy; no evidence of visual loss |
| | Grade 2 | Severe visual impairment (vision worse than 6/60; inability to count fingers at six meters), lagophthalmos, iridocyclitis and corneal opacities |

### Clinical Classification of Leprosy

The number of the anesthetic skin lesion is sufficient to diagnose and classify leprosy for starting of treatment. The most important advantage is that a community health worker can diagnose a case of leprosy with sufficient accuracy without any laboratory procedure. Treatment is initiated based on the classification.

It classifies leprosy into two as given in the **Flowchart 17G.3**:

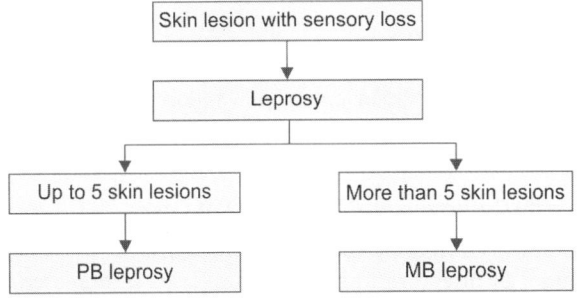

Flowchart 17G.3: Clinical classification of leprosy.

1. *Paucibacillary (PB):* Includes the less infectious types, i.e., BT, BB and TT.
2. *Multibacillary (MB):* Includes the most infectious group, i.e., BL and LL.

PB and MB leprosy are shown in **Figures 17G.14A and B**.

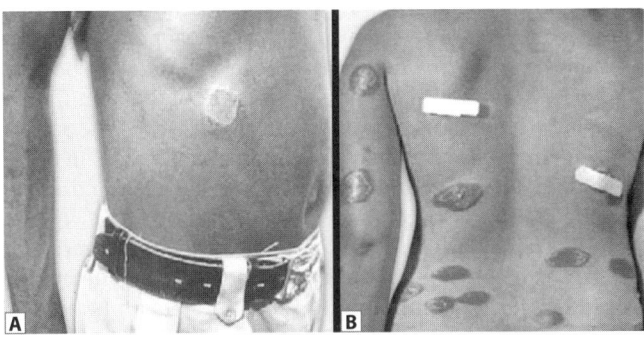

Figs. 17G.14A and B: (A) Paucibacillary; (B) Multibacillary.

## DIAGNOSIS

### Positive Skin Smear

Bacteriology is not routinely recommended for diagnosis and initiation of treatment in leprosy. Bacteriology requires sufficient laboratory facilities with trained manpower which is not possible in resource-poor countries like India.

However, the presence of bacilli in a skin smear is indicative of MB leprosy irrespective of the number of skin lesions/nerve involvement.

"Slit and Scrape" method is used to take smears from at least two sites (one active skin lesions and one earlobe). Smears can also be taken from nasal mucosa. Smears are stained by Ziehl-Neelsen technique for identification of the organism under the microscope.

The bacteriological examination includes two components.
1. *Bacteriological index (BI):* It measures the density of organism both living and dead in the smears. Leprosy is diagnosed as multibacillary or paucibacillary based on BI.
2. *Morphological index (MI):* It measures the viable bacilli which look solid and stained uniformly under the microscope. A rising MI or BI during or after full treatment indicates drug resistance or relapse.

### Lepromin Test

This is an intradermal test used to assess CMI and hence helps in classifying leprosy. It is not a diagnostic test and used in research purpose only. The test is performed by administering a specific amount (0.1 mL) of intradermal antigen (Lepromin), and the antibody response is studied by assessing the reactions at injection sites.

Two types of reactions are seen: Early and late.

### Positive Reaction (Early)

Erythema and induration >10 mm diameter that appears at 48 hours and disappears in 3–4 days. A positive reaction indicates previous exposure to leprosy, hence not an epidemiologically significant information.

### Late Reaction

Appearance of nodules >5 mm in diameter at 21 days. This indicates strong immunity against leprosy. Interpretation of lepromin test in different types of leprosy is depicted in **Flowchart 17G.4**.

### Lepra Reactions

These are hypersensitivity reactions that can occur in any type of leprosy. It may also occur in patients under treatment or

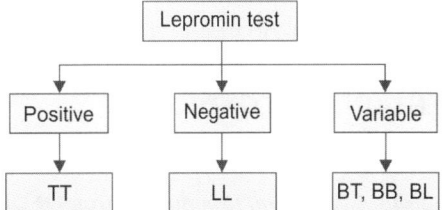

Flowchart 17G.4: Interpretation of lepromin test.

(TT: tuberculoid type, BT: borderline tuberculoid, BB: borderline-borderline, BL: borderline lepromatous, LL: lepromatous)

after completion of treatment. The exact cause of the reactions is still not known. The reactions need immediate medical interventions.

Types of lepra reactions are as follows:

***Type 1:*** It is mostly found in borderline leprosy, but may occur both in MB (Multibacillary) and PB (Paucibacillary) leprosy.
- In borderline leprosy, when the CMI is depressed, it moves towards the lepromatous end, and the reaction is termed as "downgrading". This normally happens before the start of MDT.
- Reversal reaction: The reversal reaction occurs after initiation of treatment when the CMI improves and moves towards tuberculoid type.

***Clinical presentation of type 1 reaction:*** Sudden appearance of inflammatory signs (pain, swelling, and redness) of existing skin lesions, painful nerves, etc. The patient may also develop new skin patches **(Fig. 17G.15A)**.

***Type 2 reaction:*** This is also known as erythema nodosum leprosum (ENL). This is a medical emergency and occurs only in MB leprosy.

***Clinical presentation of type 2 reaction:*** This is a sudden appearance of tender, red, and subcutaneous nodules in face and extremities. It often appears in groups. Generalized symptoms of fever, joint pain, fatigue, etc., are frequently seen **(Fig. 17G.15B)**.

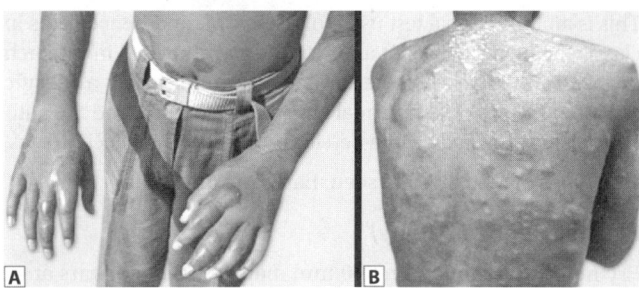

**Figs. 17G.15A and B:** (A) Type 1 lepra reaction; (B) Erythema nodosum leprosum.

> **Key Points**
> - Leprosy is transmitted mainly through droplet route.
> - Protective immunity in leprosy is CMI.
> - Weak CMI may results in lepromatous leprosy (LL), the most infectious form.
> - Strong CMI results in tuberculoid type (TT) leprosy, the least infectious form.
> - The infectivity decreases with MDT.
> - Presence of hypopigmented, anesthetic skin lesion(s) is diagnostic of leprosy.
> - Based on the number of skin lesions, leprosy is classified and treatment is started.
> - In paucibacillary, number of skin lesion is 1–5 whereas in multibacillary it is >5.
> - Bacteriology is not usually required for the diagnosis of leprosy.

## PREVENTION AND CONTROL

### Primary Prevention

- ***Information, Education, Communication (IEC):*** Society's perception of the disease greatly influences the control strategy. Sustained IEC activities regarding the disease and its curability ensure early and voluntary reporting for treatment. In spite of having the most effective antileprosy treatment, leprosy remains a problem in some areas. Community awareness and participation are crucial for early diagnosis and completion of treatment **(Fig. 17G.16)**.

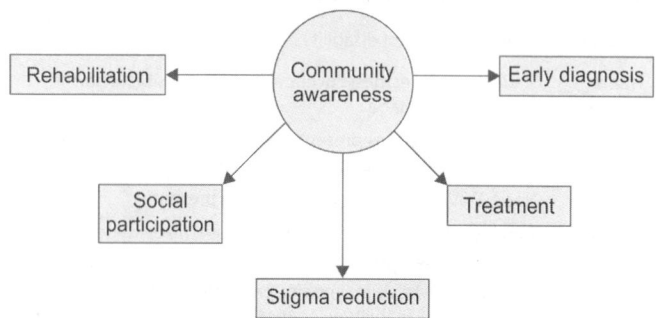

**Fig. 17G.16:** Community awareness: Key to leprosy prevention.

- ***Vaccines:*** Role of vaccines are very insignificant and still in the experimental stage. However, BCG is found to provide some degree of protection against leprosy also. However, the level of protection is variable in different research studies.
- ***Chemoprophylaxis:*** Role of chemoprophylaxis is still not established.
- ***Environmental improvement:*** Provision of adequate housing with proper ventilation and prevention of overcrowding are the few general environmental measures for prevention of transmission.

### Secondary and Tertiary Prevention

The main intervention of leprosy prevention is "Early Diagnosis and Treatment". Diagnosing the disease at the earliest prevent the advancement of the disease and subsequent disability.

### (A) Early Detection and Treatment of Cases

Detecting and treating the cases at the earliest will decrease the pool of infection in the community as undetected and untreated cases are the only sources of infection. Further, this also prevents the development of disability, since disability is one of the important reason for stigma associated with the disease.

### Different Case-detection Approaches

- ***Passive case-finding:*** This has been the conventional approach for case detection in leprosy. This approach basically relies on voluntary reporting of cases. Voluntary reporting depends on awareness and perception of the community regarding the disease and its preventability. Hence, the passive case-finding method may not capture all the cases in those communities, where misconceptions are prevalent and access to health care is low or inadequate.
- ***Active case-finding:*** Here, active house to house search for cases is being done in the high priority areas to detect the hidden cases. Community-level volunteers and frontline workers may be involved to search for the suspected skin lesions/deformities and refer them to the Primary Health

Center (PHC) for diagnosis and treatment (MDT). Three types of case-finding methods are there depending on the prevalence of the disease. These are:
- **Contact survey:** In a low prevalence area (<1 case/1,000 population), all the household contacts of leprosy case to be examined for signs and symptoms. This is the focus of case detection currently in India.
- **Group survey:** In areas where prevalence is moderate (one case/1,000 or higher), the high-risk group like slum dwellers, school children, etc., are screened for leprosy.
- **Mass survey:** In high prevalent areas (10 or more cases/1,000 population), the whole population is to be screened irrespective of their risk status. This requires extensive resources especially manpower.

### Treatment with MDT

Regular and complete treatment with MDT is the only way to cure the patient and to prevent transmission. Based on clinical classification, patients are grouped and the standard MDT regimen is to be given.

Duration of treatment is 12 months (12 Blister Packs) in MB, which has to be completed within 18 months and 6 months (6 Blister packs) in PB to be completed in 9 months **(Tables 17G.17A and B)**.

**Table 17G.17A:** MDT regimen for adults.

| Multibacillary cases (>5 skin lesions) | Paucibacillary cases (1–5 skin lesion/s) |
|---|---|
| • Rifampicin: 600 mg once monthly (supervised)<br>• Dapsone: 100 mg daily<br>• Clofazimine: 300 mg once monthly a daily dose of 50 mg | • Rifampicin: 600 mg once monthly (supervised)<br>• Dapsone: 100 mg daily |

**Table 17G.17B:** MDT regimen for children (10–14 years).

| Multibacillary cases (>5 skin lesions) | Paucibacillary cases (1–5 skin lesion/s) |
|---|---|
| • Rifampicin: 450 mg once monthly<br>• Dapsone: 50 mg once daily<br>• Clofazimine:<br>  ➤ 150 mg once in a month<br>  ➤ 50 alternate day | Rifampicin: 450 mg once monthly<br>Dapsone: 50 mg daily |

The treatment regimen of MDT for leprosy has been revised by MoHFW with approval of WHO in order to stop the transmission of Leprosy. GOI has introduced a 3-drug regimen for Paucibacillary cases in place of a 2-drug regimen for 6 months for both adults and children. Therefore, along with Rifampicin and Dapsone, 300 mg of Clofazimine in adults and 150 mg in children has been added. (Similar to Multibacillary cases). This revised regimen shall be implemented all over the country from 1st April 2025.

Under National Leprosy Eradication Programme, different case detection strategies are being followed and MDT is delivered through peripheral health institutions.

***Second line of antileprosy drugs:*** Ethionamide, Protionamide, Tetracycline (Minocycline), Quinolones, Macrolides (Clarithromycin).

***Treatment of lepra reactions:*** Patients with lepra reactions should be referred from the community to any health institution. Management of reactions include:
- Give rest to the affected part
- Symptomatic for the relief of pain and inflammation
- The drug of choice is *corticosteroid*.

MDT should not be stopped even if lepra reaction occurs during the course of MDT.

> **Note**
> - Leprosy is not hereditary.
> - It is the least infectious.
> - Leprosy is completely curable.
> - Early diagnosis and treatment completely prevent the progression of disease.
> - Treatment with MDT prevents disability.
> - Treatment makes an infectious person noninfectious.
> - *Note:* Treatment is available at all government health institution free of cost.

### (B) Disability Prevention and Medical Rehabilitation

Disability is the result of nerve damage due to leprosy or due to lepra reactions. The aim of disability prevention and medical rehabilitation (DPMR) is to maintain or restore the functioning of the patient so that the person can lead a life with full of dignity and independence.

### Disability Prevention

Different ways to prevent disabilities:
- Early diagnosis and treatment of leprosy before nerve damage sets in.
- Early identification of lepra reactions and its management.
- *Care of the wounds/ulcer:* The community must be educated about the "self-care practices" and they must be empowered enough to undertake these practices on their own. The basic practices are:
  - Care of the dry skin by applying oils
  - Use of suitable footwear
  - Prevention of injury.

### Rehabilitation

It encompasses all measures to decrease the impact of disability so that the person affected with leprosy can lead a life with the highest possible level of independence in all domains of health—physical, mental, functional, and social. Different types of rehabilitation that are applicable in leprosy:

#### Medical rehabilitation

All the medical measures for restoration of functions fall in this category. This is best achieved by the provision of MDT, use of protective aids like micro-cellulose rubber (MCR) foot ware, self-care kit, etc., re-constructive surgeries (RCS) if necessary, for correction of disability.

#### Social and psychological rehabilitation

The social impact of the disease is much more than the physical impact. The social and psychological rehabilitation plays a crucial role to create awareness, to empower the persons with disability for equal participation in every sphere of life, to promote the dignity and respect of affected person. This is only possible with the abolition of all discriminatory laws.

*Vocational rehabilitation*

This is required for encouraging livelihood and promoting economic independence. Persons with the disability needs to be employed in a safe working environment (e.g., a person with anesthetic hands or feet are not safe to be employed as cook). The person with the disability may be referred to vocational training for skill development and empowerment programs.

## ROLE OF NONGOVERNMENTAL ORGANIZATION/COMMUNITY-BASED ORGANIZATIONS/CIVIL SOCIETIES/PRIVATE CARE PROVIDERS IN LEPROSY

Leprosy control is possible only with combined and comprehensive effortts of different organizations, civil societies, nongovernmental organizations (NGOs), etc. They can be involved in:
- Awareness generation (regarding the disease, stigma reduction, implications of early diagnosis and treatment, prevention of disability, self-care at home, referral, and rehabilitation)
- Service delivery and monitoring
- Rehabilitation care
- Reconstructive surgery
- Research

Some of the organizations working for people affected with leprosy are Hind Kusht Nivaran Sangha, Gandhi Memorial Leprosy Foundation, etc.

## CURRENT APPROACHES

### Global Approach

WHO released the Towards zero leprosy: global leprosy (Hansen's disease) strategy 2021–2030 aligned to the neglected tropical diseases road map 2021–2030. The Strategy calls for a vision of zero leprosy: zero infection and disease, zero disability, zero stigma and discrimination and the elimination of leprosy (defined as interruption of transmission) as its goal.

The four strategic pillars of the strategy include:
- Implementing integrated, country-owned zero leprosy roadmaps in all endemic countries;
- Scaling up leprosy prevention alongside integrated active case detection;
- Managing leprosy and its complications and prevent new disability; and
- Combatting stigma and ensuring human rights are respected.

The Strategy also recognizes that global and national investment in research is essential to achieving zero leprosy and includes a set of key research priorities.

WHO has developed e-learning modules that aim to enhance knowledge and skills of health workers at all levels on topics related to diagnosis, treatment of leprosy and management of disabilities. These can be accessed the Open WHO platform.

India is also committed to fulfilling this goal through intensification of case detection, awareness, and rehabilitation activities.

### National Approach

The National Leprosy Eradication strategy works on the following:
- Case detection
- Disability prevention and medical rehabilitation
- IEC and BCC
- Human resource and capacity building
- Program management.

Along with the above central measures many other organizations work for leprosy which are the Hind Kusht Nivaran Sangha, Gandhi Memorial Leprosy Foundation, etc.

### National Program

The National Leprosy Eradication Programme along with support from WHO and ILEP along with NGOs is working towards the eradication of the disease, which is *further explained in Chapter 47: Health Policies and Programs in India.*

> **Why Leprosy is an Ideal Candidate for Elimination?**
>
> Following epidemiological information justify leprosy as a candidate for elimination:
> - Untreated and infected human is the only established source of infection. It is much easier to control the human source.
> - The occurrence of disease following infection is very less. Majority become immune following infection.
> - Easy and simple diagnostic tool (on clinical criteria) with sufficient accuracy. No sophisticated laboratory examination is required.
> - Effective treatment (MDT) is available to interrupt the chain of transmission.
> - Unlike TB, leprosy situation does not appear to be adversely affected by HIV infection.

## SUMMARY

- Leprosy, a chronic disease caused by *M. leprae* is one of the important causes of permanent physical disability. The disease is full of social stigma and discrimination because of disfigurement it causes. It mainly affects the skin and peripheral nerves. Damage of peripheral nerve/s causes disfigurement. Leprosy is acquired mainly through droplet route. Development of disease depends on cell-mediated immunity, which is the protective immunity in leprosy. Strong CMI results in tuberculoid leprosy, the least infectious form. Poor CMI results in lepromatous leprosy, the most infectious form. Untreated leprosy cases particularly lepromatous leprosy (LL) are the major source of infection.
- Presence of hypopigmented or erythematous skin lesion/s with definite sensory impairment is diagnostic of leprosy. Early diagnosis and treatment and disability prevention and medical rehabilitation are the two important prevention strategies. Leprosy is curable with multi-drug therapy. MDT includes dapsone, rifampicin, and clofazimine. Early and complete treatment with MDT prevents occurrence of deformities and disabilities.
- Control of leprosy is not possible only with medical management. Community awareness regarding the disease and its curability is crucial to remove the stigma, which influences the treatment seeking behavior. Based on the number of such skin lesion, leprosy is diagnosed and classified for treatment. Those having lesion/s between 1 and 5 is paucibacillary, the least infectious form and >5 is multibacillary, the most infectious form. Bacteriology is usually not required in diagnosing leprosy. Duration of treatment is 12 months and 6 months for multibacillary and paucibacillary respectively.
- Immunological and inflammatory reactions may develop during the course of the disease and these are known as lepra reactions. These also lead to disability if not identified and managed early. Medical, vocational, and social rehabilitation is an important step in promoting independence functionally, socially, and economically.

Leprosy was eliminated globally as well as from India following intensified case detection and treatment with MDT. However, high-risk pockets are still there. It is said to be eliminated when prevalence is <1 per 10,000 population. For continuation of elimination status, control activities, and surveillance is to be continued.

## SUGGESTED READING

1. Ananthanarayan and Panikers's. Textbook of Microbiology. Hyderabad: University Press (India); 2013.
2. Govt. of India. National Leprosy Eradication Programme (NLEP), Training Manual for Medical Officers; 2013.
3. National strategic plan and Roadmap for Leprosy 2023-2027, Accelerationg towards A leprosy free India January 2023, Central leprosy division, DGHS, MoHFW, GOI.
4. NLEP Annual Report. Govt. of India. 2016-17.
5. NLEP Newsletter. The House of Central Leprosy Division; 2016. pp. 11.
6. Sasakawa Memorial Health Foundation. (2002) A New Atlas of Leprosy (McDougall A, Yuasa Y). [online] Available from: https:// www.smhf.or.jp/data01/atlas_english.pdf.
7. WHO.Leprosy ; Factsheet. January 2023.
8. World Health Organization. A guide to eliminating leprosy as a public health problem. Geneva: World Health Organization; 1995.
9. World Health Organization. Global Leprosy Strategy 2016-2020: Accelerating towards a leprosy-free world. Regional Office for South-East Asia: SEARO Publications; 2016. p. 20.
10. World Health Organization. Guidelines for the diagnosis, treatment and prevention of leprosy. Regional Office for South-East Asia: SEARO Publications; 2018. p. 106.
11. World Health Organization. Leprosy: World focused on ending transmission among children. Geneva: World Health Organization; 2018.
12. World Health Organization. Weekly epidemiological record. Geneva: World Health Organization; 2018. pp. 445-56.

# EPIDEMIOLOGY OF TRACHOMA AND ITS PREVENTION AND CONTROL

*Anku Moni Saikia, Kumaril Goswami*

| | |
|---|---|
| CM7.2 | Enumerate, describe and discuss the mode of transmission and measures for prevention and control of Trachoma |
| CM8.1 | Describe and discuss the epidemiological and control measures applicable in Trachoma |

> *Case Study*
>
> *An 8-year-old child was brought to the ophthalmic department with eye issues. On examination, there was follicular inflammation of the tarsal conjunctiva. Antibiotic treatment was given and the child's eye symptoms resolved. On history, however, the doctor was able to conclude that there were many individuals around the patients area who had eye problems, and some had surgeries done for the same, some were blinded by the infection and so on. With a personal interest, the doctor tried to get more details from the area the patient belonged to and realized that the area was endemic for trachoma.*

## INTRODUCTION

Trachoma, a disease resulting from poor personal hygiene and environmental sanitation, is a disabling disease that causes blindness. Blindness is an important disability that affects all domains of health and productivity. A person with visual impairment becomes dependent both functionally and financially and has to face stigma and social discrimination. Trachoma, a leading cause of blindness in developing or underdeveloped countries is caused by the bacterium *Chlamydia trachomatis*. The impact of the disease is so tremendous that it affects not only the person with the disability but also the family and society as a whole. There is a huge economic burden on families who are already among the poorest of the poor. On one hand, the person may become unproductive because of the limitation of vision and on the other hand the cost of rehabilitation is too expensive and may not be accessible to all. In such a situation, the patient or the family may not be in a position to bear it. In a resource-scarce country like India, taking care of people with such disabilities in a meaningful way has always been a challenge. However, trachoma can be easily prevented by inexpensive, simple and highly cost-effective community-based interventions.

## PROBLEM STATEMENT

### Global

- Trachoma is a disease of poor and underdeveloped countries. In the 1950s, it was a major cause of blindness across the globe. A significant number of cases were reported even in developed countries in Europe and America during that period. The disease has decreased and gradually disappeared from the developed countries. Overall socioeconomic developments could be one reason for this achievement. The problem has remained in poor and resource constrained countries.
- Trachoma is still a problem in many countries of Asia, South and Central America, Africa, and the Middle-East. According to a recent estimate by the World Health Organization. It is responsible for the blindness or visual impairment of about 1.9 million people. Africa is the worst affected continent with 85% of all infective trachoma (active trachoma), and 44% of global trichiasis. It is responsible for 1.4% of world blindness. (WHO, Fact Sheet: Trachoma, 2022).
- WHO adopted intensive intervention package—(**S**urgery for trachomatous trichiasis, **A**ntibiotics for the organism, **F**acial cleanliness, and **E**nvironmental improvement to reduce the transmission of the disease (SAFE) in the year 1993 as a comprehensive measure of control. Following the implementation of the SAFE strategy, the burden of the disease has decreased significantly in the endemic countries. The improvement in the socioeconomic condition also contributed to the control of the disease.
- However, in spite of all these efforts, 158 million people still live in endemic areas. They may develop impairment of vision/blindness if adequate interventions are not taken in time.
- Trachoma has been reported to be eliminated in 12 countries (as of October 2018).

The global distribution of trachoma shows the prevalence of active trachoma infection across the globe as per 2018 International Trachoma Initiative report.

The prevalence is estimated based on trachoma survey report. However, information were missing from the regions where survey was not done. The actual problem may be much bigger.

As of 5 October 2022, 15 countries—Cambodia, China, Gambia, Islamic Republic of Iran, Lao People's Democratic Republic, Ghana, Malawi, Mexico, Morocco, Myanmar, Nepal, Oman, Saudi Arabia and Vanuatu—had been validated by WHO as having eliminated trachoma as a public health problem.

## Indian Scenario

It was a major problem during the 1950s. Few states like Gujarat, Rajasthan, Punjab, and Uttar Pradesh (UP) have contributed the most.

Following the introduction of the National Trachoma Control Programme in 1963, trachoma control activities were intensified. Based on the endemicity, trachoma control units were established and mass antibiotic treatment was started in children in the endemic areas.

India started the National Programme for Control of Blindness (NPCB) in 1976, where trachoma control measures were incorporated.

Currently, the disease is found in certain pockets of North India—Gujarat, Punjab, Haryana, UP, and Nicobar Islands.

*India has been declared free from "infective trachoma" among children in 2017*—with an overall prevalence found to be only 0.7% in the National Trachoma Survey which was done in 27 high-risk districts of 23 states between 2014 and 2017.

> **Note**
> Elimination of active trachoma is defined as a reduction in the prevalence of active infection among children below 10 years is less than 5%.

## EPIDEMIOLOGY

### Host Factors

#### Age

Active trachoma is a disease of children below the age of 10 years. However, chronic trachoma increases with age and seen in adults as it requires long and frequent infections and inflammations.

#### Sex

Women are at risk because they remain in more and prolonged contact with young children who might carry the infection.

#### Immunity

There is no long-lasting protective immunity following infection. The occurrence of repeated infections in an endemic area substantiates the fact.

#### Socioeconomic Status

It is a disease of low socioeconomic status. Poverty and illiteracy influence the basic sanitation and personal hygiene practices which act as important determinants of trachoma. The predominance of the disease in lower socioeconomic status could be attributed to the lack of basic provisions (clean water, sanitary latrine, and adequate sewage disposal) to interrupt the disease transmission.

### Agent Factors

*Chlamydia trachomatis* is an obligate intracellular and weakly gram-negative bacterium. The bacterium is nonspore-forming.

### Reservoir of Infection

Active trachoma cases are the sources of infection in the community. Children below 10 years of age suffering from trachoma with discharging eyes are the most common source of infection.

No animal reservoir is found until now, making the disease possible to eliminate.

### Infectious Materials

- Ocular and nasal discharge
- Fomites contaminated with the infectious discharge of active trachoma cases.

### Environmental Factors

Environmental cleanliness is the most important determinant in transmission of trachoma in the community.

#### Factors in the Physical Environment

- *Temperature and humidity:* As fly acts as transmitting vector, high temperature and humidity favors the fly survival, hence incidence of active trachoma is more during the hot and humid season of the year.
- *Overcrowding:* As trachoma is transmitted by direct contact, staying in close contacts facilitates its transmission.
- *Lack of access to adequate water:* This hampers in maintaining cleanliness and personal hygiene like face and handwashing.
- *Inadequate provision for safe disposal of excreta and refuses:* Open air defecation and unsanitary disposal of refuses lead to increase in fly population, which may act as a vector in trachoma transmission.

#### Factors in the Social Environment

Various social factors like poverty, illiteracy, ignorance, misconceptions, etc., determine the occurrence of trachoma and its progression to blindness. Customary practices like putting eye cosmetics like *Kajal* may put the children at risk in an infected environment.

### Mode of Transmission: Three "fs" (Fingers, Fomites, Flies)

#### Fingers

Direct contact with the ocular and nasal discharge (through fingers).

Indirectly contact through fomites and flies.

#### Fomites

Fomites like clothes, beddings contaminated with the ocular and nasal discharge of the patient with active trachoma.

#### Flies

Eye-seeking flies (*Musca sorbens*) which are attracted to ocular discharge and cluster around face and eyes of infected children. These particular varieties of flies feed on mucus and discharge of the eyes and transmit it through its proboscis. It can also passively transmit the organism by soiling of its feet and transmit it to uninfected children. Human feces are the main breeding sites of these flies, but it can also breed in other animal feces.

***Incubation period:*** 5–12 days.

## PATHOGENESIS

Trachoma is a disease of children, but advanced complications like blindness occur in adults. The infection involves the conjunctiva under the eyelids. In the initial stage, there is inflammatory signs and follicle formation on the bulbar conjunctiva. When the follicles resolve down, it leaves some depression on the sites, known as "Herbert's pit", which is diagnostic of trachoma. Repeated infections and inflammation can only cause severe scarring of the inside of the eyelid. Contraction of such scar tissue draws the eyelashes inside and results in a condition called as *trachomatous trichiasis* (eyelashes touching/rubbing on the eyeball). This leads to permanent corneal damage and subsequently blindness. Blindness due to trachoma is not reversible.

The extraocular mucous membrane like nasopharynx can also get infected with the organism.

## CLINICAL FEATURES

***Clinical manifestations*** can be classified into two groups depending on the stage of the disease:
1. ***Active trachoma:*** This early stage of the disease is known as "infective trachoma" which is most commonly found in children. The affected person may be asymptomatic or may have mild symptoms which are similar to any mucopurulent conjunctivitis (discharge from eyes, pain, irritation, photophobia, etc.).

   On examination, follicles and papillae can be seen over conjunctiva **(Fig. 17G.18)**. Follicles are yellow or white spots over the conjunctiva.

   An active disease is indicated by the presence of at least five follicles on the central part of the upper tarsal conjunctiva.
2. ***Chronic stage:*** Manifestations in the chronic stage are the sequelae of repeated infection during childhood. Complications like corneal opacities and blindness may occur in this stage **(Fig. 17G.17)**.

   Any patient from an endemic area with such manifestations could be a case of trachoma and should be accordingly investigated.

> **Key Points**
> - Trachoma, a leading cause of preventable blindness is caused by the bacterium *Chlamydia trachomatis*.
> - Trachoma is a disease of poor and underdeveloped countries.
> - India has declared free from "Infective Trachoma" among children in 2017.
> - Ocular and nasal secretions of an infected person are the source of infection.
> - Active trachoma is a disease of children below the age of 10 years.
> - Incubation period is 5–12 days.

## DIAGNOSIS

Diagnosis is usually made on clinical grounds. It can be diagnosed at the primary level without any sophisticated technique. For the initiation of treatment, clinical diagnosis is sufficient.

However, some laboratory tests like bacteriology and serology are also there to be used in rare circumstances.

## PREVENTION AND CONTROL

Prevention of trachoma is a multipronged strategy with coordination with various departments. These are:

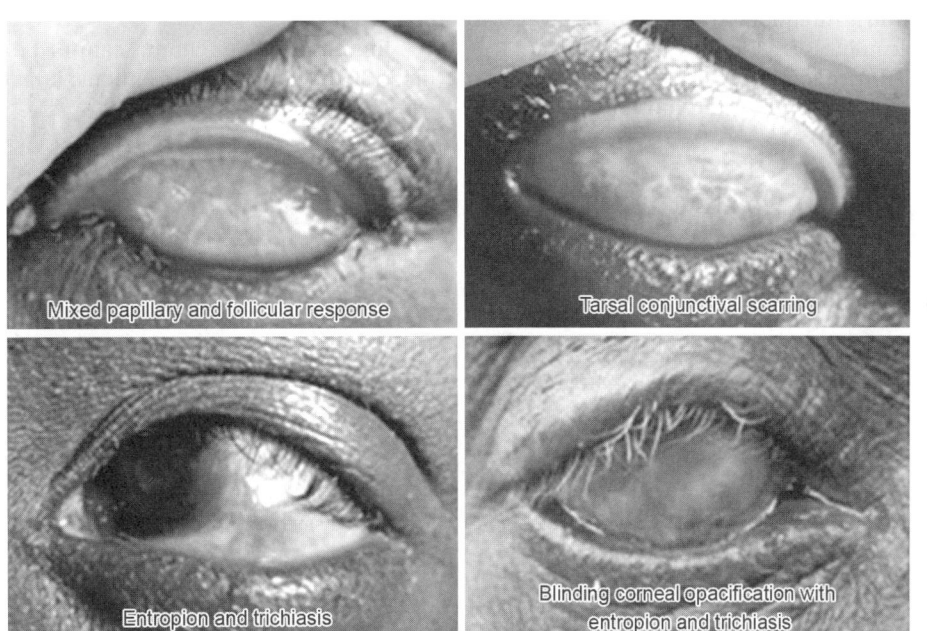

**Fig. 17G.17:** Ocular manifestation in trachoma infection.

## The Comprehensive Strategy

***The comprehensive strategy*** recommended by WHO is known by the acronym—"SAFE", a simple and low-cost interventions. This entails all the levels of prevention—primary, secondary and tertiary levels. This strategy has been implemented in the community through primary healthcare approach. The ultimate aim of all the strategies is to decrease the prevalence of active trachoma infection in children of less than 10 years of age to less than 5%.

### SAFE Strategy (Fig. 17G.18)

**S:** Surgery to correct in-turn lashes or trichiasis (both secondary and tertiary level of prevention).

**A:** Antibiotics to treat active infection with Azithromycin (can be used as both primary and secondary level).

A single oral dose of antibiotic Azithromycin (20 mg/kg body weight) is recommended by WHO. For children of less than 6 months and pregnant women, Azithromycin is not currently recommended and hence Tetracycline ointment is the treatment of choice for these two groups. Antibiotics are used as a primary prevention measure to prevent transmission or to treat the active trachoma (secondary prevention).

*Antibiotic treatment approach depends on endemicity of the diseases which is measured by the prevalence of active (infective) trachoma amongst children (>10 years) in the community*:

*Mass or blanket treatment*: If the prevalence is more than 10%, all the residents should be treated with an annual dose of antibiotic for 3 years. The aim is to bring down the prevalence to less than 5%. A repeat survey is to be done at the end of 3 years.

*Selective or targeted treatment*: If prevalence lies between 5% and 10%, selective treatment is recommended to all members of a family in whom there is a case of active trachoma.

**F:** Facial cleanliness through frequent face washing (primary level of prevention). Adequate access to clean water to maintain facial cleanliness is a must.

**E:** Environmental improvement: To interrupt the chain of transmission of trachoma infection, environmental improvement is the basic requirement which helps the people to get access to clean water and maintain basic sanitation. Removal of fecal contamination of the environment by preventing open defecation is the most effective way of fly control. This entails both primary and secondary levels of prevention.

## Information, Education and Communication

Trachoma control is not possible until and unless there is a change in behavior and practices that favors the transmission of the disease. The community must be aware of simple day to day life practices that are crucial for prevention. These practices are very simple and easy to follow. Information, education and communication activities regarding the disease and its curability ensure early reporting for seeking treatment. Interventions in early stage prevent the development of disability.

Some important health education messages are:
- Trachoma can lead to blindness if not treated
- Trachoma is preventable
- Frequent face and handwashing with clean water can prevent trachoma
- Environmental cleanliness with the sanitary disposal of excreta prevents trachoma
- Use of antibiotic in trachoma (in children) prevents blindness
- Early reporting and seeking health care in eye diseases is crucial.

## Surveillance

In areas where trachoma has been eliminated, it is very much important to sustain with the positive results achieved so far. So the monitoring and reporting of trachoma and its control activities have to be continued in those areas. A post-elimination survey is required to assess the sustainability of the activities.

Elimination of trachoma cannot be achieved only with medical and surgical interventions; it requires a broad linkage with the other sectors.

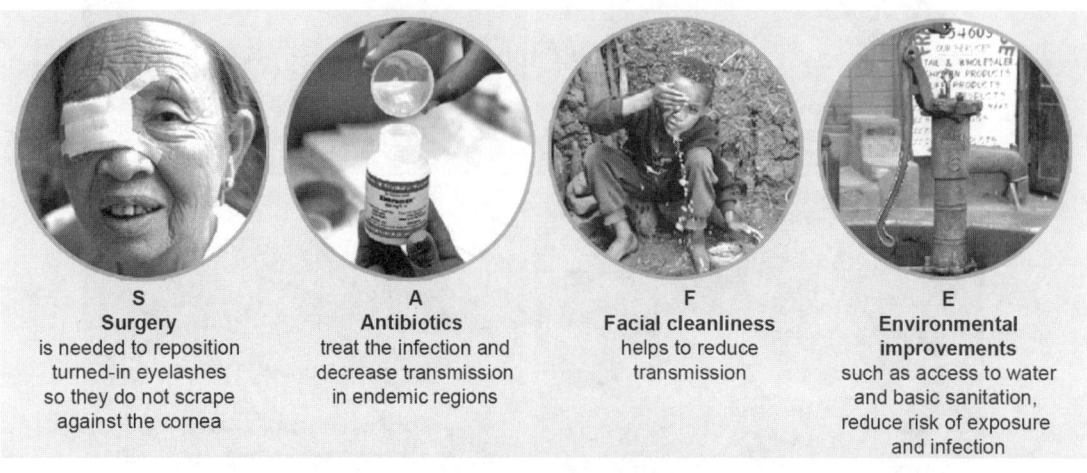

**Fig. 17G.18:** SAFE strategy.
*Source:* International Coalition for Trachoma Control.

## CURRENT APPROACHES

### Global

***GET2020:*** Following the launch of alliance for the Global Elimination of Trachoma by the year 2020 (GET2020) in 1997, World Health Assembly passed the resolution of GET2020 in the next year. To help the countries to achieve GET2020, WHO formed an alliance with the endemic countries having political commitment to end the disease. It would support and coordinate the implementation of the SAFE strategy. It supports every aspect of elimination strategy (SAFE), starting from assessing the burden (mapping), monitoring and implementation of SAFE, evaluation and technical support.

The neglected tropical diseases road map 2021-2030, endorsed by the World Health Assembly in 2020 through its decision 73(33), sets 2030 as the new target date for global elimination.

### National

India, being a part of this alliance started the campaign on SAFE strategy and achieved the goal of elimination. Eye care services have been integrated and being delivered through primary health center or community health center. The emphasis has been given on creating awareness on prevention of common eye diseases like trachoma by simple interventions like face washing and early reporting for eye diseases. Additional technical staffs have been provided for providing eye care services. Few Government of India Initiatives on the clean environment and safe water are:
- Water, sanitation and hygiene (WASH)
- Swachh Bharat.

**National Program:** The National Program for Control of Blindness was launched in 1976 as a continuation of National Program for Trachoma control when causes of preventable blindness other than trachoma came into focus. In 2017, it was redesignated as National Program for Control of Blindness and Visual Impairment. ***This is further explained in Chapter 47: Health Policies and Programs in India.***

### Key Points
- Diagnosis is usually made on clinical grounds only.
- WHO recommended a comprehensive strategy "SAFE" for the prevention and control of trachoma.
- Aim of all the strategies is to decrease the prevalence of active trachoma in children of less than 10 years of age to less than 5%.
- To interrupt the chain of transmission of trachoma infection, environmental improvement is the basic requirement.

## SUMMARY

Trachoma is one of the leading causes of preventable blindness. It is a disease of poor and underdeveloped countries. India has declared free from "infective trachoma" among children in 2017. Ocular and nasal secretions of an infected person are the source of infection. Infective trachoma occurs in children. Repeated infection in children leads to advanced complications like blindness in adults. WHO recommended a comprehensive strategy known by the acronym—"SAFE", a simple and low-cost intervention which has been implemented in the community through primary healthcare approach. Community awareness on personal hygiene and environmental sanitation are crucial for prevention of trachoma.

The ultimate aim of all the strategies is to decrease the prevalence of active trachoma infection in children of less than 10 years of age to less than 5%.

## SUGGESTED READING

1. Trachoma Atlas, International Trachoma Initiative. (2018). [online] Available from www.trachomaatlas.org.
2. WHO.Trachoma; Factsheet Oct 2022.
3. World Health Organization. (2018). Trachoma-neglected diseases. [online] Available from http://www.who.int/gho/neglected_ diseases/trachoma/en/.
4. World Health Organization. (2018). Trachoma. [online] Available from http://www.who.int/trachoma/epidemiology/en/.

# EPIDEMIOLOGY OF TETANUS AND ITS PREVENTION AND CONTROL

*Anku Moni Saikia, Kumaril Goswami*

*"It is painful for him to open his mouth. His heart beats too slowly (or weakly) for speech. You observe his saliva falling from his lips, but not falling completely...He suffers stiffness in his neck. He does not find he can look at his two shoulders and his breast".*

—(Anonymous), Circa 1500 BC

| | |
|---|---|
| CM7.2 | Enumerate, describe and discuss the mode of transmission and measures for prevention and control of tetanus |
| CM8.1 | Describe and discuss the epidemiological and control measures applicable in tetanus |

### Case Study

*Mohan and Mani of a remote village had their first child, delivered at home by an untrained "dai". The baby was feeding normally till the 6th day. On the 7th day of postpartum, the baby became unable to suck, and developed some sort of rigidity in the body. The child was taken to a local hospital and on enquiry, it was found that the poor, illiterate mother had no antenatal check-ups including any shots of a vaccine. It also came to light that as a customary practice, they applied cow dung over the umbilical stump. The child was diagnosed as a case of neonatal tetanus (NT). The child was referred to one isolation hospital where the child finally succumbed to the disease after 3 days. The following questions need to be addressed:*
- *What are the important gaps that led to the death of the newborn in the above narration?*
- *What actions must be taken in the community to prevent such newborn deaths in the future?*

## INTRODUCTION

Tetanus, particularly neonatal tetanus (NT), often a serious disease, is caused by *Clostridium tetani* (*C. tetani*) and characterized by rigidity and painful paroxysmal spasms of the voluntary muscles. Maternal tetanus (tetanus occurring during pregnancy or puerperium) and NT (tetanus in first 28 days of life) are important causes of maternal and neonatal deaths in low and middle-income countries. Neonatal tetanus is more common among the poor and disadvantaged population because of inadequate access to health services in this population. However, death due to tetanus is easily preventable with some simple community health interventions like immunization and hygienic birth practices.

Tetanus may occur at any age when there is contamination of wounds with tetanus spores in absence of adequate immunization. Tetanus occurring beyond the neonatal period is known as non-neonatal tetanus. Tetanus is a notifiable disease to the World Health Organization.

Tetanus spores are widespread in the natural environment, particularly soil, dust, and animal feces. Because of this ubiquitous distribution of spores, the disease is not amenable to eradication.

## PROBLEM STATEMENT

### Global

It is almost exclusively a disease of developing or under-developed countries. Due to extensive immunization coverage with tetanus toxoid containing vaccines (TTCV), both neonatal and non-neonatal tetanus cases as well as deaths becoming rare in developed countries. Overall socioeconomic development of these countries contributed to elimination of maternal and neonatal tetanus (MNT) even before the introduction of tetanus vaccine. During the 1980s, over one million deaths were reported every year among under-five; two-thirds of this was due to NT. A significant reduction has been observed in NT and non-neonatal cases since 1980s. In 1989, WHO passed the resolution for eliminating neonatal tetanus. Initially, elimination target was set by 1995; later it was reset by 2015. As NT is dependent on maternal immunization status and also preventive strategies for maternal and NT are same, the initiative has been renamed as MNT elimination.

Elimination has been defined as less than 1 case of NT per 1,000 live births per year in all the districts of a country.

As of March 2018, elimination status was achieved in the major part of the globe; only 14 countries have still not reached the elimination status.

The total tetanus cases have not shown a consistent declining trend. However, in 2017, cases are seen to be less than the previous year (2016). There is no robust system of reporting of non-neonatal tetanus or adult tetanus. Neonatal tetanus is mostly under-reported as it occurs mainly in inaccessible and disadvantaged population.

Tetanus cases have decreased over years due to increase immunization with TTCV.

From 1990 to 2019, the incident cases of neonatal tetanus decreased by 92.67% in global and 84.90% in low SDI regions. The global neonatal tetanus situation improved a lot from 1990 to 2019, and many low- and middle-income countries have made significant progress in eliminating tetanus. However, we must accept the fact that many newborns with tetanus are born or die at home without registration the disease; so, the true burden is unknown. Tetanus is a serious disease with a high death rate. The deaths worldwide caused by tetanus decreased by 87% from 275,379 in 1990 to 34,684 in 2019. Worldwide, the Age Standardized Death Rate (ASDR) of tetanus decreased from 4.61 (per 100,000) in 1990 to 0.49 (per 100,000) in 2019.

### Indian Scenario

- In 2019, India had the most incident tetanus cases of 16,579, followed by Pakistan, Indonesia, and Nigeria, which were all developing countries with populations of more than 200 million. In 2019, India had the most tetanus deaths of 7,332 followed by Nigeria, Pakistan, and Indonesia. Furthermore, there are 77 countries with zero deaths from tetanus compared with 58 countries in 1990.
- Documented and authentic data of non-neonatal tetanus is not available in India. Whatever statistic is available, this is just the reported cases which may not represent the actual situation.
- Although a significant number of NT deaths were reported during the 1980s, this was just the tip of an iceberg. If a large number of deaths occurring at home was reported, the actual number would have been much more. Non-reporting of neonatal deaths could be due to some prevailing misconceptions (e.g., death of newborn is the wish of God). High NT deaths in India evoked significant concern and control activities were intensified. In 1983, tetanus toxoid (TT) was introduced in the immunization program, which had boosted the effort of tetanus control. This resulted in a 95% reduction of NT in 2015 compared to 1980s.
- After having successfully eradicated the wild poliovirus, India has reached this momentous landmark in child and maternal health. Unlike polio or small pox, tetanus can not be fully eradicated as the tenacious spores of bacteria causing tetanus, clostridium tetani, are widespread in the environment. WHO considers neonatal tetanus as eliminated from a country when its incidence becomes below one case per 1,000 live births per year in every district of the country. The number dropped to about 31,500 neonatal tetanus deaths in 2005, subsequently declining to below 500 in 2013 and 2014. This has paved the way for validation of the entire country for Mother and Neonatal Tetanus Elimination by mid-April 2015 with the help of partners such as WHO, UNICEF and others. As of May 2015, globally, 22 countries are yet to be validated for MNT elimination. In the South-East Asia Region of WHO, only some districts in the eastern part of Indonesia are yet to achieve the goal.

The declining trend of NT shown in **Figure 17G.19** could be attributed to significant improvement in the following determinants:

1. ***Immunization coverage with tetanus toxoid (TT):*** Immunization of pregnant mothers was 76.3% in 2005–2006, increased to 89% in 2015–2016.
2. ***Institutional deliveries:*** The proportion of institutional deliveries has increased in successive years (81.7% in 2011–

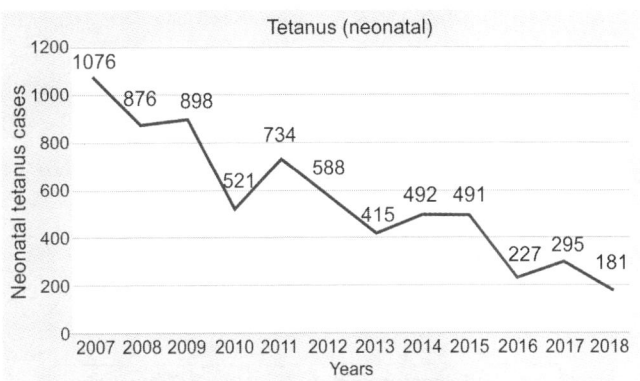

**Fig. 17G.19:** Trend of neonatal tetanus cases.
*Source:* National Health Profile (NHP) of India-2019, Central Bureau of Health Intelligence, GOI.

2012 to 90.3% in 2016–2017). Eventually, India achieved a significant milestone of MNT elimination in May 2015.

> **Key Points**
> - Tetanus is caused by *Clostridium tetani*, a spore-forming organism.
> - Maternal and neonatal tetanus is common and fatal, mostly prevalent in developing countries.
> - Spores are widespread in nature, particularly soil, making the eradication impossible.
> - Neonatal tetanus has been eliminated globally as well as from India.

## EPIDEMIOLOGY

### Host Factors

#### Age

Tetanus that occurs following injury or trauma is common in the active age group. This group has more outdoor activities; so they are more prone to injuries. Again, the protective immunity following primary immunization decreases with advancing age. The immunity can be maintained throughout the ages with adequate booster doses. The elderly population is more at risk because of this waning immunity.

Newborns and pregnant mothers obviously have a higher risk of developing tetanus.

#### Gender

More cases have been reported among males. This could be due to more involvement of males in agricultural and other fieldwork, which increases the risk of exposure to injury as well as to spores. Most often, in case of NT also, reported incidence is more in males. This could be due to gender biases in seeking health care, especially in Indian society.

#### Rural-Urban Difference

Although this is predominantly a disease of rural area, people living in urban slums are also at higher risk. In these areas, the living condition is generally poor, unhygienic practices are more and access to health care is low. The agricultural background in rural areas exposes the population to soil and animals and putting them more at risk.

### Immunity

There is no naturally acquired immunity or herd immunity. In tetanus, immunity is induced by immunizations only. Clinical disease cannot produce sufficient immunity against further infection and can be infected again. Hence, immunization with TTCV should be given to persons who already had the disease.

### Case Fatality Rate

Advanced medical care facilities like the intensive care unit (ICU) can decrease the fatality of tetanus. Without ICU, case fatality rate approaches to 100% in extreme of age.

### Agent Factors

*Clostridium tetani* is a gram-positive and spore-forming organism. Due to the anaerobic nature of the bacilli, it germinates in devitalized tissue. The spores are terminal giving a characteristic "Drumstick" or "Tennis racket" appearance under the microscope **(Fig. 17G.20)**.

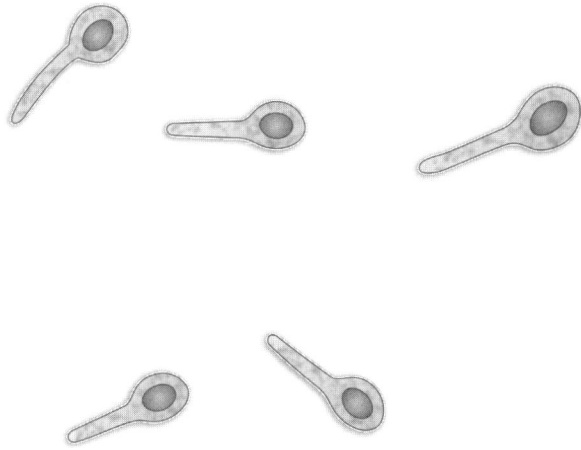

**Fig. 17G.20:** Tennis racket appearance of tetanus spores.

#### Resistance

Spores are the infective form of the organism. Neutralization of spores is difficult as spores are resistant to commonly used disinfection procedures like boiling and most of the common antiseptics.

Autoclaving at 121°C for 20 minutes is only effective for neutralizing the spores within 15–20 minutes.

### Environmental Factors

#### Physical Environment

Exposure and direct contact with soil increase the risk.

#### Social Environment

The mere presence of the organism in the physical environment is not sufficient to initiate the disease. The sociocultural behavior and practices have a great role to play. Through extensive health education and awareness program, these harmful practices can

be stopped. The factors of social environment responsible for tetanus are as follows:
- Lack of knowledge and awareness of the community regarding the disease and its preventability.
- Unhygienic delivery practices (e.g., application of cow dung over the umbilical stump).
- Lack or inadequate availability, accessibility, and utilization of primary healthcare services.

### Reservoir/Source of Infection

Soil is the main reservoir of spores. Survival of the spores in the soil for years increases the exposure risk to human. The organism is also found in the normal intestinal flora of animals and sometimes in human as commensals. These carnivores and herbivores excrete the spores in feces.

Spores are also present in dust and other inanimate substances.

Eradication of the disease is not possible considering the nature of the reservoir.

### Period of Communicability

Tetanus does not spread from one person to another. This is the only vaccine-preventable disease which is infectious but not contagious. So, herd immunity has no role in the prevention of tetanus. A person can acquire the infection only through wounds contaminated with tetanus spores.

### Mode of Transmission

Spores are transmitted from the soil through the wounds.

### Incubation Period

In non-neonatal tetanus, it is 3-21 days. The incubation period of the disease depends on the site of injury. If the site of injury is closer to the central nervous system (CNS), the incubation period becomes shorter and vice versa. Case fatality rate is more with the shorter incubation period.

In NTs, median incubation period is 7 days, ranging from 4 to 14 days.

#### Key Points
- The soil is the main reservoir of tetanus spores.
- Spores are resistant to boiling and commonly used antiseptics.
- Tetanus does not spread from one person to another.
- There is no herd immunity in tetanus.
- Immunity is acquired only through vaccination with TTCV.
- Clinical disease cannot produce sufficient immunity against further infection.

## PATHOGENESIS

*Clostridium tetani* has got two states—vegetative in the tissue and spores in the environment. Spores from contaminated soil enter into the body and germinates to vegetative form in absence of oxygen and produce powerful toxin (Tetanospasmin). Tetanolysin has no significant role in the pathogenesis **(Flowchart 17G.5)**.

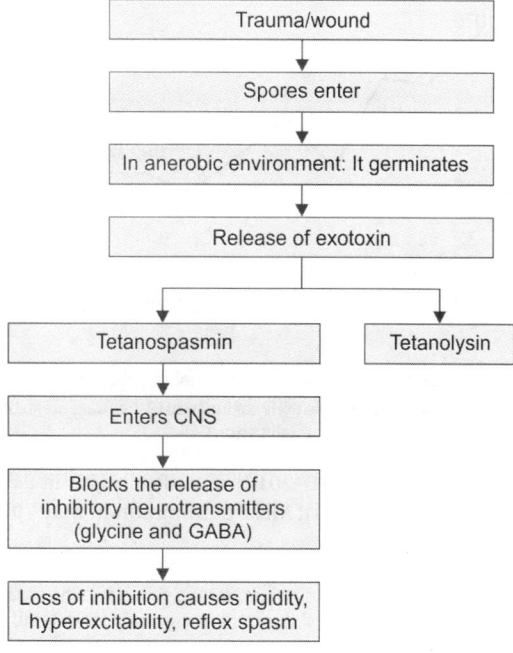

Flowchart 17G.5: Pathogenesis of tetanus.

## CLINICAL FEATURES

### Classical Clinical Presentation

***Lock jaw or Trismus (Fig. 17G.21):*** The spasm of masseter muscle leads to "trismus" which is usually the first symptom of tetanus. Rigidity then spreads to other muscles in a descending way.
- ***Sardonic Smile:*** This is due to severe spasm of facial muscles.
- ***Opisthotonus (Fig. 17G.22):*** Hyperextension of the muscles of the back and neck results in this peculiar "arching" position of the body.

Death may result from spasm of respiratory muscles or acute airway obstruction.

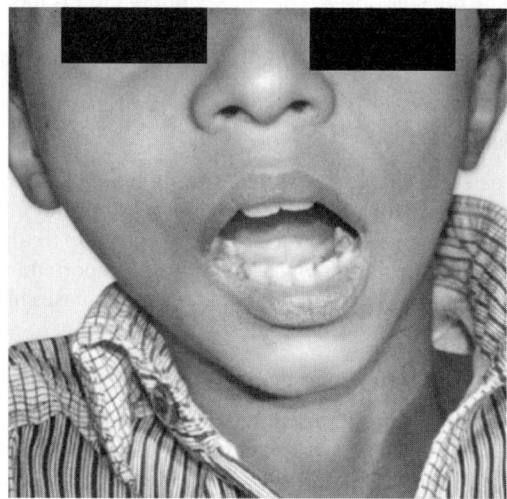

Fig. 17G.21: Trismus.

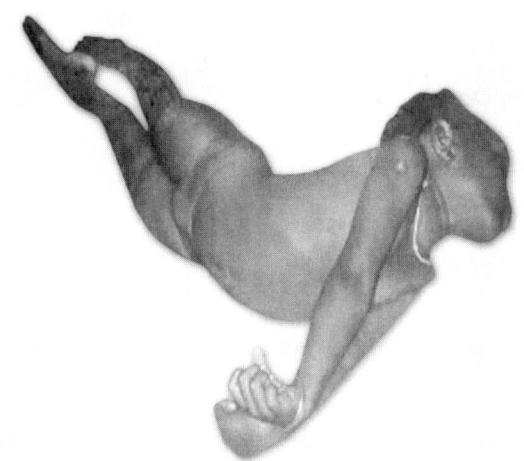

**Fig. 17G.22:** Opisthotonus.

## Types of Tetanus

Tetanus may be of different types based on the portal of entry of the organism into the human body. These are as follows:

### Traumatic

Generally, the organism enters the body through a wound. Tattooing, earlobe pricks, scalp shaving, etc., in an unhygienic environment carry the risk. It also includes the injury related to the surgical or dental procedure.

### Postabortive or Puerperal

During delivery or during puerperium (6 weeks following termination of pregnancy) spores can gain entry following unhygienic practices. This is an important cause of maternal deaths in underdeveloped countries.

### Otogenic

The organism may get entry following ear infection or ear injury. This is more common among children.

### Idiopathic

Sometimes no obvious history of injury or trauma could be elicited as a portal of entry for the organism, and in such a situation, it is known as idiopathic. This could be due to a very minute or microscopic prick which is not felt or remembered by the patient.

## DIAGNOSIS

Diagnosis is obvious from history and clinical manifestations only. No bacteriological examination is required.

History of injury, ear infection, abortion or delivery followed by typical features of the disease (trismus, rigidity, and generalized spasm) is diagnostic of tetanus.

### Neonatal Tetanus

Neonatal tetanus is a medical emergency and an important public health problem in rural, inaccessible areas as well as in urban slums. It is a consequence of inadequate immunization of pregnant women and unhygienic delivery and cord care practices. The portal of entry of the spores is through the umbilical cord stump. The disease is almost invariably fatal in absence of advanced medical facilities. Most of the cases are seen on the 8th day of birth (8th Day Disease).

Diagnosis of NT is done under the above circumstances and based on the following clinical developments:

### Baby

- Sucks or cries normally for the first 2 days after birth
- Develops following symptoms between 3 and 28 days of life. The following symptoms occur due to spasm of different muscles of mastication and swallowing:
  - Inability to suck
  - Trismus
  - Muscular rigidity
  - Convulsion

> **Key Points**
> - Tetanus is acquired through contamination of the wound with spores.
> - Only in an anaerobic environment of tissue, the spore produces the toxin.
> - History of injury followed by rigidity, spasm, and convulsion is diagnostic of tetanus.
> - Spores get entry through the umbilical stump in neonatal tetanus.
> - NT occurs due to inadequate immunization of pregnant women with tetanus toxoid and unhygienic delivery practices.

## PREVENTION AND CONTROL OF TETANUS

Curative care is expensive, difficult, and requires advanced facilities which are not feasible and practical in developing countries like India.

Primary prevention or pre-exposure prevention with tetanus toxoid containing vaccine (TTCV) is the cornerstone in combating the disease.

### Tetanus Toxoids

Tetanus toxoids are inactivated exotoxins of *C. tetani* and it induces protective antibody to tetanus exotoxin. There are two types of toxoids—adsorbed and fluid; adsorbed toxoid is preferable because of its ability to produce higher and long-lasting immune response in comparison to plain or fluid toxoid. It is the most extensively used antigen with a high degree of efficacy and safety. Although mild local reactions are common, severe adverse events are extremely rare.

The TTCV is available as:

***Monovalent tetanus toxoid:*** Used for booster doses in adolescent and pregnant women **(Fig. 17G.23)**.

***Combined:***
- *Trivalent:* Diphtheria, pertussis, and tetanus (DPT)
- *Bivalent:* Diphtheria and tetanus (DT and Td) Toxoid combination: DT vaccine is used in children (under 7 years). Td vaccine contains an equivalent amount of tetanus toxoid and reduced the amount of diphtheria toxoid in comparison to DPT or DT. Td is recommended for more than seven years of age and adults.

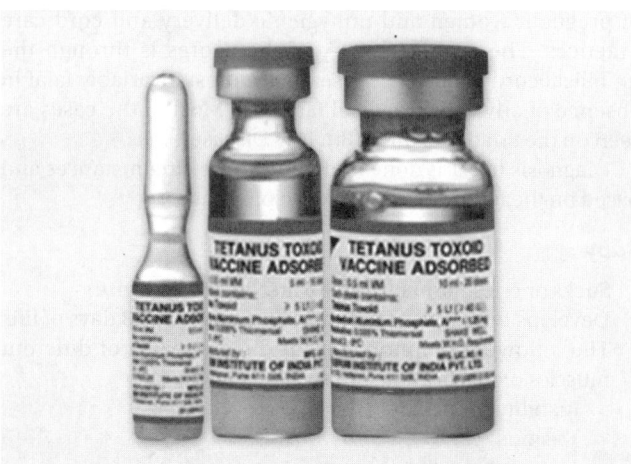

Fig. 17G.23: Tetanus toxoid vaccine (monovalent).

WHO recommended the use of Td vaccine in place of monovalent TT to boost up diphtheria immunity in the community. By 2020, WHO has planned to completely phase out of monovalent TT.
- *Pentavalent:* DPT with hepatitis B and *Haemophilus influenzae* (Hib).

***Prevention of tetanus is discussed under three headings:***
1. Prevention for the entire population.
2. Prevention of NT.
3. Postexposure prophylaxis following injury.

## Prevention for the Entire Population

In absence of herd immunity, complete immunization of all children with primary and booster doses provide immunity for the entire population.

*WHO recommends that an individual should receive six doses (three primary doses + three booster doses) of TTCV to achieve lifelong protection.* The recommended schedule for booster doses is 12–23 months, 4–7 years, and 9–15 years.

Under the National Immunization Schedule (NIS) of India, primary immunization starts at 6 weeks of age shown in **Figure 17G.25**.

A three dose primary series induces protective immunity in almost 100% of vaccinated infants.

Since 2014, DPT 1, 2, 3 have been replaced by the pentavalent vaccine in NIS **(Fig. 17G.24)**. The dose of the vaccine is 0.5 mL, given intramuscularly in the anterolateral aspect of the thigh. The main advantage of the pentavalent vaccine over DPT is widespread protection against five diseases with the same number of injections.

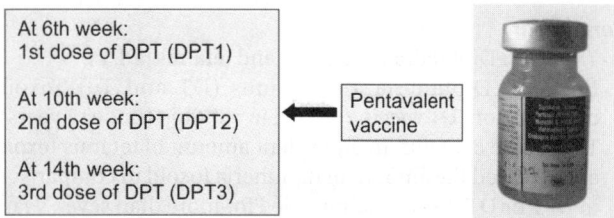

Fig. 17G.24: Replacement of DPT with pentavalent vaccine.

However, even with three primary doses, protective immunity declines if booster doses are not given in time.

### Booster Doses
- At 16–24 months: 1st booster DPT
- At 5–6 years: 2nd booster (DPT)
- At 10 years: Td
- At 16 years: Td

In India, no universal guidelines are being followed for adult immunization. Adult tetanus has not been looked as a public health priority. It is recommended that any adult with no prior immunization history against tetanus, three doses of Td/TT is recommended. First two doses are given at 4 weeks interval and the 3rd dose in 6–12 months after 2nd dose. However, with completed primary immunization history, a booster dose is given of Td every 10 years till the age of 65 years.

## Prevention of NT

The preventive strategies for maternal and NT are same; so maternal tetanus is considered to be eliminated once NT is eliminated.

### Strategies for NT Prevention
- Immunization of pregnant mother
- Clean delivery practices.

**Immunization of pregnant women:** Immunization of pregnant women with Td provides protection both for mother and her newborn. Once the mother is immunized, antibodies thus produced are transferred from mother to child and provides protection during or after delivery. This protection is short lived and to ensure long-lasting protection, the child should receive the primary immunization starting at 6 weeks of age.

Immunization of pregnant women under NIS:
- Td 1st dose (Td1): As early as possible
- Td 2nd dose (Td2): 4 weeks after Td1

If a mother received two doses of TT/Td within the last 3 years, then only one booster dose should be given.

For development of adequate maternal immunity, the minimum interval should be at least 4 weeks between the two doses of Td. The last dose of Td should be at least 4 weeks before the expected date of delivery for effective transplacental transfer of antibodies. This is the basis of giving Td as early as possible during pregnancy. However, no women should be denied of Td. Even a woman in labor, who is not previously immunized should receive a dose of Td. This is to provide long-term protection or protection in subsequent pregnancies.

**Clean delivery practices:** This can be ensured by the promotion of:
- Institutional deliveries
- *Delivery by skilled birth attendants (SBA):* In areas, where institutional access is limited and institutional delivery is not possible due to various reasons, the home deliveries are to be conducted by SBA. Training of birth attendant with special emphasis on six clean practices is an important strategy for the elimination of MNT.

The six clean practices are:
1. **C**lean surface.
2. **C**lean hands
3. **C**lean blade—a new blade should always be used for cutting the cord. As boiling does not kill the tetanus spores so the use of boiled blade is not recommended.
4. **C**lean cord tie
5. **C**lean stump—nothing should be applied on the cord stump. The reasons are:
   - Anaerobic bacteria can grow if the wound is covered
   - Drying is faster if the wound is open
   - Common antiseptics have no role in neutralization of spores
   - As universal practice
6. **C**lean perineum.

## Postexposure Prophylaxis Following Injury

Basic wound management with proper cleansing, removal of necrotic tissue, dust and foreign bodies is the primary intervention in all types of injuries. However, the modality of immunization depends on the severity of injury and history of previous immunization. WHO has classified injuries as *tetanus-prone* based on following criteria:
- Injuries more than 6 hours old
- Injuries of any duration with following characteristics: Punctured-type wound, a significant degree of devitalized tissue, contamination with soil/manure likely to contain tetanus organism, clinical evidence of sepsis, burns, frostbite, high-velocity missile injuries.

### Passive Immunization with Antitetanus Serum (ATS)

Use of ATS is indicated in tetanus-prone injuries to provide immediate protection as vaccines take up to 2 weeks for development of antibody. However, protection by ATS is short-lived. So, active and passive immunization is carried out simultaneously in such circumstances. When the simultaneous administration of toxoid and ATS are done, it should be administered using a separate syringe and at different sites. Two types of antitoxins are available: Human and equine.

*Human Tetanus Immunoglobulin (Human.Tet.Ig) is the preferred choice* for use as it is safe and does not cause the anaphylactic reaction. It gives protection for 30 days.

*Equine antitoxin* is not recommended for routine use. Being a foreign protein, it can cause anaphylactic reactions.

### Immunization in Case of Tetanus-prone Injuries

1. History of the complete course of toxoid or booster dose:
   - Within 5 years: No vaccine required
   - Between 5 and 10 years: Toxoid one dose
   - More than 10 years: Toxoid one dose + Human.Tet.Ig)
2. No history of immunization/unsure about the immunization status:
   - Toxoid complete course + Human. Tet.Ig

### Management of Nontetanus Prone Injuries

1. History of the complete course of toxoid or booster dose:
   - *Within five years:* No vaccine required
   - *Between 5 and 10 years:* Toxoid one dose
   - *More than 10 years:* Toxoid one dose

2. No history of immunization/unsure about the vaccination status: Toxoid complete course.
   - *ATS is not indicated in nonpunctured wound.*

### Role of Antibiotics

Antibiotic prophylaxis is required for wounds at high-risk of becoming infected. It kills the vegetative form of the bacilli, thereby decreasing the production of toxin. Penicillin or metronidazole is found to be useful.

With the collaborative effort of WHO, UNICEF, and UNFPA, India has made such tremendous gain towards the elimination of NT. For maintenance of the results achieved so far, the activities like immunization and clean delivery practices need to be continued with strengthening focus on community involvement and participation.

## CURRENT APPROACHES

### Global

The Maternal and Neonatal Tetanus Elimination (MNTE) initiative aims to reduce the tetanus load among mothers and newborns until it is no more a public health problem worldwide. The major strategies adopted are immunization, promoting hygiene during delivery practices.

### National

#### Strategies adopted for MNT elimination in India

The following strategies have been adopted for MNT elimination and efforts are being continued for the sustenance of elimination status.

1. ***Increasing and sustaining TT immunization of pregnant women:*** Maternal immunization with TT has been implemented in India as a part of routine immunization during antenatal visits. Universal Immunization Programme (UIP) has brought revolutionary change in immunization coverage. Through National Rural Health Mission, Govt of India has launched various activities to increase and sustain TT immunization. High-risk areas have been identified and supplementary immunization activities (SIA) are carried out to gear up the coverage. Mission Indradhanush was launched in 2014 targeting all pregnant women and children up to 2 years who are nonimmunized or partially immunized with all vaccines under UIP.
2. Ramping up immunization, safe deliveries
3. Strengthening routine immunization (RI) all over the country, particularly in low-performing as well as underserved and unreached regions has helped in MNTE. The national immunization coverage increased marginally from 61 to 65% between 2009 and 2013.
4. With Mission Indradhanush, the country has set an ambitious goal of enhancing the coverage by 5% every year, to reach the goal of full immunization coverage by 2020. Focusing on 201 low RI performing districts in the country, the initiative has reached out to all children who are either unvaccinated or are partially vaccinated against seven vaccine preventable diseases—diphtheria, whooping cough, tetanus, polio, tuberculosis, measles and hepatitis B.

6. ***Promotion of institutional delivery:*** With the launching of National Rural Health Mission (NRHM) in 2005, Govt of India in the successive years intensified the initiatives to push up the institutional delivery through different schemes like "Janani Suraksha Yojana (JSY)", "Janani Shishu Suraksha Karyakarm (JSSK)", etc. The major focus is on the economically disadvantaged pregnant women who have been given cash incentives for delivering in a public health institution. ASHAs have been entrusted to mobilize and help pregnant women and children for availing the services. Peripheral health institutions are being strengthened in a phased manner for 24 hours delivery services.
7. ***Training of birth attendants:*** Training of birth attendant with special emphasis on 'five clean practices' was started long back with Child Survival and Safe Motherhood (CSSM) Programme in 1992, is continued as an important strategy for elimination of MNT.
8. ***Ensuring adequate supply of disposable delivery kit (DDK):*** This kit contains the staffs required to maintain the 5Cs during delivery. These are: Soap (Clean hands), a plastic sheet (maintaining clean surface), new blade (Clean cutting instrument), thread (Clean cord tie), pieces of the gauge/clean clothes (Clean perineum).
9. ***Strengthening surveillance system:*** A case of NT indicates the failure in providing routine immunization, antenatal care, and clean delivery services. That is why each and every case should be reported and appropriate follow-up action is to be instituted. The surveillance system should be such that no case of NT is missed. If there is no case in an area, a NIL report should be reported.
10. ***Continuing information, education and communication activities:*** IEC activities regarding immunization, clean delivery practices, harmful ritual practices, etc., should be geared up in the community.

> **Key Points**
>
> **Strategies for NNT elimination in India:**
> - Increasing and sustaining TT immunization of pregnant women.
> - Promotion of institutional delivery.
> - Training of birth attendants.
> - Ensuring adequate supply of Disposable Delivery Kit.
> - Strengthening the surveillance system.
> - Continuation of IEC.

> **Exercise:** From a primary health center (PHC) in a hilly area, four neonatal deaths were reported during the last 6 months. All deaths occurred at home.
> 1.1. What epidemiological information will you need from the family and the community to decide that the deaths were due to neonatal tetanus? What information will you need from the institutional level?
> 1.2. What measures need to be taken to prevent such deaths at an individual, community and institutional level?
> 1.3. What measures need to be taken to prevent such deaths at an individual, community and institutional level?

## SUMMARY

Tetanus, particularly neonatal tetanus (NT), often a serious disease, is caused by *Clostridium tetani* (*C. tetani*) and characterized by rigidity and painful paroxysmal spasms of the voluntary muscles. Elimination has been defined as less than 1 case of NT per 1,000 live births per year in all the districts of a country.

As of March 2018, elimination status was achieved in the major part of the globe; only 14 countries have still not reached the elimination status. Neonatal tetanus has been eliminated globally as well as from India. The soil is the main reservoir of tetanus spores. Spores are resistant to boiling and commonly used antiseptics. Tetanus does not spread from one person to another. There is no herd immunity in tetanus. Immunity is acquired only through vaccination with TTCV. Clinical disease cannot produce sufficient immunity against further infection. Tetanus is acquired through contamination of the wound with spores. Only in an anaerobic environment of tissue, the spore produces the toxin. History of injury followed by rigidity, spasm, and convulsion is diagnostic of tetanus. Spores get entry through the umbilical stump in neonatal tetanus.

NT occurs due to inadequate immunization of pregnant women with tetanus toxoid and unhygienic delivery practices. Six clean (6 Cs): Clean surface for delivery, Clean hands, Clean blade, Clean cord tie, Clean cord stump (no applicant), Clean perineum. Strategies for NNT elimination in India: Increasing and sustaining TT immunization of pregnant women, Promotion of institutional delivery, Training of birth attendants, Ensuring adequate supply of Disposable Delivery Kit, Strengthening the surveillance system, Continuation of IEC.

## SUGGESTED READING

1. Govt. of India. Ministry of Health and Family Welfare. Immunization Handbook for Medical Officers, 3rd edition. New Delhi: Ministry of Health and Family Welfare; 2016. p. 7.
2. Govt of India. Ministry of Health and Family Welfare. Health and Family Welfare Statistics in India. New Delhi: Ministry of Health and Family Welfare; 2017. p. 78.
3. Li J, Liu Z, Yu C, Tan K, Gui S, Zhang S, Shen Y. Global epidemiology and burden of tetanus from 1990 to 2019: A systematic analysis for the Global Burden of Disease Study 2019. International Journal of Infectious Diseases. 2023 Jul 1;132:118-26.
4. National Family Health Survey (NFHS) 4 [2015–2016], India Key Indicators, India Fact Sheet, Pg-02. [Online] Available from: http:// www.rchiips.org/ nfhs.
5. Stanfield JP, Galazka A. Neonatal tetanus in the world today. Bull World Health Organ. 1984;62(4):647-69.
6. WHO. India achieves the goal of maternal and neonatal tetanus elimination (MNTE). Accessed in July 2023 available from https://www.who.int/india/footer/quick-links/media/india-achieves-the-goal-of-maternal-and-neonatal-tetanus-elimination-(mnte)
7. WHO. Maternal and Neonatal Tetanus Elimination (MNTE). [Online] Available from: www.who.int/immunization/disease/MNTE_ initiative/en/index1. html.
8. WHO. Weekly Epidemiological Record. 2017;92:205-28. [Online] Available from: http://www.who.int/wer/.
9. WHO vaccine—preventable disease: monitoring system 2018 global summary (internet). [Online] Available from: http://apps. who.int/immunization_monitoring/globalsummary.

# H. EPIDEMIC PRONE DISEASES AND INVESTIGATING THE OUTBREAKS

*Atul Trivedi, Rohit Ram*

*The world has been sharply reminded time after time of the degree to which people in all countries and on all continents remain chronically vulnerable to infectious diseases, known and unknown.*

—WHO

| | |
|---|---|
| CM 7.7 | Describe and demonstrate the steps in the investigation of an epidemic prone diseases and describe the principles of control measures |
| CM 8.4 | Describe the principles and enumerate the measures to control an epidemic prone disease |

## INTRODUCTION

Epidemic is a state of given disease, which calls for emergency response, if any disease or health-related event happens in unusual frequency, a timely response can minimize the damage to the community. With modern techniques and surveillance system, it is possible for system to respond early, provided data are regularly analyzed and interpreted and put forward for pertinent actions.

India is prone to many kinds of epidemic diseases, due to a large and diverse population, tropical climate and adverse environment. India is prone to many kinds of epidemic diseases. Historical data provides evidence for major epidemics which took a huge toll on human life. An explosive common-source epidemic of typhoid fever, most likely the world's greatest, happened in Sangli Town (Maharashtra State), India between December 1975 and February 1976. More than 9,000 cases occurred in population of about 135,000, thus giving an incidence rate of 6.59% over this 12-week period (Sathe PV Et al., Int J Epidemiol, 1983).

Conceivably dangerous changes are likewise occurring in the utilization of land, agrarian practices and food production, for example, live poultry and animal markets, and deforestation—which additionally prompts expanded contact among individuals and natural life. A portion of these animals and birds are likely sources of new pathogens. Additionally, environmental changes, for example, ecological change, likewise contribute to disease transmission **(Fig. 17H.1)**.

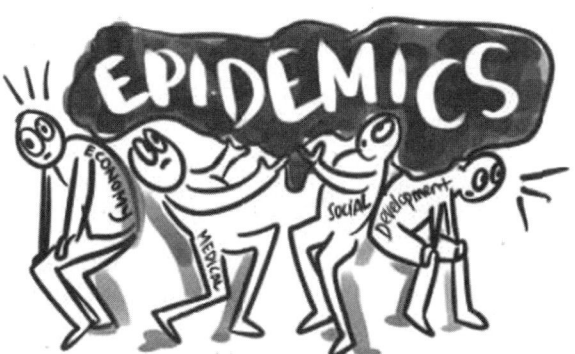

**Fig. 17H.1:** Epidemics—a burden.
*Source:* World Health Organization. Managing epidemics: key facts about major deadly diseases. Geneva: WHO; 2018. pp. 25-6.

Novice and increasingly serious risk factors enhance the transmission of diseases. In an ever-changing world, it is not always possible to completely eliminate these risk factors. Among them are the rapid movement of the population because of different business and monetary exercises. For decades, an ever-increasing number of individuals have been moving from the rural into urban areas, looking for better employments and enhanced expectations for everyday comforts. The exceptional dimensions of urbanization with impromptu and stuffed populaces of city tenants, overcrowding and poor infrastructure support present more serious dangers of disease transmission **(Fig. 17H.2)**.

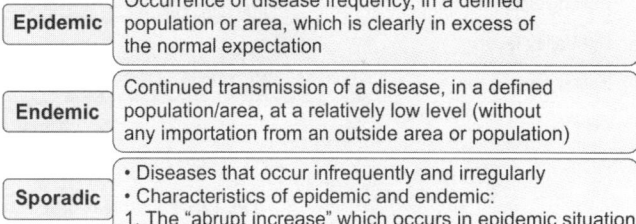

**Fig. 17H.2:** A summary of key concepts related to frequency of diseases.
*Source:* World Health Organization. Managing epidemics: key facts about major deadly diseases. Geneva: WHO; 2018. pp. 25-6.

Before anything comes, prevention is first. There are many factors and dynamics which plays an important role in the existing balance between agent, host and environment. When this balance is disturbed by any reason it will result in epidemic and as an epidemiologist, we should think "out of box" for all possibilities that may be responsible for occurrence of given epidemic. An outbreak reported from Odisha in 2008, having all characteristics of organophosphorus poisoning, which is unusual in described population, happened because of exposure through unexpected route, by water. Correct and timely diagnosis of cases is very important requirement for management of an epidemic.

The nature of transmission, the virulence of causative organisms, population immunogenicity, differential fatality and other epidemiological parameters make certain diseases more prone for epidemics than others. The following is a list of epidemic prone diseases that require a constant surveillance with strong and active control measures.

*Examples of epidemic prone diseases* **(Fig. 17H.3)**:
- Malaria
- Dengue fever [dengue hemorrhagic fever (DHF) and dengue shock syndrome (DSS)]
- Chikungunya
- Cholera
- Measles
- Diphtheria

## Section 3: Community Health Problems and Vulnerable Groups

| Disease | 2011 | 2012 | 2013 | 2014 | 2015 | 2016 | 2017 | 2018 | 2019 | 2020 | 2021 | TOTAL |
|---|---|---|---|---|---|---|---|---|---|---|---|---|
| Avian/Animal influenza | 5 | 2 | 1 | 3 |  | 5 | 5 | 3 | 2 | 5 | 16 | 47 |
| Chikungunya | 1 | 3 | 4 | 24 |  | 5 | 3 | 3 | 2 |  | 1 | 46 |
| Cholera | 24 | 24 | 11 | 1 | 19 | 16 | 14 | 23 | 19 | 4 | 12 | 167 |
| Crimean-Congo haemorrhagic fever | 1 |  | 3 |  | 4 | 2 | 8 | 4 | 8 | 3 | 3 | 36 |
| Dengue | 8 | 10 | 7 | 6 | 7 | 5 | 12 | 13 | 16 | 4 | 10 | 98 |
| Ebola virus disease | 1 | 3 |  | 3 |  |  |  | 2 | 2 |  | 1 | 12 |
| Lassa fever | 2 | 1 | 2 | 1 | 2 | 2 | 7 | 3 | 6 | 1 | 4 | 31 |
| Malaria | 2 | 2 |  |  | 3 | 3 | 11 | 4 | 8 | 3 | 7 | 43 |
| Marburg virus disease |  |  |  | 1 |  |  | 2 |  |  |  | 1 | 4 |
| Measles | 19 |  | 7 | 11 | 13 | 7 | 15 | 25 | 15 | 3 | 5 | 120 |
| Meningococcal disease/Meningitis | 11 | 11 | 3 | 4 | 4 | 8 | 10 | 7 | 2 | 2 | 2 | 64 |
| MERS |  | 3 | 5 | 9 | 2 | 1 | 1 | 5 | 4 | 1 | 2 | 33 |
| Nipah virus | 1 |  | 1 |  |  |  |  | 1 | 2 | 1 | 1 | 7 |
| Poliomyelitis | 10 | 1 | 4 | 3 | 2 | 2 | 3 | 13 | 16 | 6 | 16 | 76 |
| Rift Valley fever | 2 |  |  |  | 2 | 3 | 3 | 3 | 3 | 1 | 2 | 19 |
| Yellow fever | 2 | 3 | 3 |  | 1 | 5 | 1 | 5 | 2 | 6 | 3 | 31 |
| Zika |  |  |  | 2 | 15 | 63 | 5 | 3 | 1 |  | 2 | 91 |

**Fig. 17H.3:** Outbreak of selected infectious diseases (2011–2021).
*Source:* World Health Organization. Managing epidemics: Key facts about major deadly diseases; 2023.

- Food poisoning
- Crimean-Congo hemorrhagic fever
- Ebola virus disease
- Leptospirosis
- Whooping cough
- Influenza (pandemic, seasonal, zoonotic)
- Plague
- Severe acute respiratory syndrome (SARS)
- Yellow fever
- Zika virus disease
- Hendra virus infection
- Japanese encephalitis
- Meningococcal meningitis
- Middle East respiratory syndrome coronavirus (MERS-CoV)
- Nipah virus infection.

### ROLE OF EPIDEMIOLOGY IN AN OUTBREAK

Epidemiology has an important role in investigation of epidemic or outbreak.

The main objectives of epidemic or outbreak investigations are:
1. To define the magnitude of outbreak or epidemic
2. To find out the causes of outbreak or epidemic
3. To identify appropriate control and preventive measures.

**Flowchart 17H.1** simply explains about chronology of outbreak investigation.

Preset trigger levels for diseases will be identified with specific responses identified for various levels. The levels will depend on the epidemic potential, case fatality of the disease and the prevalence of the problem in the community.

1. *Trigger level 1:* Suspected/limited outbreak—local response
2. *Trigger level 2:* Epidemic—local and regional response
3. *Trigger level 3:* Widespread epidemic—local, regional and state level response

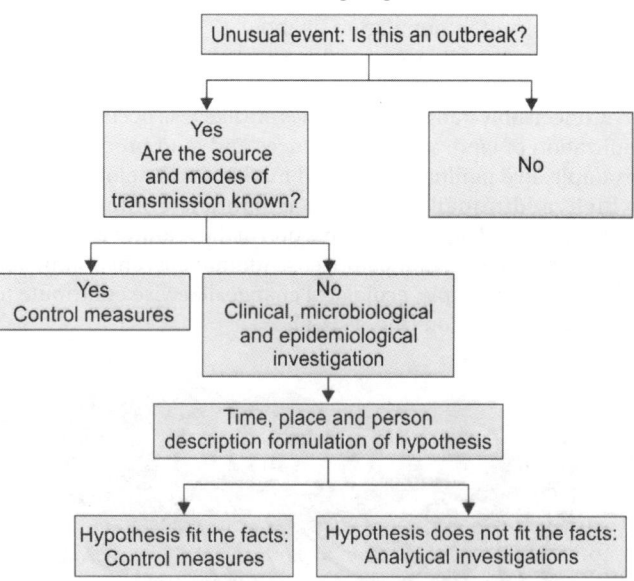

Flowchart 17H.1: Investigating an outbreak.

Table 17H.1: The balance between investigation and control while responding to an outbreak.

|  |  | Source/transmission | |
|---|---|---|---|
|  |  | Known | Unknown |
| Etiology | Known | Control +++ Investigate + | Control + Investigate +++ |
|  | Unknown | Control +++ Investigate +++ | Control + Investigate +++ |

a. In a nonendemic area, even one case of suspected epidemic prone disease should initiate a trigger response at various levels
b. In an endemic region, change in pattern of disease or evidence of clustering of disease should be considered a trigger event.

**Table 17H.1** explains about different situation in which different source versus etiology compared. Usually when both are known to us, then concentrated efforts should be made to activate full-fledged control measures. Situation is different in case of unknown etiology and unknown source of infection. When etiology is unknown and source of infection is known to us, then focus should be made on both aspects.

Graph mentioned about effective changes happened when control measures start with early identification of epidemic. It will depend on how much effectively surveillance system performing in said area **(Fig. 17H.4)**.

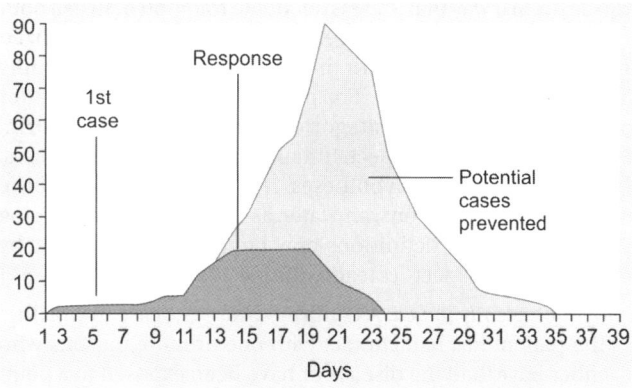

Fig. 17H.4: Natural history of an outbreak in the event of an effective response.

## INVESTIGATION OF AN OUTBREAK

Interaction between environment, agent and host is constantly going on and thus it fulfills requirement of existence of agent factors. However, change in this equilibrium, invites unexpected situation, in which agent gets dominance and results in condition called outbreak. Now, it depends on the nature of disease, agent virulence and fatality due to it determines the panic level that it generates in the community. It is necessary to understand few terminologies, which are frequently used during epidemic investigations.

*Basic reproduction number ($R_0$):* $R_0$ is defined as the expected number of other individuals that an infected individual will infect if he or she enters a population entirely composed of susceptible individuals.

*Index case:* The first case in a family or other defined group to come to the attention of the investigator.

*Primary case:* The individual who introduces the disease into the family or group under study. Not necessarily the first diagnosed case in a family or group.

*Latent period:* The period between exposure and infection is called "latent period", logic behind it is a "latent" stage of pathogen under question, without clinical symptoms or signs of infection in the host.

*Generation time:* When one person transmits an infection to another, then the time that elapses between onset of symptoms in the primary case and onset of symptoms of the secondary case is called "generation time", so, interval between receipt of infection and maximal infectivity of the host.

*Serial interval:* Gap observed in time between the onset of the primary case and the secondary case is called serial interval.

### Who Should Respond to an Outbreak?

At Primary Health Center (PHC) and Community Health Center (CHC) level medical officer of the concerned institute may be the nodal officer who will respond to an outbreak. At district, the corporation, the state and the central level special Rapid Response Teams (RRTs) are formed to investigate outbreaks. If an outbreak is suspected, the local health team should verify the same. Once this is done and if there is need to investigate, the RRT should take over and do the needful.

### Rapid Response Teams

The RRT is a multidisciplinary team that looks into various aspects of an outbreak. This team has an epidemiologist, a clinician, a microbiologist and other specialties as per requirements.

The primary job of the RRT is to examine and investigate the outbreak episodes.

Following 10 steps are essential considerations in every epidemiological investigation. Frequently, epidemic investigations are called for after the peak of the epidemic has occurred, in such cases, the investigation is mainly retrospective. No step-by-step approach applicable in all situations.

Early detection of epidemic depends on existing surveillance system in a given area. There are two types of surveillance, generally preferred to detect early outbreak.
1. **Case-based surveillance system** depends on regular data collection and analysis with close look at changing parameters and trigger levels.
2. **Event-based surveillance system** depends on events, which come to focus to authority from various sources **(Flowchart 17H.2)**.

### Steps in the Investigation of an Outbreak

1. Determine the existence of an epidemic or outbreak
2. Verify the diagnosis

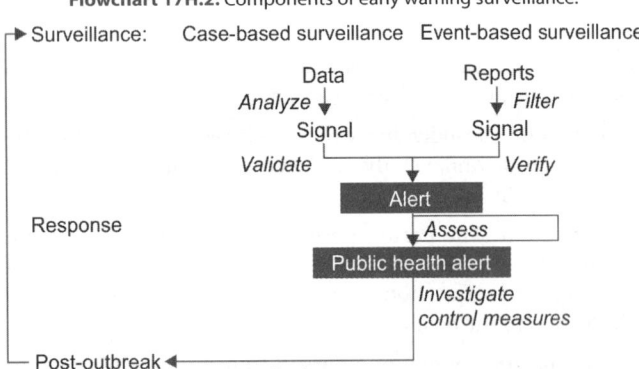

Flowchart 17H.2: Components of early warning surveillance.

3. Define a case
4. Search for cases
5. Generate hypothesis using descriptive findings
6. Test hypothesis based upon an analytic study
7. Draw conclusion
8. Compare the hypothesis with established facts
9. Communicate findings
10. Execute prevention measures.

And last important step is to document it for future use and learning.

### Determine the Existence of an Outbreak

An *outbreak* or an *epidemic* is the occurrence of more cases of disease than expected in a given area or among a specific group of people over a particular period of time. Usually, the cases are presumed to have a common cause or to be related to one another in some way. *Cluster* refers to an aggregation of cases grouped in place and time that are suspected to be greater than the number expected, even though the expected number may not be known.

One of the first tasks of the epidemiologist is to verify that a cluster of cases is indeed an outbreak. Here the observed frequency of the disease is compared with expected frequency. The expected number is usually the number from the previous few weeks or months, or from a comparable period during the previous 3 years. An arbitrary limit of two standard errors from the endemic occurrence is used to define the epidemic threshold for common diseases. Sometime, the current number of reported cases exceeds the expected number; the excess may not necessarily indicate an outbreak. Reporting may be rise because of change in the local reporting system, changes in the case definition, increasing local or national awareness, or improvement in diagnostic procedures. There could also be situations when a single case of a disease may be enough to call for investigations, e.g. a suspected case of plague, even a single case of cholera. Various factors determine whether to initiate an action and they include severity of the illness, the potential of spread, availability of control measures, political considerations, public relations, availability of resources.

### Verify the Diagnosis

The earliest report regarding an outbreak is often obtained from a health worker, lay person from community or Panchayati Raj or from media. Often the initial report is not in the form of particular diagnosis but rather in the form of a "syndromic" constellation of symptoms and signs (e.g. outbreak of diarrhea and vomiting, or fever and skin rash). It is therefore essential to verify the diagnosis of the condition that one is dealing with. At this point, information needs to be collected from patients (cases), about their signs/symptoms, their movements, about the possible exposures and what they think could have caused their present illness, and whether they know of similar cases in their neighborhood, workplace or among friends. Recording complete details at this point of time will be of value later when hypotheses are being developed. Verification of the diagnosis is usually made on clinical, laboratory and epidemiological parameters. Most important are the clinical parameters. During epidemic period, it is not necessary to confirm 100% cases by laboratory parameters; a 20–30% random sample, is adequate.

### Define a Case

Often the search for additional cases would involve a number of health team members. It is therefore important that the investigator develops case definitions which are adequately sensitive (i.e. include all those who are having the target disease, though this may entail including many who do not really have the disease) as well as adequately specific (exclude all those who do not have the target disease, though many mild or equivocal cases of the disease may also be missed out).

Apparently, the case definitions should be developed with a consensus in a way that there is adequate trade-off between both sensitivity and specificity. Development of proper, standardized case definitions is important prerequisite to ensure uniformity during the investigations. For practical purposes, it is better to have cases in three categories, viz. (1) definite/confirm, (2) probable, and (3) suspect. Initially during the investigations, while formulating the hypotheses, it may be desirable to have more sensitive definitions, and later, as the hypotheses are being refined/tested, the definitions may be made more specific by removing the "suspect" category **(Table 17H.2)**.

*Epidemiologically linked:* A confirmed case is a case in which:
1. The patient has had contact with one or more persons who either have/had the disease or have been exposed to a point source of infection.
2. Transmission of the disease-causing pathogen by the usual modes of transmission are plausible.

*For example, in case of malaria, a clinical case description: A case of fever*:

It may be accompanied with:
- Headache, backache, chills, rigors, sweating, myalgia, nausea, and vomiting

Table 17H.2: Diagnoses—particularly early in an investigation.

| Level of diagnosis for epidemic prone diseases | Where | By whom |
|---|---|---|
| Suspected case | At field level | Health worker |
| Probable case | At health center | Medical officer |
| Confirmed case | At laboratory | Laboratory technician/microbiologist/pathologist |

- Splenomegaly and anemia
- Generalized convulsion, coma, shock, spontaneous bleeding, pulmonary edema, renal failure and death (untreated *Plasmodium falciparum* infection).

*Laboratory definition of malaria*: Demonstration of malaria parasites in blood films or positive rapid diagnostic test for malaria.

*Case classification*:
- *Suspected case*: Any case of fever (in an endemic area)
- *Probable case*: Any case that meets the clinical case definition
- *Confirm case*: A suspected or probable case with laboratory confirmation of malaria parasite.

### Search for Cases

Many outbreaks are brought to the attention of health authorities by concerned health care providers or citizens. However, the cases that prompt the concern are often only a small and unrepresentative fraction of the total number of cases. Public health workers must therefore look for additional cases to determine the true geographic extent of the problem and the populations affected by it.

All efforts are to be made to ascertain cases in community of disease in question by all means of active and passive surveillance.

*Active disease surveillance:* Active disease surveillance is when state or local officials actively search for information by contacting health care providers, laboratories, schools, nursing homes, workplaces, etc. or when investigator surveys and search for cases by visit or phone or other efforts.

*Passive disease surveillance:* Passive disease surveillance begins with health care providers or laboratories initiating the reporting to state or local officials. Reportable diseases are submitted on a case-by-case basis, based on a published list of conditions.

Traditionally, the information described above is collected on a standard case report form, questionnaire, or data abstraction form. Investigators then abstract selected critical items onto a form called a line listing. Example of line listing is given in **Table 17H.3**.

### Generate Hypothesis using Descriptive Findings

Conceptually, the next step after identifying and gathering basic information on the persons with the disease is to systematically describe some of the key characteristics of those persons. Analysis specific to time, place and person (TPP) is called *descriptive epidemiology*.

When data is collected, it must be utilized to detect epidemic, types of epidemic, causative agent responsible for current epidemic and vigorous control measures.

To do all these, one must execute analysis of data with help of count, divide and compare (CDC).

- Count, divide and compare:
  - Count: Define cases to know what you count
  - Divide: Divide cases by the population denominator (the denominator must match the numerator)
  - Compare: Compare rates across groups. This step is critical for several reasons.
- This summary of data by key demographic variables provides a characterization of the outbreak—trends over time, geographic distribution (place), and the populations (persons) affected by the disease.
- This will help to identify or infer the population at risk for the disease.
- It often provides clues about etiology, source, and modes of transmission that can be turned into testable hypotheses.
- Descriptive epidemiology is very helpful to begin intervention and prevention measures.

**Time:** Traditionally, a special type of histogram is used to depict the time course of an epidemic. This graph, called an *epidemic curve*, or *epi curve* for short, provides a simple visual display of the outbreak's magnitude and time trend. The classic epidemic curve, such as the one shown in **Figure 17H.5** from an outbreak of *cholera at Parbatia* graphs the number of cases by date or time of onset of illness. There was an initial case on 10th November, followed by a rapid increase in the number of cases leading to a peak on 15th November and a progressive subsequent decrease, and the last case was on 21st November.

Epidemic curves are a basic investigative tool because they are so informative.
- The epidemic curve shows the magnitude of the epidemic over time as a simple, easily understood graph. It permits the investigator to distinguish epidemic from endemic disease. Potentially correlated events can be noted on the graph.
- The shape of the epidemic curve provides clues about the pattern of spread in the population, e.g. point versus intermittent source versus propagated (**Figs. 17H.6A to D**).

*Interpreting an epidemic curve:* The first step in interpreting an epidemic curve is to consider its overall shape. The shape of the epidemic curve is dependent on the pattern of the epidemic (for example, common source versus propagated), the period of time over which susceptible persons are exposed, and the minimum, average, and maximum incubation periods for the disease.

An epidemic curve that has a steep upslope and a more gradual downslope (known as *log-normal* curve) is characteristic of a *point-source epidemic*. In this type of epidemic, persons are exposed to the same source over a relative brief period. All the cases occur within a single incubation period (**Fig. 17H.6C**). If the duration of exposure is prolonged, the epidemic is called a *continuous common-source epidemic*, and the epidemic curve has a plateau instead of a peak (**Fig. 17H.6B**). An intermittent

**Table 17H.3:** Line listing.

| Sl. No. | Name | Age | Sex | Residential address | Workplace address | Date/time of onset of symptoms | Main symptoms/signs | Name/address of medical facility with date of admission or reporting |
|---|---|---|---|---|---|---|---|---|

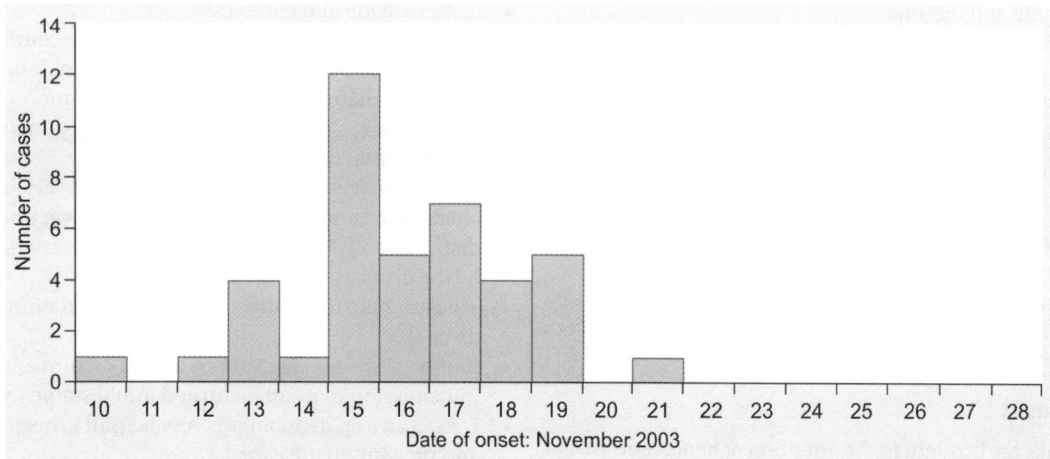

**Fig. 17H.5:** Outbreak of cholera—Parbatia, November, 2003 (epidemic curve).

common-source epidemic (in which exposure to the causative agent is sporadic over time) usually produces an irregularly jagged epidemic curve reflecting the intermittence and duration of exposure and the number of persons exposed **(Fig. 17H.6A)**. In theory, a *propagated epidemic*—is one that spread from person-to-person with increasing numbers of cases in each generation—should have a series of progressively taller peaks one incubation period apart, but in reality few produce this classic pattern **(Fig. 17H.6D)**.

The curve shows where you are in the course of the epidemic—still on the upswing, on the downslope, or after the epidemic has ended. This information forms the basis for predicting whether more or fewer cases will occur in the near future.

**Place:** In epidemic investigation, case distribution according to place, carries a meaningful clue to judge types of epidemic, source of epidemic, details about the geographic extent of epidemic as well as exhibit patterns that give important etiologic evidences. A spot map is one of the simplest and basic methods for showing clustering of cases. A **spot map**, like that used by John Snow in London in 1854 **(Fig. 17H.7)**, can give clues about mode of spread.

Spot maps are useful for demonstrating cases within a geographic area, but they do not take the size of the underlying population into account. It just reflects cases only and does not give true picture by not reflecting density of cases in population. To compare incidence between different areas with different

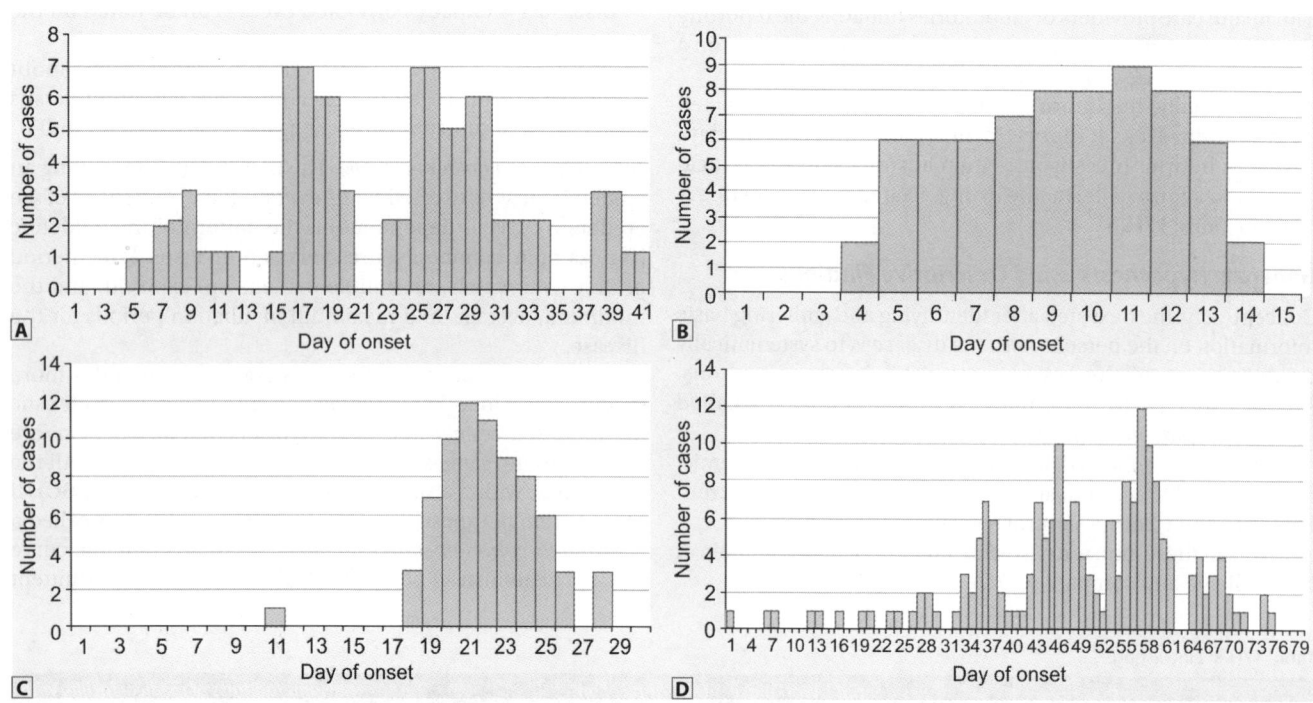

**Figs. 17H.6A to D:** Typical epidemic curves for different types of outbreaks.
*Source:* Torok M. Epidemic curves ahead. Focus on Field Epidemiology, Vol. 1. North Carolina Center for Public Health Preparedness—the North Carolina Institute for Public Health.

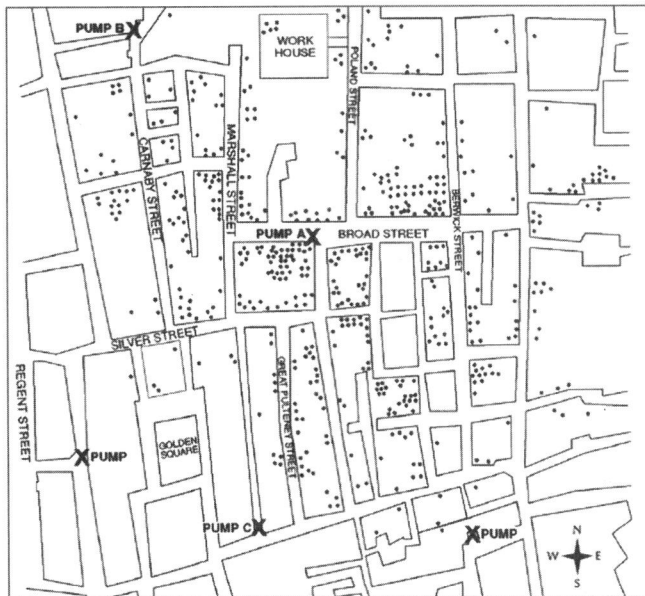

**Fig. 17H.7:** Spot map of deaths from cholera in Golden Square area, London 1854.
*Source:* Snow J. Snow on cholera. London: Humphrey Milford: Oxford University Press; 1936.

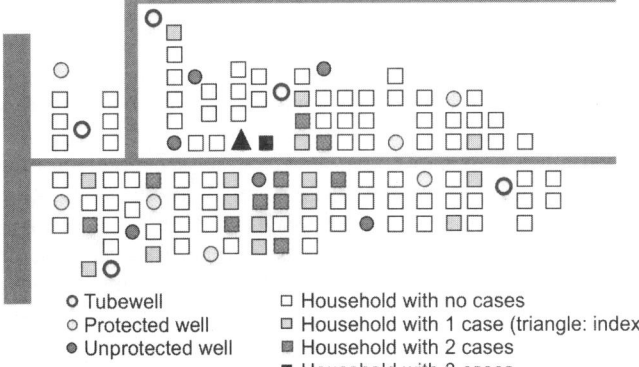

○ Tubewell
○ Protected well
● Unprotected well
□ Household with no cases
□ Household with 1 case (triangle: index)
▨ Household with 2 cases
■ Household with 3 cases

**Fig. 17H.8:** Cases of cholera at Parbatia village, November 2003.

population densities, an area map showing area-specific rates is preferable. So, in this situation **incidence maps** are more useful. **Figure 17H.8** shows the number of cases of cholera at Parbatia village in November 2003. Of the 40 case-patients, 24 (60%) were clustered around an unprotected well-located close to the residence of the index case-patient. By dividing the number of cases, by the size of the population, area-specific rates of under investigation disease can be calculated **(Fig. 17H.9)**.

**Person:** Outbreak assessment by person provides a description of actual cases as well as those who are at risk. Person characteristics that are usually described include both host characteristics (age, race, sex, and medical status) and possible exposures (occupation, diet, leisure activities and use of medications, tobacco, and drugs).

The two most commonly described host characteristics are age and gender because they are easily collected and because they are often related to exposure and to the risk of disease.

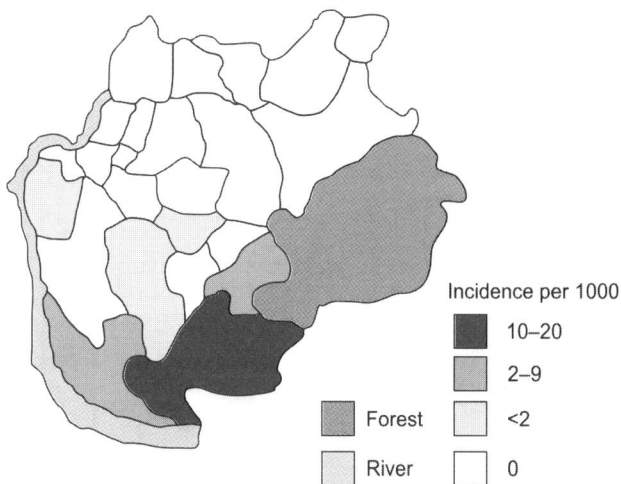

**Fig. 17H.9:** Average incidence of malaria by subcenters of Kurseong block, Darjeeling district, West Bengal, India, in 2000.
*Source:* Sharma PK, Ramakrishnan R, Hutin YJ, et al. Increasing incidence of malaria in Kurseong, Darjeeling district, West Bengal, India, 2000-2004. Trans R Soc Trop Med Hyg. 2009;103(7):691-7.

For analysis investigator should look for two type of basic analysis. CDC stands for count, divide and compare and TPP stands for time, place and person distribution. On the basis of TPP analysis, next step in the outbreak investigation is to form the hypothesis. During generating hypotheses, investigator must "think out of box" to correctly identify contributing factors behind existing outbreak. Common causes of occurrence of outbreak should be first ruled out but should not try to fix up observation into justification of outbreak.

The descriptive epidemiology may provide useful clues that can be turned into hypotheses. If the epidemic curve points to a narrow period of exposure, what events occurred around that time? Why do the people living in one particular area have the highest attack rate? Why are some groups with particular age, sex, or other person characteristics at greater risk than other groups with different person characteristics? Such questions about the data may help to generate the hypotheses that can be tested by appropriate analytical techniques.

### Test Hypothesis based upon an Analytical Study

After establishing the hypothesis, the following step is to test the plausibility of that hypothesis. Normally, hypothesis in a field survey is clinically assessed by a blend of ecological evidence, laboratory investigations, and the study of disease transmission. From an epidemiologic perspective, hypotheses are assessed in one of two different ways: either by contrasting the theories with already established factual, or by using analytical epidemiological studies to determine the causation and measure the probability of risk.

The first method is likely to be used when the clinical, laboratory, environmental, and/or epidemiologic evidence apparently supports the hypotheses that formal hypothesis testing is unnecessary.

Investigator of outbreak investigation of hepatitis E at Girdharnagar ward, Ahmedabad conducted a retrospective cohort study to test the hypothesis regarding the cause of the hepatitis outbreak (Fig. 17H.10). They have divided the area into two cohorts on the basis of suspected exposer that is contaminated drinking water (Table 17H.4).

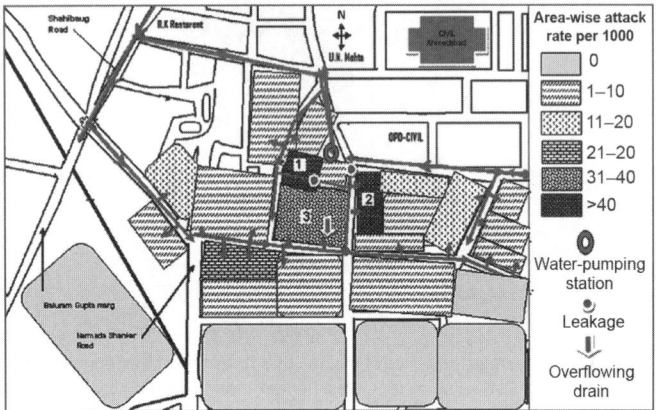

**Fig. 17H.10:** Incidence map of acute hepatitis by area in Girdharnagar, March–September 2008.
*Source:* Chauhan NT, Prajapati P, Trivedi AV, et al. Epidemic investigation of the jaundice outbreak in Girdharnagar, Ahmedabad, Gujarat, India, 2008. Indian J Community Med. 2010;35(2):294-7.

**Table 17H.4:** Incidence rate in areas consuming water from leaking pipelines and having defective drains compared to those without the leakages and overflowing drains (March–September 2008) (Chauhan NT, et al., Indian J Community Med, 2010).

| Sources of water | Number of people affected | Number of people not affected | Relative risk (RR) | 95% CI | P value |
|---|---|---|---|---|---|
| Leaking pipes and overflowing drains ($n = 8,838$) | 144 | 8,694 | 2.3 | 1.76–2.98 | <0.001 |
| Area without leakages and overflowing drain ($n = 12,525$) | 89 | 12,436 | | | |
| Total ($n = 21,363$) | 233 | 21,130 | | | |

In many other investigations, however, the circumstances are not as straightforward, and information from the series of cases is not sufficiently convincing. In such investigations, epidemiologists use analytic epidemiology to test their hypotheses. In analytical epidemiology, the *observed* pattern among case-patients or a group of exposed persons is compared with the *expected* pattern among unexposed persons. By comparing the observed with expected patterns, epidemiologists can determine whether the observed pattern differs substantially from what should be expected and, if so, by what degree. Thus, analytical epidemiology is used to test hypotheses about causal relationships. The two most common types of analytic epidemiology studies used in field investigations are retrospective cohort studies and case-control studies.

### Draw Conclusion

Conclusion is made on the basis of interpreting the results of analytical study, such as weather the suspected exposure associated with illness, what is the strength of association? Is there a statistical significance? Is there a dose response relationship? Laboratory findings are also very useful in drawing a conclusion.

### Compare the Hypothesis with Established Facts

The hypothesis that explains the epidemic must be consistent with all the facts the epidemiologist has observed. If the hypothesis does not do so, then it must be re-examined. It should do more than just strengthen speculation, explaining the cases at the peak of the epidemic.

### Communicate Findings

Development of a communications plan and communicating with those who need to know during the investigation is much necessary. The final task is to summarize the investigation, its findings, and its outcome in a report, and to communicate this report in an effective manner for preventive actions. This communication usually takes two forms, either by *An oral briefing for local authorities* or *A written report*.

Apart from it, communication strategies should be devised to address decision makers, to address media, to communicate to academician, etc.

### Execute Prevention Measures

Standard control measures may be formulated initially before the results of the investigations are available, e.g. provide safe drinking water to all residents of village in case of any waterborne disease outbreak. There are certain characteristics of good recommendations such as they should be evidence-based, specific, feasible, cost-effective and acceptable. Based on the results of investigation, short-, medium- and long-term preventive measures should be suggested. For example, if a well is the source of infection in case of outbreak of cholera, in this, the short-term preventive measure is to prevent access to the well, medium-term preventive measure is protect the well that cause the outbreak and long-term preventive measure is to ensure that all the new wells are protected.

## CASE STUDIES

### Epidemic Investigation of Jaundice Outbreak (Boxes 17H.1 and 17H.2)

Clusters of jaundice cases were reported by the civic center run by the Municipal Corporation on June 19, 2008, in the Girdharnagar ward. All the initial cases were reported from the slum area near the civic center, few of which were also admitted in Civil Hospital, Ahmedabad.

**Box 17H.1: Epidemic investigation.**
Food for thoughts?
- Before initiation of investigation, what preparation should be made by investigators?
- Which data should be on hand before starting investigation?
- Which communication to be made with local/concerned health authority?
- Is checklist required for investigation task? What kind of checklist should be with investigator?

> **Box 17H.2: Phase of investigation.**
> Food for thoughts?
> - How does investigator approach community?
> - Based on available data, which type of analysis should be done to generate hypothesis?
> - What is FIR in case of epidemic investigation?

### Details of Epidemic Investigation

An epidemic investigation was carried out in the Girdharnagar ward having a population of 66,540 (census 2001). There were 21 *chawls* located around the Girdharnagar civic center, having a population of 21,363 affected by this outbreak **(Table 17H.5)**. They searched cases using active surveillance by defining a case as an acute illness with (1) a discrete onset of symptoms and (2) jaundice or elevated serum aminotransferase levels, from March to September in the households of the Girdharnagar ward. Data were collected through (1) a door-to-door survey, and (2) hospital records. Information regarding the date of onset, age, sex, place of residence, treatment, and laboratory investigation was collected. The distribution of cases was analyzed using TPP characteristics.

After confirmation of diagnosis of disease and epidemic, investigator decided to undertake retrospective cohort study. Suspected exposure identified based on descriptive study was leaking pipelines and overflowing drains. In next step, investigator identified people who developed the disease and who did not, among the exposed and nonexposed. Blood samples of all 17 patients admitted to the Civil Hospital were subjected to serological tests for hepatitis A, B, C, and E. This is known as an epidemiological linked case, in which exposure and other determinants are same in population so, one can apply diagnosis to the group of people who shared similar characteristics. This approach is also recommended because it is not feasible to test everybody with laboratory diagnosis.

The annual incidence of viral hepatitis as per the IDSP data ranged from 0.5 to 1.2 per 1,000 in the city urban population during 2005–2006. The index case was reported to the Girdharnagar civic center on June 19 from the nearby slum. A total of 233 cases (attack rate 10.9/1,000) were reported from March to September 2008 **(Fig. 17H.11)**. There was no death due to the disease. The area-wise attack rate was higher in areas 1 (44/1,000), 2 (40/1,000), and 3 (36/1,000), respectively **(Fig. 17H.10)**. A higher incidence rate (16.3/1,000) was observed among those who were exposed to leaking pipelines and defective drains compared to those nonexposed (7.1/1,000). The relative risk for those exposed against those nonexposed was 2.3 (95% CI of RR 1.76, 2.98). The difference in the attack rate was also found to be statistically significant ($X^2 = 41.1$, $P < 0.001$).

A total of 16 out of 17 patients investigated were positive for the hepatitis E immunoglobulin M (IgM) antibody.

There was also a history of leakages in drinking water pipelines and overflowing drains in the area. **Figure 17H.10** shows the leakages and overflowing drains in the area. Residual chlorine was found in most of the water sample tested in various affected areas during the time of outbreak investigation. The timing of getting contaminated water supply coincided with the probable time period during which the possible exposure took place. Report of outbreak investigation was acknowledged to appropriate authority and necessary long- and short-term measures to control of outbreak were initiated.

**Table 17H.5:** Age- and sex-specific attack rate of jaundice cases in the Girdharnagar ward, Year 2008.

|  | Group | Cases | Population | Attack rate per 1,000 population | Z-value |
|---|---|---|---|---|---|
| Age (years) | 0–9 | 22 | 4,038 | 5.4 | |
| | 10–19 | 66 | 4,444 | 14.9 | |
| | 20–29 | 75 | 4,059 | 18.5 | |
| | 30–39 | 43 | 3,204 | 13.4 | |
| | 40–49 | 17 | 2,307 | 7.4 | |
| | 50+ | 10 | 3,311 | 3.0 | |
| Total | | 233 | 21,363 | 10.9 | |
| Sex | Male | 151 | 11,541 | 13.1 | ($P < 0.01$) |
| | Female | 82 | 9,822 | 8.3 | |

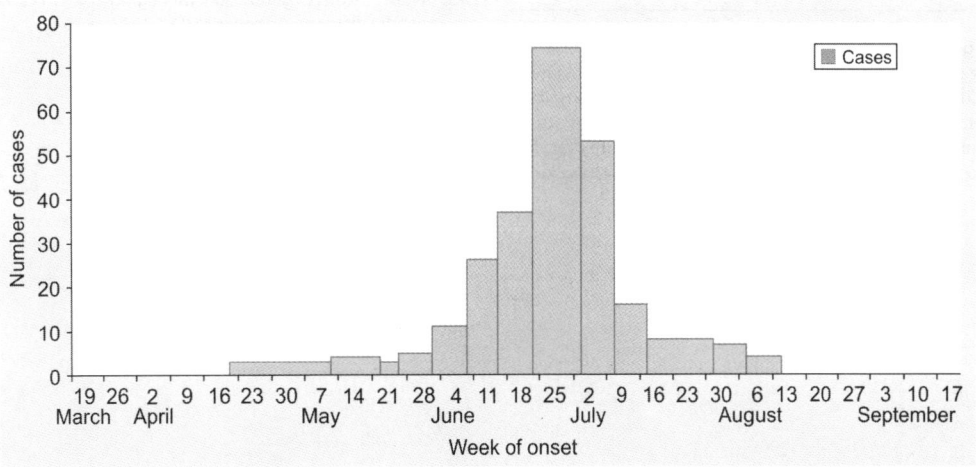

**Fig. 17H.11:** Cases of acute hepatitis by the week of onset, Girdharnagar ward, Ahmedabad, India, March–September 2008.

## CURRENT APPROACHES

### Global

- WHO provides support and help to countries in building strategies for disease control. The IHR (International Health Regulations (2005), it helps strengthen the core capacities for emergency risk management and to recover from the emergencies.
- It supports research and development activities during epidemics
- Updates on evidence based policy options
- Provides technical support and capacity building
- Maintains weekly epidemiological record

### National

The NCDC, i.e., National Centre for Disease Control (NCDC) is the nodal centre to enhance capabilities for a rapid response and laboratory surveillance.

In 2007, a Department of Health Research in the MOHFW was created to provide technical guidance during epidemics and calamities and provide tools for prevention. The department focuses on developing diagnostic tests, modules on management of case, prevention measures, establishment of new laboratories, etc.

The Indian Council of Medical Research (ICMR) is an apex body in our country for promotion of biomedical research. It also has a chain of regional institutes for the same focusing on specific infectious diseases.

### *National Program*

The Integrated Disease Surveillance Project (IDSP) which was established in 2004 has been expanded to cover all districts in the country. Each district now has an IDSP set up with a team involving epidemiologists, microbiologists, entomologist. A surveillance team and rapid response team are part each of the IDSP at district level thus helping in quick management of the outbreak. ***IDSP has been explained in details in Chapter 47: Health Policies and Programs in India.***

## SUMMARY

A disease occurring in unusual high frequency warrants urgent attention. A timely response can minimize mortalities and morbidities associated with the disease. Currently with surveillance systems in place it is possible to reduce the damage to the community at large. However, a strict vigilance with monitoring of activities is also necessary to ensure that the mechanism in place for outbreak detection and containment are working adequately.

## SUGGESTED READING

1. Case definitions for infectious conditions under public health surveillance. Centers for Disease Control and Prevention. MMWR Recomm Rep. 1997;46(RR-10):1-55.
2. Centers for Disease Control and Prevention. Principles of Epidemiology in Public Health Practice: An Introduction to Applied Epidemiology and Biostatistics, 3rd edition. Self-study Course SS1978. US Department of Health and Human Services, Centers for Disease Control and Prevention (CDC), Office of Workforce and Career Development, Atlanta, GA 30333; 2012.
3. Field Epidemiology Manual. [online] Available from https://wiki.ecdc.europa.eu/training/.
4. Holme P, Masuda N. The basic reproduction number as a predictor for epidemic outbreaks in temporal networks. PLoS One. 2015;10(3):e0120567.
5. Integrated Disease Surveillance Project (IDSP). Operational manual for district surveillance unit. IDSP, Government of India, Directorate General of Health Services, Ministry of Health and Family Welfare, Nirman Bhawan, New Delhi; Section 5:73.
6. Integrated Disease Surveillance Project. Operational manual for district surveillance unit. IDSP, Government of India, Directorate General of Health Services, Ministry of Health and Family Welfare, Nirman Bhawan, New Delhi; Section 2:23.
7. Outbreak investigation checklist: 10 steps to follow, 10 pitfalls to avoid. Indian Council of Medical Research, New Delhi; Version 6—2008. [online] Available from http://www.nie.gov.in/images/leftcontent_attach/3.A.7.PittOutb_153.pdf.
8. Panda M, Hutin YJ, Ramachandran V, et al. A fatal waterborne outbreak of pesticide poisoning caused by damaged pipelines, Sindhikela, Bolangir, Orissa, India, 2008. J Toxicol. 2009;2009:692496.
9. Porta M. A Dictionary of Epidemiology, 6th edition. Oxford: Oxford University Press. 2016. p. 343. [online]. Available from http://irea.ir/files/site1/pages/dictionary.pdf.
10. Snow J. Snow on cholera. Public Health. 1936;50:139-40. [online] Available from http://linkinghub.elsevier.com/retrieve/pii/S0033350636801115.
11. WHO. Epidemic and pandemic-prone diseases. Outbreaks Current outbreaks in the WHO Eastern Mediterranean Region. May 2023. Available from https://www.emro.who.int/pandemic-epidemic-diseases/outbreaks/index.html
12. WHO. Weekly epidemiological update on COVID-19 - 13 July 2023. Edition 151. 13 July 2023 Emergency Situational Updates.
13. World Health Organization. (2019). Disease outbreaks. [online] Available from http://www.searo.who.int/topics/disease_outbreaks/en/.
14. World Health Organization. International health regulations (2005), 3rd edition. 2016. [online] Available from http://apps.who.int/iris/bitstream/handle/10665/246107/9789241580496-eng.pdf?sequence=1.
15. World Health Organization. Managing epidemics: key facts about major deadly diseases. Geneva: WHO; 2018. pp. 25-6.

# I. EMERGING AND RE-EMERGING DISEASES OF GLOBAL IMPORTANCE

## GENERAL EPIDEMIOLOGY OF EMERGING AND RE-EMERGING DISEASES AND PUBLIC HEALTH ACTION

*Venkatrao Epari, Jyotiranjan Sahoo*

*World Health Day theme -1997:* **Emerging Infectious Diseases—Global Alert, Global Response**

| | |
|---|---|
| **CM20.1** | List important public health events of last five years |
| **MI8.4** | Describe the etiologic agents of emerging infectious diseases. Discuss the clinical course and diagnosis (vertical and horizontal integration with Internal Medicine Department) |

### INTRODUCTION

Contemplating the benefits realized from the use of antibiotics and vaccines; when victory against the risk of infectious diseases was declared by the Surgeon General William H Stewart, and proposed for diversion of devotion and resources towards chronic diseases, at a junction when the subspecialty of infectious disease was disappearing; imagine a medical resident anticipating to begin his infectious disease fellowship after completion of his formal medical training!

"Fifty years ago, people believed that the age-old battle of humans against infectious disease was virtually over. However; the events of the past few decades have shown the foolhardiness of that position. At least a dozen new diseases have been identified (e.g. AIDS, Legionnaire disease, and Hantavirus pulmonary syndrome), and traditional diseases that appeared to be on their way out (e.g. malaria and tuberculosis) are resurging. Clearly, the battle has not been won!"

In order to understand what really is going wrong, we shall review under the following headings:

### DEFINITION

**Emerging infections are defined as:**
- Those which have not been previously experienced
- Those with already known causative agents, but
  - Not known previously to infect humans or
  - Occurring in new regions, where previously they were inexistent or
  - In a new age group (e.g. previously affected old age now among the youth) with new clinical features including
  - Developing resistance to existing treatment.

AIDS is a classic example of an emerging infectious disease since its public health impact was not experienced before 1981. Similarly, a new serogroup, *Vibrio cholerae* O139 emerged in 1992 causing a large-scale outbreak in India. The emergence of drug resistance such as artemisinin-combination therapy (ACT) resistant malaria, multidrug-resistant (MDR), and extensively drug-resistant (XDR) tuberculosis are newer such challenges to the global health.

**Re-emerging infections, on the contrary, are:**
- Those which have been experienced previously, controlled or efficaciously treated
- But have recurred in a new epidemiological setting with
  - Increasing frequency and/or mortality or
  - In a more virulent form.

Pandemics of influenza-A in 1957, 1968, and 2009 are ideal examples. Similarly, India reported all-time low diphtheria cases of 2,817 in 1997 and there was a sudden increase to about 8,000 cases in 2004 with several outbreaks from various states owing to low coverage of primary immunization and boosters. An epidemiological shift was noted in these outbreaks affecting older children especially among those who were unimmunized or partially immunized (Dikid T et al., Indian J Med Res, 2013).

While the list of emerging and re-emerging diseases is endless, few that have occurred in India in the recent times are enumerated in **Table 17I.1**.

The number of reported outbreaks has progressively increased from 553 in 2008 to 1,611 in 2018 in India as shown in **Figure 17I.1**. Disease-wise outbreaks is reported in **Figure 17I.2**.

It has been almost a decade since the first PHEIC (Public Health Emergency of International Concern) was declared. WHO has declared six PHEIC till date-Swine flu in 2009, Polio in 2014, Ebola and Zika in 2016, Kivu Ebola in 2019 and the ongoing 2019-20 coronavirus pandemic. In the last decade, various viral diseases have had a serious health impact in India.

**Impact of emerging and re-emerging diseases:** *They have been enormous at socioeconomic and public health levels and it presents a great challenge for the future.* Infectious diseases contribute to approximately 30% of 1.49 billion DALYs lost every year. These diseases impose a shockingly high economic price for individuals, families, and communities in terms of healthcare cost and loss of productivity.

### FACTORS RESPONSIBLE FOR EMERGING OF INFECTIONS

**Common factors** among emerging diseases are:
- A majority (up to 70%) of these have zoonotic origin from the wildlife.
- Most are viral in origin.

### Ecological Changes and Agricultural Development

Human intrusion into wildlife territory especially in tropical regions where in people comes in contact with the natural reservoir.

Examples are
- Outbreak of Nipah virus in India owing to rapid urbanization and human intrusion into the bat infected areas.

**Table 171.1:** List of emerging and re-emerging diseases in India.

| Disease | Emergence | | Re-emergence | | Probable cause |
|---|---|---|---|---|---|
| | Year | Location | Year | Location | |
| Plague | 1896 | Mumbai | 1994 | Surat, India | Spillover from an epizootic cycle |
| Leptospirosis | 1931 | Andaman Islands | 2002 | Mumbai | Prolonged water logging due to heavy rainfall |
| Chikungunya | 1963 | India (Asian genotypes) | 2006 | Southern and central India | Multiple causes |
| Chandipura virus | 1965 | Chandipura (Nagpur) | 2003 | Andhra Pradesh, Gujarat, Maharashtra | Transmitted by sandflies, predominant in rural areas |
| Cholera (Vibrio cholerae O139) | 1992 | Southern peninsular India | — | — | Multiple causes |
| Diphtheria | — | — | 2004 | Delhi, Andhra Pradesh, Assam, Maharashtra, Chandigarh, Gujarat | Low coverage of primary immunization as well as boosters |
| Nipah | 2001 | Eastern India | 2018 | Kerala | Consumption of fruits partially eaten by the bats |
| H1N1 influenza | 2010 | Maharashtra and Gujarat (Global origin was Mexico) | — | — | Multiple causes |
| Crimean-Congo hemorrhagic fever | 2011 | Gujarat | — | — | Enzootic tick-vertebrate-tick cycle |
| Acute encephalitis syndrome (AES) | — | — | 2011 | Uttar Pradesh, Bihar, Assam and West Bengal | Multiple causes |
| COVID-19 | 2020 | Kerala (Global origin was Wuhan, China) | — | — | — |
| Norovirus | 2021 | Kerala | | | |

*Source:* Dikid T, Jain SK, Sharma A, et al. Emerging and reemerging infections in India: An overview. Indian J Med Res. 2013;138:19-31.
Chugh TD. Emerging bacterial diseases in India. J Biosci. 2008;33(4):549-55.

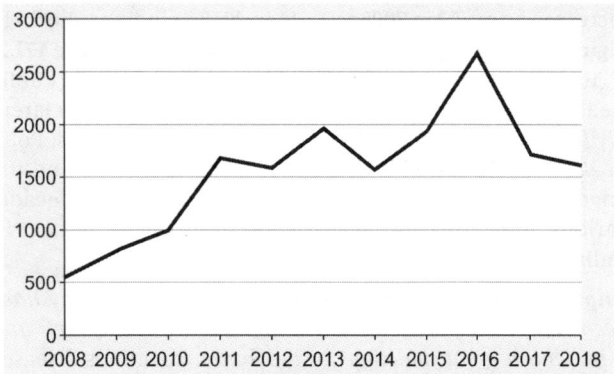

**Fig. 171.1:** Line graph showing number of reported outbreaks from 2008 to 2018.
*Source:* IDSP and Patel M et al study report.

- Lymes disease: Reforestation in the USA led greater human interaction with deer. Humans were affected as deer ticks were the natural reservoir.
- Korean hemorrhagic fever in South-East Asia, increased rice cultivation resulted in increased human contact with the field mouse which is the natural reservoir of Hantaan virus.
- Recurrences of plague epidemics – attributed to spill over from an epizootic cycle of plague in wild rodents to commensal rodents fueled by climate change.
- Several vector-borne and rodent-borne diseases—due to global warming, which in turn results in elevated rainfall, increased vegetation and creating new breeding habitats for many vectors.

Increased runoff into drinking reservoirs can also result in contamination of water bodies.

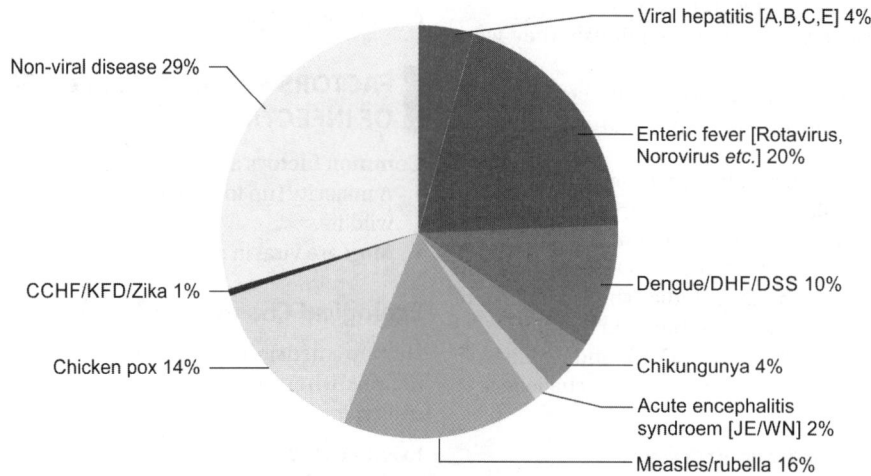

**Fig. 171.2:** Disease-wise reported outbreaks in India.
*Source:* Mourya DT, Yadav PD, Ullas PT, Bhardwaj SD, Sahay RR, Chadha MS et al. Emerging/re-emerging viral diseases & new viruses on the Indian horizon. Indian J Med Res. 2019;149(4):447-67.

### Changes in Human Demographics and Behaviors

- Scrub typhus resurgence—due to changes in the human behavior, unplanned urbanization, deforestation, and rapid transport
- Dengue fever resurgence—Use of open containers for water leading to breeding mosquitos
- Emerging infectious diseases—War refugees are exposed to new microbes from vectors and people following displacement to new areas.
- Poor infection control practices—In the context of collapsed health systems and disruption of disease control programs added with inadequate surveillance and response systems.

### International Travel and Commerce

- Humans carry pathogens, microbial flora, vectors on their body, immunological sequelae of past infections, cultural preferences, customs, and behavior along with genetic makeup to the new regions. The impact of human movement persists long afterwards especially for diseases like HIV, TB, etc.
- Slaves trade and yellow fever, Hajj pilgrimage and Cholera, Silk route and plague are other examples of international travel causing the emergence of infectious diseases.
- Movements of viruses and arthropods (especially ticks) are facilitated by transportation of livestock. Moreover, increased incidence of both tuberculosis and influenza transmission has been reported on long flight journeys.

### Technology and Industry

Advancement of technology led to mass production, which in turn increased the probability of accidental contamination.

- United States witnessed cases of hemolytic-uremic syndrome due to contamination of hamburger meat by *E. coli* strains.
- Concentrating effect of blood and nosocomial infections is also responsible for emerging infections as observed during Ebola outbreak caused by contaminated hypodermic apparatus in Congo.
- With the introduction of newer diagnostic technology identification of previously unfamiliar microbes for known ailments was made possible, e.g. *Helicobacter pylori* and peptic ulcer, human herpesvirus 6 and roseola.
- Advancement in medical technology has brought in people living longer, but with a weaker immune system predisposing to contract rare and emerging viral infections; especially following blood and organ transplantation.

### Microbial Adaptation and Transformation

Several microorganisms using different genetic mechanisms have got the ability to sustain the challenges of their environment. Rapid reproduction in RNA viruses leads to the building of rare mutations. Examples are

- Possible genetic changes in coronavirus (SARS) or "Antigenic drift" in case of influenza virus are the prototypical examples.
- Development of antimicrobial resistance by viruses (HIV), bacteria (MDR-TB) or parasites (chloroquine-resistant malaria) has been attributed to extensive and at times incorrect use of antimicrobial agents.
- Few bacteria that cause human illness which are targeted by antibiotic treatment constitute a tiny subset of the vast population in the environment (soil and other livestock). Antimicrobial resistance (AMR) to these bacteria is linked to AMR in humans thereby producing resistant strains (vancomycin-resistant enterococci, vancomycin-resistant *Staphylococcus aureus*, macrolide-resistant *S. pneumoniae*, and multidrug-resistant *Salmonella*, etc).

### Breakdown of Public Health Measures

- Outbreaks of cholera have been linked to decreased chlorination as in South America or due to lack of water supply following natural disasters.
- Non-operating water plant in Wisconsin, USA resulted in the occurrence of water-borne *Cryptosporidium*, and
- Insufficient immunization led to the emergence of diphtheria in several states of India.
- Withdrawal of mosquito control efforts have led to malaria and dengue re-emergence in many parts of the world.

## PUBLIC HEALTH ACTION

### Surveillance

An optimally functioning surveillance system (epidemiological surveillance) forms the cornerstone of controlling emerging and re-emerging diseases, along with other components of vector, serological and microbial surveillance will be able to detect outbreaks of infectious diseases early. Supporting rapid response teams can prevent further spread of the disease in the community. The Government of India established Integrated Disease Surveillance Program (IDSP) in the year 1994 following an appraisal from the National Surveillance Programme on Communicable Diseases. IDSP has captured and investigated 1,714 outbreaks in 2017 alone.

The most essential aspects of prevention of viral outbreaks lies in surveillance of agent, host and environment. WHO since long has a mandate for promoting and supervising surveillance activities which has been emphasized further in recent times as evident from International Health Regulations (IHR) and pandemics of Public Health Emergency of International Concern (PHEIC).

### Complying with IHR

International Health Regulations (IHR) ensures public health through stoppage of the spread of infections across borders. This has been revised in May 2005. Instead of traditional reporting of specific diseases, the scope has been widened to report any illness or medical condition, irrespective of origin or source that presents or could present significant harm to humans.

### Building Public Health Capacity

Improvement in public health infrastructure including special laboratories capable of accurate and rapid diagnosis forms the basis of effective public health action. In-service training programs like Field Epidemiology Training Program (FETP) of 3 months or 2 years' duration have been designed. The Government of India has also announced the training of public health leaders on Epidemic Intelligence Service (EIS) run by CDC, Atlanta in order to provide epidemiologic services to health authorities in India.

Establishing public health systems to screen the migrant population and checking for appropriate vaccination, ensuring sanitation along with urbanization and judicious use of antibiotics through public health policy are few other interventions to curb the emergence of infections.

### Research and Development

Need for conducting research to inform key policy decisions cannot be overemphasized; Rational use of drugs and pesticides; assessment of their impact on the environment; influence of climate change on disease prevention and control, Strengthening the public health laboratories and building the capacity of laboratory personnel to handle new/exotic organisms is the need of the hour.

The Department of Health Research (DHR), MOHFW, Government of India, in 2013 made a vision to establish and strengthen the network of laboratories across the country namely Viral Research and Diagnostic Laboratory Network (VRDLN). There is a network of about 100 laboratories in India with the objectives to create infrastructure and identify viruses, for capacity building, to develop diagnostics, trainings and meetings of health officials and professionals and for research.

### Information Sharing and Partnership: GOARN

A technical alliance of existing institutions and linkages has been established by the World Health Organization known as Global Outbreak Alert and Response Network (GOARN). The primary purpose is to identify, confirm and execute an appropriate response to outbreaks of international importance by pooling human and technical resources through an operational framework. Suitable subject experts reach the site of the outbreak in the least possible time to carry out a synchronized and effective outbreak control activities.

### SUMMARY

- Emerging and re-emerging diseases are infectious diseases, which have tremendous impact on the human civilization in terms of mortality, morbidity, and economic burden.
- They arise mostly due to imbalance in the ecosystem resulting from several man-made alterations.
- The control of these diseases is feasible but dependent upon collective action rather than individualistic approach.

### SUGGESTED READING

1. Agrawal V. Pandemic response and international health regulations. MJAFI. 2007;63(4):366-7.
2. Barbour AG. Fall and rise of Lyme disease and other Ixodes tick-borne infections in North America and Europe. Br Med Bull. 1998;54(3):647-58.
3. Cliff AD, Andrew D, Smallman-Raynor M. Infectious diseases: Emergence and re-emergence: A geographical analysis. Oxford University Press; 2009. pp. 763.
4. Fauci AS. Infectious diseases: Considerations for the 21st century. Clin Infect Dis. 2001;32(5):675-85.
5. Githeko AK, Lindsay SW, Confalonieri UE, et al. Climate change and vector-borne diseases: A regional analysis. Bull World Health Organ. 2000;78(9):1136-47.
6. Knobler S, Mahmoud A, Lemon S, et al. The Impact of Globalization on Infectious Disease Emergence and Control. Forum on Microbial Threats; Board on Global Health; Institute of editor. Washington, DC; 2006.
7. Kuri-Morales PA, Guzmán-Morales E, De La Paz-Nicolau E, et al. Emerging and re-emerging diseases. Gac Med Mex. 2015;151(5):674-80.
8. Mourya DT, Yadav PD, Ullas PT, Bhardwaj SD, Sahay RR, Chadha MS, et al. Emerging/re-emerging viral diseases & new viruses on the Indian horizon. Indian J Med Res. 2019;149(4):447-467.
9. Okonko IO, Donbraye E, Babalola ET, et al. Conflict and the spread of emerging infectious diseases: Where do we go from here? African J Microbiol Res. 2009;3(13):1015-28.
10. Patel M, Goel AD, Bhardwaj P, Joshi N, Kumar N, Gupta MK, Jain V, Saurabh S, Patel K. Emerging and re-emerging viral infections in India. J Prev Med Hyg. 2021;62(3):E628-E634.
11. Stenseth NC, Viljugrein H, et al. Plague dynamics are driven by climate variation. Proc Natl Acad Sci USA. 2006;103(35):13110-5.
12. Taylor LH, Latham SM, Woolhouse ME. Risk factors for human disease emergence. Philos Trans R Soc Lond B Biol Sci. 2001;356(1411): 983-9.
13. Waggoner JJ, Soda EA, Deresinski S. Rare and emerging viral infections in transplant recipients. Clin Infect Dis. 2013;57(8):1182-8.
14. Wilson ME. Travel and the emergence of infectious diseases. Emerg Infect Dis. 1995;1(2):39-46.
15. Woolhouse M, Ward M, Van Bunnik B, et al. Antimicrobial resistance in humans, livestock and the wider environment. Phil Trans R Soc B. 2015;370:1-7.
16. Woolhouse ME, Gowtage-Sequeria S. Host range and emerging and reemerging pathogens. Emerg Infect Dis. 2005;11(12):1842-7.
17. World Health Organization. Global Outbreak Alert: Response Network 2015.
18. World Health Organization. International health regulations third edition; 2005.

---

## SPECIFIC EPIDEMIOLOGY OF EMERGING DISEASES

*Madhur Verma*

*Nothing in the world of living things is permanently fixed.*
—Hans Zinsser. Rats, Lice and History (1935)

| CM8.1 | Describe and discuss the epidemiological and control measures applicable in emerging diseases |

### INTRODUCTION

With the aim of strengthening global preparedness and response of any future epidemics and pandemics, the Research and Development Blueprint continues with its mandate to accelerate research on diseases threats before they emerge and to shorten the timeline in developing safe and effective curative and preventive medical countermeasures (diagnostics, treatments and vaccines).

In order to focus research efforts, an official WHO list of priority pathogens of epidemic and pandemic potential is generated and published based on an independent, open and multidisciplinary prioritization process, using rigorous and transparent methods.

The last prioritization exercise was conducted in 2018. WHO has recently launched a global scientific process to update the list in November 2022 The prioritization exercise will draw on the lessons from COVID-19 and ensure that trust, equity and access for those at highest risk is central to future research and development efforts. WHO tool distinguishes which diseases pose the greatest public health risk due to their epidemic potential and/or whether there is no or insufficient countermeasures.

At present, the priority diseases are:
- COVID-19
- Crimean-Congo hemorrhagic fever
- Ebola virus disease and Marburg virus disease
- Lassa fever
- Middle East respiratory syndrome coronavirus (MERS-CoV) and severe acute respiratory syndrome (SARS)
- Nipah and henipaviral diseases
- Rift Valley fever
- Zika
- "Disease X"*

This is not an exhaustive list, nor does it indicate the most likely causes of the next epidemic. WHO reviews and updates this list as needs arise, and methodologies change. Based on the priority diseases, WHO then works to develop roadmaps for each one.

In this context, it becomes necessary to highlight the epidemiology and current practices for certain diseases that are important for India. Rest of the diseases are described in other sections of this book **(Table 17I.2)**.

**Table 17I.2:** Diseases and their geographical distribution.

| Disease | Year of 1st known outbreak | Country of origin | Geographical distribution includes | Case fatality rate |
|---|---|---|---|---|
| Ebola | 1976 | Democratic Republic of Congo | Central Africa and West Africa | 50% |
| Zika | 1947 | Uganda | South-east Asia, Africa, America | 8.3% |
| Nipah | 1998 | Malaysia | South-east Asia (86 countries) | 74% |
| Lassa fever | 1969 | Nigeria | West Africa | 1% |

*Source:* Ebola Outbreak Epidemiology Team, Lancet, 2018; Kindhauser MK et al., Bull World Health Organ, 2016; Chang LY et al., Nipah Virus Infection, 2013; McCormick JB et al., N Engl J Med, 1986.

## EBOLA VIRUS DISEASE

### Background

Ebola virus disease (EVD) is an acute viral hemorrhagic fever, highly fatal disease if untreated. This virus belonging to family Filoviridae has five species; Zaire, Bundibugyo, Sudan are the deadliest, and the other two are Reston and Taï forest. All species have caused disease in humans except the Reston virus (RESTV). It was initially detected in 1976 around Ebola river of Zaire that is now known as the Democratic Republic of the Congo. From that time multiple outbreaks have occurred till date. An outbreak in 2014–2016 in Africa was due to *Zaire* species. As per CDC reports, the most recent outbreak of Ebola (Sudan virus) was confirmed on September 20, 2022, by the Ugandan Ministry of Health in Mubende District, in western Uganda.

### Transmission (Fig. 17I.3)

Fruit bats serve as the natural hosts for Ebola and transmit it to animals like apes, monkeys. Virus enters the human population only when there is close contact with the infected animal, by direct contact with blood and other bodily fluids of infected people or with items contaminated with these fluids. Risk of transmission through sexual route needs more scientific evidence.

**Incubation period:** Ranges from 2 to 21 days. During incubation period humans are not known to be infectious.

**Clinical feature:** Most commonly reported symptoms include fever with malaise, myalgia with a sore throat, vomiting, loose motions, rash, bleeding diathesis that may lead to internal and external bleeding.

### Diagnosis

The EVD symptoms are very similar to many other infectious diseases like dengue. Laboratory investigations depict a leukopenia and thrombocytopenia and elevated liver enzymes. Confirmation of infection is made with the help of either antibody-capture enzyme-linked immunosorbent assay (ELISA), antigen-capture detection tests, serum neutralization test, reverse transcriptase-polymerase chain reaction (RT-PCR) assay, electron microscopy or by virus isolation by cell culture. Currently, the WHO recommends automated or semi-automated nucleic acid tests (NAT) for routine diagnostic management.

### Treatment and Vaccines

There is no specific treatment against Ebola virus till date. Supportive care mainly includes maintenance of the hydration levels of the patients. Recovery often requires months. Ebola virus continues to persist in immune-privileged sites like testicles, eye and the central nervous system, in infected pregnant women the virus continues to exist in placenta, fetus and even breast milk.

Vaccines against Ebola virus are still in different phases of drug trials, e.g., recombinant vesicular stomatitis virus–Zaire Ebola virus (rVSV-ZEBOV).

### Controlling Infection in Healthcare Settings

The healthcare workers are at a high-risk of getting infected, hence are advised to follow standard precautions while handling the patients. Refresher training focusing on universal precautions and safe disposal of dead bodies preventing contamination of the environment should be initiated. Despite following these precautions, if anybody gets exposed to virus then they should be kept under quarantine and observed for 21 days.

*Disease X represents the knowledge that a serious international epidemic could be caused by a pathogen currently unknown to cause human disease. The R&D Blueprint explicitly seeks to enable early cross-cutting R&D preparedness that is also relevant for an unknown "Disease X" (WHO 2023).

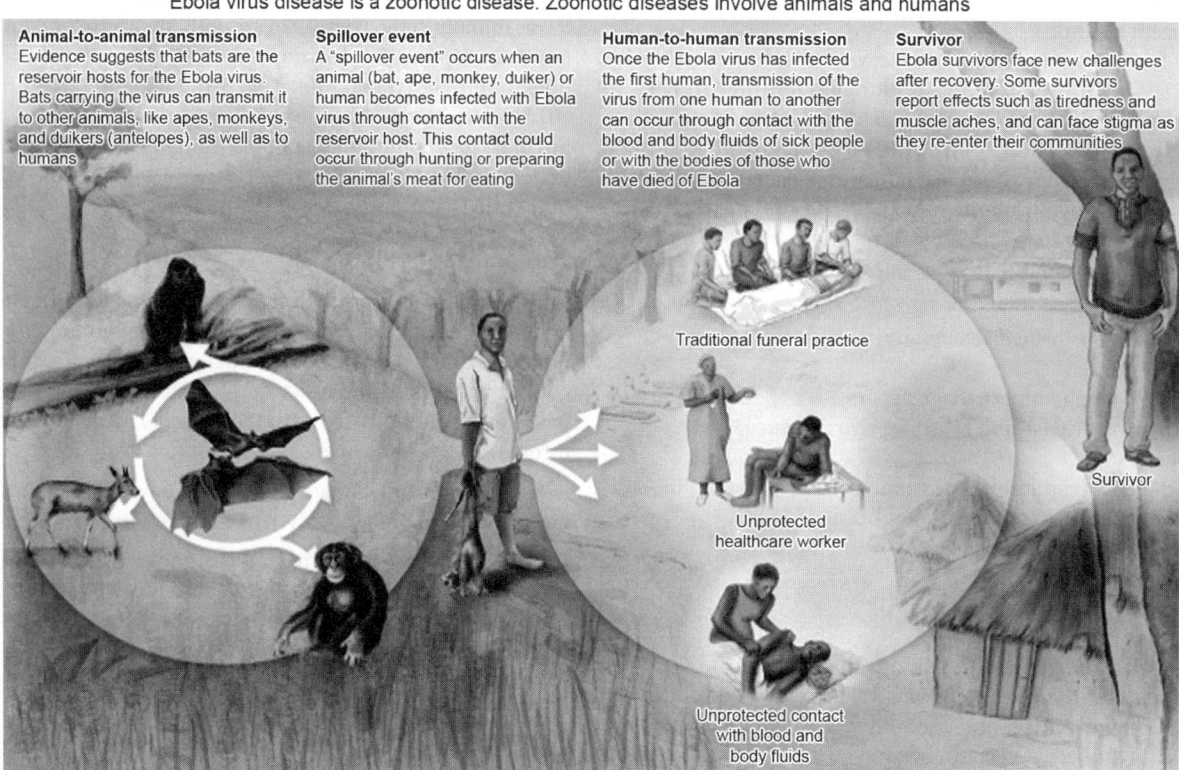

**Fig. 17I.3:** Ecology of the Ebola virus and its transmission.
*Source:* CDC Atlanta.

## Prevention and Control

Effective outbreak containment depends on a series of interventions during case management and contact tracing along with continuous surveillance and state of the art laboratory services. There is also need of health promotion and health education activities on precautions to be taken while caring the diseased family members or performing their last rituals (safe burial practices) to minimize human transmission.

## ZIKA VIRUS

### Background

Zika virus is an icosahedral, enveloped, single-stranded RNA arbovirus of *Flavivirus* genus.

Till 1952, Zika virus was known as disease-specific to the monkey, when it was first identified in humans residing in Uganda and the United Republic of Tanzania. The largest Zika outbreak was observed in 2015–2016 affected more than 33 countries with more than 1.4 million cases in Brazil alone (Jaenisch et al., Bull World Health Organ, 2018). Subsequently, this outbreak was declared as a PHEIC on February 1, 2016, after a recommendation of International Health Regulations (IHR) Emergency Committee. To date, a total of 86 countries and territories have reported evidence of mosquito-transmitted Zika infection.

India has reported the first case of ZVD from Gujarat. Subsequently, few sporadic cases (Gujarat, Tamil Nadu) and outbreaks of ZVD have been reported from Rajasthan and Madhya Pradesh states during 2017–2018. Recently, more than 100 cases Zika have been detected and confirmed with real-time reverse transcriptase-polymerase chain reaction (rRT-PCR) from the Uttar Pradesh state of India during October–November 2021.

### Transmission

Zika virus is transmitted by the *Aedes* mosquito (an arthropod), similar to other *Flaviviruses*. This mosquito commonly bites during the daytime, and bite rate is highest during the dawn and dusk. This mosquito is also responsible for the transmission of dengue, chikungunya and yellow fever. The virus can also be transmitted from pregnant mother to fetus, through sexual contact, hemo-transfusion, and organ transplantation **(Fig. 17I.4)**.

**Incubation period:** Ranges from 3 to 14 days.

### Clinical Features

The duration of viremia is approximately three days, and it is between the 3rd and 5th day after the onset of the clinical symptoms. The majority of people (80%) infected with Zika virus do not develop symptoms. Symptoms include fever, rash, conjunctivitis, muscle and joint pain, malaise, and headache, and usually last for 2–7 days.

Zika virus infection may also trigger a range of neurological complications ranging from Guillain-Barré syndrome,

## Chapter 17: Specific Epidemiology of Infectious Diseases

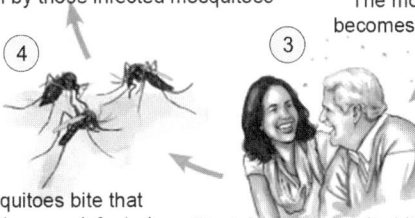
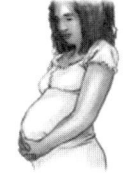
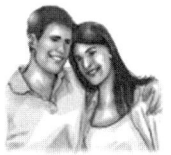
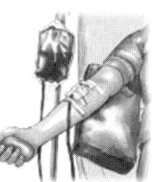

**Fig. 17I.4:** Ecology of the Zika virus and its transmission.
*Source:* CDC Atlanta.

neuropathy to myelitis, particularly in adults and older children. Transplacental transmission may lead to microcephaly, that is caused by underlying abnormal brain development or loss of brain tissue. Child outcomes vary according to the extent of brain damage. Zika virus infection during pregnancy is also responsible for other congenital abnormalities in the developing fetus and newborn such as including limb contractures, high muscle tone, eye abnormalities, and hearing loss apart from fetal loss, stillbirth and preterm birth, collectively referred to as congenital Zika syndrome. Zika-related complications are estimated to be manifested in about 5–15% of all the infants which are born to mothers who were infected during pregnancy. Congenital malformations occur following both symptomatic and asymptomatic infection.

## Diagnosis

Suspicion of Zika virus infection should be made in people who are either living in or visiting the areas in which virus transmission and vector of the disease, i.e. *Aedes* mosquitoes are identified. However, a confirmed diagnosis should be made using **nucleic acid testing (NAT) and serology for** rising titers of IgM levels **detection** using body fluids, including blood, urine or semen.

## Treatment

Due to lack of specific antiviral drug for this infection, symptomatic treatment including rest, oral hydration, medications for pain and fever is the mainstay of management for mild forms of the disease. In areas with ongoing Zika transmission, laboratory testing of infection among pregnant women should be done, and those who are symptomatic should seek medical care as early as possible. No vaccine is yet available for the prevention or treatment of Zika virus infection.

## Prevention

Like any other mosquito-borne disease, the best prevention against Zika virus disease is protection against mosquito bites. Particular attention should be given to the prevention of mosquito bites among pregnant women, women of reproductive age, and young children. Personal protection measures include wearing full sleeve clothing (dark colors to be avoided) with covering most of the body; use of window screens, keeping doors and windows closed, mosquito nets; and applying insect repellent to skin or clothing **(Box 17I.1)**.

> **Box 17I.1: The national response to the Zika virus outbreak.**
>
> The last reported Zika virus was in Jaipur city of Rajasthan state, where 157 cases were identified, including 63 pregnant women as on 2nd November 2018. After the outbreak, extensive state and national response efforts had been implemented by the Ministry of Health and Family Welfare (MOHFW). Suspected cases in the area were tested, including viral sequence analysis. Pregnant women were screened and provided information on Zika virus infection and prevention and followed by routine antenatal care and ultrasound examination. Extensive surveillance and vector control measures had been initiated, including house-to-house surveys. Community-based programs to increase public awareness, advance measures to mitigate mosquito breeding sites, and promote personal protection measures against mosquito vectors were carried out. The Government of India has maintained a laboratory-based Zika surveillance system, involving 34 laboratories to detect Zika virus infection in patients with febrile illness, developed as part of the National Zika Action Plan.

## NIPAH VIRUS

Nipah virus causes a zoonotic disease that is associated with high case fatality and virulence among people, has emerged as

> **Box 171.2: A case study from India (WHO, emergencies preparedness response, Nipah virus, India, 2023).**
>
> Between 12 and 15 September 2023, a total of six laboratory-confirmed cases of Nipah virus infection including two deaths were reported by the State Government of Kerala. All confirmed cases were males within the age range of 9 to 45 years old and were reported within the Kozhikode district of Kerala. The first case whose source of infection is unknown, had pneumonia and acute respiratory distress syndrome (ARDS) and was admitted at a hospital in late August 2023. He died a few days after admission. The other five confirmed cases were close contacts of the first case including two family members and contacts at the hospital where the first case was treated and died. The second death occurred in an individual who accompanied another patient to the hospital where the first case was being treated. He died after presenting with symptoms of pneumonia. As of 27 September 2023, 1288 contacts of the confirmed cases have been traced, including high-risk contacts and healthcare workers who treated the confirmed cases and processed their samples. All identified contacts are under quarantine for a period of 21 days. As of 27 September 2023, the four cases remain clinically stable. The Government's response measures included declaring containment zones in nine villages in the Kozhikode district with movement restrictions, social distancing, and mandatory mask-wearing in public spaces. The government restricted major public events in Kozhikode district until 1 October 2023. Alerts were issued to neighboring districts and states for enhanced surveillance.

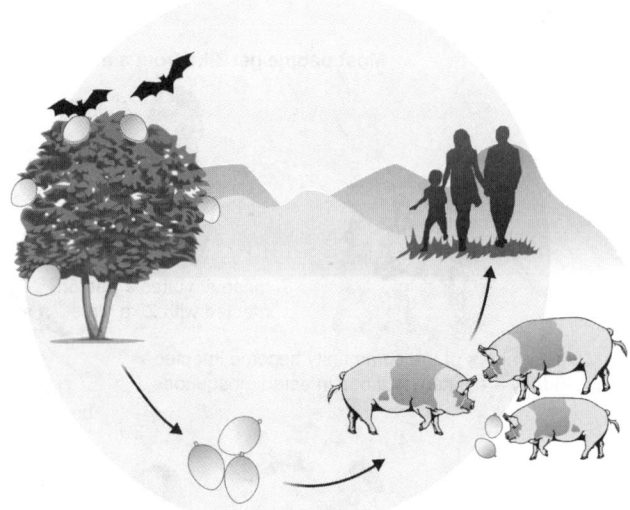

**Fig. 171.5:** Outbreaks cycle of Nipah virus. The natural reservoirs of the virus are fruit bats of Pteropid family. Pigs were infected by the bats roosting in pig farms on fruit trees. Further transmission to humans was through these pigs by close contact.

*Source:* de Wit E, Munster VJ. Nipah Virus Emergence, Transmission, and Pathogenesis. In: Global Virology Identifying and Investigating Viral Diseases. New York: Springer; 2015. pp. 125-46.

a disease of public health concern. It infects mainly pigs, along with wide range of other animals including dogs, cats, horses, and sheep. The first outbreak occurred in 1999 in Malaysia among pig farmers. In subsequent outbreaks in Bangladesh and India, consumption of fruits or fruit products (such as raw date palm juice) contaminated with urine or saliva from infected fruit bats was the most likely source of infection. During the later outbreaks in Bangladesh and India, Nipah virus spread directly from human-to-human through close contact with people's secretions and excretions. In Siliguri, India in 2001, transmission of the virus was also reported within a health-care setting, where 75% of cases occurred among hospital staff or visitors. From 2001 to 2008, around half of reported cases in Bangladesh were due to human-to-human transmission through providing care to infected patients. The disease has also been identified periodically in eastern India. Most recent outbreaks in India occurred in September 2023 in Kerala. This is the sixth outbreak of Nipah virus in India since 2001 **(Box 171.2)**.

### Transmission (Fig. 171.5)

Transmission to humans occurs either through consumption of food contaminated by infected animals or from person-to-person. In most of the outbreaks among humans, direct mode of transmission was contact with pigs harboring infection, their tissues or else from the consumption of fruits products contaminated with secretions of infected fruit bats (*Pteropus* bat species). The disease spreads among close contacts of the patients very efficiently giving evidence of human-to-human transmission. Most of the cases include hospital staff or visitors, who are involved in providing care to infected patients.

**Incubation period:** 4–14 days.

### Clinical Features

The spectrum of illness can range from asymptomatic (subclinical) infection to acute respiratory illness. The disease starts with nonspecific flu-like signs and symptoms including fever, muscle aches, headache, sore throat and vomiting. It may lead to encephalitis, which is often fatal. Recovery from encephalitis is usually complete if treated early. Still, the long-term neurologic sequel including seizure disorder and personality changes, have been reported in about 20% of the patients. Case fatality rates can range from 40%–75%.

### Diagnosis

Diagnosis often delayed due to nonspecific presentation, lag in clinical sample collection time and transfer of samples to the laboratory. During outbreaks, this hinders effective and timely interventions for infection control, resulting in high virulence, ongoing transmission and high case fatality. High level of clinical suspicion of disease is crucial during the acute and convalescent phase of the disease. For confirmation of infection, samples of body fluids for RT-PCR (real-time polymerase chain reaction) and ELISA (enzyme-linked immunosorbent assay) for antibody detection is used mainly.

### Treatment

There is no specific treatment. Symptomatic treatment for mild cases and intensive critical care for patients with severe neurological and respiratory complications are recommended measures.

### Prevention and Control

Being a zoonotic disease, control of virus transmission in animal hosts mainly pigs is the primary preventive measure. In case of an outbreak, prompt quarantine of animal premises is required. Strict infection control practices can prevent human-to-human transmission. Awareness generation among the public to reduce

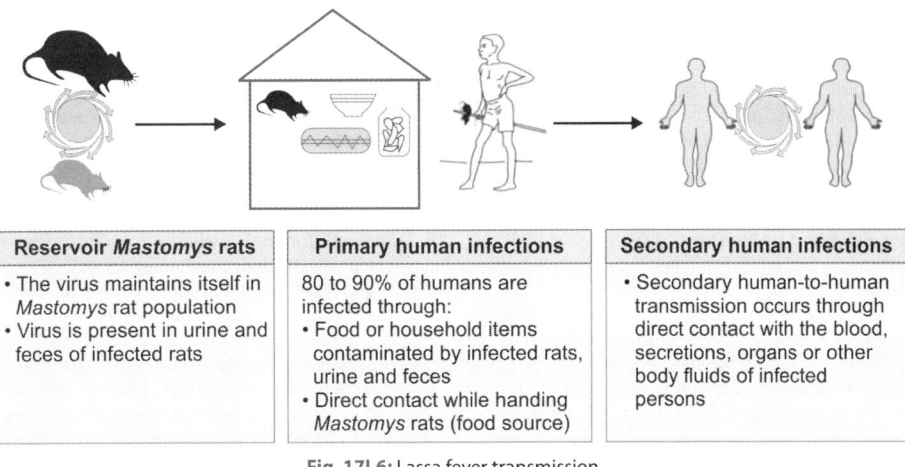

Fig. 17I.6: Lassa fever transmission.
Source: World Health Organization.

chances of exposure to the virus should parallel other preventive efforts.

## LASSA FEVER

Lassa fever is mainly a zoonotic disease causes hemorrhagic fever which was recognized in the year 1969. The virus belongs to the family *Arenaviridae* and is a single-stranded retrovirus. Lassa fever is endemic to the West African countries like Benin, Ghana, Guinea, Liberia and Mali. The transmission of disease occurs from the secretions of the infected rodent (*Mastomys* rats), infected needles and other contaminated medical equipment leads to person-to-person transmission, sexual route, poor sanitary conditions, overcrowding poses additional risk to people **(Fig. 17I.6)**.

**Incubation period:** Range from 6–21 days.

### Clinical Features

Nearly 80% of the cases are asymptomatic. The disease presents with prodromal phase includes febrile illness with weakness and malaise, followed by non-specific symptoms like headache, sore throat, cough, myalgia, chest pain and gastrointestinal symptoms of abdominal pain, diarrhea, nausea and vomiting. One-fifth of the patients may develop multiple organ dysfunctions, with the involvement of liver, spleen and kidneys that is fatal unless treated intensively. Case fatality rate is 1-15%. Disease residue is seen in the form of temporary deafness (25%), others being disturbances in gait and short-term hair loss. Most of the deaths occur within two weeks of the onset of disease. In pregnancy, more severe forms of the disease are seen, resulting in high maternal and fetal mortality.

### Diagnosis

The clinical course of the disease is varied and complex, and direct diagnosis in affected patients is challenging. Reverse transcriptase-polymerase chain reaction (RT-PCR) assay, antibody detection by enzyme-linked immunosorbent assay (ELISA), tests for detection of viral antigen and cell culture for isolation of virus are used to make the confirmed diagnosis. The specimens used for laboratory investigations are likely to be hazardous and should be handled cautiously.

### Treatment

Early containment of disease is possible through speedy isolation of patients, meticulous contact tracing and stringent infection control practices during outbreaks. Survival can be efficiently improved by prompt supportive and symptomatic care. Ribavirin is an antiviral drug, to be used in the early course of the disease.

### Prevention and Control

Key to prevention from infection is the promotion of good "community hygiene". Rodents should not be allowed to enter homes. Contact with blood and other body fluids of patients should be avoided. Special precautions should be taken by the healthcare workers while in close contact (within 1 meter) or treating the infected cases, presumptive Lassa fever or other hemorrhagic fever. Standard precautions, including personal protective equipment's use, safe injection practices should be enforced. After death, handling of corpses should be done safely.

## SUGGESTED READING

1. Centers for Disease Control and Prevention. (2005). Lassa fever. [online] Available from http://www.ncbi.nlm.nih.gov/pubmed/11987809/.
2. Chang LY, Tan, CT. Nipah virus infection. Viral Infect Hum Nerv Syst. 2013;317-36.
3. Ebola Outbreak Epidemiology Team. The outbreak of Ebola virus disease in the Democratic Republic of the Congo, April-May, 2018: an epidemiological study. Lancet. 2018;392(10143):213-21.
4. Folarin OA, Ehichioya D, Schaffner SF, et al. Ebola virus epidemiology and evolution in Nigeria. The Journal of Infectious Diseases. 2016;214 (suppl_3): S102-9.
5. Gregory CJ, Oduyebo T, Brault AC, et al. Modes of Transmission of Zika Virus. J Infect Dis. 2017;216(Suppl_10): S875-83.
6. Gurley ES, Montgomery JM, Hossain MJ, et al. Person-to-person transmission of Nipah virus in a Bangladeshi community. Emerg Infect Dis. 2007;13(7):1031-7.

7. Hageman JC, Hazim C, Wilson K, et al. Infection Prevention and Control for Ebola in Health Care Settings—West Africa and the United States. MMWR Suppl. 2016;65(3):50-6.
8. Hefferon KL. Tropical Medicine and Surgery Applications of Plant-derived Vaccines for Developing Countries. Trop Med Surg. 2013;1(1):1-4.
9. Jaenisch T, Rosenberger KD, Brady O, et al. Risk of microcephaly after Zika virus infection in Brazil, 2015 to 2016. Bull World Health Organ. 2018;95(3):191-8.
10. Kindhauser MK, Allen T, Frank V, et. al. Zika: the origin and spread of a mosquito-borne virus. Bull World Health Organ. 2016;94(9): 675-86C.
11. Krow-Lucal ER, Biggerstaff BJ, Staples JE. Estimated Incubation Period for Zika Virus Disease. Emerg Infect Dis. 2017;23(5):841-4.
12. Management C. (2017). Nigeria centre for disease control Nigeria centre for disease control standard operating procedures for Lassa Fever Case Management Standard Operating Procedures for Lassa Fever Case Management Nigeria centre ford is ease control.[online] Available from http:// www.ncdc.gov.ng/themes/common/docs/protocols/30_1502277315.pdf/.
13. Martínez MJ, Salim AM, Hurtado JC, et al. Ebola Virus Infection: Overview and Update on Prevention and Treatment. Infect Dis Ther. 2015;4(4):365-90.
14. McCormick JB, King IJ, Webb PA, et al. Lassa fever. Effective therapy with ribavirin. N Engl J Med.1986;314(1):20-6.
15. Narasiman M. Laboratory Diagnosis of Nipah Virus Infection. 2015;1999-2001.
16. Raabe V, Koehler J. Laboratory diagnosis of Lassa fever. J ClinMicrobiol. 2017;55(6):1629-37.
17. Republic U, States F, Polynesia F. (2018). Zika virus Key facts: Complications of Zika viral disease. [online] Available from http:// www.who.int/news-room/fact-sheets/detail/zika-virus/.
18. Richmond JK, Baglole DJ. Lassa fever: epidemiology, clinical features, and social consequences. BMJ. 2003;327(7426):1271-5.
19. Sullivan N, Yang ZY, Nabel GJ. Ebola virus pathogenesis: Implications for vaccines and therapies. J Virol. 2003;77(18):9733-7.
20. WHO. Prioritizing diseases for research and development in emergency contexts. Accessed in October 2023 from https://www.who.int/activities/prioritizing-diseases-for-research-and-development-in-emergency-contexts.
21. WHO. Targeting research on diseases of greatest epidemic and pandemic threat. WHO R&D Blueprint for Epidemics. Accessed in October 2023 from https://www.who.int/teams/blueprint/who-r-and-d-blueprint-for-epidemics)CDC. Key Messages–Ebola Virus Disease, West Africa. 2015; (November):1-28.
22. WHO Research and Development Blueprint. (2018). 2018 Annual review of diseases prioritized under the R&D Blueprint. (Meeting Report). [online] Available from http://www.who.int/emergencies/diseases/2018prioritization-report.pdf/.
23. World Health Organization. (2015). WHO Ebola vaccines, therapies, and diagnostics. [online] Available from http://www.who.int/medicines/emp_ebola_q_as/en/.
24. World Health Organization. (2016).Laboratory testing for Zika virus infection: Interim guidance. [online] Available from http://www.who.int/csr/resources/publications/zika/laboratory-testing/en/.
25. World Health Organization. (2018). Emergencies preparedness, response– Nipah virus—India. [online] Available from http://www.who.int/csr/don/31-may-2018-nipah-virus-india/en/.
26. World Health Organization. (2018). Nipah virus: key fact. [online] Available from www.who.int/news-room/fact-sheets/detail/nipah-virus/.
27. World Health Organization. What we know about transmission of the Ebola virus among humans. Media centre; news releases. 2014;2014(10–10):2014-6.
28. Yadav PD, Niyas VK, Arjun R, Sahay RR, Shete AM, Sapkal GN, et al. Detection of Zika virus disease in Thiruvananthapuram, Kerala, India 2021 during the second wave of COVID-19 pandemic. Journal of Medical Virology. 2022;94(6):2346.
29. Zika A, Spreads HZ, Zika C, et al. (2018). Zika basics zika: the basics of the virus and how to protect against it. Why Zika is Risky for Some People How to Prevent Zika. [online] Available from https://www.cdc.gov/zika/pdfs/fs-zika-basics.pdf/.

# CORONAVIRUS INDUCED DISEASE (COVID-19)

*Forhad Akhtar Zaman*

The COVID-19 pandemic otherwise known as the coronavirus pandemic, is an ongoing pandemic of coronavirus disease 2019 (COVID-19), caused by severe acute respiratory syndrome (SARSCoV2).

Corona viruses are a group or related RNA viruses that cause disease in mammals and birds. In humans, these viruses cause respiratory tract infections, which ranges from mild to lethal infections. Mild illness include some cases of common cold, while more lethal varieties can cause SARS, MERS and COVID-19.

They are enveloped viruses with a positive sense single stranded RNA genome and a nucleocapsid of helical symmetry. They have characteristic club shaped spikes that project from their surface, which in electron micrographs create an image resembling solar corona, from which this virus got it's name.

The COVID-19 outbreak was first identified in Wuhan, China, in December 2019. The World Health Organization (WHO) declared the outbreak a public health emergency of international concern on 30th January 2020, and a pandemic on 11th March 2020. As of 9th January 2024 more than 701.2 million cases of COVID-19 have been reported in more than 188 countries and territories resulting in more than 6.9 million deaths (worldometers.info).

## EPIDEMIOLOGY

There are three types of transmission: "droplet" and "contact", which are associated with large droplets, and "airborne", which is associated with small droplets. If the droplets are above a certain critical size, they settle faster than they evaporate, and therefore they contaminate surfaces surrounding them. Droplets that are below a certain critical size, evaporate faster than they settle; due to that fact, they form nuclei that remain airborne for a long period of time overextensive distances. Transmission occurs mainly when people are in close contact (two metres or six feet) via small droplets produced as a result of coughing, sneezing, or talking. Contaminated droplets exhaled by people who are infected are then inhaled into the lungs, or they settle on other people's faces and eyes to cause new infection. The droplets are relatively heavy, usually fall to surfaces which contaminates it and can act as fomites to further transmit the infection through hands when it comes in contact with such fomites. It does not travel far through the air. However, infection can occur over longer distances, particularly indoors.

Infectivity can begin four to five days before the onset of symptoms. The incubation period is 2 to 14 days with a mean of about 5-6 days. Infected people can spread the disease even if they are pre-symptomatic or asymptomatic. Most commonly, the peak viral load in upper respiratory tract samples occurs close to the time of symptom onset and declines after the first week after symptoms begin. Current evidence suggests a duration of viral shedding and the period of infectiousness of up to ten days following symptom onset for people with mild to moderate COVID-19, and up to 20 days for persons with severe COVID-19, including immunocompromised people.

Sputum and saliva carry large amount of viruses. Kissing, intimate contact, and feco-oral routes are also suspected to transmit the virus. Some medical procedures which are aerosol- generating transmits the virus more easily.

The virus can be transmitted in any climatic condition, hot humid or cold and evidence so far shows that it can survive and has the potential to infect in both hot and cold climatic conditions.

As of December 2021, there are five dominant variants of SARS-CoV-2 spreading among global populations: the Alpha variant (B.1.1.7, formerly called the UK variant), first found in London and Kent, the Beta variant (B.1.351, formerly called the South Africa variant), the Gamma variant (P.1, formerly called the Brazil variant), the Delta variant (B.1.617.2, formerly called the India variant), and the Omicron variant (B.1.1.529), which had spread to 57 countries as of 7 December. On December 19, 2023, the WHO declared that another distinctive variant, JN.1, had emerged as a "variant of interest." Though the WHO expects an increase in cases globally, particularly for countries entering winter, the current overall global health risk (as of December 21, 2023) remains low.

## CLINICAL FEATURES

COVID-19 is highly transmissible and the most common symptoms are dry cough, breathlessness and high-grade fever. Other symptoms that are less common and may affect some patients include aches and pains, nasal congestion, headache, conjunctivitis, sore throat, diarrhea, loss of taste or smell or a rash on skin or discoloration of fingers or toes. These symptoms are usually mild and begin gradually. Some people become infected but only have very mild symptoms. Most people (about 80%) recover from the disease without needing hospital treatment. Around 1 out of every 5 people who gets COVID-19 becomes seriously ill and develops difficulty breathing. Older people, and those with underlying medical problems like high blood pressure, heart and lung problems, diabetes, or cancer, are at higher risk of developing serious illness and high mortality rate. As per various reports, 80% of the total cases are asymptomatic, 15% with mild symptoms whereas 5% with serious condition, with an average mortality rate of 2-4%. Severe pneumonia is one of the most common complications, which may require ventilator support. Other complications include Acute Respiratory Failure, Acute Respiratory Distress Syndrome, Disseminated Intravascular Coagulation, Secondary infection and Septic shock.

## DIAGNOSIS

As the symptoms of COVID-19 is very much similar to other influenza diseases, diagnosis mainly depends on thermal screening to detect fever with other symptoms of Influenza like Illness (ILI) and history of patient (travel and contact history with confirmed COVID-19 case) but we can confirm the diagnosis only after laboratory test. Diagnostic testing has played the pivotal role for not only in disease management but also in case identification and infection control. Molecular tests like Real-time reverse transcription-polymerase chain reaction (rRT-PCR) is the gold standard for COVID-19 diagnosis. In India, True Nat, which is an indigenously developed Chip-based Real Time PCR test for *Mycobacterium tuberculosis* was also used for both screening and confirmation of covid -19 cases. Various countries have their own strategy for Covid-19 testing which have been changing as per the dynamics of evolving epidemiological information, stage of the epidemic and available resources for testing. The Covid-19 testing protocol as of September 2020 is shown in **Figure 17I.7**.

Rapid antigen testing has been included in the algorithm of coronavirus testing in India by ICMR. It is a rapid point-of-care nasopharyngeal swab test that directly detects the presence or absence of coronavirus antigen in the patient's body, generating diagnosis results within 30 minutes. These tests are designed to detect a specific protein in the virus that elicits the body's immune response. The rapid detection test kit has been able to achieve 99.3 to 100% accuracy in detecting the true negativity. However, the specificity to discover the true positive is between 50.6% to 80%. Thus, the negative results from an antigen test may need to be confirmed with a molecular PCR test. Also, the testing must be done by maintaining the kit temperature between 2° and 30°C, and so the kit will be used in containment zones or hotspots and hospital settings only.

Rapid serology testing has also been used in some countries for serosurveillance and also for determining the infection status in combination with molecular results.

## TREATMENT

The treatment and management of COVID-19 combines both supportive care, which includes treatment to relieve symptoms, fluid therapy, oxygen support as needed, and a growing list of approved medications. Highly effective vaccines have reduced mortality related to SARS-CoV-2; however, for those awaiting vaccination, as well as for the estimated millions of immunocompromised persons who are unlikely to respond robustly to vaccination, treatment remains important.

Most cases of COVID-19 are mild. In these, supportive care includes medication such as paracetamol or NSAIDs to relieve symptoms (fever, body aches, cough), proper intake of fluids, rest, and nasal breathing. Good personal hygiene and a healthy diet are also recommended. As of April 2020, the U.S. Centers for Disease Control and Prevention (CDC) recommended that those who suspect they are carrying the virus isolate themselves at home and wear a face mask. Use of the glucocorticoid dexamethasone had been strongly recommended in those severe cases treated in hospital with low oxygen levels, to reduce the risk of death. Noninvasive ventilation and, ultimately, admission to an intensive care unit for mechanical ventilation may be required to support breathing. Extracorporeal membrane oxygenation (ECMO) has

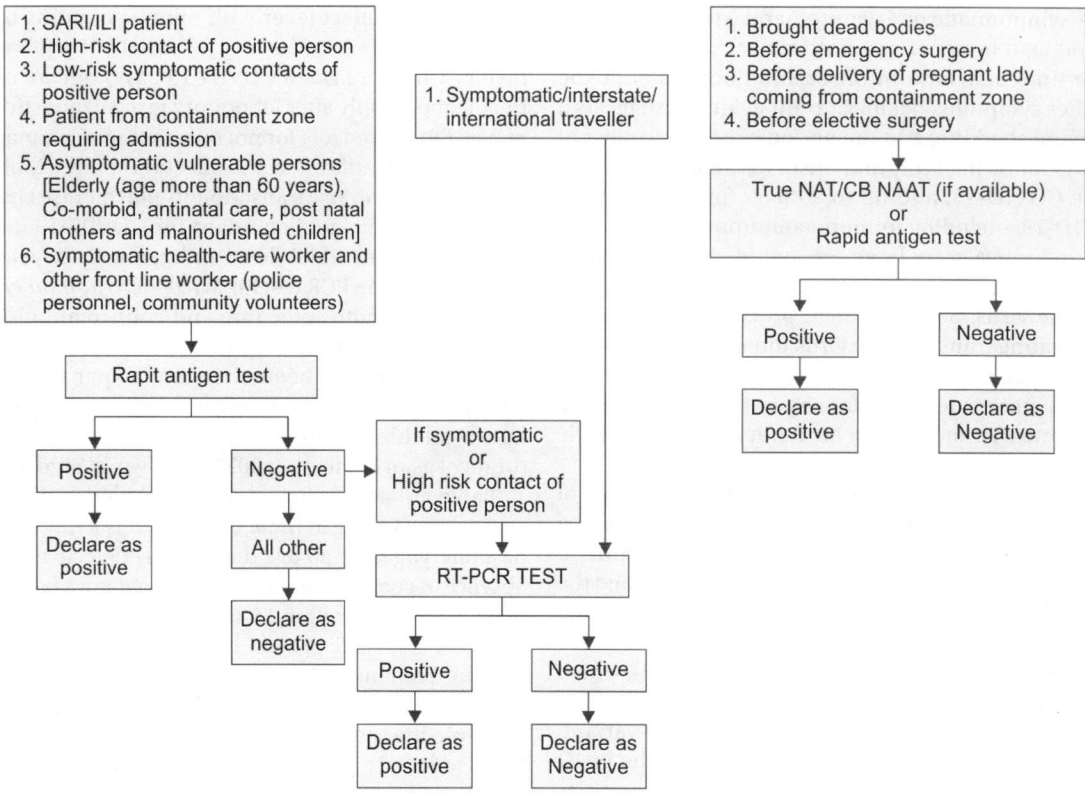

**Fig.17I.7:** COVID-19: testing protocol.

been used to address respiratory failure, but its benefits are still under consideration.

Although several medications have been approved in different countries as of April 2022, not all countries have these medications. Patients with mild to moderate symptoms who are in the risk groups can take nirmatrelvir/ritonavir (marketed as Paxlovid) or remdesivir, either of which reduces the risk of serious illness or hospitalization. Several experimental treatments are being actively studied in clinical trials. These include the antivirals molnupiravir and nirmatrelvir/ritonavir. Others were thought to be promising early in the pandemic, such as hydroxychloroquine and lopinavir/ritonavir, but later research found them to be ineffective or even harmful.

Tocilizumab, an immunosuppressive drug given in combination with other drugs was believed to prevent the cytokine release syndrome, reduce the risk of invasive mechanical ventilation and death in patients with severe COVID-19 pneumonia. Vitamin D, Vitamin C and zinc has also been tried along with the other drugs to reduce the duration of symptoms in patients.

## PREVENTION

Quarantine of people who were exposed and isolation of the infected persons after testing positive along with nationwide or area specific lockdown strategy were the common preventive measures adopted by various countries to contain the pandemic. Restricting movements of vulnerable people, prohibition of spitting in public places, immediate reporting to health authorities with symptoms of ILI, advisories to avoid any type of congregations and unnecessary travel are some other administrative measures adopted to stop spread of the infection.

Preventive measures to reduce the chances of infection include getting vaccinated, staying at home, wearing a mask in public, avoiding crowded places, keeping distance from others, ventilating indoor spaces, managing potential exposure durations, washing hands with soap and water often and for at least twenty seconds, practicing good respiratory hygiene, and avoiding touching the eyes, nose, or mouth with unwashed hands.

*Social distancing* (also known as physical distancing) which includes infection control actions intended to slow the spread of the disease by minimizing close contact between individuals was adopted by various countries to limit the transmission of infection. Methods include quarantines; travel restrictions; and the closing of schools, workplaces, stadiums, theatres, or shopping centres. Individuals may apply social distancing methods by staying at home, limiting travel, avoiding crowded areas, using no-contact greetings, and physically distancing themselves from others

### COVID-19 Vaccines

Initially, most COVID-19 vaccines were two-dose vaccines, with the sole exception being the single-dose Janssen COVID-19 vaccine. However, immunity from the vaccines has been found to wane over time, requiring people to get booster doses of the vaccine to maintain protection against COVID-19. Some of the vaccines approved for emergency use during the pandemic are:

- **Pfizer–BioNTech and Moderna vaccines,** use RNA to stimulate an immune response. When introduced into human tissue, the vaccine contains either self-replicating RNA or messenger RNA (mRNA), which both cause cells to express the SARS-CoV-2 spike protein. This teaches the body how to identify and destroy the corresponding pathogen. RNA vaccines are the first COVID-19 vaccines to be authorized in the United Kingdom, the United States, and the European Union.
- ***Oxford–AstraZeneca COVID-19 vaccine, the Sputnik V COVID-19 vaccine, and the Janssen COVID-19 vaccine*** are examples of non-replicating viral vector vaccines using an adenovirus shell containing DNA that encodes a SARS-CoV-2 protein.
- The other two vaccines—Oxford University's and Serum Institute of India's '**Covishield**' and Bharat Biotech's '**Covaxin**'— received emergency use approval from the government of India. Both are two-dose vaccines, which will have to be administered at a gap of 28 days. Covishield is recombinant COVID-19 vaccine based on Viral Vector Technology. Covaxin is whole-virion inactivated coronavirus vaccine. The efficacy of these two dose vaccines are reported to be in the range of 60–70%

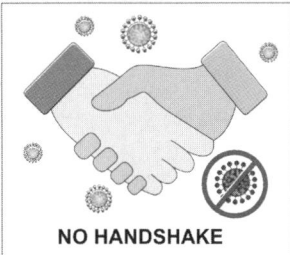
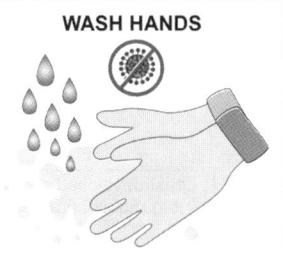
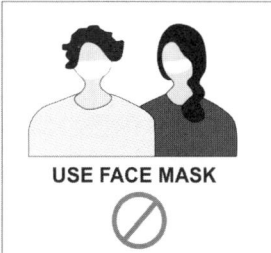
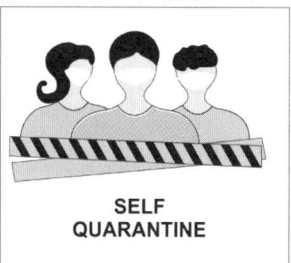
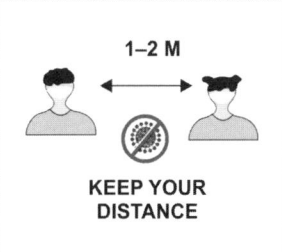
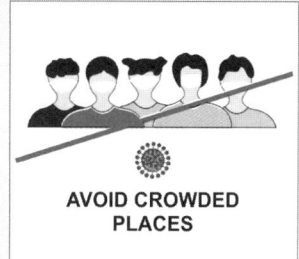

## SUGGESTED READING

1. https://www.mohfw.gov.in/pdf/GuidelinesonClinicalManagementofCOVID1912020.pdf.
2. Huang C, Wang Y, Li X, Ren L, Zhao J, Hu Y, et al. (February 2020). "Clinical features of patients infected with 2019 novel coronavirus in Wuhan, China". Lancet. 2019;395(10223): 497–506.
3. To KK, Tsang OT, Chik-Yan Yip C, Chan KH, Wu TC, Chan JM, et al. (February 2020). "Consistent detection of 2019 novel coronavirus in saliva". Clinical Infectious Diseases. Oxford University Press. doi:10.1093/cid/ciaa149. PMC 7108139. PMID 32047895.
4. Tran K, Cimon K, Severn M, Pessoa-Silva CL, Conly J (2012). "Aerosol generating procedures and risk of transmission of acute respiratory infections to healthcare workers: a systematic review". PLOS ONE. 7 (4): e35797. Bibcode:2012PLoSO...735797T.
5. "COVID-19 and Our Communities -ACON – We are a New South Wales based health promotion organisation specialising in HIV prevention, HIV support and lesbian, gay, bisexual, transgender and intersex (LGBTI) health". Acon. org.au. Retrieved 29 April 2020.
6. "COVID-19 Dashboard by the Center for Systems Science and Engineering (CSSE) at Johns Hopkins University (JHU)". ArcGIS. Johns Hopkins University. Retrieved 27 May 2020.
7. "Getting a handle on asymptomatic SARS-CoV-2 infection | Scripps Research". www.scripps.edu. Retrieved 16 May 2020.
8. "How COVID-19 Spreads". Centers for Disease Control and Prevention (CDC). 2 April 2020. Archived from the original on 3 April 2020. Retrieved 3 April2020.
9. "Naming the coronavirus disease (COVID-19) and the virus that causes it". World Health Organization (WHO).
10. "Novel Coronavirus—China". World Health Organization (WHO). Retrieved 9 April 2020.
11. "Q&A on coronaviruses (COVID-19)". World Health Organization (WHO). 17 April 2020. Archived from the original on 14 May 2020. Retrieved 14 May 2020.
12. "Q & A on COVID-19". European Centre for Disease Prevention and Control. Retrieved 30 April 2020.
13. "Sex and Coronavirus Disease 2019 (COVID-19)" (PDF). nyc.gov. 27 March 2020. Retrieved 29 April 2020.
14. "Statement on the second meeting of the International Health Regulations (2005) Emergency Committee regarding the outbreak of novel coronavirus (2019-nCoV)". World Health Organization (WHO). 30 January 2020. Archived from the original on 31 January 2020. Retrieved 30 January 2020.
15. "WHO Director-General's opening remarks at the media briefing on COVID-19—11 March 2020". World Health Organization. 11 March 2020.

# CHAPTER 18

# General Epidemiology of Noncommunicable Diseases and its Prevention and Control

*Dinesh Kumar*

*"The secret of health for both mind and body is not to mourn for the past, not to worry about the future, or not to anticipate troubles, but to live the present moment wisely and earnestly."*

—**Buddha**

**CM 7.2** Enumerate, describe and discuss the mode of transmission and measures for prevention and control of noncommunicable diseases

**CM 8.2** Describe and discuss the epidemiology and control measures applicable in noncommunicable diseases

### Activity

1. Try to recall last 10 deaths that you were involved with [As family member/relative/friend/in medicine ward]. What were the cause of death?
2. Try to recall last 10 cases admitted in general medicine ward [As seen by you during your recent medicine clinical postings]. What was the diagnosis for these cases?

Now try to classify these diseases as infectious [caused by known pathogens] or noninfectious/communicable [No known pathogen involved]. We predict that most of you would have identified more cases in non-communicable group in both cases. Does it surprise you?

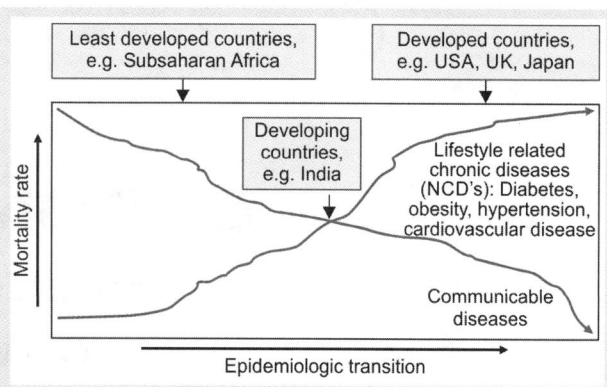

**Fig. 18.1:** A schematic representation of changes in the overall trend in the proportional mortality due to communicable and noncommunicable diseases (NCDs).

### Note

As the countries move up along the economic development ladder there is shift in the leading causes of mortality from communicable diseases to NCDs. This transition has been caused by several factors like increased longevity, changing lifestyle and environmental changes.

## INTRODUCTION

Toward the later part of 20th century, world has undergone phenomenon of "epidemiological transition". This refers to gross changes in the diseases causing morbidity and mortality from communicable to noncommunicable in nature **(Fig. 18.1)**.

Current mortality data from all over the world suggests that more deaths are due to noncommunicable diseases (NCDs) in most countries of world. Noncommunicable diseases (NCDs) kill 41 million people each year, equivalent to 74% of all deaths globally. Each year, 17 million people die from a NCD before age 70; 86% of these premature deaths occur in low- and middle-income countries. Of all NCD deaths, 77% are in low- and middle-income countries.

Cardiovascular diseases account for most NCD deaths or 17.9 million people annually, followed by cancers (9.3 million), chronic respiratory diseases (4.1 million), and diabetes (2.0 million including kidney disease deaths caused by diabetes). These four groups of diseases account for over 80% of all premature NCD deaths.

In India also, NCDs contribute to around two-thirds of mortality. Data for morbidity also follows similar trends. Overall impact of NCDs in India has been summarized in **Table 18.1**.

## CONCEPTS AND DEFINITIONS

NCDs refer to a group of diseases where there are no known pathogens that cause the disease and these cannot be transmitted from one person to another. These are usually caused by an array of internal factors (usually metabolic, immunity related, etc.) but may have a set of external factors (environmental). They are usually longstanding and caused by combination of physiological and environmental behaviors and genetic factors. As there is no specific cause-effect relationship, each of these contributing factors is referred to as risk factor. Presence of a

## Chapter 18: General Epidemiology of Noncommunicable Diseases and its Prevention and Control

Table 18.1: Impact of noncommunicable diseases (NCDs) in India.

| Health impact | Economic impact | Societal impact |
|---|---|---|
| NCDs account for 55% of disease burden and 63% of all deaths in India | Diabetes, heart diseases and stroke cost India $ 237 billion in income from 2005–15 | Overall decreased well-being of population |
| Over 20% of the population in India has at least one chronic disease | NCDs are estimated to cost India $ 3.55 trillion during the period 2012–30 | Health care expenditure eating into resources for other needs of the households |
| Probability of NCD related death during the most productive years is 26% | India could lose $ 4.8 trillion in lost economic output by 2030 due to NCDs and mental health | Premature mortality leading to problematic families and societies |
| Increased strain on the existing health systems | 60 million Indians are pushed into poverty annually due to out-of-pocket health expenditures | Increased care burden on family members leading to loss of other opportunities for development |

risk factor increases the chances of having a disease but in itself is not sufficient to cause the disease. Also, usually most NCDs have several risk factors and most risk factors are associated with several diseases. The WHO has defined risk factor as *"any attribute, characteristic or exposure of an individual that increases the likelihood of developing a disease or injury."*

## GENERAL RISK FACTORS

There are a large number of risk factors associated with NCD. The key identified factors for this transition are tobacco use, physical inactivity, the harmful use of alcohol, and unhealthy diets. Also, these risk factors are usually clustered and need to be addressed together for effective prevention of NCDs. From point of view of prevention, these risk factors may be divided as modifiable or nonmodifiable.

Modifiable risk factors, as name suggests, are amenable for changes relatively easily by the individuals concerned. Modifiable risk factors are presented in **Figure 18.2**.

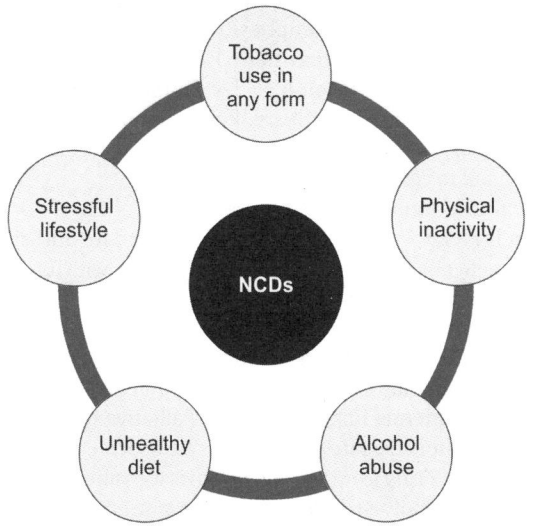

Fig. 18.2: Modifiable risk factors for noncommunicable diseases (NCDs).

Modifiable risk factors form the main content of any intervention to prevent NCD.

Nonmodifiable risk factors are not amenable to change. These include:
- Genetic make up
- Race and ethnicity
- Gender
- Increasing age
- Family history.

Nonmodifiable risk factors are usually used to identify the high-risk individual for NCD screening programs.

### Case study/Activity
Form pairs and list the risk factors identified in a family member suffering from NCDs. Facilitator to list all the identified risk factors for individual disease and summarize.

Other factors which improve the overall outcome and decrease complications in NCD include regular screening, treatment compliance, good primary healthcare, and availability of services related to NCDs in public health programs, overall health policies, etc. These factors interact to form what is commonly known as web of causation. Web of causation refers to complex interactions between various risk factors, ultimately leading to development of disease in question.

### Case study/Activity
Divide yourselves into small groups of around 10 each. Each group will prepare a web of causation for important NCDs like cardiovascular diseases, stroke, diabetes, obesity, etc. Share the activity with entire class.

### Key Points
- Epidemiological transition refers to gross changes in the diseases causing morbidity and mortality from communicable to noncommunicable in nature
- The key identified factors for the epidemiological transition are tobacco use, physical inactivity, the harmful use of alcohol, and unhealthy diet.
- From point of view of prevention, these risk factors may be divided as modifiable or non-modifiable.
- Web of causation refers to complex interactions between various risk factors, ultimately leading to development of disease in question.

## GENERAL PRINCIPLES OF PREVENTION AND CONTROL

Prevention refers to measures aimed at decreasing the occurrence of NCD or its complications, whereas control refers to decreasing the deleterious effects of the disease among individuals or communities. The terms tend to overlap in several instances as there are no clear-cut boundaries between the two. All the levels of prevention have important role in prevention and control of NCD. Given below are some examples of various levels of preventions as used for NCDs.

### Primordial Prevention

This refers to decrease the appearance of risk factors in the community or individuals. For example, a school program focusing on preventing the students from picking up habit of tobacco use or inculcating regular physical activity in school curriculum, etc.

### Primary Prevention

This refers to prevention of occurrence of disease among those who have high risk, e.g. a program among industrial workers focusing on quitting tobacco or a stress management workshop.

### Secondary Prevention

This refers to identifying the disease in very early stage and suitably managing it. For example, screening of tobacco chewers for premalignant lesions and self-monitoring of blood pressure at home among those with family history of hypertension.

### Tertiary Prevention

This refers to attempts made at limiting the disability or complications caused by disease, e.g. providing rehabilitation services for stroke patients, providing palliative care to those with advanced cancers (palliative care is an approach based at improving the quality of life of individuals and families suffering from life-threatening or life-limiting health conditions).

### Quaternary Prevention

This refers to safeguarding against the hazards that can result from over medicalization or over treatment, e.g. irrational promotion of vaccinations not proven to be effective, avoidance of rampant use of general health check-up or full body check-ups, offering end of life care options at home or hospice for terminally ill-patients. Quaternary prevention is unique in an overarching safeguard against other three levels of prevention. It aims to safeguard against irrational use of preventive, diagnostic, and curative medical interventions.

## APPROACHES FOR PREVENTION AND CONTROL OF NCDs

While these levels of prevention can be applied individually in a tailored manner, while considering these for community level interventions several factors need to be looked at. These would in turn lead to various approaches for applying preventive measures in a large community setting. These approaches could be:

- **High-risk approach**: This approach focuses on individuals with identified high risk for targeting the prevention measure, e.g. mammography for women with history of breast cancer in mother or sister or decreased salt intake by those with borderline hypertension. This approach provides high level of direct benefit to participants, usually involves lower cost, and is more acceptable in communities. This however may not necessarily be the most cost-effective approach.
- **Population approach**: This approach involves applying the preventive measures to all the individuals of a community irrespective of their risk status, e.g. teaching self-breast examination to all women of reproductive age or providing hepatitis B vaccine to all infants (to prevent hepatocellular carcinoma). This approach does not provide benefit to all the participants however overall impact on community is significant. Also overall acceptance of this approach may be lower due to absence of direct benefits. Population approaches usually tend to be cost-effective.
- **Disease-specific approach**: This approach focuses on a particular disease and involves several interventions aimed at various aspects of disease prevention and control, e.g. Erstwhile National Cancer Control Program of India. Program had provisions for early cancer screening, treatment, and community awareness activities. Such disease-specific programs are very costly to run and may lead to duplications of several activities which may be common to several diseases.
- **Life course approach**: As NCDs have several risk factors scattered across the life of individuals from womb till quite late in life, it will be imperative that any approach to control NCDs should address this aspect. The approach should start with preconception care and maternal nutrition. Scientifically sound and culturally acceptable infant feeding practices, including breastfeeding should be promoted. Promoting healthy lifestyle beginning from pre-school age right into early adulthood is key importance. This needs to be complemented with promoting healthy lifestyle, healthy aging and care for people with NCDs.

However, given the multiple common risk factors involved, an integrated approach focusing on the key services and risk factors for leading NCDs may be a better approach. Such an integrated approach should encompass evidence-based key interventions across the spectrum of prevention. Some key interventions could be:

- **Health promotion (lifestyle modification)**: For example, increased physical activity, yoga, preventing and quitting tobacco addictions, encouraging healthy diet, behavior change communication activities, and life skill education for school children.
- **Screening**: Screening for hypertension, diabetes mellitus, common cancers, mental disorders, chronic obstructive pulmonary disorder, and obesity. Screening programs may adopt high-risk approach to start with and shift to population-based approaches in later phase.
- **Early diagnosis and treatment**: Facilities for early diagnosis and treatment of common NCDs should be made available as part of primary healthcare. Point-of-care diagnostic tests and locally developed algorithm-based treatment protocols will need to be adopted.
- **Rehabilitation and palliative care**: Most of the NCDs (other than few cancers) do not have a definitive cure and available treatment needs to be continued for entire life with intermittent events of crisis needing intensive medical care. This calls for availability of rehabilitative services (to improve functional status) and palliative care services (to improve quality of life of patient and families). These are also needed to counter the social and mental impact of NCDs. Palliative care focuses on providing holistic care (physical, psychosocial, and spiritual) to those suffering from serious health issues and their families. Though initially started for cancer patients, the concept has now been extended to all diseases and even those with

unidentified serious illnesses. Experts now call for integrating palliative care for all diseases, all ages, and all stages in primary healthcare.

For integrated approach to be successful, well laid out indicators (input, process, output, outcome) need to be identified. Also, entire health system of the country will require re-orientation from communicable diseases to NCD mode. All levels of healthcare workers will need training and capacity building. The National Program for Prevention and Control of Cancer, Diabetes, Cardiovascular Diseases, and Stroke (NPCDCS) of India has incorporated most of the components of integrated approach toward NCDs.

Prevention and control of NCDs will require multipronged strategy involving multiple stakeholders.

Here are examples of key stakeholders with some strategies to control obesity **(Fig. 18.3)**.

- *Individuals*: Decide and commit to include physical activity in daily life.
- *Families*: Support individuals in adopting physical activity in daily life by allowing dedicated time and may be a pair of sports shoes!
- *Local community*: Planning for having a playground or running track or park when considering use of common area.
- *Government*: Have provision for funding of community parks or playground. Enact regulations for fat content in packed food items.
- *Commercial players*: Develop healthy packed food items. Ensure accurate information and warning on food items.
- *International bodies*: Provide technical guidance and include NCDs in their priority agenda.
- *Funding agencies*: Provide due priority in funding projects related to NCD in their grants.

> **Key Points**
> - The various levels of prevention of NCDs can be classified as primordial, primary, secondary, tertiary and quaternary
> - In a large community setting, the approaches to prevention can be classified as high risk or population or disease specific or life course.
> - The key interventions in NCD control are health promotion (lifestyle modification), screening, early diagnosis and treatment or rehabilitation and palliative care.
> - Prevention and control of NCDs will require multipronged strategy involving multiple stakeholders.

## GLOBAL EFFORTS TO TACKLE NCDs

Over last two decades or so, NCDs have gradually rightfully found place in discussions and priorities of international agencies and national governments. It started with efforts focused on specific issues of tobacco, physical activity, etc. in year at beginning of 21st century. In year 2008, World Health Organization launched action plan for the global strategy for the prevention and control of NCDs **(Fig. 18.4)**. This document marked the shifting global focus on NCDs. The document identified the four key NCDs and four key risk factors for global focus. Various strategies focusing on reorientation of primary healthcare toward NCDs were identified. The same has been emphasized in World Health Day themes related to mental health, road safety, physical activity, elderly, food safety, depression, hypertension, and diabetes. Global Noncommunicable Disease Network (NCDnet), a collaborative network comprising of United Nations agencies, intergovernmental organizations, academic institutes, research centers, nongovernmental organizations, and the business community was launched to provide guidance to the action plan.

Sustainable Development Goals (SDGs) accepted in year 2015 also focused on NCDs as an important health and development priority. SDG target 3.4 aims to reduce the NCD related premature mortality by one-third by 2030.

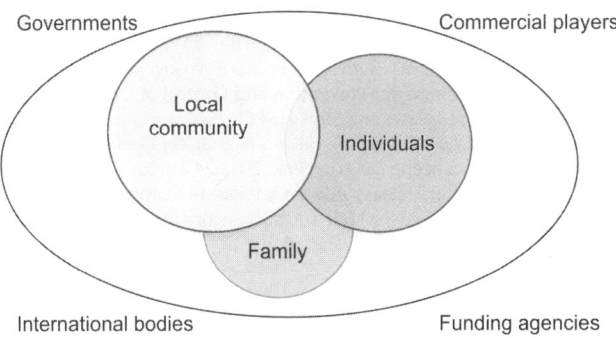

Fig. 18.3: Key players in noncommunicable disease control.

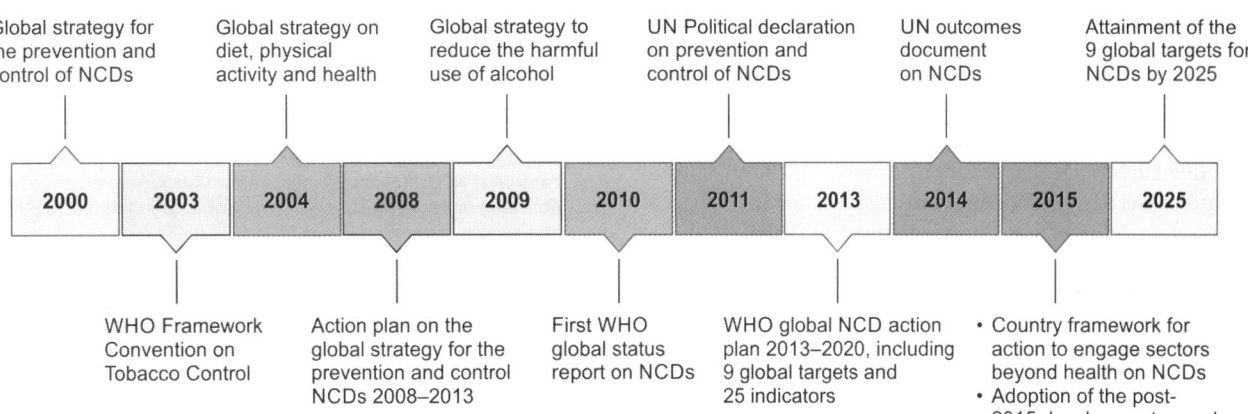

Fig. 18.4: Key global milestones in NCD control.

Current WHO efforts to control NCDs are as per the Global action plan for the prevention and control of NCDs 2013–2020. The plan visualizes a world free of avoidable burden due to NCDs. The plan envisages to raise priority, build capacity at various levels, strengthen and reorient health systems, and monitoring of trends related to NCDs.

The overarching principles of the plan are provided below:

- Life-course approach
- Empowerment of people and communities
- Evidence-based strategies
- Universal health coverage
- Management of real perceived or potential conflicts of interest
- Human rights approach
- Equity-based approach
- National action and international cooperation and solidarity
- Multisectoral action

The plan envisages reduction in the risk factors, availability of treatment, and diagnostic facilities and continues focus on four key NCDs and four risk factors. Detection, screening, and treatment of NCDs, availability of rehabilitative and palliative care services continue to be the key components.

## NATIONAL EFFORTS TO TACKLE NCDs

India, like most other developing middle-income countries, is facing the dual burden of communicable diseases and NCDs. In spite being part most of the international efforts to control NCDs, progress so far has not been adequate. Though the country has launched its Cancer Control Program in 1980s, overall it is focused primarily on increasing access to cancer treatment. This was followed by pilot projects for diabetes control in few districts. India launched its comprehensive NPCDCS in the year 2010. Key strategies adopted include health promotion through behavior change communication, outreach camps, facilities for diagnosis and treatment of NCDs at all levels of care, setting of NCD clinics, capacity building, and development of databases and surveillance system. As a part of newly launched Ayushman Bharat Scheme, Health and Wellness Center will be set up. Basic care for NCDs, palliative care, and geriatric care services will be key services provided through Health and Wellness Center. In the last few years, many new diseases or disease groups have been added to NPCDCS such as non-alcoholic fatty liver, chronic kidney disease, ST-elevation myocardial infarction (STEMI), etc. To this effect, NPCDCS has been renamed by MoHFW in May 2023 as "National Programme for Prevention and Control of Non-Communicable Diseases (NP-NCD)". *NP-NCD is explained in detail in Chapter 47: Health Policies and Programs in India.*

## SUMMARY

- NCDs contribute to about 74% of global mortality.
- Tobacco use, Alcohol use, Physical inactivity, Unhealthy diet, stress are the most important risk factors and from point of view of prevention, these risk factors may be divided as modifiable or non-modifiable.
- Prevention refers to measures aimed at decreasing the occurrence of NCD or its complications, whereas control refers to decreasing the deleterious effects of the disease among individuals or communities.
- Although high-risk approach provides high level of direct benefit to participants, this may not necessarily be the most cost-effective approach.
- Population approach involves applying the preventive measures to all the individuals of a community irrespective of their risk status; this usually tend to be cost-effective.
- Given the multiple common risk factors involved, an integrated approach involving individuals, communities, government and other agencies while focusing on the key services and risk factors is needed.
- Currently, WHO has focused on efforts to control NCDs as per the Global action plan for the prevention and control of NCDs 2013–2020 while SDG target 3.4 aims to reduce the NCD related premature mortality by one-third by 2030.
- India launched its comprehensive NPCDCS in the year 2010. It has been renamed to NP-NCD in May 2023.

## SUGGESTED READING

1. Anjana RM, Ali MK, Pradeepa R, et al. The need for obtaining accurate nationwide estimates of diabetes prevalence in India—rationale for a national study on diabetes. Indian J Med Res. 2011;133(4):369-80.
2. Directorate General of Health Services, MoHFW, Govt of India, New Delhi. National Programme for Prevention and Control of Cancer, Diabetes, Cardiovascular Diseases and Stroke (NPCDCS).
3. Martins C, Godycki-Cwirko M, Heleno B, et al. Quaternary prevention: reviewing the concept: Eur J Gen Prac. 2018;24(1):106-11.
4. PFCD India. NHSRC release Advocacy Paper to sensitize policy makers towards growing burden of NCDs, its socio-economic impact. Partnership to Fight Chronic Disease India; 2016.
5. WHO. NCD India Profile; 2018.
6. WHO. Noncommunicable diseases ; factsheet S. available from https://www.who.int/news-room/fact-sheets/detail/noncommunicable-diseases#:~:text=Noncommunicable%20diseases%20(NCDs)%20kill%2041,%2D%20and%20middle%2Dincome%20countries.
7. WHO. Noncommunicable Diseases Progress Monitor; 2020.
8. World Health Organization, South East Asian Regional Office, New Delhi. Causal-Web Analysis - A Model Approach to Joint Programme Planning; 2005.
9. World Health Organization. Global action plan for the prevention and control of noncommunicable diseases, 2013-2020.
10. World Health Organization. WHO's vision in the prevention and control of NCDs. [online] Available from http://www.emro.who.int/noncommunicable-diseases/who-work/whos-vision-in-the-prevention-and-control-of-ncds.html.

# CHAPTER 19

# Specific Epidemiology of Noncommunicable Diseases

## A. EPIDEMIOLOGY OF HYPERTENSION AND STROKE AND ITS PREVENTION AND CONTROL

### EPIDEMIOLOGY AND PREVENTION OF HYPERTENSION

*Anusha Rashmi, P Amritha Krishna, Varghese Iybu Chacko*

*One way to get high blood pressure is to go mountain climbing over molehills.*
—Earl Wilson

**CM 7.2** Enumerate, describe and discuss the mode of transmission and measures for prevention and control of hypertension

**CM 8.2** Describe and discuss the epidemiological and control measures applicable in Hypertension

## INTRODUCTION

Hypertension is a "condition in which the blood vessels have persistently raised pressure."

## GUIDELINES ON HYPERTENSION

Comparison of guidelines by American College of Cardiology (ACC)/American Heart Association (AHA) and European Society of Cardiology (ESC)/European Society of Hypertension (ESH) are shown in **Table 19A.1**.

**Table 19A.1:** Guidelines on hypertension [Whelton PK et al 2022].

| Parameters | ACC/AHA | ESC/ESH |
|---|---|---|
| Cut-off value for hypertension | <130/80 mm Hg | <140/90 mm Hg |
| Grading of normal pressure | Normal <120/80 mm Hg | Optimal <120/80 mm Hg |
| | Elevated 120-129/80 mm Hg | Normal 120-129/80-84 mm Hg |
| | | High Normal 130-139/85-89 mm Hg |
| Grading of hypertension | Grade 1, 130-139/80-89 mm Hg | Grade 1, 140-159/90-99 mm Hg |
| | Grade 2, ≥140/90 mm Hg | Grade 2, 160-179/100-109 mm Hg |
| | | Grade 3, ≥ 180/110 mm Hg |
| BP targets | < 65 Yrs, < 130/80 mm Hg | < 65 Yrs, <130/80 mm Hg |
| | >65 Yrs, < 130/80 mm Hg | > 65 Yrs, <140/80 mm Hg |

*Note:* Measurement of blood pressure has been explained at the end of the chapter.

## CLASSIFICATION OF HYPERTENSION

### Primary (Essential Hypertension)

Primary hypertension is the most common one with no identifiable cause.

### Secondary Hypertension

When hypertension occurs because of some underlying medical condition or problems then it is known as secondary hypertension.

*Secondary hypertension is caused by:*
- Kidney disorders like renovascular disease and chronic renal disease
- *Disorders of the endocrine system*—hyperthyroidism, Cushing's syndrome and pheochromocytoma, and sleep disorders
- Coarctation of the aorta and non-specific aortoarteritis.

## TRACKING OF BLOOD PRESSURE

Individuals whose pressures are low, show lower blood pressure and those with higher pressures tend to have a higher blood pressure later in life too. Therefore, blood pressure, when tracked from childhood to adulthood of an individual, makes it possible to detect high blood pressure prone individuals.

## WHY IS HYPERTENSION OF PUBLIC HEALTH IMPORTANCE?

### Problem Statement-Global

*Morbidity*

An estimated 1.28 billion adults aged 30–79 years worldwide have hypertension, most (two-thirds) living in low- and middle-income countries. An estimated 46% of adults with hypertension are unaware that they have the condition. Less than half of adults (42%) with hypertension are diagnosed and treated.

Approximately 1 in 5 adults (21%) with hypertension have it under control. One of the global targets for noncommunicable diseases is to reduce the prevalence of hypertension by 33% between 2010 and 2030. (WHO, Global Status Report on NCDs Hypertension; Factsheet, March 2023).

### Mortality

Hypertension is a major cause of premature death worldwide. Worldwide, raised blood pressure is estimated to cause 7.5 million deaths, about 12.8% of the total of all deaths. This accounts for 57 million disability adjusted life years (DALYS) or 3.7% of total DALYS.

### India

The prevalence of hypertension as per the National Family Health Survey (NFHS-4) was found to be 18.1% in 2015-2016, while 21% of females aged over 15 years had hypertension compared to 24% of males of the same age range, as estimated in NFHS-5 (2019–2021).

## RULE OF HALVES (FIG. 19A.1)

In a community half the hypertensives are not diagnosed of the morbidity. Only half of the diagnosed individuals are under treatment. Half of these patients on treatment have their hypertension under control. This concept tries to bring to notice the fact that diseases like hypertension remain undiagnosed in many individuals and even when diagnosed is not adequately treated.

Current evidences from developed countries prove that this concept is changing as the improvement in diagnosis and treatment, decreases the percentage in rule of halves. Rule of halve signifies weaker health system and awareness about the control. The strategies in the national programs are from the traditional understanding of rule of halves and emphasize increasing awareness and treatment. However, in metropolitan cities, the awareness seems to be improved and the proportion of people seeking treatment has substantially increased. Hence, specific strategies need to be emphasized in various regions depending on the level of awareness of percentage getting diagnosed, percentage getting treated, and those with adequate control.

The existing strategy works best in rural and peri-urban areas where rule of halves still holds good. In such situations capacity building of service providers and behavior change strategies to improve compliance to treatment need more emphasize while enhancing the level of awareness.

> **Key Points**
> - Hypertension is a condition in which the blood vessels have persistently raised pressure.
> - Hypertension can be classified into primary and secondary depending on underlying mechanism of causation.
> - Tracking of blood pressure refers to persistence of rank order of blood pressure with increasing age and this makes it possible to detect high blood pressure prone individuals at an early age.
> - Rule of halves is an epidemiological description of the iceberg phenomenon seen in hypertension.

## RISK FACTORS FOR HYPERTENSION

Risk factors of hypertension are classified into modifiable and non-modifiable risk factors.

### Modifiable Risk Factors

#### Behavioral Factors

- *Unhealthy diet:* Diet rich in calories, saturated and trans-fat have an excess risk for high blood pressure.
- *Harmful use of alcohol:* Alcohol reportedly increases the sympathetic system activation. An increased sympathetic outflow increases adrenoreceptor mediated reactions which is vasoconstriction and increase in heart rate. It also causes a release of endothelin 1 and 2 and angiotensin 2 which are potent vasoconstrictors.
- *Physical inactivity:* Physical activity is known to reduce arterial stiffness, vascular resistance, reduce psychosocial stress, reduce sympathetic activity, etc. thus reducing and preventing an increase in blood pressure.
- Tobacco use
- Persistent stress.

#### Metabolic Factors

- Obesity
- Diabetes
- Dyslipidemia

These risk factors have an atherosclerotic effect on the blood vessels, especially the coronary and cerebral blood vessels. The combination of abdominal obesity, uncontrolled glucose (either diabetes or insulin resistance), dyslipidemia along with hypertension, is called the *metabolic syndrome*. These conditions usually coexist and raise the risk of other events like cerebrovascular strokes.

### Non-modifiable Risk Factors

- Socioeconomic status
- Urbanization
- Aging
- Gender
- Ethnicity

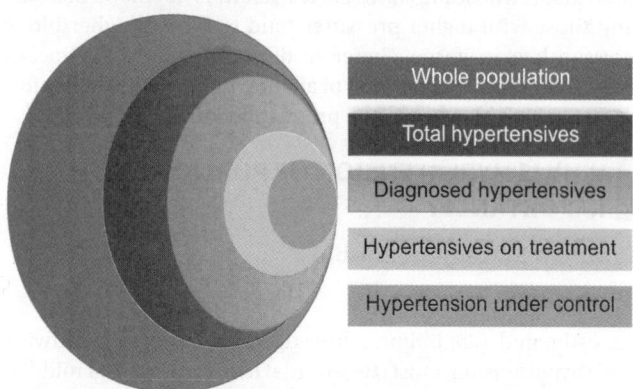

Fig. 19A.1: Rule of halves.

- Race
- Family history
- Co-existing disease like chronic kidney disease

These factors have an impact on the stress levels of an individual. They determine whether or not a person has access to timely diagnosis or treatment. Rapid urbanization develops an unhealthy environment while promoting unhealthy diet, tobacco use, and harmful use of alcohol, which in turn may lead to hypertension. Atherosclerosis in advanced age, ethnicity and sex of an individual are also an important non-modifiable risk factors.

## CLINICAL FEATURES OF HYPERTENSION

- *Asymptomatic*: Most of the patients do not have any symptoms.
- Shortness of breath, chest pain, and palpitations can be features of cardiac in sufficiency.
- *Headache*: It is more prominent in the occipital region.
- *Dizziness*: Dizziness might be associated with postural hypotension especially in older patients.
- Nosebleeds.
- *Family history*: Those with a family history of hypertension are more likely to show high blood pressure.

## COMPLICATIONS OF HYPERTENSION

Hypertension that is uncontrolled or not treated adequately can lead to complications such as aneurysms, chronic kidney disease, retinopathy, heart failure, peripheral artery disease, stroke, etc. also causing severe financial and service burden on the health system.

> **Key Points**
> - Similar to other NCDs, risk factors of hypertension may be described as modifiable which are amenable to prevention strategies and non-modifiable which cannot be changed.
> - Modifiable risk factors can be further described as behavioral (unhealthy diet, harmful alcohol use, tobacco use) and metabolic factors (obesity, diabetes)
> - Hypertension may be asymptomatic in most of the cases.
> - Complications of hypertension include multiple systems, most commonly chronic kidney disease, retinopathy and heart failure.

## MANAGEMENT AND PREVENTION

### Primordial Prevention

#### Salt Reduction Strategies

Around the world food consumption has shifted from more of vegetables and fruits to processed food. Vegetables and fruits contain potassium that helps to lower blood pressure.

"In diet one can find high amounts of salt in processed food like salami, bacon, ham, cheese, salted snacks, instant noodles, bread, etc. Salt is also added to food during cooking. Salt is also served at table as soya sauce, table salt and fish sauce."

"Sodium is also present in milk, meat, and shell fish. As a food additive sodium is present as sodium glutamate."

WHO recommendations for salt reduction are as shown in **Table 19A.2**.

**Table 19A.2:** WHO recommendations of salt reduction.

| Age group | Recommendation |
| --- | --- |
| Adults | Less than 5 g, i.e. less than a teaspoon |
| Children (2–15 years) | Less than recommended for adults |
| <2 years | Excluded as up till 6 months is the period of exclusive breastfeeding and 6–24 months is period of complementary feeding |
| Other recommendation | All salt should be iodized or fortified with iodine |

#### Broad strategies for salt reduction:

- Strict government policies and regulation enforcing manufacturers to produce healthier foods by sticking to recommended norms and acceptable levels of sodium. Also implement policies regarding putting up the recommended salt intake and sodium content in the foods on the packages.
- Involving the private sector to increase the availability of products that are low in salt.
- Increasing consumer awareness regarding intake of low salt products.

#### At home:

- Do not add salt during preparation of food.
- Do not use table salt.
- Do not consume salted food/snacks.
- Choose products with low salt content.

### Physical Activity

Regular physical activity should be advised to all individuals to keep themselves fit.

The public health recommendations presented in the WHO Guidelines (2020) on physical activity and sedentary behavior are for all populations and age groups ranging from 5 to 65 years and older, irrespective of gender, cultural background or socioeconomic status, and are relevant for people of all abilities including pregnant women are as follow:

**Children and adolescents** should do at least an average of 60 minutes per day of moderate to vigorous-intensity, mostly aerobic, physical activity, across the week. Vigorous-intensity aerobic activities, as well as those that strengthen muscle and bone, should be incorporated at least 3 days a week.

**All adults (aged 18–64 years)** should undertake regular physical activity. Strong recommendation, moderate certainty evidence, adults should do at least 150–300 minutes of moderate-intensity aerobic physical activity; or at least 75–150 minutes of vigorous intensity aerobic physical activity; or an equivalent combination of moderate- and vigorous-intensity activity throughout the week, for substantial health benefits.

**All older adults (aged 65 years and older)** should undertake regular physical activity. Strong recommendation, moderate certainty evidence older adults should do at least 150–300 minutes of moderate-intensity aerobic physical activity; or at least 75–150 minutes of vigorous intensity aerobic physical activity; or an equivalent combination of moderate- and vigorous-intensity activity throughout the week, for substantial health benefits.

**Pregnant and postpartum women** is recommended that all pregnant and postpartum women without contraindication should undertake regular physical activity throughout pregnancy and postpartum. Do at least 150 minutes of moderate intensity aerobic physical activity throughout the week for substantial health benefits.

## Primary Prevention

### Health Education

While imparting health education ill-effects of sedentary lifestyle, overweight and obesity, increased salt consumption, alcohol intake, etc., have to be stressed upon.

Also, education regarding symptoms of hypertension and timely screening especially those above 30 years should be done.

### DASH—Dietary Approach to Stop Hypertension

This includes eating vegetables, fruits and whole grains.

This diet ensures consumption of food that is less in saturated and trans-fats, low fat dairy products, food that is rich in proteins, minerals like calcium, magnesium, potassium, and fiber. This diet plan also restricts use of sweetened foods and beverages **(Table 19A.3)**.

**Table 19A.3:** Dietary approach to stop hypertension.

| Food group | Daily servings (1,600 Kcal) | Daily servings (2,000 Kcal) | Servings |
|---|---|---|---|
| Grains | 6 | 6–8 | 1 slice whole-wheat bread 1 oz. dry cereal 1/2 cup cooked cereal |
| Lean meats, poultry and fish | 3–6 | 6 or less | 1 oz. cooked lean meat, skinless poultry or fish<br>1 egg (no more than 4 per week)<br>2 egg whites |
| Vegetables | 3–4 | 4–5 | 1 cup raw leafy green vegetable<br>1/2 cup cut-up raw or cooked vegetables<br>1/2 cup (4 fluid oz) low-sodium vegetable juice |
| Fruits | 4 | 4–5 | 1 medium fruit 1/4 cup dried fruit<br>1/2 cup fresh, frozen or canned fruit<br>1/2 cup (4 fluid oz) 100% fruit juice |
| Low fat or dairy products | 2–3 | 2–3 | 1 cup (8 fluid oz) milk<br>1 cup yogurt<br>1 1/2 oz cheese |
| Fats and oil | 2 | 2–3 | 1 teaspoon soft margarine<br>1 teaspoon vegetable oil<br>1 tablespoon mayonnaise<br>1 tablespoon salad dressing |
| Sodium | 2,300 mg | 2,300 mg | |
| Food group | Weekly serving | Weekly serving | |
| Nuts, seeds, dry beans and peas | 3 | 4–5 | 1/3 cup (1.5 oz) nuts<br>2 tablespoons peanut butter<br>2 tablespoons (1/2 oz) seeds<br>1/2 cup cooked legumes (dried beans or peas) |
| Sweets | 0 | 5 or less | 1 tablespoon sugar<br>1 tablespoon jelly or jam 1/2 cup sorbet<br>1 cup (8 fluid oz) sugar-sweetened lemonade |

## Secondary Prevention

### Screening of Individuals

Following must be done to screen individuals with or at risk of developing hypertension:
- BP measurement
- BMI
- Waist circumference
- Peripheral pulses palpation
- Hearing for bruit (renal, carotid, abdominal and others)
- Eye examination.

### Routine Laboratory Tests Recommended before Initiating Therapy

- ECG
- Analysis of urine
- Blood sugar testing
- Blood urea, serum creatinine
- Fasting lipid profile.

### Treatment

Medication will be given based on:
- Level of BP
- Patient profile (like age, body weight, and occupation)
- Comorbid illness
- Organ damage
- Patient affordability.

The pharmacotherapy is based on an algorithm and must be accompanied by lifestyle modifications **(Fig. 19A.2 and Table 19A.4)**.

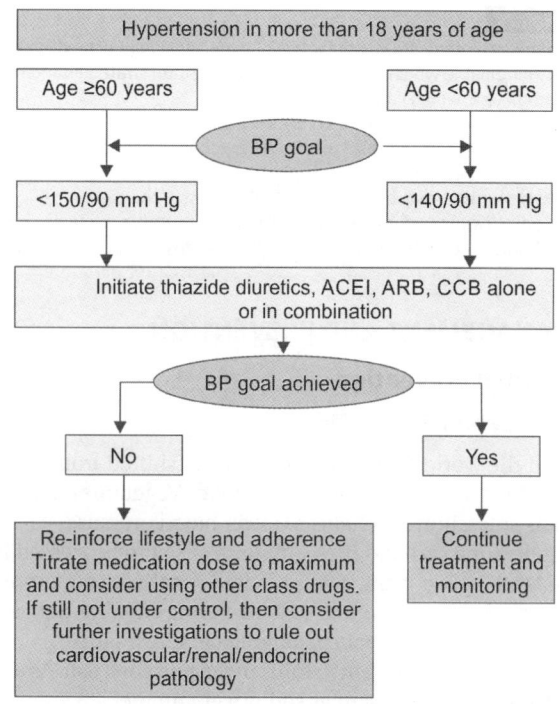

**Fig. 19A.2:** Hypertension in more than 18 years of age.

**Table 19A.4:** Pharmacotherapy for hypertension.

| Sr. no. | Drug class | Agent of choice |
|---|---|---|
| 1. | Calcium channel blockers | • Dihydropyridines—amlodipine, cilnidipine<br>• Non-dihydropyridines—verapamil, diltiazem |
| 2. | Beta-blockers | Propranolol, metoprolol, nebivolol, carvedilol |
| 3. | ACE inhibitors | Enalapril, ramipril, lisinopril |
| 4. | Angiotensin receptor blockers | Telmisartan, losartan, olmesartan, candesartan |
| 5. | Diuretics | • Thiazide—hydrochlorothiazide, chlorthalidone<br>• Potassium sparing—spironolactone, amiloride, triamterene<br>• Loop diuretics—furosemide, torsemide |
| 6. | Vasodilators | Hydralazine, terazosin |
| 7. | Centrally acting agents | Clonidine, guanfacine |

## Tertiary Prevention

The complications of hypertension include hypertensive retinopathy, hypertensive nephropathy, stroke, etc. To prevent these, regular screening needs to be done through fundoscopy and renal function tests. In an event of stroke, rehabilitative measures need to be taken.

## SURVEILLANCE IN HYPERTENSION

WHO STEPS approach is a standard surveillance tool for various non-communicable diseases (NCDs).

It includes collection of data in step-wise manner **(Table 19A.5)**:
- Information on behavior
- Information on physical measurements
- Information of biochemical tests

***Stage 1:*** Population based risk factor assessment

An annual population-based house to house survey among individuals >30 years will be done to find at-risk individuals, those already on treatment, etc. This will be done by community health workers.

***Stage 2:*** Referral

Those with or at risk will be referred to the PHCs for lab investigations in consultation with the treating doctor at the facility referred.

*Information thus obtained will contain:* At risk, number of cases—on treatment, requiring further investigations, requiring referral to a specialist, number of individuals who can be advised only lifestyle modifications, and soon.

Selected cases will be referred to CHC or district hospital for higher level investigations.

The data is recorded at each of these levels. The community health workers need to motivate the individuals on regular follow-up, adherence to treatment, and screening as well.

> **Key Points**
> - Salt reduction is important strategy for prevention of hypertension. The WHO recommends intake of less than 5 g, i.e. less than a teaspoon.
> - DASH—Dietary Approach to Stop Hypertension includes consumption of fruits and vegetables; ensures consumption of food that is less in saturated and trans-fats, low fat dairy products, food that is rich in proteins, minerals like calcium, magnesium, potassium, and fiber.
> - Secondary prevention refers to early diagnosis by screening of high-risk individuals and appropriate pharmacotherapy for diagnosed individuals.
> - Tertiary prevention refers to rehabilitative measures in the event of complications.
> - The WHO STEPS approach is a standard surveillance tool for various non-communicable diseases including hypertension.

## NATIONAL PROGRAM FOR HYPERTENSION

National Programme for Prevention and Control of Non-Communicable Diseases (NP NCD) is the national program that includes the preventive and control strategies of hypertension and other cardiovascular diseases. *NP-NCD is further discussed in Chapter 47: Health Policies and Programs in India.*

## SUMMARY

- Hypertension is a preventable disease.
- Prevention measures as in regular screening after 30 years of age, following a low salt diet, keeping oneself active with regular exercise remain the mainstay.
- Once diagnosed with hypertension, adherence to treatment with regular follow-ups are important **(Box 19A.1)**.

**Box 19A.1: How to measure blood pressure.**
- BP measurement has to be done after a minimum rest of 5 minutes during which the individual should be seated.
- BP is measured using a sphygmomanometer on the upper arm, using palpatory method followed by auscultatory method. Two readings must be taken at least 1 minute a part and average of the two readings is considered.
- If the difference between two readings is more than 5 mm Hg, then additional one or two measurements will have to be taken and an average of all the multiple readings should be used to get the final BP reading **(Fig. 19A.3)**.

*Note:* For those individuals who are at risk for postural hypertension (e.g. elderly patients with diabetes, patients on antihypertensive medications) a standing blood pressure should also betaken.

**Table 19A.5:** Method of surveillance in the community.

| Core information | Expanded information |
|---|---|
| 1. Information on behavior<br>➤ Basic details like age, gender, and literacy status<br>➤ History of:<br>♦ Tobacco use<br>♦ Consumption of alcohol<br>♦ Fruit and vegetable consumption<br>➤ Physical activity<br>2. Information of physical parameters<br>➤ Weight<br>➤ Height<br>➤ Waist circumference<br>➤ Blood pressure<br>3. Biochemical measurements<br>➤ Fasting blood sugar<br>➤ Total cholesterol | Ethnicity, marital status, household income, employment<br>History of:<br>• Use of smokeless tobacco<br>• Alcohol consumption in past seven days<br>• Oil and fat consumption<br>• Blood pressure, treatment for high BP<br>• Diabetes, treatment for diabetes hip circumference<br>High density lipoprotein (HDL)<br>Fasting triglycerides |

*(Adopted from WHO)*

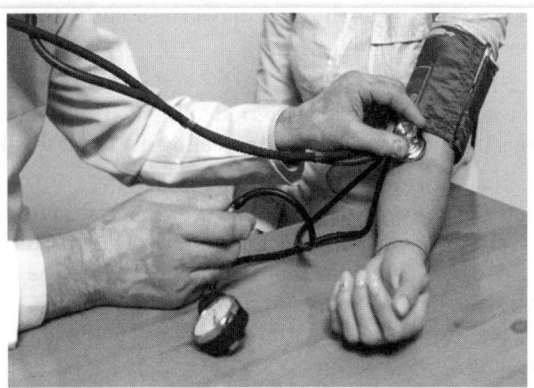

**Fig. 19A.3:** Measurement of BP.

*Source:* Frese EM, Fick A, Sadowsky HS. Blood Pressure Measurement Guidelines for Physical Therapists. Cardiopulm Phys Ther J. 2011;22(2):5-12.

## SUGGESTED READING

1. Chopra HK, Venkata C, Ram S. Recent Guidelines for Hypertension. A Clarion Call for Blood Pressure Control in India. Circulation Research. 2019;124:984–86.
2. DASH—Dietary Approaches to Stop Hypertension. [online] Available from: https://www.nhlbi.nih.gov/health-topics/dash-eating-plan.
3. Frese EM, Fick A, Sadowsky HS. Blood pressure measurement guidelines for physical therapists. Cardiopulm Phys Ther J. 2011;22(2):5-12.
4. George Bakris, Waleed Ali, Gianfranco Parati. ACC/AHA Versus ESC/ESH on Hypertension Guidelines. J Am Coll Cardiol. 2019;73(23):3018-26
5. Global Atlas on cardiovascular disease prevention and control. Published by the World Health Organization in collaboration with the World Heart Federation and the World Stroke Organization; 2011.
6. Hadaye R, Kale V, Manapurath RM. Strategic implications of changing rule of halves in hypertension: A cross-sectional observational study. J Family Med Prim Care. 2019;8(3):1049-1053.
7. India Fact Sheet: National Family Health Survey-5 (2019-21) [Jan; 2023]. 2022. http://rchiips.org/nfhs/NFHS-5_FCTS/India.pdf
8. Longo DL, Fauci AS, Kasper DL, et al. Harrison's Principles of Internal Medicine, 18th edition. New York: McGraw Hill; 2012. pp.1-340.
9. Operational guidelines. National programme for prevention and control of non-communicable diseases (2023-2030). Ministry of Health & Family Welfare Government of India; 2023
10. Surveillance of Chronic Diseases: Challenges and Strategies for India. Indian Council for Research on International Economic Relations. 2016.
11. Training Module for Medical Officers for Prevention, Control and Population Level Screening of Hypertension, Diabetes and Common Cancer (Oral, Breast & Cervical). [online] Available from nhsrcindia.org/.../Module%20for%20MOs%20for%20 Prevention%2 Control%20%2.
12. Whelton PK, Carey RM, Mancia G, Kreutz R, Bundy JD, Williams B. Harmonization of the American College of Cardiology/American Heart Association and European Society of Cardiology/European Society of Hypertension blood pressure/hypertension guidelines: comparisons, reflections, and recommendations. European Heart Journal. 2022;43(35):3302-11.
13. WHO. A Global Brief on Hypertension. Geneva: World Health Organization; 2013.
14. WHO. Hypertension. Global health observatory. Accessed in July 2023 from https://www.who.int/data/gho/indicator-metadata-registry/imr-details/3155.
15. WHO. Hypertension. Health topics Hypertension. [online] Available from:http://www.who.int/topics/hypertension/en/.
16. WHO. Hypertension; Factsheet. March 2023.
17. WHO. Surveillance in Hypertension. [online] Available from https:// www.who.int/ncds/surveillance/steps/en/.
18. WHO guidelines on physical activity and sedentary behaviour: at a glance. Geneva: World Health Organization; 2020.

---

# EPIDEMIOLOGY AND PREVENTION OF STROKE

*Anusha Rashmi, Varghese Iybu Chacko, P Amritha Krishna*

*Our greatest glory is not in never falling, but in getting up every time we fall."*
—**Confucius**

| | |
|---|---|
| **CM 7.2** | Enumerate, describe and discuss the mode of transmission and measures for prevention and control of stroke |
| **CM 8.2** | Describe and discuss the epidemiological and control measures applicable in stroke |

**Case Scenario**

*A 56-year-old high profile businessman develops weakness in the right arm, face, and legs, and is brought immediately to the emergency department of a private hospital within half an hour.*

*Examination revealed grade 3 power in the right upper limb and lower limb, and blood pressure was found to be 140/80 mm Hg. All necessary investigations along with non-contrast CT brain were done and were started on recombinant tissue plasminogen activator (rTPA) immediately.*

*The patient underwent physiotherapy and continued the same after discharge from the hospital. He was also put on anti-platelet, anti-hypertensives, and statins; comes for a general check-up. After a month the patient had improved to become independent in self-care. After 3 months his mobility had almost returned to near normal level.*

## INTRODUCTION

Stroke is a condition seen because of reduced supply of blood to brain that in turn cuts off oxygen supply to the brain and thus leading to brain tissue damage. This can lead to long-term disability or even death.

Brain is the main organ in our body that controls various body functions. To work with full capacity, the brain requires oxygen. "The brain accounts for only 2% of body weight but uses 20% of oxygen that we breathe."

The WHO definition of stroke is, "rapidly developing clinical signs of focal (or global) disturbance of cerebral function, with symptoms lasting 24 hours or longer or leading to death, with no apparent cause other than of vascular origin".

## TYPES OF STROKE

### Ischemic Stroke

This is the most common type of stroke seen when there is a block in blood supply to the brain either by a clot or a fatty deposit.

The two forms of ischemic stroke are embolic and thrombotic.
1. **Embolic stroke:** A "blood clot or plaque fragment" that is formed in the heart or the larger arteries, travels to the brain and blocks a blood vessel causing stroke.
2. **Thrombotic stroke:** It is a blood clot that develops inside the artery that supplies the brain and leads to stroke.

### Hemorrhagic Stroke

This happens when the blood vessel inside the brain bursts open causing spillage of blood.

### Transient Ischemic Attack

Transient ischemic attack (TIA) is seen when there is temporary blockage of blood flow to the brain until collaterals are formed. Hence symptoms are very transient ranging from numbness, weakness or loss of vision, loss of balance or coordination, trouble in speaking. A TIA is a serious warning sign of stroke.

## WHY IS STROKE OF PUBLIC HEALTH IMPORTANCE?

### Global Scenario

#### Morbidity

Stroke is the second leading cause of death and the third leading cause of disability."70% of strokes and 87% of both stroke-related deaths and DALYs are seen in low and middle-income countries." It occurs much earlier (15 years) in these countries (Johnson W et al, Bulletin of WHO, 2016).

Annually, 15 million people worldwide suffer a stroke. Of these, 5 million die and another 5 million are left permanently disabled, placing a burden on family and community. Stroke is uncommon in people under 40 years; when it does occur, the main cause is high blood pressure. However, stroke also occurs in about 8% of children with sickle cell disease (WHO 2023).

#### Mortality

On a global level stroke has led to 6.5 million deaths. In India, cerebrovascular accidents cause approximately 116.4 deaths per 100,000 population every year (Feigin VL et al, Global Burden of Stroke, Circ Res, 2017).

#### Disability

In 2013, stroke led to around 113 million DALYs. According to the Global Burden of Disease estimates, cerebrovascular disease causes 46,591 million DALY's (Feigin VL et al, Global Burden of Stroke, Circ Res, 2017).

### Indian Scenario

"Stroke emerged as the 5th leading cause of disease in 2016 according to reports from Global Burden of Disease." In northeast India it was seen that Manipur and Tripura had higher burden of stroke. North Indian states like Punjab and Himachal Pradesh also contributed highly towards stroke burden (India: Health of the Nation's States Report 2017).

## RISK FACTORS FOR STROKE

- High blood pressure: Stroke is mainly caused by high BP. It has been noted that when systolic and diastolic BP drops by 5 mm each, the risk of death from stroke is reduced by 50%.
- Smoking: Smoking can lead to damage of blood vessels. Passive smoking is also a risk for stroke. The risk of stroke is higher in smokers than non-smokers or in those who have quit smoking for 10 years or more by 2–4 times.
- Obesity
- Alcohol consumption
- Diabetes increases the risk of stroke because it can cause disease of blood vessels in the brain.
- Atrial fibrillation increases risk of stroke by five times.
- History of TIA
- Reduced physical activity
- Family history: History of stroke in a first degree relative.
- Age: According to Framingham Heart Study risk of stroke amongst middle aged individuals is one in six or more. The combined risk of fatal and non-fatal stroke based on study done in eight European countries had increased by 9% per year in men and 10% per year in women.
- Gender: "Women > Men partly because they live longer." Other influencers are hormonal status, exposure to birth control pills along with mental and emotional stress that is more common in women.

## SYMPTOMS OF STROKE

The most common symptom of a stroke is sudden weakness or numbness of the face, arm or leg, most often on one side of the body. Other symptoms include: "confusion, difficulty in speaking or under standing speech; difficulty in seeing with one or both eyes; difficulty in walking, dizziness, loss of balance or coordination; severe headache with no known cause; fainting or unconsciousness."

The effects of a stroke depend on which part of the brain is injured and how severely it is affected. A very severe stroke can cause sudden death.

## MANAGEMENT AND PREVENTION

### Primordial Prevention

The process of atherosclerosis is known to start during early years of life. "Maternal malnutrition acts as a predisposing factor for intrauterine growth retardation and, in turn, metabolic disorders such as insulin resistance, diabetes, hypertension, and dyslipidemia, and enhanced risk of atherosclerosis and cardiovascular death in the offspring." Hence, prevention efforts towards maternal nutrition can paveway for a healthy baby at birth. Similarly, "educating the mothers on importance of breastfeeding and proper weaning practices and developing healthy eating habits will generate lasting impact for a healthy life later."

Smoking cessation programs for pregnant women will influence maternal as well as fetal health.

### Primary Prevention

- Tobacco cessation.
- Regular physicalac tivity.
- Reduced salt consumption to <5 g per day.
- 400 g per day of fruits and vegetables.
- Those with a 10-year cardiovascular risk of >30%, aspirin, statins, and antihypertensives can be advised.
- Anti hypertensives for people with blood pressure ≥160/100.

- Anti-hypertensives for people with persistent blood pressure ≥140/90 and 10-year cardiovascular risk >20% unable to lower blood pressure through lifestyle measures.

Health education to the mass is a necessary intervention to bring about an awareness of the disease as well to motivate those with existing risk factors to get themselves screened for the same.

### Secondary Prevention

#### Early Diagnosis

***Physical examination*** evaluates whether the symptoms are still present, blood pressure recording, and auscultation of carotids.

***Investigations:*** "Blood tests, platelet, PT-INR, blood sugar, electrolytes, lipid profile, computerized tomography (CT) scan is done to look for a hemorrhage, tumor, stroke, and other conditions, magnetic resonance imaging (MRI), carotid ultrasound, echocardiogram."

***Advice on:*** Cessation of tobacco, diet that is healthy along with exercise.

#### Treatment

Medication will be given based on:
- Level of BP
- Patient profile (like age, body weight, occupation)
- Comorbid illness
- Organ damage
- Patient affordability.

***Ischemic stroke:***
- IV TPA should be administered to all eligible acute stroke patients within 3 hours of the attack
- Anti-platelets
- Lipid lowering agents
- Emergency endovascular procedures.

***Hemorrhagic stroke:*** Surgical blood vessel repair.

All stroke patients should receive early rehabilitation in the form of physiotherapy. Chest physiotherapy (if required) can be carried out by the family members.

### Tertiary Prevention

#### Rehabilitation

Rehabilitation should be intensive especially in the first 6 month's post-stroke. It is usually a multidisciplinary rehabilitation rather than just physical therapy since stroke has lasting consequences.

***Physical therapy:*** This is the most often required form of rehabilitation to improve the stiffness in the muscles and thus help the individual with improved flexibility.

***Speech therapy:*** In case the person has difficulty with words and communication then speech and language therapy will have to be considered.

***Occupational therapy:*** Occupational therapy will help to teach daily activities to the individual like bathing and dressing wherever there is a loss of memory following a stroke.

***Emotional support therapy:*** To prevent depression amongst those with stroke.

## QUALITY OF LIFE AFTER STROKE

A stroke survivor is likely to have mood swings and emotional disturbances. Depression is also seen to affect many of them as well. It should be noted that the caregivers of stroke survivors face a lot of burden as well. Hence while dealing with stroke, it is important to investigate the multidimensional factors surrounding it as well.

## NATIONAL PROGRAM FOR STROKE

The NPNCD National Programme for prevention of Non-Communicable Diseases focuses on health promotion and prevention, strengthening of infrastructure including human resources, early diagnosis and management and integration of Stroke and other non-communicable diseases with the primary health care system through NCD cells at different levels for providing optimal care." ***NPNCD is further discussed in Chapter 47: Health Policies and Programs in India***.

### National Stroke Registry Programme

The National Stroke Registry was launched in 2012 by the ICMR-National Center for Disease Informatics and Research (NCDIR).

The registry generates data on stroke incidence along with care given to stroke patients.

Two types of registries are present:
1. *Population Based Stroke Registry (PBSR):* Collects information regarding stroke from defined populations in India.
2. *Hospital Based Stroke Registry (HBSR):* Collects information from hospitals.

## 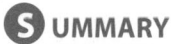UMMARY

Stroke leads to disability in individuals affected. Hence prevention is the best way to deal with stroke.

Rehabilitation is an important component to bring back the patient to near normal life following a stroke.

## SUGGESTED READING

1. American Heart Association. Stroke Factsheet. 2017. [online] Available from:http://www.strokeassociation.org.
2. Centers for Disease Control and Prevention (CDC). Women and Stroke. [online] Available from: http://www.cdc.gov/stroke/docs/women_stroke_factsheet.pdf.
3. Darnton-Hill I, Nishida C, James WP. A life course approach to diet, nutrition and the prevention of chronic diseases. Public Health Nutr. 2004;7(1A):101-21.
4. Global Atlas on Cardiovascular Disease Prevention and Control. WHO; 2011.
5. National Stroke Registry Programme (NSRP). [online] Available from:http://ncdirindia.org/stroke/BS_About.aspx#.
6. Operational guidelines. National programme for prevention and control of non-communicable diseases (2023-2030). Ministry of Health & Family Welfare Government of India; 2023.
7. Operational Guidelines – NPCDCS. [online] Available from: http://health.bih.nic.in/Docs/Guidelines/Guidelines-NPCDCS.pdf.
8. Package of Essential Noncommunicable (PEN) Disease Interventions for Primary Health Care in Low-Resource Settings. [online] Available from: http://whqlibdoc.who.int/publications/2010/9789241598996_eng.pdf.
9. Who. Stroke, Cerebrovascular accident. Accessed in July 2023 from https://www.emro.who.int/health-topics/stroke-cerebrovascular-accident/index.html

# B. EPIDEMIOLOGY OF CARDIOVASCULAR DISEASES AND ITS PREVENTION AND CONTROL

## EPIDEMIOLOGY OF CARDIOVASCULAR DISEASES—ISCHEMIC HEART DISEASE

*Ankeeta Menona Jacob, Nishanth Krishna K*

> *"I have saved the lives of 150 people by heart transplants. If I had focused on preventive medicine earlier, I might have saved 150 million people".*
> —**Christian Bernard (Heart Transplant Surgeon).**

| | |
|---|---|
| **CM 7.2** | Enumerate, describe and discuss the mode of transmission and measures for prevention and control of ischemic heart disease |
| **CM 8.2** | Describe and discuss the epidemiological and control measures applicable in ischemic heart disease |

### Case Scenario

Mr X, a 40-year-old gentleman visits you at the Primary Health Center. He works for a company as a technical support manager. Owing to his stress filled life, he smokes about 20 cigarettes per day and consumes about 90 mL of alcohol per day. He was recently diagnosed with hypertension and his blood pressure recording during the last visit was 140/80 mm Hg. His blood sugar levels however are within normal limits.
❏ What is the risk of acute cardiac event in the next few years in Mr X?
❏ What are the ways we can prevent this from happening?

## INTRODUCTION

Cardiovascular diseases are disorders that affect the circulatory system, i.e., heart and blood vessels. Cardiovascular disease (CVD) is one of the significant causes of disability and premature death. These disorders affect the most productive population, i.e., the age group 15–49 years, and significantly contribute to high mortality rates that are seen among individuals aged more than 50 years of age. Most of the cardiovascular disease related deaths occur in low and middle-income countries, thus indirectly contributing to the high costs of healthcare. The trends in the projected mortality due to CVDs predict a sharp rise in cardiovascular deaths by 2030.

## CLASSIFICATION OF CARDIOVASCULAR DISEASES (FIG. 19B.1)

Cardiovascular diseases include:
- ***Coronary artery disease***: These are diseases of the blood vessels supplying the heart.
- ***Cerebrovascular disease***: These are diseases of the blood vessels supplying the brain.
- ***Peripheral arterial disease***: These are diseases of blood vessels supplying limbs.
- ***Rheumatic heart disease (RHD)***: Diseases caused due to the damage to the heart muscle and heart valves due to rheumatic fever (RF), which will be dealt in detail in the next chapter.
- ***Congenital heart disease***: Malformations of cardiac structure existing since birth.
- ***Deep vein thrombosis and pulmonary embolism***: Blood clots in the deep leg veins that may get dislodged and get transported to the heart and lungs.
- ***Diseases of the arteries and the aorta***: This includes hypertension and also peripheral vascular disease.

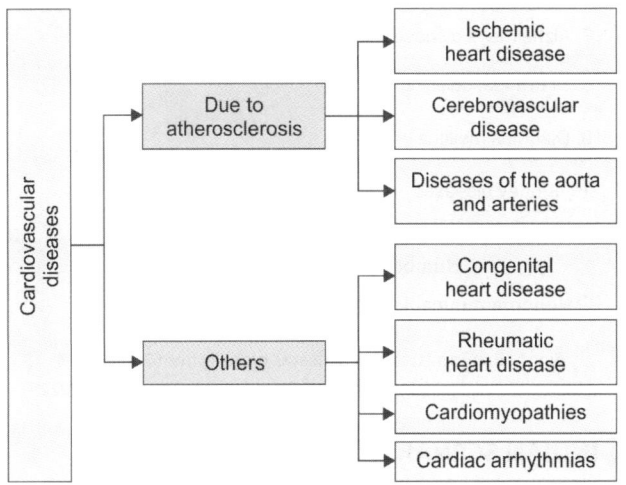

Fig. 19B.1: Classification of cardiovascular diseases.

## GLOBAL SCENARIO (BOX 19B.1)

Cardiovascular diseases (CVDs) are the leading cause of death globally. An estimated 17.9 million people died from CVDs in 2019, representing 32% of all global deaths. Of these deaths, 85% were due to heart attack and stroke. Over three quarters of CVD deaths take place in low- and middle-income countries. Out of the 17 million premature deaths (under the age of 70) due to noncommunicable diseases in 2019, 38% were caused by CVDs. (WHO, Cardiovascular diseases; Factsheet 2021) Of the 57 million deaths caused by noncommunicable diseases in 2016, CVD related deaths accounted for about 17.9 million deaths (44% of the total deaths due to non-communicable diseases). **Figure 19B.2** shows the top 10 causes of death globally from 2000 to 2019 (WHO Global Health Estimates 2022).

### Box 19B.1: Cardiovascular diseases mortality rates globally, SEA (South-East Asia) region and in India.

**Global:** Of the 57 million deaths due to noncommunicable diseases in 2016, cardiovascular disease-related deaths accounted for about 17.9 million deaths (44%).

**SEA (South-East Asia) Region:** In 2015, about 28% (3.8 million) deaths due to cardiovascular diseases and accounted for more than 43% of the total noncommunicable disease-related deaths.

**India:** Cardiovascular diseases contributed to 28.1% of the total deaths in India. Of this, ischemic heart disease and stroke contributed to 61.4% of the overall cardiovascular disease-related deaths.

## Section 3: Community Health Problems and Vulnerable Groups

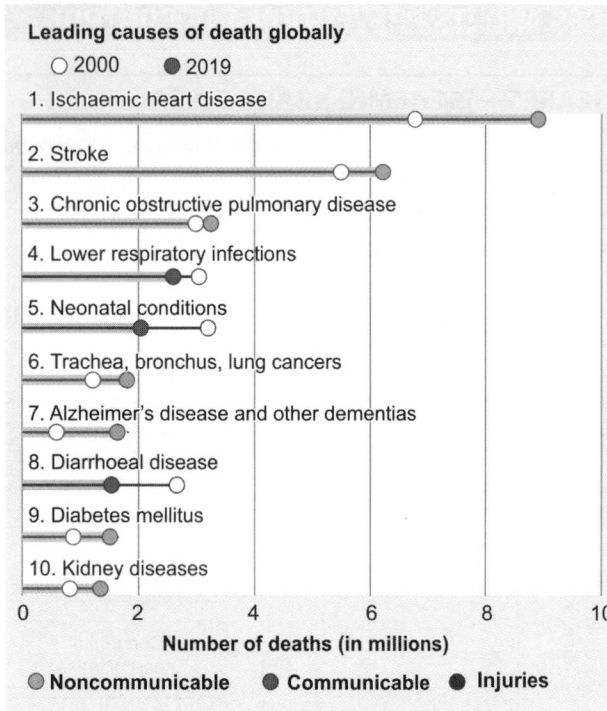

**Fig. 19B.2:** Top 10 causes of deaths globally from 2000–2019.
*Source:* Global Health Estimates 2019: World Health Organization 2022.

### INDIAN SCENARIO

Cardiovascular diseases contributed to 28.1% of the total deaths in India. Of this, ischemic heart disease and stroke contributed to 61.4% of the overall cardiovascular disease-related deaths.

### RISK FACTORS FOR CVD (BOX 19B.2)

The presence or absence of risk factors helps the healthcare professionals decide whom to subject for screening for the

**Box 19B.2: Risk factors for cardiovascular disease.**

*Major risk factors*
- Tobacco dependence
- Raised LDL cholesterol
- Low HDL cholesterol
- High blood pressure
- Elevated blood glucose
- Elevated C-reactive protein
- Overweight or obesity
- Physical inactivity
- Dietary risk factors

*Contributing risk factors*
- Socioeconomic status
- Elevated prothrombotic factors: Fibrinogen, plasminogen activator inhibitor (PAI)-1
- Markers of infection or inflammation
- Raised homocysteine
- Elevated lipoprotein (a)
- Psychological factors

*Source:* Harris R. Epidemiology of Chronic Disease.

CVDs, primarily when a high-risk approach is undertaken. The first description of the causation of atherosclerosis and ischemic heart disease depicted by McMahon and Pugh as "web of causation" is shown in **Figure 19B.3**.

The risk factors for ischemic heart disease are either *nonmodifiable* or *modifiable*.

### Nonmodifiable Risk Factors

These risk factors cannot be controlled or changed even with intervention. Thus, these factors are not amenable to prevention, but are useful in finding out which group of people who are at high-risk to develop ischemic heart disease.

- ***Age:*** The risk of cardiovascular disease is higher in men more than 45 years of age and postmenopausal women because as age advances, the exposure to risk factors and unhealthy lifestyle is longer.
- ***Sex:*** Males and postmenopausal women are at an equal or a higher risk of CVD.
- ***Family history:*** History of premature myocardial infarction or sudden death in the parents or first-degree relatives indicates high-risk.
- ***Genetic factors:*** Genetic factors determine the total cholesterol (TC) level and low-density lipoprotein (LDL) level and hence indirectly determine the risk of CVD.

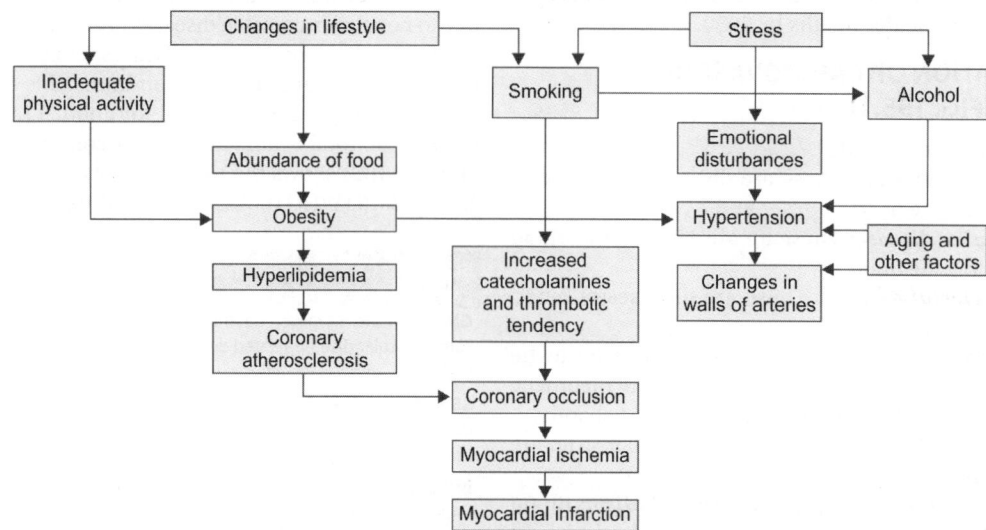

**Fig. 19B.3:** Web of causation of cardiovascular diseases.

# Chapter 19: Specific Epidemiology of Noncommunicable Diseases

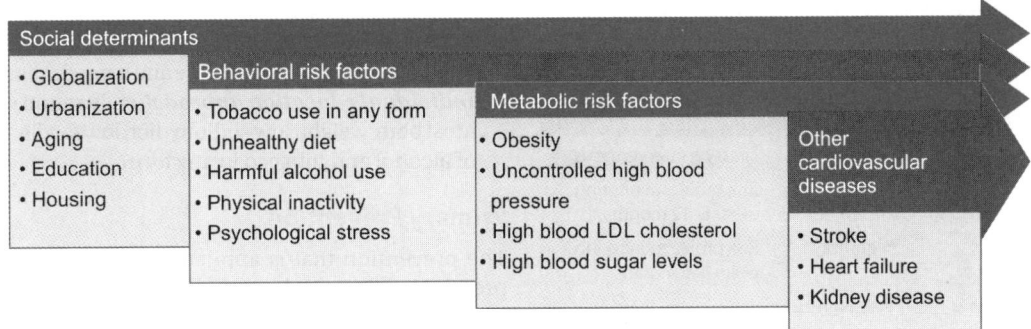

Fig. 19B.4: Determinants and risk factors for cardiovascular diseases.

## Modifiable Risk Factors

- These are behavior related traits that predispose individuals to develop ischemic heart disease. These can be reduced or controlled by modification of the lifestyle of an individual. If these factors were to be modified suitably, they can reduce the probability of cardiovascular disease in an individual.
- *Elevated blood pressure (hypertension):* Consumption of excess salt in diet, increases risk of elevated blood pressure thereby indirectly increasing the risk of heart disease and stroke.
- *Cholesterol or lipid metabolism:* High serum LDL cholesterol and low levels of HDL cholesterol are implicated in increased risk of CVDs.
- *Diet:* Consumption of diet rich in trans-fat, saturated fat, low-density cholesterol and sodium, along with low intake of vegetables, fruits, dietary salt omega-3 fatty acids, and dietary fibers increase the risk of CVDs.
- *Diabetes:* Diabetics are at two to three times higher risk of cardiovascular events. The risk in women is disproportionately higher.
- *Excessive weight or obesity:* It is associated with raised blood pressure, glucose intolerance, type 2 diabetes, and dyslipidemia, which are major risk factors for CVDs.
- *Physical inactivity:* Imbalance between the diet (energy intake) and physical inactivity (energy expenditure) leads to obesity, an integral part in the web of causation of CVDs.
- *Smoking or tobacco consumption:* Smoking is implicated in nearly 10% of CVDs. Tobacco along with other risk factors are synergistically related to death risk of CVD.
- *Socioeconomic factors and other social determinants:* IHDs are more common in upper socioeconomic classes. Poverty, poor literacy, degradation of the environment, poor housing, and unplanned urbanization lead to poor cardiovascular and general health.
- *Psychological stress:* Stress predisposes to IHD. It is associated with twice as much the risk of IHD in people with type "A" or "coronary prone" behavior pattern than normal individuals.
- *Alcohol:* Moderate drinking (up to three drinks per day) has been shown to protect against IHD in the West. However, consumption of more than two units of alcohol per day over a long period or repeated consumption of large amounts of alcohol at once (binge drinking) increases the risk of stroke, cardiac arrhythmia, and abnormalities in triglyceride metabolism.
- *Other constitutional factors:* Recent evidence suggests that hemostatic factors resulting in hypercoagulability of blood (high plasma levels of factors VII and VIII, and fibrinogen) are also associated with IHD.
- *Drugs:* Hormone replacement therapy has shown to significantly increase the risk of development of acute coronary events, venous thromboembolic phenomenon, and stroke.

The risk of CVD is not merely due to these factors occurring singly but in varying proportions of social, behavioral, metabolic and other cardiovascular disease risk factors as shown in **Figure 19B.4**, which ultimately decide the outcome of the CVD in terms of mortality and morbidity.

> **Key Points**
> - Cardiovascular diseases are disorders that affect the circulatory system, i.e., heart and blood vessels
> - CVD related deaths accounted for about 44% of the total deaths due to NCDs and trends in the projected mortality due to CVDs predict a sharp rise in CVD deaths by 2030
> - The risk factors for ischemic heart disease are either nonmodifiable or modifiable and was first depicted by McMahon and Pugh as "web of causation"
> - Modifiable risk factors are behavior related traits that predispose individuals to develop CVD and can be reduced or controlled by modification of the lifestyle

## PREVENTION OF CARDIOVASCULAR DISEASES

The common modifiable lifestyle related risk factors of major noncommunicable diseases like CVDs, cancer, diabetes mellitus, and chronic respiratory diseases are targeted for prevention and control. Intervention at this level ensures that healthy people continue to remain so. It brings about change in the behavior of individuals who are at high-risk or those with an already established cardiovascular disease.

### Total Risk Approach in Prevention of Cardiovascular Diseases

The determinants of cardiovascular risk depend on the profile of individual like age, sex, blood pressure, diet, alcohol, and tobacco consumption. This prediction of an individual's risk differs from the traditional system of exploration, identification

**Table 19B.1:** Risk stratification of fatal and non-fatal cardiovascular diseases as per WHO or ISH charts.

| Risk of cardiovascular (fatal or nonfatal event) as per WHO or ISH chart | Risk level | Intervention needed |
|---|---|---|
| <10% | Low-risk | Lifestyle interventions |
| 10 to <20% | Moderate risk | Risk profile monitoring every 6–12 months |
| 20 to <30% | High-risk | Risk profile monitoring every 3–6 months |
| ≥30% | Very high-risk | |

(ISH: International Society for Hypertension; WHO: World Health Organization)

and treatment of individual diseases like hypertension, diabetes mellitus, and hypercholesterolemia in already established CVDs. The total risk approach views the various risk factors in a logical manner to arrive at diagnostic or therapeutic interventions for an individual. This is done as early as possible using "risk prediction charts". These risk prediction charts were originally derived from the Framingham Score from the Framingham Heart Study. These charts are available for various age, sex, ethnic groups with risk factors like smoking, elevated blood sugar levels, elevated blood pressure, total cholesterol levels. These charts can be used to predict the risk level of the individual for acute cardiovascular events over the next five to ten years and suggest timely follow ups and interventions **(Table 19B.1)**.

However, these cardiovascular risk prediction charts can undermine the actual risk of an individual who has:

- An already established coronary heart disease, acute myocardial infarction, stroke, transient ischemic attacks, peripheral vascular disease, angina pectoris, with or without interventions like coronary revascularization.
- Left ventricular hypertrophy or hypertensive retinopathy (grades 3 and 4)
- Patients with type 1 or type 2 diabetes with renal compromise (microalbuminuria)
- Renal impairment or failure
- Current antihypertensive treatment
- Sedentary lifestyle
- Obesity (especially abdominal obesity)
- Premature menopause
- Family history of CVDs like stroke, in first degree relative (age cut offs include—65 years in females and 55 years in males)
- Raised C-reactive protein, prothrombotic enzymes like fibrinogen, homocysteine, and apolipoprotein B
- Fasting hyperglycemia or impaired glucose tolerance
- Not yet developed CVD but have:
  - Total cholesterol levels of more than 320 mg/dL or
  - Low-density lipoprotein of more than 240 mg/dL
  - Low high-density lipoprotein (HDL) levels lesser than 40 mg/dL in males and 50 mg/dL in females
  - Total cholesterol to HDL ratio of more than or equal to 8
  - Raised triglyceride levels of more than 180 mg/dL

## Primordial Prevention

As a part of primordial and primary prevention, the interventions for the risk factors need to be implemented through the following approaches:

The two modalities of interventions in primordial prevention:
1. ***Mass education approach:*** These measures help in postponement of development of disease and complications due to CVD's.
2. ***Individual education approach:*** Education on maintaining ideal body weight, low sodium diet, low fat diet and avoidance of alcohol and tobacco in any form.

## Primary Prevention

The prevention that is applied when risk factors are already prevalent in the population and aims at reducing the risk factors which is done by:

1. ***Population strategy:*** This refers to a mass-approach focusing on changing risk factors that are at a lower magnitude in individual. This will help in achievement in the reduction of risk factors at a faster rate in the population. These are mainly directed by specific interventions to adopt healthy dietary options, avoiding tobacco, abuse use of alcohol, decreasing the risk of developing high blood pressure by adoption of prudent or balanced diet, and improvement in physical activity as shown in **Table 19B.2**.

**Table 19B.2:** Recommendations regarding non-communicable disease risk factors prevention and control.

| Risk factor to be addressed | Description | |
|---|---|---|
| Health education on mass media via behavior change communication | | |
| Tobacco | Implementation of effective mass media campaign displays at the public places, cinema theaters, effective information, education, and communication leading to increased awareness of hazards of smoking targeted to schools and adolescents; behavior change communication through tobacco cessation health facilities and programs. | |
| | Taxation | Increase in the tax levied on tobacco and tobacco-related products |
| | Packaging | Display of health warning on tobacco and tobacco-related products |
| Smoke free areas | Elimination of second and third hand passive smoking in public areas, public modes of transport and in indoor area of work | |
| Tobacco cessation | Tobacco cessation support and measures, provision of services for those who wish to quit | |
| Unhealthy food | Behavior-change communication through mass media on salt consumption and high fat and high sugar food consumption. The following changes in diet will prevent or postpone the atherosclerotic changes:<br>• Consumption of a balanced or prudent diet<br>• Reduced salt intake by reformulation of food items and behavior change communication<br>• Implementation of nutritional labelling for salt, sodium, fats and sugar content labelling in front of the food packages<br>• Industrial food products- eliminate Trans-fat and reduction of sugar consumption<br>• Exclusive breastfeeding promotion in the first 6 months of life<br>• Subsidize rates of fruits and vegetables to improve consumption<br>• Limiting of portion/serving size<br>• Nutrition education and counseling to improve intake of prudent diet | |

*Contd...*

Contd...

| Risk factor to be addressed | Description | |
|---|---|---|
| Alcohol | Taxation | Increase in excise duties on alcoholic beverages |
| | Advertisements | Enforcement of Ban on advertisements related to alcoholic beverages |
| | Availability | Enforcement of Ban of sale of liquor on direct roads that connect state and national highways |
| | Legislative measures | To ensure laws against drunken driving, minimum age limits for alcohol consumption |
| | Supportive measures | Psychosocial intervention for individuals with harmful use of alcohol |
| Physical activity | • Awareness campaign and community-based health education programs for improvement in physical activity levels using motivation and environmental programs.<br>• Physical activity counseling and referral in primary health care<br>• Promotion of physical education, availability of adequate facilities and programs and space for physical activity<br>• Space and infrastructure for walking, cycling<br>• Workplace implementation of physical activity programs through sport and physical activity clubs, programs, events | |

2. **High-risk strategy:** This makes preventive care accessible to individuals at special risk by optimum use of clinical skills.
   - *Identification of at risk population:* Individuals educated about the risk factors will be able to approach health centers for appropriate diagnosis, follow-up, and treatment. These include individuals with strong family history of CVD, obesity, smoking and uncontrolled diabetes, which are identified using the total cardiovascular risk approach WHO/ISH risk prediction charts.
   - *Specific advice*: Trials like MRFIT (Multiple Risk Factor Intervention Trial) and North Karelia Project Oslo Heart Study have demonstrated that specific advice, related to control of risk factors significantly reduced the risk of cardiovascular event in the intervention group by the demonstration of strict observance of the CVD risk factors. However, this approach may not cover all the individuals who may experience a cardiovascular event and thus can be a limitation.

An optimum mix of these interventions among population and high-risk individuals should be implemented to shift the risk levels of cardiovascular diseases in the population as shown in **Figure 19B.5**.

## Secondary Prevention

These are the set of actions undertaken to prevent the progress of disease in its incipient stages, thus leading to prevention or postponement of complications. Secondary prevention involves adoption of aggressive preventive strategies before experiencing a cardiovascular event. The secondary prevention of CVDs includes:

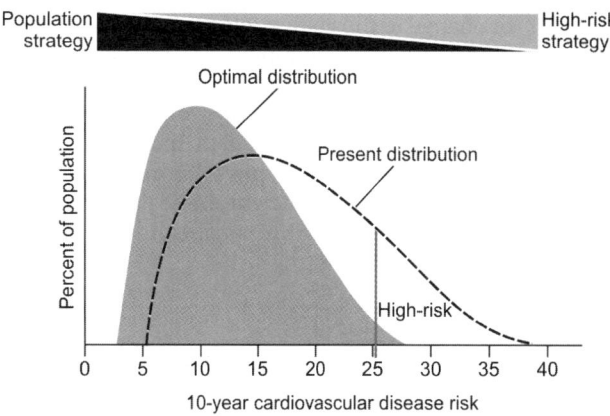

**Fig. 19B.5:** Effect of optimum implementation of individual and population level strategies.

*Source:* World Health Organization. Prevention of cardiovascular disease: guidelines for assessment and management of cardiovascular risk.

### Early Diagnosis and Treatment

Regular physical examinations and early detection of antecedent conditions that predispose people to CVD like are as follows:
- *Screening for serum cholesterol abnormalities, tracking of blood pressure and the early detection of onset of hypertension, abnormalities in blood sugars like general random blood sugar (GRBS) levels:* This is done at ages 40 and above for individuals without any risk factors and aged 30 years and above for individuals with at least one risk factor. **Screening procedures involved in cardiovascular diseases have been explained in Chapter 21: Screening for Noncommunicable Diseases in detail.**
- Treatment of conditions that may predispose to an acute cardiovascular event.
- Use of low dose aspirin (75 mg daily dose) in individuals with high-risk of acute cardiovascular event to prevent myocardial infarction and stroke.

### Noncommunicable Disease (including Cardiovascular Disease) Risk Factor Surveillance in India

Risk factors that occur in clusters in the population include abuse of alcohol, tobacco consumption in any form, unhealthy or inappropriate dietary practices, physical inactivity, obesity and hypertension, and diabetes mellitus. The presence of these risk factors is seen much before the onset of cardiovascular diseases. The demographic transition accompanied by *"risk transition"* helps to predict the trend of CVDs. This tranistion can be leveraged to make specific health service planning, monitor long-term disease prevention activities, and determine public health priorities that aid primary and secondary prevention. Health in India being a state subject, prioritization of preventive efforts and evaluation of ongoing programs will help to assess and improve the impact of preventive strategies for noncommunicable diseases. For example, impact of state and other tobacco-related policies, nutrition policies, and physical education programs at institution levels. Thus, the need of the hour is specific and focused assessment of *"risk transition*" or change in the epidemiology of CVD risk factors, at least at regional level at periodic intervals. The WHO stepwise approach for risk factor surveillance has been developed and standardized for collecting, analyzing, and dissemination of information has been developed. It has questions on noncommunicable risk factors, physical anthropometric measurements such as weight, height, waist-hip ratio, blood pressure recording, and biochemical parameters such as fasting lipid profile and glucose levels.

## Tertiary Prevention

Tertiary prevention deals with provision of critical cardiac care for acute cardiovascular events through a comprehensive strategy. This was first piloted in India at Kovai-Erode in the ST-Elevation Myocardial Infarction (STEMI) India study. Here, health centers (especially in rural areas) are equipped with facilities for initial clot lysis but without facilities for primary percutaneous coronary interventions called the "*spokes*". The health care facilities located at a distance from these centers where equipment for clot lysis, pharmacoinvasive therapy, percutaneous invasive coronary reperfusion are performed are termed as "*Hub*" hospitals as shown in **Figure 19B.6**.

The key summary of various levels of prevention and modes of intervention is shown in **Figure 19B.7**.

### Key Points
- As a part of primordial and primary prevention, the interventions for the risk factors need to be implemented through either a mass education or individual education approach.
- The prevention that is applied when risk factors are already prevalent in the population and aims at reducing the risk factors is termed primary prevention. This is by population strategy or high-risk strategy.
- An optimum mix of these interventions among population and high-risk individuals should be implemented to shift the risk levels of cardiovascular diseases in the population.
- Secondary prevention refers to the set of actions undertaken to prevent the progress of disease in its incipient stages, thus leading to prevention or postponement of complications. It mainly includes Early Diagnosis and Treatment.
- Tertiary prevention deals with provision of critical cardiac care for acute cardiovascular events through a comprehensivestrategy.

## LEVELS OF CARE FOR ACUTE CORONARY EVENTS

Medical officers at various levels would be able to diagnose IHD in a patient based on the signs and symptoms of the patients.

### Spoke Network of Healthcare Facilities: Type C or Type D Healthcare Facilities

*At primary health center level:* These usually are designated as:
1. ***Type C healthcare facility which are located within 30 min of the hub hospitals (types A or B):*** These primary health centers should be equipped with basic facilities for electrocardiogram (ECG), all drugs and oxygen. They should able to transport the patient as early as possible to perform coronary artery interventions. These interventions need to be carried out within 1 hour of the onset of symptoms of acute coronary events called "Golden Hour". The interventions should take place in less than 60 minutes (i.e. from the arrival to emergency department to performing the primary percutaneous intervention) called "door to needle time".
2. ***Type D healthcare facilities which are located more than 30 min of the hub hospitals:*** These are facilities that are equipped to thrombolyze and/or stabilize patients with acute coronary events and transfer such patients in 3–24 hours to hub hospitals (type A or type B) for further management as depicted in **Figure 19B.6**.

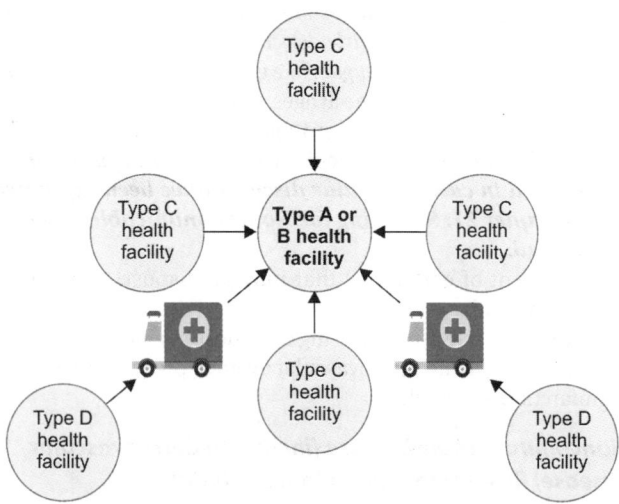

Fig. 19B.6: Hub and Spoke model for intervention in acute events of cardiovascular diseases.

Fig. 19B.7: Levels of prevention and modes of interventions in cardiovascular diseases.

## Hub/Tertiary Care Center (Type A or Type B Healthcare Facilities)

Here, the hub hospitals will have facilities available to carry out pharmacoinvasive procedures like coronary revascularization and digital catheterization.

The facilities that perform these interventions are further classified into:
- *Type A hospitals:* These health centers have round the clock (24 × 7) facilities to perform primary percutaneous interventions for cardiac catheterization and coronary artery related surgical interventions such as coronary artery bypass graft (CABG) and percutaneous transluminal coronary angioplasty (PTCA) with or without stenting.
- *Type B hospitals:* These health centers do not provide round-the-clock primary percutaneous coronary interventions.

## Follow-up of Patients with Already Established Cardiovascular Disease

- Encourage drug compliance and prompt follow-ups and required tests to ensure glycemic control for patients with diabetes mellitus, salt restricted diet, and blood pressure monitoring in patients with elevated blood pressure levels.
- Counseling patients who have already suffered a heart attack or stroke regarding the risk of fatal and nonfatal cardiac events in the future.
- Behavior and lifestyle modifications compliance to be ensured among individuals who have a high 10-year risk (≥30%) of development of fatal or non-fatal cardiovascular events.
- Prevention and prompt treatment of respiratory and other infections.
- Treatment of underlying or precipitating conditions like anemia, thiamine deficiency, and rheumatic valvular disease.

## SUMMARY

Cardiovascular diseases accounted for more than 17.9 million (32% of total deaths due to noncommunicable diseases in 2019. The majority of deaths occurring in low and middle-income countries. The increased longevity and population growth coupled with epidemiological transition, urbanization, has caused increased burden of CVDs and is expected to rise in the coming future. The risk factors are broadly classified as:
- *Modifiable risk factors:* High blood pressure, diabetes mellitus, smoking in any form or tobacco consumption, abuse of alcohol, high LDL levels, diet rich in saturated fat, trans-fat, cholesterol, sodium (salt) refined carbohydrates, physical inactivity, drugs, and other constitutional factors.
- *Nonmodifiable risk factors:* Age, gender, family history, and genetic factors.

The risk factor assessment and prevention using the total cardiovascular risk approach is necessary to reduce the burden of mortality and morbidity due to CVDs. The golden hour is important for prevention of long-term sequelae in individuals. In the primary healthcare setting with a health team approach based on the Hub and Spoke model, as piloted in India in the Kovai-Erode-STEMI-India study.

Prevention of cardiovascular diseases includes:
- *Primordial prevention:* Mass and individual education on risk factors of CVDs
- *Primary prevention:* Through health protection and health promotion by:
  **Health education:** Legislative and primary healthcare approach on risk factor prevention of tobacco, alcohol abuse, unhealthy diet, physical inactivity, and medication for hypertension and diabetes.
- *Secondary prevention:* Early diagnosis of risk factors like hypercholesterolemia, high blood pressure, diabetes mellitus and treatment of the above conditions use of low dose aspirin, WHO or ISH risk prediction charts to reduce the risk factors of the above-mentioned conditions.
- *Tertiary prevention:* By clinical diagnosis of an acute cardiac event using a health team approach with prompt referral (Hub and Spoke model) and follow-up of the patients to prevent long-term complications due to CVDs.

## SUGGESTED READING

1. Alexander T, Mullasari AS, Narula J. Developing a STEMI System of Care for Low- and Middle-Income Countries-The STEMI-India Model. Glob Heart. 2014;9(4):419–23.
2. Best buys' and other recommended interventions for the prevention and control of noncommunicable diseases-Tackling NCDs [Internet]. Geneva: World Health Organization; 2017. p. 24.
3. Harris R. Epidemiology of Chronic Disease: Global Perspectives. 1st ed. Jones and Barlett Learning; 2013. p. 725.
4. Herlitz J, Wireklint Sundström B, Bång A, Berglund A, Svensson L, Blomstrand C. Early identification and delay to treatment in myocardial infarction and stroke: differences and similarities. Scand J Trauma Resusc Emerg Med. 2010;18:48.
5. Krishnaswamy K, Sesikiren B, Laxmaiah A, Vajreswari A. DIETARY Guidelines for Indians-A Manual [Internet]. 2nd ed. Hyderabad: National Institute of Nutrition; 2010. p. 96. Available from: : http://ninindia.org/dietaryguidelinesforninwebsite.pdf
6. Prabhakaran D, Jeemon P, Sharma M, Roth GA, Johnson C, Harikrishnan S, et al. The changing patterns of cardiovascular diseases and their risk factors in the states of India: the Global Burden of Disease Study 1990–2016. Lancet Glob Health. 2018;6(12):e1339-51.
7. Prevention of cardiovascular disease: guidelines for assessment and management of total cardiovascular risk. 1st ed. Geneva: World Health Organization; 2007. p. 92.
8. Roth GA, Johnson C, Abajobir A, Abd-Allah F, Abera SF, Abyu G, et al. Global, Regional, and National Burden of Cardiovascular Diseases for 10 Causes, 1990 to 2015. J Am Coll Cardiol. 2017 Jul 4;70(1):1-25.
9. Sanchis-Gomar F, Perez-Quilis C, Leischik R, Lucia A. Epidemiology of coronary heart disease and acute coronary syndrome. Ann Transl Med. 2016;4(13):256–256.
10. World Health Organization. Non-communicable Diseases Country Profiles 2018 [Internet]. Geneva: World Health Organization; 2018. p. 224.
11. World Health Organization. Prevention of cardiovascular disease: pocket guidelines for assessment and management of cardiovascular risk: (WHO/ISH cardiovascular risk prediction charts for WHO epidemiological sub-Regions SEAR B, SEAR D). 1st ed. Geneva: World Health Organization; 2007.
12. WHO. Cardiovascular diseases: Factsheet June 2021.

# EPIDEMIOLOGY OF CARDIOVASCULAR DISEASES—RHEUMATIC HEART DISEASE

*Ekta Gupta*

**CM 7.2** Enumerate, describe and discuss the mode of transmission and measures for prevention and control of rheumatic heart disease

**CM 8.2** Describe and discuss the epidemiological and control measures applicable in rheumatic heart disease

---

*Case Scenario*

On a routine field visit, Rama an ANM in the village of Pali found that Roshni, a 12-year-old girl had not attended her school for 5 days. On enquiring, her mother reported that Roshni was having fever of 102°F and sore throat along with shortness of breath in the past 5 days. The fever occurred in bouts, persisted for few hours and then subsided on its own. In the past two days, her right knee joint was swollen and painful which subsided the next day was followed by pain and swelling of feet subsequently. She experienced shortness of breath while walking. Rama immediately took her to nearest primary health center where the medical officer examined the girl. He found that her pulse rate was 80 per minute, blood pressure was 100/60 mm Hg and respiratory rate was 32 per minute. Auscultation findings revealed a systolic murmur in the aortic area. The patient was treated with penicillin injections following which the patient recovered completely in 2 weeks.

What lead to this condition of the girl at such a young age? Could it have been prevented? Are there any precautions that she would need to take to prevent further complications? The following segment concentrates on the diagnosis, prevention and control of rheumatic fever (RF) and rheumatic heart disease (RHD).

---

## INTRODUCTION

Rheumatic heart disease is a group of heart disorders which include short-term and long-term conditions occurring due to rheumatic fever (RF). It is a condition where the heart becomes inflamed and heart valves are permanently damaged after a single or recurrent episode of acute rheumatic fever (ARF). RF affects connective tissues of heart and joints, which is preceded by throat infection caused by group A beta-hemolytic streptococci. The epidemiology of RF and RHD is almost similar. They are noncommunicable diseases, which result from a communicable disease (streptococcal pharyngitis). Around 60% of those with RF develop heart diseases during later stages of life. Following RF, the heart valves become inflamed and scarred leading to narrowing or leaking of valves and circulatory failure in later stages. The burden of ARF and prevalence and mortality from RHD in industrialized countries has declined dramatically in the late 20th century, due to changes in socio-economic conditions, improved living and hygiene standards, and increased access to appropriate health services.

## MAGNITUDE OF THE DISEASE

### World

Rheumatic fever and RHD are major public health problems particularly in low and middle-income countries and some indigenous or marginalized communities in high-income countries. RF is the leading cause of heart disease among 5–30 years age group throughout the world. Lack of reliable data pertaining to disease burden on account of RHD makes hospital morbidity data the only source for information available in some developing countries. RF and RHD account for 12–65% of hospital admissions for conditions related to heart diseases. As per the Global Burden of Disease (GBD) estimates, RHD caused 33,194,900 cases and 319,400 deaths worldwide in 2015 out of which 60% were premature deaths, i.e. before the age of 70 years. About 2% of all cardiovascular deaths, 25.5% left heart failures and 5.3% right heart failures are due to RHD. It was also responsible for loss of 11.5 million DALYs (Global Burden of Disease Study 2016). Despite measures of prevention and treatment, the mortality rate has not declined significantly between 2000 and 2015 (WHO, Disease Burden and Mortality Estimates, 2016).

### WHO Regions

All the countries in WHO regions are affected by RHD. Amongst these, the WHO African region, the South-East Asian region and the Western Pacific region are worst affected as these regions accounted for 84% of cases and 80% of total deaths due to RHD. In the South-East Asian region, the highest prevalence of RHD is seen in India (27%) while in Western Pacific region, it is mainly restricted to China and some parts of Australia, New Zealand, and the Pacific Island States inhabited by indigenous populations (Strasser T et al., WHO Chron., 1973 and Report of WHO for Rheumatic Fever and Rheumatic Heart Disease, 2004).

### India

Rheumatic fever is an endemic disease and a neglected public health problem in India affecting children living in under privileged conditions. It is responsible for 25–45% burden of acquired heart disease. In 2015, there were about 13.17 million cases and 1.19 lakhs deaths due to RHD in India. Prevalence of RHD as found in surveys in 1970's ranges from 1.2 to 2.2/1,000 in the age group of 5–30 years across India (Mathur KS et al, J Assoc Physicians India, 1971. Berry JN et al., Br Heart J, 1972. Shah B et al., Indian J Pediatr, 2013). The subsequent studies by Indian Council of Medical Research (ICMR) showed a declining trend from 2000 to 2010 with a prevalence of 0.2–1.1 per 1,000 in urban areas (Kumar RK et al., Indian J Med Res, 2013). School-based studies from 1970 to 2010 have also shown a declining trend from 5.3/1,000 in 1970 to 2.9/1,000 in 2000 and below 1/1,000 in 2010. The prevalence of RHD was reported to be 1.5–2/1,000 translating to 2.0–2.5 million cases of RHD in India **(Box 19B.3)**.

---

**Box 19B.3: Magnitude of the problem.**

- *Global*: RHD accounted for 2% of deaths due to CVDs. In 2015, RHD caused 33,194,900 cases and 319,400 deaths worldwide, out of which 60% were premature deaths, i.e. before the age of 70 years. Prevalence rates range from 0.2 per 1,000 in Havana to as high as 77.8 per 1,000 in Samoa.
- *South-East Asia (SEARO)*: In 2015, South-East Asian region accounted for 84% of total deaths and 80% of cases due to rheumatic heart disease (RHD).
- *India*: RHD is responsible for 25–45% cases of acquired heart disease. In 2015, there were about 13.17 million cases and 1.19 lakhs deaths due to RHD.

# Chapter 19: Specific Epidemiology of Noncommunicable Diseases

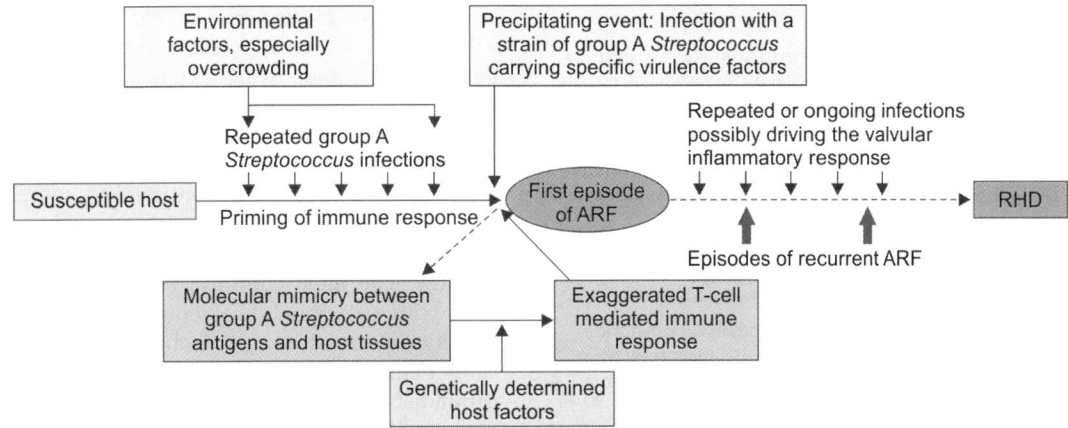

**Fig. 19B.8:** Pathogenesis of rheumatic fever and rheumatic heart disease.
*Source:* Carapetis JR, McDonald M, Wilson NJ. Acute rheumatic fever. Lancet. 2005;366:155-68.

## PATHOGENESIS OF RHEUMATIC HEART DISEASE

Rheumatic heart disease occurs due to an autoimmune response to RF. Streptococcal A carries M-proteins that are similar in structure and makeup to cardiac antigens in humans. The molecular mimicry mechanism of M proteins in group A beta-hemolytic streptococci and the muscle protein (myosin) and vascular endothelium of the heart leads to destruction of the heart tissues. This causes RHD. There is permanent damage to cardiac valves. RHD most commonly affects the mitral valve and least commonly affects the pulmonary valve. This is explained in the **Figures 19B.8 and 19B.9**.

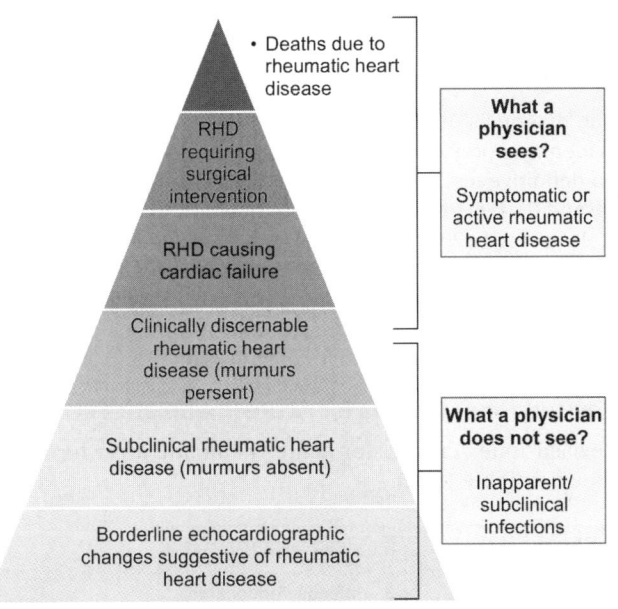

**Fig. 19B.9:** Iceberg phenomenon of rheumatic fever (RF) and rheumatic heart disease (RHD).

## EPIDEMIOLOGICAL FACTORS

### Agent Factors

The causative organism for RF is group A streptococci. Among group A streptococci, certain M serotypes beta-hemolytic streptococci (types 1, 3, 5, 6, 14, 18, 19, 24, 27, and 29) are most commonly associated with RF. However, in high incidence areas, any serotype of group A streptococci can cause ARF. All these serotypes are immunologically different with little cross immunity, thus production of an effective vaccine a difficult or an impossible task. Another difficulty in controlling this disease is existence of carriers, which are responsible for subclinical infections in the community. It is typically described as a disease that licks the joints and bites the heart.

### Host Factors

- *Age:* ARF usually affects children between 5–14 years. The initial episodes are more common in children while recurrent episodes are more common in old adolescents and young adults. People more than 30 years of age are rarely involved. In contrast, prevalence of RHD is more in 25–40 years age group.
- *Gender*: RF affects both sexes equally while RHD disproportionately affects girls and women twice as frequently as males. Females account for roughly two-thirds of the patients admitted for RHD in hospitals in India and African region. In RF/RHD endemic regions, it is an important cause of maternal and perinatal mortality and morbidity.
- *Socioeconomic status:* The role of socioeconomic conditions in causation of RF cannot be overlooked. It is a social disease linked to poverty, poor housing conditions and overcrowding, inadequate access to healthcare, and a low level of awareness of the disease in the community.
- *Immune response:* RF and RHD have an immunological basis, i.e. they occur due to an autoimmune reaction. The causative organism group A streptococci produce certain toxic products as well as some components of streptococci and host tissues have an antigenic cross-relationship. This leads to an immunological reaction, which causes an attack of RF.
- *Genetic susceptibility:* There have been reports suggesting clustering of cases and concordance among the monozygotic twins (especially in chorea) thereby confirming the role of inheritance in susceptibility to ARF. Human leukocyte antigen (HLA) class II alleles are found to be associated with this susceptibility.

## Environmental Factors

***Housing conditions:*** Poor housing conditions, overcrowding, undernutrition, poverty predispose to frequent episodes of streptococcal pharyngitis, and complications following it including RF and RHD.

***Healthcare system:*** Due to insufficient resources and expertise of manpower in healthcare system, there is either inadequate or delayed diagnosis or incomplete treatment of ARF, which leads to recurrent attacks of RF and its complications like RHD.

> **Key Points**
> - Rheumatic heart disease is a group of heart disorders which include short and long-term conditions occurring due to rheumatic fever (RF).
> - RF and RHD are noncommunicable diseases, which result from a communicable disease (streptococcal pharyngitis).
> - In 2015, about 2% of all cardiovascular deaths, 25.5% left heart failures and 5.3% right heart failures were due to RHD; WHO African region, the South-East Asian region and the Western Pacific region are worst affected.
> - Rheumatic fever is an endemic disease and a neglected public health problem in India.
> - Causative organism for RF is Group A streptococci; particularly M serotypes of the beta-hemolytic streptococci lead to an autoimmune response. It usually affects children between 5 and 14 years
> - Poor housing conditions, overcrowding, undernutrition, poverty predispose to frequent episodes of streptococcal pharyngitis, and complications following it including RF and RHD.

### Natural History of Rheumatic Fever and Rheumatic Heart Disease

The natural history of rheumatic fever and rheumatic heart disease has been shown in **Figure 19B.10**.

## CLINICAL FEATURES

Following group A streptococcal infection, a latent period of 1–5 weeks (3 weeks) precedes the appearance of clinical features of ARF. An exception is seen in carditis and chorea, where it takes up to 6 months for features to appear. In majority of cases, there is a subclinical infection of group A streptococci, which can only be confirmed by antibody tests.

- ***Fever:*** Fever is characteristically seen in acute illness and is sometimes accompanied by sweating. It lasts roughly 12 weeks and tends to recur.
- ***Joint involvement (arthritis):*** It is seen in 90% of patients. The joints are inflamed and swollen with or without tenderness. The arthritis in RHD is migratory with involvement of large joints mainly knee, ankle, hip, and elbow. Smaller joints are less commonly involved, e.g. hands and feet. The pain and swelling of the joints are transient and occur quickly and subside spontaneously within a week without any residual damage to the joint. Arthralgia (joint pain) without arthritis may also be seen involving large joints.
- ***Heart involvement (carditis):*** Around 60–70% of patients with ARF develop RHD. However, history of a previous attack of RF is not always present. There is inflammation and damage involving all layers of the heart—pericardium, myocardium, and endocardium. The hallmark of carditis in RHD is valvular damage. The most common valve affected is the mitral valve with occasional involvement of aortic valve. Carditis is clinically manifested by tachycardia, cardiac murmurs, cardiac enlargement, pericarditis, and heart failure. The most common finding on ECG is first-degree atrioventricular block.
- ***Skin involvement:*** Involvement of skin is in the form of a typical rash called erythema marginatum. It appears as a pink macule with central clearance and fades off with a serpiginous spreading edge. It usually occurs on trunk and limbs but never involves the face. Subcutaneous nodules occur as small and painless mobile lumps below the skin particularly in hands, elbows, feet, and sometimes occiput and vertebrae. They appear 2–4 weeks after the onset of disease and last up to 3 weeks and then disappear without any residual damage.
- ***Nervous system involvement (Sydenham's chorea):*** It manifests in the form of abnormal and jerky movements of the legs, arms, and body. It commonly occurs females. These are quasi purposive movements and particularly involve the head causing characteristic darting movements of the tongue. It gradually resolves within 6 weeks leaving no residual damage.

## DIAGNOSIS OF RHEUMATIC FEVER AND RHEUMATIC HEART DISEASE

The diagnosis of RF is based on clinical features along with evidence of previous group A streptococcal infection as there is no definitive test. The 2002–2003 WHO criteria for diagnosis of RF and RHD are based on revised Jones criteria (1992).

However, in 2012, American Heart Association (AHA) revised the Jones criteria further for low-risk and moderate-to-high-risk populations based on sensitivity and specificity and improved diagnosis by echocardiography and is now established as international gold standard for diagnosis of ARF.

### Revised Jones Criteria for Acute Rheumatic Fever 2015

Revised Jones criteria for acute rheumatic fever have been shown in **Table 19B.3**.

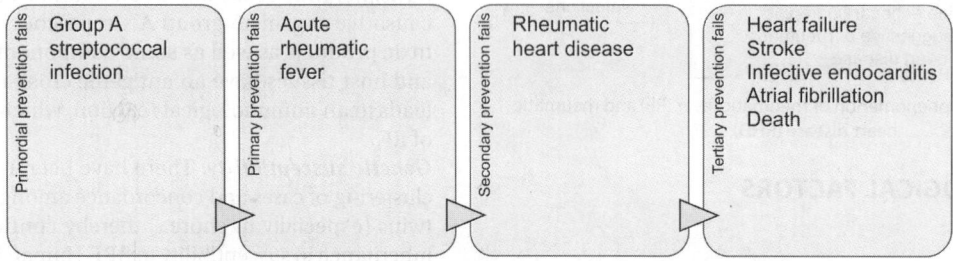

**Fig. 19B.10:** Natural history of rheumatic fever and rheumatic heart disease.

**Table 19B.3:** Revised Jones criteria for diagnosis of acute rheumatic fever and rheumatic heart disease, 2015.

### A. For all patient populations with evidence of preceding GAS infection

| | |
|---|---|
| Diagnosis: Initial acute rheumatic fever (RF) | 2 major/1 major + 2 minor manifestations |
| Diagnosis: Recurrent acute rheumatic fever (RF) | 2 major/1 major and 2 minor or 3 minor |

### B. Major criteria

| Low-risk populations* | Moderate and high-risk populations |
|---|---|
| Carditis—clinical and/or subclinical** | Carditis—clinical and/or subclinical** |
| Arthritis—polyarthritis only | Arthritis—monoarthritis or polyarthritis |
| Polyarthralgia | |
| Chorea | Chorea |
| Erythema marginatum | Erythema marginatum |
| Subcutaneous nodules | Subcutaneous nodules |

### C. Minor criteria

| Low-risk populations* | Moderate and high-risk populations |
|---|---|
| Polyarthralgia | Monoarthralgia |
| Fever (>38.5°C) | Fever (>38°C) |
| ESR ≥60 mm in first hour and/or CRP ≥3.0 mg/dL | ESR ≥30 mm in the first hour and/or CRP ≥3.0 mg/dL |
| Prolonged PR interval, after accounting for age variability (unless carditis is a major criterion) | Prolonged PR interval, after accounting for age variability (unless carditis is a major criterion) |

### Echocardiographic criteria for the diagnosis of subclinical carditis

| Pathological mitral regurgitation (meets all four criteria) | Pathological aortic regurgitation (meets all four criteria) |
|---|---|
| Seen in at least two views | Seen in at least two views |
| Jet length ≥2 cm in at least one view | Jet length ≥1 cm in at least one view |
| Peak velocity >3 m/s | Peak velocity >3 m/s |
| Pansystolic jet in at least one envelope | Pandiastolic jet in at least one envelope |

(CRP: C-reactive protein; ESR: erythrocyte sedimentation rate)
*Low-risk populations: With a rheumatic fever (RF) incidence ≤2 per 100,000 school-aged children or all-age rheumatic heart disease prevalence of ≤1 per 1,000 population per year.
**Subclinical carditis indicates echocardiographic valvulitis.

## PREVENTION AND CONTROL

Prevention and control of RF and RHD reduces the morbidity and mortality associated with RHD. It has a great public health significance because of its high incidence and prevalence and mortality especially affecting the children and young adults. The economic burden of RHD is also significant due to excess healthcare costs in treating it and indirect costs due to premature death and disability. The preventive strategies for RHD can be classified as follows **(Fig. 19B.11):**

### Primordial Prevention

The aim of primordial prevention is to eliminate risk factors for streptococcal infection, particularly poor housing conditions and overcrowding. Community health education programs should be targeted toward creating awareness regarding personal and environmental hygiene and other risk factors for streptococcal infection. Improving living conditions and breaking the poverty-disease-poverty cycle will reduce the incidence of RF in the long run.

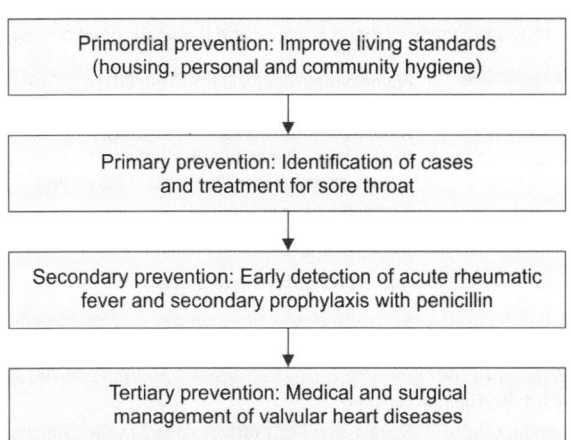

**Fig. 19B.11:** Levels of prevention of rheumatic fever and rheumatic heart disease.

### Primary Prevention

The aim of primary prevention is to prevent first episode of RF by identifying all cases of streptococcal throat infection and treating them adequately. Penicillin is the drug of choice and can prevent roughly all cases of ARF, if given within 9 days of onset of sore throat. The focus should be on "high-risk" groups, i.e. children in the age group of 5–15 years to keep them under surveillance for streptococcal pharyngitis by swabbing and culturing every case of sore throat. However, in absence of diagnostic facilities for culture of throat swab, penicillin can be given to treat sore throat without the culture report.

A single intramuscular injection of benzathine benzyl penicillin (1.2 million units) for adults and 0.6 million units for children is the drug of choice. Oral penicillin V or penicillin G can also be given as an alternative for 10 days. For patients with allergy to penicillin, erythromycin can be given.

### Secondary Prevention

Early diagnosis and treatment to prevent recurrences is a more feasible approach more so in developing countries where primary prevention of rheumatic fever is difficult. If treated adequately, 75% of people with RF recover completely without any sequelae. Because ARF patients are at higher risk of recurrence after a bout of group A streptococcal, an infection as compared to general population, long-term penicillin prophylaxis needs to be given to prevent recurrences.

The drug of choice for secondary prophylaxis of ARF is benzathine benzyl penicillin. The dose is 1.2 million units in adults and 0.6 million units in children to be administered intramuscularly every 3 weeks. This treatment must be continued for a minimum of 5 years or till the child attains the age of 18 years whichever is later **(Table 19B.4).**

For carditis patients [mild mitral regurgitation (MR) or healed carditis]—they should continue treatment with penicillin for at least 10 years after the last attack, or till the age of 25 years, whichever is longer. For patients with more severe disease or postvalve surgery cases, lifelong treatment may be needed. Since penicillin prophylaxis is a long-term affair, cardiac patient

Table 19B.4: Treatment of rheumatic fever and rheumatic heart disease.

| Acute rheumatic fever | Phenoxymethylpenicillin 500 mg BID (≥ 27 kg) 250 mg BID (≤ 27 kg) 10 days<br>Amoxicillin—50 mg/kg up to 1 g/day<br>Single dose—benzathine penicillin intramuscularly 1.2 million units in adults and 0.6 million units in children<br>Aspirin—children 80–100 mg/kg/day four to five divided doses<br>Adults (4–8 g/day) up to 2 weeks |
|---|---|
| Chorea | Severe chorea—carbamazepine or sodium valproate |
| Secondary prophylaxis for rheumatic heart disease<br>Benzathine penicillin—intramuscularly for 3 weeks, 1.2 million units in adults and 0.6 million units in children | |
| RF without carditis | 5 years after last attack or up to 21 years (whichever is longer) |
| RF with carditis | 10 years after last attack or up to 21 years (whichever is longer) |
| RF with persistent valvular disease evident clinically or on echocardiography | 10 years after last attack or up to 40 years (whichever is longer) |

*Source:* Gerber MA, Baltimore RS, Eaton CB. AHA Scientific Statement Prevention of Rheumatic Fever and Diagnosis and Treatment of Acute Streptococcal Pharyngitis. Circulation. 2009;119:1541-51.

compliance needs to be considered and it can be implemented through primary healthcare systems.

### Tertiary Prevention

The *aim* is to prevent disability and premature death in RHD patients by medical management of heart failure and heart valve related surgery. The main modalities of management are balloon mitral valvuloplasty or surgical mitral commissurotomy or valve replacement. The cost of surgical interventions, cost of prosthetic valves is quite high and because of inadequate facilities for operative procedures, developing countries face a challenge in management of RHD.

**Key Points**
- The diagnosis of RF is based on clinical features along with evidence of previous group A streptococcal infection as there is no definitive test. The 2015 WHO criteria for diagnosis of RF and RHD are based on revised Jones criteria.
- The aim of primordial prevention is to eliminate risk factors for streptococcal infection, particularly poor housing conditions and overcrowding.
- The aim of primary prevention is to prevent first episode of RF by identifying all cases of streptococcal throat infection and treating them adequately. Penicillin is the drug of choice.
- Secondary prevention refers to early diagnosis and treatment to prevent recurrences. The drug of choice for secondary prophylaxis of ARF is benzathine benzyl penicillin.
- The aim in tertiary prevention is to prevent disability and premature death in RHD patients by medical management of heart failure and heart valve related surgery.

## NATIONAL PROGRAM FOR PREVENTION AND CONTROL OF RF AND RHD

In countries like India where RF is endemic and a significant public health problem, a national program for prevention and control of RF and RHD is essential. This program should be integrated in national development plans and services delivered through the existing infrastructure. Under the platform of National Programme for Prevention and Control of Non-Communicable Diseases (NP-NCD) and Rashtriya Bal Swasthya Karyakram (RBSK), pilot projects have been launched in select districts of Bihar (Gaya), Uttar Pradesh (Firozabad), and Madhya Pradesh (Hoshangabad) for the prevention and control of RF and RHD. The scaling up of these projects in other districts will be done in a phase-wise manner. To reduce the global burden of RF and RHD, the World Heart Federation has set a goal of '**25 by 2025, in less than 25**', i.e. achieve a 25% reduction in incidence of premature deaths occurring due to RF and RHD among people aged less than 25 years by the year 2025.

The main strategies for its prevention and control are as follows:
- Improving the standards of living
- Increasing access to appropriate care
- Ensuring a consistent supply of good quality antibiotics
- Adequate monitoring and surveillance activities—schools, pregnant women
- Training health care staff in early identification of cases and appropriate management
- Procuring reliable data on incidence and burden of RF.

*A community project on control of rheumatic fever (RF) and rheumatic heart disease (RHD) known as Jai Vigyan Mission Mode project was conducted by* Indian Council of Medical Research (ICMR) in India from 2000 to 2010. The project report published in 2015 is a guide to experts or institutions involved with prevention and control of disease.

**NP-NCD is further discussed in Chapter 47: Health Policies and Programs in India.**

## CONCLUSION

Rheumatic heart disease is a serious health problem, which is preventable. For endemic countries like India, the focus on prevention and control should be on primary and secondary preventive strategies including improving the living standards of people, improving access to appropriate treatment, and ensuring regular supply of good-quality antibiotics. Lack of reliable data pertaining to RHD is a major roadblock in planning services for people. Hence, proper planning and development along with implementation of feasible national program for control of RHD should be the priority and this can be done by incorporating it in national health policy and budget. Newer advances in the field of vaccines against streptococcal infection and long-acting antibiotics for better adherence for secondary prophylaxis may go a long way in reducing the burden of RHD.

## SUMMARY

Rheumatic heart disease is a group of heart disorders leading to short-term and long-term conditions due to single or multiple episodes RF. In 2015, RHD was responsible for 305,000 deaths out of which 60% were premature deaths, i.e. before the age of 70 years accounting for about 2% of all cardiovascular deaths.

The epidemiological triad of RHD and RF is described under:
- *Agent factors:* Group A streptococci. Among group A streptococci with certain M serotypes (types 1, 3, 5, 6, 14, 18, 19, 24, 27, and 29).
- *Host factors:* ARF affects children aged 5–14 years and RHD is more frequently seen in 25–40 years of age in low and middle-income countries and some marginalized communities in high-income countries.
- *Environmental factors:* Poor housing conditions, overcrowding, undernutrition, and poverty along with inadequacies in healthcare resources for diagnosis and prompt treatment lead to recurrent attacks of RF.

The diagnosis of RF and RHD is based on the 1992 Revised Jones Criteria with 2 major/1 major + 2 minor manifestations for RF and echocardiographic criteria or the diagnosis of subclinical carditis for RHD.

The prevention of RF and RHDs is:
- *Primordial prevention:* Improvement of living standards at personal, housing and community level.
- *Primary prevention:* Identification of cases of sore throat and prompt treatment for the same.
- *Secondary prevention:* Early diagnosis and treatment to prevent recurrences of RF using benzathine benzyl penicillin. The dose is 1.2 million units in adults and 0.6 million units in children to be administered intramuscularly every 3 weeks.
- *Tertiary prevention:* Medical management of heart failure and heart valve related surgery.

## SUGGESTED READING

1. Gerber MA, Baltimore RS, Eaton CB, Gewitz M, Rowley AH, Shulman ST, et al. Prevention of rheumatic fever and diagnosis and treatment of acute streptococcal pharyngitis. Circulation. 2009;119(11):1541-51.
2. Gewitz MH, Baltimore RS, Tani LY, et al. Revision of the Jones Criteria for the diagnosis of acute rheumatic fever in the era of Doppler echocardiography: a scientific statement from the American Heart Association. Circulation. 2015;131(20):1806-18.
3. Global Burden of Disease Collaborative Network. Global Burden of Disease Study 2016 (GBD 2016) Results. Seattle, United States: Institute for Health Metrics and Evaluation (IHME), 2017. [online] Available from: http://ghdx.healthdata.org/gbd-results-tool.
4. Reményi B, Wilson N, Steer A, et al. World Heart Federation criteria for echocardiographic diagnosis of rheumatic heart disease—an evidence-based guideline. J Nat Rev Cardiol. 2012;9(5):297-309.
5. Rheumatic Fever and Rheumatic Heart Disease: Report of a WHO Expert Consultation (WHO Tech Rep Ser, 923). Geneva, World Health Organization; 2004.
6. Strasser T, Rotta J. The control of rheumatic fever and rheumatic heart disease: an outline of WHO activities. WHO Chron. 1973;27(2):49-54.
7. Watkins DA, Johnson CO, Colquhoun SM, Karthikeyan G, Beaton A, Bukhman G, et al. Global, regional, and national burden of rheumatic heart disease, 1990-2015. N Engl J Med. 2017;377:713-22.
8. WHO. (1986). Community prevention and control of cardiovascular diseases, Techn Rep. Ser. No. 732.
9. WHO. (2018). Rheumatic fever and rheumatic heart disease. Report by DG. [online] Available from: <http://apps.who.int/gb/ebwha/ pdf_ files/ WHA71/A71_25-en.pdf.
10. World Health Organization. (2016). Disease burden and mortality estimates. [online] Available from: http://www.who.int/healthinfo/global_burden_disease/estimates/en/index1.html.
11. Zühlke LJ, Steer AC. Estimates of the global burden of rheumatic heart disease. Glob Heart. 2013;8(3):189-95.

# C. EPIDEMIOLOGY OF DIABETES MELLITUS AND ITS PREVENTION AND CONTROL

*Bhanu M*

*"Let food be your medicine, and medicine your food."*
—**Hippocrates**

---

**CM 7.2** Enumerate, describe and discuss the mode of transmission and measures for prevention and control of diabetes

**CM 8.2** Describe and discuss the epidemiological and control measures applicable in diabetes

---

## INTRODUCTION

The chapter mainly focuses on the aspects of most common type of diabetes which is type 2 as compared to type 1, whose occurrence is rarely modified by primordial and primary preventive measures alone. In today's world more and more people are deviating from traditional lifestyle of consuming fresh home cooked food with healthy ingredients; the higher socioeconomic status people who consume oil, flour, and sugar in excessive amounts are at high risk. More alarming is globalization where children are exposed to various packed and processed foods. thus it is very much important to establish healthy food choices in, as dietary fat intake and obesity are closely associated with occurrence of diabetes. The other major factor influencing the initiation of type 2 diabetes is the lack of adequate age appropriate physical activity.

## CURRENT EPIDEMIOLOGICAL CONTEXT

As the years pass by, globalization and extensive international and national travel have led to an increase in risk of both infectious and noninfectious or chronic diseases across the population and regions where they were previously not seen. Following this we are now seeing a trend of "globalization" of risk factors and diseases akin to globalization of trade and travel. The disease, once considered as the problem among the rich, urban habitants, and old age, is now becoming common across most of the socioeconomic classes and age groups.

## DEFINITION

The definition accepted by both World Health Organization (WHO) and American Diabetic Association (ADA) is—diabetes is a group of metabolic disorders characterized by hyperglycemia resulting from defects in insulin secretion, insulin action or both. From the point of etiology, pathogenesis, biochemical features, and implications of diabetes mellitus, the following definition is also used—diabetes is a metabolic cum vascular syndrome of multiple etiology characterized by chronic hyperglycemia with disturbances of carbohydrate, fat, and protein metabolism resulting from defects in insulin secretion, insulin action, or both leading to changes in both small blood vessels (microangiopathy) and large blood vessels (macroangiopathy).

## CLASSIFICATION

The WHO recommends the following classification of diabetes mellitus:
- Diabetes mellitus (DM)
  - Type 1 or insulin dependent diabetes mellitus
  - Type 2 or noninsulin dependent diabetes mellitus
  - Malnutrition-related diabetes mellitus (MRDM)
  - Other types (secondary to pancreatic, hormonal, drug induced, genetic and other abnormalities)
- Impaired glucose tolerance (IGT)
- Gestational diabetes mellitus (GDM)

ADA classification of diabetes mellitus is quite elaborative and clinically oriented as compared to WHO classification.

## MAGNITUDE

### World

Diabetes is increasing to epidemic proportions across the globe. In 2019, a total of 463 million people are estimated to be living with diabetes, representing 9.3% of the global adult population (20–79 years). This number is expected to increase to 578 million (10.2%) in 2030 and 700 million (10.9%) in 2045. (International Diabetes Federation, Global and regional diabetes prevalence estimates for 2019). Diabetes was the direct cause of 1.5 million deaths and 48% of all deaths due to diabetes occurred before the age of 70 years in 2019. Another 460,000 kidney disease deaths were caused by diabetes, and raised blood glucose causes around 20% of cardiovascular deaths. Between 2000 and 2019, there was a 3% increase in diabetes mortality rates by age. (WHO. Diabetes;factsheet April 2023).

### India

In India, there are estimated 77 million people above the age of 18 years in 2019 who are suffering from diabetes (type 2), which is expected to rise to over 134 million by 2045. Approximately 57% of these individuals remain undiagnosed. There are nearly 25 million are prediabetics (at a higher risk of developing diabetes in near future). (Diabetes in India, WHO 2023)

Based on epidemiological studies, high blood glucose is defined as a distribution of fasting plasma glucose in a population that is higher than the theoretical distribution that would minimize risks to health (derived from epidemiological studies). HbA1c is used as an indicator of blood glucose level over past 3 months which may aid in diagnosing diabetes. However, it still remains a challenge to have one best cut-off at population level.

As diabetes is occurring in epidemic proportions, the economic impact it has been causing cannot be ignored. A framework on costs and economic impact of diabetes on individuals and societies was developed during a review by Yesudian et al, which is shown in **Table 19C.1**.

**Table 19C.1:** Classification of costs and economic impact on individuals and society.

| Economic impact on individual and household | | Economic impact on health sector and economic sector | |
|---|---|---|---|
| Direct costs | Hospital, transport, drug costs, foods | Direct costs (health sector) | Inpatient care, outpatient care (general physicians, district hospitals, pharmacy), long-term care |
| Indirect costs | Loss of income associated with morbidity, mortality and disability | Indirect costs (economic sector) | Costs due to absenteeism, permanent disability and mortality |

> **Key Points**
> - Diabetes is a group of metabolic disorders characterized by hyperglycemia resulting from defects in insulin secretion, insulin action or both.
> - 71% of the overall deaths in the world (2016) are attributed to NCDs, of which diabetes ranks fourth[7] and ranks seventh cause of death among all-cause mortality.
> - The more common type of diabetes is type 2 (8.5% in the adult population of the world in 2014) as compared to type 1 (3% in high income countries, less common in Asia and Latin America)
> - In India, overall prevalence of diabetes and prediabetes was found to be 7.3% and 10.3% respectively (INDIAB study).
> - In India, prevalence was higher in urban areas than in rural areas (INDIAB study).

## EPIDEMIOLOGICAL DETERMINANTS AND RISK FACTORS

An individual inherits the genetic susceptibility to develop either IDDM or NIDDM; one or more environmental factors eventually precipitate the development of overt disease. The underlying cause of diabetes is insulin deficiency which is absolute in IDDM and partial in NIDDM.

1. **Genetic factors:** Some of the genetic markers in IDDM include genes in the HLA-D (HLA-DR3 and DR4) region of the major histocompatibility complex (MHC) in the chromosome 6. NIDDM is not HLA associated. Type 2 diabetes is associated with genetic variants in the peroxisome proliferator-activated receptor-γ gene (PPARG), the ATP-sensitive potassium channel Kir6·2 (KCNJ11) and polymorphisms in the gene encoding transcription factor-7-like protein 2 (TCF7L2), especially in the Asian populations.
2. **Acquired and environmental factors:**
   a. *Infections*: Viruses implicated are rubella, mumps, and human coxsackie virus B4. Either bacterial or viral infections may precipitate over disease in both IDDM and NIDDM through nonspecific stress mechanisms.
   b. *Toxins and other mechanisms that damage bet cell function*: The role of toxins like Alloxan, pyrinuron (rodenticide), streptozotocin, certain nitrosamines in food have been explored. Malnutrition related diabetes is due to damage to islets of Langerhans of pancreas by toxins in a background of inadequate protein intake.
3. **Lifestyle factors:**
   a. *Overnutrition and obesity:* This results in reduction in the number of insulin receptors on target cells or insulin resistance through pos receptor changes (decreasing glucose transport or impeding intracellular glucose metabolism)
   b. *Physical inactivity:* Lack of exercise is seen to alter interaction between insulin and its receptors.
   c. *Severe or prolonged stress:* Several states of stress like acute MI, surgery, infections, burns, trauma lead to glucose intolerance due to hormonal effects on glucose metabolism, insulin secretion or action.
   d. *Drugs and hormones:* Some of the drugs implicated include phenytoin, thiazide diuretics, corticosteroids, oral contraceptives, etc.
   e. *Pancreatic disorders:* Inflammatory, neoplastic and other disorders like cystic fibrosis and hemochromatosis may lead to varying degrees of insulin deficiency.

Following meta-analytic study, the following independent risk factors are recognized in Asia—abdominal obesity, unfavorable changes in diet and lifestyle, cigarette smoking, impaired pancreatic beta cell function, childhood malnutrition, air pollution, certain blood dyscrasias, viral hepatitis, and tuberculosis. Gestational diabetes, poor nutrition in utero and overnutrition in later life are all known to be associated with the diabetes epidemic in Asia. Recently even smoking has been found to be associated with diabetes.

> **Key Points**
> - Most cases of type 2 diabetes are attributed to the modifiable risk factors, which can be controlled or reduced through individual and population-based strategies.
> - Risky behaviors to be avoided to prevent type 2 DM
>   ▸ Unhealthy diet
>   ▸ Physical inactivity
>   ▸ Excessive weight gain
>   ▸ Obesity
>   ▸ Overweight
>   ▸ Not managing mental and physical stress on a regular basis.

## PRINCIPLES AND APPROACHES IN PREVENTION AND CONTROL

As diabetes is becoming more and more common among the young and those with low BMI, it is imperative for a country like India to prioritize measures to prevent and control the disease where we find wide access to diverse food habits and lifestyles. The population approach should mainly focus on creating environment which promotes healthy eating, physical activity, working and playing, also make provision for healthy choices. Formulating such policies involving only the health sector would not be as effective as a "whole of government" approach which involves policy decisions in other non-health sectors too, such as education, agriculture, urban planning, trade, finance, and transport. A life-course approach is found to be best suitable for prevention of diabetes which primarily aims at preventing childhood obesity. The first 1,000 days from the point of a woman's pregnancy till the child's second birthday is the prime time to ensure adequate and healthy nutrition in mother and the child. Other key factors to consider in prevention of type 2 diabetes are provision of supportive environment for physical activity; settings-based interventions like whole of school approach, workplace interventions; fiscal, legislative, and regulatory measures for healthy diet; education, social marketing, and mobilization.

### Primordial Prevention

- *Encouraging health enhancing behaviors*, such as:
  - Participation in lifestyle exercise*
  - Healthy eating
  - Yoga
- *Avoidance of health harming behaviors*, such as:
  - Smoking
  - Excessive alcohol consumption
  - Binge eating
- *Promoting health protective behaviors*, such as:
  - Health screening
  - Clinic attendance.

Individual and mass education is the mode of intervention under primordial prevention.

### Primary Prevention

#### Population (Mass) Strategy

**Health promotion:** Promoting healthy lifestyle.

**Specific protection:** Health education on healthy eating habits, benefits of exercise and physical activity.

---

*WHO recommendations on physical activity are provided for different age groups:*
- *It is recommended that children and youth aged 5–17 years should do at least 60 minutes of moderate- to vigorous-intensity physical activity daily.*
- *It is recommended that adults aged 18–64 years should do at least 150 minutes of moderate-intensity aerobic physical activity (for example, brisk walking, jogging, gardening) spread throughout the week, or at least 75 minutes of vigorous-intensity aerobic physical activity throughout the week, or an equivalent combination of moderate- and vigorous-intensity activity.*
- *For older adults the same amount of physical activity is recommended but should also include balance and muscle strengthening activity tailored to their ability and circumstances.*

---

There have been several primary preventive and randomized clinical trials relating to type 1 diabetes, among the various interventions and factors tested are immunological approaches, monoclonal antibody, dietary modification, exposure to cows' milk, the age of introduction of solid foods, supplementation with an omega-3 fatty acid, and supplementation with vitamin D, vitamin B6 supplementation, nasal insulin, and low-dose cyclosporine.

---

*Case Scenario: Population Strategy*

The "sugar sweetened beverage tax", Mexico Focus area: Regulatory measure: In view of highest diabetes prevalence among Organization for Economic Cooperation and Development (OECD) member countries in Mexico, and with the finding of highest per capita consumption of soft drinks across the world, an increase in tax on drinks containing added sugars by over 10% was implemented nationwide in January 2014. An interim analysis showed 6% reduction in purchase of taxed sugar sweetened beverages within 1 year and estimated 11.6% decrease in quantity of drinks consumed.

---

#### High-risk Strategy

**Health promotion:** Promoting changes in the high-risk behaviors and alternate holistic healing methods.

**Specific protection:** Health education on risk factors, occurrence, and complications of diabetes.

---

*Case Scenario: High-risk Strategy*

PEN Fa'a, Samoa Island (started November 2014) Focus areas: There were three focus areas:
1. A women's committee representative from each village facilitate early detection of NCD, in liaison with government agencies.
2. A physician at district health facility initiates treatment and behavioral change measures in patients detected with hyperglycemia. The trained women representatives in the village help the patients to adhere to their treatment plans.
3. Measures are also taken to improve community awareness about various aspects of NCDs.

PEN: Package of Essential Noncommunicable (PEN), Disease Interventions for Primary Health Care.

---

### Secondary Prevention

The prime factor in ensuring quality life in patients living with diabetes is early detection and management of the disease. Later the time of diagnosis during the course of the disease, higher are the chances of suffering from complications leading to poor health outcomes. The basic diagnostics are now made available at primary healthcare settings across India through National Programme for Prevention and Control of Non-Communicable Diseases (NP-NCD). In order to ensure quick access to early diagnosis of diabetes.

#### Early Diagnosis

WHO recommends the following criteria for diagnosis of diabetes and intermediate hyperglycemia:

| Diabetes | |
|---|---|
| Fasting plasma glucose or 2-hour plasma glucose* or HbA1c | ≥126 mg/dL (≥7.0 mmol/L) or >200 mg/dL (≥11.1 mmol/L) or ≥ 6.5% |

---

*Lifestyle exercises include activities like gardening, walking with the dog, playing golf, taking the stairs instead of the elevator, i.e. any activity that gets you moving and increases your daily activity level.

Lifestyle exercises should be prescribed by the primary care doctor/treating physician based on the person's/patient's age, gender, occupation, locomotor status, any other relevant health condition, and her/his preferences, in order to gain most use out of the activity.

| Impaired glucose tolerance (IGT) | |
|---|---|
| Fasting plasma glucose and 2-hour plasma glucose* | <126 mg/dL (7.0 mmol/L) and 140 mg/dL to 200 mg/dL (7.8 to 11.1 mmol/L) |
| Impaired fasting glucose (IFG) | |
| Fasting plasma glucose and if measured 2-hour plasma glucose* | 110 mg/dL to 125 mg/dL (6.1 to 6.9 mmol/L)<br><140 mg/dL (7.8 mmol/L) |
| Gestational diabetes (GDM) | |
| One or more of the following:<br>Fasting plasma glucose<br>1-hour plasma glucose**<br>2-hour plasma glucose* | One or more of the following:<br>92 mg/dL to 125 mg/dL (5.1 to 6.9 mmol/L)<br>≥180 mg/dL (10.0 mmol/L)<br>153–199 mg/dL (8.5 to 11.0 mmol/L) |

*Venous plasma glucose 2 hours after ingestion of 75 g oral glucose load
**Venous plasma glucose 1 hour after ingestion of 75 g oral glucose load

In people who do not have symptoms, a positive test for diabetes should be repeated on another day. 1 blood glucose measurement is relatively simple and cheap and should be available at primary healthcare level.

Whereas, according to ADA, diabetes can be diagnosed in presence of one or more of the following:
- Fasting plasma glucose of more than/ equal to 126 mg/dL (fasting implies no caloric intake for at least 8 hours prior to the test).
- Symptoms of hyperglycemia with casual plasma glucose more than or equal to 200 mg/dL (casual means without regard to the time of last meal)
- 2-hour plasma glucose more than or equal to 200 mg/dL during an oral glucose tolerance test (OGTT)
- Glycated hemoglobin (HbA1C) value of 6.5% or above

We can observe that the diagnostic cutoffs are same in both WHO and ADA guidelines. However, the threshold of 100 mg/dL is recommended by ADA as normal fasting plasma glucose and 110 mg/dL by WHO. The intermediate hyperglycemic phases, where the blood glucose levels are higher than normal but not so high as to be termed diabetes are termed as impaired glucose tolerance (IGT) and impaired fasting glucose (IFG). Both WHO and ADA recognize the existence of these two stages.

Screening for diabetes can pick up the disease early and can prevent the progression of disease and complications in individuals and in a community. The following criteria are recommended by ADA for screening of diabetes.

**Screening criteria for asymptomatic individuals:**
- Age >45 years
- BMI >23 kg/m²
- Waist hip ratio >0.9 in men and >0.8 in women
- Family history of diabetes
- Sedentary lifestyle and physical inactivity
- Previously identified IFG or IGT
- BP >140/90 mm Hg in adults
- Dyslipidemia (cholesterol >200 mg/dL, TGL >150 mg/dL, LDL >100 mg/dL, low HDL: Men—<40 mg/dL, Women—<50 mg/dL).

**Screening criteria in individuals at high-risk:**
- Symptoms of hyperglycemia (polyuria, polydipsia, polyphagia, weight loss) or of complications of diabetes (e.g. tingling and numbness, burning feet, generalized/genital pruritus, recurrent infections, delayed healing or nonhealing of wounds/foot, ulcers, balanitis/vulvovaginitis, impotence, premature cataract)

- Adults with tuberculosis
- Persons on diabetogenic drugs (e.g. steroids, thiazide diuretics, oral contraceptives, etc.)
- Women with polycystic ovarian syndrome
- History of premature vascular syndrome.

**Criteria for retesting of diabetes in asymptomatic undiagnosed individuals:**
- Undiagnosed high-risk individuals with normal result—retest yearly
- Retest every 3 years if undiagnosed and not under high-risk category
- If identified to have IFG or IGT, retest yearly.

**Note**
Few examples of tools to assess the risk of having current or future diabetes:
- FINRISK
- AUSDRISK
- IDRS

## Management of Diabetes

### Nonpharmacological
Lifestyle modifications play a major role in control of blood sugar levels and diabetes.
- **Nutrition:** Appropriate diet according to a person's age, gender, ideal body weight (IBW), and occupation/physical activity is the key factor.

$$IBW = (height\ in\ cm - 100) \times 0.9$$

A person more than 120% of IBW is considered overweight and less than 90% considered underweight.

The following calorie requirement (in kcal/kg ideal body weight) is recommended:

| Activity level | Underweight | Normal | Overweight/obese |
|---|---|---|---|
| Sedentary | 35 | 30 | 20–25 |
| Moderate | 40 | 35 | 30 |
| Heavy | 45–50 | 40 | 35 |

Patient's calorie intake should be gradually altered; it should not be altered more than 500 kcal per day.
The following distribution of nutrients is recommended:

| Nutrients | % of total calories |
|---|---|
| Carbohydrate | 50–60% |
| Protein | 15–20% |
| Fat | <30% (saturated fat <10%) |
| Cholesterol | <300 mg/day |
| Fiber | 25–40 g/day—same as general population |
| Sodium | <2,000 mg/day |
| Alcohol | Not >5% of total calories |
| Vitamins and minerals | Same as general population; individualize if at high-risk |

- **Exercise:** A patient has to be thoroughly evaluated for presence of any complications or impending complications of diabetes before recommending any exercise program. The following activities are recommended based on FITT principle, i.e. frequency, intensity, time, and type.

- At least 150 min/week of moderate intensity aerobic physical activity (attaining to 50–70% of maximum heart rate or at the rate of 100 steps/minute) spread over at least 3 days/week with no more than 2 consecutive days without exercise. Shorter durations (minimum 75 min/week) of vigorous intensity or interval training may be sufficient for younger and more physically fit individuals.
- Individuals should be encouraged to reduce sedentary time, by incorporating 3 or more minutes of light activity (overhead arm stretches, walking or leg extension) every 30 minutes during prolonged sedentary activity.
- Adults with type 1 and type 2 diabetes should engage in 2-3 sessions/week of resistance exercise on nonconsecutive days.
- Flexibility training and balance training are recommended 2–3 times/week for older adults with diabetes.

### Pharmacological

The drugs used in treating diabetes are sulfonylureas, meglitinides, thiazolidinediones, alpha-glucosidase inhibitors, biguanide, dipeptidyl peptidase-4 (DPP-4) inhibitors, sodium-glucose cotransporter 2 (SGL2) inhibitors, incretin mimetics, centrally acting agent, insulin, and other injectable agent.

Success is not indicated only by early detection and initiation of diabetes treatment. There are still many challenges to be dealt with from the point of diagnosis. It is important to ensure adequate counseling to the patient with regard to periodic monitoring of appropriate and timely intake of medication, diet, physical activity, follow-up blood glucose, screening for impending complications, and self-care. Appropriate care facilities should be made available at the primary care settings, with referral services. In countries having high burden of comorbid conditions—infectious (like tuberculosis, HIV-AIDS) and NCDs (hypertension, stroke, obesity), it is essential to have facilities for integrated management of the same.

> **Case Scenario: Reversal of Disease Condition**
>
> *Barbados Diabetes Reversal Study Focus areas: Diet and physical activity*
> *Patients diagnosed with type 2 diabetes within 6 years, not on insulin were asked to stop all oral diabetic agents at beginning of 8 weeks diet strategy. They were put mainly on liquid, low carbohydrate, high fiber vegetable, and fruits diet. Repeat blood sugar after 3 months of 8 weeks diet revealed that despite several challenges 17 out of 25 participants had fasting plasma glucose levels lower than diabetic levels as compared to 3 of them at the beginning of the study.*

## Tertiary Prevention

Blood glucose levels must be monitored regularly for prevention of complications, patient should be screened for micro- and macrovascular complications and chronic cases of diabetes, especially those suffering from chronic diabetic ulcers should be provided with rehabilitation services. Picture of warning signs and impending complications of diabetes may be displayed in waiting areas of NCD clinics and primary care physicians' settings.

> **Case Scenario: Prevention of Complications**
>
> *The Ramadan initiative, Senegal*
> *Focus: Improving diabetes management using mobile technology*
> *SMS tips and advice are sent to enrolled diabetics during Ramadan to promote good health behaviors during and between fasting periods.*

> **Case Scenario: Rehabilitation**
>
> *Tajikistan*
> *Focus areas: Physical rehabilitation with external funding. Following interventions are planned in Tajikistan's only physical rehabilitation center with support from International Committee of the Red Cross:*
> ❑ *Assessment of disability and provision of assistive devices*
> ❑ *Physical rehabilitation including strengthening, endurance and gait training for those with lower limb amputations*
> ❑ *Facilitating return to work*
> ❑ *Providing education on self-management to prevent deterioration*

In India, the principles and other current aspects of prevention and control of diabetes are incorporated into NPCDCS now known as NP-NCD. **DM management guidelines (algorithms) are explained in detail in Chapter 47: Health Policies and Programs in India.**

> **Global commitment toward integrated approach to NCDs are expressed through following:**
> - WHO Global action plan for the prevention and control of NCDs 2013–2020 (WHO NCD Global Action Plan)
> - 2011 UN Political Declaration on NCDs
> - 2014 UN Outcome Document on NCDs
> - In April 2021, WHO launched the Global Diabetes Compact, a global initiative aiming for sustained improvements in diabetes prevention and care, with a particular focus on supporting low- and middle-income countries.
> - In May 2021, the World Health Assembly agreed a Resolution on strengthening prevention and control of diabetes. In May 2022, the World Health Assembly endorsed five global diabetes coverage and treatment targets to be achieved by 2030.

> **Key Points**
> - Lifestyle modifications play a major role in control of blood sugar levels and diabetes
> - Primordial prevention aims at encouraging health enhancing behaviors, avoidance of health harming behaviors and promoting health protective behaviors.
> - There are 2 strategies for primary prevention—population (mass) strategy and high-risk strategy.
> - Secondary prevention helps in ensuring quality life in patients living with diabetes by early detection and management of the disease.
> - Management of diabetes may be pharmacological or non-pharmacological.
> - Appropriate diet according to a person's age, gender, ideal body weight (IBW), and occupation/physical activity is the key.
> - Tertiary prevention targets screening for micro- and macrovascular complications and provision of rehabilitation services.

## SUMMARY

- Diabetes is a metabolic cum vascular syndrome of multiple etiology characterized by chronic hyperglycemia with disturbances of carbohydrate, fat, and protein metabolism resulting from defects in insulin secretion, insulin action, or both leading to changes in both small blood vessels (microangiopathy) and large blood vessels (macroangiopathy).
- Diabetes is increasing to epidemic proportions across the globe. Probability of an Indian aged 30–70 years dying from any of cardiovascular disease (CVD), cancer, diabetes, or chronic respiratory disease has been reported to be 23.3%.
- The population approach should mainly focus on creating environment which promotes healthy eating, physical activity, working and playing, also make provision for healthy choices.
- Screening for diabetes can pick up the disease early and can prevent the progression of disease and complications in individuals and in a community.
- Lifestyle modifications play a major role in control of blood sugar levels and diabetes.
- Global targets for prevention and control of NCDs have been set to be attained by 2025, which includes- halt the rise of diabetes and obesity.
- In India, the principles and other current aspects of prevention and control of diabetes are incorporated into NPCDCS.

### Culmination or tail end activity (to promote higher order thinking)

**Medical scenario:**
- A female patient aged about 80 years, taking medications for diabetes for the past 10 years, comes to your OPD with complaints of left upper limb swelling. How will you proceed with this case, and what further details would you look for before finalizing the treatment for this patient? How and what will you advise the patient till the execution of final treatment?
- A male patient aged about 70 years, on tablet metformin 500 mg for the past 5 years, is currently having HbA1c of 7.9 g/dL. His FBG and PPBG are 180 mg/dL and 280 mg/dL. There is a family history of diabetes in patient's father. Currently, patient is not willing to change his diet or medication, he has rigid beliefs about consumption of certain foods. He says that he goes for a walk almost every day in evening, which is apparently not brisk by way he describes it. What other conditions will you screen this patient for, what other relevant history and information would you elicit? How will you assess and take measures to address his financial constraints? How will you manage this patient? What advice(s) will you give to the patient and family? What are the socio-environmental facilities available to facilitate management of a case of diabetes in an urban and rural area?

**Nonmedical scenario**
- Interact with a postgraduate or an intern posted in an outreach center (urban and rural) to learn about the administrative-managerial-implementation issues related to NPCDS in their respective areas and the challenges faced by him/her as a primary care physician in dealing with these issues. Try to think of your own methods to overcome them and discuss the feasibility of same with your classmates.

**Worksheets to track food intake/habits and glucometer random sugar levels among yourself or an at risk or a patient of diabetes mellitus:**

| Food intake | Morning snack | Breakfast | Lunch | Evening snack | Dinner |
|---|---|---|---|---|---|
| Day 1 | | | | | |
| Day 2 | | | | | |
| Track for at least a week including quantity and nutritive values of the food consumed. | | | | | |

| GRBS | Pre-breakfast | Post-breakfast | Pre-lunch | Post-lunch | Evening | Pre-dinner | Post-dinner | Mid-night 2 am–3 am |
|---|---|---|---|---|---|---|---|---|
| Day 1 | | | | | | | | |
| Day 2 | | | | | | | | |
| Track for at least a week | | | | | | | | |

Collect the details in above format from a case of diabetes and based on that prepare a meal plan and advice the patient an appropriate treatment. Consider obtaining guidance from a dietician and a clinician while conducting this exercise. Also consider the preferences of the patient, suitable behavioral change strategy, counseling technique and other relevant issues involved.

### Note

**News titbit/Did you know?**
There was no global symbol for diabetes until 2006, and since then a blue circle is used universally to symbolize diabetes.

*History:* Diabetes was first identified as a disease as early as 3,000 years ago by Egyptians and Indians. Diabetes is a Greek word meaning siphon—to pass through, and mellitus is a Latin word meaning honeyed or sweet.

**Importance of the chapter for medical officer:**
As a primary care physician it is very essential for a medical officer to understand the life course approach of diabetes, be aware of latest diagnostic cutoffs, assessment of risk factors, importance of regular follow-ups in identifying impending complications and their prevention, various costs involved in managing diabetes, and referral services available in his/her vicinity.

## SUGGESTED READING

1. American Diabetes Association. Standards of medical care in diabetes. Diabetes Care.2017;38(Suppl 1):s1-s94.
2. Anjana RM, Deepa M, Pradeepa R, et al. Prevalence of diabetes and prediabetes in 15 states of India: results from the ICMR-INDIAB

population-based-cross-sectional study. Lancet Diabetes Endocrinol. 2017;5(8):585-96.
3. Chan JC, Malik V, Jia W, et al. Review: Diabetes in Asia: Epidemiology, risk factors, and pathophysiology. JAMA. 2009;301(20):2129-40.
4. Chen L, Magliano DJ, Balkau B, et al. AUSDRISK: an Australian type 2 diabetes risk assessment tool based on demographic, lifestyle and simple anthropometric measures. Med J Australia. 2010;192:(4)197-202.
5. Diabetes mellitus: Report of a WHO study group. Geneva, World Health Organization, 1985 (Technical report series 727).
6. Frank LL. Diabetes mellitus in the texts of old Hindu medicine (Charaka, Susruta, Vagbhata). Am J Gastroenterol. 1957;27(1):76-95.
7. Global prevalence of diabetes: estimates for the year 2000 and projections for 2030. Diabetes Care. 2004;27(5):1047-53.
8. International Diabetes Federation. Diabetes Atlas. 3rd edition. Brussels, Belgium: International Diabetes Federation; 2006.
9. Levesque C. Therapeutic lifestyle changes for diabetes. Nurs Clin North Am. 2017;52(4):679-62.
10. Lindstrom J, Tuomilehto J. The diabetes risk score: a practical tool to predict type 2 diabetes risk. Diabetes Care. 2003;26:(3)725-31.
11. Mattes R. Fat preference and adherence to a reduced fat diet. Am J Clin Nutr. 1993;57:373-81.
12. NCD Risk Factor Collaboration (NCD-RisC). Worldwide trends in diabetes since 1980: a pooled analysis of 751 population-based studies with 4 × 4 million participants. Lancet. 2016.
13. OECD. Health at a Glance 2015: OECD Indicators. Paris: OECD Publishing; 2015.
14. Operational guidelines. National Programme for Prevention and Control of Non-communicable Diseases (2023-2030). Ministry of Health & Family Welfare Government of India. 2023.
15. School Health Guidelines to Promote Healthy Eating and Physical Activity. Division of Adolescent and School Health, National Center for Chronic Disease Prevention and Health Promotion. Centers for Disease Control and Prevention. MMWR. Recommendations and Reports. 2011;60(5). [online] Available from https://www.cdc.gov/ healthyschools/npao/pdf/mmwr-school-health-guidelines.pdf.
16. Seidell JC. Review Dietary fat and obesity: an epidemiologic perspective. Am J Clin Nutr. 1998;67(3 Suppl):546S-550S.
17. Skyler JS. International Textbook on Diabetes Mellitus, 4th edition. Chichester, UK; Wiley Blackwell; 2015. pp. 541-9.
18. WHO (2012). Prevention and control of non communicable diseases: Guidelines for primary healthcare in low resource settings.
19. WHO. Diabetes: Factsheet. April 2023.
20. World Health Organization. (2010). Global recommendations on physical activity for health. [online] Available from https://www. who.int/dietphysicalactivity/factsheet_recommendations/en/.
21. World Health Organization. (2013). Global action plan for the prevention and control of noncommunicable diseases 2013-2020. [online] Available from https://www.who.int/nmh/events/ncd_ action_plan/en/.
22. World Health Organization. (2016). Diabetes country profiles. [online] Available from http://www.who.int/diabetes/country- profiles/ind_en.pdf.
23. World Health Organization. (2016). Global report on diabetes. [online] Available from http://apps.who.int/iris/bitstream/handle/10665/204871/9789241565257_eng.pdf?sequence=1.
24. World Health Organization. (2016). WHO factsheet India. Diabetes country profiles. [online] Available from http://www.who.int/ diabetes/country-profiles/ind_en.pdf.
25. World Health Organization. (2018). Global health observatory. [online]. Available from http://www.who.int/gho/mortality_ burden_disease/en/.
26. World Health Organization. (2018). Health statistics and information systems. [online]. Available from http://www.who.int/healthinfo/ global_burden_disease/estimates/en/index1.html.
27. World Health Organization. (2018). WHO methods and data sources for global burden of disease estimates 2000-2016.
28. Yesudian CAK, Grepstad M, Visintin E, et al. The economic burden of diabetes in India: a review of the literature. Globalization and Health. 2014:10:80.

# Chapter 19: Specific Epidemiology of Noncommunicable Diseases

## Annexure: Concept Map of Epidemiology of Diabetes Mellitus and its Prevention and Control

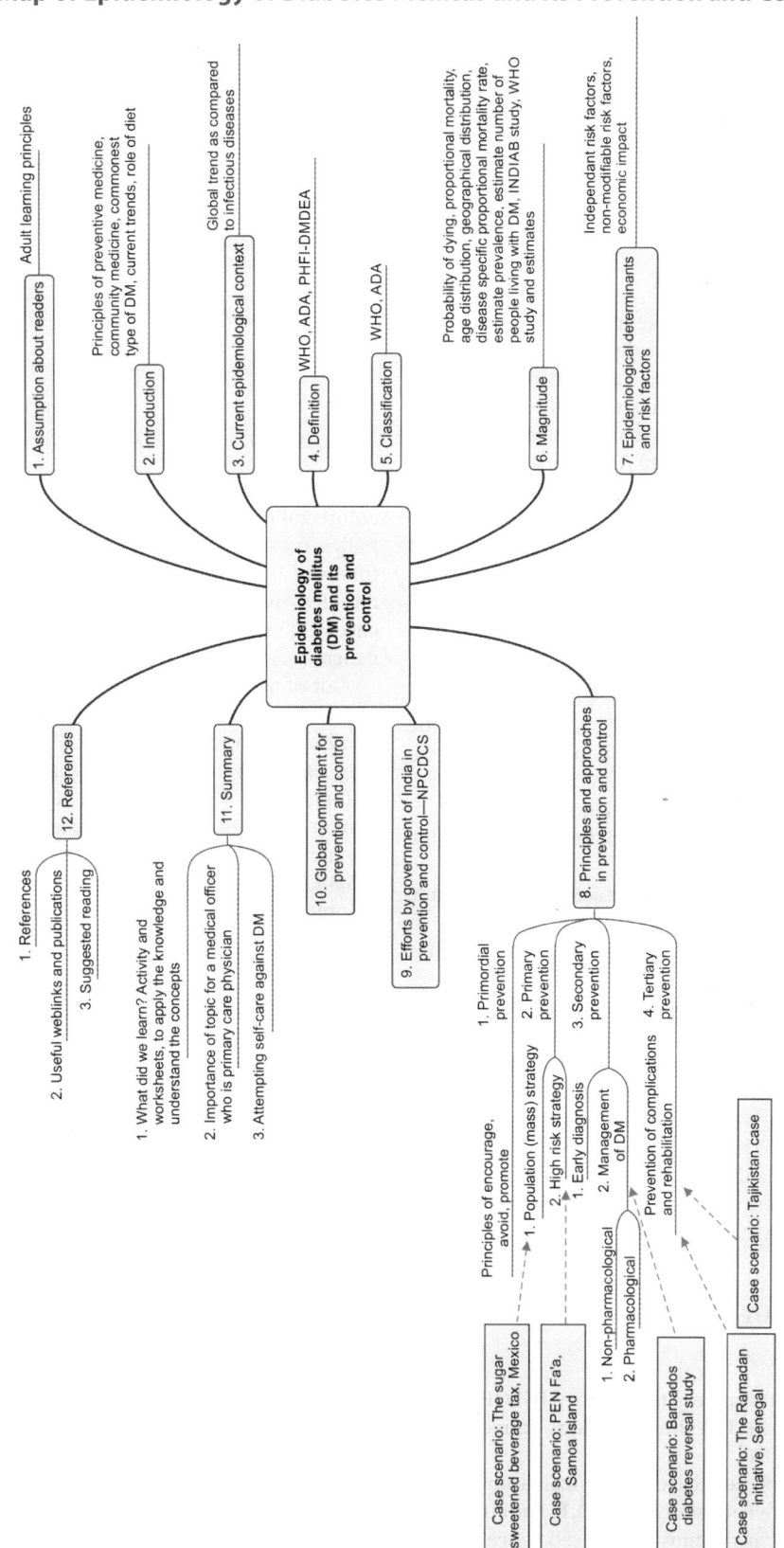

(WHO: World Health Organization; ADA: American Diabetes Association; PHFI-DMDEA: Public Health Foundation of India-Dr Mohan's Diabetes Education Academy; NPCDCS: National Programme for Prevention and Control of Cancer, Diabetes, Cardiovascular Diseases and Stroke)

# D. EPIDEMIOLOGY OF CANCER AND ITS PREVENTION AND CONTROL

*DV Bala, Animesh Jain, Pracheth R*

*You can be a victim of cancer, or a survivor of cancer. It's a mindset.*
—Dave Pelzer

| CM 7.2 | Enumerate, describe and discuss the mode of transmission and measures for prevention and control of cancer |
|---|---|
| CM 8.2 | Describe and discuss the epidemiological and control measures applicable in cancer |

## INTRODUCTION OF CANCER

Although cancer is not a new disease, interest in cancer has grown during the past century. As infectious diseases have been controlled to a large extent as the result of improved sanitation, vaccination and antibiotics resulting in increased longevity, cancer amongst other non-communicable diseases has emerged as a public health problem. They are a major public health problem in terms of morbidity, mortality and, above all, human suffering.

## DEFINITION

The term cancer represents a wide variety of heterogeneous disorders which occur in different parts of the body with different clinical manifestations. They are characterized by uncontrolled cell growth, lack of cell differentiation, ability to invade adjacent tissues, and distant spread to other organs. These are the common features that bind cancers into a single entity for the purpose of description.

There are three main types of cancers. These include
1. Carcinomas—these emerge from the epithelial cells covering the internal surfaces of organs;
2. Sarcomas—these cancers arise from mesodermal cells made up of connective tissues; and
3. Lymphomas, myelomas, and leukemias are the other types.

The term "primary tumor" is used for cancer in the organ of origin, while "secondary tumor" for cancer that has spread to regional lymph nodes and distant organs. The cancerous swelling or tumor is clinically evident as a lump or ulcer localized to the organ of origin in early stages when cancer cells multiply and reach a critical size. The symptoms and signs of invasion and distant metastases as the disease advances become clinically evident. As several cancers are, by and large, associated with different unhealthy lifestyle factors, they can be assumed to be potentially preventable.

## MAGNITUDE OF THE PROBLEM

### Worldwide

According to the Global Cancer Observatory (GLOBOCAN) estimates, there were 19.3 million incident cancer cases worldwide for the year 2020.

Estimated number of new cases of cancer among both sexes globally in 2020 are shown in **Fig. 19D.1**. For both sexes combined, breast cancer is the most diagnosed cancer (11.7% of the total cases) and closely followed by lung cancer (11.4%),

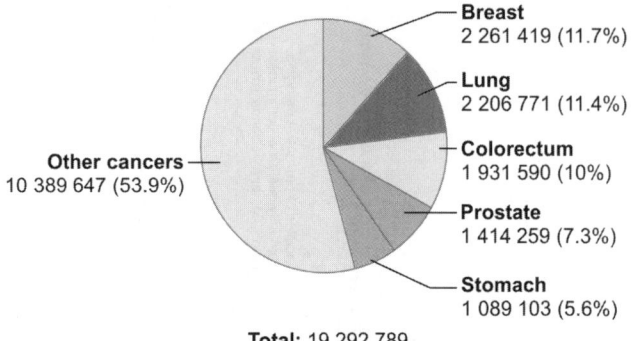

**Fig. 19D.1:** Number of new cancer cases in 2020 in both sexes (all ages).

colorectal cancer (10.0%), and prostate cancer (7.3%). Among males, most diagnosed cancer is lung (14.3% of the total cases) followed by prostate (14.1%) and colorectal (10.6%). Among females, most diagnosed cancer is breast (24.5% of the total cases) followed by colorectal (9.4%) and lung (8.4%) and cervical cancer (6.5%).

Out of all cancer related deaths, highest number of deaths globally in both sexes are due to lung cancer (18% of the total deaths), colorectal cancer (9.4%), and liver cancer (8.3%) **(Fig 19D.2)**. Among males, highest number of deaths are due to lung cancer (21.5% of the total cancer related deaths), liver cancer (10.4%) and colorectal cancer (9.3%). While among females, highest number of deaths are due to breast cancer (15.5% of the total cancer related deaths), lung cancer (13.7%), colorectal cancer (9.5%) and cervical cancer (7.7%).

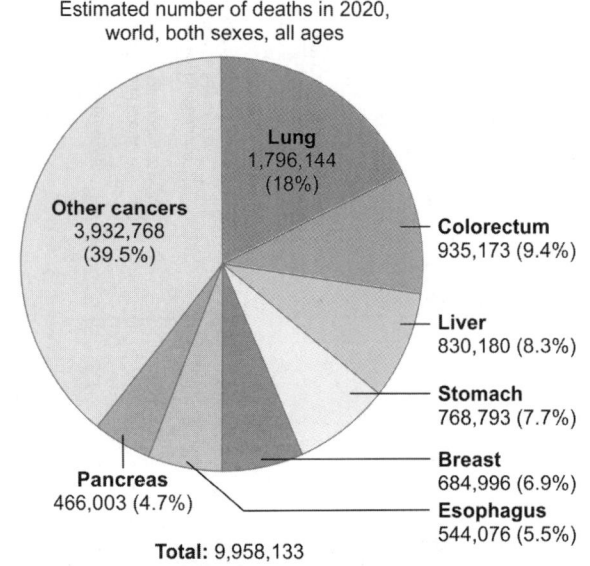

**Fig. 19D.2:** Number of deaths due to cancer in 2020 globally in both sexes.
*Source:* GLOBOCAN 2020, WHO. Global Health Observatory 2022.

## Chapter 19: Specific Epidemiology of Noncommunicable Diseases

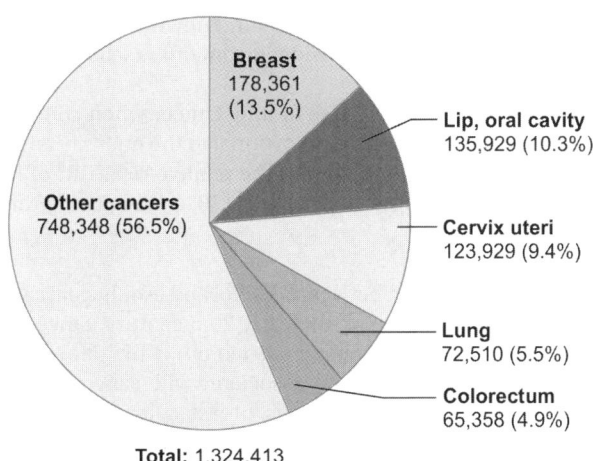

Fig. 19D.3: Number of new cancer cases in 2020 in India.

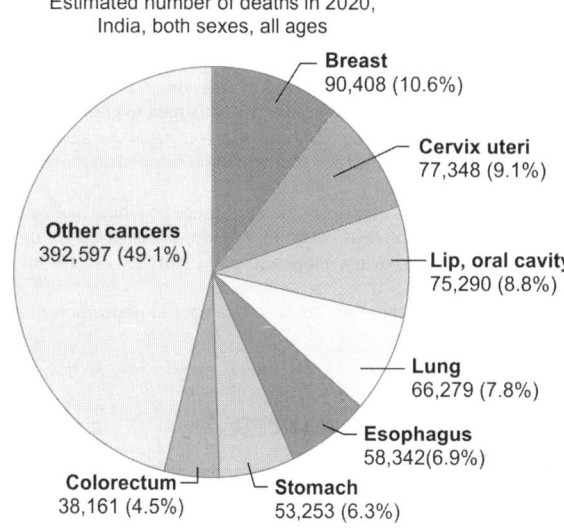

Fig 19D.4: Number of deaths due to cancer in 2020 in India in both sexes.
*Source:* GLOBOCON 2020, WHO. Global Health Observatory 2022.

### India

According to GLOBOCAN 2020 India ranked third after China and the United States of America in total number of cancer cases.

GLOBOCAN 2020 predicted that cancer cases in India would increase to 2.08 million, accounting for a rise of 57.5% in 2040 from 2020. Estimated number of new cases of cancer among both sexes in India in 2020 are shown in **Fig. 19D.3**. For both sexes combined, breast cancer is the most diagnosed cancer (13.5% of the total cases) followed by lip and oral cavity cancer (10.3%), cervical cancer (9.4%), and lung cancer (5.5%). It is worth noting that top 3 most diagnosed cancer in India occurs among females. Among males, most diagnosed cancer is lip and oral cavity (16.2% of the total cases) followed by lung (8%), stomach (6.3%), and colorectal (6.3%). Among females, most diagnosed cancer is breast (26.3% of the total cases) followed by cervical (18.3%) and ovarian cancer (6.7%).

Out of all cancer related deaths, highest number of deaths in India in both sexes are due to breast cancer (10.6%), cervical cancer (9.1%), and lip oral cavity cancer (8.8%) **(Fig 19D.4)**. Among males, highest number of deaths are due to lip oral cavity cancer (13.1% of the total cancer related deaths), lung cancer (10.9%), esophageal cancer (8.4%) and stomach cancer (8.3%). While among females, highest number of deaths are due to breast cancer (21.9% of the total cancer related deaths), cervical cancer (18.7%), and ovarian cancer (7.8%).

### CANCER PATTERNS

Global patterns show that for men and women combined, nearly half of the new cases, and more than half of the cancer deaths worldwide in 2018 are estimated to occur in Asia, in part because the region has nearly 60% of the global population. There are wide variations in the distribution of cancer throughout the world. In the South-East Asia Region of WHO, the great majority are cancers of the oral cavity and uterine cervix. Carcinoma of stomach is common in Japan, but not in United States.

The most frequently diagnosed cancer and the leading cause of cancer death, however, substantially vary across countries and within each country depending on the degree of economic development and associated social and lifestyle factors including food habits and addictions to substance use. Such international variations in the pattern of cancer can be attributed to multiple factors, such as occupational and other environmental exposures, and also genetic factors. Moreover, it is noteworthy that inadequacy in detection and reporting of cases in low resource and developing countries also result in low reporting and are responsible for variations.

Hospital data in India indicates that the sites most commonly affected are:
1. The uterine cervix and breast in women, and
2. The various sites in oral cavity and oropharynx in both sexes. These sites represent to over half of all cancer cases. They are predominantly environment related and have a strong sociocultural relationship.

Fortunately, these cancers are also easily accessible for physical examination and amenable to early diagnosis by good clinical examination and exfoliative cytology. The cure rate for these neoplasms is also very high if they are treated surgically in first two stages. However, in most of the developing countries, including India, the patients present themselves to a medical facility when the disease is symptomatic and far advanced and is not amenable to curative treatment.

Currently, over two-thirds of cancer patients are already in an advanced stage at the time of diagnosis and not amenable for curative treatment. Therefore, preventive strategies like public education for creating awareness about cancer, tobacco control would be a first step in this direction. Similarly, implementing of regular self-examination and periodical clinical examination of oral and breast by health professional for oral and breast cancers would facilitate early detection and cure. Papanicolaou (Pap) smear screening for cervical cancer would decrease the mortality due to this disease. However, paucity of facilities for screening and proper management of detected cancer patients is the crux of the problem.

> **Key Points**
> - Cancer refers to heterogenous disorders characterized by uncontrolled cell growth, lack of cell differentiation, ability to invade adjacent tissues, and distant spread to other organs.
> - Cancer is the second leading cause of death, next to coronary heart disease, in developed countries and fourth cause in the developing countries. It is the second and fourth leading cause of adult death in urban and rural India.
> - The most common cancers in men are those of lungs, oral cavity, stomach and esophagus, while in women, those of cervix uteri, breast, oral cavity, ovary, esophagus, and stomach are the most common.
> - Large majority of these are tobacco related and hence potentially preventable.

## RISK FACTORS FOR CANCER

Cancer has a multifactorial etiology. For many noncommunicable diseases, including cancer, a single disease "agent" still cannot be firmly established to the causation. Therefore, the etiology of the disease is generally discussed in terms of "risk factors". They may be truly causative (e.g. smoking for lung cancer), or merely contributory or may be predictive only in a statistical sense. The most prevalent risk factors include:
- Cigarette smoking
- Second-hand smoke
- Excess bodyweight
- Drinking alcohol
- Eating red and processed meat
- Diet low in fruits and vegetables, dietary fiber, and dietary calcium
- Physical inactivity
- Ultraviolet (UV) radiation from the sun or indoor tanning
- Six cancer-associated infections—*Helicobacter pylori*, hepatitis B virus (HBV), hepatitis C virus (HCV), human herpes virus type 8 (HHV8), human immunodeficiency virus (HIV), and human papillomavirus (HPV).

However, it is conventional to describe epidemiology with reference to modifiable and non-modifiable risk factors.

### Modifiable Risk Factors

They are responsible for 90% of all cancers. Various agents have been incriminated in the etiology of cancer. Few of the important factors are explained in detail below.

### Tobacco

India is the second largest consumer of tobacco in the world, with 10% of all smokers globally. It is in addition the third largest tobacco producer. As in other South Asian countries, there are multiple forms of tobacco consumption with 85% in noncigarette categories. The forms of smoking are also diverse—*beedis*, cigarettes, cigars, *chuttas*, cherrots, pipes, *hookahs*, dhumtis, and *chillum*. Tobacco is also chewed in a variety of forms, taken as snuff, sucked, and gargled in water.

Tobacco was first identified in 1964 in the US Surgeon General's Advisory Committee Report as a cause for cancer. It has been associated with at least 14 different types of cancer. Therefore, it is regarded as the most common risk factor for cancer. Tobacco smoking is the main known cause of human cancer-related deaths, worldwide. It contains at least 50 known carcinogens.

There is an increase in risk of lung cancer when compared to a nonsmoker and is also proportional to the quantity and the duration of smoking. In general, the relative risk (RR) of lung cancer due to smoking is of the order of 10 to as high as 20 times.

### Alcohol

Initially, an association between alcohol and esophageal cancer was confirmed way back in the early 20th century. Since then, a number of studies have been carried out, which have found alcohol drinking to be causally associated with cancers like oral cavity, pharynx, larynx, esophagus, breast, colon, lung, kidney, liver, and pancreas. Alcohol drinking is estimated to be involved in the etiology of 3% of all cancers (that is, 4% in men, 2% in women).

For all cancers caused by drinking alcohol, the risk of cancer increases with duration of drinking and the level of consumption, up to an intake of about 80 g of ethanol/day (equal to eight small pegs of hard drinks as rum or whisky). Alcohol drinking and tobacco smoking show a synergistic interaction in the etiology of cancers of the upper aerodigestive tract.

### Diet

Epidemiological studies suggest that different dietary patterns in different populations may be related to higher risk of particular types of cancer. Studies have reported that as high as 30% of all cancer cases may have some associated dietary factors.
- Consumption of red meat is known risk factors for cancers of the gastrointestinal tract particularly colorectal cancers.
- Smoked fish is closely related to stomach cancer and lack of dietary fiber to colonic cancer. The role of high-saturated fatty diet is associated with increased risk of cancer of the breast. The most consistent finding on diet as a determinant of cancer risk is the association between high consumption of vegetables and fruits and reduced risk of several cancers, also by limiting processed food or red meats. Antioxidants from fruits and vegetables may contribute to counteract some of the oxidative damage to the DNA caused by red meat and processed meat.

### Micronutrients

Role of micronutrients and their involvement in either of two metabolic mechanisms commonly called the antioxidant effect (carotenoids, vitamins C, and E) and methyl donation (folic acid and vitamin B6) and their correlation with cancer in humans has been studied extensively.

Studies have shown quite consistently that individuals with lower carotenoid levels have increased lung cancer risk. Low dietary intake of vitamin C has been found to be associated with increased risk of cancers of the stomach, mouth, pharynx, esophagus and less consistently with cancers of the lung, pancreas, and cervix.

### Food Contaminants

A variety of other dietary factors, such as food additives and contaminants are suspected as causative agents.

- The most studied food contaminants are mycotoxins and aflatoxins, are frequent among them. Aflatoxins are products of the *Aspergillus* fungi and these particularly accumulate during storage of grains in hot, humid parts of the world. Aflatoxin contaminated food and HBV infection are the two main risk factors of hepatocellular carcinoma which is most prevalent cancer in some regions of Africa, Asia, and South America.
- Certain organochlorines, dichlorodiphenyltrichloroethane (DDT) in particular has been associated with increased risk of pancreatic cancer, breast cancer, lymphoma, and leukemia in humans.
- Another group of chemicals, the polycyclic aromatic hydrocarbons (PAHs) are generated in meat when it is fried, roasted, or cooked over an open flame, and many members of this chemical class are carcinogenic.
- Similarly, N-nitroso compounds, e.g. nitrosamines may be formed by chemical reactions in foods containing added nitrates and nitrites, such as salt-processed by smoking and direct fire drying. These chemicals are proven carcinogenic.

### Infectious Agents

Infectious agents are one of the main causes of cancer accounting for 18% of cases worldwide, but are more prevalent in developing countries. The mechanism of carcinogenicity by infectious agents may be direct, e.g. mediated by oncogenic proteins produced by the agent (e.g. HPV) or indirect, through causation of chronic inflammation with tissue necrosis and regeneration.

- The most frequently incriminated viruses are hepatitis B and C, parasite liver flukes are proved to be causally related to hepatocellular carcinoma.
- HPV is attributed to cervix uteri. In fact, HPV DNA is found in virtually all invasive cervical cancers indicating that HPV is a necessary cause. About 80% of anal cancers and 30% of cancers of the vulva, vagina, penis, and oropharynx can be attributed to HPV.
- The *Epstein-Barr virus* (EBV) is associated with two human malignancies, viz. Burkitt's lymphoma and nasopharyngeal carcinoma. Hodgkin's disease is also believed to be of viral origin.
- HIV infection enhances the risk of Kaposi sarcoma by approximately 1,000-fold, of non-Hodgkin lymphoma by 100-fold, and of Hodgkin disease by 10-fold. This malignancy is seen associated with a higher prevalence of antibodies to cytomegalovirus (CMV) which is a suspected oncogenic agent. In all these cases, the role of HIV is probably as an immunosuppressive agent and hence mechanism of action is indirect.
- *Helicobacter pylori* bacteria is related to stomach cancer.
- Schistosomiasis, which is a parasitic infestation caused by *Schistosoma haematobium* also increases the risk of carcinoma of the bladder. Chronic infestation with liver fluke may cause liver cancer.

### Radiation

Exposure to ionizing radiations from natural as well as from industrial, medical, and other sources can cause leukemia, breast cancer, and thyroid cancer. Sunlight is a source of UV radiation and causes several types of skin cancer particularly in populations with fair skin, e.g. Australians of Caucasian origin.

### Physical Activity

It is reported that close to 70% of cancers have their roots in unhealthy lifestyle practices. Overweight, obesity, physical inactivity, unhealthy dietary practices, personal habits, and addictions are incriminated in the development of various cancers. Physical activity is an independent factor and it lowers the risk of several cancers (including breast and colon). About 150 minutes a week of moderate aerobic activity or 75 minutes a week of vigorous aerobic physical activity should be the target (at least 30 minutes of physical activity in daily routine). According to the American Cancer Society, obesity and physical inactivity increase the risk of breast, colon and endometrial cancers and are also associated with an increased mortality.

### Environmental Pollution

Various studies suggest that environmental pollution accounts of 1–4% of the total burden of cancer in developed countries. "Environmental pollution" refers to a specific subset of cancer-causing environmental factors namely contaminants of air, water, and soil with toxic agents. The carcinogenic pollutants for which most information is available include asbestos (referring here to non-occupational exposure).

### Occupational Exposure

Occupational exposures which include exposure to benzene, arsenic, cadmium, chromium, vinyl chloride, asbestos, polycyclic hydrocarbons, etc. are usually reported to account for 1–5% of all human cancers. Examples of occupational cancers and chemical agents are, viz. aniline dye—bladder cancer, coal tar—skin cancer, nickel, chromium, asbestos—lung cancer, ionizing radiation, and benzol—leukemia. Smoking tobacco simultaneously by the individuals who have such exposure increases the risk considerably.

### Reproductive Factors and Hormones

Metabolism of female sex hormone, reproductive factors, and menopausal status affects the development of endometrial, ovarian, and breast cancer. Use of combined oral contraceptives accounts for a slight increase in risk of breast cancer, but is protective against ovarian and endometrial cancers. Hormone replacement therapy (HRT) is associated with increases in risk of breast and endometrial cancers.

Breast cancer incidence rates increase more steeply with age before menopause than after which indicates correlation with ovarian synthesis of estrogen production. Furthermore, breast cancer risk is increased in women who have early menarche, or who have late menopause, whereas an early age at first full term pregnancy and high parity are associated with reduced risk of cancers of breast, ovary, and endometrium.

### Others

There are numerous other environmental factors, such as air and water pollution, medications (e.g. estrogen) and pesticides, which are related to cancer. Environmental factors are generally held responsible for 80–90% of all human cancers.

Both outdoor air pollution by pollutants like PAHs and indoor air pollutants like tobacco smoke, volatile compounds like benzene are linked with cancer. PAHs are associated with an increased risk of lung cancers while indoor air pollutants are reported to increase the risk of childhood leukemias and lymphomas. Furthermore, the depletion of ozone layer due to use of chlorofluorocarbons leads to skin cancer. Another environmental factor is the increased exposure to ionizing radiation exposure which may lead to skin cancer.

All the above-mentioned risk factors have been summarized in the **Table 19D.1**.

**Table 19D.1:** Modifiable risk factors in cancer.

| Risk factor | Types of cancer |
| --- | --- |
| Substance use:<br>• Tobacco: In various forms like smoking and smokeless<br>• Excessive alcohol intake | • Cancers of lung, larynx, mouth, pharynx, esophagus, bladder, and pancreas<br>• Esophageal and liver cancers |
| Dietary factors:<br>• Smoked fish<br>• High fat diet<br>• Lack of dietary fiber | • Stomach cancer<br>• Breast cancer<br>• Intestinal cancer |
| Chemicals:<br>• Aniline<br>• Coal tar<br>• Benzol | • Bladder cancer<br>• Skin cancer<br>• Leukemia |
| Viruses:<br>• Hepatitis B and C viruses<br>• Human papilloma virus | • Hepatocellular carcinoma<br>• Cervical cancer |
| Radiation: Ultraviolet radiation and excessive exposure to sunlight | • Skin cancer |

## Non-modifiable Risk Factors

They include factors that are not modifiable or preventable.

### Genetic Susceptibility and Familial Factors

Research suggests that only 5% of cancers are hereditary. There is a complex interrelationship between genetic susceptibility and environmental carcinogenic stimuli in the causation of a number of cancers.

There are some inherited cancer syndromes, e.g. retinoblastoma, neurofibromatosis, etc. that involve germline mutation in tumor suppressor or DNA repair genes. A small proportion of all breast or ovarian cancers are caused by inherited mutations of the breast cancer gene 1 (*BRCA 1*) or *BRCA2* gene, but affected family members have a 70% lifetime risk of developing breast or ovarian cancer.

### Age Incidence

Most cancers occur among middle age and elderly persons. However, no age is considered as immune to cancers. Certain cancers like Hodgkin's disease, breast cancer to some extent, exhibit bimodality and occur in young people and elderly. When there is family history, cancer usually occurs at an earlier age.

### Sex

Most cancers are more frequent among men as compared to women, except cancers of reproductive organs and breast. Nearly half of the cancers among women are associated with reproductive system as compared to 15–20% of cancers among men. Data from population-based registries under the National Cancer Registry Programme about 50–60% of all cancers among women in India are related mainly to the four organs: (1) Cervix uteri, (2) Breast, (3) Corpus-uteri, and (4) Ovaries.

It is estimated that at least one-third of all cancers are preventable, another one-third are curable, and still, one-third can be helped to alleviate pain and suffering when one presents in advanced stages of cancer and is not amenable to cure. The basic approach to the control of cancer is through primary and secondary prevention. Cancer prevention until recently was mainly concerned with the early diagnosis of the disease (secondary prevention), preferably at a precancerous stage by screening and appropriate treatment of these lesions. It is now possible to avert certain cancers by primary prevention with better understanding of the causative factors of the disease. Control of these factors in the general population as well as in particular occupational groups are major current strategies. Therefore, a comprehensive approach is needed to tackle a disease like cancer which includes a combination of steps at primary, secondary, and tertiary level.

> **Key Points**
> - The risk factors for cancer may be classified as modifiable and non-modifiable.
> - Modifiable risk factors include-tobacco, alcohol, diet, infectious agents, unhealthy lifestyle, occupational exposure and environmental factors.
> - Non-modifiable risk factors include genetic susceptibility, age and sex.
> - Usually, there is a complex inter relationship between genetic susceptibility and environmental carcinogenic stimuli; a number of risk factors may contribute in causation of cancers.

## CANCER PREVENTION AND CONTROL

Cancer control is a broad term which consists of a series of measures based on the present knowledge in the fields of prevention, early detection, diagnosis, treatment, after care, and rehabilitation. The aim is to reduce incidence of disease significantly and increase the cure rate and reducing the suffering and deformity or disability due to cancer.

### Primary Prevention

Estimated figures of cancer researchers say that nearly 50% of all cancer cases and an equal proportion of all cancer deaths in India are attributable to known risk factors. Many of these could be mitigated by effective preventive strategies, such as public education on cancer, education against all forms of tobacco and alcohol use, and vaccinations against HPV and HBV infections. Additional primary preventive measures include healthy diet, healthy weight and decreasing exposure from environmental carcinogens (radon and asbestos), protection from ionizing radiation and UV rays, etc.

Primary prevention is now regarded by the World Health Organization (WHO) as the most cost-effective step of cancer control. It includes the following steps:

### Control of Tobacco

Tobacco, as explained earlier is the single largest risk factor for cancer. If rates of tobacco usage are significantly decreased, it would be the most effective step toward cancer prevention. It is estimated that this alone would reduce cancer burden by over a million cases per year. Comprehensive tobacco control is the way forward. This would include stringent implementation of regulatory measures like the Cigarettes and Other Tobacco Products Act (COTPA), 2003 and encouraging personal commitment to avoid tobacco use. This needs concerted efforts among policy makers, professionals, and the community.

### Tackling Alcohol Use

It is a known fact that alcohol use is associated with multiple cancers. To tackle alcohol use, an approach similar to curb the menace of tobacco may be required. This includes implementation of legislations, taxations, encouraging vulnerable people to quit alcohol use, and providing professional help.

### Diet, Physical Activity, and Weight Control

Consumption of a balanced diet, practicing regular moderate intensity physical activity, and avoidance of obesity are important measures against breast and intestinal cancers. Certain measures that may be effective in this regard include— moderate intensity aerobic activity like daily brisk walking or jogging, consumption of a diet rich in fruits and green leafy vegetables, avoidance of fast or junk foods, limiting the intake of red meat and saturated fats, weight control, and preventing overweight or obesity.

### Personal Hygiene

Maintenance of personal hygiene is of paramount importance. Personal hygiene, especially sexual hygiene, may reduce the occurrence of certain cancers like cervical cancers and penile cancers.

### Preventing Excessive Radiation Exposure

Radiation is an integral component of medicine and is used both as a diagnostic and therapeutic tool. However, both ionizing and nonionizing radiation have been long recognized as causes for cancer. Therefore, radiation needs to be used judiciously and excessive exposure needs to be avoided. Diagnostic procedures involving radiation should be advised only if there is a requirement to reduce unnecessary radiation doses, particularly among vulnerable population like pregnant women and children.

### Avoidance of Occupational Exposure

It is reported that occupational cancers constitute nearly 10% of all cancers. Measures to protect workers from exposure to these occupational carcinogens are an important step to prevent occupational exposure. Measures like providing protective equipment to workers, preplacement examination, periodic medical examination, rotation of workers, and mechanization to reduce exposure to chemicals need to be adopted. These methods protect and promote the health of industrial workers.

### Reducing Environmental Pollution

Efforts need to be undertaken to reduce the extent of outdoor and indoor air pollution. Strict regulations at factories, implementation of emission standards for motor vehicles, substituting harmful substances by less harmful alternatives, and reducing exposure to tobacco smoke are some major steps.

### Controlling Infections

It is known that HBV, HCV, and HPV are associated with a high-risk for certain specific cancers. Immunization against HBV has been included in the National Immunization Schedule and is given during infancy. HBV vaccine should also be administered to those exposed to HBV individuals. Additionally, high-risk population like medical and paramedical personnel, thalassemia patients, and those on hemodialysis should be vaccinated against HBV. Similarly, HPV vaccination may be offered to girls at the onset of puberty (before 12 years of age). However, high cost remains a deterrent. Broad control measures for prevention of prevalent cancers are given in **Table 19D.2**.

Table 19D.2: Broad control measures for prevention of prevalent cancers.

| Sr. no. | Control measure | Prevention of cancers | |
|---|---|---|---|
| 1. | Control of tobacco and alcohol | Oral cavity, pharynx, larynx, lung, and esophagus | |
| 2. | Personal hygiene and barrier contraception | Cervix, penis, and vulva | |
| 3. | Prevention of radiation exposure | Leukemia | |
| 4. | Prevention of occupational exposure to industrial carcinogens | Asbestos | Mesothelioma of pleura |
| | | Benzene | Leukemia |
| | | Aniline dye—benzidine | Urinary bladder |
| 5. | Immunization—HBV and HPV | Liver (HBV), cervix, and penis (HPV) | |
| 6. | Prevention of air pollution | Lung | |
| 7. | Treatment of precancerous lesions | Oral cavity, cervix, and colon | |
| 8. | Legislation for control of tobacco, alcohol, air pollution, etc. | Lung, oral cavity, pharynx, and esophagus | |
| 9. | Cancer education to create awareness and motivate people to seek early diagnosis and Treatment | All types of cancers | |

(HBV: hepatitis B virus; HPV: human papillomavirus)

### Cancer Education

People need to be educated about certain warning signs of cancer which may enable them to report to the healthcare facility, as and when they occur. The main objective is to create awareness about cancer in the general population, motivate them for early detection which would facilitate prompt treatment. According

to the American Cancer Society, "seven" early warning signals of cancer are in the word "CAUTION", as following:
1. **C**: Change in bowel or bladder habits
2. **A**: A sore that does not heal
3. **U**: Unusual bleeding or discharge from any orifice
4. **T**: Thickening or lump in the breast, testicles, or elsewhere
5. **I**: Indigestion or difficulty in swallowing
6. **O**: Obvious change in the size, color, shape, or thickness of a wart, mole, or mouth sore
7. **N**: Nagging cough or hoarseness of voice

In addition to the above warning signals, on and off fever or persistent fever for over 2 weeks as a lone symptom, any significant loss of weight (over 10% of unintentional loss), iron deficiency anemia in elderly, and unexplained backache in any person over the age of 40 years should raise suspicion of cancer.

## Secondary Prevention

Secondary prevention in cancer generally comprises of measures like screening and early detection approaches with an aim to identify cancers at an early stage, which would go a long way in improving the treatment outcome and reducing mortality. Once diagnosed with cancer, it needs to be ensured that every individual has access to treatment, care, and support.

### Screening for Cancers

Screening programs can be effective for select cancer types when appropriate tests are used and implemented effectively. Cancer screening is an approach which facilitates early detection in apparently healthy individuals. It is defined as searching for unrecognized malignancy by applying rapidly applied tests among apparently healthy individuals. Effective screening tests are available for oral, breast, and cervical cancers which are leading cancers in our country.

Cancer screening for these sites is a feasible approach because they occur in accessible body sites and invasive cancers are usually preceded by premalignant lesions. Treatment of these precancerous lesions is relatively simple and would also prevent invasive cancer. Examples of screening methods are—visual inspection with acetic acid (VIA) for cervical cancer in low-income settings; Pap cytology test and HPV testing for cervical cancer in middle- and high-income settings; and mammography screening for breast cancer in settings with strong or relatively strong health systems.

Prostate-specific antigen (PSA) testing is now being widely used in developed countries for the early detection of prostate cancer.

Fecal occult blood test (FOBT) is a very cost-effective and quite applicable screening method available for colorectal cancer, but its specificity and sensitivity are limited. Endoscopy is more specific for diagnosis of colorectal cancer.

### Methods of Cancer Screening

- *Mass screening* by comprehensive cancer detection examination which involves rapid clinical examination by physician of one or more body sites like mass screening at specific single sites—like oral cavity, cervix, and breast.
- *Selective screening*: Examples include screening for breast cancer of those who are at high risk (e.g. clinical examination, mammography of women aged 40 years and above), Pap smear screening for all married women in the age group 35–64 years age group for cervical cancer and clinical examination of all tobacco users.

### Cancer Diagnosis

Cancer diagnosis comprises the evaluation of the patient's history, clinical examination, review of laboratory test results and radiological data, and microscopic examination of tissue samples obtained by biopsy or fine needle aspiration. Confirmation of diagnosis is mandatory for any suspected cancer diagnosis for initiating any treatment.

#### Tumor Markers

A tumor marker is a biomarker found in blood, urine, or body tissues that can be elevated by the presence of one or more types of cancer. There are many different tumor markers, each indicative of a particular disease process, and they are used in oncology to help detect the presence of cancer. An elevated level of a tumor marker can indicate cancer; however, there can also be other causes of the elevation (false positive values). They are usually not definitive diagnostic tests. The diagnosis is mostly confirmed by biopsy. Specifically, this test (in conjunction with other tests) can be used to monitor the success of a current therapy, evaluate the need for further intervention, or assess the development of recurrence.

#### Treatment

It is imperative to provide access to quality treatment to all persons diagnosed with cancer. This also includes treatment of precancerous lesions. The main goals of a diagnosis and treatment program are to cure or considerably prolong the life of cancer patients and to ensure the best possible quality of life to cancer survivors. Cancer management involves staging and treatment and starts from the moment the patient's diagnosis of cancer is confirmed.

Cancer treatment is the series of interventions including psychosocial support, surgery, radiotherapy, chemotherapy and hormone therapy, immunotherapy, biological response modifiers, etc. that is aimed at curing the disease or prolonging the patient's life considerably (for several years) while improving the patient's quality of life. A multimodality approach may be needed most of the times.

#### Surgical Prevention

Correction of precancerous conditions amenable to surgical intervention may help in primary prevention of cancers. Excision of colonic polyps, cervical premalignant lesions, and correction of undescended testes are such examples.

### Tertiary Prevention

It involves appropriate treatment in the advanced stage of disease. This includes palliative care, disability limitation, and rehabilitation.

## Palliative Care

Palliative care is one kind of tertiary prevention and is essential where many cancer patients present in advanced stages and not suitable for curative treatment. This is an approach that improves the quality of life of patients and their families facing the problems associated with life-threatening cancer, through the prevention and relief of suffering by means of early identification of associated morbidity like excruciating pain and treatment of these problems, physical, psychosocial, and spiritual.

## WHO RESPONSE

In 2013, WHO launched the Global action Plan for prevention and control of noncommunicable diseases 2013–2020 that aims to reduce by 25% premature mortality from cancer, cerebrovascular diseases, diabetes, and chronic respiratory diseases by 2025. Some of the targets are relevant for cancer prevention especially target five aimed at reducing the prevalence of tobacco use by 30%.

The prevention and control measures for cancer have been summarized in **Figure 19D.5**.

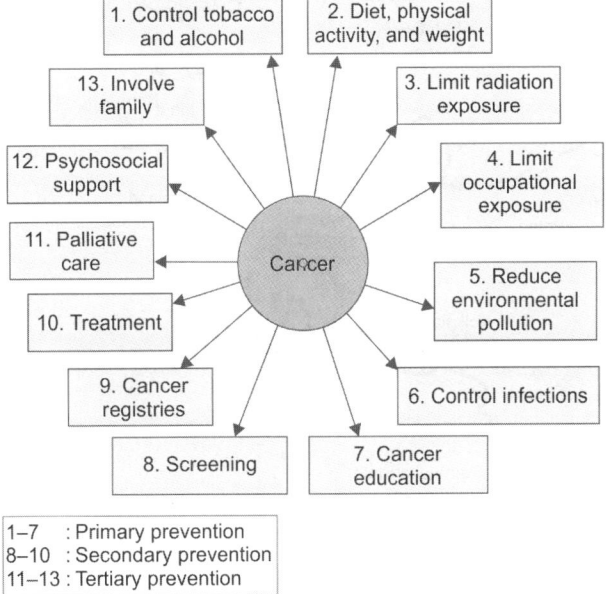

Fig. 19D.5: Depiction of the prevention and control measures for cancer.

In 2017, the World Health Assembly passed the Resolution Cancer prevention and control in the context of an integrated approach that urges governments and WHO to accelerate action to achieve the targets specified in the Global Action Plan for the prevention and control of NCDs 2013-2020 and the 2030 UN Agenda for Sustainable Development to reduce premature mortality from cancer. WHO and IARC collaborate with other UN organizations including the International Atomic Energy Agency to fight against cancer worldwide.

## NATIONAL CANCER CONTROL PROGRAMME

National Cancer Control Programme (NCCP) was launched in 1975–76 with the objectives of prevention, early diagnosis, and treatment. The program was revised in 1984–85 and subsequently in December 2004 to meet the demands and improve the availability of cancer treatment facilities across the country. During 2010, the program was integrated with National Programme on Prevention and Control of Diabetes, Cardiovascular Disease and Stroke (NPCDCS). Now renamed as National Programme for Prevention of Noncommunicable Diseases (NP-NCD) in 2023. The objectives of the program are:
1. **Primary prevention** of cancers by health education specially regarding hazards of tobacco consumption and necessity of genital hygiene for prevention of cervical cancer;
2. **Secondary prevention,** i.e. early detection and diagnosis of common cancer such as cancer of cervix, oropharyngeal cancer, breast and tobacco-related cancer by screening, and patients' education on self-examination methods; and
3. **Tertiary prevention,** i.e. strengthening of the existing institutions of comprehensive therapy including palliative care.

*This is further discussed under NP-NCD in Chapter 47: Health Policies and Programs in India.*

## CANCER REGISTRY PROGRAMME

For database of cancer cases, National Cancer Registry Programme (NCRP) was initiated in 1982 by Indian Council of Medical Research (ICMR), which gives a picture of the magnitude and patterns of cancer. In India, a network of cancer registries has been established under the NCRP.

Cancer registries refer to a systematic collection of data pertaining to cancer cases. It is an essential part of any national programme of cancer control. These are needed to assess the magnitude of cancer and plan for the services. There are two types of cancer registries; Population-based Cancer Registry (PBCR) and Hospital-based Cancer Registries (HBCR), which were started in January 1982. The population-based registries take the sample population in a geographically defined area while the hospital-based registries take the data from patients coming to a particular health institution.

### Hospital-based Cancer Registries

They record information on all cancer patients observed in a particular hospital. Their main aim is to monitor and plan patient care at an institutional level. They provide information on methods of diagnosis, stage distribution, treatment methods response to treatment, and survival at institutional level. Thus, it is beneficial in evaluation of diagnostic methods and different modalities of treatment. The data from this registry can also be used to forecast future demands for services, equipment, and manpower in a given hospital. Although these registries cannot provide incidence rates in general population, they may be used for epidemiological studies like case controls studies, to investigate etiology of a particular cancer.

### Population-based Cancer Registries

Population-based Cancer Registries (PBCR) are important resources since they provide information on the distribution of cancer in well-defined populations. They systematically collect data on all new cases of cancer occurring in a well-defined population from multiple sources such as government hospitals, private hospitals, nursing homes, clinics, diagnostic laboratories,

imaging centers, hospices, and registrars of births and deaths. The coverage is about 10% of the population of India.
- Cancer site specific incidence rates in the population can be calculated according to many different variables, such as age, sex, place of residence at the time of diagnosis, etc.
- PBCR that conduct adequate follow-up of their patients are able to estimate prevalence of cancer. Prevalence rate gives an estimate of burden of the disease in community.
- Time trend analyses are possible when data can be accumulated over long periods of time. The data of PBCR are also important in planning and evaluation of cancer control programs.
- PBCRs help in assessment and monitoring the effectiveness of screening programs. These can be used for evaluating cancer care through survival statistics. The data items collected by PBCR are determined by data collection methods and available resources (**Fig. 19D.6**).

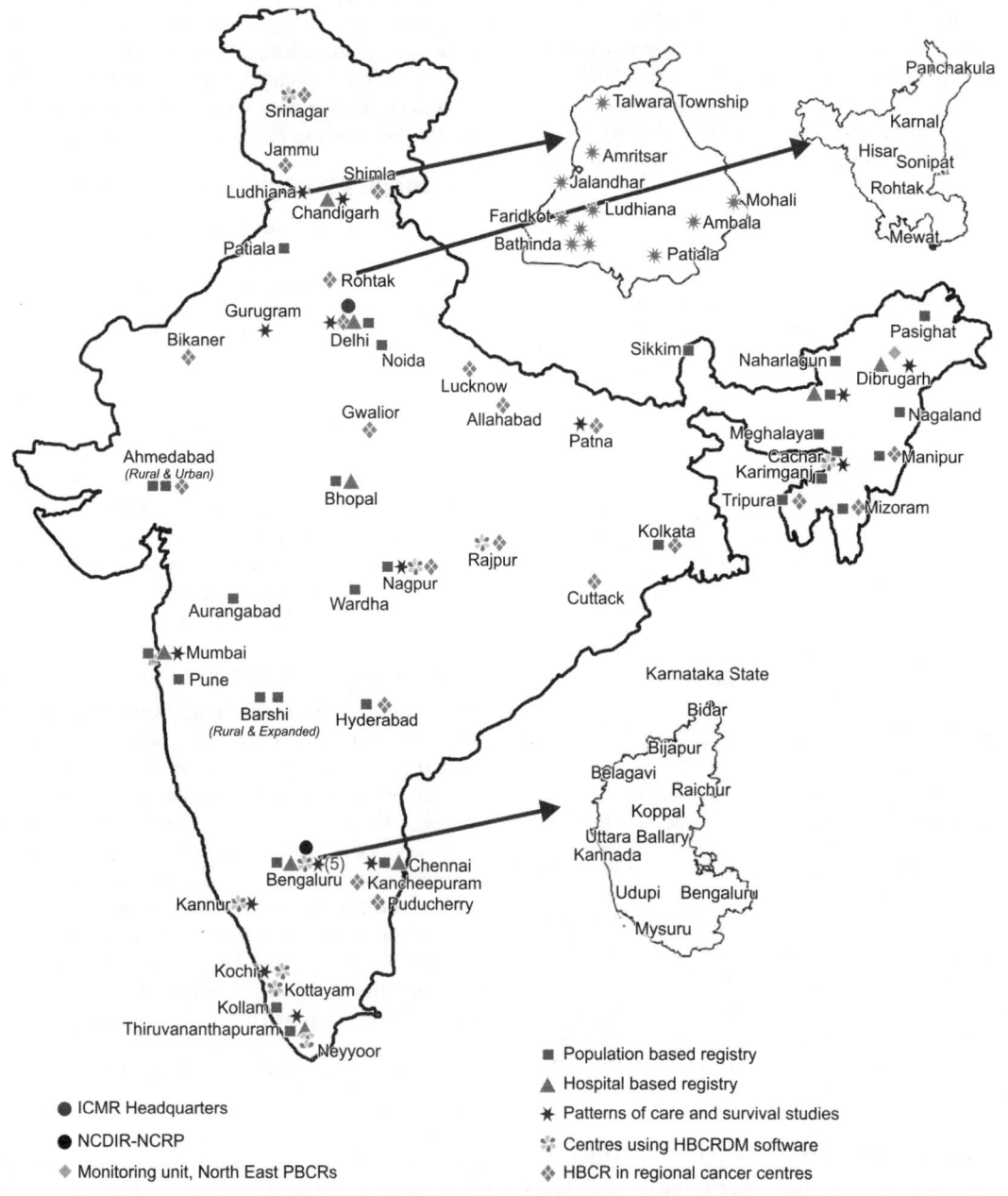

**Fig. 19D.6:** Population-based cancer registries located in India.
(HBCR: hospital-based cancer registries; ICMR: Indian Council of Medical Research; NCDIR: National Center for Disease Informatics and Research; NCRP: National Cancer Registry Programme; PBCR: Population-based Cancer Registry)
*Source:* Newsletter of NRCP CRAB 2017.

**Chapter 19:** Specific Epidemiology of Noncommunicable Diseases | 579

> **Key Points**
> - Prevention of cancer may include primary, secondary or tertiary prevention strategies
> - Primary prevention addresses the risk factors of cancer such as tobacco control, alcohol cessation, maintenance of healthy lifestyle, prevention of occupational exposure and reducing environmental pollution
> - Secondary prevention generally comprises of screening and early detection approaches with an aim to identify cancers at an early stage
> - Tertiary prevention refers to palliative care, disability limitation, and rehabilitation.
> - Cancer registry refers to a systematic collection of data pertaining to cancer cases which is needed are needed to assess the magnitude of cancer and plan for the services. At the national level, this is done by the National Cancer Registry Programme (NCRP).

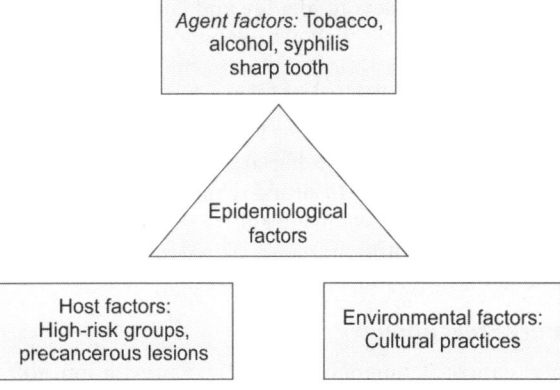

Fig. 19D.7: Epidemiological triad of oral cancer.

## EPIDEMIOLOGY, PREVENTION, AND CONTROL OF ORAL CANCER

### Problem Statement

The problem statement of oral cancer is represented in **Table 19D.3**.

Table 19D.3: Problem statement of oral cancer.

| Context | Mortality and morbidity |
|---|---|
| Global | • Oral cancer includes cancers of the lip, other parts of the mouth and the oropharynx and combined rank as the 13th most common cancer worldwide. The global incidence of cancers of the lip and oral cavity is estimated to be 377,713 new cases and 177,757 deaths in 2020.<br>• Oral cancer is more common in men and in older people, more deadly in men compared to women and it varies strongly by socio-economic circumstances.<br>• Tobacco, alcohol and areca nut (betel quid) use are among the leading causes of oral cancer. In North America and Europe, human papillomavirus infections are responsible for a growing percentage of oral cancers among young people. |
| Indian | • Oral cancer is the most common cancer in India amongst men (16.2 % of all cancers),<br>• It is the FOURTH most common cancer in India amongst women (4.6 % of all cancers),<br>• It has been reported that 135,929 new cases of the cancer of the lip and oral cavity were diagnosed in India, which amounts to 10.3%of all cancers occurring in India<br>• The 5-year prevalence of oral cancer in India is 300 413 cases<br>• A total of 75,290 deaths due to cancer of the lip and oral cavity were reported in India<br>• The mean age of oral cancer is 50 years<br>• Patients with early-stage oral cancer are 82% and with advanced stages are 27%<br>• Around 80–90% of oral cancers are directly attributable to tobacco use. |

### Epidemiological Features

Tobacco chewing is a major risk factor. However, there are other factors too.

A thorough understanding of these multiple factors is essential to reduce the incidence and mortality of oral cancer. The epidemiological features of oral cancer may be categorized into agent, host, and environmental factors. These factors are depicted in **Figure 19D.7**.

- *Agent factors:*
  - *Tobacco:* Around 90% of all oral cancers are attributed to tobacco use. It has been widely reported that oral cancer and precancerous lesion occur mostly among those who indulge in tobacco use either in the form of smoking or chewing. To substantiate this, oral cancer occurs most of the times inside the mouth on the side where the quid is kept.
  - *Alcohol:* There is strong evidence which links both alcohol use and oral cancer. It is believed that alcohol has a synergistic effect on tobacco.
- *Host factors:*
  - **Precancerous stage:** Oral cancer has a long preclinical phase with lesions like leukoplakia, erythroplakia, and oral submucous fibrosis preceding invasive cancer in majority of the cases. These precancerous lesions may be detected for up to 15 years prior to their development into invasive oral cancer. This highlights the importance of identifying precancerous lesions by screening techniques, as treatment of precancerous lesions may lead to total regression.
  - *High-risk groups:*
    ♦ These include tobacco chewers, smokers and *bidi* smokers, and betel quid users.
    ♦ Another risk group of people who sleep with the betel quid in their mouths. This behavior is associated with 37 times higher risk of developing oral cancer when compared to those who do not sleep keeping betel quid in their mouths.
- *Environmental factors:*
  **Cultural practices:** There are several cultural practices and beliefs prevalent in the community associated with oral cancer risk. Indigenous forms of smoking like *bidi, chutta, chillum,* and *hookah* are one such factor. Betel quid (mixture of betel leaf, areca nut, lime, and tobacco) is most common form of tobacco chewing in India. The mixture (khaini) is put into mouth in small amounts and slowly sucked in. Reverse smoking (smoking with burning end inside mouth) is prevalent in certain parts of Andhra and is associated with epidermoid carcinoma of hard palate. In certain communities, tobacco in powdered form inhaled as snuff. Thus, it is important for

healthcare providers to identify and address these cultural factors.

## Prevention and Control of Oral Cancer

There are different approaches for prevention of oral cancer. Health education against tobacco, alcohol, and other mouth irritants is a key message to all and school children in particular. Primary health care plays an integral role in implementing these prevention and control measures. These measures include all levels of prevention which are as follows:

### *Primary Prevention*

As oral cancer is amenable to primary prevention, tobacco chewing should be eliminated from the entire community. This would bring about a significant reduction in the incidence of oral cancer. However, this requires education of the community, including primary schoolchildren before they are initiated to tobacco use. Personal commitment to give up the unhealthy practice is more useful to those who are already habituated to any form of tobacco.

### *Tobacco Control Legislation*

A comprehensive tobacco control legislation titled "The COTPA (Prohibition of Advertisement and Regulation of Trade and Commerce, Production, Supply and Distribution) Act, 2003" was passed by the parliament in April, 2003 and notified in Gazette of India on 25th Feb, 2004.

The main provisions of the act are—a prohibition of smoking in public places; prohibition of advertisement, sponsorship, and promotion of tobacco products; prohibition of the sale of tobacco products to minors or the sale within 100 yards of an educational institution; and the display of pictorial health warnings on tobacco products and the regulation of tar and nicotine content of tobacco products.

### *Secondary Prevention*

These measures include screening and treatment. As oral cancers are almost always preceded by precancerous lesions, and can be detected early, treated easily and therefore, higher is the chance of cure of cancer or prevention of invasive cancer in premalignant lesions.
- *Screening for oral cancer:* Identification of precancerous lesions is regarded as the cornerstone for oral cancer screening. Oral cancer and its precancerous lesions may be detected by visual inspection of the oral cavity which may be performed by individuals themselves and not just by a healthcare professional. In the NPCDCS program, primary health workers like Accredited Social Health Activists (ASHAs) and Auxiliary Nurse Midwife (ANMs) are supposed to conduct visual inspection of oral cavity among those who chew tobacco or complain of ulcer or sore using a checklist during their home visits.
- *Treatment:* Oral cancer is curable cancer, if detected and treated early. The main treatment modalities include surgery and radiotherapy. Post-treatment follow-up of patients must be conducted, as there are chances of recurrence. Plastic surgery of face following cancer surgery is done simultaneously as and when necessary.

### *Tertiary Prevention*

This includes care for advanced cases and terminally ill individuals. The modalities include palliative care and rehabilitation. **Figure 19D.8** depicts a summary of prevention and control measures for oral cancer.

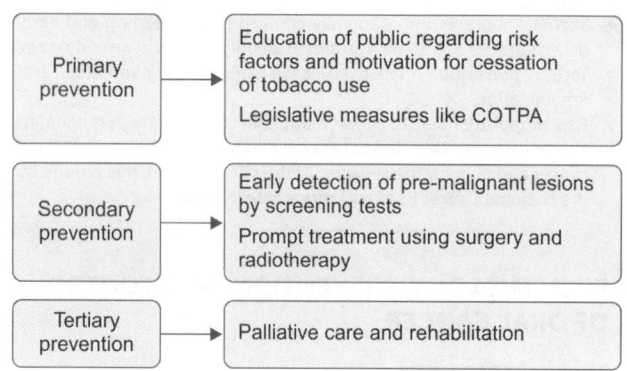

**Fig. 19D.8:** Prevention and control of oral cancer.
(COTPA: Cigarettes and Other Tobacco Products Act)

---

**Case study 1: Early Detection of Oral Cancer**

Madhav, a 36 years old mill worker, developed an ulcer on the tongue on the right lateral border. There were a few small white patches on right buccal mucosa for a year or so. One white patch started growing in size and an ulcer developed two months back. This was causing difficulty in eating and therefore he consulted a doctor in a health center. He was used to tobacco and *gutkha* chewing and he was also smoking *beedis* from his teenage years. The doctor referred him to the medical college and hospital, where partial glossectomy was done and was advised complete abstinence from tobacco. Compliance to the advice and regular follow-up helped him to prevent invasive cancer. Prevention of cancer may include primary, secondary or tertiary prevention strategies.

**Case study 2: Advanced Oral Cancer**

Asif was 57 years old and was working as a manual laborer. He came to the doctor with the complaint of inability to eat and pain on opening the mouth. He complained of a hard mass in oral cavity which did not allow him to chew. The left cheek was swollen and his face was disfigured by the huge swelling. On examination, there was a fungating mass on the left buccal mucosa occupying nearly one-third of the mouth with foul breath. Asif used to chew tobacco ever since he was 20 years old and he kept the quid in the pouch between the teeth and left buccal mucosa. He was unable to use quid since he developed these symptoms two weeks ago. Since, this is locally advanced oral cancer, it is not amenable to curative treatment, etc. only palliative care is possible in this case.

---

## EPIDEMIOLOGY, PREVENTION AND CONTROL OF BREAST CANCER

Breast cancer is the most common cancer among urban Indian women, both in terms of incidence as well as mortality. It accounts for 26.3% of all cancers in women. However, the incidence of breast cancer is significantly lower than western countries. The incidence of breast cancer is 25.8 per 100,000 women per year and is expected to rise to 35 per 100,000 women in 2026. The problem statement of breast cancer is represented in **Table 19D.4**.

Table 19D.4: Problem statement of breast cancer.

| Context | Mortality and morbidity |
|---|---|
| Global | • It is the most common malignancy among women in both developed and developing regions<br>• 2,261,419 new cases reported in 2020 in the world<br>• About 684,996 (6.9%) deaths are reported |
| Indian | • Most common cancer in women in India and accounts for 26.3% of all cancers in women<br>• Reported new cases in India are 178,361 and 90,408 (10.6%) deaths; incidence rate is 25.8 per 100,000 women per year<br>• Average age of diagnosis is 46.2 years and 48% are diagnosed in premenopausal age group<br>• Overall, 1 in 28 women is likely to develop breast cancer during her lifetime<br>• In urban areas, 1 in 22 women is likely to develop breast cancer during her lifetime as compared to rural areas where 1 in 60 women develops breast cancer in her lifetime |

## Epidemiological Features

There are multiple risk factors involved in breast cancer which are depicted in **Figure 19D.9**.

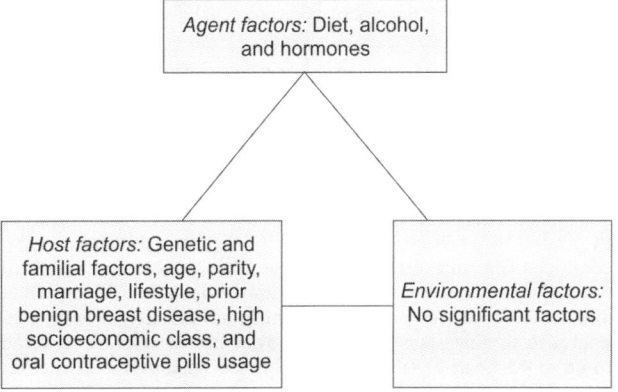

Fig. 19D.9: Epidemiological triad of breast cancer.

### Agent Factors

- **Dietary factors:** It is one of the most established risk factors for breast cancer. A diet rich in saturated fats and high calorie diets, red meat are the important etiological factors. Diets which include loads (500 g or more) of green leafy vegetables and whole fresh fruits daily are protective against breast cancer. Fiber rich diet is known to reduce the risk of breast cancer.
- **Alcohol:** High-risk of being diagnosed as breast cancer was found among women who consume alcohol. Risk depends on the quantity of alcohol consumed.
- **Hormonal factors:** Prolonged estrogen exposure is a known risk factor of breast cancer. Elevated estrogen and progesterone both increase the risk for breast cancer. About 80% of breast cancers are estrogen receptor positive.

### Host Factors

With the exception of 5-10% breast cancers where the main risk factor is genetic predisposition, in the remaining 90% of sporadic breast cancers, the identified risk factors are either reproductive, lifestyle or environmental factors, primarily through their influence on the hormonal *milieu*.

- **Genetic and familial factors:** BRCA 1 and BRCA 2 are two autosomal dominant genes which account for most inherited cases of breast cancer. Women who carry BRCA gene mutation have 60–80% lifetime risk of breast cancer development.
- **Age:** Risk of breast cancer increases with increasing age. It is more common among women aged between 35 to 50 years. Most hospital-based series in India report median age of breast cancer patients a decade younger than western series. Nearly 48% are diagnosed in the premenopausal age, which implies a more aggressive disease and negative effect on the overall prognosis and disease burden. Further, if a woman has had breast cancer before age of 40 years, the risk of cancer is doubled in the second breast.
  - There is decreased risk during menopause. Secondary rise occurs in women aged 65 years and above. Thus, a bimodal distribution of breast cancer is seen.
  - *Parity and marriage:* Early menarche and late menopause are considered as important known risk factors for breast cancer. The risk is directly related to age at which women bear their first child. Higher parity and prolonged breastfeeding are protective while nulliparity is a known risk factor.
  - *Unhealthy lifestyle practices:* Physical inactivity or sedentary lifestyle is another unhealthy lifestyle factor, which is associated with high breast cancer risk.
  - *Prior benign breast disease:* There could be a possibility of a woman who had prior benign breast disease developing breast cancer. Moreover, undergoing breast biopsy for a benign breast disease in the past is also a risk factor.

### Other Factors

- **High socioeconomic status:** Prior studies have proven that breast cancer is known to affect women who belong to an affluent background. This could be due to factors like later age at first child-birth, low parity, and usage of oral contraceptives for prolonged period which are prevalent among women of high socioeconomic background.
- **Oral contraceptive pills (OCP) use and HRT:** The evidence linking breast cancer to usage of OCPs is inconclusive. However, excessive use of OCPs before the first pregnancy, especially before the age of 25 years may increase the risk of breast cancer.
- **Exposure to radiation:** Ionizing radiation exposure is reported to be linked to breast cancer. Exposure before 20 years of age is known to carry an increased risk.

## Prevention and Control of Breast Cancer

There are many approaches to prevent and control breast cancer. However, early detection is considered as the cornerstone of breast cancer control. These measures include:

### Primary Prevention

The primary prevention measures need to be implemented from a young age. For example, age at menarche can be delayed by weight control and regular, intense physical activity. Healthy, prudent diet containing limited amount of saturated fats is important to reduce breast cancer risk.

- Cancer awareness is a key step in primary prevention of breast cancer. Women need to be taught about the importance of identifying the warning signs of breast cancer.

### Secondary Prevention

***Screening for breast cancer:*** The primary health care providers can make the general population aware about breast screening and its protocol. This includes early detection techniques like breast self-examination (BSE) and clinical breast examination of breasts by doctor/nurse/trained health worker and mammography followed by appropriate and prompt treatment. There is sufficient evidence, which suggests that screening for breast cancer may lead to a desirable treatment outcome and reduce mortality.

- ***Breast self-examination (BSE):*** This has to be carried by every woman aged 20 years and above on a fixed day every month, ideally 10 days after the menstrual period. Women need to be taught to examine all the quadrants of the breasts with flat of the hand and axillae. Every woman should also be made aware of the following signs:
  - Lump or thickening in the breast—most common
  - A change in size of breast
  - A nipple that is pulled in or retracted
  - A rash or ulcer on or around the nipple
  - Discharge from one or both nipples
  - Peau d'orange (puckering or dimpling of skin)
  - Paget's disease
  - Constant pain in the breast or armpit rarely.
- ***Palpation by physician:*** Clinical breast examination (CBE) is recommended for all women once a year after 40 years of age, preferably in the age group 40-69 years, by a healthcare professional. This involves inspection, followed by palpation of the breasts in a circular manner, clockwise, starting from the nipple and areola toward the periphery and axilla.
- ***Mammography:*** The World Health Organization (WHO) recommends mammography every 1–2 years for women aged 50–69 years. It is regarded as the most sensitive screening test. The test is less sensitive in women under 40 years as breast tissue is dense and therefore, ultrasonography (USG) is considered a better tool. USG is a useful adjunct to mammography for the diagnosis of breast abnormalities. Limitations of mammography include high cost, some risk associated with exposure to radiation and also the procedure requires special equipment and skilled technicians and trained radiologists.

***Treatment:*** The main treatment modalities of breast cancer include surgery, radiotherapy and chemotherapy. Breast conservative surgery is effective and currently it is preferred for early stages of cancer. This is followed by radiotherapy. Hormone therapy is advised as required after studying hormone receptors. Regular follow-up care is an essential component of treatment and is essential, as there are chances of recurrence among women who have undergone treatment.

### Tertiary Prevention

This refers to care for very late stages of cancer or those with distant metastasis locally advanced breast carcinoma and terminally ill individuals. This includes symptomatic care, pain relief, and psychological support. The preventive measures for breast cancer are depicted in **Figure 19D.10**.

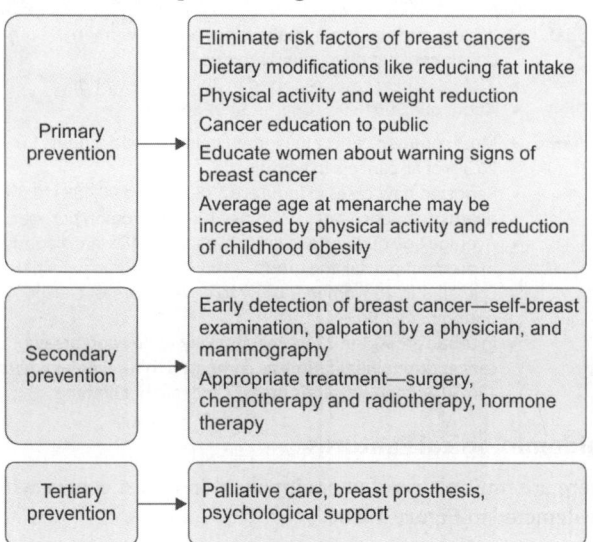

**Fig. 19D.10:** Prevention and control of breast cancer.

---

***Case study 1: Early Detection of Breast Cancer***

Rita, a married lady aged 48 years with two children, had found a small painless lump in her left breast. As she had heard someone say that a lump in breast means cancer, she discussed it with her health worker friend who took her to the doctor in the primary health center.

The doctor reassured Rita that all lumps are not cancer. However, they need to be thoroughly tested. He elicited a detailed history, conduced clinical examination and sent her to district hospital for FNAC. Cytology has revealed cells suggestive of Adeno carcinoma. Rita and her family were explained everything and was convinced by PHC doctor to comply with the medical advice promptly. She was asked to go to the nearby teaching hospital in the neighboring district for surgery to remove the lump and further treatment. She returned to PHC for regular follow-up.

***Case study 2: Advanced Breast Cancer***

- Mumtaj Begum, a 65-year-old widow, came to the local PHC doctor with a grossly enlarged right breast. She first noticed a small lump an year ago. She was living all alone with meager income sent by her two sons working in the city, she was scared to go to the doctor for she did not want to spend money on medicines.
- As the lump started growing bigger day by day, and she developed backache and swelling in the neck, she was forced to see the local doctor. On examination, the doctor found a large tumor mass which eroded the skin on the right breast and enlarged lymph nodes in right axilla and in supra clavicular region. X-ray of chest and also spine revealed metastasis in the lung and vertebra. This lady required palliative surgery, chemotherapy at the higher tertiary care hospital with subsequent follow-up with local doctor.
- Such a case should be discussed with all including health workers, who would be able to suspect and detect cases at an early stage to facilitate curative treatment and improved survival.

## EPIDEMIOLOGY, PREVENTION, AND CONTROL OF CERVICAL CANCER

Cervical cancer is one of the most preventable cancers, yet remains the world's second-leading cancer killer of women. Of the 500,000 cases diagnosed every year, more than 280,000 die.

Table 19D.5: Problem statement of cervical cancer.

| Context | Mortality and morbidity |
|---|---|
| Global | • Fourth most common cancer of women worldwide<br>• 604,127 (3.1%) new cases were reported in 2020 and about 341,831 (3.4%) deaths. |
| Indian | • In India, it is the second most common cancer in India in women accounting for 18.3% of all cancer cases in women and 9.4% of all cancer cases in both men and women.<br>• India accounts for one-fourth of global burden of cervical cancer<br>• Nearly 123,907 (9.4%) new cases in India and 77,348 deaths reported.<br>• Cervical cancer is the second largest cause of cancer mortality in India accounting for nearly 9.1% of all cancer related deaths in the country.<br>• Median age: 38 years (age 21–67 years).<br>• Rural women are at higher risk of developing cervical cancer as compared to their urban counterparts<br>• The relative five-year survival averages 42.82%. |

A joint study on cervical cancer prepared by National Institute of Cancer Prevention and Research (NICPR) revealed that India alone accounts for one-fourth of the global burden of cervical cancer.

According to NCI, infection of the cervix with HPV is the most common cause of cervical cancer. HPV is a very common infection that can spread from person to person through sexual contact. The problem statement of cervical cancer is represented in **Table 19D.5**.

## Epidemiological Features

The risk factors for cervical cancer are depicted in **Figure 19D.11**.

### Natural History of Disease

The disease follows a progressive course from epithelial dysplasia to carcinoma in situ and then invasive carcinoma. It remains at carcinoma in situ stage for around 8–10 years. However, invasive cervical cancer is mostly irreversible and left untreated, may spread locally or metastasize to distant organs in later stages.

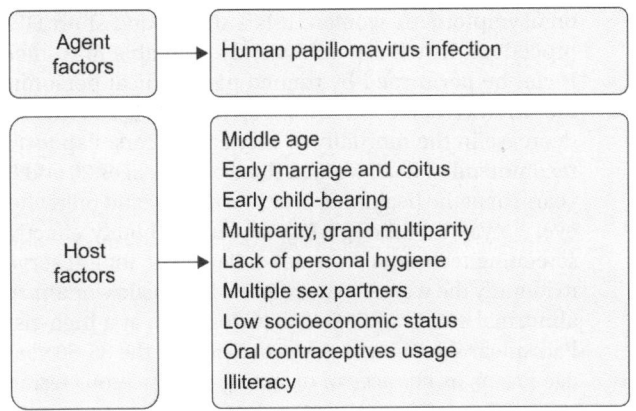

Fig. 19D.11: Epidemiological factors of cervical cancer.

The natural history of cervical cancer is depicted in **Figure 19D.12**.

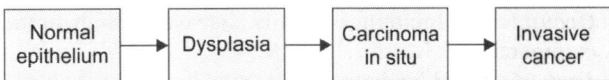

Fig. 19D.12: Natural history of cancer cervix.

### Risk Factors of Cervical Cancer

*Human papillomavirus infection (HPV):* HPV is a sexually transmitted infection and is a main cause for cervical cancer. It produces many subclinical and clinical lesions. It is associated with 50,000 new cases of cervical cancer and 250,000 associated cervical cancer deaths worldwide each year. It also causes vulvar, vaginal, anal, and penile cancers as well as precancerous lesions of vulva or vagina, genital warts, and respiratory papillomatosis. HPV infections are asymptomatic, and generally, individuals are not aware of being infected, thus facilitating the spread easily and unknowingly. At least 50% of men and women will acquire genital HPV infection during their lifetime. All sexually active women are infected with HPV at least once during their lifetime, and the highest prevalence is seen soon after the onset of sexual activities.

Till date some 100 different types of HPV have been identified but only some types have been linked to invasive cancer. Infection with certain types of HPV like HPV type 16, 18 are the most common types of HPV associated with invasive cervical cancer.

The risk factors for HPV infection include previous genital cancer, HIV infection, multiple sexual partners, and a weak immune system. Some types of HPV (type 6, and 11) cause genital warts which are easily treated and not related to cancer. However, HPV is just a necessary cause but not a sufficient cause for development of cervical cancer.

- *Age:* Highest incidence is in the age group of 35–44 years. The risk increases with increasing age, the median age being 48 years.
- *Age at marriage:* It has been identified as a key determinant for cervical cancer. Early marriage (marriage in adolescent period), early coitus, early child-bearing, and repeated pregnancies are associated risk factors for cervical cancer. Over the years, there has been a considerable increase in the socioeconomic changes in the community resulting in increase in the average age of marriage among women and reduction in parity. Concurrent improvement in personal hygiene and adoption of barrier contraception also lead to a decline in the number of cervical cancer cases.
- *Marital status:* Cervical cancer almost always occurs in married women and HPV infection, as the necessary cause, is sexually transmitted.
- *Parity:* Unlike breast cancer, the incidence of cancer cervix is higher among multiparous women when compared to nulliparous women. Repeated infections, recurrent trauma to cervix during birth, make it vulnerable.
- *Multiple sex partners:* Any type of sexual activity including only genital skin-to-skin contact or oral sex can cause HPV infection. As such, any woman, who is sexually active, is at risk for cervical cancer. The incidence of cervical cancer is higher among women with multiple sexual partners, or husband with multiple partners, as it can cause recurrent exposure to carcinogenic strains of HPV.

- **Occupation:** Incidence of this disease is high among commercial sex workers.
- **Lack of genital hygiene:** Poor genital hygiene is known to be associated at least with 80% of HPV cases. This makes the cervix vulnerable to HPV infection.
- **Socioeconomic status:** Cervical cancer incidence is known to be high among women of low-income group. Cervical cancer is a disease that has been strongly linked to poverty. The mortality rates are also known to be high among women who belong to lower socioeconomic status.
- **Genital warts:** HPV types 6 and 11 cause genital warts. Other than HPV, the presence of genital warts either in the present or past is another condition, which may predispose to cervical cancer. However, this risk factor is not as strong as HPV.
- **Other factors:** Illiteracy and ignorance are major factors leading to an increased risk of cervical cancer. OCPs usage is another risk factor for cervical cancer, as it is known to increase the risk of HPV infection. Women who have been consuming for 5 years or more have the maximum risk of cervical cancer. Smoking tobacco adversely affects the response of HPV infection to treatment, which could lead to the development of carcinoma in situ or invasive cancer.

## Prevention and Control of Cervical Cancer

### Primary Prevention

Primary prevention in case of cervical cancers has reasonable scope. HPV is necessary for the development of cervical cancer. Therefore, preventing HPV infection can prevent cervical cancer. Primary prevention involves a risk reduction approach through behavioral intervention for sexual and healthcare-seeking behavior or through mass immunization against high-risk HPV. Awareness about genital hygiene and barrier contraceptive measures are two important steps. Additional strategies include three key steps—(1) Population strategy, (2) High-risk strategy, and (3) Specific protection.

1. **Population strategy:** It includes cancer education to the entire community with emphasis on identification of specific warning signs, such as bleeding after coitus, bleeding after menopause, and unexplained vaginal bleeding.
2. **High-risk strategy:** In this case, the focus is on the vulnerable, high-risk population to obtain better yield from screening. Screening by Pap smear of this group such as multiparous women of lower socioeconomic group, commercial sex workers, women over 35 years of age, and women with multiple sexual partners is known to facilitate early diagnosis and reduce mortality significantly.
    - The objective of cervical screening is to prevent invasive cervical cancer from developing by detecting and treating women with cervical intraepithelial neoplasia 2/3 (CIN 2/3) lesions, and the effectiveness is determined by reduction in incidence and mortality. The critical components of a screening program are an acceptable good quality screening test, prompt diagnostic investigations, appropriate treatment, and post-treatment follow-up.
3. **Specific protection by HPV vaccines:**
    - Three FDA approved killed vaccines in liquid form are available to prevent HPV infection:
        1. Cervarix, bivalent vaccine which has types 16 and 18 which protects against two strains of HPV;
        2. Gardasil which is a quadrivalent vaccine protects against four strains of HPV; and
        3. Gardasil 9, which also protects against four strains of HPV.
    - All three vaccines target HPV 16 and HPV 18, the strains of HPV that cause the majority of cervical cancers.
    - The Advisory Committee on Immunization Practices (ACIP) recommends HPV vaccination for females and males at age 11 or 12. The series can start at age 9 years. For individuals who were not vaccinated at those ages, the vaccine can still be administered. Catch-up vaccines are recommended for females, men who have sex with men, and those who are immunocompromised until age 26. For men who have sex only with women, catch up vaccinations are recommended until the age of 21. Three doses are given over 3 months. HPV vaccines are very safe. Pain in the injection site is the most frequently reported adverse event.

The vaccines are most effective when administered before exposure to HPV, so it is important to give the vaccination before sexual debut. However, HPV-exposed individuals not already immunized should still receive the vaccine, as it will provide protection against strains of HPV to which the individual has not been exposed. However, the cost is quite high and those women that are at high-risk have no access to the vaccine. Vaccinated individuals should continue to have routine cervical cancer screening at age appropriate intervals.

### Secondary Prevention

There are many favorable factors with reference to cervical cancer, which makes it amenable to screening and prompt curative treatment. Cancer of cervix uteri affects an accessible site for visual inspection and it is almost always preceded by pre-invasive stage. Moreover, the lesion is slow growing and localized for around 8–10 years making it ideal for secondary prevention.

- **Screening for cancer cervix:**
    - Pap smear is a commonly practiced screening procedure on asymptomatic women. It is a simple and short OPD procedure, which is painless and acceptable to women. It can be performed by trained paramedical personnel too. In developed countries, Pap test has led to marked decrease in the mortality of cervical cancers. Pap test is recommended to all women (between the ages 20 and 65 years) or at the beginning of sexual activity and thereafter, every 3 years. Although Pap smear is a highly effective screening technique, it is not a diagnostic tool. It serves to identify the women who require diagnostic workup. An abnormal smear indicates that woman is at a high-risk. Pap smear screening has a better yield in the 35-50 years age group, as chances of detecting precancerous lesions are maximum in this group. Periodicity of test in our country is recommended at least once in five years.
    - Visual inspection using 5% acetic acid (VIA), VIA with magnification (VIAM) and visual inspection-post-application of Lugol's iodine (VILI) are alternative

screening procedures, which are easier to carry out. Present strategy includes screening women using visual inspection after application of freshly prepared acetic acid.

- **Treatment options:** It includes a multimodality approach of surgery, radiotherapy, and chemotherapy. Total hysterectomy or radical hysterectomy is advised for any invasive cancer amenable to surgery. Precancerous lesions are excised by loop excision method and carcinoma in situ by cone hysterectomy. Early stages of invasive cancer are amenable to radical surgery and advanced stages by radiotherapy. The prevention and control measures for cervical cancer are summarized in **Figure 19D.13**.

> Several important policy decisions taken by the government towards curbing cancer are highly commendable. Such policies include vaccinations health legislation measures, such as COTPA, etc., implementation of population-based screening programs for cervical, breast and oral cancer. However, the screening techniques are still not adequate and more efforts are needed keeping the feasibility and constraints in mind.

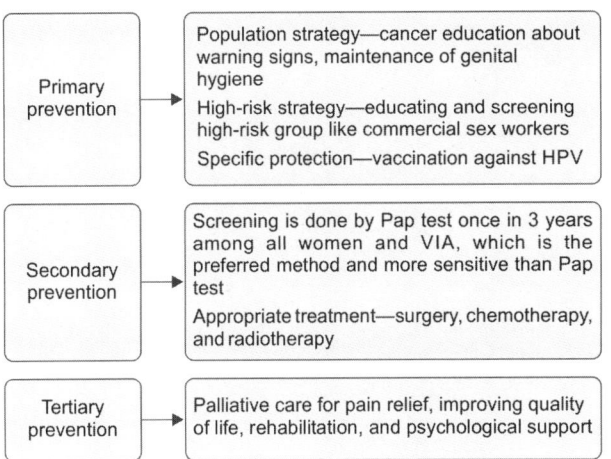

Fig. 19D.13: Prevention and control of cervical cancer.

---

*Case Study*

**1: Early Detection of Cervical Cancer**

Shanta, a 42 years old housewife accompanied her niece, who was pregnant, to the nearest health center for registration. There the nurse explained to Jyoti about the importance of the Pap test and convinced her for the test even though she had no complaints. Then, she recollected how one of their relatives in their native village had died of cervical cancer in the recent past, as it was detected very late. The Pap test was done and it was normal. She was advised regular follow-up to prevent cancer.

**2: Advanced Cervical Cancer**

Savitri, a 49 years old lady with six children had started bleeding per vagina after she stopped her regular menstruation one year ago. She thought that her periods had started again, but when bleeding and foul-smelling discharge persisted for 3 weeks, she consulted a doctor. On examination, cervix was hard and fixed. There was a large friable tumor on the cervix extending to the left lateral wall of vagina, which started bleeding on touch. It was detected as advanced cancer of cervix, amenable for palliative treatment only.

## SUMMARY

- Cancer is a major public health problem with an estimated 18.1 million cancer incident cases and 9.6 million deaths worldwide.
- India's current burden of a million incident cancers is the result of an epidemiologic transition, improved cancer diagnostics, and improved cancer data capture. The most common cancers in men are those of lungs, oral cavity, stomach, and esophagus, while in women, those of cervix uteri, breast, oral cavity, ovary, esophagus, are the most common. Oral cancer is the most common cancer in India amongst men (16.1 % of all cancers) and 80-90% of them are directly attributable to tobacco use and hence potentially preventable. Breast cancer is the most common cancer in women in India and accounts for 14% of all cancers in women. Cervical cancer is the second most common cancer in India in women accounting for 22.86% of all cancer cases in women and 12% of all cancer cases in both men and women.
- These cancers can be prevented, screened for and/or detected early and treated at an early stage which significantly reduce the death rate from these cancers.
- Common causes are cigarette smoking, chewing tobacco, alcohol drinking, dietary habits, ionizing and UV radiation, urban air pollution, indoor smoke, sexually transmitted HPV infection, infection by hepatitis or other carcinogenic infections, obesity, etc. Tobacco use is the single most important risk factor for cancer and is responsible for approximately 22% of cancer-related deaths globally. Early diagnosis of cancer is an important public health strategy in all settings. It increases the chances for successful treatment by focusing on detecting symptomatic patients as early as possible. Cancer control is a broad term which consists of a series of measures based on the present knowledge in the fields of prevention, early detection, diagnosis, treatment, after care and rehabilitation. The aim is to reduce incidence of disease significantly and increase the cure rate and reducing the suffering and deformity or disability due to cancer.
- Primary preventive measures include public education on cancer, education against all forms of tobacco and alcohol use, and vaccinations against HPV and HBV infections. Additional measures are control of occupational hazards; healthy diet, healthy weight and decreasing exposure from environmental carcinogens, protection from ionizing radiation and UV rays, etc. Vaccination against these HPV and hepatitis B viruses could prevent 1 million cancer cases each year.

Secondary prevention includes early detection and diagnosis of cancers, especially breast, cervix and oropharyngeal cancers by screening methods and patients' education on self-examination. Early detection of premalignant conditions and prompt treatment would prevent invasive cancers. Tertiary prevention involves appropriate treatment in the advanced stage of disease. This includes palliative care, disability limitation, and rehabilitation.

## SUGGESTED READING

1. Blackadar CB. Historical review of the causes of cancer. World J Clin Oncol. 2016;7(1):54-86.
2. Bray F, Ferlay J, Soerjomataraml, et al. Global cancer statistics 2018: GLOBOCAN estimates of incidence and mortality world wide for 36 cancers in 185 countries. CA Cancer J Clin. 2018;68(6):394-424.
3. Ferlay J, Soerjomataram I, Ervik M, et al. Global cancer statistics 2018: GLOBOCAN estimates of incidence and mortality worldwide for 36 cancers in 185 countries; 2018.
4. Hashemi SH, Karimi S, Mahboobi H. Lifestyle changes for prevention of breast cancer. Electron Physician. 2014;6(3):894-905.
5. Indian Council of Medical Research (ICMR) Consensus Document for Management of Breast Cancer; 2016.
6. Indian Council of Medical Research (ICMR) Newsletter of NCRP Annual Reports; 2017.

7. Kotepur M. Diet and risk of breast cancer. Contemp Oncol (Pozn). 2016;20(1):13-9.
8. Lakshmaiah KC, Guruprasad B, Lokesh KN, et al. Cancer notification in India. South Asian J Cancer. 2014;3:74-7.
9. Medical Research Council India. (2009). ICMR–MRC Workshop on Chronic Diseases. [online] Available from:https://www.icmr.nic.in/ sites/default/files/reports/Chronic_Diseases_Report.pdf.
10. Ministry of Health and Family Welfare, Government of India. (2005). National Cancer Control Programme Guidelines.
11. National Centre for Disease Control, MOHFW, GOI. National Programme for Prevention and Control of Cancer, Diabetes, Cardiovascular Diseases and Stroke Training Module for Medical Officers for Prevention, Control and Population Level Screening of Hypertension, Diabetes and Common Cancer. New Delhi: Ministry of Health and Family Welfare; 2017. pp. 4-18.
12. National Health Systems Resource Centre. National Programme for Prevention and Control of Cancer, Diabetes, Cardiovascular Diseases and Stroke (NPDCS) training manual. [online] Available from:www.nhsrcindia.org.
13. NICPR. Young Indian Women are More Vulnerable to Breast Cancer, Says CII Report. [online] Available from: http://cancerindia.org.in/ young-indian-women-vulnerable-breast-cancer-says-cii-report.
14. Peterson PE. Oral cancer prevention and control—the approach of the World Health Organization. Oral Oncol. 2009;45(4-5):454-60.
15. Sankaranarayanan R, Black RJ, Parkin DM. Cancer survival in developing countries, IARC Scientific Publication No. 145. Lyon: International Agency for Research on Cancer; 1998.
16. Sarnath D, Khanna A. Current status of cancer burden: global and Indian scenario. Biomed Res J. 2014;1:1–5.
17. Sreedevi A, Javed R, Dinesh A. Epidemiology of cervical cancer with special focus on India. Int J Womens Health. 2015;7:405-14.
18. Tota JE, Ramana-Kumar AV, El-Khatib Z, et al. The road ahead for cervical cancer prevention and control. Curr On col. 2014;21(2):e255- 64.
19. WHO. (2013). Press Release No. 223, 12 Dec. 2013, Latest World Cancer Statistics-Global cancer burden [online] Available from:https://www.iarc.fr/wp-content/ uploads/2018/07/pr223_E.pdf.
20. WHO. (2014). World Cancer Fact sheet, Cancer Research UK, January 2014. [online] Available from: https://www.cancerresearchuk.org/ sites/default/files/cs_report_world.pdf.
21. WHO. Latest global cancer data: Cancer burden rises to 18.1 million new cases and 9.6 million cancer deaths in 2018.
22. WHO. WHO Definition of Palliative Care. [online] Available from: http://www.who.int/cancer/palliative/definition/en.
23. WHO. WHO Guide for Effective Programmes: Diagnosis and Treatment Final–Cancer Module 4. [online] Available from: https://www.who.int/cancer/publications/cancer_control_diagnosis/en.
24. World Health Organization. The Global Burden of Disease: 2004 Update. Geneva, WHO, 2009.
25. www.ncdirindia.org › ncrp › Development of an atlas of Cancer in India - A project of the National Cancer Registry Programme (Indian Council of Medical Research) 2010.

# E. EPIDEMIOLOGY OF INJURIES, ACCIDENTS AND ITS PREVENTION AND CONTROL

*Shreyaswi Sathyanath M, Narayanan Namboothiri G, Jithin Daniel J*

*Quote: Better a thousand times careful than once dead*
—**Proverb**

| | |
|---|---|
| **CM 7.2** | Enumerate, describe and discuss the mode of transmission and measures for prevention and control of injuries and accidents |
| **CM 8.2** | Describe and discuss the epidemiological and control measures applicable in injuries and accidents |

## BACKGROUND

### What is an Accident?

An accident has been defined by an advisory group of World Health Organization (WHO) as an "unpremeditated event resulting in recognizable damage." An accident can also be defined as "an unfortunate incident that happens unexpectedly and unintentionally, typically resulting in damage or injury".

### What is an Injury?

The WHO states "injury" to be the "physical damage that results when a human body is suddenly or briefly subjected to intolerable levels of energy." An injury may present as a lesion in the body or as a functional impairment.

Injury can be caused by following forms of energy:
- Mechanical (collision with an object that is moving, as in case of a road traffic injury)
- Radiant (explosion leading to high intensity light or a shock wave)
- Thermal (very hot or cold water)
- Electrical
- Chemical (ingestion of a poisonous substance).

### Are Injuries and Accidents Synonymous?

Injuries are not the same as accidents. Accidents are largely chance events, without considering those that are preventable. Injuries are events that have identifiable causes and can lead to several consequences on communities and countries. Such events that are preventable and predictable cannot be called accidents; hence it is more appropriate to study them as injuries rather than accidents from the perspective of a community physician. It is important to make this distinction as "identifying these causes" and taking appropriate action is the cornerstone of injury prevention strategies. Hence, for the rest of the chapter, we will be discussing the epidemiological and preventive aspects of injuries.

## TYPES OF INJURY

Injuries have been included as "acute physical conditions" listed in Chapter XIX (injury, poisoning and certain other consequences of external causes) and Chapter XX (External causes of morbidity and mortality) under the International Statistical Classification of Diseases and Related Health Problems, Tenth Revision (ICD 10).

Chapter XX (V01-Y98) permits the coding with respect to the environmental circumstances and events, place of occurrence, and the activity which led to the occurrence of injury.

"Accidents (V01-X59)" are further divided as:
1. Transport accidents
2. Other external causes of accidental injury
   - Falls
   - Exposure to inanimate mechanical forces
   - Exposure to animate mechanical forces
   - Accidental drowning and submersion
   - Other accidental threats to breathing
   - Exposure to electric current, radiation and extreme ambient air temperature and pressure
   - Exposure to smoke, fire and flames
   - Contact with heat and hot substances
   - Contact with venomous animals and plants
   - Exposure to forces of nature
   - Accidental poisoning by and exposure to noxious substances
   - Overexertion, travel and privation
   - Accidental exposure to other and unspecified factor.

Another common method of classifying injuries for surveillance purposes by WHO is on the basis of whether the injury was inflicted deliberately or not and who has caused the injury (for instance, by self or others).
- Unintentional (or accidental)
- Intentional (or deliberate):
  - Interpersonal
  - Self-harm
  - Legal intervention
  - War, civil insurrection, etc.
- Undetermined intent.

## MAGNITUDE OF INJURIES

### Problem Statement

#### World (Table 19E.1)

Injuries due to various reasons cause more than 4.4 million deaths worldwide (8% of deaths in the world) annually and harm million more people (WHO, Injuries and Violence Facts 2021) of which unintentional injuries take the lives of 3.16 million people every year and violence-related injuries kill 1.25 million people every year. Roughly 1 in 3 of these deaths result from road traffic crashes, 1 in 6 from suicide, 1 in 10 from homicide and 1 in 61 from war and conflict.

For people age 5-29 years, 3 of the top 5 causes of death are injury-related, namely road traffic injuries, homicide and suicide. Drowning is the sixth leading cause of death for children age 5–14 years. Falls account for over 684,000 deaths each year and are a growing and under-recognized public health issue.

Injuries and violence are responsible for an estimated 10% of all years lived with disability.

Table 19E.1: Global Health Estimates 2016 summary tables: global deaths due to injuries in 2016 and projected to 2019 and 2030.

| Year | 2016 (in crores) | 2019 (in crores) | 2030 (in crores) |
|---|---|---|---|
| Population | 746 | 770 | 854 |
| Injuries | 488 | 502 | 556 |
| • Unintentional injuries | 343 | 361 | 397 |
| ➢ Road injury | 140 | 146 | 149 |
| ➢ Poisonings | 10 | 10 | 11 |
| ➢ Falls | 66 | 71 | 91 |
| ➢ Fire, heat and hot substances | 15 | 15 | 16 |
| ➢ Drowning | 31 | 31 | 33 |
| ➢ Exposure to forces of nature | 0.3 | 6 | 6 |
| ➢ Other unintentional injuries | 78 | 79 | 88 |
| • Intentional injuries | 145 | 140 | 158 |
| ➢ Self-harm | 79 | 80 | 89 |
| ➢ Interpersonal violence | 47 | 47 | 48 |
| ➢ Collective violence and legal intervention | 18 | 12 | 20 |

*Source:* WHO, GBD: Projections of Mortality and Causes of Death: 2016 to 2060.

### India

- National Crime Record Bureau report divides accidental deaths into two—(1) accidental deaths due to causes attributable to nature and (2) accidental deaths due to causes not attributable to nature, i.e., due to deliberate or negligent conduct of human beings (for e.g. drowning, explosion, falls, fire, poisoning, traffic accidents and other causes) **(Fig. 19E.1)**.
- The rate of accidental deaths (per lakh of population) has increased in 2018 as compared to 2017.

The magnitude of problem of accidents and injuries can be measured by various indicators, some of which are shown in **Box 19E.1**

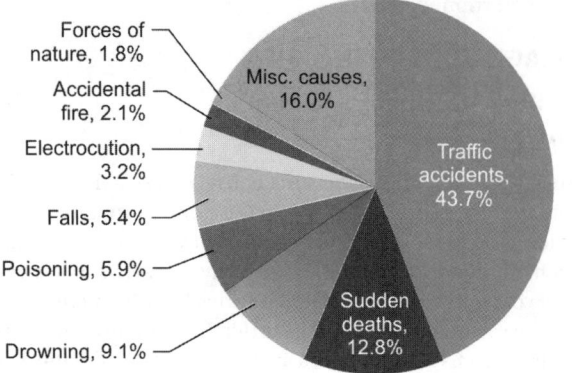

Fig. 19E.1: Percentage share of various major causes of accidental deaths during 2021 (Forces of Nature and Other Causes).
*Source:* Accidental Deaths and Suicides in India Report 2021.

**Box 19E.1: Measuring the problem.**

**Mortality:**
- It is measured in terms of deaths due to injuries
- For example, proportional mortality rate of road traffic injuries, i.e. the "number of deaths due to road traffic injuries per 100 (or 1,000) total deaths"

**Morbidity:**
- It is measured in terms of severe or mild injuries
- Abbreviated Injury Scale (AIS) is widely used to assess seriousness of the injury
- Reliability of morbidity rates is poor because of "under-reporting" (lower rates of reporting) and "mis-reporting" (wrong reporting).

**Disability:**
- It is a consequence of the injury that can occur in the accident process
- This may be classified as "temporary or permanent", "partial or total"
- This can be measured as "Disability Adjusted Life Years/ DALYs" which is a sum of "Years of Life Lost/ YLL" and "Years Lost due to Disability/ YLD".

**Key Points**
- Injuries and accidents are not synonymous; injuries refer to events that are predictable and preventable.
- Mortality is measured in terms of deaths due to injuries.
- Morbidity is measured in terms of serious and slight injuries and "Abbreviated Injury Scale" is used to assess seriousness of the injury.
- Disability measured as Disability Adjusted Life Years which is a sum of Years of Life Lost and Years Lost due to Disability.
- Transport Research Wing, Ministry of Road Transport and Highways of India provides data on road traffic injuries in India.

## EPIDEMIOLOGY OF INJURIES

Every epidemiological study is based on epidemiological triad which involves agent, host, and environment **(Fig. 19E.2)**.

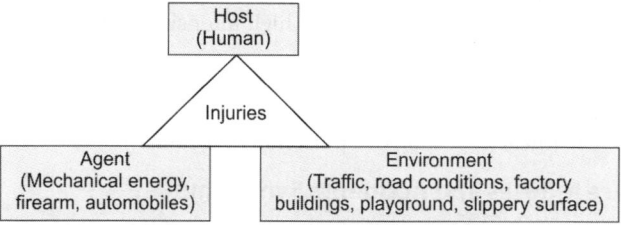

Fig. 19E.2: Epidemiological triad of injuries.

### Agent

It is the various forms of energy which is transferred to the host. The transfer of energy can be done by a vehicle which is "inanimate" (e.g. automobile) or a vector which is "animate" (e.g. a dog in case of a bite).

### Host

It refers to the person affected by the injury and his/her characteristics. For example, these characteristics include age, gender, experience, fatigue, alcohol, etc., in case of motor vehicle crashes.

### Environment

It refers to the physical surroundings (roadways or playgrounds) or social surroundings (conflicts or political unrest) that may contribute to injury.

> **Key Points**
> - Epidemiology of injuries is based on epidemiological triad which involves agent (mechanical energy, firearms, automobiles), host (human), and environment (traffic, playground, slippery conditions).
> - Haddon matrix identifies risk factors before the event, during the event, and after the event, in relation to the person, agent, and environment.
> - Main advantage of Haddon matrix: Counter measures can be developed and prioritized for implementation over short-term and long-term periods.

## PREVENTION AND CONTROL

Preventive interventions in injuries include a series of strategies aimed to prevent, reduce or alleviate injuries. They are described as follows:
- Based on the level in the injury process as primary, secondary and tertiary
- Based on the Haddon's matrix as pre-event, event or post-event phase
- Based on the method of implementation as 3 Es—education, enforcement, and engineering
- Based on the amount of action required by individual/host-active and passive.

### Primary, Secondary and Tertiary Prevention

1. **Primary prevention** means preventing the event or incidents which lead to injury, that is, to eliminate exposure to risk of occurrence of the event. This means reducing the frequency of the activity which is hazardous or reducing the hazardousness each time the activity is undertaken. For example, with respect to elderly falls, primary prevention may include identifying the risk factors that contribute to falls and modifying them, assessment of the elderly individual in depth by health professionals to look for any existing medical illness or any environmental and behavioral factors. This should be followed by treatment of the illness if identified, dose adjustment of medication, removal of hazards, introduction of exercise for muscle strength, and balance.
2. **Secondary prevention strategies** refer to prevention of injury, in case the event occurs. These range from product designs to law enforcement. For example, in case of elderly falls, injuries can be prevented by reducing bone loss using pharmacological methods like hormonal replacement therapy or bisphosphonates. Another method is hip pads that can prevent fractures even if the elderly person falls. In road traffic injuries, time is of essence for post-impact care with the aim being avoiding preventable death as well as limiting the severity of injury and ensuring the survivor's best possible recovery. In this regard, the concept of golden hour (first 60 minutes) and platinum hour (first 10 minutes) are well known.
3. **Tertiary prevention strategies** reduce or eliminate long-term disabilities and impairment, i.e., the involvement limiting the consequences of injury. Good trauma care can improve the health outcomes even if injury occurs following trauma by ensuring least delay to reach definitive care. For example, with respect to elderly falls, tertiary prevention encompasses emergency response and prompt transport of the injured elderly to the hospital without any delay. This should be followed by definitive treatment if required, e.g., orthopedic surgery. Initiating rehabilitative services are also important to prevent long-term complications as well as to minimize long-term complications/disability.

### Haddon Matrix

In injuries, William Haddon developed an extension of the "epidemiological triad" approach wherein the interaction of the agent, host, and environmental factors is plotted against the axis of time. The Haddon matrix is an analytical tool that helps to identify all factors that are associated with a crash. The advantage of combining the phases of injury **(Fig. 19E.3)** with the epidemiological model is that the matrix helps study both causation and prevention aspects of the injury. Once we identify and analyze the multiple factors that are associated with a crash, counter measures can be developed and prioritized for implementation over short-term and long-term periods.

> *Case Scenario 1*
>
> *Consider that you have been assigned the task of drawing up preventive strategies to decrease the number of falls and injuries in the local playground. How would you use the Haddon matrix to do the same?*

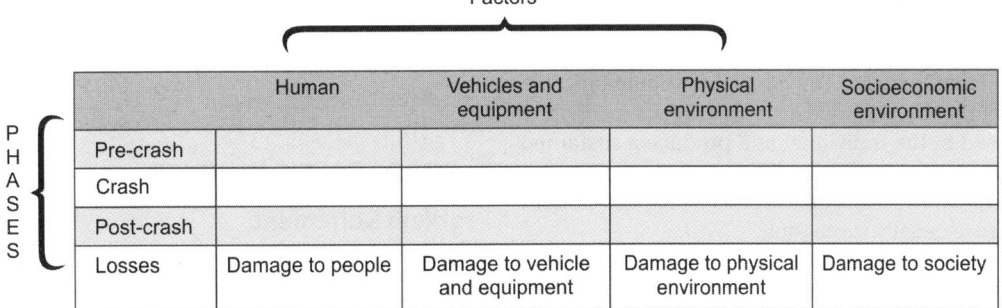

Fig. 19E.3: Phases in the Haddon matrix.

*Suggested Solution*
*The interventions that have been explained so far can be fit into the matrix as given in **Table 19E.2**.*

**Table 19E.2:** Haddon matrix to prevent falls and injuries in playground.

| | Host (child) | Agent/vehicle (equipment and devices in the playground) | Physical environment (design of the playground) | Social environment (policies and rules) |
|---|---|---|---|---|
| Pre-event (before the fall) | Safety rules to be taught to the children (e.g. prevent crowding while climbing slides) | Equipment that meets safety standards (provide good grip to prevent slipping of hands) | Build playground such that children do not climb too high | Build norms such that adults play along and keep watch over children |
| Event (during the fall and impact) | While falling, train children on ways to fall so as to minimize injury | Avoid sharp protrusions in equipments to avoid children being hit by these | Make the surfaces in the playground resilient | Monitor playground safety |
| Post-event (after the fall) | Teach the child how he/she can call for help (e.g. emergency call systems) | Do not install equipments which can prevent rescue personnel from reaching the fallen/injured child | Sitting areas for parents/caretakers with good visibility to supervise any child who might have fallen or gotten injured | Funding for emergency care and response when necessary |

### 3 Es of Implementation

The methods of implementation of prevention strategies can be categorized into 3 Es: *Education, Enforcement,* and *Engineering*.

### Education

This method is easy to implement and most commonly used. In the continuum of injury prevention, safety promotion is the first step, and this involves education to raise awareness about the need for prevention of injuries. The education should be given in such a manner that the knowledge or training once provided should be retained in the individual and produce a sustained behavioral change. Hence, those educational programs that have ongoing evaluation for the behavioral change component are the ones that are usually successful.
*Examples:* Use of social media and innovative television or media campaigns for encouraging helmet use can provide sustainable benefits. Other examples include safety awareness campaigns, alcohol, and road traffic crash education for high school students and violence prevention programs.

### Enforcement

These include legal or administrative steps for ensuring prevention of injuries. Sometimes, they may be more effective than education as it is mandatory to follow them and there is a fear of consequences among the public if not adhered to. However, the effectiveness of legislation depends upon the enforcement, presence of exemptions as well as the punishment in case of failure to comply. It is also important for the organizations or personnel (police/safety inspectors, etc.) responsible for enforcement collaborate with each other in order to have an integrated and coordinated approach.
*Examples:* These include compulsory seat belt legislations and presence of stop signals in railway crossings or intersections.

### Engineering

These are strategies which are usually passive and effective in the event phase of injury prevention. These interventions, by virtue of design, essentially ensure that the impact of transmitted energy across the host in case of the event, is minimal.
*Examples:* Better design of automobiles such that there is reduced chance of fire in case of an impact, automatic alert for medical care by sensors in the vehicle in case of emergencies and monitoring of injured person while in transit by trauma systems are some of the engineering measures for injury prevention. Other examples include helmets that are well-designed, more effective occupant restraints, barriers like grills and window bars to prevent falls among children as well as mouth guards and other protective equipment among players to prevent sports-related injuries.

## Active and Passive

These 3 E's can be further categorized into two: Active and passive.
1. **Active interventions** require the individual to actively perform the act of prevention; hence this is possible only after the change in knowledge and behavior of the concerned individual, e.g., fastening a seatbelt.
2. **Passive interventions** do not need the host (individual) to perform any act and instead the measure of prevention is built by engineering/design of the vehicle, e.g. air bags that are deployed passively in case of a crash.

> **Key Points**
> There are various methods of describing and implementing preventive interventions.
> - Primary, secondary and tertiary
> - Haddon's matrix
> - 3 E's of intervention
> - Active and passive

## ROAD TRAFFIC INJURIES

### Problem Statement

**Global**
- An estimated 1.35 million people die every year from road traffic injuries (RTIs) and more than 50 million are injured or disabled despite a first decade of action and high-level global attention. (Road Safety 2022. The Lancet Jul 2022).

- Currently, Road traffic injury is the leading cause of death among children and young adults (5–29 years old).
- It is the eighth leading cause of death for all age groups surpassing HIV/AIDS, tuberculosis and diarrheal diseases.
- There is a strong association between the risk of a road traffic death and the income level of the country.
- The burden of deaths due to RTI is disproportionately higher among the low- and middle-income countries.

***India*** (NCRB, *Accidental Deaths and Suicide in India 2022*; MoRTH, *Road Accidents in India*)
- The Transport Research Wing (TRW) of the Ministry of Road Transport and Highways of India is the nodal agency that provides information or data on road and road transport sectors.
- As reported in the Road Accidents in India 2021, India ranks first in the number of road accident deaths followed by China and US across the 199 countries and second in number of injury accidents (32/lakh people).
- Road accidents on an average decreased by 8.1 percent and injuries decreased by 14.8 percent in 2021 compared to 2019. Fatalities, however, on account of road accidents increased only by 1.9 percent in 2021 corresponds to the same period in 2019.
- In 2021, under the category of Traffic Rule Violations, over speeding is a major killer, accounting for 69.6 percent of the persons killed followed by driving on the wrong side (5.2 %) followed by driving on the wrong side/lane indiscipline, drunken driving/consumption of alcohol and drug, jumping of red light and use of mobile phones.

## Epidemiology

With respect to the epidemiological triad, the risk factors may be divided as human factors, vehicular factors and environmental factors.

**Human or host factors**: These include consumption of alcohol, medicinal or recreational drugs, fatigue, being a young male; having youths driving in the same car; being a vulnerable road user in urban and residential areas; poor eyesight of road users; human tolerance and personality factors; inappropriate or excessive speed; non-use of seatbelts and child restraints; crash-helmets not worn by users of two wheeled vehicles, etc.

**Vehicular factors**: These include factors related to braking, handling and maintenance; insufficient vehicle crash protection for occupants and for those hit by vehicles and rapid increase in motorization.

**Environmental factors**: These include defects in road design, layout and maintenance, which can also lead to unsafe behavior by road users; inadequate visibility because of environmental factors (making it hard to detect vehicles and other road users); mixture of high-speed motorized traffic with vulnerable road users and economic factors such as level of economic development and social deprivation.

Haddon described road transport as an "ill-designed man machine system" that requires comprehensive systemic treatment. We can systematically analyze each phase—pre-crash, crash and post-crash—for human, vehicle, road and environmental factors **(Table 19E.3)**.

**Table 19E.3:** Factors involved in RTI based on the Haddon matrix.

| Phase | Human | Vehicles and equipment | Environment |
|---|---|---|---|
| Pre-crash | Crash prevention | Information Attitudes Impairment Police enforcement | Roadworthiness Lighting Handling Speed management | Road design and road layout Speed limits Pedestrian facilities |
| Crash | Injury prevention during the crash | Use of restraints Impairment | Occupant restraints Other safety devices Crash protective design | Crash-protective roadside objects |
| Post-crash | Life sustaining | First-aid skill Access to medics | Ease of access Fire risk | Rescue facilities Congestion |

*Case Scenario 2*

Consider that you are working as a Medical Officer in a Primary Health Center (PHC). One morning, a road traffic accident occurs involving a car and truck that leads to the death of four people near your PHC. On further investigation it was found that for the past two years several accidents have occurred in the same spot. You are asked by the senior district officer to investigate and find the reasons for the series of accidents occurring in the place. How will you approach the given task?

**Suggested Solution**

As a community epidemiologist, we are the investigators of an epidemiological problem. So, in the given scenario, you can approach the reasons for the series of road traffic accidents as mentioned in the following four components **(Fig. 19E.4)**.

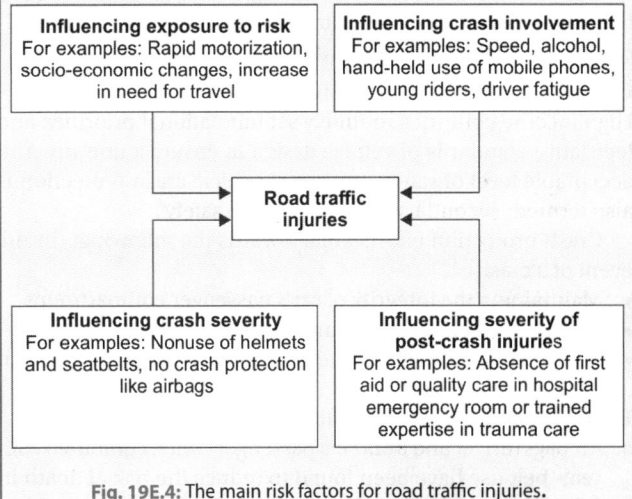

**Fig. 19E.4:** The main risk factors for road traffic injuries.

## Prevention and Control

Preventive intervention can be defined as a strategy or series of strategies that are implemented with the goal of preventing, reducing, or ameliorating road traffic injuries. Measures can include products (e.g., seat belts), environmental changes (e.g., speed bumps), behavioral and communications interventions (e.g., individual and group behavior change strategies, targeted media campaigns), and policy guidelines or laws (e.g., laws defining permissible blood alcohol levels). The three prime elements of the traffic systems to be targeted are: vehicles, road users and the road infrastructure.

Some of the strategies that have been advised by the World Health Organization include:

## *Primordial and Primary Prevention (Injury Prevention)*

### Managing Exposure to Risk through Transport and Land-use Policies

Exposure to road injury risk can be decreased by strategies that include the following:
- Reduction of motor vehicle traffic volume by implementing better land use
- Provision of efficient networks wherein the shortest or quickest routes are also the safest
- Promoting switch from higher risk to lower risk modes of transport
- Restricting motor vehicle users, number of vehicles, or enforcing better standards of road infrastructure.

### Reducing Motor Vehicle Traffic

Factors like the configuration of road network, urban population density, alternatives to private motorized transport determine the travel needs and the dependence on private motor vehicles. Measures to address these include trip reduction measures, better management of commuter transport and restrictions on vehicle parking and road use.

Road safety considerations are integral part of design and operation of the road network. Activities for safety awareness in planning road networks include:
a. Classifying road network according to primary road function
b. Setting appropriate speed limits
c. Improving road layout and design for better use.

### Crash Protective Vehicle Design

High income countries routinely set out national priorities and legislative standards of vehicle design to ensure a uniform and acceptable level of safety. Improved vehicle crash protection is also termed "secondary safety or passive safety".

Crash protection efforts aims towards the following: (in the event of a crash)
- Maintaining the integrity of car's passenger compartment
- Ensure that vehicle occupants ae properly restrained
- Reduce the probability that the occupant may be ejected from the car.

### Examples and newer technologies:

a. Air bags (driver and front seat passenger) when combined with seat- belt use have been found to reduce the risk of death in frontal crashes by 68%.
b. Measures to increase seat belt use, through legislation, information and smart audible seat-belt reminders are integral to the improvement of car safety.
c. Intelligent speed adaptation (ISA) is a system being developed that shows potential impact on incidence of road casualties. It is said that with this system the vehicle "knows" the permissible speed of the road where it is travelling.
d. Alcohol interlocks: These are automatic ignition locking systems that prevent drivers who are persistently over the legal alcohol limits from starting their car if their BAC is over the legal driving limit.
e. Speed camera: Speed cameras that record photographic evidence of a speeding offence that is admissible in a court of law, are highly effective means of speed enforcement.
f. Child restraints: The type of restraints should be appropriate for the age and weight of the child. Some types include rear-facing infant seats, forward facing child seats, booster seats, booster cushions, etc.

### Mandatory Seatbelt Use Laws

This has been one of the RTI prevention's greatest success stories. Since the law was first passed in Victoria, Australia in 1971, many countries all over the world, including India, have introduced seat belt laws that led to hundreds of thousands of lives saved worldwide.

### Motorcycle Helmets and Mandatory Laws on Helmet Wearing

This is especially important in low and middle-income countries like India, where motorized two-wheeler use is quite high.

### Setting and Enforcing Alcohol Impairment Laws

The basic element for road safety and reduction of alcohol related injuries is establishing a legal Blood Alcohol Concentration (BAC) limit. Mandatory BAC limits are an objective and simple means of detecting alcohol impairment. It also guides the drivers about safe driving practices. Upper limits of 0.05 g/dL for the general population and 0.02 g/dL for young drivers and motorcycle riders are considered best practice now.

## *Secondary and Tertiary Prevention*

### *Delivering post-crash care*

The aim of providing post-trauma care is to avoid preventable death and disability, limit the severity of injury and suffering and ensure best possible recovery and rehabilitation.

### *Golden hour concept*

According to this concept, an injured patient should receive the definitive care within 60 minutes from the time of injury for the best possible outcome, after which there is a significant increase in morbidity and mortality. Recent studies show that interventions can have impact across a longer time scale as a chain involving bystanders at the scene of the crash, emergency rescue, access to emergency care services and trauma care and rehabilitation.

I. **Pre-hospital care**

   *Role of bystanders:*
   - Contacting emergency services or other forms of help
   - Applying first aid
   - Securing the scene (e.g. preventing further crashes, crowd control etc.)

   *Emergency medical system:* Some of the aspects to be considered include standardized emergency telephone number for urgent assistance (e.g. 911), basic life support training especially in rural areas of low-income countries which lack ambulance services, police and fire fighters and safety standards in ambulances.

II. **Hospital care**

   Advanced trauma life support course training as well as other in-depth training of human resources including doctors, nurses and other professionals is important for provision of post-trauma care.

### Organization of trauma care and physical resources

Vital equipments like chest-tubes and emergency airway equipment are essential for treating life threatening chest injuries and airway obstruction. The Essential Trauma Care Project is a collaborative effort between the WHO and the International Society of Surgery that aims to improve the planning and organization of trauma care worldwide.

### Rehabilitation

Comprehensive package of initial and post-hospital care of the injured includes rehabilitation. This is important to minimize future functional disabilities and restore the person to his active role in the society.

## Global Response

- In response to this growing epidemic, in 2010 the UN General Assembly adopted Resolution 64/255 to establish the Decade of Action for Road Safety (2011–2020), the goal of which is to stabilize and reduce predicted levels of road traffic fatalities around the world.
- The Safe System approach: Safe System approach to road safety ensures that, in a crash, impact energy remains below the threshold likely to cause death or serious injury.
- A Global Plan of Action provides the roadmap towards this goal, promoting proven, cost-effective solutions for making roads safer, including those pertaining to:
  - road safety management
  - safer roads and mobility
  - safer vehicles
  - making road users safer
  - improved post-crash response and hospital care.
- The 17 Sustainable Development Goals (SDGs) include two targets that relate to road safety, one in SDG 3 (on health), and one in SDG 11 (on transport for sustainable cities).
  - Sustainable development goal 3: Ensure healthy lives and promote well-being for all at all ages:
    - 3.6. *"By 2020, halve the number of global deaths and injuries from road traffic accidents".*
  - Sustainable development goal 11: Make cities and human settlements inclusive, safe, resilient and sustainable:
    - 11.2. *"By 2030, provide access to safe, affordable, accessible and sustainable transport systems for all, improving road safety, notably by expanding public transport, with special attention to the needs of those in vulnerable situations, women, children, persons with disabilities and older persons".*

> **Key Points**
> - Over speeding is the most important factor associated with traffic accidents, accident-related deaths and injuries in 2018.
> - In 2018, India ranks first in the number of road accident deaths across the 199 countries.
> - Haddon described road transport as an "ill-designed man machine system" that requires comprehensive systemic treatment.
> - The 3 prime elements of the traffic systems to be targeted are: vehicles, road users and the road infrastructure.
> - The 17 Sustainable Development Goals (SDGs) include two targets that relate to road safety, one in SDG 3 (on health), and one in SDG 11 (on transport for sustainable cities).

## FALLS

As per the WHO, fall is defined as *"an event which results in a person coming to rest inadvertently on the ground or floor or other lower level".*

Globally, falls constitute the second leading cause deaths due to accidental or unintentional injury.

### Problem Statement

An estimated 684,000 fatal falls occur each year, making it the second leading cause of unintentional injury death. Over 80% of fall-related fatalities occur in low- and middle-income countries, with regions of the Western Pacific and Southeast Asia accounting for 60% of these deaths. About 37.3 million falls that are severe enough to require medical attention occur each year. Globally, falls are responsible for over 38 million DALYs (disability-adjusted life years) lost each year, and result in more years lived with disability than transport injury, drowning, burns and poisoning combined.

While nearly 40% of the total DALYs lost due to falls worldwide occurs in children, this measurement may not accurately reflect the impact of fall-related disabilities for older individuals who have fewer life years to lose. (WHO. Falls; Factsheet April 2021).

### Epidemiology

The age, gender and health of the individual are the important factors that determine the type and severity of injury following a fall.

- **Age:** Risk of death or injury after a fall increases with age and is highest among the elderly. This could be due to impairments in physical or cognitive domains or due to environmental factors. Children constitute another high-risk group, wherein the contributing factors include early and evolving stages of development, curiosity in their surroundings, and increasing levels of independence along with challenging 'risk taking' behaviors.
- **Gender:** Greater burden is seen among males which may be due to risk-taking behaviors and occupational hazards.
- **Other risk** factors include:
  - Occupations that include working at heights or any other hazardous environment
  - Consumption of alcohol or other substance use
  - Socioeconomic factors including poverty, poor housing, overcrowding, being/having a sole parent, young mother
  - Underlying medical conditions, such as neurological, cardiac or other disabilities
  - Side effects of medication, physical inactivity and loss of balance, particularly among older people
  - Poor mobility, cognitive or vision problems, particularly among those in an institution, such as a nursing home
  - Unsafe environments, especially for those with impairments or elderly.

### Prevention

Comprehensive and multifaceted strategies have to be laid down for fall prevention.

For older individuals, these may include:
- Screening of environment for risks of falls;
- Assessment for risk factors, such as medications; vitamin D and calcium supplementation;

- Environmental modification for those with known risk factors;
- Treatment of impairments and prescription of appropriate assistive devices;
- Muscle strengthening and balance retraining;
- Community-based programs which may incorporate fall prevention education with dynamic balance or strength training.

## DROWNING

### Problem Statement (WHO, Fact Sheets: Drowning)

Drowning a major public health problem with an estimated 236,000 deaths in 2019. Drowning is the third leading cause of unintentional injury death, accounting for 7% of all injury-related deaths. The global burden and death from drowning are found in all economies and regions, however: low- and middle-income countries account for over 90% of unintentional drowning deaths. Over half of the world's drowning occurs in the WHO Western Pacific Region and WHO South-East Asia Region; and drowning death rates are highest in the WHO Western Pacific Region and are 27–32 times higher than those seen in the United Kingdom or Germany, respectively.

### Epidemiology

**Age:** Age is one of the major risk factors for drowning as per the Global report on drowning (2014). Globally, children 1–4 years, followed by children 5–9 years have the highest drowning rates.

**Gender:** Males have high risk of drowning due to increased exposure to water and riskier behavior such as swimming alone, drinking alcohol before swimming.

**Access to water:** Increased access to water is another risk factor for drowning among occupations such as commercial fishing or using small boats in low-income countries. Children living near open water sources, such as ditches, ponds are at risk.

**Travelling on water:** Migrants or asylum seekers who travel daily often on overcrowded, unsafe vessels lacking safety equipment are at higher risk.

Other risk factors include:
- Lower socioeconomic status, and rural populations
- Infants left unsupervised
- Alcohol use, near or in the water
- Medical conditions, such as epilepsy.

### Prevention

The water hazard or exposure to drowning may be reduced significantly by installing barriers to control access.

Child care under supervision for pre-school children reduces drowning risk and also has other health benefits.

Teaching school-age children basic swimming, water safety and safe rescue skills is another approach.

Drowning prevention should also focus on effective policies and legislation.
- Safe boating, shipping and ferry
- Building resilience to flooding and managing flood risks through better disaster preparedness planning
- Developing a national water safety strategy to raise awareness of safety around water.

### Global Response

The Global report lays down recommendations to tailor and implement effective drowning prevention programs, improve data about drowning, and develop national water safety plans.

---

*Case Scenario 3*

As an MBBS undergraduate in community medicine postings, you visit an old age home, wherein you encounter Mr. Prakash, a 67-year-old resident of the home. He is on regular painkillers for left hip pain but has not been assessed by a clinician for the same. He has also had complaints of a ringing in his ears for which he has not sought any medical care. You notice that he is limping because of a fall, on a patch of wet floor. When you assess the premises, you find that corridor is dimly lit and there is a leakage in the wash basin area. Create a Haddon's matrix and identify potential areas of intervention (**Table 19E.4**).

**Suggested Solution**

Table 19E.4: Haddon matrix to prevent elderly falls.

| | *Host* | *Vehicle* | *Physical environment* | *Social environment* |
|---|---|---|---|---|
| **Pre-fall** | • Assessment of hip joint for osteoarthritic changes as well as bone density<br>• Assessment for tinnitus and balance | Use of good quality slippers which provides grip | • Repair of leaking pipes and installation of quality leak resistant plumbing system<br>• Monitoring for any defects or new leakages<br>• Well-lit corridors and prevent dark zones | Being alert for hazards and having systems in place among the management and residents for fall prevention and response |
| **Event (Fall)** | • Provision of assistive devices<br>• Use of protective pads to prevent impact during fall | Appropriate positioning and good quality hip protector | Any supportive structures to hold onto in case of fall, or thick carpeting to cushion the fall | Residential homes must meet anti-slip flooring requirements |
| **Post-fall** | • Assessment of bones for fractures or soft tissue contusions | Use of alarm systems to alert after fall | Remove physical barriers that may prevent accessing the injured after fall | Funding and coordinated system in place for the post-trauma care services and rehabilitation |

*Preventing drowning:* an implementation guide 2017 released by WHO provides concrete guidance on how to implement drowning prevention interventions for relevant stakeholders.

The WHO also organizes training programs and convenes workshops to draw together representatives of governments, NGOs and UN agencies working on drowning prevention.

In April 2021, the UN General Assembly adopted the first-ever Resolution on drowning prevention, which highlighted links to sustainable development, social equity, urban health, climate change, disaster risk reduction, and child health and well-being. The Resolution called on WHO to coordinate multisectoral drowning prevention efforts within the UN system and announced 25 July as World Drowning Prevention Day. At country level, WHO is working with Ministries of Health in several low- and middle-income countries, guiding the development of national drowning prevention strategies and supporting delivery of evidence-based drowning prevention interventions. In addition, WHO has also funded research in low-income countries exploring priority questions related to drowning prevention. At regional level, WHO organizes training programs and convenes workshops to draw together representatives of governments, NGOs and UN agencies working on drowning prevention.

# SUICIDE

## Problem Statement (WHO, Fact Sheets: Suicide, 2023)

Deaths due to suicide are about 700,000 every year; making it the fourth leading cause of death among 15-29-year-olds globally.

77% of suicides occur in low- and middle-income countries.

For every suicide there are many more people who attempt suicide. A prior suicide attempt is the single most important risk factor for suicide in the general population. For each adult death due to suicide there may be more than 20 other attempts. It is estimated that around 20% of global suicides are due to pesticide self-poisoning, most of which occur in rural agricultural areas in low- and middle-income countries. Other common methods of suicide are hanging and firearms.

## Epidemiology

There is a clear link between suicide and mental disorders (in particular, depression and alcohol use disorders). However, many suicides may occur in moments of crisis as a matter of impulse.

Further risk factors include loneliness, experience of loss, financial issues, violence, abuse or discrimination, break-up of a relationship, conflict or humanitarian emergencies.

The strongest risk factor is a previous suicide attempt.

## Prevention

WHO recommends four key interventions:
1. Restricting access to means
2. Working with the media to ensure responsible dissemination of information as well as reporting of suicide
3. Life skills education: to help young people cope
4. Early identification of those with suicide ideation or past suicide attempt; with short- and long-term follow-up contact.

## Global Response

Goal 3 of the SDGs is to ensure healthy lives and promote well-being for all at all ages.

Target 3.4 is: *"By 2030, reduce by one third premature mortality from non-communicable diseases through prevention and treatment and promote mental health and well-being".*

Within Target 3.4, suicide rate is an indicator (3.4.2).

**LIVE LIFE** refers collectively to the WHO's approach to suicide prevention, national suicide prevention strategies have to be developed based on this approach **(Table 19E.5)**.

Table 19E.5: WHO's LIVE LIFE approach.

| Cross-cutting strategies (LIVE) | Key effective interventions (LIFE) |
|---|---|
| Leadership | Less means |
| Interventions | Interaction with the media |
| Vision | Forming the young |
| Evaluation | Early identification |

### Key Points (Falls, Drowning, Suicide)
- Falls constitute the second leading cause of accidental or unintentional injury deaths.
- Risk of death or injury after a fall increases with age and is highest among the elderly.
- Age is one of the major risk factors for drowning.
- Drowning prevention strategies include installing barriers to control access and teaching school-age children basic swimming, water safety and safe rescue skills.
- There is a clear link between suicide and mental disorders; strongest risk factor being previous suicide attempt
- LIVE LIFE refers collectively to the WHO's approach to suicide prevention based on which national suicide prevention strategies have to be developed.

# POISONING

Poisoning is a result of consumption or inhalation or touching or injecting enough of a hazardous substance (poison) to cause illness or death. A poison is the substance that causes harm to a living being.

## Problem Statement

Each year suicide results in deaths of nearly a million people, and significant number of which are due to chemicals. For example, 370,000 deaths each year is estimated to be because of deliberate ingestion of pesticides.

About 5 million snake-bites occur each year resulting in 2.5 million envenomings, with 100,000 deaths and many amputations and other permanent disabilities.

The WHO estimated that unintentional poisoning caused 84 278 deaths in 2019 worldwide and a loss of five million disability-adjusted life-years (DALYs). This may be attributed largely to an exponential growth of industrialization that leads to increase of various chemicals. The abundance of such chemicals has important implications for health across the globe. Poisoning is one of the main causes of emergency visits in hospitals in many countries.

The absolute number of deaths was determined by estimating the total number of deaths that occurred due to

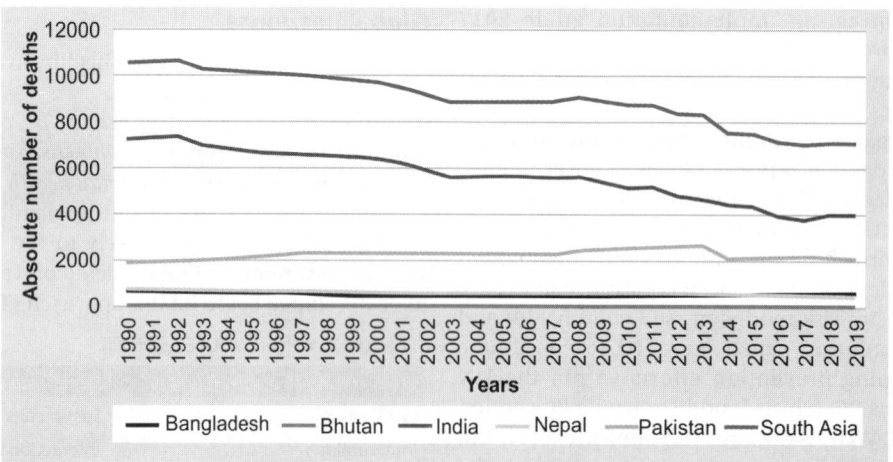

Fig. 19E.5: Absolute number of deaths due to unintentional poisoning by countries in South Asia from 1990 to 2019.
(*Source:* Khan NU, Khan U, Khudadad U, Asrar Ali, Ahmed Raheem, Shahan Waheed, et al. Trends in mortality related to unintentional poisoning in the South Asian region from 1990 to 2019: analysis of data from the Global Burden of Disease Study BMJ Open 2023;13:e062744).

poisoning in a specific year. The absolute number of deaths due to unintentional poisoning has been decreasing from 1990 to 2019 **(Fig. 19E.5)**.

## Global Response

International Programme on Chemical Safety (IPCS) on poisoning prevention and helps in capacity building.

Establishment of poison centers is an important activity under the IPCS INTOX Programme which maintains a world directory of the same.

Provision of information on chemicals, information management tools, and the development of internationally peer-reviewed guidelines concerning the prevention and clinical management of poisoning are other activities.

# VIOLENCE: SEXUAL AND INTIMATE PARTNER

Violence against women is defined by the United Nations as *"any act of gender-based violence that results in, or is likely to result in, physical, sexual, or mental harm or suffering to women, including threats of such acts, coercion or arbitrary deprivation of liberty, whether occurring in public or in private life"* (WHO, Fact Sheets: Violence against women).

Intimate partner violence (IPV) refers to *"behavior by an intimate partner or ex-partner that causes physical, sexual or psychological harm, including physical aggression, sexual coercion, psychological abuse and controlling behaviors."*

Sexual violence is *"any sexual act, attempt to obtain a sexual act, or other act directed against a person's sexuality using coercion, by any person regardless of their relationship to the victim, in any setting. It includes rape, defined as the physically forced or otherwise coerced penetration of the vulva or anus with a penis, other body part or object."*

## Problem Statement

One in three or one-third (30%) of all women have experienced physical and/or sexual violence by their intimate partner. The prevalence estimates of IPV range from 23.2% in high-income countries to 37.7% in the South-East Asia region.

In addition to IPV, globally 6% of women report having been sexually assaulted by someone other than a partner, although data for non-partner sexual violence are more limited.

Intimate partner and sexual violence are mostly perpetrated by men against women.

## Epidemiology

Gender inequality and norms on the acceptability of violence against women are a root cause of violence against women.

Risk factors for both intimate partner and sexual violence include:
- Lower levels of education (perpetration of sexual violence and experience of sexual violence)
- A history of exposure to child maltreatment (perpetration and experience)
- Family violence (perpetration and experience)
- Antisocial personality disorder (perpetration)
- Harmful use of alcohol (perpetration and experience)
- Community norms that support higher status to men than women
- Poor access of women's to paid employment.

Factors specifically associated with intimate partner violence include:
- Past history of violence
- Marital discord or dissatisfaction
- Communication issues between partners
- Controlling behaviors by males towards partners.

## Health Consequences

There can be serious short- and long-term physical, mental, sexual and reproductive health issues for women as given below:
- Death due to homicide or suicide
- Injury due to the violence
- Unintended pregnancies, induced abortions, gynecological problems, and STIs, including HIV

- Poor pregnancy outcomes like miscarriage, stillbirth, pre-term delivery and low birth weight babies
- Mental health issues such as depression, post-traumatic stress and anxiety disorders, eating disorders, sleep difficulties
- Physical complaints like headaches, back pain, abdominal pain, gastrointestinal disorders and poor overall health
- Sexual violence especially during childhood, can lead to smoking, drug and alcohol use, and risky sexual behaviors in later life; perpetration of violence (for males) and being a victim of violence (for females).

### *Impact on children*

a. Children who grow up in families with violence may have several behavioral and emotional disturbances including perpetrating or experiencing violence in later life
b. Higher rates of infant and child mortality.

## Prevention

Advocacy and counseling interventions may improve access to services for survivors of intimate partner violence.

The most promising prevention strategies in low resource settings, include:

- Empowering women economically and socially through a combination of skills training and microfinancing
- Improvement of communication and relationship skills within couples and communities
- Reduction in access to, and harmful use of alcohol
- Transformation of gender and social norms through community mobilization.

It is also important to enact and enforce legislation; develop and implement policies to improve gender equality by:

- Enforcement of marriage, dowry, divorce and custody laws for ending discrimination against women.
- Modification and enforcement in inheritance laws and ownership of assets for ending discrimination.
- Improving women's access to paid employment.
- Developing and resourcing national plans and policies to address violence against women.

The health sector can:

- Play a role in advocacy to make violence against women unacceptable and bring out the public health response
- Provide training and sensitization to health care providers on how to respond to survivors
- Prevent recurrence of violence through early identification of women and children in need, appropriate referral and support
- Comprehensive sexuality education curricula taught to young people
- Carrying out population-based surveys, or including violence against women in demographic and health surveys.

## Global Response

Global plan of action on strengthening health systems in addressing IPV was developed at the World Health Assembly in 2016.

WHO, in collaboration with partners, is:

- Building the evidence base on the size and nature of violence against women in different settings and improving the methods for measuring violence against women in the context of monitoring for the Sustainable Development Goals
- Strengthening research and capacity to assess interventions to address partner violence
- Undertaking research to test and identify effective health sector interventions
- Developing guidelines and implementation tools for strengthening the health sector response to intimate partner and sexual violence and synthesizing evidence on what works to prevent such violence
- Collaborating with international agencies and organizations to reduce and eliminate violence globally through initiatives such as the Sexual Violence Research Initiative, Together for Girls, the UN Women-WHO Joint Programme on Strengthening Violence against Women, the UN Joint Programme on Essential Services Package for Women Subject to Violence, and the Secretary General's political strategy to address violence against women and COVID-19.
- In 2019, WHO and UN Women with endorsement from 12 other UN and bilateral agencies published RESPECT women— a framework for preventing violence against women aimed at policy makers. Each letter of RESPECT stands for one of seven strategies: Relationship skills strengthening; Empowerment of women; Services ensured; Poverty reduced; Enabling environments (schools, workplaces, public spaces) created; Child and adolescent abuse prevented; and Transformed attitudes, beliefs and norms. For each of these seven strategies there are a range of interventions in low and high resource settings with varying degree of evidence of effectiveness. Examples of promising interventions include psychosocial support and psychological interventions for survivors of intimate partner violence; combined economic and social empowerment programs; cash transfers; working with couples to improve communication and relationship skills; community mobilization interventions to change unequal gender norms; school programs that enhance safety in schools and reduce/eliminate harsh punishment and include curricula that challenges gender stereotypes and promotes relationships based on equality and consent; and group-based participatory education with women and men to generate critical reflections about unequal gender power relationships.

## SUMMARY

- ❖ Injuries and accidents ae not the same; injuries are largely predictable and preventable
- ❖ Injuries are classified as-unintentional, intentional and of undetermined intent
- ❖ The Indian National Crime Record Bureau report classified deaths due to injuries as natural, un-natural and other causes of accidental deaths
- ❖ Epidemiological triad of injuries can be explained in terms of agent (mechanical energy transferred by animate or inanimate object), host (human and his/her characteristics) and environment (conditions of physical/social environment)
- ❖ Haddon's matrix is an analytical tool that helps to understand all factors associated with an injury in terms of 3 phases: pre-event, event and post event which is further systematically analyzed for agent, host and environmental factors

- There are various methods of describing and implementing preventive interventions which include:
  - Primary, secondary and tertiary
  - Haddon's matrix
  - 3 E's of intervention
- The most common component of injuries is road traffic injuries
- With respect to the epidemiological triad of RTIs, the risk factors may be divided as human factors, vehicular factors and environmental factors
- SDG target 3.6 is to halve the number of global deaths and injuries from road traffic accidents
- Age and gender are important risk factors for fall and drowning
- There is a clear link between suicide and mental disorders with the strongest risk factor being a previous suicide attempt
- LIVE LIFE refers collectively to the WHO's approach to suicide prevention
- The WHO has established an International Programme on Chemical Safety (IPCS) on Poisoning Prevention
- Intimate partner and sexual violence are mostly perpetrated by men against women.

## SUGGESTED READING

1. Accidental deaths and suicides in India 2018. Available from: http://ncrb.gov.in/StatPublications/ADSI/ADSI2015/adsi-2018-full-report.pdf.
2. Disability-adjusted life years (DALYs). World Health Organization. Available from: https://www.who.int/data/gho/indicator-metadata-registry/imr-details/158
3. Drowning. Available from: https://www.who.int/news-room/fact-sheets/detail/drowning.
4. Falls. Available from: https://www.who.int/news-room/fact-sheets/detail/falls.
5. Global status report on road safety 2018. Available from: https://www.who.int/publications-detail/global-status-report-on-road-safety-2018
6. Guidelines for Essential Trauma Care. World Health Organization. June 2012. Available from: https://www.who.int/publications/i/item/guidelines-for-essential-trauma-care
7. Haddon's Matrix. Information Sheet. Available from: http://www.npaihb.org/images/epicenter_docs/injuryprevention/HaddonMatrixBasics.pdf.
8. ICD-10 Version:2016. Available from: http://apps.who.int/classifications/icd10/browse/2016/en#/XX.
9. Injuries and Violence: Key Facts. World Health Organization. March 2021. Available from: https://www.who.int/news-room/fact-sheets/detail/injuries-and-violence
10. Injury Surveillance Guildelines. World Health Organization. March 2001. Available from: https://www.who.int/publications/i/item/9241591331
11. Model Core Program Paper: Prevention of Unintentional Injury. Canada: British Columbia Health Authorities; 2009.
12. Nicholl PJ. Optimal use of resources for the treatment and prevention of injuries. British Medical Bulletin. 1999;55 (No 4):713-25.
13. Pless I, Hagel B. Injury prevention: a glossary of terms. J Epidemiol Community Health. 2005;59(3):182–5.
14. Post-crash response: supporting those affected by road traffic crashes. Available from: https://www.who.int/publications-detail/post-crash-response-supporting-those-affected-by-road-traffic-crashes.
15. Prevention and management of cases of poisoning. World Health Organization. Available from: https://www.who.int/teams/environment-climate-change-and-health/chemical-safety-and-health/incidents-poisonings/prevention-and-management-of-cases-of-poisoning
16. Prevention of injuries to children and young people: the way ahead for the UK | Injury Prevention. Available from: https://injuryprevention.bmj.com/content/4/suppl_1/S17.
17. Road Accidents in India | Ministry of Road Transport & Highways, Government of India. Available from: https://morth.nic.in/road-accident-in-india
18. Road traffic deaths per 100,000 population – Indicators and a Monitoring Framework. Available from: http://indicators.report/indicators/i-25/
19. Road traffic injuries: Factsheet. World Health Organization. December 2023. Available from: https://www.who.int/news-room/fact-sheets/detail/road-traffic-injuries
20. Rogers FB, Rittenhouse KJ, Gross BW. The golden hour in trauma: Dogma or medical folklore? Injury. 2015;46(4):525–7.
21. Runyan CW. Introduction: back to the future—revisiting Haddon's conceptualization of injury epidemiology and prevention. Epidemiol Rev. 2003;25:60–4.
22. Suicide. Available from: https://www.who.int/news-room/fact-sheets/detail/suicide
23. Violence against women. Available from: https://www.who.int/news-room/fact-sheets/detail/violence-against-women
24. WHO | Decade of Action for Road Safety 2011-2020. World Health Organization; [cited 2020 Apr 22]. Available from: http://www.who.int/roadsafety/decade_of_action/en/
25. WHO | Road safety training manual. Available from: http://www.who.int/violence_injury_prevention/road_traffic/activities/training_manuals/en/

# F. BLINDNESS

*Deepthi R, Manjula R, Shashi Kumar M*

*The only thing worse than being blind is having sight but no vision.*
—Helen Keller

| CM 7.2 | Enumerate, describe and discuss the mode of transmission and measures for prevention and control of blindness |
| --- | --- |
| CM 8.2 | Describe and discuss the epidemiological and control measures applicable in blindness |

## INTRODUCTION

According to World Health Organization, 80% of blindness in the world is avoidable: These are conditions that could be prevented or controlled if timely application of the available knowledge and interventions were taken. Blindness causes tremendous human suffering for the affected individuals and their families. For developing countries, where 9 out of 10 of the world's blind live, this represents a social, economic and community health problem. It is important to understand the scope of the problem; the time has arrived to focus and concentrate all international efforts on combating avoidable blindness.

## DEFINITION OF BLINDNESS UNDER NPCB

'The definition of Blindness under the National Programme for Control of Blindness (NPCB)' is hereby modified in line with WHO Definition as: *"Presenting distance visual acuity less than 3/60 in the better eye and limitation of field of vision to be less than 10 degrees from center of fixation" (Table 19F.1)*.

### Other Definitions

- **Economic blindness:** Level of blindness that prevents an individual from earning his wages
- **Social blindness:** Is the degree of disability that hampers an individual from socially interacting with the family and peer in satisfactory manner
- **Manifest blindness:** Visual acuity if 1/60 or just perception of light in the better eye
- **Absolute blindness:** Inability to perceive light in any eye
- **Curable blindness:** Blindness is reversible by prompt management
- **Preventable blindness:** Loss of vision that could have been completely prevented by effective measures
- **Avoidable blindness:** Sum total: Curable blindness + Preventable blindness. 80% of blindness are avoidable.

**Table 19F.1:** Revised categories of visual impairment.

| Presenting distance visual acuity | | |
| --- | --- | --- |
| Category | Worse than | Equal to or better than |
| Mild or no visual impairment **0** | | 6/18 |
| Moderate visual impairment **1** | 6/18 | 6/60 |
| Severe visual impairment **2** | 6/60 | 3/60 |

*Contd...*

*Contd...*

| Presenting distance visual acuity | | |
| --- | --- | --- |
| Category | Worse than | Equal to or better than |
| Blindness **3** (Social blindness) | 3/60 | 1/60* |
| Blindness **4** (Manifest blindness) | 1/60* | Light perception |
| Blindness **5** (Absolute blindness) | No light perception | |
| **9** | Undetermined or unspecified | |

*\* Or counts fingers at one meter. Category **6–8**, involves blindness of monocular visual impairment of various degrees.*

### Definition of Visual Impairment and Blindness

The currently used definition includes the term "best Corrected Vision" in the better eye. The methodology followed for measuring visual acuity, particularly in population-based studies, is to use a "pin hole" in patients whose "presenting" vision is below a certain cut off point (currently 6/18). Many recent studies have shown that the use of "best corrected" vision overlooks a large proportion of persons with visual impairment, including blindness, due to uncorrected refractive error, a common occurrence in many parts of the world.

### Nomenclature

The current ICD uses the words "LOW VISION" for categories 1, 2 and 3 of Vision impairment. In the practice of eye care "LOW VISION" has a specific meaning as defined by WHO. This is as follows: "A person with low vision is one who has impairment of visual functioning even after treatment and/or standard refractive correction, and has a visual acuity of less than 6/18 to light perception, or a visual field of less than 10 degree from the point of fixation, but who uses, or is potentially able to use, vision for planning and/or execution of a task".

> **Case Scenario 1**
>
> *Consider that you are a medical officer in the PHC and a patient comes to you with complaints of loss of vison.*
> *On examination with the Snellen chart visual acuity is detected as worse than 1/60. He is also unable to work as a manual laborer and earn his wages. How would you classify him?*
>
> *Suggested Solution*
>
> *As per the revised Categories of Visual impairment, the patient is said to have manifest blindness and as he is unable to earn, he would also be said to have economic blindness.*

## PROBLEM STATEMENT

The International Classification of Diseases 11 (2018) classifies vision impairment into two groups, distance and near presenting vision impairment. **Distance vision impairment** is further categorized into Mild – presenting visual acuity worse than 6/12 to 6/18, *Moderate* – presenting visual acuity worse than 6/18 to 6/60, *Severe* – presenting visual acuity worse than 6/60 to 3/60 and *Blindness* – presenting visual acuity worse than 3/60. **Near vision impairment** is when presenting near visual acuity worse than N6 or M.08 at 40 cm.

### Global

Globally, at least 2.2 billion people have a near or distance vision impairment. In at least 1 billion – or almost half – of these cases, vision impairment could have been prevented or has yet to be addressed. This 1 billion people include those with moderate or severe distance vision impairment or blindness due to unaddressed refractive error (88.4 million), cataract (94 million), age-related macular degeneration (8 million), glaucoma (7.7 million), diabetic retinopathy (3.9 million), as well as near vision impairment caused by unaddressed presbyopia (826 million).

In terms of regional differences, the prevalence of distance vision impairment in low- and middle-income regions is estimated to be four times higher than in high-income regions. With regards to near vision, rates of unaddressed near vision impairment are estimated to be greater than 80% in western, eastern and central sub-Saharan Africa, while comparative rates in high-income regions of North America, Australasia, Western Europe, and of Asia-Pacific are reported to be lower than 10%. (WHO World report on vision (2019)).

### India

In India most of the blindness (92.9%) and visual impairment (96.2%) cases were due to avoidable causes. India is close to achieving the World Health Organization's goal of reducing it to 0.3% of the total population by 2020.

Most (81%) of them are aged 50 years and above. Among children, an estimated 19 million children are vision impaired. Of these, 12 million children have vision impairment due to refractive error. Highest prevalence of blindness was seen in age group of above 80 (11.6%), followed by 70–79 age group (4.1%), 60-69 age group (1.6%) and 50-59 age group (0.5%).

## ETIOLOGY

**Global scenario:** Chronic eye diseases like cataract, uncorrected refractive error and glaucoma constitutes the main cause of blindness with significant reduction in infectious diseases, such as trachoma and onchocerciasis. Majority, i.e., 80% of all vision impairment, vision can be restored **(Table 19F.2)**.

Table 19F.2: Global causes of vision impairment.

| Major global causes of moderate to severe vision impairment | Major global causes of blindness (Fig. 19F.1) |
|---|---|
| 1. Uncorrected refractive errors 53% | 1. Unoperated cataract 39.1% |
| 2. Unoperated cataract 25% | 2. Uncorrected refractive error 18.2% |
| 3. Age-related macular degeneration 4% | 3. Glaucoma 10.1% |
| 4. Glaucoma 2% | |
| 5. Diabetic retinopathy 1%. | |

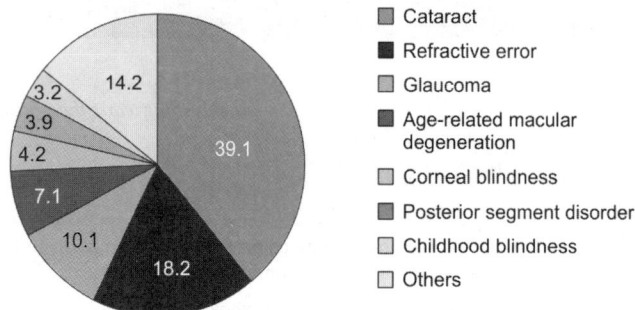

Fig. 19F.1: Global causes of blindness.
*(Source:* WHO estimates 2004).

**Indian scenario:** The main causes for blindness in India are Cataract (62.6%), Refractive Error (19.70%), Glaucoma (5.80%) **(Fig. 19F.2)**.

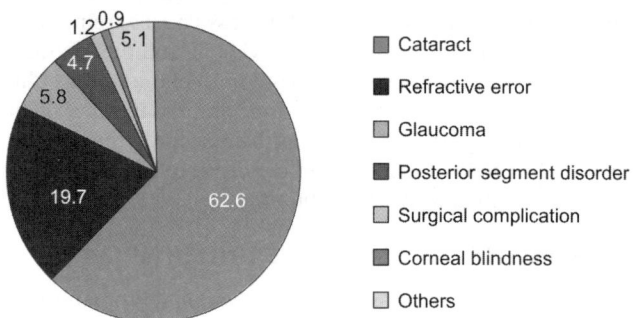

Fig. 19F.2: Causes of blindness in India.
*(Source:* NPCB 1999-2001 survey).

> **Key Points**
> - According to World Health Organization, 80% of blindness in the world is avoidable- conditions that could be prevented or controlled if timely application of the available knowledge and interventions were taken.
> - Blindness under the National Programme for Control of Blindness (NPCB) is defined as: "Presenting distance visual acuity less than 3/60 (20/400) in the better eye and limitation of field of vision to be less than 10 degrees from center of fixation.
> - Uncorrected refractive errors and Un-operated cataract are the 2 most common causes of vision impairment and blindness globally and in India.

## EPIDEMIOLOGICAL DETERMINANTS OF BLINDNESS

**Age:** Various diseases causing blindness affect different age groups. *Cataract* in developed countries is observed between 60-70 years of age, however in developing countries cataract is seen as early as 40 years. *Glaucoma* especially angle closure glaucoma is seen after 40 years of age. Blinding *nutritional blindness* is commonly observed in children under five years of age. *Trachoma* is most prevalent under two-year-old children, which declines after 5 years of age. However, blinding complications like inverted lids appear only after fourth decade of life. *Age-related macular degeneration* is observed after 65 years of age.

**Gender:** Studies quote women are affected with *cataract* more than that of males, but men are 1.6 times more likely to undergo cataract surgeries than compared to women. Blinding *Trachoma* is also commonly observed among females.

**Region:** Blindness is commonly seen in developing countries than compared to developed countries. People living in rural areas and urban slums have high prevalence of blindness due to *nutritional blindness, cataract and trachoma*.

**Malnutrition:** Low socioeconomic status, blindness following any natural disasters, early withdrawal of breast milk and late supplementation of weaning foods are associated with nutritional blindness.

**Environmental factors:** Exposure to sunlight is an important determinant of *Cataract*. An ultraviolet ray at 295 nm is proven to be caterogenic. Cigarette smoking has a positive correlation with *Cataract*. Poor environmental sanitation, overcrowding, poor personal hygiene, inadequate water supply, flies are commonly associated in *Trachoma* cases. *Age-related macular degeneration* is commonly seen among people with hyperopia with cigarette smoking.

**Predisposing diseases:** Diabetic retinopathy is one of the leading causes of blindness. Improper control of diabetes leads to early cataract formation and diabetic retinopathy. Dehydration crisis and post-measles attack are associated with blindness.

**Social factors:** Low social class is associated with risk factors like poor general nutrition, use of biofuel, low literacy status and other factors are instrumental in occurrence of blindness. Low socio-economic status is associated with blindness due to *Cataract, Nutritional Blindness and Trachoma*.

Other social factors responsible for high prevalence of blindness in India include:
- Increase in population
- Increase in life expectancy
- Poor access to eye care facilities
- Underutilization of available ophthalmic manpower
- Compromised nutritional status of mother, infant and children
- Lack of awareness regarding eye health
- Environmental factors predisposing to high infection rate.

# PREVENTION AND CONTROL OF BLINDNESS

## Primary Prevention

Trained primary level (Grassroot) workers should provide promotive and preventive services for eye care. This also includes services provided for the minor ailment of Eyes through primary healthcare approach.

- Health education of the community regarding eye care, hygiene and sanitation and frequent washing of eyes in trachoma endemic areas, regarding proper nutrition especially in context of vitamin A rich foods and availability of eye care services.
- Upliftment of socio-economic status, general standards of living and general condition.
- Nutritional supplementation program especially with vitamin A.
- Fortification of certain foods with vitamin A (addition of vitamin A to *dalda* in India). Many other foods have also been considered for vitamin A fortification (sugar, salt, tea, margarine and dried skimmed milk).
- Immunization of children against common diseases particularly measles, since measles aggravates the effects of an existing vitamin A deficiency state.
- Provision of eye care services, as a part of primary health care system.
- Personal protection using goggles/eye shield in high-risk occupations.
- Social actions during fairs and festivals by keeping children at a safe distance from places where crackers are burst.
- Health education of personal hygiene of the Eyes.
- Eye care in the early neonatal care, includes cleaning of the eyes with separate sterile swabs, followed by use of tetracycline drops/freshly prepared silver nitrate solution for the suspected neonates who are at risk of ophthalmia neonatorum conditions.
- Treatment of minor eye ailments, such as superficial foreign-bodies, conjunctivitis, etc.
- Health promotive measures to prevent eye complications due to *Diabetes Mellitus* and *Hypertension* by adopting self-care practices such as maintaining normal blood sugar levels and blood pressure, undergoing screening for early detection of retinopathy.

## Secondary Prevention

This includes early diagnosis and treatment of curable blindness, such as refractive errors, cataract, glaucoma, trichiasis, entropion, ocular trauma, etc. These services are provided through community health centers, and district hospitals by a qualified Ophthalmologist.

Secondary prevention, by way of early diagnosis and treatment, is the mainstay of programs for prevention and control of blindness. These services are to be provided by Medical Officers at primary health centers, with assistance of ophthalmic assistants and optometrists. The major conditions which would be resolved by this approach are cataract, glaucoma, trachoma, refractive errors, diabetic eye complications besides providing early emergency treatment for injuries.

- **Cataract:** Surgical removal of the opacified lens followed by intraocular lens implantation is the way to restore vision. Early diagnosis and provision of surgery using eye camp approach is the cornerstone.
- **Trachoma:** The 'SAFE' Strategy includes Surgery, Antibiotics, Facial cleanliness and Environmental improvements has been recommended by WHO to control Trachoma.
- **Glaucoma:** Early diagnosis and treatment is to be offered to glaucoma patients to avoid irreversible blindness.
- **Diabetic eye complications:** Early detection of diabetic eye complications like cataract, retinopathy by screening programmes and referral to higher centers for the management of complications.
- **Refractive errors:** This refers to early detection of refractive errors through school health programs and offering the corrective glasses, which would also improve the school

performance by children. These services should also be provided in the primary health centers.
- **Special screening examinations:** Retinopathy of prematurity and Retinitis pigmentosa are to be screened during early childhood.
- In case of early stages of vitamin A deficiency conditions, vitamin A therapy can be advised.
  - All patients >1 year of age: 200,000 IU vitamin A orally or 100,000 IU by IM, immediately on diagnosis and repeated the following day and 4 weeks later.

Procedures, such as retinal detachment surgery, laser surgeries for retinopathy and refractive errors, corneal grafting, corrective procedures for squints, etc., the tertiary level of care is provided through super-specialty hospitals, medical colleges, national institutes and high-tech hospitals.

> **Key Points**
> - Malnutrition, environmental and social factors are the usual modifiable risk factors for blindness.
> - Primary prevention refers to promotive and preventive services for eye care and services for minor ailment of eyes through primary health care approach.
> - Secondary prevention includes early diagnosis and treatment of curable blindness, such as refractive errors, cataract, glaucoma, etc. provided at community health centers, and district hospitals.
> - Tertiary prevention encompasses early detection of complications and rehabilitation through more complicated procedures at the tertiary level of care.

> **Case Scenario**
>
> A 40-year-old banker with history of Type II DM x 5 years presents to the PHC for his annual visit. He has been experiencing progressive blurring of vision in the left eye since his last visit one year ago. His glycemic control has been poor. He is also a chronic smoker and has not made any attempts to quit the same. No eye examinations have been made in the last visit and patient was not advised regarding the importance of medication adherence or smoking cessation in the past. What level of prevention would be most applicable in this scenario?
>
> **Suggested Solution**
>
> Diabetic retinopathy is the leading cause of blindness in working age individuals and it is very important that individuals with diabetes have a dilated fundus exam at least yearly to monitor for diabetic retinopathy. However, in this case this has not been done in the last visit.
> There is no role of primary prevention in the left eye currently. Secondary prevention for early diagnosis has also failed. At present, only tertiary prevention by referral to a higher center for determining the extent of retinopathy and management by laser surgery can be done.

## COMMUNITY OPHTHALMOLOGY

The concept of primary ophthalmic care consisting of standalone ophthalmic services and integrated community health services is included in Community Ophthalmology.

**Origin:** Bath in 1978 proposed community ophthalmology for promoting eye health and blindness prevention. This can be achieved through planning programs using methodologies of community health and ophthalmology.

**Need:** The high rate of avoidable blindness is a failure of hospital-based eye care services. This did not provide preventive services for the populations in need. Trained health care personnel and adequate infrastructure at primary health care level are the basic needs which were not equipped in public health facilities. There is no effective delivery of health education regarding eye care to the needy. Ophthalmology services were delivered solely by Ophthalmologists at tertiary care centers. Primary level and secondary level care hospitals did not have ophthalmology services due to lack of ophthalmologists.

**Actions:** Creation and training of the new cadre of health care personnel known as eye health care workers, eye health care educators or ophthalmic assistants. They are trained to provide eye care and blindness prevention services at the grassroots level.

For example, in trachoma endemic villages, these eye care health workers would provide access to eye drops and also educate families about the importance of hand washing and sanitation. These eye care workers identify cataract, educate families about the cure for blindness due to cataract with simple eye surgery. Community Ophthalmology has played a major role in changing the belief among general population that blindness can be identified and treated effectively and is not an inevitable consequence of aging.

Curative ophthalmology can make a significant impact on the general population only in conjunction with community ophthalmology. It includes community activities like need assessment, planning, and appropriate use of resources to curative and rehabilitative eye services. Principles of community ophthalmology are incorporated in the flagship eye program "Vision 2020: The Right to Sight".

## GLOBAL AND NATIONAL RESPONSE

### Vision 2020–The Right to Sight

It is a global initiative with a goal to eliminate avoidable blindness by the year 2020.

**World sight day**, celebrated on October 11th every year is the most important advocacy event to focus global attention on blindness and visual impairment and about eye care to prevent them. This event is coordinated by International Agency for the Prevention of Blindness (IAPB).

Glaucoma is a silent painless contributor for avoidable blindness. **World glaucoma awareness week** is celebrated from March 11th to March 17th is an annual event globally to work on elimination of glaucoma blindness by advocating people to have regular eye checkups and prevent blindness.

In India, the National Program for Control of Blindness was launched in 1976 as a continuation of National Program for Trachoma control when causes of preventable blindness other than trachoma came into focus. In 2017, it was redesignated as National Program for Control of Blindness and Visual Impairment. **The further details of Vision 2020 and Nation Program is explained in Chapter 47: Health Policies and Programs in India.**

### Eye Donation

It is an act of donating eyes after the death of a person. Only corneal blindness can be benefited in this process. Corneal blindness is responsible for 7.1% of blindness in India.

## SUMMARY

According to WHO, 80% of the Blindness is avoidable that includes the sum of curable and preventable blindness. Major causes of blindness globally are Cataract (39.1%), Refractive error (18.2%), Glaucoma (10.1%), Age-related macular degeneration (7.1%) and Corneal blindness (4.2%). Top five causes of blindness in India are Cataract (62.6%), Refractive error (19.7%), Glaucoma (5.8%), Posterior segment disorder (4.7%) and Surgical complications (1.2%).

Cataract and age-related macular degeneration are seen among elderly, however trachoma and refractive errors are common among young children. Blindness is common among females, in developing countries, children suffering with under nutrition and low socioeconomic status.

Prevention and control of the blindness can be implemented at different levels of health care, depends on the sophistication of the center, availability of ophthalmologist and superspecialists. Altogether, by appropriate management at each levels and appropriate referrals could achieve the VISION 2020.

Avoidable blindness is on a rise as a result of concentration of hospital based eye care services dependent solely on ophthalmologists, lack of trained health care personnel, infrastructure and ineffective delivery of health education regarding eye care to the needy. Curative ophthalmology can make a significant impact on the general population only in conjunction with community ophthalmology. It includes community activities like need assessment, planning, and appropriate use of resources to curative and rehabilitative eye services.

Vision 2020 is a global initiative with a goal to eliminate avoidable blindness by the year 2020. World sight day, celebrated on October 11th every year for advocacy on blindness and visual impairment.

## SUGGESTED READING

1. Bath PE. Cataract surgery training of residents in an urban and virtual environment. J Cataract Refract Surg. 1998;24(6):727-9.
2. Bourne RRA, Flaxman SR, Braithwaite T, Cicinelli MV, Das A, Jonas JB, et al. Vision Loss Expert Group. Magnitude, temporal trends, and projections of the global prevalence of blindness and distance and near vision impairment: a systematic review and meta-analysis. Lancet Glob Health. 2017;5(9):e888–97.
3. http://dghs.gov.in/content/1354_3_National Programme for Control of Blindness Visual. aspx.
4. Jose R, Rathore AS, Sachdeva S. Community ophthalmology: Revisited. Indian J Community Med. 2010;35:356-8.
5. National Programme for Control of Blindness in India. Achievements. Ophthalmology Section, Directorate General of Health Services, Ministry of Health and Family Welfare, Government of India. New Delhi: Nirman Bhavan; 2004. p. 23.
6. Report of the 11th meeting of the WHO Programme Advisory Group on the Prevention of Blindness: WHO PBL /95.51.
7. Resnikoff S, Pascolini D, Etya'ale D, Kocur I, Pararajasegaram R, Pokharel GP, et al. Global data on visual impairment in the year 2002. Bull World Health Organ. 2004; 82: 844-51
8. Vision 2020: The Right to Sight Global initiative for the elimination of avoidable blindness, Action plan 2006-2011, WHO 2007, Geneva.
9. WHO (2018). International Classification of Diseases, Injuries and Causes of death, 11th Ed. WHO, Geneva, 2018.
10. World Health Organization, Global Data on Visual Impairments 2010, 2012.
11. WHO. Blindness and vision impairment; Factsheet; 2022.

# G. EPIDEMIOLOGY OF CHRONIC OBSTRUCTIVE PULMONARY DISEASE (COPD) AND ITS PREVENTION AND CONTROL

*Sandeep Kumar Panigrahi, Venkatarao Epari*

*Breathing is the greatest pleasure in life.*
—Giovanni Papini

| | |
|---|---|
| CM 7.2 | Enumerate, describe and discuss the mode of transmission and measures for prevention and control of chronic obstructive pulmonary diseases |
| CM 8.2 | Describe and discuss the epidemiology and control measures applicable in chronic obstructive pulmonary diseases |

> **Case Scenario 1 (historical perspective)**
>
> In 1901, King Edward VII of England became the king after the death of Queen Victoria. He died just within 10 years of becoming the king.
> He was suffering from severe chronic bronchitis, a form of COPD (being a lifelong smoker, he used to smoke a mix of 20 cigarettes and 12 cigars per day). As on date COPD patients in the United Kingdom are treated at a hospital bearing his name – King Edward VII Hospital in Windsor, England.

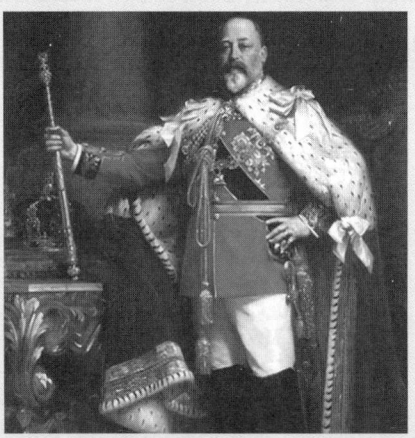

## INTRODUCTION

The most common non-malignant respiratory conditions characterized by airway dysfunction are collectively known as obstructive airway diseases that includes chronic obstructive pulmonary disease (COPD) and asthma. COPD is usually defined as *"an irreversible and progressive airflow obstruction due to inflammation of the peripheral airways and lung parenchyma"*. On the other hand, airflow limitation in asthma may be variable and reversible, and is critical in distinguishing between the two. However, recent evidence shows that reversibility cannot be used as a distinguishing feature making both of them described together as 'overlap syndrome'.

COPD is not a communicable disease, and is incurable. It is diagnosed usually in middle-aged or older adults. Estimates of 2015 show that COPD is the fourth largest among the killers globally. It is also a major cause of gradual disability which people might be unaware of. Once strongly established changes become irreversible in nature.

COPD is sometimes considered as a systemic disease. COPD is an umbrella term and covers both 'Chronic bronchitis' and 'Emphysema'. Most patients with COPD are known to have features of both emphysema and chronic bronchitis. Various hypothesis (Dutch and British) have suggested that COPD may be a phenotypic response of an individual's genetic predisposition for atopy and airway hyper-responsiveness to environmental factors (like allergens, tobacco and air pollutants) **(Fig. 19G.1)**.

COPD presents usually in fifth and sixth decades of life with excessive cough (called as smoker's cough) which is productive in nature along with shortness of breath (with physical activity), wheezing or whistling or squeaky sound on breathing, and chest tightness. Dyspnea initially is progressive and initially present on exertion but gradually starts appearing at rest. Symptoms have been present for more than 10 years usually at presentation. Concomitant factors like sleep disorders may be present in many patients. Pulmonary hypertension and cor pulmonale mark the late stage of the disease.

Japanese Respiratory Society classifies COPD into two phenotypes on the basis of Forced Expiratory Volume$_1$ (FEV$_1$) – PP (Pink Puffers) and BB (Blue Bloaters). PP may be underweight and present with pink complexion, dyspnea, emphysema predominant lesions and an increase in lung tidal volume. Retraction of respiratory muscles may be seen for compensation. BB may be normal or overweight, present with cyanotic features, right heart failure, non-emphysematous distal airway disease. They have normal or decreased lung capacity and an increase in residual volume.

> **Key Points**
> - COPD is usually defined as "an irreversible and progressive airflow obstruction due to inflammation of the peripheral airways and lung parenchyma"
> - COPD is an umbrella term and covers both 'chronic bronchitis' and 'emphysema'
> - It usually presents as excessive cough (called as smoker's cough) along with shortness of breath in fifth and sixth decades of life
> - COPD is classified into two phenotypes on the basis of Forced Expiratory Volume 1 (FEV1) – PP (Pink Puffers) and BB (Blue Bloaters).

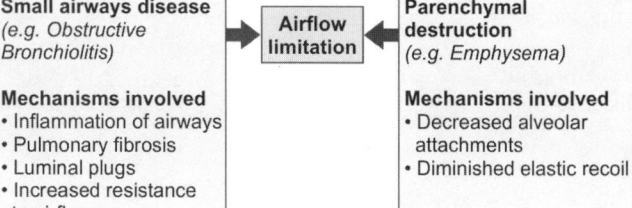

**Fig. 19G.1:** Mechanisms underlying airway limitation in COPD. *Modified and adapted from Agusti A. Chronic obstructive pulmonary disease: a systemic disease [Internet]. Vol. 3, Proc Am Thorac Soc. 2017. pp478-481. Available from: http://www.ncbi.nlm.nih.gov/pubmed/16921116*

## Chapter 19: Specific Epidemiology of Noncommunicable Diseases

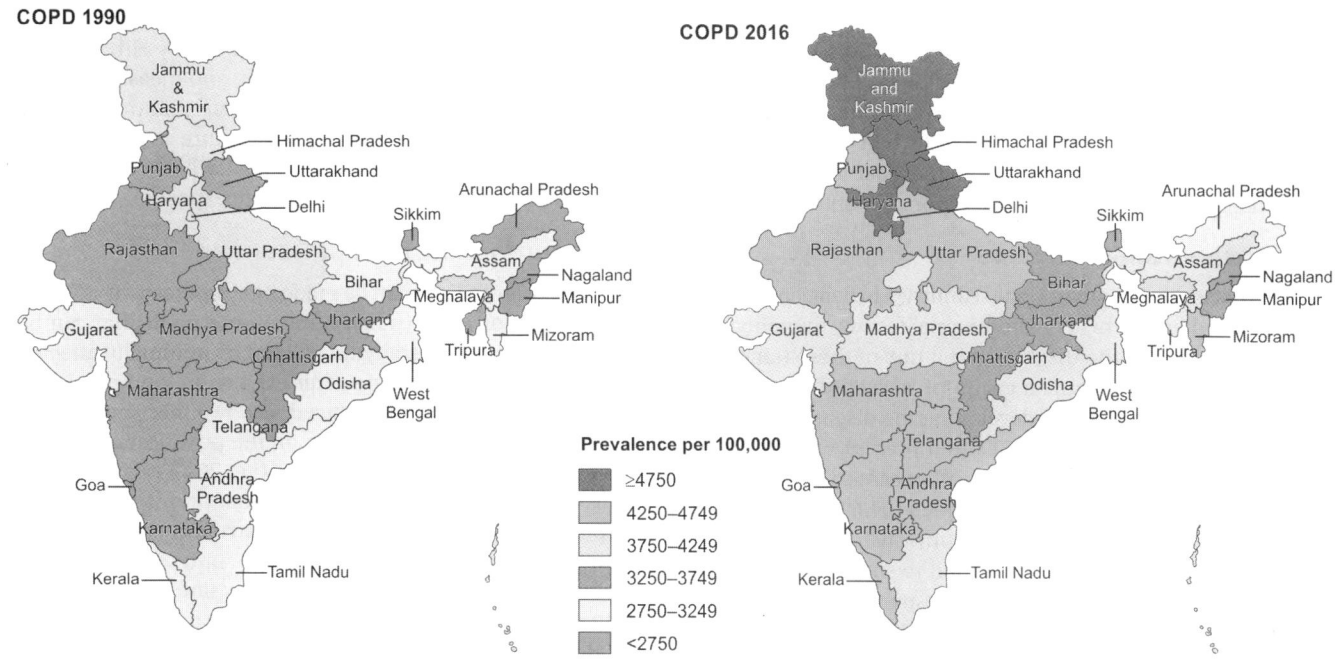

Fig. 19G.2: COPD burden in India: Situation past and present.
*Courtesy:* The burden of chronic respiratory diseases and their heterogeneity across the states of India: The Global Burden of Disease Study 1990–2016.

## MAGNITUDE OF PROBLEM

Chronic obstructive pulmonary disease (COPD) is the third leading cause of death worldwide, causing 3.23 million deaths in 2019.

Around 90% of deaths due to COPD globally are contributed by low and middle-income countries. COPD is the seventh leading cause of poor health worldwide (measured by disability-adjusted life years).

Prevalence of COPD ranges from 0.2% to 37% across countries. There has been an increase in mortality due to COPD by 11.6% compared to 1990 levels. It is however estimated that COPD may become the third leading cause of death globally by the year 2030 from fourth position in 2015.

Tobacco smoking accounts for over 70% of COPD cases in high-income countries. In LMIC tobacco smoking accounts for 30–40% of COPD cases, and household air pollution is a major risk factor.

A systematic review consisting of 101 prevalence studies across 28 countries from 1990-2004, showed that the pooled prevalence of COPD was 7.6%, with chronic bronchitis having a prevalence of 6.4% and emphysema of 1.8%. Whereas, pooled prevalence for COPD estimated using spirometry (used for screening purpose) was 8.9%. In India, chronic respiratory diseases were responsible for 10.9% of the total deaths and 6.4% of the total DALYs in 2016. They also account for 32% of the total global DALYs in 2016. COPD and asthma were responsible for 75.6% and 20.0% of the chronic respiratory disease. The crude prevalence of COPD in 2016 was 4.2%. The crude prevalence was highest in Jammu and Kashmir, Himachal Pradesh, Uttarakhand, and Haryana. The highest DALY rates for both COPD and asthma in 2016 were in the states of Rajasthan and Uttar Pradesh **(Fig. 19G.2)**.

## EPIDEMIOLOGY

### Risk Factors: Modifiable

Smoking (especially tobacco smoking) followed by ambient particulate matter are the major risk factors for COPD.

These are followed by household air pollutants (or HAP like using biomass fuels like wood and crop residues, and coal fuels), occupational particulates (like coal dust, silica dust, welding fumes, and organic dusts including cotton, grain, and wood), ozone levels, and second-hand smoke in decreasing order of DALYs. Smoking contributes largely to COPD burden in countries with high socio-developmental index (SDI), whereas in countries having low SDI, this high proportion of COPD is contributed by environmental factors.

WHO estimates that indoor smoke emanating from biomass fuels may be responsible to as much as 35% of all COPD cases in low and middle income countries. Researches as on today have established the causal association of $PM_{2.5}$ (particulate matter ≤ 2.5 nm) with COPD, with an average exposure of as little as 5 years linked to the onset of COPD.

A large burden on COPD still remains unexplained and even could not be explored in GBD study. History of asthma is now a known risk factor in never smoking COPD cases and may increase the risk of COPD by as much as 10-30 fold.

With no gender discrepancy in use of tobacco, COPD is no more common in men now in developed countries. In fact, the prevalence is same in both men and women, except in older age where more men are affected. Reasons may be attributed to increase in tobacco consumption among women in high-income and higher exposure to biomass fuel (source of indoor air pollution) in low-income countries. In India, the age-specific prevalence of COPD was found to increase rapidly after 30 years, with a greater increase in men. The highest prevalence among men was in the 80 years or older age group (37·8%) and among women in the 75–79 years age group (19.7%).

Frequent lower respiratory infections during childhood is another factor which cannot be left out when considering the causes of COPD. Other risk factors are occupational dust exposure and exposure to chemicals like vapors, irritants, and fumes.

### Risk Factors: Non-Modifiable

Carriers having deficiency of alpha-1 antitrypsin deficiency (AAT) may not need exposure to environmental factors, thus showing a genetic linkage of the disease, and a mix of these (smoking and genetic linkage) forms a group of 'susceptible smokers' who actually at more risk of developing the disease among all the smokers. These cases of AAT often present with COPD at an early age (before 40 years) unlike other cases. Genome-wide Association (GWA) studies have identified *CHRNA3/5* [a variant in the nicotinic acetylcholine receptor (nAChR) subunit gene located on 15q25, known to be related to smoking habits and addiction], and a new locus on chromosome 19q13 (including regions associated with smoking behavior) as having association with COPD and sometimes severe COPD.

> *Case Scenario 2*
>
> Mr Mohan, 58 years old presented to the PHC with shortness of breath for the past week. He is a chronic smoker for the past 35 years and he has been smoking 20 beedis per day. He also complains of production of mucoid sputum but there is no hemoptysis. He has been having similar symptoms on and off for the past 10 years. He was a worker in a coal mine in the past, but has been unable to work for few years because of his illness.
> The patient was diagnosed to be a case of COPD. Identify the risk factors for his disease?
> **Suggested solution**
> Modifiable risk factor: Tobacco smoking is the major culprit in this case. Patient gives a history of chronic smoking.
> There could also be a role of exposure to occupational particulates of coal dust in the past in the disease causation.

> **Key Points**
> - Around 90% of deaths due to COPD globally are contributed by low and middle-income countries.
> - In India, chronic respiratory diseases were responsible for 10·9% of the total deaths and 6·4% of the total DALYs in 2016
> - Smoking (especially tobacco smoking) followed by ambient particulate matter are the major risk factors for COPD.
> - Indoor smoke emanating from biomass fuels may be responsible to as much as 35% of all COPD in LAMIC.
> - Carriers having deficiency of alpha-1 antitrypsin deficiency (AATD) may not need exposure to environmental factors, thus showing a genetic linkage of the disease.

## PREVENTION AND CONTROL

### Health Promotion and Specific Protection

Health promotional measures should aim at avoiding risk factors at individual and community levels, and including factors such as tobacco smoke, environmental exposures (both at home and at work), etc. Personal hygiene, vaccination by Hib vaccine, pneumococcal vaccine, influenza vaccine and measles vaccine will decrease recurrent respiratory infections and thus may be crucial in specifically protecting against future cases of COPD. Personal protective equipment during work where environment is not conducive is also required to reduce exposure.

### Early Diagnosis and Prompt Treatment

Early diagnosis of COPD can be made by spirometry. The forced vital capacity (or FVC) (maximum volume of air that can be forcibly expired) is generally unaffected or minimally affected in COPD; while $FEV_1$ (volume of air exhaled in the first second of expiration) is significantly reduced. COPD is therefore defined only after excluding asthma based on the post-bronchodilator $FEV_1/FVC$ ratio. A cut-off value of 0.7 (i.e. 70%) is widely used for classification. Bronchodilator treatment prior to spirometry is important to establish nature of obstruction as reversible (asthma) or irreversible (COPD). Recent revised GOLD guidelines state that along with spirometry one has to consider symptoms and history of exacerbations while diagnosing COPD.

GOLD Criteria classifies the severity of COPD further into four categories based on post-bronchodilator $FEV_1$ in spirometry:
- GOLD 1 category: Mild (more than 80% of the predicted $FEV_1$)
- GOLD 2 category: Moderate (50% to 80% of the predicted $FEV_1$)
- GOLD 3 category: Severe (30% to 50% of the predicted $FEV_1$)
- GOLD 4 category: Very severe (less than 30% of the predicted $FEV_1$).

Risk of COPD patients is currently categorized using GOLD guidelines with symptoms and history of exacerbations. Symptoms are assessed using Modified British Medical Research Council (mMRC) or COPD assessment test scale (CAT). Fewer symptoms group have an mMRC of 0 to 1 or CAT of less than 10, while those with more symptoms have an mMRC of more than 2 or CAT score of more than 10. Similarly, low risk of exacerbations is those who have 0 to 1 exacerbation a year, and high risk have 2 or more exacerbations a year. Low risk group do not require hospitalization while high risk require. High-risk patients must be on the radar.
- Group A: Low risk with fewer symptoms
- Group B: Low risk with more symptoms
- Group C: High risk with fewer symptoms
- Group D: High risk with more symptoms

Quitting smoking is the single most modality of treatment of COPD. Exacerbations can be controlled with vaccinating against influenza and *S. pneumoniae*. Similarly macrolides (like Azithromycin) may show promising results for controlling exacerbations. Bronchodilators such as fluticasone propionate, salmeterol or a combination may be of help at the time of exacerbation.

### Disability Limitation and Rehabilitation

Quality of life has to be maintained in patients where disease has progressed to a greater extent with symptoms such as dyspnea even at rest or cor pulmonale has set in. Regular follow up visits should be done. Lung functions using spirometry is to be monitored at least once a year. During other follow up visits, any change in symptoms, like those of cough and sputum production, dyspnea, fatigue, limitation in daily activity, and/or any sleep disturbances are to be assessed. Smoking cessation is very useful to decrease the deterioration. Adherence to pharmacotherapy (usually fluticasone propionate, salmeterol or a combination of both give good results) should be monitored. This monitoring can also point out the increase need of bronchodilators indicating exacerbation of symptoms. Acute exacerbation can be prevented by vaccination with influenza vaccine.

## GLOBAL AND NATIONAL RESPONSE TO COPD: A PUBLIC HEALTH PROBLEM

In population-based surveys, COPD is often defined on the basis of:
1. Self-report of a doctor diagnosis of COPD, bronchitis or emphysema;
2. Self-report of respiratory symptoms; and
3. Spirometry with or without prior bronchodilator treatment.

But these self-reports may significantly underestimate the true disease prevalence. This is probably largely due to under-diagnosis of COPD by most general practitioners. Use of post-bronchodilator spirometry to determine the diagnosis of COPD in population-based studies is strongly recommended, as otherwise this may overestimate the prevalence of COPD and may also include asthma in the diagnosis and result in envisaging a larger public health problem.

Health policies of the country regulating sale and consumption of tobacco products is of primary help in decreasing the burden of the disease. India was one of the few countries for ratifying WHO Framework on Tobacco Convention and there have been many policies and legislations restricting smoking in public areas. National Tobacco Control Programme is an important initiative taken by India to implement tobacco control strategies in the country.

United States has realized public health importance of COPD and formulated a COPD National Action Plan with five major goal areas—empower COPD families, improve prevention and management of COPD, improve collection and utilization of analyzed COPD data, increase research in COPD field, and translate into national policies and program recommendations.

COPD is included in the WHO Global Action Plan for the Prevention and Control of Noncommunicable Diseases (NCDs) and the United Nations 2030 Agenda for Sustainable Development. WHO is taking action to extend diagnosis of and treatment for COPD in a number of ways. Rehabilitation 2030 is a new strategic approach to prioritize and strengthen rehabilitation services in health systems. Pulmonary rehabilitation for COPD is included in the Package of Interventions for Rehabilitation, currently under development as part of this WHO initiative. Reducing tobacco smoke exposure is important for both primary prevention of COPD and disease management. The Framework Convention on Tobacco Control is enabling progress in this area as are WHO initiatives such as MPOWER and mTobacco Cessation. Further prevention activities include the WHO Clean Household Energy Solutions Toolkit (CHEST) to promote clean and safe interventions in the home and facilitate the design of policies that promote the adoption of clean household energy at local, programmatic and national levels.

The Global Alliance against Chronic Respiratory Diseases (GARD) contributes to WHO's work to prevent and control chronic respiratory diseases. GARD is a voluntary alliance of national and international organizations and agencies from many countries committed to the vision of a world where all people breathe freely. (WHO. Chronic obstructive pulmonary disease (COPD); factsheet. 16 March 2023).

In India, prevention and management of chronic respiratory diseases are covered through a health program called as National Programme for Prevention of Non Communicable Diseases (NPNCD) *which is explained in detail in Chapter 47: Health Policies and Programs in India.*

### Key Points
- Health promotional measures should aim at avoiding risk factors at individual and community levels.
- Early diagnosis of COPD can be made by spirometry.
- Recent revised GOLD guidelines state that along with spirometry one has to consider symptoms and history of exacerbations while diagnosing COPD.
- GOLD Criteria classifies the severity of COPD further into four categories based on post-bronchodilator FEV1 in spirometry.
- Quitting smoking is the single most modality of treatment of COPD.

## SUMMARY

- Most common non-malignant condition represented by chronic bronchitis and emphysema.
- Fourth largest killer among all diseases globally.
- Around 90% of deaths due to COPD is in low- and middle-income countries.
- Presents in middle to older age, with a large burden of disease being hidden.
- Symptoms may include cough with lot of mucus, shortness of breath on exertion, wheezing or whistling or squeaky sound on breathing, and chest tightness.
- Smoking is the most important cause (even second-hand smoke). Others include lung irritants (air pollution PM 2.5), chemical fumes and dusts from the environment or workplace.
- Quitting smoking is the most important preventive measure. Exacerbations can be controlled by other modalities like influenza vaccination, antibiotics, etc.
- Covered under NPCDCS (National Programme for Prevention and Control of Cancer, Diabetes, Cardiovascular Diseases and Stroke) in India.

## SUGGESTED READING

1. Alvar A, Decramer M, Frith P. Global Initiative for Chronic Obstructive Lung A Guide for Health Care Professionals Global Initiative for Chronic Obstructive Disease. Glob Initiat Chronic Obstr Lung Dis. 2010;22(4):1–30.
2. BMJ. BMJ Best Practice-COPD [Internet]. BMJ Best Practice. 2017. Available from: https://bestpractice.bmj.com/topics/en-us/7
3. British Medical Journal. COPD Criteria. In: BMJ Best Practices [Internet]. BMJ Publ. Group; 2017 [cited 2018 Jul 23]. Available from: https://bestpractice.bmj.com/topics/en-us/7/criteria#referencePop1
4. Chronic obstructive pulmonary disease (COPD). Keyfacts. World Health Organization. March 2023. Available from: https://www.who.int/news-room/fact-sheets/detail/chronic-obstructive-pulmonary-disease-(copd)#:~:text=Smoking%20and%20air%20pollution%20are,gets%20 vaccines%20to%20prevent%20infections.
5. Douwes J, Boezen M, Brooks C, Pearce N. Chronic Obstructive Pulmonary Disease and Asthma. In: Detels R, Gulliford M, Karim AQ, Tan CC, editors.

Oxford Text Book of Global Public Health [Internet]. 6th ed. United States of America: Oxford University Press; 2015. p. 945–69.
6. Gibson PG, Simpson JL. The overlap syndrome of asthma and COPD: what are its features and how important is it? Thorax. 2009;64(8):728–35.
7. Guo C, Zhang Z, Lau AKH, Lin CQ, Chuang YC, Chan J, et al. Effect of long-term exposure to fine particulate matter on lung function decline and risk of chronic obstructive pulmonary disease in Taiwan: a longitudinal, cohort study. Lancet Planet Heal. 2018;2(3):e114–25.
8. Halbert RJ, Natoli JL, Gano A, Badamgarav E, Buist AS, Mannino DM. Global burden of COPD: systematic review and meta-analysis. Eur Respir J. 2006;28(3):523–32.
9. Jo YS, Lim MN, Han YJ, Kim WJ. Epidemiological study of PM2.5 and risk of COPD-related hospital visits in association with particle constituents in Chuncheon, Korea. Int J Chron Obstruct Pulmon Dis. 2018;13:299–307.
10. Kaur J, Jain DC. Tobacco control policies in India: implementation and challenges. Indian J Public Health. 2011;55(3):220–7.
11. National Heart Lung and Blood Institute, National Insitute of Health, US Department of Health and Human Services. COPD National Action Plan 2017.
12. Papadakis M, McPhee SJ, Rabow MW. CURRENT Medical Diagnosis and Treatment 2016. 55th ed. Papadakis M, McPhee SJ, editors. United States of America: McGraw Hill Education; 2016;pp.1–2093.
13. Papaioannou AI, Bania E, Alexopoulos EC, Mitsiki E, Malli F, Gourgoulianis KI. Sex discrepancies in COPD patients and burden of the disease in females: A nationwide study in Greece (Greek obstructive lung disease epidemiology and health economics: GOLDEN study). Int J COPD. 2014;9:203–13.
14. Rycroft CE, Heyes A, Lanza L, Becker K. Epidemiology of chronic obstructive pulmonary disease: a literature review. Int J Chron Obs Pulmon Dis. 2012;7:457–94.
15. Salvi S, Kumar GA, Dhaliwal RS, Paulson K, Agrawal A, Koul PA, et al. The burden of chronic respiratory diseases and their heterogeneity across the states of India: the Global Burden of Disease Study 1990–2016. Lancet Glob Heal. 2018;6(12):e1363–74.
16. Soriano JB, Abajobir AA, Abate KH, Abera SF, Agrawal A, Ahmed MB, et al. Global, regional, and national deaths, prevalence, disability-adjusted life years, and years lived with disability for chronic obstructive pulmonary disease and asthma, 1990–2015: a systematic analysis for the Global Burden of Disease Study 2015. Lancet Respir Med. 2017;5(9):691–706.
17. The top 10 causes of death. World Health Organization. December 2020. Available from: https://www.who.int/news-room/fact-sheets/detail/the-top-10-causes-of-death
18. WHO. Chronic obstructive pulmonary disease (COPD); factsheet.16; 2023.
19. World Health Organization (WHO). Global Health Observatory Data | WHO [Internet]. WHO. World Health Organization; 2018.
20. World Health Organization (WHO). WHO | Burden of COPD [Internet]. WHO. World Health Organization; 2013.

# CHAPTER 20

# Primary Health Care Approach to Noncommunicable Diseases

*Baridalyne Nongkynrih\*, Cherian Varghese\**

*It is health that is real wealth, not pieces of gold and silver*
—**Mahatma Gandhi**

**CM 8.5** Describe and discuss the principles of planning, implementing and evaluating control measures for disease at community level bearing in mind the public health importance of disease

## WHAT ARE NONCOMMUNICABLE DISEASES?

Non-Communicable Diseases (NCDs) are chronic diseases that are not transmissible from one person to another. Taking this definition into account, NCDs may thus include wide spectrum of medical disorders both acute and chronic like Cancers, Diabetes, Hypertension, Cardiovascular Diseases and Stroke, Chronic Kidney Diseases (CKDs), Chronic Obstructive Pulmonary Diseases (COPDs) and Asthma, Non-Alcoholic Fatty Liver Disease (NAFLD), and a gamut of other diseases (NPNCD 2023).

They share multiple risk factors, prolonged period of disease development, and often lead to complications and death. The World Health Organization (WHO) defined them as a four-by-four set considering the shared risk factors and this approach is constantly evolving. In 2018, mental health was added as the fifth NCD and air pollution as the fifth risk factor making it a 5 × 5 matrix, which has further evolved through the inclusion of oral diseases as a sixth disease group and of sugars as a sixth risk factor **(Table 20.1)**.

Table 20.1: 6 × 6 Approach of non-communicable diseases.

| 6×6 | Oral disease and conditions | Sugars |
|---|---|---|
| 5×5 | Mental disorder and conditions | Air pollution |
| 4×4 | Cardiovascular diseases | Tobacco |
| | Diabetes | Alcohol |
| | Cancers | Unhealthy diet |
| | Chronic respiratory disease | Physical inactivity |

## WHAT IS THE BURDEN OF NCDs?

At a global level, 7 of the 10 leading causes of deaths in 2019 were noncommunicable diseases (*See* **Figure 19B.2 from Chapter 19**). The four main NCDs (CVD, cancer, diabetes and chronic respiratory disease) are responsible for almost 74% of all deaths annually worldwide. NCDs shorten the lifespan of billions of adults and land many into a life of poor quality or economic struggle (WHO 2022). NCDs are emerging as the leading cause of premature mortality globally. Each year, 17 million people die from a NCD between the ages of <70 years; over 86% of these "premature" deaths occur in low- and middle-income countries.

In India and other Southeast Asian countries, NCDs affect relatively younger population as compared to the Western countries.

In India, NCDs are estimated to account for 63% of all deaths **(Fig. 20.1)**. Cardiovascular diseases [coronary heart disease, stroke, and hypertension (HT)] contribute to 27% of all NCD

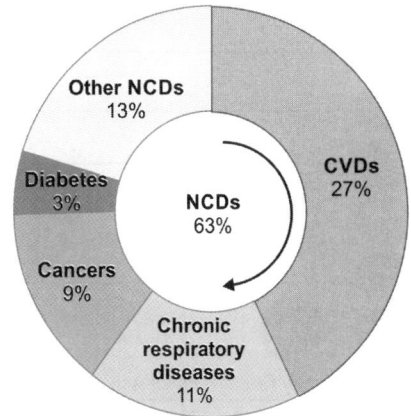

Fig. 20.1: Proportion of deaths related to NCDs in India.
*Source:* WHO non-communicable diseases Country Profiles, 2018.

---

*\*The views expressed in this commentary are solely the responsibility of the authors and they do not necessarily reflect the views, decisions or policies of the institution with which they are affiliated.*

deaths followed by chronic respiratory disease (11%), cancers (9%), and diabetes (3%) (WHO, NCD Country Profiles, 2018).

## WHAT IS THE GLOBAL AGENDA FOR NCDs?

Noncommunicable diseases are part of the Sustainable Development Goals (SDGs) and SDG 3.4 targets NCDs—reduce premature mortality from NCDs by one-third by year 2030 **(Fig. 20.2)**. There are also targets for year 2025 for NCDs and their risk factors.

Following the Political Declaration on NCDs adopted by the UN General Assembly in 2011, WHO developed a global monitoring framework to enable global tracking of progress in preventing and controlling major NCDs—cardiovascular disease, cancer, chronic lung diseases, and diabetes—and their key risk factors **(Box 20.1)**.

## APPROACH TO NONCOMMUNICABLE DISEASE: PREVENTION AND CONTROL

To reduce the growing burden of NCDs, it is important not only to detect and treat the diseases but also their key underlying risk factors, namely tobacco use, unhealthy diet, harmful use of alcohol, physical inactivity, air pollution and sugar consumption. The WHO has developed a set of evidence-based and cost-effective interventions covering the four risk factors and four diseases **(Box 20.2)**.

Reducing modifiable risk factors for NCD and underlying social determinants are to be undertaken through creation of health-promoting environments.

> **Note**
> Noncommunicable disease prevention is a continuum and needs primary health care (PHC) and referral services. Heart attacks, stroke, complication of diabetes and asthma, and cancers need to be addressed at referral care.

## WHY DO WE NEED A PRIMARY HEALTH CARE APPROACH TOWARD NCDs?

The core principles of PHC which are: equitable distribution of health services, community participation, intersectoral coordination, and use of appropriate technology are highly relevant in NCD prevention and control. PHC offers a way to provide equitable access to those in need and promotes efficient use of resources.

### Equitable Distribution

Traditionally, NCDs or "lifestyle diseases" used to be thought of as diseases of the affluent. However, NCDs are now seen across all sections of the population. Diabetes, hypertension, heart disease, and cancer afflict the poor as well as the rich, urban as well as rural population. The only way to reach out to all sections of the population is through a wide network of health centers providing universal access to health care to all.

### Community Participation

The principle of community participation is perhaps most applicable to NCDs. Risk factors for NCDs are very closely linked to health behavior, they are multifactorial and deeply intertwined

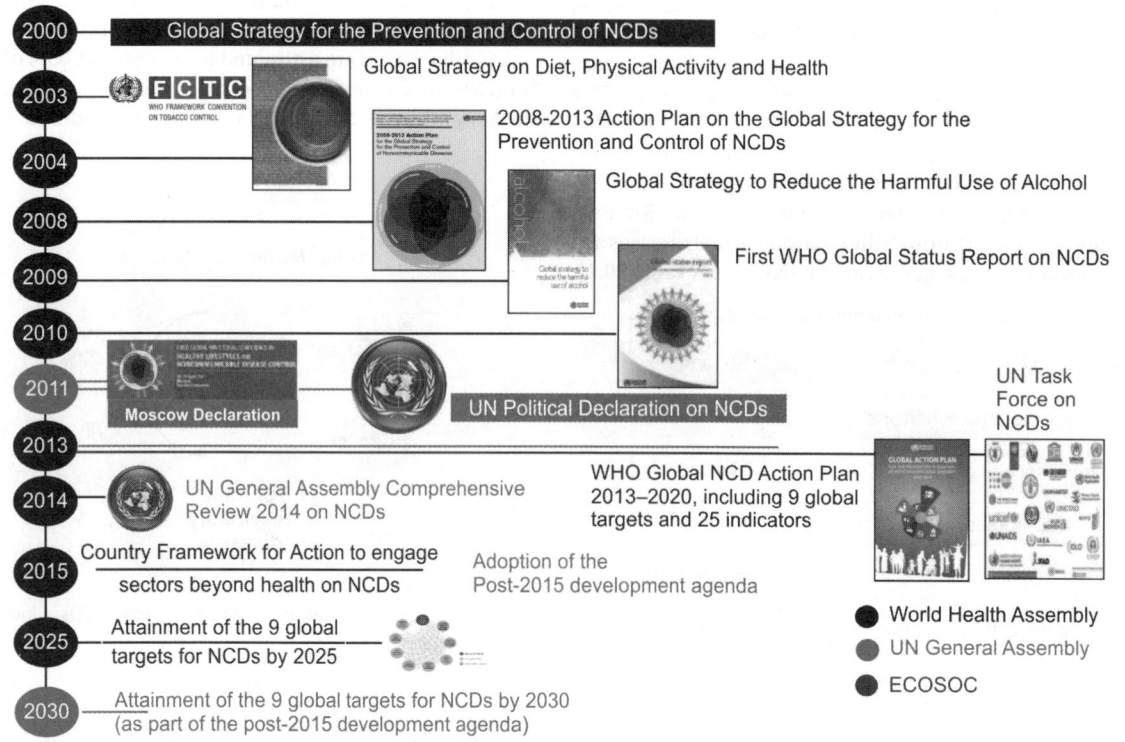

Fig. 20.2: Global milestones in the prevention and control of noncommunicable diseases.
(ECOSOC: Economic and Social Council; NCDs: noncommunicable diseases; WHO: World Health Organization).

## Chapter 20: Primary Health Care Approach to Noncommunicable Diseases

**Box 20.1:** Voluntary global targets for prevention and control of noncommunicable diseases (NCDs) to be attained by year 2025.

(1) A 25% relative reduction in the overall mortality from cardiovascular diseases, cancer, diabetes, or chronic respiratory diseases

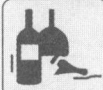
(2) At least 10% relative reduction in the harmful use of alcohol, as appropriate, within the national context

(3) A 10% relative reduction in prevalence of insufficient physical activity

(4) A 30% relative reduction in mean population intake of salt/sodium

(5) A 30% relative reduction in prevalence of current tobacco use

(6) A 25% relative reduction in the prevalence of raised blood pressure or contain the prevalence of raised blood pressure, according to national circumstances

(7) Halt the rise in diabetes and obesity

(8) At least 50% of eligible people receive drug therapy and counseling (including glycemic control) to prevent heart attacks and strokes

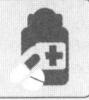
(9) An 80% availability of the affordable basic technologies and essential medicines, including generics, required to treat major noncommunicable diseases in both public and private facilities

**Box 20.2:** World Health Organization (WHO) "best buys"—(very cost-effective interventions that are also high impact and feasible for implementation even in resource-constrained settings).

**Tobacco**
- Reduce affordability of tobacco products by increasing tobacco excise taxes
- Create by law completely smoke-free environments in all indoor workplaces, public places and public transport
- Warn people of the dangers of tobacco and tobacco smoke through effective health warnings and mass media campaigns
- Ban all forms of tobacco advertising, promotion and sponsorship

**Harmful use of alcohol**
- Regulate commercial and public availability of alcohol
- Restrict or ban alcohol advertising and promotions
- Use pricing policies such as excise tax increases on alcoholic beverages

**Diet and physical activity**
- Reduce salt intake
- Replace trans fats with unsaturated fats
- Implement public awareness programs on diet and physical activity
- Promote and protect breastfeeding

**Cardiovascular disease and diabetes**
Drug therapy (including glycemic control for diabetes mellitus and control of hypertension using a total risk approach) and counseling to individuals who have had a heart attack or stroke and to persons with high risk (≥30%) of a fatal and nonfatal cardiovascular event in the next 10 years

**Cancer**
- Prevention of liver cancer through hepatitis B immunization
- Vaccination against human papillomavirus (2 doses) of 9–13 years old girls
- Prevention of cervical cancer by screening of women aged 30–49 years with either through VIA, PAP smear (every 3–5 years) or HPV test (every 5 years) linked with timely treatment of precancerous lesions.

with customs and traditions, e.g. dietary habits, use of tobacco, and alcohol. Therefore, an active involvement of the community is vital for bringing about changes in health behavior.

### Intersectoral Coordination

Intersectoral refers to the collaboration of various health and non-health sectors. NCD prevention includes a wide spectrum of activities, most of which are in the non-health sector, e.g. tobacco, alcohol, healthy diet, and physical activity. Hence to address these problems, involvement of different sectors will be crucial.

### Appropriate Technology

There is often a misconception that primary care is suboptimal care. However, it is important to remember that primary care follows evidence-based recommendations. Scientific and reliable diagnostic tools, evidence-based treatment guidelines, and essential medicines are recommended to ensure that everyone has access to good quality healthcare whether a patient is managed in a primary health center or a tertiary hospital.

## WHAT IS A PRIMARY HEALTH CARE APPROACH TOWARD NCDs?

The rise of NCDs has been driven by primarily four major risk factors: (1) tobacco use, (2) physical inactivity, (3) the harmful use of alcohol, and (4) unhealthy diets. While prevention of NCDs is important, management of patients who have developed NCDs is equally important. The focus of NCD prevention and control should, therefore, address both these areas **(Fig. 20.3)**.

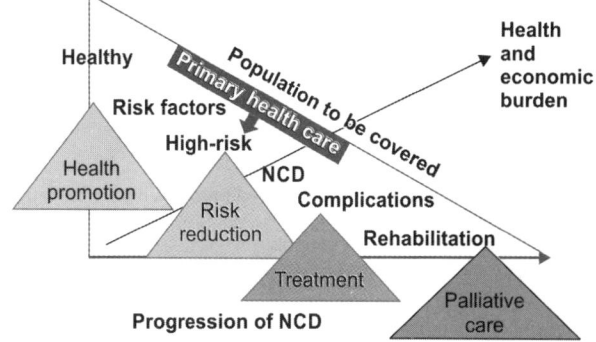

**Fig. 20.3:** Progression of noncommunicable diseases (NCDs) and role of primary health care.

Hence, a PHC approach toward NCD includes:
- Prevention of NCDs through control of risk factors
- Management of NCDs in primary care settings
- Referral.

## Prevention of Noncommunicable Diseases Through Control of Risk Factors

Preventive strategies focus on the common underlying behavioral risk factors for NCDs including tobacco and harmful alcohol use, physical inactivity, and unhealthy diet. Rapid changes in diet and lifestyle have occurred with industrialization, urbanization. This is having a significant impact on the health and nutritional status of populations, particularly in developing countries. While standards of living have improved, food availability has expanded and become more diversified, and access to services has increased, there have also been significant negative consequences in terms of inappropriate dietary patterns, decreased physical activities and increased tobacco use, and a corresponding increase in diet-related chronic diseases, especially among poor people.

These will help in controlling the metabolic risk factors like raised blood pressure, blood sugar and cholesterol, and obesity.

Comprehensive public health approaches for prevention and control of NCDs should target the human lifespan through a life course approach. Health interventions, which target the population starting from infancy through childhood, adolescence, and adulthood, would be the most effective measures **(Box 20.3)**.

### Health Promotion

Noncommunicable disease activities should move beyond hospitals and health centers to involve non-health departments, e.g. education, agriculture, food industry, traders, media, youth groups, women's groups, etc. The term multisectoral is also used interchangeably to refer to health action carried out simultaneously by a number of sectors within and outside the health system. **Figures 20.4 and 20.5** show the various sectors which can work together for providing a healthy environment.

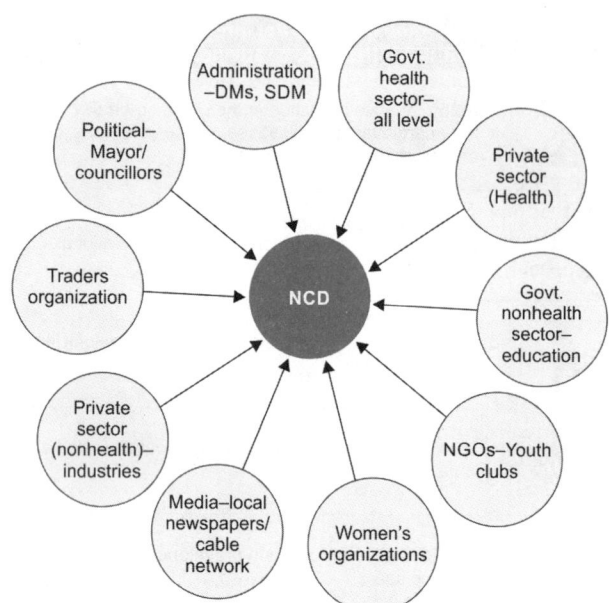

Fig. 20.4: Important sectors involved in noncommunicable disease (NCD) control activities.

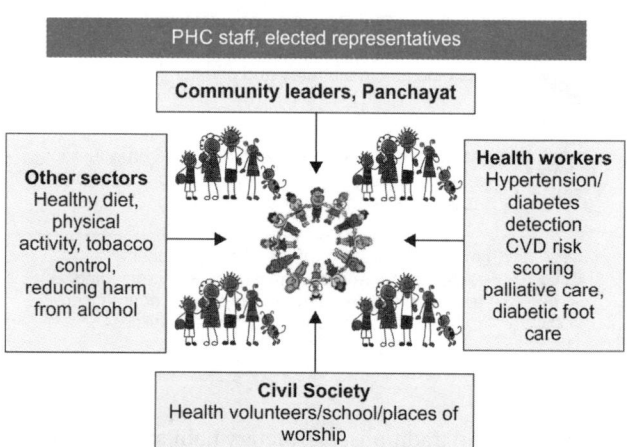

Fig. 20.5: Stakeholders in a community for health promotion activities.
(CVD: cardiovascular disease; NCDs: noncommunicable diseases)

---

**Box 20.3: Comprehensive life-course interventions for prevention and control of noncommunicable diseases (NCDs).**

**Infancy**
- Exclusive breastfeeding for 6 months
- Complementary feeding starting from the age of 6 months with continued breastfeeding up to 2 years of age or beyond.

**Childhood and adolescence**
- Improve life skills education
- Promote physical activity in school and society
- Safe and healthy foods in schools
- Restrict marketing of and access to food products high in salt/sugar/unhealthy fats
- Institute tobacco and alcohol controls.

**Adulthood**
- Improve maternal nutrition
- Implement tobacco prevention and cessation programs
- Improve availability and affordability of food
- Encourage physical activity
- Provide access to effective prevention and care of risks and diseases.

*Source*: World Health Organization (WHO). (2010). Package of Essential Noncommunicable (PEN) Disease Interventions for Primary Health Care in Low-Resource Settings.

---

### Examples of Convergence with Other Sectors in Health Promotion Activities

#### Engaging Panchayati Raj Institutions in Noncommunicable Disease Programs

Involvement of Panchayati Raj Institution (PRI) will improve the work at the grassroots level. They could also be sensitized to include NCD issues in village health and sanitation committees (VHSCs). PRIs can also facilitate and promote IEC activities related to NCD prevention.

#### Convergence with Education Department

We all know that schools are the most effective medium for behavioral change. So, it is very important to involve schools, both government and private and all *Zilla Saksharata Samitis*

(District Education Committees). NCD activities can be a part of school health by involving school teachers, parents, and adolescents in awareness programs, organize competitions, sports activities, health day celebrations, etc.

*Other Social Groups*

Social groups like NGOs, women's groups, and youth groups who are interested to work in the field of health can be included. Liaising with such groups and planning combined activities for NCD prevention will be useful.

## Management of Noncommunicable Diseases in Primary Health Care

It is imperative that patients with NCDs should be provided with standard, evidence-based management options to prevent complications. It is important to emphasize that there is no difference in the management of uncomplicated HT or diabetes whether in the tertiary hospital or in a primary health center as long as standard guidelines are followed. Uncontrolled diabetes mellitus (DM), HT will lead to end-organ damage; therefore, the goal of management is to prevent the patient from developing complications due to long-standing disease.

It is, however, crucial to understand that the basis of management of chronic NCDs are different from those of acute infectious diseases. A comparison to explain this concept is given here in **Table 20.2**.

> **Key Points**
> - Noncommunicable diseases (NCDs) are a group of conditions, which share multiple risk factors and the four main NCDs are responsible for almost 74% of all deaths worldwide.
> - The core principles of PHC which are: equitable distribution of health services, community participation, intersectoral coordination, and use of appropriate technology are highly relevant in NCD prevention and control.
> - Comprehensive life-course interventions are needed for prevention and control of noncommunicable diseases (NCDs).
> - There is a need for convergence of multiple sectors for NCD prevention and control.
> - Patients with NCDs should be provided with standard, evidence-based management options at primary health care.

### Why are NCDs Services Needed in Primary Health Care?

- The silent epidemic of NCDs is gradually overwhelming the health systems of the world resulting in high costs to both the health system and to individuals.
- The enormity of the burden of NCDs is too large to be controlled by health promotion measures alone.
- Moreover, the scale of the NCD burden means that it is no longer feasible to manage these diseases through specialists or in hospitals alone.
- Primary care, therefore, represents a feasible, affordable, and equitable option for reaching people in need of health care for NCDs.

### What are the Barriers for Delivering NCD Services in Primary Health Care Settings?

There are barriers and challenges for delivery of NCD interventions at the primary care level.

- First, all major health programs in India and other developing countries have focused on maternal and child health (MCH) services and infectious diseases. Not much emphasis was given to NCDs which were so far looked upon as diseases of the affluent and developed countries. However, due to epidemiologic transition, as a result of aging, rapid unplanned urbanization and globalization, there is a gradual increase of NCDs. India is witnessing a surge of NCDs in urban and rural areas as well.
- Second, a common perception is that the management of NCDs requires super-specialists and high-end technology for diagnosis and treatment. The delivery of NCD services in primary care has not been established.
- Third, the skills needed for delivery of all NCD interventions are too complex to be learnt by the primary care workforce. NCDs rarely occur as a single condition. A patient with diabetes is also likely to have HT and have multiple risk factors. Management of such complex situations needs skills and support from a strong health system.
- Fourth, NCDs are chronic diseases which require ongoing monitoring and often lifelong adherence to treatment. Patients with NCDs will continue to remain in the health system. Hence, unlike infectious disease, the goals of NCD care are not generally to cure but to enhance functional status, minimize symptoms, and prolong and enhance the quality of life.
- Finally, as there are many competing priority conditions that our country needs to address at the primary care level, other conditions with high mortality infectious diseases, disease outbreaks, and disasters often take priority over NCD care

## ORGANIZING NONCOMMUNICABLE DISEASE SERVICES IN A PRIMARY HEALTH CARE

Noncommunicable disease management services in a primary care level consist of screening activities and management of

Table 20.2: Differences between the management of acute infectious diseases (diarrhea) compared to chronic diseases [e.g. diabetes mellitus (DM)].

| | Diarrhea | Diabetes mellitus |
|---|---|---|
| Diagnosis | Simple to diagnose | Multiple tests needed for confirmation |
| Disciplines involved | Only one discipline needed | Many disciplines involved, good referral system needed |
| Specialist treatment | No need for specialized treatment | Specialists needed |
| Duration of treatment | Short duration of treatment (days/weeks) | Prolonged, often lifelong for DM and hypertension (HT) (decades) |
| Recovery | Immediate recovery | No complete recovery; improvement in quality of life |
| Return to normalcy | Quick return to normalcy after cure | Needs continuous care instead of cure |
| Follow-up | Short follow-up | Lifelong follow-up and rehabilitation |

diagnosed cases. Most NCDs are not symptomatic until late in the development of the disease. A syndromic approach alone, therefore, is not appropriate for NCDs. As far as possible, opportunistic screening is recommended. All patients diagnosed with HT, diabetes, chronic obstructive pulmonary disease (COPD), and asthma needs to be managed as per standard protocols.

## Patient Flow Pathway

As shown in the **Flowchart 20.1**, an indicative plan is given for organizing opportunistic screening activities and management of diagnosed patients at the PHC which include:

- Screening of adults above 40 years should be treated as a routine activity in the outpatient department (OPD) at a PHC. For this purpose, a separate room/counter needs to be identified at the PHC. If there is no possibility for a separate room, screening needs to be setup in the existing OPD room.
- All patients diagnosed with HT and diabetes needs to be managed as per standard protocols.
- Ideally, each patient should be given a unique ID number to avoid duplication during multiple visits.
- A record of patients' BP, height weight, and blood sugar, if indicated, etc. will be recorded in a treatment card.
- If resources permit, patients should deposit the treatment card in the PHC. This will enable patient tracking, follow-up and identification of dropouts and patients lost to follow-up.
- All patients should be counseled on lifestyle changes, treatment compliance, and regular follow-up.

## Plan for Patient Follow-up

Patients must be informed to come for follow-up in the PHC regularly. Patients with NCDs need not go to a secondary or tertiary hospital for a refill of drugs. Once a patient is diagnosed and started on treatment, he/she can collect the medicines from a primary health center. Six monthly or annual checkups can be done in a CHC or district hospital. This will help to decongest the overburdened hospitals.

## Essential Requirements for Noncommunicable Disease Services Delivery in Primary Care Settings

To ensure smooth NCD delivery services, adequate resources must be available which include:

- Adequate manpower, e.g. trained health worker, nurse, pharmacist, counselor, and medical officer
- Availability of standard protocols (described here)
- Availability of essential drugs and technologies (described here)
- Establish a good referral system
- Establish a good data recording and reporting system.

## Evidence-based Clinical Protocols

Evidence-based clinical protocols have been developed for addressing the four major NCDs (cardiovascular disease, cancer, diabetes, and chronic respiratory diseases). The purpose is to provide guidance for healthcare providers working in a primary health center. They are designed as simple flowcharts with clear referral criteria.

### *Why do We need Standard Protocols?*

There is a need for standard protocols because:

- There are no standard guidelines for management of NCDs in primary care level

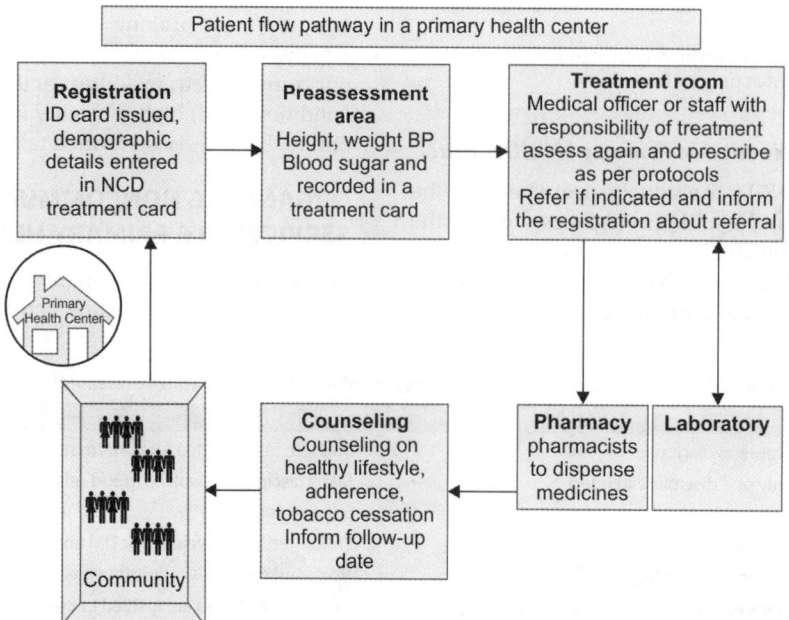

**Flowchart 20.1:** Patient flow pathway in a PHC.

(NCD: noncommunicable disease; PHC: primary health care)

- Due to lack of appropriate prevention and care, many people are unnecessarily suffering from preventable NCDs and their complications
- Healthcare costs are rising because the cost of treatment of complications (e.g. coronary bypass surgery, amputations, heart attacks, and strokes)
- In most regions of the world, the four major NCDs (cardiovascular disease, cancer, diabetes, and chronic respiratory diseases) contribute to at least 50% of the NCD burden.

## Availability of Essential Medicines, Equipment, and Technology for Noncommunicable Disease Management

One of the main reasons for poor adherence to medications is unavailability of medicines in a PHC, and inability of patients to purchase medicines. WHO provides a list of essential medicines to be available in the PHC **(Table 20.3)**. The presence of an essential drugs list will help the medical officer to procure medicines and to ensure that there are no stock-out of medicines. Similarly, there is a list of equipment and technology to be used for diagnosis and management of NCD in a PHC **(Table 20.4)**.

**Table 20.3:** Core list of medicines required for implementing essential noncommunicable disease (NCD) interventions in primary care.

| For Primary Care facilities with Physicians (For PC facilities with only nonphysician health workers most of the medicines below are required for refill of prescriptions issued by physicians at a higher level of care) | |
|---|---|
| • Hydrochlorothiazide<br>• Calcium channel blocker (amlodipine)<br>• Beta-blockers (atenolol and Metoprolol)<br>• Angiotensin inhibitor (enalapril)<br>• Statin (simvastatin)<br>• Insulin<br>• Metformin<br>• Glimepiride<br>• Teneligliptin<br>• Diltiazem<br>• Isosorbide dinitrate<br>• Glyceryl trinitrate<br>• Furosemide<br>• Spironolactone<br>• Salbutamol<br>• Prednisolone<br>• Alteplase<br>• Aspirin<br>• Paracetamol | • Ibuprofen<br>• Morphine<br>• Penicillin<br>• Amoxicillin<br>• Hydrocortisone<br>• Epinephrine<br>• Heparin<br>• Diazepam<br>• Magnesium sulfate<br>• Dextrose infusion<br>• Glucose injectable solution<br>• Sodium chloride infusion<br>• Oxygen |

*Source:* World Health Organization (WHO). (2009). WHO Model List of Essential Medicines, 16th List. [online] Available from http://apps.who.int/iris/bitstream/handle/10665/70642/a95055_eng.pdf;jsessionid=389C6066CB7788E2B70F95277E2552D2?sequence=1.

**Table 20.4:** List of essential technologies and tools for implementing essential NCD interventions in primary care.

| Technologies | Tools |
|---|---|
| Thermometer | WHO/ISH risk prediction charts |
| Stethoscope | Evidence-based clinical protocols |
| Blood pressure measurement device | Flow charts with referral criteria |

*Contd...*

| Technologies | Tools |
|---|---|
| Measurement tape | Patient clinical record |
| Weighing machine | Medical information register |
| Peak flow meter | Audit tools |
| Spacers for inhalers | |
| Glucometer | |
| Blood glucose test strips | |
| Urine protein test strips | |
| Urine ketones test strips | |
| **Add when resources permit:** | |
| Nebulizer | |
| Pulse oximeter | |
| Blood cholesterol assay | |
| Lipid profile | |
| Serum creatinine assay | |
| Troponin test strips | |
| Urine microalbuminuria test strips | |
| Tuning fork | |
| Electrocardiograph (if training to read and interpret electrocardiograms is available) | |
| Defibrillator | |

(NCD: noncommunicable disease; WHO: World Health Organization)

> **Key Points**
> - Some of the barriers and challenges for delivery of NCD interventions at the primary care level include competing priority conditions and undue focus on maternal and child health or infectious diseases with a resulting neglect in strategies to tackle NCDs as well as the need for ongoing monitoring and often lifelong adherence to treatment.
> - To ensure smooth NCD delivery services, adequate resources must be available which include: Adequate manpower, Availability of standard protocols, Availability of essential drugs and technologies, Good referral system, as well as a Good data recording and reporting system.

## INTEGRATION WITH OTHER HEALTH PROGRAMS

There should be an integration of NCD control interventions with other existing programs [e.g. tuberculosis (TB), human immunodeficiency virus (HIV), maternal and child health, and school health]. There is evidence of a close link between TB and diabetes because those with diabetes have—two to three times the risk of developing TB. Collaboration in screening for diabetes in TB clinics and for TB in diabetes clinics could enhance case finding. Similarly, there is evidence to show that women with gestational diabetes have a greater risk of poor outcome of pregnancy. Control of gestational diabetes in the MCH programs, therefore, can help **(Fig. 20.6)**. Similarly, integrating NCD long-term or palliative care with HIV care program is a win-

win situation since both cater to long-term care and support as a part of the program.

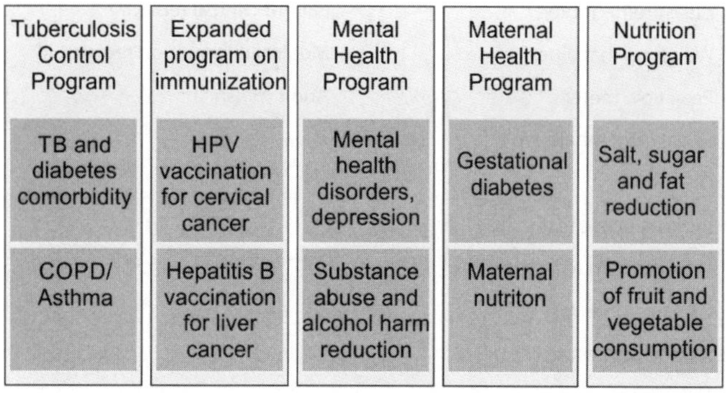

| Tuberculosis Control Program | Expanded program on immunization | Mental Health Program | Maternal Health Program | Nutrition Program |
|---|---|---|---|---|
| TB and diabetes comorbidity | HPV vaccination for cervical cancer | Mental health disorders, depression | Gestational diabetes | Salt, sugar and fat reduction |
| COPD/Asthma | Hepatitis B vaccination for liver cancer | Substance abuse and alcohol harm reduction | Maternal nutriton | Promotion of fruit and vegetable consumption |

**Fig. 20.6:** Existing programs which can contribute to NCD prevention.
(COPD: chronic obstructive pulmonary disease; HPV: human papillomavirus; NCD: noncommunicable disease)

## DATA RECORDING AND REPORTING SYSTEM

A good system of data collection and recording is essential for monitoring the program. Data collection and recording could be:
- **Paper-based**: This is based on a system of paper-based individual health records, registers, and data collection forms.
- **Hybrid (paper and electronic)**: A data collection model using a longitudinal register (paper-based or electronic).
- **Electronic:** The electronic system should collect and aggregate the facility data similar to the paper-based system.

Data system essentials:
- A good recording and reporting system is very important to monitor the activities
- Assign unique ID, developed for NCD specifically
- Responsibility for data entry and record keeping should be fixed—by whom, how often, etc. needs to be clear
- As far as possible, the health facility should have an electronic data management system
- Compiling reports should be done as required by the health system—monthly, quarterly, and annually

## MONITORING OF NONCOMMUNICABLE DISEASE PROGRAM

### What is Monitoring and Why is it Important?

*Monitoring* is an ongoing function where data is collected on specified indicators to provide managers of an ongoing program with indications of the extent of progress, achievement of objectives, and use of resources. Relevant indicators for monitoring NCD control programs include estimation of treatment rate and control rate **(Table 20.5)**. Other indicators can also be used depending on the objectives of the program.

**Table 20.5:** Examples of indicators for monitoring NCD program.

| Term | Definition | Calculation |
|---|---|---|
| Treatment rate | Out of those diagnosed with disease by the public health facilities, how many are currently on treatment within the system | Number currently on treatment in government health facilities divided by total patients diagnosed |
| Control rate | Those currently being treated with medication who have achieved control values as defined for HT or DM | Number of those currently being treated who are controlled |

(DM: diabetes mellitus; HT: hypertension; NCD: noncommunicable disease)

## SUMMARY

Noncommunicable diseases affect the poor as well as the affluent. Strokes, heart attacks, diabetes, and obstructive lung diseases entrench people in poverty as a result of catastrophic health expenditure, loss of gainful employment due to chronic ill health, and premature death of breadwinners of families.

Cost-effective interventions for prevention and management of NCDs are available. However, these interventions are often not accessible to the poor particularly in resource-constrained settings.

There is an urgent need to build up NCD care services in the primary level, so as to decongest the already burdened tertiary healthcare centers in the country and to provide equitable access.

## SUGGESTED READING

1. National List of Essential Medicines 2022. Government of India. Ministry of Health and Family Welfare. Nirman Bhavan, New Delhi 13 September, 2022.
2. Operational guidelines. National programme for prevention and control of non-communicable diseases (2023-2030). Ministry of Health & Family Welfare Government of India. 2023
3. World Health Organization (WHO). (2008). Primary Health Care: Now More Than Ever. [online] Available from https://www.who.int/whr/2008/whr08_en.pdf.
4. World Health Organization (WHO). (2010). Package of Essential Noncommunicable (PEN) Disease Interventions for Primary Health Care in Low-Resource Settings.
5. World Health Organization (WHO). (2011). From Burden to "Best Buys": Reducing the Economic Impact of Non-Communicable Diseases in Low- and Middle-Income Countries.
6. World Health Organization (WHO). (2014). Global Status Report on Noncommunicable Diseases 2014.
7. World Health Organization (WHO). (2016). Management of noncommunicable diseases in primary health care.
8. World Health Organization (WHO). (2018). Global Monitoring Framework for NCDs: About 9 voluntary global targets.

# CHAPTER 21

# Screening for Noncommunicable Diseases

*Rizwan Suliankatchi Abdulkader, Kathiresan Jeyashree*

*"The trick to seeing the future is to know where and how to look for it."*

| CM 8.2 | Use of essential laboratory tests at the primary care level for Non communicable diseases |
|---|---|
| CM 10.2 | Enumerate and describe the methods of screening high-risk groups and common health problems |

## INTRODUCTION

The burden of noncommunicable diseases (NCDs) is increasing worldwide. NCDs have become the major causes of mortality and morbidity, and their prevention and control has become a major public health concern. NCDs affect the developed and developing world disproportionately, with the latter bearing 86% of the burden of NCD related premature deaths (deaths in those aged <70 years) (WHO, NCD Key Facts, September 2023).

Developing countries like India are challenged with the dual burden of infectious diseases on one hand and noncommunicable diseases on the other. In India, NCDs that cause the most mortality and morbidity are cardiovascular diseases, hypertension, diabetes, and cancers. Without careful investment and implementation of preventive and control strategies, NCDs could soon overwhelm the healthcare system of the country.

For most NCDs, their natural history from—(1) exposure to risk factors, (2) risk factors to asymptomatic and symptomatic disease, and (3) manifest disease to development of complications, is fairly well understood. This knowledge is useful to a public health expert who is keen to identify targets for preventive interventions. Further, even though NCDs are distinct pathological entities, most of them share common modifiable risk factors. Thus, cost-effective and efficient preventive strategies targeting these few risk factors can be implemented to control many NCDs. A large study in the United States (Ford FS et al 2007) demonstrated that 61% reduction in the burden of coronary heart diseases between 1980 and 2000 was achieved through screening and control of high BP, tobacco smoking, raised cholesterol, and physical inactivity.

It is essential to be able to detect the risk factors/diseases at earlier stages when, if intervened, the course of the disease and its outcome can be changed positively. This detection is facilitated by screening—for the risk factors, for the NCDs themselves and their complications. Such screening should be ideally followed by confirmatory investigations and interventions to prevent or treat NCDs.

Deriving from your knowledge of the general principles of screening, it should be clear that most, if not all, NCDs might lend themselves to effective screening and subsequent preventive strategies. Though mental health and injuries also fall under the realm of NCDs, their screening and prevention are not discussed here. In the current chapter, screening will be discussed in the context of the most common NCDs in the Indian programmatic scenario namely, cardiovascular disease (CVD), obesity, hypertension, diabetes mellitus, and cancers (of breast, cervix and oral cavity).

## RISK FACTORS: PREVENTION CONTINUUM OF NCDs

Tobacco use, unhealthy diet, physical inactivity and harmful use of alcohol are the most common and important risk factors by virtue of their prevalence and attributable fraction. Raised blood pressure, raised blood sugar, and obesity, besides being intermediate risk factors for some NCDs, are also considered diseases themselves.

As depicted in **Figure 21.1**, CVDs provide more than one opportunity during their pathogenesis for early detection and management. Preventive efforts can begin prior to the development of risk factors in which case it would constitute primordial prevention. Early detection of the NCD itself by screening is usually considered secondary prevention. Interestingly for NCDs, it would also act as primary prevention if we were screening for certain risk factors. For example, screening for raised blood pressure or blood glucose to prevent future development of CVDs could be interpreted as primary prevention in the context of CVDs and secondary prevention in the context of hypertension or diabetes.

> **Reflection corner**
>
> Can you construct the risk factor continuum, as in **Figure 21.1**, for cervical cancer and identify points of possible screening?

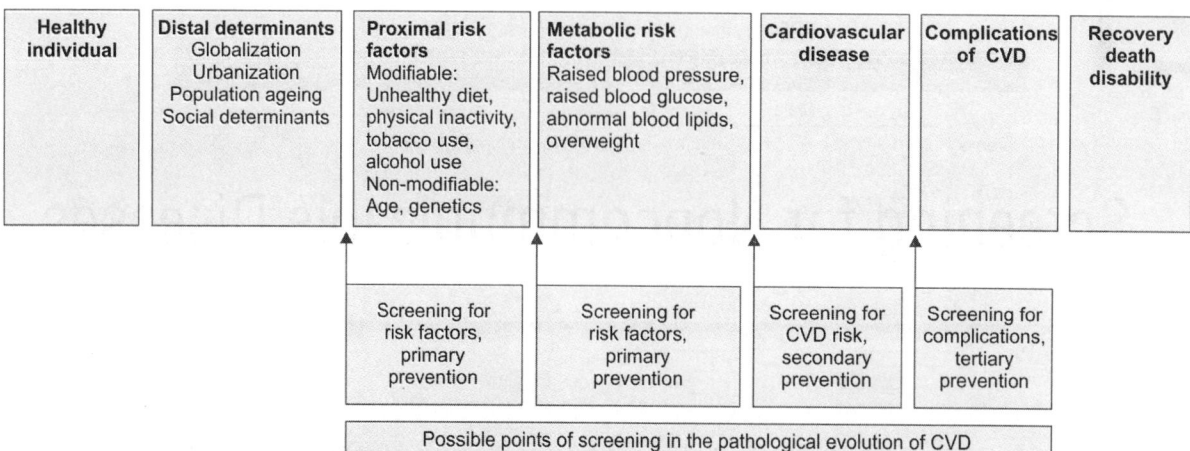

Fig. 21.1: Continuum of risk factors in NCDs—an example of cardiovascular diseases.

## APPLYING THE GENERAL PRINCIPLES OF SCREENING TO NCDs

NCDs satisfy most of the prerequisites for screening. They are an important health problem in the community, and their natural history is well understood. They have an early detectable stage and, if treated at this stage, the course of the disease changes and the outcome improves. In addition to cost-effective, acceptable, valid and reliable screening tests being available, mechanisms to follow-up, control or treat them are also in place in most situations. A good risk-benefit ratio has been established for most of these screening techniques.

### NCDs and their Screening Methods

There are several tests that can be used for detecting the presence of NCDs or their risk factors **(Table 21.1)**.

Screening can be carried out by clinical instruments (e.g. BP, waist circumference) or laboratory tests (e.g. blood sugar or serum cholesterol). It could also combine the above with self-reported history recorded using checklists to detect people at a high risk for NCD. For example, the WHO/ISH cardiovascular risk prediction charts are easy to use graphs that predict a 10-year risk of cardiovascular event **(Fig. 21.2)**. Another example of a simple screening tool is the community-based assessment checklist for early detection of NCDs used in the national program by Accredited Social Health Activists (ASHAs) and Auxiliary Nurse Midwives (ANMs) **(Fig. 21.3)**. An individual who scores >4 in this checklist is at high risk for NCDs and should be prioritized for check up in the primary health center (PHC).

> **Reflection corner**
> What are the components of the Indian Diabetes Risk Score? Can it be used as a screening tool?

The choice of a screening test depends on a number of factors such as properties of the test (validity and reliability), its availability, affordability, acceptability, and ease of use by less skilled persons. **Table 21.2** evaluates the commonly used screening tests for NCDs. Many of the tests are low cost, easily available, relatively accurate, and easy to perform, making them the ideal choice for screening.

Table 21.1: Screening methods for noncommunicable diseases and their risk factors.

| Risk factor/disease | Screening method |
|---|---|
| Tobacco use | Interview/self-reporting |
| Problematic use of alcohol | Interview/self-reporting |
| Raised blood pressure | BP estimation using digital sphygmomanometer |
| Raised blood glucose | Glucose estimation in blood/urine |
| Dyslipidemia | Serum lipid profile |
| Obesity | Body mass index, waist circumference, skinfold thickness |
| Cardiovascular diseases | World Health Organization/International Society of Hypertension (WHO/ISH) charts, biomarkers (C-reactive protein, BNP) |
| Cervical cancer | Pap smear, visual inspection with acetic acid |
| Breast cancer | Clinical breast examination, mammography, genetic testing (BRCA1 and BRCA2) |
| Oral cancer | Oral cavity visual examination by trained health workers |

(BP: blood pressure; WHO: World Health Organization; ISH: International Society of Hypertension)

> **Key Points**
> - It is essential to be able to detect the risk factors/diseases at earlier stages when, if intervened, the course of the disease and its outcome can be changed positively. This detection is facilitated by screening—for the risk factors, for the NCDs themselves and their complications.
> - NCDs satisfy most of the prerequisites for screening. A good risk-benefit ratio has been established for most of these screening techniques.
> - The choice of a screening test depends on a number of factors such as properties of the test (validity and reliability), its availability, affordability, acceptability, and ease of use by less skilled persons.

### Population-based Screening for NCDs in India

In India, screening for NCDs comes under the umbrella of the "National Program for Prevention and Control of Diabetes, Cardiovascular Disease and Stroke (NPCDCS)" renamed as NP-NCD (National Program for Prevention and Control of Non Communicable Diseases) of the Ministry of Health and Family Welfare. This screening program is integrated into the three-level primary health care system.

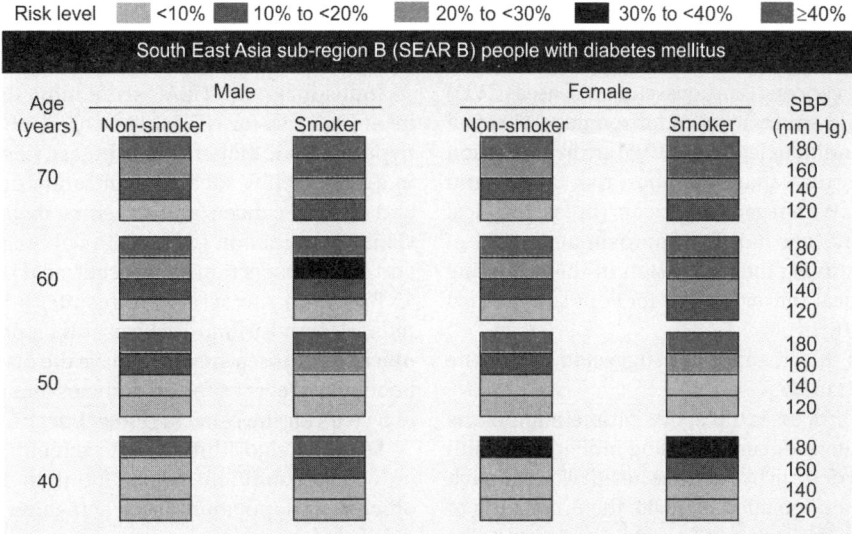

Fig. 21.2: WHO/ISH cardiovascular risk prediction chart.

| Part A: Risk Assessment | | | |
|---|---|---|---|
| Question | Range | Circle any | Write score |
| 1. What is your age? (in complete years) | 30–39 years | 0 | |
| | 40–49 years | 1 | |
| | ≥50 years | 2 | |
| 2. Do you smoke or consume smokeless products such as Gutaka; or Khaini ? | Never | 0 | |
| | Used to consume in the past/ sometimes now | 1 | |
| | Daily | 2 | |
| 3. Do you consume Alcohol daily? | No | 0 | |
| | Yes | 1 | |
| 4. Measurement of waist (in cm) | Female / Male | | |
| | <80 cm / <90 cm | 0 | |
| | 80–90 cm / 90–100 cm | 1 | |
| | >90 cm / >100 cm | 2 | |
| 5. Do you undertake any physical activities for minimum of 150 minutes in a week? | Less than 150 minutes in a week | 1 | |
| | At least 150 minutes in a week | 0 | |
| 6. Do you have a family history (anyone of your parents or siblings) of high blood pressure, diabetes and heart disease? | No | 0 | |
| | Yes | 2 | |
| Total Score | | | |
| A score above 4 indicates that the person may be at risk for these NCDs and needs to be prioritized for attending the weekly NCD day | | | |

Fig. 21.3: Community-based assessment checklist (CBAC) form used in the national NCD Control Programme in India.

Table 21.2: Characteristics of different screening tests available for NCDs.

| Test name | Availability in primary health centers | Accuracy | Cost-effectiveness | Technical feasibility | Diseases prevented/controlled |
|---|---|---|---|---|---|
| Digital Sphygmomanometer to measure BP | +++ | +++ | +++ | +++ | Hypertension, CVD |
| Glucometer to measure blood glucose | +++ | +++ | +++ | +++ | DM, CVD |
| WHO/ISH cardiovascular risk prediction charts | +++ | +++ | +++ | +++ | CVD |
| Visual inspection using acetic acid by trained health professionals | + | ++ | ++ | ++ | Cervical cancer |
| Clinical breast examination by trained health professionals | +++ | ++ | ++ | ++ | Breast cancer |
| Oral cavity visual examination by trained health professionals | +++ | ++ | ++ | ++ | Oral cancer |

(BP: blood pressure; WHO: World Health Organization; ISH: International Society of Hypertension; NCD: noncommunicable diseases; CVD: cardiovascular disease)

Population-based screening of NCDs under this program targets apparently healthy individuals aged >30 years. The diseases currently prioritized for screening are diabetes, hypertension and breast, cervical and oral cancers. Cardiovascular diseases (CVD) such as heart attacks and stroke account for roughly 25% of all deaths and the major conditions leading to CVD are hypertension and diabetes, which in turn share common risk factors and prevention approaches. With regard to cancers (breast, cervical and oral cavity cancers) account for approximately 34% of all cancers in India justifying their inclusion in the screening program MoHFW, Medical Officer Module for Population based Screening for NCDs, 2016).

The following steps of screening are suggested under the NCD control program in India:

The first step in this process is the active enumeration of the population and registration of families using individual health cards. This activity is carried out by frontline health workers such as ASHAs or ANMs. In a population of 1,000, the proportion of people in the age group more than 30 years, is assumed to be approximately 37%, i.e. 370 people, women constituting 49% (182) and men 51% (188). This gives a rough estimate of the number of beneficiaries for screening; 370 for hypertension, diabetes and oral cancer and 182 for cervical and breast cancers (MoHFW, Module for multi-purpose workers on prevention, screening and control of common NCDs, 2005).

Then, the ASHA/ANM completes the community-based assessment checklist (CBAC) for all women and men aged more than 30 years in their community. This checklist collects information on age, family history, waist circumference, physical inactivity, tobacco exposure, and alcohol use, and assigns a risk score.

Individuals with CBAC score more than 4 are considered to be at high risk for NCDs. They are mobilized for screening for hypertension, diabetes and breast, cervical and oral cancers in a fixed facility such as a subcenter or PHC. For oral, breast, and cervical cancers, the screening methods employed are oral visual examination (OVE), clinical breast examination (CBE), and visual inspection using acetic acid (VIA), respectively.

Based on the screening results, further management, or referral for those found to be positive is done by the PHC medical officer. For those who do not have the disease, the screening is to be repeated every year for diabetes and hypertension and once in 5 years for the cancers **(Flowchart 21.1)**.

Detailed algorithms for the screening and management of individual conditions can be found in the module for medical officers on population-based screening for noncommunicable diseases.

WHO Country Office has been an integral part of the PBS initiative since its inception and roll out, and further support is being provided for its convergence with HWCs Intensive trainings have been held to provide quality services, including screening of communities against diabetes, hypertension, oral cancers, and the two most common cancers among women (breast and cervical cancer), for early detection and management. PBS has potential to reach 500 million adults by 2022. It also prioritizes screening and referral services to individuals who have a higher

**Flowchart 21.1:** Process of screening and further action under national NCD Control Programme in India.

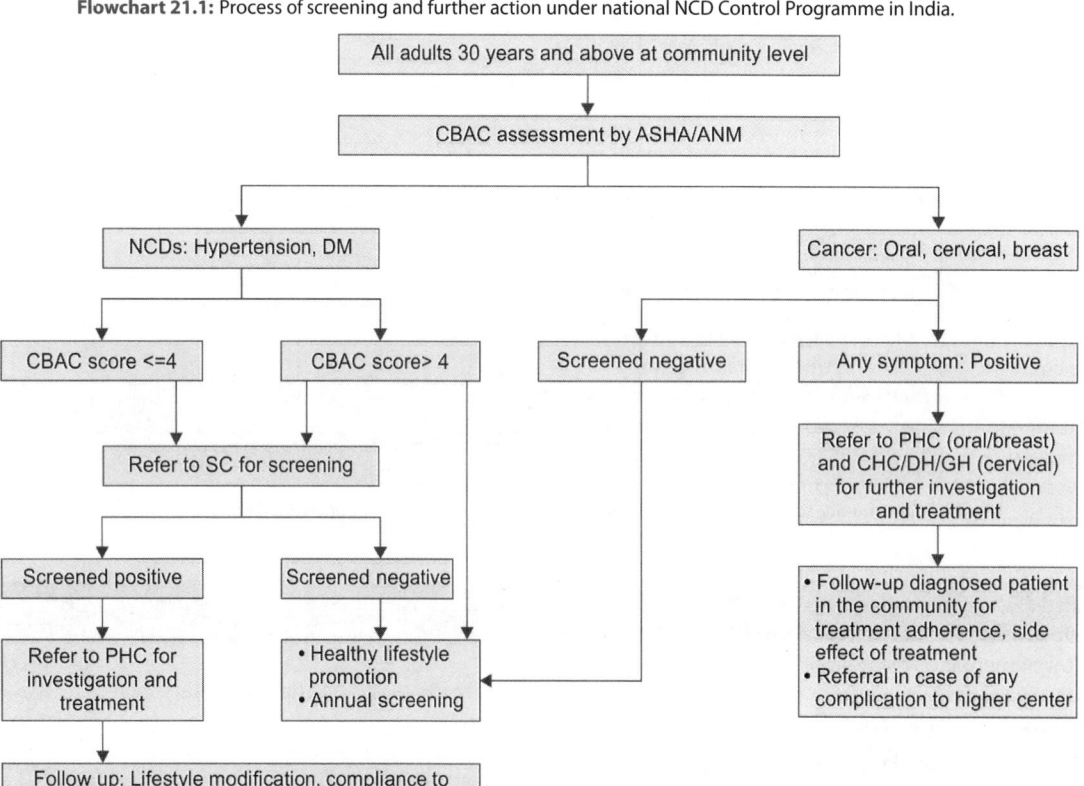

risk of developing NCDs—such as users of smokeless tobacco that raises the risk of oral cancers—through risk assessment scores. Till March 2021, more than 25 000 medical officers, 24 000 staff nurses, 100 000 female multipurpose workers, and 400 000 ASHAs have been trained to provide screening and referral services. In the same period, PBS has covered 64 million individuals above the age of 30 years, and close to 4.3 million women have been referred for cervical cancer screening based on the risk assessment at the primary health care level.

(WHO. INDIA: Grassroots screening to prevent and control non-communicable diseases. 7 April 2021. Available on https://www.who.int/india/news/feature-stories/detail/grassroots-screening-to-prevent-and-control-non-communicable-diseases)

> **Reflection corner**
> What skills would an ANM and ASHA require to be able to perform NCD screening in the community?

Opportunistic screening is also envisioned under this program where all patients visiting a PHC are screened for hypertension, diabetes mellitus, and certain cancers. The program has linkages with other programs to screen for NCDs among high-risk individuals, e.g., the NP-NCD and the National Tuberculosis Elimination Programme practice bidirectional screening where all newly registered TB patients are offered blood glucose testing, and their smoking and alcohol habits are documented.

## EVALUATION OF NCD SCREENING PROGRAMS

Evaluation of screening programs is complicated and costly, but an essential exercise. Effectiveness of screening programs might be confounded by biases namely healthy volunteer, lead-time or length time bias. Also, the follow-up required to generate conclusive evidence on the impact of a screening program is time and resource consuming.

To understand how effective an NCD screening program has been in a community, periodic monitoring and evaluation must be incorporated into the design of the screening program itself. Evaluation can be internal or external. These evaluations are done for quality control of the program or sometimes even to justify the continued implementation of the program.

- The evaluation may focus on the implementation (coverage and quality indicators), outcome (yield of new cases) or impact (averted deaths, disability adjusted life years, and cost effectiveness) of the screening program. It is anticipated that there will be a paradoxical increase in disease incidence in the short term. This is only due to the earlier detection of the disease. Other impact measures that can be assessed are prevalence of advanced disease stages and disease specific mortality.
- Cost effectiveness studies, a type of evaluation, evaluate if the cost of implementation of the screening program outweighs the benefits in terms of lives saved or disability adjusted life years averted (*see* Case Study below). Analysis of the opportunity cost of the screening program tries to understand the benefits foregone by not implementing some other competing strategy. These costing studies have to be conducted in the country where the screening program will be ultimately implemented.

Finally, newer advances in diagnostics and therapeutics necessitate that evaluation of a screening program be a dynamic process. Cost effectiveness of the screening program has to be assessed in comparison with the newer alternatives and not older standards of care. If more effective alternatives to screening are discovered, a decision to discontinue the screening program may be considered.

> **Reflection corner**
> Can you think of indicators you may use to evaluate a population-based screening program for diabetes among adults aged >30 years using capillary blood glucose measurement?

> **Key Points**
> - In India, screening for NCDs comes under the umbrella of the "National Programme for Prevention and Control of Non-communicable Diseases" of the Ministry of Health and Family Welfare.
> - Population-based screening of NCDs under this program targets apparently healthy individuals aged >30 years.
>   - First step in this process is the active enumeration of the population and registration of families using individual health cards.
>   - In the next step, the ASHA/ANM completes the community-based assessment checklist (CBAC).
> - Individuals with CBAC score >4 are considered to be at high risk for NCDs.
> - Opportunistic screening is also envisioned where all patients visiting a PHC are screened for hypertension, diabetes mellitus, and certain cancers.
> - Evaluation of screening programs is an essential exercise—can be internal or external.

## Case Study: Impact Evaluation of a Screening Program

The Trivandrum Oral Cancer Screening Study Group conducted a cluster-randomized controlled trial during 1996–2004 in Trivandrum to assess the effect of visual screening on oral cancer mortality. Healthy participants aged >35 years were randomized to either receive three rounds of visual inspection of oral cavity by trained health workers at 3-year intervals or to a control group. Screen-positive persons were referred for clinical examination by doctors, biopsy, and treatment. The authors reported that there was a 38% reduction in oral cancer incidence and an 81% reduction in oral cancer mortality in the screening group. Sustained reduction in oral cancer mortality during the 15-year follow-up was also observed. The authors recommended the introduction of population-based screening programs for oral cancer in high-incidence countries like India.

## Case Study: Economic Evaluation of a Screening Program

A study assessed the cost-effectiveness of various screening strategies for cervical cancer in five different countries, including India. The authors assessed the direct and indirect costs of the different strategies and considered reduction in lifetime risk of cancer and cost per year of life saved as outcomes. They found that the various screening strategies reduced the lifetime risk of cancer by 25–36% and cost less than $500 per year of life saved. Among the many strategies examined, the most cost-effective strategy was the Indian one-visit visual inspection strategy, which cost $10 per year of life saved (Goldie SJ et al., N Eng J Med, 2005).

## SCREENING AND SURVEILLANCE

Surveillance is often confused with screening. However, these two activities are fundamentally different. Screening is usually performed for the purpose of early detection of disease after which the test results are conveyed to the patients and is followed by appropriate management. On the other hand, surveillance is primarily carried out to quantify the prevalence and analyze disease trends over time through large surveys. There is usually no intention to convey the results to or treat the patients. In other words, feedback to the individual is not part of surveillance. An example of NCD surveillance is the WHO STEP wise survey that is conducted regularly to assess the burden of NCD risk factors in the population.

### Issues in Screening

1. Screening programs have to be ethical and equitable. The principle of non-maleficence is an overarching issue in disease screening given that this activity is performed on "healthy" persons. Protection of the individual's interests, autonomy, and health, reigns supreme over anything else. Vested interests in screening programs, like that of pharmaceutical companies or practitioners or other players like the Government itself, need to be carefully ruled out before rolling out any screening program. It has to be ensured that only proven and evidence-based screening tests are offered in these programs.
2. Further, these tests must be evaluated for their effectiveness and quality of their implementation before they are incorporated into routine health care practice. While the validity of screening techniques for detecting a particular disease are well established, the benefits of large-scale screening programs implemented in community settings have been poorly evaluated. This is true for NCD screening programs as well. Uncertainty clouds many steps in the NCD screening program (e.g. eligibility criteria, screening technique, frequency of testing, and cut-offs for diagnosis).
3. Ethically responsible NCD screening programs must ensure that those who are screened receive maximum benefit and experience minimal harm and anxiety. It has to be remembered that framing and adhering to clear guidelines for management of individuals detected with high risk for NCDs is vital. For example, for a person who tests positive in diabetes mellitus screening, the guidelines for confirmatory testing, cut-offs for diagnosis, line of management, level of healthcare where she or he will be managed, referral links for management of emergencies and complications should be identified before the screening is done and must be integral to the design of the screening program.
4. One has to anticipate the additional burden on the existing services that a screening program may pose by virtue of detecting "new" cases and plan accordingly. An NCD screening program without proper support health infrastructure and manpower will be ineffective and pointless regardless of the validity of the tests it employs because it would fail to show measurable impact. Worse, it can lead to anxiety among those screened and loss of public trust in the system. Accurate detection of burden of disease is not the sole aim of a screening program. It should ultimately result in the decline of that burden.
5. Individuals may face stigmatization in the process of screening. For example, a healthy person detected with cancer through a screening program may be at risk for stigmatization at workplace or personal life.
6. Other equally grave concerns are the false assurance given to false negative persons and the unnecessary anxiety caused by false positive results. Careful and sensitive planning may avoid such undesirable effects. Proper health communication activities are required to avoid such issues.
7. Equity in an NCD screening program means that the benefits of the program reach all those who are in need of it, particularly, the sections of population that bear an unfair share of the NCD burden. Such a screening program should also pave way for fairness in allocation of resources to even out this inequitable distribution. An inefficient screening program will be counterproductive and use up essential and limited resources. This, in turn, can diminish the overall health of a community and worsen pre-existing inequities.

### Prevention Paradox

Consider the distribution of a parameter, e.g., blood pressure, in the population. Screening will detect individuals with raised BP and follow them up with treatment to prevent CVD. This is called high-risk strategy. Another approach is to focus on the whole population and employ an intervention (e.g. reduce salt content of packaged foods) that shifts the distribution of the population's BP. This is called population/mass strategy.

Prevention paradox (or Geoffrey Rose's paradox) states that any prevention strategy applied on the entire population may bring huge gains for the entire population but it is likely to be of little benefit to the individual. In other words, large numbers of people must participate in a preventive strategy in order to benefit a few. Focusing only on those with high risk might not be able to prevent the larger number of deaths occurring among the many with smaller risk. Therefore, it is always prudent to employ an optimal combination of these two approaches.

### Recent Advances in NCD Screening

With the advancement of technology, it has become easier to screen for many types of diseases in the population. In the context of NCDs, mobile based applications have been developed by private firms that can connect the user in a remote place to doctors situated hundreds of miles away. Miniature sensors such as glucometer, blood pressure monitor, ECG and cholesterol analyzers can be connected to smart phones and they, in turn, can relay this information to the doctor for interpretation and management. It remains to be seen how such telemedicine technology will benefit NCD control.

> **Reflection corner**
> Reflect on how smartphones can be used to screen for NCDs

## SUMMARY

- Globally and nationally, noncommunicable diseases pose a major health burden in terms of attributable morbidity and mortality.
- Primary and secondary prevention of NCDs and their common risk factors provide the most sustainable and cost-effective approach to their prevention and control.
- Most NCD screening programs target diabetes, hypertension, CVD and breast, cervical, and oral cancers.
- These NCDs have a well-defined natural history and share certain common risk factors. Valid and reliable screening tools, such as blood sugar estimation, WHO/ISH risk prediction charts or Pap smears can detect them at an early stage. Also, effective treatments are available which can improve health outcomes, if administered at an early stage.
- Adequate health manpower and infrastructure should be in place before initiation of any screening program. This will ensure that those detected with the disease will receive the appropriate standard of care.
- In India, under the National Programme for Prevention and Control of Diabetes, Cardiovascular Disease and Stroke (NPCDCS), population-based screening for diabetes, hypertension and breast, cervical, and oral cancers is performed for apparently healthy individuals aged >30 years.
- ASHAs and ANMs use a community-based assessment checklist for NCD screening in the community. High-risk individuals thus identified are referred to health centers for further management.
- NCD screening programs should be equitable and ethical. The benefits of the program should be equitably distributed among the population providing maximum benefits to the vulnerable sections of the community. At the same time, the programs should ensure no/minimal harm to the beneficiaries.
- Evaluation of a screening program is vital, though resource intensive. Studies evaluating cost, implementation, and impact of a screening program have to be periodically conducted and should be an integral part of the program itself.
- NCD screening programs, if implemented efficiently, can reduce the nation's NCD burden.

## SUGGESTED READING

1. Detels R, Gulliford M, Karim QA, et al. (Eds). Population screening and public health. In: Oxford Textbook of Global Public Health, 6th edition. Oxford: Oxford University Press; 2017. pp. 1715-9.
2. McQueen DV (Ed). Global handbook on non-communicable diseases and health promotion. New York: Springer; 2013.
3. Ministry of Health and Family Welfare. Medical officer module for population-based screening for non-communicable diseases. New Delhi: Government of India; 2016.
4. Ministry of Health and Family Welfare. Module for multi-purpose workers on prevention, screening and control of common non-communicable diseases. New Delhi: Government of India; 2005.
5. Ministry of Health and Family Welfare. Operational guidelines prevention, screening and control of common non-communicable diseases: Hypertension, diabetes, and common cancers (oral, breast, cervix). New Delhi: Government of India; 2004.
6. Ministry of Health and Family Welfare. Training module for staff nurses on population based screening of common non-communicable diseases. New Delhi: Government of India; 2004
7. Rayner M, Wickramasinghe K, Williams J, et al. An introduction to population-level prevention of non-communicable diseases. Oxford: Oxford University Press; 2017.
8. Sankaranarayanan R, Ramadas K, Thara S, et al. Long term effect of visual screening on oral cancer incidence and mortality in a randomized trial in Kerala, India. Oral Oncol. 2013;49(4):314-21.
9. Strong K, Wald N, Miller A, et al. Current concepts in screening for non-communicable disease: World Health Organization Consultation Group Report on methodology of non-communicable disease screening. WHO Consultation Group. J Med Screen. 2005;12(1):12-9.
10. Wilson JMG, Jungner G, World Health Organization. Principles and practice of screening for disease. Geneva: WHO; 1968.
11. World Health Organization. Implementation tools: Package of essential non-communicable (PEN) disease interventions for primary health care in low-resource settings. Geneva: WHO; 2013.
12. World Health Organization. WHO/ISH cardiovascular risk prediction charts. Geneva: WHO; 2007.

# CHAPTER 22

# Noncommunicable Disease Surveillance

*Roopa Shivashankar*

*"Chance favors the prepared mind."*
—**Louis Pasteur**

| CM 8.6 | Educate and train health workers in disease surveillance |

## WHAT IS THE ROLE OF SURVEILLANCE IN NONCOMMUNICABLE DISEASE (NCD) CONTROL?

In the previous chapter, we have learnt that NCDs are the most common cause of deaths across the world. There are many levels of interventions that can be done to control NCDs. It is crucial not only to understand the burden and trends of NCD risk factors, diseases, and their impacts (disability and mortality) but also to monitor the uptake and effectiveness of interventions or programs to prevent and control NCDs. Surveillance systems provide such information to the relevant stakeholders regularly so as to take necessary action in a timely manner. World Health Organization (WHO) defines Public Health Surveillance as "the continuous, systematic collection, analysis and interpretation of health-related data needed for the planning, implementation, and evaluation of public health practice". The same definition applies to NCD surveillance system.

### Uses of NCD Surveillance System (Box 22.1)

Planning a program to prevent and control NCDs needs continued input on dynamic changes in the burden of diseases and risk factors levels, regional distribution and status of current control measures. NCD surveillance system provides this information to the program. For instance, the information on the burden of diseases is crucial for planning (funds, human resources, and other logistics) the NCD care system. For example, the budget for the purchase of blood pressure-lowering medications will need information on the number of patients with hypertension being treated at the healthcare facilities.

> **Box 22.1: Uses of NCD surveillance system.**
> - Ascertain the burden of NCDs and trend in risk factor prevalence
> - Understand geographical distribution
> - Monitor the spread and uptake of control programs
> - Evaluate the effectiveness of preventive and control measures

(NCD: noncommunicable disease)

As planning is cyclical and continuous the surveillance system needs to continuously collect, analyze, interpret, and disseminate data for planning actions. ***Planning cycle is explained in detail in Chapter 42B: Health Planning.***

## WHAT FACTORS SHOULD BE CONSIDERED UNDER NCD SURVEILLANCE?

There are three major aspects of diseases that need to be considered under surveillance systems—Deaths, Diseases, and Determinants. NCDs are a large group of diseases and there is multitude of determinants for these diseases. Therefore, countries or regions should decide on which factors under each of these aspects should be under NCD surveillance.

### Deaths or Mortality Surveillance

Mortality surveillance is relatively simpler to implement and interpret. The indicators of mortality surveillance include total, age- and sex-specific NCD death rates and cause-specific death rates for major NCDs.

### Diseases or Morbidity Surveillance

Cardiovascular diseases, diabetes mellitus, respiratory conditions—asthma and chronic obstructive pulmonary diseases and cancers make a major part of the NCDs in most countries. NCD disease surveillance system of most countries includes them. Disease prevalence, incidence, and trend over time are the most common indicators for disease surveillance. Additionally, common complications of diseases can also be a part of a surveillance system that measures the health system response, e.g. the number of cases of amputations (as an indicator for untreated diabetes mellitus).

### Determinants or Risk Factor Surveillance

There is a long latent period between exposure to risk factors and the occurrence of NCDs, therefore, it is all the more crucial to have a risk factor surveillance in an NCD surveillance system. Timely information on these factors will help design the programs to prevent and control the risk factors which in

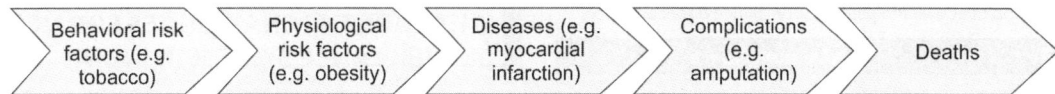

Fig. 22.1: Aspects of noncommunicable disease surveillance system.

turn will help in the reduction of NCD burden. However, NCDs are multifactorial, and these risk factors are at several levels embedded in web of causation. The NCD surveillance system should at the least have structures to measure population levels of common physiological risk factors (obesity, high blood pressure, high blood glucose, dyslipidemia) and behavioral risk factors (tobacco and alcohol use, low physical activity, unhealthy diet and air pollution) **(Fig. 22.1)**.

In addition to the three aspects, the NCD surveillance system should also include indicators of national health system capacity and response—infrastructure, human resources, accessibility, and availability of medications and other interventions.

### Key Points

- Public Health Surveillance is defined as "the continuous, systematic collection, analysis and interpretation of health-related data needed for the planning, implementation, and evaluation of public health practice
- There are three major aspects of diseases that need to be under surveillance systems—Deaths, Diseases, and Determinants
- NCD surveillance system should have structures to measure population levels of common physiological risk factors (obesity, high blood pressure, high blood glucose, dyslipidemia) and behavioral risk factors (tobacco and alcohol use, low physical activity, unhealthy diet and air pollution)

## WHAT ARE THE COMPONENTS OF NCD SURVEILLANCE SYSTEMS?

As in any surveillance system, there are three major components of NCD surveillance system—population, data collection, and dissemination of information **(Fig. 22.2)**.

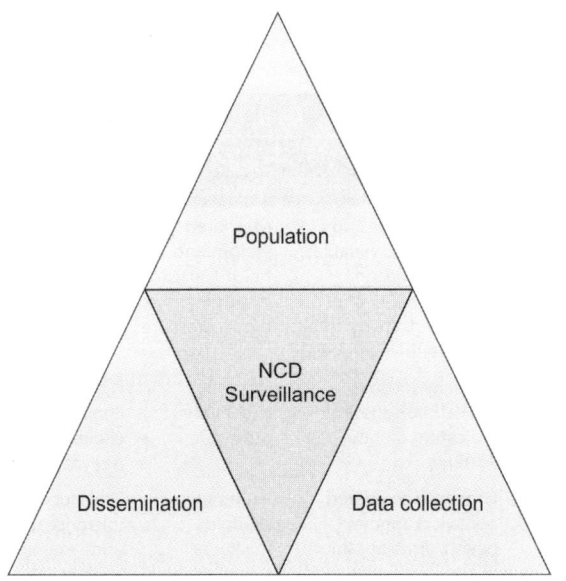

Fig. 22.2: Components of noncommunicable disease (NCD) surveillance system.

### Population

One needs to understand "what population does the surveillance system covers". Some parts of the system may cover all the population such as death registration. However, most part of the surveillance system covers specific or some selected population in the country. For example, public health system reports cover only those populations who receive care from public health clinics.

### Data Collection, Analysis, and Interpretation

The information needed by NCD surveillance may be collected from various sources. Some examples of the sources of data are described in **Table 22.1**. Note that many of the risk factors information uses non-health data sources.

Table 22.1: Data sources and examples for noncommunicable disease surveillance in India.

| Aspect of surveillance | Sources of data | Examples in India |
|---|---|---|
| Mortality surveillance | Vital registration | • Death registry<br>• Million Deaths Study (MDS) |
| Morbidity | Disease registry | • Regional Cancer Registries |
| | Clinical information system | • Reporting from National Programme for Prevention of Non-Communicable Diseases (NP-NCD) |
| | Periodic surveys | • District Level Health Survey (DLHS) |
| Physiological risk factors | Periodic surveys | • National Family Health Survey (NFHS)<br>• District Level Health Survey (DLHS) |
| | Sentinel surveys | • WHO-STEPS Survey at In-Depth sites |
| Risk factor surveillance | Periodic surveys | • Global Adult Tobacco Survey (GATS)<br>• Global Youth Tobacco Survey (GYTS)<br>• Physical activity surveillance<br>• Global School-based Student Health Survey (GSHS)<br>• National Nutrition Monitoring Bureau Surveys (NNMB) |
| | Sentinel surveys | • WHO-STEPS Survey at In-Depth sites<br>• Cervical cancer surveillance |
| | Non-health sources | • Sales data of tobacco<br>• Household expenditure surveys by National Sample Survey Organization (NSSO) |

(*Source:* WHO. Noncommunicable Disease Surveillance, Monitoring and Reporting AVAILABLE FROM https://www.who.int/teams/noncommunicable-diseases/surveillance/systems-tools)

### *Types of Data Collection System*

The data collection system may be active or passive **(Table 22.2)**.
The collected data will be analyzed and reported as predefined indicators for dissemination.

**Table 22.2:** Comparison of active and passive surveillance data collection.

| Active surveillance | Passive surveillance |
|---|---|
| • Collection of new data<br>• Examples: WHO-STEPS survey; GATS survey<br>• Advantages:<br>  ➢ Standardized data collection with better data<br>  ➢ Complete data<br>• Disadvantages:<br>  ➢ Expensive<br>  ➢ Covers limited population<br>• Example: WHO-STEPS survey | • Using existing sources of data collected for other purposes<br>• Examples: Vital registration; health systems reports<br>• Advantages:<br>  ➢ Covers large population<br>  ➢ Inexpensive<br>• Disadvantages:<br>  ➢ High missing data and errors<br>  ➢ Risk factors data is not collected<br>• Example: Cancer registries |

## Dissemination

The major differentiating factor of public health surveillance from epidemiological surveys is that the findings from the surveillance system, by design leads to actions. Therefore, the dissemination of the information to the decision-makers is the most crucial aspect of the public health surveillance system. These disseminations may be provided as forms of report or policy briefs. Surveillance findings may also be reported to other stakeholders (e.g. medical doctors at clinics who provided reports) and the general population (e.g. via media).

Note that the surveillance system is not just a data collection system. It is a cycle where data collection is followed by analysis and interpretation and disseminated to decision-makers so that action is taken and then the cycle is repeated **(Fig. 22.3)**.

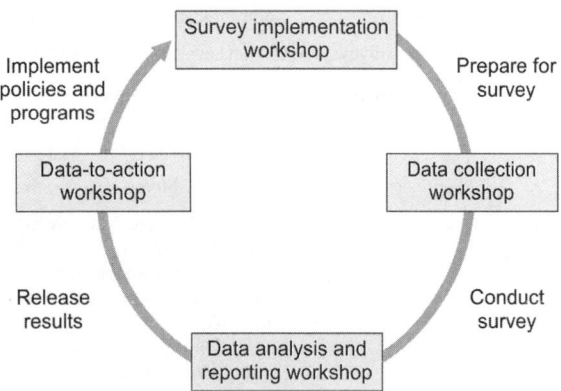

**Fig. 22.3:** Surveillance as a cycle.

> **Key Points**
> - There are three major components of NCD surveillance system—population, data collection, and dissemination of information.
> - The data collection system may be active (e.g., WHO-STEPS survey; GATS survey) or passive (e.g., Vital registration; health systems reports).
> - The collected data will be analyzed and reported as predefined indicators for dissemination.
> - The dissemination of the information to the decision-makers is the most crucial aspect of the public health surveillance system.

## WHAT ARE THE CHALLENGES FOR NCD SURVEILLANCE SYSTEM IN INDIA?

In low- and middle-income countries such as India, the health systems mainly cater to maternal-child health and infectious diseases. The program to combat NCDs and surveillance systems is in early stages and therefore there are several challenges in establishing a well-functioning surveillance system. The challenges include—low priority or lack of resources, lack of capacity in human resources, and low use of technology for data transmission.

## EXAMPLE OF NCD SURVEILLANCE—WHO STEPS APPROACH

World Health Organization's STEPS (STEP wise approach to NCD risk factor surveillance) approach aims to build NCD surveillance systems in countries and provides standardized tools to obtain the basic data on the burden and trends of NCD and risk factors. STEPS approach is population-based and involves an active collection of data **(Table 22.3)**. STEPS instruments are administered in three levels—questionnaires (self-reported data), physical measurements, and biochemical parameters (blood samples). The risk factor assessment at all the three levels is divided into three modules based on the variables on which the data is to be collected—core, expanded, and optional. The STEP wise approach states that the countries should collect data on a minimum set of core variables that predict the major risk factors for chronic diseases. The approach allows for flexibility to obtain data on expanded and optional modules that are adopted in context-specific to the region. The optional variables provide more detailed information on the risk factors that are required for the local level. Collection of data on standardized variables allows for both intra- and inter-country comparison and to draw the trends of NCD risk factors among the member states.

**Table 22.3:** STEPS approach to risk factor assessment.

| | Level | | |
|---|---|---|---|
| Measures | Step 1 (self report) | Step 2 (physical) | Step 3 (biochemical) |
| Core | Socioeconomic and demographic variables, years of education, tobacco and alcohol use, physical inactivity, intake of fruit and vegetables | Measured weight and height, waist circumference, blood pressure | Fasting blood sugar, total cholesterol |
| Expanded | Ethnicity, income, education, household indicators, dietary patterns | Hip circumference, pulse rate | High-density lipoprotein-cholesterol, triglycerides |
| Optional | Other health-related behaviors, mental health, disability, injury | Pedometer, skinfold thickness | Oral glucose tolerance test; urine examination |

## SUMMARY

World Health Organization (WHO) defines Public Health Surveillance as "the continuous, systematic collection, analysis and interpretation of health-related data needed for the planning, implementation, and evaluation of public health practice". The same definition applies to NCD surveillance system.

As planning is cyclical and continuous, the surveillance system needs to continuously collect, analyze, interpret, and disseminate data for planning actions.

There are three major aspects of diseases that need to be under surveillance systems—Deaths, Diseases, and Determinants.

- The indicators of mortality surveillance include total, age- and sex-specific NCD death rates and cause-specific death rates.
- Disease prevalence, incidence, and trend over time are the most common indicators for disease surveillance.
- Population levels of common physiological risk factors (obesity, high blood pressure, high blood glucose, dyslipidemia) and behavioral risk factors (tobacco and alcohol use, low physical activity, unhealthy diet and air pollution) also need to be measured.

There are three major components of NCD surveillance system—population, data collection, and dissemination of information.

- Population refers to what population does the surveillance system covers.
- The data collection system may be active or passive.
- The dissemination of the information to the decision-makers is the most crucial aspect of the public health surveillance system. These disseminations may be provided as forms of report or policy briefs.

## SUGGESTED READING

1. CGHR. Million Death Study (MDS). [online] Available from http://www.cghr.org/projects/million-death-study-project/.
2. Chapter 3: Monitoring NCDs and their risk factors: a framework for surveillance, WHO NCD report.
3. David Stuckler D, Siegel K. Sick Societies: Responding to the global challenge of chronic diseases.
4. Global Adult Tobacco Survey. [online] Available from https://www.wto.org/english/tratop_e/serv_e/gatsqa_e.htm.
5. Government of India. (2018). Household Consumer Expenditure: National Sample Survey. Open Government Data (OGD) Platform India.
6. London School of Hygiene and Tropical Medicine. (2009). Types of surveillance [Internet]. The use of epidemiological tools in conflict-affected populations: open-access educational resources for policy-makers.
7. Ministry of Health and Family Welfare, Department of Health and Family Welfare G of I. National Programme for Prevention and Control of Cancer, Diabetes, Cardiovascular Disease and Stroke (NPCDCS). Ministry of Health and Family Welfare. GOI.
8. National Cancer Registry Programme. (2013). [online]. Available from http://www.ncdirindia.org/NCRP/index.aspx.
9. Roth GA, Abate D, Abate KH, et al. Global, regional, and national age-sex-specific mortality for 282 causes of death in 195 countries and territories, 1980–2017: a systematic analysis for the Global Burden of Disease Study 2017. Lancet. 2018;392(10159):1736–88.
10. Stuckler D, Siegel K. Sick Societies: Responding to the global challenge of chronic disease. Oxford University Press; 2012. pp. 1-376.
11. Surveillance of major noncommunicable diseases in the South-East Asia Region. Report of an Intercountry Consultation, WHO/SEARO, New Delhi, 2-4 August 2000.
12. World Health Organization. (2003). WHO STEPwise approach to NCD surveillance.
13. WHO. Noncommunicable Disease Surveillance, Monitoring and Reporting Accessed in July 2023 available from https://www.who.int/teams/noncommunicable-diseases/surveillance/systems-tools

# CHAPTER 23

# Epidemiology of Nutrition and Food-related Diseases and its Prevention and Control

## EPIDEMIOLOGY OF NUTRITION-RELATED DISEASES AND ITS PREVENTION

*Amir Maroof Khan, Paras Agarwal, Shveta Lukhmana, Charu Kohli*

| CM 5.2 | Describe and demonstrate the correct method of performing a nutritional assessment of individuals, families and the community by using appropriate method |
| --- | --- |
| CM 5.3 | Define and describe common nutrition-related health disorders, their control and management |
| CM 5.5 | Describe the methods of nutritional surveillance |
| CM 5.8 | Describe and discuss the importance and methods of food fortification and effects of additives and adulteration |

> *Case Scenario*
>
> *You are the medical officer at a primary health care setting. A pregnant woman comes to you for her antenatal checkup. You detect conjunctival pallor in the woman. What all dietary advices will you give to the pregnant woman?*

## NUTRITIONAL EPIDEMIOLOGY

Food provides nutrition and it also plays an important role in health and disease. Nutritional epidemiology is the application of epidemiological principles and tools to understand the relationship between nutrition and health and to prevent nutrition-related diseases. It can be considered as a subspecialty of epidemiology. It encompasses three things: (1) dietary assessment, (2) diet-related exposures, and (3) statistical modeling to find diet-disease relationships. However, it is nearly impossible to undertake epidemiological studies to study nutrition and health, as robust as we do for drug trials. One reason is that measuring food intake accurately is a challenge in community settings. Another reason is the wide variety of food items, their nutrition-related constituents, and the interactions between them, all these vary a lot between individuals.

## NUTRITION-RELATED DISORDERS

### Malnutrition

Malnutrition can either be due to inadequate intake or an excess intake of calories. Malnutrition, in all its forms, includes **undernutrition** (underweight, wasting and stunting), micronutrient deficiency (vitamin and mineral deficiency) and **overnutrition** [including obesity and diet resulting noncommunicable diseases (NCDs)].

### Undernutrition (Underweight, Wasting and Stunting)

#### How to Measure Undernutrition?

The nutritional status of under-five children is assessed by the following indicators—stunting, wasting and underweight **(Table 23.1)**.

**Table 23.1:** Indicators of undernutrition in children.

| Indicator | Numerator | Denominator | Definition |
| --- | --- | --- | --- |
| Stunting | Number of under-fives falling below minus 2 standard deviations (moderate and severe) and minus 3 standard deviations (severe) from the median height-for-age of the reference* population | Children under the age of 5 years in the surveyed population | Stunting refers to a child who is too short for his or her age. It results from undernutrition over long period of time. Stunting can lead to severe irreversible physical and cognitive impairment |
| Wasting | Number of under-fives falling below minus 2 standard deviations (moderate and severe) and minus 3 standard deviations (severe) from the median *weight-for-height* of the reference* population | Children under the age of 5 years in the surveyed population | Wasting refers to a child who is too thin for his/her height. Wasting occurs due to recent rapid weight loss or the failure to gain weight. A child who is moderately or severely wasted has an increased risk of death, but it can be treated |
| Under-weight | Number of under-fives falling below minus 2 standard deviations (moderate and severe) and minus 3 standard deviations (severe) from the median *weight-for-age* of the reference* population | Children under the age of 5 years in the surveyed population | Weight for age (W/A) is a composite indicator of both long-term malnutrition (deficit in height/"stunting") and current malnutrition (deficit in weight/ "wasting") |

*Reference population is based on WHO Child Growth Standards, 2006.

- ***Stunting (height for age):*** The child is too short for his/her age. This is the result of chronic undernutrition.
- ***Wasting (weight for height):*** The weight of the child is too less for his/her height. It indicates acute nutritional deficiency or sudden weight loss due to an illness. It has been shown that wasting increases the risk of death in childhood from infectious diseases such as diarrhea, pneumonia and measles.
- ***Underweight (weight for age):*** The weight of the child is too low for his/her age. This can result from stunting, wasting, or both.

First 1,000 days of life is a critical window in terms of growth and development as inadequate and insufficient nutrition coupled with multiple bouts of infection may impact physical as well as cognitive development reduces individual's productive capacity and increases the risk of various degenerative diseases. World Bank estimates that childhood stunting may result in a loss of height among adults by 1% which may further lead to a reduction in individual's economic productivity by 1.4% (World bank, Repositioning Nutrition as central to development, 2006).

### Classification of Wasting of Acute Malnutrition

| Moderate acute malnutrition | Moderate wasting and/or mid-upper arm circumference (MUAC) ≥ 115 mm and < 125 mm |
| --- | --- |
| Severe acute malnutrition | Severe wasting and/or MUAC < 115 mm and/or bilateral pitting edema |

### Magnitude of Problem

UNICEF-WHO-World Bank Group Joint Malnutrition Estimates (2023) shows that stunting prevalence has been declining since the year 2000, more than one in five (22.3% or 148.1 million) children under 5 were stunted in 2022, and at least 45.0 million (6.8%) suffered from wasting and 13.7 million (2.1%) suffered from severe wasting at any given point of time in the year. At 14.8 per cent, South Asia's wasting prevalence represents a situation requiring a serious need for intervention with appropriate treatment programs. Meanwhile, the number of children under 5 affected by overweight worldwide has increased from 33.0 million in 2000 to 37.0 million in 2022 **(Fig. 23.1)**.

According to the National Family Health Survey (NFHS-5) estimates (2019–2021), 19.3% are wasted, 32.1% are underweight and 35.5% are stunted **(Fig. 23.2)**.

A set of six global targets have been endorsed by the WHO for improvement of maternal, infant and young child nutrition which are shown in **Table 23.2**.

The alarming rate of undernutrition, among under-five children reiterates the synergistic relationship between infections and malnutrition which is shown in **Flowchart 23.1**.

The "1,000 days" initiative underscores the importance of first critical "1,000 days" between women's pregnancy and child's 2nd birthday. Initiatives taken toward good nutrition and care during these 1,000 days facilitates cognitive development, reduces the risk of chronic diseases later in life and improves education and earning potential thereby benefitting the individual, country and economy at large.

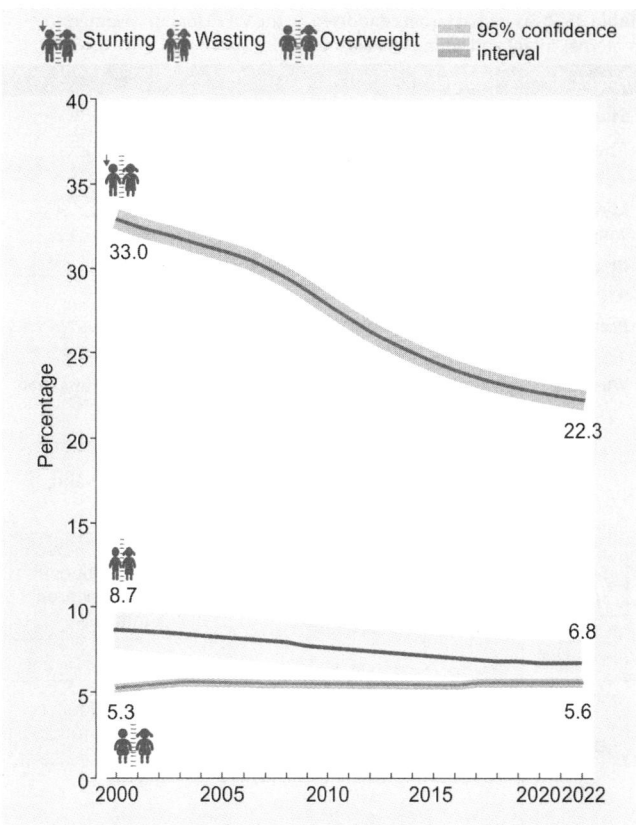

**Fig. 23.1:** Percentage of stunted, overweight and wasted children under-five, global, 2000–2022.

*Source:* UNICEF, WHO, World Bank Group joint malnutrition estimates, 2023 edition.

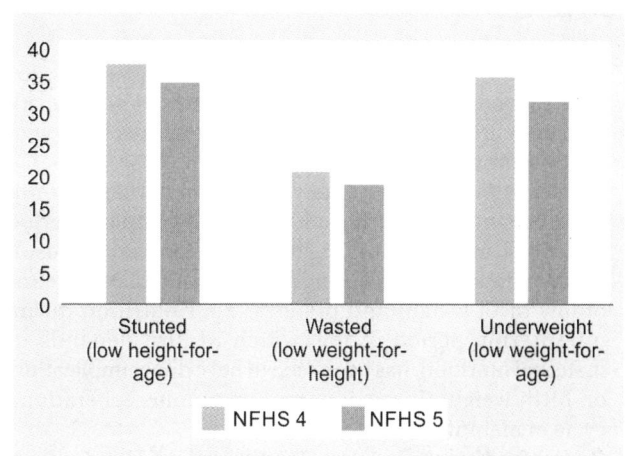

**Fig. 23.2:** Prevalence of undernutrition in India.

*Source:* National Family Health Survey-5 (2019–2021).

### Risk Factors for Undernutrition

Undernutrition occurs as a result of a complex interaction between various physiological, sociocultural, demographic and economic factors which are as follows:

Table 23.2: Six global targets endorsed by the WHO for improvement of maternal, infant and young child nutrition.

| Factor | Target |
|---|---|
| Stunting | 40% reduction in under-five stunting |
| Anemia | 50% reduction among women of reproductive age group |
| Low birth weight | 30% reduction |
| Childhood overweight | No increase in childhood overweight |
| Breastfeeding | Increase up to at least 50% the rate of exclusive breastfeeding |
| Wasting | Reduce and maintain the childhood wasting to less than 5% |

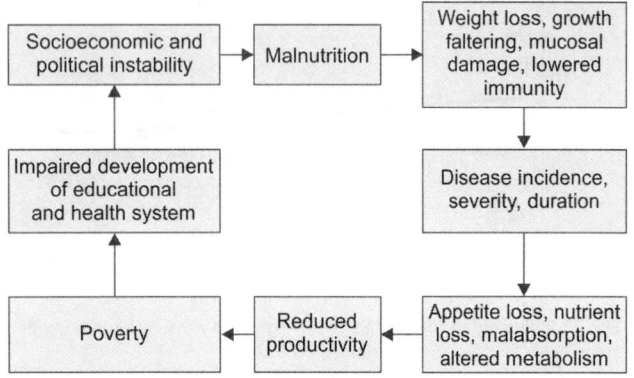

Flowchart 23.1: Synergistic relationship between infections and malnutrition.

Source: Adapted from Fenn B. (2009). Malnutrition in humanitarian emergencies. [online] http://www.who.int/diseasecontrol_emergencies/publications/idhe_2009_london_malnutrition_fenn.pdf.

- *Sociodemographic factors*: Mother's literacy status, low socioeconomic status coupled with household poverty, and food insecurity result in lack of awareness and access to good quality nutrition.
- *Maternal factors*: Short-stature, poor maternal nutrition preconceptionally, during antenatal and postnatal period, infections, mental health, maternal smoking and exposure to secondhand smoke during pregnancy increases the risk of low birth weight and preterm. Poor nutrition during intrauterine period of life, which in turn depends on maternal nutrition, has been seen to have direct implications on birth weight. It sets into motion an intergenerational cycle of malnutrition.
- *Breastfeeding practices*: Inappropriate, inadequate, insufficient, delayed or complete lack of breastfeeding perpetuates a cycle of malnutrition. Children who are breastfed are far more resilient to infections as compared to those who are not breastfed. In addition, the time of initiation of complementary feeding is a critical window for malnutrition to set in, if not done properly. Around the same time, i.e. around 6–9 months, the child begins to crawl and creep and is predisposed to infections, particularly those transmitted through fecal-oral route.
- *Gender*: Malnutrition in India has a skewed distribution with respect to gender. Women, across all ages, are particularly vulnerable to severe malnutrition due to poor feeding, child rearing and health seeking practices. The socio-cultural milieu of our country is such that it accords selective responsibility of childbearing and child rearing to a woman without empowering her for the same. This coupled with a huge gender gap in terms of food security and accessibility sets into motion a vicious intergenerational cycle of malnutrition which gets passed on from a malnourished mother to her child.
- *Home environment*: Poor child rearing practices including nonresponsive feeding, large family size, unsatisfactory sanitation and poor water supply, food insecurity, inappropriate allocation of food and lack of female empowerment result in child neglect and thereby, malnutrition more often than not.
- *Quality of foods*: Poor quality of micronutrients and macronutrients, low dietary diversity and presence of antinutrient component in the diet makes jack a dull boy.
- *Dietary practices*: Infrequent and inadequate feeding, inappropriate food consistency, insufficient quantity and nonresponsive feeding can compromise the growth of the child making them more susceptible to infections and malnutrition.
- *Food and water safety*: Unsafe, unhygienic and/or contaminated food and water, unsatisfactory sanitation, poor hygiene, unsafe preparation and storage of food serve as a proxy marker of pathogenic environment.
- *Poor hand hygiene*: Hand hygiene is an often underestimated and underrated technique for prevention of infections and thereby malnutrition. Six simple steps of hand washing practiced regularly before preparation, serving and eating meals and after going to the toilet can go a long way in prevention of malnutrition.
- *Food (in) security*: Problem of malnutrition in India is a case of inequitable distribution and poor purchasing parity. Lack of food grain production, ill-equipped public distribution system (PDS), poor literacy rates, unemployment and poor per capita purchasing power parity comprise an important cause of malnutrition.
- *Other factors*: Adolescent pregnancy, high fertility and lack of birth spacing increase the chances of intrauterine growth restriction (IUGR) and preterm. This coupled with other factors like poverty, low socioeconomic status, poor knowledge and means of livelihood to make ends meet often results in malnutrition.

## Monitoring of Growth

Growth standards offer an insight about the extent of growth and development during the critical growth periods during childhood and enable appropriate and timely action in order to address malnutrition.

**Anthropometric Assessment**
- *Weight*:
  - Salter (spring hanging) scale can weigh up to 25 kg.
    - Hook the scale to a tripod or horizontal stick placed at eye level
    - Suspend the weighing pants from the lower hook and readjust the zero on the scale
    - Undress the child and place him/her in the weighing pants
    - Take the reading to the nearest 100 g, after the child has stabilized in the pants.
- *Electronic scale*: Scale should be placed on a flat surface, readjust the zero error (if any), undress the child and remove their shoes.
  - If the child can stand: The child should be made to stand on the scale with feet slightly apart and record the weight to the nearest 100 g
  - If the child cannot stand: Firstly, weigh the caregiver and then weigh the caregiver and child together. Subtract the caregiver's weight to determine child's weight.
- *Length/height*:
  - Length should be measured for infants and children less than 24 months of age in lying down position using a length board called as "infantometer".
    - Position the baby on the board supine with eyes looking up, such that board is perpendicular to the lower border of the eye and ear canal
    - Ensure that the spine should be straight and shoulders should touch the board. Caregiver should hold the head in this position from behind the headboard
    - Straighten the child's legs by applying gentle pressure to the knees and place the child's feet such that the plantar surface of the feet is flat against the footboard and toes are pointing upward.
  - Height should be measured for children over 24 months of age in standing position using a height board called as "stadiometer".
    - Child should be made to stand on a stadiometer such that back of the head, shoulder blades, buttocks, calves and heels touch the vertical board, trunk should be balanced over waist such that the child is neither leaning forward nor backward and feet are slightly pulled apart.
  - All the measurements should be recorded to the nearest 0.1 cm.
- *Edema*:
  - Grasp the foot such that it should rest in investigators hand.
  - Place the thumb on the dorsum of the foot and press it gently for a few seconds.
  - If a pit remains in the foot after the thumb has been removed, it indicates edema.

The National Center for Health Statistics (NCHS)/WHO reference curves have been used since late 1970s. These curves had some limitations and they did not reflect early childhood growth as the anthropometric measurements were done quarterly, which is insufficient to illustrate the growth rate among under-five children. In addition, the data used to develop NCHS reference curves was obtained from a longitudinal study among 0- to 3-year-old children of European ancestry. The data was not representative as these children were selected from a single community in the United States of America. Statistical models, to understand variability and pattern of growth, were not available at the time of development of NCHS/WHO curves. To overcome these limitations, WHO Multicentre Growth Reference Study (MGRS) was conducted among 9,440 children from diverse backgrounds including Brazil, Ghana, India, Norway, Oman and the USA between 1997 and 2003.

This was done to generate a *"standard"*, which showed how children *should* grow as against a *"reference"* (NCHS/WHO) that merely described *how* children grew in a particular timeframe and place. This made it an internationally applicable standard. The MGRS study was conducted among healthy and privileged children who were living under favorable conditions and the data was in congruence with the "best" health-related practices. The mothers of these children were following health-promoting practices, i.e. they were nonsmokers and were breastfeeding (i.e. exclusive or predominantly breastfeeding for at least 4 months and partial breastfeeding was continued up to at least 12 months, initiation of complementary feeding at 6 months of age). Gross motor developmental milestones (six in number) were also included in the MGRS study **(Table 23.3)**.

Table 23.3: Difference between old and new growth chart standards.

| New growth chart standards | Old growth chart standards |
|---|---|
| 1. Six countries across different continents were included, which made this an internationally acceptable standard | 1. Children of European ancestry from a single community from USA were included, which was not representative |
| 2. It established breastfeeding as a norm | 2. It was based on growth of artificially fed children |
| 3. It describes how children should grow by taking into account health promoting behaviors | 3. It merely described how they grew at a particular place and time |
| 4. It generated "Standards" | 4. It generated "References" |
| 5. It includes new innovative growth indicators, e.g., skinfold thickness, which are useful for monitoring childhood obesity | 5. It does not include any such indicators |
| 6. It includes a window of achievement for six key motor development milestones | 6. Not included |

Impact of introduction of new standards on estimates of undernutrition is as follows:
- A substantial increase in underweight rates during 0–6 months of age and a decrease thereafter
- Higher rates of wasting during infancy
- Increase in rates of stunting throughout childhood.

### Impact

Malnourished children fail to reach their optimum potential in terms of size, physical capacity to work and economic productivity. It results in delayed enrolment and higher absenteeism along with poor school performance and higher repetition of class. Cognitive impairment due to malnutrition also results in lack of productivity. It predisposes to diseases like diarrhea, acute respiratory infections, malaria and measles.

### Prevention and Control

Measures to prevent and control malnutrition can be stratified into multiple levels such as individual, family and community level.
- ***Using the lifecycle approach to address malnutrition***
  *Among women*: A woman often comprises a neglected and vulnerable cohort, who is given all the responsibilities of

housekeeping, childbearing, child rearing, etc. but is usually not empowered for the same. Simple proactive measures, as detailed below, can help avert and address malnutrition in all its forms.

- **Breastfeeding**:
  - *At individual level*: Every child should be exclusively breastfed, irrespective of gender. This becomes especially important in case of a preterm or low birth weight child. Early initiation and exclusive breastfeeding for 6 months provide essential nutrients and offer protection against gastrointestinal infections. If for some reasons (working mother, active infection in mother, mother dies during childbirth, etc.), the child cannot be put to breast, expressed mother's milk can be given using a "katori and spoon" instead of bottle. In case mother's milk is not available, then other women in the family can also be trained to feed the child. Artificial feeding is best avoided or should be used as a last resort.
  - *At family level*: Familial support during breastfeeding is pivotal. The mother has to be taught, encouraged and assisted to breastfeed regularly and correctly.
  - *At community level*: Various breastfeeding support groups can network together and identify new mothers or pregnant women and encourage them to breastfeed (exclusive breastfeed for 6 months). People can share positive experiences so as to instill determination among new mothers who wish to do the same.
- **Prelacteal feeds**: The sociocultural milieu of our country is such that a child is often given honey or gripe water as the first feed following which breastfeeding is initiated, and this, as a matter of fact, is considered auspicious. Prelacteal feeds predispose the child to various infections. It is during pregnancy that a woman is most receptive to all forms of advice. Therefore, pregnant women and their family during the antenatal period should be counseled against prelacteal feeds and other alternatives should be discussed with them.
- **Timely introduction of complementary feeding:** At the age of 6 months, complementary feeding should be initiated gradually.
  - *At individual level*: Timely introduction of adequate and appropriate complementary feeding coupled with dietary diversification can help prevent undernutrition from setting in. Mother can be taught various simple recipes so as to make the food more interesting and appealing.
  - *At family level*: The family should be encouraged to feed the child from the family pot. Feeding is a collective responsibility and each family member should be encouraged to take on that role.
  - *At community level*: Role of Anganwadi and community health workers is paramount when it comes to nutrition counseling. The lactating mother and child should be enrolled in Anganwadi and be given nutrition counseling and (age-appropriate) nutrition to children to address malnutrition. Anganwadi workers (AWWs) should regularly weigh the child and pick up growth faltering, if any, at the first instance and take remedial measures for the same.
- **Developmental milestones and predisposition to infections:**
  - *Individual/Family level*: The child begins to crawl and creep around the same time as complementary feeding is initiated, wherein he/she picks up infections that go unnoticed. This coupled with poor hand hygiene practices results in acute malnutrition. In addition, teething starts at around 9 months of age. This is a critical window in terms of growth faltering. This is the age when artificial teats/teethers are introduced to facilitate teething, which may potentially introduce infections. Parents and family should be counseled and advocated preventive measures.
  - Community health workers should ensure that age appropriate immunization is given to the child and any symptom suggestive of acute infection should be picked up and referred to higher center, if required. Auxiliary workers should be trained, time and again, about early identification and measurement of malnutrition and be sensitized toward impact of malnutrition.
- **Adolescence**: This is another critical window in the paradigm of nutrition wherein a lot of hormonal changes take place, which impact both physical and mental growth. It is during this time that habits are formed. It is also a phase when body dysmorphic disorders take shape among both adolescent boys and girls. This is a crucial period, which if capitalized properly can result in a healthy demographic dividend.
- **Antenatal women**: A healthy mother shall give birth to a healthy baby. Every antenatal woman should receive adequate nutrition, iron prophylaxis, prophylaxis against worm infestation and other supplements, as indicated. She should be registered as a beneficiary in her respective Anganwadi in order to receive supplemental nutrition and birth counseling. Special focus on the critical 1,000-day window from a woman's pregnancy to her child's second birthday is critical.

- *Growth monitoring*: Especially for under-five children should be done at regular intervals at Anganwadi centers. Growth faltering, if any, should be picked up at the first instance as the weight of the child begins to plateau. High-risk children identified during growth monitoring or otherwise should be promptly referred to higher center or nutritional rehabilitation center, whichever appropriate.
- *Immunization*: Immunization against vaccine preventable diseases offer protection against common diseases of childhood, which may perpetuate a cycle of malnutrition. Therefore, every child should be offered complete immunization at Anganwadi centers and every dropout child in the community should be traced and immunized. Clients who refuse immunization to their under-five children should be counseled about the benefits of immunization and the protection that it offers. If required nongovernmental organizations (NGOs) or community-based organizations

can also help conduct health education sessions to educate and motivate such non-utilization clients.
- **Covariates of malnutrition:**
  - **At individual/family level:** Parents/families should be sensitized toward hand hygiene through six simple steps of hand washing, before cooking, serving, eating or feeding a child and after using toilet. They should also be made aware about importance of sanitary latrines and its role toward prevention of infection. They should be able to pick up signs of growth faltering, passage of worm in stools, etc. and be able to report to the nearest health facility.
  - **At community level:** Village health and sanitation committee should ensure construction of sanitary latrines in their respective areas. Health workers should organize health education sessions to spread awareness about importance of using sanitary latrines and use such platforms to dispel myths about toilets in residential premises.

"Comprehensive implementation plan on maternal, infant and young child nutrition" clearly spells out global nutrition targets that are to be achieved by 2025, which are as follows:
- Achieve 40% reduction in the number of under-five children who are stunted.
- Reduce and maintain childhood wasting to less than 5%.

## Overweight (Obesity)

Obesity is considered as an abnormal or excessive fat accumulation in the body that may impair health. A body weight higher than the expected weight for a particular age and sex is referred to as "obesity" and "overweight". Obesity is itself becoming a public health problem in India. It is considered as a disease as well as a risk factor for other diseases.

### Pathogenesis

Etiopathogenesis of obesity is multifactorial, with overnutrition or excess of calories being the most common cause. Both genetic and environmental factors interact to the development of obesity in an individual. The rapidly changing lifestyle toward sedentary habits and the trend of processed and junk foods is a major risk factor. There is a growing trend of consuming a high salt, high-fat diet in the community and less of vegetables, fruits and fiber-rich diet.

### Burden

***Global:*** As per WHO factsheet on obesity in 2016, more than 1.9 billion adults (39%) aged 18 years and older were overweight. Of these, over 650 million adults (13%) were obese. Over 115 million people suffer from obesity-related problems in developing countries. According to the WHO, rates of overweight and obesity are increasing in both developed and developing countries around the world. In many countries, prevalence of obesity has doubled or tripled over the past decades. The worldwide prevalence of obesity nearly tripled between 1975 and 2016.

Obesity is also increasing among children and adolescents. The prevalence of overweight and obesity among children and adolescents aged 5–19 has risen dramatically from just 4% in 1975 to about 18% in 2016. There is also an increase of chronic diseases related to obesity especially in urban settings.

In SEARO, an estimated 8.8 million children aged 0–5 years and between 2% and 24% of adolescent girls are overweight. Among adult women, prevalence of overweight or obesity ranges between 18% and 30%.

***India:*** The prevalence of obesity and overweight is showing a rapid increase in past years. Age standardized prevalence of obesity [body mass index (BMI) ≥ 30] has increased by 22% in the span of 4 years (2010–2014). According to Global Nutrition Report 2017, prevalence of obesity among under-five children is 2% and among adolescents, overweight and obesity is 13%. Among adult males, 18% are overweight and 2% are obese while among females, 22% are overweight and 5% are obese.

### Epidemiology of Obesity

#### Agent Factor

**Nutrition:** The most important agent factor of obesity is food. Consuming more quantity of food than required amount leads to deposition of excess fat in the body. Quality of foods consumed also plays a major role. Among different foods, some foods items contribute most to obesity like food having high fat content and high-sugar foods like ice-creams, candies, etc. On the other hand, salads, whole grains, cereals, etc. play a protective role in obesity.

#### Host Factor

There are some demographic risk factors for obesity among adults and children.
- **Age:** Older age people are more prone to develop obesity. As age increases, physical activity decreases which leads to higher risk of obesity and overweight. Children and adolescents who are overweight/obese have a higher risk of remaining obese in adulthood.
- **Gender:** Obesity is more common among females than males. This may be due to hormonal changes, weight gain during pregnancy and difference in physical activity level.
- **Marital status:** People who are married have higher probability of obesity than unmarried and single.
- **Geographical distribution:** People in Europe, the United States of America, and Australia have a higher probability of developing obesity. Also, those who are residing in Atlantic Provinces are at higher risk.
- **Physical inactivity:** Individuals who have sedentary lifestyle due to behavior or any other reason like work profile tend to develop obesity.
- **Education:** Less educated people have higher probability of developing obesity than those who are educated.
- **Endocrine disorders:** Some endocrine disorders like Cushing's syndrome, polycystic ovarian disease (PCOD), hypothyroidism, diabetes, etc. are associated with obesity.
- **Psychological state:** Some studies have showed that stress, depression and anxiety are associated with obesity among adults due to increased food consumption during such states. Excess food intake provides a nonspecific sense of stress relief and escape from intolerable circumstances.
- **Genetics:** Some genetic disorders or chromosomal abnormalities in genes cause obesity in children. One of the most well-known forms of syndromic obesity is Prader-

Willi syndrome (PWS), which is caused by a chromosomal abnormality.
- **Lifestyle:** Habits like binge eating, sedentary lifestyle, liking for fast foods, etc. play a major role in obesity. Snacking habit of packaged food items like chips, burgers, noodles, etc. also contributes to calorie intake, and thus risk of developing obesity.
- **Breastfeeding:** Children who are fed formula milk instead of breast milk are more prone to develop obesity than breastfed babies.
- **Socioeconomic status:** People in higher socioeconomic strata have higher rates of obesity than in lower strata.

*Environment*
- **Seasonal variation:** People tend to eat more during winters than summers due to increased consumption of calories to maintain body temperature.
- **Food economics:** Availability of fast foods items which are affordable and ready to eat also has an impact on obesity development in the population.
- **Social factors:** Meal patterns are socially affected. In India, urban communities are more prone to consuming easily accessible junk food.
- **Marketing factors:** Intense marketing of fast food items using mass media, print media and use of celebrities for publicity also impact eating habits among the population, most vulnerable being children and adolescents.
- **Physical environment:** The physical infrastructure surrounding the people has a direct impact on the lifestyle practices. Urban spaces with no cycling or walking tracks, no parks restrict the physical activity of the people living in that environment.

### Assessment of Obesity

There are different methods of measuring obesity. Ideal measure is by estimating body fat. Most common measures are weight-for-height, BMI, waist circumference, waist-hip ratio (WHR), skinfold thickness. Most commonly, it is expressed in terms of BMI.
- **Body mass index** (Quetelet index) = Weight (kg)/Height (in meter)
- **Ponderal index** = Height (cm)/Cube root of body weight (kg)
- **Broca index** = Height (cm) minus 100
- **Corpulence index** = Actual weight/Desirable weight. This should not exceed 1.2
- **Waist-hip ratio:** Greater than 1.0 in male and greater than 0.85 in female are considered as abdominal fat accumulation.

Body mass index is the standard measure used to diagnose overweight and obesity in adults requiring measurement of weight and height. Adults with BMI measures greater than 30 are considered obese, while those with BMI measures greater than 25 are classified as overweight as given in **Table 23.4**.

Body mass index provides a useful measure of overweight and obesity at the individual and population level as it is the same for both genders, and all ages for adults. However, it is not considered as an absolute indicator from a clinical point of view as different individuals may have different fat content.

**Table 23.4:** Classification of obesity.

| Classification | International (WHO standards) | Asian population (proposed by Asia Pacific report—WHO, IASO, IOTF 2000) | Remarks |
|---|---|---|---|
| Underweight | <18.5 | <18.5 | WHO has retained international classification, but their expert consultation identified further potential public health action points (23.0, 27.5, 32.5, and 37.5) for Asian population |
| Normal BMI | 18.5–24.9 | 18.5–22.9 | |
| Overweight | ≥25.0 | ≥23.0 | |
| Pre-obese (at risk) | 25.0–29.9 | 23.0–24.9 | |
| Obesity grade I | 30.0–34.9 | 25.0–29.9 | |
| Obesity grade II | 35.0–39.9 | ≥30.0 | |
| Obesity grade III | ≥40.0 | | |

In children, age is considered while defining overweight and obesity.

For children under-five years of age:
- Overweight is weight-for-height greater than 2 standard deviations above the WHO Child Growth Standards median
- Obesity is defined as weight-for-height greater than 3 standard deviations above the WHO Child Growth Standards median.

Overweight and obesity are defined as follows for children aged between 5 years and 19 years:
- Overweight is BMI-for-age greater than 1 standard deviation above the WHO Growth Reference median.
- Obesity is defined as greater than 2 standard deviations above the WHO Growth Reference median.

### Consequences of Obesity

Being overweight or obese (indicated by a raised BMI) is a major risk factor for NCDs like cardiovascular diseases (heart disease and stroke), musculoskeletal disorders especially osteoarthritis of joints (commonly knee joints), and some cancers (endometrial, ovarian, breast, prostate, liver, gallbladder, kidney and colon).

Obesity is a morbid profile, with consequential limited ability for physical activity and thus a vicious cycle of poor lifestyle measures. Obesity early in onset (childhood obesity) is seen to be associated with greater incidence of premature deaths and disabilities in adulthood. Obese children are more prone to breathing difficulties, higher risk of fractures, hypertension, insulin resistance, and even psychological effects like depression.

### Prevention and Control of Obesity

Prevention of obesity is the key solution at community level. It is largely preventable and creating enabling and supportive environments in the communities would have the greatest impact. Healthier food choices, encouraging regular physical activity right from school level would definitely shape and influence long-term behavior. Health education measures including advice on limiting intake of total fat and sugars, following a balanced diet, avoiding so-called junk food, increasing consumption of good quality fruits and vegetables including whole grains, nuts and legumes are important at the individual level.

Encouraging healthy habits, including regular physical exercise and discouraging unhealthy choices like sweetened beverages, processed high calorie foods, etc. is very important. Policy level decisions like higher taxes on sugar sweetened beverages and foods, policy and guidelines for nutrition content of foods manufactured, restriction of marketing of unhealthy food items specifically targeting children and adolescents are other measures. Recent evidence has shown presence of Bisphenol A (BPA) in plastics being used to store or carry food has been associated with increased risk of insulin resistance and obesity. Bisphenol is a suspected endocrine disrupter and use of BPA-free plastics is advisable.

Any obesity that may have a medical basis, should be referred to an appropriate Physician/Diabetologist/Endocrinologist for an evaluation and management of underlying cause. These referrals may include suspected diabetes, thyroid disease (hypothyroidism), Cushing's disease, PCOD, etc. Suspicion should be more in individuals with a typical clinical history or a strong family history of such conditions.

The WHO has developed a "Global Action Plan for the Prevention and Control of NCDs 2013–2020". It intends to achieve the commitments of the UN Political Declaration on NCDs which was endorsed by Heads of State and Government in September 2011. The "Global Action Plan" will contribute to progress on 9 global NCD targets to be attained by 2025, including a 25% relative reduction in premature mortality from NCDs by 2025 and a halt in the rise of global obesity to match the rates of 2010.

# MICRONUTRIENT DEFICIENCIES

## Iron Deficiency Anemia

Iron deficiency is one of the most common forms of malnutrition across the globe. Iron deficiency anemia results from inadequate amount of red blood cells caused by lack of iron. It is defined by low hemoglobin or hematocrit, and is commonly used to assess the severity of iron deficiency in a population **(Table 23.5)**.

**Table 23.5:** Hemoglobin levels (g/dL) to diagnose anemia at sea level (Guidelines for control of iron deficiency anemia, MoHFW).

| Population, age | No anemia | Mild | Moderate | Severe |
|---|---|---|---|---|
| Children, 6–59 months | ≥11.0 | 10.0–10.9 | 7.0–9.9 | <7.0 |
| Children, 5–11 years | ≥11.5 | 11.0–11.4 | 8.0–10.9 | <8.0 |
| Children, 12–14 years | ≥12.0 | 11.0–11.9 | 8.0–10.9 | <8.0 |
| Nonpregnant women, 15 years and above | ≥12.0 | 11.0–11.9 | 8.0–10.9 | <8.0 |
| Pregnant women | ≥11.0 | 10.0–10.9 | 7.0–9.9 | <7.0 |
| Men, 15 years and above | ≥13.0 | 11.0–12.9 | 8.0–10.9 | <8.0 |

## Functions of Iron

As part of myoglobin and hemoglobin, it is required for storage and transport of oxygen from lungs to tissues. Iron is used as a cofactor in deoxyribonucleic acid (DNA) synthesis and repair. Its role as an electron acceptor/donor as a component of cytochromes is vital for energy reduction and detoxification of endogenous metabolites, drugs and toxins.

## Iron Absorption

Dietary iron mainly exists in the form of "heme" and "nonheme". Heme iron is found in meat, seafood and poultry and has a better bioavailability as compared to nonheme iron which is mainly found in foods of plant origin, e.g., amaranth, spinach, turmeric, whole Bengal gram, bajra, etc. The absorption of iron occurs in the duodenal and proximal jejunum and depends on the state of iron atom, presence of inhibitors and promoters in the diet and disorders of duodenum and jejunum like celiac disease and tropical sprue. The absorbable form of iron is "ferrous" state or when it is bound by a protein such as heme. Certain dietary compounds that inhibit dietary absorption of iron are phytates (found in plant-based diets), polyphenols (present in black and herbal tea, coffee, wine, legumes, cereals, fruit and vegetables), calcium, animal protein (casein, whey, egg whites), soy protein and oxalic acid (in spinach, beans and nuts). Ascorbic acid increases the dietary absorption of iron by overcoming the effects of all dietary inhibitors.

Iron is required among all age groups across both genders for behavioral and cognitive development and better child survival. Iron deficiency results in low birth weight, perinatal mortality, maternal mortality, obstetric complications, poor work capacity, poor cognition, etc.

## Problem Statement

In 2019, global anaemia prevalence was 29.9% in women of reproductive age, equivalent to over half a billion women aged 15–49 years. Prevalence was 29.6% in non-pregnant women of reproductive age, and 36.5% in pregnant women. In 2019, global anaemia prevalence was 39.8% in children aged 6–59 months, equivalent to 269 million children with anaemia. The prevalence of anaemia in children under five was highest in the African Region, 60.2% (WHO Global Anaemia estimates, 2021 Edition).

India has a very high prevalence of anemia with nutritional anemia being a major public health problem in India. According to NFHS-5, anemia is prevalent among both men and women across all age groups. Approximately 57.2% non-pregnant women and 52.2% of pregnant women were found to be anemic (<12.0 g/dL). In addition, 25% men were found to be anemic. Among under-five children, prevalence of anemia was found to be 67.1%. To make matters worse, only 44.1% antenatal women had reportedly consumed iron-folic acid for 100 days or more while they were pregnant.

## Factors

Anemia develops through three main mechanisms: (1) ineffective erythropoiesis, (2) hemolysis and (3) blood loss. Nutritional anemia is one of the most important contributors to anemia and iron deficiency being the most important cause of the same, which results due to following factors:

- ***Increased requirement***: The requirement of iron increases in certain physiologic and metabolic states, e.g., during pregnancy (owing to expanded blood volume), lactation and menstruation (increased blood loss), and among vulnerable groups like infants, children and adolescents (growth spurts). Adolescent girls are particularly vulnerable owing to an

increased demand of iron for growth as well as an increased loss due to menstruation, which is further exacerbated if an adolescent female becomes pregnant.
- ***Decreased intake***: Decreased intake due to low socioeconomic status, poor dietary practices, consumption of monotonous diet with no or lack of dietary diversification often results in iron deficiency.
- ***Decreased absorption and utilization***: Poor dietary practices including overcooking of food, food handling and eating practices which result in loss of micronutrients, presence of dietary factors like tannins, phytates and divalent ions in tea, coffee, carbonated drinks, fiber and milk may result in poor absorption and utilization of iron.
- ***Increased loss***: Presence of comorbidities like malaria, schistosomiasis, hookworm infestation, menorrhagia, chronic gastritis, celiac disease, Crohn's disease, duodenal pathology, etc. predisposes individuals to an increased risk of developing anemia.

Various high-risk groups which are particularly vulnerable to iron deficiency anemia are:
- Children especially under-five children
- Pregnant women
- Adolescent girls
- Elderly (>60 years).

### Clinicopathologic Picture

The classic symptoms are conjunctival or palmar pallor, fatigue, headache, dyspnea, etc.; however, in severe cases, skin and hair may become dry, rough and damaged, alopecia, koilonychia or atrophic glossitis. It has a negative effect on physical performance, especially on work productivity, endurance and energetic efficiency. Iron deficiency during neurogenesis in infancy may result in poor motor development and cognition among children resulting in low productivity later in life. Anemia is an important predictor for maternal and perinatal mortality and is often associated with poor birth outcomes like prematurity and low birth weight. Among elderly, anemia is associated with muscle weakness, impairment of executive functions, dementia, increased risk of falls, disability and hospitalizations.

### Prevention and Control

- ***Promotion of infant and young child feeding (IYCF) practices***: Promotion of IYCF practices including exclusive breastfeeding at birth can prevent iron deficiency. Iron stores at birth are usually adequate until 4–6 months of age, except in low birth weight and premature infants, who require iron supplements in the first 6 months. Exclusive breastfeeding for 6 months takes care of the iron requirement owing to its higher bioavailability in breast milk. This coupled with adequate, appropriate and timely introduction of complementary feeding.
- ***Dietary practices***: Improved dietary practices including cooking, food handling and consumption of a balanced diet with emphasis on locally available iron-rich foods go a long way in preventing iron deficiency.
- ***Proxy markers of malnutrition***: Improved hygiene and sanitation, including hand washing practices and addressing comorbidities like malaria, schistosomiasis, hookworm infestation, etc., which result in decreased absorption and increased loss of iron, can go a long way in preventing iron deficiency from setting in.
- ***Increasing awareness and correct knowledge*** among caregivers such as auxiliary nurse midwife (ANM), accredited social health activists (ASHAs), AWWs, teachers, peer educators, parents and adolescents in order to address the issue of iron deficiency anemia among adolescent boys and girls as part of AFHSs under Rashtriya Kishor Swasthya Karyakram (RKSK).

Besides this, various other steps have been taken by the government of India to address the problem of iron deficiency anemia like food fortification, National Iron-plus Initiative, biannual deworming, etc.

- ***Iron supplementation***: In order to address management of anemia across various life stages and at different levels of care "*National Iron-plus Initiative*" was launched wherein the following groups are covered for supplementation of iron and folic acid:
  1. **6–59 months**: Biweekly 20 mg of elemental iron and 100 µg folic acid for 100 days in 1 year. This is usually administered as liquid formulation. Age-appropriate deworming using albendazole tablets wherein a dose of 200 mg is given to children between 1 year and 2 years of age and 400 mg is given to children aged 2 years and above.
  Iron-folic acid syrup shall be administered twice every week on fixed days under direct supervision of ANM/ASHA, after ruling out severe acute malnutrition (SAM).
  2. **6–10 years**: 45 mg elemental iron and 400 µg folic acid is given once every week to children studying in 1st to 5th grade in government and government-aided schools. For out of school children (including dropouts and those who are not enrolled in schools), the same is administered through Anganwadi centers.
  3. **10–19 years**: Under weekly Iron-Folic Acid Supplementation (WIFS), 100 mg elemental iron and 500 µg folic acid is given to adolescents once every week along with biannual deworming, in school through teachers and at Anganwadi centers for school dropouts.
  4. Iron supplementation for women in reproductive age group, pregnant women and lactating mothers.
- ***Deworming***: Biannual deworming is done among 1–19 years old children at all schools and Anganwadi centers using chewable tablet to address iron deficiency caused by hookworm infestation. In addition, spreading awareness about general cleanliness and personal hygiene, importance of footwear, avoiding open defecation, hand washing before eating and after using toilet, properly washing fruits and vegetables with clean water before consumption are some other ways to prevent worm infestation and subsequent iron deficiency anemia.
- ***Food fortification***: Double-fortified salt (DFS) has been introduced in mid-day meal (MDM) and Integrated Child

Development Services (ICDS) program, wherein ferrous sulfate and ferrous fumarate is used along with a stabilizer to prevent reaction between iodine and iron.

Fortification of wheat flour with iron (NaFeEDTA), folic acid, zinc, vitamin B has been attempted in States of Madhya Pradesh, Gujarat, Mumbai and Haryana to assess feasibility, cost implications and logistical issues before introducing the same in ICDS, MDM and PDS in future.

States of Karnataka and Odisha (formerly Orissa) have introduced fortified rice with iron, folic acid, zinc, vitamins A and B fortification through pilots in their MDM programs and other States like Gujarat, Haryana, Tripura, Maharashtra, Chandigarh, Dadra and Nagar Haveli shall follow soon.

Classification of anemia as a problem of public health significance has been shown in **Table 23.6**.

**Table 23.6:** Classification of anemia as a problem of public health significance.

| Prevalence of anemia (%) | Category of public health significance |
|---|---|
| ≤4.9 | No public health problem |
| 5.0–19.9 | Mild public health problem |
| 20.0–39.9 | Moderate public health problem |
| ≥40 | Severe public health problem |

Various positive initiatives that have been taken to address the issue of iron deficiency anemia across all age groups are as follows:

1. Administration of iron and folic acid (iron ki "neeli goli") once weekly to 6–19 years old children in school and to dropouts in Anganwadi centers. This is being done under WIFS.
2. Iron supplementation to antenatal women in prophylactic or therapeutic doses as advisable.
3. Biannual deworming among children aged 1–19 years to address hookworm infestation.
4. Use of double fortified salt (DFS) in preparation of MDM and food served under ICDS programs.
5. Dietary supplementation at Anganwadi centers under ICDS to antenatal women and children between 6 months and 6 years of age to address micronutrient malnutrition.

### Vitamin A Deficiency

Vitamin A is an essential nutrient needed in small amounts for normal functioning of visual system, for growth and development, maintenance of epithelial integrity, immune function, and reproduction. It is essential for somatic function, which encompasses growth, development and differentiation of epithelial structures and bone. It is essential for spermatogenesis, oogenesis, placental development, fetal and embryonic growth. Retinol is essential for formation of rhodopsin by the rods, which are responsible for vision in dark. Vitamin A also has anti-infective properties.

#### Problem Statement

Vitamin A deficiency (VAD) is one of the leading causes of preventable childhood blindness. Globally about 30% of under-five children are vitamin A deficient (WHO, Global Prevalence of Vitamin A Deficiency in Population at Risk 1995–2005, 2009) and about 2% of all deaths are attributable to VAD in this age group (Stevens GA et al., Lancet Global Health, 2015). Southeast Asia had the highest burden of VAD among preschool children wherein 91.5 million preschool children in Southeast Asia were found to have serum retinol concentrations less than 0.70 µmol/L and 82.4% reported night blindness **(Fig. 23.3)**. The most recent nationally representative data is from a survey done by National

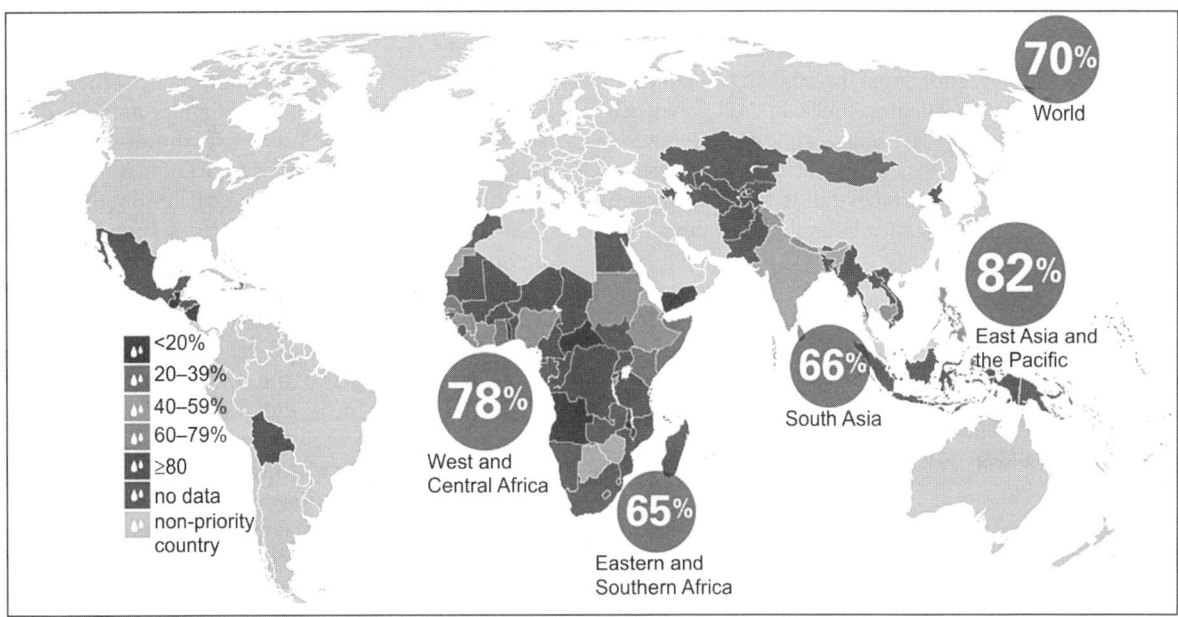

**Fig. 23.3:** Prevalence of vitamin A deficiency, global.
*Source:* UNICEF global nutrition database, 2017, based on administrative reports from countries for 2015.

Nutrition Monitoring Bureau (NNMB) in eight States, wherein prevalence of Bitot's spots among rural preschool children, from eight States, was found to be 0.8%, prevalence of blood VAD [serum retinol < 0.70 μmol/L was 61% (52–88%) and that of severe blood VAD (<10 μg/dL)] was 21.5% in all these States (NNMB, VAD Final Report, 2006).

### Sources

Vitamin A or retinol, found in animal foods such as liver, egg yolk, fish, meat and dairy products like butter, cheese, whole milk, is a fat soluble vitamin. Beta-carotene, provitamin A precursor is present in green leafy vegetables, yellow fruits like papaya, mango, pumpkin, etc., is biologically less active than retinol. Vitamin A is stored in liver, which forms an important buffer during lean periods of vitamin A intake.

Recommended dietary allowances or retinol in various age groups [Indian Council of Medical research (ICMR)] have been shown in **Table 23.7**.

**Table 23.7:** Recommended dietary allowances (ICMR–2020 guideline).

| Group | | Retinol (μg) |
|---|---|---|
| Infants | 0–6 months | 350 |
| | 6–12 months | 350 |
| Children | 1–6 years | 390–510 |
| | 7–9 years | 630 |
| Adolescents | 10–17 years | 770–1000 |
| Adults | Man | 1000 |
| | Woman | 840 |
| | Pregnancy | 900 |
| | Lactation | 950 |

### Deficiency

Vitamin A deficiency is a systemic disease that affects cells and organs throughout the body and causes "keratinizing metaplasia" of respiratory, urinary and intestinal epithelia. In VAD, goblet cell numbers are reduced in epithelial tissues resulting in reduction of mucus secretion leading to loss of antimicrobial properties. Cells lining protective tissue surfaces fail to regenerate and differentiate. These changes precede ocular manifestations, but remain largely undetectable.

Gradual depletion of vitamin A stores results in xerophthalmia, which may manifest as night blindness, conjunctival xerosis, Bitot's spots, corneal xerosis, ulceration, scarring and keratomalacia **(Tables 23.8 to 23.10)**.

**Table 23.8:** Classification of xerophthalmia.

| XN | Night blindness |
|---|---|
| X1A | Conjunctival xerosis |
| X1B | Bitot's spots |
| X2 | Corneal xerosis |
| X3A | Corneal ulceration/keratomalacia < 1/3rd corneal surface |
| X3B | Corneal ulceration/keratomalacia ≥ 1/3rd corneal surface |
| XS | Corneal scar |
| XF | Xerophthalmic fundus |

**Table 23.9:** Indicators of vitamin A deficiency.

| Criteria | Group | Public health importance | | |
|---|---|---|---|---|
| | | Mild | Moderate | Severe |
| Night blindness | Children (24–71 months of age) | <1% | 1–5% | ≥5% |
| | Pregnant women[a] | ≥5% | | |
| Serum/plasma retinol <0.70 μmol/L | Preschool[b] children/ pregnant women[c] | ≥2–<10% | ≥10–<20% | ≥20% |

[a]Based on history of night blindness during a woman's most recent pregnancy in the previous 3–5 years that ended in a live birth.
[b]6–71 months of age.
[c]The cut-off used here is similar to that used for children.

**Table 23.10:** Prevalence criteria for determining the public health significance of spectrum of vitamin A deficiency in children aged 6 months to 6 years.

| Indicator | Minimum prevalence, % |
|---|---|
| Night blindness (XN) | >1 |
| Bitot's spots (X1B) | >0.5 |
| Corneal xerosis/corneal ulceration/keratomalacia (X2/X3A/X3B) | >0.01 |
| Corneal scar (XS) | >0.05 |

- **XN—Night blindness**: It is the earliest manifestation of VAD wherein function of "rods" is impaired and affected child is unable to move around the house or neighborhood after dusk and is unable to find their toys or food. It is also known as "chicken eyes". It is difficult to recognize among young children who have not yet begun to crawl.
- **X1A, X1B—Conjunctival xerosis and Bitot's spots**: Vitamin A deficiency results in loss of goblet cells and transformation of conjunctival epithelium to stratified squamous type. As a result, the conjunctiva becomes dry, roughened and corrugated with fine droplets or bubbles on the surface and appears like "sandbanks at receding tide". Conjunctival xerosis appears as a whitish yellow triangular patch and is usually seen in both the eyes. It is most commonly located in the temporal bulbar conjunctiva adjacent to the limbus.
  Further changes over the area of conjunctival xerosis can lead to the development of "Bitot's spots". The proposed pathogenesis of these lesions is keratinization of the xerotic conjunctiva and colonization by saprophytic bacilli.
- **X2—Corneal xerosis**: Corneal xerosis is essentially dryness of the cornea. Absence of tear cells is most obviously manifest in the inferonasal part of the cornea as that is the part which is covered last by the eyelids while blinking. This dryness is clinically apparent as punctate white spots over the cornea which stains brightly with fluorescein.
- **X3A, X3B—Corneal ulceration/keratomalacia**: Corneal ulcer is defined as loss of corneal epithelium with or without underlying stromal defect. Xerosis predisposes cornea to infection due to loss of tear film. These infections subsequently penetrate beneath the surface and erode the stromal tissue. Extensive infections can eventually lead to complete erosion of stromal tissue at the site of the ulcer, a condition called "keratomalacia", and lead to corneal perforation. Significant

corneal thinning can also lead to bulging out of the cornea and result in corneal ectasia.
- **XS—Scars**: Healing response at the site of ulceration leads to development of corneal opacity, which is known as corneal scar. Depending on the severity of the opacity, it may be graded as a nebular, macular or leucomatous opacity. Occasionally, the iris becomes adherent to the corneal scar leading to the development of staphyloma. These lesions, however, are not specific for xerophthalmia.

## Causes
- **Demographic features**: It is commonly seen among people with low socioeconomic status, illiterate, poor health seeking behavior and those living in impoverished environment like overcrowded slums, where environmental sanitation and personal hygiene is compromised.
- **Age**: VAD can affect any age group but it primarily affects children of preschool age due to their increased susceptibility to infections coupled with increased bodily requirements of the same.
- **Feeding practices**:
  - Vitamin A deficiency is rare among children who are breastfed as breast milk contains readily absorbable form of retinol.
  - Vitamin A deficiency begins to set in at the time of initiation of complementary feeding among children whose diet is deficient in vitamin A-rich foods.
  - Insufficient intake or dietary deprivation that is usually common in Southern and Eastern Asia where rice, which is devoid of beta-carotene, is the staple food.
- Decreased bioavailability of provitamin A carotenoids such as in fat malabsorption, liver disorders, etc.
- Interference with absorption or storage is likely in celiac disease, cystic fibrosis, pancreatic insufficiency, duodenal bypass, bile duct obstruction. Concomitant intestinal and respiratory infections often result in poor absorption, and utilization of vitamin A thereby predisposing to VAD.

## Prevention and Control
- **Promoting consumption of vitamin A-rich food**
  - Exclusive breastfeeding for 6 months and timely introduction of complementary feeding should be encouraged and ensured. Breastfeeding may be continued for up to 2 years. In addition, care should be taken that colostrum is not discarded and should be given to the neonate.
  - Promote regular consumption of foods rich in vitamin A like green leafy vegetables and yellow and orange vegetables and fruits like papaya, mango, pumpkin, carrots, oranges, dairy products like milk, cheese, paneer, ghee, eggs, liver, etc., by pregnant and lactating mothers and by children under-five years of age.
  - Health education regarding VAD and preventive measures about the same should be given to women and children visiting Anganwadi, antenatal and immunization clinics.
  - They should also be made aware of the importance of dietary diversification in order to prevent micronutrient deficiency.
- **Fortification of edible oil**: Food Safety and Standards Authority of India (FSSAI) recommends fortification of edible oil sold in packaged form for consumption at household level and all toned and double-toned milk should be fortified with vitamin A.
- **Administering supplemental dose of vitamin:** The supplemental dose of vitamin A should be administered to under five children the recommended schedule of which is as shown in **Table 23.11**.

Table 23.11: Administration of vitamin A supplements to under-five children according to recommended schedule.

| Age (in completed months) | Dose of vitamin A (per oral) |
|---|---|
| 9 months | 100,000 IU |
| 18 months | 200,000 IU |
| 24 months | 200,000 IU |
| 30 months | 200,000 IU |
| 36 months | 200,000 IU |
| 42 months | 200,000 IU |
| 48 months | 200,000 IU |
| 54 months | 200,000 IU |
| 60 months | 200,000 IU |

- **Administering measles containing vaccine:** Ocular complications of measles are more likely to occur among vitamin A deficient children. Therefore, it is pivotal to administer two doses of measles containing vaccine to every eligible child.
- **Address concomitant illness** like diarrhea and measles, which can result in VAD, which further worsens the preexisting disease, thereby setting a self-perpetuating cycle into motion.

Vitamin A supplementation to children between 6 months and 59 months of age at every 6 months through universal immunization program and concomitant immunization against measles is being given to under-five children to protect against VAD disorders.

### Iodine Deficiency Disorders

Iodine is an essential micronutrient required for synthesis of thyroid hormones, thyroxine ($T_4$) and tri-iodothyronine ($T_3$) for normal thyroid functioning, growth and development. Insufficient and suboptimal intake results in inadequate production of thyroid hormone collectively termed as iodine deficiency disorders (IDDs).

### Problem Statement

Iodine deficiency poses a major global threat to health and development because it is the most common cause of preventable mental impairment worldwide. Globally, 1.88 billion people are at risk of iodine deficiency. About 241 million school-age children (6–12 years old) have reportedly poor iodine intake, of which nearly 32% (approximately 76 million) live in South East Asia (Andersson M et al., J Nutr, 2012). In India, the most recent sample surveys done in 390 districts across all the States/UTs showed that 333 districts are endemic

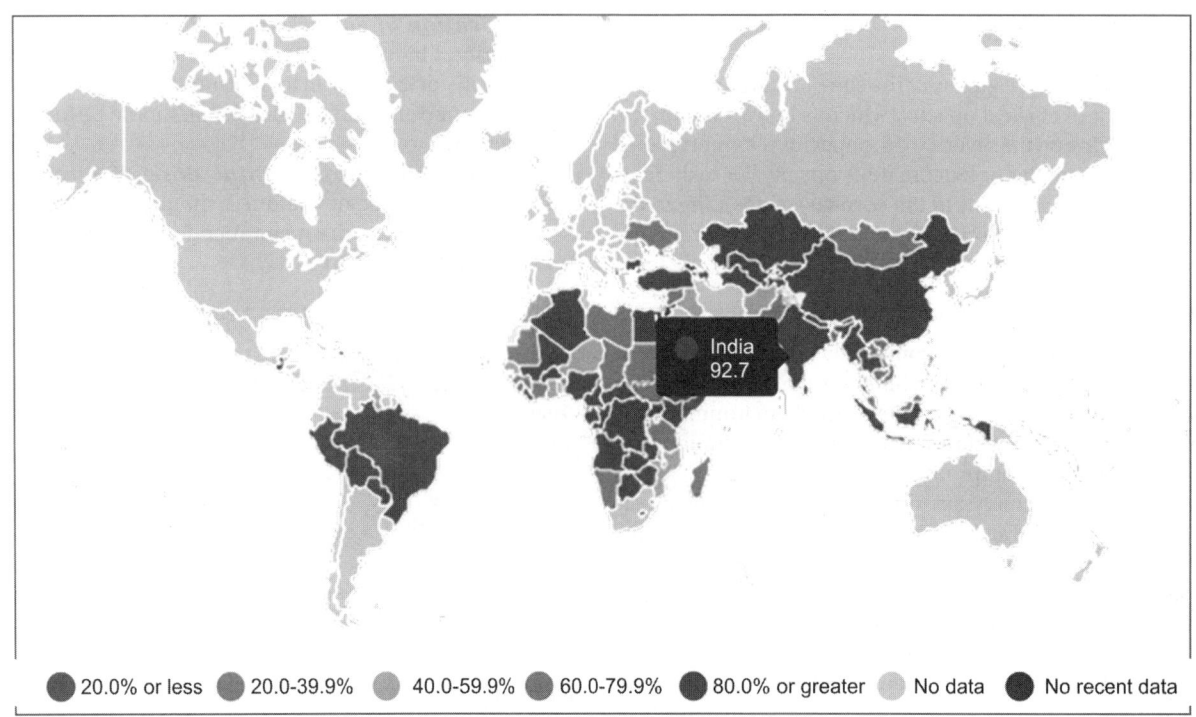

**Fig. 23.4:** Percentage of households consuming salt with any iodine, 2018.

*Source:* Global database, 2018, based on Multiple Indicator Cluster Surveys (MICS), Demographic and Health Surveys (DHS) and other nationally representative surveys, 2011– 2018. [online] Available from UNICEF Data. Monitoring the situation of children and women. https://data.unicef.org/topic/nutrition/iodine-deficiency/#status.

for prevalence of IDDs where the prevalence is more than 5%. It further states that iodine deficiency is not confined to the sub-Himalayan belt and is prevalent across the country with no state/UT being free from IDD **(Fig. 23.4)** (NIDDCP Annual Report, 2016–17).

### *Iodine Requirement*

The average daily requirement of an adult is about 100–150 µg/day. Iodine is normally present in soil and water.

Therefore, the crops grown on iodine-rich soil are sufficient to fulfill the normal requirement, except in iodine deficient areas.

### *Factors*

Iodine deficiency is a multifaceted problem with ecological, socioeconomic and developmental connotation.
- *Ecological factors*: Increasing deforestation, heavy rainfall, melting of glaciers leads to increased flooding and erosion of the topsoil, which washes away the iodine, thereby making the soil and eventually the crop grown in that soil deficient in iodine.
- *Intake and absorption*: Iodine metabolism is adversely affected by insufficient intake of iodine from foods, interaction with possible goitrogens, e.g., cassava, sorghum, sweet potato, cabbage, cauliflower, broccoli, turnip, soy and millets and exposure to cyanogenic compounds. It must, however, be understood that goitrogens are usually active only if iodine supply is limited and/or goitrogen intake is of longer duration.
- *Other factors*: In addition, unregulated use of pesticides, unclean drinking water and exposure to endocrine disruptors and industrial pollutants (like resorcinol and phthalic acid) have also been implicated as potential factors resulting in iodine deficiency.

Deficiency of micronutrients like selenium, iron and vitamin A may also exert goitrogenic effect in areas of iodine deficiency.

### *Clinicopathologic Picture*

Iodine deficiency disorders form a spectrum of abnormalities ranging from goiter, hypothyroidism, impaired mental function, mental retardation, and physical subnormality, myxedematous cretinism, dwarfism, psychomotor defects, deaf mutism, spastic diplegia, squint to abortions, stillbirths, congenital anomalies, increased perinatal and infant mortality, which are completely preventable, but usually not treatable **(Table 23.12)**. Intelligence quotient (IQ) among people living in iodine deficient areas has been found to be lower (by up to 13.5 points) as compared to those living in iodine sufficient areas.

Iodine deficiency among pregnant women, especially during first and second trimester, may adversely impact fetal and perinatal outcomes including thyroid function and neurogenic development.

**Table 23.12:** The spectrum of iodine deficiency disorders (IDD).

| Physiological groups | Health consequences of iodine deficiency |
|---|---|
| All ages | Goiter hypothyroidism<br>Increased susceptibility to nuclear radiation |
| Fetus | Spontaneous abortion<br>Stillbirth<br>Congenital anomalies<br>Perinatal mortality |
| Neonate | Endemic cretinism including mental deficiency with a mixture of mutism, spastic diplegia, squint, hypothyroidism and short stature, infant mortality |

*Contd...*

*Contd...*

| Physiological groups | Health consequences of iodine deficiency |
|---|---|
| Child and adolescent | Goiter<br>Impaired mental function, delayed physical development<br>Iodine-induced hyperthyroidism |
| Adults | Goiter hypothyroidism<br>Impaired mental function<br>Iodine-induced hyperthyroidism |

*Source*: Hetzel BS. Iodine deficiency disorders (IDD) and their eradication. Lancet. 1983;2:1126-9.

### Prevention and Control

- Due to near-universal penetration of "salt", the most preferred strategy for control of IDD remains universal iodization of "salt". But higher salt intake has been implicated in the pathogenesis of cardiovascular diseases. Therefore, an "Expert Consultation in 2007 on salt as a vehicle for fortification" concluded that policies for universal iodization of salt are in coherence with that for prevention of cardiovascular diseases. Under the Prevention of Food Adulteration Act 1954, sale of non-iodized salt has been banned by the Government of India since 17th May 2006. As a result consumption of non-iodized salt has come down to 9%. In addition, 71% population has access to iodized salt, as reflected by the survey conducted by the United Nations International Children's Emergency Fund (UNICEF) and Ministry of Health and Family Welfare. The recommended adult requirement of iodine is 150 μg/person/day. Common salt is fortified with potassium iodate with iodine content of salt being 30 ppm at production and 15 ppm at consumption levels.
- In order to provide access of iodized salt to below the poverty line (BPL) population, Salt Commissionerate has coordinated with State Food and Civil Supplies Commissionerates in various states to distribute iodized salt under PDS at reasonable rates.
- In addition, DFS (iron + iodine) to be used in the preparation of MDM.
- Iodized oil injections have also been used to correct iodine deficiency among pregnant and lactating women in Papua New Guinea, Latin America, Africa and some parts of Asia.

### Community Assessment of Iodine Status

Urinary iodine excretion (UIE), a well-accepted, operationally feasible and sensitive biochemical indicator, is used to assess status of iodine at population level. Ideally 24-hour urine collection should be done to account for individual and day to day variability, but because of operational feasibility spot samples are taken. Besides this, WHO has prescribed a set of epidemiological indicators for classifying IDDs as significant public health problem, which includes goiter grade, thyroid volume, serum thyroid-stimulating hormone (TSH) and serum thyroglobulin (Tg) **(Table 23.13)**.

Neck inspection and palpation, done as part of goiter surveys, is used to describe goiter grade. To assess goiter, volume of lateral lobe is compared to the terminal phalanx of the subject under investigation. If the volume of each lateral lobe is greater than the phalanx being compared thyroid gland is labeled as goitrous.

According to the WHO, goiter is classified into three grades upon local physical examination which is as follows:
- *Grade 0*: Thyroid that is neither palpable nor visible
- *Grade 1*: Goiter that is palpable but not visible. Examination is done with neck held in normal position
- *Grade 2*: Thyroid that is clearly visible with neck held in normal position.

In addition, volume of thyroid is measured using ultrasonography.

**Table 23.13:** Epidemiological criteria for assessing the severity of iodine deficiency disorders.

| Indicator | Target population | Severity of public health problem | | |
|---|---|---|---|---|
| | | Mild | Moderate | Severe |
| Goiter grade[a] >0 | SAC (6–12) | 5–19.9% | 20–29.9% | ≥30% |
| Median UIE[b] (μg/L) | SAC | 50–99 | 20–49 | <20 |
| Thyroid volume[c] (>97th centile) by USG | SAC | 5–19.9% | 20–29.9% | ≥30% |
| TSH[d] > 5 mU/L | Neonates | 10–19.9% | 20–39.9% | ≥40% |
| Median Tg[e] ng/mL serum | C/A | 10–19.9% | 20–39.9% | ≥40% |

[a]A thyroid gland is considered goitrous when each lateral lobe has a volume greater than the terminal phalanx of the thumbs of the subject being examined.
[b]Median UIE is used because it is not normally distributed.
[c]It is taken as a function of age, gender and body surface area.
[d]TSH levels are increased in iodine deficient population in first few weeks of life, which is known as transient thyrotropinemia, owing to increased iodine turnover due to iodine deficiency.
[e]Serum thyroglobulin levels reflect iodine nutrition over a period of months or years, which is increased in thyroid hyperplasia and goiter.

(SAC: school-age children; C/A: children and adults; UIE: urinary iodine excretion; USG: ultrasonography; TSH: thyroid-stimulating hormone)

Thyroid-stimulating hormone serves as a sensitive indicator of iodine levels among newborns. In the first few weeks of life, iodine deficient infants have raised serum TSH concentrations, which are known as transient newborn hypothyroidism or hyperthyrotropinemia, owing to increased iodine turnover due to iodine deficiency.

Levels of serum Tg indicate iodine balance in the body over the last few months or years, which is increased in thyroid hyperplasia and goiter.

Under the National Iodine Deficiency Disorder Control Programme (NIDDCP), efforts are being made to increase the uptake of adequately iodated salt at household level to 100% in order to bring down the prevalence of IDD to below 5% in the country. For successful implementation of the same, surveys have been conducted to assess the magnitude of IDD in various districts. In addition, extensive information, education and communication (IEC) activities have been conducted to create awareness about effects of using iodized salt.

## ASSESSMENT OF COMMUNITY NUTRITIONAL STATUS

### Nutritional Assessment

It is a systematic way to establish nutritional status of an individual after objectively measuring the energy-requirements.

An appropriate nutritional assessment done with objective parameters in relation to specific health indications helps to prepare an adequate nutritional management for the patient. The purpose of nutritional assessment is to understand the distribution and geography of nutritional disorders in an area. It helps to identify individuals or population groups who are at-risk of becoming malnourished, or are actually malnourished. Also, it will determine other epidemiological factors responsible or associated with nutritional deficiencies. All this will guide to develop health care programs to meet the community needs regarding prevention of malnourishment. It is also useful to measure the effectiveness and impact of the nutritional programs and interventions.

## Methods of Nutritional Assessment

There are two types of methods to assess nutrition: (1) direct and (2) indirect. Direct methods deals with the individual and are based on objective criteria. Indirect methods are based on use of community health indices which reflect nutritional influences **(Flowchart 23.2)**.

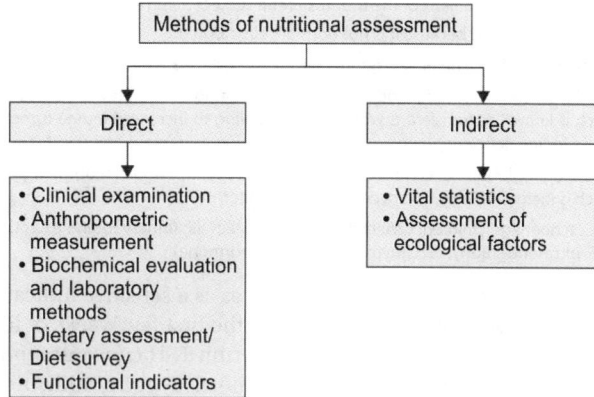

Flowchart 23.2: Methods of nutritional assessment.

### Direct methods

- **Clinical examination**: It is a very important part of all nutritional surveys. It is considered as the simplest and most practical method of determining nutritional status of an individual or a group of individuals. A number of physical signs that are known to be associated with malnutrition are assessed in this method which is observed during clinical examination. A thorough clinical examination is done with special attention to hair, angles of the mouth, gums, nails, skin, eyes, tongue, muscles, bones and thyroid gland where signs of nutritional deficiency or excess are most commonly present. Presence of relevant signs helps in establishing the nutritional diagnosis. If a community physician is well trained, it is rapid, easy to perform, inexpensive and noninvasive method. The disadvantages are that it may not detect early cases, malnutrition cannot be quantified, and many deficiencies can be missed if they are unaccompanied by physical signs.

Clinical signs are classified into three categories.

1. **Signs not related to nutrition**: Signs that have no nutritional significance, e.g. pterygium.
2. **Signs that need further investigation**: They are of probable nutritional significance, e.g., corneal vascularization.
3. **Signs known to be of value**: These signs are nutritionally significant and strongly suggest dietary deficiency or excess like Bitot's spots.

- *Anthropometric methods*: Anthropometry is the measurements of body height, weight and calculating related proportions. It is a crucial component of clinical examination of infants, children and pregnant women. It is used to evaluate both undernutrition and overnutrition. The commonly used methods are body weight, height, crown-heel length, and mid-upper arm circumference. Head and chest circumference are also commonly measured in children less than 5 years of age. Other anthropometric measurements are skinfold thickness, WHR and waist circumference.

**Common measurements:**
- *Height*: The person stands erect and bare footed on a stadiometer which is fixed with a movable headpiece. The headpiece is leveled with vault of skull and height is recorded to the nearest 0.5 cm. There are disadvantages of taking height as a measure of nutritional status because it does not indicate present nutritional status of the individual since height of the individual is affected only in long-term illness or deficiency and remains unaffected in acute stages.
- *Body weight* is the most commonly used anthropometric measure for the evaluation of nutritional status of an individual. A calibrated electronic or balanced-beam scale is used to measure weight. Weight should be taken in minimal clothing with no shoes.

**Anthropometric indicators:**
- Weight-for-age (%) = (Weight of child/Weight of "normal child" of same age) × 100
- Weight-for-height = (Weight of child/Weight of "normal child" of same height) ×100

Weight-for-height classification does not take age into consideration, i.e. it is an age independent parameter.

When weight-for-height is less than 80% of normal, it indicates wasting.
- *Body mass index:* The internationally accepted standard for assessing body size in adults is the BMI. It is computed using the following formula:

$$BMI = Weight\ (kg)/Height\ (m^2)$$

High BMI is associated with type 2 diabetes mellitus and is associated with high risk of cardiovascular morbidity and mortality.

Anthropometry is objective and easy method of nutritional assessment. Readings are also reproducible. It is inexpensive and needs minimal training. Anthropometry has some limitations like interobserver's errors in measurement, difficulties with reference standards, i.e. local versus international standards and different statistical cut-off levels.

- ***Biochemical evaluation and laboratory assessment***: These are investigations done in laboratories like hemoglobin estimation, stool examination for the presence of ova or cyst for intestinal parasites and urine examination for albumin and sugar. Measurements of individual nutrients in body fluids, e.g., serum iron, vitamin D, $B_{12}$ levels are also included in this method. They are useful in detecting early changes in body metabolism and nutritional status. They may appear before overt clinical signs. If the tests are performed correctly using calibrated machines, it will give precise, accurate and reproducible results. It is usually used to validate data obtained from clinical examination. However, it is time consuming, expensive and needs trained personnel and facilities.
- ***Functional indicators***: These are investigations which measure the functionality of the body cells or tissues. They can help deduce the possible deficiency state like vitamin E and selenium deficiency causing erythrocyte fragility, vitamin K deficiency leads to increased prothrombin time, vitamin $B_{12}$ can affect nerve conduction, etc.
- ***Dietary assessment***: Dietary assessment is the best approach for identifying nutrients which are consumed in lesser amount or in excess by an individual or group of individuals. Assessment of nutritional intake of an individual, family or a population is important to have an idea about existing pattern of dietary habits and deficiencies prevalent among the population, especially vulnerable groups like pregnant and lactating women, under-five children and adolescents. With different regions or populations having varying food habits, dietary assessment becomes a challenging task. Currently, there are no single "gold standard" method of dietary assessment. All available methods differ in their reliability, accuracy, costs, participant burden, and susceptibility to bias. However, dietary assessment makes it possible to recognize problems related to eating patterns and constitute a valuable tool for evaluating the best way to deliver the most suitable nutritional education and policy decisions in a country.

Dietary assessment can be done at individual, household, state or national level by detailed history taking, computerized dietary assessment and by chemical analysis of food eaten. Assessment method will depend on requirement of data like dietary patterns, nutritional status, behaviors, adequacy of macronutrient and micronutrient intakes, or the effects of an intervention on dietary intakes and/or nutritional status.

**Dietary assessment methods at individual level (Table 23.14):**

**Table 23.14:** Comparison of dietary assessment techniques.

| Instrument | Advantages | Disadvantages |
|---|---|---|
| 24-hour dietary recall | Intake is quantified<br>Less bias for nonresponse<br>Low burden on respondent<br>No effect on eating behavior | High cost<br>Time consuming<br>Intake is underreported due to varying factors |
| Food record | Intake is quantified<br>Could affect and increase self-monitoring of dietary intake among individuals<br>No recall bias | High cost<br>Respondent burden<br>Extensive training and motivation of respondent needed<br>Time consuming |

*Contd...*

*Contd...*

| Instrument | Advantages | Disadvantages |
|---|---|---|
| Diet history | Easy for respondent to report "usual" intake<br>Low cost<br>No effect on dietary behavior | Imprecise method<br>Difficult task for respondent, intake may be misreported |
| Food frequency questionnaire | Usual individual intake is assessed<br>Low cost<br>No effect on dietary behavior | Imprecise<br>Difficult for respondent<br>Intake may be misreported |

- *24-hour recall technique*: It is asking the food intake of the individual in the last 24 hours by dietitian or a trained interviewer. Sometimes it is repeated at different days of the week and seasons to get a complete picture of dietary behavior and remove bias arising from day-to-day variation. It is critical for evaluation of usual intake especially in populations with a varied diet. However, it could be more useful in non-industrialized countries where the diet is simpler. Strengths of this method include low respondent burden, suitability for large scale surveys and ease of administration even by telephone. Limitations of this method are its dependence on memory, difficulty in estimating portion sizes, bias since single observation provides very limited information of an individual's intake and tendency of people to hide poor dietary habits.
- *Multiple 24-hour recalls or multiple days of diet records*: Dietary intake is collected for a number of days to be more comprehensive of nutritional preferences. At least 3 days of data is required. Some researchers are of opinion that multiple days of diet records to be a gold standard method for collection of individual dietary data. Seven days of dietary record is considered as a dietary cycle. Strengths include better precision, low burden on respondents and suitability for large scale surveys. Weaknesses are that it is expensive, memory dependent, difficulty in estimating portion sizes, and reluctance of people to reveal poor dietary habits.
- *Food records*: Here, individuals are asked to record all foods which are eaten for usually 3-7 days. Quantification of food is estimated rather than weighed. Quantification of the food intake is done by measuring frequencies of standard portion sizes, estimating weight with household measures, with help of diagrams or photographs or photographic record. Strengths of this method are low respondent burden and memory independent. Weaknesses include misreporting and higher cost associated.
- *Weighed-food records*: In this method, an individual or an investigator weighs each item of food and drink prior to consumption by the individual for a period of 3-7 days. Seven-day weighed food record is taken as the "gold standard". Two investigators should be available for this method—one for taking history and weighing and other to records observations. Strengths of this method include its wide use and precision of portion sizes. Weaknesses are high respondent burden, misreporting, high cost and limited data is provided for food composition.
- *Food frequency questionnaire (FFQ)*: It is frequently used method in Western countries which consists of a list of

food items and a corresponding set of frequencies like daily, three times a week or monthly. It can be interviewer administered or self-completed and is mostly qualitative together with portion sizes history. Some information about quantity can be assessed, however for quantifying calories it is not a valid method. It is easy to conduct, and gives an information about the "food types" consumed in various communities.

- *Video and photographic method*: It is a newer method of dietary assessment. The photography of food items is done either by the individual whose data is being collected or by the study team and supplementing it the FFQ. Strength of this method is that it allows direct visualization of quality of food and there is no need of presence of a person for data collection, but it is not feasible for conducting large surveys and pictures taken are unclear to ascertain accurately, making food contents difficult to identify.

**Dietary assessment among infants and young children**: The above-mentioned dietary assessment methods are suitable for adults. For assessing the dietary assessment of infants and young children in the community, the following indicators are used. These are minimum diet diversity, minimum meal frequency, and minimum adequate diet.

- *Minimum diet diversity*: It is proportion of children aged 6–23.9 months of age who receive foods from four or more food groups.

  *Dietary diversity refers to the child receiving 4+ of the following food groups*:
  - Cereals, roots and tubers
  - Legumes and nuts
  - Dairy products (milk, yogurt, cheese)
  - Meat, fish, poultry, etc.
  - Eggs
  - Vitamin A-rich fruits and vegetables
  - Other fruits and vegetables.

- *Minimum meal frequency*: It is proportion of breastfed and non-breastfed children who are 6–23.9 months of age who receive solid, semisolid, or soft foods or milk feeds the minimum number of times or more.

  *Minimum meal frequency is defined as*:
  - Two times for breastfed infants 6–8 months
  - Three times for breastfed children 9–23 months
  - Four times for non-breastfed children 6–23 months.

- *Minimum adequate diet*: Children who meet both the above-mentioned minimum meal frequency and minimum diet diversity are considered to have minimum adequate diet.

**Dietary assessment at the household level:**

- *Food account method:* An individual in the household keeps a daily record of all food items which are purchased in the household during a given time period, usually 7 days. Those food items which are consumed outside of the home are not counted or if the food is discarded as plate waste, or fed to pets. It gives information about the mean food consumption. Strengths of this method are low respondent burden and inexpensive to use for a larger population survey. Weaknesses are food eaten outside by members are not taken in assessment which may give an incorrect picture of dietary pattern.

- *List-recall method*: Here, an interviewer asks a person in the household to recall all food items utilized by whole household. The quantity and price of foods are noted for a specified period of time like 1–7 days. It is relatively simple method but memory dependent.

- *Inventory method*: A specified record of stock of food items is prepared in a household at the beginning and end of a specified period, usually 1 week. Average intake of food per person per day is calculated as stocks at beginning of week minus stocks at end of the week divided by total number of persons taking meal and divided by number of days. It is used for hostels, army barracks, orphanages, etc. Advantages of this method are that a large sample can be covered in short period of time, but holidays and attendance affect the estimation of nutrients and it is not a direct measurement of food.

- *Household food record method*: In this method, either members of the household or field staff keeps a records of all foods consumed at each meal by weight. This is then measured into individual servings.

- *Telephone survey*: Information on household food consumption or of specific foods is gathered by telephone surveys. It is less expensive than other methods.

*Utilization of data:* In many countries, household methods are used for their national food consumption surveys. Data is also collected about socioeconomic status, purchasing practices, number of meals and snacks consumed outside of the home, and food-assistance program participation, etc. to have a comprehensive picture of the nutritional practices. Other information like eating patterns, use of dietary supplements, weight, height, and general health status can also be collected simultaneously.

**Dietary assessment at the national level:**

- *Food balance sheets*: The gross national food supply is calculated by adding values of domestic food production, food taken from stocks *minus* exports, food added to stocks, food diverted for nonhuman food, and estimated waste. Per capita availability per day is calculated as: stocks at beginning of year plus food produced plus imports, minus stocks at end of year plus exports plus cattle or poultry feeds, divided by mid-year population, multiplied by 365 days. It is useful for administrators, planners to monitor food position in the country and to take appropriate decisions but it is of little use to health workers and does not give actual diet consumption.

- *Market databases*: Database of commercial market reports consisting of projected sales of packaged foods sold in

grocery stores is utilized. This data is used to analyze trends in consumer preferences of foods.
- *Computerized dietary assessment*: A software based on composition of foods is developed and is used for nutritional analysis. The nutrient values are usually averages of several chemically analyzed samples of food items.
- *Nutrient analysis systems*: It is also based on computer software programed on the basis of the ability to enter foods as eaten and produce an analysis of nutrient intakes by days or week. Many computer programs have been designed for use by consumer, an interviewer, or researcher.

### *Indirect methods*

- **Vital statistics**: Under-five mortality rate, prevalence of anemia in pregnant women, etc. are some of the statistical indicators which give a picture of nutritional status of population.
- **Ecological studies**: Malnutrition is the result of complex interaction of varying ecological factors like socioeconomic factors, health and educational services, sociocultural factors and food production. All these factors are assessed to get an indirect idea of nutritional status of the population.

## Nutritional Surveillance

It is a process of continuous scrutiny of all the nutritional factors and burden of nutritional states and its application in the public health interest. It gives information about health and development planning and is crucial for program implementation and evaluation. If performed well, it also provides timely warning signals and possible interventions to predict any food crisis and thereby help in better planning for long-term action. Information gathered in the surveillance process assists in providing baseline information on nutrition and related factors of socioeconomic factors, demography, food security and cultural aspects in a population.

### *Goal*

The goal of a food and nutrition surveillance system is to provide regular and updated information on the nutritional conditions of a population and the influencing factors. This information shall provide the basis for decisions for policy planning and management of programs relating to improvement of food consumption patterns and nutritional status.

### *Objectives*

The immediate objectives of a food and nutrition surveillance system are:

- To describe the nutritional status of the population, with particular reference to defined subgroups at risk including defined age groups and geographic areas. This enables the targeting of risk groups for action
- To provide information on the causes and associated factors (which may or may not be nutrition related) of nutritional problems in order to facilitate the adoption of preventive measures
- To promote decisions by governments concerning priorities and resource allocation, to formulate policies and programs
- To enable predictions on the basis of current trends of nutritional problems, provide early warning signals of impending crisis and emergencies
- To monitor nutritional programs and to evaluate their effectiveness.

### *Methods*

The following common methods are recommended for a food and nutrition surveillance system:

- **Large-scale food and nutrition surveys**: The surveillance system should make an inventory of all large national surveys related to health, food and nutrition that could act as a basis by breaking data down at subregional, district and village levels namely Demographic Health Survey, National Nutrition Survey or National Food Security Surveys.
- **Repeated small-scale surveys**: Repeated small-scale surveys are population-based surveys that use standard methods to collect quantitative and qualitative data. They assess the type, severity and extent of malnutrition and its causes among a representative sample of the population (children and/or adults). Repeated surveys include national surveys, which are periodically conducted at national level, and small-scale surveys, which are carried out at local level to gather nutrition information at a suitable time.
- **Sentinel site surveillance**: Sentinel site surveillance involves surveillance in a limited number of sites to detect trends in the overall well-being of the population. The sites may be specific population groups or villages that cover populations at risk. Trends are monitored for various indicators, including nutritional status, morbidity, dietary issues, coping strategies and food security. Data can be collected and analyzed centrally (centrally-based sentinel site surveillance) or by trained members of the community (community-based sentinel site surveillance).
- **School census data**: Nutritional assessment is occasionally undertaken in schools, where children are measured through censuses every 2–3 years. The objective is to identify high-risk children with poor health, malnutrition and low socioeconomic status. Results can be used to target school feeding programs and support policy-making in food-based strategies. The need for monitoring obesity among school aged children is becoming more important.
- **Growth monitoring**: It is a continuous monitoring of growth in children. Its aim is to identify slowing or faltering of growth at the individual level, and thus help to correct the problem promptly. Formerly, growth was usually measured as weight-for-age once per month. However, the WHO new growth curve (weight/height or length) is now recommended. Growth monitoring can either be conducted by health professionals at maternal and child health clinics (clinic-based growth monitoring) or by trained members of the community in villages

(community-based growth monitoring). Community-based growth monitoring is a function of the Anganwadis in India.

## Types of Indicators

They used for nutritional surveillance include:
- *Nutritional status indicators*, e.g. low birth weight indicates maternal nutritional status, infant and young child nutrition is indicated by the proportion of infant being breastfed, infant and child mortality rates, anthropometric parameters like weight-for-age, height-for-age, weight-for height
- *Indicators of causes/risk factors*, e.g., indicators related to socioeconomic status, food supply, food security
- *Indicators for monitoring and evaluating nutrition programs*, e.g., percentage of children utilizing the food supplementation from Anganwadi, percentage of children enrolled in MDM program.

## Steps of Nutritional Surveillance

- *Planning the survey*: Arrange for required funds, administrative formalities and permissions, recruit the surveyors and validate the tools.
    - Define—What is the problem status? → Define and describe the type of nutritional problem, e.g. malnutrition, micronutrient deficiency, etc.
    - Who are the population groups at risk? → Describe the population characteristics which make certain groups at risk of condition like geography, socioeconomic status, etc.
    - Why is the population group at risk? → Determine and identify the causal and associated factors. The causes could be immediate (shortage of food, poor health of individual, etc.) or presence of any other contributing factor like inequitable resource distribution, poor sanitary conditions and infections.
    - Where to get the relevant data from? → Identify the data sources. There can be many data sources which are decided depending upon the purpose for which surveillance has been undertaken.
- *Identify goals:* Identify survey goals and objectives, study population and methodology, outcomes variables and data analysis tools.
- *Training*: Training of staff is done followed by pretesting of tool.
- *Review information:* A review of the available information or literature related to the anticipated survey area.
- *Identify relevant indicators*: Demographic information like household details, residence, socioeconomic profile like per capita income, food source, water source, anthropometric indicators, coverage of nutritional intervention, morbidity rates on the area, food consumption patterns, etc.
- *Selecting survey methodology*: Most commonly used survey designs are as follows:
    - **Longitudinal survey**: Data is collected over a period of time for the same population in a defined geographic area. It helps in establishing trends of nutritional status over a period of time.
    - **Cross-sectional surveys**: One of the commonly used methods that takes a snapshot of the population at a defined point of time. They are used in emergency situations also.
- *Select survey sample*
- *Data collection tools and instrument*
- *Data collection*
- *Compilation of data and report writing.*

Nutritional surveillance differs from growth monitoring essentially in the fact that while growth monitoring is a tool for preserving and promoting an individual's nutritional status, nutritional surveillance is for the community nutritional status. Nutrition monitoring differs from surveillance because the former is not accompanied by intervention. The ICMR established the National Nutritional Monitoring Bureau in 1972 with the objective of nutrition monitoring in the country.

> **Note**
> The paucity of reliable and comparable data from all parts of the country is a definite obstacle toward a realistic and disaggregated problem definition. This calls for a nationwide monitoring system.
> *National Nutrition Policy, Government of India, 1993.*

## GLOBAL TARGETS FOR NUTRITION

"Comprehensive implementation plan on maternal, infant and young child nutrition" was endorsed by the World Health Assembly to address the dual burden on malnutrition. It spells out global targets for nutrition that are to be achieved by 2025 which are as follows:

> 1. Achieve *40%* reduction in the number of under-five children who are *stunted*
> 2. Achieve *50%* reduction of *anemia* among women in reproductive age group
> 3. Achieve *30%* reduction in *low birth weight*
> 4. Ensure that there is *no increase in childhood overweight*
> 5. Increase the rate of *exclusive breastfeeding* in the first 6 months up to at least *50%*
> 6. Reduce and maintain childhood *wasting* to less than *5%*.

We will fail miserably in the achievement of the above-mentioned targets if the current trends continue to prevail. Therefore, concerted efforts are needed in the thrust priority areas, so as to address malnutrition in all its forms.

In order to address the issue, continuum of care approach has to be adopted and integrated with life cycle approach so as to interrupt the vicious intergenerational cycle of malnutrition. Various action points that have been suggested are:

1. To foster enabling environment for the implementation of comprehensive food and nutrition policies.
   Food and nutrition policies should be a cross-cutting theme across various sectors and stakeholders so as to comprehensively address the nutrition challenges. Political commitment of the highest level shall be required for it to emerge as a central theme in the existing policy framework.
2. Integration of all forms of health interventions that have an impact on nutrition in national nutrition plans.

Evidence-based cost-effective interventions should be integrated into existing health care delivery system and be linked with existing programs so as to have good visibility and utilization by the community. Concurrently, strengthening of the health systems and promotion of universal coverage of nutritional interventions should also be done.
3. To encourage development and implementation of cross-cutting policies and programs which may be outside the purview of health sector yet identify and include nutrition in an all-encompassing form.
4. Convergence of food and nutritional policies with other factors which impact malnutrition such as gender equality, peace, security, education, food production, social security, unemployment, strengthening of PDSs and overcoming the challenges of food insecurity shall go a long way to make food of good nutritional quality available and accessible to all those who need it the most. Encourage and promote breastfeeding by creating enabling environment for the same, especially at the work place. Strict implementation and regulation of Infant and Milk Substitutes Act.
5. To ensure provision of manpower and financial resources for the implementation of nutritional interventions.
Strengthening of human and financial capital is of utmost priority so as to deliver effective and quality interventions.
6. To regulate monitoring and evaluation of policies and programs and their implementation.
Strengthening of health management and information system so as to ensure regular and timely collection, collation, analysis and interpretation of data. To identify the strengths and gaps in the delivery system based on the data so as to bring about a policy change, if required.

## SUGGESTED READING

1. Andersson M, Karumbunathan V, Zimmermann MB. Global iodine status in 2011 and trends over the past decade. J Nutr. 2012;142:744-50.
2. Bagcchi S. Hypothyroidism in India: more to be done. Lancet Diabetes Endocrinol. 2014;2(10):778.
3. Control of vitamin A deficiency and xerophthalmia. Report of a Joint WHO/ USAID/Helen Keller International/IV ACG Meeting Geneva, World Health Organization, 1982 (WHO Technical Report Series, No. 672).
4. Food Safety and Standards Authority of India. [online] Available from http:// ffrc.fssai.gov.in/ffrc/icds_progress.
5. Gaskell H, Derry S, Andrew Moore R, et al. Prevalence of anaemia in older persons: systematic review. BMC Geriatr. 2008;8:1.
6. ICMR. Nutrient Requirement and Recommended Dietary Allowances for Indians. A report of the Expert Group of the ICMR; 2020.
7. National Institute of Nutrition. Nutrition Atlas. [online] Available from http://218.248.6.39/nutritionatlas/iron.php.
8. National Iodine Deficiency Disorder Control Programme. Annual report (2016-17). Ministry of Health and Family Welfare, Government of India, New Delhi. pp. 78-80.
9. National iron plus initiative for anaemia control among 6 months onwards population. [online] Available from http://www.nrhmhp.gov.in/sites/default/files/files/Iron%20plus%20initiative%20 for%206%20months%20-5%20years.pdf.
10. Rashtriya Kishor Swasthya Karyakram. Operational framework, 2014 Ministry of Health and Family Welfare, Government of India, New Delhi.
11. Sommer A, Davidson FR. Assessment and control of vitamin A deficiency: the Annecy Accords. J Nutr. 2002;132:2845S-50S.
12. Sommer A. Vitamin A Deficiency and its Consequences. A Field Guide to Detection and Control, 3rd edition. Geneva: WHO; 1995.
13. Stevens GA, Bennett JE, Hennocq Q, et al. Trends and mortality effects of vitamin A deficiency in children in 138 low-income and middle-income countries between 1991 and 2013: a pooled analysis of population-based surveys. Lancet Glob Health. 2015;3:e528-36.
14. The state of the world's children 2013. Children with disabilities. New York: United Nations Children's Fund; 2013.
15. WHO. Global nutrition targets 2025: low birth weight policy brief (WHO/NMH/NHD/14.5). Geneva: World Health Organization; 2014.
16. WHO. Global nutrition targets 2025: stunting policy brief (WHO/NMH/NHD/14.3). Geneva: World Health Organization; 2014.
17. WHO Child Growth Standards. Length/height-for-age, weight-for-age, weight-for-length, weight-for-height and body mass index-for-age. Methods and development. Geneva: World Health Organization; 2006.
18. World Health Organization, United Nations Children's Fund. (2009). WHO child growth standards and the identification of severe acute malnutrition in infants and children. A joint statement.
19. World Health Organization (2018). Child growth standards. Frequently asked questions. [online] Available from http://www. who.int/childgrowth/ faqs/how_different/en/.
20. World Health Organization. Born too soon. The Global Action Report on preterm birth. Geneva, WHO; 2012.
21. World Health Organization. Comprehensive implementation plan on maternal, infant and young child nutrition (WHO/NMH/ NHD/14.1). Geneva: WHO; 2014.
22. World Health Organization. Food and nutrition surveillance systems: technical guide for the development of a food and nutrition surveillance system for countries in the Eastern Mediterranean Region. WHO Regional Publications, Eastern Mediterranean Series (33). WHO; 2013.
23. World Health Organization. Global Nutrition Policy Review 2016- 2017: country progress in creating enabling policy environments for promoting healthy diets and nutrition. Geneva: World Health Organization; 2018.
24. World Health Organization. Global nutrition targets 2025. Policy brief series (WHO/NMH/NHD/14.2).
25. World Health Organization. Global prevalence of vitamin A deficiency in populations at risk 1995–2005. Geneva, Switzerland: World Health Organization; 2009.
26. World Health Organization. Indicators for assessing vitamin A deficiency and their application in monitoring and evaluating intervention programmes. Geneva: World Health Organization; 1996 (WHO/NUT/96.10).
27. World Health Organization. MCEE-WHO methods and data sources for child causes of death 2000-2016. Geneva, WHO; 2018.
28. World Health Organization. Nutritional anaemias: tools for effective prevention and control. Geneva: World Health Organization; 2017.
29. World Health Organization. Salt as a vehicle for fortification. Report of a WHO Expert Consultation, Luxembourg, 21–22 March 2007. Geneva: World Health Organization; 2008.
30. Zimmermann MB, Jooste PL, Pandav CS. Iodine-deficiency disorders. Lancet. 2008;372:1251-62.

# EPIDEMIOLOGY OF FOOD-RELATED DISEASES AND ITS PREVENTION

*Abhishek Singh*

## FOOD ADDITIVES

Most of us have seen in our childhood, mothers and grandmothers pickling the mango and lime by the adding the oil, salt, and spices in order to preserve them for fairly long periods. In fact, these were natural additives. Thus, idea of adding nonfood elements to food items was first introduced centuries ago.

Industrialization and increasing population changed the pattern of food demand. The food processing industry is using modern techniques and chemical additives to meet increasing demand of "ready to eat food".

Food additives are *nonnutritious* elements added deliberately to food, usually in little quantities, to enhance its appearance, texture, and flavor, etc. Food additives can be derived from flora, fauna or minerals, or may be synthetic.

Food additives can be grouped into two broad categories:
1. ***Additives intentionally added to food:***
   - *Coloring agents*, e.g., saffron, turmeric
   - *Flavoring agents*, e.g., vanilla essence
   - *Sweeteners*, e.g., saccharin, cyclamate
   - *Preservatives*, e.g., sorbic acid, sodium benzoate
   - *Acidity imparting agents*, e.g., acetic acid, etc.
   - *Thickening agents*, e.g., alginate (from seaweed) and casein used in ice creams, cheese, yogurt, etc.
   - *Emulsifiers*: Retain water and oil mixed together, e.g., lecithin, monoglycerides and diglycerides are used in margarine, baked goods, and ice cream
   - *Antioxidants*: Check spoilage, change in taste, and color loss due to exposure to air, e.g., vitamin C and vitamin E.
   
   Human beings can consume food additives safely but certain preservatives like nitrites and nitrates can produce nitrosamines, a toxic substance that has been linked to cancer.
2. ***Contaminants:*** Incidental entry at various stages like packing, processing, and farming practices (insecticides).

**Remember:** List of frequently used food additives (emulsifiers, stabilizers, thickeners, and gelling agents).

| Names | Food articles |
|---|---|
| Lecithins | Chocolates, margarine, and potato snacks |
| Citric acid | Pickles, dairy products, and baked products |
| Tartaric acid | Baking powder |
| Alginic acid | Ice creams, desserts |
| Agar | Ice cream, soups, and tinned ham |
| Gums | Ice creams, soups, and confectionery |
| Pectin | Jellies |

**Remember:** Some commonly used food preservatives.

| Antioxidants | |
|---|---|
| Ascorbic acid | Beer, soft drinks, fruits, meat, and powdered milk |
| Tocopherols | Vegetable oils |
| Gallates | Vegetable oils, fats, and margarine |
| BHA and BHT | Fats, margarine in baked products |
| **Other preservatives** | |
| Sorbic acid | Cheese, yogurt, and soft drinks |
| Acetic acid | Pickles, sauce |
| Lactic acid | Sauce, confectionery |
| Propionic acid | Bread, cakes, and flour |
| Benzoic acid | Soft drink, pickles, fruit products, and jams |
| Sulfur dioxide | Soft drinks, fruit products, beer, cider, and wine |
| Nitrites | Cured meats, cooked meats, and meat products |

(BHA: butylated hydroxyanisole; BHT: butylated hydroxytoluene)

### Law and Regulations Related to Food Additives

A matter of great concern to the public and health administrators is the effects and consequences of food additives on human beings. Possible harmful effects of food additives on health of human beings need to be explored before allowing its usage. Throughout the world, there are various laws to regulate the set of food additives. In India, two such legal provisions related to food additives are: (1) the Prevention of Food Adulteration (PFA) Act and (2) the Food Products Order. Food additive is labeled as an adulterant in case law does not permit its use. The food is also considered adulterated if maximum permissible limits are voided for any food additive. As per the law, it is mandatory to print the quantity of the additive on the label affixed to the container. The word "artificially colored" must be printed on the label if any extraneous coloring agent is added to a food.

The Joint FAO/WHO Expert Committee on Food Additives (JECFA) is an international agency that evaluates the safety profile of food additives. Every food additive has to get safety clearance from JECFA then the Codex Alimentarius Commission (CAC) provides maximum use levels. Only such food additives can be used in foods.

## FOOD PRESERVATIVES

One cannot consume food immediately on production in routine hectic life. The process of food decay and deterioration sets in as food is cooked due to the enzymes and other chemicals present in it, which start the process of decay. Both bacteria and fungi cause food decay in favorable circumstances. Environmental factors like temperature and humidity amplify the decay. This food decay and deterioration renders the food unfit for human consumption. Preserving food, therefore, becomes imperative.

> **Food Preservation**
> - Enhances the keeping quality of food
> - Preserves its nutritional characteristics
> - Retains the appearance, color, and texture of food.

Examples of commonly used preservatives are as follows:
- ***Natural preservatives:*** Most commonly used natural preservatives are the naturally occurring and easily available items such as table salt and sugar. High osmotic pressure does not permit bacteria to propagate. Salt has been used to make pickles. Sugar is added in the syrup form to fruits to increase their shelf life and to conserve them. Jams and jellies are preserved as solutions of high osmolarity using sugars. Another set of natural preservatives are the ones that target enzymes that are present in fruits and vegetables; these enzymes are the ones that continue to act or metabolize even after the fruits are cut. For example, citric and ascorbic acids present in lemon juice, inhibits the enzyme phenolase that is responsible for browning of the cut surface of apples and potatoes. Herbs, spices, and vinegar are other examples of natural preservatives.
- ***Antioxidants:*** Antioxidants preserve food articles by preventing spoilage and limit changes in flavor and color loss caused by atmospheric exposure. Vitamin C and vitamin E are such examples. There are various other antioxidant preservatives such as butylated hydroxyanisole (BHA).
- ***Antimicrobial preservatives:*** These preservatives play an important role in the prevention of microbial growth and multiplication. Examples of such preservatives are benzoic acid, sulfur dioxide ($SO_2$), ethanol, sodium nitrate, sulfites, and disodium ethylenediaminetetraacetic acid (EDTA) **(Table 23.15)**.
- ***Microbes as preservatives:*** Some of the microbes due to their microbial activity are used for the production of food as well as in the preservation of food items. Examples of such are cheese, flavoring agents, Sauerkraut processed, and preserved by lactobacilli. Fungi such as yeast ferment sugars and produce alcohol, which in turn, leads to food preservation.
- ***Irradiation:*** One of the modern methods of food preservation is use of radiations such as radioactive rays or high-intensity X-rays or streams of electrons. As the food irradiated is done when it is already in the packets, there is minimal person-to-food contact thus, reducing contamination. Irradiation may cause some change in the color; however, the food is not turned radioactive. Irradiation may also prolong the shelf lives of perishable foods items such as strawberries, potatoes, etc.

**Table 23.15:** Suspected toxic effects of food preservatives.

| Classes | Preservatives | Toxic effects |
|---|---|---|
| Antimicrobials | Benzoic acid | Allergies |
| | Sorbic acid | Contact allergy |
| | Sulfites | Allergies |
| | Nitrites, nitrates | Carcinogenesis (nitrosamines), methemoglobinemia |
| Antioxidants | BHT | Mouse liver carcinogen |
| | BHA | Rat stomach carcinogen |
| | Alkyl gallates | Allergy, fetal, and neonatal toxicity |

(BHA: butylated hydroxyanisole; BHT: butylated hydroxytoluene)

### Health Concerns on Food Preservatives

Health concerns have been raised with usage of food preservatives such as bronchial asthma on exposure to $SO_2$ used to preserve wines, and allergic reactions because of preservatives, implications of nitrites as carcinogens.

## FOOD FORTIFICATION

Fortification of food is cost-effective, public health measure to add additional nutrients to the food item aiming to reduce nutritional disorders in the population. Food fortification is defined as "the process whereby nutrients are added to foods in relatively small quantities to maintain or improve the quality of diet of a group, a community, or a population". In fortification, the level of nutrients added surpasses their natural level in the food item.

### Need for Fortification

India harbors nearly one-third of the population suffering from vitamin and micronutrient deficiencies across globe. Almost 70% of Indian population consumes less than 50% of recommended dietary allowance for micronutrients resulting in high incidence of anemia, vitamin A deficiency, and iodine deficiency disorder (IDD), etc. Food fortification is a very cost-effective and scalable public health intervention to address micronutrient malnutrition.

It dates back to 400 BC when Persian physician Melampus mentioned nutrient supplementation of foods for the first time. In order to boost the mythical sailors' resistance to spears and arrows, he gave him sweet wine mixed with iron filings. The French Physician Boussingault recommended adding of iodine with salt to avoid goiter in year 1831. However, it was introduced as a strategy to address micronutrient malnutrition in 1920s. Ever since the paradigm of food fortification has evolved in terms of coverage of micronutrient and food products and has led to near eradication of various micronutrient deficiencies in many countries.

The process of fortification helps the community to overcome selected micronutrient deficiency. A food fortification program is generally started in the population where the deficiency is endemically present in the diet. Some of the fortification programs of demonstrated effectiveness are:
- ***Wheat flour (atta):*** Launched by Government of India in February 1970, in Bombay for fortification of atta with edible groundnut flour to improve its vitamin, minerals, and protein content.
- ***Iodization of salt:*** For prevention and control of endemic goiter, 30 ppm of iodine (potassium iodate) at manufacturer level and 15 ppm at the consumer level, must be present in the edible salt, under the PFA Act.
- ***Fortification of vanaspati ghee, butter, and milk:*** Compulsory vitamins A and D, 2,500 IU of vitamin A, and 175 IU of vitamin D per 100 g of vanaspati by the Government of India.

- **Addition of iron salts** to common salt for the prevention of nutritional anemia.
- **Fluoridation** of water for prevention of dental caries.
- Twin (double) fortification of common salt with iodine and iron.

> **Restoration versus Enrichment**
>
> *Restoration* means the bringing up the level of nutrients to the preprocessing, storage, or handling level. The essential nutrients that gets lost during the process of manufacturing, or normal storage and handling procedures.
>
> *Enrichment* means bringing the nutrients to the preprocessing level solely, though the term has been used interchangeably with fortification.

For fortification, the following criteria must be fulfilled by the nutrient and the vehicle:
- The vehicle fortified has be taken consistently as portion of the regular daily diet
- The nutrient should not be hazardous
- The addition of the nutrient should not change taste, odor, or appearance of the food, and
- The cost of fortification should not be beyond the reach of the population.

> **Benefits and advantages of food fortification**
> - *Cost-effective:* Avoids main micronutrient deficiencies at a minor cost
> - No need to change the dietary habits of the end-users
> - *Population-based approach:* Benefits large number of people
> - Relatively quick implementation and easily sustainable.

## ADULTERATION OF FOODS

Section 3(a) of Food Safety and Standards Act, 2006 defines adulterant as: *any material which is or could be employed for making the food unsafe or substandard or misbranded or containing extraneous matter*. Extraneous matter means any matter contained in an article of food which may be carried from the raw materials, packaging materials, or process systems used for its manufacture or which is added to it, but such matter does not render such article of food unsafe.

Any article is considered as adulterated in case it does not possess the substance or quality as required by the customer, if food contains other substances degrading the matter and quality of food, if food is replaced by low quality substance, or if any ingredient of the food has been taken away, or if it contains any poisonous element, the food is considered to be adulterated (PFA Act).

**Remember:** Some common food adulterants.

| Food items | Adulterants |
|---|---|
| Cereals | Mud, grits |
| Dal | Kesari dal, dyes |
| Dhania powder | Horse dung or cow dung powder |
| Haldi powder | Lead chromate powder |
| Black pepper | Dried papaya seeds |
| Chili powder | Brick powder |
| Tea | Used tea dust, gram husk, and tamarind seeds powder |
| Milk | Addition of starch and water, fat extraction |
| Honey | Sugar, jaggery |
| Mustard seeds | Prickly poppy seeds—*Argemone* |
| Sweets | Non-permitted colors |
| Ghee | Vanaspati |
| Edible oils | Mineral oils, argemone oil |
| Icecream | Cellulose, starch, and nonpermitted colors |

### Prevention of Food Adulteration Act

The Indian Parliament passed the PFA Act in 1954 with the main objectives of safeguarding unadulterated and wholesome food to consumers and to guard consumers from dishonest trade practices. In 1955, the "Central Committee for Food Standards" framed the PFA Rules. It was amended three times, respectively during 1964, 1976, and 1986 to make it more stringent.

In states, the state government enforces the Act through the government appointed public analyst and food inspectors, who has power to check the supply, storage, and marketing of food. The food inspector should draw and send the sample of food article to the laboratory for testing in case of suspected food adulteration. With the amendment of the Act in 1986, now consumer and the voluntary organizations can take food samples.

### Sample Collection, Disposal, and Analysis

The food inspector informs the vendor in advance regarding sample collection and its analysis as per the PFA Act. The vendor is paid for the cost of food sample. The signature of the vendor is also taken. This sample is packed and sealed in three packets. One sample is sent to public analyst. Another two samples are submitted to the local health authority for safe custody. The local government public analyst conducts analysis of sample. Local health authority receives the report. In case the sample is proved as adulterated, court of law takes appropriate action. The vendor reserves the right to appeal in the court within 10 days asking for analysis of reserve samples. Court may send reserved samples for reconfirmation to any of the four reference laboratories located at Mysore, Kolkata, Pune, and Ghaziabad.

### Punishment

If the adulteration is proved, as per the Act fine of 1,000 with a minimum imprisonment of 6 months is imposed. For the cases of adulteration, which may result in grievous health problem or even death [within the meaning of Section 320 of Indian Penal Code (IPC)], the punishment of life imprisonment and a fine not be less than 5,000 is imposed.

## FOOD TOXICANTS

A toxic or poisonous substance might be present in anybody's food. In small doses, a substantial toxic effect may not be there, but in a higher dose or chronic consumption, it may prove fatal. A lot of toxic effects of foods are well-known. **Table 23.16** explains a wide range of ill effects of natural food poisons.

Table 23.16: Toxic ingredients and their effects present in common foods.

| Food stuffs | Active toxic ingredients | Effects on |
|---|---|---|
| Some bananas | 5-hydroxytryptamine, adrenaline, and noradrenaline | Central and/or peripheral nervous systems (CNSs) |
| Some types of cheese | Tyramine | Blood pressure |
| Almond, cassava | Cyanide | Tissue respiration |
| Some fish/meat | Nitrosamines | Cancers |
| Mustard oil adulterated with argemone oil | Sanguinarine | Epidemic dropsy |
| Kesari dal (Lathyrus) | β-N-oxalylamino-L-alanine and others | Neurolathyrism |
| Brassica species (seeds) | Glucosinolates, thiocyanate | Goiter |
| Green potato | Solanine | Gastrointestinal upset |
| Mushrooms (Amanitamuscaria, Amanitaphalloides) | Various toxins | CNS effects |
| Groundnuts | Aflatoxin | Aflatoxicosis |

## Lathyrism

*Lathyrus* is traditionally considered as poor man's crop. In India, in mixed cropping, *Lathyrus sativus* is intentionally planted with wheat in the dry areas. In good rainfall, wheat grows nicely compared to the *Lathyrus* (and it is not harvested); however, poor rainfall leads to a poor crop of wheat and more crop of *Lathyrus* is reaped. *Lathyrus* does not show any signs of toxicity if consumed in small amount but in larger amounts (providing more than 50% of energy), it can damage the nervous system resulting in spastic paralysis. Earlier, it was common practice that laborers were paid *Khesari dal* as kind and not in cash by some landlords (*zamindars*). Thus, poor laborers used it as staple diet and became victims of neurolathyrism.

The term lathyrism coined by *Cantani* in Italy. It is a neurodegenerative disorder that causes neurolathyrism in human beings and osteolathyrism or odoratism in animals. Neurolathyrism occurs mostly in those consuming it as a staple pulse, i.e. diets containing over 30% of this dal consumed for more than 6 months may result in this disease.

### Problem Statement

Bangladesh, Nepal, Pakistan, Ethiopia, Canada, and China have reported several epidemics. During World War II, 400 g of grass pea boiled in salt water with 200 g barley bread and chopped straw were given to Rumanian Jewish inmates. Out of 1,350–1,400 inmates, 800 developed paralysis within a period of 90 days. In India, in districts of Madhya Pradesh (Satna and Rewa), Maharashtra, Uttar Pradesh, Bihar, Rajasthan, Assam, and Gujarat, cases of lathyrism have been reported (Shibamoto F et al., Academic Press, 2009).

### Agent Factors

*Lathyrus sativus* (Khesari dal) is also referred to as *Teora dal, Lak dal, Batra, Matra*, and grass pea, etc. It appears similar to Arhar dal (Toor dal), red gram, or Bengal gram. If carefully examined, the *Lathyrus* seeds are triangular in shape and grayish in color. It is cheap but good source of protein.

*Lathyrus sativus* contains BOAA, a neurotoxin responsible for the neurolathyrism. Content of BOAA toxin in seeds varies from 0.2 g% to 1.0 g%. These are water soluble. This property can be made use for removing the toxin. First soak the pulse in hot water and then discard the soak water.

> Beta-N-oxalylamino-L-alanine was extracted in 1962 from the common vetch (*Vicia sativa*) that normally grows as a weed in *Lathyrus sativus*. BOAA causes neurolathyrism in humans. The toxin in the pulse, which causes osteolathyrism or odoratism in animals, is β-aminopropionitrile (BAPN).

### Host Factors

a. *Age and sex:* Commonly affects the men in the age group of 15–45 years
b. *Occupation:* Incidence is high among agricultural laborers
c. *Pathogenesis:* BOAA is a neurotoxin that has affinity for nerve cells of upper motor neurons. The toxin-induced degeneration of spinal motor tracts (pyramidal tracts) and sclerosis is the underlying pathology. There is loss of axis cylinders with gliosis of crossed pyramidal tracts in the lumbar and lumbosacral spinal cord leading to paraplegia. The sensory system and the motor nerves to muscles of trunk, upper limbs, and sphincter are spared. Lesions are reversible only in early latent stages of the illness.

### Latent Period

It varies from 1 month to 3 months depending on the amount of the pulse consumed.

### Clinical Features

The clinical symptoms of the disease lathyrism are acute in onset, often preceded by exertion or exposure to cold. A patient may often report as being paralyzed on getting up in the morning. Some cases may give history of backache and stiffness of legs preceding the paralysis of legs. It causes spastic paralysis of lower limb. *Acton (1922)* described following stages of the disease: (a) **Latent stage:** In this stage, when person is subjected to physical stress, it exhibits ungainly gait. Spasmodic muscular contractions of calf muscles are earliest symptom. This stage is considered important from the prevention point of view, since at this stage, withdrawal of the pulse from the diet, it will result in widespread diminution of the disease, (b) **No-stick stage:** The subject takes short jerky steps without using walking stick. Babinski sign is absent, (c) **One-stick stage:** The subject walks on toes with a crossed gait and uses stick to make the balance. On examination, ankle clonus and Babinski sign are present, (d) **Two-stick stage:** The subject walks with crossed legs (scissors gait) with the support of two crutches because of excessive bending of knees. The subject gets tired easily on walking a small distance. Ankle clonus and Babinski sign are present, and (e) **Crawler stage:** In this stage, knee joints cannot support the weight of the body making erect posture difficult. The thigh and leg muscles show atrophic changes. The patient is able to move by crawling, carrying his weight on his hands. The person is crippled. Pyramidal signs are present.

## Prevention and Control of Lathyrism

- *Removal of toxin:* The BOAA toxin can be removed by two methods:
  1. **Steeping method:** This method can be used at household level. In this method, pulse is soaked (before boiling) in hot water for 120 minutes. Since the toxins are water soluble, BOAA toxin steeps into the water. After 2 hours, soaked water is drained off completely. Pulse is again washed using clean water and sun dried. The pulse is then used for consumption. The drawback with this method is that water-soluble vitamins and minerals are also lost along with toxin.
  2. **Parboiling:** This method is more suitable for large-scale operations. This is an improved method of removal of toxin from pulse. It can be done by two ways—(1) The pulse is soaked in lukewarm water, like parboiling the rice, and then subjected to steam for 15 minutes, (2) Soaking the pulse in limewater overnight and next day it is washed and cooked.
- *Vitamin C prophylaxis:* In early stages of the illness, 500–1,000 mg ascorbic acid given daily for a week or so heals the damages well.
- *Genetic approach:* Cultivation of strains of *Lathyrus sativus* having lesser amount of BOAA toxin (<0.1%) may be an effective approach to prevent lathyrism while keeping same food habits. The Indian Agricultural Research Institute, New Delhi, has developed low toxin strains of *Lathyrus sativus*.
- *Health (nutritional) education:* People in the areas where *Khesari dal* is cultivated and consumed, should be educated about the hazards of using this pulse as part of meal and methods of removal of toxin before cooking.
- *Banning the crop:* The PFA Act in India has banned cultivation, harvesting, and consumption of *Lathyrus* in any form like whole, split, or flour; however, it is practically nonexistent where the need is utmost such as in the states of Madhya Pradesh, Bihar, Odisha, and Gujarat where the pulse is widely cultivated and consumed. As practically, it is not feasible to avoid consumption of *Khesari dal*, so the proportion of *Lathyrus* should be limited to less than 25% of the total cereals and pulses consumed every day.

## Aflatoxins

This is a special group of fungal mycotoxins produced under conditions of improper storage, namely *Aspergillus flavus* and *Aspergillus parasiticus*. Aflatoxicosis is characterized by hepatitis, cirrhosis of liver, and enteritis caused by ingestion of infested food grains. The fungi responsible are present everywhere and can affect many of the dietary staples of rice, corn, nuts, chilies, and spices in developing countries.

> In 1974, an outbreak of hepatitis due to aflatoxicosis was reported confirming 106 deaths. It was limited to the tribal population residing in approximately 200 villages of Banswara district (Rajasthan) and Panchmahal district (Gujarat). All of a sudden, people developed ascites, edema of lower limbs, and portal hypertension. The outbreak lasted for 2 months. Laboratory analysis disclosed that meals of affected people had maize infected with a fungus, *Aspergillus flavus* in the range of 6.25–15.6 ppm. It was estimated that affected people might have consumed 2,000–6,000 µg/kg or parts per billion (ppb) of aflatoxins, daily within a month period (Abbas HK, CRC Press, 2009).

### Problem Statement

Aflatoxins were first isolated in 1960 in England after reports of death of Turkeys fed on infested peanut and cottonseed meal came in limelight. They suffered from hepatitis and enteritis. Human cases have been reported since then.

### Agent and Environmental Factors

*Aspergillus flavus* or *Aspergillus parasiticus* are fungi that commonly affect foods in suboptimal storage settings such as high temperature (30–37°C) and high humidity (moisture levels above 16%). These are commonly seen in the rainy season, during floods, and near sea regions.

### Foods Infested

The fungus has been observed to infest improperly stored foods like maize, groundnut, jowar, rice, wheat, sunflower, tree nuts, spices, etc.

### Toxins

"Aflatoxins" are causative agent. *Aflatoxin B1* is the most powerful known natural hepatocarcinogen. Another toxin *Aflatoxin G1* is also known. They can cause hepatitis (jaundice), ascites, portal hypertension, liver cirrhosis, and even cancer of liver.

### Clinical Features

Illness is characterized by jaundice, rapidly developing ascites, commonly associated with bilateral pedal edema.

### Prevention and Control

Main issue is to confirm proper storage of food items after drying in dry containers to prevent fungal contamination of food grains; the moisture content should be kept as low as 10%. Foods contaminated by aflatoxin are not fit for human consumption. This problem can be addressed by educating the general population about the health hazards of consuming contaminated food grains.

## Ergot

While aflatoxicosis is a storage fungus, *Claviceps* are field fungi because most of infestation of crops occurs during the flowering or seeding stages. This fungi looks like a black mass. Its seeds are black in color and irregular in shape. Seeds get harvested with food grains. Ergotism is caused by ingestion of food grains like *bajra*, rice, wheat, and *rye* infested by *Claviceps fusiformis* and *Claviceps purpurea*.

A toxin called ergotamine causes the illness. In some African countries, scientists have succeeded in isolating the toxin from the blood of pregnant females, the breast milk blood of pregnant females, the breast milk and also from the cord blood with marked seasonal variations. Generally, 0.05 mg/100 g of the food is considered safe limit for the ergot alkaloids.

> Term "ergot" is derived from a French word "argot" that means spur. Sacred Persian literature (400–300 BC) comments on grass causing pregnant women to drop the womb and die in childbirth. Ancient Greeks and Romans did not consume rye. Use of rye probably commenced with beginning of Christian era that got introduced into Western Europe at that time. Evidence of ergot poisoning began to be found since then.

> **St. Anthony's fire**
>
> In the 11th century, epidemics of ergot poisoning were termed as *St. Anthony's fire*. This term explains the intolerable burning limb pain perceived by the affected persons. Hand and feet of affected people turned black due to dry gangrene. Mummified limbs got separated from the joints in due course. Latin term "Ignis Sacer" meaning holy fire expressed the burning sensation in early phase. The Order of Hospitallers of St. Anthony was instituted in 1093 in southern France to relieve the sufferings. Patients reported improvement in their condition on visiting the St. Anthony's shrine located a distance away. It was, perhaps, because of interruption of consumption of ergot-affected cereals, due to relocation to a new area, the shrine.

### Clinical Features

The clinical symptoms include nausea and vomiting, abdominal cramps, and drowsiness extending up to 24–48 hours after consumption of infested grain. In chronic cases, painful cramps in digits and limbs associated with burning, itching, and peripheral gangrene have been documented.

### Prevention

Floating the ergot-infested grains in 20% salt water is a method to remove the infested grains. Hand picking or air floatation can also remove the infested grains.

## Epidemic Dropsy (Argemone Poisoning)

Epidemic dropsy results from consumption of mustard oil adulterated or contaminated with the oil of *Argemone mexicana* seeds (prickly poppy seeds). The Mexican prickly poppy grows wild in India. Large prickly leaves and bright yellow or white flowers are characteristics of this plant. Mustard (*Brassica nigra*) and argemone seeds look alike. Mixing of these two seeds may be deliberate or accidental. Deliberate adulteration is profit oriented. In our country, the highest incidence is observed in July-August and lowest in the month of April.

### Problem Statement

As per records, first case of epidemic dropsy from India was reported from Kolkata in year 1877. Several outbreaks have been reported from all over India since then. Most recently epidemic has been reported from New Delhi in year 1999 causing over 3,000 hospitalization and more than 60 deaths. Epidemiological investigations disclosed that almost all the affected subjects were using mustard oil as cooking media and that was purchased loose from local vendors.

> **1998 Delhi oil poisoning: "Dropsy epidemic"**
>
> In 1998, the capital of India witnessed mustard oil poisoning in the form of dropsy, which left over 60 people dead and 3,000 people ill. Considered one of the most tragic cases, raids were conducted at several places. Samples of mustard oil "Dhara" were collected from various grocery shops. The National Dairy Development Board (NDDB) released advertisements requesting consumers not to buy its trusted brand of "Dhara" mustard oil. Laboratory investigations confirmed the mixing of mustard oil with Argemone oil, an adulterant that can cause dropsy, glaucoma, and even blindness in humans.

### Pathogenesis

Mukherjee et al. isolated sanguinarine, a toxin from argemone oil in 1941. Sarkar et al. described two toxins namely: (1) sanguinarine and (2) dihydrosanguinarine in argemone oil in 1948. Sanguinarine is 2.5 times more toxic than dihydrosanguinarine. The toxin is absorbed from the gut into the circulation. Sanguinarine interferes with the carbohydrate metabolism leading to accumulation of pyruvic acid. Argemone oil mainly affects blood vessels. Sanguinarine increases the capillary permeability that leads to edema. The duration of exposure is also important. Sanguinarine binds to plasma proteins and this property helps it to retain in the body for up to 96 hours after ingestion. This may cause cumulative toxicity even with exposure in very small dose.

### Clinical Features

Patients usually present with complaints of watery diarrhea and vomiting of subacute or insidious onset. This may persist for 7–10 days. Most patients have bilateral pitting edema of the lower limbs. Some patients may give history of burning sensations, itching, and paresthesias too. Mild to moderate anemia and hypoproteinemia are commonly observed. Renal azotemia and retinal hemorrhages are also common. Glaucoma is found in 0–12% of cases. Dyspnea, cardiac failure, and death may follow.

### Detection of Toxin

- *Nitric acid test:* To perform this test, 5 mL of oil to be tested and 5 mL of nitric acid are taken in a test tube and shaken well. On standing, layer of nitric acid changes its color depending upon quantity of argemone oil. As quantity of argemone oil increases, color changes from yellow to orange-yellow or crimson. The test can detect adulteration with more than 0.25% concentration of oil. Major drawback of this test is high false-positive rate. A positive test should be confirmed.
- *Ferric chloride test:* In this test, 2 mL each of oil to be tested and concentrated hydrochloric acid are taken in a test tube and mixed well. This solution is heated in a water bath at 33.5–35°C for 2 minutes. At this stage, it is reheated again for 1 minute after adding 8 mL of ethyl alcohol. Now, 2 mL of ferric chloride is mixed and the tube is heated again in the bath for 10 minutes. If there is argemone oil in test oil, an orange-red precipitate forms.
- *Paper chromatographic method:* It is the most sensitive method as this method can detect as low as 0.0001% argemone oil adulteration.

### Prevention and Control Measures

Following measures may be adopted:
- General public should be sensitized about dangers of argemone plant. Its growth should be discouraged and deweeding of argemone plant should be done.
- Education and motivation of farmers about careful selective cultivation of yellow-seeded mustard. Farmers can easily detect argemone seeds even with the naked eye as they are black or dark-brown color.

- There should be ban on the sale and purchase of unpacked mustard oil. Strict enforcement of the PFA Act to handle dishonest dealers.

## Endemic Ascites

It occurs due to the contamination, either deliberate or accidental, of the millet *Panicum miliare* (popular as Gondhali among local people) with weed seeds of *Crotalaria* (popular as Jhunjhunia among local people). Jhunjhunia seeds contain pyrrolizidine alkaloids which are hepatotoxic in nature.

During the years 1973 and 1976, an outbreak of a disease in Nagesia tribals of Madhya Pradesh (Kusmi block of Surguja district) was reported. People suddenly developed ascites and jaundice, affecting people of all age groups except infants and both the sexes with high mortality rate of approximately 40%. A team from the National Institute of Nutrition, Hyderabad, conducted outbreak investigations. They concluded that this outbreak was due to intake of millet seeds contaminated with *Crotalaria* seeds, which form their main diet (Bhar RV, Indian J Pediatr, 1987).

Main preventive and control measures are educating and sensitizing general public regarding this disease and causative plant especially in affected areas, removal of Jhunjhunia plants growing with staple, and sieving of millet at the domestic level to remove the seeds of Jhunjhunia as these seeds are smaller compared to those of millet.

## Fusarium Toxins

*Fusarium incarnatum* is a field fungus that affects crops like sorghum, rice, and maize and may pose health hazards to livestock and man. *Fusarium* is commonly found in the subtropical and temperate areas. *Fusarium* is known to produce deoxynivalenol and fumonisin toxins, which causes vomiting and diarrhea.

During the World War II, in Russia consumption of *Fusarium* infected millet containing trichothecene group of mycotoxins produced an alimentary toxic aleukia characterized by hemorrhagic rash, bleeding from nose, leukopenia, necrotic angina, and nonfunctioning of bone marrow. In India during 1929, consumption of *Fusarium* infected food grains resulted in "moldy ragi poisoning" causing episodes of vomiting and diarrhea among affected people.

## PREVENTION AND CONTROL OF FOOD ADULTERATION DISEASES IN INDIA

- *Establishment of food standards:*
  - **Codex Alimentarius Commission (CAC):** The CAC is the main structure of the joint FAO/WHO Food Standards Programme. The CAC has framed food standards for markets at international level. The basis of Indian food standards as well as other countries is more or less than the standards of the CAC.
  - **Prevention of Food Adulteration Standards:** These standards are established as per the PFA Act (1954), to set minimum level of quality of food articles possible in Indian scenario. Any food article is deemed adulterated if it does not confirm to the minimum standards.
  - **Agmark Standards:** The Directorate of Marketing and Inspection of the Government of India prescribe Agmark Standards. The Agmark offers the consumer a guarantee of quality of food article as per the set standards.

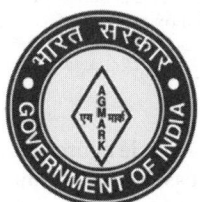

  - **Indian Standards Institution (ISI) Standards:** The ISI mark on food article is an assurance of good quality as per the standards laid down by the Bureau of Indian Standards for that product.

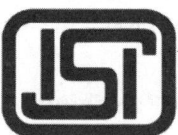 

  The Agmark and ISI standards are not mandatory, but purely voluntary. They express degrees of excellence above PFA standards and norms.
  - **Food Safety and Standards Authority of India (FSSAI):** The FSSAI was founded in year 2008 under Food Safety and Standards Act, 2006. The aims of this authority are to place the scientific standards for food articles, to control and standardize not only the manufacture and storage but also the distribution, sale, and import of food articles. It is responsibility of FSSAI to safeguard the public health by regulating and supervising the food safety.

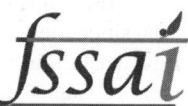

- *Legislative measures:*
  - The Vegetable Oil Products (Control) Order, 1947
  - The PFA Act, 1954
  - The Essential Commodities Act, 1955 (in related to food)
  - The Fruit Products Order, 1955
  - The Solvent Extracted Oil, De-oiled Meal and Edible Flour (Control) Order, 1967
  - The Meat Food Products Order, 1973
  - The Milk and Milk Products Order, 1992
  - The Edible Oils Packaging (Regulation) Order, 1998
  - The Food Safety and Standards Act, 2006.

## SUGGESTED READING

1. Abbas HK. Aflatoxin and Food Safety. Boca Raton: CRC Press; 2005.
2. Allen LH, De Benoist B, Dary O, et al. (2006). Guidelines on food fortification with micronutrients. [online] Available from http:// apps.who.int/iris/bitstream/handle/10665/43412/9241594012_ eng.pdf?ua=1.
3. Anand SP, Sati N. Artificial preservatives and their harmful effects: looking toward nature for safer alternatives. Int J Pharma Sci Res. 2013;4:24-96.
4. Bamji MS, Krishnaswamy K, Brahmam GN. Textbook of Human Nutrition. New Delhi: Oxford & IBH; 2016.
5. Bhat RV, Rao RN. Foodborne diseases in India. Indian J Pediatr. 1987; 54:553-62.
6. De Costa C. St. Anthony's fire and living ligatures: a short history of ergometrine. Lancet. 2002;359:1768-70.
7. Dudeja P, Gupta RK, Minhas AS. Food Safety in the 21st Century: Public Health Perspective. New York: Academic Press; 2016.
8. Food Safety and Standards Authority of India (FSSAI). (2010). Food Safety and Standards Regulation, 2010.
9. Food Safety and Standards Authority of India (FSSAI). (2017). Large Scale Food Fortification in India: The Journey So Far and Road Ahead.
10. Gandy JW, Madden A, Holdsworth M. Oxford Handbook of Nutrition and Dietetics. New Delhi: Oxford University Press; 2007.
11. Hakim SA. Argemone oil, sanguinarine, and epidemic-dropsy glaucoma. Br J Ophthalmol. 1954;38:193-216.
12. Ikhlas AK, Abourashed EA. Leung's Encyclopedia of Common Natural Ingredients: Used in Food, Drugs and Cosmetics. United States: John Wiley & Sons; 2011.
13. Joint FAO/WHO Expert Committee on Food Additives (JECFA). (2005). Summary and Conclusions of the Sixty-fourth Meeting. [online] Available from http://www.fao.org/3/a-at877e.pdf.
14. Leung AY. Encyclopedia of Common Natural Ingredients Used in Food, Drugs, and Cosmetics. United States: Wiley; 1980.
15. Mejia LA. (1994). Fortification of Foods: Historical Development and Current Practices. [online] Available from http://archive.unu.edu/unupress/food/8F154e/8F154E03.htm.
16. Parke DV, Lewis DF. Safety aspects of food preservatives. Food Addit Contam. 1992;9:561-77.
17. Passmore R, Eastwood MA. Human Nutrition and Dietetics, 8th edition. London: Churchill Livingstone; 1986.
18. Peraica M, Radić B, Lucić A, et al. Toxic effects of mycotoxins in humans. Bull World Health Organ. 1999;77:754-66.
19. Russell NJ, Grahame WG. Food Preservatives. New York: Springer Science & Business Media; 2003.
20. Shibamoto M, Takayuki F, Bjeldanes LF. Introduction to Food Toxicology. New York: Academic Press; 2009.
21. Shukla S, Shankar R, Singh SP. Food safety regulatory model in India. Food Control. 2014;37:401-13.
22. Smith J. Food Additive User's Handbook. Glasgow: Blackie; 1991.
23. Spencer PS, Roy DN, Ludolph A, et al. Lathyrism: evidence for role of the neuroexcitatory aminoacid BOAA. Lancet. 1986;2:1066-7.
24. Stob M. Naturally occurring food toxicants: estrogens. In: Stob M (Ed). Handbook of Naturally Occurring Food Toxicants. Boca Raton: CRC Press; 2018.
25. Trienekens J, Zuurbier P. Quality and safety standards in the food industry, developments and challenges. Int J Prod Econ. 2008;113:107-22.
26. Wiedenfeld H. Toxicity of pyrrolizidine alkaloids–a serious health problem. Clin Exp Health Sci. 2011;1:79-87.
27. World Health Organization, Food and Agriculture Organization of the United Nations. (2001). General Standard for Contaminants and Toxins in Food and Feed.
28. World Health Organization, Food and Agriculture Organization of the United Nations. (2007). Codex Alimentarius Commission: Procedural Manual.

# CHAPTER 24

# Reproductive Health and Family Welfare

*Pooja Goyal, Mitasha Singh, Shveta Lukhmana*

*"It is easy to add but difficult to maintain."*

| CM 9.4 | Enumerate and describe the causes and consequences of population explosion and population dynamics of India |
|---|---|
| CM 9.5 | Describe the methods of population control |
| CM 10.1 | Describe the current status of reproductive health |
| CM 10.6 | Enumerate and describe various family planning methods, their advantages and shortcomings |

## REPRODUCTIVE HEALTH

The concept of **reproductive health was** introduced at the International Conference on Population and Development in 1994. The Conference emphasized the fundamental role of women's interests in population matters and introduced the concept of sexual and reproductive health and reproductive rights.

The reproductive health is defined as a state of complete physical, mental and social well-being and not merely the absence of disease or infirmity, in all matters relating to the reproductive system and to its functions and processes. Its core components are promotion of reproductive health, voluntary and safe sexual and reproductive choices for individuals and couples, including decisions on family size and timing of marriage. Sound reproductive health is integral to the vision that every child is wanted, every birth is safe, every young person is free from HIV, and every girl and woman is treated with dignity. Implicit in this vision is the idea that men and women will be able to exercise their rights to information on and access to safe, affordable and acceptable methods of fertility regulation as well as quality health care services.

### Milestones in Reproductive Health

**1952:** India became the first country in world to launch Family planning program with a clinic base approach.

**1992:** Child Survival and Safe Motherhood (CSSM) Programme was launched in the month of August.

**1994:** International Conference on Population and Development (Cairo) prompted a paradigm shift in population program, with the advocacy of client-centered and quality-oriented reproductive health approaches.

**2000:** The National Population Policy was formulated which reiterated the government's commitment to promote voluntary and informed choice, and continuation of the target-free approach in family planning service delivery.

**2005:** The National Rural Health Mission (NRHM) was launched to revamp the public healthcare delivery system and seeks to provide accessible, affordable and quality healthcare to rural population.

**2005:** Reproductive and Child Health Programme II (RCH II) was introduced and focuses on addressing reproductive health needs of the population.

**2005:** Conditional Cash Transfer schemes like Janani Suraksha Yojana (for promoting institutional deliveries) were introduced to help address economic barriers for access to services.

**2012:** Family Planning 2020 was launched to intensify family welfare measures and reproductive health.

**2013:** NHM launched in 2013 included RMNCH +A and control of CD and NCD.

> **Note**
> **Twelve Pillars of Reproductive Health**
> 1. Status of women
> 2. Family planning
> 3. Maternal care and safe motherhood
> 4. Abortion
> 5. Reproductive tract infections and HIV/AIDS
> 6. Infertility
> 7. Nutrition
> 8. Infant and child health
> 9. Adolescent reproductive health and sexuality
> 10. Sexual behavior and harmful sexual practices
> 11. Environmental and occupational health
> 12. Reproductive tract malignancies.

**Reproductive health care** can be understood from the concept of reproductive health. It is the group of services including methods and techniques that contribute to reproductive health and wellbeing. It also includes sexual health, which means enhancement of life and personal relations.

Over the years, women's health needs have been addressed through maternal and child health program, focusing primarily

# Chapter 24: Reproductive Health and Family Welfare

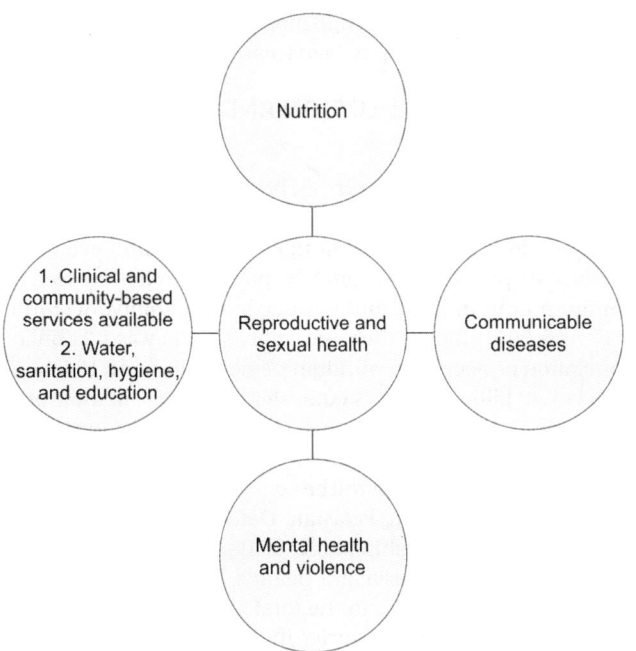

Fig. 24.1: Determinants and consequences of reproductive and sexual health.

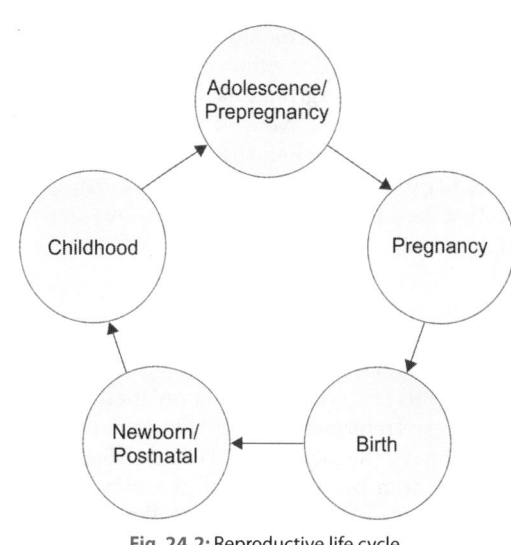

Fig. 24.2: Reproductive life cycle.

on narrow aspect of their lives. With new knowledge and changing perspectives, women's health is now being viewed in a holistic perspective as a continuum of care that starts before birth and progresses cumulatively through childhood and adolescence to adulthood and old age. The determinants and responses to women's health profile must consider all factors along with biological ones; such as the economic, social and cultural factors that affect their status, as well as gender relations between women and men (**Figs. 24.1 to 24.3**).

## Reproductive Rights

Woman empowerment is vital to attainment of reproductive health. Reproductive right refers to women's right to decide

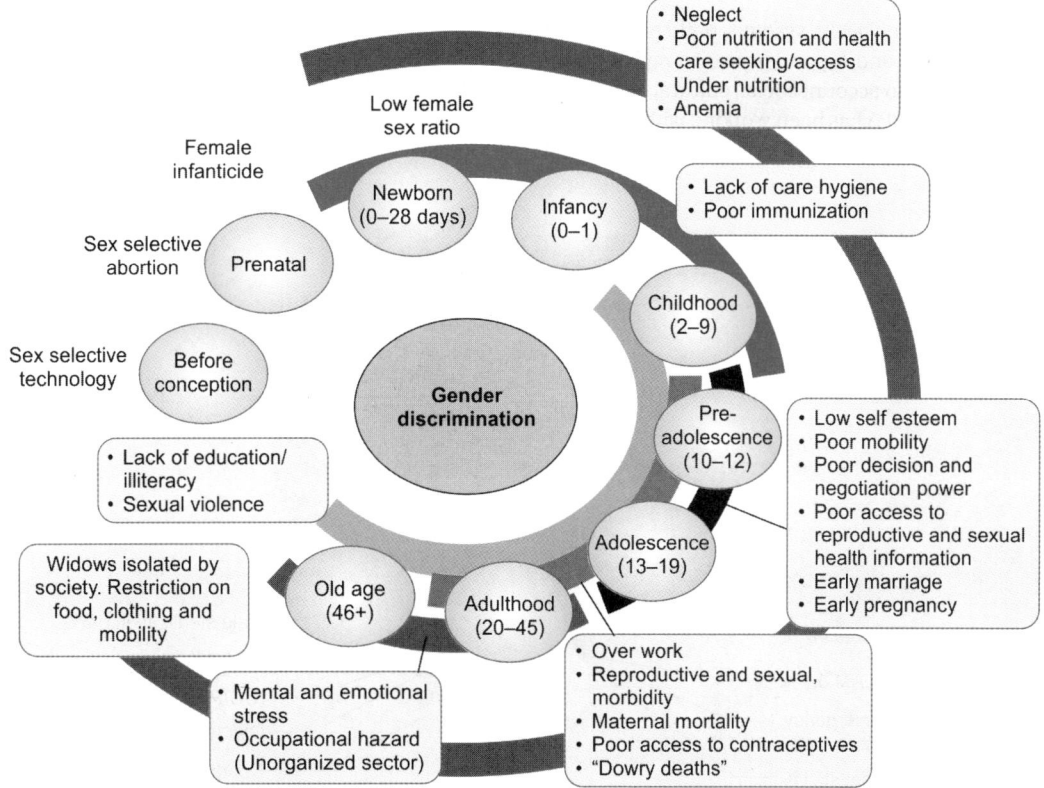

Fig. 24.3: Determinants of reproductive health at all stages of life.

whether, when and how to have children regardless of nationality, class, age, religion, ethnicity, race, disability, marital status and sexuality in the given social, economic and political conditions. Women Global Network for Reproductive Rights further elaborates that women should have full information about sexuality and reproduction, access to comprehensive reproductive health services that meet women's needs including right to safe and legal abortion, safe pregnancy and childbirth.

### Current Status of Reproductive Health in India

As per National Family Health Survey (NFHS-5, 2019-21) total fertility rate (TFR) of country is 2.0. Population in 24 states of India has achieved replacement level TFR. According to Sample Registration Survey (SRS, 2016) the TFR in 12 States has fallen below two children per woman and 9 States have reached replacements levels of 2.1 and above. Delhi, Tamil Nadu and West Bengal have reported lowest fertility rates. Fertility has declined even among the poor and illiterate (National Health Profile, 2018). The couple protection rate by any method of contraception according to NFHS-5 is 66.7%. Unmet need for family planning is 9.4%. As per NFHS-5, male participation in sharing responsibility for contraception is only 7.9% among currently married couples. Family planning methods used by currently married women aged 15-49 years is shown in **Figure 24.4**. India's current maternal mortality ratio is 97 per lakh live births (SRS Special bulletin for maternal mortality 2018-2020). Incidence of sexually transmitted and reproductive tract infections in India is found to be 5–6% (National Health Profile of India 2018).

It is imperative to strengthen health systems, build trust among the communities they serve and expand access to reproductive health programs that take into account social, cultural, economic and gender dimensions. UNFPA has been working with a range of partners to promote reproductive health in India with the aim to reduce maternal mortality, child mortality, as well as provision of range of quality contraceptive services.

## POPULATION EXPLOSION AND NEED FOR ITS STABILIZATION

The population of a country is both an asset and liability. Population explosion is the phenomenon of increase in growth of population up to the extent that it fails to fulfill even basic needs of its people. Unfortunately, population has crossed the optimum limit in India and has become a liability. According to Census 2011 (India), the population of India was 1.21 billion. Population projected on worldometer for India as on 15 January 2024 is 1.43 billion which is equivalent to 17.76% of the world's population, and ranks number 1 in the list of countries by population. It is expected that during 2015-2050, half of the world's population growth will be concentrated in nine countries including India, Nigeria, Pakistan, Democratic Republic of the Congo, Ethiopia, United Republic of Tanzania, United States of America (USA), Indonesia and Uganda, listed according to the size of their contribution to the total growth. China and India remain the two largest countries in the world, each with more than 1 billion people, representing 19% and 18% of the world's population, respectively. In April 2023, the population of India surpassed that of China. Effective implementation of population policy, family planning and family welfare measures are essential to stabilize population explosion.

In India, due to uncontrolled population growth the progress achieved in the economic field has been eroded. Factors responsible for population explosion is given in **Table 24.1**

### Measures for Population Control/Population Stabilization

- Family welfare measures
- Social welfare measures

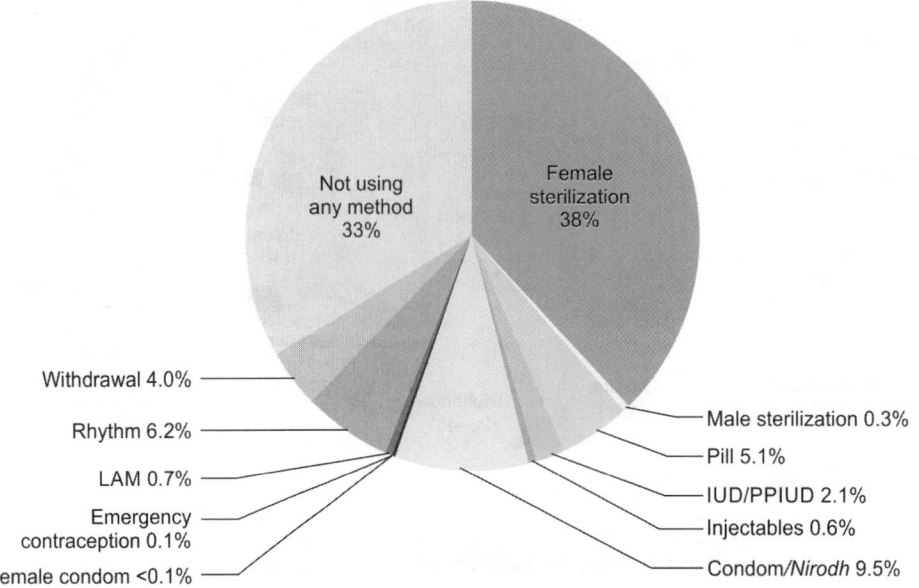

Fig. 24.4: What contraceptive methods do women use [National Family Health Survey (NFHS)-5].

Table 24.1: Factors and possible reasons behind each factor for population explosion.

| High birth rate | Low death rate | Migration |
|---|---|---|
| • Universal marriage norm<br>• Early age at marriage<br>• Teenage pregnancies<br>• Poverty and illiteracy<br>• Preference for a male child<br>• Role of women in decision making | • Advancement in medical science including improved diagnostic facilities, better healthcare infrastructure<br>• Health awareness and increased investment on health by people<br>• Political will for universal health coverage | Illegal migration from neighboring countries |

## FAMILY PLANNING AND FAMILY WELFARE

- Family planning is a cost-effective investment, which if done in time, can help to reduce the impact of high population growth.
- It can help women to achieve the desired family size and avoid unintended and untimely pregnancies.
- Timely use of contraceptives can prevent unsafe abortion and reduce maternal deaths.
- Sustainable Development Goal calls for universal access to family planning by 2030, and the Family Planning 2020 (FP 2020) initiative.
- Sustainable Development Goal 3.7 reaffirms this commitment by emphasizing improved access to reproductive health.

## Family Planning

India has been a pioneer in formulating a National Family Planning Programme in 1952 in order to accelerate the path to demographic transition. An Expert Committee (1971) of the WHO defined family planning as "a way of thinking and living that is adopted voluntarily, upon the basis of knowledge, attitudes and responsible decisions by individuals and couples, in order to promote the health and welfare of the family group and thus contribute effectively to the social development of a country". Main objectives of family planning practices are:
- To avoid unwanted births
- To bring about wanted births
- To regulate the intervals between pregnancies
- To control the time at which births occur in relation to the ages of the parent
- To determine the number of children in the family.

### Why Focus on Unwanted Pregnancies

Unwanted pregnancy is one where either the woman, or man, or both did not desire a child at the time of conception. Interruption of pregnancy in India could be due to medical, personal or social reasons where conception is unwanted. The consequences of abortion outside medical setting are dangerous both in terms of physical and mental health. Hence, the primary aim of family planning is to avoid such unwanted pregnancies.

### Why Focus on Number of Pregnancies and Birth

Complications of pregnancy and delivery are associated with high parity. It has been observed that maternal mortality increases with each subsequent pregnancy and significantly beyond the fifth. There is also a significant correlation between increased parity with fetal death rates and recurrent infection among infants.

### Why Focus on Spacing

Spacing is interval between conceptions or births. It has been proved that closely spaced pregnancies are associated with anemia, lactational insufficiency in mother and complications during pregnancy and delivery. A rise in infant mortality has been observed as birth interval decreases. Poorly spaced pregnancies result in poor and early weaning which is associated with increased diarrheal disease episodes in first two years of life.

### Why Focus on Timing of Birth with Respect to Maternal Age

Timing refers to time at which first and last birth occurs after the woman's marriage. This also takes into account the mother's age. Women who get pregnant before the age of 20 years or beyond the age of 35 years are at a higher risk of poor maternal and fetal outcomes including pregnancy related death, fetal loss and prematurity. Incidence of congenital anomalies like Down's syndrome increases as the age of mother increases above 35 years.

## Family Welfare

The concept of welfare is very comprehensive and is basically related to quality of life. Promotion of contraception purely on a voluntary basis, without any force, and with provision of due information about the various contraceptive alternatives is the central philosophy of our national family welfare program.

It was only in the fourth Five Year Plan (1969-1974) that the targets for population control were given to health workers and forced sterilization were made. But this approach was unacceptable to the people. As a result, from 1st April 1996, the Family Welfare Programme was implemented all over India based on Target Free Approach (TFA). The basic characteristics of TFA were to provide services according to client needs and eliminate centrally determined targets. In 1997, GOI realized that the term 'target free Approach' (TFA) was misinterpreted by health workers as TFA with no targets so no work. To communicate clear guidelines to health workers the TFA was renamed as Community Need Assessment approach (CNAA) in 1997. The practice of setting centrally defined, method-specific targets for contraception was abolished. It was replaced by decentralized; area-specific need assessment known as **Community Needs Assessment Approach (CNAA)**. In this approach health workers estimated felt health care needs of the population and prepared plan in order to meet these needs. Workers were also expected to involve community leaders in preparing these plans and promote community participation. Depending on the report generated by the health workers, Medical officer at PHC used to prepare the "Action plan". This is a document which mentions activities to be carried out in a specified time frame including the resource requirements, timetable and venue for each action.

> **Family Planning to Family Welfare**
>
> In 1977, the then ruling government in India developed a new population policy which was to be accepted not by compulsion but voluntarily. Hence, the term 'family planning' was replaced by 'welfare' which had following characteristics:
> - Voluntary and Informed Choice
> - Addressing unmet needs
> - Improve range and quality of services available
> - Removal of Demographic goals and targets
> - Increased participation of men Women's Participation in management
> - Prevention and control of abuse by program managers and providers

## Women in Reproductive Age (WRA)

Women in reproductive age in India is defined as those between 15–49 years age group. They contribute to 25.74% of total population of the country (Census 2011). The currently married women among the 15–49 years age group women are 73.84% (Census 2011).

## Eligible Couple

The primary purpose of Maternal and Newborn Health (MNH) Registry is to quantify and understand the trends in primary outcomes in defined geographic areas in order to provide population-based statistics on Stillbirth, Neonatal and Maternal Mortality and to know the causes and to take remedial action. Eligible couple is defined as a currently married couple with wife aged between 15 and 49 years who is in need of family planning services. Eligible couple (EC) in any area is calculated using following formula:

No. of EC in a population per year = (Projected population during that year) × (Rate)

(Where rate is the estimated number of eligible couple per 1000 population on the basis of census)

The basic document for organizing family planning program in India is the "Eligible Couple Register". It has to be updated regularly by the family planning program staff for a particular area.

### Target Couple

The priority couples within the broad definition of "eligible couples" are those who have had 2–3 living children. Family planning was initially largely directed to such couples. The definition of a target couple has been gradually enlarged to include families with one child or even newly married couples with a view to develop acceptance of the idea of family planning from the earliest possible stage. The term target couple, however, is no more used.

## CONTRACEPTIVE METHODS

Contraceptive methods can broadly be classified into:
A. Spacing methods (Temporary)
    I. Barrier method
        a. Physical
        b. Chemical
        c. Combined
    II. Intrauterine device
    III. Hormonal methods
    IV. Post-Conception Methods
    V. Natural/Miscellaneous
B. Terminal methods (Permanent)
    I. Male sterilization
    II. Female sterilization

## Spacing (Temporary) Methods

Birth spacing refers to the time interval between two successive pregnancies. After a live birth, the recommended interval before attempting the next pregnancy is at least 24 months in order to reduce the risk of adverse maternal, perinatal and infant outcomes. However, recent studies have suggested that longer birth spacing (3–5 years) may be more beneficial.

*Benefits of contraception:* Contraception allows and empowers a woman to make strategic life choices about her sexual and reproductive health and places her as a crucial stakeholder in the decision-making matrix. It reduces maternal mortality, child mortality, abortions and risk of sexually transmitted diseases like HIV transmission. Studies reveal that without contraceptive use the number of maternal deaths would have been 1.8 times higher than at present. Family Planning can avert more than 30% of maternal deaths and 10% of child death if couples spaced their pregnancies more than 2 years apart. A UNFPA Study has estimated that if the current unmet need for family planning could be fulfilled within the next five years, the country can avert 35,000 maternal deaths and 12 lakhs infant deaths. Constant efforts by the government have resulted in the decline of unmet need for family planning from 25.4% (DLHS-I) to 21.3% (DLHS-III) but approximately 4.2 crore couples still have an unmet need for contraception (1.6 crore for spacing and 2.6 crore for limiting). It favorably impacts the fertility rates and stabilizes population. Hence, it is prudent to increase the basket of choices as well as the service coverage simultaneously in the National Family Welfare Programme.

### Barrier Method

1. *Male condom:* It is a thin sheath made of latex or other material **(Fig. 24.5)**.
   **Mechanism of action:** The male condom acts as a physical barrier. It covers the penis and protects the wearer's partner from deposition of semen in vagina, thus prevents conception as well as transmission of sexually transmitted diseases. Condom is a very useful method of contraception where coital act is infrequent or irregular. Each condom can only be used once. **Benefits** of using a male condom are that it is inexpensive, easily available, do not require any prescription and easy to use. It protects against sexually transmitted diseases and HIV and has a lower risk of dysplasia and cancer. **Contraindications and/or side effects:** Specifically, no contraindications except that it may result in an allergic reaction among individuals suffering from latex allergy. It may also, sometimes, reduce sensitivity and pleasure and can slip or get torn during the act. **Failure rate:** 2–3 to 14 per hundred women years in typical users. Three varieties of condoms are

1. Handle with care

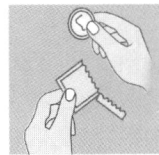

- The condom comes rolled up in a small package
- Open the package carefully
- Teeth, fingernails or sharp objects can damage the condom
- Once you have taken it out of the package, look to see which way it unrolls

2. Put the condom on

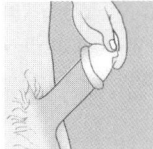

- Put condom on as soon as penis is hard and erect
- Pinch the top of the condom between your thumb and first finger to keep air out
- Leave about ½ inch of room at the tip. This allows space to catch the semen, so the condom would not break

3. Roll it down

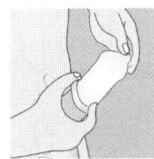

- Hold condom against the head of the penis
- Use your other hand to carefully unroll the condom over the penis, all the way down to the base

4. After sex

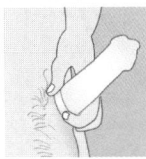

- After ejaculation, take the penis out while it is still hard
- Hold the rim of the condom around the base of the penis as it is pulled out
- Be careful not to spill any semen

5. Take it off

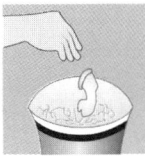

- Make sure the penis is away from your partner's body before your remove the condom
- Throw the used condom away. Never use a condom more than once

**Fig. 24.5:** How to use a condom.

available in India: dry types (non-lubricated), deluxe types (lubricated) and super deluxe types (colored, thinner and lubricated with spermicidal agents).

2. ***Sponge***: Shaped like a mushroom cap, it is made of polyurethane and contain one gm of nonoxynol-9. The sponge should be moistened with water (and not saliva), just before inserting and then placed over cervix. Once applied, it can be used for 24 hours. However, it should not be removed for 6 hours after intercourse. It is marketed under the brand name 'Today'. It may sometimes cause allergic reaction, toxic shock syndrome, vaginal irritation and fungal infection. It has a high failure rate of up to 20–40 per hundred women years **(Fig. 24.6)**.

3. ***Diaphragm:*** The diaphragm fits over the cervical opening, thereby preventing sperm from entering the uterus. It may be inserted for up to 6 hours before the intercourse and can safely be used during breastfeeding. It is best avoided in case of frequent urinary tract or bladder infections or if there is an allergy to rubber or latex. Insertion and removal of diaphragm requires skill, and it may lead to vaginal irritation and urinary tract infection in some cases. It has a failure rate of up to 6–12 per hundred women years **(Figs. 24.7A and B)**.

4. ***Female condom:*** It is made from soft thin plastic, polyurethane and is worn inside vagina. It has two rings, a thick inner ring with closed end, which is placed in the vagina, and thin outer ring that remains outside the body, covering the vaginal opening. Its insertion is similar to that of a tampon. It can be worn anytime before the act, i.e. before the penis comes in contact with the vagina. It should be used only once and removed immediately after the act by gently pulling it out. Difficult and incorrect use often results in failure rates of up to 5–21 per hundred women year. Female and male condom should not be used simultaneously **(Figs. 24.8A and B)**. *Merits*: Prevents pregnancy as well as STDs including HIV/AIDS, controlled by woman and can be used even during menstruation. *Demerits*: Relatively expensive and not a very popular choice among women.

5. ***Spermicides:*** It includes foam, creams, jellies, suppositories, etc. which contain active surface agents that damage sperm cell membrane and inhibit oxygen uptake by sperms and

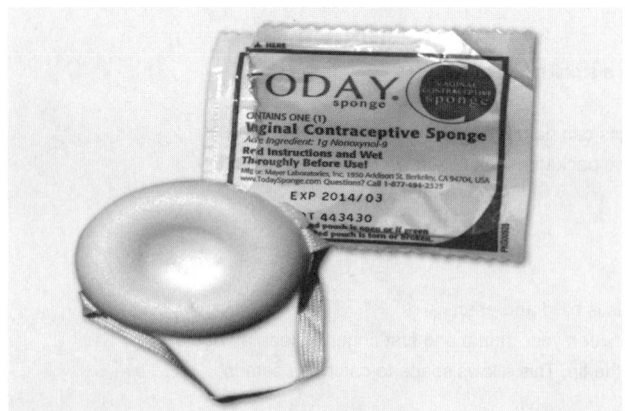

**Fig. 24.6:** Vaginal sponge.
*Source:* Available from http://teenhealthsource.com/birthcontrol/sponge-details/.

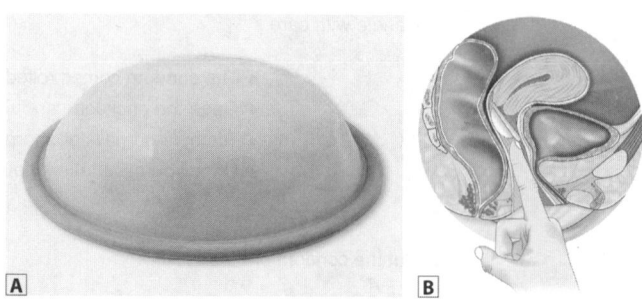

**Figs. 24.7A and B:** (A) Vaginal diaphragm; (B) Cervical cap after insertion.
*Source of 24.9A:* Available from https://www.istockphoto.com/in/photo/diaphragm-gm493174657-40698996.

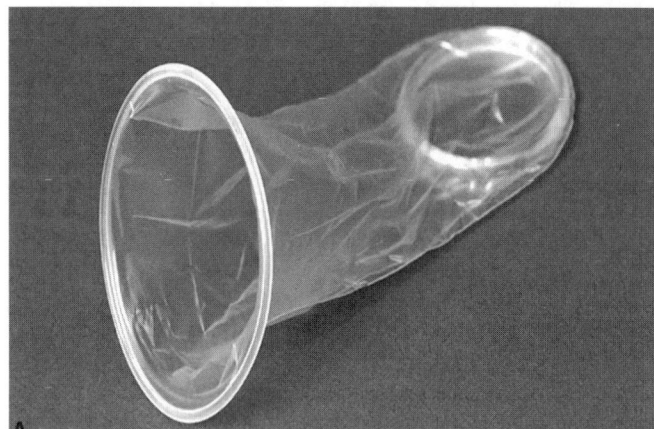

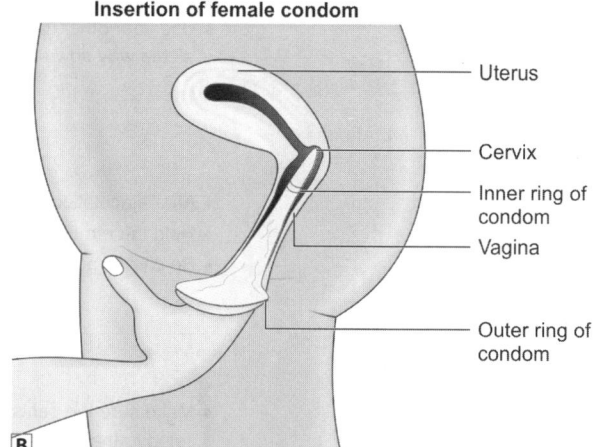

**Figs. 24.8A and B:** Female condom and its insertion.
*Source of Fig. 24.8A:* Available from http://www.vibe.ng/comfortably-wearing-a-female-condom.
*Source of Fig. 24.8B:* Available from http://www.womens-health-advice.com/birth-control/female-condom.html.

kill them. The main drawbacks of the spermicides are that they should be used almost immediately before the act and should be applied in areas where sperm deposition is likely, is associated with burning and irritation and have a high failure rate. This can be reduced by using spermicides in conjunction with physical barrier methods.

### Intrauterine Contraceptive Devices (IUCD)

It is a highly effective, long acting, reversible family planning method, comprising of a small device made of plastic and copper, and is inserted into the uterus. It can be classified on the basis of:

### Shape:
- Closed (e.g. Grafenberg's ring, Birnberg bow, Ota ring), and Closed IUCDs have a circumscribed aperture of <5 mm, therefore loop of intestine or omentum may get strangulated if the device accidentally ruptures through the uterus into the peritoneal cavity. Closed IUCDs have become obsolete nowadays.
- Open (e.g. CuT, Cu7, Lippes loop, etc.).

*Contents:*
- ***Non-medicated (first generation):*** Government of India introduced Lippes loop, a non-medicated, biologically inert IUCD, in 1965 under the national family planning programme, which has also become obsolete.
- ***Medicated,*** which can further be classified into copper containing and hormone releasing devices.
  - Copper based (second generation) (e.g., CuT200B, Cu7 (Gravigard), CuT 380A (Paragard) and Nova T, CuT 375: Radio-opaque copper wire is wrapped around the stem and arm of polypropylene frame. In CuT 380A, 314 mm$^2$ of copper wire is wrapped on the vertical stem and 33 mm$^2$ of wire is wrapped on each arm of IUCD. CuT 380 A has a life of 10 years and CuT 375 has 5 years. In Nova T, silver is added to copper wire, thereby, increasing its lifespan to five years **(Figs. 24.9 and 24.10)**.

**Mechanism of action:** CuT does not inhibit ovulation. It acts predominantly in the uterine cavity causing metabolic, enzymatic and nonspecific inflammatory

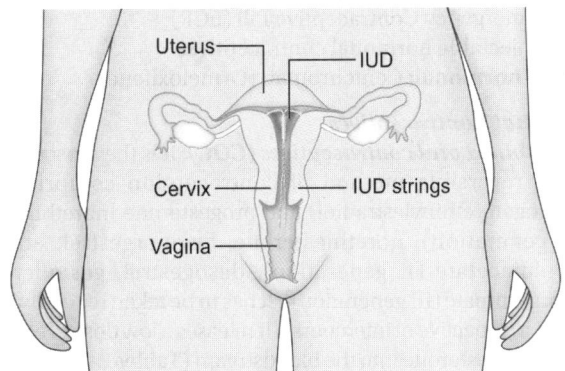

**Fig. 24.9:** CuT after insertion.
(IUD: intrauterine device)

*Timing of Insertion:* It can be inserted during or soon after menstruation, immediately following delivery within 48 hours, after 6 weeks postpartum and immediately after legally induced first trimester abortion. Immediate insertion is not recommended after second trimester abortion. It is preferably inserted during the follicular phase as the diameter of the cervical canal is greater and uterus is relaxed which increases the chances of its take up by the uterine cavity.

*Insertion of IUCD:* It should be inserted using gentle 'withdrawal technique.'

*Follow Up After Insertion:* Client should be asked to check the thread after every menstrual cycle to ensure that it is *in situ*. They must return for follow up after the first menstruation following IUCD insertion. The client should be advised to report immediately in case any of the following warning signs appear: missed periods, abdominal pain, pain during intercourse, local infection or foul smelling discharge, fever, chills and spontaneous expulsion. In absence of any complaints she must report for the examination after one year and two years of insertion.

Depending upon the type of IUD it has to be removed after the specific lifespan is over.

reaction in endometrium. Therefore, if fertilized ovum reaches the uterine cavity for implantation, it is engulfed by the macrophages. It also acts a foreign body in the uterine cavity, thereby, making it difficult for sperm to ascend the uterine cavity. In addition, it also increases the tubal motility and uterine contractibility.

Due to this, fertilized ovum reaches the uterine cavity before the development of chorionic villi and is unable to implant.

It has a low expulsion rate as compared to other IUCD and lower incidence of side effects

- **Hormone based (Third generation)** (e.g., Progestasert, LNG IUCD): Hormone releasing IUCD's are more efficacious with lower expulsion rates and have reduced risk of ectopic pregnancy and pelvic inflammatory disease as compared to copper carrying IUCD.

**Mechanism of action:** Hormone releasing IUCD increases viscosity of cervical mucus, thereby preventing sperm penetration. It also causes endometrial atrophy making it unfavorable for implantation. 38 mg progesterone is present in silicone oil reservoir in the vertical stem of Progestasert. In levonorgestrel IUCD, polydimethylsiloxane membrane is present around the stem, which acts as steroid reservoir.

*Ideal Candidate for IUD Insertion*

Women in the reproductive age group, women who has given birth to a child (should be avoided in nullipara) and not suffering from pelvic inflammatory disease, willing to check thread, willing for follow up.

IUCDs have a failure rate of 1 per hundred women year in the first year of insertion. Over 10 years of use, failure rate has been seen to be 2 per hundred women year.

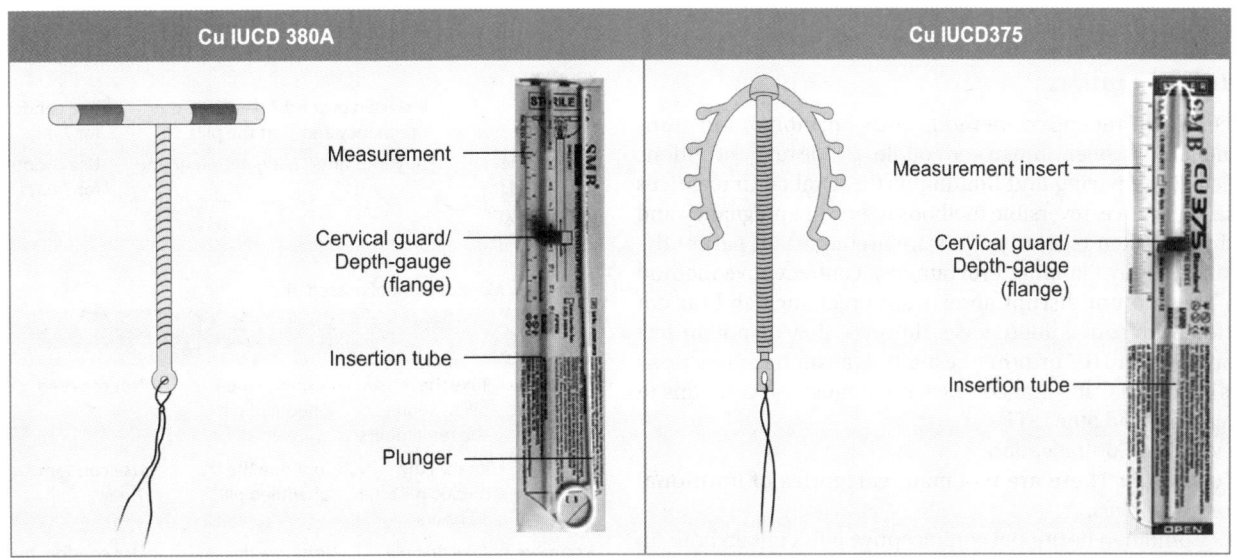

**Fig. 24.10:** Copper T 380A and 375.

### Advantages

IUCDs are simple and easy to insert, have a longer life, highest continuation rates and offer reversible protection against pregnancy. It is effective immediately after insertion and does not require daily attention by the user. It can safely be offered to lactating woman and once removed, return of fertility is almost immediate. It does not have hormonal side effects neither does it have any drug interaction.

### Non-Contraceptive Uses

IUCDs are used to prevent formation of adhesions following excision of uterine septum. Levonorgestrel IUCD is used to treat menorrhagia, dysmenorrhea, endometrial hyperplasia, endometriosis, adenomyosis and fibroid.

### Side Effects

The common side effects usually encountered after IUCD insertions are bleeding and pain. It may lead to an increased risk of pelvic inflammatory disease, actinomyces infection, ectopic pregnancy and dysmenorrhea. Incidence of uterine perforation is usually low and most perforations occur at the time of insertion. Expulsion rates are usually of the order of 5–15%, which is low. They do not, however, have systemic effects and return of fertility is almost immediate. IUCD does not protect against tubal and ovarian pregnancy, chances of which are highest with progestasert and lowest with levonorgestrel IUCD.

### Contraindications

**Absolute contraindications** to use of IUCD are acute pelvic inflammatory disease, dysfunctional uterine bleeding, known or suspected pregnancy, cancer of cervix, uterus or adnexa or any other pelvic tumor, previous ectopic pregnancy. **Relative contraindications** are fibroid uterus, congenital malformations or uterine prolapse, within 6 weeks following cesarean section, nulliparous women, history of heart disease or diabetes, severe anemia, conditions associated with increased susceptibility to infections, e.g., HIV positive patients not on ARV, leukemia, intravenous drug abuse, etc.

## Oral Contraceptives

An Oral Contraceptive method, both hormonal and non-hormonal ones, offer women and couples a wide range of options for delaying, spacing and limiting births. Oral contraceptives are safe, effective, reversible methods to prevent pregnancy and need to be taken regularly. They are an important part of the National Family Planning Programme's contraceptive method mix. They do not disrupt an existing pregnancy and do not interfere with sexual intercourse. However, they do not protect a woman from HIV or other Sexually Transmitted Infections (STIs). Women using oral contraceptives must use condoms to prevent HIV and other STIs.

Types of Oral Contraception:

A. **Hormonal:** There are two main categories of hormonal contraceptives:
   1. Combined hormonal contraceptive pills contain both an estrogen (usually ethinylestradiol) and a progestin
   2. Progestin-only contraceptive pills contain only progesterone a synthetic analogue (progestin).
   3. Emergency Contraceptive Pill (ECP)
   4. Injectable hormonal contraceptives

B. **Non-hormonal:** Centchroman (Ormeloxifene)

### Hormonal Contraceptives

- **Combined oral contraceptives (COC):** It is the most effective and reversible method of contraception comprising of estrogen (ethinylestradiol) and progesterone [norethindrone (I generation), norethiesterone, levonorgestrel, ethynodioldiacetate (II generation), desogestrel, gestodene or norgestimate (III generation)]. It has to be taken regularly every day, irrespective of intercourse. It releases a low dose of estrogen and progesterone into the bloodstream **(Tables 24.2 and 24.3)**.

Table 24.2: How to prescribe the pill?

| Women's situation | When to start | Back up method |
|---|---|---|
| Having regular menstrual cycle | Within first 5 days of starting the menstrual cycle | Not required |
| | If started after 5 days of starting the menstrual cycle, rule out pregnancy | Use a condom for first 7 days |
| **Breastfeeding** | | |
| Within first 6 months of child birth | Not recommended | Barrier contraceptive/POP |
| Beyond 6 months after childbirth | Anytime after resuming normal menstrual cycles, as specified above | Not required |
| | If menstruation not resumed, rule out pregnancy and start the pills | Use condoms for first 7 days |
| **Not breastfeeding** | | |
| Within first 4 weeks of childbirth | Any time on days 21-28 days after giving birth | Not required |
| Beyond 4 weeks after child birth | Any time after resuming normal menstrual cycles, as specified above | Not required |
| | If menstruation not resumed, rule out pregnancy and start the pills | Use condoms for first 7 days |
| After first or second trimester abortion | Immediately within 7 days | Not required |
| | If started beyond 7 days, rule out pregnancy and start the pills | Use condoms for 7 days |
| Amenorrhea (unrelated to pregnancy or breastfeeding) | Anytime, after ruling out pregnancy | Use condoms for 7 days |

Table 24.3: Management of missed pills.

| Missed pills | How to manage | How to continue | Back up method |
|---|---|---|---|
| 1 or 2 pills in the first week | Take the missed pill as soon as she remembers | Continue the scheduled pill | Not required |
| | If takes the missed pill after 12 hours | Continue the scheduled pill | Use condom for first 7 days |
| 3 or more pills in first 14 days | Take first pill as soon as possible | Continue the scheduled pill | Use condom for first 7 days/consider ECP if had sex in last 72 hours |

*Contd...*

*Contd...*

| Missed pills | How to manage | How to continue | Back up method |
|---|---|---|---|
| 3 or more pills in third week | Take first pill as soon as possible | Continue the hormonal pills as scheduled. Discard the nonhormonal pills. Start a new pack the very next day. | Use condom for first 7 days/ consider ECP if had sex in last 72 hours |
| Missed any nonhormonal pill | Discard the missed pill | Continue the scheduled pill. Start the new pack as usual | Not required |

- **Mechanism of Action:** COCs act by inhibiting ovulation and interfering with tubal motility. Estrogen inhibits FSH increase and progesterone inhibits LH surge. It causes atrophy of endometrium, thereby, preventing implantation. In addition, it causes thickening of cervical mucus making it viscous and tenacious preventing sperm penetration.

  COCs are available as 'standard dose pill' (EE ≥ 50 micro gm), 'low dose pill' (EE 30–35 micro gm), 'very low dose pill' (EE 20 micro gm). The combined OCP in government supply is available as 'Mala N' which has 21 'active' (hormonal) and 7 'inactive' (Do global "nonhormonal" contain ferrous fumarate) pills **(Fig. 24.11)**.

  First pill should be taken on the first day (or within first five days) of starting the menstrual cycle and should be taken once daily orally for 28 days without a break, preferably at the same time irrespective of the intercourse and the next pack should be started the very next day without a break. Additional contraception is required with antibiotics, e.g., cephalosporin, ampicillin and with enzyme inducing drugs like rifampicin, griesofulvin, phenobarbitone, spironolactone, ketoconazole, meprobamate, etc.

  COCs have a failure rate of 0.3 per HWY with perfect use and up to 8 per HWY with typical use.

- **Contraindications: Absolute contraindications** to use of combined pills are past or present thromboembolic disorder, coronary artery disease, known or suspected breast, endometrial or any other estrogen dependent neoplasia, pregnancy, hepatic adenoma, carcinoma or benign liver tumors, undiagnosed abnormal genital tract bleeding, markedly impaired liver function. **Relative contraindications** are migraine, gestational diabetes or diabetes, hypertension, depression, varicose veins, age >35 years, smoker, recent history of hepatitis, asthma, gall-bladder disease, ulcerative colitis, concomitant use of drugs that interfere with OCP, lactating women, etc.

- **Noncontraceptive benefits of COCs:** COCs have several noncontraceptive benefits, e.g., it reduces menorrhagia, polymenorrhea and dysmenorrhea and prevents anemia. It improves endometriosis, hirsutism, acne, autoimmune disorders of thyroid and rheumatoid arthritis and reduces the risk of PID, ectopic pregnancy, benign breast disease, fibroid uterus, carcinoma endometrium and ovary and protects against osteoporosis.

- **Side effects:** There are certain side effects associated with the use of OCP's like nausea, vomiting, headache, weight gain, mastalgia, chloasma, leucorrhea, breakthrough bleeding, hypomenorrhea, mood changes, sleep disturbances, psychotic manifestations, vascular manifestations like thromboembolism, cholestatic jaundice, hepatocellular adenoma, cervical carcinoma. OCP use also increases the chance of urinary tract infection, cervicitis, candidiasis and chlamydia trachomatis.

  COC available in public sector is Mala N, which contains 21 hormonal tablets containing 0.15 mg of levonorgestrel and 30 micro g of ethinyl estradiol and 7 nonhormonal iron tablets.

- **Progesterone only Pill/Micro Pill/Mini Pill:** Contain very low doses of progesterone (levonorgestrel or desogestrel). POPs can be safely used among lactating women, as they do not affect quality and quantity of milk. It can also be offered to women with history of hypertension, obesity, diabetes, fibroid, epilepsy and thromboembolic disorders.
  - **Mechanism of action:** It causes thickening of cervical mucus and endometrial atrophy.

    How to prescribe the pill?: It has to be taken one tablet daily, without any break, starting from first day of the menstrual cycle. It can be started at any time if it is reasonably certain that she is not pregnant. Failure rate of POP with perfect use among women who are breastfeeding is 0.3 per HWY and that among nonlactating women is 0.9 per HWY. However, it increases up to 1 per HWY among lactating and up to 3–10 per HWY among nonlactating women with typical use.
  - **Side effects:** It may lead to breakthrough bleeding (irregular, unexpected and heavy), ordinary headaches (usually non-migranous), mood changes and breast tenderness.
  - **Contraindications:** To use of POPs are previous ectopic pregnancy, ovarian cyst, breast and genital cancer, abnormal vaginal bleeding, active liver disease, porphyria and hepatic tumor.

- **Emergency contraception/postcoital contraception/morning-after pill:** emergency contraceptive pill is used to prevent pregnancy after unprotected sexual intercourse, sex was coerced or contraceptive accidents like condom rupture or missed pills. In the National Program, An EC pill contains only progestin—Levonorgestrel (1.5 mg per tablet). However, combined oral contraceptive pills containing an estrogen and a progestin can also be used as EC pills. ECPs are also called "morning-after pills" or postcoital contraceptives. This, however, is not an abortifacient and has no effect on the existing pregnancy. These are not appropriate for regular use as a contraceptive method because of the higher possibility of failure compared to other contraceptive method. In addition, frequent use of emergency contraception can result in side-effects such as menstrual irregularities. The repeated use poses no known health risks but is less effective than a regular method in preventing pregnancy.

  The following have been used as part of emergency contraception (some of which are now obsolete):

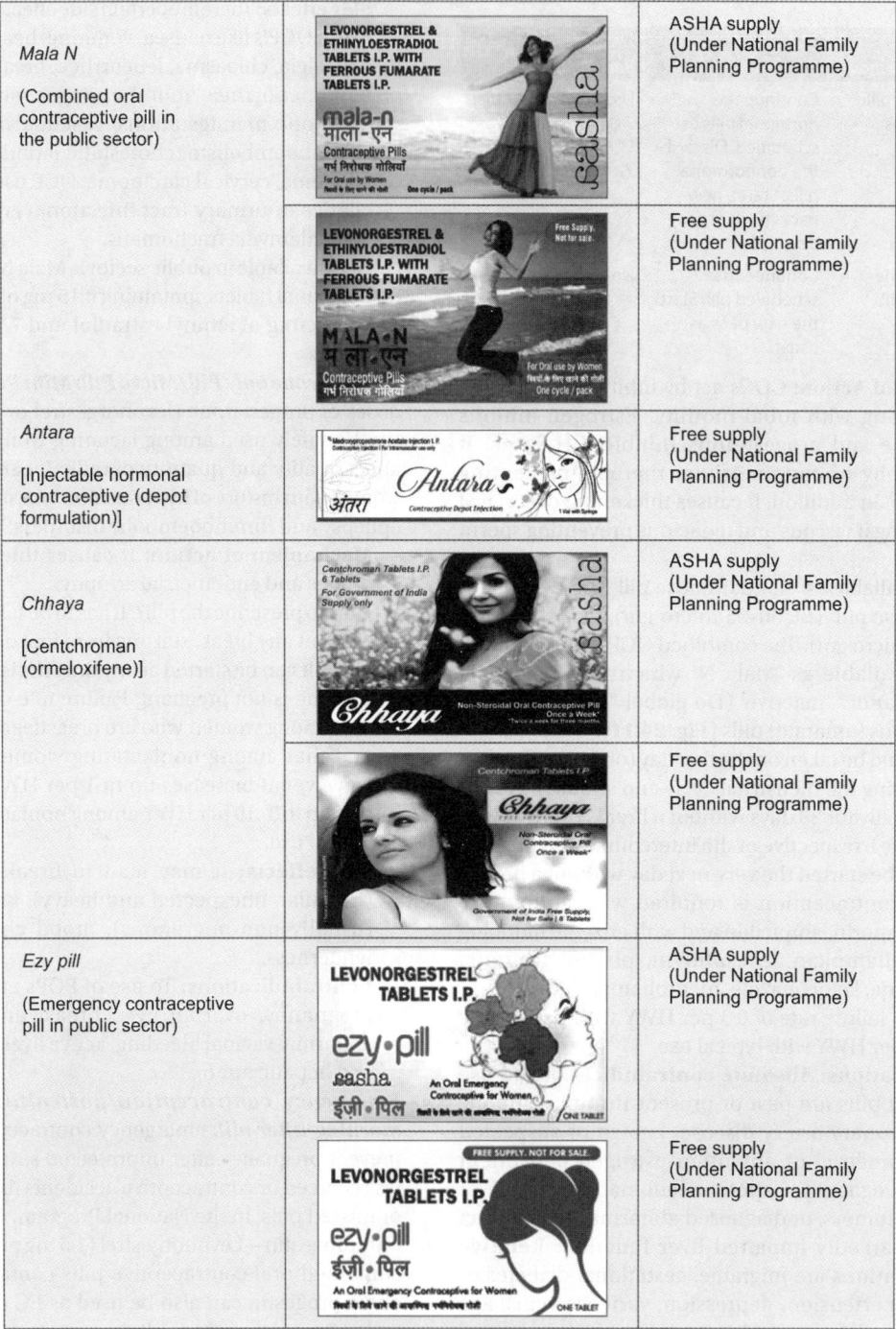

**Fig. 24.11:** Hormonal contraceptives.
*Source:* Reference Manual for Oral Contraceptive Pills. Family Planning Division, MoHFW.GoI, March 2016.

- Diethylstilbestrol (DES)-25 mg twice daily for a period of 5 days
- Ethinyl estradiol (EE)-2.5 mg twice daily for a period of 5 days.
- Premarin (conjugated estrogen) 5 mg twice daily for 5 days.
- Yuzpe method (Combined estrogen progesterone regimen): It is the most commonly used regimen wherein first dose is taken as early as possible but within the 72 hours of unprotected intercourse. Second dose should be taken twelve hours after the first dose.
- Ezy pill: It contains one tablet of 1.5 mg of levonorgestrel per tablet. Take the pill immediately after unprotected/ accidental intercourse or as soon as possible within next 3 days (72 hours). If not available, the woman can take four

tablets of Mala-D at the earliest followed by four more tablets after 12 hours of the first dose **(Fig. 24.11)**.
- IUCD: Can be inserted within 5 days of unprotected intercourse. CuT is the best postcoital contraceptive due to lowest failure rate and it can be left in the uterine cavity for ongoing contraception for next few years.
- **Injectable hormonal contraceptives:** These are contraceptives containing estrogen, progestins or both and are administered intramuscular or subcutaneous. There are two main types of injectable contraceptives:
  a. Progestogen only injectable: Contain only progesterone
     i. Depot Medroxy Progesterone Acetate (DMPA): This has been added to the basket of choice under National Family Planning Programme.
     ii. Norethisterone enanthate (NET-EN)
  b. Combined Injectable Contraceptive: Contain both estrogen and progesterone.
  - **Mechanism of action:** It acts by inhibiting the ovulation by suppressing the midcycle LH peak, causes endometrial atrophy and thickens the cervical mucus. It need not be taken daily unlike an OCP and does not have estrogenic side effects. It reduces menorrhagia and dysmenorrhea and is safe during lactation. It can be used as an interim contraception before vasectomy becomes effective. However, it does not protect against STI/RTI and HIV and may cause headache, breast tenderness, nausea, acne, irregular bleeding, amenorrhea and delayed return of fertility after discontinuation.
  - **When to Start DMPA:** It can be started anytime during the menstrual cycle (preferably within seven days of menstruation, ideally on the first day), immediately after abortion and childbirth, if the woman is not lactating. However, if the woman is lactating, start after six weeks.
  - **Site of Injection:** It is given through intramuscular route in the upper arm in deltoid or in upper and outer part of gluteus muscle (buttocks) or in anterolateral part of thigh. It can safely be given to any woman irrespective of age, parity and smoking status. It can be safely administered to lactating women except during first six weeks, women at risk of STI/HIV or HIV infected.
  - **Contraindications:** Injectable steroids are contraindicated if there is an active thrombophlebitis, thromboembolic disorder, undiagnosed abnormal genital tract bleeding, known or suspected pregnancy, acute liver disease, benign or malignant liver tumor and known or suspected carcinoma breast or blood pressure more than 160/100 mm Hg.
  - **Side effects:** The client may experience irregular or prolonged and heavy bleeding, amenorrhea, weight gain, headache, mood changes.

## Non- Hormonal Oral Contraceptive Pill

### Chhaya (Centchroman) (Fig. 24.11)

Ormeloxifene, a non-hormonal, non-steroidal, non-carcinogenic, non-teratogenic pill, is a selective estrogen receptor modulator, which acts by increasing the movement of the fertilized ovum through the fallopian tubes to the endometrial cavity, before it is ready for implantation. It also increases the rate of maturation of ovum and inhibits the fertilized ovum from implantation. It was developed indigenously by the Central Drug Research Institute (CDRI), Lucknow. It is safe for lactating women and is not known to cause any side effects except for prolongation of menstrual cycles in few women. It causes prompt return to fertility and can be given to women of all age groups. It should be taken twice a week for first 3 months and once a week thereafter. It has a failure rate of about 1–2 per HWY with perfect use. However, given the little experience, failure rate with typical use has not been documented so far.

## Post Conception Methods

1. **Menstrual regulation**
   It is a procedure which intends to aspirate uterine contents within 6 to 14 days of a missed period but before pregnancy is confirmed with the help of a pregnancy test. This is carried out as an outpatient procedure without requiring any anesthesia. Complications like uterine perforation and trauma may arise. After the procedure woman may suffer increased risk of abortion, infertility, menstrual disorders and ectopic pregnancies as late complications.

2. **Menstrual induction**
   It consists of intrauterine application of medical agents like prostaglandin (2.5 to 5 mg solution of PG F2) to induce menses in woman in whom menses is delayed.

3. **Abortion**
   Abortion is defined as removal of fetus before the period of viability (before 28 weeks of gestation). Modern methods use medication or surgery for abortions. The optimal time for abortion is up to the 8th week of gestation. The Indian Law (MTP Act 1971) allows abortion only up to 20 weeks.

## Natural Methods

This involves identifying signs and symptoms of fertility during menstrual cycle so as to plan a pregnancy. The various indicators which can help monitor the fertility are:

1. **Standard days method:** This method should be used if the menstrual cycles are regular and 26 to 32 days long. A woman with more than two longer or shorter cycles should opt for another method. Considering first day of menstrual bleed as the first day, the fertile period begins on day 8 and continues through day 19 of the cycle. This is the time when a couple should consider abstinence or practice safe sex for this method to be effective.

2. **Calendar rhythm method:** It takes into account the duration of cycles in the last one-year. To estimate the fertile period, subtract 18 from the total duration of shortest recorded cycle and 11 from that of the longest recorded cycle in last one year. For example, if a shortest cycle is 26 days long and longest cycle is 32 days long; subtract 18 from 26 and 11 from 32, which equal 8 and 21 respectively. Therefore, the fertile period extends from 8th day to 21st day of the cycle, considering first day of the cycle as first day of the menstrual bleeding. The disadvantage with these methods

is that the menstrual cycles are often not regular. They offer effective contraception only if the couple is motivated and understands the implications of failure which amount to 9 per hundred women year.

3. **Basal body temperature (BBT):** There occurs a physiological rise of BBT at the time of ovulation by 0.3 to 0.5 degree C as a result of an increase in the production of progesterone. Temperature should be recorded every morning before getting out of bed and before eating, drinking and smoking, preferably at the same time every morning. Unsafe intercourse should be avoided from first day to 3 days after the temperature rise. This method has high failure rates of up to 20 per hundred women year.

4. **Billing's method/Cervical mucus secretions:** There occur some changes in the consistency of cervical mucus during menstrual cycle, due to hormonal variations, which can be observed by touch or by toilet paper. Appearance of mucus marks the beginning of fertile period, which is usually 4–7 days prior to ovulation. Mucus secretions are moist, sticky, white and creamy which becomes clearer and slippery with 'egg white' consistency immediately before ovulation, which is also called the 'peak day'. The mucus consistency becomes thicker 3 days after ovulation indicating that the fertile period is over.

5. **Lactational amenorrhea method (LAM):** Exclusive breastfeeding suppresses woman's fertility in early months after delivery due to an increase in prolactin, which inhibits ovulation. It uses three parameters: Return of menstrual period after childbirth, patterns of breastfeeding and the time postpartum. LAM is effective until her menstrual period has not returned since delivery (bleeding or spotting during the first 56 days is not considered as menstrual bleeding), if she is breastfeeding exclusively and on demand, both during day and night and the baby is less than six months old.

Some other traditional methods are abstinence and coitus interruptus (also known as withdrawal method). These methods are difficult to practice and have high failure rates (25 per hundred women year). The client should be given adequate and correct information and training regarding traditional methods and repeated follow-up should be done to ensure regular and correct usage.

## Permanent/Terminal Methods

As the name suggests, these methods are generally irreversible.

### Female Sterilization

An MBBS doctor or DGO MD/MS in obstetrics and gynecology or specialist in other surgical field trained in minilap or laparoscopic sterilization can perform these procedures.

a. **Mini laptubectomy**
   *Timing:* It can be performed anytime within 7 days after the start of her menstrual bleeding (interval sterilization), within 7 days or after 6 weeks or more postpartum after ruling out pregnancy, post abortion (at the time of abortion or within 7 days).
   The procedure is determined by the size of the uterus and timing of last delivery.

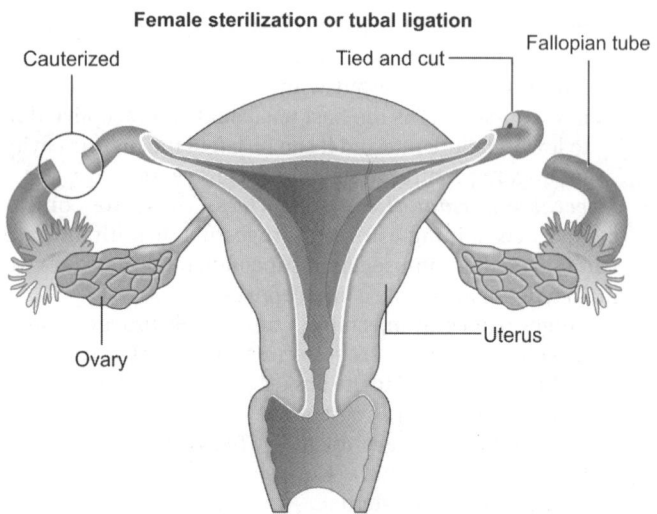

**Fig. 24.12:** Tubal ligation.

b. **Laparoscopic tubal occlusion**
   *Timing:* It is usually performed as an interval procedure or after first trimester abortion (concurrently).
   It involves inserting a long thin tube with a lens in it into the abdomen through a small incision. It enables the doctor to see and block or cut the tubes (**Fig. 24.12**).
   *Ideal Candidate:* Ever-married woman between 22 to 49 years of age having at least one living child more than one-year of age with no history of previous sterilization procedure(s) and be able to understand implications of sterilization (mentally fit).

### Male Sterilization

Vasectomy is a safe, effective and simple contraceptive method with low complication and failure rate. The two procedures that are currently being done are: (1) incisional vasectomy and (2) no-scalpel vasectomy (NSV). In incisional vasectomy scalpel incisions are made in the scrotum, which requires multiple stitches as compared to NSV wherein a small skin puncture is made which reduces the risk of bleeding and hematoma. Further, it does not require closure with stitches, which aids in quick recovery and fewer complications.

*Complications:* It may, however, cause swelling of the scrotal tissue, bruising and pain that usually subsides within 24 to 48 hours with ice packs, scrotal support and analgesics. Other complications may include hematoma, stitch abscess, scrotal infection, sperm granuloma and orchitis. There is also a possibility that the procedure may fail either due to technical failure or spontaneous re-canalization in some cases. There is, however, no association of vasectomy with prostatic or testicular cancer and cardiovascular disorder.

*Postoperative advice:* An individual can resume normal work within 48 hours and sexual intercourse within two to three days. However, another contraceptive method should be used for at least 3 months. Manual labor and strenuous work should be avoided for at least 48 hours and cycling should be resumed only after 7 days. The operated area should be kept clean and dry and the dressing should not be opened or disturbed until 48 hours after the procedure. There are no dietary restrictions. Bath can be taken after 24 hours.

A trained MBBS doctor can perform vasectomy in government and accredited private institutions **(Fig. 24.13)**.

***Eligible Candidate:*** An ever-married man between 22 to 60 years of age with at least one living child of more than one year of age with no past history of sterilization and the client should be mentally sound.

Vasectomy is not effective immediately. The couple should use an alternative method of contraception for first three months after sterilization until no sperms are detected in semen.

***Advantages:*** It is a very safe procedure, which does not involve stitches/incisions. It takes about 5–10 minutes to perform the procedure and does not entail prolonged pre- or postoperative admission. It does not reduce or affect the masculinity in any way does not cause any weakness. NSV does not protect against STI or HIV. It only prevents pregnancy. Rarely, failure may occur due to occlusion of a structure other than vas deferens, risk of which is 1–4 per 5,000 vasectomies.

## Postpartum Family Planning

In addition to postpartum sterilization and postpartum IUCD currently available under the National Programme, other postpartum family planning options can be: (i) Progestin only Pills (POPs) which is a well-recognized non-invasive option for spacing births in the postpartum period particularly for breastfeeding women and (ii) Centchroman (Ormeloxifene) as once-a-week contraceptive, a promising non-hormonal option for spacing, as it is safe for lactating women **(Table 24.4)**.

## Cafeteria Approach

This approach has been adopted by the Family Welfare Programme since 1960s. In this, clients are provided with a choice of contraceptive methods. It provides the clients with basket of choices that includes five official methods—female sterilization, male sterilization, intrauterine contraceptive device (IUCD), oral contraceptives, and condoms. This approach recognizes that different people have different needs, based on their age, family size preferences, economic conditions, religion and other factors. Cafeteria approach emphasizes on limitation of family size rather than on contraception.

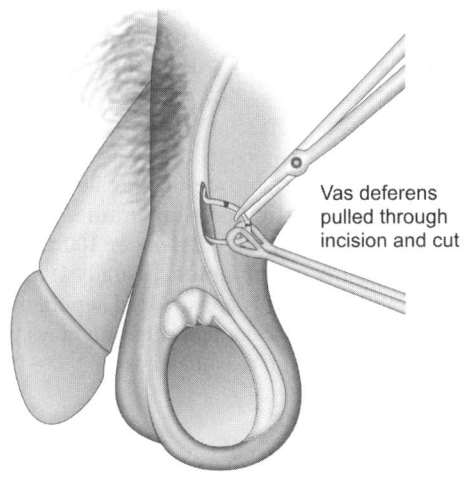

**Fig. 24.13:** No-scalpel vasectomy.

**Table 24.4:** The public sector provides the following contraceptive methods at various levels of health system.

| Family Planning Method | Service Provider | Service Location |
|---|---|---|
| **Spacing Methods** | | |
| IUCD 380 A, IUCD 375 | Trained and Certified ANMs, LHVs, SNs and Doctors | Sub center and higher levels |
| Injectable Contraceptive MPA (Antara Programme) | Trained ANMs, SNs and Doctors | Sub center and higher levels |
| Oral Contraceptive Pills (OCPs) | Trained ASHAs, ANMs, LHVs, SNs and Doctors | Village level sub center and higher levels |
| Condoms | Trained ASHAs, ANMs, LHVs, SNs and Doctors | Village level sub center and higher levels |
| **Emergency Contraception** | | |
| Emergency Contraceptive Pills (ECPs) | Trained ASHAs, ANMs, LHVs, SNs and Doctors | Village level sub center and higher levels |
| **Limiting Methods** | | |
| Minilap | Trained and certified MBBS Doctors and Specialist Doctors | PHC and higher levels |
| Laparoscopic Sterilization | Trained and certified MBBS Doctors and Specialist Doctors | Usually CHC and higher levels |
| NSV: No-scalpel Vasectomy | Trained and certified MBBS Doctors and Specialist Doctors | PHC and higher levels |

*Note: Contraceptives like OCPs, Condoms are also provided through Social Marketing Organizations.*

## Counseling for Contraceptives

It is imperative to help women and their spouses to gain increased control over their reproductive health. One of the main ways to achieve this is through counseling on family planning methods during late pregnancy, the postpartum and the post-abortion periods. Special emphasis is placed on interpersonal communication (IPC) and use of local traditional media for increasing acceptance and understanding of messages and thereby their effect and impact through behavior change. **GATHER Approach** is used for contraceptive counseling. There are 6 steps to it which can be remembered by the Mnemonic "GATHER".

**G:** Greet clients—with a smile and in a friendly manner

**A:** Ask their contraceptive requirements by asking open ended questions

**T:** Tell them about available methods under RCH program

**H:** Help them to choose the method most suitable to them by providing correct information

**E:** Explain use, side effects (if any), and failure rate of the method chosen

**R:** Return visit, follow up explained

A counselor should be empathetic, patient, understanding, supportive, helpful and encouraging to motivate his/her clients to express their emotions and health problems.

### Role of Social Marketing in Family Welfare

The social marketing of contraceptives was conceived by Peter King and his colleagues at Calcutta's Indian Institute of Management in 1964. Using commercial marketing techniques, social marketing makes a product available, affordable and seeks to influence social behaviors not intended to benefit the marketer, but to benefit the target audience and society at large. The Government of India (1968) became the first country to initiate a social marketing program for contraceptives with the launch of condoms under the brand name of "Nirodh". It helps in increase in choices, awareness and acceptability of contraceptives.

Currently the Ministry of Health and Family Welfare is providing condoms and OCPs under the social marketing scheme by the brand names Nirodh and Mala-D which contributes to 1/3rd of the total distribution of contraceptives.

### Adolescents and Reproductive Health

Sexual activity and unmet need for contraception are common among married as well as unmarried adolescents. According to the latest 2015-16, National Family Health Survey (NFHS-4) data, one in four Indian women (26.8%) is married before 18, and 7.9% of women aged 15 to 19 are pregnant or mothers. Contraception prevalence among adolescents is less due to lack of sex education and adolescent friendly health services. Condoms are the recommended contraceptives available for adolescents. It provides dual protection against unwanted conception and STDs/HIV. Although female condoms are relatively expensive than male condoms but may be opted where male partner is resistant. Emergency contraceptive pills (ECPs) can reduce the risk of unintended pregnancy when taken after unprotected sexual intercourse and offer women an important second chance to prevent pregnancy when a regular method fails or when no contraceptive method was used or sex was forced. ECPs contain either progesterone alone or progestin and estrogen combined together to prevent ovulation.

While menstrual hygiene and problem of anemia among adolescents is recently recognized as well as addressed by the government, sexual and reproductive health is still a relatively neglected area. If addressed adequately this will reduce unwanted teenage pregnancies, unsafe abortions, transmission of STD/HIV among adolescents and school drop outs.

### Evaluation of Effectiveness of Contraceptive Methods

The degree to which contraceptive method produces desired result depends on a number of factors including fertility, age of woman, correct usage of method, and natural strengths of the method. Effectiveness of contraception is presented in terms of failure rates.

- *Perfect use failure rate:* The number of pregnancies occurring when the method is used consistently and correctly at all times.
- *Typical use failure rate:* The number of pregnancies occurring when the method is used both correctly and incorrectly, reflecting contraceptive practice in real life. Pills and barrier methods have higher typical use than perfect use failure rates as they are user dependent.
- Methods which do not need dependency on user like Intrauterine devices have similar perfect and typical use failure rates. Other methods (e.g. abstinence) have very different perfect and typical use failure rates.

### *Pearl Index*

Historically, contraceptive efficacy has been calculated by the Pearl index named after Raymond Pearl. The Pearl Index is recorded as a statistical estimation of pregnancy risk per year. The formula used is:

$$\text{Pearl index} = \frac{\text{Number of pregnancies} \times 12}{\text{Number of women in the study} \times \text{duration of study in months}} \times 100$$

For example, if during a test 100 women use a certain contraceptive method and during a period of 12 months, 2 unintended pregnancies occur, the Pearl index is 2. The period of pregnancy (10 months) and abortion (4 months) are deducted from the 'duration of study in months' in denominator. The unit of Pearl Index is HWY (hundred women years). If the Pearl Index is 2, it means a failure rate of 2 per 100 women years of use (or 2 accidental pregnancies per 100 women years of use). Since, the average reproductive period of women is 25 years, Pearl Index of 2 HWY means 0.5 accidental pregnancies will occur if a woman uses particular contraceptive method for entire reproductive period. The higher the Pearl index, the lower the effectiveness/the higher the failure rate of the contraceptive method. This index can range from '0' when no pregnancy occurred among any women during period of follow up to 1200 when all women become pregnant if they are using that particular method in given time (one year). The drawback of this formula is that the calculation is based on the observation of only a sample population. If the test is applied on different populations the same contraceptive can perform differently. Also the duration of the study may impact the result as it was statistically found that the longer a couple uses a certain method, the lower the registered failure rate.

### *Life Table Methods*

Recent researchers use life table method to calculate cumulative failure rates over a particular time frame. They present failure rate as number of pregnancies per 100 women years, standardized by yearly cut-off points (usually 1, 3 or 5 years). The daily life-table method is constructed separately for each reason for discontinuation, considering only days in which a discontinuation for a certain reason occurs.

### Couple Protection Rate

Couple protection rate (CPR) is an indicator of the prevalence of use of contraceptive services in the community. It is one of the output indicators of family welfare program at local level. It is defined as the percent of eligible couples effectively protected against childbirth by one or the other approved methods of family planning, viz. sterilization, IUD, condom or oral pills. Sterilization as per the latest national data accounts for over 60 per cent of effectively protected couples.

Alternate term used is contraceptive prevalence rate which is defined as the percentage of women (in 15-49 years age group) currently using any contraceptive method. The modern contraceptive prevalence rate is limited to women using modern contraceptive methods, viz. sterilization, condoms, oral hormonal pills, intrauterine devices, injectable, implants, vaginal barrier methods, and emergency contraception. Contraceptive Prevalence Rate is a ratio, not a rate. (Prevalence is measured by a ratio and incidence by a rate.)

Demographers are of the view that the demographic goal of net reproductive rate (NRR) = 1 can be achieved only if the CPR exceeds 60 per cent.

As per NFHS-5 (2019-21), 67% currently married women (15-49 years age) use any method of contraception (*see* **Fig. 24.4**). Among the states, the use of contraceptive methods is the lowest in Meghalaya (27%), Mizoram (31%), and Bihar (56%), and highest in West Bengal, Odisha, and Himachal Pradesh (74% each) (NFHS-5).

## Effective couple protection rate (ECPR)

ECPR is percentage of eligible couples protected against one or other methods of family planning, viz. condoms, OCPs, IUDs, sterilizations taking into account their effectivity.

Effectivity of approved contraceptive methods:
1. Condoms: 50%
2. IUDs: 95%
3. OCPs: 100%
4. Sterilization (vasectomy or tubectomy): 100%

For a given contraceptive use by couple in an area, multiply the effectivity of contraceptive method and the resulting number will be the effectively protected couples with that particular contraceptive.

Effectively protected couples = no. of couples using a particular contraceptive in an area × effectivity of contraceptive method.

$$ECPR = \frac{\Sigma \text{ effectively protected couples from all contraceptives}}{\text{Number of Eligible couples in that area}}$$

## Concept of Unmet Need for Family Planning

A sizeable proportion of pregnancies in India are unplanned (mistimed or unwanted). It is anticipated that if all unwanted births could be eliminated, the total fertility rate would drop to the replacement level of fertility.

Unmet need for family planning is defined as the percentage of women of reproductive age, either married or in a union, whose need for family planning has not been met. These women are those who either want to stop or delay childbearing but are not using any method of contraception.

$$\text{Unmet need} = \frac{\text{Women of reproductive age (15-49 years) who are married or in a union and who have an unmet need for family planning}}{\text{Total number of women of reproductive age (15-49) who are married or in a union}} \times 100$$

The numerator includes women who are productive and sexually active but are not using any method of contraception. But they report of not wanting any more children or wanting to delay the birth of their next child for at least two years. The gap between women's reproductive intentions and their contraceptive actions is actually the unmet need. The indicator is useful for tracking progress towards the target of achieving universal access to reproductive health.

Total demand for family planning = contraceptive prevalence + unmet need

Unmet need for modern methods = unmet need for family planning + prevalence of modern methods

Unmet need in India for different age groups can be summed up as:
- Unmet need in <20 years old women: spacing the births
- Unmet need in 20-24 years old women: spacing the births
- Unmet need in >30 years old women: limiting the births

### Magnitude

India contributes to 20% of world's eligible couples with unmet need. According to NFHS-5 (2019-21) 9 percent of currently married women have an unmet need for family planning, including 4 percent who have an unmet need for spacing births and 5 percent who have an unmet need for limiting births. Unmet need for family planning methods is highest in Meghalaya (27%) and Mizoram (19%).

### Trends

The women with an unmet need declined slightly (by 19%) during the six years between NFHS-1(35%, 1992-93) and NFHS-2 (16%, 1998-99). The decline was more marked in the case of unmet need for spacing (25%) than for limiting (12%). It further decreased to 13.9% as per NFHS 3 (2005-06). However, the decline was only by 1% in a decade from NFHS-3 (2005-06) to NFHS-4 (2015-16). Decline of 7% noted from NFHS-4 to NFHS 5 (2019-21).

### Barriers to Contraceptive Needs

The barriers to contraceptive choice and meeting contraceptive needs in the country are evidence based and have been summed up as:
- Low awareness regarding reversible contraceptives among males and females.
- Incomplete or incorrect information on where to obtain methods and how to use them.
- Gender inequalities in decision making and limited male participation in use of contraceptives.
- Limited access to a wider choice of methods.
- Sometimes providers do not counsel women and men about variety of methods to exercise their right to contraceptive choice.
- Stock-outs and irregular supplies of reversible contraceptives.

- Service providers tend to pay no attention to women's need for privacy, and are callous about women's dignity. This compromises the quality of services.

## SOCIAL WELFARE MEASURES AND INITIATIVES TO CONTROL POPULATION

Population change often has long-term consequences throughout the society. Hence it is the combined responsibility of the government as well as society to take appropriate measures to check the population growth. To control excessive population growth contraceptive measures have been discussed earlier and social measures are as follows **(Table 24.5)**:

**Table 24.5:** Social welfare measures and Initiatives by GOI to control population.

| Measures Required | Initiatives taken by Government of India |
|---|---|
| 1. Raising age at marriage | Child marriage Restraint Act,1978 fixing minimum age at marriage for girls to 18 years and boys to 21 years |
| 2. Increase in literacy level | 1. Establishment of Anganwadi and primary schools<br>2. Encouraging adult education |
| 3. Reduce poverty | **Rural areas**<br>1. National Rural Livelihood Mission (NRLM)-Deen Dayal Antayodaya Yojana<br>2. Mahatma Gandhi National Rural Employment Guarantee Act (MGNREGA)<br>3. Mahila Kisan Sashaktikaran Pariyojana<br>**Urban areas**<br>1. Swarna Jayanti Shahri Rozgar Yojna |
| 4. Women empowerment | The Women's Reservation Bill 2008 was introduced by UPA-I government which proposed to amend the Constitution of India to reserve 33% seats in the Lower House of Parliament of India, the Lok Sabha and in all state legislative assemblies for women. It was introduced but lapsed. |
| 5. Raising standards of living | 1. Indira Awaas Yojana<br>2. Bharat Nirman Scheme |

### United Nations Fund for Population Activities (UNFPA) Strategic Plan 2018–21

This is aligned with the 2030 Agenda for Sustainable Development and its 17 Sustainable Development Goals. The goal of the strategic plan, 2018–2021, is to "achieve universal access to sexual and reproductive health, realize reproductive rights, and reduce maternal mortality to accelerate progress on the agenda of the Programme of Action of the International Conference on Population and Development, to improve the lives of women, adolescents and youth, enabled by population dynamics, human rights and gender equality".

UNFPA will organize its work around three transformative and people-centered results in the period leading up to 2030. These include: (a) an end to preventable maternal deaths; (b) an end to the unmet need for family planning; and (c) an end to gender-based violence and all harmful practices, including female genital mutilation and child, early and forced marriage.

### Family Planning 2020

India is one of the chief protagonists in the global Family Planning 2020 action plan formulated in 2012. Aim is to drive access, choice, and quality of family planning services. Since FP2020 commitment in 2012, India has continued its efforts to expand the range and reach of contraceptive options through rolling out new contraceptives and delivering a full range of family planning services at all levels. Mission Parivar Vikas was launched in 2016 initially for 146 high priority districts in the 7 high focus states, is scaled up in all districts of the seven high focus states as well as six north-eastern states of the country with an aim to ensure availability of contraceptive products to the clients at all the levels of Health Systems. *This is further explained in Chapter 47: Health Policies and Programs in India.* India has integrated family planning into the Reproductive, Maternal, Newborn, Child, and Adolescent Health Plus Nutrition (RMNCAH+N) Strategy. The Government of India has enhanced its supply chain system through rolling out Family Planning Logistics Management Information System (FP-LMIS). Increasing awareness and generating demand for family planning services through comprehensive media campaigns have been priorities. The Government of India has increased domestic investment for family planning.

## ASSISTED REPRODUCTIVE TECHNOLOGY (ART)

India faces a high burden of infertility and over the last few years, Assisted Reproductive Treatment/Technology (ART) has turned out to be a boon for those deprived of progeny. **Assisted Reproductive Technology (ART)** refers to procedures used to assist people in achieving conception.

### Methods of ART

- ***In vitro fertilization (IVF):*** Here fertilization occurs outside the body. It is the most effective ART and is usually used when a woman suffers blockade of fallopian tubes or when a man produces very few sperm.
  **Method:** In IVF the ovaries are stimulated with the help of drugs to produce multiple eggs. Once mature, the eggs are removed from the woman and are allowed to fertilize with the man's sperm in a dish in the laboratory. After 3 to 5 days, healthy embryos are implanted in the woman's uterus.
- ***Zygote intrafallopian transfer (ZIFT) or Tubal embryo transfer:*** In this method fertilization occurs in the laboratory and fertilized embryo is transferred to the fallopian tube instead of the uterus.
- ***Gamete intrafallopian transfer (GIFT):*** Involves transferring eggs and sperm into the woman's fallopian tube. So fertilization occurs in the woman's body.
- ***Intracytoplasmic sperm injection (ICSI):*** It is indicated in case of couples experiencing male factor infertility, especially problems with the quality or quantity of sperm. It is also recommended for older couples or for those with failed IVF attempts.

**Method:** A single sperm is injected into a mature egg. After fertilization, the embryo is transferred to the uterus or fallopian tube.

*Newer ARTs:* Many newer techniques like, Artificial reproduction, Cloning, Cytoplasmic transfer, Cryopreservation of (sperm, oocytes, embryos), Embryo transfer, Fertility medication, Hormone treatment have came into existence.

### Challenges in ART

- Lack of awareness regarding availability of such fine and promising techniques.
- Lack of regulation of ART Clinics: The ART Bill which was originally drafted in 2008 and then revised in 2010 and 2014 is still pending in the parliament. There is an urgent need for this bill to be made into a law.

## SUMMARY

Concept of sexual and reproductive health came into existence during International Conference on Population and Development (ICPD) in 1994. There are several reproductive health concerns in India like high unwanted fertility, high maternal mortality, STI/RTI and poor access to health services which need to be addressed in order to improve reproductive health status of people. Contraception allows and empowers a woman to make strategic life choices about her sexual and reproductive health. It favorably impacts the fertility rates and stabilizes population. To raise contraceptive prevalence, Ministry of Health and Family Welfare is putting best of its efforts to increase the basket of choices as well as the service coverage simultaneously in the National Family Welfare Programme. Currently, contraceptive choices available at various levels of public health institutions are Condoms, IUDs, OCPs (hormonal and non-hormonal), emergency contraceptives, injectable MPA for spacing between pregnancies and tubectomy and vasectomy services as terminal methods of contraception. Enactment of Medical Termination of Pregnancy Act, 1971 and PCPNDT Act, 2003 further helps to reduce maternal mortality due to unsafe abortions. Amalgamation of family welfare measures with social welfare measures is the key to improve women health.

## SUGGESTED READING

1. Centers for Disease Control and Prevention. (2016). Condom effectiveness. [online] Available from https://www.cdc.gov/condomeffectiveness/Female-condom-use.html.
2. Cleland J, Bernstein S, Ezeh A, Faundes A. Family planning the unfinished agenda. Lancet. 2006; 368(9549): 1810-27
3. Conde-Agudelo A, Rosas-Bermúdez A, Kafury-Goeta AC. Birth spacing and risk of adverse perinatal outcomes: a meta-analysis. JAMA. 2006;295: 1809-23.
4. Government of India. Census of India. Annual Health Survey report: A Report on Core and Vital Health Indicators. Part I. New Delhi: GOI; 2014.
5. Government of India. District Level Health Survey III (2006–2007). IIPS, Mumbai: Ministry of Health and Family Welfare; 2008.
6. Government of India. District Level Health Survey IV (2012-13). IIPS, Mumbai: Ministry of Health and Family Welfare;2015.
7. Government of India. Handbook on Medical Methods of Abortion to Expand Access to New Technologies for Safe Abortion. New Delhi: MoHFW;2016.
8. Government of India. IUCD Reference Manual for Medical Officers and Nursing Personnel. MoHFW, GOI;2013.
9. Government of India. Manual on Target-free Approach in Family Welfare Programme. New Delhi: Ministry of Health and Family Welfare; 1996.
10. Government of India. National Family Health Survey (NFHS-4) (2015–2016). India fact sheet. IIPS, Mumbai: Ministry of Health and Family Welfare; 2017.
11. Government of India. National Family Health Survey III (2005-06). India fact sheet. IIPS, Mumbai: Ministry of Health and Family Welfare; 2007.
12. Government of India. Press Information Bureau. Ministry of Health and Family Welfare. Health Ministry to launch "Mission Parivar Vikas" in 145 High Focus districts for improved family planning services. [online] Available from http://pib.nic.in/newsite/PrintRelease.aspx?relid=151049..
13. Government of India. Press Information Bureau. Ministry of Health and Family Welfare. Initiatives under the Family Planning Programme. [online] Available from http://pib.nic.in/newsite/PrintRelease.aspx?relid=159064.
14. Government of India. Sample registration survey statistical report, 2016. New Delhi: Office of the Registrar General and Census Commissioner, India; 2016.
15. https://main.mohfw.gov.in/sites/default/files/NFHS-5_Phase-II_0.pdf
16. Pearl R. Factors in human fertility and their statistical evaluation. Lancet. 1993;222(5741):607-11.
17. Review of implementation of Community Needs Assessment approach for family welfare in India. Policy Project II. The Futures Group International. New Delhi: MoHFW;1998.
18. Special Bulletin on Maternal Mortality in India, 2016-18. Sample Registration System, Vital Statistics Division. New Delhi: Office of the Registrar General and Census Commissioner, India.
19. Trussell J, Hatcher RA, Cates W Jr, et al. A guide to interpreting contraceptive efficacy studies. Obstet Gynecol. 1990;76(3 Pt2):558-67.
20. Trussell J. Methodological pitfalls in the analysis of contraceptive failure. Stat Med. 1991;10(2):201-20.
21. United Nations. Executive Board of the United Nations Development Programme, the United Nations Population Fund and the United Nations Office for Project Services. (2017). UNFPA strategic plan, 2018-2021.
22. United Nations. Programme of Action of the International Conference on Population and Development. New York: United Nations;1994.
23. United Nations 2015: World Population Prospects: the 2015 Revision. DVD edition. New York: United Nations, Department of Economic and Social Affairs, Population Division; 2015.
24. United Nations Population Division (UNPD), Department of Economic and Social Affairs. World contraceptive use: 2015. [online] Available from http://www.un.org/en/development/desa/ population/publications/dataset/contraception/wcu2015.shtml.
25. United Nations Population Division. 2017 Revision of World Population, India Population. [online] Available from https://esa. un.org/unpd/wpp/.
26. World Health Organization. Family planning in health services: report of a WHO expert committee [meeting held in Geneva from 24 to 30 November 1970]. WHO technical report series no. 476. Geneva: WHO;1971.

# CHAPTER 25

# Maternal Health

*Pragti Chhabra*

CM 10.1 Describe the current status of maternal health
CM 10.2 Enumerate and describe the methods of screening of high-risk group (maternal health) and their common health problems
CM 10.3 Describe customs and practices during pregnancy

### Case Scenario

*Mrs. P, a mother of two children aged 30 years with primary school education, belonging to Below Poverty Line (BPL) family was pregnant with 8 months amenorrhea. She was a housewife and her husband a factory worker. She was pregnant for the fourth time. First time, she delivered in a private hospital. Second time, she delivered at home and third pregnancy terminated in a spontaneous abortion. This was her 4th pregnancy for which the first ANC was done at 6th month of pregnancy at the local dispensary. A 2nd ANC check-up was done at 8th month of pregnancy during which she had hemoglobin of 7.5 g/dL. She was prescribed Iron and Folic acid tablets to be taken 2 times a day. At the end of 9 months of pregnancy, she experienced labor pains at 10 am. A Dai in the slum conducted the delivery by 1 pm. The placenta was not expelled completely and she started bleeding profusely. There was no one to take her to the hospital immediately. The husband returned from work at 6 pm and by that time she had gone in shock. She was taken to a maternity home that was not equipped to handle the complication. She was referred to the Medical College Hospital, but she died on the way.*

The above case study shows us how various medical, social, behavioral and health system factors that could have been avoided or acted upon to prevent the death.

## INTRODUCTION

Maternal health as the name suggests refers to the health of the mother. However, the term mother means not only a woman who is pregnant or has given birth, but also includes all women in the child bearing age or reproductive age namely 15–49 years. This is because all women in this age group are prospective mothers. This group is constituted by 24% of the population that is almost one-fourth of the population of India as per the Census 2011. Similar to the definition of health, it includes the physical, mental and social aspects of the health of the mother.

Women in this age group are critical for the social and economic development of any country. The health and wellbeing of women is important not only for themselves, their families and the communities they belong to, but also for the future generations to come. Motherhood is an important function that encompasses bearing and raising children that shape the future of the nation. Along with the function of childbearing that is maintaining and sustaining the human race, women are involved in the functions of income generation, growing and cooking food, household work, taking care of the children, elderly and the sick.

The health of the mother plays a very important role in the wellbeing of the offspring. Mother's health affects health of a person from preconception, fetal, neonatal, infancy, childhood to adulthood. If the mother is malnourished, i.e. undernourished or has a micronutrient deficiency such as anemia, the child is likely to have intrauterine growth retardation (IUGR), low birthweight (LBW), premature birth or other complications. Infections such as syphilis, human immunodeficiency virus (HIV), Hepatitis B, etc. can be transmitted from mother to child. Behaviors such as smoking, alcohol and drug intake during pregnancy can be detrimental to the fetus. Mothers form a vulnerable group due to high morbidity and mortality especially during pregnancy, childbirth and postnatal period. They also face a higher risk of poor health due to the lower status accorded to women in certain sections of the society. However, morbidity and mortality in this group is mainly due to preventable and treatable causes. There are strategies available to manage these problems and reduce the morbidity and mortality.

### Note

**Taj Mahal: Reminder of Maternal Death**

Taj Mahal of Agra is recognized as one of the Wonders of the World and a United Nations Educational, Scientific and Cultural Organization (UNESCO) world heritage site, but sadly, it is also reminder of a maternal death. Mumtaz Mahal was an empress, wife of Shah Jahan who died during childbirth in postpartum hemorrhage following birth of her 14th child in 1631 at the age of 38 years.

In modern times too Smita Patil, a famous actress died due to childbirth complications in 1986 at the young age of 31. These tell us that so many young lives of women in their productive years are lost in pregnancy and childbirth every year.

## CURRENT STATUS OF MATERNAL HEALTH: MAGNITUDE OF MATERNAL MORTALITY AND MORBIDITY

Various indicators have been suggested to measure maternal health. However, maternal mortality is the most widely used indicator and is used to compare the status of maternal health. Sustainable Development Goal for maternal health is to reduce global maternal mortality ratio to less than 70 per 100,000 live births. Maternal mortality refers to deaths due to complications from pregnancy or childbirth. From 2000 to 2020, the global maternal mortality ratio (MMR) declined by 34 per cent—from 339 deaths to 223 deaths per 100,000 live births, according to UN inter-agency estimates.

Though there has been a reduction in the absolute number of maternal deaths occurring around the world, still a large number are dying due to causes that are preventable. According to the data compiled by WHO and UNICEF 295,000 maternal deaths occurred in the year 2017. Of these 130,000 deaths occurred in the least developed countries. The sub-Saharan Africa accounted for approximately 66% and Southern Asia nearly 20% of maternal deaths.

Though the MMR at the global level is estimated to be 223 per 100,000 births, there is a wide variation in different parts of the world. The highest MMR was reported from South Sudan at 1223 and the lowest MMR was reported from Australia and New Zealand at 4 and Europe at 13 per 100,000 births, reaffirming a great disparity within countries of the world. (*Trends in Maternal Mortality: 2000 to 2020 WHO*, Geneva, 2023, World Health Organization, UNICEF, United Nations Population Fund and The World Bank.)

In India too, a steady decline in maternal mortality ratio **(Fig. 25.1)** has been recorded from 398 per 100,000 live births in 1998 to 97 per 100,000 live births in 2018-20. However, there is lot of variation within states with Kerala having the lowest maternal mortality ratio of 19, next being 33 for Maharashtra and 43 per 100,000 live births for Telangana. The state with the highest MMR is Assam (195), followed by Madhya Pradesh (173), and Uttar Pradesh (167) (Special Bulletin on Maternal Mortality in India, 2018–20).

Maternal mortality does not reflect the whole picture, it is just the tip of the iceberg; there are 20-30 cases of acute or chronic *maternal morbidity* for every maternal death. Many of these lead to sequelae that are detrimental to women's physical, mental or sexual health and affect their quality of life.

> **Note**
> **Maternal morbidity** is defined as any health condition attributed to and/or complicating pregnancy and childbirth that have a negative impact on the woman's well-being and/or functioning.

There is not much information on the prevalence of maternal morbidity due to lack of standard definitions and identification criteria. There are few studies on maternal morbidity, those too are mainly hospital based, disease specific. It is estimated that approximately 27 million morbidity episodes occur in a year, if we consider only the five most common direct obstetric complications namely eclampsia, preeclampsia, postpartum hemorrhage, puerperal infection and abortion complications. Maternal morbidity conditions can be visualized as a spectrum with the most severe known as '*maternal near miss*' at one end to nonlife-threatening morbidity at the other end. As expected, the prevalence of conditions increases as we move from severe to less severe.

> **Note**
> '**Maternal near miss**' defined by the World Health Organization (WHO) as the near death of a woman who has survived a complication occurring during pregnancy or childbirth or within 42 days of the termination of pregnancy.

## MATERNAL MORTALITY: INDICES, CAUSES AND PREVENTION

Maternal mortality is listed as an indicator to measure health status by WHO. It is also used as a measure of inequalities and reflects the level of healthcare available to mothers. According to the International Classification of Diseases-10 (ICD-10), the definitions related to maternal mortality are given below:

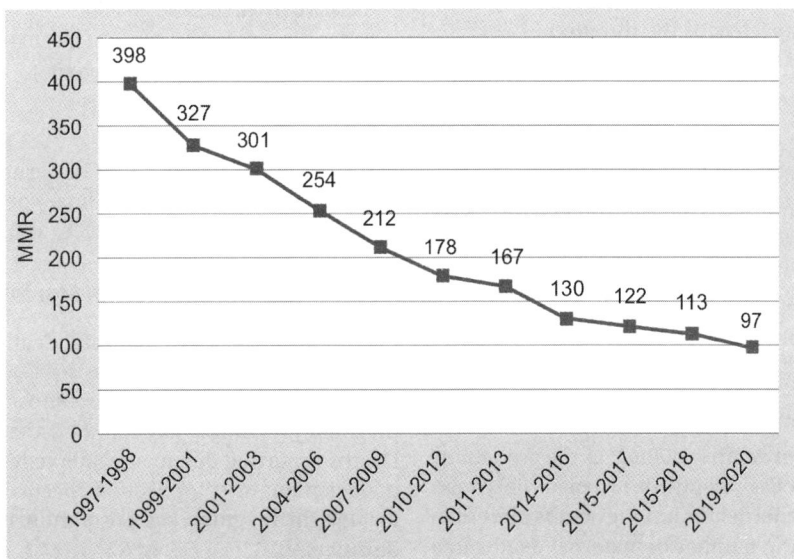

**Fig. 25.1:** Maternal mortality ratio in India from 1997 to 2020.
*Source:* Special bulletin on Maternal mortality in India 2018–20. New Delhi: Office of the registrar general, India; 2020.

> **Note**
>
> **Maternal death** is defined as:
>
> The death of a woman while pregnant or within 42 days of termination of pregnancy:
> - Irrespective of the site or duration of pregnancy
> - From any cause related to or aggravated by the pregnancy or its management
> - Not from accidental or incidental causes.
>
> **Pregnancy-related death** is defined as:
>
> The death of a woman while pregnant or within 42 days of termination of pregnancy:
> - Irrespective of the cause of death.
>
> **Late maternal death** is defined as:
>
> The death of a woman from direct or indirect obstetric causes:
> - More than 42 days, but less than 1 year after termination of pregnancy.

## Indices of Maternal Mortality

Various measures of maternal mortality are used to assess the burden of maternal deaths. The number of maternal deaths in a population is determined by two factors, one the risk of death associated with a single pregnancy or childbirth and second, the number of pregnancies, a woman has on an average in the 15–49 year age period that is fertility of the population. Thus, the number of maternal deaths can be high either due to high risk of death in each pregnancy or high fertility or both.

Maternal mortality is measured by the following indices:

- **Maternal mortality ratio (MMR)** is defined as number of maternal deaths in women (15–49 years) per 100,000 live births. It is a measure of risk of maternal death per livebirth. It is the most commonly used measure of maternal mortality. The formula is given as:

$$\text{MMR} = \frac{\text{Number of maternal deaths from any cause related to or aggravated by pregnancy or its management (excluding accidental or incidental causes) during pregnancy and childbirth or within 42 days of termination of pregnancy, irrespective of the duration and site of the pregnancy}}{\text{Number of live births}} \times 100{,}000$$

- **Maternal mortality rate (MM rate)** is defined as the number of maternal deaths in women (15–49 years) per number of living women (15–49 years). It is a measure of both the risk of death per pregnancy or childbirth and the level of fertility of the population. The formula is given as:

$$\text{MM rate} = \frac{\text{Number of maternal deaths in women (15–49 years)}}{\text{Number of living women (15–49 years)}} \times 100{,}000$$

- **Lifetime risk of maternal death** is defined as the probability of a woman 15–49 years of age dying due to a maternal cause.
- **The proportion of maternal deaths among deaths of women of reproductive age** is the number of maternal deaths in a given time period divided by the total deaths among women aged 15–49 years.

> **Note**
>
> **The sample registration system**: It is a dual record system for enumeration of births and deaths in a national sample. Continuous enumeration of the births and deaths is done by the enumerator in a sample unit. In addition to this, a full time supervisor independently conducts half-yearly survey in each sample. After completion of the half-yearly surveys, data obtained by the enumerator and supervisor are matched. Every unmatched or partially matched data is again verified by visit to the respective household. It also records the causes of death using Verbal Autopsy instrument. A maternal mortality report was released for 1997–2003, thereafter special bulletin on maternal mortality is being released based on SRS data compiling the data of 3 years. The first was based on data of the years 2011–13, and the latest for years 2018–20.
>
> The **Annual Health Survey (AHS)** is conducted under the National Rural Health Mission to monitor core vital and health indicators on an annual basis. AHS is conducted in the states of Assam, Bihar, Chhattisgarh, Jharkhand, Madhya Pradesh, Odisha, Rajasthan, Uttar Pradesh and Uttarakhand. The AHS States account for about 50% of the total population of India, 61% of births, 71% of infant deaths, 72% of under 5 deaths and 62% of maternal deaths. In these surveys information on key household and demographic characteristics, status of maternal health, health care services and many important mortality and morbidity indicators are obtained.

## Causes of Maternal Mortality

It is difficult to pinpoint a single cause of maternal death as other than medical causes there are social, behavioral and health system factors that may contribute to the occurrence of maternal death.

> **Note**
>
> **Some famous people who died due to maternal causes:**
> **Grand Duchess Alexandra Georgievna**, wife of Grand Duke of Russia: 1861–84
> **Alice Hathaway Lee Roosevelt**, wife of President Theodore Roosevelt of America: 1861–84
> **Gianna Beretta Molla**, Italian Pediatrician: 1922–62
> **Maria Leopoldina** of Austria, Empress Consort of Brazil: 1797–1826
> **Isabella Becton**, English author: 1836–65
> **Nadine Shamir**, American singer: 1972–2004
> **Paula Modersohn Becker**, German artist
> **Smita Patil**, Indian actress: 1955–86

The above list shows that maternal death was a common tragedy that not only killed ordinary people but also the women of the privileged section of society also.

### Medical Causes of Maternal Mortality

The medical causes of maternal death are classified as **direct obstetric** and **indirect causes**.

Direct obstetric causes are those that result due to the pregnancy including labor and postnatal period up to 6 weeks. Deaths occurring due to any interventions, omissions, incorrect management or complications occurring due to these are also included in this group, e.g., postpartum hemorrhage, hypertensive disorders.

Indirect causes include diseases that were present prior to or developed during pregnancy.

The main direct causes of maternal deaths reported globally are hemorrhage, hypertensive disorders, sepsis, obstructed labor and abortion.

### Hemorrhage

Depending on the stage of pregnancy, it is classified as antepartum and postpartum hemorrhage.

- ***Antepartum hemorrhage (APH)***: It refers to bleeding from the genital tract after 20 weeks of pregnancy but before the delivery of the baby. It is mainly due to 3 causes namely:
  1. *Placenta previa*: It is implantation of placenta in the lower segment of the uterus
  2. *Abruptio placentae*: It is separation of placenta from uterus before labor
  3. Rupture uterus.
  
  Management of this requires starting an intravenous line at the PHC. These women cannot be treated at the primary level and are referred to the First Referral Unit (FRU) for further management.

- ***Postpartum hemorrhage (PPH)***: It is defined as blood loss of more than 500 mL following delivery or hemorrhage leading to hemodynamic disturbances in the form of tachycardia and/or hypotension. A woman can bleed up to 500 mL/min and die within 5–10 minutes of onset. It may be difficult to estimate the exact blood lost, therefore for operational reasons PPH may be defined as soaking of more than one pad per hour or bright red bleeding with or without clots. Even a lower amount of blood loss can cause the condition of the woman to worsen in diseases such as anemia, preeclampsia and certain medical conditions.

  If the PPH occurs within 24 hours of delivery, it is called *primary PPH*. Secondary PPH is defined as excessive vaginal blood loss or heavy lochial discharge occurring at least 24 hours after the end of the third stage of labor up to 42 days post delivery. Uterine atony is the most common cause of PPH, but genital tract trauma (i.e. vaginal or cervical lacerations), uterine rupture, retained placental tissue, or maternal coagulation disorders may also result in PPH.

  Intramuscular oxytocin is the recommended uterotonic drug for the treatment of PPH. If bleeding is not controlled after use of oxytocin, the next uterotonic IV methergine fixed dose or sublingual misoprostol 800 mg is to be given. Isotonic crystalloids are given for the management of shock. If oxytocin and other uterotonics fail to stop the bleeding or the bleeding may be partly due to trauma, use of tranexamic acid is recommended for the treatment of PPH. If bleeding continues the patient is transferred to higher facility with ongoing uterotonic infusion.

***Prevention:*** There are certain conditions that predispose to hemorrhage, however in 90% of cases, no risk factors are present. By ensuring that all pregnant women have access to a skilled birth attendant the risk can be minimized. This is done by:
- Active management of third stage of labor
- Use of uterotonic drug during third stage of labor: Oxytocin is the drug of choice, if oxytocin is not available, oral misoprostol can be given. In home birth, oral misoprostol is recommended.

### Hypertensive Disorders

Hypertensive disorders of pregnancy **(Table 25.1)** include gestational hypertension, preeclampsia and eclampsia and chronic hypertension. These are important causes of maternal mortality and perinatal morbidity and mortality.

**Table 25.1:** Classification of hypertensive disorders in pregnancy.

| Condition | Definition | Prevalence |
|---|---|---|
| Gestational hypertension | Hypertension that:<br>• Develops beyond 20 weeks of gestation<br>• Returns to normal within 42nd postpartum day and is not associated with any other features of preeclampsia | 6–7% of pregnancies |
| Preeclampsia/eclampsia | Hypertension presenting beyond 20 weeks of gestation with >300 mg protein in a 24-hour urine collection or 1 + (0.3 g/L) on urine dipstick. Eclampsia is the occurrence of seizures in a pregnant woman with preeclampsia | 5–7% of pregnancies |
| Chronic hypertension | Blood pressure 140/90 mm Hg present before pregnancy, before the 20th week of gestation, or persisting beyond the 42nd postpartum day | 1–5% of pregnancies |
| Preeclampsia superimposed on chronic hypertension | The onset of features diagnostic of preeclampsia in a woman with chronic hypertension beyond 20 weeks of gestation | 20–25% of chronic hypertension pregnancies |

Early detection and management of preeclampsia can avoid its serious complication eclampsia. The woman is advised to visit to the health care facility or a home visit by the health worker. During each visit the following is specially looked for:
- Weight gain
- BP measurement
- Check for body edema
- Urine for protein
- Fetal well-being: Fetal movement and heart rate.

She is advised to rest as much as possible preferably in the left lateral position. She is referred for induction at 37 weeks of gestation.

Warning signs and symptoms of impending eclampsia are explained with the advice to report to the health facility.

> **Note**
> **Warning signs and symptoms of impending eclampsia are:** Headache, epigastric pain, vomiting, oliguria, visual disturbances and diminished fetal movements.

***Management of eclampsia:*** Check that the woman can breathe. She should be placed on her left side. Clean her mouth and nostrils and remove secretions. Give her oxygen.

***Control fits:*** Magnesium sulfate is the drug of choice; it is given by slow intravenous (IV) infusion. Diazepam can also be given, but only if magnesium sulfate is not available.

***Control BP:*** By giving hydralazine, the next drug of choice is nifedipine.

***Control fluid balance:*** By monitoring the urinary output.

If the woman is in early labor, referral to FRU is made. If she is in late first stage or second stage of labor, delivery to take place at primary health care, then refer for further management.

### Sepsis

Sepsis remains an important cause of maternal mortality and morbidity in the developing countries. It can occur during the post abortion and postpartum period.

> **Note**
> **Predisposing factors** that can lead to sepsis are:
> - Anemia
> - Poor nutrition
> - Prolonged rupture of membranes
> - Repeated vaginal examination
> - Intrauterine manipulation
> - Genital tract lacerations
> - Hemorrhage or hematoma formation.

A diagnosis of sepsis is suspected if a woman presents with the following in the postpartum or postabortal period:
- Oral temperature >38°C
- Foul smelling vaginal discharge
- Excessive and continuous bleeding after 24 hours
- Continuous lower abdominal pain
- Subinvolution of uterus.

**Management:** If the woman is not very sick, i.e. no high-grade fever, pulse not very high and conscious, she is given broad spectrum antibiotics and referred.

If the woman is sick, i.e. has high-grade fever, rapid pulse and appears confused, she is given injectable antibiotics and referred. Her general condition is assessed and managed symptomatically.

### Abortion

Abortion is defined as the loss of products of conception before the period of viability, i.e. before 20 weeks of gestation. It could be:
- ***Spontaneous abortion***: It presents with bleeding per vaginum.
- ***Induced abortion***: It is deliberate termination of pregnancy before the period of viability. If it performed by persons lacking the necessary skills or at facilities that are not certified to conduct abortion it is said to be unsafe abortion. It can lead to sepsis and other complications.

Management of abortion depends on the type of abortion and the presence of complications.

### Obstructed Labor

Obstructed labor is defined as a condition where though strong uterine contractions are present, the fetus is unable to descend due to mechanical factors. The most common cause is fetopelvic disproportion or cephalopelvic disproportion, as in majority of births the head is the presenting part. This means that the fetal head is large compared to pelvis or the pelvis is small for the fetal head or a combination of both. Other reasons for obstructed labor can be abnormal presentation, twins, hydrocephalus or rarely abnormalities in reproductive tract such as large tumor in the pelvis.

Obstructed labor can lead to premature rupture of membranes leading to fetal/maternal infection that can be fatal. It can lead to uterine rupture leading to hemorrhage and death. Diagnosis of this condition is made by the presence of a history of prolonged labor; on examination signs of physical and mental exhaustion, dehydration, fever, pain and shock are present.

***Management:*** Rehydrate the patient by intravenous infusion and start broad spectrum antibiotics. Refer as operative intervention which is usually required to relieve obstruction and deliver the baby.

### Anemia

Anemia is a condition in which the number of red blood cells (RBCs), and consequently their oxygen-carrying capacity, is insufficient to meet the body's physiological needs. It is one of the most important indirect causes of maternal mortality or morbidity in India. It is also an important cause of low birth weight, prematurity and perinatal mortality.

It is diagnosed by measuring the Hemoglobin (Hb) level in the blood. According to WHO, the diagnosis and classification of anemia is shown in **Table 25.2**.

**Table 25.2:** Classification of anemia.

| Group | No anemia | Mild | Moderate | Severe |
|---|---|---|---|---|
| Non-pregnant women | ≥12 g/dL | 11–11.9 g/dL | 8–10.9 g/dL | <8 g/dL |
| Pregnant women | ≥11 g/dL | 10–10.9 g/dL | 7–9.9 g/dL | <7 g/dL |

The prevalence of anemia is higher in women due to menstrual loss and poor intake of iron rich foods. According to the WHO global database on anemia, 42% of pregnant women and 30% of non-pregnant women in the age group 15–45% have anemia. Majority (85%) of this burden is contributed by Asia and Africa. (MoHFW, National Guidelines for Control of Iron Deficiency Anemia: National Iron+ Initiative, 2018). The NFHS-5 data shows that the prevalence of anemia in women is 57%, it is highest at 58% in lactating women, 57% in pregnant and 57.5% in non-pregnant women. The prevalence of anemia is more (58%) in women belonging to higher wealth index as compared to those from lower wealth index (48%).

Pregnant women with no anemia are given 60 mg of elemental iron and 500 mcg of folic acid daily for 180 days after first trimester at 14–16 weeks of gestation; repeated for 180 days in postpartum period. Those with Hb 7–11 g/dL are given 60 mg of elemental iron and 500 mcg of folic acid twice daily. Hb levels should be assessed monthly to look for the response of the treatment. In women with Hb 8 or less than 8 g/dL, the cause of anemia should be determined. In women with Hb level of 5–6.9 g/dL and those not responding to treatment should be referred to PHC/FRU (First Referral Unit)/DH and receive intravenous Iron Sucrose or Ferric Carboxy Maltose.

### Social and Health System Factors Contributing to Maternal Mortality

Social and health system factors also contribute significantly to the occurrence of maternal mortality. The important factors that affect maternal mortality are as follows:

- **Age**: Mothers with age less than 18 years and more than 35 years at pregnancy are at higher risk of maternal mortality and morbidity.
- **Parity**: Primipara and women with parity 4 or more are at a higher risk and the risk increases with parity.
- **Socioeconomic status**: Women belonging to lower socio-economic status are more at risk.
- **Education**: Women with no or lesser education are more at risk.
- **Age at marriage**: Women married at age less than 18 years are more likely to experience unsafe pregnancy.
- **Inadequate spacing between pregnancies**: Women who conceive with inadequate spacing between pregnancies are at higher risk of maternal mortality.
- **Poor environmental sanitation**: Women living in poor environmental conditions with lack of safe water and sanitation are more susceptible to infections.
- **Maternal mortality is higher in the rural area** as compared to urban area.
- **Cultural practices** such as food taboos, myths about pregnancy, childbirth and postnatal period that may be harmful to the mother.
- In communities that accord low status to women and domestic violence is present; there is a higher risk of maternal mortality.
- **Availability of services**: Poor availability of antenatal care, skilled attendance at delivery, emergency obstetric care increases the chances of maternal mortality
- Lack of access to skilled and competent maternal health staff contributes to maternal deaths.

A significant number of maternal deaths occur due to **'three delays'.**

> **Note**
> **The three delays:**
> 1. **Delay in deciding** to seek care at the family level that is due to lack of knowledge about the complication or lack of support to the mother
> 2. **Delay in reaching** the appropriate health facility is due to lack of access due to inadequate transport or socioeconomic factors
> 3. **Delay in receiving** quality care on reaching the facility due to inadequate skilled manpower or infrastructure.

## Prevalence of Causes of Maternal Mortality

WHO has used various datasets namely civil registration, reports, special surveys and published studies to provide the cause of maternal deaths at the global level. As per this review 73% of the maternal mortality is due to direct obstetric causes, with hemorrhage being the cause in 27%, hypertensive disorders 14%, sepsis 10.7% and abortion 7.9% **(Fig. 25.2)**. About two-thirds of the hemorrhage deaths are due to postpartum hemorrhage. In the developing countries hemorrhage and hypertensive disorders of pregnancy are the main direct causes of maternal mortality. There are regional variations; hemorrhage contributes to about 30% of maternal deaths in Africa and Asia while hypertensive disorders are the leading cause in Latin America and Caribbean. Among the indirect causes, Anemia is important in Asia while HIV/AIDS in Africa.

Globally, the greatest reduction in deaths due to hemorrhage and sepsis has been reported.

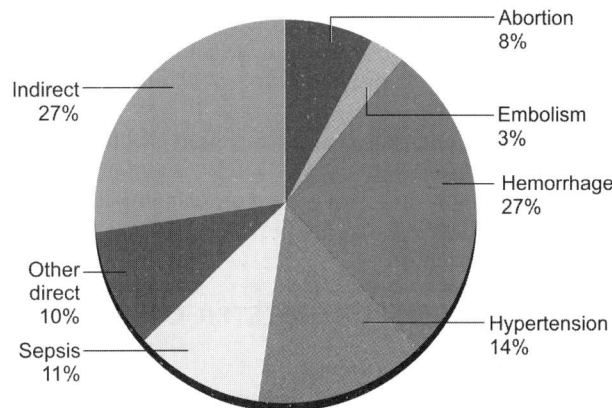

**Fig. 25.2:** Worldwide causes of maternal mortality.
*Source:* Say L, Chou D, Gemmill A, et al. Global causes of maternal death: a WHO systematic analysis. Lancet Glob Health. 2014;2.

In India, as per the special survey on Causes of Death by the Sample Registration System, hemorrhage (37%) was the most common cause followed by sepsis (11%), abortion (8%), hypertensive disorders (5%) and obstructed labor (5%) **(Fig. 25.3)**.

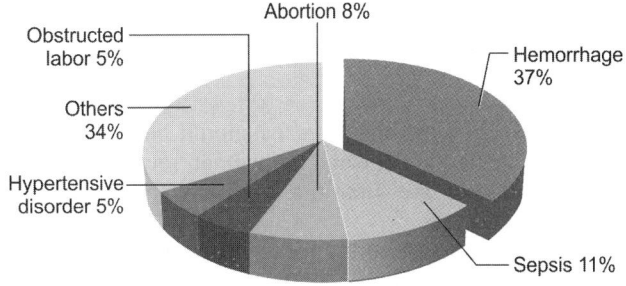

**Fig. 25.3:** Causes of maternal mortality in India.
*Source:* Causes of maternal deaths in India, SRS 2001-03.

## Prevention of Maternal Mortality

There is evidence which shows that majority of the maternal deaths can be prevented. This can be done by the following mechanisms:

- **Prevention of unwanted births,** i.e. reduction in infertility and promotion of wanted births by improving the access and use of contraceptives. Practice of adequate spacing of 3 years between births can reduce maternal deaths.
- **Prevention of unsafe abortions**: Access to safe abortion services can prevent maternal deaths due to abortions.
- **Access to skilled care in pregnancy and childbirth:** Every woman should have access to skilled care during pregnancy and childbirth.
  For example, the risk of postpartum hemorrhage is effectively reduced on injecting oxytocin immediately after childbirth.
- **Clean delivery:** Infection after childbirth can be eliminated by the practice of a clean delivery. **This includes five cleans that are: clean hands, clean surface, clean cord tie, clean razor blade and clean cord stump.**
- **Early recognition** of signs of complications and their treatment in a timely manner.

The three delays can be avoided by:
1. Delay in deciding to seek care at the family level: Improving knowledge about the complication and providing support to the mother
2. Delay in reaching the appropriate health facility: Providing transport to mother
3. Delay in receiving quality care on reaching the facility: Improving quality of care by provision of skilled manpower and infrastructure.

## INTERVENTIONS FOR OBSTETRIC CARE

### Antenatal Care

Antenatal care is the health care provided to the mother during pregnancy. It is an important component of the continuum of care. Timely and quality antenatal care improves the maternal and fetal outcome of pregnancy.

> **Note**
> **Objectives of Antenatal Care**
> - Promote and maintain the physical, mental and social health of mother and baby by detecting and managing complications during pregnancy
> - Develop birth preparedness and complication readiness plan
> - Help prepare mother to breastfeed successfully, explain mother regarding normal puerperium and danger signs in puerperium, and how to take good care of the child.

*Early registration:* All pregnancies should be registered as early as possible ideally when the woman recognizes she is pregnant and not later than the first trimester (before 12th week of pregnancy).

A minimum of 4 health checkups with the provision of services should be done.
1st visit: It is recommended as soon as the pregnancy is suspected and not later than 12 weeks
2nd visit: Between 14 and 26 weeks
3rd visit: Between 28 and 34 weeks
4th visit: Between 36 weeks and term.

**On the 1st antenatal visit,** the socio-demographic details that include identification details, age, address, etc. are noted. The obstetric history that includes previous pregnancies, their outcome and any complications are recorded. The date of last menstrual period (LMP) of the woman is recorded and the expected date of delivery (EDD) is calculated. This is done by applying the Neagle's rule that is adding 9 calendar months +7 days to the LMP for a woman with regular menstrual periods. If LMP is forgotten the date of positive pregnancy test or record of vaginal examination or date of quickening is used to calculate the EDD. At the first and every subsequent visit, history of complaints and past history of illness is enquired. General physical examination, systemic and abdominal examination is done at each visit.

*General physical examination:* Height and weight, pulse rate, blood pressure, respiratory rate, temperature, pallor, pedal edema, icterus is recorded.

*Systemic examination:* Cardiovascular system, respiratory system.

*Per abdomen examination:* Fundal height of uterus, presentation and position of fetus, fetal heart rate is measured.

The following investigations are done: Hemoglobin estimation, blood group including Rh factor, urine for albumin and sugar, venereal disease research laboratory (VDRL)/rapid plasma reagin (RPR), human immunodeficiency virus (HIV), hepatitis B surface antigen (HBsAg) test and blood glucose level.

> **Note**
> **Importance of ANC**
> - Women with **height <145 cm** or 4'10" are high-risk pregnancy
> - **Weight gain:** On an average there is 9–11 kg weight gain during pregnancy. It is minimal in the 1st trimester, after 1st trimester there should be weight gain of 2 kg per month or 0.5 kg per week. If it is less than this, it points towards intrauterine growth retardation that will result in low birth weight. Give her dietary advice and refer to Anganwadi for food supplementation. If the **weight gain is more than 3 kg per month** it could be due to preeclampsia or twins.
> - **Blood pressure**: If the systolic blood pressure (SBP) >140 mm Hg or diastolic blood pressure (DBP) >90 mm Hg after 20 weeks, it is suggestive of preeclampsia. **SBP ≥160 mm Hg or DBP ≥110 mm Hg** is a danger sign indicating severe preeclampsia.

### Services Provided

**Iron and folic acid supplementation**: Anemia is defined as Hb< 11 g/dL during pregnancy.

If there is no anemia, the pregnant women to receive prophylactic dose of 60 mg of elemental iron and 500 µg of folic acid for 180 days. If Hb <11g/dL, 60 mg of elemental iron and 500 µg of folic acid is given twice a day.

**Calcium supplementation**: All pregnant women are given calcium tablets to be taken twice a day (total 1 g calcium/day), starting from 14 weeks of pregnancy up to six months postpartum.

**Immunization against Tetanus and Diphtheria**: Two doses of Tetanus toxoid Td vaccine that contains Tetanus and Diphtheria toxoids are given; 1st dose at 16–20 weeks or first contact and 2nd dose at 20–24 weeks. There should be minimum gap of 4 weeks between 2 doses of Td injections and second dose should be preferably given at least 4 weeks before estimated delivery date (EDD). If a woman who had received two doses becomes pregnant again within 3 years, then 1 booster is given. Earlier Tetanus Toxoid (TT) vaccine was given during pregnancy which has been replaced with Td vaccine which protects against maternal and neonatal Tetanus as well as Diphtheria.

### Dietary Advice

There is an increased energy requirement of additional 350 calories during pregnancy and 600 calories during first 6 months of lactation and 520 calories in 6–12 months of lactation. The estimated average protein requirement during pregnancy increases by 7.6 g/day in 2nd trimester and 17.6 g/day in 3rd trimester for every 10 kg gestational weight gain. (However, the RDA or safe levels of additional protein intake increases by 9.5 g/day and 22 g/day in 2nd and 3rd trimester respectively). For 0–6 months lactation, the average requirement increases by 13.6 g/day and safe intake increases by 16.9 g/day, while from 7–12 months lactation former increases by 10.6 g/day and latter increases by 13.2 g/day respectively. The RDA for pregnant and lactating women for iron is 40 and 23 mg, calcium is 1,000 and 1,200 mg, and folic acid is 570 and 330 µg respectively.

In terms of foodstuffs, an additional 35 g of cereals, 15 g of pulses, 300 mL milk, green leafy vegetables and fruits should be added to the mothers diet.

## Other Advice

- *Adequate rest,* i.e. 8 hours at night and 2 hours in afternoon
- *Birth preparedness:* Prepare the necessary items for birth
  - Identify a skilled attendant and arrange for presence at birth
  - Identify appropriate site for birth, and how to get there
  - Encourage for institutional delivery
  - Identify support people, including who will accompany the woman and who will take care of the family
  - Establish a financing plan/scheme.
- Importance of breastfeeding
- Danger signs.

> **Note**
> **Danger signs during pregnancy:** These are warning signs about which the woman is told to visit the doctor/health facility immediately.
> - Fever
> - Headache, blurring of vision
> - Generalized swelling of the body and puffiness of face
> - Palpitations, easy fatigability and breathlessness at rest
> - Pain in abdomen
> - Vaginal bleeding/watery discharge
> - Reduced fetal movements.

## Intranatal Care

The intranatal period or childbirth is a normal physiological process; however, complications can arise during this period leading to severe morbidity and mortality in both the mother and the newborn.

## Normal Labor

This begins with the onset of labor which is divided into three stages. The first stage starts with onset of labor pains and ends with full dilatation of the cervix. The second stage starts with full dilatation of cervix to the delivery of the baby. The third stage starts after delivery of baby and ends with delivery of the placenta.

The progress of labor should be assessed by monitoring the onset and duration of uterine contractions, cervical dilatation, fetal and maternal condition. This is done by using a **partograph**. The partograph as the name suggests is a graphic recording of the progress of labor. It is the most important tool for health workers at all levels to monitor progress of labor and take appropriate action.

> **Note**
> **Partograph includes:**
> - **Progress of labor:** Record of the uterine contractions and cervical dilatation with time
> - **Maternal condition:** Pulse rate and blood pressure
> - **Fetal condition:** Fetal heart rate is counted and recorded half hourly
> - **Condition of amniotic membranes** and color of amniotic fluid
> - **Interventions:** Drug or intravenous fluid before delivery.

> **Note**
> **Indications for referral to FRU: Interpreting a Partograph**
> - Fetal heart rate <120 beats/min or >160 beats/min
> - Meconium and/or blood stained liquor
> - Cervical dilatation plotting crosses the alert line
> - Uterine contractions not increasing in duration, intensity or frequency.

Thus, the partograph is a useful tool for the health workers as it helps in early identification of complications and deciding on appropriate care and referral during the intranatal period.

During the second stage, the baby is delivered and the umbilical cord is cut and tied using sterile instruments.

Active management of third stage of labor (AMTSL) should be only done by skilled birth attendant/trained staff to prevent postpartum hemorrhage (PPH).

> **Note**
> **Active management of third stage of labor** includes:
> - Giving a uterotonic drug: This is given to enhance uterine contraction and prevent PPH. Injection Oxytocin is the drug of choice. In settings where oxytocin is unavailable, Misoprostol (600 µg) orally is recommended.
> - Controlled cord traction (CCT): This is used to assist the expulsion of placenta. However, CCT is contraindicated in settings where skilled birth attendants are not available.

Majority of deliveries are uncomplicated but 3/4th of maternal deaths occur during labor. These complications are not always predictable or preventable. It is essential to promote deliveries by **skilled birth attendant.**

## Skilled Birth Attendant

Professionally trained health worker with skills necessary to manage normal pregnancy, delivery, immediate postnatal period, diagnose and refer obstetric and newborn complications. It includes doctor, midwife or nurse who has midwifery skills to recognize onset of complications, perform essential interventions, start treatment and supervise referral of mother and baby.

## Traditional Birth Attendants (TBAs)

Also known as Dai is a traditional, independent, non-formally trained community based providers of care during pregnancy, childbirth and postnatal period. Earlier TBAs were provided training at the Primary Health Centers to conduct deliveries. However, since the launch of the Reproductive and Child Health Programme in 1997, there is promotion of institutional deliveries and births by skilled birth attendants.

*Quality ANC* includes minimum of at least 4 ANCs including early registration and 1st ANC in first trimester along with physical and abdominal examinations, Hb estimation and urine investigation, 2 doses of Tetanus Diphtheria (Td) Immunization and consumption of IFA tablets (180 days during ANC and 180 days during PNC).

## Postnatal Care

Postnatal period or puerperium begins after 3rd stage of labor to 6 weeks after delivery. It is the most neglected aspect of maternity care and contributes to maternal mortality. Rapid changes take place in this period in the body especially the genital organs. The uterus contracts immediately after the delivery of the placenta.

> **Note**
> **The objectives of postnatal care are to:**
> - Check general well-being of the mother and baby
> - Detect and treat postpartum complications in the mother and baby
> - Discuss breastfeeding, birth spacing and child care issues with the mother
> - Inform mother about the importance of immunization and immunization schedule of the child

In institutional deliveries, it is recommended that the mother and baby are discharged after at least 48 hours after delivery in a normal birth. This ensures that the above objectives are met with.

In case of home delivery, the 1st postnatal visit should be conducted within 24 hours of delivery by Accredited Social Health Activist/Auxiliary Nurse Midwife (ASHA/ANM).

- During the first visit details about the childbirth are enquired, any complaints about heavy bleeding per vaginum, convulsions, abdominal pain, fever, bowel and bladder functions, sleep and lactation is elicited.
- *A general physical examination* including measurement of pulse rate, temperature, BP and pallor is done.
- *Per abdomen examination* for height of uterus is undertaken.
- *Examination of site of episiotomy* if conducted and lochia is done.
- *Examination of breast* is done for any lump or tenderness.

Second visit is done on 3rd day and third visit on 7th day of birth.
- Ask about bleeding per vaginum, foul smelling discharge, breast tenderness or pain, fever or any other complaint during the visit.
  Subsequently, the visits are conducted on 14, 21, 28 and 42 day of birth.
- *Advice:* Early ambulation is advised but she is told to avoid strenuous activity.
- *Diet:* There is an increased requirement of 600 calories during first six months of lactation. She is advised a light diet on first day then diet rich in calories, proteins, iron, calcium and vitamins.
- *Iron 60 mg and Folic acid 500 μg* tablets are given for at least 180 days postpartum.
- *Personal and perineal hygiene* is important to prevent infection.
- *Breastfeeding:* Explain mother about the importance of feeding child with colostrum rich in antibodies. Exclusive breastfeeding is advised for first six months.
- *Contraception:* Lactation gives protection against conception for about 6 weeks. Beyond this, the woman should be counseled regarding use of appropriate contraceptive methods. She can be advised about both terminal and spacing methods. The spacing methods available are postpartum Intrauterine Contraceptive Devices (IUCD) and barrier methods such as condoms. Combined oral contraceptives containing estrogens and progesterone are contraindicated for the first six months as they affect both the quality and quantity of breast milk.
- She is informed about the following danger signs:

> **Note**
> **Danger signs:** Excessive bleeding, convulsions, fever and excessive weakness, breast engorgement, severe pain abdomen, painful micturition or pain in chest or legs.

## High-risk Pregnancy

It is defined as pregnancy that is complicated by factors that adversely affect the maternal or perinatal outcome of pregnancy. Every pregnancy should be screened for these factors:
- Age of mother more than 35 years or less than 18 years at first pregnancy
- Height of mother is less than 140 cm
- Grand multiparity
- Two or more previous miscarriages or induced abortions
- Previous stillbirth, neonatal death or birth of babies with congenital anomalies
- Previous cesarean section or hysterotomy
- Complications in previous pregnancy
- Systemic disease, viz. cardiovascular disease, kidney disease, asthma, liver disease, thyroid disease, epilepsy in mother
- Infections such as tuberculosis, HIV, malaria, hepatitis, sexually transmitted infections (STI), reproductive tract infection (RTI), etc. in mother
- Multiple pregnancies
- Preeclampsia, eclampsia
- Anemia
- Gestational hypertension.

## Essential Obstetric Care

There are certain risk factors that if present increase the likelihood of complications during pregnancy and childbirth. However, these cannot be used to predict complications as evidence has shown that women labeled as 'high-risk' may not develop the complication while those with 'low-risk' may present with complications. The 'risk approach' followed earlier that meant special management for the high risk has been replaced by the principle that all women are at risk to develop a complication and thus essential obstetric care must be available to all. This is being done by operationalizing the primary health cares (PHCs) for 24 × 7 services and also training the SNs/LHVs/ANMs in Skilled Attendance at Birth.

> **Note**
> **Essential obstetric care** includes:
> - Early registration
> - Minimum 4 antenatal checkups
> - Anemia prophylaxis and treatment
> - Mebendazole for deworming
> - Tetanus toxoid vaccine
> - Skilled care at birth
> - Postnatal care
> - Birth spacing

## Emergency Obstetric Care

Majority of the maternal mortality and morbidity can be avoided by the provision of basic obstetric care to all the women and comprehensive obstetric care to those with complications.

> **Note**
> **Basic obstetric care** is defined as the availability of the following services by a skilled health personnel:
> - Administration of antibiotics
> - Administration of uterotonic drugs (Oxytocin)
> - Administration of anticonvulsants (Magnesium Sulfate)
> - Manual removal of the placenta
> - Removal of retained products following miscarriage or abortion
> - Assisted vaginal delivery, preferably with vacuum extractor
> - Basic neonatal resuscitation care.
>
> **Comprehensive obstetric care** includes all the above functions and:
> - Performing cesarean sections
> - Safe blood transfusion
> - Provision of care to sick and low-birth weight newborns, including resuscitation.

It is recommended by the WHO and United Nations Population Fund (UNFPA) that there should be at least 5 facilities per 5,00,000 population that are fully equipped and available 24 × 7 to provide basic obstetric care. There should be at least one facility available for 5,00,000 population that is available for provision of comprehensive obstetric care.

## OTHER INDICATORS OF MATERNAL HEALTH (TABLE 25.3)

**Table 25.3:** Maternal health indicators in India.

| Indicators | NFHS 4 (2015–16) | NFHS-5 (2019-21) |
|---|---|---|
| Mothers who had antenatal check-up in the first trimester (%) | 58.6 | 70 |
| Mothers who had at least 4 antenatal care visits (%) | 51.2 | 58.1 |
| Mothers whose last birth was protected against neonatal tetanus (%) | 89 | 92 |
| Mothers who consumed iron folic acid for 100 days or more when they were pregnant (%) | 30.3 | 44.1 |
| Mothers who had full antenatal care^ (%) | 21 | |
| Institutional delivery (%) | 78.9 | 88.6 |
| Births assisted by a doctor/nurse/LHV/ANM/other health personnel (Safe deliveries) (%) | 81.4 | 78 |

^ Full antenatal care is at least four antenatal visits, at least one tetanus toxoid (TT) injection and iron folic acid tablets or syrup taken for 100 or more days.

## MATERNAL DEATH REVIEW (MDR)

Review of maternal death is a process to identify factors at various levels namely community, facility, district, regional and national level that may have contributed to the maternal mortality. It aims to provide a detailed analysis of these factors so that the lacunae at various levels in the health system catering to the requirements of pregnancy and childbirth can be identified. These need to be addressed so as to improve the quality of obstetric care and reduce maternal mortality and morbidity. Analysis of maternal deaths also provide information about the delays that may have contributed to these so that appropriate action can be taken for the factors that are avoidable or preventable and hence there is improvement in the provision of care from home to the health facility.

The process of **maternal death surveillance and response (MDSR)** has been instituted for identification, notification and review of maternal deaths that would lead to action for preventing maternal deaths in the future and improve maternal healthcare. It is important to note that the purpose of the review is not to find faults or blame any one but to point the lacunae and institute measures to address them.

All the maternal deaths occurring in the area will be reviewed at both the community and facility level.

**Community based MDSR:** This is done to identify personal, family or community factors that may have contributed to the maternal death. It is conducted by interviewing the family members, neighbors and others who may be aware about the events preceding the death. The verbal autopsy format is used for the review.

**Facility-based MDSR:** This is conducted in all the Government teaching hospitals, referral hospitals, secondary level hospitals, district hospital, sub-district and CHCs with more than 100 deliveries in a year.

The purpose is to improve the quality of services of the facility by identifying the gaps in provision of care and take action for improvement. A facility-based MDSR (FBMDSR) format is filled up by the treating medical officer and the same is analyzed by the FBMDSR committee.

**Confidential Review** is done to investigate the line of management in cases of maternal mortality and morbidities. This is done by a multidisciplinary team in an anonymous manner to observe the management protocols and guidelines are adhered to or not. For this a confidential review committee is formed to review all the records related to the death and submit a report. Action is taken to address the deficiencies and improve the health system.

*Maternal Death Review is further explained in detail under the Chapter 51D: Medical Certification for Cause of Death and Verbal Autopsies.*

## CURRENT APPROACHES IN HEALTH CARE SERVICES

**The Millennium Development Goals (MDGs)** were set to monitor the progress of important development and health outcomes around the world between 1990 and 2015. Maternal health was an important part of the MDGs. It was included in MDG 5 that dealt with sexual and reproductive health.

> **Note**
> **Target 5.A:** To reduce the maternal mortality ratio by three quarters between 1990 and 2015
> **Indicator 5.1:** Maternal mortality ratio
> **Indicator 5.2:** Proportion of deliveries attended by skilled health personnel.

**The Sustainable Development Goals** were constituted to further build on the successes of MDGs with emphasis on equality, harmony, environmental protection, partnership and peace.

Goal 3 relates to health which is 'ensure healthy lives and promote well-being for all at all ages.'

> **Note**
> 
> **The target 3.1 relates to maternal health**, with a goal to reduce the maternal mortality ratio to less than 70 per 100,000 live births by 2030.
> 
> The related indicators are:
> - **Indicator 3.1.1:** Maternal mortality ratio
> - **Indicator 3.1.2:** Proportion of births attended by skilled health personnel.

To achieve the target of less than 70 maternal deaths per 100,000 live births by 2030, an annual rate of reduction of at least 7.5% is required, which is more than double the annual rate of progress achieved from 2000 to 2015. Thus, considerable efforts shall be needed to achieve the goal.

**The Global Strategy for Ending Preventable Maternal Mortality aims towards:**

- Reducing the inequalities in access to the reproductive, maternal, and newborn healthcare services and their quality is improved
- Universal health coverage for comprehensive reproductive, maternal, and newborn healthcare is available
    - All causes of maternal mortality, reproductive and maternal morbidities are addressed
    - High quality data is available from the health systems so that the needs and priorities of women and girls are known
    - Accountability to improve quality of care and equity is ensured.

The risk of maternal and neonatal mortality is very high around the period of childbirth. Majority of the causes of maternal and newborn mortality can be prevented by appropriate care of mothers during labor, and of mother and newborn immediately after birth. There is enough evidence globally on the importance of skilled care at birth in reducing maternal mortality and morbidity. On the same lines, the Government of India for more than a decade has focused on increasing institutional deliveries through programs such as Janani Suraksha Yojana (JSY) and Janani Shishu Suraksha Karyakram (JSSK). There has been a marked increase in the proportion of institutional births over the past decade from 38.7% in 2005–06 (NFHS-3) to 80% in 2015–16 (NFHS-4) and 88.6% in 2019–21 (NFHS-5). However, the decline in the MMR is not as much as the rise in institutional deliveries. This may be due to sub-optimum quality of services during institutional deliveries which include inadequate material resources, skilled manpower, etc. These are being improved by provision of resources and training to improve skills of the health providers.

*Maternal health has been integrated into Reproductive, Maternal, Newborn, Child, and Adolescent Health Plus Nutrition (RMNCAH+N) Strategy which is further explained in detail in Chapter 47: Health Policies and Programs in India.*

## SUGGESTED READING

1. Alkema L, Chou D, Hogan D, et al. Global, regional, and national levels and trends in maternal mortality between 1990 and 2015, with scenario-based projections to 2030: a systematic analysis by the UN Maternal Mortality Estimation Inter-Agency Group. Lancet. 2016;378: 462-74.
2. Firoz T, Chou D, von Dadelszen P, et al. Measuring maternal health: Focus on maternal morbidity. Bull World Health Organ. 2013;91:794-6.
3. https://main.mohfw.gov.in/sites/default/files/NFHS-5_Phase-II_0.pdf
4. International Institute for Population Sciences (IIPS) and ICF. (2017). National Family Health Survey (NFHS-4), 2015-16: India.
5. International Institute for Population Sciences (IIPS) and Macro International. (2007). National Family Health Survey (NFHS-3),2005- 06: India.
6. International Institute for Population Sciences. (2008). District Level Household and Facility Survey 3, 2007-8.
7. Kassebaum NJ, Bertozzi-Villa A, Coggeshall MS, et al. Global, regional, and national levels and causes of maternal mortality during 1990–2013: a systematic analysis for the Global Burden of Disease Study 2013. Lancet. 2014;384(9947):980-1004.
8. Ministry of Health & Family Welfare, Government of India. Guidelines for pregnancy care and management of common obstetric complications by medical Officers. Maternal Health Division, Ministry of Health & Family Welfare Government of India. New Delhi. 2005.
9. Ministry of Health and Family Welfare, Government of India. (2014). National Guidelines for Calcium Supplementation during Pregnancy and Lactation. [online]. Maternal Health Division, Ministry of Health and Family Welfare, Government of India, 2014.
10. Ministry of Health and Family Welfare, Government of India. Anemia Mukt Bharat-intensified National Iron Plus Initiative (I-NIPI) Operational Guidelines for Programme managers. Ministry of Health and Family Welfare Government of India, New Delhi, 2018.
11. National Health Mission. (2017). Guidelines for Maternal Death Surveillance & Response.
12. National Health Mission. Guidance Note on Prevention and Management of Postpartum Haemorrhage. [online]. Available from http://rmncha.in/wp-content/uploads/guidelines_img/1487588659.pdf.
13. Registrar General of India. Special Bulletin on Maternal Mortality in India, 2010-12, 2014-16, 2015-17, 2016-18.
14. Say L, Chou D, Gemmill A, et al. Global causes of maternal death: a WHO systematic analysis. Lancet Glob Health. 2014;2:e323-33.
15. UNICEF. United Nations Children Fund (UNICEF) Coverage Evaluation Survey. (2009).
16. USAID. (2013). A Strategic Approach to Reproductive, Maternal, Newborn, Child and Adolescent Health (RMNCH+A) in India. [online]. Available from https://www.mchip.net/sites/default/files/ RMNCH+A%20in%20India.pdf.
17. World Health Organization. Trends in maternal mortality 2000 to 2017: estimates by WHO, UNICEF, UNFPA, World Bank Group and the United Nations Population Division. World Health Organization; Geneva, Switzerland, 2019.

# CHAPTER 26

# Child Health

*Ravneet Kaur, Akhil Dhanesh Goel*

| | |
|---|---|
| CM 10.1 | Describe the current status of newborn and child health |
| CM 10.2 | Enumerate and describe the methods of screening of high-risk group (Neonate and Child) and their common health problems |
| CM 10.3 | Describe customs and practices during childbirth, lactation and child feeding practices |
| CM 10.5 | Integrated Management of Neonatal and Childhood Illness and other co-existing programs |

## INTRODUCTION

Childhood is a crucial period in life. This is the formative stage for sound physical, mental, and social development. The dynamic process of growth and development is the essence of childhood. *Growth* refers to an increase in the physical size of the body, and is associated with an increase in cell size and cell number. *Development* which is complementary to physical growth, indicates acquisition of skills for optimal functioning and is related to myelination of the nervous system. The physical, psychological, and emotional domains of the child development are responsible for shaping child into an independent adult. As children represent the future generation, it is of the utmost importance to ensure good health for them.

However, this age group is exposed to many health risks and is vulnerable to high morbidity and mortality. A large number of children suffer from poor health and nutrition. Globally, the under-five mortality rate (U5MR) is very high. Every year, more than 10 million children die in developing countries before they reach their fifth birthday. A large majority of these deaths are due to acute respiratory infections (ARIs), diarrhea, measles, malaria, or malnutrition. Most of the children suffer from a combination of these illnesses. Thus, most of the children suffer from and die from a few common conditions, which are largely preventable with simple interventions. Apart from causing deaths, childhood morbidities hinder normal physical growth and neurocognitive development. Repeated illnesses also lead to undernutrition, which further predisposes the child to infections. A number of factors, such as sociodemographic background, economic status, education of the parents, and household environment, access to healthcare, etc., are associated with exposure and outcome of diseases among children.

Continuum of care provided to children at birth (even before birth), throughout childhood and adolescence will have an effect on their immediate health and well-being, as well as on their overall health and development throughout the later years of life.

Under the life course approach, the childhood period is divided into three subgroups: (1) Under-five children, (2) older children (5–9 years), and (3) adolescents (10–19 years).

The under-five period is further grouped into—neonatal period (first 28 days of life), infancy (first year of life), and preschool years (1–5 years) **(Table 26.1)**.

According to Census 2011, children (0–6 years) constitute 13% of the total population in India. The proportion of children (0–18 years) is 39% of the country's total population.

In the present chapter, we shall learn about the status of health problems among children, particularly those under-five years of age, the magnitude and causes of morbidities and mortality among children in India, and various measures for their prevention and control.

**Table 26.1:** Age subgroups as defined by the World Health Organization.

| Terminology | Definition* |
|---|---|
| Under-five | First 5 years of life |
| Neonatal period | First 28 days of life |
| Early neonatal period | First 7 days of life |
| Postneonatal period | 28 days to first year of life |
| Infancy | First year of life |
| Preschool | 1–5 years |
| Older child | 5–9 years |
| Adolescent | 10–19 years |

*The upper limit of the interval refers to completed days, months, or years.
*Source:* World Health Organization. Strategic directions for improving the health and development of children and adolescents. Geneva: WHO; 2002.

## GLOBAL BURDEN OF CHILD MORTALITY AND MORBIDITY

According to World Health Organization (WHO) 2020, 5 million children under-five years of age died in 2020 across the globe. Deaths in the neonatal period constitute 2.4 million. In 2018, 4.0 million (75% of all under-five deaths) occurred within the first year of life. Out of these, about 75% of all under-five deaths occur in Africa and South-East Asia. The risk of under-five mortality is highest in the sub-Saharan African region [74 (68–86) per 1,000 live births] which is nearly 14 times higher than the Europe and North America. SDG target 3.2 is to reduce child mortality to at least as low as 25 per 1,000 live births by 2030 **(Fig. 26.1)**. [Child mortality (under 5 years) 28 January 2022 and WHO Infant mortality, The Global Health Observatory, Explore a world of health data].

In addition to the differences in the mortality rates among different countries, there are inequities within countries that lead to substantially high mortality among populations belonging to poor socioeconomic strata, those living in rural areas, and having low literacy among mothers.

According to the latest Global Health Estimates for 2016 from the WHO, three quarters of children aged 0–14 years are dying from communicable, perinatal, and nutritional conditions which disproportionally affect children in poorer settings.

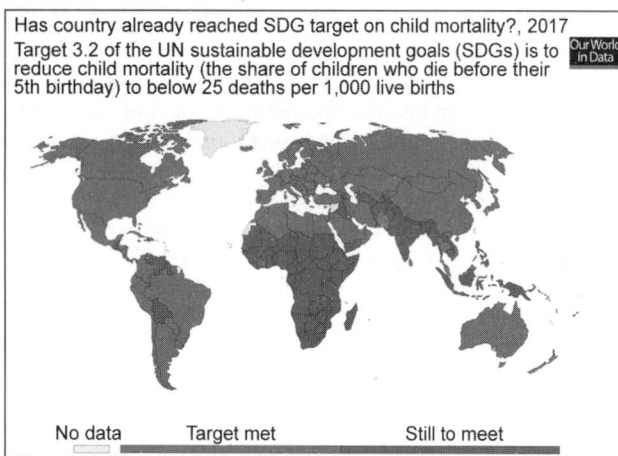

**Fig. 26.1:** Under-five mortality rate (deaths per 1,000 live births), 2020 with Sustainable Development Goal (SDG) target status.
*Source:* Estimates Developed by the UN Inter-agency Group for Child Mortality Estimation (UNICEF, WHO, World Bank, UN DESA Population Division), 2020.

## MORBIDITY IN UNDER-FIVE CHILDREN

Although the measurement of morbidity is more complex than measurement of mortality among under-five children, however, it is known that main causes of morbidity are directly correlated with major causes of deaths in this age group. Diarrhea and ARI with their associated symptoms, such as fever, cough, and difficulty in breathing are among the most common forms of childhood morbidity which lead to millions of deaths worldwide each year. The common factors affecting growth and development in children are shown in **Figure 26.2**.

The common health problems among under-five children are:
- Low birth weight (LBW)
- Malnutrition – already discussed in *Chapter 23: Epidemiology of Nutrition and Food-related Diseases and its Prevention and Control.*
- Childhood infections
- Disability and deformity.

### Low Birth Weight

Low birth weight (LBW) is defined as birth weight less than 2,500 g (up to and including 2,499 g) irrespective of gestational age. This may be further stratified into "very low birth weight" (<1,500 g) and "extremely low birth weight" (<1,000 g).

### *Magnitude of Problem*

Low birthweight affects 1 in 7 newborns worldwide. In 2020, 19.8 million newborns, an estimated 14.7 percent of all babies born globally that year, suffered from low birth weight. These babies were more likely to die during their first month of life and those who survived face lifelong consequences including a higher risk

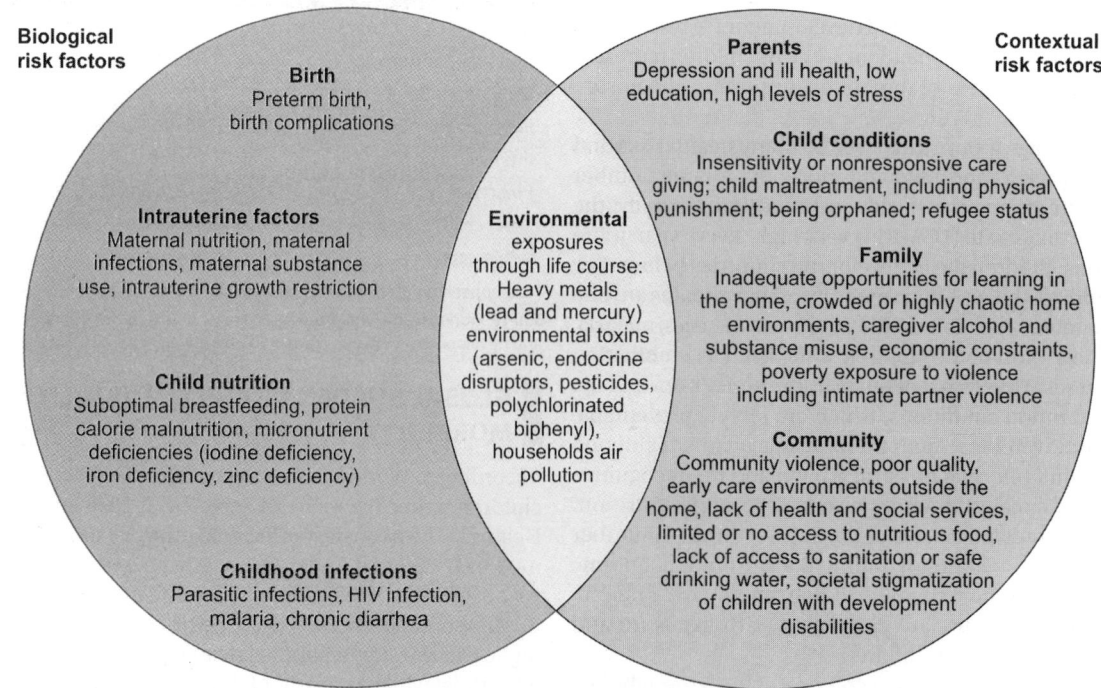

**Fig. 26.2:** Factors affecting growth and development.

of stunted growth, lower IQ and adult-onset chronic conditions such as obesity and diabetes. In Southern Asia, the prevalence of low birthweight was 24.9% in 2020 (UNICEF-WHO low birth-weight estimates 2023).

As reported by National Family Health Survey-5 (2019–21) in India, 91% of live births in 5 years preceding the survey had written record available for birth-weight. Out of these, 18% had LBW, the same as in 2015–16.

Low birth weight is a heterogeneous group of infants comprising of:
- Preterm children
- Children with IUGR
- Children born preterm along with growth restriction.

Preterm refers to a child born before 37 completed weeks of gestation. These are the babies "born too soon". An estimated 13.4 million babies were born too early in 2020. That is more than 1 in 10 babies. Approximately 900,000 children die in 2019 of complications of preterm birth. Many survivors face a lifetime of disability, including learning disabilities and visual and hearing problems. Prematurity accounts for 16% neonatal deaths and about 2% postneonatal deaths and the target is to achieve 30% reduction in prevalence of LBW. Preterm births can be further classified into:
- Extremely preterm (<28 weeks)
- Very preterm (28–<32 weeks)
- Moderate to late preterm (32–37 weeks).

## Causes of Preterm Births

### Maternal Causes
- Age: Preterm births are very common among adolescents and elderly women
- Short stature women
- Lack of birth spacing due to poor uptake, lack of awareness or difficult access to available contraceptives and feminization of reproductive health. There has been a lot of feminization when it comes to family planning practices and childbearing and child rearing practices. Male participation in the same is almost negligible as is indicated by the dismal statistics of male sterilization (0.03%).
- Malaria, urinary tract infections, syphilis, human immuno-deficiency virus (HIV) and bacterial vaginitis, sometimes result in cervical insufficiency and eventually preterm births.
- Undernutrition, obesity, micronutrient deficiency like anemia
- Lifestyle-related factors: Smoking (including exposure to secondhand smoke), alcohol, recreational drug use among women during pregnancy or otherwise often results in preterm births and LBW. This occurs due to placental vasoconstriction.
- Grand multiparity
- Maternal conditions such as cervical incompetence, multiple pregnancy, placental insufficiency, antepartum hemorrhage, pre-eclampsia and eclampsia, uterine rupture, diabetes, hypertension, renal disease, malaria, toxemia
- Multiple gestation, intrauterine infections, chromosomal abnormalities.

### Health System related
- Provider initiated: Many a times preterm birth are provider initiated
- Accessibility and affordability to health services
- Delay in reaching appropriate health facility equipped to manage LBW.

### Prevention of Low Birth Weight

*Strengthening healthcare delivery system*: Making appropriate, culturally and gender sensitive healthcare available, affordable and accessible to all those in need.

- ***Interventions targeted to address maternal health:***
    - Strict implementation of regulations pertaining to legal age at marriage and right to education should be ensured in order to prevent adolescent pregnancy and promote literacy and reduce dropout rate among girls.
    - Prevent unplanned and ill-timed pregnancy by promoting planning for pregnancy and adequate birth spacing of at least 3 years. Birth spacing using appropriate contraceptive methods improves maternal and perinatal outcomes and allows woman to replenish her bodily reserves and also reduces neglect of elder child.
    - Increasing access to and uptake of family planning services as a spacing method and increasing male participation in family welfare.
    - Improved maternal nutrition: All pregnant and lactating women should be registered at the *Anganwadi* centers and should receive supplemental nutrition. In addition, iron and folic acid should be given to all pregnant women for at least 100 days to address anemia and strict compliance should be ensured. Nutritional education regarding healthy foods, food habits and preparation, dietary diversification should be given to all adolescent girls, women of reproductive age group and pregnant women. PDS should be strengthened to address food insecurity. Access to clean and safe water should be ensured.
    - Identification of high-risk cases: Antenatal women at extremes of age, short stature women, women with poor lifestyle habits, etc., should be screened at primary healthcare level and referred to the nearest higher center.
    - Antenatal registration: All antenatal women should register for a hospital delivery/delivery by a skilled birth attendant in order to get best intrapartum facilities and a favorable postnatal outcome.
    - Infections, if any, should be first and foremost prevented, identified and treated such as malaria during pregnancy.
    - Proactive management of pre-eclampsia, cervical incompetence.
    - Promotion of healthy lifestyle: Cessation of smoking, alcohol and recreational drug use and promotion of hand hygiene, etc., can alleviate the incidence of LBW.
    - Strengthen referral facilities in order to improve the perinatal and postnatal outcome.
    - Social protection (e.g., conditional cash transfer programs) in order to incentivize healthcare visits.

- *Adolescent-friendly health services (AFHSs)* for counseling of adolescents on reproductive and sexual health in order to increase correct use of contraceptives and reduce adolescent pregnancy.
- *Increasing access to antenatal healthcare services*:
    - At least one antenatal checkup per month by a gynecologist, under Pradhan Mantri Surakshit Matritva Abhiyan (PMSMA), to identify high-risk pregnancy and counseling regarding nutritional intake, breastfeeding, birth spacing and appropriate child care.
    - Screening of high-risk pregnancy for preterm such as those with previous preterm birth, grand multipara, adolescent pregnancy, multiple gestation, etc.
    - Early detection and treatment for infections in pregnancy including urinary tract infections, malaria, bacterial vaginosis, syphilis, sexually transmitted infections (STIs) and HIV.
    - Management of pre-existing chronic conditions and screening for diseases such as diabetes, anemia, hypertension, renal disease, etc.
    - Timely identification of IUGR and referral to higher center wherein the referral center should be equipped to manage children who are preterm or small for gestational age.
    - Strengthening healthcare facilities, through infrastructure and skilled manpower, for proactive management of pre-eclampsia, eclampsia, cervical incompetence, placental insufficiency, antepartum hemorrhage, uterine rupture, etc.

### *Management of Low Birth Weight*

- Essential newborn care.
- Tocolytics to slow down labor and administration of corticosteroid for fetal lung maturity.
- Antibiotics for preterm premature rupture of membranes (PROM) to prevent infection.
- Kangaroo mother care: It offers thermal protection, facilitates breastfeeding and ensures bonding between mother and child. It includes skin-to-skin contact by placing the baby between the mother's breast in an upright position, chest-to-chest with head slightly extended, arms flexed, hips flexed and extended in a "frog" position and abdomen at the level of mother's epigastrium. Skin-to-skin contact can be continued till the baby reaches gestational age of 40 weeks or attains 2,500 g of weight. A LBW baby is rarely able to suck and may not be able to take oral feeds. Therefore, they have to be fed intravenously or through a nasogastric tube. A LBW baby is rarely able to suck due to poorly developed reflexes. Therefore, the mother should be encouraged to express breast milk and feed the baby using a cup and spoon until the baby is able to breastfeed. In addition, the baby also needs love, care and attention to be able to grow effectively.
- Case management of preterm babies with complications such as infection, jaundice and respiratory distress syndrome.
- Child should be adequately immunized for age. Efforts should be made to minimize the dropout rate and delays in immunization. Parents should be counseled and encouraged for regular and timely immunization.

Under "Comprehensive implementation plan on maternal, infant and young child nutrition", we aim to achieve 30% reduction in LBW by 2025 globally. Under the Ministry of Health and Family Welfare, various flagship programs have been initiated and strengthened to deliver comprehensive maternal and child healthcare to improve perinatal outcomes, one of which is LBW.

- Cash transfer under Janani Suraksha Yojana (JSY) to promote institutional deliveries for improved outcomes.
- Identification of high-risk antenatal woman and timely referral to an equipped higher center.
- Transport services (ambulance services) are provided to patients under Janani Shishu Suraksha Karyakaram (JSSK) to and from the health facility.
- Under Adolescent-Friendly Health Initiatives (AFHI), adolescents are given sex counseling and premarital counseling. In addition, adolescent girls who get married before the age of 18 years are encouraged to postpone their first pregnancy and use appropriate family welfare methods.

## Childhood Infections

Infectious diseases cause a considerable morbidity in under-five children. In some cases, these diseases can lead to long-term disability.

Children under 5 are especially vulnerable to infectious diseases like malaria, pneumonia, diarrhea, HIV and tuberculosis. Pneumonia, diarrhea and malaria were responsible for approximately 30% of global deaths among children under the age of 5 in 2019. Common diseases leading to morbidity in this age group are ARI, pneumonia, diarrhea and malaria.

Vaccine preventable diseases such as measles, polio, diphtheria, tetanus, pertussis, and pneumonia due to *Haemophilus influenzae* type B and Streptococcus pneumonia are other important causes of under-five morbidity. Although safe and effective vaccines are available for these diseases, they can occur among children belonging to regions with low levels of routine immunization.

### *Magnitude of Problem*

- As reported by United Nations International Children's Emergency Fund (UNICEF), an under-five death occurs every minute due to pneumonia and nearly every minute, a child dies from malaria (WHO/UNICEF, Childhood diseases 2023).
- There are over 2 billion cases of diarrheal disease every year and is the leading cause of malnutrition amongst children under-five. Nearly a quarter of under-five deaths occur due to pneumonia and diarrhea.
- Frequent episodes of diarrhea lead to vicious cycle of undernutrition, impaired immune function, and increased susceptibility to infections.

### *Causes and Associated Factors*

- Poor socioeconomic status, low literacy, and lack of safe water and sanitation are closely associated with childhood infections.

- Deaths due to pneumonia and diarrhea are disproportionately high among children below the age of 2 years. Nearly 80% of mortality due to pneumonia and approximately 70% due to diarrhea occur in this age group.

### Prevention and Control of Childhood Infections

- Promoting exclusive breastfeeding for the first 6 months of life, and continued breastfeeding until 2 years of age or longer, with age-appropriate complementary feeding
- Vitamin A supplementation
- Immunization for all vaccine preventable diseases
- Promoting good hygiene, practices including handwashing with soap
- Ensuring safe drinking water and sanitation
- Reducing household air pollution and promoting the use of clean fuels
- Timely and effective treatment of pneumonia and diarrhea
- Provision of essential medicines and supplies—antibiotics and oxygen (for pneumonia) and low osmolarity oral rehydration solution (ORS) and zinc (for diarrhea).

## Birth Defects

Birth defects are one of the major contributors in child mortality. *Birth defects can be defined as structural or functional abnormalities including metabolic disorders, which are present from birth.* These are also known as *congenital disorders* or *congenital malformations.* Congenital anomalies are the major cause of newborn deaths within 4 weeks of birth and can result in long-term disability with a significant impact on individuals, families, and healthcare systems.

### Magnitude of Problem

- An estimated 240,000 newborns die worldwide within 28 days of birth every year due to congenital disorders. Congenital disorders cause a further 170,000 deaths of children between the ages of 1 month and 5 years. (WHO: Congenital disorders-Factsheet, Feb 2023).
- According to joint WHO and March of Dime (MOD) report, birth defects account for 7% of all neonatal mortality. Nearly 7.9 million (6%) births worldwide occur with serious birth defects. Out of these, 94% occur in the middle and low-income countries (WHO, Management of birth defects and hemoglobin disorders: Report, 2006).
- The prevalence of birth defects in India is 61–69.9 per 1,000 live births (NHP, congenital anomalies).
- Epidemiology of birth defects in India: The country reports 24 million births, that is, nearly one-fifth of births occurring worldwide. Health and demographic data reflect evidences of epidemiological transition. Neonatal mortality rate is 24 per 1,000 live births and shows a similar urban-rural difference (14 for urban and 27 for rural areas). The infant mortality rate is 33 per 1,000 live births with a large urban (23)-rural (38) difference. (Government of India Ministry of Health and Family Welfare 2019).

- Major birth defects include:
  - Congenital heart defects (8–10 per 1,000 live births)
  - Neural tube defects (4–11.4 per 1,000 live births)
  - Congenital deafness (5.6–10 per 1,000 live births)
  - Down syndrome (1.4 per 1,000 live births)
  - Hemoglobinopathies
  - Glucose-6-phosphate dehydrogenase deficiency.

### Causes of Congenital Birth Defects

These can be caused by single gene defects, chromosomal disorders, multifactorial inheritance, environmental teratogens (an agent which can cause a birth defect), and micronutrient deficiencies.

### Risk Factors for Congenital Birth Defects

- *Maternal age at conception:* Incidence of Down syndrome is related to fertility status of older (>35 years)
- *Maternal nutritional status and medical conditions:*
  - Iodine deficiency (neonatal hypothyroidism)
  - Folic acid deficiency (high-risk of having a baby with a neural tube defect)
  - Diabetes mellitus, obesity, and seizure disorders.
- *Environmental factors:*
  - Exposures to teratogens before and after conception
  - Maternal exposure to certain medications, psychoactive drugs, tobacco, alcohol, radiation, and pesticides during pregnancy may increase the risk of congenital anomalies in fetus or neonate.
  - Working or living near, or in, waste sites, smelters or mines may also be a risk factor.
- *Infections:* Some maternal infections during pregnancy can increase the risk of birth defects, such as:
  - Rubella infection during pregnancy can result in miscarriage, deafness, intellectual disability, heart defects, and blindness in newborn.
  - Toxoplasmosis infection during pregnancy can cause birth defects, such as hearing loss, vision problems, and intellectual disability.
  - Sexually transmitted infections, such as syphilis, cytomegalovirus can cause serious birth defects.
  - *Zika virus infection*: During pregnancy can cause birth defects like microcephaly and other abnormalities.
- *Parent's carrier status of a genetic disorder:* Carrier status for various genetic disorders such as thalassemia, sickle cell anemia, and metabolic disorders can lead to these disorders in the offspring.

### Prevention of Birth Defects

- *Primary prevention:* It aims to ensure that newborns are free of birth defects. This can be achieved by following interventions:
  - *Family welfare services*—enabling couples to space pregnancies and plan family size, define the ages at which they wish to complete their family and reduce the proportion of unintended pregnancies.

- *Preconceptional health of women*—ensuring good diet throughout the reproductive years with adequate amount of macronutrients and micronutrients (vitamins and minerals—iron, iodine, and folic acid). Preconceptional intake of folic acid supplementation to prevent neural tube defects.
- *Promoting healthy dietary habits and lifestyle*—avoiding the intake of harmful substances (such as alcohol and smoking including passive smoking).
- *Safe environment*—avoiding environmental exposure to hazardous substances at home and workplace (e.g., heavy metals, pesticides, and radiation exposure).
- Detecting, treating, and preventing **maternal infections**.
- **Control of diseases**, such as insulin-dependent diabetes mellitus and epilepsy.
- **Rubella vaccination** to all school-aged children and adolescents. The rubella vaccine can also be given (at least 1 month prior to pregnancy) to women who have not been vaccinated and do not have a history of rubella in childhood (two doses of rubella vaccine at an interval of 4 weeks).
- Avoiding use of teratogenic drugs during pregnancy and prior to conception (in women planning for the pregnancy). No medication should be taken in pregnancy without consulting a doctor.
- **Prevent mosquito bites** and sexual transmission of Zika virus among those either living in or traveling to areas where Zika virus is reported.
- *Sensitization and capacity building of healthcare personnel* involved in maternal and child health and promoting prevention of congenital anomalies.
- *Secondary prevention:* It aims to reduce the number of children born with birth defects.
  - With the use of medical genetic screening and prenatal diagnosis, birth defects are detected and the couple offered genetic counseling and therapeutic options.
- *Tertiary prevention:* It is directed toward the early detection and management in a child born with congenital birth defects.

## Childhood Disability

A large number of children suffer from some form of disability that affects their quality of life and has an impact on the parents and families.

Fifteen percent of the world's population – at least one billion people – have some form of disability, whether present at birth or acquired later in life. Nearly 240 million of them are children [UNICEF, June 2023].

### Common Types of Disabilities

- Visual impairment
- Hearing impairment
- Locomotor impairment
- Cerebral palsy
- Mental retardation and mental illness
- Children with learning disabilities:
  - Dyslexia
  - Dysgraphia
  - Dyscalculia
- Attention deficit and hyperactivity disorder (ADHD).

As per 2011 census of India, there are 7,862,921 children with disability in the below 19-year age group including 1,410,158 visual impairment, 1,594,249 hearing impairment, 683,702 speech disorder, 1,045,656 movement disorder, 595,089 intellectual disability, 678,441 multiple disability, and 1,719,845 other disabilities.

The children with disabilities have special needs, including need for special education. Hence, it is imperative that correctable causes of disability be identified early, and children with disability be rehabilitated in such a manner that they can reach their optimal development potential.

### Prevention of Childhood Disability

Early detection and timely intervention of medical conditions that cause disability can lead to reduction in mortality, morbidity and lifelong disability.

The Government of India has taken many initiatives for early detection of disabilities among children.

- **Rashtriya Bal Swasthya Karyakram (RBSK)** was launched in 2013, it focuses on extensive health services and covers 30 conditions including screening, diagnosis, and treatment for defects at birth, diseases, deficiencies developmental delays, and disabilities (4Ds) among all children from birth up to 18 years of age.
- Vision screening of schoolchildren for detecting correctable causes of poor vision especially refractive errors, and in minimizing long-term permanent visual disability.
- Screening for ear diseases and hearing impairment.
- District early intervention centers (DIEC) at district hospitals to provide referral support to children detected with health conditions following health screening.

In the census of India conducted in the year 2011, the questions regarding disability were included for the first time.

The **India Newborn Action Plan (INAP)** formulated in September 2014, has integrated the approaches for the prevention and care of newborn with birth defects into primary healthcare.

### Other Priorities for Children's Health

Congenital anomalies, injuries, and noncommunicable diseases (NCDs) (chronic respiratory diseases, acquired heart diseases, childhood cancers, diabetes, and obesity) are the emerging priorities in the global child health agenda.

Besides injury and NCDs, behavioral problems and child delinquency are other emerging child health problems. This highlights the need for social support, child guidance clinics, and counseling services for children with behavioral problems.

## MORTALITY IN UNDER-FIVE CHILDREN

The mortality among children is an important indicator of a country's development. Worldwide the burden of childhood mortality is huge.

> **Definitions:**
> - *Neonatal mortality:* The probability of dying within the first month of life
> - *Postneonatal mortality:* The probability of dying between the first month of life and on the first birthday. It is calculated as the difference between infant and neonatal mortality
> - *Perinatal mortality:* The probability of death of fetus after 28 weeks of gestation (or fetus having weight of 1,000 g) and within first week of life
> - *Infant mortality:* The probability of dying between birth and the first birthday
> - *Child mortality:* The probability of dying between the first and fifth birthdays
> - *Under-five mortality:* The probability of dying between birth and the fifth birthday

## Current Status and Trend—Global

### Current Status

As reported by the UNICEF nearly 13,800 under-five deaths occur in a day worldwide. The global U5MR in 2019 was 38 deaths per 1,000 live births [UNICEF, Jan 2023].

The risk of death is highest in the first 28 days of life. Among all under-five deaths, 47% were contributed by the newborn deaths in 2021.

During the first month of life, nearly half of the deaths occur within the first 24 hours of and three quarters (75%) occur in the first week. Immediately after the birth, the first 48 hours is the most crucial period for newborn survival.

In 2021, the global neonatal mortality rate was estimated to be 18 deaths per 1,000 live births, the global postneonatal mortality rate was 11 per 1,000 live births, and the probability of dying after the age 1 and before the age 5 was 10 per 1,000 live births. Thus, the U5MR which includes all the above-mentioned three groups was 38 deaths per 1,000 live births **(Fig. 26.3)**.

### Trends

Substantial progress has been made in reducing under-five mortality since 1990. The global U5MR has dropped by 59% from 93 deaths per 1,000 live births in 1990 to 38 in 2021 **(Fig. 26.4)**. Worldwide, the number of neonatal deaths decreased from 5.1 million in 1990 to 2.4 million in 2019. However, the decline in neonatal mortality from 2000 to 2019 has been slower (41%) than that in postneonatal mortality (60%) globally.

A very mild direct mortality impact of COVID-19 on child and youth mortality has been observed. Still, indirect mortality among children and youth resulting from obstacles like exhausted healthcare systems, interrupted vital interventions and services like vaccination and nutrition, and household income loss remain of great concern to the global public health community.

In 2021, 5.0 million children died before reaching their 5th birthday. This is an immense, intolerable and mostly preventable loss of life [Levels and Trends in Child Mortality. Report 2022 Estimates developed by the United Nations Inter-agency Group for Child Mortality Estimation].

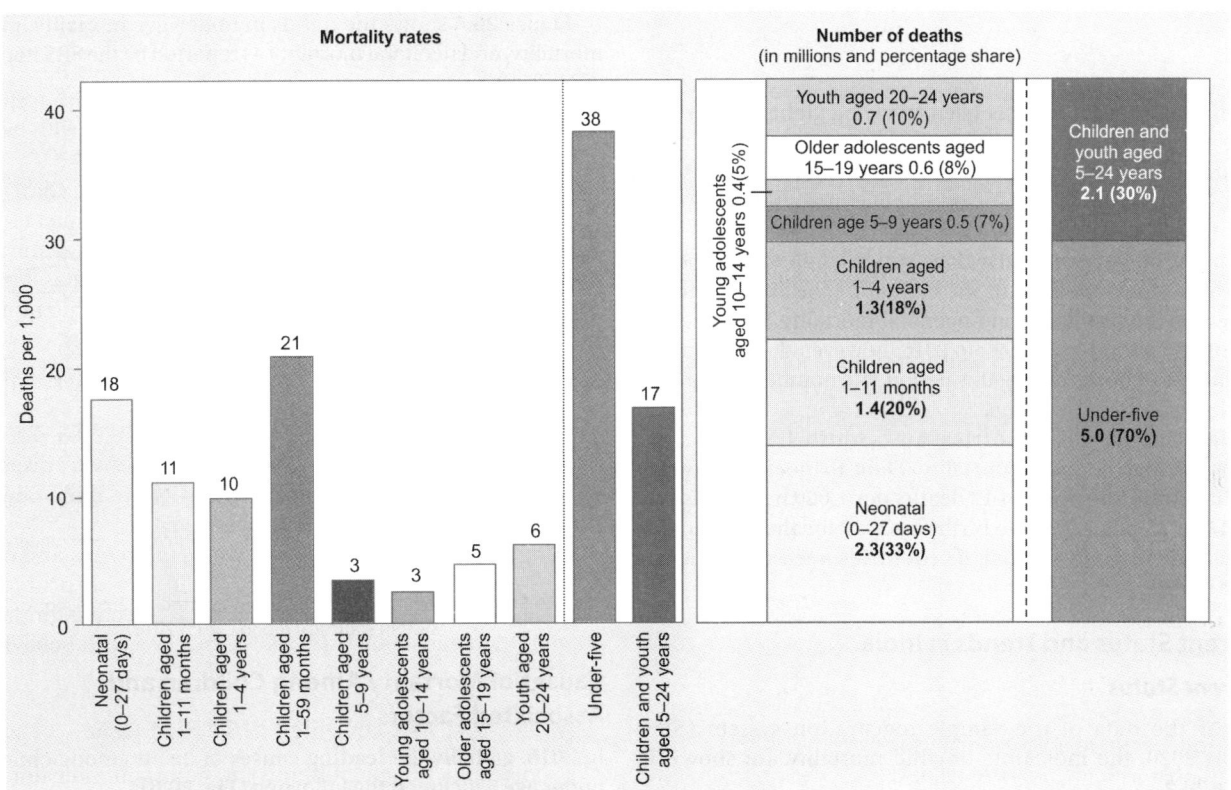

**Fig 26.3:** Global childhood mortality rate and number of deaths y age (UN IGME Estimates 2021).

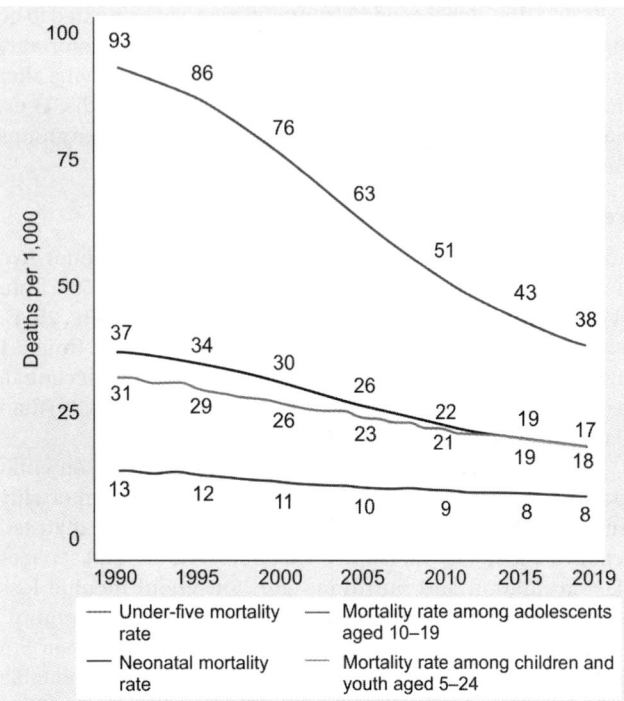

**Fig. 26.4:** Global trends in neonatal and under-5 mortality (1990–2018).
*Source:* UNICEF. Levels and trends in childhood mortality: Report 2020 - Estimates developed by the UN Inter-agency Group for Child Mortality Estimation (UN IGME).

Although the U5MR has been reducing globally, there are wide disparities across different regions and countries. Sub-Saharan Africa has the highest U5MR in the world. Besides this, there are geographic and socioeconomic inequities within the countries.

Among the geographical regions, sub-Saharan Africa reported relatively slower decline in the neonatal mortality. Although there was modest decline in neonatal mortality in this region during the period from 1990 to 2016, however, due to increase in number of births during this period, the number of neonatal deaths was almost the same.

Many countries in Africa and South-East Asia are reporting high neonatal mortality. Thus, to meet the target of neonatal mortality rate of 12 deaths per 1,000 live births and U5MR to 25 per 1,000 live births by 2030 for the sustainable development goals (SDGs), 53 countries need to accelerate their efforts.

## Current Status and Trends in India

### Current Status

As per the data of the sample registration system (SRS) report 2020, the indicators of child mortality are shown in **Table 26.2**.

**Table 26.2:** Indicators of child mortality in India [SRS 2020].

| Indicator | No. of deaths (per 1,000 live births) | | |
| --- | --- | --- | --- |
| | Total | Rural | Urban |
| Early neonatal mortality rate (number of deaths less than 7 days of life per 1,000 live births) | 15 | 17 | 9 |
| Neonatal mortality rate | 20 | 23 | 12 |
| Infant mortality rate | 28 | 31 | 19 |
| Perinatal mortality rate | 18 | 21 | 12 |
| Stillbirth rate | 3 | 4 | 3 |
| Under-five mortality rate | 32 | 36 | 21 |

*Source:* Registrar General of India. SRS statistical Report—May 2018. [online] Available from: http://www.censusindia.gov.in/vital_statistics/SRS_Statistical_Report.html.

### Trends

Historically, the infant and child mortality in India have been very high. In 1921, the infant mortality rate (IMR) was nearly 225/1,000 live births. At the time of independence, the IMR was very high being 161/1,000 live births. There was some decline in the sixties (146/1,000) and 130/1,000 live births in mid-seventies.

The under-five mortality also declined from 200 in sixties to 167 in the mid-seventies.

However, since 1978, there has been a decline in both IMR and U5MR.

**Figure 26.5** shows the trends in under-five mortality, infant mortality, and neonatal mortality as reported by the SRS Reports 2011–2018.

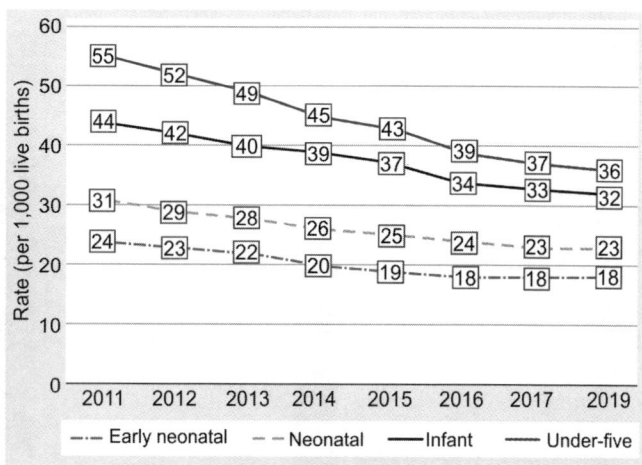

**Fig. 26.5:** Trends in childhood mortality as reported in sample registration system statistical reports 2011–2018.

## Causes of Mortality Among Children and Associated Factors

In 2018, globally the leading causes of death among children under age 5 included the following **(Fig. 26.6):**

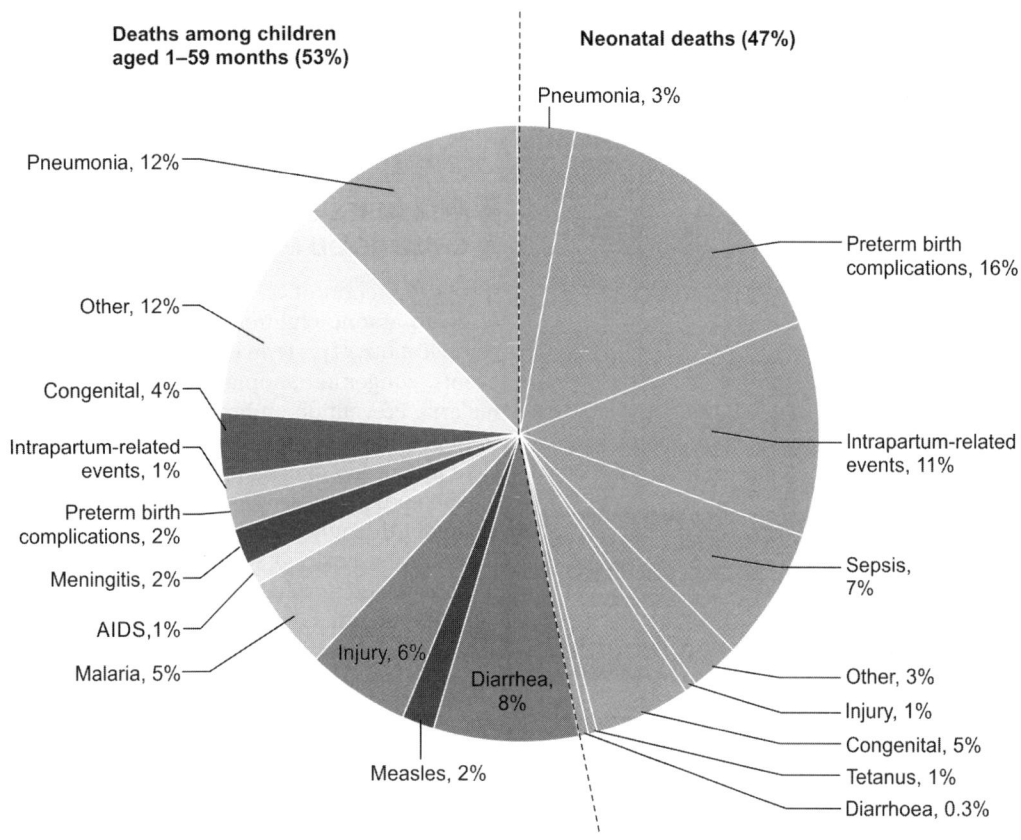

Fig. 26.6: Causes of deaths among children under-five years of age (2018).
Source: UNICEF. Levels and trends in childhood mortality: Report 2019 - Estimates developed by the UN Inter-agency Group for Child Mortality Estimation (UNIGME). [online] Available from: http://www.un.org/en/development/desa/population/publications/mortality/child-mortality-report-2019.shtml.

- Preterm birth complications (18%)
- Pneumonia (16%)
- Intrapartum-related events (12%)
- Congenital anomalies (9%)
- Diarrhea (8%)
- Neonatal sepsis (7%)
- Malaria (5%).

It has been found that a small number of conditions lead to majority of the deaths. Leading causes of death in children under-five years are preterm birth complications, pneumonia, birth asphyxia, diarrhea, and malaria.

- **Among the neonates,** majority of the deaths are caused by preterm birth, intrapartum-related complications such as birth asphyxia, hypothermia, and sepsis.
- **After the neonatal period and during the first 5 years of life,** the main causes of death are pneumonia, diarrhea, and malaria. Undernutrition is an important contributing factor making children more vulnerable to severe disease and death.
- Common childhood illness, such as diarrhea, pneumonia, and malaria leads to higher mortality among children with undernutrition especially those with severe acute malnutrition (SAM).
- As much as 45% of deaths in children below the age of 5 years are related to undernutrition (WHO 2020).

## Factors Associated with Child Mortality

- *Place of residence (rural or urban):* It has been shown that mortality is relatively lower in urban areas as compared to rural areas. Since 1981, estimates have revealed a higher level of neonatal, infant, and under-five mortality in rural areas as compared to urban areas. NFHS-5 also shows that the U5MR is higher (45.7/1,000) in rural areas as compared to 31.5 deaths per 1,000 in urban areas.
- *Mother's education:* Numerous studies have proved that increase in mother's year of schooling reduces the risk of mortality throughout the childhood. Education is important as it exposes the mother to information regarding nutrition, contraception, immunization, as well as increases the demand and utilization of healthcare services.
- *Social group:* The U5MR for scheduled castes, scheduled tribes, and other backward classes are considerably higher than for those who are not from these social groups.
- *Household wealth:* The U5MR is inversely related to household wealth. As per the data of NFHS-5, the U5MR was 59 deaths per 1,000 live births and 20 deaths per 1,000 live births in the lowest wealth and the highest wealth quintiles, respectively.
- *Demographic factors (Fig. 26.7):* Other sociodemographic factors associated with high-risk of infant mortality are:

- *Maternal age at child birth:* Less than 18 years and more than 30 years
- *Sex of the baby:* Male sex
- *Birth order:* More than three
- *Birth interval (previous as well as succeeding):* Less than 2 years.

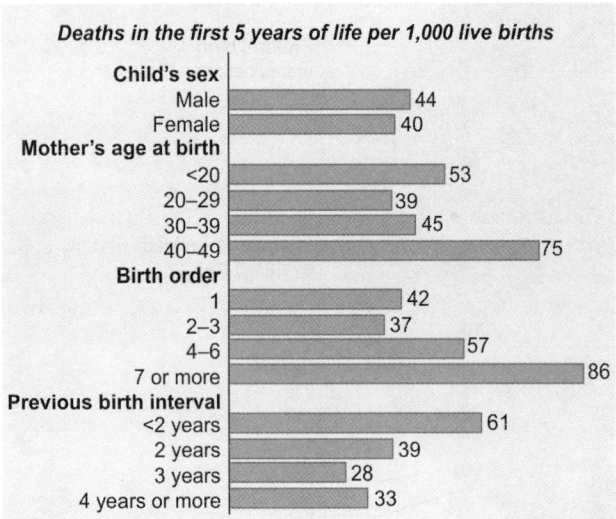

Fig. 26.7: Sociodemographic factors associated with under-five deaths (NFHS-5).

## INFANT MORTALITY

It is a very sensitive and comprehensive indicator of health because it reflects quality of maternal and child health services as well as availability and utilization of services. It also indicates the socioeconomic conditions under which the infants live.

The current status and trends of infant mortality are already discussed above.

### Causes of Infant Mortality

Broadly, the causes of infant mortality can be divided into neonatal causes (*refer* **Figure 26.6**) and postneonatal causes.

**Neonatal causes:**
- Low birth weight
- Hypothermia
- Birth injury
- Obstructed labor
- Birth asphyxia
- Congenital anomalies
- Neonatal tetanus
- Acute respiratory distress syndrome
- Diarrheal diseases

**Postneonatal causes (1 month–1 year):**
- Acute respiratory infections
- Diarrheal diseases
- Other communicable diseases
- Malnutrition
- Congenital anomalies
- Accidents

Risk factors for infant mortality are same as discussed in factors associated with childhood mortalities.

### Prevention and Control of Infant Mortality

Since infant mortality is multi-causation in nature, prevention and control is also aimed at multiple levels. This is discussed in elaboration below along with prevention and control of other childhood mortalities.

## MEASURES FOR PREVENTION AND CONTROL OF CHILDHOOD MORBIDITIES AND MORTALITY

As per the report of WHO in 2021, globally the leading causes of death among children under the age of 5 years included complications of preterm birth, pneumonia, intrapartum-related events, congenital anomalies, diarrhea, neonatal sepsis, and malaria. Prevention and treatment of these causes are critical to improving newborn, child, and young adolescent survival. High proportion of neonatal deaths is the result of diseases and conditions that are associated with quality of care around the time of childbirth. Thus, strengthening of health services is essential. It should be ensured that every birth is attended by skilled personnel, and hospital care is available in times of emergency. Cost-effective interventions for newborn health should cover the antenatal period, the time around birth and the first week of life, as well as care for small and sick newborns.

### Global Goals and Targets

The United Nations Millennium Development Goals (MDG) 2000 had reduction of child mortality as one of its main goals. The aim was to reduce U5MR by two-third in the period between 1990 and 2015. In this 25 years period, the global U5MR reduced by more than 50% from 90 to 43 deaths per 1,000 live births per year in 2015. However, this trend is insufficient as essential care is still elusive to a bulk of children in underprivileged and vulnerable situations. Preventable causes like diarrhea, pneumonia, and malaria still kill about 16,000 children every day in 2015.

In 2016, the UN Statistical Commission proposed the indicator framework for SDGs wherein, by 2030, all countries will aim to reduce the **neonatal mortality rate to 12/1,000 live births and U5MR to 25/1,000 live births (SDG Goal 3, Target 2)**.

### Targeting Childhood Morbidities and Mortalities in India

India is a major contributor of the global under-five mortality and the government of India has progressively introduced a gamut of strategies to target the various childhood morbidities and mortalities **(Box 26.1)**. The first of the various programs in this line was the Child Survival and Safe Motherhood (CSSM) program in 1992 launched with support from World Bank and UNICEF addressing issues like universal immunization program, management of diarrhea, and respiratory infections along with emergency obstetric care. This was further upgraded to Reproductive and Child Health (RCH) programme in 1997 by adding in additional components for management of reproductive tract infections and STIs. Later, "Integrated Management of Neonatal and Childhood Illnesses" (IMNCI 2003) was adopted from WHO Integrated Management of Childhood Illness (IMCI) strategy in 1995 for syndromic management of common diseases seen in under five children population. Navjaat Shishu Suraksha

> **Box 26.1: Major strategies and policies targeting childhood morbidities and mortality in India.**
> - 1978: Expanded program of immunization (EPI) launched to vaccinate the children for BCG, OPV, DPT, and typhoid
> - 1985: Universal Immunization Program (UIP) when measles vaccine was added and typhoid vaccine was discontinued
> - 1990: Vitamin A supplementation added to the UIP
> - 1992: Child Survival and Safe Motherhood (CSSM)
> - 1997: Reproductive and Child Health phase I (RCH-I)
> - 2003: Integrated Management of Neonatal and Child Illnesses (IMNCI)
> - 2005: Janani Suraksha Yojana and RCH-II under National Rural Health Mission (NRHM)
> - 2011: Facility Based Newborn Care (FBNC), Navjaat Shishu Suraksha Karyakram (NSSK), and Janani Shishu Suraksha Karyakram (JSSK)
> - 2013: Reproductive maternal newborn child and adolescent health (RMNCAH+N), enhancing optimal IYCF practices
> - 2014: Home-based Newborn Care Guidelines, India Newborn Action Plan
> - 2016: Promotion of Infant and Young Child feeding practices (IYCF)- Mother's Absolute Affection (MAA) programme
> - 2018: Anaemia Mukt Bharat (AMB)-POSHAN Abhiyaan
> - 2018–19: National De-worming Day (NDD)-10th Feb every year
> - 2023: Reproductive maternal newborn child and adolescent health plus nutrition (RMNCAH+N)

(BCG: Bacillus Calmette-Guerin; DPT: diphtheria, pertussis, and tetanus; IYCF: infant and young child feeding; OPV: oral poliovirus vaccine)

Karyakram (NSSK) has further endeavored in training health personnel in basic newborn care and resuscitation.

The **RMNCH+A** (Reproductive, Maternal Child and Adolescent health) strategy launched in India in 2013 which is renamed recently as RMNCAH+N involves linking key interventions across the continuum of care from prepregnancy to the postpartum period focusing on the inter-relationships between maternal, reproductive, neonatal, child and adolescent healthcare and linking the nutrition related strategies to all the life stages. *All the major strategies and policies targeting childhood morbidities and mortality in India in Box 26.1 are explained further in Chapter 47: Health Policies and Programs in India.*

## Birth Preparedness and Complication Readiness

The care of the newborn baby starts with educating and training the prospective mother and other family members to be prepared for an ideal care of the new guest in the family.

Birth preparedness and complication readiness (BPCR) is a globally accepted antenatal counseling strategy that encourages pregnant women, their families, and communities to effectively plan for births and deals with emergencies, if they occur. BPCR programs generally include counseling for women and their families to—(1) encourage them to take decisions before the onset of labor and potential occurrence of obstetric complications; (2) inform them about the signs of complications so they will know and be able to react promptly if needed; (3) inform them about the locations of emergency services to make the care-seeking process more efficient; and (4) encourage them to save the money needed to pay for services and to plan their transportation to a health facility during labor and in case of emergency. BPCR interventions have been shown to reduce neonatal mortality by almost 18%.

## Essential Newborn Care

All babies need basic care to support their survival and well-being at birth and postnatal period which has been bundled as essential newborn care (ENC).

The key components of ENC are:
- Warmth
- Immediate breathing
- Breastfeeding
- Infection prevention
- Active look out for danger signs.

*Warmth:* The newborns' skin temperature tends to rapidly fall within seconds of birth by conduction (through contact with solid objects such as cloth, surface, etc.), convection (through cold air currents from an open window), radiation (to nearby colder objects, e.g., walls) or evaporation (of the amniotic fluid from the surface)—all of which can cause hypothermia and eventual death, if not managed in time. Placing the baby between the mother's breasts maintains the baby's temperature at the correct level. The first skin-to-skin contact should last uninterrupted for at least 1 hour after birth or until after the first breastfeed. The mother and baby should be covered with a warm and dry cloth, especially if the room temperature is lower than 25°C. "Warm chain" for temperature maintenance should be a continuous process starting from the time of delivery and continued throughout the early and late neonatal period **(Box 26.2)**.

> **Box 26.2: Warm chain.**
> - Warm delivery room (>25°C) with no draught (direct cool air)
> - Immediate drying and removal of wet cloths
> - Skin-to-skin contact between baby and mother and cover with dry cloth
> - Early initiation of breastfeeding
> - Postpone bathing until umbilical cord stump heals (around 1 week)
> - Cover the baby with appropriate clothing especially the head
> - Warmth during transportation and rooming-in
> - Kangaroo mother care for stable low birth weight babies and rewarming of stable bigger babies
> - Training of mothers and healthcare providers in preventing hypothermia by timely recognition and ensuring that the baby's feet are warm to touch

*Immediate breathing:* Any baby can have a breathing difficulty at birth. Neonatal resuscitation using a bag and mask resuscitator is a basic technique which every doctor or staff nurse is required to know. Apart from this, if meconium has been passed, then immediate suction of mouth and nose should be done after birth. If the baby is crying or the chest movements are regular with respiratory rate 30–60 per minute, there is no need of resuscitation or suctioning.

*Breastfeeding:* Breastfeeding is a simple and effective public health intervention. It has been shown that breastfed children have better growth and development and are less likely to suffer from asthma, gastroenteritis, skin, and respiratory diseases. Recommended practices include early initiation of breastfeeding within 30 minutes of birth, exclusive breastfeeding till 6 months of age and complimentary feeding along with breastfeeding after 6 months of age.
- All mothers should be counseled about proper attachment and positioning for initiating breastfeeding. The key points in **proper positioning** are:

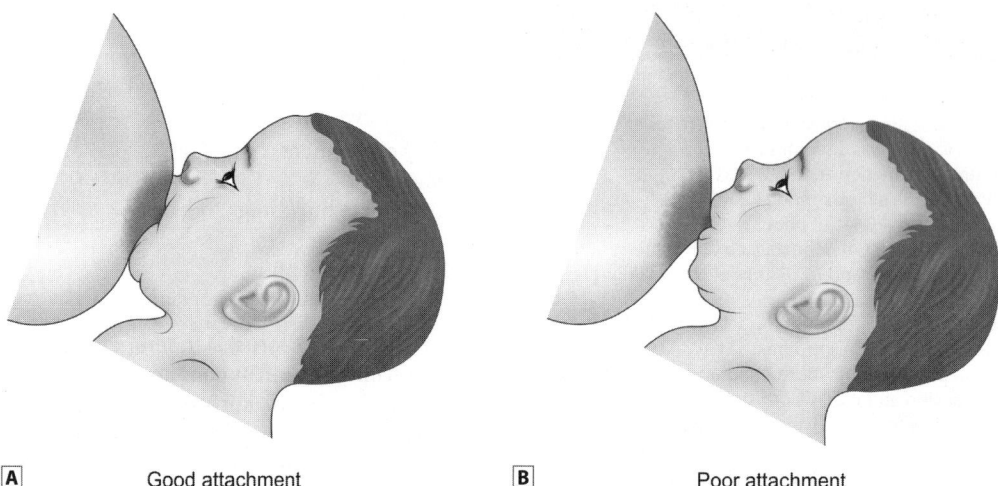

**Figs. 26.8A and B:** Signs of good and bad attachment.
*Source:* UNICEF/WHO Breastfeeding and Support in a baby-friendly hospital.

- Baby's head and body should be straight
- Baby's face should face mother's breast
- Baby's body should be close to mother's body
- Mother should support the baby's whole body with one hand. She should support her breast with other hand, put her fingers below the breast and thumb above the areola to help shape the breast.
- The signs of **good attachment** are **(Figs. 26.8A and B)**:
  - More areola is visible above the baby's mouth than below it
  - Baby's mouth is wide open
  - Baby's lower lip is turned outwards
  - Baby's chin is touching the breast.
- Poor attachment may occur due to inexperience of mother, lack of skilled support, or inverted nipples or bottle feeding. After ascertaining proper attachment, the next step is to assess if the baby is sucking effectively where the baby takes several slow deep sucks followed by swallowing and then pauses. If the suckles are of shorter duration and the baby tires out or is unable to continue long enough, he/she will need to be fed expressed milk using spoon or cup. Breastfeeding is considered adequate, if the baby passes urine six to eight times a day, sleeps for 2–3 hours after feeds and crosses birth weight by 10–14 days **(Box 26.3)**.

---

**Box 26.3: Advantages of breastfeeding.**

**Benefits to baby:**
- Complete nutrition
- Easily digestible and well absorbed
- Prevents infections and decreases risk of gastrointestinal and respiratory infections
- Promotes emotional bonding
- Better brain growth

**Benefits to mother:**
- Helps in involution of uterus
- Lactational amenorrhea and natural contraception
- Lowers risk of breast and ovarian carcinoma

**Benefits to society:**
- Cost-effective
- Promotes family planning
- Decreases need for hospitalization and
- Contributes to child survival

---

***Infection prevention:*** Sepsis is a leading cause of neonatal mortality and can be easily prevented by maintaining cleanliness and handwashing practices **(Box 26.4)**. As always, prevention is more cost-effective than treatment of infections in neonates. Handwashing is the simplest and relatively cheap intervention for infection prevention. The six recommended steps of handwashing include sequential cleaning of palms and fingers and web spaces, back of hands, fingers and knuckles, thumbs, fingertips and wrists, and forearms up to elbow.

---

**Box 26.4: Interventions to prevent infections and sepsis.**

**The six cleans at the time of delivery:**
1. Clean hands (washed with soap and water)
2. Clean delivery surface
3. Clean blade for cord cutting
4. Clean string or rubber band to tie cord
5. Clean cloth to wrap the baby
6. Clean clothes for the mother

**The six cleans in postnatal period:**
1. Handwashing with soap and water by all caregivers before touching baby
2. Restrictive handling, i.e., minimize the number of persons who touch and care for the baby
3. Clean cloth or diaper or napkins
4. Handwashing after changing clothes or diapers or napkins
5. Clean cord—do not apply anything
6. Exclusive breastfeeding

---

***Active look out for danger signs:*** Early diagnosis of sick newborn is of paramount importance especially since many signs could be very nonspecific, for example—lethargy. The various danger signs that should be actively look out for are:
- Baby is not feeding well
- Convulsions
- Drowsy or unconscious
- Decreased or no movement on stimulation
- Fast breathing (>60 breaths per minute)
- Grunting
- Severe chest in drawing
- Hypothermia
- Hyperthermia

- Central cyanosis
- Bleeding or discharge from cord, ear or eyes
- Jaundice.

Essential newborn care can be chronologically divided into five distinct time phases:
1. Preparation for birth
2. Immediate newborn care (first 60 minutes of birth)
3. Early newborn care (1–6 hours of birth)
4. Care before discharge (6–48 hours of birth)
5. Care at discharge.

*Phase 1: Preparation for birth:* The delivery room where the baby is born into should have a designated newborn care corner (vide infra).
- Ensure warm (~25°C) and draught free delivery room
- Switch on radiant warmer half an hour before
- Availability of suction machine
- Keep at least two warm and dry towels ready
- Availability of soap and running water for handwashing
- Availability of sterile gloves
- Availability of sterilized delivery kit
- Ensure functional bag and mask.

*Phase 2: Immediate care of newborn (first 60 minutes):*
- Call out time of birth
- Check for meconium. If there is meconium and/or baby is not crying, perform suction immediately before drying
- Deliver the baby on mother's abdomen and congratulate her. Show her the baby's genitals to identify the gender
- Check for breathing and start to dry the baby with warm towels
- Change the wet towel. Ensure skin-to-skin contact with mother
- Cover baby with dry and warm towel
- Clamp the cord at two places and cut the cord between the two clamps within 1–3 minutes of birth
- Look for major malformations and birth injuries
- Support mother to initiate breastfeeding
- Place an identity tag on the baby.

*Phase 3: Early newborn care:*
- Record weight of the baby
- Administer 1 mg vitamin K intramuscularly
- Examine for vital signs and look-out for danger signs
- Vaccinate with Bacillus Calmette-Guérin (BCG), oral polio vaccine (OPV), and Hepatitis B birth dose
- Practice rooming-in.

*Phase 4: Care before discharge:*
- Monitor breathing, temperature, cord stump, eyes, skin, and look out for danger signs
- Ensure successful establishment of breastfeeding
- Counsel mother for exclusive breastfeeding
- Postpone bathing till umbilical cord stump heals (around 1 week)
- Continue to keep the baby warm.

*Phase 5: Care at discharge:*
- Examine in detail for danger signs
- Counsel mother for exclusive breastfeeding
- Counsel mother to be on look-out for danger signs
- Counsel mother for timely vaccinations of the child.

## Infant and Young Child Feeding Recommendations

For optimal growth and development, nutrition practices during the first 1,000 days of life (270 days in utero and first 2 years after birth) have been emphasized by WHO/UNICEF.
- Exclusive breastfeeding till end of six months, i.e., 180 days
  - Every mother, especially first-time mothers, should be supported by doctors, nursing and other health staff for correct positioning, latching and treatment of problems, such as engorgement, nipple fissures and delayed "coming-in" of milk.
  - Often mothers may begin to doubt their ability to fulfill the needs of the growing baby. She should be counseled and motivated during all health contacts and at home through home visits by trained community worker.
  - Working mothers often discontinue breastfeeding after returning to work following maternity leave. Such mothers should be assisted with:
    - Obtaining adequate maternity/baby care/breastfeeding leave
    - Encouraged to carry the baby to a work place/crèche wherever such facility exists.
    - Continuing EBF by expressing milk while they are out at work.
    - Consider the concept of "Hirkani's rooms" at work places (dedicated room at the workplace where working mothers can express milk and store in a refrigerator during their work schedule).
  - If the breastfeeding was temporarily discontinued due to an inadvertent situation, re-lactation should be tried as soon as possible using the WHO recommended Supplemental Suckling Technique (SST) technique.
  - Mothers should feel comfortable to nurse in public-hurdles impeding breastfeeding in public places should be removed. Special areas/rooms need to be established in places such as bus stands, railway stations, air-ports, etc.
- After six months, introduce optimal complementary feeding with energy dense home-made food.
  - Complementary feeding should be projected as the bridge that the mother has to make between liquid to solid transition and to empower the baby to "family pot feeding".
  - Breastfeeding should be actively supported and the term "weaning" should be avoided
  - Appropriately thick homogenous complementary foods home-made from locally available foods should be introduced at six completed months while continuing breastfeeding as frequently as possible.
  - Some recommendations for preparing dense foods:
    - Use staple home-made food (as these are fresh, clean, cheap and easily available), e.g., cereal-pulse mixture in 2:1 ratio.
    - Add sugar/jaggery and ghee/butter/oil to provide more calories from smaller volumes.
    - Fermented porridge, use of germinated or sprouted flour and toasting of grains before grinding can enrich the food.
  - Easily available, cost-effective seasonal uncooked fruits, green and other dark colored vegetables, milk and milk

products, pulses/legumes, animal foods, oil/butter, sugar/jaggery may be added in the staples gradually.
- Consistency of foods should be appropriate to the developmental readiness of the child in munching, chewing and swallowing. Avoid foods which can pose choking hazard. Introduce lumpy or granular foods and most tastes by about 9–10 months.
- Continue breastfeeding for minimum two years and even beyond.
- Mother should communicate, look into the eyes, touch and caress the baby while feeding. Practice responsive feeding.

### Baby-friendly Hospital Initiative

Although breastfeeding and timely complementary feeding is recognized as crucial for infant growth, development, and protection from infections, there was a need recognized by WHO/UNICEF to reinforce "breastfeeding culture", defend against "bottle-feeding culture", and reinforce mothers confidence in their ability to breastfeed. Such empowerment required an advocacy for social mobilization and comprehensive communication strategy at all levels of society. Obstacles to breastfeeding, which may exist within the health system, workplace, and community needed to be identified and addressed in a culturally sensitive manner.

### Monitoring Growth and Development

There is a predictable weight gain in a healthy baby—around 800 g each month during the initial 2 months of life, then 600 g in 3rd and 4th months, about 400 g in 5–6 months, and thereafter around 200 g per month up to 3 years. Similarly, from birth to 1 year of age, normal infants increase their length by 50%.

**Monitoring growth:** Growth monitoring is a regular measurement of growth, which enables mothers to visualize growth, or lack of it, and obtain specific, relevant and practical guidance to ensure continued regular growth and health of children. It is classically done using growth charts (developed by David Morley) which serve the dual purpose of identifying malnourished children (or those at risk of becoming malnourished) as well as helps in educating mothers and caregivers regarding child feeding and care practices. Growth charts have made the phenomenon of undernutrition visible, which was otherwise not identified before becoming severe. **Box 26.5** gives a summary of various methods that can be used for assessment of physical growth. Weight-for-age is the most frequently used globally accepted parameter for growth monitoring.

During the first 5 years of life, children all over the world grow in a similar fashion under optimum physiological conditions and supportive healthy environment. Hence, an internationally representative growth standard was envisaged by WHO to promote maximum growth potential in children along with allowing intercountry comparability. WHO growth standards 2006 are based on the multi-growth reference study and adopted in Indian guidelines since August 2008.

The innovative aspects of the new WHO growth standards are:
- Using a prescriptive approach, i.e., giving a "standard" rather than a "reference"
- Using breastfed infant born to nonsmoking mothers as a normative model

**Box 26.5: Summary of various growth indicators.**
- Height-for-age (H/A), is an indicator of *chronic malnutrition*. A child exposed to inadequate nutrition for a long period of time will have a reduced growth and therefore a lower height compared to other children of the same age (stunting).
- Weight-for-age (W/A), is a *composite indicator* of both long-term malnutrition (deficit in height or "stunting") and current malnutrition (deficit in weight or "wasting").
- Weight-for-height (W/H), is an indicator of *acute malnutrition* that tells us if a child is too thin for a given height (wasting).
- In *emergencies*, W/H is the best indicator as:
  ➢ It reflects the present situation;
  ➢ It is sensitive to rapid changes (problems and recovery);
  ➢ It is a good predictor of immediate mortality risk;
- It can be used to monitor the evolution of the nutritional status of the population.
- Bilateral edema is an indicator of Kwashiorkor. All children with edema are regarded as being severely acutely malnourished, irrespective of their W/H.
- Mid-upper arm circumference (MUAC) is *simplest*, fast and is *age-independent*. It is a good predictor of immediate *risk of death*, and can be used to measure acute malnutrition from 6 to 59 months (although it overestimates rates in the 6–12 month age groups). The risk of measurement error is very high, therefore MUAC is only used for quick screening and rapid assessments of the nutritional situation of the population mostly in emergency humanitarian situations.
- Head circumference-for-age is often used as part of health screening for potential developmental or neurological disabilities in infants and young children. Very small and very large circumferences are both indicative of health or developmental risk.
- *Skin-fold thickness*: Triceps and subscapular skin fold measurements assess the thickness of subcutaneous tissue and reflect fatness primarily. The skin fold indicators are thus a useful addition to the battery of growth standards for assessing childhood obesity.

- Excluding children affected by morbidities that affect growth like repeated bouts of infectious diarrhea and Crohn's disease
- Using an international sample of children
- Using skin-fold thickness for assessing tissue growth and childhood obesity
- Using growth velocity standards
- Measuring universal motor development milestones like sitting without support, hands-and-knees crawling, standing with assistance, walking with assistance, standing alone, and walking alone.

### *Growth Chart*

Also called as the "road to health" chart, these were initially developed by David Morley in Nigeria and are now used universally for growth monitoring. The growth chart is a plot of age on the X-axis from birth to 5 years and weight on the Y-axis from 0 to 22 kg. The X-axis is divided into five blocks representing a year—each is further divided into 12 months by vertical lines. Similarly, the weight on Y-axis is divided into 500 g units by thick horizontal lines and 100 g units by thin horizontal lines. There are three color coded zones—(1) green representing normal, (2) yellow representing moderately underweight (–2SD to –3SD) and (3) red (below –3SD). It is included in the postnatal care section of the Mother and Child Protection card for early identification of growth faltering and undernutrition. The steps in using the growth chart include:

- Correct determination of age calculated from date of birth.
- Correct determination of weight using standard calibrated weighing scale.
- Selecting the correct gender and age appropriate chart and plotting the weight-for-age accurately on it. Join the previous point with the current plotted point.
- Interpreting the direction of the growth curve and recognizing inadequate growth if any.
- Inform and educate the parents about the growth assessment and follow-up action as needed.

The Weight-for-Age Growth charts are integrated with the Mother and Child Protection card. *Anganwadi* worker, with the support of ASHA and ANMs are primarily involved with community-based monitoring of growth and development through the *Anganwadi* centers. All infants below 6 months of age are followed at monthly intervals and thereafter at 3 monthly intervals **(Figs. 26.9A and B)**.

**Monitoring development:** The early years of life are critical because this is the time when the brain develops, have a high capacity for change, and the foundation is laid for health and well-being throughout life. And therefore, proper monitoring of this development is essential. In fact, 43% of children in low- and middle-income countries are unable to realize their full development potential.

A *"comprehensive development assessment"* involves a detailed evaluation by a trained pediatric psychologist using standardized tools like the Bayley Scale for Infant Development. *"Development screening"* on the other hand involves search for developmental delay in otherwise asymptomatic population followed by a more comprehensive diagnostic assessment. In India, the RBSK aims at screening for developmental delays in 0–18 years population.

Development assessment is classically done across four domains although there is considerable overlap. These are:
1. *Gross motor:* Neck and body control, sitting, standing, walking, and running
2. *Fine motor and vision:* Coordinated action of fingers such as pincer grasp, dressing, writing, playing instrument, and visual development
3. *Speech, language, and hearing:* Both verbal and nonverbal communication skills, hearing development.
4. *Social behavior and play:* Feeding, toileting, and social interactions.

A screening tool as compared to a comprehensive assessment tool, should be brief, simple and usable by laypersons with short training. There are more than 20 screening tools available for development screening across various countries. However, none are suitable to be used globally across different population like the growth chart. The most well-known and widely used methods are the Bayley Infant Neurodevelopment Screen (BINS), Denver Developmental Material II, British Ability Scales, Stanford Binet Intelligence Scale, Ages and Stages Questionnaire (ASQ). However, these are developed for western population and may not be directly applicable to the Indian children due to sociocultural differences.

A summary of various development screening scales that have been used in Indian settings are presented in **Table 26.3**.

**Table 26.3:** Screening tools which can be used for screening of developmental delay in community settings by frontline workers.

| Sr. no. | Name of screening tool | Length | Type of screening | Age group | Validity |
|---|---|---|---|---|---|
| 1. | Baroda development screening test for infants | 54 items | Child testing and parent interview | 0–30 months | Sensitivity 65–93% and specificity 77.37–94.44% |
| 2. | The Trivandrum Developmental Screening Chart | 17 items | Child testing and parent interview | 0–2 years | Sensitivity 66.8% and specificity 78.8% |
| 3. | ICMR psychosocial developmental screening test battery | 66 items | Child testing | 0–6 years | NA |
| 4. | 10 questions screening instrument | 10 questions | Parent report | 2–9 years (modified TQSI for 0–2 years) | Sensitivity and specificity >80% |
| 5. | Lucknow development screen | 27 questions | Parent report | 0–2 years | Sensitivity 95.9% and specificity 73.1% |
| 6. | Ages and stages questionnaire | 30 per questionnaire (21 different questionnaires at various ages) | Parent report | 0–60 months | Sensitivity 83.3% and specificity 75.4% |

## Childhood Immunization

Vaccines stimulate the body's own immune system to protect the person against subsequent infection or disease. Immunization is a proven tool for controlling and eliminating life-threatening infectious diseases and is estimated to avert between 2 and 3 million deaths each year. It is one of the most cost-effective health investments, with proven strategies that make it accessible to even the most hard-to-reach and vulnerable populations. It has clearly defined target groups; it can be delivered effectively through outreach activities; and vaccination does not require any major lifestyle change.

The Universal Immunization Program in India is currently providing vaccine against the following vaccine preventable diseases:
- Severe form of childhood tuberculosis
- Hepatitis
- Polio
- Diphtheria
- Pertussis
- Tetanus
- *Haemophilus influenzae* type b
- Rotavirus
- Measles
- Pneumococcal pneumonia
- Rubella
- Japanese encephalitis

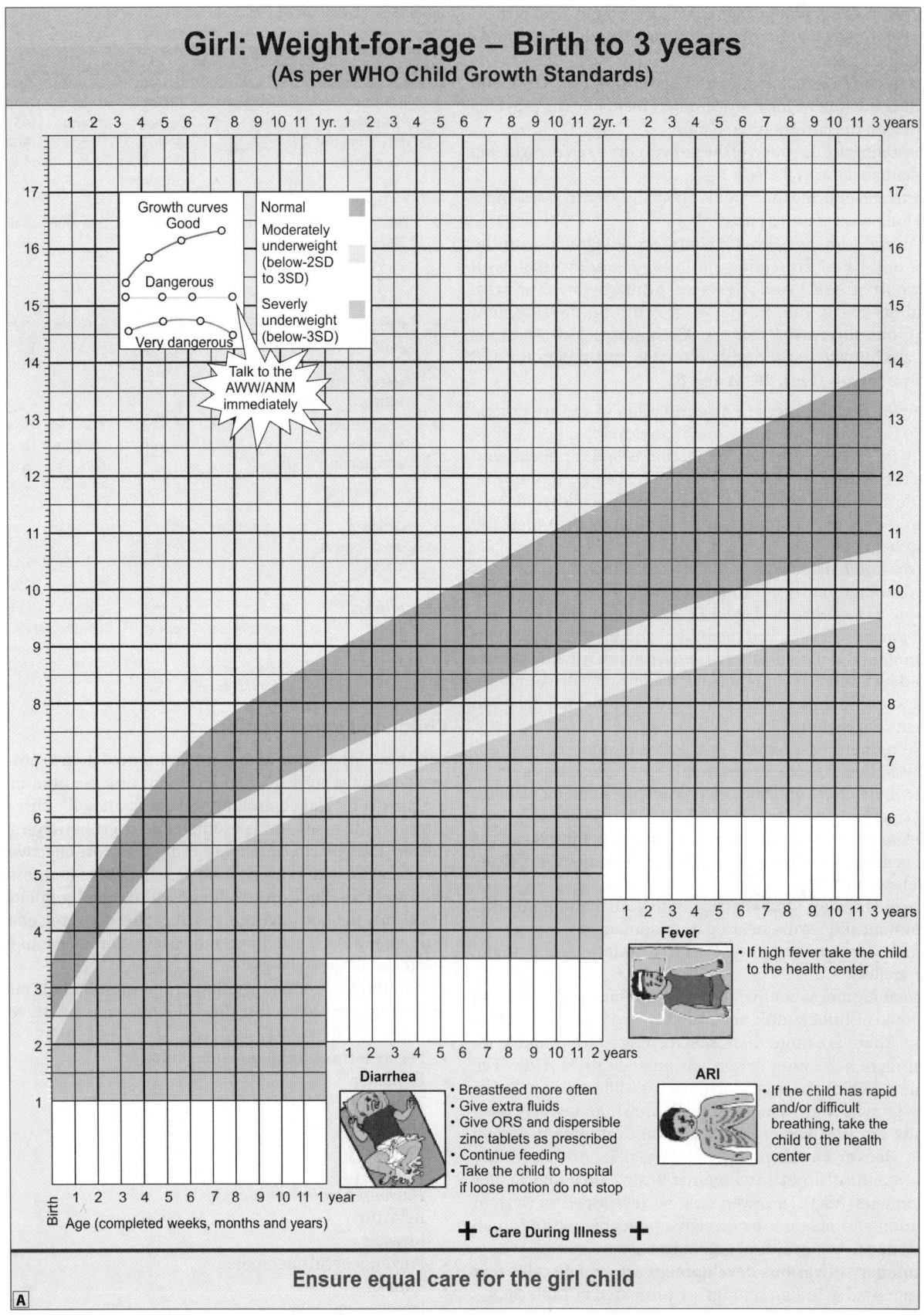

Fig. 26.9A

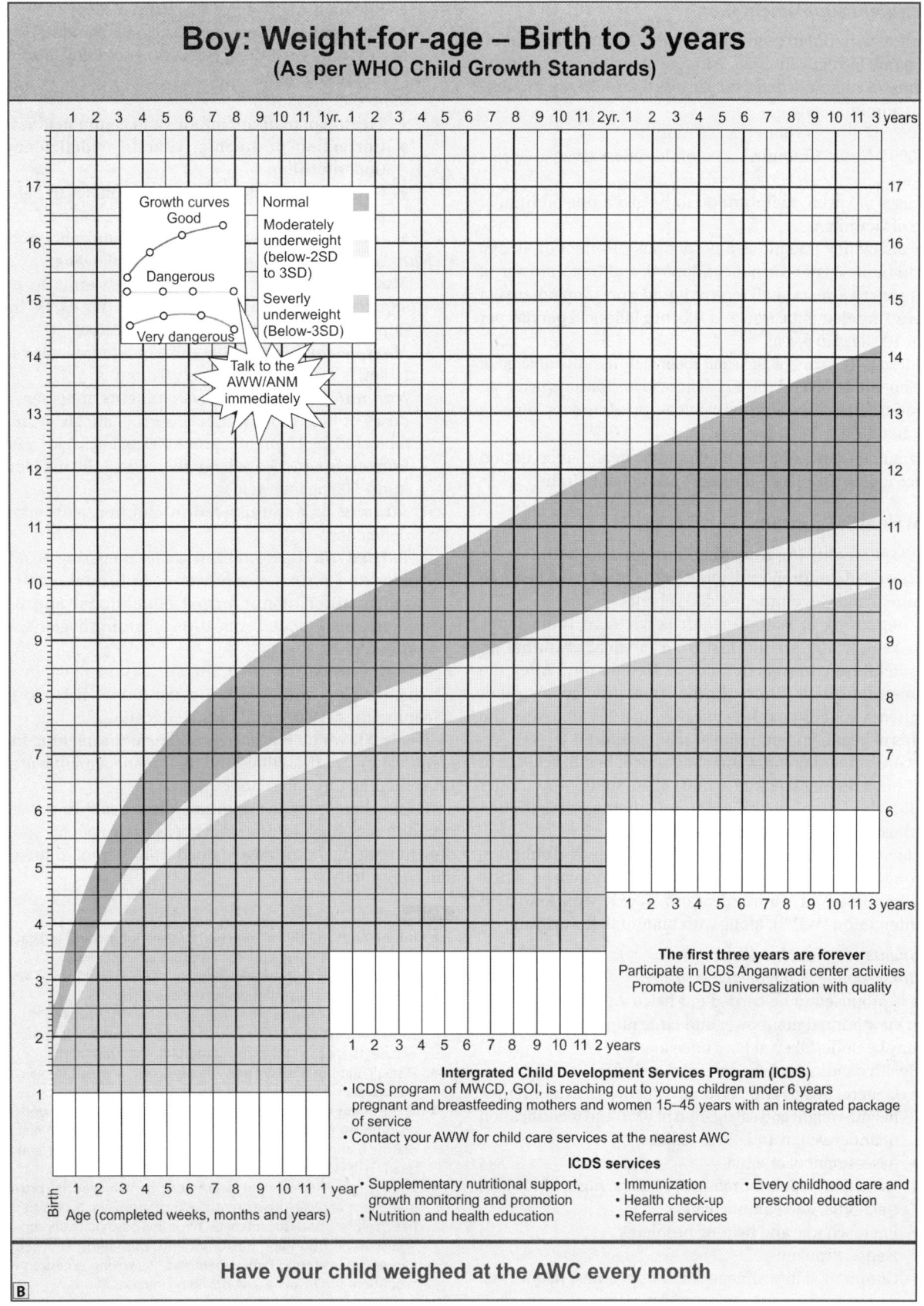

**Fig. 26.9B**

**Figs. 26.9A and B:** Growth chart. (*For color version, see Plates 2 and 3*)

### Micronutrient Supplementation

Currently, vitamin A, iron and folic acid (IFA) supplementation programs are in vogue in India. With the objective to reduce the prevalence of vitamin A deficiency to less than 0.5%, the strategy includes administering:

- 100,000 IU dose of vitamin A at 9 months
- 200,000 IU (after 9 months) at 6 monthly intervals up to 5 years of age
- All cases of severe malnutrition to be given one additional dose of vitamin A.

Iron deficiency anemia is a pernicious problem of all age groups in India. As per the policy adopted, children from age of 6 months up to 5 years shall receive liquid iron supplements in doses of 20 mg elemental iron and 100 mcg folic acid per day per child for 100 days in a year.

Children 6–10 years of age shall receive iron in the dosage of 30 mg elemental iron and 250 mcg folic acid for 100 days in a year.

Children above this age group would receive iron supplements in the adult dose.

Iodization of salt is another major public health intervention to reduce iodine deficiency disorders prevailing in India.

## School Health Program

The School Health Program was launched to address the health needs of children and adolescents aged 6–18 years in Government and Government-aided schools.

The beginning of school health services in India dates back to 1909, when for the first time medical examination of schoolchildren was carried out in Baroda city. After the recommendation of Bhore Committee, the government constituted a school health committee in 1960 to assess the standards of health and nutrition of schoolchildren.

The Government of India launched school health scheme in 1996–97 but it did not fare well in most of the states. Now, under the NHM, the school health program is being strengthened within the context of RMNCH+A program.

The focus is on physical and mental health needs of children, nutritional interventions, promotion of physical activity, counseling, fixed-day immunization, weekly iron folic acid supplementation (WIFS), along with biannual deworming.

### Components of school health program:

- *Health screening and remedial measures*:
  - It is proposed to be carried out twice a year, but keeping in view limited manpower and large number of students, may be undertaken at least once a year.
  - Health conditions to be screened include:
    - General health and personal hygiene, measurement of height, weight and calculation of BMI, and identification of underweight and obese children.
    - Assessment of anemia
    - Eye examination for refractory errors, night blindness, trachoma, and conjunctivitis
    - Ear discharge and hearing problems
    - Dental problems
    - Common skin problems such as scabies, pyoderma, and lice
    - Rheumatic and congenital heart disease
    - Disabilities—visual, hearing, and locomotor
    - Learning disorders, behavior problems, and mental health problems.
  - Remedial measures:
    - Treatment of minor injuries and common illnesses
    - Correction of anemia, vitamin A deficiency, and undernutrition
    - Counseling for children with disabilities or behavioral problems
    - Immunization as per National Immunization Schedule.
- *Nutritional interventions*—include the following:
  - **Mid-day meal (MDM) program:** It aims to provide supplementary nutrition to children. The MDM has also improved school enrolment and retention.
  - **Mass deworming:** Single dose of albendazole (400 mg tablet) is recommended every 6 months.
  - **Iron and folic acid tablets:** Students are given weekly doses of IFA. Those from class 1 to 5 are given small IFA tablet (45 mg elemental iron + 400 µg folic acid) and those from class 6 to 12 are large IFA tablet (100 mg elemental iron + 500 µg folic acid)
  - **Vitamin A:** Administered in children with vitamin A deficiency
  - **Iodized salt:** Using iodized salt for preparing MDMs.
- *Health and nutrition education:* In formal curriculum-based manner or nonformal educational approaches, students are provided education regarding hygiene, health, and nutrition.
- *Safe and supportive environment:* To ensure environment, which is safe from injuries, clean toilets, first aid rooms, counseling services, and health education.

The RBSK which envisages child health screening for early identification of disabilities and their management will also be implemented through schools.

Thus, schools play an important role in health and well-being of children. Schoolchildren also act as agents of change as they disseminate the knowledge gained from school to their home and community.

> **Note**
> - Infant and childhood mortality is an important indicator of socioeconomic development of a country.
> - The mortality is high among countries of Africa and South-East Asia.
> - There are wide disparities within the countries.
> - Children belonging to rural areas, households with poor socioeconomic status, marginalized social groups, and low education of parents are at a higher risk of morbidity and mortality.
> - A small number of easily preventable conditions lead to majority of the deaths.
> - The leading causes of morbidity and mortality among under-five children are preterm birth and/or LBW, acute respiratory infections, diarrhea, and congenital anomalies. Neonatal deaths account for nearly half (46%) of the under-five deaths.
> - Ending preventable child deaths can be achieved by providing immediate and exclusive breastfeeding, improving access to skilled health professionals for antenatal, birth, and postnatal care, improving access to nutrition and micronutrients, promoting knowledge of danger signs among family members, improving access to water, sanitation, and hygiene, and providing immunizations.

## SUGGESTED READING

1. Child Health - Governnment of India [Internet]. NHM Components: RMNCH+A. [online] Available from: http://nhm.gov.in/nrhm-components/rmnch-a/child-health-immunization.html.
2. Development Initiatives. (2018). 2018 Global Nutrition Report: Shining a light to spur action on nutrition. Bristol, UK: Development Initiatives.
3. Gera T, Shah D, Garner P, Richardson M, Sachdev HS. Integrated management of childhood illness (IMCI) strategy for children under five. Cochrane Database Syst Rev. 2016;(6):CD010123.
4. Hack M, Klein NK, Taylor HG. Long-term developmental outcomes of low birth weight infants. Future Child. 1995;5:176-96.
5. International Institute for Population Sciences (IIPS) and ICF. National Family Health Survey (NFHS-4), 2015-16. India, Mumbai: IIPS. 2017.
6. Ministry of Health and Family Welfare, Government of India. HOME BASED NEWBORN CARE—Operational Guidelines (revised 2014).
7. Ministry of Health and Family Welfare, Government of India. Facility Based Newborn Care: Operational Guidelines For Planning and Implementation.
8. Ministry of Home Affairs. Registrar General of India. Census 2011. [online] Available from: www.censusindia.net.
9. National Health Mission. Rashtriya Bal Swasthya Karyakram (RBSK) New Delhi. [online] Available from: http://nhm.gov.in/images/pdf/programmes/RBSK/For_more_information.pdf.
10. National Health Portal. Congenital Anamolies (Birth Defects). [online] Available from: https://www.nhp.gov.in/disease/gynaecology-and-obstetrics/congenital-anomalies-birth-defects.
11. NIMS, ICMR, and UNICEF. Infant and Child Mortality in India: Levels, Trends and Determinants. New Delhi: National Institute of Medical Sciences (NIMS), Indian Council of Medical Research (ICMR), and UNICEF India Country Office; 2012.
12. Sachs M, Dykes F, Carter B. Feeding by numbers: an ethnographic study of how breastfeeding women understand their babies' weight charts. Int Breastfeed J. 2006;1(1):29.
13. Sharma R. Birth defects in India: Hidden truth, need for urgent attention. Indian J Hum Genet. 2013;19(2):125-9.
14. Soubeiga D, Gauvin L, Hatem MA, Johri M. Birth Preparedness and Complication Readiness (BPCR) interventions to reduce maternal and neonatal mortality in developing countries: Systematic review and meta-analysis. BMC Pregnancy Childbirth. 2014;14(1):129.
15. United Nations Children's Fund (UNICEF). Levels and trends in childhood mortality: Report 2019– Estimates developed by the UN Inter-agency Group for Child Mortality Estimation (UNIGME).
16. United Nations Children's Fund (UNICEF). The state of the world's children. 2016: A fair chance for every child.
17. United Nations Children's Fund (UNICEF): Global database. Monitoring the Situation of Children and Women. 2014. Low birthweight.
18. World Health Organization. Global Health Observatory data. Trends in childhood mortality. 2016. [online] Available from: www.who.int/gho/child_health/en.
19. World Health Organization. International statistical classification of diseases and related health problems, Tenth revision, Second edition. Geneva: World Health Organization; 2004.
20. World Health Organization. Management of birth defects and haemoglobin disorders: Report of a Joint WHO-March of Dimes meeting. Geneva, Switzerland: WHO; 2006.
21. World Health Organization. Strategic directions for improving the health and development of children and adolescents. Geneva: WHO; 2002.
22. World Health Organization. World Report on Disability. 2011. [online] Available from: http://www.unicef.org/protection/ World_ report_on_ disability_eng.pdf.
23. World Health Organization/The United Nations Children's Fund (UNICEF). Ending preventable deaths: Global Action Plan for Prevention and Control of Pneumonia and Diarrhoea; 2013.

# CHAPTER 27

# Adolescent Health

*Shaili Vyas, Deepshikha, Rakesh Kakkar*

*"Adolescence is the period of development from childhood to adulthood."*

> **CM 10.8** Describe the physiology, clinical management and principles of Adolescent including ARSH

## INTRODUCTION

Adolescents or, more generally, young people represent an important segment of society; particularly in developing countries, where they are the bulk of the population. They form the majority in terms of size, and also as the reservoir for future leaders, and are the promise of a better life for the community.

By definition, the term, "adolescence", is applied to the age group, usually between 10 and 19 years, in which children undergo rapid changes in body size, physiological, and psychological and social functioning. This is the result of surging hormones and social expectations designed to foster the transition from childhood to adulthood. True to the literal meaning of the term (the Greek word, *adolescere* denotes "to grow and to mature"), the sentinel occurrence during the period of adolescence is, "rapid growth", not just physical and biological (sexual) but also emotional, cognitive, psychological, and social. This phase of life is full of opportunities and healthy adolescents are a great asset for contributing to national development. However, adolescents are also exposed to risks and vulnerabilities at the same time.

There are 1.3 billion adolescents in the world today, more than ever before, making up 16% of the world's population (UNICEF, April 2022)

Adolescence is generally perceived to be a healthy period of life because mortality is relatively low in this age group. This is, however, deceptive, since adolescents face many challenges in their life and several of these challenges relate to their health. These health challenges are, of course, different from what they faced when they were younger.

> **Note**
> Adolescence means "to emerge" to achieve "identity". Adolescent age group is 10–19 years.

## ADOLESCENTS PROFILE IN INDIA

According to the WHO, adolescents are those persons who are in the age group of 10–19 years, "youth" who are from 15–24 years and "young people" are from 10–24 years. Adolescents (10–19 years) constitute about one-fourth (21.4% or 243 million) of India's population and young people (10–24 years) about one-third (or 350 million) of the population. This represents a huge opportunity that can transform the social and economic fortunes of the country (Strategy Handbook, RKSK, Adolescent Health Division MoHFW, 2014).

Adolescents are not a homogeneous population. They exist in a variety of circumstances and have diverse needs. The transition from childhood to adulthood involves dramatic physical, sexual, psychological and social developmental changes, all taking place at the same time. In addition to opportunities for development this transition poses risks to their health and well-being.

> **Note**
> - Adolescents comprise around *21.4%* of the total population which means every *fifth* person in India is an adolescent.
> - There are *243 million* adolescents comprising nearly one-fifth of the total population.
> - *India has the largest adolescent population in the world.*
> - On the basis of different needs, adolescence has been divided into two phases: (1) "early" (10–14 years) and (2) "late" (15–19 years).

## ADOLESCENTS AND THEIR NEEDS FOR HEALTH SERVICES

Adolescence is an important phase in life as it gives a second chance to improve the health and well-being of a child in their second decade as well as an opportunity to alleviate emergence of risk factors that may lead to diseases in adulthood. The health status of adolescents reflects on the health and well-being of the next generation. Although adolescence is considered to be a healthy phase, more than 33% of the disease burden and almost 60% of premature deaths among adults can be associated with behaviors or conditions that begin or occur during adolescence for example, tobacco and alcohol use, poor eating habits, sexual abuse, and unsafe sex.

They pose different challenges for the healthcare system than children and adults, due to their rapidly evolving physical, intellectual, and emotional development.

The special characteristics that demarcate adolescence are as follows:
- Rapid physical growth and development
- Physical, mental and psychosocial maturity (may be at different times)
- Sexual development and maturity with start of sexual activity
- Inquisitive and experimenting behavior
- Transition from dependent to independent phase
- Search for adult identity.

# GROWTH AND DEVELOPMENT

Prompt and considerable physical growth and development demarcate adolescence, including sexual development. Beginning of biological growth and development during adolescence is signified by the onset of puberty, which is often defined as the physical transformation of a child into an adult. A myriad of biological changes occurs during puberty including sexual maturation, increases in height and weight, completion of skeletal growth accompanied by a marked increase in skeletal mass, and changes in body composition.

## Emotional Development

Emotion is derived from Latin word *emover* meaning "stir up".

Adolescents have to withstand, not only with their physical alterations, but also with associated emotional changes. Changes in physical appearance leads to emotional stress, strain, abrupt and rapid mood swings. Getting emotionally disturbed by apparently unimportant and trivial matters is a common feature of this period. Hormonal changes results in restlessness, irritability, anger, sex, and stress. It becomes almost necessary for adolescents to learn how to face and deal patiently with the turbulence they face and requires development of a sense of balance and self-imposition of limits on expression of one's needs and desires. This phase also leads to development of abstract thinking enabling them to think and evaluate systematically and detect and interrogate deviation. People around them often neglect this deviation in behavior because of "generation gap".

- Emotion can be positive or negative, constructive or destructive
- Searching for identity, influenced by gender, peer group, cultural background, and family expectations, which includes self-concept and self-esteem
- Seeking more independence
- Seeking more responsibility, both at home and at school
- Looking for new experiences. May engage in more risk-taking behavior
- Thinking more about "right" and "wrong"
- Influenced more by friends' behavior—sense of self and self-esteem
- Starting to develop and explore a sexual identity
- *Communicating in different ways*: Communication with peers through internet, mobile phones, and social media.

**Daniel Goleman dimensions of emotional intelligence are:**
- Self-awareness
- Self-regulation
- Motivation
- Empathy
- Social skills

# HEALTH ISSUES OF ADOLESCENCE

Key health issues of adolescence are discussed in Table 27.1.

**Note**
- Estimated over 3,000 per day, i.e., 1.2 million adolescents died in 2015, mostly from preventable or treatable causes.
- Road traffic injuries were the leading cause of death in 2015. Other major causes of adolescent deaths include lower respiratory infections, suicide, diarrheal diseases, and drowning.
- Globally, there are 44 births per 1,000 girls aged 15–19 per year.
- Half of all mental health disorders in adulthood start by age 14, but most cases are undetected and untreated.

## Early Marriage, Pregnancy, and Childbirth

*Globally, this is the leading cause of mortality for 15–19 years females.*

NFHS-5 data shows that 15% of the girls and 1.5% of boys were married at the age of 15–19 years and 6.8% of the girls already have a child. Out of total pregnancies about 16–19% are teenage pregnancies. The risk of maternal death is about three times higher in girls of 15–19 years age group and five times higher in those younger than 15 years compared to women in their 20s, which is mainly due to unsafe abortion and postpartum hemorrhage.

One of the specific targets of the health Sustainable Development Goal (SDG 3) is that by 2030, the world should ensure universal access to sexual and reproductive healthcare services, including for family planning, information and education, and the integration of reproductive health into national strategies and programs. Better access to contraceptive information and services can reduce the number of teenage pregnancies. Laws that specify a minimum age of marriage at 18 and which are enforced can help.

**Table 27.1:** Health issues of adolescence.

| Communicable diseases | Noncommunicable diseases | Accidents/injuries | Addictions | Psychosocial problems |
|---|---|---|---|---|
| • HIV<br>• STIs/STDs<br>• Tuberculosis<br>• Hepatitis<br>• Respiratory infections<br>• Other infections | • Mental disorders such as depression, suicide, homicide<br>• Malnutrition/undernutrition<br>• Obesity<br>• Menstrual disorder | • Violence<br>• Injuries both unintentional and self-injury<br>• RTA | • Drug use/abuse<br>• Smoking/nicotine use/tobacco use<br>• Alcohol use | • Trafficking and prostitution<br>• Teen and unintended pregnancies<br>• Illegal abortions<br>• Homelessness<br>• Academic problems and dropping out of school<br>• Eating disorders |

## Sexually Transmitted Infections (STIs), Including Human Immunodeficiency Virus (HIV)

Initiation of sexual activity while they lack adequate knowledge and skills for protection places adolescents at a higher risk of unwanted pregnancy, unsafe abortion and STIs including HIV/AIDS. In 2019, about 1.7 million adolescents between the ages of 10 and 19 were living with HIV worldwide (Adolescent HIV UNICEF Data, 2019).

One of the specific targets of the health SDG 3 is that by 2030 there should be an end to the epidemics of AIDS, tuberculosis, malaria and neglected tropical diseases, hepatitis, water-borne diseases and other communicable diseases. Young people need to know how to protect themselves and must have the access to means. This includes being able to obtain condoms to prevent sexual transmission of the virus and clean needles and syringes for those who inject drugs. Better access to HIV testing and counseling, and stronger subsequent links to HIV treatment services for those who test HIV positive.

## Communicable Diseases

Improved vaccination services, hygienic conditions, sanitation, safe water, and health promotion activities worldwide showed marked reduction in adolescent deaths and disability from preventable causes.

## Mental Health

Prevalence of mental disorder is rising day-by-day. The third leading cause of morbidity and disability among adolescents is depression, while suicide is the third leading cause of mortality among adolescents aged 15–19 years.

Adolescents are facing increased risk of developing mental health problems due to violence, humiliation, poverty, and feeling devalued. Good mental health can be promoted by building life skills and providing psychosocial support in schools and other community settings.

## Tobacco, Alcohol, and Drugs

Tobacco, alcohol, and substance abuse are current serious issues concerned with adolescents as they are ignorant about its long-term effects.

Harmful use of tobacco, alcohol, and drugs among adolescents is a major concern in many countries. It reduces self-control and increases risky behaviors, such as violence, unsafe sex or dangerous driving. It is a primary cause of injuries and premature deaths. It can also lead to health problems in later life and affect life expectancy.

Setting a minimum age for buying and consuming tobacco and alcohol are among the strategies for reducing their use.

Drug abuse among 15–19-year-old adolescent is also an important global concern. Drug control may focus on reducing drug demand, drug supply, or both, and successful programs usually include structural, community, and individual-level interventions.

## Injuries

Unintentional injuries are the leading cause of death and disability among adolescents. In 2015, over 115,000 adolescents died as a result of road traffic accidents. Young drivers need advice on driving safely and laws prohibiting driving under the influence of alcohol and drugs need to be strictly enforced. Drowning is also a major cause of death among adolescents—57,000 adolescents are estimated to have drowned in 2015, out of two-thirds were boys, and an essential intervention to prevent these deaths is teaching children and adolescents to swim (WHO, Adolescents: health, risk and solutions, 2018).

## Nutritional Problems

Nutritional requirement are higher in adolescence phase than any other phase of life. Inadequate dietary intake at this phase leads to hindered growth and delayed sexual maturation.

Many adolescents in developing countries enter this phase as undernourished, making them more vulnerable to disease and early death. At the other terminus of the spectrum, the number of adolescents who are overweight or obese is incrementing in low, middle and high-income countries.

Propensities such as counting calories, dieting and exercising inspired by celebrity cannot be taken as a positive impact, often they do it in an incorrect way which may lead to complications. Instead of taking balanced diet they starve and end up in anorexia nervosa. These issues can be reduced by routine screening and nutritional education.

Iron deficiency anemia is the leading cause of years lost to death and disability in 2015. Iron and folic acid supplements are a solution that additionally avails to promote health afore adolescents become parents.

Customary deworming in areas where intestinal helminths such as hookworm are prevalent is recommended to avert micronutrient (including iron) deficiencies.

### Nutritional Anemia

The need for iron increases with rapid growth, expansion of blood volume and muscle mass. As boys gain lean body mass at a faster rate than girls, they require more iron than girls. Iron deficiency in diet leads to nutritional anemia (**Figs. 27.1 and 27.2**).

### Prevention of Nutritional Anemia

- **Health promotion:**
  - Adequate nutrition
  - Nutritional education to improve dietary habits
  - Breastfeeding and appropriate and timely weaning
  - Iron rich diet

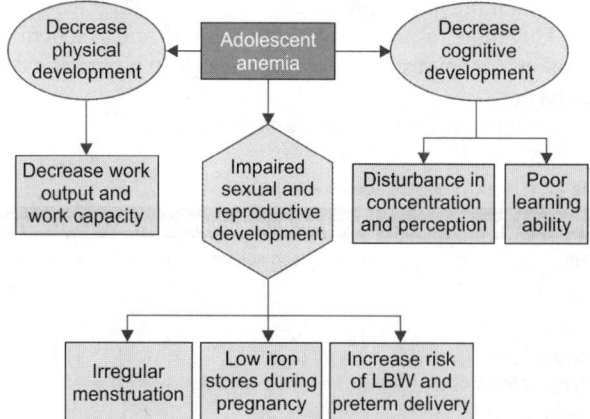

**Fig. 27.1:** Effects of anemia.

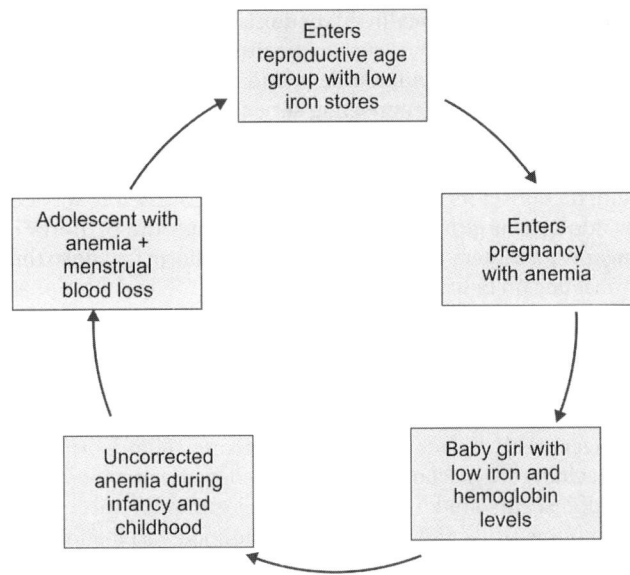

**Fig. 27.2:** Vicious cycle of anemia.

- Increase enhancers of iron absorption in daily diet (e.g., vitamin C)
- Health education
- Periodic deworming during childhood and pregnancy
- Footwear use
- Safe drinking water
- **Specific protection:**
  - Food fortification
  - National nutritional anemia prophylaxis program (NNAPP)
  - Deworming
  - National nutritional anemia control program (NNACP)
- **Treatment of iron deficiency anemia (IDA):**
  - Oral iron therapy
  - Parenteral iron therapy

| Age group | Intervention/dose | Regime | Service delivery |
|---|---|---|---|
| 10–19 years | 100 mg elemental iron and 500 µg of folic acid | Weekly throughout the period 10–19 years of age and biannual deworming | In school through teachers and for those out-of-school through AWC mobilization by ASHA |

## Addiction in Adolescent

### Causes

*Adolescents are more vulnerable to addiction because of:*
- Lack of knowledge about the dangers of consuming addictive substances
- Peer influence and pressure to try something new
- They are highly influenced by their friends and try to mimic their behaviors like experiment with cigarettes, alcohol, and other harmful substances. Hence, parents should always be aware of their children's peer group.
- They think that substance use can help overcome boredom, depression, stress, and fatigue. Also, media images that glamorize these products may also mislead them.
- They may feel under pressure to perform beyond their capacity in academics, sports or winning over friends and under the false impression that drugs may help them, which leads them to fall into the vicious cycle of substance abuse.
- They do what they see, means if an elder in their family indulges in substance abuse, they are more likely to start the same.
- On the other hand, easy availability of these substances, community norms, and adverse family situations may push them into addictions.
- Managing peer pressure by being aware of the ill effects of drug abuse and developing skills to overcome peer pressure. Also persuade the peers not to engage in unhealthy and risky behaviors.
- Empowered with adequate information and skills, they should be able to decide what is good for their body, their life and hence, they should be taking well-informed and responsible decisions.
- As unhealthy habits and risky behaviors are formed during early adolescence, so preventive measures should be focused at this age by imparting health education and health promotion activities.

## ADOLSCENT REPRODUCTIVE AND SEXUAL HEALTH

Health care needs for reproductive health exists throughout the reproductive years (15–45 years) and therefore access and availability to these services is required in all the phases of life starting from the adolescence phase. Reproductive health services include provision of contraceptives, safe abortion services, diagnosis and management of RTI/STI, including HIV, etc.

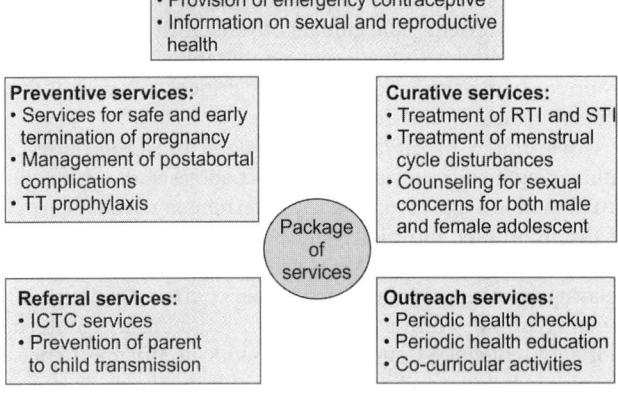

### Menstrual Hygiene

In India, menstrual practices are still clouded by taboos and sociocultural restrictions for adolescent girls and women. Various evidence suggests that besides having limited access to products of sanitary hygiene, and lack of safe sanitary facilities (which includes sanitary napkins, toilets in schools, availability of water, privacy and safe disposal) which could restrict school attendance leading to unachievable SDG target 4. Secondly, it would also contribute to local infections, i.e., PID during this period leading to infertility and nonattainment of motherhood, a highly crucial phase in a women's life.

The Ministry of Health and Family Welfare (MoHFW) has launched a scheme as part of the adolescent reproductive and sexual health (ARSH) component under RCH II for promotion of menstrual hygiene among adolescent girls. The scheme aims at ensuring that adolescent girls have adequate knowledge and information about menstrual hygiene and the use of sanitary napkins, so that high quality, safe products are made available to them, and environmentally safe disposal mechanisms are readily accessible. Initially the scheme was implemented in certain selected states/districts where a pack of 6 sanitary napkins was provided under the brand name "Freedays".

These napkins are sold at ₹ 6/- for 6 sanitary napkins by ASHA through door-to-door sale and by also utilizing the platform of schools and *Anganwadi* centers. Out of the sale, ASHA gets an incentive of ₹ 1 besides getting a free packet of sanitary napkins per month.

Menstrual Hygiene Day is yet another initiative by WHO and UNICEF and is celebrated every year on 28th May so as to create awareness and gain confidence to manage menstruation with safety and dignity using safe hygienic material, secondly to have adequate water and space for washing and bathing and thirdly to dispose of sanitary products with privacy. Ready for RED is yet an innovative e-learning platform about menstruation and menstrual hygiene products for teenagers aged 11–16 years.

## HEALTH EDUCATION AND COUNSELING

### Background

According to 2011 census data, there are 253 million adolescents in the age group 10–19 years, which comprise little more than one-fifth of India's total population. This age group comprises of individuals in a transient phase of life requiring nutrition, education, counseling and guidance to ensure their development into healthy adults. Considering demographic potential of this group for high economic growth, it is critical to invest in their education, health, and development.

Government of India has recognized the importance of influencing health-seeking behavior of adolescents. The health situation of this age group is a key determinant of India's overall health, mortality, morbidity and population growth scenario. Therefore, investments in ARSH will yield dividends in terms of delaying age at marriage, reducing incidence of teenage pregnancy, meeting unmet contraception need, reducing the maternal mortality, reducing STI incidence and reducing HIV prevalence. It will also help India realize its demographic dividends, as healthy adolescents are an important resource for the economy.

### Need for Health Education and Counseling

As most of the adolescents are shy in nature, they hardly disclose their doubts or confusion due to lack of trust, privacy, etc. They often fear exploitation, discrimination on the basis of age, sex, rural/urban, school/non-school going, etc. Most of the time they are reluctant in seeking help from others. Also, there is lack of knowledge as in from where to seek help regarding their physical/physiological and emotional needs.

Counseling is a process which empowers one to analyze a particular problem and to find out the best possible option to solve it. Adolescent health education and counseling is being provided at adolescent friendly health clinics (AFHC), at all levels of care on stipulated days and time with due referral linkages. Adolescent counseling services on important health issues as nutrition, puberty, RTI/STI prevention, contraception, delayed marriage and child bearing are being provided through trained counselors. Health education and counseling services for adolescent girls is also provided through the platform of Anganwadi centers. Schools also acts as a platform for adolescent counseling on behavior risk modification.

## IMMUNIZATION IN ADOLESCENTS

Vaccine coverage in adolescents in general is inadequate as they have less contact with the physicians as compared to younger children, lack access to health care, and opportunities to vaccinate are most of the times missed by the provider.

Adolescents are an important target group for vaccination as immune protection provided by childhood vaccination may not provide adequate protection to this group as the effect of vaccination gradually wanes off. The initial vaccination in childhood maybe given in inadequate doses. Thirdly, it provides recent vaccines available for immunization. Certain risk groups also demand vaccination, as adolescence is a time for exploration and experimentation, adolescents engage in high-risk activities which increases their risk for various infectious diseases, such as hepatitis B and human papillomavirus (HPV). Three important infections: (1) *Neisseria meningitidis*, (2) pertussis, and (3) HPV, for which effective vaccination now is available, are especially prevalent in the adolescent years, making the adolescent age group the ideal target age for prevention.

*Adolescent vaccinations are of two types:*

| Routine | Catchup |
|---|---|
| • HPV<br>• Tdap (Tetanus, Diphtheria and Pertussis)<br>• Influenza | • Hepatitis A<br>• Hepatitis B<br>• Varicella<br>• Japanese encephalitis<br>• Measles, mumps and rubella<br>• Typhoid |

### Vaccination Schedule for Adolescents

| Vaccine | Recommended age of vaccination |
|---|---|
| Tdap/Td | • Tdap is always preferred over Td at the age of 10 years followed by repeat Td every 10 years only when an adolescent immunized earlier with three doses of DPT below 1 year and booster at the age of 1.5 years and at 5 years |
| MMR | • One dose at 12–13 years of age, if not received earlier |
| Rubella | • One dose to girls at 12–13 years of age, of MMR or rubella if not given earlier |
| Hepatitis B | • Three doses 0-1-6 months, if not received earlier |
| Hepatitis A | • Two doses 0-6 months, if not received earlier |
| Typhoid | • Single dose intramuscular Vi polysaccharide or three doses of oral typhoid vaccine on alternate day empty stomach. Booster is given every 3 years |
| Varicella | • 1 dose up to 2–12 years and two doses after 12 years of age |

| Vaccine | Recommended age of vaccination |
|---|---|
| JE vaccine | • The recommended age for Japanese encephalitis (JE) vaccination if raised to 18 years in endemic regions |
| HPV | • Only two doses of either of the two HPV vaccines for adolescent/preadolescent girls aged 9–14 years<br>• For girls 15 years and older, and immunocompromised individuals 3 doses are recommended<br>• For two-dose schedule, the minimum interval between doses should be 6 months.<br>• For three-dose schedule, the doses can be administered at 0, 1–2 (depending on brand) and 6 months |

## ADOLESCENT FRIENDLY HEALTH SERVICES

*Adolescents fail to access health services because of the following key factors*:
- Lack of information about availability of services and means to access it.
- Social and cultural restrains
- Lack of need of adolescent health as assessed by the parents as physically they appear to be healthy
- Lack of trust on the health system
- Lack of privacy or confidentiality
- Inaccessible services, i.e., either too far way or too expensive
- Unfriendly noncooperative staff.

With this background in mind, MoHFW has launched AFHC across the country. The aim is to provide clinical and counseling services to adolescents by modifying the existing health system.

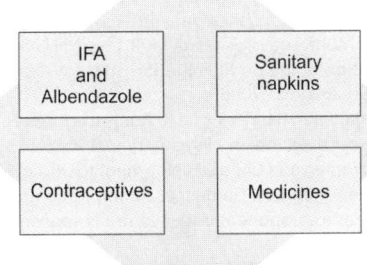

## Commodities Available at AFHC

*Services available at AFHC*:

| Curative services | Counseling services |
|---|---|
| **Treatment of:**<br>• Severe malnutrition<br>• RTI/STI problems<br>• Menstrual disorders<br>• Sexual concerns of males and female<br>• Management of depression<br>• Noncommunicable diseases and other common ailment<br>• Injuries related to accidents and violence<br>• Management of substance misuse<br>• Treatment of noncommunicable diseases such as hypertension, stroke, cardiovascular diseases, and diabetes | **Counseling on:**<br>• Nutrition<br>• Menstrual disorders<br>• Personal hygiene, menstrual hygiene, use of sanitary napkins<br>• Use of contraceptives, sexual concerns, sexual abuse<br>• Gender violence, depression<br>• Substance misuse/abuse<br>• Promoting healthy behavior to prevent noncommunicable diseases |

## Life Skill/Family Life Education

In current scenario, adolescents are facing many challenges in their daily lives. Many critical issues arise during adolescence such as puberty, dealing with sexuality issues, tackling emotional turbulence, completing education, choosing career options, facing responsibilities as an adult, etc. Majority of the schools in India focus mainly on the development of scholastic, reading and writing skills of the children. It is felt that good academic performance of the students would help in developing confidence and personality of students at par with today's world. The schools are not able to satisfy their psychological needs, unable to communicate with them, identify their risk factors, unable them to make good decisions and finally ended up in frequent failures and suicidal attempts by the adolescents. Hence, Life Skills Development Program is being recommended for 30–45 days for both school-going and out of school adolescents.

Five core life skills and examples of life skill activity has been presented in **Figure 27.3**.

## CURRENT APPROACHES IN HEALTHCARE SERVICES (GLOBAL AND NATIONAL)

*Current approaches in healthcare services are of two types:*
1. Global approach, goals, and targets
2. Health programs and schemes, legislation, etc.

### Global Approach, Goals, and Targets

#### Global Strategy for Women's, Children's, and Adolescents' Health

The strategy sets out to ensure every woman, child and adolescent, in any setting, anywhere in the world, is able to both survive and thrive by 2030. To achieve the above certain evidence-based health interventions are:
- Routine vaccinations (e.g., HPV, hepatitis B, diphtheria-tetanus, rubella, measles)
- Promotion of healthy behavior (e.g., nutrition, physical activity, no tobacco, alcohol or drugs)
- Prevention, detection and management of anemia, especially for adolescent girls
- Counseling and services for sexual and reproductive health including contraception
- Psychosocial support for adolescent mental health
- Prevention and response to sexual and other forms of gender-based violence
- Prevention and response to harmful practices such as female genital mutilation and early and forced marriage
- Prevention, detection and treatment of communicable and noncommunicable diseases and STDs and RTIs including HIV, TB, and syphilis
- Diagnosis and management of substance abuse
- Skill training of parents, for managing behavioral disorders in adolescents
- Assessment and management of adolescents who present with unintentional injury, including alcohol-related injury
- Prevention of suicide and management of self-harm/suicide risks.

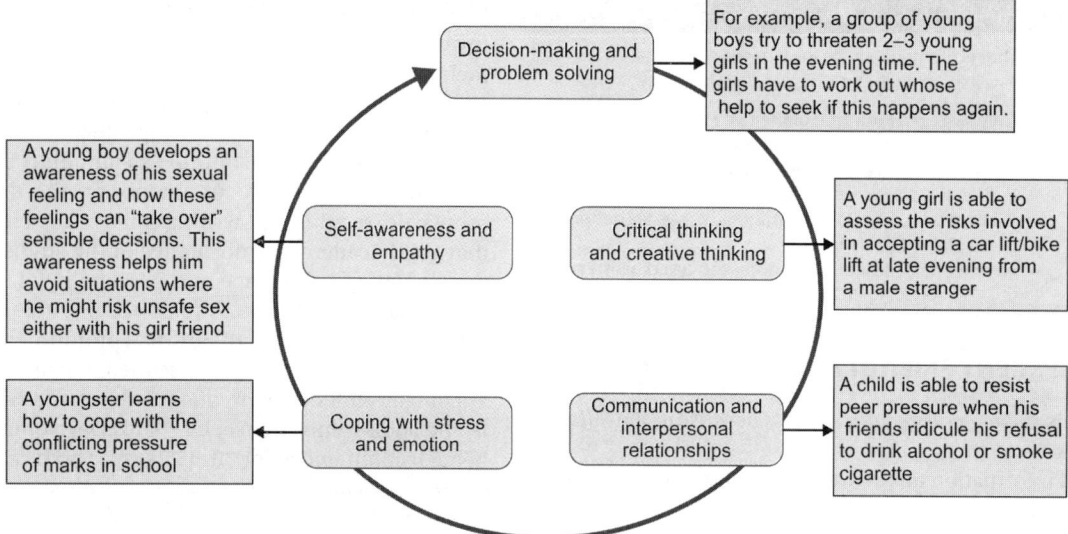

**Fig. 27.3:** Five core life skills and examples of life skill activity.

## Monitoring Framework for the Global Strategy for Women's, Children's, and Adolescents' Health (2016–2030)

The global strategy for women's, children's and adolescents' health (2016-2030) was launched in September 2015. It was set with an objective to improve women's, children's, and adolescents' health in alignment with the Sustainable Development Goals (SDGs) along with three axes:
1. Survive (end preventable deaths)
2. Thrive (ensure health and well-being) and
3. Transform (expand enabling environments).

### Key Indicators

- *Survive:* Adolescent mortality rate
- *Thrive:*
  – Adolescent birth rate (10–14, 15–19) per 1,000 women in that age group
  – Current country health expenditure per capita (including specifically on RMNCH+A) financed from domestic sources
  – Number of countries with laws and regulations that guarantee women aged 15–49 access to sexual and reproductive health care, information, and education
- *Transform:*
  – Proportion of children and young people in schools with proficiency in reading and mathematics
  – Proportion of women, children, and adolescents subjected to violence (SDG 5.2.1, 16.2.3).

**Note**

Equity is a cross-cutting consideration aligned with SDG 17.18.1, with disaggregation of indicators when relevant, including by age, sex, education, wealth, and settings—rural, urban, humanitarian.

## Health Programs and Schemes

*The health programs and schemes related to adolescent health including adolescent reproductive and sexual health, nutrition related schemes, School health program, schemes under ICDS and Rashtriya Kishor Swasthya Karyakram are explained in detail in Chapter 47: Heath Policies and Programs in India.*

## SUGGESTED READING

1. A strategic approach to reproductive, maternal, newborn, child and adolescent health (RMNCH+A) in India. For healthy mother and child. (2013).
2. Department of Women and Child Development (GOI). (2010). [online]. Available from wcd.nic.in/sites/default/files/1-SABLAscheme_0.pdf.
3. https://main.mohfw.gov.in/sites/default/files/NFHS-5_Phase-II_0.pdf.
4. Implementation guide on RCH II ARSH strategy. For state and district programme managers. (2006).
5. Ismail S, Shajahan A, Rao TS, Wylie K. Adolescent sex education in India: Current perspectives. Indian J Psychiatry. 2015;57(4):333-7.
6. Ministry of Women and Child Development (GOI). (2000). Kishori Shakti Yojana—A new initiative. Guidelines for implementation of adolescent girls scheme as a component under centrally sponsored ICDS (general) scheme.
7. MoHFW (GOI). (2013). NRHM Component: Reproductive & Child Health: Adolescent Health: WIFS.
8. MoHFW (GOI). (2013). School Health Programme. National Health Mission.
9. MoHFW (GOI). (2014). Rashtriya Kishor Swasthya Karyakram (RKSK). National Health Mission.
10. Morrison MA. Addiction in adolescents. West J Med. 1990;152(5):543-6.
11. Orientation programme for medical officers to provide adolescent-friendly health services. [online]. Available from: http://www.nhm.gov.in/images/pdf/programmes/RKSK/Medical_Officer_Training_ Manual/Resource_Book_Medical_Officer.pdf.
12. Samal J, Dehury RK. Salient Features of a Proposed Adolescent Health Policy Draft for India. J Clin Diagn Res. 2017;11(5):LI01-LI05.
13. Scheme for promotion of menstrual hygiene among adolescent girls in Rural India. (2013). [online]. Available from: www.nhm.gov. in/nrhm-components/rmnch-a/adolescent-health-rksk/menstrual-hygiene-scheme mhs/background.html.
14. UNESCO. (2002). Adolescence Reproductive Health. Module 6. [online]. Available from: http://www.unesco.org/education/ mebam/module_6.pdf.
15. WHO. (2018). The global strategy for women's, children's and adolescents' health (2016-2030). Survive Thrive Transform.

# CHAPTER 28

# Geriatric Health

*Rakesh Kakkar, Gouri Sen Gupta*

*"You do not heal old age. You protect it; you promote it; you extend it".*
—**Sir James Sterling Ross**

| | |
|---|---|
| **CM 12.1** | Define and describe the concept of geriatric services |
| **CM 12.2** | Describe health program for aged population |
| **CM 12.3** | Describe the prevention of health problems for aged population |

## INTRODUCTION

The word "geriatrics" was derived from the Greek word "*Geras,*" meaning old age, and "*Iatrike*" meaning medical treatment. Ignatz Leo Nascher coined it in 1909. The world is witnessing increasing life expectancies at global level due to global improvement in health care and living conditions thus geriatric healthcare is a global focus area for all. The world is slowly aging and so is its population. In 2001, India has joined the rank of a "greying nation," i.e., nation with 7% or more of its population in the 60 plus years segment and there is also increase in the number of the "older old" population. (Population and aging in Asia, The growing elderly population, 2018). This reflects increase in life expectancy and is also a good indicator of improvement in healthcare services. However, with an increase in elderly population several medical, social and economic concerns are also brought in which has become a major challenge for health departments all around the world.

## DEMOGRAPHY OF THE ELDERLY

People over 60 years of age or above were 5.6% of the total population in 1961, 7.7% in 2001, while 8.6% population in 2011 census **(Fig. 28.1)**. By 2050, the projected older adult population would be 19%. Population experts believe that in next 25–30 years people over 65 years of age would be twice the number of children less than 5 years of age. Thus more geriatric care experts would be needed than pediatricians.

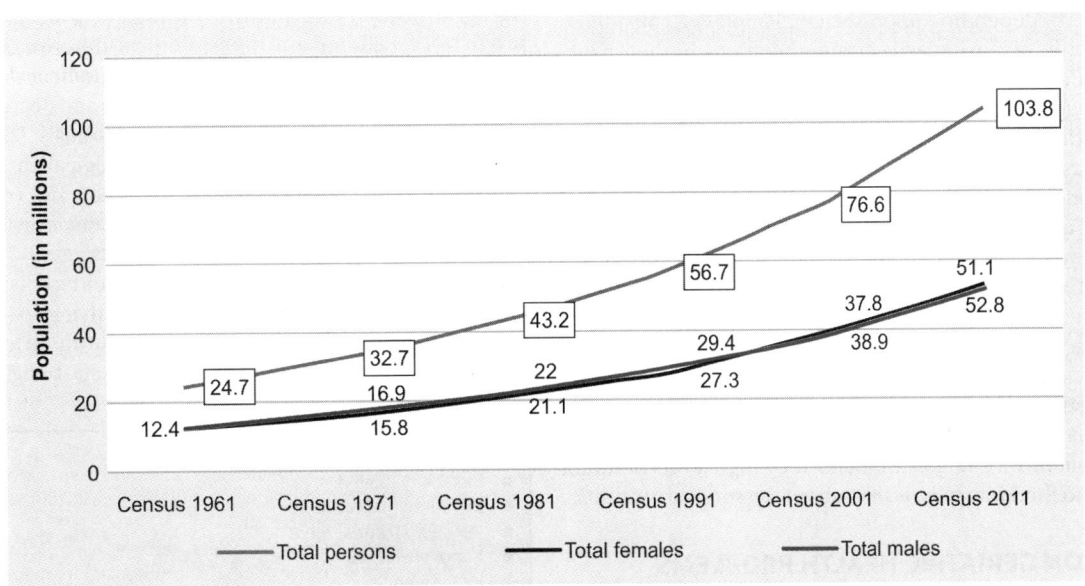

**Fig. 28.1:** Graph shows elderly population (aged 60 years and above) in India.
*Source:* Population Census Data 2011.

## Population Census Data 2011

As per census statistics 2011, only 29% of elderly population resides in urban area while remaining resides in rural areas which may make service delivery a challenge. The ratio of women/men over 85 years is 2:1 that indicates feminization of elderly population. Recorded sex ratio was 1,033 for older adults, i.e., over 60 years of age in census 2011.

The age sex population structure of most developing countries is pyramid in shape with broad base representing infants due to high birth rate and top (apex) of pyramid tapers off sharply representing old age population. Developed countries shows pillar shaped age sex pyramid because of rapidly increasing life expectancy and decline of fertility and mortality rates, thus all age represent almost equally.

Literacy rates are up trending among the older adult population from 27% (1991) to 44% (2011), literacy plays a crucial role, because patients, too, have educational needs related to health literacy and understanding treatment options. But the potential support ratio or dependency ratio is rising from 10.9% (1961) to 14.2% (2011) in our country and approximately 30% of older adults are below poverty line, all these figures indicate need of socioeconomic support required for this age group. (Ministry of Social Justice and Empowerment, 2018).

## DEFINITION

Common agreed definition of aging is "progressive process associated with declines in structure and function, impaired maintenance and repair systems, increased susceptibility to disease and death, and reduced reproductive capacity." Geriatrics is branch of medicine which deals with the healthcare of the aging people. While "gerontology" refers to the "study of physical, biological, psychological and sociological changes which are incident to old age." Senility is the physical and mental weakness associated with old age. While "senescence" is the process of growing old.

The cut off for old age is difficult to define as "old age" or "aged" is relative term depending upon society. People are considered old when with increasing age certain alterations in their usual activities or social roles are observed. From the social point of view, old age commences with retirement from service. For uniformity United Nations defines an aged person as who is more than 60 years of age. In January, 1999 as per "National Policy on Older Persons" Government of India has adopted "senior citizen" or "elderly" as a person who is 60 years of age or above. People between 60 years and 74 years are "young old" and 75–84 years as "middle old" and people above 85 years as "oldest old" or "infirm."

Life expectancy at 60 is the average number of years that a person at that age can be expected to live, assuming that age-specific mortality levels remain constant. This is a better estimate of survival within the adult life course than life expectancy at birth, particularly for low- and middle-income countries. Life expectancy at birth is hugely influenced by high levels of infant mortality and therefore tells us little about the survival of adults.

## COMMON GERIATRIC HEALTH PROBLEMS

Normal aging causes no symptoms unless associated with disease and is usually with only few restrictions. Any abrupt decline in function is usually pathological and not due to aging. Aging is multifactorial process depends on amount of care, consumed diet, environmental factors, personal habits, genetic factors and also neglect of body in previous years of life. Normal aging can be retarded by modification of risk factors. There is a wide gamut of social, psychoemotional and physical correlates which determine the medical problems. It is cumulative effect of illnesses, stresses, accidents and trauma in individual health and nutritional status in early years of life. It is pertinent to understand that aging is a continuous process and is always associated with physiological and biological decline **(Table 28.1 and Fig. 28.2)**.

**Table 28.1:** Health problems of elderly.

| Both the genders | Male | Female |
|---|---|---|
| Ocular diseases | Benign prostatic hypertrophy (BPH) | Menopausal problems |
| Hearing defects | Prostatic cancer | Urinary incontinence |
| Reduced muscular strength and coordination | Male sexual dysfunction | Cancers and other disease of female genital tract |
| Accidents and injuries | | Osteoporosis |
| Nutritional deficiencies | | |
| Dental problems | | |
| Cardiovascular diseases | | |
| Increased susceptibility to adverse effects of physical environment | | |
| Increased susceptibility to infections | | |
| Degenerative neurological diseases | | |
| Complication of diabetes | | |
| Cancers | | |

### Biological

Aging is predictable natural biological process, involving progressive cellular and physiological deterioration related to mental, physical, behavioral and biomedical domains and increased susceptibility to various diseases and decreased ability to adapt to stress because of impaired homeostasis. These changes are nonreversible, independent of pathological conditions and contribute to loss of function or death. It depends on numerous factors and occurs at different rates in different individuals. Thus, it is difficult to say when an individual starts aging.

Ensuring proper timely treatment to elderly is sometimes challenging as due to social factors, cognitive impairment, and decreased hearing they develop uncaring attitude towards their health and care givers at family level also start neglecting their health.

**The I's of geriatrics morbidities**
- Instability (frailty)
- Inanition (malnutrition)
- Intellectual impairment
- Impoverishment
- Incontinence
- Incoherence (delirium)
- Insulin resistance (diabetes mellitus)
- Immobility

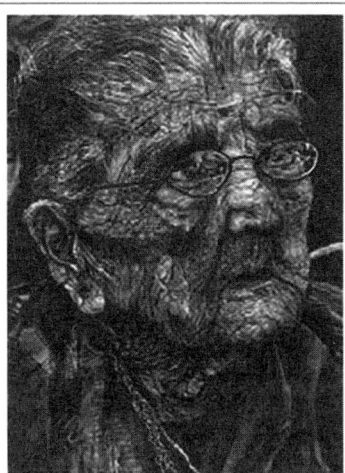

**Neurological system**
- Brain changes with age
- Clinical depression common
- Altered mental status common.

**Cardiovascular system**
- Hypertension common
- Changes in heart rate and rhythm.

**Gastrointestinal system**
- Constipation common
- Deterioration of structures in mouth common
- General decline in efficiency of liver
- Impaired swallowing
- Malnutrition and result of deterioration of small intestine.

**Musculoskeletal system**
- Osteoporosis common
- Osteoarthritis common.

**Respiratory system**
- Cough power is diminished
- Increased tendency for infection
- Less air and less exchange of gases due to general decline.

**Renal system**
- Drug toxicity problems common
- General decline in efficiency.

**Skin**
- Perspires less
- Tears more easily
- Heals slowly.

**Immune system**
- Fever often absent.
- Lessened ability to fight disease.

**Fig. 28.2:** Changes in the body systems of the elderly.

### Psychological

Physical, physiological, psychological conditions, social prestige, financial status, personal lifestyle, family support system are some of influencers of health of elders. This is period of critical changes in body, mind and spirit. Loneliness, boredom, depression, dejection, grief and worrying about the future which are common in this age group alter the normal physiological processes. Many of them also complain of loss of memory, loss of confidence, and a sense of hopelessness. Some of them suffer from senile dementia, Alzheimer's disease and other mental disorders. The prominent thrust areas resulting in sociopsychological frustration among the elderly are general attitude towards old age, degradation of their status in community, problems of isolation, loneliness and generation gap.

*Elder abuse* is also quite common among elderly. The prevalent patterns of elder abuse include psychological abuse in terms of verbal assaults, threats and fear of isolation, physical violence and financial exploitation. More women than men complain of maltreatment in terms of both physical and verbal abuse. Person suffering from physical or mental impairment and dependent on the caretakers for most of his or her daily needs is likely to be the victim of elder abuse. Old people with high educational background and sufficient income are also found to be subjected to abuse.

### Social

Many elderly people after retirement from their job feel reduction in income, social status, authority, power, respect and importance. Similarly, after loss of spouse, friends and colleagues, social isolation of person may sometimes occur. The loss of the decision-making power by those who have surrendered their property in favor of younger members and loss of status and decision-making power is felt more by aging women than men. Ageism is accusing them as inefficient and discriminating, against elderly people on the basis of their age. They are disregarded for employment, and are forced towards restricted social activity, thus it marginalizes and excludes older people in their communities.

Years of life lost due to premature deaths, in adults aged 60 years or more due to various disease conditions is shown in **Figure 28.3**.

## PREVENTIVE AND COMMUNITY GERIATRICS

Preventive geriatrics is the art and science of preventing diseases in the geriatric population and promoting their health and efficiency. It implies that process of ageing should be smooth and physiological rather than pathological thus focus is mainly on primary prevention rather than on secondary prevention. Certain principles mentioned in **Box 28.1** are essential for providing preventive geriatric healthcare services.

### Health Promotion: Healthy Aging

As per World Health Organization "healthy aging is the process of developing and maintaining the functional ability that enables well-being in older age." Functional ability comprises the health-related attributes that enable people to be and to do what they have reason to value. Healthy aging starts at birth with our genetic inheritance. So, care of old age should begin right from early childhood. Adoption of healthy lifestyle and promotive measures undertaken during childhood and adulthood are to ensure healthy aging which constitute pregeriatric care. Preventive gerontology suggests adopting healthy lifestyle inclusive of healthy diet, exercise and avoidance of substance abuse.

Supportive, "age-friendly" environments allow older people to live fuller lives and maximize the contribution they make. Healthy aging starts with healthy behaviors in earlier stages of life, i.e., childhood, adolescent and young adulthood. Pregeriatric care includes regular moderate physical activities. Walking, cycling and swimming and Yoga are some of activities that can be included on daily basis for well-being of elderly.

Older people have small appetite, hence small frequent, nutrient dense (with micronutrient) foods should be included,

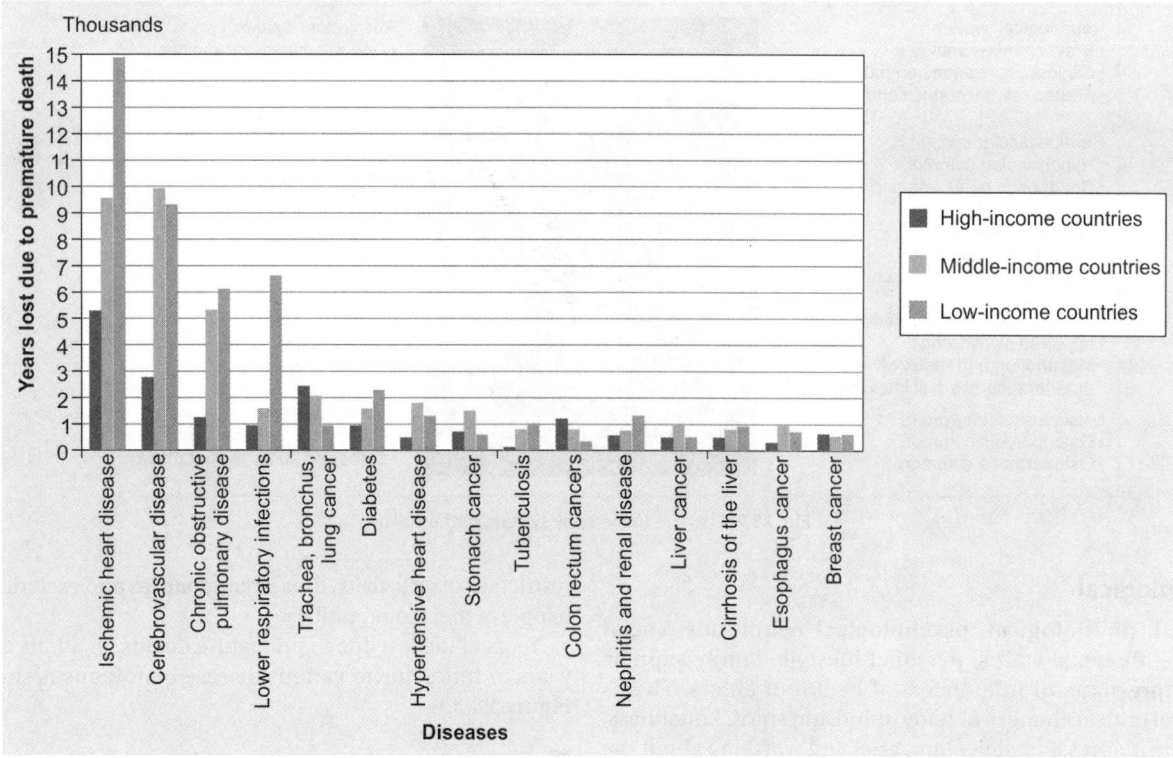

**Fig. 28.3:** Years lost due to premature death. Years of life lost due to death per 100,000 adults aged 60 years and older by country income group.
*Source:* World Health Statistics 2011. Geneva WHO.

> **Box 28.1: Principles of geriatric healthcare includes.**
> - Individuals become more and more heterogeneous or dissimilar as they age
> - Aging does not produce an abrupt decline in organ function but disease always does
> - Aging process is accentuated by disease and attenuated by modification of risk factors such as smoking, sedentary lifestyle and obesity
> - Investigation is essential tool for diagnosis but under or over investigation are to be avoided

keeping not only quantity but also the quality. Nourishing, digestible, easy to chew and easy to swallow foods and beverages are preferred. Ensure 4–5 serving of fruits and vegetables and cut down on fried foods containing saturated and trans-fats.

Preferred diet is with less fat (less than 30 g/day), sugar and salt and high in protein (0.8–1 g/kg/day), fibers (complex carbohydrates instead of refined sugars) and calcium.

## Early Diagnosis and Treatment

Early detection and treatment of disease developing in young age, diabetes mellitus, hypertension or early stages of cancer, are likely to give rise to decreased morbidity and mortality in geriatric age group.

### Screening

Special health and screening camps should be organized for detection of hypertension, diabetes through simple diagnostic procedures and identification of "early warning signs" for cancer, training women about breast self-examination for presence of lump in breast and exfoliative cytology of vaginal smear in elderly women. By conducting health assessment of elderly and collecting information related to vision, joints, hearing, chest, blood pressure (BP), blood sugar, etc. in a questionnaire during health center visit and thereafter data can be updated and maintained on subsequent visits. Screening procedures for maintaining healthy and active aging has been described in **Table 28.2**.

### Periodic Health Check-up

Early diagnosis and treatment of diseases is preferred strategy for conditions detected in elderly to minimize or eliminate residual damage. Unlike the other age groups, elderly or older person comprise a group whose needs are multidisciplinary and require not only medical but also social, environmental and mental support. Annual health check-up includes vision, hearing, and laboratory examination of blood test, stool for occult blood and ECG. Adequate advice on chronic morbidities like chronic obstructive pulmonary disease, arthritis, diabetes, hypertension, etc. including lifestyle modification and dietary recommendations.

> **Components of comprehensive geriatric assessment**
> - Physical
> - Functional
> - Psychological: Cognitive, affective
> - Socioeconomic: Financial status, social support and care facility
> - Environmental

**Table 28.2:** Screening procedures for health conditions in elderly.

| | |
|---|---|
| Breast cancer | Mammography |
| Cataract | Medical examination of eye |
| Cervical cancer | Cervical Pap smear |
| Colorectal cancer | Stool for occult blood |
| Coronary artery diseases | Analysis of risk, electrocardiogram (ECG) |
| Deafness | Medical evaluation (Whisper test) and audiometry |
| Dementia | Minimental state examination (MMSE) |
| Diabetes mellitus | Blood glucose estimation |
| Diabetic retinopathy | Fundoscopic examination, fluorescein angiography |
| Dyslipidemia | Lipid profile |
| Glaucoma | Tonometry for intraocular pressure |
| Hypertension | Recording of blood pressure |
| Lung cancer | X-ray (Chest) |
| Osteoporosis | Bone densitometry after risk assessment |
| Prostate cancer | Rectal examination, prostrate specific agent (PSA) level |

### *Rehabilitation*

Tertiary level prevention strategies focus on detection and treatment of debilitating chronic conditions with aim of minimizing residual disability and rehabilitation. Rehabilitation in elderly is done by enabling person to acquire skills that is needed to live independent life. Preventive geriatrics focuses on prevention and reduction of disability and improvement of quality of life (QOL) of old age people. Spectacles, dentures, sun glasses and hearing aids are given free to the needy aged persons.

Rehabilitation is multidisciplinary effort by combination of medical, social, educational and vocational training to achieve highest possible level of functional ability. Physiotherapist, clinical psychologist, social workers or person trained in rehabilitation work can help in physiotherapy and medical rehabilitation. They can visit bed ridden elderly and counsel the care providers at family level. Resettlement is done by restoration of patient in his or her own conducive atmosphere.

Day care centers provide excellent atmosphere where recreational activities (carom, table tennis, etc. or bhajans, yoga camps and other spiritual activities) can be organized. Provision of old age homes or senior citizen club can provide facilities to its members in the form of training in yoga, meditation, aerobics and fulfillment of hobbies, etc. for enhancing physical and mental health.

### *Geriatric Healthcare Centers*

Treatment of all old persons suffering from medical and psychological diseases including sensory loss is done at a dispensary or a general hospital. There is provision of package of geriatric services available at different levels under National Program for Health Care of Elderly (NPHCE) that is at subcenter, primary health center, community health center, district hospital and regional geriatric center (RGC) level.

## CURRENT APPROACHES IN GERIATRIC HEALTH CARE SERVICES

### Global Approach

Over a period of 50 years the domain of geriatrics and gerontology has changed immensely from curative and rehabilitative to prevention and promotion. WHO had introduced the concept of active aging in 2002. Based on "the world report on aging 2015" it was changed to concept of *healthy aging from 2015-2030*. WHO describes *"healthy aging"* as "the process of developing and maintaining the functional ability that enables well-being in older age." *Functional ability* is "the abilities which enable all elderly people to meet their basic needs and to learn, grow and make decisions, remain mobile, to build and maintain relationships; and to effectively contribute to society."

For healthy and active aging there is a need to focus on action at numerous sectors and aiding elderly people to contribute effectively not only to their families, but also to communities as well as economies. 1st October is celebrated as International Day of Older Persons across the globe to propagate various cross cutting sectors best practices. Also, 15th June every year is set aside as world elder abuse day to create awareness regarding the various types of abuse faced by elderly.

Recently, World Health Assembly adopted *"The Global Strategy and Action Plan for Aging and Health (GSAP)"* in May 2016. Objectives of this strategy are *"a framework to achieve healthy aging* for all **(Table 28.3)**."

*2020-2030 has been declared by WHO, as the decade of the elderly.* The 10 priorities identified by GSAP for collaborative effort of various stakeholders provide the plan for substantial activities that are required to achieve the objectives of the "WHO global strategy and action plan on aging and health."

### National Approach: Major Government of India Initiatives for Elderly Population

Many ministries are catering to the needs of elderly, the Ministry of Social Justice and Empowerment (MoSJE) deals with the social issues of elderly while Ministry of Health and Family Welfare (MoHFW) addresses the health concerns. Between these two ministries the key initiatives of government to address the issues of persons above 60 years age are:
- National Policy on Older Persons (NPOP)–1999, 2011
- Maintenance and Welfare of Parents and Senior Citizens Act–2007
- National Program for Health Care of Elderly (NPHCE)—2010

### *National Policy on Older Persons*

They adopted by MoSJE in 1999, focuses on well-being of elderly. The policy which was revised in 2011 to value an age integrated society, has a number of provisions for support to elderly people. The principal areas of intervention are as follows:
- Financial security
- Healthcare and nutrition
- Shelter, education, welfare
- Protection of life and property

**Table 28.3:** The global strategy and action plan for aging and health.

| Vision | A world in which everyone can live a long and healthy life |
|---|---|
| Strategic objectives | • Commitment to action on healthy aging in every country<br>• Developing age-friendly environments<br>• Aligning health systems to the needs of older populations<br>• Developing sustainable and equitable systems for providing long-term care (home, communities and institutions)<br>• Improving measurement, monitoring and research on healthy aging |
| Action plan 2016–2020 goals | • 5 years of evidence-based action to maximize functional ability that reaches every person<br>• By 2020, establish evidence and partnerships necessary to support a Decade of Healthy<br>• Aging from 2020 to 2030 |

- Involvement of nongovernment organizations
- Training of manpower
- Establishment of a National Council for Senior Citizens.

### Maintenance of Senior Citizens Act, 2007

"As per Maintenance of Senior Citizens Act 2007 there is a legal compulsion for children and successors to offer maintenance to senior citizens and parents, by monthly allowance. This act also provides simple, immediate and economical instrument for the protection of life and property of the older persons. A senior citizen, who is not capable to maintain himself from his own earning or out of the property owned by him, is entitled to get relief under this act. Children or grandchildren or relative are under obligation to look after his or her parent either father or mother or both or relative. If such children or relative is not maintaining his parents or senior citizen respectively, then the parents or senior citizen can seek the assistance of a Tribunal constituted under this act."

### National Program for Health Care of Elderly

As per the National Policy on Older Persons (1999), MoHFW was assigned with the program to address the health care needs of the elderly. Hence to address various health-related problems of elderly people, The MoHFW had launched the "National Program for the Health Care of Elderly" (NPHCE) during 2010–11. *The program is further explained in detail in Chapter 47: Health Policies and Programs in India.*

## SOME OTHER INITIATIVES

### Integrated Program for Older Persons

Integrated program for older persons is a scheme by the MoSJE for maintenance of old age homes, day care centers, mobile medicare units and multifacility care center for older widows, etc. Aim of the program is to improve the quality of life of elderly person by provision of elementary facilities such as housing, food, medical or health care and recreation activities, etc. through local bodies, nongovernmental voluntary organizations, etc.

### Rashtriya Vayoshri Yojana

Rashtriya Vayoshri Yojana (RVY) is a scheme funded from the "senior citizens" Welfare Fund since 2016. Under the RVY scheme, devices to assist in living with disability to elderly person of BPL category who are facing age-related disabilities such as decreased vision, hearing impairment, loss of teeth and locomotors disabilities. The aids and assistive devices, viz. walking sticks, elbow crutches, walkers or crutches, tripods or quadpods, hearing aids, wheelchairs, artificial dentures and spectacles are provided to eligible beneficiaries. RVY is being executed by Artificial Limbs Manufacturing Corporation of India (ALIMCO), which is under the MoSJE. The beneficiary identification will be done by a committee at the district level headed by the district collector and kits will be distributed in camps.

### Indira Gandhi National Old Age Pension Scheme (IGNOAPS)

The Ministry of Rural Development's National Social Assistance Program (NSAP) extends social assistance for poor households—for the aged, widows, disabled, and in cases of death where the breadwinner has passed away. Under this scheme, financial assistance is provided to person of 60 years and above and belonging to family living below poverty line as per the criteria prescribed by Government of India. Central assistance of ₹200 per month is provided to person in the age group of 60–79 years and ₹500 per month to persons of 80 years and above.

### The Pradhan Mantri Vaya Vandana Yojana

The Pradhan Mantri Vaya Vandana Yojana (PMVY) was launched in May 2017 to ensure provision of social security in elderly person. This is a simplified version of the Varishtha Pension Bima Yojana and will be implemented by the Life Insurance Corporation (LIC) of India. Under the scheme, on payment of an initial lump sum amount ranging from ₹1.5 lakhs for a minimum pension of 1,000 rupees per month to a maximum of ₹15 lakhs for a maximum pension of ₹10,000 per month, beneficiary will get an guaranteed rate assured pension based on return at 8% per annum and is payable on monthly or quarterly or half-yearly or annually basis. This scheme has been extended up to 31st March 2020.

## SUGGESTED READING

1. Elderly in India. (2016). Elderly in India Profile and Programmes 2016. New Delhi: Ministry of Statistics and Programme Implementation. Government of India.
2. Introduction to sociology—1st Canadian https://opentextbc.ca/introductiontosociology/chapter/chapter13agingandtheelderly/
3. Ministry of Health and Family Welfare. (2018). Operational Guidelines, National Programme for Health Care of the Elderly (NPHCE).
4. Northern Illinios Public Health. Proceeding of NIPHC/HCPT Seminar on services for aged—a national commitment; 1996 Oct: New Delhi.
5. World Health Organization. (2015). World Report on Ageing and Health.

# CHAPTER 29

# Occupational Health

*Pankaja Raghav, Manoj Kumar Gupta, Ankit Sheth*

*"Safety and Health is not only second economic policy; it is a basic human right"*
—**Kofi Annan, UN Secretary General, 2003**

| | |
|---|---|
| CM 11.1 | Enumerate and describe the presenting features of patients with occupational illness including agriculture |
| CM 11.3 | Enumerate and describe specific occupational health hazards, their risk factors and preventive measures |
| CM 11.4 | Describe the principles of ergonomics in health preservation |

## INTRODUCTION—CONCEPT, NEED, AND SCOPE

Almost every individual is involved in some or the other occupations. Workers represent 50% of the global population. The health of workers is an essential prerequisite for productivity and economic development. Place of work is an important environment for the workers. It has becomes imperative to provide healthy and safe working environment. But it is interesting to note that there is no occupation which is 100% safe and without any hazards. There is a wide spectrum of occupational morbidity ranging from minor occupational injuries to malignancies.

The modern occupational health started after the industrial revolution. To keep up with the demands, these large-scale manufacturing industries came up with a unique set of problems such as use of dangerous machinery and chemicals which leads to hazardous factory conditions, long working hours for employees, child labor, etc. Certain progressive thinkers started challenging the risk and danger for the workers and started working in this direction. Eventually the first Factory Act came into force in 1833, which later passed through a number of subsequent updates and revisions.

Following three objectives are of prime importance in occupational health:
1. Promotion and maintenance of health of the worker to improve the capacity of working
2. Improvement in work environment so that health and safety are not compromised
3. Induction of healthy work culture to improve health and safety of worker as well as to improve the productivity by culminating positive social climate at workplace.

## DEFINITION OF OCCUPATIONAL HEALTH

Bernardino Ramazzini, the father of occupational medicine (OM), in his publication in 1700, De Morbis Artificaum advised the doctors to ask, "what your occupation is?" Occupational health has been defined by the International Labour Organization (ILO) and WHO in 1950 and updated as follows by the ILO/WHO Joint Committee on Occupational Health in 1995:

*"Occupational health aims at: the promotion and maintenance of the highest degree of physical, mental and social well-being of workers in all occupations; the prevention amongst workers of departures from health caused by their working conditions; the protection of workers in their employment from risks resulting from factors adverse to health; the placing and maintenance of the workers in an occupational environment adapted to his physiological and psychological capabilities; and, to summarize, the adaptation of work to man and of each man to his job".*

According to ILO, an occupational disease is *"Any disease contracted as a result of an exposure to risk factors arising from work activity"*. In most countries, a disease is defined "occupational" when the national authorities acknowledge its occupational origin.

## WORKFORCE AND HEALTH

### Organized and Unorganized Sector (Table 29.1)

In a highly populated country like India, people opt for many types of jobs in different sectors for their livelihood. Broadly these sectors are divided into three categories—primary, secondary, and tertiary.
1. *Primary sector jobs* are mainly agriculture related and include the activities which are directly dependent on environment, as these refer to utilization of earth's resources such as land, water, minerals, and vegetation. It thus includes agriculture, mining, hunting, fishing, forestry, etc. Due to the outdoor nature of the work, people engaged in primary sector activities are called red collar workers.
2. *Secondary sector jobs* are mainly industry related and include the activities which add value to natural resources by transforming

raw materials into valuable products. People who are involved in secondary activities are termed as blue collar workers.

3. *Tertiary sector jobs* are white collar jobs, as these are mainly service related and include production and exchange activities.

As per the result of labor force survey conducted by National Sample Survey Office (NSSO), Ministry of Statistics and programme implementation on employment and unemployment, Labour Force Participation Rate (LFPR) for persons of age 15 years and above was 60.8% in rural areas and 50.4% in urban areas in 2022–2023 the number of estimated employed persons in 2022 were 523.8 million in the country, of (Labor force, World bank data 2022).

**Table 29.1:** Difference between organized and unorganized sector.

| | Organized sector | Unorganized sector |
|---|---|---|
| Definition | The sector in which the employment terms are fixed and people have assured jobs | The sector that is constituted by the small and scattered units which are not registered with the government |
| Regulations | Government laid rules and regulations to follow, which are given in various laws such as the factories act, minimum wages act, bonus act, Provident Fund act, payment of gratuity act, shops and establishments act, etc. | There are rules and regulations, but are not followed strictly |
| Payment | The salaries are paid as per Basic Wage act. There is a system of regular monthly salary and regular increment | The wages are low and irregularly paid. Usually follow daily wages system and salary increment is rare |
| Security | The employee enjoys the security of employment | There is no such job security |
| Benefits | Employees in organized sector enjoy add-on benefits such as medical facilities, pension, leave travel compensation, paid leave, medical leaves, overtime pays, provident fund and insurance and medical claims and benefits, etc. | Workers do not have any such benefits |
| Termination | The employees cannot be forced to leave the job without any valid and strong reason | The workers can be asked to leave the job without any valid reason |
| Insights | The employee of the organized sector is only 17% of the total people but constitute 50% of the GDP of India | Unorganized sector constitutes 83% of the employed people and constitutes only 50% of the GDP of India |
| Examples | Employees of central government, railways, banks, etc. Factories, enterprises, industries, schools, hospitals and units which are registered with the government | House-hold manufacturing activity and small scale and tiny sector of the industry such as construction workers, domestic workers, people working in small size enterprises which are not affiliated with the government |

## AGRICULTURE AND HEALTH

Agriculture and health have two-way interactions with each other; agriculture affects health and similarly health affects agriculture. Although agriculture is considered to promote good health through production of food, material (for shelter) and medicinal plants, yet it has close association with many health problems including a range of occupational health hazards, under-nutrition, food-borne diseases, AIDS and other diet related chronic diseases. The interesting part is that agriculture can be responsible for both alleviation as well as spread of these health-related conditions. This two-way connection between agriculture and health provides an opportunity for these two different sectors/departments to work together and move towards a positive vicious cycle of interaction to prevent health and agricultural problems.

The flow diagram in **Figure 29.1** shows a conceptual framework to represent the linkages between health and agriculture. Across the top are the core knots related to the agricultural supply chain, which includes producers, systems, and outputs related to agriculture. At the bottom there are important health problems affecting the poor in developing countries such as undernutrition, vector-borne diseases, HIV/AIDS, foodborne diseases, diet-related chronic diseases, and occupational health hazards. In the middle are the most critical intermediary processes linking agriculture and health in both directions: the labor process, environmental change, income generation, and access to food, water, land, and health-related services. As shown on the left side of the figure, these interactions are all influenced by policies, policy processes, and governance.

### Health Hazards in Agriculture

Perhaps more than any other occupational group, agricultural workers are exposed to a tremendous variety of environmental hazards that are potentially harmful to their health and well-being. Six **"Hazard Zones"** for workers that are directly attributable to changes in climate:

1. **Heat:** Workers exposed to hotter temperatures are more vulnerable to heat-related illnesses (HRIs) such as heat stroke and heat exhaustion.
2. **Extreme weather:** Violent rain, extreme drought, flash floods and mudslides all expose workers to dangerous conditions.
3. **Ozone:** Warmer temperatures lead to an increase in ground-level ozone, which can be associated with serious respiratory issues such as lung damage, pneumonia and Chronic Obstructive Pulmonary Disease (COPD).
4. **Polycyclic aromatic hydrocarbons:** Burning coal, gasoline, oil, trash or other materials releases polycyclic aromatic hydrocarbons (PAHs) that are linked to certain types of cancer.
5. **Workplace violence:** Multiple studies have found a relationship between heat and crime, or aggressive and violent behavior.
6. **Pathogens and vector-borne diseases:** Standing water created by extreme rain or flooding can be a breeding ground for certain pathogens. It can also contribute to an increase in vector-borne diseases such as Zika virus, Lyme disease or West Nile virus.

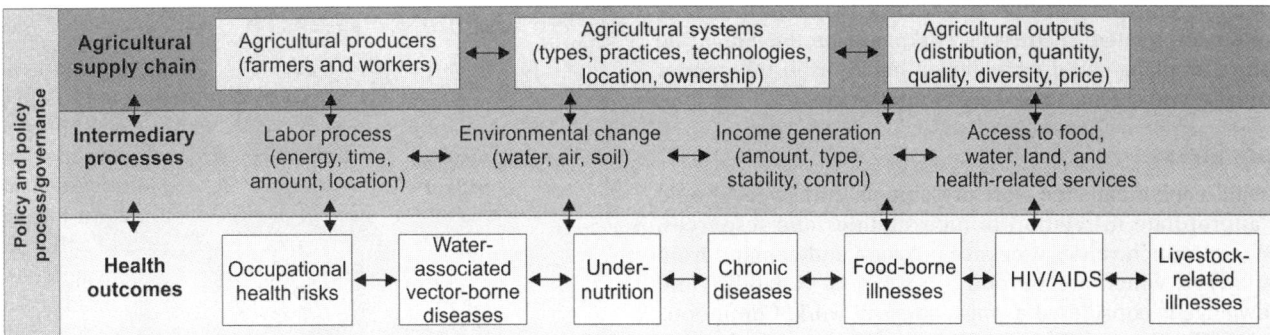

Fig. 29.1: A conceptual framework to represent the linkages between agriculture and health.
*Source:* Hawkes C et al., Int Food Policy Res Inst, 2006.

Following are major health hazards of agricultural workers:
- **Respiratory hazards:** Agricultural workers are usually at greater risk of developing respiratory problems. Cough and congestion are very common among agricultural workers and their family members. Reaction to both immunologic (e.g., pollens, cereal grain and grain dust, livestock dander, fungal antigens and mites in organic dusts) and nonimmunologic (e.g., due to organic insecticides and organic dust) agents is responsible for precipitation of asthmatic symptoms among farmers. Pre-existing bronchial hyperactivity has a synergistic effect with these agents in developing bronchospasm. Organic dust toxic syndrome (ODTS), which occurs after heavy organic dust exposure, is a common respiratory illness among farmers and is manifested by influenza-like illness with fever, headache, nausea and muscle aches. "Farmer's lung" is an immunologically mediated pneumonitis caused by inhaled dust of fungal spores from moldy hay or grain. Certain gases that are highly reactive (e.g., ammonia, sulfur dioxide, chlorine, hydrogen sulfide and ozone) cause mucous membrane irritation and pulmonary edema. Low level exposure of these gases causes lung and eye irritations, dizziness, drowsiness, and headaches. Nitrogen dioxide and phosgene, which are water in-soluble chemicals also causes toxic pulmonary damage. Exposure to silo gases (a mixture of NO, $NO_2$ and $CO_2$) causes silo filler's disease, in which pulmonary edema is main feature.
- **Accidents:** Challenging work environment, laborious work, use of hand tools and negligence towards use of safety measures and precautions are some of the factors responsible for occupational injury. The risk of accidents and injuries among farmers has increased with time due to intensive use of machinery and other equipment. Among nonfatal accidents, musculoskeletal injuries are predominant. Bruises, fractures, lacerations, penetration by foreign bodies, contusions and sprains or strains are the most frequent type of occupational injuries.
- **Zoonotic diseases:** Zoonotic diseases may be transmitted to livestock farmers through contamination during production, processing, and handling of food products of animal origin. Lack of awareness about the occurrence of zoonotic diseases has been a major problem in commencing adequate and effective control measures.
- **Noise:** Noise-induced hearing loss (NIHL) is another common preventable health hazard on the farm. Prolonged exposure to noise produced by machinery used for farming such as tractors, grain dryers, choppers, etc., can also cause permanent hearing loss.
- **Skin disorders:** Exposure to different chemicals such as pesticides, long working hours in hot and humid climates, and working with dangerous machinery make working conditions hazardous in the farms and predisposes farmers to occupational skin diseases. Chemicals such as pesticides, disinfectants, and rubber have been identified as possible offending agents. The most common skin problem among farmers is contact dermatitis. The most common parts affected are hands, which are vital for performing their work duties.
- **Cancers:** Due to long working hours under the bright sun rays, skin and lip cancers are among the most common concerns of the farmers. Besides that, exposure to different types of chemicals used for agriculture purpose may also be associated with lymphomas.
- **Chemical hazards:** On a daily basis farmers are exposed to different types of chemicals like fertilizers, pesticides and insecticides. These chemicals can enter the body through many routes, but the most common ways are through the skin and by inhalation. These chemicals can cause toxic hazards to agriculture workers.
- **Heat stress:** Exposure to excessive heat in workplace can cause various health problems starting from mild skin rash to fatal heat stroke. Some of the health impacts are sweating, dehydration, salt loss, loss of perceptual and motor performance, heat exhaustion, loss of ability to work and increased accident risk. As, farmers work for long hours outdoor with long-term sun exposure, they are at potential risk of developing heat stress.

## OTHER SERVICE SECTORS

White collar jobs are considered as relatively safe, clean and easy jobs, as there are the least chances of life-threatening accidents in these jobs. But with time various factors have come up which are affecting the health of office employees/workers. These factors cannot be neglected as with prolonged exposure; these can be life threatening for the workers.

Major factors responsible for affecting health of the office workers are related to stress at workplace, prolonged sitting posture, smoking and drug addiction habits, exposure to poor air quality and chemicals and ergonomic factors.

### Work Stress

A healthy job means the work pressure on employees should be appropriate in relation to their abilities and resources. The work which values excessive pressure and demand from employees, which are beyond the workers' capability and knowledge is considered as most stressful work. Continuous working in stressful situations may lead to some unhealthy practices and health issues like sleeping disorders, anxiety, headache, depression, digestion problems, etc., which can lead to noncommunicable diseases at an early age. Family and social issues such as fighting with partners, beating and unnecessary scolding children and spoiling relations with neighbors may also be consequences of working constantly in stressful conditions.

### Air Quality

If the air quality at work is improved, productivity will increase. Proper indoor ventilation removes pollutants and smell which originates inside the building. It also prevents the accumulation of moisture and controls the relative humidity. The presence of moisture or very high relative humidity contributes to the development of molds and other biological contaminants to thrive. It can further lead to "sick building syndrome". Very low relative humidity also irritate mucous membrane and causes dry eyes and sinus discomfort.

### Chemicals

Many types of chemicals are used in the office on daily basis such as toners for photocopiers and faxes, correction fluids, liquid detergents, etc. Constant exposure to these chemicals for a long time can be responsible for skin and eye disorders and allergies.

> **Points to ponder**
> - Occupational health aims at the promotion and maintenance of the highest degree of physical, mental and social well-being of workers in all occupations.
> - In organized sector the employment terms are fixed and people have assured jobs, while unorganized sector is constituted by the small and scattered units which are not registered with the government.
> - Industrialization has led to migration of people in huge numbers from rural areas to urban regions and has resulted in overpopulation and overcrowding in urban areas and in development of slums.
> - Agricultural workers are exposed to variety of environmental hazards that are potentially harmful to their health and well-being.
> - White collar jobs are considered as relatively safe, clean and easy, as there are least chances of life-threatening accidents. But with time various factors have come up which are affecting the health of office employees/workers.

## OCCUPATIONAL ENVIRONMENT AND HEALTH HAZARDS (FIG. 29.2)

As per American Public Health Association, "Environmental health focuses on the relationships between people and their environment. Improving environmental health promotes the

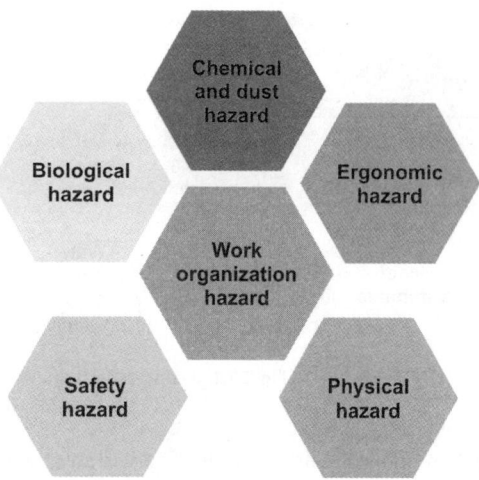

**Fig. 29.2:** Occupational environment and health hazards.

healthy and safe communities". Occupational environment has lot of impact on the health of workers, the term "occupational environment" is the sum of external conditions and influences which prevail at the workplace and have impact on the health of workers. Occupational environment has adverse health effects for the workers. These effects have been caused either by exposure to hazards and harmful agents, or by environmental degradation. Many of these exposures are involuntary.

**Occupational environment and health hazards can be classified as follows:**

*Physical agents and hazards:* The factors in the environment which are harmful without even coming in close contact with it, such as radiation (including ionizing, nonionizing) magnetic fields, extreme pressures (high pressure, vacuum), exposure to sunrays, extreme temperature, loud noise, vibration, etc. Besides that, lighting conditions such as working in extreme dark or in excessive glare can also be harmful.

*Chemical agents and hazards:* In the workplace, workers are exposed to chemical preparations in different forms (solid, liquid or gas). There can be a varied range of problems due to chemical solutions depending on the toxic properties, e.g., irritation of the skin and respiratory problems due to inhalation of the chemicals. These chemical hazards may be due to liquids such as cleaning products, acids, paints, solvents, vapors and fumes that come from welding or exposure to solvents, flammable materials such as gasoline, gases such as acetylene, propane, carbon monoxide and helium, solvents, pesticides, and explosive chemicals.

*Biological agents and hazards:* Biological agents may be hazards in occupations where the workers are working with animals, or infectious materials. Places such as hospitals, laboratories, emergency response, nursing homes, outdoor occupations, etc. may expose to biological hazards. Blood, body fluids, bacteria and viruses, fungi/mold, plants, insect bites, animal and bird droppings, etc. may be the types of exposure.

*Ergonomics hazards:* These are because of wrong body positions and working conditions leading to strain on the body parts. The ergonomic hazards range from mild muscle pain to serious long-term illnesses depending on the duration of exposure. Improperly adjusted workstations and chairs, poor posture, frequent lifting, awkward (especially repetitive) movements, frequent use of force, vibration, etc. are some of the ergonomic hazards.

***Psychosocial agents and hazards (work organization hazards):*** Psychosocial agents are also called stressors. They cause either short-term effects (stress) or long-term effects (strain). Most of the psychological hazards are associated with workplace related issues such as workload and lack of control/respect, workplace violence, lack of flexibility in working, lack of social support/relations, sexual harassment, etc.

***Safety hazards:*** They include unsafe conditions, which may be responsible for injury, illness and sometimes death. Safety hazards include spills on floors or tripping hazards, such as blocked aisles or cords running across the floor, working from heights, working near unguarded machinery and moving machinery parts, electrical hazards due to frayed cords or improper wiring, confined spaces and machinery-related hazards (lockout/tagout, boiler safety, forklifts, etc.).

## Physical Health Hazards

### Heat Stress

In heat stress the heat-regulating mechanisms of the body is disturbed. It can't simply eliminate enough heat. So, the internal body temperature rises above 98.6°F. It affects the physiological processes and results in strain on the body. This situation is called heat stress. This heat stress produces different symptoms which are called HRIs. These symptoms are categorized based on their severity **(Fig. 29.3)**.

Outdoor workers such as farmers, construction workers, miners and workers who constantly work in hot environments such as firefighters, bakery workers, boiler room workers and factory workers are at more risk of developing heat stress. Conditions such as old age (65 years and above), obesity,

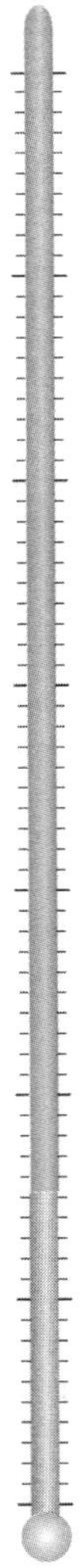

| | | | |
|---|---|---|---|
| **Heat rash prickly heat** | Signs and symptoms: | Red spots on the skin that resemble blisters; prickly or itchy sensation |
| | What's happening: | Sweat glands become clogged and inflamed when sweat cannot evaporate; happens in humid conditions and/or when clothing traps sweat against the skin |
| **Heat cramps** | Signs and symptoms: | Spasms of the legs, arms or abdomen; often accompanied by heavy sweating and thirst; happens after physical labor |
| | What's happening: | A loss of body salt, through sweat, cause water to rush into the muscles, resulting in cramping or spasms |
| **Early heat illness** | Signs and symptoms: | Fatigue; dizziness; irritability; inability to concentrate; impaired; judgment |
| | What's happening: | Blood flow to the brain is reduced as the body redirects blood to release heat from the skin |
| **Heat syncope** | Signs and symptoms: | Sudden dizziness; pale complexion; moist skin; normal body temperature |
| | What's happening: | Blood flow to the brain is reduced as the body redirects blood to release heat from the skin |
| **Heat exhaustion** | Signs and symptoms: | Excessive sweat; dry mouth; extreme thirst; headaches or feeling dizzy; lightheadedness; mood change or irritability; rapid breathing; chills; fainting or weakness; heat cramps; nausea; decreased or dark-colored urine; pale; moist skin; fatigue |
| | What's happening: | Less blood flow to the brain, resulting from blood flow to the body's surface; this results in less oxygen reaching the brain and therefore lightheadedness, headaches, and mood changes; body's temperature regulator is still functioning trying to cool the body |
| **Heat stroke** | Signs and symptoms: | Often occurs suddenly; extremely high body temperatures; lack of sweating; confusion or aggressive behavior; seizures or convulsions; coma in severe cases; unresponsiveness to clapping; dizziness; fast pulse; dry, hot, red skin |
| | What's happening: | Over 150°F, the body stops sweating and the temperature-regulating system stops functioning due to too much heat; blood flow to the brain is significantly reduced; rising internal temperatures risk damage to organs including the heart, brain, central nervous system, liver and kidney; brain damage or death can result |

**Fig. 29.3:** Heat-related illnesses and their symptoms.

cardiovascular diseases, hypertension, etc. increase the risk of developing heat stress.

### Risk Factors for the Development of Heat-related Illnesses

*Personal risk factors*
- **Weight:** Overweight or obese people retain more heat due to more fat and less physically fit muscles, which generates heat.
- **Pregnancy:** An increase in their core temperatures may have negative health effects on the fetus in pregnant women.
- **Age:** People in extreme age groups are more susceptible. Old age people have less capacity of pumping blood and less efficient sweat cooling mechanism. Infants and young children have larger body surface area as compared to body mass. The central nervous system, which helps in regulating body temperature is not fully developed in children, it also usually deteriorates in old people.
- **Existing medical conditions:** Chronic health conditions affect the normal physiological functioning of the body including response to heat stress. Diseased heart has less capacity of pumping blood in body which is required for cooling of the body. Other NCDs such as hypertension and diabetes affect blood vessels restricting the blood flow. Skin diseases or other skin conditions also affect the heat releasing process of the body.
- **Physical fitness:** A person who is physically fit, has acclimatized muscles to physical activity. These muscles generate less heat.
- **Acclimatization:** Not being habitual of working in extreme heat, increases the risk of heat stress, as the heat regulating system of body does not function properly.
- **Drinks:** Alcohol causes dehydration of the body and increases the risk of HRIs.
- **Attitudes:** Few people have risky behavior as they are bounded by certain cultural or personal beliefs. This increases the risk of developing heat stress.

*Environmental risk factors*
The body eliminates heat by evaporation, conduction, convection, and radiation.
- **Temperature:** Body cannot release heat through radiation when outside temperature is high. This increase the risk of heat stress.
- **Heavy machinery:** Heavy machinery produces heat in lager amount which increases environmental temperature and leads to risk of heat stress for the worker.
- **Time of day:** In the afternoon temperature is higher than morning hours.
- **Shade or cloud cover:** Absence of any shade exposes the worker to sunlight.
- **Wind:** Good air circulation/wind flow causes heat release from the body by convection and evaporation of the sweat.
- **Humidity:** Humidity interferes in evaporation of sweat.
- **Workload:** Strenuous and long hours' physical activity generate more heat.
- **Heavy clothing:** Certain cloths trap heat and prevent heat release through convection or radiation, such as personal protective equipment.
- **Pesticide exposure:** Certain pesticides cause excessive sweating.

### Prevention and Management of Heat Disorders
- **Heat stress:** Should wear loose-fitting, light-colored cotton clothes and hat with a brim or cap. Use of bandana under the hat and placing a wet bandana on the neck to keep body cool **(Fig. 29.4)**. Drink lot of water before going to work and drink one cup of water every 15 minutes. Always drink before getting thirsty.
- **Heat exhaustion:** Immediate management at place of work include remove worker from hot area and give plenty of liquids to drink, remove unnecessary clothing, cool the worker with cold compresses or have the worker wash head, face, and neck with cold water and encourage frequent sips of cool water and take worker to a clinic or emergency room for medical evaluation and treatment.
- **Heat rash:** Workers with heat rash should be shifted to a cooler, less humid work environment, rash area should be kept dry, powder may be applied, but ointments and creams should be avoided.
- **Heat cramp:** Workers with heat cramps should drink water and have a snack and/or carbohydrate-electrolyte replacement liquid (e.g., sports drinks) every 15–20 minutes, avoid salt tablets, get medical help if the worker has heart problems, is on a low sodium diet, or if cramps do not subside within an hour.
- **Rhabdomyolysis:** A medical condition associated with heat stress and prolonged physical exertion, resulting in the rapid breakdown, rupture, and death of muscle. When muscle tissue dies, electrolytes and large proteins are released into the bloodstream that can cause irregular heart rhythms and seizures and damage the kidneys. Workers with rhabdomyolysis will present with muscle cramps/pain, abnormally dark (tea or cola colored) urine, weakness, exercise intolerance, asymptomatic. Workers with symptoms of rhabdomyolysis should: stop activity, increase oral hydration (water preferred), seek immediate care at the nearest medical facility, and checked for rhabdomyolysis (i.e., blood sample analyzed for creatine kinase).
- **Heat syncope:** Workers with heat syncope should be asked to sit or lie down in a cool place and slowly drink water, clear juice, or a sports drink.

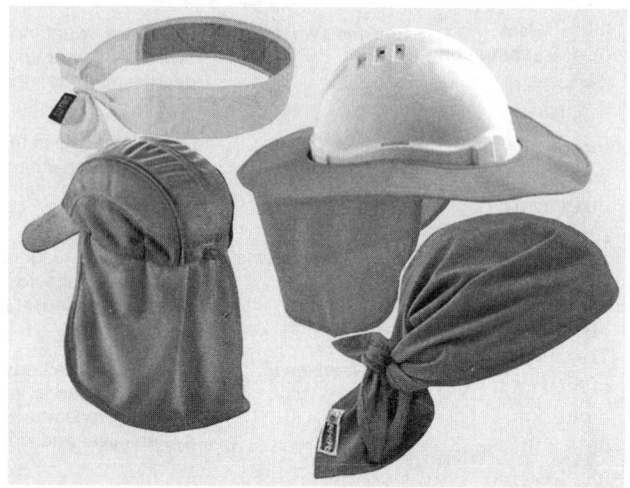

**Fig. 29.4:** Bandana to be used under the hat for temperature control.

- **Heat stroke:** Immediate management will include moving the worker to a shaded, cool area and remove outer clothing, cool the worker quickly with a cold water or ice bath if possible; wet the skin, place cold wet clothes on skin, or soak clothing with cool water, circulate the air around the worker to speed cooling, place cold wet clothes or ice on head, neck, armpits, and groin; or soak the clothing with cool water.

## Cold Stress

Outdoor workers, and those who work in an area that is poorly insulated or without heat are more susceptible to cold stress. Following are cold related illnesses:

- **Hypothermia:** It is an abnormally low body temperature. After exposure to cold temperatures, the body starts losing heat faster than it can be produced. Stored energy gets utilized after prolonged exposure to cold. The worker will not be able to identify the occurrence of hypothermia as it affects the brain, and the worker will not be able to do anything about it. This makes hypothermia particularly dangerous. The early symptoms are shivering, fatigue, loss of coordination, confusion and disorientation. Late Symptoms are no shivering, blue skin, dilated pupils, slow pulse and breathing, loss of consciousness. Immediate management will include shifting of the worker to warm place, removal of wet clothing, warm the center of their body first-chest, neck, head, and groin-using an electric blanket, if available; skin-to-skin contact, dry layers of blankets, clothing, towels, or sheets, warm beverages may help increase the body temperature. Alcohol should not be given. Nothing should be given to an unconscious person. After their body temperature has increased, keep the victim dry and wrapped in a warm blanket, including the head and neck. If the victim has no pulse begin cardiopulmonary resuscitation (CPR).
- **Frostbite:** It is an injury to the body that is caused by freezing. It affects the nose, ears, cheeks, chin, fingers, or toes. It can permanently damage body tissues leading to amputation. In extremely cold temperatures, the risk of frostbite is increased in workers with reduced blood circulation and among workers who are not dressed properly. Symptoms are due to reduced blood circulation to hands and feet (fingers or toes can freeze) numbness, tingling or stinging, aching, bluish or pale, waxy skin. Immediate management includes taking the workers to a warm room as soon as possible, walking on frostbitten feet or toes should be avoided as it will increase the damage, immerse the affected area in warm-not hot-water, warm the affected area using body heat, e.g., the heat of an armpit can be used to warm frostbitten fingers, do not rub or massage the frostbitten area; doing so may cause more damage, do not use a heating pad, heat lamp, or the heat of a stove, fireplace, or radiator for warming. Affected areas are numb and can be easily burnt.
- **Trench foot:** It is also known as immersion foot, is an injury of the feet resulting from prolonged exposure to wet and cold conditions. Trench foot can occur at temperatures as high as 60°F if the feet are constantly wet. Injury occurs because wet feet lose heat 25-times faster than dry feet. As there will be no circulation, lack of oxygen and nutrients and buildup of toxic products at the affected site leading to tissue damage. Symptoms are Reddening of the skin, numbness, leg cramps, swelling, tingling pain, blisters or ulcers, bleeding under the skin, gangrene (the foot may turn dark purple, blue, or gray). Immediate management will include Removal of shoes/boots and wet sock, drying of feet. Workers suffering from trench foot should avoid walking on affected feet, as this may cause tissue damage.
- **Chilblains:** They are caused by the repeated exposure of skin to temperatures just above freezing to as high as 60°F. The cold exposure causes damage to the capillary. This damage is permanent, and the redness and itching will return with additional exposure. The redness and itching typically occurs on cheeks, ears, fingers, and toes. Symptoms: redness, itching, possible blistering, inflammation, possible ulceration in severe cases. Immediate management includes workers suffering from chilblains should be advised to avoid scratching, slowly warm the skin, use corticosteroid creams to relieve itching and swelling, and keep blisters and ulcers clean and covered.

## Noise

It is essentially any unwanted or undesirable sound. Occupational noise induced hearing loss (NIHL) is caused by exposure to sound levels or durations that damage the hair cells of the cochlea. Initially, the noise exposure may cause a temporary threshold shift—that is, a decrease in hearing sensitivity that typically returns to its former level within a few minutes to a few hours. Repeated exposures lead to a permanent threshold shift, which is an irreversible sensorineural hearing loss. Depending on the cause of your NIHL, symptoms may be immediate, or you may develop them over time. Some of the most common noise-inducing hearing loss symptoms include inability to hear high-pitched sounds, muffled or distorted speech, tinnitus, and a feeling of fullness or pressure in the ear. Combined exposures to noise and certain physical or chemical agents (e.g., vibration, organic solvents, carbon monoxide, ototoxic drugs, and certain metals) appear to have synergistic effects on hearing loss. Noise exposure is also associated with nonauditory effects such as psychological stress and disruption of job performance and possibly hypertension. Noise may also be a contributing factor in industrial accidents.

Preventing and treating NIHL involves a combination of proactive measures to avoid exposure to loud noises and, when necessary, medical interventions. To prevent NIHL, individuals should use ear protection, such as earplugs or earmuffs, in noisy environments or workplaces. Noise-canceling headphones can also be employed to reduce ambient noise. Treatment for NIHL focuses on early detection through regular hearing check-ups. Hearing aids may be recommended for mild to moderate hearing loss, while cochlear implants can be an option for severe cases. Tinnitus, often associated with NIHL, can be managed through counseling and sound therapy. Once hearing loss occurs, it is crucial to avoid further noise exposure. Seeking professional advice is important for personalized recommendations and long-term auditory health.

### Vibration

Occupational exposure to vibration can be due to hand-arm vibration (HAV) and whole-body vibration (WBV).

- **Hand-arm vibration:** It leads to "hand-arm vibration syndrome" (HAVS) leading to following disturbances: (**Refer Figs. 29.5 to 29.7**)
  - *Vascular disturbances:* Vibration white fingers (VWF) secondary Raynaud's phenomenon
  - *Neurological disturbances:* Numbness reduced tactile sensitivity, reduced manual dexterity
  - *Effect on the locomotor system:* Muscles, bones, joints, tendons
  - Comfort and performance
- **Whole-body vibration:** It is transmitted to the whole body by the surface supporting it, e.g., through a seat or the floor. It is commonly experienced by drivers, operators and passengers in mobile plant when travelling over uneven surfaces. WBV may also be experienced while standing, e.g., standing on platforms attached to concrete crushing plant. WBV includes sharp impacts like shocks and jolts. Exposure to WBV mainly occurs in vehicles used off-road or on unsealed roads, e.g., on farms and construction, mine and quarry sites. It can also occur in other places like in small, fast boats and in helicopters. Long-term exposure to WBV show evidence of risks to health, mainly musculoskeletal disorders involving the lower spine, neck and shoulders. High WBV exposure increases the risk of lower-back pain, herniated discs and early degeneration of the spine.

Exposure to WBV may cause or make worse:
- Cardiovascular, respiratory, neurological, endocrine and metabolic changes
- Digestive problems
- Reproductive organ damage in both men and women, and
- Impairment of vision, balance or both.

### Radiation Hazards

Radiation can cause biological effects that may be harmful to the exposed person and the magnitude or probability of these effects is directly proportional to the dose. Approximately 20% of people die from various forms of cancer whether or not they ever receive occupational exposure to radiation. These effects may be classified into three categories:

- **Somatic effects:** Physical effects occurring in the exposed person. These effects may be early or late. Early effects occur shortly after a large exposure that is delivered within hours to a few days. They are observable after receiving a very large dose in a short period of time, e.g., 300 rads (3 Gy) received within a few minutes to a few days. This type of dose is called an acute dose or acute exposure. The same dose received over a long time period would not cause the same effect. It is important to distinguish between whole body and partial body exposure. A localized dose to a small volume of the body would not produce the same effect as a whole body dose of the same magnitude. Delayed effects may occur years after exposure. These effects are caused indirectly when the radiation changes parts of the cells in the body, which causes the normal function of the cell to change, e.g., normal healthy

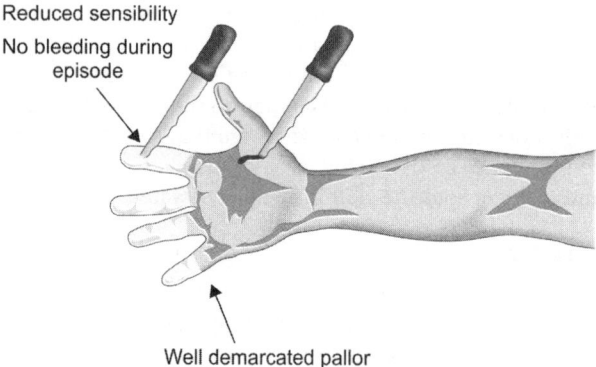

Fig. 29.5: Vibration white fingers.

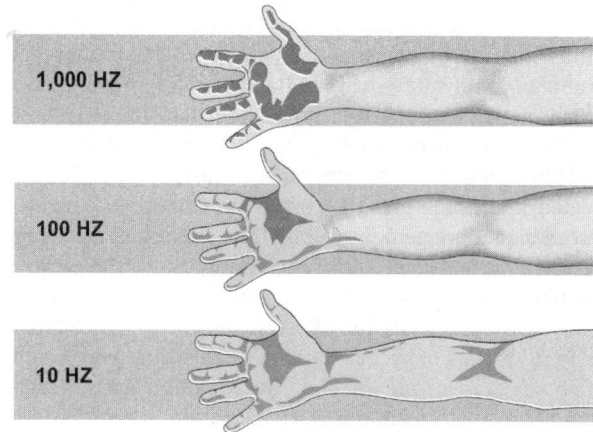

Blue color indicate area under impact of vibration.

Fig. 29.6: Vascular disturbances.

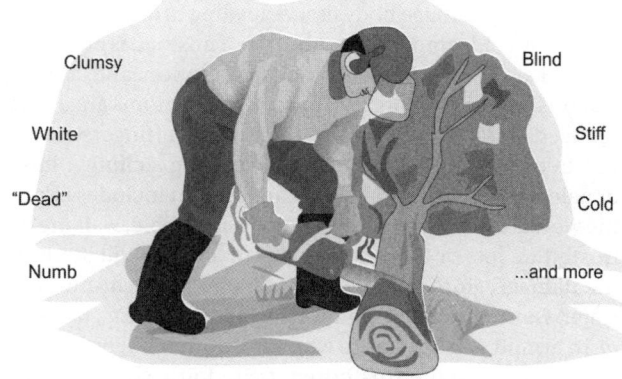

Fig. 29.7: Hand-arm vibration.

cells turn into cancer cells. The potential for these delayed health effects is one of the main concerns addressed when setting limits on occupational doses. A delayed effect of special interest is genetic effects.
- **Genetic effects:** Genetic effects may occur if there is radiation damage to the cells of the gonads (sperm or eggs). These effects may show up as genetic defects in the children of the exposed individual and succeeding generations.

- ***Teratogenic effects:*** Effects such as cancer or congenital malformations that may be observed in children who are exposed during the fetal and embryonic stages of development.

### Barometric Pressure

Conditions which can develop due to barometric pressure include hypoxia (due to decreased barometric pressure at high altitude and the resultant decrease in ambient oxygen), acute mountain sickness (headache mostly at night, loss of appetite, nausea and vomiting, disturbed sleep, fatigue, shortness of breath, cough and neurological symptoms such as memory deficits and auditory or visual disturbances), high-altitude pulmonary edema (symptoms similar to acute mountain sickness along with decreased exercise tolerance, increased recovery time after exercise, shortness of breath on exertion, and persistent dry cough), high-altitude cerebral edema (extreme form of acute mountain sickness that includes generalized cerebral dysfunction), and retinal hemorrhages (usually asymptomatic). Patients with sickle cell disease are more prone to develop painful vaso-occlusive crisis at high altitude.

*Note:* **Chemical and biological hazards have been covered in section of occupational diseases.**

## SICKNESS ABSENTEEISM

Word sickness—is derived from the concept of the "sick role", a role that carries certain privileges (to stay away from work), as well as obligations (to seek medical help and to "get well"). Absenteeism is a habitual pattern of absence from a duty or obligation. It is the practice of regularly staying away from work or school without good reason. It can be voluntary or involuntary.

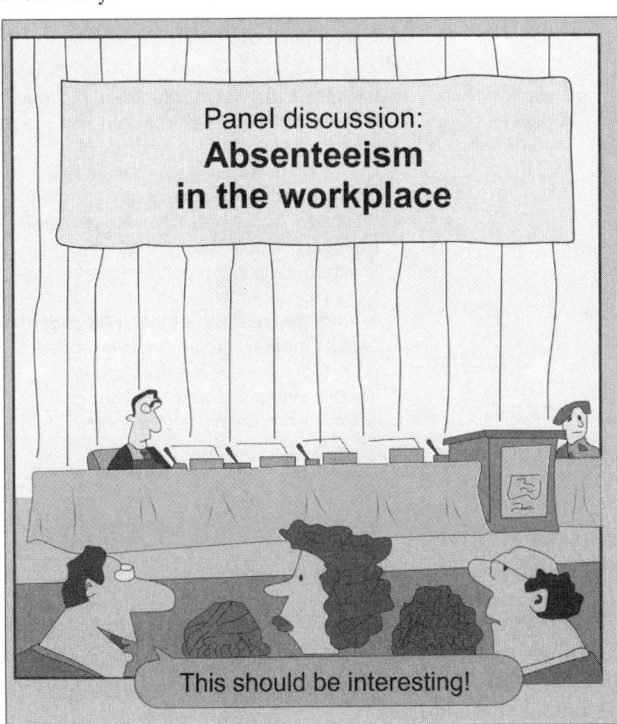

Voluntary is an employee's deliberate or habitual absence from work without valid reason. In involuntary absenteeism employees can be absent from work for several reasons such as illness, death in the family, and the personal reasons which are unavoidable and understandable. Many employers have sick-leave policies that allow employees a certain number of paid absent days per year.

Long hours of work, bad working conditions, lack of co-operation and understanding between management and workers, sickness, accidents and occupational diseases are the major causes of sickness absenteeism. Other causes may be low wages, lack of proper medical aid and health programs, lack of canteen services, rest rooms, etc., bad housing conditions, evil of drinking, lack of marketing facilities, social or religious festivals, marriages, education of children, problem of transport facilities and sometimes workers from rural areas go back to villages, for short or long periods, during sowing and harvest season.

Labor absenteeism is harmful to both employee and workers:
- Normal workflow in the factory is disturbed.
- Overall production in the factory goes down.
- Casual workers may have to be employed to meet production schedules such workers are not trained properly.
- Forceful unwilling replacement of employee.
- Impede production with serious cost repercussions.
- Overtime allowance will increase considerably because of higher absenteeism.
- When several workers absent themselves, there is extra pressure of work on their colleagues who are present.
- Workers lose wages for the unauthorized absence from work.
- Habitual absentees may be removed from service causing them great hardship.

Following approaches can be used to reduce voluntary absenteeism:
- Good factory management and practices
  - Disciplinary approach
  - Positive reinforcement
  - Combination approach
  - No fault absenteeism
  - Paid time-off (PTO) programs
- Adequate pre-placement examination
- Good human relations
- Application of ergonomics

> **Points to ponder**
> - In heat stress the heat-regulating mechanisms of body is disturbed. So, the internal body temperature rises above 98.6°F. It affects the physiological processes and results in strain on the body.
> - Outdoor workers, and those who work in an area that is poorly insulated or without heat are more susceptible to cold stress.
> - Occupational exposure to vibration can be due to hand-arm vibration and whole-body vibration.
> - Sickness absenteeism is the practice of regularly staying away from work or school without good reason. It can be voluntary or involuntary.

## OCCUPATIONAL DISEASES

According to WHO an "*occupational disease is any disease contracted primarily as a result of an exposure to risk factors arising from work activity*". The ILO and the WHO have estimated that 5–7% of global fatalities are attributable to work-related illnesses and occupational injuries. The list contains the definition of each occupational disease and is the basis for the fundamental occupational safety and health legislation. (ILO and WHO, Occupational Safety and Health, 2006) **(Table 29.2)**.

## Pneumoconiosis

Pneumoconiosis is a group of interstitial lung diseases caused by lung parenchyma's reaction to the certain inhaled dust. Silicosis, asbestosis and coal workers' pneumoconiosis, which are caused by inhalation of silica dust, asbestos fibers and coal mine dust, respectively are considered as primary pneumoconiosis. As a typical process, these diseases take many years to develop. But sometimes only a short period of intense exposure is sufficient to develop the disease, e.g., rapidly progressive forms of silicosis. In severe forms these diseases often cause lung impairment, permanent disability and death.

Some dusts are biologically inert but radiologically alarming, as they are visible on chest radiographs and CT scan. They hardly progress in clinical disease or deficit in pulmonary functions. But dusts like silica and asbestos are fibrogenic, and causes damage to lung parenchyma by inducing fibrosis rather than the dust itself. So, they develop characteristic radiological patterns and restrictive deficits in lung functions. They may progress even after exposure to the causative mineral has stopped.

Inhalation of dust containing coal (anthracosis), aluminum, barium, beryllium (berylliosis), antimony, iron (siderosis), cobalt (hard metal disease), graphite, kaolin, mica, talc, etc. may cause other forms of pneumoconiosis. But these are rare compared to primary pneumoconiosis. Sometimes pneumoconiosis may be caused by exposure to organic dust such as cane fibers (bagassosis), cotton dust (byssinosis), tobacco (tobaccosis), hay or grain dust (farmer's lung), etc.

In developed countries such as UK and similar countries, asbestosis is the most common form of pneumoconiosis. But in developing countries such as India silicosis is most prevalent pneumoconiosis followed by asbestosis and coal workers' pneumoconiosis.

## Silicosis

Exposure to crystalline silica dust causes multiple diseases such as silicosis, pulmonary TB, lung cancer, chronic obstructive pulmonary disease (COPD) and autoimmune and renal diseases. But silicosis and silicotuberculosis are the two high priority occupational diseases of concern in low and middle income countries. Respirable crystalline silica dust particles which are less than 7 microns, are invisible to naked eyes. These silica particles are comprised of an atom of silicon and two atoms of oxygen ($SiO_2$) uncombined with other elements, hence sometimes called "free silica".

***Epidemiology:*** Silicosis occurs everywhere in the world, but is especially prevalent in low and middle income countries. China has the most patients with silicosis among the world. In India, large mining industries are concentrated in states such as Jharkhand, Chhattisgarh, West Bengal and Odisha. Around 3.0 million workers are at high risk of exposure to silica; of these, 1.7 million work in mining or quarrying activities. (Gupta A, Silicosis, 1999). The burden of silicosis is often under-reported due to poor surveillance.

**Table 29.2:** List of occupational diseases (as per ILO 2010).

| 1. | Occupational diseases caused by exposure to agents arising from work activities | |
|---|---|---|
| | a. Chemical agents | Beryllium, cadmium, phosphorus, chromium, manganese, arsenic, mercury, lead, fluorine, carbon disulfide, halogen derivatives, benzene, etc. |
| | b. Physical agents | Noise, vibration, compressed or decompressed air, ionizing radiations, optical (ultraviolet, visible light, infrared) radiations including laser, extreme temperatures, etc. |
| | c. Biological agents | Brucellosis, hepatitis viruses, HIV, tetanus, tuberculosis, toxic or inflammatory syndromes, anthrax, leptospirosis, etc. |
| 2. | Occupational diseases by target organ systems | |
| | a. Respiratory diseases | • Pneumoconiosis caused by fibrogenic mineral dust (silicosis, anthraco-silicosis, asbestosis), silicotuberculosis<br>• Pneumoconiosis caused by nonfibrogenic mineral dust, siderosis<br>• Bronchopulmonary diseases caused by hard-metal dust<br>• Bronchopulmonary diseases caused by dust of cotton (byssinosis), flax, hemp, sisal or sugar cane (bagassosis)<br>• Asthma caused by recognized sensitizing agents or irritants inherent to the work process<br>• Extrinsic allergic alveolitis caused by inhalation of organic dusts or microbially contaminated aerosols, arising from work activities<br>• Chronic obstructive pulmonary diseases<br>• Diseases of the lung caused by aluminum<br>• Upper airways disorders caused by recognized sensitizing agents or irritants inherent to the work process |
| | b. Skin diseases | Allergic contact dermatoses and contact urticaria, irritant contact dermatoses, vitiligo, etc. |
| | c. Musculoskeletal disorders | • Radial styloid tenosynovitis due to repetitive movements, forceful exertions and extreme postures of the wrist<br>• Olecranon bursitis due to prolonged pressure of the elbow region<br>• Prepatellar bursitis due to prolonged stay in kneeling position<br>• Epicondylitis due to repetitive forceful work<br>• Meniscus lesions following extended periods of work in a kneeling or squatting position<br>• Carpal tunnel syndrome due to extended periods of repetitive forceful work, work involving vibration, extreme postures of the wrist, or a combination of the three |
| | d. Mental and behavioral disorders | Post-traumatic stress disorder |
| 3. | Occupational cancer | |
| 4. | Other diseases | Miners' nystagmus |

*Causes:* Silicosis is caused by exposure to crystalline silica, which originates from drilling, crushing, braking, grinding, hammering and sand blasting of earth's crust. Silica exists in nine different crystalline forms or polymorphs with the three main forms being quartz, which is by far the most common, tridymite and cristobalite. It also occurs in several cryptocrystalline forms. Multiple occupations such as mining, stone cutting, construction work, tunnel work, masonry, sand blasting, glass manufacturing, ceramics work, steel industry work, quarrying, etc. are associated with silicosis **(Fig. 29.8)**.

*Pathophysiology:* There are four pathological variants of silicosis namely—(1) simple (nodular) silicosis, (2) progressive massive fibrosis, (3) silico-proteinosis, and (4) diffuse interstitial fibrosis. Discrete hard nodules with upper-lobe predominance is usual finding in the gross pathological examination of the lung. Most frequent lymph nodes to enlarge are hilar and peribronchial. On microscopy, silicotic nodules can be seen in hilar lymph nodes and lung parenchyma. In progressive massive fibrosis, lung nodules become confluent, resulting in lesions of one cm or more in diameter.

*Clinical features:* Silicosis is a progressive interstitial lung disease. It does not produce symptoms itself. Depending on the progression, it can be acute, accelerated and chronic. If it progresses to progressive massive fibrosis, tuberculosis (TB), COPD, emphysema, chronic bronchitis or lung carcinoma, then exertional dyspnea and productive cough may develop due to lung function impairments. Systemic sign and symptoms such as clubbing, fever, weight loss, etc. should be attributed to lung cancer or TB until proven otherwise. Accelerated silicosis and chronic silicosis have similar kind of symptoms. In acute silicosis, patients may become disable within few months of exposure.

*Diagnosis:* Most common presentation is classic silicosis, which typically develops after 10–20 years of work exposure in dust-generating industries and during that time patient remains asymptomatic. The duration of exposure may be lower depending on the socioeconomic status and environmental conditions. So, a thorough and comprehensive occupational history of exposure is of utmost importance in the case of silicosis. After history, radiological features (X-ray chest or CT) are characteristic for diagnosis of silicosis **(Fig. 29.9)**. The typical plain chest X-ray appearances are similar to those of coal worker's pneumoconiosis, with a profusion of small nodules in the upper and mid zones.

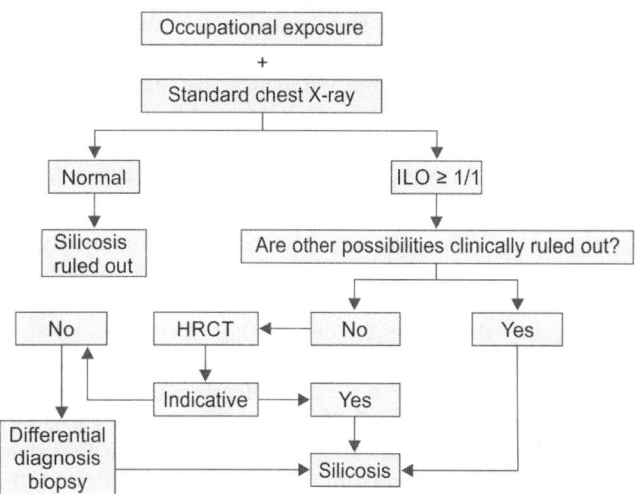

**Fig. 29.9:** Algorithm for diagnosis of silicosis.
(ILO: International labor Organization; HRCT: high-resolution computed tomography)

Hilar and mediastinal lymph node enlargement may be present **(Fig. 29.10)**. Lung biopsy is rarely required to distinguish silicosis (especially PMF) from lung cancer or TB.

*Management:* Silicosis is invariably progressive disease even after cessation of exposure, so regular assessment through detailed lung function tests and serial chest X-rays are required. There are no effective pharmacological treatments for silicosis. But it is 100% preventable disease with simple cost effective interventions of dust suppression and use of personal protective measures while working. The main challenge of eliminating silicosis in India is lack of preventive efforts especially in unorganized sectors of industry which do not fall under the Factory Act of India (1948). This Act mandates a well-ventilated working environment, provisions for protection from dust, reduction of overcrowding and provision of basic occupational healthcare.

Smoking cessation is important in silicosis patients, as silica is a carcinogen, so they are at greater risk of lung cancer. Silicosis also increases the risk of developing pulmonary TB, which is termed

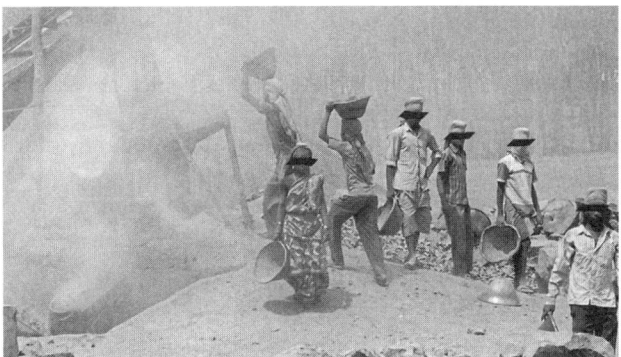

**Fig. 29.8:** Exposure to crystalline silica during working in stone mine.

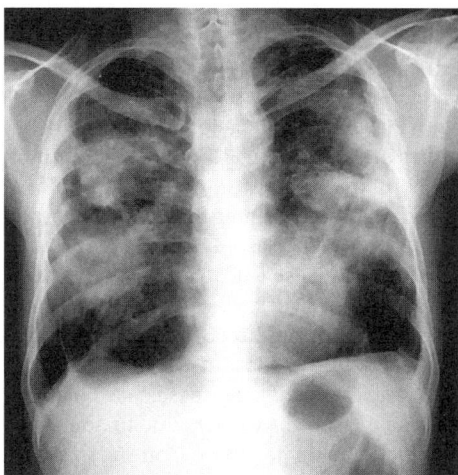

**Fig. 29.10:** Typical plain chest X-ray of silicosis patient (PA view).

silicotuberculosis. So, TB should also be thoroughly assessed for the silicosis patients where TB is endemic. This TB typically affects upper lobe of the lung and same is visible in chest X-rays. But it may be masked by silicosis. Other complications related to silicosis may be related to the development of connective tissue diseases such as systemic lupus erythematosus (SLE), scleroderma and glomerulonephritis.

***Compensation for silicosis:*** The National Human Rights Commission, India Commission recommended the offering of financial assistance to all those certified silicosis patients and to the next of the kins of the deceased of silicosis by the State Government. This amount varies State to State, e.g., a sum of rupees 2 lakhs is offered to certified silicosis patient and rupees 3 lakhs each to the next of the kins of the deceased of silicosis by the State Government of Rajasthan. Rajasthan is the first state to launch a policy on pneumoconiosis on 3rd October 2019 (NHRC, Intervention on Silicosis, 2016).

## Asbestosis

Asbestos, which are naturally occurring hydrated silicate fibers are used in variety of construction and insulation purposes due to their tensile strength and resilience. Based on their chemistry and fiber morphology asbestos minerals are divided into two groups: amphibole and serpentine. The amphibole group includes crocidolite, amosite, tremolite, actinolite, and anthophyllite asbestos. The serpentine group is comprised solely of chrysotile asbestos. Thus, there are a total of six types of asbestos minerals. The first case of asbestosis was detected in the early 1900s, and the term "asbestosis" was coined by Cooke in 1927.

***Epidemiology:*** According to WHO estimates, globally around 125 million people are exposed to asbestos at the workplace and at least 107,000 people die each year from occupational exposure to asbestos. In India, an estimated 100,000 people are exposed to asbestos at work. It was being mined in India at places such as Andhra Pradesh (Pulivendula), Jharkhand (Roro), Rajasthan (Ajmer, Bhilwara, Udaipur, Rajsamand). In 2011, India banned asbestos mining and asbestos waste. But it continues to trade in raw asbestos and asbestos-based products, commonly found in the roofs of houses, especially in poorer regions of the country.

***Causes:*** All the six types of asbestos minerals (chrysotile, amosite, crocidolite, tremolite, anthophyllite and actinolite) are carcinogenic **(Fig. 29.11)**. Inhalation and ingestion both are the primary routes of exposure to asbestos. Inhalation of asbestos fibers from contaminated air in the working place, or from ambient air in housing containing friable asbestos materials are major kinds of exposures to asbestos. Damage to buildings due to natural disasters can also lead to asbestos exposure. Soil and water (both ground and surface) can also be contaminated by asbestos from natural and anthropogenic sources such as human made chances in nature, disposal of asbestos containing wastes in landfill, etc. Asbestos related diseases have been reported in family members of asbestos workers due to domestic exposure of fibers carried home on hair or on clothing by workers. Dose, duration of exposure, size, shape, and chemical composition of asbestos fibers, source of the exposure and individual risk factors

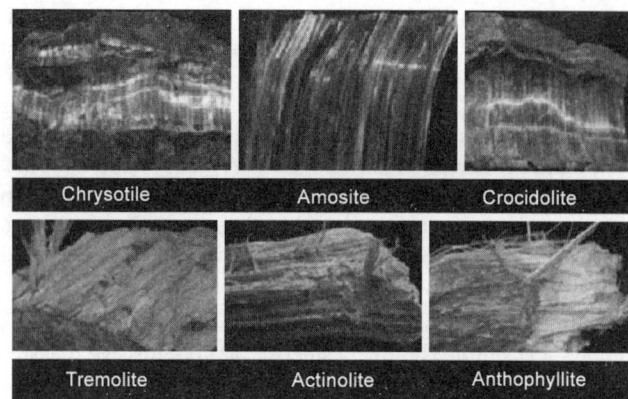

**Fig. 29.11:** Six types of asbestos fibers.

such as smoking and pre-existing lung disease are the factors which affect the risk of developing asbestos related diseases.

***Clinical features:*** Asbestos exposure can lead to fibrosis of the lungs, pleural plaques, pleural effusion and thickening of pleura. It can directly cause four distinct malignancies viz; mesothelioma, lung carcinoma, ovarian cancer and laryngeal cancer. Other cancers which may be associated with asbestos exposure include esophageal cancer, gallbladder cancer, kidney cancer and throat cancer. The symptoms of asbestos related diseases may be apparent after many decades of exposure, such as:

- Shortness of breath, wheezing, or hoarseness
- Persistence of cough, which gets worse over time
- Blood in sputum
- Pain or tightening in the chest
- Swelling of the neck or face
- Difficulty in swallowing
- Weight loss
- Loss of appetite
- Fatigue and anemia

The disease is progressive even after removal of the exposure. In advanced stage clubbing of fingernails, distress, and cyanosis may also develop.

***Diagnosis:*** Similar to silicosis, a thorough and comprehensive occupational history of exposure is of utmost importance. A thorough physical examination is recommended for diagnosis with the following tests.

- *Lung function test:* Reduced vital capacity and forced expiratory volume
- *Sputum examination:* Asbestos bodies (which are asbestos fibers coated with fibrin)
- *Chest X-ray:* A ground glass appearance in the lower two thirds of the lung fields **(Fig. 29.12)**
- *Ultrasonography of lungs:* For pleural effusions and evaluating pleural thickening
- CT scan of lungs
- Bronchoscopy
- Lung biopsy

***Management:*** There is no specific therapy for asbestos related diseases. Withdrawal from further exposure and cessation of

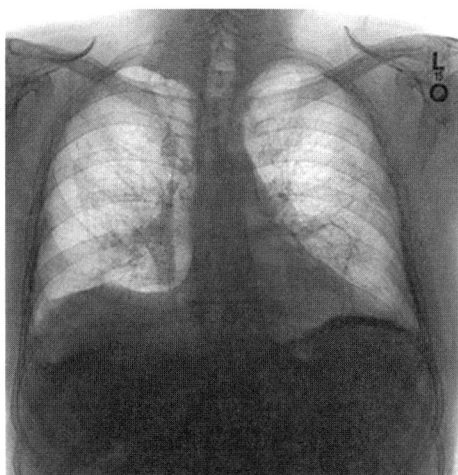

**Fig. 29.12:** Chest radiograph illustrating parenchymal abnormalities in asbestosis.

smoking are recommended measures. WHO has recommended following public health action:
- Most efficient way is to stop the use of all types of asbestos
- Replacing asbestos with safer substitutes
- Taking measures to prevent exposure to asbestos in workplace such as dust control measures, use of breathing protection measures, protective gloves, protective clothing, safety goggles, rotation of workstation for the employees, good ventilation facilities at workplace, avoiding eating and drinking during work.
- Improve methods of early diagnosis, treatment, and rehabilitation including periodic medical examination of employees, vaccination against influenza and pneumococcal pneumonia, antimicrobial therapy for respiratory infections and the use of oxygen, if necessary, surgery, radiotherapy, and chemotherapy may be considered in cancer cases.
- Establishing registries and organizing medical surveillance for lung cancer, mesothelioma and other asbestos related diseases of exposed workers.
- Raising awareness about the hazards associated with asbestos and asbestos related diseases
- Encourage healthy lifestyle among workers.

## Anthracosis

Anthracosis is the milder type of pneumoconiosis which is usually asymptomatic. It is caused by the accumulation of carbon in the lungs. Repeated exposure to air pollution or inhalation of smoke or coal dust particles can lead to this accumulation of carbon. It is caused by occupational exposures to carbon, silica, and quartz particles, which are deposited in the macrophages, mucosa, and submucosa and causes bronchial anthracosis.

Anthracosis usually presents with symptoms very similar to COPD, except for the history of smoking. Most common symptoms are cough and dyspnea. Association of TB may add onset of weight loss or fever. On auscultation wheezing usually appears and less frequently rales or decreased breath sounds. It may also present with complications of enlarged mediastinal lymph nodes such as vocal cord paralysis or broncholithiasis.

Diagnosis can be confirmed with bronchoscopy, X-ray lung and CT scan. Empirical treatment includes bronchodilators, corticosteroids and antibiotics.

### Farmer's Lung Disease

Farmer's lung disease (FLD) is the most prevalent form of hypersensitivity pneumonitis. This was first described by Campbell in 1932. It is considered as a significant cause of morbidity among farmers in some countries. It is caused by the inhalation of microorganisms (most commonly the bacteria thermophilic actinomycetes) from hay and the dust from grain or straw stored in very damp conditions with high levels of humidity and at temperatures of between 40 and 60°C. Besides that, this disease is influenced by many other factors such as climatic conditions, geographical locations, local customs and practices, and intensity of exposure to antigens.

Farmer's lung disease causes three kinds of hypersensitivity reactions; (1) acute, (2) subacute and (3) chronic. An acute attack is an intense reaction which develops within 4–8 hours of exposure to antigen. The common symptoms are dry irritating cough, fever and chills, fast breathing, tachycardia and shortness of breath. A subacute attack is less intense and takes lone time to develop symptoms than an acute attack. The common symptoms are muscle ache, joint pain, cough, mild fever with chills, loss of appetite, shortness of breath and weight loss. These symptoms of acute and subacute FLD can be misdiagnosed with flu. Chronic attack follows many repeated acute attacks and represents the stage of permanent lung damage. Common symptoms are persistent cough, depression, body ache, joint pain, fever, night sweat, shortness of breath, loss of appetite, weight loss and weakness. These symptoms of FLD get worse in winter season.

Like other interstitial pulmonary diseases, the diagnosis can be made based on clinical suspicion, backed up by a detailed history of workplace and environmental exposure, clinical symptoms, pulmonary function tests, radiological findings (X-ray and CT), cytological evidence on bronchoalveolar lavage (BAL), and consistent pathology results.

The treatment of FLD is based mainly on prevention part by avoiding exposure to the antigen by withdrawal of the patient from the farming environment. Development and implementation of new techniques for drying the hay, and ventilation and mechanization of stock feeding is another way of prevention of FLD. Besides that, respiratory protective equipment should also be used to avoid exposure. In acute forms treatment with glucocorticosteroids accelerates recovery. Lung transplantation is indicated in case of progressive disease with respiratory failure.

### Byssinosis

It is an occupational lung disease which affects workers in cotton processing, hemp or flax industries. These raw cotton and other textile materials have biological materials that trigger allergic reactions in the body. This is also known by other names such as Monday fever, brown lung disease, mill fever or cotton workers' lung. Because it causes breathing difficulty (like asthma) in the initial part of the week and improves as the work-week progresses or dust exposure stops. Cough, difficulty in breathing and chest tightness are common symptoms of the disease. In severe cases, patient may experience flu-like symptoms, such as fever, shivering, muscle ache, joint pain, tiredness along with a dry cough. Prolonged exposure may cause lung damage that resembles irreversible COPD. The diagnosis is made based on the history of work exposure and suggestive symptoms. If early diagnosis is made and exposure to cotton dust is stopped, most people will not develop permanent lung damage and symptoms may also reverse.

### *Bagassosis*

Bagassosis is also a form of hypersensitivity pneumonitis, which is caused due to inhalation of sugarcane fiber waste (called bagasse). It is believed that a fungus is possibly involved in development of Bagassosis. Shortness of breath, cough, hemoptysis and low-grade fever are the common symptoms of the disease. The disease may also lead to diffuse bronchiolitis. Diagnosis is made based on occupational history and chest X-ray, which shows mottling of lungs or shadows. Dust control measures with good ventilation at workplace, use of facemask and periodic medical examinations of employees who are at risk for exposure are the preventive measures for the disease. Addition of propionic acid to sugar cane waste also reduces the exposure.

## Occupational Dermatitis

Dermatitis or eczema is an inflammation of the skin. Occupational dermatitis is a type of contact dermatitis, which occurs due to contact with certain substances at the workplace. There are two types of contact dermatitis which can occur due to occupational exposure, contact irritant dermatitis and allergic contact dermatitis (ACD). Usually, the majority (80%) of the cases are of contact irritant dermatitis, and only 20% of the cases are of allergic type.

### *Irritant Contact Dermatitis*

In contact irritant dermatitis, the substance which irritates the skin and is responsible for development of dermatitis is called irritant, or corrosive if it is highly irritant. Irritant dermatitis is analogs to chemical burn, as it acts by eroding or burning the outer protective layers of the skin. If it is a strong acid or alkali substance, then corrosion will occur early. If the irritant concentration is very high, the damage will be more. If duration of exposure is long or if it is a repeated exposure, the effect will be more. If a person is more susceptible such as childhood allergy, dry skin, very fair complexion, etc. then the irritant will affect early. To develop irritant contact dermatitis (ICD), direct exposure is required. So, it usually occurs on hands, forearm and face. Acute ICD is manifested by red, swollen, itchy, painful and ulcerated skin. While chronic ICD is characterized by eczematous skin eruption, erythema, dryness, cracking and fissuring of the skin. It mainly involves the back of the hands including the fingers and the finger webs and subsequent involvement of the palm.

### *Allergic Contact Dermatitis*

As name suggests, the worker becomes sensitized and develop allergic reaction to certain substance used in his occupation. It is a kind of type IV or delayed hypersensitivity. This development of allergy is a gradual process, and the duration of exposure may vary from days to years. A few substances are very allergic in nature and called sensitizers. If there is repeated exposure, the chances of developing allergies are more. Person having history of allergy to some other substances are less vulnerable, while individuals who do not have any kind of allergy are more sensitive to develop ACD. Unlike contact irritant dermatitis it is not dose related. Once the person becomes sensitized, it remains for the whole life. Most common sensitizers are chromates (in cement), nickel (in artificial jewellery), formaldehyde, epoxy resins, wood dust, flour, adhesives and printing chemicals.

A worker can be exposed to both irritants and sensitizers at a time and can develop both irritant and ACD simultaneously. In a usual sequence irritant dermatitis develops first and leaves the skin exposed to sensitizers and irritants simultaneously. But the reverse also happens sometimes. ACD is characterized by redness, itching and scaling of the skin at the site of the contact, but very frequently involvement of the eyelids occurs.

### *Management*

Prevention is the key to managing contact dermatitis. It includes the following:
- *Primary prevention:* It aims to isolate potential irritants or allergens. Local and general ventilation may be sufficient if skin exposure occurs through air in the form of particulate dust or vapor. Protective clothing such as gloves, boots and aprons are also helpful. Many water-resistant (contain hydrophobic substance such as silicone) and oil resistant barrier creams can also be used which can protect against water soluble substances such as acids, alkali, dye and oil solvent substances such as dust, oils and greases, respectively. Personal hygiene in reference to washing hands with mild soap and water is also of utmost importance. Eating, drinking and smoking at the workplace should also be completely prohibited. Certain changes in work practices in the form of covering the work surface with absorbent sheets, cleaning the work surface with industrial cleaner and sweeping or vacuuming of dust and particulate matter also help. Promoting awareness about exposure to allergens, recognition of early symptoms and signs through health education and both employee and employer motivation to use preventive measures also have tremendous beneficial effects.
- *Secondary prevention:* Diagnosis of occupational dermatitis obtaining the detailed work exposure history and clinical examination of the patient is of paramount importance. Patch tests with a standard tray and a special environmental allergen will verify the allergic components of occupational dermatitis and can form the basis for prevention through

screening. Workplace provocation test can be carried out if the patch test is still negative and ACD is suspected. The treatment of occupational dermatitis depends on its stage. The acute phase is best treated with steroids (topical or systemic) and an antihistamine. Surgical debridement and skin grafting may be needed in very rare cases specifically when big ulcers develop. The chronic phase can be managed by moisturizing creams along with topical steroids. Antibiotics may be required sometimes if there is evidence of secondary infection.

- *Tertiary prevention:* Assessment of skin impairment and disability should be carried out. Rehabilitation efforts are required to restore the economic and vocational usefulness of the affected worker. The worker may also be supported in receiving compensation and disability benefits after establishing occupational causation.

## Occupational Cancers

Occupational cancers are caused by exposure to carcinogens at workplace. Some of the carcinogens, which are known include chemical carcinogens (e.g., benzene), viruses (e.g., hepatitis B), hormones (e.g., estrogens), natural minerals (e.g., asbestos), alcohol and radiation (e.g., ultraviolet radiation). It is a very complicated process to identify and classify the carcinogens. International Agency for Research on Cancer (IARC), an agency of the World Health Organization, has published the most authoritative lists of carcinogens **(Table 29.3)**.

The latest global data released by the ILO (based on information from 2010 to 2011) indicate that some 666,000 fatal work-related cancers occur every year. These estimates also varies with the type of cancer. The most common types of cancer due to occupational exposure are lung cancer, bladder cancer and mesothelioma.

### Lung Cancer

Lung cancers contribute 54–75% of all occupational cancers. As per IARC, Agents classified as known Group 1 lung carcinogens are listed in **Table 29.4**.

**Table 29.3:** Agents classified by the IARC monographs, Volumes 1–122.

| Group 1 | Carcinogenic to humans | Sufficient evidence of carcinogenicity in humans and in experimental animals | 120 agents |
|---|---|---|---|
| Group 2A | Probably carcinogenic to humans | Limited evidence of carcinogenicity in humans and sufficient evidence of carcinogenicity in experimental animals | 82 |
| Group 2B | Possibly carcinogenic to humans | Limited evidence of carcinogenicity in humans and less than sufficient evidence of carcinogenicity in experimental animals | 302 |
| Group 3 | Not classifiable as to its carcinogenicity to humans | Inadequate evidence of carcinogenicity in humans and in experimental animals | 501 |
| Group 4 | Probably not carcinogenic to humans | Evidence suggesting lack of carcinogenicity in humans and in experimental animals | 1 |

(IARC: International Agency for Research on Cancer)

**Table 29.4:** Group 1 IARC carcinogens with sufficient evidence of causing lung cancer in humans.

| S. No. | Agent category | Agents |
|---|---|---|
| 1. | Ionizing radiation-all types | |
| 2. | Chemicals and mixtures | Ether, coal-tar pitch, soot, sulfur mustard, diesel exhausts |
| 3. | Occupations | Aluminum production, coal gasification, coke production, hematite mining (underground), iron and steel founding, painting, rubber production industry |
| 4. | Metals | Arsenic, beryllium, cadmium, chromium, nickel |
| 5. | Dust and fibers | Asbestos and silica dust |
| 6. | Personal habits | Indoor emissions from household combustion Tobacco smoke |
| 7. | Other exposures | MOPP (vincristine-prednisone-nitrogen mustard-procarbazine mixture) |

(IARC: International Agency for Research on Cancer)

For most of the carcinogenic agents responsible for the development of lung carcinoma, a dose-response relationship between cumulative exposure and the risk for lung cancer has been estimated. Besides that, there is usually a lag period of 10–30 years from initial exposure to the time point when relative risk increases to statistical significance level.

### Bladder Cancer

Bladder carcinoma is the tenth most common cancer globally, and occupational exposure has been identified as the important risk factor for the development of bladder cancer second to smoking. As per the estimates, around 20% of all bladder cancers in industrialized countries are due to occupational exposure. Several occupational carcinogens have been found associated with increased risk of bladder carcinoma **(Table 29.5)**.

**Table 29.5:** Group 1 IARC carcinogens with sufficient evidence of causing bladder cancer in humans.

| Urinary bladder | • Aluminum, arsenic, auramine, magenta<br>• 4-aminobiphenyl, benzidine, chlornaphazine, cyclophosphamide, 2-naphthylamine, ortho-toluidine<br>• Painting, rubber production industry<br>• Tobacco smoking, X-radiation, gamma-radiation |
|---|---|

(IARC: International Agency for Research on Cancer)

### Mesothelioma

Mesothelioma is a very aggressive kind of malignancy, which affects the pleura, peritoneum, and sometimes pericardium. In 1950 it was found to be linked with occupational exposure of asbestos and classified as occupational disease. Mesothelioma has a long latency period (up to 40 years and has very poor prognosis, as most patients die within 1 year of diagnosis). It is mostly associated with exposure to the amphibole family of asbestos. So far, other than asbestos exposure no connection has been scientifically proved between mesothelioma and any other occupational exposure like air pollution.

### Leukemia

Leukemia is a malignant transformation of hematopoietic cells, which produces abnormal leukemic cells, which in turn suppresses the production of normal blood cells. It has varied clinical presentations, prognosis and response to treatment. Exposure to ionizing radiation, benzene and alkylating agents have been substantiated as the only hazards for leukemia. In the early 20th century, an association between ionizing radiation and leukemia was assumed, due to uncontrolled exposure of medical personnel and patients to the radiations, used for diagnostic and therapeutic purposes. After radiation exposure, Benzene is considered as the second most documented risk factor for leukemia. Other than Benzene, Cytostatic drugs, especially chemotherapeutic regimens which contain alkylating agents such as Busulfan, Cyclophosphamide, Chlorambucil, etc. are another documented risk factor for developing leukemia. Workers may expose to these cytostatic drugs at any level starting from production, transportation, distribution, preparation and administration to patients.

### Skin Cancers

The London surgeon Sir Percival Pott observed the occurrence of squamous cell carcinoma of the scrotum among chimney sweepers and first time highlighted the link between occupational exposure and skin cancer in 1775. Exposure to the products of distilling tar and pitch, which are also responsible for occupational skin cancers, was increased with time due to industrial revolution. The association between skin cancers and ionizing radiation was recognized in the early 20th century, when frequent occurrence of skin cancers were observed on the hands of doctors and technicians who were exposed to X-rays.

### Prevention of Occupational Cancers (Table 29.6)

At present, scrotal cancer caused by PAHs, liver cancer caused by vinyl chloride, nasal cancer caused by nickel or wood dust, bladder cancer caused by aromatic amines and leukemia caused by exposure to benzene, have practically disappeared from developed countries due to adoption of preventive measures. Even lung cancer and mesothelioma caused by asbestos are gradually decreasing in countries where early and appropriate measures are taken. The prevention of occupational cancer is specific because it mainly relies on legislative efforts, since the population at risk can be relatively easily identified.

### Occupational Injuries and Accidents

Occupational injury can be defined as any personal injury, disease or death resulting from an occupational accident. These occupational accidents are unexpected and unplanned incidences, including acts of violence arising out of or in connection with occupation, which may also include training or traveling as a requirement of the occupation. Injuries at the workplace can be considered as proxy indicator of inadequate working environment. These injuries impose large damages to the active manpower of our society and annually a significant amount of money is spent to compensate those work-related injuries, diseases, and disabilities. Occupational injuries are the leading cause of death of workers at age up to 37 years, and are in third place in the total population. As per the global estimates of fatal occupational injuries, the mean rate of fatal occupational accidents worldwide is 14 per 100,000 employees in a year. The maximum rate (23.1) has been recorded in Asia.

**Table 29.6:** Hierarchy of preventive measures.

| Implementation step | Suggested interventions |
|---|---|
| Step 1 Core | • Develop regulatory and enforcement control of carcinogens<br>• Avoid introducing known carcinogens to the workplaces |
| Step 2 Expanded | • Monitor and reduce occupational exposure to carcinogens<br>• Organize health surveillance of exposed workers |
| Step 3 Desired | • Develop comprehensive worker's health programs based on primary prevention to improve working and living conditions<br>• Substitute carcinogens with less dangerous substances |

Following are different types of occupational injuries:
- Superficial injuries and open wounds
- Fractures
- Dislocations, sprains and strains
- Traumatic amputations
- Concussion and internal injuries
- Burns, corrosions, scalds and frostbite
- Acute poisonings and infections
- Other specified types of injuries such as effects of radiation, effects of heat and light, hypothermia, effects of air pressure and water pressure, drowning and nonfatal submersion, effects of noise and vibration, etc.

There are multiple risk factors which are responsible/contribute for occupational accidents and injuries as:
- Extreme age groups (young age and old age) workers are more susceptible.
- Males are more prone for injuries as compared to females.
- Lower educational status and poor safety training are associated with more incidences of injuries.
- Workers with less than 6 months of experience showed higher relative risk compared with workers who have job tenure of more than 2 years.
- A positive association has been observed between smoking and occupational injuries.
- Alcohol consumption increases the risk of work accidents.
- Accidents are less in morning hours and gradually the rate increases as the fatigue sets in.
- Psychological factors such as overconfidence, carelessness, too fast working, etc. increase the risk.
- Permanent workers are less susceptible to occupational injuries than temporary workers.
- *Job stress:* Demanding high physical and mental workloads increases the risk.
- Not using or improper use of protective equipment also increases the risk of occupational injuries.
- Hazardous worksite conditions (e.g., loud noise, extreme temperatures, vibration).

- Associated comorbidities such as chronic heart disease, diabetes, depression or other health problems.
- Certain occupations such as construction, agriculture, manufacturing, hunting and forestry, etc.

### *Prevention of Occupational Injuries and Accidents*

Recognizing the risk factors is of utmost importance to plan, develop, implement and evaluate safety regulations to reduce the incidence of occupational injuries. Implementation of occupational health and safety management system in the workplace are some of the protective factors for prevention of occupational injuries. The traditional public health approaches to prevent the occupational injuries includes following phases:
- ***Surveillance:*** Identify and prioritize problems through injury surveillance
- ***Risk factor identification:*** Quantify and prioritize risk factors through analytic injury research
- ***Intervention development and evaluation:*** Identify existing or develop new strategies to prevent occupational injuries, including evaluation and confirmation of effectiveness
- ***Implementation:*** Of the most effective injury control measures through dissemination and technology transfer
- ***Monitoring and evaluation:*** Evaluate and monitor the results of intervention efforts.

In a crude sense, implement the measures of technical protection, provide a technically perfect equipment and tools, provide optimal illumination, protection against noise, customize job environment to its purpose, protective clothes, and optimization of microclimate are necessary at the workplaces for prevention of occupational accidents and injuries.

## Occupational Burnout and Stress

Occupational stress is considered as a mental and physical response/reaction, which generates due to interaction of an individual with his working environment, and due to mismatch between work needs with his abilities and demands. Stress is not a disorder, and it usually happens in all kinds of jobs with special emphasis on jobs which deal with human health. As a typical phenomenon, stress is a starting phase of burnout. Burnout is nothing but adding up of the stress with time. Thus, burnout cannot develop without stress, but the other way round is possible. Burnout is considered as a disorder which has significant effect on physical and psychosocial well-being of the worker. Similarly, depression, which is also a psychological stress, may sometimes overlap with burnout. However, burnout is apparently work related, whereas depression is more multifactorial in origin and pervasive in nature. But burnout is one of the strongest predictors of depression. These days, occupational burnout is a common problem among all the occupational settings and especially in healthcare settings, and based on the available data, one in every seven person suffer with occupational burnout at the end of the day.

### *Difference between Stress and Burnout (Table 29.7)*

**Table 29.7:** Difference between stress and burnout.

| Stress | Burnout |
|---|---|
| Worker put too much effort | Little or no input/effort |
| Experience emotions more strongly | Experience flattening of emotions |
| Causes hyperactivity | Causes a helpless feeling |
| Have less energy | Have less motivation and hope |
| Can lead to anxiety | Can lead to depression |
| Mostly physical consequences | Mostly emotional consequences |
| Higher chances of early death | Higher chances of early hopelessness |

### *Prevention of Occupational Stress and Burnout*

Prevention and management of occupational stress begins at the level of organization. An organization which is committed to protecting its workers in reasonable and appropriate ways, is actually investing in the future. It is important because it aims towards changing the environment and thus addresses the workplace stressors and risk factors. There are several tools to reduce stress at workplace such as cognitive behavioral intervention (CBI), relaxation and meditation techniques, and communication trainings.

Beside the efforts from the organization side, there are requirements of supplemental efforts at individual level, because occupational stress has different impacts throughout a working population. Preventive stress management at individual level can be of following three types:
1. ***Primary prevention*** is stressor directed and aims at alleviating the sources of stress. It works by helping individuals to manage personal perceptions of stress, promote her/his personal work environment, and maintain work-life balance. The leading tool for primary prevention is good social support.
2. ***Secondary prevention*** is response directed and aims to alter the responsibility to inevitable stress. It works by helping individuals to regulate stress-induced energy, emotions, and physical fitness. Physical fitness programs and activities have widely come up in occupational settings to employees to prevent distress.
3. ***Tertiary prevention*** is symptom directed and help in alleviating any suffering that may arise. It focuses on treatment therapies and counseling interventions to restore physical mental and emotional health and function.

## ERGONOMICS

Ergonomics is considered as "the scientific study of human work and the application of this scientific information to the design of objects, systems, and environments concerning human beings". In the field of occupational health, this can be easily understood as the implementation of multiple scientific measures to improve the compatibility between employee and its workplace. These measures are designed considering the potential of the worker and restrictions within the workplace environment, so that, safety and workers related parameters (such as comfort, job satisfaction, efficiency, productivity, quality, personal development, etc.) can be significantly restored.

Ergonomics is not limited to examining only the passive ambient situation at workplace, but also encourages the employee to make the best use of his or her abilities. All the ergonomic-related changes are recommended after evaluating the type of work and the demands on the worker. Ergonomics allows designing of appropriate workplace layout; enablement of healthy work culture (by addressing issues of workload management and manpower shortage); reduction in job related psychological stress; minimizing medication errors; enhancing safety of patients; and marketing of medicinal commodities. In the modern era, this science is primarily used to negate work related stressors (such as abnormal postures, poor workstation designs, forceful extension of joints, etc.), which increases the risk of multiple musculoskeletal disorders.

Good posture at workplace is illustrated in **Figures 29.13 and 29.14.**

The Indian Society of Ergonomics is the only professional body representing ergonomics/human factors in India. It is affiliated to the International Ergonomics Association (IEA) and nominates members to its committees. It was established in 1983 with the objective to promote and enhance ergonomics and allied studies, research and training particularly in India, for the benefit of the people at work, to improve their welfare and quality of life.

# ANATOMICAL, PHYSIOLOGICAL, PSYCHOLOGICAL-BASED PREVENTION AND CONTROL OF OCCUPATIONAL MORBIDITIES, AND MORTALITIES

The intervention can be clinical (e.g., clinical examinations) as well as nonclinical (e.g., workplace risk assessment). The interventions can be categorized as preventive and therapeutic interventions. Preventive intervention is further divided into primary, secondary and tertiary prevention. In occupational health, primary preventive interventions involve exposure prevention and specific protection by vaccination.

The basic strategies for controlling injury and occupational diseases in decreasing order.
- Substitute more hazardous materials/processes with less hazardous materials/processes
- Engineering controls to separate workers from hazards
- Administrative controls to minimize contact with hazards (uncontrollable by engineering)
- Using personal protective equipment.

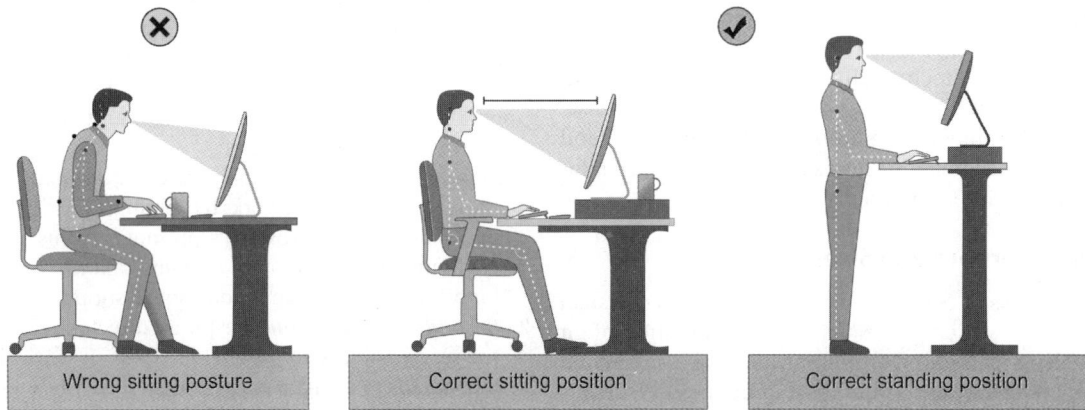

**Fig. 29.13:** Designing of appropriate workplace layout.

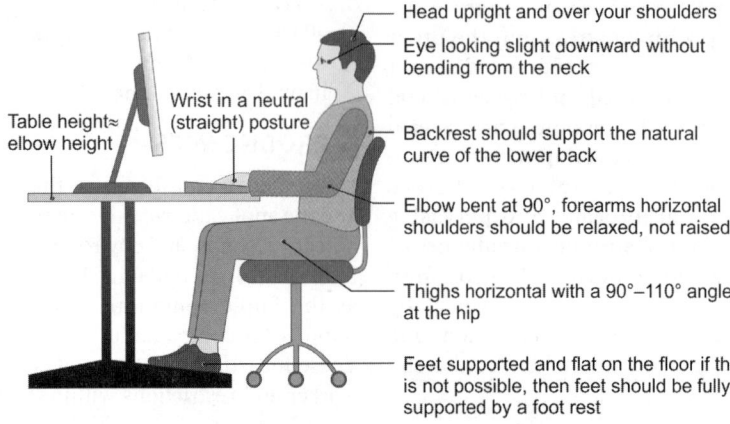

**Fig. 29.14:** Good sitting posture.

## Strategies to Improve Working Conditions

Broadly, interventional strategies to reduce occupational morbidities and mortalities can be applied at international, national, workplace, and individual level.

### International Interventions

ILO-WHO Joint Committee on Occupational Health has recommended the following priorities to ILO and WHO regarding international occupational health issues.
- Guide and support national occupational safety and health programs
- Enhance regional collaboration and coordination
- Coordinate and enhance information and educational programs and materials
- Provide awareness-raising activities and instruments through campaigns, events, and special days.

### National/Government Interventions

As a regulatory framework, development and implementation of laws and rules for workplace, and their dissemination and enforcement are major role the government can play for prevention and control of occupational morbidities and mortalities. The strict monitoring of implementation at the workplace is also an essential part in which government can support. Compensation regulations for workers and stipulations in regard to the number of employees to be engaged in a particular occupation are other forms of government intervention which may indirectly improve the working conditions.

### Workplace-based Interventions

Substitution of more hazardous materials (e.g., asbestosis) and processes with less hazardous ones, increasing awareness through trainings, behavior change communications, etc. are some of the examples of workplace-based interventions. Training and awareness generation activities are the ones with no compelling economic hindrance. Even elementary knowledge of employer and workers about risks and their prevention measures is beneficial.

### Individual Interventions

The general principle is that most public health interventions are more effective when they are applied at an organizational level rather than individual level. This holds true for workplace interventions also. Maintaining personal hygiene and vaccination are strategies to be managed at individual level. Healthcare workers should receive influenza and Hepatitis-B vaccination regularly when taking care of patients. Employees should adopt a healthy lifestyle by taking adequate rest, balanced diet, regular exercises, using self- relaxation techniques and abstaining from smoking and alcohol.

## Healthy Workplace Concept

In an average day, a person spends more of his time in working than any other routine activity. So, the workplace becomes an important setting to protect and promote health. It is the responsibility of industries to promote worker's health and foster healthy workplaces to protect health through various measures including providing safe and hazard-free work environments. The concept of healthy workplace is an old concept, which has improved with time, starting from an exclusive focus on occupational safety (protection from physical, chemical, biological, and ergonomic hazards) to include the factors which profoundly influence worker health such as organization, culture, lifestyle and the community at workplace.

WHO Regional Office for the Western Pacific defines a healthy workplace as *"A healthy workplace is a place where everyone works together to achieve an agreed vision for the health and well-being of workers and the surrounding community. It provides all members of the workforce with physical, psychological, social and organizational conditions that protect and promote health and safety. It enables managers and workers to increase control over their own health and to improve it, and to become more energetic, positive and contented."*

There are four arenas in which actions towards a healthy workplace can best be taken (**Fig. 29.15**).

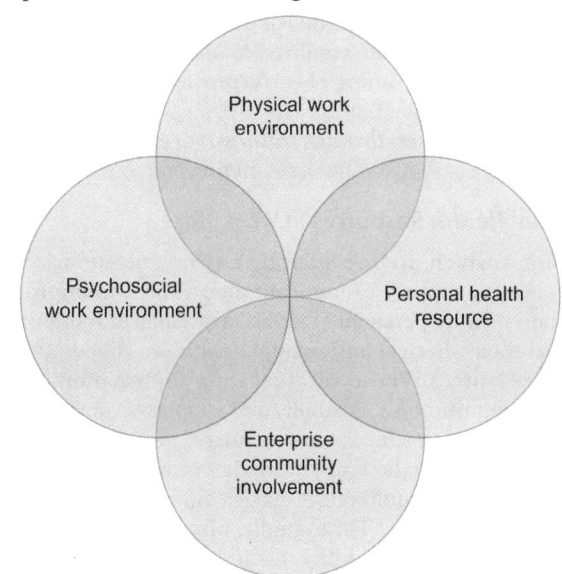

Fig. 29.15: Avenues of influence for a healthy workplace.

### Physical Work Environment

Hazards in physical work environment typically have the maximum potential to harm the workers, so, the occupational health and safety laws and codes primarily focus on these factors. These hazards must be identified and controlled through following hierarchy of control processes which influence the physical work environment.
- ***Elimination of harmful agents/hazards:*** For example, prohibiting asbestos use or use of asbestos insulation material
- ***Substitution of harmful agents:*** For example, benzene can be replaced with toluene or another less toxic chemical
- Engineering controls such as wet drilling of stones, installing noise buffers, isolating infectious patients, setting up local exhaust ventilation

- **Administrative controls:** For example, formulation, provision and monitoring of safety management system and guidelines, regular repair and maintenance of assisting devices, job rotation and appropriate rest break, provision of information and training, formulating contingency plan, etc.
- **Use of personal protective equipment:** For example, masks, gloves
- **Environmental monitoring:** Regular monitoring of noise level at workplace, taking air and water samples regularly to assess the quality of air and water.

### Psychosocial Work Environment

Culture, ethics, values, beliefs and attitudes of organization makes the psychosocial work environment for worker. Following are examples to control hazards which influence psychosocial work environment:

- **Eliminate or modify at the source:** For example, reallocation of the work to reduce workload, train supervisors in leadership and communication skills, zero tolerance policy for workplace discrimination and harassment.
- **Lessen impact on workers:** For example, allowing flexibility to deal with work/life conflict situations, allow flexibility in the location and timing of work, provide timely, open, and honest communication.
- **Raising awareness through trainins:** For example, awareness regarding conflict and harassment prevention.

### Personal Health Resources in Workplace

Resources which are provided by any organization to their employees to support or motivate their efforts, to improve or maintain healthy personal lifestyles, as well as to monitor and support their physical and mental health are called personal health resources. These resources are information, health services, opportunities, flexibility and supportive environment. These personal resources are required to create a healthy workplace because lack of knowledge of workers synergizes with employment conditions to make it difficult to adopt healthy lifestyle by any worker. For example, physical inactivity due to long working hours, poor diet due to lack of access to healthy meals at work, smoking at workplace, undiagnosed or untreated illness due to lack of accessible and affordable healthcare, high levels of HIV infections among workers due to lack of knowledge for prevention of HIV/AIDS, etc. Personal health resources at the workplace can be enhanced by providing appropriate information and trainings, medical services, policy and financial supports and other facilities to promote healthy lifestyle.

### Enterprise Community Involvement

Enterprise community involvement refers to the activities by any enterprise in such a way that it goes above and beyond its day-to-day offerings for a community in which it operates. The spouses, children and other family members of the workers also share the common exposures and adverse conditions including noise, chemicals, and biohazards with workers due to existence of their residences in the same community where industries exist. Poisoning due to pesticides and other harmful chemicals, and exposure to carcinogens and neurotoxins due to pollution of drinking water and air, are some of the examples of these kinds of nonoccupational exposures. So, besides having engineering and environmental solutions, there is need to extend the efforts to provide accessible and affordable quality healthcare to families of the workers. The enterprise may choose to provide support and resources in following ways:

- Provide clean air and water to the community by controlling air and water pollution due to industrial byproducts
- Initiate and support screening programs for communicable and noncommunicable diseases
- Extending accessible and affordable healthcare to the family members of the workers through supporting the establishment of healthcare facilities in the community
- Instituting and ensuring gender equality policies at the workplace to protect and support women employees
- Provide free or affordable elementary education to workers and their family members
- Provide subsidized public transportation to workers and help in building good roads, sidewalks, etc.

## Medical Examinations

Following are the major objectives of medical examinations:

- To detect early abnormalities and prevent workers from developing occupational diseases
- To verify the effectiveness of existing preventive strategies
- To provide occupational health education and advice to workers.

### Pre-employment/Pre-placement Medical Examinations

There are two main purposes of pre-employment medical examinations:

1. To provide base-line health data against which subsequent changes after employment can be evaluated
2. To ensure medical fitness of work

### Periodic Medical Examinations

Periodic medical examinations aim to detect susceptible workers for whom corrective actions are required before they develop overt occupational diseases. For example, a lead worker with a high blood lead level should be suspended from work temporarily to stop further exposure to lead and to receive necessary medical treatment. Meanwhile, safety and health measures at work should be reviewed for necessary remedial actions. The frequency of periodic medical examinations depends on the nature of the occupational hazards. For most hazardous exposures, these examinations are conducted annually. Law stipulates that employee engaged in mines, quarries, compressed air conditions, radiation exposure conditions should undergo pre-employment and periodic medical examinations including X-rays and blood tests.

# SURVEILLANCE AND REPORTING

Occupational diseases surveillance and reporting requires systematic monitoring of health events among workers to prevent and control occupational hazards and their associated diseases and injuries. This surveillance has the following four essential components.

1. Gather information on cases of occupational diseases and injuries.
2. Clean and analyze the data.
3. Disseminate the results to workers, employers, governmental agencies and the public.
4. Intervene based on data to alter the factors that produced these health events.

Surveillance commonly refers to two broad sets of activities in occupational health. Public health surveillance and medical surveillance. *Public health surveillance* refers to activities undertaken by central, state or local governments within their respective jurisdictions to monitor and to follow up on occupational diseases and injuries. This type of surveillance is based on the working population. The recorded events are suspected or established diagnoses of occupational illness and injury. *Medical surveillance* refers to the application of medical laboratory tests and procedures to individual workers who is at risk for occupational morbidity, to determine whether an occupational disorder may be present. Medical surveillance is generally broad in scope and represents the first step in ascertaining the presence of a work-related problem.

Strategies for surveillance and reporting is usually limited to recording of acute injuries at workplace even for industrialized countries. Unfortunately, it is in incomplete form in developing nations. This component is usually ignored unless it is required by law or by a parent company (for multinational companies). Lack of reporting affects workers' compensation for accidents and injuries.

# CURRENT APPROACHES IN HEALTHCARE SERVICES

## International Labour Organization

The International Labour Organization was established in 1919. ILO is the tripartite UN agency which brings together governments, employers and workers of 187 member States, to set labor standards, develop policies and devise program. ILO is devoted to promoting social justice and internationally recognized human and labor rights, pursuing its founding mission that social justice is essential to universal and lasting peace. ILO support its goals and society as a whole in a variety of ways, including;

- Formulation of international policies and programs to promote basic human rights, improve working and living conditions, and enhance employment opportunities
- Creation of international labor standards backed by a unique system to supervise their application
- An extensive program of international technical cooperation formulated and implemented in an active partnership with constituents, to help countries put these policies into practice in an effective manner
- Training, education and research activities to help advance all of these efforts.

India, a Founding Member of the ILO, has been a permanent member of the ILO Governing Body since 1922. The first ILO Office in India started in 1928. The ILO's overarching goal is Decent Work (DW), i.e., promoting opportunities for all women and men to obtain decent and productive work in conditions of freedom, equity, security and dignity. The DW concept is translated into Decent Work Country Programmes (DWCPs), prepared and adopted by the tripartite constituents and ILO, at country levels. The DWCP-India (2007–2012), aligned to the 11th Plan and the United Nations Development Assistance Framework. The Decent Work Technical Support Team for South Asia (DWT) in New Delhi with the team of international specialists is working very closely with the ILO Offices in the subregion. The DWT provide technical support to seven countries in the subregion: Afghanistan, Bangladesh, India, Maldives, Nepal, Pakistan, and Sri Lanka.

## Occupational Health Safety Legislation

The basic aim of the concerned law making and amending authorities is to devise laws which provide safety standards to protect the basic needs of workers and take care of their welfare. These laws are flexible enough to create rather than destroy jobs and increase the overall wellbeing of workers.

The main objectives of Occupational Health Safety (OHS) related legislation are:

- Providing a statutory framework including the enactment of general enabling legislation on OHS in respect of all sectors of economic activities, and designing suitable control systems of compliance, enforcement and incentives for better compliance.
- Providing administrative and technical support services.
- Providing a system of incentives to employers and employees to achieve higher health and safety standards.
- Establishing and developing research and development capabilities in emerging areas.
- Reducing the incidence of work related injuries, fatalities and diseases.
- Reducing the cost of workplace injuries and diseases.
- Increasing community awareness regarding areas related to OHS.

## Relevant Legislation in India

- The Factories Act
- Workmen's Compensation Act, 1923
- Maternity Benefit Act
- Employment State Insurance Scheme (ESIS)
- Central Government Health Scheme (CGHS).

*Note: Details about the provision of the acts are further discussed in Chapter 49: Health Legislations in India.*

## SUMMARY

- Occupational health aims at the promotion and maintenance of the highest degree of physical, mental and social well-being of workers in all occupations.
- In organized sector the employment terms are fixed, and people have assured jobs, while unorganized sector is constituted by the small and scattered units which are not registered with the government.
- Agricultural workers are exposed to a variety of environmental hazards that are potentially harmful to their health and well-being.
- White collar jobs are considered relatively safe, clean and easy, as there are least chances of life-threatening accidents. But with time various factors have come up which are affecting the health of office employees/workers.
- In heat stress the heat-regulating mechanisms of the body is disturbed. So, the internal body temperature rises above 98.6°F. It affects the physiological processes and results in strain on the body.
- Outdoor workers, and those who work in an area that is poorly insulated or without heat are more susceptible to cold stress.
- Occupational exposure to vibration can be due to hand-arm vibration and whole-body vibration.
- Sickness absenteeism is the practice of regularly staying away from work or school without good reason. It can be voluntary or involuntary.
- An occupational disease is any disease contracted primarily because of exposure to risk factors arising from work activity.
- Pneumoconiosis is a group of interstitial lung diseases caused by lung parenchyma's reaction to certain inhaled dust. Silicosis, asbestosis and coal workers' pneumoconiosis, which are caused by inhalation of silica dust, asbestos fibers and coal mine dust, respectively are considered as primary pneumoconiosis.
- Farmer's lung disease is the most prevalent form of hypersensitivity pneumonitis.
- Occupational dermatitis is a type of contact dermatitis, which occurs due to contact with certain substances at the workplace. There are two types of contact dermatitis which can occur due to occupational exposure, contact irritant dermatitis and allergic contact dermatitis.
- Lung cancers contribute 54–75% of all occupational cancers.
- Occupational stress is considered as a mental and physical response/reaction, which generates due to interaction of an individual with his working environment, and due to mismatch between work needs with his abilities and demands.
- Burnout is nothing but adding up of the stress with time.
- Ergonomics is considered as the scientific study of human work and the application of this scientific information to the design of objects, systems, and environments concerning human beings.
- In occupational health, primary preventive interventions involve exposure prevention and specific protection by vaccination.
- Interventional strategies to reduce occupational morbidities and mortalities can be applied at international, national, workplace, and individual level.
- A healthy workplace is a place where everyone works together to achieve an agreed vision for the health and well-being of workers and the surrounding community.
- Periodic medical examinations aim to detect susceptible workers for whom corrective actions are required before they develop overt occupational diseases.
- ILO is the tripartite UN agency which brings together governments, employers and workers of 187 member States, to set labor standards, develop policies and devise program.

## SUGGESTED READING

1. About the ILO. Available from: https://www.ilo.org/global/about-the-ilo/lang--en/index.htm.
2. Acute silico-proteinosis. A new pathologic variant of acute silicosis in sandblasters, characterized by histologic features resembling alveolar pro.- PubMed - NCBI. Available from: https://www.ncbi.nlm.nih.gov/pubmed/ 5775743.
3. Adams RM. Occupational skin cancer. In: Adams RM (Ed). Occupational Skin Disease. New York: Grune and Stratton; 1983. pp. 82-98.
4. Adisesh A. 1658c. The ILO list of occupational diseases and the WHO ICD. In BMJ Publishing Group Ltd; 2018. p. A230.3-A230. Available from: http://oem.bmj.com/lookup/doi/10.1136/oemed-2018-ICOHabstracts.653
5. Adverse effects of crystalline silica exposure. American Thoracic Society Committee of the Scientific Assembly on Environmental and Occupational Health. Am J Respir Crit Care Med. 1997;155(2):761-8.
6. Applebaum KM, Graham J, Gray GM, et al. An Overview of Occupational Risks From Climate Change. Curr Environ Health Rep. 2016;3(1):13-22.
7. Asbestos-related diseases | National Health Portal Of India. Available from: https://www.nhp.gov.in/disease/non-communicable-disease/asbestos-related-diseases.
8. Austin H, Delzell E, Cole P. Benzene and leukemia. A review of the literature and a risk assessment. Am J Epidemiol. 1988;127(3):419-39.
9. Babović P. Occupational accidents as indicators of inadequate work conditions and work environment. Acta Medica Median. 2009;48(4):22-6.
10. Bena A, Giraudo M, Leombruni R, et al. Job tenure and work injuries: a multivariate analysis of the relation with previous experience and differences by age. BMC Public Health. 2013;13:869.
11. Burton J. WHO Healthy Workplace Framework and Model: Background and Supporting Literature and Practices. WHO; 2010. Available from: http://www.who.int/occupational_health/healthy_workplace_framework.pdf
12. CDC - Heat Stress - Heat Related Illness - NIOSH Workplace Safety and Health Topic. 2018. Available from: https://www.cdc.gov/niosh/topics/heatstress/heatrelillness.html.
13. CDC - NIOSH Workplace Safety and Health Topic - Cold Stress - Cold Related Illnesses. 2018. Available from: https://www.cdc.gov/niosh/topics/coldstress/coldrelatedillnesses.html.
14. CDC - Pneumoconioses - NIOSH Workplace Safety and Health Topic. 2017. Available from: https://www.cdc.gov/niosh/topics/pneumoconioses/default.html.
15. Choobineh AR, Amirzadeh F. General occupational health. 6th ed. Shiraz: Publishers of Shiraz University of Medical Sciences; 2003.
16. Cullinan P, Reid P. Pneumoconiosis. Prim Care Respir J. 2013;22(2):249-52.
17. Fernández Álvarez R, Martínez González C, Quero Martínez A, et al. Guidelines for the Diagnosis and Monitoring of Silicosis. Arch Bronconeumol Engl Ed. 2015;51(2):86-93.
18. Gainer RD. History of ergonomics and occupational therapy. Work Read Mass. 2008;31(1):5-9.
19. Government of Canada CC for OH and S. Occupational Cancer: OSH Answers [Internet]. 2018. Available from: http://www.ccohs.ca/.
20. Hawkes C, Ruel MT. Understanding the Links between Agriculture and Health. Int Food Policy Res Inst. 2006;3(6):36.
21. Heat Stress: Farmworker Health and Safety [Internet]. Association of Farmworker Opportunity Programs; 2010. Available from: https://www.osha.gov/dte/grant_materials/fy09/sh-19485-09/trainer_guide.pdf.
22. Holness DL, Beaton D, Harniman E, et al. Hand and Upper Extremity Function in Workers With Hand Dermatitis: Dermatitis. 2013;24(3):131-6.
23. Joshi TK, Gupta RK. Asbestos-related morbidity in India. Int J Occup Environ Health. 2003;9(3):249-53.
24. Leung CC, Yu ITS, Chen W. Silicosis. The Lancet. 2012;379(9830):2008-18.
25. Mechanisms in the Pathogenesis of Asbestosis and Silicosis | American Journal of Respiratory and Critical Care Medicine. Available from: https://www.atsjournals.org/doi/full/10.1164/ajrccm.157.5.9707141.
26. Murray CJL, Lopez AD, Organization WH, Bank W, Health HS of P. The Global burden of disease: a comprehensive assessment of mortality and disability from diseases, injuries, and risk factors in 1990 and projected to 2020: summary. 1996; Available from: http://apps.who.int/iris/handle/10665/41864.
27. Neira M. Healthy Workplaces: a model for action. For employers, workers, policy-makers and practitioners. Switzerland: World Health Organization; 2010.

28. Occupational Dermatitis Frequently Asked Questions - Health and Safety Authority. Available from: http://www.hsa.ie/eng/Workplace_Health/Occupational_Asthma_and_Dermatitis/Occupational_Dermatitis_Frequently_Asked_Questions/
29. Occupational exposure to vibration from hand-held tools: A teaching guide on health effects, risk assessment and prevention [Internet]. WHO; Available from: http://www.who.int/occupational_health/pwh_guidance_no.10_teaching_materials.pdf.
30. Occupational silica exposure and lung cancer risk: a review of epidemiological studies 1996-2005. - PubMed - NCBI. Available from: https://www.ncbi.nlm.nih.gov/pubmed/16403810.
31. Prevention of Occupational Cancer. The Global Occupational Health Network, WHO; 2006. Available from: http://www.who.int/occupational_health/publications/newsletter/gohnet11e.pdf.
32. Rosenstock L, Cullen M, Fingerhut M. Occupational Health. In: Jamison DT, Breman JG, Measham AR, Alleyne G, Claeson M, Evans DB, Jha P, Mills A, Musgrove P (Eds). Disease Control Priorities in Developing Countries [Internet]. 2nd ed. Washington (DC): World Bank; 2006. Available from: http://www.ncbi.nlm.nih.gov/books/NBK11750/.
33. Selman M, Pardo A, King TE. Hypersensitivity pneumonitis: insights in diagnosis and pathobiology. Am J Respir Crit Care Med. 2012;186(4):314-24.
34. Slattery DA. Occupational medicine as a specialty. Postgrad Med J. 1989;65(760):89-93.
35. Subramanian V, Madhavan N. Asbestos problem in India. Lung Cancer Amst Neth. 2005;49 (Suppl 1):S9-12.
36. WHO | Global strategy on occupational health for all: The way to health at work. WHO. Available from: http://www.who.int/occupational_health/publications/globstrategy/en/index5.html.
37. WHO | Occupational and work-related diseases [Internet]. WHO. Available from: http://www.who.int/occupational_health/activities/occupational_work_diseases/en/.
38. WHO | Silicosis and silicotuberculosis in India [Internet]. WHO. Available from: http://www.who.int/bulletin/volumes/94/10/15-163550/en/.
39. Wilson JR. Fundamentals of systems ergonomics/human factors. Appl Ergon. 2014;45(1):5-13.
40. Workforce in Organised/Unorganised Sector. Available from: http://pib.nic.in/newsite/PrintRelease.aspx?relid=147634.
41. World Cancer Report 2008. Available from: http://www.iarc.fr/en/publications/pdfs-online/wcr/2008/.

# CHAPTER 30

# Mental Health

*Harshal Ramesh Salve*

*"The voice of the intellect is a soft one. But it does not rest until it has gain a hearing"*
—**Sigmund Freud**

CM 15.1 Define and describe the concept of mental health
CM 15.2 Describe warning signals of mental health disorders

## INTRODUCTION

Mental health is a non-negotiable component of community health. The World Health Organization (WHO) defines mental health as a positive sense of well-being encompassing the physical, mental, social, basic economic, and spiritual aspects of life; not merely absence of disease. Mental health is considered as a barometer of the social life of a population and the rising level of morbidity and mortality is a sign of social as well as individual malaise. It is much more than hospital-based treatment of severe mental illness. Interventions for improvement of mental health comprises of range of activities, such as promotion of healthy lifestyle, coping up strategies and detection of covert mental illness. Like other illness mental illness is also attributed to interaction between various biological (age, gender, etc.), social (urbanization, low socioeconomic status, domestic violence, homelessness) and psychological (stressful events in life) factors.

Unfortunately, mental health and mental illness does not receive due importance from society and the policy makers like other noncommunicable diseases. On the contrary, mental illness is often ignored both by the sufferer and care provider. This adds to the increasing burden of mental illness and widening of "treatment gap".

## CHARACTERISTICS OF MENTALLY HEALTHY PERSON

Mentally healthy person has following characteristics:
- Positive attitude towards oneself
- Do not become overwhelmed by emotions, such as fear, anger, love, jealousy, guilt, or anxiety
- Having meaningful, lasting and satisfying personal relationships
- Feel comfortable with company of other people
- Ability to take life as it comes and master it
- Capability to take own decisions

## CLASSIFICATION OF MENTAL ILLNESS

According to **American Psychiatry Association**, following are the warning signs of mental illness:
- ***Withdrawal***: Recent social withdrawal and loss of interest in others.
- ***Drop in functioning***: An unusual drop in functioning, at school, work or social activities, such as quitting sports, failing in school or difficulty performing familiar tasks.
- ***Problems thinking***: Problems with concentration, memory or logical thought and speech that are hard to explain.
- ***Increased sensitivity***: Heightened sensitivity to sights, sounds, smells or touch; avoidance of over-stimulating situations.
- ***Apathy:*** Loss of initiative or desire to participate in any activity.
- ***Feeling disconnected***: A vague feeling of being disconnected from oneself or one's surroundings; a sense of unreality.
- ***Illogical thinking***: Unusual or exaggerated beliefs about personal powers to understand meanings or influence events; illogical or "magical" thinking typical of childhood in an adult.
- ***Nervousness***: Fear or suspiciousness of others or a strong nervous feeling.
- ***Unusual behavior:*** Odd, uncharacteristic, peculiar behavior.
- ***Sleep or appetite changes***: Dramatic sleep and appetite changes or decline in personal care.
- ***Mood changes***: Rapid or dramatic shifts in feelings.

Presence of one or more of these signs at same time raises the suspicion of deranged mental health of the person. Such person should seek help of the mental health professional.

Mental illness is characterized by alteration in mood, behavior, and thinking causing personal distress and affecting daily/routine functions of an individual. International Classification of Diseases, 10th Revision (**ICD-10**) classified mental illness as follows:
- ***Organic (pathological changes in the brain are evident)***: Dementia, Alzheimer's diseases, delirium, etc.
- ***Neurosis (behavioral disorders with insight)***: Mood disorders, anxiety disorders, phobic disorders, obsessive compulsive disorders, etc.
- ***Psychosis (behavioral disorders with loss of insight)***: Schizophrenia, delusional disorders, psychosis, etc.

- **Other illness**: Personality disorders, childhood developmental disorders, eating disorders, conduct disorders.

Goldberg introduced the concept of Common Mental Disorders (CMDs). **Common Mental Disorders** includes mood disorders and "Neurotic, Stress related and Somatoform disorders" as per ICD 10th revision. These disorders constitute majority of the burden of mental illness in the community and at the primary care. CMDs are easy to diagnose, treat and these are also amenable for prevention. Hence, identification and treatment of CMDs are essential in improving mental health status of the population.

## EPIDEMIOLOGY OF MENTAL ILLNESS

### Global Scenario

In 2019, 1 in every 8 people, or 970 million people around the world were living with a mental disorder, with anxiety and depressive disorders the most common. In 2020, the number of people living with anxiety and depressive disorders rose significantly because of the COVID-19 pandemic (WHO factsheet, Mental Disorders, June 2022). They caused 7% of all global burden of disease as measured in DALYs and 19% of all years lived with disability in 2017. Depression was associated with most DALYs for both sexes, with higher rates in women as all other internalizing disorders, whereas other disorders such as substance use had higher rates in men. Mental and addictive disorders affect a significant portion of the global population with high burden, in particular in high- and upper-middle-income countries. The relative share of these disorders has increased in the past decades, in part due to stigma and lack of treatment. (Global Burden of Diseases, Institute for Health Metrics and Evaluation, 2017 Report).

In addition, mental illness has been linked to other health problems in developing countries like maternal depression with low birth-weight and growth failure of child, diabetes mellitus, hypertension, myocardial infarction, asthma, metabolic syndrome, increased risk for HIV and tuberculosis. Evidence of higher burden of CMDs during pregnancy is also available. Social cost attributed to mental illness and associated social stigma may be much more and not quantifiable.

### Indian Scenario

Since last few decades, Indian population is going through the process of the development, which is responsible for rapid urbanization, growth of urban slums, widening inequalities in economic status and widespread poverty. All these factors are responsible for stressful life, which is causing an increase in mental illness in the population.

In 2017, 197.3 million people had mental disorders in India, including 45.7 million with depressive disorders and 44.9 million with anxiety disorders. Thus, one in every seven Indian suffered from one or another mental illness. The contribution of mental disorders to the total DALYs in India increased from 2.5% in 1990 to 4.7% in 2017. In 2017, depressive disorders contributed the most to the total mental disorders DALYs (33.8%), followed by anxiety disorders (19.0%), idiopathic developmental intellectual disability (IDID; 10.8%), schizophrenia (9.8%), bipolar disorder (6.9%), conduct disorder (5.9%), autism spectrum disorders (3.2%), eating disorders (2.2%), and attention-deficit hyperactivity disorder (ADHD; 0.3%); other mental disorders comprised 8.0% of DALYs. Almost all (>99.9%) of these DALYs were made up of YLDs. (India State-Level Disease Burden Initiative Mental Disorders Collaborators, adapted from Global Burden of Disease, 2019).

National Mental Health Survey (NMHS), the first of its kind multi-state survey in India carried out by National Institute of Mental Health and Neurosciences (NIMHANS), Bengaluru in the year 2015-16. Overall prevalence of mental illness in lifetime was 13.7% and current was 10.6%. Current prevalence of anxiety disorders and depressive disorders were 3.6%, and 0.8% respectively. (National Mental Health Survey of India, NIMHANS, 2015-16).

Prevalence of mental illness was reported almost similar in both males and females. However, alcohol use disorders and bipolar and affective disorders (BPAD) were common in males. While, depressive disorders were reported more among females. Mental illnesses were more common in urban metro areas as compared to rural area. Prevalence of other mental illness among adults reported in NMHS is mentioned in **Table 30.1**.

**Table 30.1:** ICD-10 DCR prevalence (%) of mental morbidity among adults in NMHS.

| | Lifetime | Current |
|---|---|---|
| F10–F19: Mental and behavioral problems due to psychoactive substance use | Data not available | 22.4 |
| F10: Alcohol use disorder | Data not available | 4.7 |
| F11–19: Except 17 other substance use disorder | Data not available | 0.6 |
| F17: Tobacco use disorders | Data not available | 20.9 |
| F20–F29: Schizophrenia, other psychotic disorders | 1.4 | 0.4 |
| F30–F39: Mood (affective) disorders | 5.6 | 2.8 |
| F30–31: Bipolar affective disorders* | 0.5 | 0.3 |
| F32–33: Depressive disorder | 5.3 | 2.7 |
| F40–F48: Neurotic and stress-related disorders | 3.7 | 3.5 |
| F40: Phobic anxiety disorders** | | 1.9 |
| F41: Other anxiety disorders*** | 1.3 | 1.2 |
| F42: Obsessive compulsive disorder | | 0.8 |
| F43.1: Post-traumatic stress disorder (PTSD) | | 0.2 |

\* Includes single mania and hypomania episodes
\*\* Includes agoraphobia and social phobia
\*\*\* Includes panic disorder and generalized anxiety disorder

### Burden at Primary Care

Mental Illness contributes to substantial amount of morbidity at primary care level in India. Studies reported 17–46% of patients present with mental illness at primary care setting in India. CMD constitutes majority of mental illness burden at primary care. Most of the time diagnosis of mental illness at primary care remains undiagnosed due to covert nature of symptoms.

## RISK FACTORS OF MENTAL ILLNESS

Mental illness usually attributed to multifactorial causality. Poverty and social exclusion are the proven independent risk

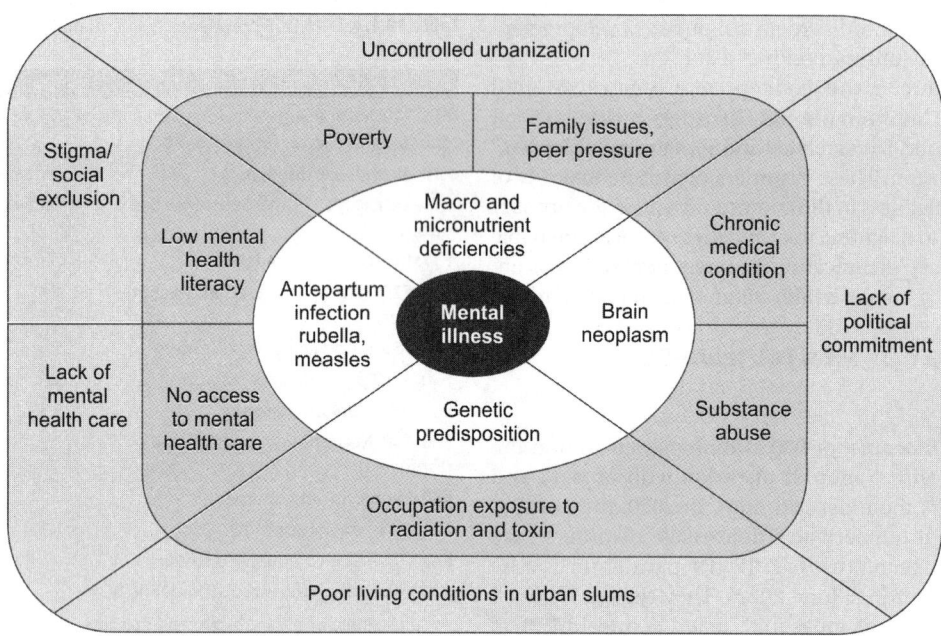

**Fig. 30.1:** Socio-politico-developmental model of occurrence of mental illness.

factors for the development of mental illness both in high-income countries and low- and middle-income countries (LAMIC). Poverty due to its association with unemployment and lack of affordable housing, is responsible for mental illnesses, such as depression and anxiety. Other risk factors for mental illness are described in **Box 30.1**. Stressors during crucial stages of lifetime are mostly responsible for precipitation of mental illness in most of the cases. Antenatal, childhood, adolescence and old age are crucial phases in the lifetime. Possible socio-politico-developmental model for causation of mental illness is described in **Figure 30.1**.

---

**Box 30.1: Risk factors and causes of mental illness.**

**Organic**
- Brain neoplasms
- Cerebral arthrosclerosis
- Metabolic diseases
- Neurological diseases
- Infectious diseases affecting brain
- Infections—rubella, measles during antepartum period have impact on cognition of new-born

**Hereditary**
- Genetic predisposition for autism, schizophrenia, alcohol abuse (to some extent)

**Social and environmental**
- Poverty
- Illiteracy
- Peer pressure, work-related stress
- Family issues—domestic violence, broken homes, nuclear families
- Experience of natural disaster
- Nutritional—iodine deficiency, pyridoxine and thiamine deficiency, malnutrition

**Physical**
- Trauma
- Toxicity due to mercury, manganese, lead
- Radiation exposures

---

## DETECTION AND TREATMENT OF MENTAL ILLNESS

Evaluation by psychiatrist remains the gold standard for diagnosis of mental illness. Detection of severe mental illness is relatively easier and needs to be managed by psychiatrist. There is paucity of psychiatrist in both secondary and primary care health facility in India. At the primary health care, CMD presents with other non-specific symptoms. Hence, training general physicians in diagnosis, treatment and referral of CMDs is essential in India. Efforts are also being made to train health workers or Accredited Social Health Activists (ASHAs) to screen individuals in the community for CMDs. All available tools help nonspecialist physicians to screen and diagnose mental illness as per International Classification of Diseases (ICD) and Diagnostic and Statistical Manual for Mental Disorders (DSM). Currently ICD version 10 and DSM version IV are in use.

National Mental Health Programme (NMHP) envisaged integration of primary health care with mental health care services. District Mental Health Programme (DMHP) is part of NMHP. Under DMHP, trained manpower, drugs for treatment and referral services for mental illness are being made available at both primary and secondary health care facility in selected districts India.

## MENTAL ILLNESS AND STIGMA

Persons with mental illness suffers stigma in the society in many ways. Firstly, they themselves and their family members refused to acknowledge the problem. Secondly, affected person and their family members often face neglect, harassment and violence in the society. Crime against mental challenged individuals is not uncommon in the society. Stephen M Lawrie documented that patients with mental illness were stigmatized since long in all communities and this stigmatization was more than just "labeling" the patients. Common attitudes towards mental illness include considering the condition as frightening, shameful, imaginary, feigned and incurable and the patients are labeled as dangerous, unpredictable, untrustworthy, unstable, lazy, weak, worthless and/or helpless in the community. This attitude of the society all across the communities is attributed to failing to acknowledge biomedical causality of mental illness.

Stigma towards mental illness are linked to the Mental Health Literacy (MHL) in the community.

Concept of MHL was introduced by Jorm et al. an Australian Psychologist in 1997. MHL is defined as "knowledge and beliefs about mental illness which aid their recognition, management or prevention" MHL is critical component of mental health care services particularly in the country with poor overall health literacy.

Improving mental health literacy in a community improves the overall attitude of a community, reduces in stigma towards person with mentally illness, improve health seeking behavior and eventually emotional and mental well-being of the community.

In India, due to lack of awareness about the scientific cause, mental illness usually attributed to supernatural beliefs. Stigma associated with mental illnesses has also been reported to be high. Healthcare providers are also reported to be stereotypical but nonstigmatizing with regard to person with the mental illness in India. Major four strategies responsible for successful stigma reduction program are listed in **Figure 30.2**.

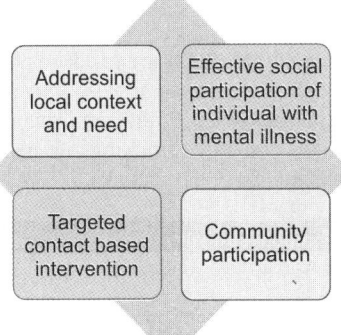

**Fig. 30.2:** Core strategies for successful stigma reduction program for mental health.

## SUICIDE AND SELF-HARM

According to National Crime Record Bureau (NCRB), Annual suicide rate in India is 10.6 per 1 lakh populations. Most of the suicide deaths are reported from young population (18–30 years). Family problems and medical illness are the most common reasons reported for suicides in India. NMHS reports high suicidal risk among middle age (40–49 years), among females and in urban metro population. Most of the suicides are preventable if its attempts and risk are best monitored.

## PREVENTION OF MENTAL ILLNESS

### Primary Prevention

As true for any noncommunicable diseases, exact cause of mental illness is still subject of research. Hence, healthy physical and social environment remains the only option available for prevention of stressors leading to precipitation of mental illness. Reducing the stigma in the society is the cornerstone of prevention of mental illness. Creating awareness at various levels through all available resources is necessary to reduce stigma about mental illness. Awareness generation in the community regarding mental health should focus on following points:

- Biomedical concept of medical illness
- Identification of common symptoms of mental illness in daily life
- Availability of treatment options, health care facilities to improve health seeking
- Nonhereditary, non-communicability of mental illness
- No use of tobacco, alcohol, any other substance
- ***Promoting healthy lifestyle:*** Adequate physical activity, healthy diet, adequate sleep, yoga
- Coping up techniques in post disaster or stressful events

Major policy level intervention for reduction of suicide was made through Mental Health Care Bill 2017 by decriminalizing the act of suicide. Stress reduction, and coping up strategies remains the key suicide prevention intervention at the community level. Coping up training, stress reduction techniques, healthy lifestyles should be promoted through schools so that these skills get inculcated during early childhood. Support of the family and peers are quintessential for person dealing with mental illness in the community.

### Secondary Prevention

Early diagnosis, referral and effective treatment are also applicable for mental illness. Training of primary level health care providers in identification and treatment of mental illness is needed. As discussed above, there are tools available for screening and diagnosis of mental illness at primary care settings. Use of ASHA in community awareness generation, screening and patient referral could be possible option in India. Ensuring availability of drugs used in treatment is critical for sustained management of CMD at primary care level.

### Tertiary Prevention

Aim of tertiary prevention in case of mental illness is rehabilitation both physically and socially. Psychiatric rehabilitation is essential for all person with severe and persistent mental illness. More than 50% of severe mental illness requires rehabilitation. The aim of the rehabilitation is to make person with mental illness live physically, emotionally and social productive life in the community with minimal external aid. Focus of rehabilitation is on changing attitude and perception of the person and their caregiver about the illness, so that person can cope up with the disease in a better way. It also includes developing suitable environment for person with mental illness to reduce stressors.

Residential continuum with shelter home, trained staff is traditional way of psychiatric rehabilitation but uncommon these days. Vocational rehabilitation initially limited to hospital now has expanded to other set up with more real situation and environment. Community-based rehabilitation for mental illness is ideal but its challenging even in today's modern world due to social stigma.

## SUBSTANCE USE AND DEPENDENCE

### Definition and Burden of Substance Use

According to WHO, substance abuse refers to the harmful or hazardous use of psychoactive substances, including alcohol and illicit drugs. Psychoactive substance use can lead to dependence syndrome. It is characterized by cluster of behavioral, cognitive, and physiological symptoms, such as strong desire to take the drug, difficulties in controlling its use, persisting in its use despite harmful consequences, a higher priority given to drug use than to other activities and obligations, increased tolerance, and sometimes a physical withdrawal state. Experience taking action mostly under peer pressure during young age leads to substance use.

Substance abuse has multifactorial causality. Documented risk factors of substance use can be classified as below:
- ***Biological***: Genetic makeup, ethnicity, mental illness
- ***Environmental***: Peers, poverty, stress, physical and sexual abuse, family environment

ICD 10 identifies following psychoactive drug potential for abuse with serious health hazards:
- Alcohol
- Cannabinoids
- Cocaine
- Caffeine
- Hallucinogens
- Opioids
- Sedatives
- Tobacco
- Volatile solvents
- Others

Common identifying symptoms of person with substance abuse are as follows:
- Loss of interest in daily routine activities and reduction of leisure activities, such as sports, hobby
- Loss of body weight, appetite
- Change in gait, posture
- Change in sleep-wake cycle
- Sudden change in mood
- Impaired memory and poor concentration
- Withdrawal from social activities

Alcohol use and tobacco use are most commonly substance abused globally. Annually 3.3 million deaths are attributed to harmful alcohol use globally. Harmful use of alcohol and tobacco use are established risk factors for cardiovascular diseases, metabolic syndrome, stroke, liver cirrhosis, carcinoma of liver, pancreatic carcinoma.

Tobacco kills half of its users globally as per WHO estimates. More than 7 million deaths attributed to tobacco use in a year globally. Harmful effect of tobacco mentioned in the **Figure 30.3**.

Global Adult tobacco Survey (GATS 2) reported decline in use of tobacco in India in last five years. As per survey, 10.7% and 21.4% adults use smokeless tobacco and smoked tobacco respectively. Smokeless tobacco includes *gutkha, khaini, pan masala, jarda*, raw tobacco, etc. Clear gender differential towards male are reported with respect to both smoke and smokeless tobacco use.

## Passive Smoking or Second-hand Smoking

Exposure to tobacco smoke to the nonsmoker in closed environment, such as home, work place, transport is called as exposure to passive smoke or second-hand smoking. In 1981, Scientist from Japan demonstrated effect of second-hand smoke

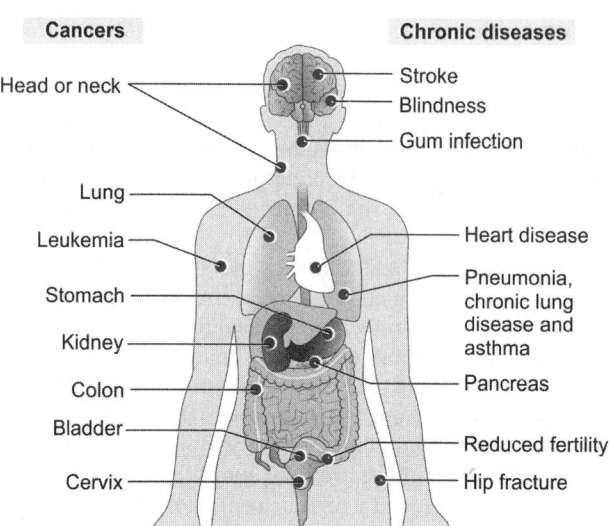

**Fig. 30.3:** Harmful effect of tobacco in human health.

on human health. Tobacco not only affects user but also people surrounding the user.

In India, among adults, 38.7% are exposed at home, 30.2% at work place and 7.4% are exposed at closed public places to the second-hand smoking. Recent meta-analysis reported strong evidence of linkages of passive smoking and health conditions. (Cao S et al., PloS One, 2015) **(Box 30.2)**.

> **Box 30.2: Health conditions strongly associated with passive smoking.**
> - Invasive meningococcal disease in children
> - Cervical cancer
> - Pharyngeal carriage for meningitis and streptococcal pneumonia
> - Food allergy
> - Lower respiratory tract infections
> - Childhood asthma
> - Lung cancer
> - Stroke

## Prevention and Rehabilitation for Alcohol and Tobacco Users

- ***Regulate availability of the substances***: Age restrictions, public places ban.
- ***Restriction of advertising***: Warning/caution on packaging.
- ***Using pricing policies***: High taxation on products.
- ***Raising awareness about harmful effect of substance use***: Public places, schools, health facilities, social gatherings.
- ***Strict implementing motor vehicle driving law:*** Prohibition of drink and drive.
- ***Support community action for prevention of substance use***: Community support groups, discouraging use of tobacco, alcohol in society by name of customs, rituals, etc. Involvement of opinion makers, local leaders and religious leaders in the community outreach activities.
- ***Community-based rehabilitation of substance dependent person:*** Creating self-help groups, creating shelter homes for people recovering from substance dependence, ensuring community support to family of affected person, providing earning opportunities for person recovered from substance dependence.

- *Develop surveillance system for substance use and policy formulation:* Establish surveillance mechanism in routine health care.

## INTERVENTIONS FOR PROMOTION OF MENTAL HEALTH

### Global Level Intervention

WHO dedicated two World Health Days to Mental Health. In the year 2001 it was "Mental Health: Stop Exclusion dare to care" advocating elimination of stigma related to mental illness. In the year 2017, it was "Depression—Let's Talk" focusing on second most common cause of DALY.

Mental Health Gap Action Programme (mhGAP) was launched by WHO in the year 2008 to reduce the treatment gap for mental illness globally. It envisaged evidence-based mental health care in nonspecialized care for resource poor settings. MhGAP programme focus on priority conditions depending on its burden, economic aspect, disability and violation of human rights. These conditions include depression, psychosis, bipolar disorders, dementia, epilepsy, developmental and behavioral disorders, substance use disorders and self-harm. MhGAP programme gives protocols for management of these priority conditions. These protocols are based on assessment, decision and management of the condition. October 10 is celebrated as World Mental Health Day.

### National Level Interventions

India launched National Mental Health Programme (NMHP) in the year 1982 in India. Major objective of this program was to create awareness and reduce stigma about mental illness. District Mental Health Programme is part of NMHP, which aims to decentralize mental health care to the district level in the country. Under this program specialized manpower was provided at district health care facility. Community participation, training of nonspecialized manpower in mental health care are pillars of DMHP. *This is further explained in detail in Chapter 47: Health Policies and Programs in India.*

Effective and sensitive health care delivery system is the key to prevention of mental illness in the community. Mental Health Policy of India 2014 gives following principles for effective mental health care services in the country:

- *Equity:* More for the needy without any discrimination
- *Justice*: Reaching most vulnerable
- *Integrated care*: Within existing health care system
- *Evidence-based care*: Decision making based on research evidences
- *Quality:* As per international and national standards
- *Participatory rights-based approach*: Involvement of person and caregiver in decision making for management of illness and follow-up
- *Governance and effective delivery*: Intersectoral coordination between government, private and NGO partners in delivery interventions
- *Value base in all training and teaching program*: Value-based medical and paramedical teaching
- *Holistic approach:* Recognizing connection between mind, body and soul.

Government of India enacted The Mental Health Care Act, 2017. "The Act aimed to provide mental health care services to person with mental illness to protect, promote and fulfill the right of such persons during delivery of mental health care and services and matters connected therewith or incidental there to." This Act empowers mental ill person with right for health care and right to decide treatment modalities.

## SUMMARY

- Mental health is an integral part of concept of holistic health
- High undiagnosed burden with high treatment gap for mental illness
- CMDs are most common preventable and treatable mental illness
- High stigma for mental illness in the community affects health seeking
- Tobacco use in all form are hazardous to health
- Integration of mental health care at primary care is effective approach to reduce burden of mental illness in the community

## SUGGESTED READING

1. Goldberg DP, Blackwell B. Psychiatric illness in general practice: a detail study using a new method of case identification. Br Med J. 1970;2(5707):439-43.
2. Gururaj G, Varghese M, Benegal V, et al. and NMHS collaborators group. National Mental Health Survey of India, 2015-16: Prevalence, patterns and outcomes. Bengaluru, National Institute of Mental Health and Neuro Sciences, NIMHANS Publication No. 129, 2016.
3. Hasler G, Gergen P, Kleinbaum D. Asthma and panic in young adults: a 20-year prospective community study. Am J Respir Crit Care Med. 2005;171(11):1224-30.
4. Hemingway H, Marmot M. Evidence based cardiology: psychosocial factors in the aetiology and prognosis of coronary health disease: Systematic review of prospective cohort studies. Br Med J. 1999;318: 1460-67.
5. Jahoda M. Current concepts of positive mental health. Joint commission on mental health and illness monograph series: Vol.1. New York, NY, US: Basic Books; 1958.
6. Jha S, Salve HR, Goswami K, et al. Burden of common mental disorders among pregnant women: a systematic review. Asian J Psychiatr. 2018;36: 46-53.
7. Jorm AF. Why we need the concept of "Mental Health Literacy". Health Commun. 2015;30:1166–8.
8. Kumar A. District Mental Health Programme in India: A Case Study. J Health Dev. 2005;1(1):24-35.
9. Mathias K, Kermode M, San Sebastian, et al. Under the banyan tree-exclusion and inclusion of people with mental disorders in rural North India. 2015, BMC Public Health, 15:446.
10. Math SB, Chandrashekar CR, Bhugra D. Psychiatric epidemiology in India. Indian J Med Research. 2007;126(3):183-92.
11. Meng L, Chen D, Yang Y, et al. Depression increases the risk of hypertension incidence: a meta-analysis of prospective cohort studies. J Hypertens. 2012;30(5):84251.
12. Patel V, Kleinman A. Poverty and common mental disorders in developing countries. Bull World Health Organ. 2003;81:609-15.
13. Patel V. Mental health in low- and middle-income countries. Br Med Bulletin. 2007:1-16.
14. Rahman A, Iqbal Z, Bunn J, et al. Impact of maternal depression on infant nutritional status and illness: a cohort study. Arch Gen Psychiatry. 2004;61(9):946-52.
15. Rossler W. Psychiatric rehabilitation today: an overview. World Psychiatry. 2006;5(3):151-7.
16. Roy T, Lloyd CE. Epidemiology of depression and diabetes: a systematic review. J Affect Disord. 2012;142:S8-S21.
17. Sayers J. The World health report 2001-Mental health: new understanding, new hope. Bull World Health Organ. 2001;79(11): 1085.
18. The Mental Health Care Act. 2017. [online] Available from https://indiacode.nic.in/bitstream/123456789/2249/1/A2017-10.pdf.

# CHAPTER 31

# Urban Health, Rural Health and Tribal Health

*Manish Rana, Harsh Bakshi, Anjali Modi, Priscilla Kayina, Gneyaa Bhatt, Madhurjya Baruah*

## URBAN HEALTH

### GLOBAL SCENARIO

Globalization of urbanization is one of the most important social changes of the 20th century. Globally, more people live in urban areas than in rural areas, with 55 per cent of the world's population residing in urban areas in 2018. In 1950, 30 per cent of the world's population was urban, and by 2050, 68 per cent of the world's population is projected to be urban. Just three countries—India, China and Nigeria are expected to account for 35 per cent of the growth in the world's urban population between 2018 and 2050. India is projected to add 416 million urban dwellers, China 255 million and Nigeria 189 million (UN, World Urbanization Prospects, 2018). In general, the process of urbanization has been associated with economic and social transformations like greater geographic mobility, lower fertility, increased life expectancy, increased level of literacy, better health, greater access to social services, and enhanced opportunities for cultural and political participation. However, unplanned or inadequately managed urban expansion leads to pollution and environmental degradation, unsustainable production and consumption patterns leading to more inequality in urban areas than rural areas and many of the world's urban poor live in substandard conditions. Looking to that, Sustainable Development Goals has also dedicated one goal (SDG 11) to urban health: "Making cities inclusive, safe, sustainable and resilient". It presents a serious challenge for government authorities to cope with this "new urban revolution".

### INDIAN SCENARIO

Population residing in urban area in India, according to 1901 census, was 10.8%. This count increased to 27.8% according to 2001 census and as per census 2011, this count is more than 377 million constituting 31.16% of the total population (Census of India, Primary Census abstract for slum, 2011) **(Fig. 31.1)**.

Urban growth has led to rapid increase in number of urban poor population, many of whom live in slums and other squatter settlements. More than 17% of total households in urban areas lived in slums (Census of India, Primary Census abstract for slum, 2011). As per United Nations projections, 53% of the total

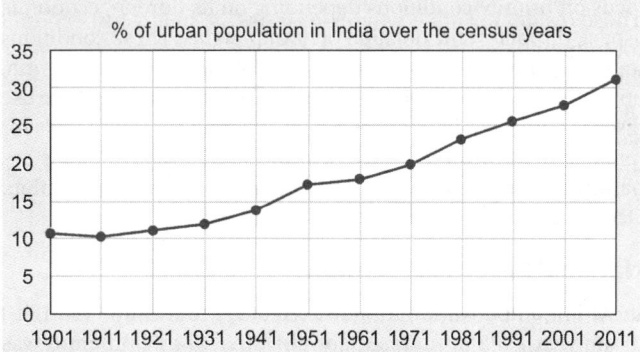

Fig. 31.1: Urban population in India over the census years 1901–2011.

population of India will be in urban regions by 2050 (UN, World Urbanization Prospects, 2018).

### VARIOUS DEFINITIONS WITH REGARDS TO URBAN AREA IN INDIA

#### Towns or Urban Area

- All places with a municipality, corporation, cantonment board or notified town area committee, etc.
- All other places which satisfy the following criteria:
  - A minimum population of 5,000
  - At least 75% of the male working population engaged in nonagricultural pursuits
  - A density of population of at least 400 persons per sq km.

#### Urban Agglomeration

It is a continuous urban spread constituting a town and its adjoining outgrowths (OGs) or two/more physically contiguous towns together with/out OGs of such towns. OGs are railway colony, university campus, port area, military camps, etc., which have come up near a statutory town outside its statutory limits but within the revenue limits of a village or villages contiguous to the town. Urban agglomeration (UA) must consist of at least

**Table 31.1:** Type of town/urban agglomeration (UA) as per their population.

| Type of town | Population criteria | No. of towns as per census 2011 | Remarks, if any |
|---|---|---|---|
| Class I UAs/towns | 1 lakh or above | 468 | |
| Million plus UAs/towns | 1 million or above | 53 out of above 468 | |
| Mega cities | More than 10 million | 3 out of above 53 | Greater Mumbai UA, Delhi UA, Kolkata UA |

a statutory town and its total population should not be less than 20,000 as per the 2001 Census. In varying local conditions, there were similar other combinations which have been treated as UA, for example, Greater Mumbai UA, Delhi UA, etc. **(Table 31.1)**.

## Slums (Slum Census 2011, Under Section 3 of the Slum Area Improvement and Clearance Act, 1956)

Those residential areas where dwellings are in any respect unfit for human habitation by reasons of dilapidation, overcrowding, faulty arrangements and designs of such buildings, narrowness or faulty arrangement of streets, lack of ventilation, light, sanitation facilities or any combination of these factors which are detrimental to safety, health and morals.
- Probable reasons for upcoming slums in India may be urbanization, industrialization, more earning opportunities, more economic growth and higher standard of living resulting in large-scale migration from rural to urban areas.
- Although in general, slum dwellers are worse off than non-slum dwellers, this pattern is not consistent for all indicators in every city and there are large disparities in health and living conditions between the poor and nonpoor in cities.
- Not all slum dwellers are below poverty line and non-slum residents are not always better off than slum residents are. Therefore, health and other interventions targeting only slum areas will not cover all urban poor.
- *Household living conditions in slums*:
  - Slums have much poorer housing conditions than non-slum areas in all respect, i.e., construction material, residential crowding, or ventilation of the dwelling.
  - Not much difference between slum and non-slum households in access to piped drinking water in almost all cities.
  - In almost all cities, the accessibility to proper sanitation facility is much worse in slum areas than in non-slum areas. Open defecation is highest among the poor in every city.

## VULNERABLE POPULATION REQUIRING HIGH FOCUS IN URBAN AREA

- Urban poor population living in listed and unlisted slums
- Homeless, ragpickers, street children, rickshaw pullers, construction/brick/lime kiln workers, sex workers, and other temporary migrants.

## STATUS OF HEALTH IN URBAN AREA WITH COMPARISON TO RURAL AREA AND TRIBAL AREA

The vital statistics of urban and rural area are shown in **Table 31.2**. In general, all health indicators are better in urban area as compared to rural area and tribal area **(Table 31.3)** except for sex ratio which is better in rural area and tribal area both.

**Table 31.2:** Vital statistics (SRS 2020).

| Rates | Urban | Rural |
|---|---|---|
| Birth rate (per 1,000 population) | 16.1 | 21.1 |
| Death rate (per 1,000 population) | 5.1 | 6.4 |
| Infant mortality rate (per 1,000 live births) | 19 | 31 |
| Under-five mortality rate (per 1,000 live births) | 21 | 36 |

**Table 31.3:** Other demographic and reproductive and child health indicators (NFHS-5, 2019–21).

| Indicators | Urban | Rural | Tribal |
|---|---|---|---|
| Sex ratio, age 0–6 (females per 1,000 males) | 924 | 931 | 990 |
| Literacy rate (F) (15–49 age group) | 83% | 65.9% | 49.4% |
| Literacy rate (M) (15–49 age group) | 89.6% | 81.5% | 68.5% |
| Children age 12–23 months fully immunized | 83% | 84% | 55.8% |
| Institutional delivery | 93.8% | 86.7% | 68% |
| Children under 5 years who are stunted (height-for-age) | 30.1% | 37.3% | 43.8% |
| Children under 5 years who are underweight (weight-for-age) | 27.3% | 33.8% | 45.3% |
| Children under 5 years who are wasted (weight-for-height) | 18.5% | 19.5% | 27.4% |

However, when it comes to the health of urban poor, it is very low as compared to overall urban indicators **(Box 31.1)**.

**Box 31.1:** Health indicators of urban poor (GOI, NUHM: Framework for implementation, 2013).
- Under-five mortality rate of 72.7
- 46% underweight children among urban poor
- 46.8% women with no education
- 44.4% institutional deliveries
- 60% miss total immunization before completing 1 year

## Causes of Deaths in Urban and Rural Area (Table 31.4)

**Table 31.4:** Top 10 causes of death in rural and urban areas (all ages): 2010–2013 (Census of India, Primary Census abstract for slum, 2011).

| Rank | Causes of death (rural) | Causes of death (urban) |
|---|---|---|
| 1 | Cardiovascular diseases | Cardiovascular diseases |
| 2 | Ill-defined/other symptoms, signs and abnormal clinical or laboratory findings | Ill-defined/other symptoms, signs and abnormal clinical or laboratory findings |
| 3 | Respiratory diseases | Malignant and other neoplasms |
| 4 | Perinatal conditions | Respiratory diseases |
| 5 | Malignant and other neoplasms | Digestive diseases |
| 6 | Diarrheal diseases | Perinatal conditions |
| 7 | Unintentional injuries: Other than motor vehicle accidents | Unintentional injuries: Other than motor vehicle accidents |
| 8 | Digestive diseases | Diarrheal diseases |
| 9 | Respiratory infections | Genitourinary diseases |
| 10 | Tuberculosis | Unintentional injuries: Motor vehicle accidents |

## CHALLENGES IN URBAN HEALTH

- Until recently, urban health was not the main focus of public health policies because of following reasons:
  - Majority of the population was living in rural areas.
  - It was assumed that the heavy concentration of health facilities and personnel in urban areas, particularly private sector would automatically take care of the increasing urban population and their health needs.
- However, with rapid urbanization, most of the cities have been divided into two parts—one part who have access to all the amenities and conveniences that make life comfortable and pleasant, whereas the other part (slum dwellers) that fail to meet even people's most basic needs, and live in poor condition.
- Broadly following are the challenges in tackling urban health:
  - *Housing and sanitation*: Most urban poor live in slums and squatter settlements lead to problems of overcrowding and are at risk of getting exposed to various hazards, such as living near hillsides subject to landslides, living near riverbanks and water basin locations subject to flooding, or sites near industrial hazards. No access to toilets lead to open defecation.
  - *Food and water*: Most of the time, urban poor people live in the midst of pathogenic microorganisms. They often rely on street food, fast food, processed and cheap food, leading to various nutritional problems. Risks of water contamination is also there in slums due to the unreliability of supplies or illegal connections and related water storage practices.
  - *Urban transport*: Lack of public transport infrastructure and services, lack of good networks for cycling and walking, and attraction to a more affluent lifestyle have led to a rapid transition to cars or motorcycles which lead to problems of road traffic accidents and air pollution.
  - *Noise*: It is a consequence of transportation, construction, and industrialization.
  - *Air pollution (outdoor or indoor)*: The sources can be vehicle exhaust, road dust, domestic solid fuel combustion, food kiosks, generator usage in multiple venues (such as hospitals, hotels, markets and apartment complexes), industrial emissions including those from brick kilns and rock quarries, construction activities in the city, and waste burning along the roadside and at the landfills.
  - *Climate change*: Urban temperatures is said to be as much as 5–11°C higher than in surrounding rural areas due to the greater heat absorption of dense urban built spaces and lowered capacity for evaporative cooling (urban heat island effect).
  - *Demanding urban life*: Leads to living with stress of all kinds. Therefore there is rising levels of risk factors, such as tobacco use, unhealthy diet, lower amount of physical activity, the harmful use of alcohol and drugs, and risky sexual behavior.
  - *Health and social services—intraurban differences*: Though available, they are inadequate and insufficiently accessible to people living in slum areas or for urban poor leading to health and social inequities. There is large private sector but poor cannot access them. Many slums are not having primary healthcare facility. Ineffective outreach and weak referral system.
  - *Service delivery challenges*: Multiplicity of urban local bodies, state government, etc., for management of health needs of urban people. It requires clarity of responsibilities of all stakeholders for urban health. Many slums or settlements are not notified, reaching them is a challenge.
  - *No convergence* among wider determinants of health.
  - *Others*: Problems of child labor, domestic violence, and sexual abuse.

## PUBLIC HEALTH PROBLEMS

- Infectious diseases exacerbated by poor living conditions, such as tuberculosis (TB), acute respiratory infections (ARIs), vector-borne diseases (VBDs), and human immunodeficiency virus (HIV)
- Noncommunicable diseases, such as heart disease, cancers, and diabetes and conditions fuelled by various risk factors as described in challenges above
- Mental health problems
- Accidents, injuries, and road traffic accidents
- Nutritional problems, i.e., malnutrition, vitamin or mineral deficiencies, dental problems and obesity which in turn is associated with diabetes and cardiovascular problems.
- Potential health impacts of climate change, e.g., ill-health from heat exposure, spread of infectious diseases to new locations through ecological changes
- Health consequences due to air pollution range from premature mortality due to aggravated morbidity effects, such as asthma, chronic bronchitis, and oxygen deficiency in blood. Other health impacts include eye irritation, respiratory illness, and impacts on reproductive health.
- Noise-induced hearing loss and other consequences of noise pollution
- Violence and crime.

### What can be done and How?

World Health Organization in its document of healthy cities project mentioned qualities of a healthy city as below:

A city should strive to provide:

- A clean, safe physical environment of high quality (including housing quality)
- An ecosystem that is stable now and sustainable in the long-term
- A strong, mutually supportive and nonexploitive community
- A high degree of participation and control by the public over the decisions affecting their lives, health, and well-being
- The meeting of basic needs (for food, water, shelter, income, safety, and work) for all the city's people
- Access to a wide variety of experiences and resources with the chance for a wide variety of contact, interactions, and communication
- A diverse, vital, and innovative city economy

- The encouragement of connectedness with the past, with the cultural and biological heritage of city dwellers and with other groups and individuals
- An optimum level of appropriate public health and sick care services accessible to all
- High health status (high levels of positive health and low levels of disease)

World Health Organization also recommended the following five calls to action to build a healthy and safe urban environment:

| 1. Promote urban planning | • Design cities to promote physical activity<br>• Make healthy food available, safe, and affordable<br>• Provide adequate health services for all<br>• Improve road safety |
|---|---|
| 2. Improve urban living conditions | • Locate houses in safe places<br>• Improve housing conditions<br>• Control indoor and outdoor pollution<br>• Ensure safe water and improved sanitation |
| 3. Ensure participatory urban governance | • Share information about city planning for health<br>• Encourage public dialogue<br>• Involve communities in decision-making<br>• Create opportunities for participation |
| 4. Build inclusive cities that are accessible and age-friendly | • Make public transport accessible to disabled people<br>• Develop safe walkways for those with special needs<br>• Build public places and buildings for easy access<br>• Promote active city life and sports for all |
| 5. Make urban areas resilient to emergencies and disasters | • Locate health facilities in safe areas<br>• Build more resilient health facilities to withstand known dangers<br>• Strengthen community preparedness and response capacity<br>• Improve disease surveillance |

## URBAN HEALTH EQUITY ASSESSMENT AND RESPONSE TOOL (HEART)

Urban health equity assessment and response tool (HEART) is a guide to **(Table 31.5)**:
- Identify and analyze inter- and intra-city inequities in health
- Facilitate decisions on viable and effective strategies, interventions, and actions to reduce them.

**Table 31.5:** Core indicators of urban HEART.

| Health outcomes | Summary indicators, i.e., infant mortality<br>Disease-specific mortality and morbidity indicators, i.e., for diabetes, tuberculosis, and road traffic injuries |
|---|---|
| Social determinants of health | **Physical environment and infrastructure:**<br>Access to safe water and improved sanitation<br>Social and human development<br>Education<br>Skilled birth attendance<br>Full immunization<br>Prevalence of tobacco smoking<br>**Economics:**<br>Level of unemployment<br>**Governance:**<br>Government spending on health |

(HEART: health equity assessment and response tool)

## VARIOUS SCHEMES/PROGRAMMES BY GOVERNMENT OF INDIA FOR URBAN HEALTH

### Jawaharlal Nehru National Urban Renewal Mission (JNNURM)

It was started in 2005 and ended in 2014. It is replaced by Atal Mission for Rejuvenation and Urban Transformation (AMRUT) 2015. The purposes of the mission are to: (1) Ensure that every household has access to a tap with assured supply of water and a sewerage connection; (2) Increase the amenity value of cities by developing greenery and well-maintained open spaces (parks); and (3) Reduce pollution by switching to public transport or constructing facilities for nonmotorized transport (e.g., walking and cycling).

### National Urban Housing and Habitat Policy 2007

This policy has "affordable housing for all" as its motto with a focus on the urban poor.

### Rajiv Awas Yojna 2013

It works toward a "Slum Free India" with objective that every citizen gets access to basic infrastructure and social amenities.

### National Urban Livelihood Mission (NULM) 2013

To reduce poverty of urban poor by enabling them to access gainful self-employment and skilled wage employment opportunities.

### Smart Cities Mission 2015

The purpose is to drive economic growth and improve the quality of life of people by enabling local area development and harnessing technology, especially technology that leads to smart outcomes.

The core elements in a smart city would include:
- Adequate water supply
- Assured electricity supply
- Sanitation including solid waste management
- Efficient urban mobility and public transport
- Affordable housing especially for the poor
- Robust IT connectivity and digitalization
- Good governance especially e-governance and citizen participation
- Sustainable environment
- Safety and security of citizens, particularly women, children and the elderly
- Health and education

### Pradhan Mantri Awas Yojna 2015

It is housing scheme for people belonging to lower income group, economically weaker section, and middle income group.

### Swachh Bharat Urban

Objectives are: (1) Elimination of open defecation; (2) Eradication of manual scavenging; (3) Modern and scientific municipal solid waste management; (4) To effect behavioral change regarding healthy sanitation practices; (5) Generate awareness about sanitation and its linkage with public health; and (6) Capacity augmentation for urban local bodies to create an enabling environment for private sector participation. It includes swachh survekshan, construction of individual/community/public toilets, door-to-door waste collection, waste to energy conversion, and waste to compost conversion.

### Heat Action Plan

It provides a framework for implementation, coordination, and evaluation of extreme heat response activities in cities or town in India that reduces the negative impact of extreme heat. Its primary objective is to alert those populations at risk of heat-related illness in places where extreme heat conditions either exist or are imminent, and to take appropriate precautions which are at high-risk.

## SUGGESTED READING

1. Atal Mission for Rejuvenation and Urban Transformation. [online] Available from http://amrut.gov.in/#.
2. Forgotten voices: The world of urban children in India. [online] Available from https://www.pwc.in/assets/pdfs/publications/ urban-child/urban-child-india-report.pdf.
3. Guidelines for Preparation of Action Plan—Prevention and Management of Heat-Wave. 2016. National Disaster Management Authority, Government of India.
4. Gupta K, Arnold F, Lhungdim H. 2009. Health and Living Conditions in Eight Indian Cities. National Family Health Survey (NFHS-3), India, 2005-06. Mumbai: International Institute for Population Sciences; Calverton, Maryland, USA: ICF Macro.
5. Guttikunda S, Jawahar P. (2011). Urban Air Pollution Analysis report-India; September 2011. Urban Emissions Info. New Delhi, India.
6. https://censusindia.gov.in/nada/index.php/catalog/44376.
7. https://main.mohfw.gov.in/sites/default/files/NFHS-5_Phase-II_0.pdf.
8. International Institute for Population Sciences, Mumbai and Ministry of health and Family Welfare, Government of India. National Family Health Survey 4 (2015-16): India Fact Sheet.
9. National Urban Health Mission: Framework for implementation. Ministry of Health and Family Welfare, Government of India, May 2013.
10. National Urban Housing and Habitat Policy 2007. Government of India. Ministry of Housing & Urban Poverty Alleviation, New Delhi.
11. National Urban Livelihood Mission (NULM)-Mission document. Government of India. Ministry of Housing and Urban Poverty Alleviation New Delhi.
12. National Urban Renewal Mission–NURM. [online] Available from http://mohua.gov.in/cms/JNNURM.php.
13. Pradhan Mantri Awas Yojna-2015. [online] Available from https://www.pradhanmantriyojana.co.in/pm-awas-yojana/.
14. Rajiv Awas Yojana. [online] Available from https://www.india.gov. in/information-rajiv-awas-yojana.
15. Smart cities mission. Ministry of Housing and Urban Affairs, Government of India. [online] Available from http://smartcities.gov. in/content/innerpage/what-is-smart-city.php.
16. Sustainable Development Goals. [online] Available from https://sustainabledevelopment.un.org/sdg11.
17. Swachh Bharat Urban. Ministry of Housing and Urban Affairs, Government of India. [online] Available from http://swachhbharaturban.gov.in.
18. The challenge of slums: global report on human settlements, 2003. United Nations Human Settlements Program.
19. Twenty steps for developing a Healthy Cities project 3rd Edition, 1997 World Health Organization Regional Office for Europe 1997.
20. Urban Health. [online] Available from http://www.who.int/gho/urban_health/en.

# RURAL HEALTH

## INTRODUCTION

'Rural' means in, of or like the countryside. The census of India defines rural areas as 'areas which do not fall in category of urban'. All places with a municipality, corporation, cantonment board or notified town area committee, etc. (known as statutory town) were classified as urban and not rural areas. In addition, areas having population of less than 5,000, more than 25% engaged in agricultural pursuits and a population density of less than 400 per square km are defined as rural (Gramin Bharat, India.gov.in). Compared to 1960 when 82% of Indian population lived in rural areas; currently 66% population is rural. Globally, 3,476 million, 45% of total world population lives in countryside (rural areas) (World bank, UN Population division's World Urbanization Prospects, 2018; Global urban and rural population in 1995, 2010 and 2025, Statista). Out of this 830 million live in India (Census of India: Rural urban distribution of population, 2011).

Culture is deep rooted in rural societies and villagers love their cultural heritage. Villagers confirm their behavior to established norms of behavior, some of which are good (consuming freshly prepared home-based foods, close social interaction with other villagers, etc.) while some are bad (tobacco addiction, open air defecation, etc). Various factions develop in villages based on thinking, ideology, occupation, caste and other factors having differentiated approach to health services. Villages provide a simple life, pure environment, fresh air to breathe and enough opportunities for thinking and mental development with reduced stress levels and healthy life. Lack of quality educational opportunities as well as ignorance and prejudices (avoiding papaya and banana during pregnancy, avoiding colostrum to infants, preference for male child) exposes them to poor health and well-being. Certain superstitions like isolation of women during menstruation, visit to deity (goddess) temple along with offerings during pregnancies and sacrifices in temples for children or to cure health problems are still present in rural communities.

Rural health or rural medicine is the interdisciplinary study of health and healthcare delivery in rural environments. It is explored that the people of rural areas have comparatively different healthcare needs from those living in urban areas. More than often, the lack of access to healthcare services is prime reason for poor health status of the rural community. Moreover, disparity in other factors, such as geography, socioeconomic conditions, work environment, infrastructure and support as well as individual well-being between urban and rural areas also lead to different health status in both these communities. Rural areas have a higher dependency ratio, as most of the populace is composed of children and elderly. Many health-related problems in rural areas are due to poor socioeconomic condition, lower literacy levels, higher prevalence of tobacco and alcohol addicts, and high mortality due to lack of proper health care. Rural areas in general have high poverty rate, and as we know poverty is one of the largest social determinants of health.

Recently, determining health status of the rural areas is one of the major areas of research in many countries. These efforts have led to the development of several research institutes globally focusing on rural health including the Centre for Rural and Northern Health Research in Canada, Countryside Agency in the United Kingdom, the Institute of Rural Health in Australia, the New Zealand Institute of Rural Health and ICMR–Model Rural Health Research Units in India. The principal objective of such studies is to identify the health care needs of the individuals residing in rural areas, and to provide policy level suggestions to meet those demands. Rural proofing is the concept of incorporating the needs of rural communities into services offered by the government.

Households in rural area comprise 67% of total households in India. 83.3% of households in rural India cook food inside their house of which 46% of households do not have a kitchen and 7% of rural households despite having a kitchen in home, cook food outside their home. Majority of women are exposed to smoke while cooking predisposing them to respiratory illness like chronic obstructive pulmonary disease (COPD).

Around the world, the health status of rural areas is worse than urban (world rural health). With the concentration of poverty, low health status and high burden of disease in rural areas, there is a need to focus specifically on improving the health of people in rural and remote areas. This is essential where migration of rural people to urban areas in need of better situations is very high and has to be reversed. The main issue in rural health is access to care. Generally, the rural people prefer to be taken care of or treated in their local environment with conventional therapies.

According to national census 2011, the rural population constitutes approximately 70% of Indian population, while 91% of country area is rural with a average household size of 4.9 members per household. Like other developing countries, though India has also not been able to provide required number (quantitative) and quality of rural health services, lot has been done to improve demographic indicators of rural health.

About 75% of health infrastructure, medical manpower and other health resources are concentrated in urban areas where 31% of the population live. Infectious diseases, such as diarrhea, amoebiasis, typhoid, infectious hepatitis, worm infestations, measles, malaria, tuberculosis, whooping cough, respiratory infections, pneumonia and reproductive tract infections dominate the morbidity pattern especially in rural areas. A rising trend of noncommunicable diseases especially hypertension, diabetes and cancers has been observed.

## GROWTH RATE

The growth rate of India has declined from 21.5 (2001 census) to 17.6 in (2011 census). This slowing of overall growth rate is attributable to sharp fall of growth rate in rural area from 18.2 to 12.2, while urban area shows no change in the decadal growth rate of 31.5.

The urban infant mortality rate is 23 in comparison 36 per thousand live births in rural. The birth rate in urban and rural areas are 16.1 and 21.1 per thousand respectively (SRS Statistical Report, 2020).

## SOCIODEMOGRAPHIC INDICATORS OF RURAL HEALTH (TABLES 31.6 TO 31.8)

### Literacy Rate

The literacy rate in males and females between 15–49 years of age is 81.5% and 65.9%, respectively for rural areas compared to national literacy of 71.5% and 84.4% among men and women respectively. Almost 41% women of India have 10 or more years of schooling. In rural India only 33% women had completed 10 or more years of school. Women complete primary education as each village has a primary school but secondary school are located in selected villages and insecurity of traveling to another village averts parents from allowing female children to have secondary education. Women education has been neglected since ages with priority for household chores in India. Literacy rates are much lower among SC and ST communities which are predominantly in rural areas. Gender gap in literacy has improved drastically for rural sector 19.8 (census 2011) to 15.6 (NFHS-5, 2019–21).

**Table 31.6:** Summary of household parameters of urban and rural India from census 2011.

| Sl. No. | Parameters | India | Rural | Urban |
|---|---|---|---|---|
| 1 | Condition of occupied households: | 246,740,228 | 167,874,291 | 78,865,937 |
| 1a | Good | 53.1% | 45.9% | 68.4% |
| 1b | Livable | 41.5% | 47.5% | 28.7% |
| 1c | Dilapidated | 5.4% | 6.5% | 2.9% |
| 2 | Type of wall of house: | | | |
| 2a | Kutcha/semi-pucca | 48.4% | 57.6% | 28.7% |
| 2b | Pucca | 51.6% | 42.4% | 71.3% |
| 3 | Type of fuel used for cooking: | | | |
| 3a | Smoke-emitting fuel (firewood, crop residue, cow dung cake, coal, lignite, charcoal, kerosene) | 70.1% | 87.3% | 33.7% |
| 3b | Smokeless fuel (LPG, PNG, electricity, biogas, others) | 29.5% | 12.5% | 65.7% |
| 4 | Drinking water: | | | |
| 4a | Tap water from treated source | 32% | 17.8% | 62% |
| 4b | Tap water from untreated source | 11.6% | 13% | 8.6% |
| 4c | Well, hand pump, tube well, bore well | 52.9% | 65.2% | 26.9% |
| 4d | Spring, river, tank or other source | 3.5% | 4% | 2.5% |
| 4e | Within premises | 47% | 35% | 71% |
| 4f | Near or away from premises | 53% | 65% | 29% |
| 5 | Latrines: | | | |
| 5a | Latrine within premises | 46.9% | 30.7% | 81.4% |
| 5b | Public latrines | 3.2% | 1.9% | 6% |
| 5c | Open | 49.8% | 67.3% | 12.6% |
| 6 | Lighting in house: | | | |
| 6a | Electricity | 67.3% | 55.3% | 92.7% |
| 6b | Kerosene or oil | 31.6% | 43.4% | 6.6% |

(LPG: liquefied petroleum gas; PNG: piped natural gas)

**Table 31.7:** General health indicators (NFHS-5, 2019–21).

| Indicators | Rural | India |
|---|---|---|
| Sex ratio, age 0–6 year (females per 1,000 males) | 931 | 990 |
| Sex ratio at birth for children born in last 5 years (females per 1,000 males) | 931 | 929 |
| Infant mortality rate (IMR) per 1,000 live births (SRS May 2020 Bulletin) | 36 | 32 |
| Under-5 mortality rate per 1,000 live births (SRS May 2020 Bulletin) | 40 | 36 |
| Current use of family planning (currently married women 15–49 years) | 65.6 | 66.7 |
| Female sterilization (currently married women 15–49 years) | 38.7 | 37.9 |
| Unmet need for family planning (currently married women 15–49 years) | 9.9 | 9.6 |

**Table 31.8:** Maternal and child health (NFHS-5, 2019–21).

| Indicators (in percentages) | Rural | India |
|---|---|---|
| At least four antenatal care visits | 54.2 | 58.1 |
| Mothers protected against neonatal tetanus | 91.7 | 92.0 |
| Mothers who consumed iron folic acid for 100 days or more | 40.2 | 44.1 |
| Institutional deliveries | 86.7 | 88.6 |
| Mothers who received postnatal care within 2 days of delivery | 75.4 | 78.0 |
| Children age 12–23 months fully immunized | 76.8 | 76.4 |
| Children underage 6 months exclusively breastfed | 65.1 | 63.7 |
| Children underage 3 years breastfed within an hour of birth | 40.7 | 41.8 |
| Children age 6–8 months receiving solid or semisolid food and breast milk | 43.9 | 45.9 |
| Prevalence of ARI in children | 3.0 | 2.8 |
| Prevalence of diarrhea in children | 7.7 | 7.3 |
| Prevalence of fever in children | 67.8 | 69.0 |

(ARI: acute respiratory infection)

## Households with Amenities

Approximately 90% of rural India have an improved drinking water source and utilize iodized salt. Household members covered by a health scheme or health insurance are less than 30% in rural areas.

## Nutrition

Compared to nutritional status of Indian population at national level and urban areas, rural people have poor nutritional status in almost all parameters, such as body mass index and anemia. Children and women (both pregnant and nonpregnant) were slightly more anemic in rural areas. Among all women between 15–49 years of age, 57% Indian women are anemic and having hemoglobin levels below 11 g/dL, while 58.5% rural women are anemic. During pregnancy, 54.3% rural women are anemic against 52.2% overall national prevalence of anemia in pregnant women.

## Sex Ratio

A higher sex ratio at birth in rural areas (931 females/1,000 males) is attributable for migration of males to urban areas for work, leaving their family in villages.

IMR, U5MR and MMR are higher in rural areas for lack of accessibility to quality health services and poor health seeking behavior.

The health care infrastructure in rural India has been developed as a three tier system and is based on population norms. Subcenters are the most peripheral and first contact point between the primary health care system and community; while primary health centers are the first point of contact between community and medical officer.

## SUGGESTED READING

1. Global urban and rural population in 1995, 2010 and 2025 (in millions). Statista. The statistics portal.
2. https://censusindia.gov.in/nada/index.php/catalog/44376
3. https://main.mohfw.gov.in/sites/default/files/NFHS-5_Phase-II_0.pdf
4. Patil AV, Somasundaram KV, Goyal RC. Current health scenario in rural India. Aust J Rural Health. 2002;10:129-35.
5. Rural population (% of total world population). World Bank staff estimates based on the United Nations Population Division's World Urbanization Prospects: 2014 Revision.
6. World's population increasingly urban with more than half living in urban areas. Available from: http://www.un.org/en/development/desa/news/population/world-urbanization-prospects-2014.html

# TRIBAL HEALTH

## INTRODUCTION

Tribal communities are defined as those communities which have primitive traits, distinctive culture, geographical isolation, shyness of contact with the community at large, and backwardness according to Lokur Committee. Although tribal groups are defined by certain common features, such as similar modes of living, each living in defined areas, having a common dialect within them, having cultural homogeneity and a unifying social organization, each tribal group differs from one group to the other in terms of race, language, culture and beliefs, health practices, etc. As per Constitution of India different tribal groups are specified under Article 366 (25) and Article 342.

India has the second largest tribal population in the world, representing 8.6% of India's population, occupying about 15% of country's total land area. According to Census 2011, there are 705 different tribes identified in India from 30 States and Union Territories. Geographically, they reside mostly in two geographical areas, i.e., Central India and North East India with 89.97% living in rural areas and 10.03% in urban (Ministry of Tribal affairs, Statistical profile of STs of India, 2013). Madhya Pradesh has the highest number of scheduled tribe population in terms of numbers, and Lakshadweep has the highest state ST percentage among the different states and union territories of India.

In India, the tribes can be broadly categorized into five regional groups based on ecological, social, economic, administrative, and ethnic factors:

1. *Himalayan region:* It has three subregions: (A) North-Eastern Himalayan region, (B) Central Himalayan region, and (C) North-Western Himalayan region.
2. *Middle region:* It is constituted by the States of Bihar, Jharkhand, Chhattisgarh, West Bengal, Odisha, and Madhya Pradesh; where more than 55% tribal population lives.
3. *Western region:* It includes the states of Rajasthan, Gujarat, Maharashtra, Goa, Dadra and Nagar Haveli.
4. *Southern region:* It is comprised of the states of Andhra Pradesh, Tamil Nadu, Karnataka, and Kerala.
5. *Island region:* The Islands of Andaman and Nicobar in the Bay of Bengal and Lakshadweep in the Arabian Sea.

The tribal communities in India belong to three races viz. Proto-Australoids, Mongoloids, and Negroids and speak four major families of languages viz.—Austro-Asiatic Family, Tibeto-Chinese family, Dravidian family, and Indo-European Family.

The tribal population are distinct groups of people who are dependent on their land for their livelihoods, largely self-sufficient and self-reliant, and generally isolated and not integrated into the national society. In general they faired worst in all kinds of growth and development indicators, including health indicators among the different groups of society. The disease patterns and health seeking behavior in them are different as compared to the general population due and among certain tribes because of their isolation, a mere contact with the outside world can often set off deadly epidemics which has the capacity to exterminate the whole tribe as seen among India's Jarawa tribes with measles and malaria outbreaks.

The distribution of scheduled tribe population in various states of India is shown in **Figure 31.2**.

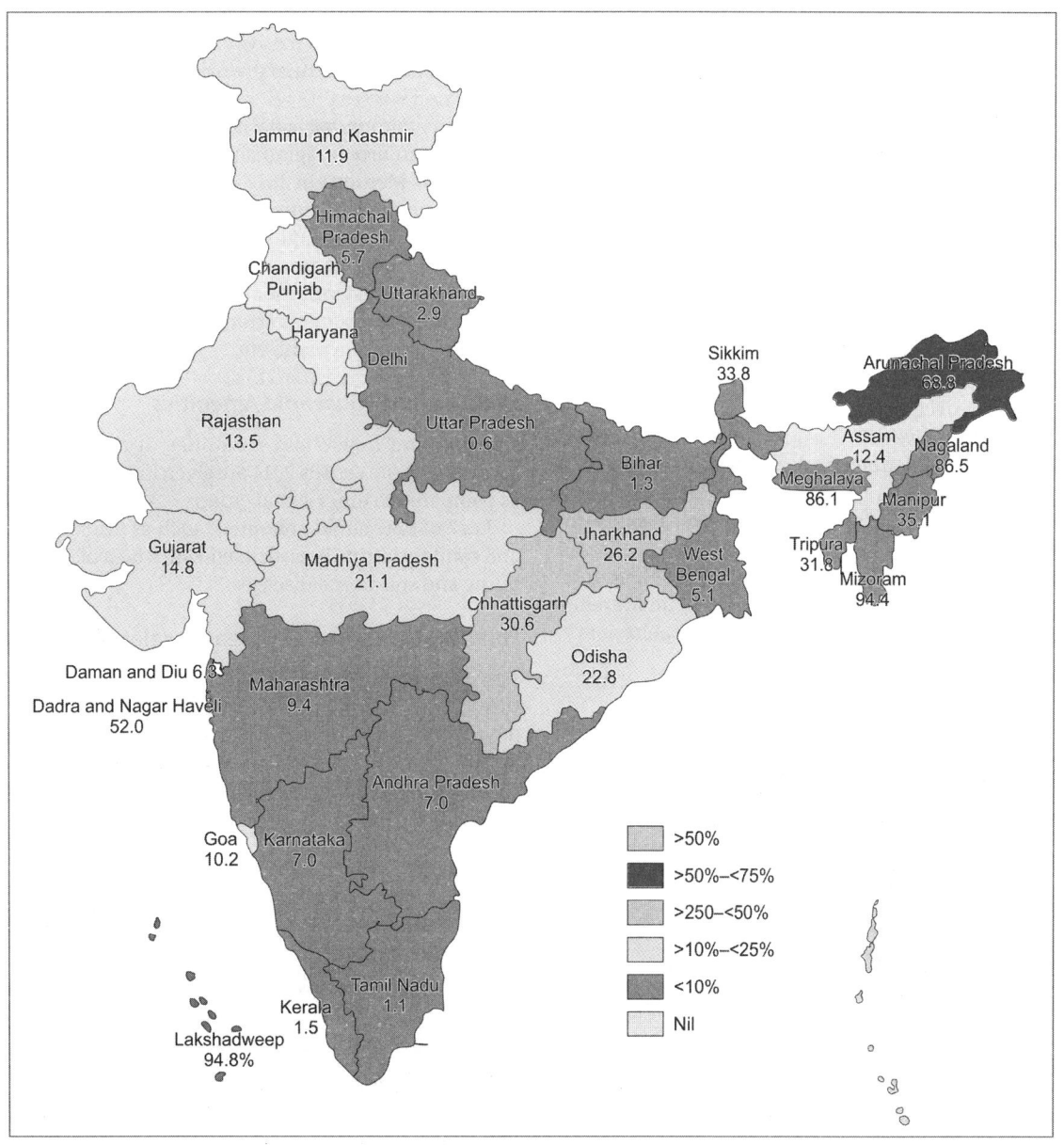

**Fig. 31.2:** Percentage of state-wise schedule tribe population.

## SOCIODEMOGRAPHIC, ECONOMIC AND HEALTH STATUS OF TRIBAL POPULATION IN INDIA

### Demography and Extinction

An increasing trend in the population size is seen among the tribal communities as in the rest of India, but the growth rate is slower among some tribes and in some, there is negative population growth leading to extinction. In India, Jarawa tribe in the Andamans, Khairwar and Korku tribes of Madhya Pradesh, Dhimal tribe of North Bengal, etc., are designated as Particularly Vulnerable Tribal Groups, who has worst socioeconomic and health indicators compared to other tribes, and they are at risk of going into extinction along with their languages and there are currently such 75 recognized communities (Planning Commission, 12th five year plan, 2012). To counter declining population among the tribal population, certain states in India have put a ban on sterilization among tribal population (Madhya Pradesh, now Chhattisgarh).

### *Sex Ratio*

Sex ratio among tribal population in India is 990, and they have the best sex ratio across all social groups currently (Census, 2011). Child sex ratio is still highest across social groups, although it is showing a declining trend as observed in the rest of population of India.

### *Literacy*

Literacy among tribal is the lowest in India as shown in **Figure 31.3**. Although improvement is seen in the literacy rate over the years, with declining trend in school dropout rates, the quality of education received remain questionable. Annual Status of Education Report (ASER) from tribal rural districts reported 93% of students studying in Class V could not read Class II textbook (Ministry of Tribal affairs, Report of High level Committee, 2014).

Lack of education and quality education makes them more vulnerable to superstitious beliefs and practices, unawareness about health issues, and unhealthy health seeking behaviors.

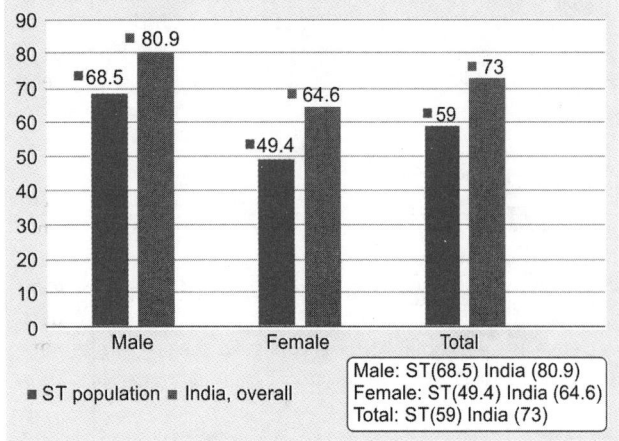

**Fig. 31.3:** Bar diagram comparing literacy among schedule tribe population with overall population of India.
*Source:* Census of India: 2011

### *Economic Typology and Poverty*

According to Vidyarthi, economic typology of the Indian tribes can be grouped into eight groups and they are:
1. Forest hunting type
2. Hill cultivation type
3. Plain agriculture type
4. Simple Artisan type
5. Pastoral and cattle Herder type
6. Folk-artist type
7. Agricultural and nonagricultural type (the tribe working in manufacturing industry)
8. Skilled, white collar job and traders type (some individuals, of the families of tribal communities are working in the State and Central Government services owing the facilities of reservation for the tribes) and so on.

According to the census 2001, 44.70% of the scheduled tribe (ST) population were cultivators, 36.9% agricultural laborers, 2.1% household industry workers, and 16.3% were other occupation workers.

Poverty rate among tribal is highest with 45.3% in rural region and 24.1% in urban region according to Planning Commission (Tendulkar Method) in 2011–2012 as against 25.7% and 13.7% in the general population during the same period (Planning Commission of India, 12th Five year Plan, 2012).

The availability of funds directly affects the kind and extend of health services. A family or individual avails in times of ill-health and indirectly through various factors, such as malnutrition, illiteracy, unemployment, etc.

### *Housing and Household Amenities*

Housing and household amenities of the tribal population according to the census 2011 are given in **Table 31.9**, faring lower as compared to other social groups.

Lack of household amenities, such as drinking water source and sanitary latrine is associated with a host of infectious water-borne and soil-borne diseases.

### Health Status and Key Health-related Indicators

The general health status of the tribal population is far from satisfactory with high morbidity and mortality. The key health indicators among the tribal communities are given in **Table 31.10**. They performed poorer compared to other social groups and are among the most disadvantaged social groups in India.

**Table 31.9:** Housing and household amenities among tribal population.

| Housing and household amenities | Schedule tribe | Others |
|---|---|---|
| Good house condition | 40.6% | 57.2% |
| Within premises drinking water source | 19.7% | 52.8% |
| Household using electricity | 59% | 67% |
| Latrine facilities within premises | 23% | 47% |
| Fuel for cooking—firewood/crop residue, cow dung cake | 87% | 66% |

Others: Other social groups

Table 31.10: Key health indicators among tribal population (NFHS-5, 2019-21).

| Health indicators | Schedule tribe | India |
|---|---|---|
| Under 5 mortality rate per 1,000 live births | 50.3 | 41.9 |
| IMR per 1,000 live births | 41.6 | 35.2 |
| Neonatal mortality rate per 1,000 live births | 28.8 | 24.9 |
| All basic immunization (BCG, MCV/Measles/MMR/MR, and three doses each of DPT/Penta and Polio vaccine) | 76.5% | 76.5% |
| Life expectancy at birth | 60* | 68 |
| Total fertility rate (TFR) | 2.09 | 1.99 |

Source: National Family Health Survey-5.

The diseases seen among the tribal population are varied as the tribal groups themselves. Common conditions which are seen in them are given below.

- **Nutritional disorders:** The proportions of men and women who are thin are 25.2% and 31.7%, respectively, while the percentage of overweight or obesity is 9.8% in men and 10% in women highlighting undernutrition as a major problem among them along with anemia and other micronutrients, such as vitamins and minerals.
  - The prevalence of anemia is high with 64.6% in women and 32.7% in men (National Family Health Survey-5, 2019-21).
  - The consumption of essential vitamins and minerals among the scheduled tribes is lowest among all social groups. It also has been seen that the consumption of different nutrients is consisted below the recommended dietary allowances.
  - *Undernutrition among children:* The nutritional status of the children is given in **Table 31.11**. The prevalence of malnutrition specifically undernutrition is high among them. The percentage of children who are anemic is 76.8%, the highest across all social categories.

Table 31.11: Nutritional status among tribal children (NFHS-5, 2019-21).

| Social groups | Stunted | Wasted | Underweight |
|---|---|---|---|
| Schedule tribe | 40.9% | 23.2% | 39.5% |
| India | 35.5% | 19.3% | 32.1% |

Source: National Family Health Survey-5.

  - Percentage of ST children consuming foods rich in vitamin A is at 43.8% which is lower than the national average. The tribal population are considered as "Son of soil" and they consume what is produced and foraged in their surroundings, which makes them more vulnerable to nutritional deficiencies.
  - The vicious cycle of malnutrition and infection is well known; inadequate dietary intake leading to weight loss, lowered immunity making them more prone to different morbidities both in childhood and adulthood.
- **Communicable diseases:** The incidence of communicable diseases among the tribal population is high. Diseases such as tuberculosis, malaria, human immunodeficiency virus (HIV) or acquired immunodeficiency syndrome (AIDS), hepatitis, sexually transmitted diseases (STDs), filariasis, diarrhea and dysentery, hepatitis, parasitic infestation, viral and fungal infections, conjunctivitis, yaws, scabies, measles, leprosy, acute respiratory infections, etc., are common in them.

Poverty, poor hygiene with poor environmental sanitation, lack of safe drinking water, low literacy, and poor health care delivery services are major factors associated with prevalence of communicable diseases.
  - *Malaria:* The prevalence of malaria is varied, and is as high as 50% in certain places with *Plasmodium falciparum* accounting for 30–90% of the infections in the forested areas (ICMR, Tribal Bulletin, 2004). Proximity to forest in their habitation is considered as one of the major factors leading to high number of cases of malaria.
  - *Tuberculosis:* Prevalence of tuberculosis is as high as 1,500 per 1 lakh population among the tribal population with an average estimate of 703 per 1 lakh population. Inaccessibility to health care service, prevalent malnutrition, and HIV infections could be some of the reasons contributing to the rise in the number of tuberculosis (Thomas BE et al., Indian J Med Res, 2015).
  - *HIV:* HIV prevalence rate is 0.46% among the STs according to National Family Health Survey-4, and is same in both men and women. Different sexual practices with high prevalence of sexually transmitted diseases, prevalent injectable drug users, poor health care services and their utilization are some reasons which have led to high prevalence of this disease among the tribal population.
- **Noncommunicable diseases and risk factors:** The incidence of chronic noncommunicable diseases is on the rise among the tribal population also and is seen in the rest of the population.
  - *Hypertension:* The prevalence of hypertension among adult men varies from 14.8–19.9%, and that of female is 10.8–18.5%. The prevalence of hypertension does not vary much across the social groups but the health seeking behavior is poorer among tribal communities.
  - *Diabetes mellitus:* According to study by the National Institute of Nutrition, the prevalence of diabetes mellitus is 6.6% in men and 5.5% in women (National Nutrition Monitoring Bureau, ICMR, 2012).
  - *Cancers:* In northeast region which has high percentage of tribal in each state also has the two districts which have the highest incidence of cancer in India, i.e., Aizawl in Mizoram and Papumpare in Arunachal Pradesh. The factors which are thought to be responsible are excessive consumption of tobacco and betel nut, consumption of large amount of hot beverages, with different food habits, such as consumption of smoked meat.
  - The prevalence of overweight and obesity is 10.9% in men and 10.6% in women, and excess in waist circumference is 6.9% in men, and 11% in women.
  - Tobacco use among tribal men is 56.8% and among tribal women is 16.9% highest across all social groups. Alcohol use among tribal women is 6.5%, whereas in other women it is less than 1%. Among men the alcohol use is 41.3%, and it is still the highest across all social groups (Census, 2011). One of the reasons considered for the high consumption is its acceptance culturally and traditionally especially in the northeastern region of the country.

- ***Diseases common in tribal population:*** Hemoglobinopathies are commonly seen among the tribal population.
  - Sickle cell disease and trait are conditions which are common among tribal communities with a prevalence of up to 40% is seen among the tribes residing in central, western, eastern, and southern region (Balgir RS, Int Public Health J, 2011; Naidy KV, IJMART, 2015).
  - Glucose-6-phosphate dehydrogenase deficiency is seen among Kondh, Bhatra, Gond, Pajara with prevalence of 16%. Higher prevalence of up to 27.9% is seen in certain tribal communities (Balgir RS, OJHAS, 2011; Chakma T, Glimpses of Tribal health in India, ICMR).
  - Hemoglobin E is a common condition seen in southeast Asia, and is most commonly prevalent among the people belonging to northeast region of India.
  - *Thalassemia* gene is seen in among tribal communities of Parajan Bhuyan, Kutia Kondh, Lodha, etc., with prevalence of up to 12.7% among them (Balgir RS, Indian National Confederation and Academy of Anthropologists: Jhargram; 2013).
  
  The practice of endogamy or consanguineous marriage prevalent in their culture and customs may be one of the important reasons for the common prevalence of these diseases.
- ***Maternal and child health:*** The indicators of maternal and child health among the scheduled tribes have continued to improve over several years. As compared to NHFS-4, the indicators like pregnancy registration, antenatal care through skilled health attendant, two tetanus toxoid injection, 100 tablets of iron-folic acid, prevalence of acute respiratory infection in children, etc. have improved and now at par with India level.

---

*A story from a poor remote tribal village of northeast India*

Doing strenuous physical activities during term pregnancy till development of labor pains and getting back to work right after delivery is a common scene in the poor tribal regions. The short narration below tells the everyday story of the poor tribal women.

One fine day, a term pregnant lady climbed the treacherous mountains to work in the fields alone, a place far away from the village for livelihood. As she toiled in the fields, her labor started. There were no health facilities in the vicinity nor were there anyone who responded to her cry of help. She was all on her own. Upon realizing that the delivery was eminent, she prepared herself to deliver her child in the field. She got a blade of a variety of "tall grass" which grows commonly in the region to cut the umbilical cord with its sharp edge, and got a small cloth to tie it. She delivered her 8th child in the field, cut the cord, and wrapped the child up in her working clothes and after resting for a while walked back home with the child in her arms.

Fortunately for her family, both the mother and child survived.

---

- ***Others:*** Injuries due to accidents, snake bites, and animal bites are common among the tribal population because of their close proximity to the forests.

### Health Care Delivery in Tribal Population

Public health care infrastructure for healthcare delivery in the tribal population of rural setting follows a different population norm, where one subcenter is for 3,000 populations, and one primary health center for 20,000 population. According to rural health statistics there is a huge shortfall of doctors at primary health centers and physicians, pediatricians, or any other specialist at community health centers in tribal areas making healthcare unavailable to majority of the tribal. The problems are compounded by lack of essential drugs and equipment, difficult terrain and lack of transport facilities and communication, and traditional healers and practices. These factors make the health care delivery to the tribal population poor and inefficient.

Health is a function of different sectors working effectively together with different groups of people enjoying equal health. The tribal population as seen lacks behind in any type of indicators or growth and development and to improve their health and well-being, special emphasis is required. Although different schemes targeted to tribal population are provided by the government of India, the progress seen is not substantial.

There is also a huge deficit in researches carried out among the tribal population. Availability of information is crucial for the planning and development of any community.

## POLICIES AND PROGRAMMES

In India, the Nehruvian Panchsheel of 1952 are the five guiding principles for the administration of tribal affairs for socioeconomic development as there is no National Tribal Policy at present. The Scheduled Castes and Tribes (Prevention of Atrocities) Act 1989 is an act to prevent atrocities against the scheduled castes and tribes of the country and the Scheduled Tribes and Other Traditional Forest Dwellers Act 2006 is to address the historical injustice committed against forest dwellers and restore their right to the land and forest produce. Ministry of Tribal Affairs is the nodal agency for looking after the affairs of the tribal but this Ministry along with Ministry of Health and Family Welfare has largely ignored the health component of the tribal population.

The first national policy on identifying the importance of tribal health recommended various schemes and modifications in population norms for tribal population and Medical Care for Remote and Marginalized and Nomadic Communities was also launched in the 9th 5-year plan targeting the "primitive tribal groups" now called particularly vulnerable tribal groups and nomads. But there are no concrete health development plans laid down for the tribal population.

## SUMMARY

Major factors associated with increased risk of development of disease among the tribal populations are:
- Poverty
- Malnutrition
- Difficult geographical terrains and isolation
- Low literacy
- Poor environmental sanitation and lack of safe drinking water
- Lack of health infrastructure and manpower
- Lack of researches
- Lack of concrete development plan and policies
- Sociocultural barriers and taboo
- Beliefs in taboos, spiritual powers and faith healing, invalidated tribal remedies, compounded with lack of availability, and access to established system of medicine contributed to the failure of delivery of health services to the tribal population.

## SUGGESTED READING

1. Balgir RS. Biomedical anthropology in contemporary tribal society of India. In: Behera DK, Pfeffer G (Eds.) Contemporary Society: Tribal Studies (Tribal Situation in India). New Delhi: Concept Publishing Company. 2005;6: 292-301.
2. Basu S. Dimensions of tribal health in India. Health Population Perspect Issues. 2000;23(2):61-70.
3. Guha BS. The Racial Affinities of People of India. Census, of India 1931, Vol. I Part 1MB, Government Press, Shimla.
4. ICMR Bulletin. Health status of primitive tribes of Orissa. Indian Council of Medical Research. 2003;33(10).
5. ICMR Bulletin. Tribal Malaria. Indian Council of Medical Research. 2004:34(1).
6. Lokur BN. The report of the advisory committee on the Revision of the lists of scheduled castes and scheduled tribes. New Delhi: Department of Social Security; 1965.
7. Ministry of Health and Family Welfare. Rural health statistics. 2017.
8. Ministry of Tribal Affairs. Annual Report 2016-17. New Delhi.
9. Ministry of Tribal Affairs. Report of high level committee on socio-economic, health and educational status of tribal communities of India. New Delhi; 2014.
10. MOHFW. (2012). Indian Public Health Standards (IPHS) guidelines for primary health centers. New Delhi: Directorate General of Health Services, Ministry of Health and Family Welfare, Government of India. (online) Available from http://mohfw.nic.in/NRHM/IPHS_Revised_Guidlenes_2012/Primary_Health_Centres.pdf.
11. Murhekar MV, Chakravarty R, Murhekar KM, et al. Hepatitis B virus genotypes among the Jarawas: a primitive Negrito tribe of Andaman and Nicobar Islands, India. Archives of Virology. 2006;151(8):1499-510.
12. Naidy KV. Tribal health care problems in India: An Overview. IJMART. 2015;2(3):49-54.
13. National Centre for Disease Informatics and Research. Annual report 2016-17. Bangalore: Indian Council of Medical Research; 2017.
14. National Nutrition Monitoring Bureau. Diet and Nutritional Status of Rural Population, prevalence of hypertension, and diabetes among adults and infant and young child feeding practices. Hyderabad: National Institute of Nutrition-Indian Council of Medical Research; 2012.
15. Planning Commission. Twelfth Five Year Plan. New Delhi; 2012.
16. Statistics Division. Statistical profile of Scheduled Tribes of India. Ministry of Tribal Affairs. 2013.

# CHAPTER 32

# Traveler's Health

*Yogita Bavaskar, Sumit Aggarwal, Alka Kaware, Manoj Talapalliwar, Poonam Sancheti*

> "The world is a book and those who do not travel read only one page".
> —St. Augustine

| | |
|---|---|
| CM8.1 | Describe and discuss the epidemiology of traveler's health problems and prevention. |
| CM18.1 | International health—international health regulations for travelers. |

## INTRODUCTION

The medical specialty dealing with traveler's health is called as Travel medicine or Emporiatrics (In Greek, "Emperos" meaning traveler, "iatrics" means medicine). It is a specialized branch of medicine which is concerned with the prevention and management of traveler's related various health issues. This branch of medicine deals with the epidemiology of the health risks to the traveler globally, prevention of disease, vaccination and pretravel counseling.

In the era of globalization, traveling is inevitable. Globally there is an increase in number and speed of traveling from one geographical part to another geographic part of the world. International travel is increased for tourism, personal meetings, ecotourism, medical tourism, commerce, trade, academic, research, political, etc. International tourism showed resilience throughout 2022 despite major headwinds such as the emergence of the Omicron variant at the end of 2021, the Russian invasion of Ukraine and a challenging economic environment, especially high inflation. Some 963 million tourists travelled internationally in 2022, more than double those in 2021, though 34% fewer than in 2019, meaning 66% of pre-pandemic visitors were recovered (International Tourism Highlights, 2023) **(Figs. 32.1 and 32.2)**.

Globally, the power of tourism could be and should be used as a driving force to achieve sustainable development by the year 2030. It is included as a target in 3 out of 17 SDG (target 8.9, 12.b, 14.7).

The importance of traveler's health in India came into focus in February 2003, the respiratory illness SARS spread beyond China, when several international travelers became infected and within 4 months, 8,000 cases of SARS and nearly 800 deaths occurred in 29 countries. It generated widespread

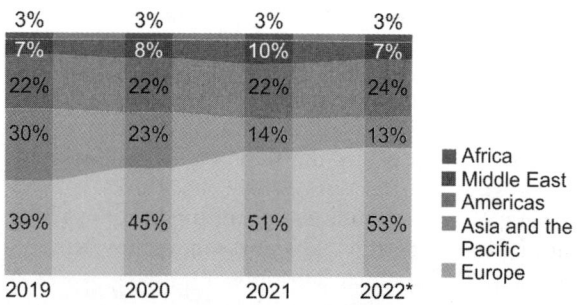

**Fig. 32.1:** International tourism receipts (share of world, %), Data as of June 2023.

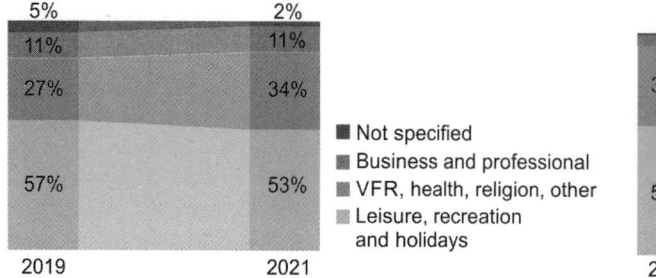

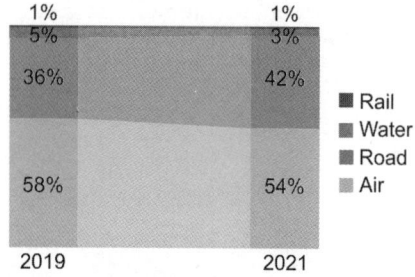

**Fig. 32.2:** Purpose of visit and mode of transport in world, 2019 and 2021.
(VFR: visiting friends and relatives)
*Source:* UNWTO, international tourism highlights, 2023.

panic, affecting travel and threatened global economy. The international concern is to eliminate or minimize the risk of transporting endemic diseases and travel-related conditions to nonendemic geographical areas without affecting trade, tourism and other sectors of life.

India being growing economy has major concern in traveler's health. The number of Indian nationals who undertook foreign trips during 2022 were 21.09 million.

In year 2022, India recorded Foreign Tourist Arrivals (FTAs) of 6.19 million with a growth of 305.4% over same period of the previous year and there were 677.63 million Domestic Tourist Visits (DTVs) 10.55 million Foreign Tourist Visits (FTVs) all over the country during the year 2021 (Ministry of Tourism, GOI, Annual Report 2022–23).

## TRAVEL EPIDEMIOLOGY

### Burden of Travel-related Diseases

- The exact burden of travel-related diseases is difficult to calculate. It's very hard to get a precise numerator (number of cases with the disease/event in the travelers) and denominator (number of travelers altogether or travelers for a particular destination). The major problem is that most of the travelers who get infected would have come back to their native countries before developing symptoms so would not be recorded in the surveillance data of traveled country. Similarly, diseases having short incubation periods or of less durations may have been cured before a traveler returns one's own country and thus might not be reflected in surveillance data of that country.
- Post-travel illness surveillance information collected from 2007 to 2011 by the Geo Sentinel network around the world shows that majority of travel-related illnesses were contracted in the Asia (33%) followed by sub-Saharan Africa (27%). Whereas in 2013 diarrhea, fever, and acute respiratory infection (ARI) were the most common diseases reported.
- Infectious diseases are the main cause of illness among travelers but, they account for only 1–4% of deaths in travelers. Geographical distribution of acquiring infectious diseases shows that falciparum malaria was more prevalent in West Africa, typhoid in Indian subcontinent whereas leptospirosis and scrub typhus in Southeast Asia.
- Cardiovascular problems were the most common single cause of death, contributing for nearly 50% of all deaths among international travelers, followed by other medical causes 25% and injuries 13%. The most common cause of injury were vehicle accidents, followed by drowning **(Figs. 32.3 and 32.4)**.

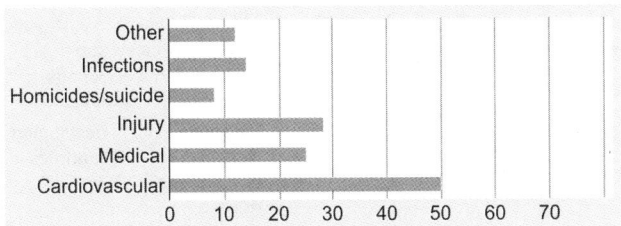

**Fig. 32.3:** Causes of death in travelers.

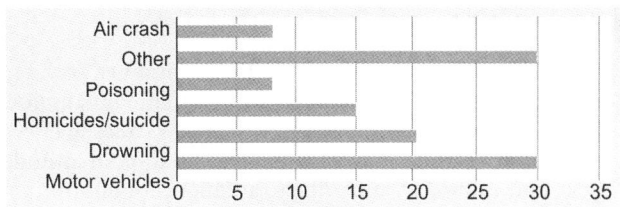

**Fig. 32.4:** Injury-related causes of death in travelers.
*Source:* International travel and health, WHO, 2012 Report.

## DETERMINANTS OF HEALTH RISK DURING TRAVEL

The risk of travel-related illness varies among the travelers, depending on traveler's characteristics and destination. The determinants of health risks are as follows **(Fig. 32.5)**:

- **Pre-existing health issues of the traveler:** Health status of traveler before starting travel is the important determinant of health during travel period. Whether traveler has any history of health problem, allergies or previous immunizations; and in case of a female traveler, whether she is pregnant or breast-feeding. Infants, chronically ill, immunocompromised and old age travelers may have more risk.
- **Destination(s), standards of accommodation, food hygiene and sanitation:** Poor quality and unhygienic accommodation at destinations, inadequate medical services and nonaccess to clean water can cause serious risks to health of travelers. So, travelers traveling into remote area must take precautions to prevent illness.

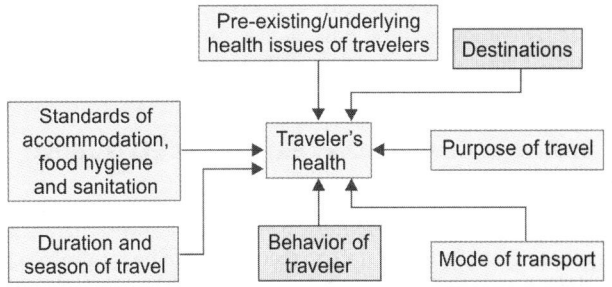

**Fig. 32.5:** Key determinants of health risk.

- **Purpose of travel and behavior of traveler:** Travelers going for field works and staying in temporary shelters are at higher risk due to exposure to natural physical and biological environments. If someone goes outside in malaria-endemic area without practicing proper precautions to avoid mosquito bites may result in getting malaria.
- **Season and duration of travel:** Season of travel will determine the exposure to infectious diseases and ultimately the necessity of some vaccines or drugs, such as antimalarial drugs. The duration of travel determines whether traveler is exposed to noticeable fluctuations due to altitude, humidity and temperature or to sustained exposure to pollution.
- **Mode of transport:** Cruise/ship where large number of people from different regions of the world travel together was a determinant in several influenza outbreaks.

## TRAVEL HEALTH RISKS

- **Health Risk Factors Related to Environment:** Travelers frequently experiences sudden and dramatic fluctuations in the environmental situations, which may cause ill effects on health. Traveler may have to face variation in altitude, heat and humidity, ultraviolet radiation, foodborne and waterborne health hazards, intestinal parasites, animals and insects bites, etc.
- **Exposure to Blood or Other Body Fluids:** For travelers, blood transfusion may be required during a medical emergency due to sudden massive blood loss, i.e., road traffic accident, surgery, severe gastrointestinal hemorrhage, gynecological or obstetric emergency.
- **Infectious Diseases of Potential Risk:** Travelers may get exposed to prevalent infection in area visited, i.e., vector-borne diseases, enteric fever and nonspecific viral syndromes, etc. Modes of transmission can be foodborne and waterborne, vector-borne, zoonosis, sexually transmitted diseases, bloodborne, airborne or transmission via soil.
- **Injuries and Violence:** Travelers may get injured due to violence or unintentional injuries. Road traffic accidents, injuries during recreational activity, such as swimming, diving, sailing and other activities pose a serious threat. Evidence show that, how traveling in holiday significantly increases risk of violence due to alcohol and illicit drug uses.
- **Psychological Health:** Some times international travel may be stressful due to various reasons. Travelers may feel separated from family and social support system, to face foreign cultures, languages and unexperienced threats to health and well-being. This may eventually lead to physical and psychological problems, such as anxiety, mood disorders and suicide attempts. Pre-existing psychological disorders may get exacerbated.

## VARIOUS CONDITIONS EXPERIENCED DURING TRAVEL

- **Jet lag:** Older people are more likely to have severe jet lag and generally takes longer time to recover. It can be minimized by adapting to the local schedule as early as possible. Jet lag can be avoided by prior adjusting sleep schedules before traveling.
- **Traveler's diarrhea:** It is caused by contaminated food, water along with contributing factors, such as anxiety, jet lag, etc. It often comes abruptly and leads to four to five episodes of loose motions. In most of the cases, traveler's diarrhea will subside in a day or two without taking medical treatment.
- **Motion sickness:** Travelers who are susceptible to motion sickness must consult a physician for medications to prevent motion sickness.
- **Altitude sickness:** At higher altitude, presence of dry air, reduced oxygen concentration and low barometric pressure results in altitude sickness. It causes headache, shortness of the breath and dehydration. Mostly one can face altitude sickness at 10,000 feet or more, but a few individuals may get affected at 5,000 feet.
- **Middle east respiratory syndrome (MERS):** It's a viral respiratory illness which was first reported in year 2012 in Saudi Arabia. Causative agent is a corona virus known as MERS-CoV. Most people develop severe acute respiratory illness having fever, cough and shortness of breath, while mortality is 50%.

## PREVENTIVE MEASURES AND PRECAUTIONS

To prevent the travel related health issues following precautions can be followed:

### General Precautions

Travelers, travel organizations, medical professionals and host governments are accountable to provide health care services to travelers who are traveling between different countries and continents. Travelers should have health insurance for destinations with major health risks and where medical care is costly or is not easily available. Travelers should carry a basic medical kit and personal health information card every time they are traveling. Health information card in the local language stating blood group, chronic diseases or allergies, and medications being taken.

### Specific Precautions

#### Vaccines for Travelers (Table 32.1)

- **Routine vaccination:** DPT, hepatitis B, *H. influenzae* type b, MMR, pneumococcal, OPV, rotavirus, BCG, HPV.
- **Selective use for travelers:** Hepatitis A, Japanese encephalitis (JE), meningococcal, rabies, typhoid, yellow fever.

### Vaccination for Special Disease Conditions

Additional vaccinations includes influenza and pneumonia vaccines for individuals having asthma, respiratory, cardiac diseases, diabetes and over 65 years of age. Vaccination for young travelers—Meningococcal vaccine, HPV.

**Table 32.1:** Vaccine recommendations for specific diseases.

| Diseases | Vaccine | Dose | Remark | Mandatory for these countries |
|---|---|---|---|---|
| Hepatitis A | Hepatitis A vaccine | 0.02–0.05 mg/kg body weight, every 4 months | It should not be given 3 weeks prior and up to 2 weeks after giving live vaccine | Developing countries |
| Meningococcal meningitis | Meningococcal vaccine-serogroups (A, C, Y and W135) | 0.5 mL IM | | Saudi Arabia during the Hajj pilgrimage, sub-Saharan Africa |
| Japanese encephalitis | JE vaccine | 0.5 mL SC, 3 doses | | Asian countries |
| Yellow fever | Yellow fever vaccine | 0.5 mL, IM | Single dose can give life long immunity | Sub-Saharan Africa |
| Rabies | Anti-rabies vaccine, pre-exposure | 0.1 mL ID on 0, 3, 7 days | For adults and children, occupational risk (e.g., veterinarians) | Developing countries |

(IM: intramuscular; SC: subcutaneous; JE: Japanese encephalitis; ID: intradermal)

## Malaria

Chemoprophylaxis complemented by personal protective measures and vector control measures are used.

### Short-term Prophylaxis (Less than 6 Months)

Daily antimalarial have to be initiated the day before arrival to destination area. Chloroquine (weekly) should be started 1 week before travel and mefloquine (weekly) should be started 2-3 weeks before travel, to achieve higher pretravel blood levels and to know side effects if any. These prophylactic medications have to be taken regularly for the whole duration of stay in the malaria endemic area, and continued for 4 weeks after departure.

### Long-term Chemoprophylaxis (More than 6 Months)

Follow-up screening is recommended twice-yearly for early retinal changes, for a person who has taken 300 mg of chloroquine weekly for more than 5 years and after 3 years if chloroquine has been taken daily in dose of 100 mg. Mefloquine is contraindicated in persons with history of convulsions, neuropsychiatric problems and cardiovascular diseases **(Table 32.2)**.

Table 32.2: Drug regimens for prophylaxis of malaria.

| Drugs | | Usual amount per tablet/capsule | Adult dose |
|---|---|---|---|
| Generic name | Trade name | | For prophylaxis |
| Chloroquine[a] | Aralen Avlochlor Nivaquine Resochin | 100 or 150 mg (base) | 3 tablets of 100 mg or 2 tablets of 150 mg once a week or 1 tablet of 100 mg daily for 6 days per week |
| Proguanil[b] | Paludrine | 100 mg | 2 tablets (200 mg) once a day |
| Mefloquine[c] | Laraim Eloquin Mephaquin | 250 mg | 1 tablet (250 mg) once a week on the same day each week |
| Doxycycline[d] | Vibramycin | 100 mg | 1 capsule (100 mg) once a day |

[a]Also available as suspension
[b]Recommended only in association with chloroquine
[c]The use of higher treatment dose regimen is recommended for infections acquired in areas on the Thailand/Cambodia and Thailand/Myanmar borders only
[d]There is little experience with this drug and knowledge of its efficacy and toxicity is limited

## Infectious Diseases for which there are no Vaccines

Infectious diseases, such as acute gastroenteritis, traveler's diarrhea, amoebic dysentery and giardiasis are treated by drugs like trimethoprim-sulfamethoxazole, doxycycline, ciprofloxacin (500 mg), norfloxacin (400 mg), imidazole group antibiotics as directed by physician.

## Preventive Measures Against Fecal-Oral Disease

Bottled water is safe otherwise water can be boiled before drinking. Hand washing should be done often and always before handling and having food. Ensure to have thoroughly cooked food and consume it when it's still hot. Avoid roadside food. Carry ORS in medical kit.

## Measures to Reduce Jet Lag

Old age travelers may experience severe jet lag. Eat light meals and limit consumption of alcohol and caffeine. At least 4-hour sleep during the local night, i.e., "anchor sleep" is important to adapt the body's internal clock to new time.

## Conditions Requiring Blood Transfusion

Travelers with chronic medical diseases, such as thalassemia or hemophilia should get medical advice before traveling.

### Pre-exposure Vaccination

Travelers should get vaccinated with Hepatitis B vaccine for protection against hepatitis B.

### Post-exposure Prophylaxis

It is carried out as an emergency medical response for protection against HIV and hepatitis B infection. During accidental exposure to infected blood and/or other body fluids, immediate first-aid care and post-exposure prophylaxis (PEP) should be provided.

## Measures to Prevent Road Traffic Collisions and Injuries

Travelers should know the formal and local traffic rules of destination countries. Beware of wandering animals. Do not drive after drinking alcohol. Do not drive on unfamiliar roads.

## Measures for Adaptation to the Environment

Excessive sun exposure can cause erythema, chemical hypersensitivity, eye damage, bleaching of the skin and skin cancers including malignant melanoma. Clothing made of natural fibers, such as cotton having light colors is preferable to dark fabrics. One should drink at least 2 liters of fluid/day.

## Preventive Measures to Ensure Mental Health During Travel

Travelers with a significant history of mental disorder should receive specific medical advice and self-monitoring techniques. Almost 1 in 10,000 travelers taking mefloquine prophylaxis against malaria develop neuropsychiatric problems, such as seizures, encephalopathy as well as psychosis.

# INTERNATIONAL HEALTH REGULATIONS

The International Health Regulations (IHR) is an agreement among 196 countries, including all WHO Member countries, to work together for health security of the world. Under the IHR, all countries need to report all events of international public health impact. The IHR were adopted in 1969, amended in 1973 and 1981 and completely revised in 2005. The purpose of the regulations is to prevent, protect against, control, and provide public health responses to the international spread of disease in ways that are

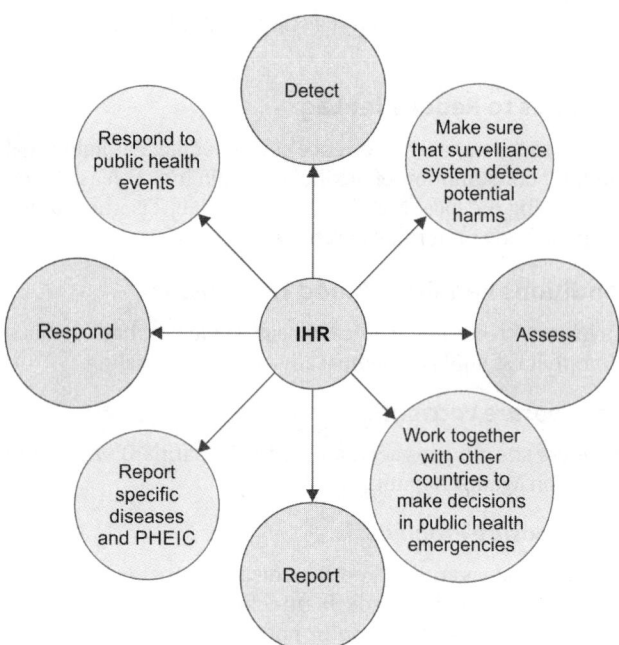

**Fig. 32.6:** International health regulations (IHR) mandates.
(PHEIC: public health emergencies of international concerns)

commensurate with and restricted to public health risks, and that avoid unnecessary interference with international traffic and trade.

The IHR mandates **(Fig. 32.6)** all countries to:
- **Detect:** Ensure surveillance systems and laboratories are able to detect public health threats.
- **Assess:** Work in collaboration in case of public health emergencies.
- **Report:** Report any other potential public health emergency of international concern.
- **Respond:** Responding to the public health events.

The goal of the IHR is "to stop events in their tracks before they become emergencies".

## Principles of International Health Regulations

The regulations shall be implemented:
- With full respect for dignity, human rights and fundamental freedom of persons
- Guided by the charter of the United Nations and the constitution of the WHO
- Guided by the goal of their universal application for the protection of all people of the world from the international spread of disease
- States have right to legislate and to implement legislation in pursuance of their health policies.

## PUBLIC HEALTH EMERGENCIES OF INTERNATIONAL CONCERN

The revised IHR outlines the assessment, management and information sharing for public health emergencies of international concerns (PHEICs).

An extraordinary public health event:
- A public health risk to other countries through the international spread of disease
- Potentially requires a coordinated international response
- Determined by WHO after consultation with Emergency Committee.

### Notification
- Each State Party shall notify WHO, within 24 hours about assessment of public health information of all events accurately and in detail which constitutes a PHEIC.
- Four decision criteria to assess public health events:
    1. Is the public health impact of this event potentially serious?
    2. Is this event unusual or unexpected?
    3. Is there the potential for international spread?
    4. Is there the potential for travel and trade restrictions?

If 2 of the 4 criteria are met, countries are required to notify WHO within 24 hours.

**Following chapters in IHR (2005) deal with public health measures related to traveler's health:**

### Chapter I—General Provisions
**Article 23: Health measures on arrival and departure.**
A State Party may require information about traveler's destination, itinerary and a non-invasive medical examination. Any medical examination, procedure, vaccination or other prophylaxis shall only be performed with their informed consent or that of their parents or guardians.

### Chapter III—Special Provisions for Travelers
**Article 30: Travelers under public health observation.**
**Article 31: Health measures relating to entry of travelers.**

Invasive medical examination, vaccination or other prophylaxis are required only when necessary to determine whether a public health risk exists; and for travelers seeking temporary or permanent residence. If a traveler refuses to provide the information or the documents, the State Party may deny entry.

**Article 32: Treatment of Travelers:** State Parties shall treat all travelers with courtesy and respect; taking into consideration the gender, sociocultural, ethnic or religious concerns of travelers; and providing adequate food and water, accommodation and clothing, protection for baggage and other possessions, medical treatment, etc.

### Part VI—Health Documents
**Article 36: Certificates of vaccination or other prophylaxis.**
A traveler in possession of a certificate of vaccination/other prophylaxis shall not be denied, even if coming from an affected area, unless the competent authority has verifiable indications and/or evidence that the vaccination or other prophylaxis was not effective.

In India, Yellow fever is specifically designated under these regulations for which proof of vaccination or prophylaxis is required for entry from countries with risk of yellow fever transmission.

## TRAVEL NOTICE (TABLE 32.3)

Centers for disease control (CDC) has issued different types of notices for international travelers on 5th April, 2013. They describe both levels of risk for the traveler and recommended preventive measures to take at each level of risk.

**Table 32.3:** Travel notice.

| Notice level | Traveler action | Risk to traveler |
|---|---|---|
| Level 1: Watch | Reminder to follow *usual* precautions for this destination | Usual baseline risk or slightly above baseline risk for destination and limited impact to the traveler |
| Level 2: Alert | Follow *enhanced* precautions for this destination | Increased risk in defined settings or associated with specific risk factors; certain high-risk populations may wish to delay travel to these destinations |
| Level 3: Warning | Avoid all nonessential travel to this destination | High risk to travelers |

## SUMMARY

- Travel medicine or Emporiatrics is a specialized branch of medicine that is concerned with the prevention and management of travelers related to various health issues.
- Infectious diseases are the main cause of illness among travelers but, they account for only 1–4% of deaths in travelers. Cardiovascular problems were the most common single cause of death, contributing for nearly 50% of all deaths among international travelers, followed by other medical causes (25%) and injuries (13%).
- There are few defined determinants of travelers' health and risk factors for their health during travel. Preventive measures can be adopted to have healthy travel.
- The IHR is an agreement among 196 countries, including all WHO Member countries, to work together for the health security of the world. Under the IHR, all countries need to report all events of international public health impact.
- The IHR mandates all countries to detect public health threats, assess work in collaboration in case of public health emergencies, to report any potential public health emergency of international concern and responding to public health events.
- The revised IHR outlines the assessment, management, and information sharing for PHEICs. That is a public health risk to other countries through the international spread of disease, potentially requires a coordinated international response and it is determined by WHO after consultation with Emergency Committee.

## SUGGESTED READING

1. Annual Report January 2018-March 2019. Ministry of Tourism. Government of India. [online] Available from http://tourism.gov.in/annual-report-2018-19.
2. Causes of death for travelers in developing countries. [online] Available from https://www.cdc.gov/traveltraining/local/ Pre Travel Consultation and Best Practices/page23599.html.
3. Do you need vaccinations while travelling abroad? Available from http://www.medicinenet.com/script/main/art.asp?articlekey=61178.
4. Gubler DJ. Epidemic dengue/dengue hemorrhagic fever as a public health, social and economic problem in the 21st century. Trends Micro Biol. 2002; 10(2):100-3.
5. Huang DB, Okhuysen PC, Jiang ZD, et al. Entero aggregative *Escherichia coli*: an emerging enteric pathogen. Am J Gastroenterol. 2004;99(2):383-9.
6. International Health Regulations. World Health Organization. 2005. 3rd edition.
7. International travel and health. World Health Organization.[online] Available from http://www.who.int/ith/en/.
8. Lawson JM. Update on Escherichia coli O157:H7. Curr Gastro enteral Rep. 2004; 6(4):297-301.
9. Mackenzie JS, Gubler DJ, Petersen LR. Emerging flaviviruses: the spread and resurgence of Japanese encephalitis, West Nile and dengue viruses. Nat Med. 2004;10:S98-S109.
10. Travel Epidemiology—Chapter 1—2018 Yellow Book. Travelers' Health. CDC [online]. Available from https://wwwnc.cdc.gov/travel/yellowbook/2018/introduction/travel-epidemiology.
11. Travel Notice. CDC. [online] Available from https://wwwnc.cdc.gov/travel/notices.
12. World Tourism Organization (UNWTO). International Tourism Highlights, 2019 edition.

# CHAPTER 33

# Genetics and Health

*Manju Toppo*

*"We all know interspecies romance is weird".*
—**Tim Burton**

### Case Scenario

*Miss X, a third order Muslim girl child was born to her parents belonging to low socioeconomic and educational status at a private hospital, where she was suspected of suffering from Down's syndrome and was then advised for karyotyping, which revealed positive findings. Later on, she was diagnosed with atrial septal defect (ASD), following repeated respiratory tract infections and got operated at the age of 5 months. She later went on to develop hyperopia, for which correction was done at 4 years of age. At the age of 7 years, she is significantly long sighted and has the typical dysmorphic features of Down's syndrome face. She is moderately built with mild degree of mental retardation, moderate speech and language difficulty. She is advised physical exercise as a part of her daily routine and is under physical therapy program in tertiary care hospital.*

## INTRODUCTION

Genetics is defined as the study of inheritance, dealing with the transmission of hereditary characters from generation to generation. Human genetics is therefore concerned with the inheritance of human traits and their relationship to the human health. Most of the burden of disease and the variations in prevalence of disease including genetic diseases, among populations is mainly due to environmental factors.

The father of genetics is *"Gregor Johann Mendel"*, a late 19th-century scientist. Mendel's most popular study was "trait inheritance", in which he depicted the patterns of transmission of traits from parents to offspring. Mendel observed that organisms (pea plants) inherited the traits of parental plant by way of discrete "units of inheritance". This term maybe considered as an ambiguous definition of gene. Later in 1953, James Watson and Francis Crick determined the structure of the DNA molecule. In 1966, Marshall Nirenberg, Har Gobind Khorana and Robert W Holley solved the genetic code, in which they showed that 3 DNA bases code for one amino acid. They got the Nobel Prize in 1968. In 1990, first gene therapy was performed by Dr W French Anderson. So in the present day too, there is great amount of human genetic variation and the concept to genetic disease is still in revision.

## PROBLEM STATEMENT

In the world, approximately more than 3 million children born with a serious genetic defect die per year and majority of these deaths occur in developing countries. Globally, an estimated 8 million newborns are born with a birth defect every year. Nine out of every ten children born with a serious birth defect are in low- and middle-income countries. In the WHO South-East Asia Region, birth defects are the third most common cause of child mortality, and the fourth most common cause of neonatal mortality, accounting for 12% of all neonatal deaths and between 2010 and 2019, birth defects increased as a proportion of child mortality from 6.2 to 9.2% (WHO, 2023). In India, children with birth defect is estimated to be 6–7 per hundred per year, which may be translated to 1.7 million birth defects annually out of 26 million births (WHO Report, 2006). Approximately 5% of the world's population is estimated to carry trait genes for hemoglobin disorders, such as sickle-cell disease and thalassemia. Each year >300,000 babies with severe hemoglobin disorders are born.

According to WHO, the worldwide incidence of Down's syndrome is estimated to be between 1 in 1,000 to 1 in 1,100 live births. Each year in the United States of America, approximately 3,000–5,000 children are born with Down's syndrome affecting around 250,000 families. India has the highest number of people suffering from Down's syndrome in the world with an incidence of 1 per 850–900 live births. Neural tube defects are also the most common malformation having an incidence of 1–5 per thousand live births.

## PUBLIC HEALTH IMPORTANCE

Genetic disorders affect physical, psychological and social well-being of patients as well as their families.

Understanding the role of genetic information and anticipating the due course of genetic tests and diagnoses can help minimize distress amongst both patient and family and maximize the benefits.

In the developing countries like India, establishment of comprehensive medical genetic services, where proper genetic testing and screening can be done is need of the hour. Also the people are not aware about the treatment, management and care options available for individuals with genetic conditions.

## GENES

Gene is the essence that makes every individual unique. They are the code of instructions, inside cells, that control the physical appearance and looks of individual. Different gene composition of every individual renders different instructions. Genes are arranged in structures called chromosomes that are 23 pairs in humans. Chromosomes are made up of DNA in which the instructions in an individual gene are written as the special code. Based on different combinations of genes, each individual has unique set of genes. These genes can matchup in many ways to make different combinations. An individual inherits two copies of each gene, one from each parent. This is why many family members look a lot alike and others do not look like each other at all. Genes can also increase the risk in a family for getting certain health conditions.

## GENOTYPE AND PHENOTYPE

The genetic constitution, of a cell, an individual or organism is known as genotype. It is that hereditary information that has percolated to an individual by their parents and know his or her genetic makeup. Modalities such as biological assay (PCR) can be used to determine what genes are on an allele. The interaction of one's genetic makeup and his/her environment results in the appearance or characteristic of an individual, which is known as the phenotype. As the phenotype also depends upon the environment, which can alter from person to person, phenotype cannot be inherited. It is the observation made in an individual such as skin, hair, and eyes, etc. Examples are shown in **Figures 33.1A and B**.

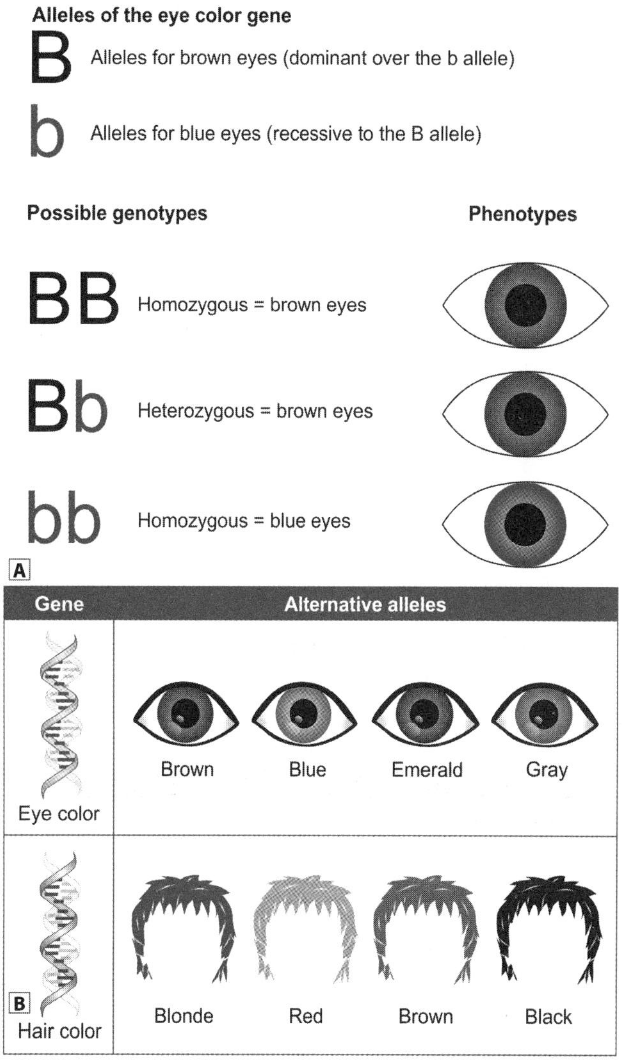

### The Hardy–Weinberg Equilibrium

*Hardy-Weinberg law* can be defined as a fundamental principle of population genetics: population gene frequencies and genotype frequencies remain constant from generation to generation if mating is random and if mutation, selection, immigration, and emigration do not occur.

The Mendelian genetics, which consist of populations of diploid and sexually reproducing individuals, is dealt with the use of Hardy–Weinberg theorem.

This theorem states the following:
- Moving from generation to generation, allele frequencies do not change.
- If two alleles at a locus are $p$ and $q$, then $p^2$, $2pq$ and $q^2$ are the expected genotype frequencies. Once the population is in Hardy–Weinberg equilibrium, the frequency distribution does not change **(Fig. 33.2)**.

Hardy and Weinberg, amongst the other population geneticists came to a conclusion that to prevent a population from evolution, the following conditions should be met:
- No mutation occurs
- No natural selection occurs
- Infinitely large population size
- Breeding occurs amongst all members
- Mating occurs randomly
- Number of offspring produced by everyone should be the same
- No migration of population should take place, either in or out

All of the above states that if in a population, no mechanisms of evolution are acting, evolution will not occur. As this is impossible that all of the above occurs in a population, the evolution is a definite outcome.

## MUTAGENS

It refers to any agent that can alter the structure or sequence of DNA. It can be both natural or manmade, physical or chemical.

| Physical factors | Chemical factors |
|---|---|
| • High temperature<br>• Various types of radiation<br> ➢ X-rays<br> ➢ UV radiation<br> ➢ Ionizing radiation<br> ➢ Cosmic radiation | • pH changes<br>• Certain chemicals—benzene, phenol, etc. |

Figs. 33.1A and B: Example of genotype and phenotype.

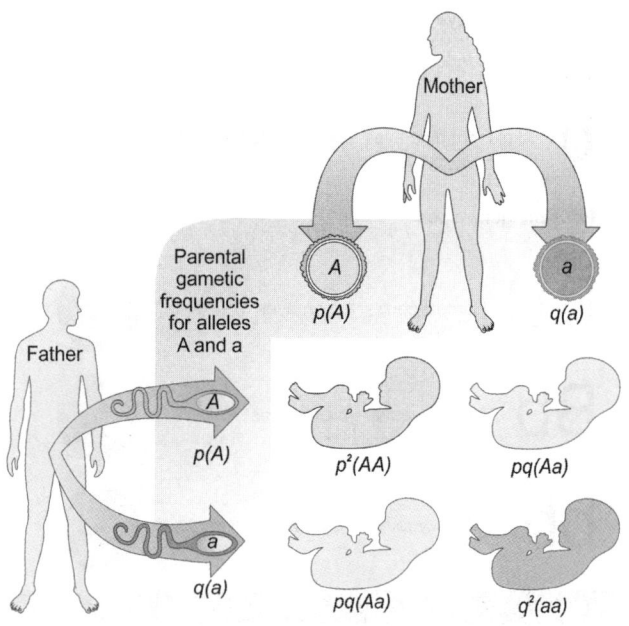

**Fig. 33.2:** The Hardy–Weinberg law applied to 2 alleles.
*Source:* Encyclopedia Britannica.

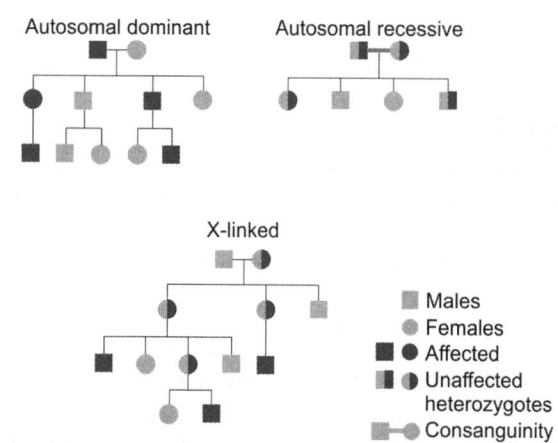

**Fig. 33.3:** Mendelian inheritance.

*Mutagens:* Types, effects and examples

| Mutagens | Effects | Examples |
|---|---|---|
| Carcinogens | Carcinogenesis and tumor formation | *Chemical:* Aflatoxins<br>*Biological:* Retroviruses<br>*Physical:* X-ray irradiation |
| Clastogens | Chromosome breaks, deletions and rearrangements | *Chemical:* Bleomycin<br>*Biological:* HIV virus<br>*Physical:* UV waves |
| Teratogens | Congenital malformations | *Chemical:* Valproate<br>*Biological:* Toxoplasma gondii<br>*Physical:* X-ray irradiation |
| Nonspecific mutagens | Nonspecific damage to the genetic material | *Chemical:* Innumerable types<br>*Biological:* Toxoplasma virus<br>*Physical:* X-ray irradiation |

## GENETIC DISORDERS

There are many types of genetic inheritance and the classification of diseases based on their genetic basis is:
- Monogenic (Mendelian) disorders
- Chromosomal abnormalities
- Multifactorial inheritance or polygenic disorders
- Mitochondrial inheritance

### Single Gene Inheritance

Mendelian or monogenic inheritance both are synonyms to single gene inheritance. Changes or mutation occur in the DNA sequence of a single gene results is this type of inheritance.1 out of every 200 birth suffers from any of the 6,000 known single gene disorders, e.g., Marfan syndrome, cystic fibrosis, Huntington's disease, sickle cell anemia and hemochromatosis. Single-gene disorders are inherited in recognizable patterns: autosomal dominant, autosomal recessive, and X-linked **(Fig. 33.3)**.

### Chromosomal Abnormalities

Chromosomes carry the genetic material, and thus, any abnormalities in chromosome number or structure can result in genetic disease. This may be in the form of alternations in the number or structure of chromosomes, autosomes or sex chromosomes.

The change in number is brought by nondisjunction which occurs when either *homologue fail to separate* during anaphase I of meiosis, or *sister chromatids fail to separate* during anaphase II. This results in defective gamete, one having an extra copy and other having a missing chromosome. When this takes part in fertilization, it results in aneuploidy (abnormal chromosome number) either monosomy or trisomy, e.g., Down syndrome or trisomy 21 is a common disorder occurring as a result of three copies of chromosome 21. Other chromosomal abnormalities include Turner syndrome (45, X) and Klinefelter syndrome (47, XXY) **(Fig. 33.4)**. The structural changes in the chromosomes are in the form of deletion (e.g., the cat cry syndrome 46, XX or XY, 5p-), duplication (e.g., Fragile X syndrome) and translocation (e.g., acute myelogenous leukemia).

### Multifactorial Inheritance

It is also known as complex or polygenic inheritance. This type of in heritance results from a combination of mutations in multiple genes with environmental factors contributing to outcomes. They include mainly the noncommunicable diseases, e.g., cardiovascular diseases, diabetes, cancer, hypertension, Alzheimer disease, arthritis and obesity. Different genes present on chromosomes 6, 11, 13, 14, 15, 17 and 22 influence breast cancer susceptibility. Heritable traits, such as fingerprint patterns, height, eye color and skin color are also influenced by multifactorial inheritance.

### Mitochondrial Inheritance

This type of genetic disorder is caused by mutations occurring in the nonchromosomal DNA of mitochondria. Number of circular pieces of DNA in each mitochondrion may vary from 5 to 10, e.g., Leber's hereditary optic atrophy; myoclonus epilepsy

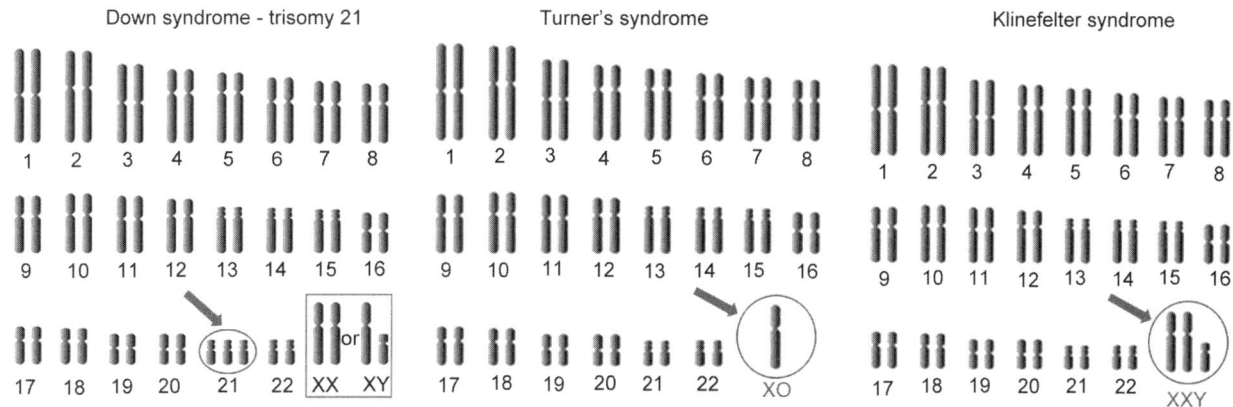

**Fig. 33.4:** Chromosomal abnormalities.
*Source:* Prenatal Testing for Down syndrome: Understanding Two New Studies ...Parents Magazine.

with ragged red fibers and a form of dementia: mitochondrial encephalopathy lactic acidosis and stroke-like episodes.

Our genetic heritage is holistically viewed as a sequential arrangement of chromosomes. The research in this field is dynamic and continuous and thus brings us closer to a complete human genome reference sequence. Human chromosomes are 23 pairs: 22 pair autosomal chromosomes and 2 sex chromosomes. A total of 46 chromosomes house almost 3 billion base pairs of DNA which again contain about 30–40,000 protein-coding genes. The function of almost 95% of the genome is not clear and the coding regions make <5%. The density of genes amongst chromosome may vary. Most genetic diseases are the direct result of a mutation in one gene. Finding out how genes contribute to diseases having a complex pattern of inheritance such as in the cases of diabetes, asthma, cancer and mental illness are the most difficult problem ahead. Amongst these diseases, the disease occurrence is not decided by the presence or absence of single gene alone. The above mentioned diseases manifest as a result of more than one mutation. Also, many genes together may each make small contribution to persons' susceptibility to a disease and affect how they react to environment.

## GENE-RELATED HEMOGLOBINOPATHIES

Hemoglobinopathies are disorders affecting the structure, function, or production of hemoglobin. The outcomes of these hemoglobinopathies range in severity from asymptomatic laboratory abnormalities to death in utero.

### Sickle Cell Anemia

Sickle cell anemia is an autosomal recessive disorder occurring as a result of change in amino acid from glutamic acid to valine (point mutation) at 6th position in the β-globin gene. The above change brings about morphological changes in the RBC, which becomes sickled and loses the characteristic pliability needed to traverse small capillaries. These now possess "sticky" membranes that are unusually adherent to the endothelium of small venules resulting in unpredictable episodes of microvascular vaso-occlusion and premature RBC destruction (hemolytic anemia).

The function of spleen is to destroy the abnormal RBC and these cells get hemolyzed here. The rigid adherent cells clog small capillaries and venules, causing manifestations, such as episodes of ischemic pain (i.e., painful crises) and ischemic malfunction or frank infarction in the spleen, central nervous system, bones, liver, kidneys, and lungs. The concentration of hemoglobin S (HbS) in the RBC of affected individual decides the rate of sickling. The disease is common among people of sub-Saharan Africa, South America, the Caribbean, Central America, Saudi Arabia, India and Mediterranean countries, such as Turkey, Greece and Italy. Sickle cell anemia is common in areas in which malaria is endemic. In India, the sickle gene is widespread among many tribal population groups with prevalence varying from 1 to 40% of heterozygotes [(ICMR), 1987]. As per the international nomenclature, instead of commonly used term, sickle-cell anemia, the term, sickle cell disease, must be used since major complication of the disease is vascular obliterations and the organ damage they cause, not anemia.

Though the manifestations begin to appear during first year of life, where instead of HbA2, HbS begin to replace HbF, the onset of disease occurs in fetal life. The clinical features include sickle-cell crises in the form of pain, involving back, extremities, thorax, abdomen and central nervous system (CNS) in particular.

Patients are chronically ill and present with jaundice, hepatomegaly and cardiomegaly. Death occurs due to acute thoracic syndrome (ATS), spleen crises, and strokes. Patients with sickle cell syndromes requires continuous care. There is no specific treatment, only symptomatic care along with proper hydration and comprehensive medical management is helpful in improving quality of life. Continuous research in the field of gene therapy for sickle cell anemia is being done, but no safe measures are currently available yet.

### Thalassemia

It is an autosomal recessive disorder. It is caused by reduction or lack of synthesis of globin chains [alpha (α) or beta (ß) chains] resulting in hereditary form of anemia. Carrier status also confers some resistance to malaria.

Two main types of thalassemia:
1. ***Alpha thalassemia*** occurs when a gene or genes related to the alpha globin protein are missing (gene deletion). These diseases occur in persons from Southeast Asia, the Middle East, and China and in those of African descent. Thalassemia is by far the most common hemoglobinopathy in India, but because of serious genetic risk, it is the milder form (-α/aα) of alpha-thalassemia which is predominant. Knowing the alpha-genotype is useful for genetic counseling for prenatal diagnosis in couples where one of the parents may have reduced indices coupled with a raised RBC count and normal HbA2 levels.
2. ***Beta thalassemia*** occurs when a beta globin gene is changed (point mutation)so as to affect production of the beta globin protein. Beta thalassemia affects persons of Mediterranean origin. To a lesser extent, Chinese, other Asians and African Americans can be affected.

The disease starts manifesting after 6 months of age, when hemoglobin synthesis switches from HbF to HbA. This group of disorders ranges from mild blood abnormalities to fatal anemia. Presently, blood transfusion is the only mode of treatment for severe thalassemia. Only a few patients are cured by bone marrow transplantation. Since it is autosomal recessive disease, genetic counseling and avoiding consanguineous marriage may help in reduction of severe form of thalassemia.

### Hemophilia

It is an X-linked chromosomal bleeding disorder which was the first diseases recognized as being genetically determined occurring with a frequency of about 1:10,000 male newborns. Hemophilia A and B results from a deficiency of clotting factors VIII and factor IX respectively. Factor VIII (synthesized mainly in the liver) is one of the many factors involved with blood coagulation. The severity of hemophilia and the frequency of bleeding depend upon the degree of residual factors VIII or IX activity. According to National Health Portal of India (2018), hemophilia A (clotting factor VIII deficiency) is the most common form of the disorder present in about 1 in 5,000–10,000 births and hemophilia B (factor IX deficiency) occurs, in around 1 in about 20,000–34,000 births. It is estimated that 10–80% of people with hemophilia are present in developing countries such as India (Haemophilia Federation of India, 2010). However, hemophilia cases remain under diagnosed, and many cases are not registered.

Hemophilia is more likely to occur in males than females. The females are usually carriers. Since the factors which help in blood clotting are deficient, the disease manifest as excessive, prolonged and delayed bleeding. In severe hemophiliacs the bleeding can occur in areas such as the brain or inside joints, this can be fatal or permanently debilitating.

## ADVANCES IN MOLECULAR GENETICS

### Human Genome Project

This project was a herculean project initiated as joint effort of US Department of Energy and the National Institutes of Health in the year 1990. In April 2003, Human Genomic Project sequencing was completed. This project is an initiative to create a complete mapping of human genome with each coding gene defined and sequenced. This project helps in designing "custom drugs" (pharmacogenomics) based on individual's genetic constitution so that gene therapy can be used for treatment. This may also help in identifying suspect of a crime with the help of DNA matching.

*Factors contributing to the high rates of congenital disorders in low and middle income countries:*
- No or reduced availability of public health measures towards prevention and care of congenital disorders.
- Nonavailability of quality genetics services and inadequate health care prior to and during pregnancy.
- High rates of consanguineous marriages in many countries especially Southeast Asia regions which contribute significantly to the expression of autosomal recessive diseases.
- Advanced maternal age at first conception (primipara) have increased incidence of chromosomal trisomies such as Down syndrome and advanced paternal age has been found to show increased risk of occurrence of new mutations leading to certain autosomal dominant disorders.
- Large family size is also found to contribute to high numbers of affected children especially with autosomal recessive conditions.

### Gene Therapy

Gene therapy is a scientific technique that helps in formation of missing protein by introduction of a normal gene in place of a defective gene. It is also helpful in correcting a deficient phenotype which helps in synthesis of sufficient amounts of a normal gene to improve a genetic condition. This can be achieved through transfer of the desired gene sequences into the genome and hence modification of cells. Gene therapy are of two types: In-vivo gene therapy in which normal genes are delivered inside the body and Ex-vivo in which the genes are inserted in the cells outside the body, and the treated cells are placed back into the body. In in-vivo technique, viral vectors are utilized to cripple its ability to cause disease. Ex-vivo manipulation techniques are electroporation, calcium phosphate gold bullets (fired within helium pressurized gun) and human artificial chromosomes.

Gene therapy is used in the treatment of cystic fibrosis, hemophilia, muscular dystrophy and sickle cell anemia.

## PREVENTIVE AND SOCIAL MEASURES

### Primary Prevention—Health Promotion and Specific Protection

1. **Eugenics:** In 1883 Francis Galton coined the word 'Eugenics' from the Greek, good ("eu") and born ("genics"). It is defined as "the science of improvement of the human race through better breeding". It is of two types—positive eugenics and negative eugenics.
   - ***Positive eugenics:*** Promotes marriage and breeding between people considered "desirable" to create good breed for future generations.
   - ***Negative eugenics:*** Improving the quality of the human race by eliminating or excluding biologically inferior people from the population. This goal required severe restrictions on reproductive rights, for those with "defects" had to be kept from reproducing, if necessary through the

forceful sterilization. Example is elderly and sick people were killed under Hitler's policy of eugenics.
2. **Euthenics:** Euthenics is a science concerned with improving the well-being of mankind through improvement of the environment. Mere improvement of genotype is of no use unless the improved genotype is given access to a suitable environment which will enable the gene to express themselves readily, e.g., children with mild mental retardation when placed in an encouraging environment showed improvement in their IQ.
3. **Genetic Counseling:** The process by which patients or relatives at risk of genetic disorder are advised regarding the consequences of the disorder and thus the probability of developing or transmitting it and the ways this may be prevented or avoided is called genetic counseling. It may also be defined as an educational process that assist the affected and/or at-risk individuals and their families to understand the nature of the genetic disorder, modes of transmission and the available options for management, prevention and family planning. An authorized health professional person is called genetic counselor who is academically and clinically trained to provide genetic services to individuals and families. The genetic counselor provides client-centered services regarding the issues, the occurrence, the risk of occurrence of a genetic condition or birth defect. He also responds to queries, concerns, and experiences meaningful to the client's circumstances. The genetic counselor communicates about the genetic, medical and technical information in comprehensive and in language understandable to the client and acceptable in terms of psychosocial and cultural background of each client and their family. If conception fails even after genetic counseling, the couples must be counseled to conceive from sperm donation, or couple can opt for adoption. Genetic counseling can be both prospective counseling and retrospective counseling.
   - *Prospective Genetic Counseling*
     - In this type of counseling, the genetic disorder has not yet expressed itself.
     - To assess the probability of having a child with genetic disorders, it is done in heterozygotic individuals.
     - If a person is identified as heterozygotic for a genetic condition, he/she should be advised against marrying another heterozygotic individual as there is increased risk of the trait expressing itself in the phenotype.
   - *Retrospective Genetic Counseling*
     - In this type of counseling, the disease has already occurred in the family.
     - This is more common as compared to prospective genetic counseling.
     - This is because, after having a child with congenital anomalies/mental retardation/inborn errors of metabolism people usually come for genetic counseling only.
     - The interventions as a part of retrospective genetic counseling are—contraception, sterilization and termination of pregnancy.

## Specific Protection

- Individuals as well as community protection against mutagens, such as X-rays or other ionizing radiations.
- Protection of gonads to radiation in patients undergoing X-ray must be ensured.
- Prevention of Rh hemolytic disease of newborn by immunization with anti-D globulin.

## Secondary Prevention

Once the defective gene is acquired by an individual, nothing can be done except for secondary or tertiary level of prevention which are costly and cumbersome and quality of life of an individual is also affected. Efforts must be made for prevention of genetic disorders by reproduction options since primary prevention techniques also are difficult and have their own limitations. In prevention by reproductive options couples at risk are identified and are offered voluntary options to avoid having an affected child. Such options include:

- ***Detection of carriers for autosomal recessive conditions:*** The purpose of testing of carrier genes is to help at risk couples to plan their reproduction to reduce the chances of birth of an affected child. These testing services may be voluntary or mandatory by law, depending on the country for example premarital testing for thalassemia in Cyprus and Iran. The paternal and maternal chromosomal study should be done and if both spouses are found to be carriers then voluntary genetic counseling services regarding the reproductive options available must be offered to avoid having an affected offspring. The options must be provided in detail and possible effect of not following the advice must be explained. The clients may be encouraged to choose the options voluntarily but should not be forced. The options include: (a) if detection is premarital the client must be advised not to marry with the carrier, (b) abstinence from reproduction, (c) testing the genetic risk, or (d) undergoing prenatal diagnosis and if found abnormal then providing the option of continuing or interrupting an affected pregnancy, depending on gestational size and the Medical Termination of Pregnancy Act. The reproductive options approach has multiple ethical issues—firstly it must be voluntary and not forced or mandatory, secondly it requires social consensus, organization and resources.
- ***Prenatal screening:*** The noninvasive prenatal screening to rule out Down syndrome and other possible chromosomal abnormalities could be done in positive screens if desired by the couple.

### *Prenatal Diagnosis*

*Noninvasive [Known as Noninvasive Prenatal Testing (NIPT)/ Noninvasive Prenatal Screening (NIPS)]*

| Sl. No. | Noninvasive screening test | Gestational age for screening | Conditions screened |
|---|---|---|---|
| 1. | Cell free DNA | After 9–10 weeks | Trisomy 21, 18,13 (and in some cases X and Y) |
| 2. | First-trimester screen (Nuchal translucency, Papp-A, hCG) | 10–13 weeks | Trisomy 21 |
| 3. | Triple screen (hCG, AFP, uE3) | 15–22 weeks | Trisomy 21 |
| 4. | Quadruple screen (hCG, AFP, uE3, DIA) | 15–22 weeks | Trisomy 21 |

(DNA: deoxyribonucleic acid; AFP: alpha-fetoprotein; DIA: dimeric inhibin-A; hCG: human chorionic gonadotropin; Papp-A: pregnancy-associated plasma protein A; uE3: unconjugated estriol)

***Invasive screening:*** Increased risk for fetal chromosome abnormalities such as advanced maternal age (35 years old or older), a positive maternal serum analyte screen, or previous child with a chromosome abnormality or a parental chromosome rearrangement are the most common indication for consideration of invasive prenatal testing. Increased risk for a detectable mendelian disorder (earlier birth of an affected child or family member, positive screening outcome), structural fetal anomalies detected by ultrasound, increased risk for polygenic/multifactorial disorder (neural tube defect); positive screen, abnormal ultrasound, family history or exposure to teratogens that increase the risk for detectable abnormalities (e.g., valproic acid and neural tube defects) are amongst the other indications for consideration of invasive prenatal testing. The indication for invasive testing may designate the type of procedure available for diagnosis like in cases of increased risk for fetal neural tube defects; chorionic villus sampling is not an appropriate test as this technique cannot obtain amniotic fluid for the α-fetoprotein (AFP) and acetylcholinesterase analyses.

| Sl. No. | Invasive screening test | Gestational age for screening | Conditions screened |
|---|---|---|---|
| 1. | Chorionic villous sampling | 10–14 weeks | Chromosomal disorders (e.g. Down syndrome) or other genetic diseases (e.g. cystic fibrosis, sickle cell disease) |
| 2. | Amniocentesis | 15 weeks or greater | Chromosomal abnormalities, sex determination |
| 3. | Fetal blood sampling | Second trimester | Blood factor abnormalities, such as hemophilia A, hemophilia B, or von Willebrand disease; to diagnose autosomal recessive or X-linked immunologic deficiencies, including severe combined immunodeficiency, Chédiak–Higashi syndrome, Wiskott–Aldrich syndrome and chronic granulomatous disease |
| 4. | Fetal tissue sampling | 17–20 weeks | Severe hereditary skin diseases (genodermatoses) |

- Newborn screening is the "head" of genetic screening program. The concept of newborn screening began with screening for phenylketonuria (PKU) in developed nations in the 1960. Soon this was followed by screening for congenital hypothyroidism (CH). The rationale for newborn screening is in accordance with the concept of early diagnosis and (preventive) treatment before symptoms appears. Thus, newborn screening can be considered as secondary prevention of congenital disorders. For example, when a family is informed about the diagnosis of a severe or fatal defect in fetus after conception then following must be considered:
  - Preparation of family for the challenges they will be facing when they have a baby.
  - Possible options regarding effective treatment if any must be suggested as well as surgical options must also be looked for if affordable, e.g., surgery can only be used to treat some defects, such as spina bifida or congenital diaphragmatic hernia.
  - Terminating the pregnancy: this is the only option for some families.
  - The family may be referred for cardiologist opinion regarding heart surgery, and a neonatologist opinion regarding the care of a postoperative newborn.
- *Predictive genetic testing:* Screening of carriers for thalassemia and other hemoglobinopathies must be offered to a couple preconceptionally or as early as possible during pregnancy if they have a positive family history of such diseases.
- *Follow-up of children:* For children born with congenital disorders and genetic diseases, interventions to prevent complications and improve quality of life of the affected individual is the only option available (e.g., hemoglobinopathies, deafness).

## Tertiary Prevention (Surgical Repair and Rehabilitation) (Fig. 33.5)

### *Disability Limitation*

Much can be done to limit disability caused by genetic diseases, even though they may not be amenable to permanent cure at present, like children suffering from mental deficiency due to phenylketonuria can be prevented to a large extent by keeping them on a low phenylalanine diet from the very beginning. Diseases, such as hemophilia, sickle cell anemia and thalassemia can be controlled by appropriate therapeutic and preventive measures.

### *Rehabilitation*

- Defects, such as congenital heart defects, cleft lip and palate, neural tube defects, surgical treatment is the only option.
- Early referral of children with genetic disorders which are known to cause physical or mental disability.
- Learning disabilities and cognitive impairment, rehabilitation programs such as teaching skills through aids to improve psychomotor function for diseases like muscular dystrophy, Friedreich ataxia, phenylketonuria and retinitis pigmentosa.

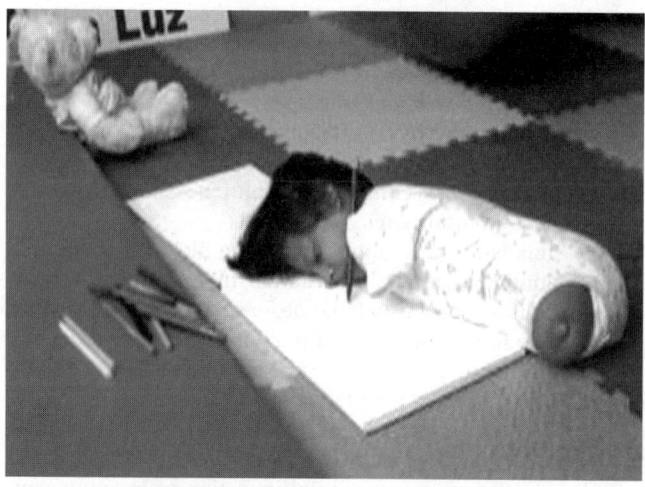

**Fig. 33.5:** An example of tertiary prevention.

## COMMUNITY GENETICS

Community genetics is a field of research in biology that helps in analyzing evolutionary genetic processes that occur among interacting populations in communities. It is the art and science of the responsible and realistic application of health and disease-related genetics and genomics knowledge and technologies in human populations and communities to the benefit of individuals therein. Community genetics in the fraternity of medicine providing tools to deal with genetic diseases (hereditary diseases) via identification of the diseases and the syndromes, identification of the changes in chromosomes or in genes, diagnosis and screening of populations having higher incidence of certain genetic diseases. Community genetics" reflects attempts of clinical geneticists to apply their counseling methods to the whole population. Community genetics and clinical genetics are interlinked yet different. Though individual's benefit is the central theme for community genetics and clinical genetics, community genetics seeks to locate people within the wider community who may be at increased risk of a genetic problem, but have not yet been identified or helped. Whereas clinical geneticists deal with persons or families with a particular problem or concern who have requested or been referred for a consultation.

### Public Health Challenge

It is evident that in the decades to come, scientific advances in molecular genetics will have great impact on prevention and health care. For community doctors who are aware about all relevant developments in sufficient detail, close communication between the community doctor and clinical genetic specialist is necessary to keep pace with the progress. With regard to genetic counseling and reproductive medicine, working agreement between primary care and specialist centers are important. There are other competing health priorities, such as infectious disease, malnutrition, prenatal care, labor and delivery care and neonatal care. Medical profession and public health officials opine that genetics is not a health priority and misconceptions that genetic services are expensive and relevant only to rare diseases. People are still not aware about the full range of options available for prevention of genetic disease, with prevention often misperceived as being limited to the abortion of affected fetuses, lack of public education about genetic risks and the range of preventive options. The prevalence and burden of genetic diseases is under estimated hence health planners are not unable to weigh fairly the demands generated about genetic disease control against other health needs. Lastly the importance of sound epidemiological data of genetic diseases should be emphasized to convince policy makers of the need for wide availability of genetic services, affordable and accessible to common man. It is a neglected sector and requires much attention as the national policy for the treatment of rare diseases and Rashtriya Bal Swasthya Karyakram (RBSK) incorporates only a component of it.

## CONCLUSION

Genetic disorders have powerful impact on families of affected individuals requiring continual attention in absence of treatments. Once a family member is diagnosed with a genetic disorder, means that other blood relatives are also at risk, even though presently they are asymptomatic. Apart from medical implications, emotional challenges and reproductive implications are at stake. Major concern amongst the family members is that their progeny might inherit the disease which would further lead to seeking multitude of tests and various treatment options.

- The father of genetics is *"Gregor John Mendel".*
- Each cell has genes which determine the physical appearance and the bodily functions of an individual.
- Genotype refers to the genetic constitution, phenotype is an appearance or characteristic of an individual
- Human genome project is an initiative to create a single linear map of human genome with each coding gene defined and sequenced.
- Gene therapy is a scientific technique helps in formation of missing protein by introduction of a normal gene in place of defective gene.
- Eugenics is defined as "the science of improvement of the human race through better breeding". It is of two types: positive eugenics and negative eugenics.
- Point mutation of sixth amino acid (glutamic acid to valine) in the $\beta$-globin gene results in sickle cell anemia which is an autosomal recessive disorder.
- Reduction or lack of synthesis of globin chains [alpha ($\alpha$) or beta($\beta$) chains] results in thalassemia which is a hereditary form of anemia.
- Chromosomal inheritance is inheritance of a mutated gene of which Hemophilia A is a classic example.
- Deficiency of clotting factor VIII in the body leads to hereditary bleeding disorder: Hemophilia A
- For early diagnosis of congenital disorders and genetic diseases, genetic counseling should be done along with clinical examination and laboratory investigations (biochemical assays, cytogenetics, DNA testing, etc.).
- More research should be encouraged to collect epidemiological data related to genetic disorders.

## SUGGESTED READING

1. A Strategic Approach to Reproductive, Maternal, Newborn, Child and Adolescent Health (RMNCH+A) In India.
2. Benn P, Cuckle H, Pergament E. Non-invasive prenatal testing for aneuploidy: current status and future prospects. Ultrasound Obstet Gynecol. 2013;42(1):15-33.
3. Bertolino F, Ratto A. On the Bayesian Inference of the Hardy-Weinberg Equilibrium Model. In: di Bacco M, d'Amore G, Scalfari F. (Eds.) Applied Bayesian Statistical Studies in Biology and Medicine. Springer; 2011:pp. 25-40.
4. Bhatia HM, Rao VR. Genetic Atlas of Indian Tribes, Bombay Institute of Haemotolgy (ICMR);1987.

5. Carlson LM, Vora NL. Prenatal diagnosis: Screening and diagnostic tools. Obstet Gynecol Clin North Am. 2017;44(2):245-56.
6. Community genetics services: report of a WHO consultation on community genetics in low- and middle-income countries. Geneva, Switzerland, 13-14 September 2010.
7. Control of hereditary diseases. Report of a WHO Scientific Group. World Health Organ Tech. Rep. Ser. 1996;865:1-84.
8. Cook L. The Hardy-Weinberg principle. Biological Sciences Review. 2003;15(4):7-9.
9. Creary M, Williamson D, Kulkarni R. Sickle cell disease: current activities, public health implications, and future directions. J Women's Health (Larchmt). 2007;16(5):575-82.
10. Ghosh K, Shetty S, Sahu D. Haemophilia care in India: innovations and integrations by various chapters of haemophilia federation of India (HFI). Haemophilia. 2010;16:61-65.
11. Hans JTD, Martin L, Akira H. Clinical Neuroembryology: Development and Developmental Disorders of the Human Central Nervous System, 2nd Edition. Heidelberg: Springer;2014.
12. Harper PS. Practical Genetic Counselling, 7th edition. CRC Press; 2010.
13. Hoots WK. The registry and surveillance in hemoglobinopathies: improving the lives of individuals with hemoglobinopathies. Am J Prev Med. 2010;38(4):S510-1.
14. Human Genomics in Global Health, World Health Organization. Accessible at-https://www.who.int/genomics/en/.
15. Kelly TE. Autosomal dominant and recessive traits. Clinical Genetics and Genetic Counselling, 2nd edition. Year Book Medical Publishers Inc., Chicago. 1986:67.
16. Leo P, Al-Gazali L, Anand S, et al. Community genetics. Its definition 2010. J Community Genet. 2010;1(1):19-22.
17. Limwongse C. Medical genetic services in a developing country: lesson from Thailand. Current Opinion in Pediatrics. 2017; 29(6):634-9.
18. Orel V. Gregor Mendel: the first geneticist. Oxford University Press, USA;1996.
19. Sawicki MP, Samara G, Hurwitz M, Passaro E. Human genome project. The Am J Surg. 1993;165(2):258-64.
20. Shulman LP, Simpson JL, Elias S. Invasive prenatal genetic techniques. In: Sciarra J (Ed). Gynecology and Obstetrics. Lippincott, Philadelphia; 1992.
21. Stern C. The Hardy-Weinberg Law. Science. 1943;97(2510):137-8.
22. Verma IC, Bijarnia S. The burden of genetic disorders in India and a framework for community control. Community Genet. 2002; 5(3):192-6.
23. Vieweg J. Basic principles of gene therapy. Der Urologe. Ausg. A. 1996;35(5):378-89.
24. Watkins AE. Heredity and evolution. John Murray; London;1935.
25. WHO (2006). Medical genetic services in developing countries: the ethical, legal and social implications of genetic testing and screening.

# CHAPTER 34

# Special Topics

## A. CLIMATE CHANGE AND HEALTH

*Praveen Kulkarni, Sunil Kumar D*

| CM 3.1 | Describe the health hazards of pollution |

### INTRODUCTION

Climate change is a major public health challenge of the current century. Climate change poses a serious threat to the health of mankind, particularly those who reside in lower income countries. It has implications for the production of food, the quality of water and air, coastal settlements, and animal health. Climate change leads to a spectrum of health problems lasting from a few days to life-threatening conditions like cancer. Thus, it is important to take all possible steps to prevent the factors that lead to and aggravate the negative impacts of climate change. India is experiencing rapid demographic and epidemiological transitions along with rampant globalization, industrialization and urbanization. All these factors, combined with the exponential growth of the population make India prone to being a victim of climate change.

### CLIMATE CHANGE

#### What is Climate Change?

Before going into definition of climate change, let us understand the difference between weather and climate.

Weather is the atmospheric condition that prevails at a given moment and in a given geographical area and may change within days or even hours. On the other hand, climate is the state of the atmosphere over several years in a larger geographical area. In simple terms, weather may change on a minute, hourly, daily, or seasonal basis, but climate is the average of weather changes over a long period of time.

According to the United Nations Framework Convention on Climate Change (UNFCCC), climate change is defined as a change in climate that is attributed directly or indirectly to human activity, which alters the composition of the global atmosphere and is in addition to natural climate variability observed over comparable time periods.

### Causes of Climate Change

Causes of climate change can be categorized into natural and manmade ones. Natural causes contribute little to the overall effects of climate change, while the anthropogenic factors, also known as human-related factors contribute to climate change to a larger extent. These causes are summarized in **Flowchart 34A.1**.

### Driving Forces for Climate Change

These are the factors that drive people to engage in various activities leading to climate change. Mainly there are five driving

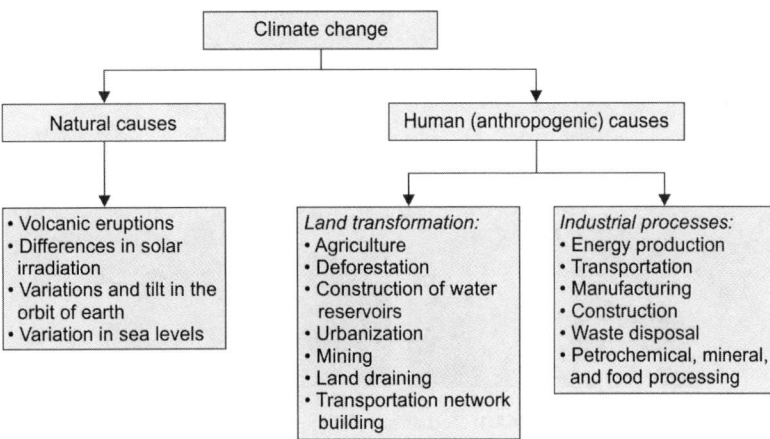

**Flowchart 34A.1:** Causes of climate change.

*Source:* Adapted with modification from IPCC, 2007: Climate Change 2007: Synthesis Report.

forces, such as—(1) technological advancements, (2) population growth, (3) economic development, (4) industries and (5) attitudes and beliefs.

Soaring population growth across the world has increased the requirement for energy, which is supplied by technological advances resulting in climate change. Rapid economic growth and industrialization have led to rampant emissions from factories resulting in increased carbon dioxide concentration. Increased purchasing capacity among people has brought in the belief in luxury, comfort, and an attitude of richness leading to negligence of mass transport and the purchase of their cars and automobiles, further enhancing the burden of climate change.

## Greenhouse Effect

This is a natural process that warms the surface of earth. When the energy from sun reaches the earth's atmosphere, a proportion of it is reflected back to space and the rest is absorbed by greenhouse gases (GHGs). With increase in the concentration of GHGs, the larger amount of solar energy is trapped into the atmosphere resulting in greenhouse effect **(Table 34A.1)**.

**Table 34A.1:** Sources of greenhouse gases.

| Water vapor | Natural |
|---|---|
| Methane | Decomposition of wastes in landfills, agriculture, ruminant digestion, and manure management |
| Carbon dioxide ($CO_2$) | Respiration, volcano eruptions, deforestation and burning of fossil fuels |
| Nitrous oxide | Commercial and organic fertilizers, combustion of fossil fuel, nitric acid production, and burning of biomass |

## Mechanism of Climate Change

The land transformation and industrial processes will produce large amount of GHGs, such as methane, carbon dioxide, nitrous oxide, water vapor, etc., leading to enhanced greenhouse effect. This results in increased atmospheric temperature, warming of oceans, melting of ice caps, rise in the level of sea, changes in rain patterns, and abrupt changes in climatic conditions like flood, tornadoes, cyclone, heat waves, etc. All these changes directly or indirectly influence the health and lifestyle of human beings **(Fig. 34A.1)**.

## Magnitude of Climate Change

### Global Scenario (Pachauri RK, Climate Change 2014: Synthesis Report)

- **Atmosphere:** Earth's surface has been successively warmer in last three decades than any time since 1850. In last 800 years, the period from 1983 to 2012 was likely to be the warmest 30-year period. On an average, the atmospheric temperature has increased by 0.85°C in the period from 1850 to 2012.
- **Cryosphere:** Ice sheets in Greenland and Antarctic have been losing their mass since last 20 years.
- **Ocean:** Warming of oceans contributes to more than 90% of energy on the climate system. Globally, the warming of ocean is largest near the upper 75 m by 0.11 (0.09–0.13) degree Celsius per decade.
- **Sea level:** In the period between 1901 and 2010, the average sea level rose by 0.19 m. The rate of rise in sea level since the mid of 19th century has been larger in last two millennia.

### Indian Scenario (GOI, National Action Plan for Climate Change, 2007)

- **Surface temperature:** In India, level of surface temperature has increased by approximately 0.4°C over last century.
- **Rainfall:** Even though the overall monsoon rainfall has not shown much significant change at national level, regional variations in monsoon are recorded. West coast and northern Andhra Pradesh have recorded increased monsoon rainfall. A trend of decreased monsoon rainfall has been recorded in Madhya Pradesh, Kerala, Gujarat, and North Eastern India.

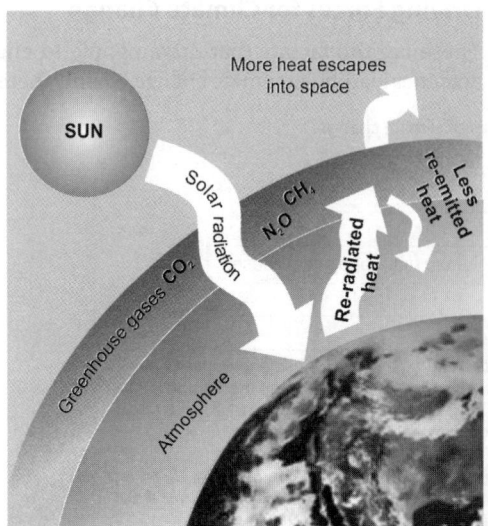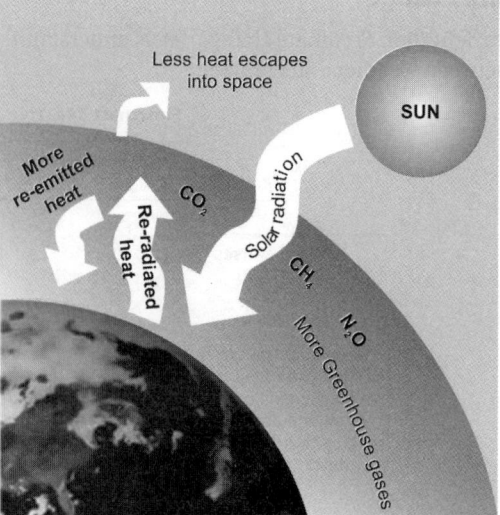

**Fig. 34A.1:** Mechanism of climate change.

- ***Extreme weather events:*** In last 130 years, the incidence of severe storm along the coast has increased by 0.011 events per year. West Bengal and Gujarat states have reported increased trends while Odisha has recorded decreased trend in storm incidence.
- ***Rise in sea levels:*** There have been reports of increase in the sea level at the rate of 1.06–1.75 mm per year.

# IMPACT OF CLIMATE CHANGES ON HEALTH (FIG. 34A.2)

- ***Extreme weather-related illnesses:***
  - *High temperature:* Heat hyperpyrexia, health exhaustion, heat stroke, dehydration, syncope attacks, cerebrovascular accidents, respiratory illnesses, etc.
  - *Low temperature:* Hypothermia, frostbite, trench foot, respiratory illnesses, etc.
- ***Air pollution-related illnesses:*** Accumulation of gases produced out of industrial processes and human activities will lead to air pollution, which increases the burden of allergy, asthma, acute and chronic respiratory diseases, cardiovascular diseases, etc.
- ***Waterborne diseases:*** Alterations in pattern of rainfall related to climate change, availability of water and water quality could influence the magnitude of water-related diseases, such as acute gastroenteritis, cholera, typhoid, amebiasis, ascariasis, etc. Water washed diseases illnesses like scabies, skin infections can result due to lack of water for taking care of personal hygiene.
- ***Vector-borne diseases:*** Dynamics of vector population and disease transmission are affected by change in atmospheric temperature and humidity. Thus, there will be increase in the incidence of vector-borne diseases, such as malaria, dengue, lymphatic filariasis, chikungunya, leishmaniasis, and Japanese encephalitis.
- ***Mental illnesses:*** Abrupt changes in the weather and increased incidences of natural calamities will lead to socioeconomic disruption among people residing in these zones. These critical incidents will increase the risk of an array of mental illnesses, such as stress, anxiety, depression, etc.
- ***Nutritional deficiencies:*** Extremes of weather conditions like flood and drought may influence the food production leading to protein energy malnutrition and micronutrient deficiencies, etc.
- ***Food-borne diseases:*** Higher atmospheric temperatures can lead to increase in incidence of *Salmonella* and other bacteria-related food poisoning as bacteria can grow rapidly in warmer environments. Extreme weather events, such as flood and drought pose major challenge for food distribution, especially when waterways and roads are damaged.
- ***Trauma:*** The increasing incidents of natural calamities like hurricane, cyclone, flood, etc., may lead to accidents and trauma requiring immediate attention from health authorities.
- ***Skin diseases:*** Due to depletion of ozone and exposure to ultraviolet (UV) rays, there will be increase in the incidence of skin diseases like malignant melanoma, nonmelanocytic skin cancer—squamous cell carcinoma, basal cell carcinoma, sunburn, photodermatoses, chronic sun damage, etc.
- ***Ophthalmic diseases:*** Exposure to excessive solar irradiation and UV rays may result in increased incidence of eye problems such as, photoconjunctivitis and acute photokeratitis, climatic droplet keratopathy, cancer of the cornea and conjunctiva, pterygium, cataract, uveal melanoma, macular degeneration, acute solar retinopathy, etc.
- **Suppression of cell-mediated immunity** leads to increased susceptibility to infection and reactivation of latent infections.

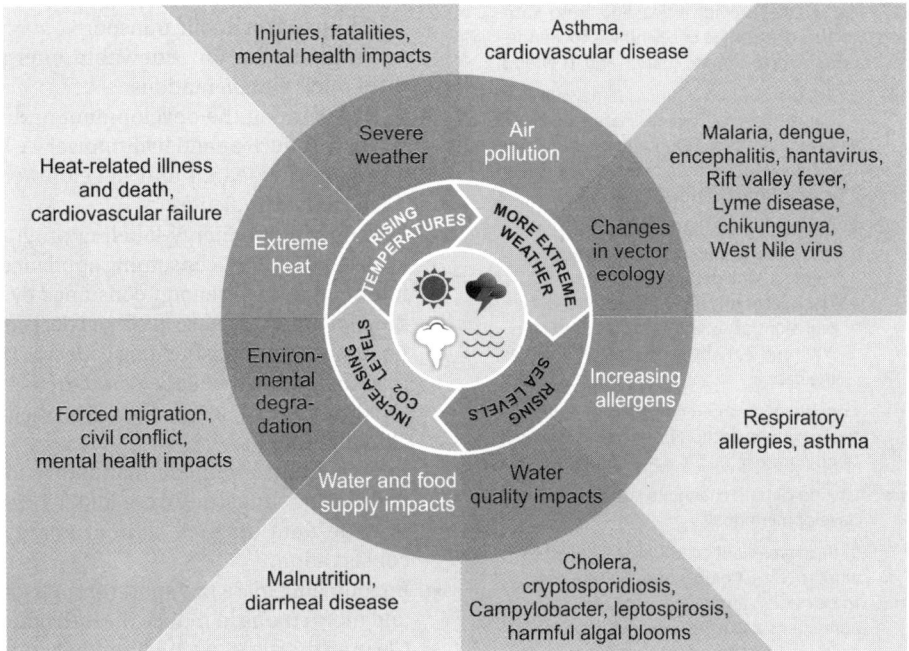

**Fig. 34A.2:** Pathways by which climate change affects human health.

## Deadly Dozen

The health experts from Wildlife Conservation Society released a report on health impacts of climate change in the year 2008 and named it as "Deadly Dozen: Wildlife Diseases in the Age of Climate Change". This report lists 12 infectious diseases that have potential to spread into new regions of the world due to climate change. These include:

> (1) avian influenza, (2) babesia, (3) cholera, (4) ebola, (5) intestinal and external parasites, (6) plague, (7) lyme disease, (8) red tides, (9) rift valley fever, (10) sleeping sickness, (11) tuberculosis and (12) yellow fever

## STRATEGIES TO COMBAT THE HEALTH IMPACTS OF CLIMATE CHANGE

While learning about the strategies to combat the health impacts of climate change, it is important to understand the following important terminologies:

1. ***Adaptation:*** Adjustments in natural or anthropogenic systems in response to actual or expected climatic stimuli or their effects, which moderates harm or exploits beneficial opportunities.
2. ***Adaptive capacity:*** The ability of a system to adjust the climate change (including climate variability and extremes) to moderate potential damages, to take advantage of opportunities, or to cope with consequences.
3. ***Mitigation:*** Preparing ourselves to combat the impacts of climate change.

## INTERNATIONAL RESPONSE TO CLIMATE CHANGE CLIMATE CHANGE

| Year | Effort | Salient features |
|---|---|---|
| 1988 | Intergovernmental Panel on Climate Change (IPCC) was formulated | The IPCC's mandate was to regularly publish reports that provide a clear and up-to-date picture of the state of scientific knowledge pertaining to climate change and its effects. |
| 1992 | Rio Earth Summit at Brazil | • Adapted United Nations Framework Convention on Climate Change (UNFCCC)<br>• Decided to organize Conference of Parties (COP) annually to share the progress made in reducing the impact of climate change |
| 1997 | Kyoto protocol | • Also known as international emission reduction, production, and sharing contract (or agreement)<br>• The goal of this protocol was to reduce emissions of six GHGs by 5.2% between 2008 and 2012 by keeping 1990 levels as the base |
| 2009 | Copenhagen Climate Change Conference | Copenhagen conference officially defined the maximum acceptable increase in global temperature to be 2°C above preindustrial era |
| 2012 | Rio+20 Conference | Linking climate change to sustainable development goals |
| 2015 | Paris agreement | In this agreement, all countries agreed to work to restrict global temperature rise to below 2°C, and to strive for 1.5°C. This agreement also provides a roadmap for collaborative and comprehensive climate actions that will reduce emissions and enhance climate resilience. |

## Climate Change and Sustainable Development Goals

> **Sustainable Development Goal-13: Take Urgent Actions to Combat Climate Change and its Impacts**
>
> *Targets*
> - Strengthening of resilience and adaptive capacity to climate change related hazards and natural disasters across all the countries.
> - Integrate climate change measures into national policies, strategies, and planning.
> - Improve education, awareness generation, capacity building of human resource and institutions on climate change mitigation, adaptation, early warning, and impact reduction.
> - Implementation of the commitment undertaken by developed countries to the UNFCCC for mobilizing jointly USD 100 billion annually by 2020 to address the needs of developing countries for ensuring meaningful mitigation actions.
> - Promote mechanisms for capacity building toward effective planning and management of climate change in developing countries and small island developing states, by focusing on women, youth, local, and marginalized communities.
> - Acknowledging that the UNFCCC is the primary international, intergovernmental forum for negotiating the global response to climate change.

## INDIA'S EFFORTS TO COMBAT CLIMATE CHANGE

India is the third largest emitter of GHGs and contributes to 5.3% of global emissions. In October, 2015, India made a commitment to reduce the emissions intensity of its GDP by 20–25% from its base levels in 2005 by 2020 and 33–35% by 2030. On October 2nd, 2016, India formally ratified the Paris agreement (UN in India, SDG Goal 13: Climate Change, 2016).

*India's efforts to combat climate change are:*

- India has adapted *Integrated Energy Policy in 2006* to reduce the intensity of emission of GHGs. Provisions under this policy are:
  - Promoting efficient management of energy in all sectors
  - Emphasis on public transport
  - Emphasizing on renewable energy sources, such as biofuels and plantations
  - Accelerating the development and use of clean energy, such as nuclear and hydropower
  - Focused research and development on clean energy-related technologies.
- Introduction of energy-labeling program for appliances in 2006 for all energy-consuming appliances. The label provides information on the energy consumed by the appliance, so that the consumer can make informed decision while purchasing it.
- Energy conservation building code was launched in May, 2007 to address design of large commercial buildings to optimize building's energy demand based on their locations in different climatic zones.
- Energy audits are made mandatory for large scale energy consuming industries from 2007. These industries should provide data on their annual energy consumption and conservation.
- Encouraging mass transport through city buses, local trains, and metro trains to reduce the individual use of vehicles.
- Clean air initiatives, such as introduction of compressed natural gas, retiring old and polluting vehicles, and emission test for vehicles.

- Ujjwala Scheme to promote use of LPGs among families of lower socioeconomic status by giving up subsidies by people who can afford.

## NATIONAL ACTION PLAN ON CLIMATE CHANGE

The Ministry of Health and Family Welfare, Government of India, has proposed a "National Action Plan on Climate Change and Human Health", a policy aimed at protecting people against climate-sensitive illnesses, such as cardiorespiratory diseases, cancers, and allergies. The mission and strategies under this plan include:

- *National Solar Mission:* Encouraging utilization of solar energy
- *National Mission for Enhanced Energy Efficiency:* Enhance the energy efficiency in various industries and appliances
- *National Water Mission:* Ensure integrated water resource management
- *National Mission for Strategic Knowledge for Climate Change:* Establish open platform to share knowledge and expertise on climate change
- *National Mission for Green India:* Preservation of forests and afforestation
- *National Mission for Sustainable Agriculture* to protect agriculture and crops from effect of climate change
- *National Mission for Sustaining Himalayan Ecosystem*

## SUMMARY

Climate change is a major public health challenge of the current century. Technological advancements, population growth, economic development, industries, attitudes and beliefs of people are considered to be five major anthropogenic driving forces for climate change. Greenhouse gases, such as water vapor, methane, carbon dioxide and nitric oxide are the major contributors to climate change. Raising temperature, change in the rainfall patterns, increasing sea level, melting of ice sheets, etc. are the major impacts of climate change. Major health consequences of climate change on human health are related to respiratory illnesses, vector-borne diseases, cancers, mental illnesses, skin diseases, waterborne diseases, food borne infections, trauma, ophthalmic illnesses, etc. Adaptation, adaptive ability and mitigation are the major strategies to combat climate change. There are many concerted efforts undertaken at international level to gather the commitment of global community on this emerging issue. Encouraging use of clean energy sources, afforestation, water conservation, controlling combustion of fuel are some of the adapted by India to prevent the consequences of climate change.

## SUGGESTED READING

1. Australian Government. Department of Environment and Energy. Green House Effect. [online] Available from http://www. environment.gov.au/climate-change/climate-science-data/climate-science/greenhouse-effect.
2. Government of India. (2007). National Action Plan for Climate Change. Prime Minister's Office for Climate Change 2007. [online] Available from http://www.moef.nic.in/downloads/home/Pg01-52.pdf.
3. Joon V, Jaiswal V. Impact of Climate Change on Human Health in India: An Overview. Health Population Persp Issues. 2012;35(1):11-22.
4. National Aeronautics and Space Administration. (2018). NASA—Global Climate Change, Vital Signs of Change. Blanket around the earth. [online] Available from https://climate.nasa.gov/causes/.
5. NCDC. (2016). Draft National Action Plan for Climate Change and Human Health NAPCCHH. [online] Available from https://www.ncdc.gov.in/index1.php?lang=1&level=1&sublinkid=120&l id=146.
6. Pachauri RK, Meyer LA. Climate Change 2014: Synthesis Report. Contribution of Working Groups I, II and III to the Fifth Assessment Report of the Intergovernmental Panel on Climate Change. Geneva, Switzerland: IPCC; 2014. p. 151.
7. United Nations Climate Change. Paris Agreement. [online] Available from https://unfccc.int/process-and-meetings/the-paris-agreement/the-paris-agreement.
8. United Nations Framework Convention on Climate Change. (2007). Climate Change: Impacts, Vulnerabilities and Adaptation in Developing Countries. [online] Available from https://unfccc.int/resource/docs/publications/impacts.pdf.
9. United States Environmental Protection Agency. (2017). Climate Impacts on Human Health.
10. US Department of Climate Change. (2010). Transportation's role in reducing US Green House Gas Emissions, Volume 1: Synthesis Report 2010.
11. Wilson G, Fairén V, García-Sanz J, et al. (2012). T869 Module 1: Introduction to climate change in the context of sustainable development. Climate Change: from science to lived experience.
12. World Health Organization. (2003). Climate change and human health: risks and responses. Summary 2003.

# B. DISASTER MANAGEMENT

*Jyotiranjan Sahoo, Venkatarao Epari*

*"While it is impossible to control the forces of nature; however, the health sector has precise responsibilities, interests & opportunities in reducing the consequences of disaster"*

| CM13.1 | Define and describe the concept of disaster management |
| CM13.2 | Describe disaster management cycle |
| CM13.3 | Describe man made disasters in the world and in India |
| CM13.4 | Describe the details of the National Disaster management Authority |

## CONCEPT AND DEFINITION

The term disaster *(meaning 'bad star'; Greek origin)* refers to any sudden catastrophic event resulting in an insurmountable loss, destruction of life and resources, directly or indirectly affecting the socioeconomic, cultural, political and mental state of people; may be of a country as a whole.

Typical characteristics of a disaster are unpredictability, unfamiliarity (of the event to inhabitants), uncertainty (of occurrence and damage it causes), and urgency (or speed at which it occurs).

The most accepted definition by the United Nations International Strategy for Disaster Reduction, which is recognized by the World Health Organization is that:

*"A serious disruption of the functioning of a community or a society involving widespread human, material, economic or environmental losses, and impacts, which exceeds the ability of the affected community or society to cope using its own resources."*

An event in order to qualify as a disaster, one of the following criteria is usually met. If more than or equal to 10 people are killed; 100 or more affected; the state declares an emergency, or an international assistance is called for.

Often the term disaster is used synonymously with hazard. However, there is a subtle difference. Hazard can be defined as *"any dangerous phenomenon, human activity, or a condition that has a potential to cause loss of life or injury, property damage, loss of livelihoods and services, social and economic disruption, or environmental damage"*. In disaster management hazards are identified and targeted to reduce the consequences of any disaster. Poor building construction code is one such example of hazard, which is targeted in disaster management.

The outcome and impact of the disaster depends broadly on three factors.
1. **The risk or the frequency:** It is the probability of occurrence of a particular event or disaster and the losses each would cause.
2. **The vulnerability:** It measures the extent of services or infrastructure of a community or geographic area is likely to be disrupted or damaged by the disaster.
3. **The capacity of the community:** It measures the availability of resources within a community, strengths, and attributes that are needed to recover from losses.

There is a direct relation between these factors, which can be expressed by the following equation.

$$\text{Disaster risk} = \text{Hazard} \times \text{vulnerability}$$

**Table 34B.1:** Classification of disaster.

| Natural disaster | Manmade disaster |
|---|---|
| 1. *Acute/rapid*<br>➢ Geophysical<br>  ♦ Earthquake<br>  ♦ Volcanic eruption<br>  ♦ Tsunami<br>➢ Hydrological<br>  ♦ Flood<br>  ♦ Avalanche or landslide<br>➢ Meteorological<br>  ♦ Cyclone<br>  ♦ Strom<br>  ♦ Tornado<br>  ♦ Extreme temperature<br>  ♦ Cold wave<br>➢ Climatological<br>  ♦ Drought<br>  ♦ Extreme heat or cold<br>  ♦ Forest fire<br>➢ Biological<br>  ♦ Epidemic or pandemics<br>2. Slow or gradual<br>➢ Drought<br>➢ Pest infestation (e.g., locus)<br>➢ Desertification | 1. *Unintentional*<br>➢ Industrial accident<br>  ♦ Explosion<br>  ♦ Fire<br>  ♦ Hazardous material release<br>➢ Structural collapse<br>➢ Transportation crash<br>2. Intentional<br>➢ Civil strife<br>➢ Terrorism<br>➢ War or complex emergencies |

## TYPES OF DISASTER

Generally, disasters are classified according to the hazard they are associated with. Mainly, it is of two types, natural and manmade disasters. A complete list of the types of disasters with their subtypes is given in **Table 34B.1**.

## BURDEN DUE TO DISASTER

According to World Disaster Report 2016, on an average 600 natural or manmade disasters occurred every year in the world. More than 1,420 million people were affected and more than 700,000 people died worldwide from disasters during 2006–15. The worst affected continent was Asia followed by Africa. In 2016 alone, a total of 102 countries were affected by disasters distressing 411 million people, causing around 8,000 deaths with an economic loss of 97 billion US dollars. Countries having low human development index were the worst affected by disasters. While only one quarter (25.7%) of total disasters occurred in countries having low human development, but they accounted for more than half (56.8%) of the deaths (IFRC, World Disaster Report, 2016). **Figure 34B.1** shows the occurrence of the different types of disasters with associated mortality (CRED, Preliminary data: Human impact of natural disasters, 2016).

The vulnerability of India to disasters is higher as more than half of the land is prone to earthquakes, more than one-tenth of land is prone to floods and river erosions, more than

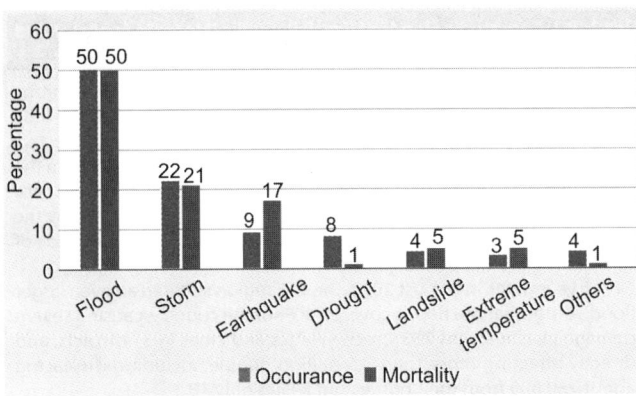

Fig. 34B.1: Worldwide occurrence and mortality according to disaster type in 2016.

three-fourths of the coastline is prone to cyclones or tsunami and more than two-thirds of the agricultural land is prone to droughts. Since the 1970s, 30 major disasters have occurred in India. Most recent being Uttarakhand flood and landslides, which had reported around 4,094 deaths (NDMA, Disaster Data and Statistics, 2018). India reported 17 natural disasters in 2016 alone, affecting 331 million people and causing 884 deaths, thus ranking at first place in the list of countries by the number of people affected (Centre for research on Epidemiology of Disasters, 2016).

## FACTORS CONTRIBUTING TO THE IMPACT ON HEALTH FOLLOWING DISASTER

Every disaster is unique, but few factors are common in all disasters and if these are recognized well in advance then they can be used to optimize the use of resources for management of public health. Postdisaster health problems are determined by the following factors:

### Social Reaction

Panic or waiting in shock is generally expected following a disaster but it rarely occurs. It is seen that survivors rapidly recover from the initial shock and begin search and rescue within minutes of a disaster. Rumors are the major phenomenon after a disaster, particularly of epidemics, which hampers the humanitarian actions. Sometimes people intentionally refuse to evacuate the disaster site or unwilling to submit to the action taken by the authority. Since the survivor or unaffected people are the first to respond to a disaster, adequate information, and capacity building for appropriate humanitarian activities should be directed towards meeting the needs of survivors.

### Communicable Disease

Risk of disease transmission is increased following disaster resulting in major outbreaks. Most commonly seen outbreaks are due to fecal contamination of food and water. In the long run, vector-borne disease transmission increases, especially after the flood and heavy rain. Zoonotic disease transmission is also increased due to the displacement of wild animals near human settlements.

### Population Displacements

After a disaster, rapid population movement occurs, which is mostly unorganized. This leads to importation of newer diseases, overcrowding and compromised basic sanitation facilities, which along with the lack of public services can increase the morbidity and mortality.

### Climatic Exposure

Exposure to extreme climatic conditions, such as heavy rain, cold storms, etc., occurs mostly during the disaster. After the disaster, these climatic exposures can be minimized, if proper clothing and shelter are provided to the affected individuals.

### Food and Nutrition

Disruption of food stock and public distribution system during a disaster is the major causes of food shortage and hunger following a disaster. Although short-term food shortage is not severe to cause malnutrition but in conditions like extreme drought may result in malnutrition especially among communities completely dependent upon help from outside. Most commonly affected are the vulnerable groups of any society like children, lactating mothers, and elderly people.

### Water and Sanitation

Damage to the water distribution and sewage drainage system results in a shortage of drinking water and disruption of excreta or waste disposal. Such conditions lead to deterioration of basic sanitation and contribute to spreading of gastrointestinal and other illnesses.

### Mental Health

Depression and anxiety which occur immediately following disaster but they are not major public health problems. Mental health problems were largely seen in the industrialized or the urban areas of developing countries during postdisaster rehabilitation or reconstruction phase. Post-traumatic stress disorder (PTSD) is the most common manifestation.

### Damage to the Health Infrastructure

Natural disasters, such as earthquakes or floods can cause severe structural damage to health facilities or make them structurally unsafe. Such a situation can jeopardize the life of inpatients or health personnel and hamper the capacity of the facility to provide services to the affected community. Indirectly, it causes an increase in mortality rate after a disaster. For example, in 1985 Peru witnessed earthquake, destroying 13 hospitals with 866 deaths; among them, 100 were health professionals. The World Health Day 2009 theme was "Save lives: Make hospitals safe in emergencies" and it highlighted the crucial role of a safe health infrastructure in times of disasters.

All these common health outcomes can occur in all types of natural disasters with varying degree. **Table 34B.2** shows the short-term health outcome depending on the type of disaster.

**Table 34B.2:** Short-term health outcome according to type of disaster.

| Effect | Earthquakes | Cyclones without flood | Floods | Landslides |
|---|---|---|---|---|
| Death | +++ | + | +++ | +++ |
| Injuries | +++ | ++ | + | + |
| Damage to health facilities | +++ | +++ | ++ | ++ |
| Damage to water supply | +++ | + | ++ | +++ |
| Shortage of food | + | ++ | ++ | + |
| Population displacement | +/− | + | + | +/− |
| Communicable disease | ++ | ++ | ++ | ++ |

+++ indicate severe/more common; ++ indicate moderate; + indicates low; +/− indicates rare

## DISASTER MANAGEMENT CYCLE

Disaster management can be defined as *"the systematic process of using administrative directives, organizations, and operational skills and capacities to implement strategies, policies and improved coping capacities in order to lessen the adverse impacts of hazards, and the possibility of disaster"*. From a public health point of view, disaster has three key phases (1) predisaster, (2) disaster, and (3) postdisaster phase and management is based on these three phases. The detail steps of the disaster management cycle are presented in **Figure 34B.2**. **Box 34B.1** shows a case study showing importance of disaster management.

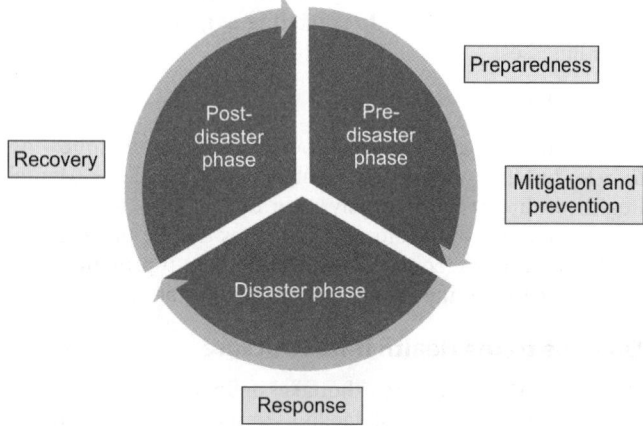

**Fig. 34B.2:** Disaster management cycle.

### Predisaster Phase

#### Preparedness

The objective is to develop measures that enable individuals, communities, and government to respond rapidly and effectively to a disaster situation. Following measures should be taken in the preparedness phase:
1. Risk analysis of health sector of a particular country or geographical region to different types of disaster is the first step of preparedness.

> **Box 34B.1:** Case study: Floods of Czech Republic (Moore M Et et al., Rand Center for Domestic and International Health Security, 2007).
>
> In July 1997, countries in Central and Eastern Europe (CEE) were hit by heavy rains, hailstorms, and high winds that led to what was at the time the worst flooding in a century. Over 1 million people were directly affected, buildings, roads, agricultural land, and infrastructure was destroyed. In the Czech Republic, floods hit 538 villages and cities in total of 34 districts, covering approximately 40% of the country. 50 people were killed by the flooding, more than 60,000 people evacuated, and several hundreds of thousands more were directly affected.
> Only 5 years later, in August 2002, the CEE region suffered an even larger flood. Altogether the floods covered 40% of the country, causing severe damage in as many as 753 Czech villages and cities in 31 districts, and directly affecting more than 1.5 million people, including displacing about 230,000 from their homes but killing only 18.
>
> **Key practices that avoided deaths:**
> - *Early warning:* In response to the devastation of the 1997 floods, the Czech Hydrometeorological Institute (CHMI) restructured itself into a network of forecasting offices to better offer actionable information for the prevention and mitigation of future disasters.
> - *Emergency medical care:* Another innovation implemented in the Czech Republic following the 1997 floods was the increased emphasis placed on emergency and disaster medical care in the country.
> - *Coordination:* Finally, by the end of 2000, the Czech Republic had established three general laws related to disaster situations—the Saw establishing an Integrated Rescue System, the Law on Crisis Management, and the Law on Economic Measures for Crisis States.

2. Institutionalization of proper health policy or plan and legislation on disaster. For example, legislation to ensure every health facility have hospital disaster response plan.
3. Development of a proper coordination mechanism with internal or external agencies who can help in a disaster situation like armed forces, united nations, red cross, NGOs, etc.
4. Relation with the media is critical as they play a pivotal role in disseminating information about simple measures to be taken in order to reduce the postdisaster effects. The health sector conveys such messages to the community through media.
5. Strengthening the health programs and services in order to respond quickly and appropriately to a disaster situation.
6. A proper administrative decision to ensure adequate manpower and logistic supply to the health facility should be undertaken beforehand.
7. Mock drills should be undertaken with the active participation of health staff and keep disaster plans up to date.

### Mitigation and Prevention

Mitigation is defined as *"measures taken to reduce both the effects of the disaster itself and the vulnerable conditions leading to it in order to reduce the scale of a future disaster"*. Use of the term prevention in a disaster is not entirely appropriate, as most natural disasters cannot be prevented while certain manmade disasters are preventable.

Following are the activities undertaken in the mitigation program:
- Identification of risk and determination of vulnerability of areas exposed to hazards.
- Developing proper design and building codes that will protect the water supply, sewage system, and the health infrastructure in the event of a disaster.

- The inclusion of mitigation measures, such as proper planning, designing, and choosing an appropriate site for new health facilities and maintenance of existing facilities.
- Identification of the priority or critical health facilities and to make them fit for a disaster situation.
- Dissemination of information, sensitization, and training of personnel involved in an operation, administration, and maintenance of facilities.
- Provision of early warning system in high-risk areas.

## Disaster Phase

This phase denotes the time during which an actual event of a disaster takes place, affecting the elements and population at risk. The duration of the event will depend on the type of disaster, e.g., within seconds in case of earthquake and days in case floods. During the disaster, the immediate response is to set up control rooms, putting the contingency plan in to action, issuing warning, action for evacuation, taking people to safer areas, rendering medical aid, food, drinking water, and clothing to the victims. The emergency relief activities were undertaken during and immediately after a disaster, which includes immediate relief, rescue, and the damage needs assessment and debris clearance.

## Postdisaster Phase

It is the implementation phase and also called as recovery phase. The outcome of a disaster in terms of morbidity and mortality relies upon the actions taken in this phase. Postdisaster phase directly depends on preparedness and mitigation process undertaken during the predisaster phase. Following general measures are important in the postdisaster phase.

- *Search, rescue, and first aid:* It is the first step following a disaster. Most immediate help in this step will come from the uninjured survivors. Provision of a prompt and quality first aid service depends on preparedness and training.
- *Care at the disaster site:* Generally, the transport of victims to hospital immediately following a disaster is not possible. Thus, appropriate care or treatment at the disaster site is necessary. This can be achieved by a fixed first aid facility at the disaster site along with the mobile team.
- *Triage:* After a disaster, the proportion of individuals seeking medical care generally exceeds the capacity of the health facility. In an emergency situation, the general principle of "first come, first served" to the patient cannot be applied. Triage is an approach adopted in an emergency situation, where patients are classified on the basis of injuries and their severity. Most commonly used and internationally accepted classification is the color-coding system. Red indicates high priority to be transferred immediately to a health facility. This category of patients has critical injuries and they are more likely to survive, if simple life-saving measures are applied. Yellow indicates medium priority or urgent cases; they are likely to survive, if care is given within hours. The green color code is used for an individual with minor injuries or for ambulatory patients, where treatment can be delayed. The black code is used for the dead or moribund patients, where the chance of survival in minimum. It basically determines the transportation and admission priority of victims to the hospitals. Ideally, triage should be carried at the disaster site and by the trained local health worker.
- *Tagging:* It is the process of identifying patient through a tag attached to them describing their name, sex, age, triage category, and treatment received. It is to provide care on a priority basis.
- *Hospital reception and treatment:* At the healthcare facility, an expert clinician should once again prioritize patients according to the injuries as it may determine the survival of patients.
- Standardized simple therapeutic procedures: ***Standard and simple therapeutic measures should be applied to an emergency situation, as it aims to save lives and prevent further complications.***
- *Epidemiological surveillance and control of epidemics:* The objective of surveillance and control of epidemics is to:
  - Reduce the risk of disease transmission through appropriate public health measures.
  - Establishing a disease reporting system to identify and manage outbreaks promptly.
  - Rapid investigation of outbreaks to clarify rumors and proper distribution of resources.
- *Vaccine and vaccination:* Mass vaccination programs should be discouraged. WHO does not recommend vaccination against typhoid and cholera following an outbreak in endemic countries rather supports the provision of safe potable water and proper sanitation as the most effective strategy. Natural disasters do not increase the chance of tetanus significantly, thus mass vaccination against tetanus is also usually unwanted. Strengthening and maintenance of the existing routine immunization program along with cold chain maintenance must be given priority rather than mass vaccination programs.
- *Water supply:* Following a disaster, it is vital to establish the physical integrity, capacity, bacteriological, and chemical quality of the water supply. Microbial contamination of water is the major threat to public health. Chlorination is the recommended process to ensure water quality in emergency situations due to its effectiveness, availability and cost. The recommended level of free residual chlorine in emergency situations is 0.7 mg/L. If normal water sources are disrupted then consider alternate sources.
- *Mass distribution of disinfectants:* As discussed chlorination is the first measure but the mass distribution of disinfectants should only be considered if affected persons have prior experience in their use. Appropriate water storage containers are distributed.
- *Food safety:* Contamination of food due to inadequate sanitation is the major cause of foodborne illnesses. Kitchen and personal hygiene are of utmost importance during feeding programs in temporary shelters.
- *Basic sanitation and personal hygiene:* Latrines for the residents, refugees, displaced people, and relief workers should be provided in the disaster-hit area. Communal trench latrines are the alternatives in disaster.
- *Vector control:* Leptospirosis, malaria, dengue, typhus, and plague are some of the important vector-borne diseases

following a disaster. Areas endemic to these diseases are particularly at risk. Thus, control programs should be intensified in the postdisaster phase.
- **Burial of the dead:** Since most of the deaths in a disaster are due to trauma, corpses are less likely to cause a disease outbreak. Victims of a disaster, even carriers of transmissible diseases, are in fact, a far lesser threat to the public than while they were alive. If the corpses contaminate the water bodies, they can pose a problem. Apart from the risk of disease, dead bodies represent a sensitive social issue. Burial is the best method for dead body disposal, if it is culturally acceptable and feasible.
- **Temporary settlements and camps:** Population movement or displacement leads to the creation of temporary settlements. The objective of these settlements is to provide the inhabitant acceptable standard of living and to minimize the cost. Few important criteria should be followed before setting up a camp.
  – The site should be located in close proximity to the main road and should have good drainage facility.
  – Camps should be planned in a such a fashion that few families are grouped together to form a cluster around communal services.
  – Sanitation services should be appropriate and adequate. It is recommended that for every 20 individuals, at least one latrine should be there.
  – Provision of safe water is also a major criterion for setting up camps. At the campsite, every individual should be provided with a minimum of 15 liters of clean water for domestic purposes.

In nutshell, Health Sector has precise responsibilities, interests, and opportunities in reducing the consequences of a disaster.

## NATIONAL DISASTER MANAGEMENT AUTHORITY OF INDIA

Recognizing the importance of disaster management as a National priority, Government of India set up a High-Powered Committee (HPC) in August 1999 and a National Committee following Gujarat earthquake in order to make recommendations for preparing disaster management plans and suggest effective mitigation mechanisms. In December 2005, through enactment of Disaster Management Act, National Disaster Management Authority (NDMA) headed by the Prime Minister, and State Disaster Management Authorities (SDMAs) headed by respective Chief Ministers was created with a vision

"To build a safer and disaster resilient India by a holistic, proactive, technology driven, and sustainable development strategy that involves all stakeholders and fosters a culture of prevention, preparedness, and mitigation".

The NDMA has the following few important responsibilities to ensure timely and effective response to disasters.
- Lay down policies on disaster management; approve the National Plan and plans prepared by the Ministries or Departments of the Government of India.
- Lay down guidelines for the State Authorities in drawing up the State Plan.
- Coordinate the enforcement and implementation of the policy and plans.
- Recommend provision of funds for the purpose of mitigation.

## SUGGESTED READING

1. Centre for Research on the Epidemiology of Disasters. 2016 preliminary data: Human impact of natural disasters. Centre for Research on the Epidemiology of Disasters. [online] Available from: https://www.cred.be/publications.
2. International Federation of Red Cross and Red Crescent Societies (IFRC). World disasters report 2016: resilience: saving lives today: investing for tomorrow. Genève: Fédération internationale des sociétés de la Coix-Rouge; 2016.
3. Moore M, Trujillo HR, Lawson BS, Basurto-Davila R, Evans DK. Models of Relief: Learning from Exemplary Practices in International Disaster Management. Santa Monica, CA: RAND Center for Domestic and International Health Security; 2007.
4. National Disaster Management Authority, Government of India. Disaster Data and Statistics. New Delhi: National Disaster Management Authority; 2018.
5. National Disaster Management Authority, Government of India. Vulnerability Profile. New Delhi: National Disaster Management Authority; 2018.
6. National Disaster Management Authority Govt. of India. National Disaster Management Plan (NDMP). India: National Disaster Management Authority Govt. of India; 2016.
7. National institute of disaster management. Disaster management—terminology. [online]. Available from: http://www.nidm.gov.in/PDF/Disaster_terminology.pdf.
8. Pan American Health Organization. Natural disasters: protecting the public health. Washington, DC: Pan American Health Organization; 2000.
9. Pfefferbaum B, Houston JB, North CS, et al. Youth's Reactions to Disasters and the Factors that Influence their Response. Prev Res. 2008;15(3):3-6.
10. United Nation International Strategy for Disaster reduction. UNISDR terminology on disaster risk reduction. Geneva: United Nation International Strategy for Disaster reduction; 2009.
11. Watson JT, Gayer M, Connolly MA. Epidemics after Natural Disasters. Emerg Infect Dis J. 2017;13.

# C. HOSPITAL-ACQUIRED INFECTIONS AND ITS PREVENTION AND CONTROL

*Jay K Sheth*

| CM 11.5 | Describe occupational hazards of health professionals and their prevention and management |
|---|---|
| CM8.1 | Describe and discuss Hospital acquired infections |

## BACKGROUND

In spite of great progress in medical care and community health measures, infections still continue to develop in hospitalized patients and these may also affect the healthcare staff and even the individuals accompanying the patients. The hospital-acquired infections or healthcare acquired infections, which are also known as nosocomial infections, are still major cause of increased morbidity as well as death among hospitalized patients. They increase the duration of hospital stay and thereby significantly contribute in the increased cost of care as well. Such infections are a major economic burden not only for healthcare institutions but also for individual patients, their family and society at large.

To correctly spell-out an infection as hospital-acquired infection, it must not be present nor be incubating at the time of hospital admission. *A hospital-acquired infection is "an infection acquired in hospital by a patient who was admitted for a reason other than that infection. This includes infections acquired in the hospital but appearing after discharge and also occupational infections among staff of the facility".* Clarifying this further, these infections are those infections acquired in hospital or healthcare service unit that first appear 48 hours or more after hospital admission or within 30 days after discharge following in-patient care. This should also include infections appearing to individuals accompanying the patient at the healthcare institution.

## EPIDEMIOLOGY OF HOSPITAL-ACQUIRED INFECTIONS

Hospital-acquired infections occur worldwide and are reported not only from the resource-poor developing countries but from developed countries as well. The risk of hospital-acquired and healthcare related infections is 2–20 times higher in developing countries as compared to developed countries.

According to WHO hospital-acquired infections are a major cause of death and disability for patients. A prevalence study conducted by WHO representing 4 WHO regions (Europe, Eastern Mediterranean, Southeast Asia and Western Pacific), 14 countries and 55 hospitals showed an average of 8.7% of hospitalized patients had hospital-acquired infections. At any time, over 1.4 million people worldwide suffer from infectious complications acquired in hospital. The highest prevalence of such infections was reported from the Eastern Mediterranean and Southeast Asia regions (11.8 and 10.0% respectively).

Incidence of nosocomial infection in India shows a wide variation from 15% to as high as 50% depending on the healthcare setup, type of patients treated, type of setup (government/private), patient load, unit/section of the healthcare setup, site of infection studied, duration of hospital stay required for the given condition, qualification of the healthcare staff and resources available for quality barrier nursing.

Infections of surgical wounds, urinary tract infections and lower respiratory tract infections are amongst the most frequent nosocomial infections. As documented by various studies, nosocomial infections occur most frequently in the intensive care units (ICUs) as well as acute surgical/orthopedic wards. Increasing variety of investigations, invasive medical procedures creating potential routes of infection, increasing drug-resistant among microorganisms and their transmission, crowded population at the hospitals, decreased immunity of patients, etc., play a vital role in promoting infection in hospital settings.

> Poorly followed infection control practices amplify the effect of all such risk factors and convert the potential risk situation into a reality.

Risk of nosocomial infection can be categorized by the type of patient and type of procedure **(Table 34C.1)**.

**Table 34C.1:** Categorization of nosocomial infection risk.

| Risk of infection | Type of patients | Type of procedures |
|---|---|---|
| Minimal | • Not immunocompromised<br>• No significant underlying disease | Noninvasive<br>No exposure to biological fluids |
| Medium | Infected patients or patients with some risk factors | Exposure to biological fluids<br>or<br>Invasive nonsurgical procedure (e.g. peripheral venous catheter or urinary catheterization) |
| High | Immunocompromised patients, multiple trauma, severe burns, organ transplant, etc. | Surgery<br>or<br>High-risk invasive procedure (e.g. central venous catheter, endotracheal intubation) |

## PREVENTION OF NOSOCOMIAL INFECTIONS

> Prevention of nosocomial infection is a collective responsibility of each and everyone involved in patient care. Isolation strategies, barrier nursing, sterilization and disinfection practices, evidence-based optimum and rational use of antimicrobials, etc., have crucial role for the prevention and control of nosocomial infection.

**Cleaning, disinfection** and **sterilization** must be followed properly to minimize the risk of transmitting microorganisms from various surfaces, instruments, equipment's and the overall hospital environment.
- Prior to disinfection or sterilization, all instruments, equipment's and surfaces must be cleaned. This can be done manually with detergent and water, automatic washers, enzymatic cleaners or ultrasonic cleaners.
- Disinfection is a process of removing microorganisms without complete sterilization. Disinfection can be achieved

by thermal or chemical disinfection and is not a substitute for sterilization. There is no single ideal disinfectant and its selection must take into account instrument, purpose, heat sensitivity, desired level of disinfection, etc.
- Sterilization is destruction of all the microorganisms and is required for anything and everything that penetrates sterile body parts. Sterilization can be achieved by moist heat (steam under pressure), dry heat, through chemical or even through irradiation.

Written policies and procedures must be prepared and regularly updated appropriately for each and every facility, procedure and activity. All the important standard operating procedures (SOPs) must be properly visible at prominent locations where such procedures are routinely or most likely to be performed (e.g., hand washing protocol near the washbasin, biomedical waste management protocol near the colored dustbin, etc.). A compilation of all such protocols in the form of infection control manual should be easily available and strictly followed in a healthcare setup.

**Table 34C.2** enlists recommended measures for different risk categorization of nosocomial infection.

**Table 34C.2:** Recommended measures for different risk categorization of nosocomial infection.

| Risk of infection | Asepsis | Antiseptics | Hands | Cloths | Devices |
|---|---|---|---|---|---|
| Minimal | Clean | None | Simple hand washing | Street cloths | Clean or disinfected |
| Medium | Asepsis | Standard antiseptic products | Hygienic hand washing | Protection against blood and biological fluids | Disinfected and sterile |
| High | Surgical asepsis | Specific major antiseptic products | Surgical hand washing | Surgical cloths, dress, mask, caps, sterile gloves | Disinfected and sterile |

## Universal Precautions

All healthcare workers must assume that every patient can be a source of infection and their blood/body fluids are potential source of their infection irrespective of their signs, symptoms, investigation status or diagnosis. Apart from blood, various body fluids are potential sources of infection as they carry the blood-borne pathogens; these are semen, vaginal secretions, amniotic fluid, pericardial fluid, pleural fluid, cerebrospinal fluid, synovial fluid or any body fluid that is visibly contaminated with blood or body fluid. Every possible precaution must be applied to blood, all these body fluids and excretions as they have the potential to transmit the infective pathogen.

Universal precautions are nothing but universally taking all the precautions in all the patients, i.e., treating all patients in the healthcare facility with the same basic level of "standard" precautions. It involves a set of basic work practices that are essential to provide a high level of protection to patients, healthcare workers and visitors.

> Since, familiarity affects perception of risk, knowing the risk provides motivation to follow preventive advices!!!

## Standard Precautions for all Patients

- Wash hands promptly after contact with infective material
- Use no touch technique wherever possible
- Wear gloves when in contact with blood, body fluids, secretions, excretions, mucous membranes and contaminated items
- Wash hands immediately after removing gloves
- All sharps should be handled with extreme care and as per guidelines
- Clean up spills of infective material promptly as per the guideline
- Ensure that patient-care equipment, supplies and linen contaminated with infective material is either discarded, or disinfected or sterilized between each patient use
- Ensure appropriate biomedical waste handling as per the law

## Handwashing and Antisepsis

Hand hygiene has been well documented and demonstrated as an important factor for the prevention of transmission of nosocomial infections. However, hand washing practices are frequently ignored inviting easy transmission of infections particularly in a healthcare setup **(Table 34C.3)**. Many infectious diseases (particularly with colonization, enteric infection, skin infections, etc.) are transmitted through contact transmission.

Washing or decontaminating hands is recommended using a plain soap, antimicrobial agent, such as an alcoholic hand rub or waterless antiseptic agent. This must be strictly followed before any direct contact with patients, between contact with different patients, immediately after removing gloves and even between task and procedure on the same patient (to prevent cross contamination). Finger nails should be cut regularly and kept short and clean. Artificial finger-nails are not recommended. Wearing of watch, bracelet, ring or other jewelry is strongly discouraged. Steps of hand washing are shown in **Figure 34C.1**.

**Table 34C.3:** Major forms of hand hygiene.

| Technique | Main purpose | Influence on hand flora | Agents | Rapidity of action | Residual effect |
|---|---|---|---|---|---|
| Social hand washing | Cleansing | Reduces transient flora | Non-medicated soap | Slow | Short |
| Careful hand washing | Cleansing after patient contact | Partly removes transient flora | Non-medicated soap | Slow | Short |
| Hygienic hand disinfection | Disinfection after contamination | Kills transient flora | Alcohol | Fast | Short |
| Surgical hand disinfection | Preoperative disinfection | Kills transient flora and inhibit resident flora | Antibacterial soap, alcoholic solutions | Slow (soap) or fast (alcohol) | Long |

## Rub hands for hand hygiene! wash hands when visibly soiled

 Duration of the entire procedure: 20–30 seconds

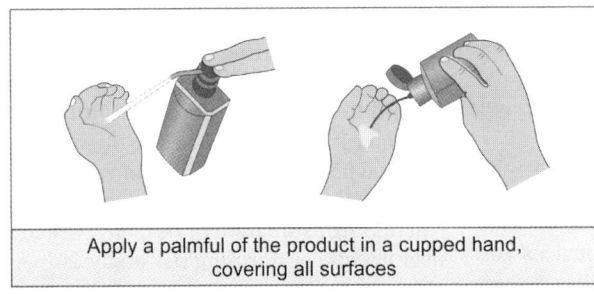

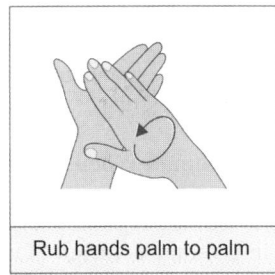

Apply a palmful of the product in a cupped hand, covering all surfaces

Rub hands palm to palm

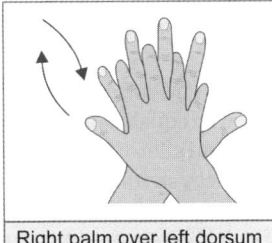

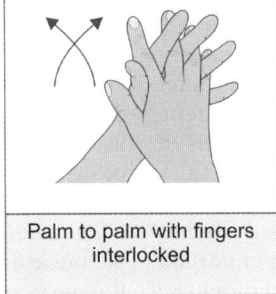

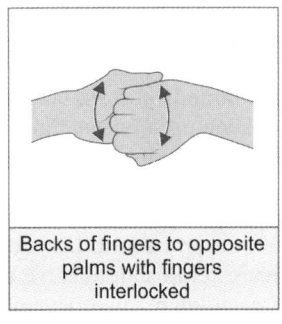

Right palm over left dorsum with interlocked fingers and vice versa

Palm to palm with fingers interlocked

Backs of fingers to opposite palms with fingers interlocked

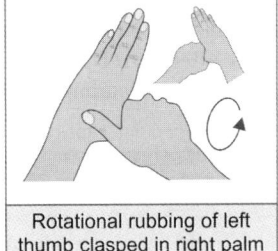

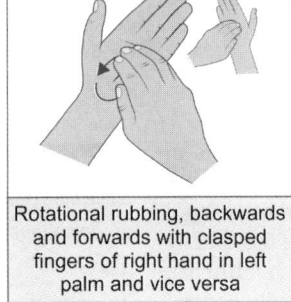

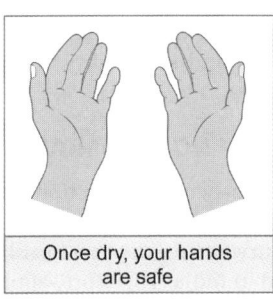

Rotational rubbing of left thumb clasped in right palm and vice versa

Rotational rubbing, backwards and forwards with clasped fingers of right hand in left palm and vice versa

Once dry, your hands are safe

**Fig. 34C.1:** Steps of handwashing.
*Source:* Adapted from WHO brochure on hand hygiene

> **Interesting Historical Perspective**
>
> Ignaz Semmelweis observed the differential rates of maternal deaths due to puerperal infections in postnatal divisions where students were taught. He proposed the theory of transmission of infection by the students through direct contact and ordered everyone to wash their hands in a solution of chlorinated lime before each examination. The drastic reduction in deaths thus resulted into discovery of the cause of puerperal fever and became instrumental in introducing the antisepsis into medical practice.

## Personal Protective Equipment

Personal protective equipment (PPE) serves as a physical barrier in preventing contact of the microorganisms with the susceptible host/healthcare worker. It must be remembered that PPE reduces but does not completely eliminate the risk of acquiring an infection and so, it must be very clear that it must be used effectively, correctly and at all times whenever and wherever there is a potential risk of transmission of infection. Since, complacency is likely when PPE are used, everyone must also be aware that use of PPE does not replace the need to follow any of the basic infection control measures such as hand hygiene. Continuous availability of personal protective equipment and adequate training for its proper use is essential (For more detailed description on use of personal protective equipment, refer to Hospital Infection Control Guidelines by ICMR, GoI).

Personal protective equipment should be used by:
- Healthcare workers including medical and paramedical staff who provide direct care to patients.
- Laboratory staff, who handle patient specimens.
- All the support staff who are indirectly involved in providing healthcare but are at risk of acquiring infections through contact with blood, body fluids, secretions and excretions.
- Family members who provide care to patients and are in a situation where they may have contact with blood, body fluids, secretions and excretions.

## INFECTION CONTROL COMMITTEE

Since prevention of nosocomial infection is a collective responsibility, a common platform is required for sharing of information and data related to nosocomial infections, establishing effective surveillance system including drafting and implementing SOPs or guidelines, discussing prospective plans for infection prevention, etc.

An Infection Control Committee should essentially consider continuous review of data, recalculation of risks, advocacy for appropriate changes in SOPs, suggesting and implementing proactive and timely interventions, review of new devices and newer technologies from infection control point of view, review of nosocomial infection cases/outbreaks, etc. The committee is usually headed by the administrative head/superintendent of the hospital. Adequate representation of management team, medical staff, paramedical staff, laboratory and other establishments, housekeeping services, training department, etc., is crucial to include and discuss all the dimensions of infection control.

A compilation of all the recommended infection control activities, information, evidences and instructions as well as practices in a healthcare setup should serve as an important tool as an infection prevention manual. The manual should be not only be developed but must also be updated frequently by the Infection Control Committee taking into account the data, experiences, evidences and availability of newer resources/techniques/technologies.

## SURVEILLANCE OF NOSOCOMIAL INFECTION

The ultimate aim of nosocomial infection surveillance is to prevent all the nosocomial infections. However, the quality and consistency of surveillance data on healthcare associated infections are limited in India. Therefore, applying the quality assurance and quality control checks on the healthcare sectors using the evidence-based data holds the key to control and prevent hospital-acquired infections. Activities, such as accreditation of healthcare institutions takes into account the standardization of the treatment and infection control practices which reflects the key to reduce the hospital-acquired infections.

### Specific objectives of surveillance:
- Improve awareness of medical and paramedical staff
- Monitor trends and changes in nosocomial infections
- Identify need to formulate new guidelines, SOPs
- Find out scopes of improvement in current practices and guidelines
- Evaluate effectiveness of existing preventive measures
- Suggest improved practices for prevention of infection.

### Surveillance system must be:
- Applied consistently across various sections and at different times
- As simple as possible, using minimal resources so as not to lose consistency
- Flexible to allow changes to meet changing needs
- Sensitive to catch nosocomial infections even at low incidence
- Specificity of confirming as nosocomial infection using standard definitions, procedures and testing
- And last but not the least surveillance system must not be only on paper. It must be implemented and practiced routinely.

Nosocomial infection rate is an important indicator of safety and quality of care in a healthcare facility. However, since the passive reporting of cases has limited importance, active surveillance of nosocomial infection is recommended. Focus should be paid not only to the number of people acquiring nosocomial infections but also on the denominator of the non-infected patients, calculation of various risk factors, comparing suspected risk factors, statistical analysis of risk factors and calculating estimation of risk, etc., which may prove to be very useful while performing risk analysis.

## DISINFECTION PROCEDURES

### Feces and Urine

Feces and urine should be collected in impervious vessels and disinfected by adding an equal volume of one of the disinfectants listed in **Table 34C.4** and allowed to stand for 1–2 hours. To allow proper disinfection feces should be first broken up with a stick. If the disinfectants listed in **Table 34C.4** are not available, an equal amount of quicklime or freshly prepared milk of lime (1 of lime to 4 of water) may be added, mixed and left for 2 hours. If none is available, a bucket of boiling water may be added to the feces which is then covered and allowed to stand until cool. After disinfection, the excreta matter may be emptied into water closet or buried in ground. Bedpans and urinals should ideally be steam disinfected. Alternatively, they may be disinfected with 2½% cresol for an hour after cleaning.

Table 34C.4: Agents suitable for disinfection of feces and urine.

| Disinfectant | Amount per liter | Percent |
| --- | --- | --- |
| Bleaching powder | 50 g | 5 |
| Crude phenol | 100 mL | 10 |
| Cresol | 50 mL | 5 |
| Formalin | 100 mL | 10 |

### Sputum

This is best received in gauze or paper handkerchiefs and destroyed by burning. If the amount is considerable (as in TB hospitals), it may be disinfected by boiling or autoclaving for 20 minutes at 20 lbs pressure. Alternatively, the patient may be asked to spit in a sputum cup half-filled with 5% cresol. When the cup is full, it is allowed to stand for an hour and the contents may be emptied and disposed off.

### Air

To reduce the risk of nosocomial infections through respiratory route, the air must be as clean as possible, particularly in high risk sections of the healthcare setup.

Modern day operation theaters are usually under positive air pressure to minimize the inflow of air from other areas into the operating units. Positive air pressure is created by mechanically supplying more air in an area which is removed by an exhaust, forcing the fast replacement rate. For effective air ventilation, inlets should be located high on wall or on ceiling and away from ventilation discharge outlets which should be on a low wall so that contaminated air is effectively filtered out. Bacteria free clean air is provided with vertical flow air pressure and air velocity of at least 0.25 m/sec through high efficiency particulate air (HEPA) systems which provides 20–25 air changes in an hour. The same principle is also applied to special ICU, microbiological laboratories handling highly infectious culture media and similar high-risk areas.

On the other hand, negative air pressure is important in areas where patients with infections transmitted by respiratory route are kept. For negative air pressure, the area must be a closed one and is negative air pressure is created by supplying less air to the area than the amount of air which can be sucked out/removed by the ventilation system. This produces an inflow around the air entry points and reduces the outward movement of the contaminated air from the suspended area.

> For nosocomial infections which spread through respiratory route, appropriate air ventilation system is very important. Positive and negative air pressure gradient, laminar air flow, unidirectional air flow hoods, HEPA system, air velocity and air exchange rate in a closed unit are important in controlling the spread of nosocomial infections.

## SUGGESTED READING

1. Chartier Y, Emmanuel J, Pieper U, et al. Safe management of wastes from health-care activities, 2nd edition. Geneva: World Health Organization; 2014.
2. Ducel G, Fabry J, Nicolle L. Prevention of hospital-acquired infections: A practical guide. Geneva: World Health Organization; 2002.
3. Favero MS. CDC guideline for handwashing and hospital environmental control, 1985. Infect Control. 1986;7:231-43.
4. Larson E. 1994 APIC Guidelines Committee. APIC guidelines for handwashing and hand antisepsis in health care settings. Am J Infect Control. 1995;23(4):251-69.
5. Samuel SO, Kayode OO, Musa OI, et al. Nosocomial infections and the challenges of control in developing countries. Afr J Clin Exp Microbiol. 2010;11(2):102-10.
6. Swaminathan S, Prasad J, Dhariwal AC, et al. Strengthening infection prevention and control and systematic surveillance of healthcare associated infections in India. BMJ. 2017;358:j3768.
7. Wenzel RP. The economics of nosocomial infections. J Hospit Infect. 1995;31(2):79-87.
8. WHO. Hand Hygiene: How, Why & When. 2009 Available on http://www.who.int/gpsc/5may/Hand_Hygiene_Why_How_and_When_ Brochure.pdf.
9. World Health Organization. (2011). Report on the burden of endemic health care-associated infection worldwide.

# D. BIOMEDICAL WASTE AND ITS MANAGEMENT

*Ashok Mishra, Manoj Bansal, Sasmita Mungi, Priyesh Marskole*

| CM14.1 | Define and classify hospital waste |
|---|---|
| CM14.2 | Describe various methods of treatment of hospital waste |
| CM14.3 | Describe laws related to hospital waste management |

## INTRODUCTION

Biomedical waste management is an important public health issue. After so many years of formulation of Biomedical Waste Management and Handling Rules (1998), indiscriminate disposal of hospital waste is still a major challenge. The common reasons behind are lack of awareness on recommended segregation methods, safe disposal methods and ignorant behavior of hospital authorities. In this chapter, we included Biomedical Waste Management and Handling Rules Amendment 2016, types of hospital waste, steps of safe biomedical waste management, hazards associated with biomedical waste and their prevention.

Hospital is an establishment which provides various preventive, diagnostic, curative, rehabilitative and research services. "Bio-medical waste" means any waste, that is generated during the diagnosis, treatment or immunization of human beings or animals, or research activities pertaining thereto, or in the production or testing of biological waste in health camps, including the categories mentioned in Schedule I of the Biomedical Waste Management and Handling Rules 1998.

Management of hospital waste needs special attention and any negligence can contaminate hospital environment and spread infections to the hospital staff, visitors, persons engaged in supportive services and most importantly to the patients. It is the responsibility of hospital authorities to maintain handling and disposal of generated waste in the safest and most effective way to minimize health risk and keep the hospital environment as clean and hygienic as possible.

## QUANTUM OF WASTE

Waste generation in any hospital depends on numerous factors, such as the type of hospital, the proportion of reusable items, the proportion of indoor and outdoor patients and existing waste management methods. In middle- and low-income countries, healthcare waste generation is usually lower than in high-income countries.

Waste generation varies in the developed and developing countries with sizeable intercountry and interspecialty variations. It varies from 1 to 5 kg/bed/day in developed countries to 1 to 2 kg/bed/day in developing countries.

World Health Organization reported that in high-income countries the waste generation is higher, i.e., 0.5 kg/bed/day as compared to low-income countries where average waste generation is 0.2 kg/bed/day. But in reality, the condition is grave in low-income countries due to lack of segregation between hazardous and nonhazardous wastes and also poor waste management and waste handling practices (WHO, 2018).

## TYPES OF HOSPITAL WASTE

- ***Infectious waste:*** This includes culture and microbial stocks from laboratory, surgical waste of patients with infectious disease, waste generated in infectious disease or isolation ward, instruments or materials that have been in contact with infected persons and animals, etc.
- ***Pathological waste:*** This includes body fluids, such as blood, urine, CSF, etc., and organ sample for histological examination.
- ***Sharps:*** These wastes are potentially much hazardous and can be a source for pricks or cuts. Needle, blade, broken glass ampoules and nails, etc., are some examples of sharp waste.
- ***Pharmaceutical waste:*** This includes expired, discarded or unused drugs and vaccines.
- ***Genotoxic or cytotoxic waste:*** This type of waste mainly comprises of cytotoxic or antineoplastic drugs.
- ***Chemical waste:*** This consists of useless or dumped chemicals generated due to diagnostic or experimental procedures, cleaning or disinfection.
- ***Radioactive waste:*** This can comprise any form of waste contaminated with radionuclide substances.
- ***Pressurized containers:*** Examples are pressurized cylinders, cartridges and aerosol cans. Pressurized gas containers need special care for handling and should never be incinerated as they may explode.

## AT RISK GROUPS

The main groups at risk are:
- Persons working in the hospital and hospital support services
- Patients attending hospital
- Attendants of the patients
- Staff engaged in waste handling and waste disposal process

## ADVERSE CONSEQUENCES OF POOR BIOMEDICAL WASTE MANAGEMENT

Improper management of biomedical waste can cause:
- Injuries from sharps to medical and paramedical personnel and waste handlers
- Increased risk of infections particularly HIV, hepatitis B and C
- Risks associated with hazardous chemicals or drugs
- Organic component ferments and attracts flea breeding
- Repacking and reuse of disposables.

## BENEFITS OF BIOMEDICAL WASTE MANAGEMENT

- Positive health and environment effects:
  - Reduces or eliminates the potential to transmit disease
  - Eliminates dispersal of infectious waste into the environment
- Enhanced community image:
  - Demonstrates environmental consciousness
  - Conveys a proactive process in meeting Biomedical Waste Laws and regulation

- Economic advantages:
  - Volume reduction
  - Savings in reduced cost and handling time
  - Less personnel resources and storage space required.

## BIOMEDICAL WASTE (MANAGEMENT AND HANDLING) RULES

The Ministry of Environment and Forests, Government of India issued notification on July 28, 1998. These rules impart guidelines and regulations for biomedical waste management in the country. These were further amended in 2000, 2003 and 2016 for wider and more effective implementation to improve the waste management system and to minimize its impact on environment.

These rules shall be applicable to all persons involved in any step of biomedical waste management and handling. BMW Rules 2016 has 4 Schedules.
- Schedule I: Biomedical wastes categories and their segregation, collection, treatment, processing and disposal options
- Schedule II: Standards for treatment and disposal of biomedical wastes
- Schedule III: List of prescribed authorities and the corresponding duties
- Schedule IV:
  - Part A: label for biomedical waste containers or bags
  - Part B: label for transporting biomedical waste bags or containers.

### Schedule I: Segregation of Biomedical Waste (Fig. 34D.1)

Segregation means "separation of different types of waste by sorting or the systematic separation of biomedical waste into designated categories".

It is the most important step as it helps to minimize the quantities of hazardous waste, thereby we can minimize the associated risk as well as cost of management.

The best method to classify different categories of biomedical waste is by putting the waste in the color coded bags or bins. Segregation of biomedical waste should ideally be as near to the site of waste generation as possible.

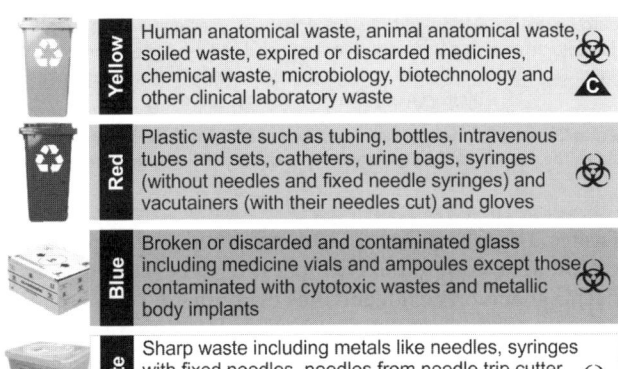

**Fig. 34D.1:** Segregation of biomedical waste as per BMW Rules 2016.
*(For color version, see Plate 1)*

*Part-1 of schedule I:* Biomedical wastes categories and their segregation, collection, treatment, processing and disposal options **(Table 34D.1)**.

*Part-2 of schedule I:*
- Nonchlorinated plastic bags shall be used for the storage and transportation of biomedical waste, as per Bureau of Indian Standards (BIS).
- For chemical treatment 10% sodium hypochlorite having 30% residual chlorine for 20 minutes or any other equivalent chemical reagent as given in Schedule III.
- Chemical treatment before incineration is required only for microbiological and potentially infectious waste.
- Dead fetus before the age of viability (as per MTP Act 1971) can be viewed as human anatomical waste and transported in yellow bag for disposal along with a copy of MTP certificate issued by competent authority.
- The hub of syringes should be cut, and needles should be either destroyed or placed in puncture proof containers.

### Collection, Storage and Transportation

It is the responsibility of hospital workers that bags should be filled only three-fourth with biomedical waste and then tied and removed. It should never be stapled, to avoid the risk of tear. The containers or bags shall be labeled as specified in Schedule IV.

Storage means "the holding of biomedical waste for such period of time, at the end of which waste is treated and disposed of". **Untreated biomedical waste should not be stored more than 48 hours**. If it becomes necessary to store beyond such a period, information to prescribed authority should be given and appropriate measures should be taken to avoid any ill effect associated with biomedical waste.

Transportation means "movement of biomedical waste from the point of generation or collection to the final disposal". The waste carrying vehicle should be in accordance with the guidelines given by Pollution Control Board and Motor Vehicle Act, 1988. The waste carrying vehicle should be adequately labeled and provide information as specified in Schedule IV.

### Schedule II: Standards for Treatment and Disposal of Biomedical Wastes

Biomedical waste should be treated and disposed of as per Schedule I and standards mentioned in Schedule II by all the health facilities and common biomedical waste treatment facility.

No occupier shall establish onsite treatment and disposal facility, if a service of common biomedical waste treatment facility is available within a distance of 75 km. Waste treatment equipment, such as incinerator, autoclave or microwave, shredder and effluent treatment plant (ETP) should be available at common biomedical waste treatment facility (described later).

### Incineration

Incineration comes from a Greek word meaning "burn to ashes". Incineration was first introduced in the mid-fifties. Incineration must be specifically selected, designed and built to meet the needs of each hospital or healthcare facility on an individual basis. It depends upon type of waste, calorific value, quantities and volume of waste.

**Table 34D.1:** BMW categories and their disposal options.

| Category | Type of waste | Type of bag or container to be used | Treatment and disposal options |
|---|---|---|---|
| Yellow | • *Human anatomical waste:* Human tissues, organs, body parts and fetus below the viability period (as per the MTP Act 1971 and its amendments)<br>• *Animal anatomical waste:* Experimental animal carcasses, body parts, organs, tissues, including the waste generated from animals used in experiments | Yellow colored non-chlorinated plastic bags | Incineration or plasma pyrolysis or deep burial* |
| | • *Soiled waste:* Items contaminated with blood, body fluids, such as dressings, plaster casts, cotton swabs and bags containing residual or discarded blood and blood components | | Incineration or plasma pyrolysis or deep burial.* In absence of above facilities, autoclaving or microwaving/hydroclaving followed by shredding or mutilation or combination of sterilization and shredding |
| | • *Expired or discarded medicines:* Pharmaceutical waste, such as antibiotics, cytotoxic drugs including all items contaminated with cytotoxic drugs along with glass or plastic ampoules, vials, etc. | Yellow colored nonchlorinated plastic bags or containers | Expired cytotoxic drugs and items contaminated with cytotoxic drugs to be returned back to the manufacturer or supplier or to common biomedical waste treatment facility for incineration at temperature >1,200°C. All other discarded medicines shall be either sent back to manufacturer or disposed by incineration |
| | • *Chemical waste:* Chemicals used in production of biological and used or discarded disinfectants | | Incineration or plasma pyrolysis or encapsulation in hazardous waste treatment, storage and disposal facility |
| | • *Chemical liquid waste:* Liquid waste generated due to use of chemicals in production of biological and used or discarded disinfectants, silver X-ray film developing liquid, infected secretions and body fluids, liquid from floor cleaning and house-keeping activities, etc. | Separate collection system leading to effluent treatment system | After resource recovery, the chemical liquid waste shall be pretreated before mixing with other wastewater. The combined discharge shall conform to the discharge norms given in Schedule III |
| | • *Discarded linen, mattresses, beddings contaminated with blood or body fluid* | Nonchlorinated yellow plastic bags or suitable packing material | • Nonchlorinated chemical disinfection followed by incineration or plasma pyrolysis<br>• In absence of above facilities, shredding or mutilation or combination of sterilization and shredding. Treated waste to be sent for energy recovery or incineration or plasma pyrolysis |
| | • *Microbiology, biotechnology and other clinical laboratory waste:* Blood bags, laboratory cultures, specimens of microorganisms, live or attenuated vaccines, residual toxins, dishes and devices used for cultures | Autoclave safe plastic bags or containers | Pretreat to sterilize with nonchlorinated chemicals on-site as per National AIDS Control Organization or World Health Organization guidelines thereafter for Incineration |
| Red | *Contaminated waste (recyclable):* Wastes generated from disposable items, such as tubing, bottles, intravenous tubes and sets, catheters, urine bags, syringes (without needles and fixed needle syringes) and vacutainers with their needles cut and gloves | Red colored nonchlorinated plastic bags or containers | • Autoclaving or microwaving/hydroclaving followed by shredding or mutilation or combination of sterilization and shredding. Treated waste to be sent to registered or authorized recyclers or for energy recovery<br>• Plastic waste should not be sent to landfill sites |
| White (translucent) | *Waste sharps including metals:* Needles, syringes with fixed needles, needles from needle tip cutter or burner, scalpels, blades, or any other contaminated sharp object that may cause puncture and cuts<br>This includes both used, discarded and contaminated metal sharps | Puncture proof, leak proof, tamper proof containers | Autoclaving or dry heat sterilization followed by shredding or mutilation or encapsulation; combination of shredding cum autoclaving; and sent for final disposal to iron foundries (having consent to operate from the State Pollution Control Boards or Pollution Control Committees) or sanitary landfill or designated concrete waste sharp pit |
| Blue | • *Glassware:* Broken or discarded and contaminated glass including medicine vials and ampoules except those contaminated with cytotoxic wastes<br>• *Metallic body implants* | Cardboard boxes with blue colored marking | Disinfection (by soaking the washed glass waste after cleaning with detergent and sodium hypochlorite treatment) or through autoclaving or microwaving or hydroclaving and then sent for recycling |

*Disposal by deep burial is permitted only in rural or remote areas where there is no access to Common Biomedical Waste Treatment Facility. This will be carried out with prior approval from the prescribed authority and as per the standards specified in Schedule-III. The deep burial facility shall be located as per the provisions and guidelines issued by Central Pollution Control Board from time to time.

## Principles of Incineration

Incineration is a process using very high temperature to reduce organic and flammable waste to inorganic and nonflammable matter resulting in great reduction in the total volume and weight of this waste. This is particularly useful for non recyclable, nonreusable waste items.

The combustion of organic compounds produces mainly gaseous emissions, toxic substances (e.g., metals, halogenic acids), and particulate matter, plus solid residues in the form of ashes. The ash and waste water produced by the process also contain toxic compounds, which have to be treated to avoid adverse effects on health and the environment.

## Types of Incinerator

Three basic kinds of incineration technology are of interest for treating healthcare waste:

1. Double-chamber pyrolytic incinerators, which may be especially designed to burn infectious healthcare waste **(Fig. 34D.2)**

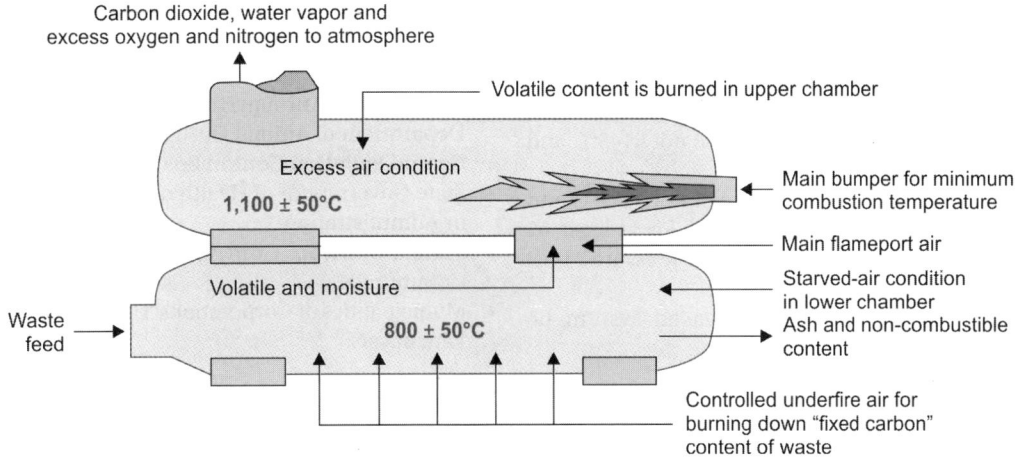

Fig. 34D.2: Double chamber incinerator.

2. Single chamber furnaces with static grate, which should be used only if pyrolytic incinerators are not affordable
3. Rotary kilns operating at high temperature, capable of causing decomposition of genotoxic substances and heat resistance chemicals.

***Standards for Incineration***

- The temperature for the primary chamber shall be a minimum of 800°C and for the secondary chamber a minimum of 1050°C +/- 50°C.
- Combustion efficiency (CE) shall be at least 99.00%.
- Particulate matter shall be below 50 mg/Nm³.
- Nitrogen oxides (NO) and $NO_2$ shall be below 400 mg/Nm³.
- HCl shall be limited to 50 mg/Nm³.
- Total Dioxins and Furans shall be limited to 0.1ng TEQ/Nm³ (At 11%$O_2$).
  - All upcoming and existing incinerators shall comply with the above stated standards. Operator of common biomedical waste treatment facility shall monitor gaseous emission once in three months through an approved laboratory.
  - Ash from the incineration of biomedical waste shall be disposed of at common hazardous waste treatment and disposal facility. However, it may be disposed of in municipal landfill, if toxic metals are within limit defined under hazardous waste (Management and Handling and Transboundary Movement) Rules, 2008.

***Waste Types not to be Incinerated***

- Pressurized gas containers
- Large amount of reactive chemical wastes
- Silver salts and photographic or radiographic wastes
- Halogenated plastics, such as PVC
- Waste with high mercury or cadmium content, such as broken thermometers, and used batteries
- Sealed ampoules or ampoules containing heavy metals.

***Advantages and Disadvantages of Incineration***
***Advantages:***

- It reduces waste volume and weight
- It renders the waste unrecognizable
- Suitable for all types of waste
- Energy recovery potential
- Can treat chemotherapeutic waste

***Disadvantages:***

- High capital costs
- High maintenance and repair costs
- High energy input and low efficiency
- Sitting difficulties
- Permission difficulties
- Public opposition

### Plasma Pyrolysis

Plasma pyrolysis is an alternate method to incinerator. Plasma pyrolysis treatment technology can be installed for disposal of biomedical waste categories as per BMWM Rules wherein destruction of biomedical waste similar to incineration can be achieved.

### Autoclave (Fig. 34D.3)

The autoclave is a process of steam sterilization under pressure and used for the purpose of disinfecting and treating biomedical waste.

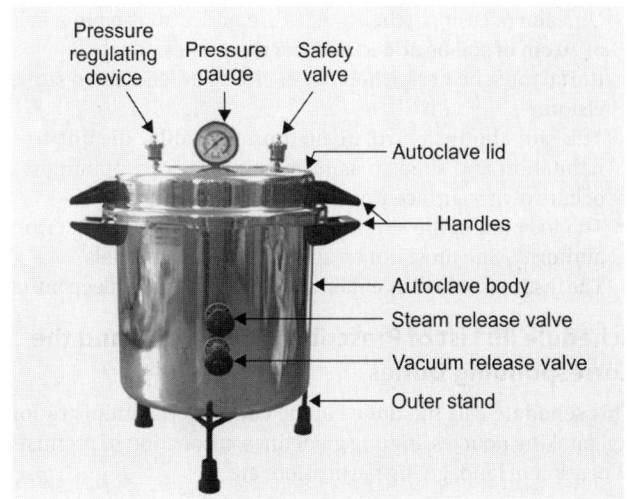

Fig. 34D.3: Autoclave.

### Standards for Autoclaving

- For *gravity flow autoclave*, a temperature of not <121°C and pressure 15 pounds per square inch (psi) for at least 60 minutes; *or* a temperature of not <135°C and pressure 31 psi for at least 45 minutes; *or* a temperature of not <149°C and pressure 52 psi for at least 30 minutes.
- For *prevacuum autoclave*, a temperature of not <121°C and pressure 15 pounds per square inch (psi) for at least 45 minutes; *or* a temperature of not <135°C and pressure 31 psi for at least 30 minutes.
  - For optimum results, prevacuum-based system be preferred against the gravity type system.

### Microwave

Most microorganisms are destroyed by the thermal effect of electromagnetic radiation spectrum lying between 300–300,000 MHz. The water contained within the wastes is rapidly heated by the microwaves and the infectious components are destroyed by heat conduction.

Microwave treatment shall not be used for cytotoxic, hazardous or radioactive wastes, contaminated animal carcasses, body parts and large metal items.

The microwave should completely and consistently kill the bacteria and other pathogenic organisms that are ensured by approved biological indicator, i.e., *Bacillus atrophaeus spores* using vials or spore strips with at least $1 \times 10^4$ spores per detachable strip.

### Shredder

Shredding is a process by which waste (such as syringes, blades, catheters, intravenous sets/bottles, and blood bags) is deshaped or cut into smaller pieces to make the waste unrecognizable. This helps prevent the reuse of biomedical waste and also serves as an identifier that the waste has been disinfected and is safe to dispose of.

### Standards for Deep Burial

- A pit or trench which is about 2 meters deep. It should be half filled with waste and then covered with lime within 50 cm of the surface, before filling the rest of the pit with soil.
- On each occasion, when wastes are added to the pit, a layer of 10 cm of soil be added to cover the wastes.
- Burial must be performed under close and dedicated supervision.
- The site should be relatively impermeable, distant from habitation and sited so as to ensure that no contamination occurs of any surface water or ground water.
- The location of the site will be authorized by the prescribed authority. Site must not be accessible to the animals.
- The institution shall maintain a record of all pits for deep burial.

### Schedule III: List of Prescribed Authorities and the Corresponding Duties

This schedule lists the duties of the concerned administration, e.g., making policies, issuing guidelines, inspection of premises, allocation of land, giving permission, etc.

- Ministry of Environment, Forest and Climate Change, Government of India
- Central or State Ministry of Health and Family Welfare, Central Ministry for Animal Husbandry and Veterinary or State Department of Animal Husbandry and Veterinary
- Central Pollution Control Board
- State Government of Health or Union Territory Government or Administration
- State Pollution Control Boards or Pollution Control Committees
- Municipalities or Corporations, Urban Local Bodies and Gram Panchayats.

### Schedule IV

*Part A:* Label for biomedical waste containers or bag

 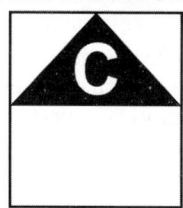

*Part B:* Label for transporting biomedical waste bags or containers

These are forms in which information is entered regarding (a) category, (b) sender's name and (c) contact person.

## COMMON BIOMEDICAL WASTE TREATMENT FACILITY

It is a place where waste generated from various health facilities is imparted necessary treatment. It means any facility wherein treatment, disposal of biomedical waste or processes incidental to such treatment and disposal is carried out, and "operator of a common biomedical waste treatment (CBWTF) facility" means a person who owns or controls a facility for the collection, reception, storage, transport, treatment, disposal or any other form of handling of biomedical waste. Operator must establish bar coding and global positioning system (GPS) for handling of biomedical waste.

The CBWTF shall be located:
- As near as possible to its area of operation in order to minimize the transportation distance in waste collection, thus enhancing its operational flexibility.
- Far away from residential and sensitive area and should have a buffer zone of at least 500 meters.
- At least 1 kilometer away from the surface water body.

A CBWTDF shall be allowed to cater healthcare units with 10,000 beds situated at a radial distance of 75 km. However, in an area where 10,000 beds are not available within a radial distance of 75 km, existing CBWTF in the locality may be allowed to cater the healthcare units situated outside the said 75 km radius, provided there is no other facility in the next 75 km radial distance.

## OCCUPATIONAL SAFETY MEASURES

- All the healthcare workers and other staff involved in handling of biomedical waste shall be provided appropriate and adequate personal protective equipments, such as head gear, apron, hand gloves, etc.
- Conduct health check-up at least once a year and maintain the records for the same.
- Provide training to all the workers involved in handling of biomedical waste at the time of induction and at least once a year thereafter.
- Immunization of all the workers involved in handling of biomedical waste for protection against the diseases, including hepatitis B and tetanus and maintain the records for the same.
- Report major accidents caused during handling of biomedical waste and the remedial action taken and the records relevant thereto, (including nil reporting) in Form I to prescribed authority.

## SUMMARY

"Biomedical waste" means any waste, which is generated during the diagnosis, treatment or immunization of human beings or animals or research activities.

It is estimated that 80–85% waste is general or domestic or non-infectious waste, 10% is infectious and 5% is other hazardous waste. According to WHO high-income countries generate on an average up to 0.5 kg of hazardous waste per bed per day; while low-income countries generate on an average 0.2 kg.

Hospital waste can be classified as infectious waste, pathological waste, sharps, pharmaceutical waste, genotoxic or cytotoxic waste, chemical waste, r**adioactive waste and pressurized containers.**

The Ministry of Environment and Forests, Government of India notified Biomedical Waste Management and Handling Rules on 28th July 1998, under the provision of Sections 6, 8 and 25 of the Environment (Protection) Act, 1986. Rules provided a regulatory framework for management of biomedical waste generated in the country. These rules were subsequently amended. Latest amendment was made in 2016. These rules shall apply to all persons who generate, collect, receive, store, transport, treat, dispose or handle biomedical waste in any form.

Various steps involved in the management of biomedical waste are segregation, collection, storage, offsite and onsite transportation and final disposal as per the Biomedical Waste Management and Handling Rules, 2016.

Common Biomedical Waste Treatment Facility is a place where waste generated from various health facilities is imparted necessary treatment.

For occupational safety all the workers involved in the handling of hospital waste must be provided appropriate PPEs, conduct health check-up at least once a year, provide training, immunization for protection against the diseases, such as hepatitis B and tetanus, report major accidents caused during handling of biomedical waste and the remedial action taken and the records relevant thereto, (including nil reporting) in Form I to prescribed authority.

## SUGGESTED READING

1. Acharya DB, Singh M. The Book of Hospital Waste Management. Minerva Press, New Delhi; 2000: pp. 5-98.
2. Bio-medical Waste Management Rules, 2016 (Amended), Central Pollution Control Board, Ministry of Environment, Forest and Climate Change, Government of India.
3. Health-care Waste. World Health Organization. 2018. [online] Available from https://www.who.int/en/news-room/fact-sheets/detail/health-care-waste.
4. Manual on Hospital Waste Management. Central Pollution Control Board, Delhi; 2000.
5. Pruss A, Giroult E, Rushbrook P. Safe management of waste from health-care activities. WHO; Geneva.1999:20-74.
6. Standard operative procedure, Manual for Control of Hospital Associated Infections, NACO New Delhi; 50-66.

# E. BIOTERRORISM

*Ashok Mishra, Priyesh Marskole, Manoj Bansal, Sasmita Mungi*

*"Bioterrorism is a threat to every nation that loves freedom"*
—**George W Bush**

## INTRODUCTION

Bioterrorism or biological warfare can be defined as "intentional use of living organisms or their toxic products to cause death, disability or disease in man, animals or plants or to poison food and water supplies".

The term bioterrorism and biological warfare are generally used synonymously but bioterrorism is an action of a sub-national entity rather than a state as a whole. With the passage of time biological warfare has come up as an attractive way in military tactics as compared to conventional warfare because it can kill more massively and effectively with relatively lesser cost and efforts. Biological weapons (BWs) can be defined as "any microorganism, virus, infection, substance or biological product having the capability to cause death, disease or other biological dysfunction in man, animals or plants to cause large scale casualty and suffering". Such microbes can be natural, wild type strains or genetically engineered organisms.

To enumerate a few factors that keep BWs at par with other modern weapons:
- It is cheaper (sometimes called *poor man's atomic bomb*) and easier to prepare.
- It can be produced and stored in ample amount for a long time.
- It can be produced in simple laboratory setup.
- Biological toxins are one of the most toxic substances known.
- It can cause large scale casualty with minimum input especially in crowded areas.
- It remains undetected by routine security (biosensor), agent dispersal can be done silently without being noticed.
- The culprits can save themselves easily as it takes time for the disease to arise in the target population from the time of attack (owing to latent and incubation period).
- It destroys the enemy leaving his infrastructure intact as booty for the attackers.

*Biological weapons have limitations too:*
- There is difficulty in protecting workers during production, transportation and delivery of biological agents.
- It is difficult to maintain quality control and prevent contamination during growth and harvesting.
- It needs a very efficient delivery system.
- It may be dispersed in unexpected and self-harming ways, if not controlled properly.
- It needs specific conditions of temperature, humidity and other climatic conditions for production and storage.
- Very difficult to control and regulate its impact once released on enemies.

*Broadly, different varieties of biological weapons are:*
- *Microorganisms:* These are ones which infect and spread in the target population. These can be natural strains or may be genetically formed. Agents in this group are of diseases like anthrax and plague.
- *Biologically derived bioactive substances (BDBS):* These are mostly products of metabolism like biological toxins, hormones, neuropeptides, cytokines, etc.
- *Manually designed biological toxin like substances:* It includes nerve gases (tabun—a cholinesterase inhibitor) and pesticides.

*An ideal biological weapon:*
A biological agent to be called ideal should have following characteristics:
- It should be highly infectious and fatal.
- It should be produced readily in huge quantities.
- It should be dispersed in air or water easily.
- It should withstand the change in atmospheric conditions.
- It should remain stable for long duration for storage.
- Its effect should not be easily treatable by antibiotics and other regular therapy.

## MODES OF APPLICATION

The different modes of application of BWs are:
- Catapulting **(Fig. 34E.1)** the dead bodies of human or animals, infected with specific disease to turn rival forces or population infected with that disease.
- Artificial cloud or as aerosol spray: It is the most common route of disseminating the agents and aerosols can be dissipated in two ways:
  1. *Point source munitions:* Aerosol is dispersed through stationary aerosol generator, bomblets, etc.
  2. *Line source munitions:* The aerosols are dispersed through the low lying aircraft or speed boats along with coastlines.

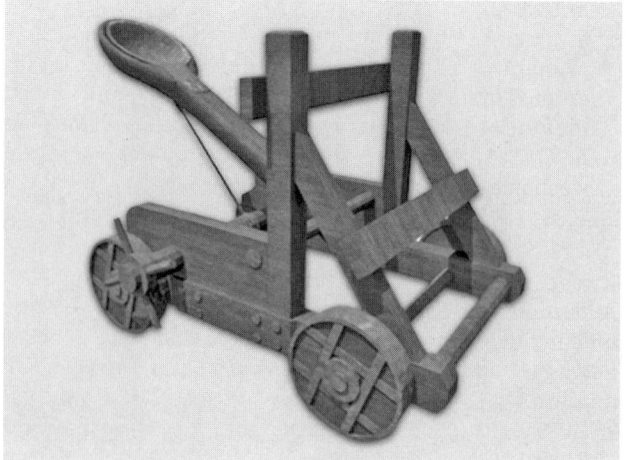

**Fig. 34E.1:** A catapult.

- Contaminating drinking water or food products
- Distributing clothes with infectious agent to the target population
- Through postal system or book

- Using bomb clusters, guided missiles, spray tanks or guns
- Remote control devices, motor vehicles or robots
- Using scorpions or poisonous snakes
- Deliberate infiltration of infected animals, pests or vectors.

***Different phases of evolution of chemical and biological weapons:***
- *Phase I:* World War I witnessed the use of gaseous chemicals, such as chlorine and phosgene.
- *Phase II:* Anthrax and plague bombs used in World War II. Use of nerve agents, e.g., tabun—a cholinesterase inhibitor.
- *Phase III:* Vietnam War in 1970 constituted this phase. Use of lethal chemical agent "agent orange" a mix of herbicides causing defoliation and crop destruction.
- *Phase IV:* Era of biotechnological revolution and the use of genetic engineering.

## HISTORICAL BACKGROUND

Humans have used BWs in disputes for hundreds of years. A few instances are given here.

### Ancient Times

- In 6th century BC Assyrian poisoned the wells of their enemies using rye ergot, a poisonous fungus.
- Solon, an Athenian law giver repeated the same act by poisoning the water supply with hellebore, a herb purgative during the siege of Krissa.
- In 184 BC, Hannibal's force hurled earthen pots filled with poisonous snakes at the ships of King Eumenes II of Pergamon to win a naval battle.

### Medieval Times

- In 1340 AD, the castle of Thun-lÉvêque in Hainault (presently in North France) was hurled upon with dead horses and other animals by catapult.
- In 1346 AD during the historic siege of Kaffa (now Feodosiya in Ukraine), a Seaport City, the Tatar forces catapulted the plaque infected cadavers into the sieged city. Plague epidemic erupted in the city, which also affected the entire Europe in the form of dreadful plague epidemic killing 25 million people.
- In 1785 Tunisian forces used plague tainted clothing as a weapon in the siege of La Calle.

### Modern Times

It was Germany which weaponized the infectious agents, such as *Anthrax bacillus* and *Pseudomonas mallei* (Glanders) for the first time in modern era. Germans also developed new generation nerve gas (tabun, sarin and suman), 200 times more lethal than mustard gas.
- In 1930s Japan came out as the leader in acts of bioterrorism. They used the Chinese prisoners of war (POW) as guinea pigs to test the lethality of agents, such as anthrax, cholera, typhoid and plague. Japanese dropped 'paper bags' field with plague-infested fleas over several Chinese cities, such as Chuhsien, Ninpo, Chhinhua, Quzhou, etc., resulting in mass casualty. It is worth notice that bioterrorist attack backfired and killed 1,700 persons in Japanese troops itself.
- In 1984, in Dalas, Oregon members of a religious cult contaminated salads in restaurants with *Salmonella typhimurium* in an attempt to influence the results of elections.
- In 1995, the Japanese cult Ann Shimriky released nerve gas in a Tokyo subway.
- In the recent past anthrax bacillus contaminated letters were posted to politicians causing massive panic. Overall, 18 people got infected and 5 people died.

## CATEGORIES OF BIOLOGICAL DISEASE OR AGENTS

According to Centers for Disease Control and Prevention (CDC), BWs have been categorized in following groups:

| | |
|---|---|
| *Category A:* These are high-priority agents posing a risk to national security, can be easily transmitted and disseminated, result in high mortality, have major public health impact, cause panic in public and require special action for public health preparedness. | *Agents/Diseases include:* Anthrax (*Bacillus anthracis*), botulism (*Clostridium botulinum* toxin), plague (*Yersinia pestis*), smallpox (*Variola major*), tularemia (*Francisella tularensis*), viral hemorrhagic fevers (Filoviruses, e.g., Ebola, Marburg) |
| *Category B:* These are second highest priority agents and include those agents which are moderately easy to disseminate, cause moderate and low mortality rates and require specific diagnostic capacity and upgraded disease surveillance. | *Agents include:* Brucellosis (*Brucella* species), Epsilon toxin of *Clostridium perfringens*, food safety threats (e.g., *Salmonella* species, *E. coli* O157:H7, shigella, *Staphylococcus aureus*), glanders (*Burkholderia mallei*), melioidosis (*Burkholderia pseudomallei*), psittacosis (*Chlamydia psittaci*), Q fever (*Coxiella burnetii*), ricin toxin from *Ricinus communis* (castor beans), abrin toxin from *Abrus precatorius* (rosary peas), Staphylococcal enterotoxin B, Typhus (*Rickettsia prowazekii*), Viral encephalitis (alphaviruses, for example, *Venezuelan equine* encephalitis, eastern equine encephalitis, western equine encephalitis), water supply threats (*Vibrio cholerae*, *Cryptosporidium parvum*) |
| *Category C:* The third priority agents comprise of emerging pathogens that could be engineered for massive destruction in the future. These are easily available, easier to be produced and disseminated but also have capacity to cause huge public health impact. | *Examples include:*<br>• Nipah virus<br>• Hanta virus<br>• Severe acute respiratory syndrome (SARS) virus<br>• $H_1N_1$ (a strain of influenza)<br>• *Mycobacterium tuberculosis* (Multidrug resistant strains) |

## MAGNITUDE OF THREAT WITH BIOLOGICAL WEAPONS

Though the exact quantity and whereabouts of stockpiled BWs by nations or other entities are not precisely known but their production has been in reports time and again.

US began its research of BW in 1942. In 20th century between 1949 and 1969 it is said that the US Military developed BW and investigated their effects at its army's laboratories in Camp Detrick, Maryland. In 1970s the former Soviet Union stockpiled tons of smallpox virus and maintained production capabilities at least until 1990. It also sponsored an anthrax weapon program despite being a signatory to biological and toxin weapons convention (BTWC) [An agreement to end the development and production of BWs ratified by more than 100 nations including USA in 1975].

Though USSR claimed that it dismantled the BW program and destroyed its stock in late 1980s, but experts are doubtful if all stocks, equipment and records are really destroyed.

On a similar note, in the 1990s Iraq accepted before UN inspectors that it had produced concentrated botulinum toxin and had developed bombs to deploy large quantities of botulinum toxin and anthrax. Though the Iraqi government dismantled its bioweapon program after the first Iraq war, the details and whereabouts of the material they developed is still unknown.

An unclassified US department of state report in 2005 states that many nations still are suspected of continuous biological warfare programs in violation of the biological and toxin weapons convention like China, Iran, North Korea, Russia, Syria and possibly Cuba.

# MAJOR BIOLOGICAL WEAPONS

## Common Features of Selected Potential Bioterrorism Agents

| Incubation period | Mode of transmission | Mortality rate | Diagnosis | Signs and symptoms | Treatment |
|---|---|---|---|---|---|
| **Anthrax** | | | | | |
| 4–6 days. Spores can remain dormant for up to 60 days | Cutaneous, inhalation, gastrointestinal (rare) | Cutaneous: 20% if untreated. Inhaled: 45% | Gram stain, blood or wound culture rapid ELISA test | Flu-like symptoms, abrupt onset of respiratory distress, cyanosis, shock, septicemia | Ciprofloxacin or doxycycline |
| **Smallpox** | | | | | |
| 12–14 days | Aerosolization, direct contact, fomite exposure | 30% | Clinical presentation of lesions, electron microscopy of vesicular fluid, virus cell culture | High fever, cutaneous eruptions in the stages of macules, papules, vesicles and pustules, which on drying leave behind permanent pockmarks | • No antiviral treatment<br>• Vaccination immediately or up to 4 days reduce mortality |
| **Plague** | | | | | |
| 2–8 days | Aerosolization, flea vector | Pneumonic: almost 100% if untreated | Clinical gram stain of sputum, blood or CSF. Wright's stain for bipolar (safety pin) staining | There are three forms of plague—bubonic, pneumonic and septicemic | Streptomycin or gentamicin with ciprofloxacin or doxycycline |
| **Tularemia** | | | | | |
| 1–14 days | Aerosolization, rodent vector | < 2% | Sputum or blood culture, sputum and blood for direct fluorescent antibody or immunohistochemical stain | Fever, dry cough, pneumonia, pulse-temperature dissociation | Streptomycin or gentamicin |
| **Botulism** | | | | | |
| 2 hours to 8 days | Aerosolization, food contamination | Treated: < 5% untreated: up to 60% | Clinical serum bioassays | Paralysis of parasympathetic system (ptosis, dysphagia, dysarthria, diplopia and constipation) | Supportive treatment and antitoxin |
| **Viral hemorrhagic fever (VHF) (i.e., Lassa, Ebola, Marburg, Crimean-Congo)** | | | | | |
| 2–21 days | Aerosolization, rodent, mosquito, and tick vectors | 10–90% | ELISA or IgM antibody detection RT-PCR, viral isolation | Conjunctival hemorrhage and multiorgan failure (Ebola) | Consider ribavirin |

(ELISA: enzyme-linked immunosorbent assay; CSF: cerebrospinal fluid; IGM: immunoglobulin M; RT-PCR: reverse transcription polymerase chain reaction)

# PREVENTION AND CONTROL

Bioterrorism is an outcome of various associated factors. Therefore, it needs a multifaceted approach involving various sectors in the community.

The prominent ones being:
1. The community
2. Health system
3. Communication and transportation
4. Administration and legal provisions

## The Community

In any disaster, early detection is the key to prevent mass casualties therefore the general public needs to remain vigilant and should know when to suspect a bioterrorist attack. Some epidemiological clues which can assist in early detection of a possible bioterrorist attack are listed below:
- Manifestation of a disease in more severe than its usual form or failure of disease to respond to its regular therapy.
- Too many cases of unexplained diseases or deaths in a particular region.
- Differentiation between natural and bioterrorist infections:
  – *Natural*: There is gradual rise in cases.
  – *Terrorist*: There is sudden rise in cases, in hours or days.
- Unusual route of exposure for a particular pathogen than its usual route, e.g., reporting of inhalational route for diseases that usually occur through other exposure route.

- Occurrence of a disease, which is unusual for the given geographic area or transmission season.
- Disease transmitted by a vector that is usually not present in the given area.
- Unusual strains or variants of organisms or antimicrobial resistance patterns different from those already known.
- Disease outbreaks of the same illness occurring in non-contiguous areas.
- Multiple disease entities in one patient, indicating that mixed agents have been used in the event.
- Claim of attack made by a terrorist group.
- Any discovery of munitions or bioterrorist agents.

All of the above mentioned clues, if encountered, should be minutely examined by authorized agencies. After verification of a bioterrorist attack and confirmation of diagnosis initiation should be made for appropriate prevention and control measures and management of specific infection as per the standard protocol of its treatment.

### Health System

Regular and proper training of medical personnel, laboratory technicians, public health officials, epidemiologists and veterinary personnel should be conducted in advance with a special focus on individual care management, essential provisions to be maintained in an emergency room, how to arrive quickly at a presumptive diagnosis of agents involved and also to manage large and suspected exposures.

Various departments in health facility, such as medicines, surgery, neurology, anesthesia, ICU, radiology, nursing, pharmacy, store, transport and referral services and supportive staff need to work in close coordination for efficient management. A permanent team of experts for bioterrorist hazard can also be formed beforehand.

Desirable precautions to be taken by health personnel while dealing with a victim of a bioterrorism attack are as follows:
- Should wear gloves before touching blood secretions, excreta or any other body fluid.
- Should wear mask, glass and face shield during sample collection or other procedure particularly while working within 3 feet of patient's vicinity following standard precautions.
- All the materials used by the victim should be disposed off properly and safely.
- Injuries to self and patient should be avoided from sharps.
- Mouth to mouth resuscitation should be avoided, rather ventilation devices should be used.
- Patient can be placed in a private room or in ward with patients affected by same infections.
- Movement and transportation of the patient should be restricted. Mask to be placed on the patient, if transported.

### *Role of Clinical Laboratories in Bioterrorism*

The clinical microbiologists and laboratories hold a crucial significance in episodes of Bioterrorist attacks. These are the first line of defense who can timely detect the occurrence of biological attack, water-borne or food-borne infection outbreak, and can notice resistance to antibiotics.

As per the Centres for Disease Control (CDC) laboratories are classified into four levels for the purpose of detecting biological agents.
1. **Level A laboratories:** Routine pathogens are cultured and identified here. The organisms are then referred to higher level laboratories for confirmation.
2. **Level B laboratories:** Tests done here are confirmatory tests, antibiotic susceptibility tests and rapid presumptive identification (with the help of fluorescent antibody reagents).
3. **Level C laboratories:** Provision of molecular level testing is present in these more sophisticated laboratories.
4. **Level D laboratories:** Also named "hot lab" is highest in expertise and conduct very highly specialized tests, such as culture or molecular identification of highly infectious viral agents.

To further save the invaluable time consumed by laboratory tests, a uniform diagnostic protocol can be formulated following a syndrome based diagnostic criteria for the suspected infections.

### Communication and Transport

An efficient, clear and fact based communication is a key element for strengthening a prompt response capability and preparedness against a bioterrorist attack. It can also help in alienating fear, panic and unfounded rumors.

The safety and law enforcement agencies, public health sectors, private and public organizations and all forms of media should join hands to actively disseminate relevant information to the public regarding how to avoid exposure along with medical advice relevant to the nature of the incident.

The key points which communication should focus on:
- The details of probable source, time, place and nature of exposure
- The determinants and potential risks of acquiring the infection
- Self-precaution and safety measures
- The available treatment and control facilities in nearby health units
- Reduction of anxiety and panic in unexposed persons
- Avoidance of unnecessary isolation or quarantine of people
- Reduction in apprehension of health staff by providing bioterrorism readiness education with self-protection skills

### *Surveillance*

An early detection mechanism should be in place to recognize patterns of syndromes or other clues that can indicate the early manifestations of a bioterrorist attack with due promptness.

Some early detection systems are:
- *Biological integrated detection system (BIDS):* It conducts both genetic and antibody based detection on the suspected aerosol particles dispersed in the environment.
- *Long range biological stand-off detection system (LRBSDS):* It can detect aerosol clouds from a distance up to 30 km and can thereby provide "early warning".
- *The short range biological standoff detection system (SRBSDS):* Still in experimental stage in a newer generation detection system. It uses ultraviolet and laser induced fluorescence to detect biological aerosol clouds.

Along with the communication sector, a well organized transport system also has a pivotal role in smoother movement of victims, affected community towards appropriate health facilities and also the movement of relief providers towards the affected sites.

Police and fire control teams are also ones which are mostly first to be called at affected site, therefore they all need to be well informed and equipped to provide best possible assistance.

## Administration, Government Policies and Legal Provisions

The National Disaster Management Authority (NDMA) of our nation works for the prevention and control of bioterrorism attacks. To the existing eight battalions of the National Disaster Response Force, each consisting of 1,000, two more battalions have been sanctioned. Half of the present force is specifically trained to deal with chemical, biological, radiological and nuclear (CBRN) threats. To work with NDMA a more cooperative and collaborative approach is needed from all sectors and sections of the society to eliminate bioterrorism and its lethal impacts.

### Legal Provisions

The two principal international treaties in this field are:
1. The 1925 Geneva Protocol
2. The 1972 Biological Weapons Conventions

1. **Geneva Protocol:** After the extensive use of chemical weapons, such as chlorine and mustard gas, during the First World War, the international community came together to formulate legislation on these kinds of weapons and to prohibit their further use. The member states of the League of Nations came up with a protocol for the prohibition of the use in war of asphyxiating poisonous gases and of bacteriological methods of warfare on 17 June 1925.

   This treaty, referred to as the Geneva Protocol of 1925, came into force on 8 February 1928. At the time of its inception, it had 130 states parties, including the five permanent members of the present United Nations Security Council but did not include 64 WHO member states.

   The Geneva protocol prohibits "the use in war of asphyxiating poisons or other gases and of all analogous liquids, materials or devices" and also "extends this prohibition to the use of bacteriological methods of warfare".

   The limitations of Geneva protocol included:
   1. It only prohibited the use of such weapons, but not their possession.
   2. Not all nations were its signatory.
   3. Many states reserved the right to use the weapons in retaliation if they are attacked by such weapons.

   Some state parties also reserved the right to use these weapons against states not party to this protocol.

2. **Biological weapons convention:** Biological weapons convention (BWC) is a convention on the prohibition of the development, production and stockpiling of bacteriological (biological) and toxin weapons and on their destruction. It was signed on 10 April 1972 and came into force on 26 March 1975. Presently BWC has 151 states parties, including the five permanent members of UNSC but it does not include 42 WHO member states.

Article I of the convention identifies items that each state party "undertakes never in any circumstances to develop, produce, stockpile or otherwise acquire or retain". These items have been defined as:
- *Microbial or other biological agents, or toxins*: Whatever their origin or method of production, of types and in quantities that have no justification for prophylactic, protective or other peaceful purposes.
- Weapons, equipment or means of delivery designed to use such agents or toxins for hostile purposes or in armed conflict. Article II mandates states parties to destroy or divert to peaceful purposes all agents, toxins, weapons, equipment and all means of delivery within nine months of entry into the convention.

## UPCOMING TRENDS

Emergence of relatively new and unknown pathogens, such as Middle-East respiratory syndrome coronavirus and Zaire ebola virus is a concern. Manipulation of pathogens by biotechnological advancement is a constant threat, e.g., "designer substances" which affect particular organ or specific group of enemies and "ethnic bombs" are believed to be under development.

"*Terrorism and deception are weapons not of the strong, but of the weak.*"

—Mahatma Gandhi

## SUMMARY

Bioterrorism, i.e., the deliberate use of biological product or pathogen to harm human, animal or other living creature to destabilize a government or to intimidate a civilian population has been reported historically and still pose a serious threat to human civilization. Biological weapons are easier to develop and cheaper and have lethal consequences. It is not only a public health menace but also a concern of international security.

## SUGGESTED READING

1. Arizona Department of Health Services. History of Biowarfare and Bioterrorism. Available from https://www.azdhs.gov/preparedness/emergency-preparedness/bioterrorism/.
2. Biological warfare and Terrorism, Medical issues and response, satellite Broadcast, September 26-28, 2000.
3. CDC (2000). Biological and Chemical terrorism: Strategic Plan for Preparedness and response. Available from https://www.cdc.gov/mmwr/preview/mmwrhtml/rr4904a1.htm
4. Centers for disease control and prevention (CDC). (1999). Bioterrorism Readiness Plan.
5. Centers for disease control and prevention (CDC). Emergency preparedness and response.
6. Christopher GW, Cieslak TJ, Pavlin JA, et al. Biological warfare, a historical perspective. JAMA. 1997;278:412-7.
7. Darling RG, Catlett CL, Huebner KD, et al. Threats in Bioterrorism. I: CDC Category A agents. Emerg Med Clin North Am. 2002;20(2):273-309.
8. Etzel RA. Mycotoxins. JAMA. 2002;287(4):425-7.
9. Franz DR, Jahrling PB, Friedlander AM, et al. Clinical recognition and management of patients exposed to biological warfare agents. J Am Med Assoc. 1997;278:399-411.
10. Galwankar S. Bioterrorism: A war with Infectious weapons. Indian Pract. 2001;54(12):851-6.
11. Glass TA, Schoch-Spana M. Bioterrorism and the people: How to vaccinate a city against panic. Clin Infect Dis. 2002;34:217-23.

12. Hamilton JD, Baron EJ, et. al. Role of clinical microbiology Laboratories in the management and control of Infectious disease and the delivery of health. Clin Infect Dis. 2001;32:605-11.
13. Hari Prasad K. The medical Implication of Biological and Chemical Terrorism. Indian Pract. 2001;54(12):916-33.
14. International Committee of the Red Cross. Meeting of the states parties to the convention on the prohibition of the development, production and stockpiling of bacteriological (Biological) and Toxin.
15. Jermigan DB, Raghunathan PL, Bell BP, et al. Investigation of bioterrorism related anthrax, United states, 2001: Epidemiologic findings. Emerg Infect Dis. 2002;8(10):101-28.
16. Johnson TJ. A History of Biological warfare from 300 B.C. to the present. Available from http://www.haadi.ir/Upload/Image/2016/10/Orginal/f8c8c444_e249_404f_ abc0_16da4f33acb5.pdf
17. Jortani SA, Snyder JW, Valdes R Jr. The Role of the Clinical Laboratory in Managing Chemical or Biological Terrorism. Clin Chem. 2000;46:1883-93.
18. Mayor A. Dirty Tricks in Ancient warfare. Mil Hist Quart. 1997:10(1):37.
19. Richmond JY, McKinney RW. Biosafety in Microbiological and Biomedical Laboratories' 3rd edition. Washington, DC: US Department of health and human services; 1993.
20. Roberts A, Guelff R. Documents on the laws of war, 3rd edition. Oxford, Oxford University Press; 2000.
21. The Biological bomb. The Lancet. 1968;291(7540):465.
22. The text of the Biological weapons convention. Available at http://www.opbw.org/convention/conv.html.
23. Torok TJ, Birkness KA, Foster LR, et al. A large community outbreak of salmonellosis caused by intentional contamination of restaurant salad Bars. JAMA. 1997;278:389-95.
24. United Nations Office For Disarmament Affairs. Available from https://www.un.org/disarmament/wmd/bio/1925-geneva- protocol/.
25. US Department of health and human services (2002). Hospital preparedness for mass casualties. Available from https://www.phe.gov/preparedness/planning/hpp/Pages/default.aspx.
26. US Department of State. Text of the Biological Weapons Convention. Available from https://www.state.gov/t/isn/bw/c48738. htm.

# SECTION 4

# Community Health Management

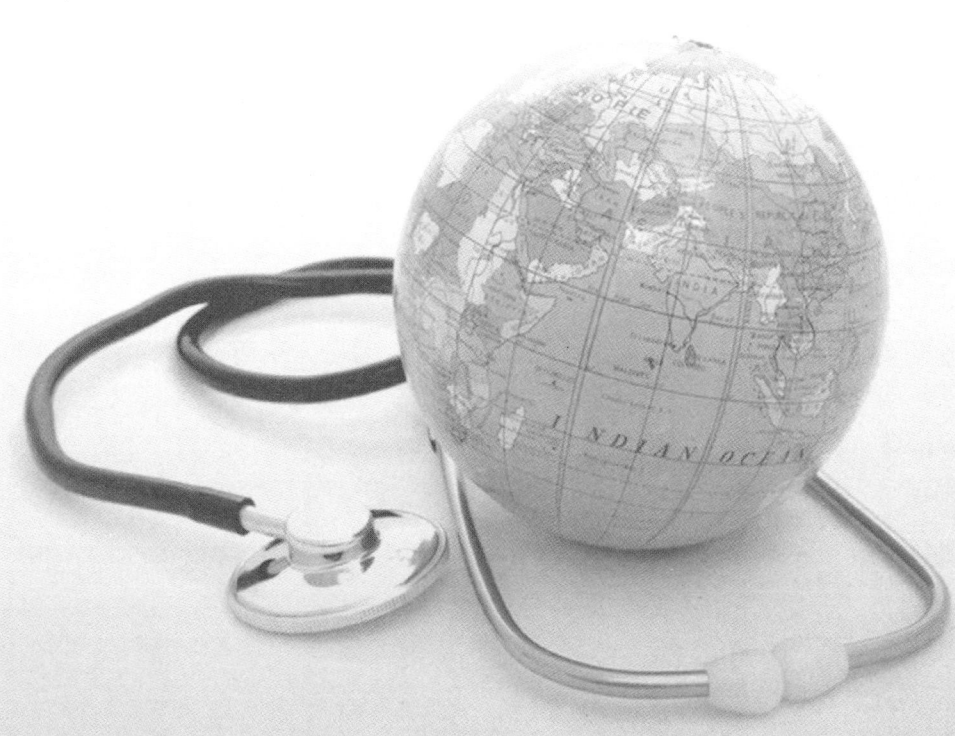

*"Put on the coat of manager over your apron, you are out in the community to manage the health of millions."*

# SECTION OUTLINE

35. Great Achievements in Community Medicine
36. Global Health Situation
37. Community Health
38. Managing Community Health
39. Healthcare Delivery System Across Nations
40. Human Resources for Health
41. Health Financing
42. Health Management
43. International Healthcare Agencies
44. Special Topics

# CHAPTER 35

# Great Achievements in Community Medicine

*Liaquat Roopesh Johnson*

**CM 20.2** Describe various issues during outbreaks and their prevention
**CM 20.3** Describe event important to health of community

## INTRODUCTION

Today, we live in a world where the population has crossed 8 billion. Much of this increase occurred between 1900 and 2000, when the global population increased from 1.5 to 6.1 billion people. Yet, today, fewer people die of communicable diseases than 100 years ago, and more people enjoy a reasonable standard of living than in the past. For instance, the average life expectancy at birth (LEB) in India in 1900 was 23 years—a third of today's value. Most of this premature mortality was due to communicable diseases like plague, influenza, and cholera—conditions that have long ceased to decimate entire populations. Globally, a hundred years ago, every 100–200th woman died due to pregnancy-related causes (500–1,000/100,000 live births)—that value is now around 200/100,000 live births.

Clearly, something changed around 1900 that allowed more people to survive, and for longer. It was not so much a single change, but several changes that occurred simultaneously—control of pandemics; decrease in maternal, child, and general mortality; better food, living conditions and work environment, etc. Much of that change has to do with the adoption of simple practices like clean water and good sanitation; healthier environments; better hygiene, etc.—interventions that continue to form the foundations of community medicine practice over 100 years later. In this chapter, we will examine the role community medicine has played in increasing lifespans and living conditions, as well as reducing sickness and death to date.

## INCREASE IN LONGEVITY

Longevity simply indicates having a long life, while lifespan measures the number of years lived. However, merely measuring the duration of one's life does not help answer the question, "How long will I live"? The answer to that question can be obtained by examining life tables. These are estimates of how many years a person can be expected to live from any age onward, and are constructed by determining the probability of death at each age (These probabilities are obtained from past mortality statistics, and are compiled to generate a single probability value for each year of life). The estimates are based on the assumption that the prevailing mortality patterns will persist unchanged throughout a person's lifetime. Since the mortality patterns are constantly changing, the estimates are just an approximation. Life expectancy at birth (LEB), perhaps the most commonly cited estimate of longevity is defined as "the average number of years that a newborn is expected to live if current mortality rates continue to apply".

As per the WHO and World Bank Report, the global LEB for children born in 2015 was 71.4 years (69.1 years for males and 73.8 years for females). However, this was not always the case. The LEB for our hunter–gatherer ancestors was probably 25 years. There was little, if any, progress by the Roman Empire, and even as recently as 1700, the LEB in England— the second richest country in the world at the time was only 37 years (Cutler D et al., J Econ Perspect, 2006). Until 1850, regardless of where one was born, the average LEB was around 30 years with the highest being 40 years **(Figs. 35.1 and 35.2)** (Roser M et al., Our World in Data, 2018). Most of the mortality was on account of what we now consider preventable causes—communicable diseases, pregnancy-related, and environmental causes.

From **Figure 35.1**, it is clear that global life expectancy remained between 20 and 40 years till the middle of the 20th century. Most of the increase in life expectancy is fairly recent, with rapid increase occurring in the last 75–80 years.

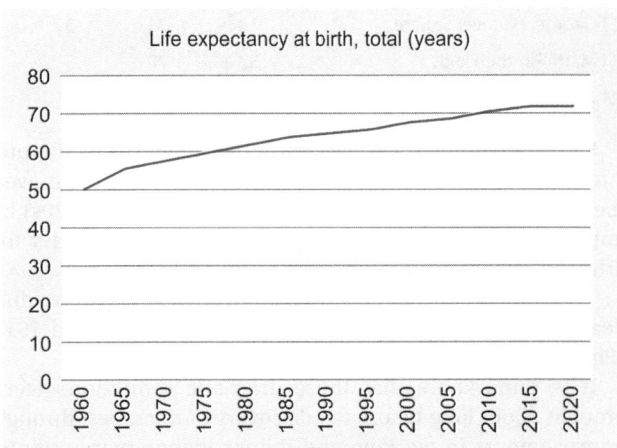

**Fig. 35.1:** Global life expectancy.
*Source:* Data.worldbank.org based on 2022 revisions.

> **Putting Increased Life Expectancy in Perspective**
>
> Before 1850, on an average, children were 14 years old when one parent died. Traditionally, parents died before their youngest children completed education.
>
> Today, an average child may be 55–60 years old at their father's death.

In **Figure 35.2**, it is evident that we have made tremendous progress in terms of life expectancy in the last 250 years. In the absence of community medicine interventions, it is likely that we would still be experiencing similar life expectancy rates as our forefathers in the 19th century.

There are health records from England and Wales dating back to the 19th century that allow us to determine the factors responsible for the decline in mortality. The Great Sanitary Awakening resulted in a rapid improvement in water, hygiene, and sanitation across England and Wales. The impact of this change can be seen in the decrease in deaths due to typhoid during that period.

Death rate due to typhoid in England and Wales was reduced after the construction of sewers. A similar reduction was seen in the deaths due to cholera during the same period. William Farr showed the dramatic difference in cholera death rates between the East and West Ends of London **(Table 35.1)**. While the East End received sewage contaminated downstream water, their West End counterparts received relatively cleaner upstream water.

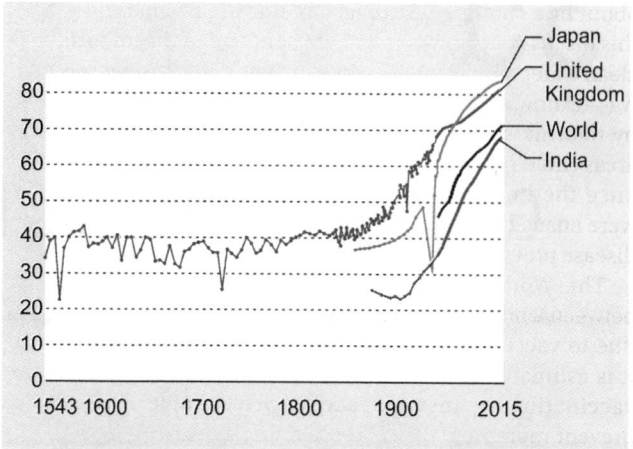

**Fig. 35.2:** Life expectancy at birth in selected countries.
*Source:* Clio-Infra estimates until 1949; UN Population Division from 1950 to 2015
OurWorldinData.org/life-expectancy-how-is-it-calculated-and-how-should-it-be-interpreted.

**Table 35.1:** Cholera deaths per 10,000 population in London (Bryer H., Human Development, 2006).

| Description | 1849 | 1853–4 | 1866 |
|---|---|---|---|
| All London average | 62 | 46 | 18 |
| *East End* | | | |
| Bermondsey | 161 | 179 | 6 |
| St George, Southwark | 164 | 121 | 1 |
| Newington | 144 | 112 | 3 |
| Rotherhithe | 205 | 165 | 9 |
| *West End* | | | |
| Kensington | 24 | 38 | 4 |
| St George, Hanover Square | 18 | 33 | 2 |
| St Martin-in-the-Fields | 37 | 20 | 5 |
| St James, Westminster | 16 | 142 | 5 |

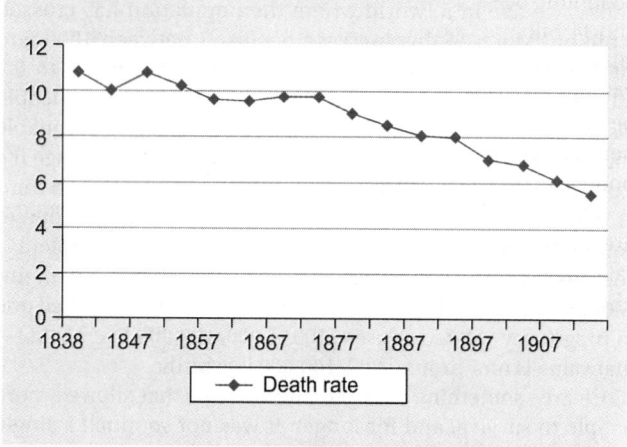

**Fig. 35.3:** Adult death rate (per 1,000 population) in England and Wales (1838–1912).
*Source:* Bryer H., Human Development, 2006.

Since cholera is transmitted through the fecal-oral route, a reduction in cholera deaths could have only been achieved (before effective immunization was available in the 1920s) by improved sanitation, and the availability of clean water for drinking, cooking, domestic, and personal hygiene.

The effect of sanitary reform can be clearly seen on adult death rates in England and Wales between 1838 and 1912 **(Fig. 35.3)**.

It is remarkable that these dramatic reductions were brought about long before the discovery of microbes, through improvements in working and indoor living environments, cooking, sewage treatment and waste removal, refrigeration, medical interventions (e.g. vaccination), clean water, and hand-washing at the community level. The importance of such general measures cannot be understated—water, sanitation, and hygiene are responsible for around 2.4 million deaths (4.2% of all deaths), and 6.6% of disability-adjusted life years (DALYs) globally. 90% of this burden is borne by under-5 children (73% in just 15 developing countries), costing households US$340 million; and national health systems US$7 billion. According to one estimate, water purification alone explains half the reduction in mortality (in the US) in the first third of the 20th century (Cutler D et al., J Econ Perspect, 2006). Many water, sanitation, and hygiene interventions yield a net benefit of US$3–46 for every dollar spent. Ironically, attitudes toward hygiene and water were largely responsible for both the decline in public sanitation before the 19th century; and the Great Sanitary Awakening in the 19th century. Prior to the Great Sanitary Awakening, bathing was considered immoral; thereafter, it was considered central to moral and physical health. The shift in attitude was brought about by a combination of factors that are beyond the scope of this discussion. However, one must note that the importance of clean water; public and personal hygiene; and proper sanitation was acknowledged by governments after many years of activism by reformers—they failed to see how improvements in these areas could possibly save lives or reduce diseases. Nevertheless, once the link was established, several pieces of legislation were enacted that covered water, sanitation, public health, and disease prevention (Bryer H., Human Development, 2006).

The World Health Organization (WHO) estimates that between 2 million and 3 million deaths are prevented each year due to vaccination (Vanderslott S, Our world in data, 2018). It is estimated that in 73 low- and middle-income countries, vaccination against 10 vaccine-preventable diseases will prevent more than 20 million deaths and save US$350 billion in cost of illness over 20 years. Lifelong productivity gains from the prevention of deaths and disability during the 20 years are estimated to be US$330 billion and US$9 billion, respectively. Over the lifetime of the vaccinated cohorts, these vaccinations will save around US$5 billion in treatment costs; and yield broader economic benefits of US$820 billion—all for an investment of US$34 billion (Ozawa S et al., Bulletin World Health Organ, 2017; Orenstein WA, PNAS, 2017). A recent study estimates that 24 million cases of impoverishment due to medical cost would be averted by vaccines administered in 41 developing countries between 2016 and 2030, with the greatest benefits in the two poorest quintiles (Chang AY, Health Affairs, 2018).

The economic and social impacts of increased life expectancy are many—later marriages, delayed childbirth, reduced fertility rate, increased duration of marriage, and opportunities for longer engagement in economically productive work. This is why many of the broad interventions mentioned previously are essential for the achievement of Sustainable Development Goals. Although a direct effect of life expectancy on economic growth is doubted, it has substantially improved living standards.

## INCREASE IN LIVING STANDARDS

There is no single measure that can effectively capture standard of living. Therefore, composite measures (that combine more than one measure) have been developed. The two most frequently used indicators of living standards are human development index (HDI) and physical quality of life index (PQLI).

We have already seen how life expectancy has increased tremendously in the last 200 years. The relationship between life expectancy and standard of living has also been described—an increase in the former is significantly associated with improvements in the latter. Therefore, it is easy to see how historical HDI levels were the result of poor life expectancy, and the accompanying low standards of living. As mentioned earlier, increased life expectancy has several social and economic impacts. Together, these drive social and economic development.

Human development index includes three measures: life expectancy, knowledge, and standard of living. Life expectancy significantly impacts the latter two—literacy rates improve with child survival; and better literacy increases the potential for economic productivity; increased economic productivity leads to better per capita income, and therefore, improved standards of living. Therefore, an increase in life-expectancy mirrors an increase in HDI.

**Figure 35.4** clearly shows how HDI values for India were stagnant till 1920, after which they rose considerably. While the

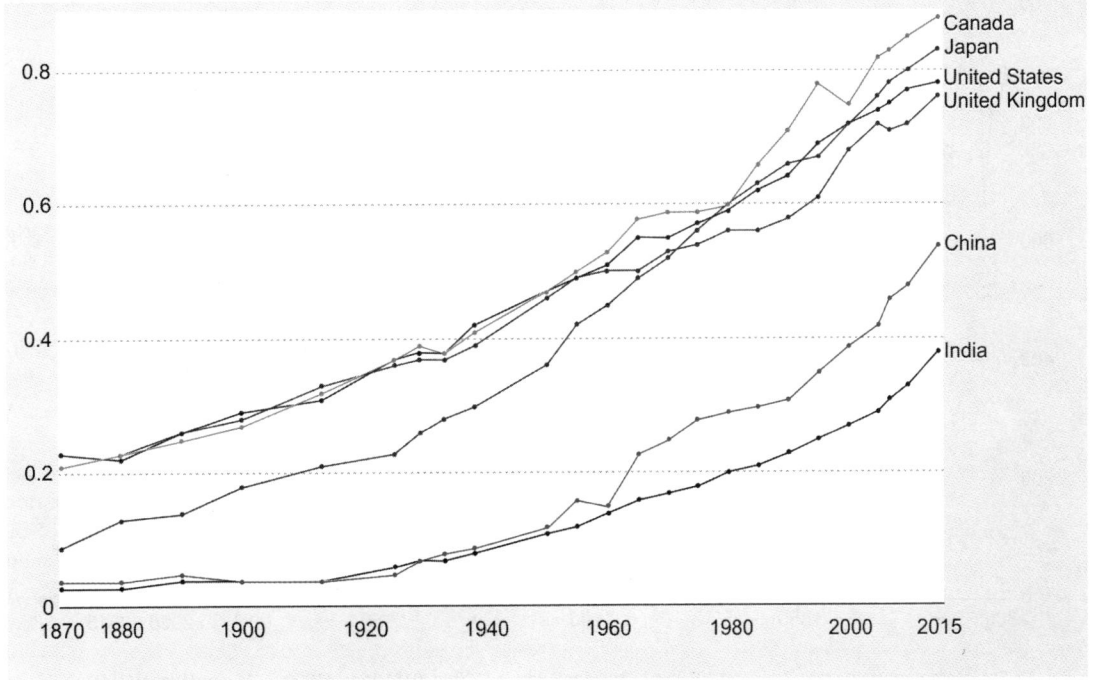

**Fig. 35.4:** Historical index of human development.
*Source:* Prados de la Escosura (2018).

improvements in HDI are linear, the rate of improvement is not uniform.

In general, the countries with low HDI also have low life expectancy, and vice versa. As mentioned previously, most of the increase in life expectancy has resulted from the community-wide adoption of basic interventions—clean water and good sanitation, immunization, better nutrition, better care during pregnancy and at delivery, improved personal and environmental hygiene, etc.

It is evident that any discussion on living standards is incomplete without mentioning the role of increased life expectancy on the same. Therefore, one can rightfully claim the increase in living standards as an achievement of community medicine.

## IMPROVEMENT IN MATERNAL AND CHILD HEALTH

In the absence of any intervention, the "natural" maternal mortality is around 1,500/100,000 live births (Larberghe W Van et al., 2000). Most of this mortality is on account of hemorrhage, sepsis, and difficulties during labor. An examination of historical maternal mortality rates indicates when, and by how much these values have declined.

Sweden is one of the few countries with records dating back to the 18th century. From **Figure 35.5**, we can see that it experienced a significant decline in maternal mortality ratio by the year 1900. During the 19-20th centuries, Sweden was a thinly populated country that was not as affluent as some of the other European countries. Despite this economic disadvantage, it managed to achieve a much lower maternal mortality ratio long before other countries did. How did a small country with scarce resources (at the time), manage such an impressive feat? The answer lies in the approach. In the 18th century, the Swedish government introduced for the first time in the world, the notion of "avoidable maternal mortality", by reporting that at least 400 out of 651 women dying in childbirth could have been saved if there had been enough midwives (Larberghe W Van et al., 2000).

This resulted in the enactment of a policy of training enough midwives to ensure that all deliveries (home deliveries were the norm) would be attended by qualified personnel. Although training so many midwives was a slow process—100 years after the report, 40% births were attended by midwives; increasing to 78% over the next 40 years. Traditional birth attendants at delivery declined from 60% (1861) to 18% by 1900, by which time only 2-5% of all deliveries took place in hospitals.

Midwives would be supervised by the public health doctor; and they were allowed considerable autonomy. The doctor could be involved in case of major complications, and was accountable for official reports. Sweden was quick to adopt and generalize aseptic techniques by 1881—just a few years after its introduction in hospitals.

Maternal mortality rates declined at much slower rates in other countries (including England and Wales and the USA) because of a reluctance to follow Sweden's example. In the US and UK, for instance, doctors opposed and obstructed the work of midwives in many locations. Further, midwives often lacked the support needed from the system, and were isolated. Delayed acknowledgement of "avoidable maternal mortality" and enactment of appropriate legislation; lack of funding; and inefficient implementation of applicable legislative measures, all served to delay progress. Many of the same factors operate in some countries even today.

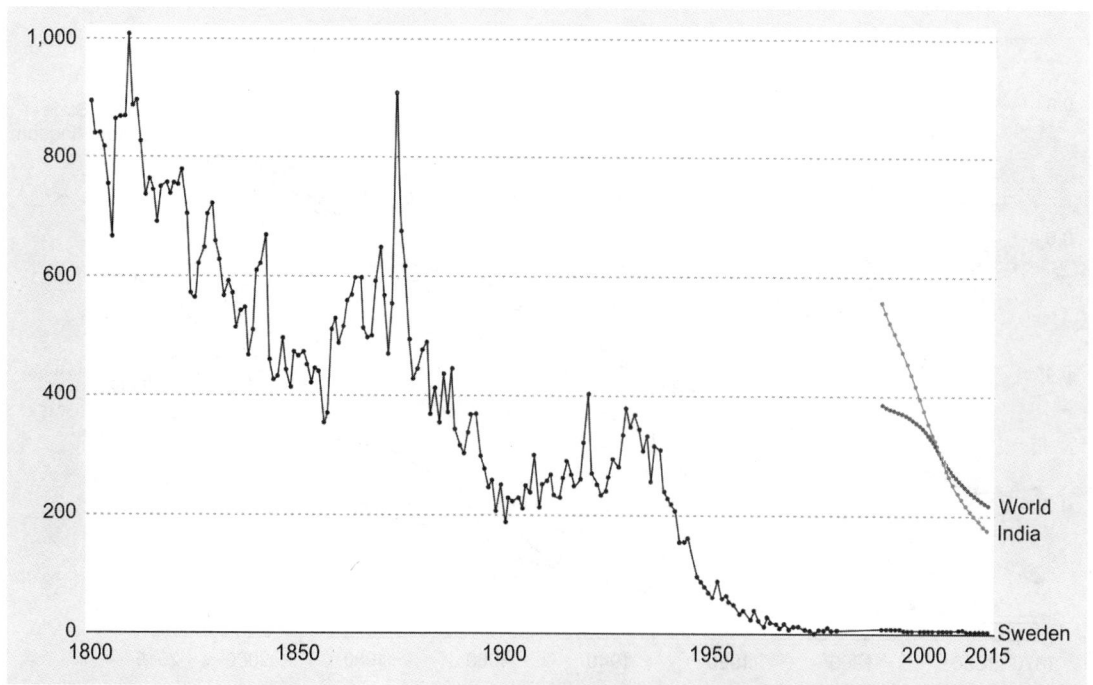

**Fig. 35.5:** Maternal mortality ratio (per 100,000 live births) for Sweden (1800–2015), India (1990–2015) and World (1990–2015).
*Source:* Gapminder (2010) and World Bank (2015) OurWorldinData.org/human-development-index.

Child mortality, or deaths of children less than 5 years of age, was a significant contributor to overall mortality in the 18–19th centuries. During the 18th century, every third child died in Sweden; in 19th century in Germany, every other child died. From that level, global child mortality declined to 23% in 1950; and further fell to 4.3% in 2015 **(Fig. 35.6)** (Roser M., Our World in Data, 2018). The reason this remarkable improvement does not make headlines is because it has occurred over many decades—too slowly for us to realize. The reduction of child and infant mortality is defined as "the measure of all things", since it is directly affected by the availability of clean water and safe sanitation; income and education of parents; prevalence of malnutrition and disease; efficacy of health services; and the health and status of women.

As can be seen in **Figure 35.7**, Sweden had considerably lower child mortality rates than other countries long before global efforts to reduce child mortality were initiated. This is attributed to four strategies implemented in 18th century in Sweden:

- The distribution of pamphlets and leaflets on childcare and treatment of illnesses
- State-sponsored increase in the number of doctors trained; and regulation of their activities
- Provision of specialized training in medicine and childcare to clergymen with requirements to maintain records, announce public health measures, maintain a small pharmacy, and keep medical books.
- Centralized training, licensing and regulation of midwives, with responsibility for postnatal care (including the promotion of breastfeeding).

Despite the impressive gains in child survival over time, progress has been nonuniform, with some countries taking much longer to achieve similar improvements.

The reason why Sweden took so long to achieve a child mortality rate of 1 in 20, is because of patchy implementation of the four strategies mentioned earlier. Some counties (=districts) in Sweden had higher child mortality rates due to nomads;

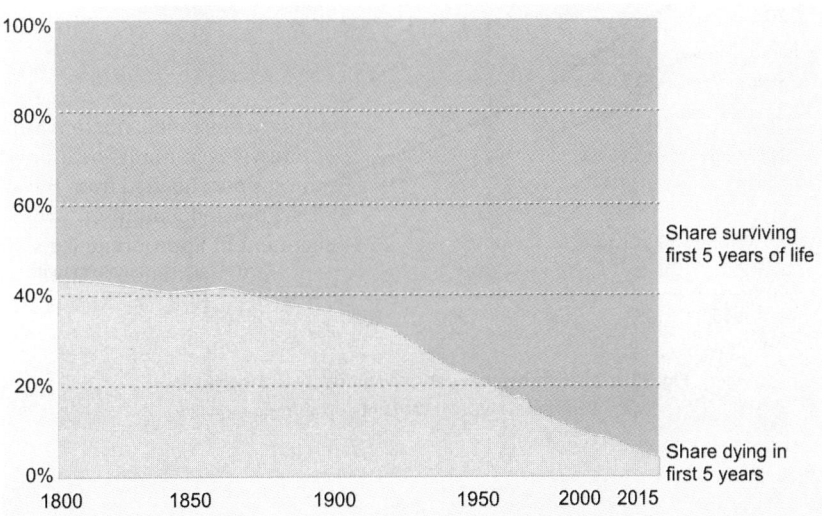

Fig. 35.6: Historical and modern global child mortality (expressed as proportion surviving the first 5 years of life).
*Source:* Gapminder and the World Bank OurWorldinData.org/a-history-of-global-living-conditions-in-5-chart.

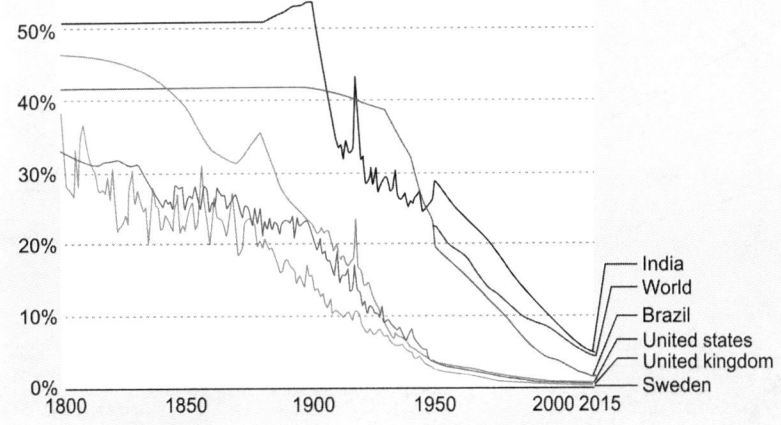

Fig. 35.7: Child mortality rates for selected countries from 1800–2015.
*Source:* Gapminder estimates up until 1949 and UN Population Division from 1950 to today OurWorldinData.org.

reluctance to send women for midwife training; improper breastfeeding practices, etc.

Naturally, one wonders what factors resulted in the global reduction in child mortality. The reasons are unsurprisingly: improvement in living conditions (better living standards) **(Fig. 35.8)**; increases in female literacy; and increase in (public) healthcare spending.

We have already seen how increase in life expectancy directly enhanced living standards at the global level. This drove improvements in child mortality through better living standards, as well as the consequent increase in female literacy.

Most of the preventable mortality was on account of common childhood illnesses like pneumonia. With better living conditions, improved healthcare facilities and female literacy, there was a substantial decline in deaths due to these causes **(Fig. 35.9)**. This meant that most of the under-5 mortality began happening during infancy. However, with the provision of better antenatal care, and trained personnel at delivery, a substantial proportion of infant and neonatal mortality was also reduced **(Fig. 35.10)**.

Much of infant mortality is due to neonatal mortality; reducing the latter will reduce the former. Further, such reductions may be brought about through basic community medicine interventions, and are not a function of income status.

The importance of female literacy cannot be understated. Even within very poor countries, regions with higher female literacy rates have lower child mortality rates. The relationship

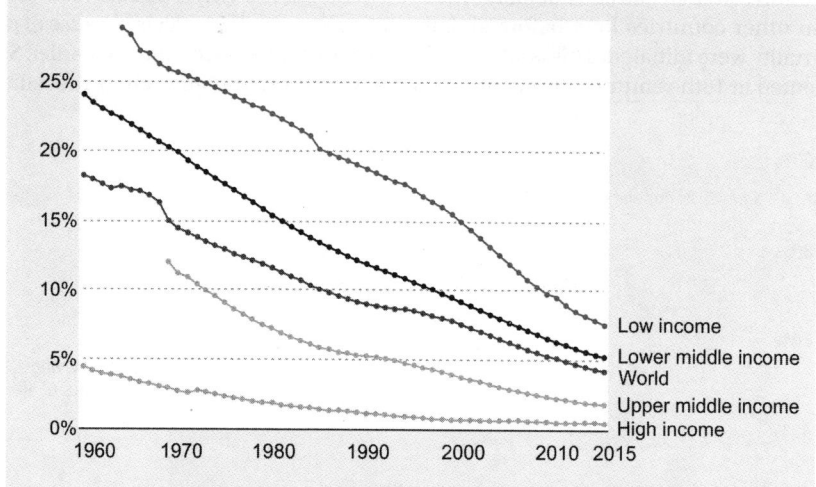

**Fig. 35.8:** Relationship between child mortality and income level.
*Source:* World Bank—WDI OurWorldinData.org/child-mortality.

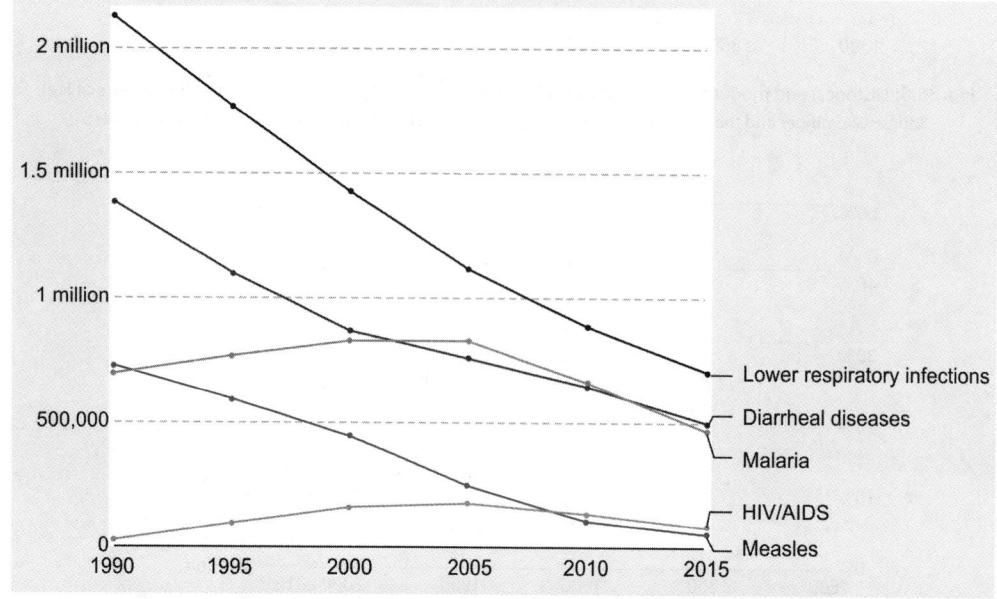

**Fig. 35.9:** Global childhood deaths from the five most lethal infectious diseases.
*Source:* IHME Global Burden of Disease (child deaths by disease) (2017). https://ourworldindata.org/child-mortality.

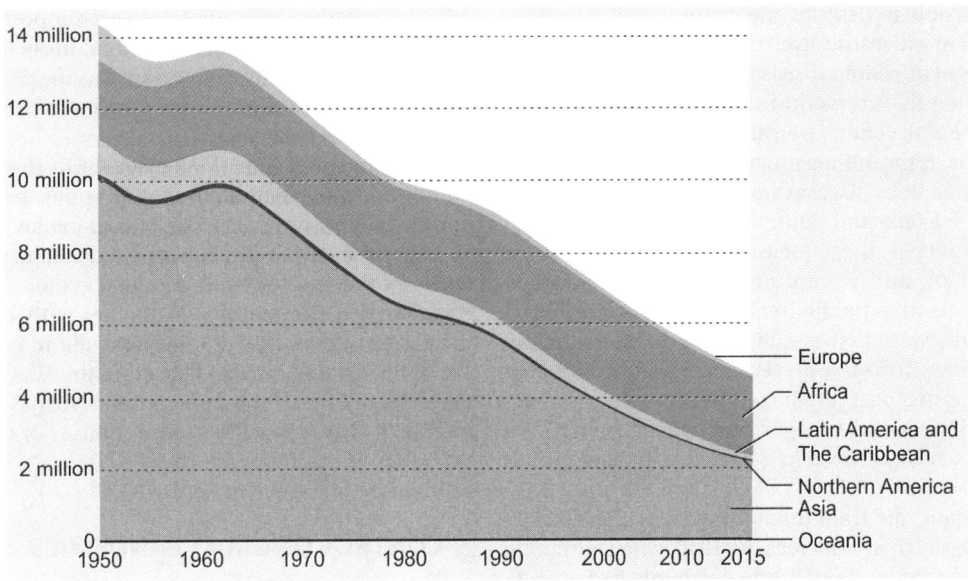

**Fig. 35.10:** Decline in absolute number of infant deaths by world region.
*Source:* UN Population Division (2017 Revision). https://ourworldindata.org/child-mortality.

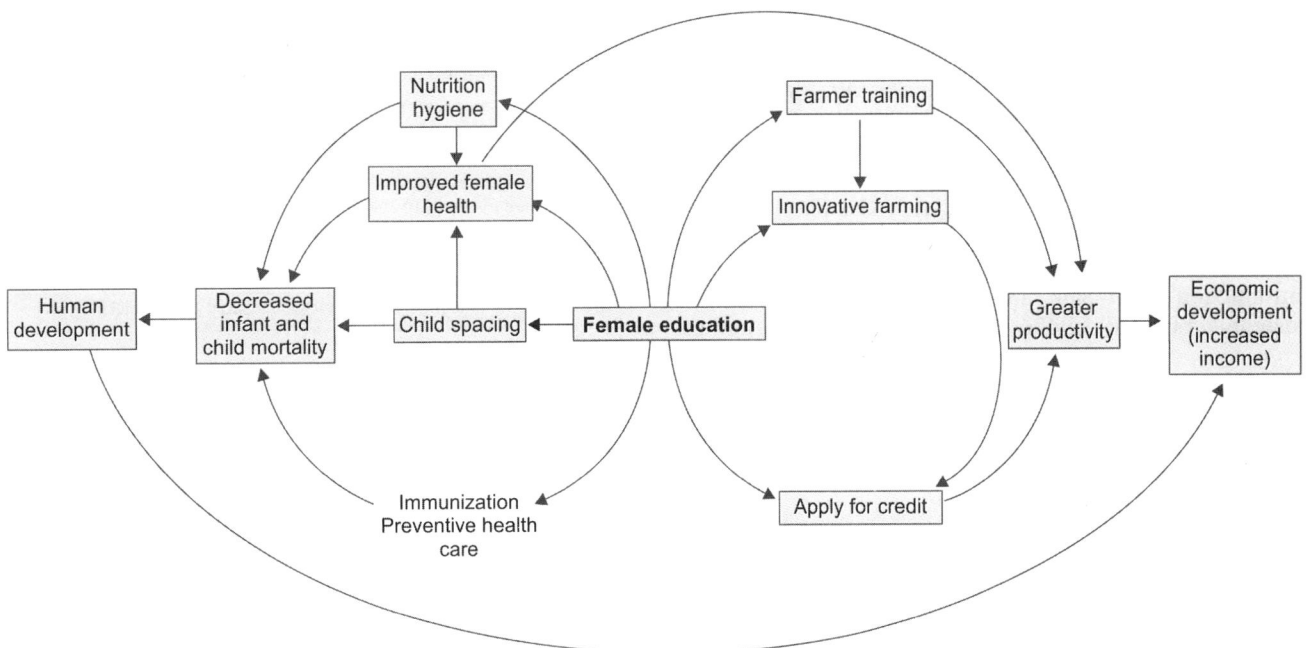

**Fig. 35.11:** The relationships between female literacy, economic, and human development.

between female literacy and child mortality is shown in **Figure 35.11**.

The decline in child mortality has had a significant impact on fertility. While women in India on average had around six children till the middle of the 20th century, typically, only around half of them survived the first 5 years of life. Thereafter, when a greater proportion of children began surviving 5 years, the total number of children born by a woman declined to around 3.

This decline in fertility rate accompanied declining infant mortality rates the world over. Together, these two factors enabled rapid improvements in life expectancy with some countries experiencing a 10 years increase in life expectancy over a short time period.

## CONTROL OF INFECTIOUS DISEASES

One of the major contributors to increase in life expectancy was the control of infectious diseases. In 1900, diarrhea, enteritis, pneumonia, and tuberculosis were the leading causes of death in the USA accounting for one-third of all deaths. 40% of these were among under-5 children (CDC, Morb Mortal Weekly Rep, 1999).

Since, it is not possible to describe the control of all infectious diseases, this section will restrict itself to a discussion of the most important aspects of infectious disease control.

Community health interventions to control infectious diseases during the 20th century were informed by the discovery of microorganisms in the 19th century. Considerable progress in the control of infectious diseases was made by 1,900 through improvements in hygiene and sanitation; and the provision of clean water. In the USA, these measures were implemented through local, state, and federal agencies, and reinforced the concept of collective public health action. County level health departments were first established in 1908, and made considerable progress in disease prevention measures like water treatment, sewage disposal, organized solid waste disposal, food safety, public education regarding hygienic practices, and chlorination. These resulted in a decrease in incidence of waterborne diseases.

In 1900, the death rate from tuberculosis was 194/100,000 US population, mostly in urban areas. By 1940, when antibiotic therapy was introduced in the USA, the death rate had already declined to 46/100,000 US population. This was a result of the general measures mentioned earlier, and improvements in housing (CDC, Morbidity Mortality Weekly Report, 1999).

The US initiated universal vaccination campaigns targeting common diseases like smallpox, mumps, measles, diphtheria, tetanus, poliomyelitis, and *Haemophilus influenzae* type b meningitis. When a combined diphtheria-tetanus toxoid and pertussis vaccine was licensed in 1949, state and local health departments implemented immunization programs mainly focused on poor children. This strategy was possibly based on the fact that historically the greatest burden of infectious diseases fell on the poorest especially the urban poor. The introduction of the Salk poliovirus vaccine in 1955 lead to government funded childhood vaccination programs, and the 1962 Vaccination Assistance Act that supports the purchase of several childhood vaccines. Together, these measures resulted in the near elimination of common vaccine preventable diseases **(Fig. 35.12)**, and inspired the concept of disease eradication through global cooperation.

The control of infectious diseases in the USA was further enhanced by the institution of state sponsored national animal and pest control programs. These programs helped eliminate dog-to-dog transmission of rabies, and reduced malaria to negligible levels by the late 1940s. Rodent and vector-control operations enabled the elimination of plague, with the last outbreak occurring during 1924–25. Perhaps the most telling statistics are of the leading causes of death in the USA in 1900 and 1997 **(Fig. 35.13)** that show how chronic diseases have replaced infectious diseases as the leading causes of death. The factors influencing the decrease in infectious diseases in the 20th century are presented in **Figure 35.14**.

## CONTROL OF GREAT PANDEMICS

For a large part of human history, epidemics of plague, smallpox, leprosy, syphilis, cholera, typhoid fever, yellow fever, and other infectious diseases were the norm. Therefore, the fact that all great acute epidemic catastrophes happened before 1950 is truly remarkable. We will examine two of the greatest pandemics in human history—Black death and Spanish flu here.

> The term "Black death" first appeared in the 16th century, long after the pandemic had ceased—it was called the great mortality or the great pestilence by contemporary (14th century) writers. For long, the disease involved was a matter of speculation. Then, an outbreak of bubonic plague in Hong Kong in 1894 leads to the discovery of the plague bacillus (*Y. pestis*), and the realization that the Black death was probably caused by plague. Subsequent examination of 14th century documents has convinced experts that the Black death was, indeed, caused by (bubonic) plague.

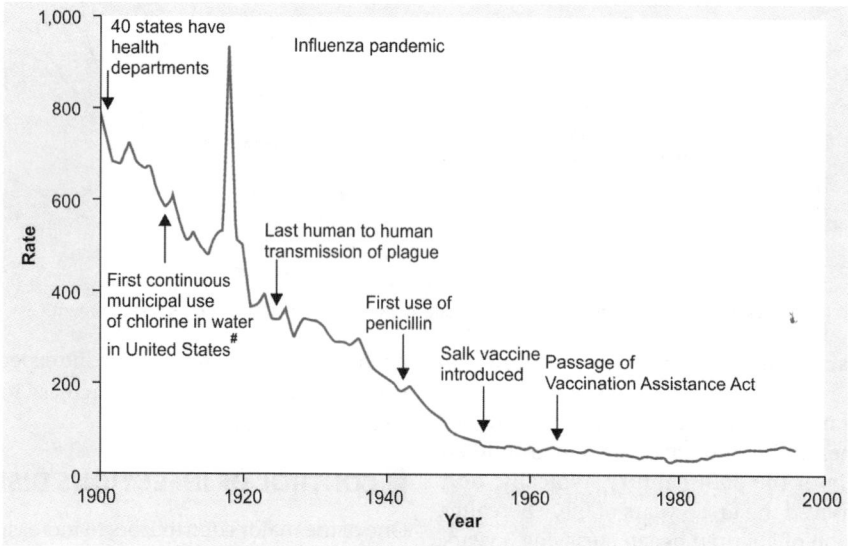

Fig. 35.12: Crude death rate* for infectious diseases in the USA, 1900–1996.

*Per 100,000 population per year.
#American Water Works Association. Water chlorination principles and practices: AWWA manual M20. Denver, Colorado: American Water Works Association, 1973.
Source: Adapted from Armstrong GL. Conn LA. Pinner RW. Trends in infectious disease mortality in the United States during the 20th century. JAMA 1999:281;61–6.

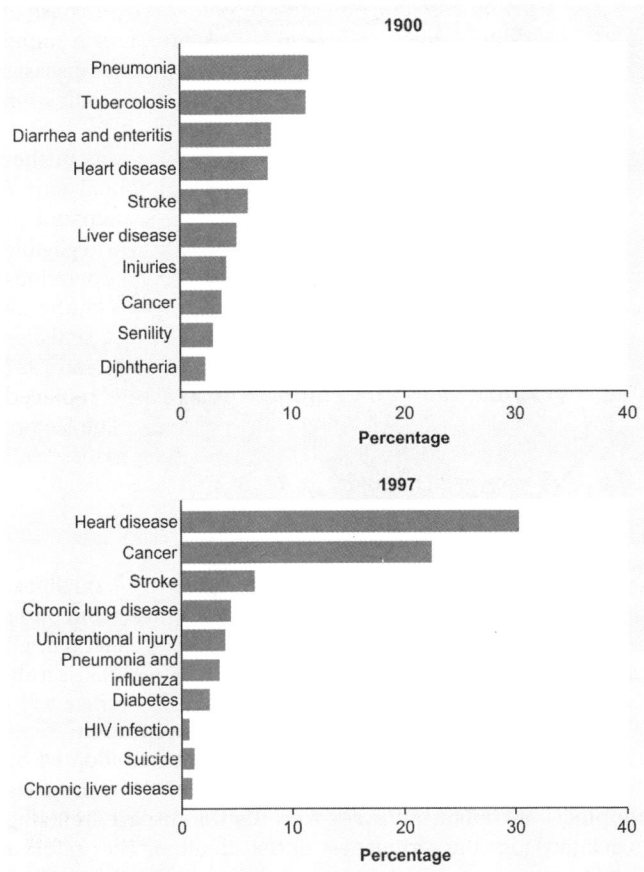

Fig. 35.13: Ten leading causes of death as a proportion of all deaths in the USA, 1900 and 1997.

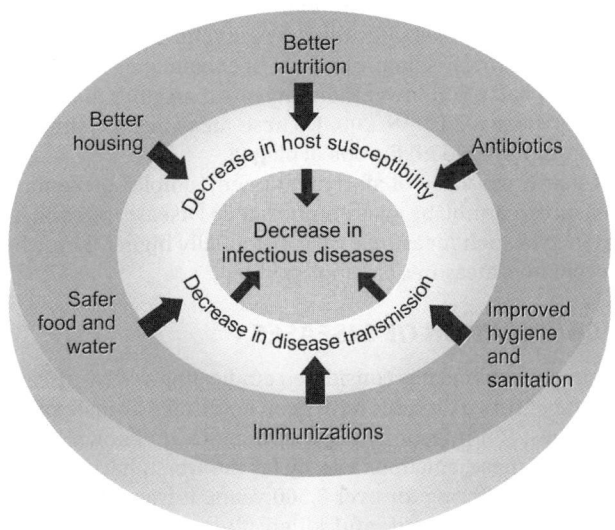

Fig. 35.14: Factors influencing the decrease in infectious diseases.

The great plague pandemic of 1347-1350 (Black Death) was one of the greatest demographic catastrophes in human history causing extensive depopulation in Europe, Northern Africa, and the Middle East. One estimate suggests that black death killed almost one-third of Europe's population **(Fig. 35.15)**. Other estimates suggest an average mortality of 50% (40-70%), or between 25 million to 45 million individuals (Slavicek LC, The Black Death, 2008).

Fourteenth century Europe was very different from today's Europe: The catholic church reigned supreme, and pervaded every aspect of human life; Latin was the main language; serfdom was prevalent; personal hygiene and sanitation were very poor—bathing was a rarity, and fecal matter was practically everywhere; diseases were thought to be caused by the inhalation of noxious fumes or vapors; medicine was intertwined with astrology—disease was attributed to celestial events—and religion—the wrath of God; bloodletting—the process of bleeding a person by making a cut in the vein was one of the main therapeutic interventions, as was the practice of consuming concoctions made of herbal and animal products. Although the population of Europe was only around 77 million, it was overpopulated relative to available resources.

The Black death caused so many deaths that corpses lay rotting everywhere, filling the air with a putrid stench. People were so frightened of contracting the disease that parents abandoned their sick children, locking them outdoors. Across all strata of society, people avoided contact with the dying and the dead, refusing to carry the dead to the cemetery. Most of the gravediggers, clergy, lawyers, apothecaries (pharmacists), and doctors perished. This lead to the use of petty criminals for disposing the dead- often in mass graves. Even these proved inadequate, and corpses were simply left to rot. In many cities, the number of dead outnumbered the living. The survivors were so shocked that they simply waited for their own deaths, convinced that the end of the world was at hand.

For around 350 years, the response to plague was fleeing the area. However, this only served to further spread the disease. Gradually, community health interventions of surveillance, quarantine, isolation, disinfection, and creation of public health boards were instituted. Quarantine and other barrier technologies lead to the disappearance of plague from Western Europe, and are invoked to this day.

Influenza is unique in that unlike other pandemic causing diseases mentioned previously, it continues to cause epidemics and pandemics. Despite the lack of records of ancient influenza pandemics in China, it is suspected that China is the birthplace of modern influenza epidemics. The first well documented influenza epidemic occurred in 1173 in modern-day Italy and France. This was followed by epidemics in 1414, 1557, 1675-1676, 1788-1790, 1789-1790, and 1830-1832.

The pandemic of 1847 was the first truly global epidemic of influenza. Thereafter, the Russian flu occurred from 1889-1893, and affected Great Britain as well. At one point, one-third of London's population was incapacitated by the flu, and caused substantial deaths and economic damage. There were 125,000 influenza deaths in Great Britain in 1891; and 250,000 influenza deaths in 1892.

The worst influenza pandemic occurred in 1918-1919, when the "Spanish flu" killed over 20,000,000 people globally. Some historians suspect that this number may have perished in India alone, where reliable records were unavailable, and estimate global mortality at over 100 million (Laver G, Microbes Infect, 2002; Kupperburg P, Chelsea House Publishers, 2008).

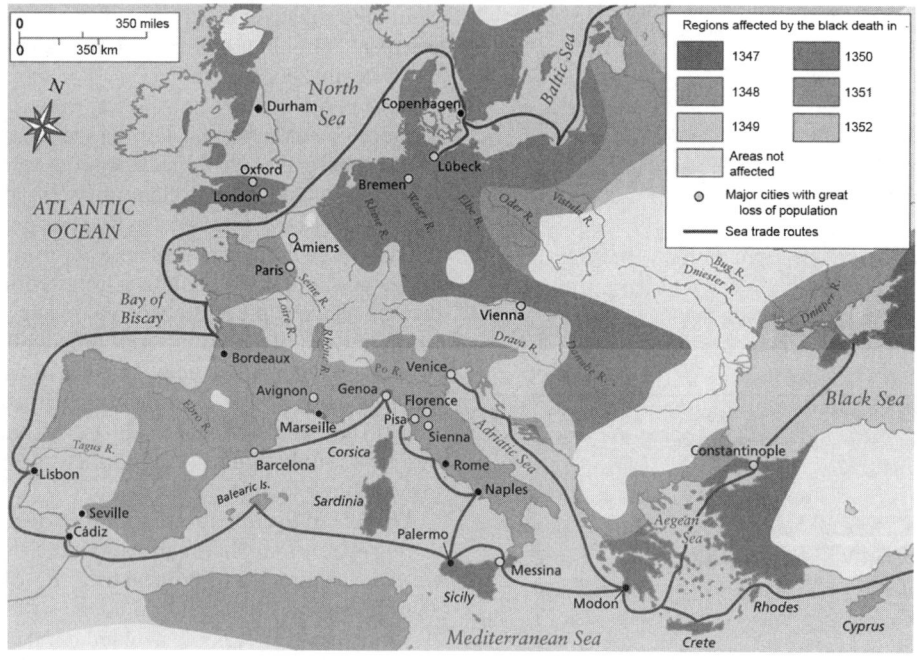

**Fig. 35.15:** Map showing the chronological spread of the Black death in Europe (1347–1352).

The pandemic occurred in multiple waves, with temporary returns to normalcy in between. One of the major reasons for the global spread of disease was the mobilization of vast troops and supplies for World War I. The pandemic probably began in the USA, then spread to Europe, South America, Asia, Africa, Australia and New Zealand. Several accounts report that more soldiers died of disease than battle. The warring nations—USA, Germany, Great Britain, France and Italy—deliberately suppressed reports of disease to avoid creating panic among the general population. However, Spain which was not participating in the war, did the opposite, resulting in the disease being named the "Spanish flu". Even in the USA, the sheer magnitude of cases was so high that officials quickly lost count. Many countries in Asia and Africa had practically nonexistent recordkeeping. Therefore, there are few reliable statistics of cases and deaths worldwide.

> **What was the impact of 'Spanish flu'?**
>
> The USA lost approximately 0.65% of its population; Italy, around 1%; Mexico, 4% of its total population, and 5–9% of its young adults. 4% of the African population of Cape Town died within 4 weeks. One-third of Japan's population fell ill; 10% of the population of Guam died; Russia and Iran both lost 7% of their respective populations. 14% of Fiji's population died in a mere 16 days; 22% of Western Samoa's population died.
>
> India was one of the worst affected with around 20 million deaths. 9% of European troops in India died; 10% of natives died; and 21% of Indian troops perished. In a single week, nearly 1,500 people died in erstwhile Bombay. Industries came to a halt because 60% of laborers were too sick to work. Although several parts of India were experiencing crop failure, the decreased crops also could not be harvested as workers were affected by illness. Consequently, food production declined by 20%, and prices doubled. So many people died in Punjab, that survivors ran out of firewood for cremation.
>
> Considering that the global population in 1918 was 1.8 billion, the influenza pandemic killed a staggering 5% of the world's population. If the same death toll were experienced today, around 350 million would be dead.

What is interesting, is the knowledge that mortality rates varied between cities, and reflected the strategies adopted by individual cities to control the epidemic. In the USA, some cities adopted nonchalant attitudes towards the disease, refusing to acknowledge the seriousness of the situation. They refused to institute preventative measures, and suppressed reports of illness and deaths to portray a picture of normalcy. Cities that initiated "social distancing" measures early, and implemented multiple such measures simultaneously (wearing of surgical masks; closing of schools, theaters and churches; prohibiting public gatherings; isolating patients or encouraging them to stay at home) had a 50% lower mortality rate than cities that did not do so (Morse SS, PNAS, 2007). These measures are similar to those employed to rid Europe of plague.

Clearly, the value of aforementioned "simple" preventative measures cannot be overemphasized. Disease rates in the absence of such measures are substantially higher than when preventative measures are implemented.

# ERADICATION OF DISEASES

Although mankind has considered eradicating several diseases, till date only two diseases have been eradicated—smallpox and rinderpest (an infectious disease in cattle, no known human cases). Of these, smallpox was by far the worst, having caused death and suffering for over 3,500 years. It was much feared, as it blinded, maimed, and killed; there was no treatment, and eventually affected everyone. Between 15% and 30% of its victims died within 1–2 weeks in Asia and Africa, brought about in no small measure by the difficulty in drinking and eating due to pustules on the tongue and inside the mouth. In the 20th century alone, smallpox killed an estimated 300 million—more than twice the number killed in military wars of that century (Henderson DA, Vaccine 2011). Several decades have passed since the eradication of smallpox, and later generations do not fully appreciate the importance and magnitude of that achievement. This section will attempt to shed light on what must be the greatest achievement of community health in the 20th century.

To appreciate the magnitude of the achievement, one needs to understand the background against which the WHO launched the Smallpox Eradication Programme (SEP) in 1966. At the time, over 30 countries were endemic with importations reported from an additional 12 countries; and around 10 million cases were estimated in 1967 (Henderson DA, Vaccine 2011; Strassburg MA, Am J Infect Control, 1982). The cold war between the USA and erstwhile USSR was underway, but the plan called for universal cooperation and collaboration. The program was unprecedented in its scale, but suffered from a lack of funds, as well as support—including many developed and developing countries; even then WHO Director-General, Marcelino Candau, who opposed it fearing it would fail. The fear of failure stemmed from the imminent failure of the much publicized (and well-funded) Malaria Control Programme which received widespread support globally. The UNICEF decided not to be involved with the program based on its experience with the malaria program.

Mass vaccination campaigns had not been previously attempted in developing countries, as they often lacked proper health service systems, and suffered from severe resource shortages. A heat-stable vaccine had only recently become available, as also a bifurcated needle for vaccination. India continued to use the liquid (heat-sensitive) vaccine for many years after the freeze-dried vaccine was developed. The liquid vaccine had to be maintained at low temperatures, and was viable for only 48 hours. At a time when electricity was unavailable in most parts of the country, this was a major challenge. Further, only a small proportion of those vaccinated were protected. Vaccine failure was common and well known, causing much reluctance toward vaccination. Prior to the bifurcated needle, vaccination was via a painful rotary lancet that required multiple punctures, and resulted in considerable vaccine wastage. India accounted for 60% of global smallpox burden, but a National Smallpox Eradication Program (NSEP) had failed within 5 years of its launch in 1962. There were several reasons for this failure: Lack of accurate data on the number of smallpox cases with gross under-reporting (only between 1 and 10% of all cases were reported); dependence on liquid vaccine in the presence of unsatisfactory procurement, distribution, storage and handling of vaccine; widespread concealment of cases due to fears of vaccination among the general population, and punishment among healthcare workers; lack of central monitoring of vaccine quality produced by vaccine units; overdependence on mass vaccination as the strategy for smallpox eradication; lack of support or enthusiasm for the SEP among healthcare personnel and administrators at all levels (Thanks to the gross under-reporting of smallpox cases, few believed that smallpox was a major public health problem in India. In addition, there was a feeling that smallpox eradication was more of a foreign priority than a national necessity. This lead to further antagonism toward the eradication program. Since several previous attempts to control smallpox had failed, many believed that eradication was impossible.); the scale of operations required to successfully eradicate smallpox through mass vaccination (each of India's 600 million people would have to receive primary vaccination; and a further 12 million infants would have to be vaccinated each year. Even if primary vaccinations were carried out at a rate matching the annual population growth, 25% of the population would remain unprotected); lack of adequate leadership and planning at the highest level (NSEP was hampered by severe staff shortage— there were only three officials available to implement the program at the national level. There was no operational plan either—that came much later, when the WHO got involved); disparities in performance between states (In India, health is a state subject, and NSEP was implemented differently in various states. While the Southern states made great progress, states in Northern and Central India did not). There was mistrust between Indian healthcare personnel and the WHO representatives due to experiences during the 1950s and early 1960s.

> One of the most important developments in smallpox eradication occurred in 1966 in Nigeria, where less than 50% of the population had a vaccination scar. Dr William Foege had to control smallpox outbreaks in Eastern Nigeria, but there was a delay in supplies for mass vaccination. With limited resources, he resorted to intensive vaccination only in the houses immediately surrounding newly reported cases. Outbreaks ended within 2–3 weeks after vaccination began. This demonstrated that outbreaks could be extinguished by vaccinating people in a limited area around every new case, even if the general area had many unvaccinated people. The subsequent surveillance-containment strategy of actively searching for cases, and vaccinating everyone around the case was based on this experience.

Remarkably, SEP was able to garner the cooperation and collaboration of both Soviet Russia and the USA; obtain funding from various sources; avert India's withdrawal from the campaign; and develop and implement plans across the world.

The essential program strategy consisted of three parts:
1. Undertaking of mass vaccination programs in endemic countries to assure protection of 80% of the population.
2. Surveillance-containment with reporting of all cases of smallpox each week by all health units.
3. Distribution of regular and frequent surveillance reports to everyone participating in the program; and health officials.

The program achieved its earliest successes in 20 West African countries rendering over 100 million people smallpox free within 3.5 years. This dramatic success demonstrated the effectiveness of the new smallpox strategy, and provided a boost to the program. However, India and modern-day Bangladesh presented the greatest challenge—more than 700 million people at the time; bureaucratic complexities; tens of millions of people traveling daily; and scores of refugees associated with civil war, famine, and massive floods (Henderson DA, Vaccine, 2011). Nevertheless, the goal was achieved, with substantial assistance—economic, political, and material—from JRD Tata during epidemic outbreaks in Tatanagar, Bihar in 1974. Considering the challenges, the success of the SEP program was almost miraculous.

> How large an operation was the search for smallpox cases in India? In April 1976, out of a scheduled 692,189 villages, 682,151 villages and 1,322 municipal areas were searched. A staff of 142,176 personnel was mobilized to visit each house in every village. This was repeated 6 months later by 152,441 health workers including malaria and family-planning staff who searched 668,332 villages. One of the strategies for case detection was the investigation of rumors of smallpox cases. By the end of November 1976 a total of 1,951,487 cases had been entered as suspected fever-with-rash cases, visited, and examined; 833,412 cases of chickenpox and zero cases of smallpox were found.

The lessons learned from the global campaign for eradication of smallpox have helped inform programs to eradicate poliomyelitis, dracunculiasis, and measles to name a few. Of the 3 strains of wild poliovirus (type 1, type 2 and type 3), wild poliovirus type 2 was eradicated in 1999 and wild poliovirus type 3 was eradicated in 2020. As of 2022, endemic wild poliovirus type 1 remains in two countries: Pakistan and Afghanistan.

India has already eradicated yaws, dracunculiasis, and poliomyelitis—a phenomenal achievement. India's later success in eradicating poliomyelitis owes much to the SEP—it first established a healthcare monitoring and surveillance system; provided training to key personnel at the national and sub-national levels; galvanized the healthcare workers into action; gave the confidence to undertake massive interventions—the Pulse Polio Immunization Programme is the largest in the world; and firmly established a working relationship between Indian healthcare personnel and international agencies like WHO.

## SUMMARY

Public health actions and interventions are responsible for most of the improvements in life expectancy; maternal and child health; control of infectious diseases and pandemics; and eradication of diseases like smallpox. However, most of these improvements took place over a long time period, making it inapparent to casual observers. Despite subsequent advances in technology, the value of basic, simple community health interventions to improve health cannot be discounted. These form the basis for plans to achieve the Sustainable Development Goals, and remain relevant to our quest for healthy and long lives. To claim that community medicine transformed the world is not a hollow boast, but the unacknowledged truth.

## SUGGESTED READING

1. Aberth J. The Black Death: The Great Mortality of 1348-1350. New York, NY: Palgrave Macmillan US; 2005.
2. Acemoglu D, Johnson S. Disease and Development: The effect of life expectancy on economic growth [Internet]. Cambridge, MA; 2006. Report No.: 12269.
3. Bartram J, Cairncross S. Hygiene, sanitation, and water: Forgotten foundations of health. PLoS Med. 2010;7(11):e1000367.
4. Bhattacharya S, Dasgupta R. Smallpox and polio eradication in India: Comparative histories and lessons for contemporary policy. Cien Saude Colet. 2011;16(2):433-44.
5. Brachman PS. Infectious diseases—past, present, and future. Int J Epidemiol. 2003;32(5):684-6.
6. Brilliant LB. The Management of Smallpox Eradication in India. The University of Michigan Press: Rodale, John Wiley & Sons Canada Limited; 1985.
7. Bryer H. Morbidity and Improvements in Water and Sanitation : Some Lessons from English History. Human Development; 2006.
8. Carmichael AG. Infectious Disease and Human Agency: An Historical Overview. Scr Varia. 2006;106.
9. Centers for Disease Control and Prevention. Achievements in Public Health. 1900-1999: Control of Infectious Diseases. Morb Mortal Wkly Rep. 1999;48(29):621-9.
10. Chang AY, Riumallo-Herl C, Perales NA, et al. The equity impact vaccines may have on averting deaths and medical impoverishment in developing countries. Health Aff. 2018;37(2):316-24.
11. Corsini CA, Viaozzo PP. The historical decline of infant mortality: An overview. The decline of infant mortality in Europe: 1800-1950-Four National Case Studies; 1993.
12. Cutler D, Deaton A, Lleras-muney A. The Determinants of Mortality. J Econ Perspect [online]. 2006;20(3):97-120.
13. Haacker M. Contribution of increased life expectancy to living standards. London; 2010.
14. Henderson DA. Eradication: Lessons from the past. Bull World Health Organ. 1998;76(Suppl. 2):17-21.
15. Henderson DA. The eradication of smallpox – An overview of the past, present, and future. Vaccine [Internet]. 2011;29(Suppl. 4):D7-9.
16. Kupperberg P. The Influenza Pandemic of 1918-1919, 1st edition. New York, NY: Chelsea House Publishers; 2008. pp. 1-121.
17. Morse SS. Pandemic influenza: Studying the lessons of history. Proc Natl Acad Sci. 20071;104(18):7313-4.
18. Orenstein WA, Ahmed R. Simply put: Vaccination saves lives. Proc Natl Acad Sci. 2017;114(16):4031-3.
19. Ozawa S, Clark S, Portnoy A, et al. Estimated economic impact of vaccinations in 73 low- and middle-income countries, 2001–2020. Bull World Health Organ. 2017;95(9):629-38.
20. Slavicek LC. The Black Death, 1st edition. Chelsea House Publishers; 2008.
21. Suresh P, Johnson LR. The post-2015 agenda: from millennium development goals (MDGS) to sustainable development goals. Int J Curr Res Rev. 2015;7(15):62-7.
22. UNDP. Human Development Index (HDI). Human Development Reports. 2018. Available from http://hdr.undp.org/en/content/ human-development-index-hdi.
23. United Nations Development Programme. Human development report 2016. United Nations Development Programme. 2016;193.
24. World Health Organization (WHO). [2006]. Life expectancy at birth. [online] Available from http://www.who.int/whr/2006/en/.

# CHAPTER 36

# Global Health Situation

*Prakash Patel*

## INTRODUCTION

The world has made remarkable progress in the last century to improve health of the human beings. Despite this, many health problems need to be addressed to achieve sustainable developmental goal (SDG). Major health problems include high maternal and child mortality, poor nutritional status, communicable diseases [importantly HIV/AIDS, tuberculosis (TB), and malaria], noncommunicable diseases and their risk factors (tobacco, alcohol, etc.) and harmful environmental conditions. Natural disasters and human conflicts/wars are also important contributors in mortality and morbidity globally. Important global health issues are highlighted in the following section. Top 10 leading causes of death globally are shown in **Figure 36.1**.

## GLOBAL HEALTH SITUATION

### Reproductive and Maternal Health

Maternal and child health situation of a community indirectly reflects overall health and healthcare services of the community. Maternal health is the health status of a woman

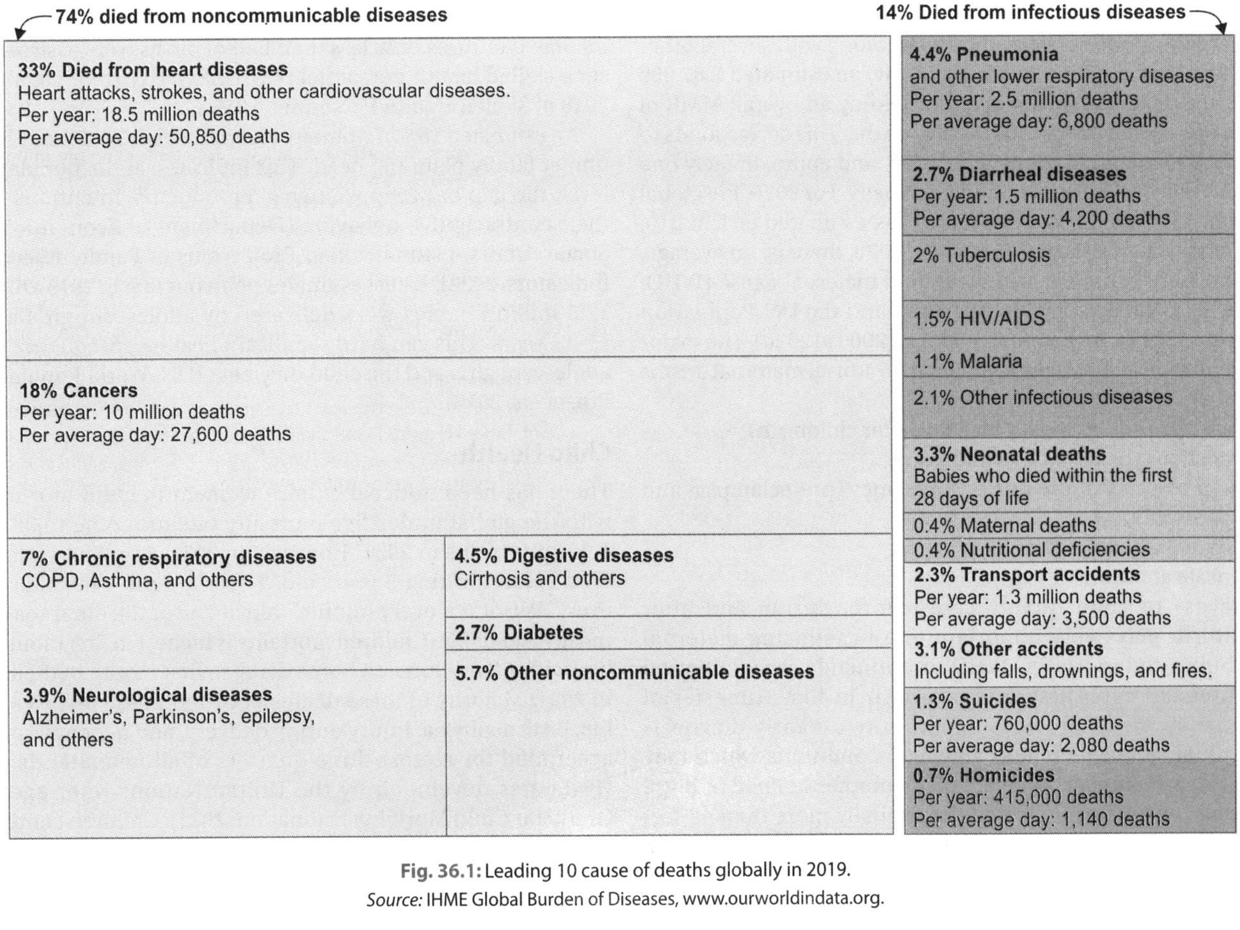

**74% died from noncommunicable diseases**

**33% Died from heart diseases**
Heart attacks, strokes, and other cardiovascular diseases.
Per year: 18.5 million deaths
Per average day: 50,850 deaths

**18% Cancers**
Per year: 10 million deaths
Per average day: 27,600 deaths

**7% Chronic respiratory diseases**
COPD, Asthma, and others

**3.9% Neurological diseases**
Alzheimer's, Parkinson's, epilepsy, and others

**4.5% Digestive diseases**
Cirrhosis and others

**2.7% Diabetes**

**5.7% Other noncommunicable diseases**

**14% Died from infectious diseases**

**4.4% Pneumonia**
and other lower respiratory diseases
Per year: 2.5 million deaths
Per average day: 6,800 deaths

**2.7% Diarrheal diseases**
Per year: 1.5 million deaths
Per average day: 4,200 deaths

**2% Tuberculosis**

**1.5% HIV/AIDS**

**1.1% Malaria**

**2.1% Other infectious diseases**

**3.3% Neonatal deaths**
Babies who died within the first 28 days of life

**0.4% Maternal deaths**

**0.4% Nutritional deficiencies**

**2.3% Transport accidents**
Per year: 1.3 million deaths
Per average day: 3,500 deaths

**3.1% Other accidents**
Including falls, drownings, and fires.

**1.3% Suicides**
Per year: 760,000 deaths
Per average day: 2,080 deaths

**0.7% Homicides**
Per year: 415,000 deaths
Per average day: 1,140 deaths

**Fig. 36.1:** Leading 10 cause of deaths globally in 2019.
*Source:* IHME Global Burden of Diseases, www.ourworldindata.org.

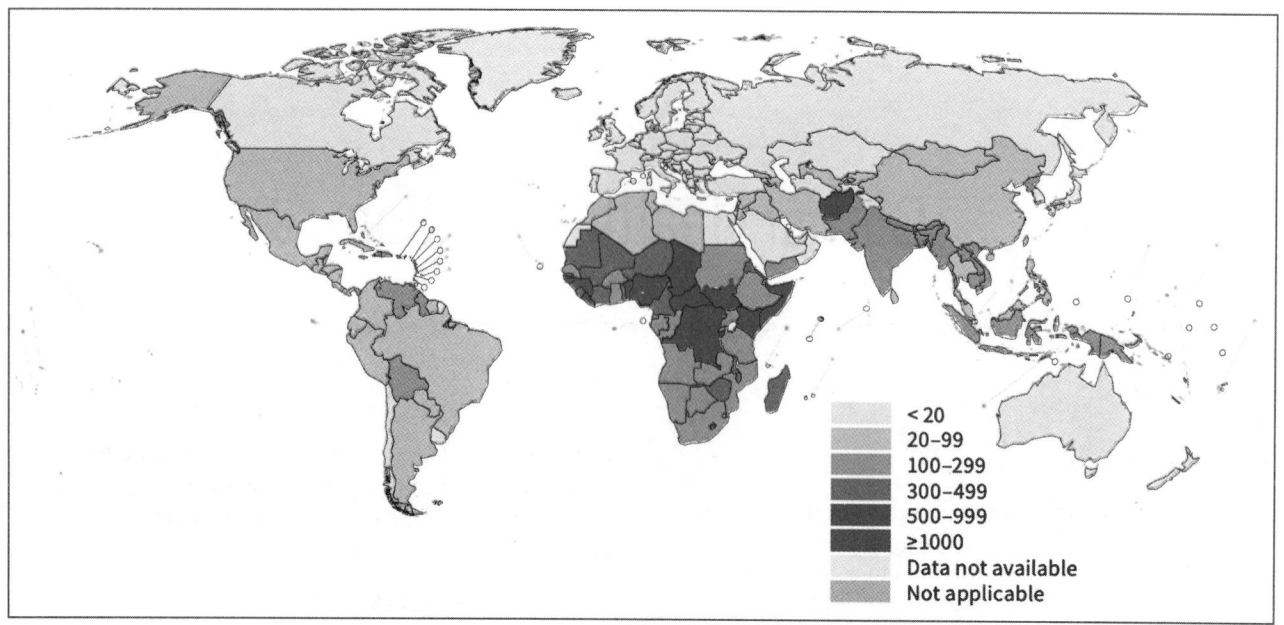

**Fig. 36.2:** Maternal mortality ratio (Maternal deaths per 100,000 live births), 2020.
*Source:* Trends in maternal mortality 2000 to 2020: estimates by WHO, UNICEF, UNFPA, World Bank Group and UNDESA/Population Division. Geneva: World Health Organization; 2023.

during pregnancy, childbirth and postnatal period. Morbidity and mortality in women due to pregnancy and childbirth is mainly concentrated in low- and middle-income countries **(Fig. 36.2)**. A report released by WHO along with several other UN organizations reported that globally, an estimated 2,87,000 maternal deaths occurred in 2020, yielding an overall MMR of 223 maternal deaths per 100 000 live births. This corresponds to almost 800 maternal deaths every day, and approximately one maternal death every two minutes globally. For 2020, the global lifetime risk of maternal mortality was estimated at 1 in 210; this means for a girl aged 15 years in 2020, there is, on average, a 1 in 210 risk that she will die from a maternal cause (WHO, UNICEF, UNFPA, World Bank Group and the UN Population Division, Trends in maternal mortality: 2000 to 2020). The major complications that account for nearly 75% of all maternal deaths are:

- Severe bleeding (mostly bleeding after childbirth)
- Infections (usually after childbirth)
- High blood pressure during pregnancy (pre-eclampsia and eclampsia)
- Complications from delivery
- Unsafe abortion

Access to good quality care before, during and after childbirth plays very important role in reducing maternal morbidity and mortality. WHO recommends early initiation of antenatal care, first antenatal visit in first trimester of pregnancy which provides opportunity for early diagnosis and timely management of antenatal conditions which may have adverse impact on health of the mother or child or both. However, estimates indicated that globally more than 40% of pregnant women did not receive early antenatal care (Moller AB et al., Lancet Global Health, 2017). Available data indicate that more than 90% of all births were attended by a trained midwife, doctor or nurse in most high-income and upper-middle-income countries while in several low- and middle-income countries only less than half of births were assisted by such skilled health personnel (UNICEF/WHO, Joint Database 2018 of Skilled Health Personnel, 2018).

An estimated 16% of women of reproductive age globally have unmet family planning need. This indicates, at the population level, the gap between women's reproductive intentions and their contraceptive behavior. (Department of Economic and Social Affairs, Estimates and Projections of Family Planning Indicators, 2022). Latest estimates point out that in 2015 around 12.8 million babies were delivered by adolescent girls aged 15–19 years. This can have significant health consequences on adolescent girls and the child they bear (UN, World Population Prospects, 2018).

## Child Health

There has been noticeable improvement in child mortality, with the global under-five mortality rate dropping to 38 per 1,000 live births in 2021. However, in 2021, 5 million children died before turning 5 years old. That's around 14,000 deaths every day, or ten every minute, due to one or the other reason, mostly avoidable. Children mortality is highest in first month of life, with 2.3 million newborns dying in first month of their life in 2021. Majority of these deaths occurred in the first week of life. Birth asphyxia, injury during delivery, and neonatal sepsis accounted for almost three quarters of all neonatal deaths (Estimates developed by the United Nations Inter-agency Group for Child Mortality Estimation, 2022). Children continue to face widely differing chances of survival based on where they are born **(Figure 36.3)**.

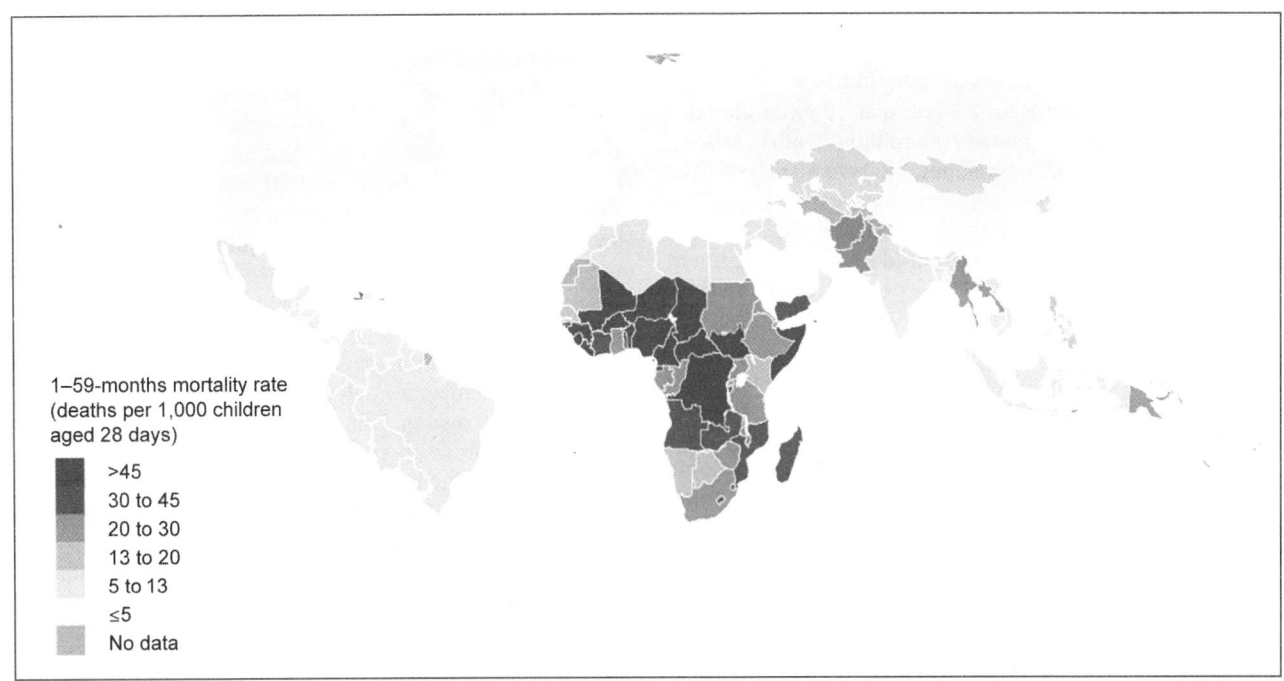

**Fig. 36.3:** Child mortality rate (Under five deaths per 1000 live births), 2021.
*Source:* Estimates developed by the United Nations Inter-agency Group for Child Mortality Estimation, 2022.

Under nutrition is a great challenge to health of the children, especially in WHO South East Asia region and WHO African region. Globally in 2022, estimated 148 million children below 5 years (22%) were stunted (short height for their age), with 3 out of 4 living in the WHO South East Asia region or WHO African region. In the same year, 45 million children below 5 years (6.8%) were wasted (low weight for their height), while 37 million (5.5%) were overweight (overweight for their height). In WHO Eastern Mediterranean region both undernutrition and overnutrition (obesity) coexist in a population (UNICEF/WHO/World Bank Group Joint Child Malnutrition Estimates, Levels and Trends in Child Malnutrition, 2022).

## Aging

Populations across the globe are rapidly aging. An estimated 524 million people (8% of world's population) were aged 65 years or above. This number is projected to rise about 1.5 billion (16% of world's population) by 2050 (WHO, Global Health and Aging, 2018). Increase in proportion of aged population in low- and middle-income countries is mainly due to gross decrease in mortality at younger ages, especially during childbirth, infancy and childhood period. Increase in aged population in high-income countries is mainly a result of declining mortality among those who are older. Aging presents unique challenges to the healthcare infrastructure and demand a comprehensive community health response. Two facts worth noting are: (1) Not only is the absolute number of old people increasing, but also the pace of this change is very high, which means countries have lesser time to cope with the changing population structure. (2) Larger proportion of this increase in geriatric population is going to take place in low- and middle-income countries, which already have limited resources to deal with existing health problems of their population. Other than cardiovascular diseases and geriatric syndrome (comprising of pathological states typical of aging like dementia, delirium, incontinence, vertigo, falls, spontaneous bone fractures, failure to thrive, etc.), psychosocial issues, such as depression, neglect, isolation and elder abuse, bear a huge burden on geriatric population.

## Infectious Diseases

Globally, HIV, TB and malaria remain the leading causes of death among the infectious diseases. There were approximately 39 million people living with HIV/AIDS worldwide at the end of 2022, and 1.3 million people becoming newly infected globally in 2022. Most affected region is the WHO African Region followed by Southeast Asian region. In 2022, 6,30,000 people died from HIV-related causes. When considering all people living with HIV, 86% knew their status, 76% were receiving antiretroviral therapy and 71% had suppressed viral loads (WHO, HIV-AIDS Key Facts, 2023).

Another important infectious disease is Tuberculosis (TB) which is present in humanity since ancient times. TB is a preventable and usually curable disease. Yet in 2022, TB was the world's second leading cause of death from a single infectious agent, after coronavirus disease (COVID-19), and caused almost twice as many deaths as HIV/AIDS. Globally, the estimated TB incidence rate (new cases per 1,00,000 population per year) was 133 in 2022. The net reduction from 2015 to 2022 was 8.7%, far from the WHO End TB Strategy milestone of a 50% reduction by 2025. The reported global number of people newly diagnosed with TB was 7.5 million in 2022. This is the highest number since WHO began global TB monitoring in 1995 and up from 6.4

million in 2021. The number in 2022 probably includes a sizeable backlog of people who developed TB in previous years, but whose diagnosis and treatment was delayed by COVID-related disruptions. India accounts for 27% of total TB cases globally. In 2022, TB caused an estimated 1.30 million deaths globally. In 2022, 55% of people who developed TB were men, 33% were women and 12% were children (aged 0 -14 years). About 50% of TB patients and their households face total costs that are catastrophic (>20% of annual household income). Treatment success rates have improved: to 88% for people treated for drug-susceptible TB and 63% for people with MDR/RR-TB (Global TB Report, WHO, 2023).

Malaria also remains important cause of mortality and morbidity globally. There is no significant improvement in the situation since last many years. Globally in 2022, there were an estimated 249 million malaria cases in 85 malaria endemic countries and areas. In 2015, the baseline year of the Global technical strategy for malaria 2016 -2030 (GTS), there were an estimated 231 million malaria cases. In 2022, malaria case incidence was 58 per 1000 population at risk as against 81 per 1000 population at risk in 2000. In 2022, India accounted for 66% of cases in the southeast region. Almost 46% of all cases in the region were due to P. vivax. Sri Lanka was certified malaria free in 2016 and remains malaria free. Globally, malaria deaths declined steadily from 8,64,000 in 2000 to 6,08,000 in 2023. Globally, the malaria mortality rate (i.e. deaths per 1,00,000 population at risk) halved from about 29 in 2000 to 14.3 in 2022. Lack of consistent funding, civic conflict in endemic area, irregular climate patterns, resistance to insecticides and anti-malarial drugs are the main challenges in control of malaria (World Malaria Report, WHO, 2023).

Viral hepatitis accounts for a significant global disease burden and high mortality from liver cancer and cirrhosis. In 2019, 296 million people were living with chronic hepatitis B virus infection and 58 million people with chronic hepatitis C virus infection worldwide. New estimates show that total 3.0 million people newly acquire hepatitis B and hepatitis C virus infection each year. Viral hepatitis caused 1.1 million deaths in 2019, 96% of which were caused by hepatitis B and C virus. Most of these deaths result from chronic liver disease and liver cancer. People from economically disadvantaged regions, displaced people and migrants, and rural populations are more severely affected. Further, injecting drug use is a major contributor to the hepatitis C epidemic globally. Other affected population groups include health-care workers exposed through needle-stick injuries, people in prisons and closed settings, and men who have sex with men. Among people living with HIV, untreated hepatitis coinfection promotes more rapid progression of hepatitis B - and/or C -related liver disease, hepatocellular cancer, and untimely death, undermining the gains of effective HIV treatment. HIV coinfection doubles the risk of mother-to-child transmission of viral hepatitis (Global Progress Report on Viral Hepatitis, 2021).

Apart from above mentioned diseases, neglected tropical diseases (NTDs) are another group of diseases which, as the name suggests, neglected over the years. Due to negligence, their estimated are highly under-reported.

## Noncommunicable Diseases

Noncommunicable diseases (NCDs) kill 41 million people each year, equivalent to 74% of all deaths globally. Each year, 17 million people die from a NCD before age 70; 86% of these premature deaths occur in low- and middle-income countries. Cardiovascular diseases account for most NCD deaths, or 17.9 million people annually, followed by cancers (9.3 million), chronic respiratory diseases (4.1 million), and diabetes (2.0 million including kidney disease deaths caused by diabetes). These four groups of diseases account for over 80% of all premature NCD deaths. (Global Health Estimates, WHO, 2023).

These diseases are driven by forces that include rapid unplanned urbanization, globalization of unhealthy lifestyles and population ageing. Unhealthy diets and a lack of physical activity may show up in people as raised blood pressure, increased blood glucose, elevated blood lipids and obesity. These are called metabolic risk factors and can lead to cardiovascular disease, the leading NCD in terms of premature deaths.

Tobacco use is a major and important risk factor for cardiovascular disease, cancers, and chronic respiratory disease. The tobacco epidemic is one of the biggest public health threats the world has ever faced, killing over 8 million people a year around the world including an estimated 1.3 million non-smokers who are exposed to second-hand smoke. Around 80% of the world's 1.3 billion tobacco users live in low- and middle-income countries. In 2020, 22.3% of the world's population used tobacco: 36.7% of men and 7.8% of women. Along with individual health, tobacco has enormously negative social, environmental and economic impact (WHO Report on Global Tobacco Epidemic, 2023).

The worldwide level of alcohol consumption trends varies widely across WHO regions. Consumption of alcohol in the WHO South-East Asia region rose by almost 30% since 2010, while that of the WHO European region declined by 12%, but remaining the highest in the world (WHO, GISAH, 2018).

## Mental Health

Pre-pandemic, in 2019, an estimated 970 million people (13% of global population) in the world are living with a mental disorder, 82% of whom were in low- and middle-income countries. The prevalence of mental disorders varies with sex and age. In both males and females, anxiety disorders and depressive disorders are the two most common mental disorders. Anxiety disorders become prevalent at an earlier age than depressive disorders, which are rare before ten years of age. They continue to become more common in later life, with highest estimates in people between 50 and 69. Among adults, depressive disorders are the most prevalent of all mental disorders (World Mental Health Report, WHO, 2022). It is obvious that psychiatric illnesses are often disabling, and this is reflected in the markedly higher proportion of overall disease burden caused by the mental disorders. Untreated mental disorders also cause mortality due to suicide. Worldwide, suicide is a major cause for concern. According to the WHO, every year, almost 1 million people lose their life in suicide; a "global" mortality rate of 16 per 100,000 population or 1 death every 40 seconds and rising every year

(WHO Mental Health: Suicide Prevention). The biggest risk for suicide is poorly diagnosed and untreated mental disease.

### Injuries and Violence

Worldwide approximately 1.19 million people were killed by road traffic accidents every year and another 50 million were injured (WHO, Global Health Estimates, 2023, WHo Factsheet). The death rate due to road traffic accidents was 2.6 times higher in low-income countries compared to high-income countries.

Violence against children and women has lifelong impacts on the health and well-being of individual, families, communities and nations. Recent estimates indicate that globally almost one out of four adults (23%) suffered physical abuse in childhood and about one in three women (35%) experienced physical and/or sexual violence at some point of time in their life (WHO, Global and regional estimates of violence against women, 2013).

### Environmental Risks

Poor access to clean fuels and efficient technologies for cooking forced over 3 billion people cooking with polluting fuel and inefficient stove combinations in 2016. The resulting household air pollution has caused estimated 3.8 million deaths from NCDs (including heart disease, stroke and cancer) and acute lower respiratory infections in 2016. In 2016, across the world more than half of population living in urban area were exposed to outdoor air pollution leading to 4.2 million deaths. Combined, indoor and outdoor, air pollution leads to an estimated 7 million deaths, one out of eight deaths, globally every year (WHO, GHO data, Public Health and Environment, 2022, WHO Fact Sheets).

Unsafe drinking water, unsafe sanitation and lack of hygiene are also other important causes of death, with approximately 829,000 associated deaths occurring every year (March 2023, UNICEF Report). Unintentional poisonings were responsible for over 100,000 deaths in 2016 relatively higher in low-income countries (Jacob KS et al., Lancet, 2014).

### Occupational Health and Safety

Health and safety at workplace are important contributors of overall health status of the global population, especially adult. Workplace Safety and Health Institute estimated annual 2.78 million deaths globally attributed to work and workplace environment in 2015. Work-related mortality contributed 5% of the world total deaths. Work and workplace environment related mortality accounted for 86.3% of the total estimated deaths and fatal accidents at workplace accounted for the remaining 13.7%. Health and safety of worker have improved a lot in most high-income countries. However, a lot needs to be done in middle- and low-income countries to improve workers' safety (Ministry of Social Affairs and Health, Global Estimates of Occupational Accidents and work related illnesses 2017).

### Other Important Causes of Mortality and Morbidity

Natural disaster accounted for approximately 11,000 annual deaths globally. Low- and lower-middle-income countries typically have higher burden. Murders account for estimated 477,000 deaths globally in 2016, with highest rate in the WHO Region of the Americas (31.8% per 100,000 population). Estimated 180,000 people were killed in wars and conflicts directly in 2016. The death due to conflicts in last 5 years is almost double that the previous 5-year period (WHO, Global Health Estimates 2016, 2018).

## SUMMARY

| Sr. No. | Indicator | Current global status |
|---|---|---|
| 1. | Maternal deaths | 2.87 lakhs (2020) |
| 2. | Infant deaths | 39 lakhs (2021) |
| 3. | Neonatal deaths | 23 lakhs (2021) |
| 4. | Under 5 mortality rate | 50 lakhs (2021) |
| 5. | Children under 5 years who are stunted | 1,480 lakhs (2021) |
| 6. | Children under 5 years who are wasted (weight-for-height) | 450 lakhs (2021) |
| 7. | Children who are overweight | 370 lakhs (2021) |
| 9. | People living with HIV | 390 lakhs (2022) |
| 10. | Total AIDS related deaths till date | 404 lakhs (2019) |
| 11. | Newly diagnosed TB cases | 75 lakhs (in 2022) |
| 12. | Deaths due to TB | 13 lakhs (2022) |
| 13. | Malaria cases | 2,490 lakhs (2022) |
| 14. | Malaria deaths | 6.08 lakhs (2023) |
| 15. | Hepatitis cases | 3,540 lakhs (2019) |
| 16. | Hepatitis deaths | 11 lakhs (2019) |
| 17. | NCD mortality | 410 lakhs (2023) |
| 18. | Deaths from road traffic accidents | 11.9 lakhs (Estimated Every Year, 2023 WHO factsheet) |
| 19. | Unintentional poisoning deaths | 1 lakh (2016) |
| 20. | Deaths due to air pollution | 70 lakhs (Estimated Every year, WHO factsheet 2022)) |
| 21. | Deaths due to unsafe drinking water and sanitation | 8.2 lakhs (Estimated Every year, 2023 UNICEF) |

## SUGGESTED READING

1. Ministry of Social Affairs and Health. (2017). Global Estimates of Occupational Accidents and Work-related Illnesses 2017. Workplace Safety and Health Institute. Singapore 2017.
2. Trends in maternal mortality: 2000 to 2017. Estimates by WHO, UNICEF, UNFPA, World Bank Group and the United Nations Population Division. Geneva: World Health Organization; 2019.
3. United Nations Children's Fund. (2017). Levels and Trends in Child Mortality. Report 2017. Estimates developed by the UN Inter-agency Group for Child Mortality Estimation. United Nations Children's Fund, World Health Organization, World Bank and United Nations. New York (NY): United Nations Children's Fund; 2017.
4. WHO global report on trends in prevalence of tobacco smoking 2000–2025, second edition. Geneva: World Health Organization; 2018.
5. World Health Organization. (2015). Global status report on road safety 2015. Geneva: World Health Organization; 2015.
6. World Health Organization. (2018). Global Health and Aging.
7. World Health Organization. (2018). Global Health Estimates 2016: Deaths by cause, age, sex, by country and by region, 2000–2016. Geneva: World Health Organization; 2018.

8. World Health Organization. (2018). HIV/AIDS [online database]. Global Health Observatory (GHO) data. Geneva: World Health Organization.
9. World Health Organization. (2018). Levels and trends in child malnutrition: UNICEF/WHO/World Bank Group Joint child malnutrition estimates; Key findings of the 2018 edition. New York (NY), Geneva and Washington (DC): United Nations Children's Fund, World Health Organization and World Bank Group; 2018.
10. World Health Organization. (2018). Public health and environment [online database]. Global Health Observatory (GHO) data. Geneva: World Health Organization.
11. World Health Organization. (2018). WHO Global Information System on Alcohol and Health (GISAH) [online database]. Global Health Observatory (GHO) data. Geneva: World Health Organization.
12. World Health Organization. (2019). Global tuberculosis report 2019. Geneva: World Health Organization; 2019.
13. World Health Organization. (2019). World malaria report 2019. Geneva: World Health Organization; 2019.
14. World Health Organization: The Global Burden of Disease: 2004 Update. Geneva: World Health Organization; 2008.
15. World Health Organization [Internet]. Mental health: suicide prevention (SUPRE).

# CHAPTER 37

# Community Health

*Manish Kumar Singh*

| | |
|---|---|
| CM 1.7 | Enumerate and describe health indicators regarding community health |
| CM 17.1 | Define and describe the concept of health care to community |
| CM 17.2 | Describe community diagnosis |

## INTRODUCTION

A community is a diverse group of people living in a defined geographical area with common goals, interests, experiences, norms, values, and organization. People living in a nearby residential apartment, people in slums, migrant laborers, people with a common occupation (i.e., doctors, healthcare workers) or common interests (environmentalists) all constitute a community. Community influences the health status of an individual.

McKenzie and his colleagues in 2005 defined community health as "health status of a group of people and the actions/conditions both private and public to promote, protect, and preserve their health". Community health requires multisectoral and multidisciplinary collaboration for health promotion, disease prevention, diagnosis, treatment, and rehabilitation. Community health can be described as health of the people, by the people, and for the people. It is influenced by developments in other sectors/disciplines such as agriculture, education, science and technology, power, and human resource development, etc.

Community health activities such as maintenance of birth/death records, provision of food and water supply, building of household/community toilets, clean surroundings, and safe disposal of animal/human waste influence the health of the overall community. Each community has a different health status determined by various factors, some of which can be modified to bring about a positive change in health status of the community.

## FACTORS INFLUENCING COMMUNITY HEALTH (FIG. 37.1)

### Physical Factors

It comprises the influence of geographical location (altitude, latitude, and climate), environment, community size, and industrial growth, etc. In tropical countries, parasitic and infectious diseases, and malnutrition is a common community health problem. The warm, humid climate and rainfall throughout the year favors spread of parasitic/infectious diseases and the poor soil conditions contribute to inadequate food production and consequently malnutrition. In temperate climate countries non-communicable diseases such as obesity, cardiovascular diseases, etc. are important community health problems.

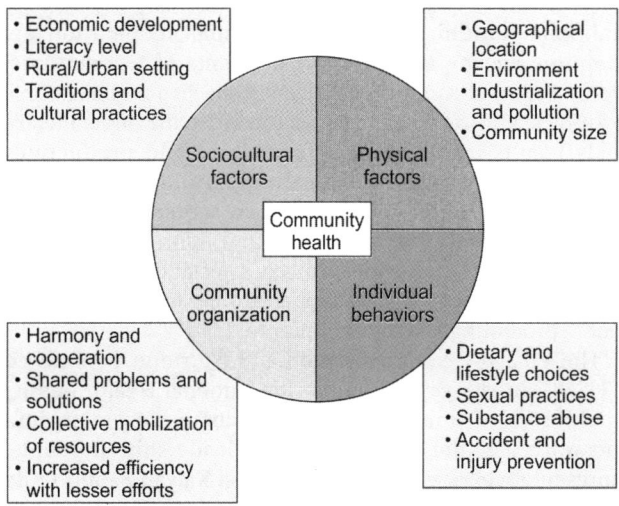

**Fig. 37.1:** Factors influencing community health.

Environmental pollution resulting from community practices and industrial growth has been documented to lead to cardiovascular and respiratory mortality and morbidity.

Community size and industrial development can impact community's health either way. Community size is an advantage, if the community can plan, organize, and use its resources in an effective manner. Larger communities have a greater range of health problems, but at the same time also have adequate health professionals and better facilities compared to smaller communities. Industrial development generates additional resources for community health programs, but at the same time also leads to environmental pollution, overcrowding, occupational injuries, and illness.

### Socioeconomic and Cultural Factors

A community with poor socioeconomic status has poverty, illiteracy, people are deprived of basic necessities, lack access to proper nutrition, sanitation, quality health care, etc. Such communities have increased likelihood of being exposed to environment hazards, and also more likely to be subject to crime and violence. Economically developed communities with good living conditions have problems such as increase in incidence of cardiovascular diseases, cancers, road traffic accidents, etc. that mostly result from modifiable risk factors. Urban community has higher stress-related illnesses compared to rural community. Rural communities lack access to quality health care. Cultural factors such as giving prelacteal feed, not feeding colostrum contribute to infant mortality. Traditions like child marriage lead to increased risk of maternal mortality and bigger family size. Some cultural practices like brushing teeth before the first meal of the day have a positive impact on health. Cultural practices determine policy decisions and regulations. High preference for male child and female feticide in the community led to the regulation of Pre-conception and Prenatal Diagnostic Techniques Act (PCPNDT). Religion also has impact on health care and health behavior.

## Community Organization

Mahatma Gandhi believed that mutual cooperation and common sharing are the basic elements of a community. Identification of common problems, collective mobilization of resources, and working together toward achieving collective goals results in increased effectiveness and productivity. Community organization reduces duplication of efforts and avoids imposition of solutions not in agreement with local culture and needs. Various formal and informal community organizations of authorities, citizen, special groups, socially-culturally-intellectually like-minded groups, etc. can contribute a lot in promoting healthy community.

The Village Health Sanitation and Nutrition Committees (VHSNC) at village level under the National Health Mission (NHM) seek to promote ability of the community to organize and work together under the active leadership of people's representatives at grass root level. Rogi Kalyan Samiti under NHM involves community members, Panchayati Raj Institution members, and NGOs in the management of services at public sector hospitals.

## Individual Behavior

Individual behavior issues that are of concern include diet and physical activity, tobacco and alcohol consumption, drug intake, sexual activity, use of personal road safety measures, etc. Personal activities such as exercise, balanced diet, and wearing seat belt, etc. promote or protect one's own health.

The factors discussed above are all key determinants for community health. However, each of them has different impact on the health of the community. This can be best explained by the Centers for Disease Control and Prevention (CDC) 5-tier *health impact pyramid* (**Fig. 37.2**). As we move up the pyramid interventions have progressively lesser impact and require more individual effort. Actions and interventions at the socioeconomic factors level that form the base of the pyramid such as education, housing, employment, poverty alleviation, etc. have the maximum impact on community health and require very less individual effort.

The second level of the pyramid comprises interventions that seek to change the environment context, so as to make healthy life options the choice by default regardless of the socioeconomic and other factors. Fluoridated water supply, sale of only iodized salt, clean air/water/food, etc. not only improves health and but also reduces loss of productivity and health expenditure.

The third level of pyramid comprises long-lasting protective interventions applied either once or frequently (e.g., immunization, colonoscopy at regular intervals, smoking cessation programs, etc.). Fourth level of pyramid refers to evidence-based clinical care interventions. The overall impact of these interventions is limited due to lack of accessibility, unpredictable effectiveness, and adherence. At the top of the pyramid are counseling and educational interventions. They have the smallest impact on community health, although if applied consistently and repeatedly may bring considerable change. This model needs to be kept in view when designing interventions for community health.

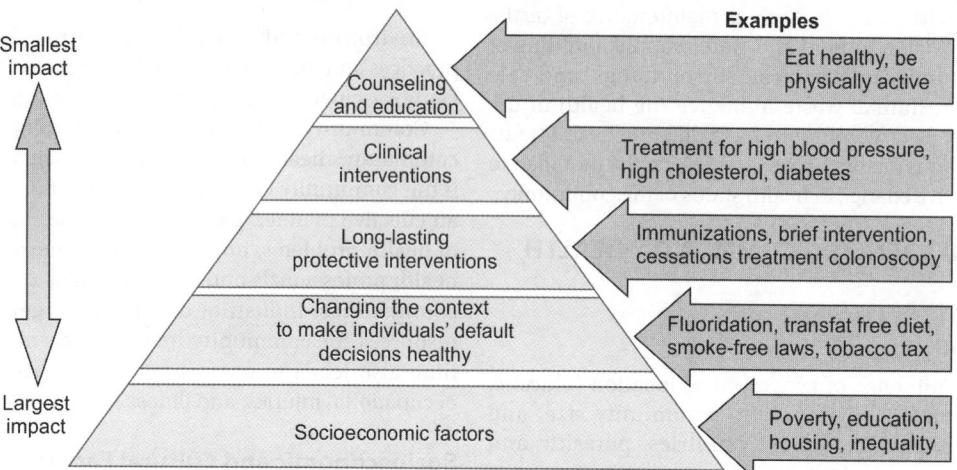

**Fig. 37.2:** CDC 5 Tier health impact pyramid.

## HEALTHY COMMUNITY

Healthy community is defined as "A community where people come together to make their community better for themselves, their family, their friends, their neighbors and others". A healthy community exerts control over the decisions affecting their life, health, and well-being. Healthy community has the following characteristics (**Fig. 37.3**):

- *Stable, sustainable ecosystem, and safe environment:* Ecosystem imbalance affects climate, environment, agriculture, and availability of natural resources thus directly and indirectly influencing health of community. Communities need to maintain a safe environment to keep them healthy. Changing ecological system leads to emergence of diseases not seen by the native community.
- *Healthy policies:* Healthy policies guide the government to develop and implement various programs and legislations for making healthy community. Healthy policies mean policy on health and related sector such as environment, nutrition, etc. or policies on vulnerable groups such as children, women, occupational worker, geriatric people or tribal group, etc.
- *Community participation:* It helps the community to identify its health problems and needs, develop culturally and socially acceptable solutions, strategies to problems, take responsibility for their health and welfare thus ensuring its sustainability.

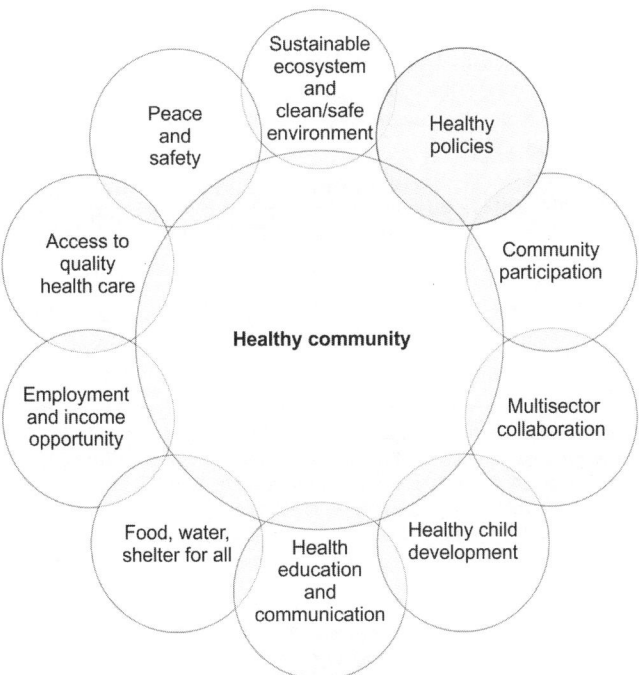

Fig. 37.3: Characteristics of a healthy community.

- *Multisectoral collaboration:* Sectors other than health, such as education, industry, and agriculture, etc. also have an impact on health. Multisectoral collaboration helps achieve effective, efficient, and sustainable health outcomes.
- *Healthy child development:* Healthy community has a good system for child nutrition and educational opportunities. Healthy child development sustains the healthy community.
- *Health education and communication:* It provides new knowledge, arouses interest, brings about change in attitude, leads to acquisition of skills, and finally adoption of health promoting life style and practices. It also promotes the use of health services.
- *Availability of food, water, and shelter:* A community with access to safe source of water and good nutrition is immune to infections and nutritional deficiency disorders, and enjoys life to its full potential. Community health is threatened by contaminated and polluted water.
  People are at constant threat from environment surrounding them. Hence, they require a safe and secure shelter from which they can access basic amenities, education, and vocational opportunities.
- *Employment and income opportunity:* Ample income and employment opportunities for individuals in a community result in better access to and availability of the basic amenities, i.e., food, housing, education, and healthcare services.
- *Access to quality health care:* Every year thousands of people die because of preventable and curable health problems such as diarrhea, tuberculosis, etc. The reason being lack of access to quality healthcare services. A healthy community has access to affordable and acceptable quality healthcare for prevention and promotion of health, diagnosis, and cure of disease/illness and rehabilitation.
- *Peace and safety:* War, riots, internal conflicts, insurgency, political instability, arson, loot, and high crime rate in the community adversely affects the community health. It directly affects with injuries and death and indirectly affects with disruption of services and reduction of educational and economical opportunities. To be a healthy community; peace and safety are equally important as safe and clean environment.

> **Hiware Bazaar: Story of a village transformation to a healthy community.**
>
> Hiware bazaar is a village in Ahmed Nagar district of Maharashtra. It is an inspirational example about how community organization and working together toward a common goal can transform individual lives in a community. Before 1989, it was drought prone and facing migration of villagers, high crime and water scarcity. Majority of its population lived below the poverty line. By the year 2010, the average income of the villagers increased many folds. 50 villagers had an average annual income between INR 1,000,000 and 1,200,000 and only three families were below the poverty line.
>
> This became possible due to community ownership and participation. The community started drip-irrigation, rainwater harvesting, and switched to alternate crops that needed less water. The community imposed ban on liquor, adopted family planning, and promoted voluntary labor for development of the village. This led to improved socioeconomic status in the village. The village was declared as an "ideal village" by the Government of Maharashtra and received the "National Water Award" by the Government of India in 2007.

*Source*: The greening of Hiware Bazaar in Maharashtra, The Hindu, March 25, 2017.

## MEASURING COMMUNITY HEALTH: CONCEPT AND PURPOSE

To determine the health status of an individual, we often use a battery of tests that give various measurements, e.g., blood pressure, respiratory rate, temperature, hemoglobin level, blood counts, renal function test, pulmonary function test, liver function test, and so on. Some tests give idea about a specific organ or system affected while some tests give information about the general health status.

Similarly, to determine the health status of a community, a set of indicators of basic demographic, socioeconomic, environmental characteristics, health status, and health services, e.g., infant mortality, maternal mortality, incidence/prevalence rate of tuberculosis/HIV, etc., are used. Some of these indicators give an idea regarding health status of a specific vulnerable population group or burden of a specific health problem in a community. To know the overall health status of a community often a set of various indicators are combined to get a composite index.

Community health is measured to identify major health issues, prevalent risk factors/cause and to plan delivery of effective health care to address these issues. It helps to apply principles of equity and social justice in designing and implementation of health programs accessible and acceptable to the community.

Community health measurement indicators can be broadly classified as shown in **(Table 37.1)**. *Disease specific, group specific and health status indicators are already discussed in Chapters 9, 24 and 25.*

## Socioeconomic Indicators

While overall community health indicators give idea about the health status of community, specific indicators for disease and vulnerable groups help in reducing the burden of specific diseases affecting community health and improving health status of vulnerable groups. Socioeconomic status has an impact on utilization of health care services as well as susceptibility to diseases and thus overall health of the community. Hence, the knowledge regarding the socioeconomic status of the community and collective measures to improve it is very essential for a healthy community.

### People Living Below Poverty Line

Poverty line is the minimum income/expenditure needed to purchase a set of goods and services necessary to satisfy basic human needs.

In India, "*Poverty line*" prior to 2005 was based on food security and was defined as expenditure needed for a daily calorie intake of 2,400 and 2,100 per person in rural and urban areas, respectively. It did not take into account other basic requirements of the poor, such as housing, clothing, education, health, etc.

The Tendulkar Committee revised poverty line in 2011-2012 and defined poverty line as income of INR 228.9 per capita per month or INR 27 per person per day in rural area and INR 264.1 per capita per month or INR 33 per person per day in urban area (at 1993-1994 prices). As per the Tendulkar Committee, 21.9% (269.78 million) of India's population lived below the "poverty line".

This was further revised by the Rangarajan Committee that suggested the urban poverty line as income of INR 47 per person per day (INR 1,407 per person per month or INR 7,035 per family of five per month) and rural poverty line as INR 32 per person per day areas (INR 972 per person per month or INR 4,860 per family of five per month). As per this report, 29.5% of India's population lived below the "poverty line".

In 2015, World Bank defined *International poverty line* as USD 1.90 per head per day of purchasing power parity. As per 2012 estimates, about 900 million people (12.8% of global population) lived in extreme poverty. The SDGs target is to bring down the number of people living in extreme poverty to less than 3% of the world population by 2030.

### Literacy Level

Literacy level in a community is an indicator of its level of development. Higher level of education and literacy contribute to improvement in socioeconomic conditions. A literate is a person 7 years and more in age, who can read, write, and understand any language. As per 2011 census, literacy rates in India stand at 74%.

$$\text{Crude literacy rate} = \frac{\text{Number of literate persons}}{\text{Total population}} \times 100$$

$$\text{Effective literacy rate} = \frac{\text{Number of literate persons aged 7 years and above}}{\text{Total population aged 7 years and above}} \times 100$$

> Gender-wise male literacy stands at 81% and female literacy stands at 65%. The gap between male and female literacy rates has declined from 21.6% in 2001 to 16.7% in 2011, but is still short of the target set by planning commission of 10% for the year 2011-2012. State wise, Kerala has the highest literacy rates at 93.9%, whereas Bihar has the lowest literacy rates at 62%.

**Table 37.1:** Indicators used for community health measurement under various categories.

| Diseases specific | Group specific | General health status | Socioeconomic status | Health service delivery related | Overall community well-being |
|---|---|---|---|---|---|
| • Incidence<br>• Prevalence<br>• DALY<br>• QALY<br>• Case fatality rate<br>• Survival rate | • IMR<br>• MMR<br>• Under 5 mortality rate<br>• Neonatal mortality rate | • Crude death rate<br>• Standardized death rates<br>• Life expectancy at birth<br>• HALE | • People living below poverty line<br>• Literacy level<br>• Villages/town with availability of safe drinking water<br>• Household with toilet | • Doctor-population ratio<br>• Immunization rate<br>• Couple protection rate<br>• Out of pocket expenditure | • Standards of living<br>• Level of living and quality of life<br>• PQLI<br>• HDI<br>• MPI |

(DALY: disability adjusted life year; HALE: health-adjusted life expectancy; HDI: human development index; IMR: infant mortality rate; MMR: maternal mortality ratio; MPI: multidimensional poverty index; PQLI: physical quality of life index; QALY: quality-adjusted life year)

## Household with Toilet

As per the census 2011, 46.9% households had toilet (Latrine) facility available within the premises and only about 3.2% households used public latrine. Nearly 50% households still practice open defecation. To achieve universal sanitation coverage, "Swachh Bharat Mission" was launched on 2nd October, 2014. About 7.8 crore household toilets have been built since then. 4 lakh villages are now open defecation free. 19 states/UT and 417 districts have become open defecation free.

## Availability of Safe Drinking Water

As on 1st April 2017, about 13 lakh habitations across India had access to safe drinking water under the National Rural Drinking Water Programme.

As per census 2011, about 46.6% households had a drinking water source available within their premises and about 35.8% households had a drinking water source available near the premises. About 17.6% households had to travel away to get water.

A major issue with safe drinking water availability is the maintenance of the source and many sources get nonfunctional with use. This is mainly due to lack of community participation, lack of ownership by the people, resulting in neglect in maintenance.

## Health Service-related Indicators

They measure the availability, accessibility, expenditure on health, coverage, and utilization of health services. It helps in effective work force and program planning and management.

### Doctor-population Ratio

As per, World Health Organization, doctor-population ratio should be of 1:1,000. In India, currently there are 13.08 lakh registered allopathic doctors. Assuming 80% availability of registered allopathic doctors and 5.65 lakh active AYUSH doctors, the doctor-population ratio in the country is 1:834 (Press Information Bureau, MoHFW, GoI, July 2022).

### Out of Pocket Expenditure

OOPE is usually incurred when an individual's visit to healthcare provider (clinic/hospital/pharmacy/laboratory etc.) is not provided for `free' through a government health facility or a facility run by a not-for-profit organization or if this individual is not covered under a government/private health insurance or social protection scheme.

OOPE are a burden to all households as they are incurred during a health event when the household is already in distress. Household's OOPE usually higher than 10% of total household consumption expenditure is catastrophic and it might push the household below the poverty line leading to impoverishment.

In 2019-20, Household's Out of Pocket Expenditure on health (OOPE) was 47.07% of total health expenditure for India (which is 1.54% of GDP, and Rs. 2,289 per capita). Private Health Insurance expenditure was 6.99% of total health expenditure for India. (National Health Accounts 2019-2020).

# OVERALL COMMUNITY WELL-BEING INDICATORS

## Standards of Living/Level of Living

*Standard/level of living* is a measure of level of wealth, comfort, goods, necessities, and services available to a population belonging to a particular socioeconomic class in a community. Standard of living includes (as per WHO)—(1) income and occupation, (2) standards of housing, sanitation and nutrition, and (3) level of provision of health, educational, recreational and other services.

## Quality of Life

It is one's own perception of his/her position in life with regards to the culture and values of the community he/she lives and to his/her goals, expectations, standards, and concerns.

> Standard of living and level of living are objective component of well-being, whereas quality of life is a subjective component of well-being.

## Physical Quality of Life Index

*Physical quality of life index (PQLI)* is a composite index of three indicators—*infant mortality rate, life expectancy at 1-year age, and level of literacy* with equal weightage to each of them. *Per capita gross national product (GNP)*, a measure of economic growth, is not taken into consideration. It measures results of socioeconomic and political policies and seeks to complement GNP. PQLI value ranges from 0 to 100. (0 = worst performance and 100 = best performance). Ultimate objective is to attain a PQLI of 100. *PQLI is applicable for international and national comparison. PQLI of India is 65.*

## Human Development Index

Human development index (HDI) summarizes average achievement in three key dimensions of human development:
1. Long and healthy life (Indicator—life expectancy at birth)
2. Knowledge (Indicator—mean years of schooling for adults aged 25 years and more and expected years of schooling for children of school going age). The expected years of schooling is capped at 18 years
3. Decent standard of living (Indicator—gross national income per capita). For calculating HDI logarithm of income is used. It shows the decrease in importance of income with increasing GNI. GNI per capita is capped at USD 75,000.

*Each of the above three components of HDI has a maximum and minimum values* **(Table 37.2)**:

$$\text{Dimension index} = \frac{\text{Actual value} - \text{minimum value}}{\text{Maximum value} - \text{minimum value}}$$

Table 37.2: Maximum and minimum value of key human development index components.

| Dimension | Maximum value | Minimum value (Subsistence values) |
|---|---|---|
| Life expectancy | 85 | 20.0 |
| Mean year of schooling | 15 | 0 |
| Expected year of schooling | 18 | 0 |
| Gross National Income per capita (PPP$) | 75,000 | 100 |

Human development index is the geometric mean of indices for each of the three dimensions, with equal weightage to all. Its value ranges between 0 and 1.

Human development index does not reflect on inequality, poverty, human security, empowerment, etc. Norway, Switzerland, and Australia rank the top 3 globally on HDI. India ranks 132 (With an HDI of 0.633) of the 189 countries globally in 2021.

Countries are also classified on basis of HDI as developed (HDI ≥ 0.8), developing (HDI 0.5–0.799), and underdeveloped country (HDI < 0.5) (UNDP, Human Development Report, 2019).

| HDI (0-1) mainly input indicators | | | PQLI (0-100) mainly outcome indicators | | |
|---|---|---|---|---|---|
| Life expectancy at birth | Schooling years | GN income | Life expectancy at 1 year | IMR | Literacy |

## Multidimensional Poverty Index (UNDP, Human Development Report, 2019)

It identifies how people are being left behind across three key dimensions: health, education, and standard of living. It comprises 10 indicators. People who are deprived of at least one-third of these weighted indicators fall into the category of multidimensionally poor. The global multidimensional poverty index (MPI), revised and updated in September 2018, now covers 105 countries in total, which are home to 77% of the world's population. In 2015-16, more than 364 million people were poor as per MPI in India **(Table 37.3)**.

**Table 37.3:** Multidimensional poverty index.

| Dimension | Indicator | Deprived if living in the household where | Weight |
|---|---|---|---|
| Health | Nutrition | An adult under 70 years of age or a child is undernourished | 1/6 |
| | Child mortality | Any child has died in the family in the five-year period preceding the survey | 1/6 |
| Education | Years of schooling | No household member aged 10 years or older has completed six years of schooling | 1/6 |
| | School attendance | Any school-aged child is not attending school up to the age at which he/she would complete class 8 | 1/6 |
| Standard of living | Cooking fuel | The household cooks with dung, wood, charcoal or coal | 1/18 |
| | Sanitation | The household's sanitation facility is not improved (according to SDG guidelines) or it is improved but shared with other households | 1/18 |
| | Drinking water | The household does not have access to improved drinking water (according to SDG guidelines) or safe drinking water is at least a 30-minute walk from home, round trip | 1/18 |
| | Electricity | The household has no electricity | 1/18 |
| | Housing | Housing materials for at least one of roof, walls and floor are inadequate: the floor is of natural materials and/or the roof and/or walls are of natural or rudimentary materials | 1/18 |
| | Assets | The household does not own more than one of these assets: radio, TV, telephone, computer, animal cart, bicycle, motorbike or refrigerator, and does not own a car or truck | 1/18 |

## COMMUNITY HEALTH NEEDS ASSESSMENT PROCESS

Community health needs assessment is a continuous ongoing developmental process that involves describing the state of health of local people, identifying major risk factors/causes of ill health, and choosing appropriate steps to address these. It helps to plan effective healthcare delivery and public health program in lines with the principles of equity and social justice. Local community members are considered the key resource in assessment of community health needs. "Needs" are those felt and expressed by local people and also those defined by professionals.

Community health needs assessment involves the following steps **(Fig. 37.4)**:

- *Profiling:* It is collection of relevant information regarding health status and needs of the population, factors affecting health, gaps, and strengths in services and resources that can be mobilized to address population health issues

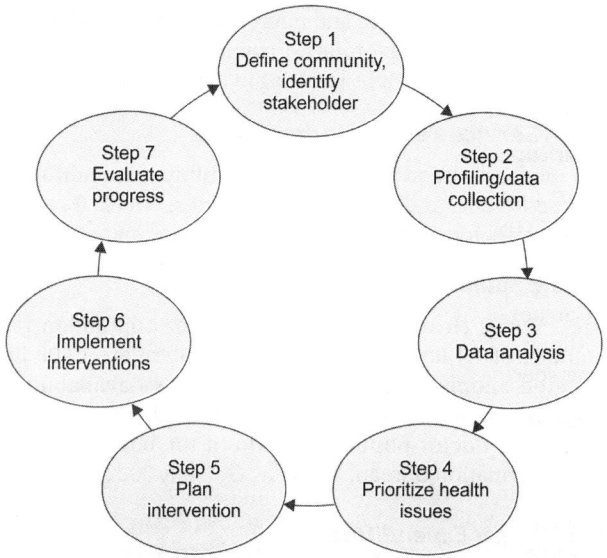

**Fig. 37.4:** Community health need assessment, implementation, and evaluation cycle.

- Analysis of community profile to identify major health issues and contributory factors
- Decide on priorities for action
- Plan interventions to address priority issues
- Implement planned evidence-based interventions engaging community members and stakeholders to build in them a sense of ownership and shared responsibility
- Evaluation of health outcomes/program and reviewing them with community members to consider what worked well and strategize on improvement and scale up.

To assess community needs we use specific techniques. A single technique may sometimes yield limited information and a combination of techniques may have to be used. Choosing a technique or a combination is also governed by constraints of time, money, and other resources. Some of the important *community need assessment techniques* are as follows:

- Key informant approach
- Public forum approach
- Nominal group process technique
- Delphi technique
- Survey approach.

### Key Informant Approach

It involves interview of "key informants". Key informants are people in the community who because of their training/educational status or affiliation to an organization, agency or population are in a good position to know about needs of the community. Key informants can be elected officials (e.g., mayor), religious leaders, school administrators, hospital administrators, representatives of local NGO, physicians, lawyers, school teachers, etc. Data obtained gives a comprehensive idea about community needs.

#### Steps

- Identify "key informants"
- Decide and design study tool to gather information on community needs—questionnaire/interview form
- Data collection
- Analysis and interpretation
- Feedback and further refinement by sharing study findings with key informants and discussion.

#### Advantages

- Easy and can be used by community volunteers
- Inexpensive
- Helps establish rapport, trust, and community involvement
- Allows clarification on conclusion
- Can be combined effectively with other techniques
- Allows input from multiple key informants with varied perspective on community needs.

#### Disadvantages

- Information obtained may be biased if selection of key informants is not proper (e.g., information is obtained from "service providers" and "consumers" are ignored).
- Personal relation of researcher and informants may influence type of data.
- Representativeness of total community is difficult to achieve.

### Public Forum Approach

It involves a series of public meetings, where participants (community members and key informants) discuss community needs, priority, and solutions.

#### Steps

- A set of questions (What/Why/Where/How) pertinent to most community residents are developed to help the discussion.
- Selection of a site *geographically* and *socially* acceptable to all segments of population conducive to open interchange of ideas.
- Communication of purpose, date, time, and place of meeting.
- Introduction of purpose, objective, rules for discussion, ask questions, and encourage open discussion and interchange of ideas.
- Record ideas and suggestions during the meeting.

#### Advantages

- We get opinions from a wide range of participants
- We get solutions/ideas to help decision makers on needs assessed
- A dialogue is initiated between "providers" and "consumers" of services
- Easy, inexpensive and quick approach
- Design is flexible and other techniques can be incorporated.

#### Disadvantages

- Requires good leadership and advance planning and organization
- Opinions may be of those who attend and viewpoints of all may not be heard
- Participants in the forums may represent some "vested interest" groups
- Poor advertising may result in limited participation
- Participants in forums may use the sessions to publicize their grievances
- If not facilitated well, only a few vocal participants will be heard
- In case of a large turnout, everyone does not get to speak and time for each speaker is also cut down
- May generate more questions than answers
- Forums may generate unrealistic expectations among participants.

### Nominal Group Process Approach

It seeks to maximize creative participation of group members taking into consideration the advantage of each person's knowledge and experience to generate ideas, seek clarification, reach consensus, prioritize, and make decisions on alternative actions in a face-to-face nonthreatening situation.

#### Steps

- Participants are divided into small groups of 6 to 20 persons
- Each participant writes his/her idea on piece of paper
- Each participant discusses his/her ideas and all concerns are listed on a chart
- Each idea is discussed, clarified, and evaluated by the group
- Each participant then assigns his/her priority by silent ballot
- Group priorities are compared
- Final group priorities are discussed.

#### Advantages

- A definite conclusion can be reached by a heterogeneous group
- Motivates all group members to participate and get involved
- Generates many ideas in a short time
- We get input from people of different backgrounds and experiences

- Stimulates creative thinking and effective dialog
- Ideas generated are clarified and prioritized.

*Disadvantages*
- Difficult to organize. Requires advance preparation and training group facilitators
- Facilitator has a tough job encouraging agenda building
- Assertive persons may dominate unless the facilitator has leadership skills.

## Delphi Technique

It generates ideas, seeks clarifications, builds consensus, prioritizes, and helps decision-making on alternative actions using a series of questionnaires and summarized feedback reports from preceding responses. There is no physical interaction between the participants and they do not know who all the other respondents are. It allows exchange of opinions and priorities and result in change in opinion and priorities of respondents based on summarized feed backs.

*Steps*
- A questionnaire is developed on issues, causes, solutions/actions, and is shared with a group of respondents
- Each respondent gives his ideas/answers independently
- Response to the questionnaires are summarized into a feedback
- Based on feedback, a second questionnaire seeking to prioritize the input from first round is developed and administered to the same respondents
- Respondents review feedback independently and rate priority ideas and return
- The process is repeated until a general agreement is reached on problems, causes, solutions, and actions.

*Advantages*
- Allows participants to remain anonymous. Hence, there is no individual dominance or social pressure
- Inexpensive
- Conducive to independent thinking
- A well-selected respondent panel provides a broad analytical perspective on local problems and concerns
- Helps reach consensus between groups that are hostile to each other.

*Disadvantages*
- Tendency to eliminate extreme positions and force a middle of road consensus
- Time consuming
- Requires skill in written communication
- Requires adequate time and participant commitment.

## Survey Approach

Data is collected from a sample of individuals in the community (selected using appropriate sampling techniques) on issues and community needs using any of the following methods:
- Personal interviews
- Self-administered questionnaires completed by respondents
- Telephone interviews
- Mailed questionnaires.

> National Family Health Survey (NFHS) is a large-scale, multi-round survey carried out in a representative sample of households throughout India. The information enables government to monitor and evaluate policies and programs related to population, health, nutrition, and HIV/AIDS.
> NFHS-1 (1992–1993) collected extensive information on population, health, and nutrition, with emphasis on women and young children. NFHS-2 (1998–1999) added data on quality of health and family planning services, domestic violence, reproductive health, anemia, nutrition, and the status of women. NFHS-3 (2005–2006) tested more than 100,000 women and men for HIV and more than 200,000 adults and young children for anemia. NFHS-4 (2015–2016) provided estimates of indicators at district level for all 640 districts in the country. In addition to data collected in NFHS-4, NFHS-5 has collected data on target population in alignment with Sustainable Development Goals (SDGs), expanded age range will be considered for diabetes, hypertension and also for its risk factors, inter-alia questions on disability, collection of blood samples for carrying out tests for malaria, HbA1c and Vitamin D and measurement of waist and hip circumference, pre-school education, death registration, etc. has been carried out. However, the HIV testing component has been dropped from NFHS-5.

*Advantages*
- Results are valid and reliable
- Helps assess behaviors, opinions, attitudes, knowledge, and beliefs.

*Disadvantages*
- Costly and time-consuming
- Training on sample size/sampling and survey instruments is desired
- Requires expertise to develop survey, train interviewers, conduct interviews, and analyze results.

## SUMMARY

> Community health involves multisectoral and multidisciplinary collaboration to promote, protect, improve, and preserve the health of people in a community. It is determined by physical factors, social and/or cultural factors, community organization, and willingness to work together and individual behaviors of community members.
>
> Measurement of community health is a systematic process of collecting information on health status of people, important health issues, prevalent risk factors/causes of poor health and actions needed to address these issues. It helps to plan better allocation of scarce resources and to deliver accessible, acceptable, and effective health care to the local community. Community health is measured by a set of indicators summarizing mortality, morbidity, disability, burden of disease, socioeconomic status, and health service delivery.
>
> A healthy community has multisectoral collaboration, inclusive, equitable, and broad community participation and control over the decisions affecting life, health, and well-being. It also has additional attributes like safe environment, optimum and accessible healthcare services.
>
> Community needs can be assessed using a variety of individual techniques or their combination. Key informant approach, public forum approach, nominal group process technique, Delphi technique, and survey are a few important community need assessment techniques. Choosing a technique or a combination also depends on the available time, money, and resources.

## SUGGESTED READING

1. Central Bureau of Health Intelligence, Directorate General of Health Services, Ministry of Health & Family Welfare, Government of India. National Health Profile. (2018).
2. Frieden TR. A Framework for Public Health Action: The Health Impact Pyramid. Am J Public Health. 2010;10(4):590-5.
3. Health resources in action. Advancing public health and medical research. [online] Available at www.hria.org.
4. McKenzie JF, Pinger RR, Kotecki JE. An Introduction to Community Health. Boston: Jones and Bartlett Publishers; 2005. p. 5.
5. Office of the Registrar General & Census Commissioner, India, Ministry of Home Affairs, Government of India. (2011). Provisional Population Totals: India: Census 2011.
6. UNDP. Human development report, human development for everyone. (2019).
7. United Nations Development Programme, Human Development Reports. (2018). The 2018 Global Multidimensional Poverty Index (MPI).

# CHAPTER 38

# Managing Community Health

*AM Kadri, Ankit Sheth, Anupam Banerjee*

| | |
|---|---|
| CM 1.1 | Define and describe the concept of Public Health |
| CM 17.2 | Describe community diagnosis |
| CM 17.3 | Describe primary healthcare, its component and principles |
| CM 17.4 | Millennium development goals |

## INTRODUCTION

Every community wishes to enjoy better health and lead a good quality life. An individual wants to lead a long healthy life free from suffering. One wants to enjoy physical strength and have a good family, professional and social life throughout one's entire lifetime. Every community and country wants its citizens to be healthy. Healthy citizens contribute to the better productivity of the country, while those who are diseased become liabilities, usurping the resources that could have been used for various developmental activities in education, infrastructure, irrigation, agriculture, power generation, etc. Coupled with the following three developments in the field of pure science as well as social science modern medicine has been compelled to widen its focus from being just 'exclusively disease oriented'.

1. ***Rise of scientific era:*** During last four to five centuries' an environment created for the scientific understanding of the occurrence of diseases which led to gradual efforts in direction of their prevention.
2. ***Advancement in medical science:*** Better treatment and control over the diseases resulted in increase of longevity. With increase in the life expectancy, people started shifting their focus towards a better 'quality of life'.
3. ***Stabilization of the country borders:*** In the ancient times, invasion and acquisition of geographical territories was considered as the means of gaining prosperity. Following the devastating World War I (1914-1918) and World War II (1939-1945), the world leaders developed the wisdom to create various international agencies for maintaining peace and attaining prosperity through international cooperation. Stabilization of the geographical boundaries of countries ensured. Gradually the focus shifted on to the development of the community as a means for overall development of the country hence health gained the status as the most important determinant for growth and progress of the country.

## EVOLUTION OF SCIENCES FOR MANAGING COMMUNITY HEALTH

Conventional medical services were focused on curative medicine, being delivered *only* to those who were sick and *reached* the hospitals. It offered very little for those who were out in the community and also wished to live a healthy life. The focus of modern medical science gradually broadened from just treating and curing the diseased to improving the quality of life of individuals, people and ultimately that of a community. To meet the goal of improving people's health, modern medicine has tried to seek the answer to the following questions.

1. Why do some groups or communities enjoy better health compared to others?
2. Why are some diseases seen more often in specific groups or community?
3. How are people may be protected from diseases?
4. How can health of the community be improved so that they can enjoy good quality life?

The search for answers for the above four questions led to the formation of a formal discipline, concerned with managing the health of the community. This evolved through various phases of disease prevention and health promotion. It witnessed expansion and amalgamation of different sciences and practices. The various concepts, approaches and sciences evolved for managing community health are given as follows.

### Hygiene

As a part of evolution, human learnt the importance of bathing and personal cleanliness. The importance of bathing gradually shifted from being one of pure aesthetic to that of being helpful in the prevention of diseases. During the development of Greek medicine (1200-100 BC), importance of personal cleanliness in the health was noted. One of the early leaders of Greek medicine, Asclepius stressed it and legend is that one of his daughter Hygeia was worshiped as goddess of health (another daughter Panacea was worshiped as goddess of medicine). The seeds of the *preventive medicine* were sowed in medical sciences as *hygiene*. However, *hygiene, per se,* was seen as the responsibility of an *individual* and not as a part of medical science for community health or centuries.

## Public Health

The seeds of preventive care which were sowed three thousand years back, could only foster as scientific practice in the mid-nineteenth century. It was in the post-industrial revolution (1760–1840) period in the early 19th century that the primitive scientific approach for *preventive medicine* emerged in England. The period of the industrialization revolution saw huge migrations, overcrowding in cities, formation of unsanitary slums, and accumulation of filth around. Large number of illnesses and deaths were reported in the industrial workers which affected industrial productivity. A high morbidity and mortality in children and women (especially of lower social status) were reported. During this time period, the life expectancy in the professional and elite group of England was 44 years, while that of the working class was 22 years. This was point of worry for industrialists and Government of Great Britain. Following the great cholera epidemic in 1832 in England, Edwin Chadwick, a lawyer, was asked to investigate the health of the inhabitants of large towns. Chadwick identified that the filth spread across the cities and towns, was the major cause behind the ill health of the people, especially those of the labor class. Following his report, antifilth crusade began in Great Britain. A law *'Public Health Act of 1848'* was enacted to improve sanitation. This concept of *'sanitation awakening',* which started in Great Britain, gradually spread across Europe and into the United States of America and then across the world. Improving sanitation and provision of safe drinking water became a most important approach in the practice of preventive medicine as a part of government responsibility.

During this phase of evolution, measures were largely generic and targeted towards protecting health of the public: hence these measures named as *public health actions*. This was first ever attempt in medical science to manage the health of the community at a large.

## Preventive Medicine

While efforts to prevent diseases via improvement in sanitation were going on, in other places across the world, some other path breaking inventions happened. There were three important events which changed the future course of disease prevention and health promotion.
1. **Addition of fresh lime and vegetables** to prevent the occurrence of scurvy in sailors during their long voyage. This was discovered by a French naval surgeon, James Lind in the year 1753.
2. **Inoculation of fluid from cowpox lesion to prevent smallpox.** This developed the concept of vaccination by a British physician Edward Jenner in year 1796.
3. **Discovery of germ theory** by French bacteriologist Louis Pasteur in the year 1860.

The first two discoveries charted another path for *preventing* specific diseases by specific measures which was later on known as *'preventive medicine'*. With the discovery of germ theory, the understanding about the dynamics of disease transmission and use of specific measures to *prevent* diseases became known.

With invention of numerous vaccines, discovery of antibiotics and identifying the interventions to break the chain of specific disease transmission, the role and importance of *preventive medicine* in medical care and management of the health of the community increased. Antirabies treatment (1883), cholera vaccines (1898) diphtheria antitoxin (1894), antityphoid vaccine (1898) and antiseptics and disinfectants (1827–1911) consolidated the practice of preventive medicine.

The term *'preventive medicine'* is to be applied against specific diseases in contrast to the *'public health measures'*, which are a general approach like environmental health management, nutrition promotion, etc.

*Preventive medicine* differs from *conventional public health* as it is being practiced at three levels:
1. On healthy people
2. On high-risk groups (vulnerable groups)
3. At community (mass) level but specifically aiming to prevention of transmission of specific disease.

The eradication of smallpox (1980), reducing cases of dracunculiasis, yaws, and poliomyelitis to the verge of eradication and reduction in morbidity and mortality of diseases, such as malaria, tuberculosis, measles, diphtheria, HIV are some of the success stories of preventive medicine.

## Social Medicine

Though the world was reaping the health benefits of public health actions and preventive medicine measures it was being gradually realized that for improvement of people's health, mere preventive medicine and conventional public health actions were not sufficient. It was observed that the levels of health and patterns of diseases were unequally distributed among different socioeconomic groups. Benefits of improved nutrition, good housing, access and utilization of health services were determined by economic conditions, social status, educational levels, social-support mechanisms, etc. The role of social factors in disease occurrence (social pathology) emerged and the importance of social factors in modifying health outcomes was realized. This approach is known as *social medicine.*

However, social medicine had little say in medical science until the International Public Health Conference held at Alma-Ata (1978), in which the world leaders unanimously recognized the inter-relationship and interdependency between health and socioeconomic development. The leaders made a declaration, popularly known as the *Alma-Ata declaration*, under which *'health goal was defined as a social goal'* and *'health development was integrated with overall social-economical goal of community'*. It declared "Health for All by 2000 AD" as a global agenda and recommended *primary healthcare (PHC) approach,* to attain this goal. The Millennium Development Goals (MDGs, 2000) and the Sustainable Development Goals (SDGs 2015) still ratify the importance of social development as an important approach towards managing health of the community.

Though the approaches being used in managing community health by all three different sciences, (conventional public health, preventive medicine and social medicine) were different, their scope of application and aim were same with overlapping in practices. Hence in the 1900s a subject namely Preventive and Social Medicine (PSM) encompassing all the three approaches emerged as a part of medical curriculum.

## Community Medicine

During the 1970s, the concept of *'community oriented primary care'* to bring preventive, promotive and clinical care closer to community, emerged in various parts of the world. This can be termed as the very initial form of practice of Community Medicine. It is concerned with organizing the preventive, promotive and primary clinical care for a defined community. In this practice, use of epidemiology, newer approaches such as surveillance, and disease control measures were interposed into the primary clinical care. In India too, the discipline of Preventive and Social Medicine, was changed to Community Medicine discipline during the mid-1970s.

Community Medicine is a specialty which deals with the health of the community. In other words, Community Medicine is community-oriented healthcare. Community Medicine is developed as a specialist branch in the medical science which is concerned with the managing health of the Community. The Indian Association of Preventive and Social Medicine (IAPSM) has defined Community Medicine as "*a science and art of promoting health, preventing diseases and prolonging life by range of interventions (promotive, preventive, curative, rehabilitative and palliative) in close partnership and association with healthcare delivery system and with active community participation and intersectoral coordination.*"

Community Medicine is involved in delivering the preventive, promotive, clinical and rehabilitative healthcare to the community by use of sciences of epidemiology, health system and healthcare services with focus on community. The relationship and interaction between them is known as the Triad of Community Medicine **(Fig. 38.1)**.

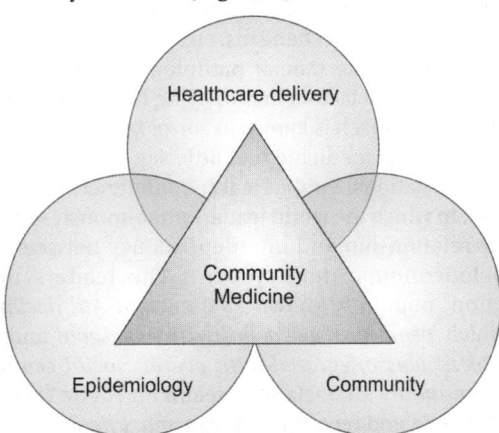

**Fig. 38.1:** Triad of Community Medicine.

As per IAPSM's definition, Community Medicine has three broad areas of interventions.

1. **Promoting health of the community:** This envisages promoting health of members of community to the highest attainable level where an individual or community enjoys full physical, psychological and social well-being.
   - *Physical well-being* means members of the community are enjoying the level of health, which is expected at their age. Their biological systems are working at optimum level, and they can physically carry out all activities expected of their age.
   - *Psychological well-being* means members of community are having a state of mind, where they have balance with self, situation and surroundings. They have optimum cognitive and rational judgmental abilities, possess inner peace, are contented in life and share a harmonious relationship with others.
   - *Social well-being* means enjoying a good standard of life. The members of community have access to safe water, adequate foods, proper shelters with good surroundings and basic services and adequate social support.

   Seven key interventions for health promotion:
   1. Provision of adequate and safe drinking water
   2. Provision of adequate and safe food
   3. Good housing and sanitary surroundings
   4. Improving the education level of community
   5. Improved health literacy and healthy behaviors
   6. Reduction of poverty and better opportunities of livelihood.
   7. Social and financial security and support mechanisms

   Many of the above interventions are out of domain of healthcare. Nonetheless, by developing better coordination with the responsible sectors, the overall health of the community can be improved.

2. **Preventing diseases in community:** The second objective of the Community Medicine is protecting the health of community members from the ever-present threat of diseases in the surrounding. Identifying the existing threat, eliminating them, creating shield against them are the key approaches in the preventing the disease **(Table 38.1)**.

3. **Prolonging longevity of community:** The third area under focus of Community Medicine is to increase the longevity of the members of the community. Early detection and prompt treatment of diseases, increasing the availability and accessibility of the medical care, establishing good referral linkages for serious cases are some of the ways to prevent premature deaths along with promoting health and preventing the diseases.

**Table 38.1:** Health threats to the community.

| Threats | Potential adverse outcomes[#] |
|---|---|
| Cases and carriers (human) | Various infectious/communicable diseases |
| Contaminated water | Waterborne diseases |
| Stale foods/contaminated foods | Foodborne diseases |
| Arthropod* | Malaria, filarial, dengue, gastroenteritis, etc. |
| Rodent* | Plague, leptospirosis, nipah fever |
| Animals/birds* | Zoonotic diseases |
| Birds* | Psittacosis, allergic alveolitis, etc. |
| Polluted air | Obstructive and carcinogenic respiratory diseases |
| Chemical polluted foods and soils and water | Chemical and toxin-related diseases |
| Adulterated foods/toxins/chemical in food | Chemical and toxin-related diseases |
| Deficient macro- and micro-nutrients in food and diets | Nutritional-related diseases |

*Contd...*

*Contd...*

| Threats | Potential adverse outcomes# |
|---|---|
| Collection of water and waste water | Arthropod borne diseases |
| Insanitary waste disposal (foods) | Rodent borne diseases |
| Insanitary human excreta disposal | Soil helminths and water/food diseases |
| Unsafe behavior (e.g., sexual behavior, tobacco chewing, smoking alcoholism, rash driving) | Sexually transmitted infections including HIV, cancers, liver failure, accidents, etc. |

*Not all but some of them act as vehicle or carrier of the pathogens and facilitate transmission of infections.
#List is indicative only.

## SUMMARY OF EVOLUTION OF SCIENCE IN MANAGING COMMUNITY HEALTH (TABLE 38.2)

There is no clear-cut demarcation of time when one phase ended and another phase started. With increase in wisdom of understanding about the health and diseases, various attempts were made to adopt methodological techniques and scientific approaches towards managing community health with overlapping period of time and overlapping approaches. In all phases and forms of evolution the goal and objectives remained the same: promoting health, preventing disease transmission and prolonging life of members of the community for sake of the better understanding, the progression can be shown as step ladder pattern as given in **Figure 38.2** with predominance of particular phase during specific period (Kadri AM, Indian Journal of Community Health, 2017).

Table 38.2: The phases of managing community health, discipline and corresponding time period.

| Phase | Discipline/science evolved | Probable period of evolution |
|---|---|---|
| Cleanliness and personal care | Hygiene | 1200 BC |
| Sanitation awakening | Public health | 1830s AD |
| Disease control | Preventive medicine | 1780s AD |
| Health development | Social medicine | 1900s AD |
| Primary healthcare and health system reform | Community medicine | 1970s AD |

## KEY CONCEPTS IN THE MANAGEMENT OF COMMUNITY HEALTH

Over the years, key concepts which emerged in managing health of the community are as follow:
1. **Health** is a considered as a human right. Health is no more is the responsibility of an individual but has become the responsibility of the government.
2. **Treatment** is viewed as an '*expenditure*' while **disease prevention** is viewed as an '*investment*'.
3. Social and environmental factors are important determinants for health and disease outcomes.
4. Health is a *social goal rather than a medical goal*'.
5. *Community oriented healthcare:* Healthcare closer to the community is a more cost-effective approach and has wider reach to the members of community. Curative healthcare is a complex, technology controlled, institution-based expensive strategy as compared with community-oriented approach.
6. *Community-based health workers and community participations* have larger role in managing health of community and making the community healthy.

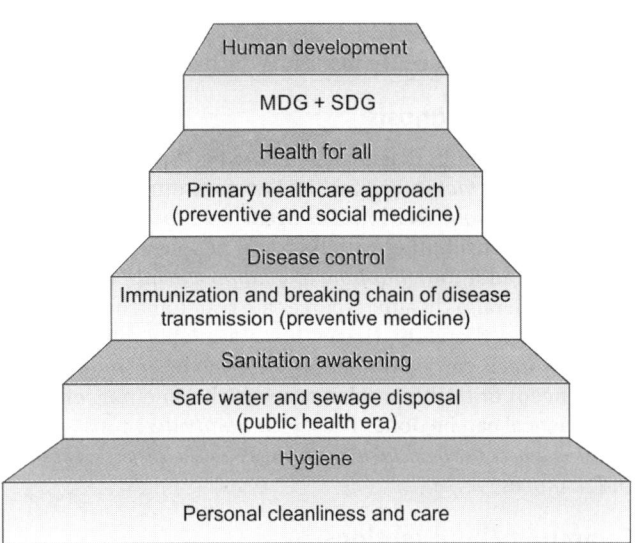

Fig. 38.2: Step ladder model: Evolution of sciences and approaches in managing community health.

Disease prevention is more economically and socially rewarding than treatment of the diseases hence preventive and promotive services became part of modern medical sciences.

As currently mix of all approaches are used in managing community health, the term '*public health*', '*preventive and social medicine*', and '*community medicine*' are often used interchangeably. The main responsibility for health of community is that of the government, which is working towards protecting and promoting the health of the community it is commonly referred to as *public health*. But one should not be confused and has to remember that the ultimate aim of all the disciplines, by whatever name it is known, is improving the health of people living in the defined community.

## MANAGING COMMUNITY HEALTH

Globally, health is viewed as a fundamental human right and it is the duty of the government to protect and preserve it. World Health Organization (WHO) has mentioned it as one of the important basic rights in its constitution. Promoting, protecting and restoring health of the people is the responsibility of the government. Principles in managing community health are Community Oriented healthcare, i.e., PHC for everyone and special care for those at risk. Approaches in managing health of community are delivering preventive, promotive and primary (essential) healthcare to the members of the community (up to their door step), by involving the trained community healthcare workers and integrating the health development of the people with community's (socioeconomic) development. Two important methods in managing community health are "community diagnosis" and "community intervention" which can be equated with "clinical diagnosis" and "clinical interventions" practiced in managing the patient.

## Community Diagnosis

Making a community diagnosis is *identifying the health problems and causative factors behind it*. For community diagnosis, *information about local health needs and local diseases are gathered* in consultation with the local people and the health workers. In addition, *mapping of available health resources* is done. In general, as health resources are scarce and health needs are manifold, therefore, (based upon available information), *prioritization* is carried out. Priorities are to be accorded to the health needs or health problems for which something effective and practical can be done. Thus, *community diagnosis helps in deciding where the healthcare providers should target their efforts and resources.*

## Community Interventions

Community diagnosis helps in identifying the health problems affecting the community and reasons behind it. Based on them, health interventions are planned. These are called community interventions. It is related with the clinical interventions instituted by conventional clinician in managing patient's diseases condition. However, it differs from clinical interventions in three aspects.

1. It contains large number of preventive and promotive interventions. Many of them are applied in the community settings, e.g., community level water purification and disinfection, health awareness, antimosquito measures, etc.
2. Many clinical services are imparted in the community setting (at doorstep of people) by use of trained community health workers, e.g., immunization, home-based child care, antenatal care, etc.
3. Some interventions, though carried out in the healthcare institutional settings, are strategized and aimed towards improvement of the health of the community, e.g., family planning operations, diagnostic procedures for diseases, *Anganwadi*, Nutritional Rehabilitation Center (NRC), etc.

## Steps in Managing the Community Health

There are seven steps in managing the health of community (Table 38.3).

**Table 38.3:** Seven steps in managing the community health.

| Steps | Actions | Purpose |
|---|---|---|
| 1 | Gathering health information of the community | Community diagnosis |
| 2 | Measurement of the health conditions | |
| 3 | Planning and organizing healthcare services | Community interventions |
| 4 | Monitoring community health | |
| 5 | Integrating with health system | Supportive community interventions |
| 6 | Intersectoral coordination | |
| 7 | Community involvement | |

## Gathering Community Health Information

Every community is at different stages of health development. They have different socioeconomic, demographical, geographical, environmental and climatic conditions. They have different health issues, varied opportunities and availability of resources, and institutional support mechanisms. Hence, they have different types and levels of risk factors towards potential health demanding conditions. Hence for managing the health of every community, we need to first understand the community.

It includes gathering information about:
- Health needs and demands of a community
- Factors influencing health and disease in the community
- Health resources available
- Vulnerability of community and 'at-risk groups' of people

This is like the complete history taking and general examination of a patient in the clinical scenario.

Most of the community health information is readily available from various sources, such as:
- Census, population data, Civil Registration System (CRS), Sample Registration System (SRS), National Family Health Survey (NFHS), etc.
- Data from Revenue Department giving information about the age, sex, caste, religion, educational status, below poverty line (BPL) status of the people, etc.
- List of hospitals, doctors and healthcare providers
- Medical records and interactions with local hospital administrators and doctors
- List of institutions, such as school, voluntary agencies, government welfare and rehabilitation centers
- Agencies, such as water supply and sewage management, public distribution system, women and child development, etc.
- Meteorological department
- Customs, culture and local festivals and traditions

Information which are missing can be gathered by special studies or surveys. Based on the information, health profile and epidemiological situation (locally prevalent disease and factors associated with them) are prepared. This information acts as the base (foundation/baseline data) for listing health needs and prioritizing, planning and organizing health services.

## Measurement of the Health Conditions

In conventional clinical practice for clinical diagnosis (as a part of managing an individual patient), inspection (observation), palpation, auscultation and investigations are carried out and vitals (temperature, pulse, respiratory rate, etc.). These help in objectively recorded individual's health status. Similarly, in community diagnosis, certain vitals (health indicators) are measured, such as birth rate, death rate, infant mortality rate, maternal mortality ratio, incidence and prevalence of diseases.

For diagnosis of diseases, the *'etiology of the disease;'* is searched for, similarly in managing community health, we need to identify *'the causation' (associated factors and their attribution in health outcomes) need to be identified*. But unlike patient management, where clinicians try to investigate pathogens and pathology only, in managing the community health, positive factors (*determinants*) and their positive influence in health promotion are also identified along with risk factors which pose threat to health.

For managing community health some of the common measurements are as follows:

Measurements of:
- Mortality
- Morbidity
- Disability
- Fertility
- Healthcare services, their needs, availability, accessibility, coverage, utilization, quality, etc.
- Social services (related with health) their needs, availability, accessibility, coverage, utilization, quality, etc.
- Health-related knowledge, beliefs, attitude, behavior (practices)
- Health status, standard of living, burden of disease, disability adjusted life years, etc.
- Effectiveness of interventions in desired health outcomes.

For making community diagnosis, knowledge and skills of general epidemiology, epidemiology of specific health problems and diseases and biostatistical methods are necessary.

## *Planning and Organizing Healthcare Services*

Even a richest of rich country does not have enough money and human resources to meet all the health needs of its community. Furthermore, available resources have a cut throat competition with needs of other sectors, such as: education, agriculture, infrastructure, defense, etc. Hence prioritization of health needs amongst all health needs is a prerequisite before planning and organizing any healthcare service. In managing health of community, health services are planned and organized in a way that they encompass basic (preventive, promotive and primary) health services targeting everyone and selected special services to those at risk (vulnerable) group with a robust referral linkage between secondary and tertiary care hospitals. Three approaches for interventions in managing community health are as below.

1. **Public interventions:** These interventions are targeted to large sections of the population with the aim to promote overall health or control the diseases in general. Safe drinking water, waste management, pollution control, improved dietary habits, improved food supply and distribution are examples of such interventions.
2. **High-risk group interventions:** Interventions are targeted to specific groups (such as mothers, women, children, adolescents, geriatrics, occupational workers, tribal) who are chosen for their greater vulnerability. These are often *cost-effective interventions* are aimed towards targeting the health needs and problems related to specific vulnerable group.
3. **Health problem specific approach:** Certain interventions are specially focused towards specific health issues *(vertically targeted interventions),* such as tuberculosis, leprosy, HIV, measles, malaria, anemia, nutritional deficiency, hypertension, sickle cell anemia, substance abuse, high fertility, adverse sex ratio, etc. When health problem needs to be tackled aggressively due to its large impact on the community health, such an approach needs to be adopted. The *effectiveness* of such interventions is high in managing the health problem, but they are comparatively *cost intensive*. They are integrated with high-risk group interventions or at times with general interventions, depending upon burden of the disease locally.

## *Monitoring Health of Community*

In conventional clinical practice to monitor the health conditions, follow-up visits/rounds are carried out. Besides comparing the changes in signs and symptoms, change in the vitals (such as temperature, pulse, blood pressure, respiratory rates) and other biological markers (through laboratory or radiological investigations) are done as a part of patient monitoring protocol. These guide the clinicians to make decision about further course of treatment.

Similarly, during monitoring of community health situation it is required to make mid-course correction for managing health of the community. The purpose of monitoring community health situation is to know the effect of community health interventions, identify the reasons behind failure or poor effect (if any), and make any change in community interventions to attain the goal.

For monitoring community health, different epidemiological and community health indicators are monitored. Periodical surveys, such as Sample registry surveys, HIV sentinel surveillance, tuberculosis incidence study, National Family Health Surveys (NFHS), District Level Household Survey (DLHS) etc., are some of the ways of monitoring community health. Periodicity of such surveys and studies vary from yearly to five yearly depending upon the health outcomes to be monitored. They are known as *'health outcome indicators'* (to monitor short-term effect) and help to assess the *'health impact'* (to monitor long-term effect).

## *Integrating with Health System*

The best result of management of the community health can be attained if it is integrated with the local health system. *Health system is the network of institutes which is involved in planning, organizing and delivering the healthcare services.* Government health system is the principal player of healthcare delivery system. Besides government health system, there are other institutes such as private hospitals, international healthcare agencies, charitable health institutes, voluntary health agencies, local nongovernment agencies working in health, academic and research in health. Partnership should be developed with such related agencies working in the community.

## *Intersectoral Coordination*

For management of the health of community, along with health services, social determinants, such as provision of safe water, education, good nutrition, and proper housing and sanitation conditions must be addressed. The healthcare team, is not directly involved in the delivery of these services. However, their interaction with these departments would provide timely warning, ensure optimum management of resources, and prevent reduplication of efforts.

## Community Involvement

It is believed that for sustaining the good health of the community *'people's health should be put into the hands of the people'*. Merely generating awareness about 'health and its determinants' is not sufficient. Members of the community need to get involved in each and every process of community health intervention, such as assessment of health needs, planning of health services, mobilization of resources, organizing healthcare services, monitoring health situation and services, coordinating with other sectors.

The differences between managing an individual's health and healthcare of the community have been discussed in **Table 38.4**.

Conventional medical practices (managing patients) and community medicine practices (managing health of community) are not opposite but are complimentary to each other. Community Health Management is a broadening of the medical science from individual patient centric medical care to the healthcare which includes community-oriented preventive and promotive care besides conventional curative care. The scope and role of both the approaches can be better understood through **'Torch Light Model'** as shown in the **Figure 38.3**.

Table 38.4: Differences between managing an 'individual's health' and 'community health.

|  | *Managing individual's disease* | *Managing community health* |
|---|---|---|
| Branch | General and specialist branches under traditional modern medicine, e.g., general practice, internal medicine, surgery, pediatrics, etc. | Community medicine/preventive and social medicine/social and preventive medicine/public health |
| Goal | To make the patient disease free | To improve health of the whole community so that they can enjoy quality life as an individual, group and community |
| Objectives | Restore the normal biological pathology in bodily system | Health promotion, diseases prevention and prolonging life |
| Focus on health | Nil | Improving health |
| Focus on disease | Cure | Control, elimination, eradication |
| Scope of actions | Patients | Community, high-risk groups, vulnerable groups, family and individual and their socio-politico-economical and physical environment |
| Approach | • Biomedical<br>• Human body, fragmented into body system, organ, cells and biochemical process | Holistic (human beings with their complete surroundings involving biological, environment and social determinants and available health system) |
| Strategies | Diagnosis of the disease and treatment of the patient | Primary healthcare, health system strengthening, health programs and schemes, health legislation |
| Types of care | Medical care (curative services only) | Healthcare (preventive, promotive, curative, rehabilitative services) |
| Areas of operations | Clinics and hospitals | Community to clinics |
| Interventions | At individual level:<br>• Patient history taking<br>• Physical examination<br>• Mainly medical or surgical therapy | At community level:<br>• Health surveillance system<br>• Disease screening<br>• Health promotion through public health measures, such as nutritional improvement, provision of safe drinking water, proper sewage system, scientific waste management, integrated vector control, etc.<br>• Integrating health development with community development through intersectional coordination and community participation<br>At individual/vulnerable group level:<br>• Health promotion<br>• Specific protection<br>• Screening for early diagnosis and treatment<br>• Treatment of common illnesses and management of diseases having epidemic potentiality<br>• Referral linkages with specialist medical care<br>• Disability limitations<br>• Community based rehabilitation |
| Knowledge and skills used | Conventional subjects under medical sciences | • Basics of medical science<br>• Basic to good understanding of various other disciplines<br>• Epidemiology<br>• Biostatistics and research methodologies<br>• Nutrition<br>• Environmental health<br>• Medical entomology<br>• Sociology<br>• Communication and health education<br>• Health system and management |

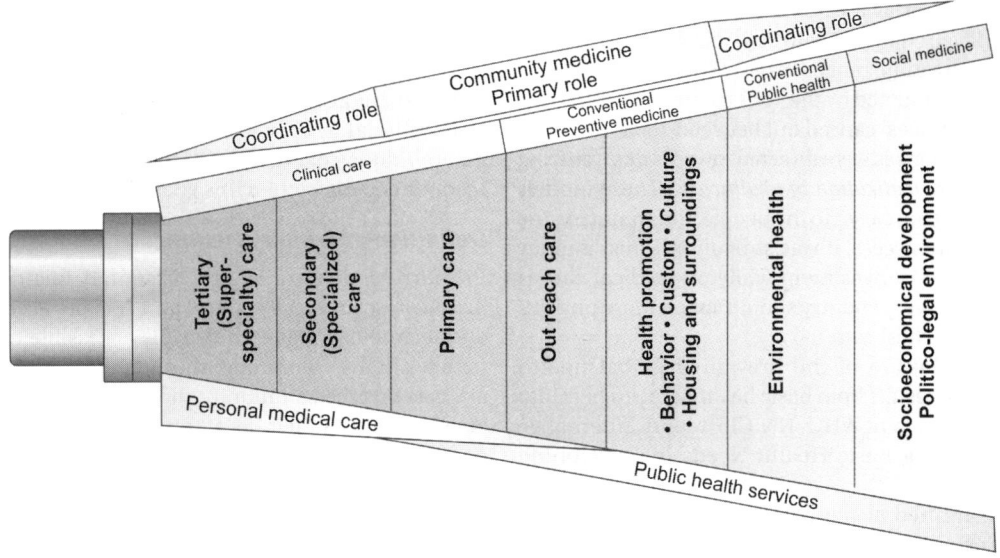

**Fig. 38.3:** 'Torch Light Model' for healthcare and role of clinical medicine and other disciplines in managing community health.
*Source:* Kadri AM, Indian Journal of Community Medicine, 2017

## GLOBAL APPROACHES IN MANAGING HEALTH OF COMMUNITY

In 1948, a specialized health agency, looking into the global health perspectives was established by the United Nations (UN): it was named as the World Health Organization (WHO). The role of WHO is to provide directions, technical assistance and promote coordination and cooperation between the member countries and help them in attaining the highest level of health of people living therein. In the year 1978, the first ever attempt was made to 'develop a health system' in the member countries with the aim of managing the global health. The *'Primary Healthcare approach'* was recommended as a strategy followed by recommendation of two other strategies: *'health system reform'* and *'universal health coverage (UHC)'* with the focus on managing health of the entire country.

### Primary Healthcare

Though the formal declaration of PHC was made by the WHO in 1978 (as a part of Alma-Ata declaration during International Conference of Public Health), it's concept had already emerged during late 1960s and early 1970s. During this period, it was felt by the world health leaders that science and technology had advanced and better health could have been achieved with available technical knowledge. Until then, that the provision of medical care was only by specialist doctors (with use of complex and costly medical technologies). Unfortunately, this could only be accessed and afforded by a privileged few. It was estimated that around four-fifths of the world's population were deprived of basic health needs. Key observations on the world health situation were as follows:
- Hospital-based healthcare system was widely prevalent.
- Healthcare was increasingly complex and costly with low social relevance.
- In most countries, the best use of advanced science and technology could not be made for most of the citizens.
- Tremendous disparities in health conditions existed both: among countries (inter-countries) and within country (intra-country).
- Lack of emphasis on preventive care.
- Vertical health approaches (disease control) used in malaria control, smallpox eradication could not meet overall health needs of the people.
- Availability of health personnel, equipment and supplies against requirement were inadequate.
- Health resources were predominantly allocated mainly for sophisticated medical care.
- Medical facilities were clustered largely in urban areas.

The gloomy global health situation has highlighted the failure of prevailing health systems. In this backdrop of growing dissatisfaction with the existing hospital-based, medical care driven, complex, costly, and technologically loaded health system, some experiences from community-based basic healthcare projects in a number of countries were found promising. Some of these to be promising examples are as follows:
- Indian rural medical care system based on the Bhore Committee's recommendations (1943) established on basic healthcare philosophy.
- Medical missionaries working in developing countries, under The Christian Medical Commission (a specialized organization of the World Council of Churches and the Lutheran World Federation, created in the late 1960s).
- Experience of rural medical services with the use of *'barefoot doctors'* in Communist China (1964–1976). They were village health workers who lived in the community they served, with stress on rural healthcare and preventive rather than curative services, using combined western and traditional medicines.
- Community-oriented primary care by Sydney Kark in South Africa where nurses and paramedics were involved in providing basic care in community settings.
- Use of medical auxiliaries in developing countries, such as Bangladesh, China, Cuba, India, Niger, Nigeria, Tanzania,

Venezuela, and Yugoslavia where trained village workers at the grass roots level, equipped with essential drugs and simple methods, were providing ranges of basic services.
- Several projects conducted by the WHO for the development of 'basic health services' carried out between 1965–1970.

All the above experiences were directed towards demystifying the dominance of *'medicalization of healthcare'*. These models thus brought medical care closer to the people: thus reducing the disparity in healthcare access. It was strongly felt that "money spent on primary care is investment while on medical care is the expenditure" and every country should spend more on PHC than cost intensive medical care.

Considering the failure of the prevailing global health situation and positive results from basic healthcare projects into consideration, in 1975 a joint WHO-UNICEF report, 'Alternative Approaches to Meeting Basic Health Needs in Developing Countries', was released.

The report examined successful PHC experiences from across the world and identified the key factors for their success. The report recommended that social and developmental dimensions needed to be incorporated in the basic healthcare model.

Two key observations in this report were:
1. Health problems and socioeconomic problems are interwoven but social determinants (such as economical condition, safe water and proper sanitation, shelter, nutrition) was unfortunately, not focused upon for health promotion.
2. Health systems worked outside the main stream of social and economic development.

This report led to the shaping of the concept of PHC.

### First International Conference on Public Health and Alma-Ata Declaration

To discuss about the prevailing health situation, develop strategies and advocate actions towards improving the levels of global health, an "International Conference on Public Health" was held at Alma-Ata, the erstwhile capital of Kazakhstan (then part of Soviet Union) during 6–12th September, 1978. Delegates from 134 governments and representatives of 67 United Nations organizations, specialized agencies and nongovernmental organizations in official relations with WHO and UNICEF attended this conference.

*The objectives of the conference were to:*
- Promote the concept of primary healthcare in countries
- Exchange experience and information on the development of primary healthcare within the framework of comprehensive national health systems and services
- Evaluate the present health and healthcare situation throughout the world and as it relates to, and can be improved by, primary healthcare
- Define the principles of primary healthcare as well as the operational means of overcoming practical problems in the development of primary healthcare
- Define the role of governments, national, and international organizations in technical cooperation and support for the development of primary healthcare
- Formulate recommendations for the development of primary healthcare

At the end of the conference; an Alma-Ata Declaration was released, signed by the all leaders from various countries, international agencies and developmental partners, setting an ambitious goal of *'Health for All'* by 2000 AD. The strategy recommended to attain this goal was 'Primary Healthcare'.

### Definition of Primary Healthcare

Primary healthcare is the "essential healthcare based on practical, scientifically sound and socially acceptable methods and technology made universally accessible to individual and families in the community through their full participation and at a cost that the community and country can afford to maintain at every stage of their development in the spirit of self-reliance and self-determination".

### Principles of Primary Healthcare

The International Conference on Primary Healthcare and Alma-Ata's Declaration brought a revolutionary change (*referred to as paradigm shift*) in the concept of health. Four key ideas floated in this conference were:
1. Equity in the healthcare
2. Use of appropriate technology
3. Community participation
4. Intersectoral coordination

These four ideas became the 'Pillars for the Primary Healthcare' and are referred to as *'Principles of Primary Healthcare'*.

**Equitable distribution:** It was observed that there were gross inequalities in health outcomes between the countries as well as within a country **(Table 38.5)**. This was due to inequalities of availability and utilization of healthcare services. Health services were mainly concentrated in urban areas and within reach of the affluent people. To bridge this gap, it was needed that axis of healthcare be shifted towards rural and urban slums with the strategy to cater to those who needed the most. As per this principle, primary care and other services must be accessible to residents irrespective of their financial status, gender, age, caste, color, location (urban/rural), and social class. Thus, under equitable distribution resources are invested more in areas where it is needed more. Higher priority is given to high risk groups, such as women, children, under-privileged segments and underserved areas. Equitable distribution is the key to attain health for all.

**Table 38.5:** Inequalities in health and socioeconomic indicators in the world around 1980.

| | Least developed countries | Other developing countries | Developed countries |
|---|---|---|---|
| Number of countries | 29 | 90 | 37 |
| Total population (millions) | 283 | 3,001 | 1,131 |
| Infant mortality rate (per 1,000 liveborn) | 160 | 94 | 19 |
| Life expectancy (years) | 45 | 60 | 72 |

*Contd...*

*Contd...*

|  | Least developed countries | Other developing countries | Developed countries |
|---|---|---|---|
| Newborn with birth weight of ≥2,500 g | 70% | 83% | 93% |
| Coverage by safe water supply | 31% | 41% | 100% |
| Adult literacy rate | 28% | 55% | 58% |
| GNP per capita | $170 | $520 | $6,230 |
| Per capita public expenditure on health | $1.7 | $6.5 | $244 |
| Public expenditure on health as % of GNP | 1.0% | 1.2% | 3.9% |

*Note:* The figures in the table are weighted averages, based on data for 1980 or for the latest available year.

*Source:* WHO, Global Strategy for health for all by year 2000, 1981

***Appropriate technology:*** The poor people often remain deprived of the benefits of sophisticated disease oriented medical technology, due to the prohibitively high cost involved and its limited reach. Under primary healthcare approach, the provision of medical techniques, equipment and drugs which are based on the technology that are simple, effective, affordable by the community in their spirit of self-reliance, is recommended. The key point to remember is that, 'appropriate technology' should be simple, effective, socially acceptable without posing any economical and operational burden on the country which is using them.

Appropriate technology may be soft technology or hard technology. *Soft technology* brings about a change in an individual's or community's behavior through advocacy and social participation. *Hard technology* refers to preparing engineering designs, manufacturing materials and equipment using affordable resources and locally available technology without succumbing to prohibitively exorbitant costs. Appropriate health technologies range from simple products, such as oral rehydration solution, growth charts, Shakir's tape, use of breath counting to detect pneumonia, use of shake test, vaccine vial monitor (VVM), to highly sophisticated products, such as manufacturing of polyvalent vaccines, Electronic Vaccine Intelligence Network (eVIN) to monitor vaccine storage temperature, etc.

***Community participation:*** 'Medical elitism' was one of the causes of inequalities in health conditions in the society. Over specialization of health personnel and top-down healthcare delivery system siphoned off large chunks of limited fund. However, it could only cater to a privileged few. Community participation is the principle accepted in a befitting reply to stub out medical elitism: its *motto* is *'putting people's health in people's hand.'*

Awareness of the community regarding their own health needs and development of self-reliance to fulfill the needs, are key determinants for community development. For achieving it, the members of the community should have all the *rights* to participate in their *duties* towards improvement of standards of health. Disseminating relevant information, increasing health awareness and establishing appropriate institutional arrangements through communities, families and individual, are some of the ways that the community can take up the responsibilities for their health and well being.

For ensuring adequate community participation, trained community health workers are placed under the guidance of a qualified health team to deliver preventive, promotive and primary clinical care. The community health workers act as the first contact between the people and the health system for various health needs of the community. They are also trained to assess the health needs, plan and organize resources for various healthcare community healthcare activities as well as monitor and report them in real time. Involving community representative in delivery of healthcare as a Village Health Guides, ASHA, creation of Village Health and Sanitation Committee, Mahila Aarogya Samiti are some examples of community participation or involvement.

***Intersectoral coordination:*** There are many determinants of health which lie outsides of the domain of health department. Departments of Public Works and Engineering (for housing, safe water and sanitation), electricity, agriculture and animal husbandry, pollution control board, social welfare, roads and transport, labor, women and child development, food safety are some examples with which the health department needs to have proper coordination to ensure optimum delivery of healthcare services to address the social determinants of health as well as in delivering specific healthcare in coordination with related sectors.

### Eight Elements of Primary Healthcare

Eight components to be fulfilled towards the delivery of PHC were:
1. *Health education* on locally prevailing health problems and ways to prevent and control them
2. Promotion of *good nutrition* and development of an adequate food supply
3. Improvement of the *health of mother and children*, as well as family planning
4. Provision of adequate, *safe water and proper sanitation*
5. *Immunization* against major infectious diseases
6. Prevention and control of *locally endemic diseases*
7. Appropriate *treatment* for common diseases and injuries
8. Provision of *essential medicines*

### Challenges Faced in the Implementation of Primary Healthcare Concept

- Lack of political commitment after the initial enthusiasm in Alma-Ata.
- Lack of vision to reform and giving priority to primary care over medical care.
- Comprehensive PHC was viewed as too idealistic, expensive and unachievable in its goals of achieving total population coverage, hence the commitment reduced over time.
- The concept of *'selective PHC'* largely focusing on reducing child (<5 year) mortality and improving maternal care overtook the proposed *'comprehensive PHC'*.
- *Vertical programs* dominated under PHC at the cost of comprehensive PHC.
- The core PHC principle of community participation, could not be fulfilled in many countries.
- Due to lack of availability of infrastructure, staff, drugs and facilities in the newly created Primary Health Centre set-up, people felt that the Primary Health Center was a cheap,

substandard form of healthcare. They were thus not attracted to it.
- Civil war, natural disasters, political instability, changing demographic and epidemiological scenario adversely affected the ability of Primary Healthcare to maintain comprehensive services in many countries (especially, Sub-Saharan countries).

### Salient Outcomes of Primary Healthcare Movement

In spite of all challenges and criticism for not attaining the target health for all 2000 by AD, PHC concept made many significant changes on the global health front. *'PHC movement'* initiated across the world. Governments, civil society organizations, professionals, researchers and grass roots organizations all joined hands to improve the global health. Some of the salient outcomes of this movement are as follows:
- The interrelationship and interdependence between health, social and economic development was globally recognized.
- Health goal was established as social goal rather than a medical goal and it was put as an important determinant for the overall human development.
- Primary healthcare strategy was adopted by many developing countries and was made an integral part of the health system and of overall social and economic development of the community.
- For the first time global health goal "health for all by 2000 AD" was proclaimed: the world was viewed as one global community. This laid the foundation for managing community health globally.
- Combined efforts and coordination between different agencies and countries for managing the health of the people of the world was started.

### India and Primary Healthcare

India was already having a healthcare system based on delivery of basic healthcare services to rural population, supported by the village health guide scheme and auxiliary functionaries. Keeping the recommendations of the Alma-Ata declarations, India subsequently prepared its first ever health policy (as a statement) in the year 1983, to attain the goal of health for all by 2000 AD, keeping primary healthcare as the principal core strategy.

## Health Sector System Reforms

The concept of *'health system reform'* which originated among international health experts and developmental agencies was the result of changes in economic philosophy based on market forces and the economic benefits of better health.

The term 'Health systems' includes all the organizations, institutions and resources that are devoted for producing health actions. A *'health action'* is any effort, through personal healthcare, public health services, intersectoral initiatives, whose primary purpose is to improve health.

The World Bank in its World Development Report (1993) advocated three pronged strategies for improving health in the developing countries.
1. Governments need to foster an economic environment that enables households to improve their own health.
2. The spending of governments on health should be redirected towards more cost-effective programs that focus more on helping the poor.
3. Governments need to promote greater diversity and competition in the financing and delivery of health services.

*'Reducing the health inequalities'* was the focus in primary healthcare concept. In the concept of health sector reforms, *'improving performance'* became the keywords. It was emphasized that effectiveness of health systems plays a greater role in the attainment of the highest possible level of health, by all people.

### Four Sets of Primary Healthcare Reforms

In the year 2008, WHO revisited the ambitious vision of PHC. The World Health Report (2008), suggested a change in approach from 'Primary Healthcare" to "Health System Reform". It advocated four sets of reforms that reflect a convergence between the values of PHC, the expectations of citizens and the common health performance challenges **(Fig. 38.4)**. They are as follows:
1. ***Universal coverage reforms:*** There should be universal access to health, equity and social justice to ensure social health protection.

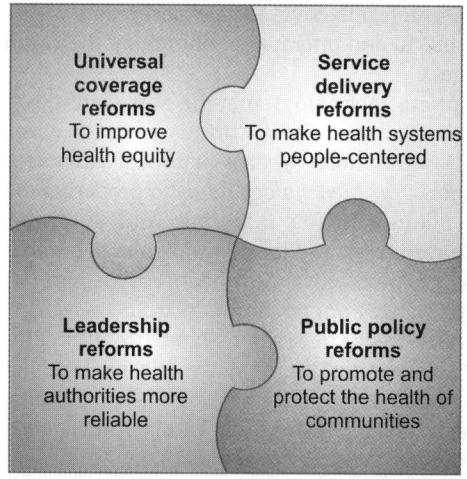

**Fig. 38.4:** Four sets of health sector reforms.
*Source:* Van Lerberghe W, The World Health Report, 2008.

2. ***Service delivery reforms:*** Health services need to be reorganized as per people's needs and expectations. This will make them more socially relevant and responsive to the changes in world and produce better outcomes.
3. ***Public policy reforms:*** This will help in framing policies which have a wider reach for various sectors and strengthen health interventions by encompassing public health actions into primary care.
4. ***Leadership reforms:*** Suggests moving away from *'centralized and authoritarian leadership'* to *'laissez-faire type'* of leadership. In Laissez faire type of leadership, the leaders try to give the *least possible guidance* to subordinates, and try to achieve control throu23gh less obvious means. This promotes the inclusive, participatory, negotiation-based work culture.

Under the health system reform approach, the performance of healthcare services, dominated over the socioeconomic development agenda. Management of health system to deliver effective and efficient health services became the focus. The availability, accessibility, acceptability and affordability of health services were stressed upon, to improve the performance of health system. Gradually various concepts of management and human resource management were brought into to improve the performance of the health system.

## Universal Health Coverage

The end of the 20th century saw landmark movements like the 'Health for All by 2000', the introduction of the 'Health System Reforms' approach. However, when a situational analysis of health was carried out in the year 2005 findings concerning the aspect of service coverage were alarming.
- In some countries <10% births were attended by a skilled health worker.
- Poor children were dying earlier and rich children were living longer.
- Certain groups (such as migrants, ethnic minorities and indigenous people) were using health services far less that than others, even though their health needs were more.
- Around 150 million people suffered financial hardship annually and 100 million were pushed below the poverty line. In many countries up to 11% of the population faced financial hardships every year due to illness and up to 5% to them were forced to extreme poverty.

Looking to the gloomy picture of health in spite of the all global attempts, it was realized that *access* to preventive, promotive, curative and rehabilitative health services was critical. In the year 2005, the WHO recommended the *Universal Health Coverage (UHC) strategy* with an emphasis on sustainable health financing.

Universal health coverage is defined as *'access to key, promotive, preventive, curative, rehabilitative and palliative health interventions for all at an affordable cost, thereby achieving equity in access.'* It means that all people and communities can use various promotive, preventive, curative, rehabilitative and palliative health services as per their need. These services need to be of sufficient quality (to be effective), while also ensuring that their use does not expose the user to financial hardships.

Three objectives proposed to achieve the goal under UHC are:
1. *Reducing mortality/morbidity:* To reduce morbidity and mortality among the financially and socially underprivileged, *'equity in access to health services'* is to be ensured. This would enable that anyone who needs healthcare services, gets them, irrespective of their paying capacity.
2. *Ensuring patient satisfaction:* The mere coverage of promotive, preventive, curative, rehabilitative and palliative health services is not sufficient. They should also have *'sufficient quality'* to achieve improvement of the health of the community.
3. *Preventing financial impoverishment from catastrophic costs of illness:* Every year globally, approximately 44 million households (around 150 million individuals), throughout the world face catastrophic health expenditure: about 25 million households (100 million individuals) are pushed into poverty by their need to pay for health services. WHO has proposed that health expenditure be viewed as *'catastrophic'* whenever it is ≥40% of a household's *'nonsubsistence income'* (income available after basic needs of food clothing and shelter) have been met. Using the poverty line, *nonsubsistence income* is equivalent to the remaining income after subtraction of total household's income with the poverty line income. For simple calculation, out-of-pocket expenditure (on healthcare) which is >10% of total household income is considered as the catastrophic effect of illnesses.

### *Coverage Box of Universal Health Coverage*

The above three objectives of UHC are demonstrated as three dimensions of a box; named as a 'coverage box' **(Fig. 38.5)**.

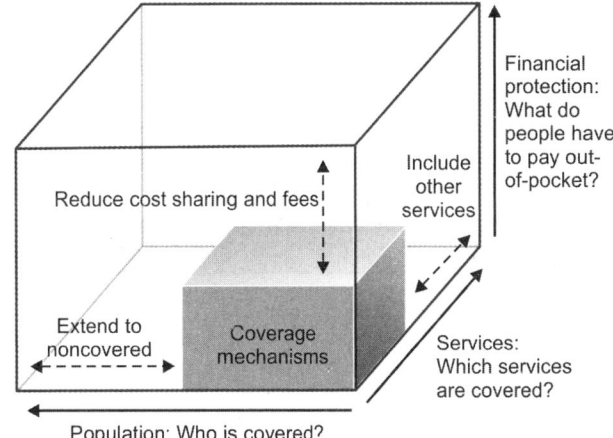

**Fig. 38.5:** Coverage box towards achieving Universal Health Coverage.
*Source:* WHO, Global Strategy for health for all by year 2000, 1981

Universal health coverage is having *three key elements*:
1. Health service coverage
2. Financial protection coverage
3. Whole population

These are demonstrated through three dimensional coverage box **(Fig. 38.5)**. Every country needs to assess the gap on all three dimensions and should try to organize the health system to bridge the gap between current coverage and expected universal coverage.

The key strategies recommended by WHO in the year 2005 for developing health system towards UHC are as follows:
- **Health insurance** to protect individual or family against catastrophic effect of out of pocket health expenditure.
- Adequate and equitable distribution of **good quality healthcare** facilities, healthcare manpower and essential services.
- All funds and activities under specific health programs are to be managed and organized in an integrated way so that it may help in developing a **sustainable financing system**.
- **Planning keeping in mind international development goals** and achieving agenda of health for all.
- Development of the health scenario should be **contextual to the sociocultural, political and economic scenario** of the country.
- Development of **public private partnership (PPP)** wherever possible through strong overall government stewardship.

### Resolution of the United Nations for Promoting Universal Health Coverage

On 12th of December, 2012, the United Nations adopted a resolution promoting Universal Health Coverage as a tool to promote human development. The UN unanimously resolved and urged all countries to provide affordable, quality healthcare to the citizens, by accelerating progress toward universal health coverage as an essential priority for international development. The 12th of December is now celebrated globally as the Universal Health Coverage Day.

### Universal Health Coverage and Sustainable Development Goals

The Sustainable Development Goals [a set of 17 global goals set by the United Nations Development Programme (UNDP), to be achieved by 2030], also lays importance on the concept of Universal Health Coverage. The goal 3 of the SDG is "ensure healthy lives and promote well-being for all at all ages" which in short is referred to as "good health". It has also identified two indicators (**Box 38.1**).

---
**Box 38.1: Indicators of universal healthcare under the Sustainable Development Goals.**

**Target 3.8:** Achieve universal health coverage, including financial risk protection, access to quality essential healthcare services and access to safe, effective, quality and affordable essential medicines and vaccines for all.

**SDG indicator 3.8.1:** Coverage of essential health services (defined as the average coverage of essential services based on tracer interventions that include reproductive, maternal, newborn and child health; infectious diseases; noncommunicable diseases; and service capacity and access; among the general and the most disadvantaged population).

**SDG indicator 3.8.2:** Proportion of population with large household expenditures on health as a share of total household expenditure or income.

---

Under SDG, UHC is defined as *'all people receive the health services they need, including public health services designed to promote better health, prevent illness, and to provide treatment, rehabilitation and palliative care of sufficient quality to be effective, while at the same time ensuring that the use of these services does not expose the user to financial hardship.'*

### Universal Health Coverage and India

As a signatory to the SDGs, India is committed towards achieving Universal Health Coverage. The government of India has taken steps to ensure equitable access to affordable, accountable and appropriate health services of assured quality (promotive, preventive, curative and rehabilitative) for every citizen of India, irrespective of their income, social status, gender, caste, region and religion. The government is the main guarantor and enabler, although not necessarily the *only* provider, of health and related services. Three important steps towards achieving UHC by the Government of India:
1. National Health Policy, 2017
2. National Health Protection Schemes for 10 crore families
3. Creation of 1.5 lakh health and wellness centers

## GLOBAL HEALTH: STRATEGIES AND AGENDAS

Three strategies to improve the global health are:
1. Primary healthcare
2. Health sector reforms
3. Universal health coverage

Three agendas for managing global health are:
1. **Health for all (HFA) by 2000:** Set in 1977 with targets to be achieved by 2000.
2. **Millennium development goals:** Set in 2000 with targets to be achieved by 2015.
3. **Sustainable development goals:** Set in 2015 with targets to be achieved by 2030.

### Health for All by 2000 AD

In 1977, the World Health Assembly decided that the main social target of the World Health Organization as well as individual government should be *'the attainment of a highest possible level of health by all the people of the world, by the year 2000 AD that permits every individual to lead a socially and economically productive life.'* It was the first time ever that a global target for health was framed with the ambition to make the changes in health of the global community through coordinated efforts. In 1978, at an International Conference on Primary Healthcare, held in the city of Alma-Ata (of the former USSR), PHC was recommended as the key to attaining HFA by 2000 AD.

***Understanding health for all:*** The goal of HFA 2000 by AD was made with the view to attain of WHO's objective *'the attainment of the highest possible level of health by all peoples that will permit every individual to lead a socially and economically productive life.'*

Health for All by 2000 AD does not mean that at the end of 20th century every person would become healthy and would not have any disease. HFA by 2000 AD meant that *all* people in *all* countries would have at least such a level of health that they would be capable of working productively and actively participate in the social life of the community where they lived. Every country was at their liberty to achieve this keeping their individual social, political, economic and health scenario into consideration.

***Global strategy for health for all by 2000 AD:*** After the Alma-Ata declaration in 1981, the WHO recommended a broad framework, based on which, every country or region could develop local and national strategies as per the prevailing health situation. The strategies recommended to manage the health of world with the goal to attain HFA by 2000 AD were:

- Establish the health system by *developing infrastructure*, starting from the level of primary healthcare.
- Deliver healthcare services and programs (which incorporate preventive, promotive, diagnostic, therapeutic and rehabilitative dimensions) to reach the whole population.
- *Use technology that is appropriate* (scientifically sound, adaptable to local circumstances, affordable and acceptable for providers and users).
- *Involve individuals, families, communities and other stakeholders.*
- Use and mobilize resources the country can afford and maintain.
- *Create international support mechanism* (for exchange of information, promoting research and development, technical support, training and intersectoral coordination for facilitating establishment of PHC in countries).

*Global Indicators for monitoring Health for All by 2000 AD goal:* For monitoring the progress toward achieving the goal of HFA by 2000 AD 12 indicators were fixed under the global strategy. Out of these 12 indicators, 6 indicators were to monitor the establishment and functioning of the governance and health delivery system, while 1 indicator was to specifically monitor the 4 key performance outputs under PHC, while 3 indicators were to monitor the health outcomes. Last 2 indicators were focusing on two key elements of social-economical development. They were as follows:

1. **Indicators for assessing Governance and Health System:**
   - Presence of an official health policy (statement or declaration of commitment by the highest level of country).
   - Formation of community involvement mechanisms for the implementation of strategies and their functionality (use in real life day to day scenario).
   - Allocation of at least 5% of the gross national product (GNP) to health by government.
   - Reasonable allocation (percentage wise) of the national health expenditure towards local healthcare (PHC *excluding* hospitals).
   - Equitable distribution (in contrast to equal distribution) of various resources (human, facility, materials, etc.) as per the need of special groups and geographical areas (such as urban, rural, tribal).
   - Presence of well-defined strategies for health for all in the developing country.

2. **Indicators for assessing performance of healthcare system (output indicators):** Availability of PHC to entire population, with at least the following:
   - Safe water in the home or within 15 minutes' walking distance, and adequate sanitary facilities in the home or immediate vicinity.
   - Immunization against diphtheria, tetanus, whooping-cough, measles, poliomyelitis, and tuberculosis.
   - Local healthcare, including availability of at least 20 essential drugs, within one hour's walk or travel.
   - Trained personnel for attending pregnancy and childbirth, and caring for children up to at least 1 year of age.

3. **Indicators for assessing outcome of healthcare system (outcome indicators):**
   - The nutritional status of children is adequate, in that:
     ♦ A birth weight of at least 2,500 g for at least 90% of newborn infants.
     ♦ A weight for age that corresponds in at least 90% of children.
   - For all identifiable subgroups, the infant mortality rate should be below 50 per 1,000 live births.
   - Increasing the life expectancy at birth more than 60 years.

4. **Indicators for assessing socioeconomical levels:**
   - For both men and women, the adult literacy rate should reach to 70% or more.
   - Per capita gross national product should be more than US $500.

## Millennium Development Goals

At the dawn of a new millennium, members and representatives of 189 countries met at the headquarters of the United Nations in New York between 6th and 8th September 2000 in the 'Millennium Summit'. They discussed the world situation and recognized that, there is a collective responsibility of all societies and community to uphold the principles of human equality, human equity and human dignity at the global level.

To fulfill the responsibilities and duties toward the people of the world, they set a global development agenda with 8 goals to be achieved by 2015, which are known as *MDGs*. As a commitment to world's development, all world leaders at the Millennium Summit signed a declaration, known as the United Nations Millennium Declaration.

The *original* declaration had *8 international development goals with 18 measurable targets and 48 indicators to monitor progress.* A *revised* indicator-framework on MDGs came into effect from January 2008. This framework had 8 goals, 21 targets and 60 indicators.

These goals were set to measure against situation of 1990 and to be achieved by the year 2015.

The 8 *goals* were **(Fig. 38.6)**:
1. Eradicate extreme poverty and hunger
2. Achieve universal primary education
3. Promote gender equality and empower women
4. Reduce child mortality
5. Improve maternal health
6. Combat HIV/AIDS, malaria and other diseases
7. Ensure environmental sustainability
8. Develop a global partnership for development

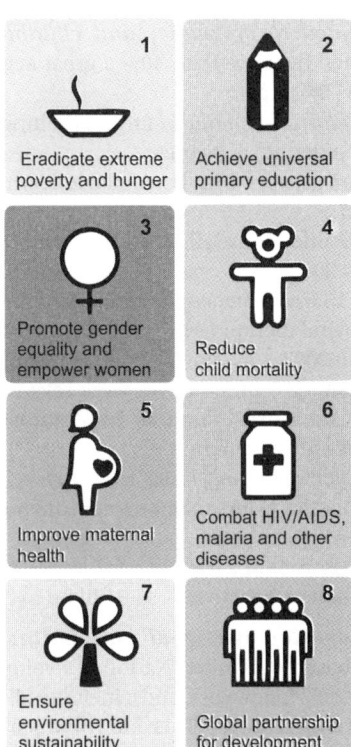

Fig. 38.6: Eight millennium development goals.

*Millennium development goals and health:* Under MDGs, three goals (goal 4, 5 and 6) were *'direct health goals'* but all other goals were related with health. For example, health can be positively influenced by reducing poverty, hunger and environmental degradation, while better health provides enabling environment for both children and adults to learn and earn. Gender equality is essential to the achievement of better health. In fact, MDGs put health at the center of development of all countries; all the MDGs influence health, and health influences all the MDGs.

***Millennium development goals—What we achieved:*** MDGs led to one of the most successful antipoverty movement in history. The global mobilization and landmark commitment by world leaders were translated into an inspiring action plan and practical steps that have enabled people across the world to improve their lives and future prospects.

**Though all the set targets could not be achieved:** Nonetheless, some of the salient achievements were as follows (MDG Report 2015, United Nations):
- Since 1990, the number of people living in extreme poverty has declined by more than half, falling from 1,900 million in 1990 to 836 million in 2015.
- The *primary school enrolment rate* in the developing countries has reached 91%, and enrolment rate of girls has also increased.
- *Child mortality* decreased from 100 million in 2000 to 57 million in 2015, witnessing a fall of 43%, but fell short of the 67% target.
- The *global prevalence of underweight among children aged less than* 5 nearly achieved a 50% reduction between 1990 and 2015, declining from 25% to 14%.
- *Deaths related to pregnancy and childbirth (maternal mortality)* fell by more than 40% a great achievement, but short of the 75% target.
- *HIV, tuberculosis and malaria targets* (halting and reversing the global epidemic) were met.
  - Reduction of over 6.2 million malaria deaths between 2000 and 2015.
  - New HIV infections fell by approximately 40% between 2000 and 2013.
  - By 2014, 13.6 million people living with HIV were receiving antiretroviral therapy (ART) globally, an increase from 0.8 million in 2003.
  - An estimated 37 million lives were saved between 2000–2013 by measures, such as tuberculosis prevention, diagnosis and treatment.
- The *target for drinking water was met*, with 91% of the global population using an improved drinking water source, compared to 76% in 1990.
- Official development assistance for health increased from US$11.6 billion in 2000 to US$ 35.9 billion in 2014.

***Millennium development goal and India:*** India's MDG framework is based on United Nations Development Group's (UNDG) MDG 2003 framework, and it includes all the eight goals, 12 out of the 18 targets (targets 1–11 and 18) which are relevant for India and related 35 indicators. Some of the targets and related indicators were not relevant for India and sufficiently reliable data was not readily available. Hence, these were either dropped or modified to suit Indian context. India developed its National Health Policy in the year 2002 as a political commitment to health goals under MDGs and guide the various initiatives to achieve it.

## Sustainable Developments Goals

**Birth of the sustainable development goals:** In 2015 the MDGs came to the end of their term. During the course of realizing the MDGs, several limitations became apparent:
- Lack of interlinkages between different goals
- Focus was more *'target oriented'*, and the emphasis was on a *'one-size-fits-all'* development planning approach
- Progress towards MDGs varied both, within and between individual countries.

Five years before the completion of the MDG (in 2010), the member states of the UN gave their first mandate to start to look ahead beyond 2015. At the UN Conference on Sustainable Development in Rio de Janeiro in 2012 *(Rio+20)*, a second approval was given. This conference initiated an inclusive intergovernmental process to prepare a proposal on *SDGs*. It was decided that the SDGs should be integrated into the UN post-2015 development agenda, to set the world on a more prosperous and sustainable path by 2030.

The Agenda included four key components:
1. **The declaration:** A *'vision statement'* of what we want to achieve in the next development agenda.
2. **Goals and targets:** A new set of goals and targets to build on and succeed the MDGs.
3. **Financing and the means of implementation:** The *'how'* of delivering the post-2015 development agenda.
4. **Monitoring and review:** Defining a process to track progress on commitments made by all stakeholders.

At the headquarters of the United Nations in New York, the member countries met between 25th and 27th September 2015 to look ahead beyond MDG and to set global agendas and discuss plan of actions with a vision to transform the world. The UN General Assembly adopted the new development agenda "Transforming our world: the 2030 agenda for sustainable development". They declared 17 SDGs of the 2030. Agenda for sustainable development and 169 interlinked targets to be attained by collaborative partnership between countries and stakeholders were spelt out. These SDGs came into force on 1st January, 2016.

Sustainable development has been *defined* as *"development that meets the needs of the present without compromising the ability of future generations to meet their own needs"*. Sustainable development has *three core elements:*
1. Economic growth
2. Social inclusion
3. Environmental protection

The 17 SDGs are broader and more ambitious than the MDGs, and relevant to all people in all countries to ensure that "no one is left behind". SDGs are integrated and indivisible. These agendas are focusing on *five "Ps", i.e., people, planet, prosperity, peace and partnership.* These five principles are to guide activities under each specific goal to be achieved for next 15 years, i.e., 2030.

> **Note**
> - **Theme of SDG:** No one is left behind
> - **Core elements:** Economic growth, social inclusion, environmental protection
> - **Five principles (5P's):** People, planet, prosperity, peace and partnership

*Arching principles (these principles are covering various dimensions to achieve the ultimate goal and hence are referred to as arching principles):*
- **People:** SDGs are determined to completely curb poverty and hunger, to ensure that all human beings can fulfill their potential in dignity and equality and in a healthy environment.
- **Planet:** SDGs are designed to support the needs of present and future generations by taking urgent actions on climate change—sustainable consumption, production and sustainably managing the planet's natural resources.
- **Prosperity:** SDGs are determined to ensure that all human beings can enjoy prosperous and fulfilling lives and that economic, social and technological progress occurs in harmony with nature.
- **Peace:** SDGs are determined to foster peaceful, just and inclusive societies which are free from fear and violence. There can be no sustainable development without peace and no peace without sustainable development.
- **Partnership:** SDGs are determined to mobilize the means required to implement this 2030 Agenda through a revitalized global partnership for sustainable development. This would require participation of all countries, all stakeholders and all people.

While the SDGs are not a law to abide by, it is expected that governments take ownership and establish national taskforce for the achievement of the 17 goals **(Fig. 38.7 and Box 38.2)**. A core feature of the SDGs is their strong focus on "means of implementation"—the mobilization of financial resources, capacity building and technology, as well as data management. Difference between millennium development goals and sustainable development goals is discussed in **Table 38.6**.

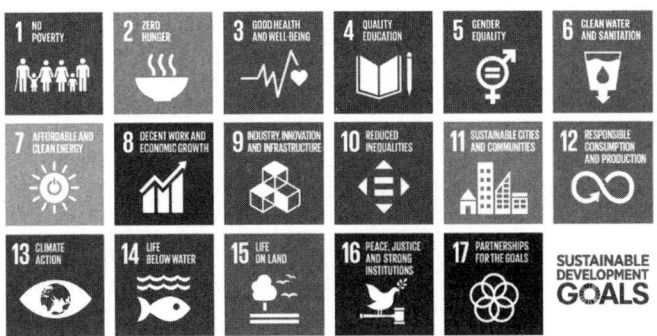

**Fig. 38.7:** The 17 core areas of sustainable development goals of the 2030 Agenda for Sustainable Development.

**Table 38.6:** Millennium development goals (MDGs) vis-à-vis sustainable development goals.

| Millennium development goals | Sustainable development goals |
|---|---|
| • MDGs reflected a narrower range of development outcomes (in poverty, education and health), and had limited set of human development targets | • SDGs by declaration are "integrated and indivisible, global and universally applicable". SDGs cover economic, social and environmental pillars of sustainable development with a strong focus on equity |
| • Mainly relevant to *developing* countries | |
| • MDGs were relatively silent about the impact of politics, security and global peace for human development | • SDGs are relevant to all countries |
| • All MDGs were mostly independent of each other, though health was given due importance in almost all of the MDGs | • SDG explicitly recognizes the importance of peace and security as necessary conditions for sustainable development |
| | • SDGs are cross-cutting and inter-linked by design |

> **Box 38.2: The 17 sustainable development goals (effective 1st January, 2016).**
>
> **The 17 SDGs:**
> 1. End poverty in all its forms everywhere
> 2. End hunger, achieve food security and improved nutrition and promote sustainable agriculture
> 3. Ensure healthy lives and promote well-being for all at all ages
> 4. Ensure inclusive and equitable quality education and promote lifelong learning opportunities for all
> 5. Achieve gender equality and empower all women and girls
> 6. Ensure availability and sustainable management of water and sanitation for all
> 7. Ensure access to affordable, reliable, sustainable and modern energy for all
> 8. Promote sustained, inclusive and sustainable economic growth, full and productive employment and decent work for all
> 9. Build resilient infrastructure, promote inclusive and sustainable industrialization and foster innovation
> 10. Reduce inequality within and among countries
> 11. Make cities and human settlements inclusive, safe, resilient and sustainable
> 12. Ensure sustainable consumption and production patterns
> 13. Take urgent action to combat climate change and its impacts
> 14. Conserve and sustainably use the oceans, seas and marine resources for sustainable development
> 15. Protect, restore and promote sustainable use of terrestrial ecosystems, sustainably manage forests, combat desertification, and halt and reverse land degradation and halt biodiversity loss
> 16. Promote peaceful and inclusive societies for sustainable development, provide access to justice for all and build effective, accountable and inclusive institution at all levels
> 17. Strengthen the means of implementation and revitalize the global partnership for sustainable development

***Health and sustainable development goals:*** Almost all the SDGs are directly related to health or will contribute to health indirectly. One of the goals (SDG 3), "ensure healthy lives and promote well-being for all at all ages" with 13 measurable targets specifically sets out for health. One of the targets is UHC which provides an overall framework for the implementation of agenda in all countries. UHC is the only target that cuts across all targets of the health goals, as well as links health-related targets in the other goals.

The health-related indicators among different SDGs may be grouped into the seven thematic areas:

**Section 4:** Community Health Management

1. Reproductive, maternal, newborn and child health
2. Infectious diseases
3. Noncommunicable diseases (NCDs) and mental health
4. Injuries and violence
5. UHC and health systems
6. Environmental risks
7. Health risks and disease outbreaks

While the only SDG explicitly focused on health is SDG3, there are 10 other goals addressing health-related issues.

***Sustainable development goals in India:*** Sustainable development goals provide India with a valuable opportunity to adopt development pathways that will enable it to stand shoulder to shoulder with its Asian peer countries. The government is working on the principle of *'Sabka Sath, Sabka Vikas'* to gain achievements in poverty reduction, education, gender equality, health, safe water and sanitation as well as climate change. This strategy is in line with that being advocated by Member States at the United Nations. Strengthening of health system any many new initiatives in the health are part of India's strategies to achieve the health goals under SDG.

***Sustainable Development Report for India 2023:*** The Sustainable Development Report 2023 marks the eighth edition of the annual assessment of progress for all UN member states towards the Sustainable Development Goals. India stands at SDG Index rank 112 out of 166 member countries, with SDG Index score of 63.5. The overall score measures the total progress towards achieving all 17 SDGs. The score can be interpreted as a percentage of SDG achievement. A score of 100 indicates that all SDGs have been achieved. The overall performance of India towards achieving all SDGs in shown in **Figure 38.8**, while performance indicators for SDG3 is shown in **Table 38.7**.

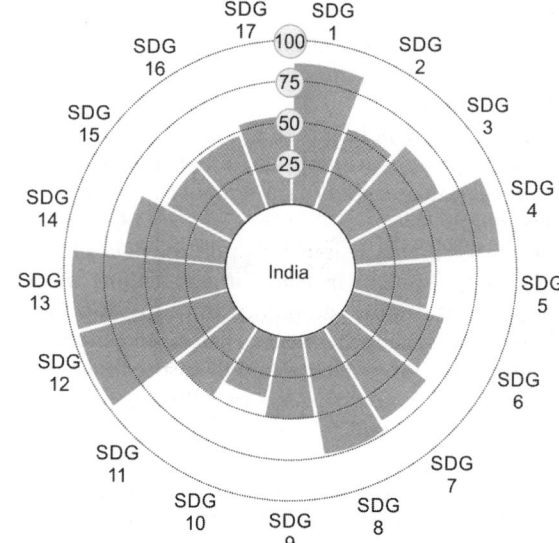

**Fig. 38.8:** Average performance by SDG for India.
*Source:* Sustainable Development Report 2023.

**Table 38.7:** Performance of SDG3 by indicators, India.

| SDG3—Good health and well-being | | | |
|---|---|---|---|
| Maternal mortality rate (per 100,000 live births) | 102.7 2020 | ○ | ↑ |
| Neonatal mortality rate (per 1,000 live births) | 19.1 2021 | ● | ↑ |
| Mortality rate, under-5 (per 1,000 live births) | 30.6 2021 | ○ | ↑ |
| Incidence of tuberculosis (per 100,000 population) | 210.0 2021 | ● | → |
| New HIV infections (per 1,000 uninfected population) | 0.1 2021 | ● | ↑ |
| Age-standardized death rate due to cardiovascular disease, cancer, diabetes, or chronic respiratory disease in adults aged 30–70 years | 21.9 2019 | ○ | → |
| Age-standardized death rate attributable to household air pollution and ambient air pollution (per 100,000 population) | 139.3 2019 | ○ | ● |
| Traffic deaths (per 100,000 population) | 15.6 2019 | ● | → |
| Life expectancy at birth (years) | 70.8 2019 | ○ | ↗ |
| Adolescent fertility rate (births per 1,000 females aged 15–19) | 12.2 2018 | ● | ● |
| Births attended by skilled health personnel (%) | 89.4 2021 | ● | ↑ |
| Surviving Infants who received 2 WHO-recommended vaccines (%) | 85 2021 | ○ | → |
| Universal health coverage (UHC) index of service coverage (worst 0–100 best) | 61 2019 | ● | ↗ |
| Subjective well-being (average ladder score, worst 0–10 best) | 3.9 2022 | ● | ↓ |

Dashboards: ● SDG achieved ○ Challenges remain ● Significant challenges remain ● Major challenges remain ● Information unavailable
Trends: ↑ On track or maintaining SDG achievement ↗ Moderately improving → Stagnating ↓ Decreasing •• Trend information unavailable

*Source:* Sustainable Development Report 2023.

*(For color version, see Plate 4)*

**Goals and targets (from the 2030 agenda for sustainable development).**

*Goal 3. Ensure healthy lives and promote well-being for all at all ages*

3.1 By 2030, reduce the global *maternal mortality ratio* to <70 per 100,000 live births

3.2 By 2030, end preventable deaths of newborns and children under 5 years of age, with all countries aiming *to reduce neonatal mortality* to at least as low as 12 per 1,000 live births and *under 5 mortality* to at least as low as 25 per 1,000 live births

3.3 By 2030, end the epidemics of *AIDS, tuberculosis, malaria and neglected tropical diseases and combat hepatitis, water-borne diseases and other communicable diseases*

3.4 By 2030, reduce by one-third *premature mortality from noncommunicable diseases* through prevention and treatment and promote mental health and well-being

3.5 Strengthen the prevention and treatment of *substance abuse*, including *narcotic drug abuse* and harmful use of *alcohol*

3.6 By 2020, halve the number of global deaths and injuries from *road traffic accidents*

3.7 By 2030, ensure universal access to *sexual and reproductive healthcare services*, including for family planning, information and education, and the integration of reproductive health into national strategies and programs

3.8 *Achieve UHC*, including financial risk protection, access to quality essential healthcare services and access to safe, effective, quality and affordable essential medicines and vaccines for all

3.9 By 2030, substantially reduce the number of deaths and illnesses from *hazardous chemicals and air, water and soil pollution and contamination*

3.a Strengthen the implementation of the World Health Organization Framework Convention on *Tobacco Control* in all countries, as appropriate

3.b Support the research and development of *vaccines and medicines* for the communicable and noncommunicable diseases that primarily affect developing countries, provide access to affordable essential medicines and vaccines, in accordance with the *Doha Declaration on the Trade-Related Aspects of Intellectual Property Rights (TRIPS) Agreement and Public Health*, which affirms the right of developing countries to use to the full the provisions in the agreement regarding flexibilities to protect public health, and, in particular, provide access to medicines for all

3.c Substantially increase *health financing and the recruitment, development, training and retention of the health workforce* in developing countries, especially in least developed countries and small island developing states

3.d Strengthen the capacity of all countries, in particular developing countries, for *early warning, risk reduction and management of national and global health risks*

**Sets of challenges for India for realizing SDGs**

- *Completing the unfinished MDG agenda*
- *Strengthening critical development drivers*, such as economic growth, industrialization, employment creation and reduction of inequality within and between countries, basic infrastructure including energy and institutions, along with good governance
- *Developing capacity to address new and emerging challenges*, such as deteriorating environment, irrational consumption and production patterns that are rapidly depleting natural resources, and develop liveable urban areas
- *Accessing the means of implementation* including transfer of advanced sustainable technologies from developed countries as well building capacities of our own technological and engineering resources.

## SUGGESTED READING

1. Cueto M. The origins of primary healthcare and selective primary healthcare. Am J Public Health. 2004;94:1864-74.
2. Djukanovic V, Mach EP. Alternative approaches to meeting basic health needs in developing countries: a joint UNICEF/WHO study. Geneva: World Health Organization; 1975.
3. Hall JJ, Taylor R. Health for all beyond 2000: The demise of the Alma-Ata Declaration and primary healthcare in developing countries. Med J Aust. 2003;178:17-20.
4. India UN (2015). India and the MDGs: Towards a Sustainable Future for All. [online] Available from https://www.unescap.org/resources/ india-and-mdgs-towards-sustainable-future-all.
5. Joseph A, Kadri AM, Krishnan A, et al. IAPSM declaration 2018: Definition, role, scope of community medicine and functions of community medicine specialists. Indian J Community Med. 2018;43:120-1.
6. Kadri AM. Managing effective reform for Community Medicine subject: Vision to actions. Indian J Comm Health. 2017;29:337-9.
7. Kadri AM. Reforming community medicine in line with the country's health priorities-Let's make it relevant and rational. Indian J Community Med. 2017;42:189.
8. Lawn JE, Rohde J, Rifkin S, et al. Alma-Ata 30 years on: revolutionary, relevant, and time to revitalise. Lancet. 2008;372:917-27.
9. Mahler H. Present Status of WHO's Initiative," Health For All by the Year 2000". Ann. Rev. Public Health. 1988;9:71-97.
10. Millennium Development Goals. [online] Available from: http:// www.undp.org/content/undp/en/home/sdgoverview/mdg_goals. html.
11. Ministry of Statistics and Programme Implementation (2015). Millennium Development Goals: India Country Report; 2015.
12. United Nations. (2000). United Nations millennium declaration. [online] Available from http://www.un.org/millennium/ declaration/ares552e.htm.
13. United Nations. (2015). Transforming our world: The 2030 agenda for sustainable development. Resolution adopted by the General Assembly.
14. United Nations Development Programme: Human development report 2003. Millennium Development Goals: A compact among nations to end human poverty. New York: Oxford University Press; 2003.
15. United Nations Foundation. Post-2015 Development Agenda. [online] Available from: http://www.unfoundation.org/what-we- do/working-with-the-un/post-2015-development-agenda.
16. Van Lerberghe W. The world health report 2008: Primary healthcare: now more than ever. Geneva: World Health Organization; 2008.
17. World Bank. World development report 1993: Investing in health: World development indicators. New York: Oxford University Press; 1992.
18. World Health Organization. (2000). The world health report 2000: Health systems: Improving performance.
19. World Health Organization. (2016). Health in 2015: From MDGs, millennium development goals to SDGs, sustainable development goals. Geneva: World Health Organization.
20. World Health Organization. The Declaration of Alma Ata. Presented at. International Conference on Primary Healthcare. Alma Ata. 1978.

# CHAPTER 39

# Healthcare Delivery System Across Nations

*Rashmi Kundapur, Harshitha HN, Rahul Hegde*

## PREREADING ACTIVITY

- Visit different healthcare system and talk to the people working there about the system of health care
- Identify good system and bad system by talking to the clients attending the system
- Prepare a list of doubts/questions that you wish to clarify about healthcare system.

*Suggested environment and method for learning from the following text*:
- Silent, independent, at self-paced, reading followed by immediate mental recall.
- The students are also suggested to learn about the other locally relevant, practical aspects of the topic from his/her seniors and teachers.
- Self-directed learning or problem-based learning can also be used under the guidance of seniors, teachers, or mentors.

## HEALTH SYSTEM: STRUCTURE AND FUNCTIONS

To meet the health needs of the community a country or community requires a good and efficient robust health system. The health system consists of all organizations, people and actions whose primary intent is to promote, restore or maintain health. This includes efforts to influence determinants of health as well as more direct health-improving activities or curative care.

Health system includes government, charity or private hospitals and healthcare centers. It also includes health programs, health schemes, teaching and training institutes in health and medical care, health care research institutes, health care regulation authorities; vector-control campaigns; health insurance organizations; occupational health and safety legislation, etc. Health system includes intersectoral action by health staff, for example, encouraging the ministry of education to promote female education, a well-known determinant of better health. Any system is designed to cater the specific health care need of the community. But due to limitation of the resources, priorities have to be set for the requirements. This envisages proper planning so that the resources are not wasted. It is designed to meet the health needs of the community through the use of available knowledge and resources. The service provided through healthcare delivery system should be comprehensive and community based. The resources should be distributed according to the needs of the community. The healthcare system is intended to deliver the health care services. It constitutes the management sector, and involves organizational matters. Health systems have multiple goals. The World Health Report 2000 defined overall health system outcomes or goals as: improving health and health equity, in ways that are responsive, financially fair, and make the best, or most efficient, use of available resources.

## Conventional Model of System

Conventional model of any system is *input-process-output (IPO) model* (**Flowchart 39.1**). The inputs are the resources put into the system. Process represents various preventive, promotive, curative, palliative and rehabilitative activities carried out through use of the resources put into. Output is the services delivered out of the system. They are like vaccinations carried out, patient treated, health center-hospitals built, doctors-health personnel produced, etc.

The healthcare services are designed to meet the health needs of the community through the use of available knowledge and resources. The service provided should be comprehensive and community based. The resources should be distributed according to the needs of the community.

The final desired outcome or output impact of healthcare delivery system is to attain the changed health status or improved health status of the community which is expressed in terms of lives saved, deaths averted, diseases prevented, cases treated, expectation of life prolonged, etc.

World Health Organization (WHO) has proposed a health system framework keeping the specific nature of health care. It consists of six health blocks and four outcomes. The six building blocks of a health system are given in **Figure 39.1**.

### Good Health Services

Good health services are the ones which deliver safe, effective, quality personal and non-personal health interventions to the people in need with minimal waste of resources.

**Example:** A comprehensive PHC Programme has been in place in the remote Sayaboury province in Laos since 1991. It has achieved impressive results. Between 1996 and 2003 health facility utilization tripled, maternal mortality dropped 50%, and by 2003 infant and child mortality were less than one-third of the national average.

Flowchart 39.1: World Health Organization health system strengthening framework.

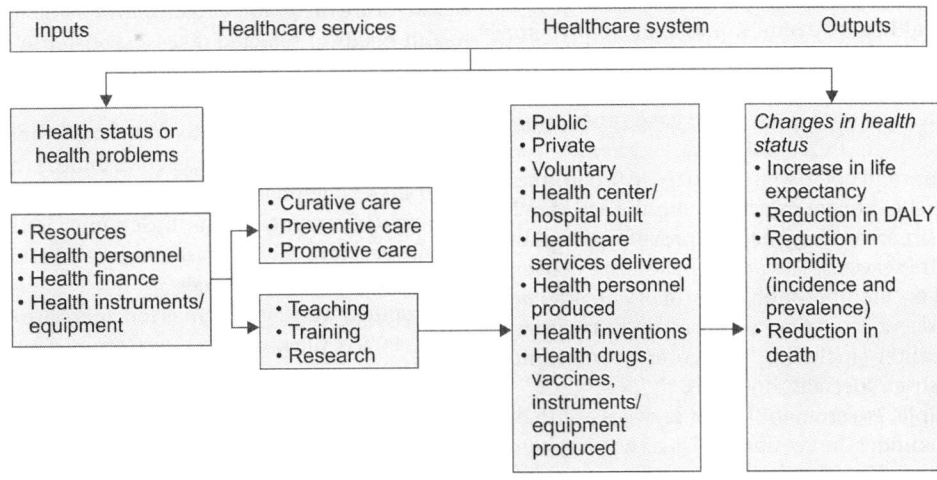

(DALY: disability-adjusted life-year)

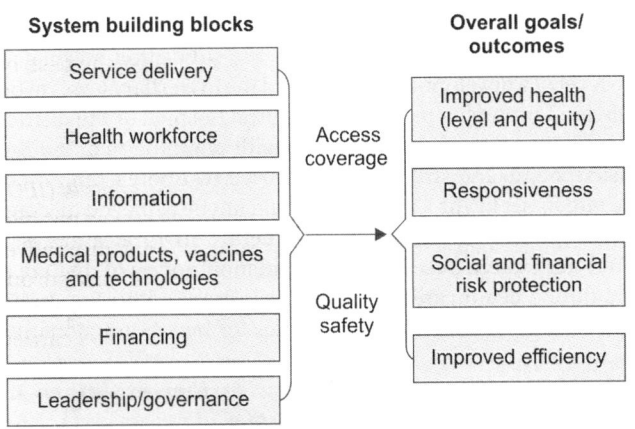

Fig. 39.1: World Health Organization health system framework.
Source: www.who.int.net.

## A Well-performing Health Workforce

It refers to one which works in ways that are responsive, fair and efficient to achieve the best possible health outcomes, with available resources and prevailing circumstances. In this system there are sufficient numbers and mix of staff, fairly distributed; they are competent, responsive and productive.

**Example**: Lady Health Workers (LHWs) in Pakistan. Evaluations of this program have found that in areas with LHWs, there are a higher proportion of deliveries conducted by a skilled attendant; more babies exclusively breastfed; more mothers who know about oral rehydration, and who give it to children with diarrhea; and more children fully vaccinated, compared with areas without LHWs.

## A Well-functioning Health Information System

It is one that ensures the production, analysis, dissemination and use of reliable and timely information on health determinants, health systems performance and health status.

## A Good Health Financing System

It is able to generate adequate funds for health, in ways that ensure people can use needed services, and are protected from financial catastrophe or impoverishment associated with having to pay for them.

**Example:** Social and financial protection in Colombia. Colombia's national health insurance scheme was part of a package of health reforms introduced nationwide in 1993. The subsidized regime played a key role in increasing coverage for the poor and people living in rural areas. Coverage of people increased over a period of time from 3 to 57% and also increased utilization of healthcare facilities was observed.

## TYPES OF HEALTHCARE SYSTEM

*Every country develops the health system as per their health needs, availability of resources and vision for health care.*

Health systems are always characterized according to the source of health care finance of the system. They can be broadly classified into three categories:

1. *Public*: Run on government (public) fund. Developed and managed by government agencies. Many countries are having healthcare system, which is completely or predominantly funded and managed by government. Health system of United Kingdom is the example of such system.
2. *Private*: Run on private fund. Developed and managed by private agencies. Many countries are having healthcare system, which is completely or predominantly funded and managed by private players. Health system of United States is the example of such system.
3. *Mix*: Countries, which are not having any of predominant public or private healthcare providers. Health needs of the community are being catered by mix of public or private healthcare providers. India is example of such mixed healthcare system.

## INDIAN HEALTHCARE SYSTEM (FLOWCHART 39.2)

India has a mixed healthcare system. In India, preventive and promotive care are being taken care of largely by public healthcare system with tiny contribution by private healthcare providers who majorly function on charity cause. Even government plays major role in clinical care. Public healthcare system is well developed in rural areas and not so well organized in urban areas, while most of private healthcare providers in India are largely concentrated in urban area. They majorly provide secondary and tertiary healthcare services. The public healthcare delivery system is developed on the philosophy of primary health care (PHC) and developed as a three-tier healthcare delivery system consisting of PHC center (including subcenter), community health center and district/specialist hospitals.

In India, in principle, government health services are to be available to all citizens under the tax-financed healthcare system. However, in practice bottlenecks are present in accessing such services which compel households to seek private health care. This results in high out-of-pocket expenditure for households. The public health sector in India covers 18% of total outpatient care and 44% of total inpatient care.

In recent past, the key initiative for making health care affordable and accessible to all citizens through partnership with private providers at national and state levels have stepped in, e.g., the Rashtriya Swasthya Bima Yojana (RSBY) and Pradhan Mantri Jan Arogya Yojana (PM-JAY) are such initiatives. Besides that, many other programs are also initiated, which began in 2008 under the Ministry of Labor and Employment to provide health insurance coverage to families below the poverty line.

In 2015–2016, 41.3 million families were enrolled which constituted 57% of the target. The scheme now also includes unorganized workers (11 other categories), aiming to cover maximum number of people. For example, in Gujarat such as Mukhyamantri Amrutam Yojana, Chiranjeevi Yojana and Balsakha are the *public-private partnership* to meet the curative health needs of selected diseases, obstetric care and pediatric diseases, respectively for identified poor or marginalized communities.

The true social health insurance scheme in India for which both employee and employer contribute is the Employees State Insurance Scheme for factory workers. The civil servants have Central Government Health Scheme. Railway and defense employees have their own schemes, and many states also have schemes for their employees.

Despite of various schemes too, there are evidences to say in 2014, <20% of the population was covered by any form of health coverage.

The foundation of India's public health system was laid on the basis of the recommendations made by the "Health Survey and Development Committee", popularly known as the "Bhore Committee", in its report submitted in 1946. "The Committee specified three levels of health care—(1) *primary* (to be delivered by "Primary Health Center" and its associated subcenters), (2) secondary level (to be delivered by a subdistrict hospital at the level of a development block), and the (3) tertiary level (to be delivered through a tertiary care referral hospital at the district level)." Even though subsequent health planning retained the basic scheme and structure as proposed by Bhore Committee, the targets set by the Committee, could not be achieved till date.

The public health care infrastructure in rural areas is a three-tier system based on the population norms of that area. The public healthcare system varies in rural and urban India with respect to the population norms for health functionaries appointed.

***Healthcare system in India is further explained in Chapter 46: Indian Healthcare System.***

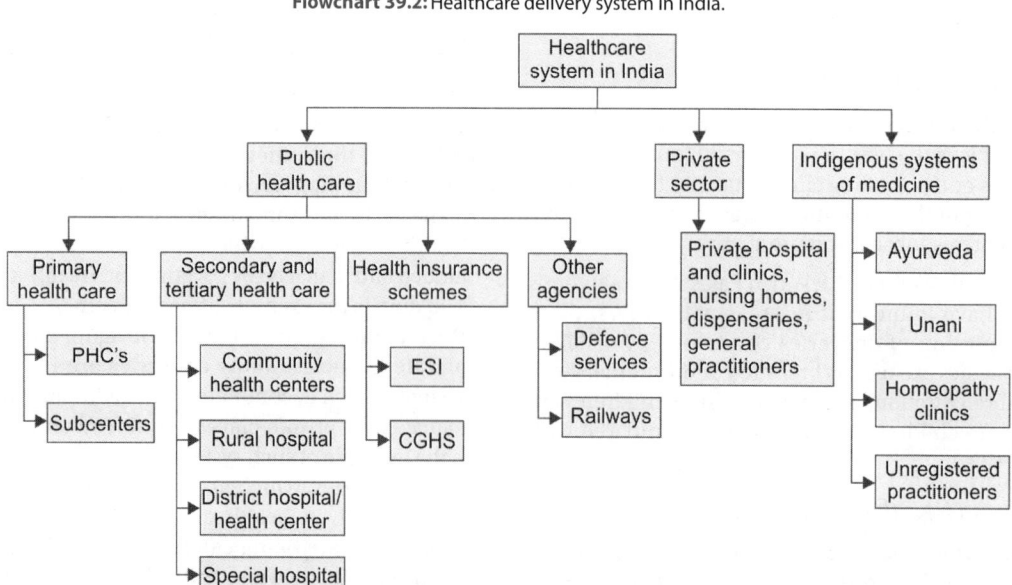

**Flowchart 39.2:** Healthcare delivery system in India.

(PHC: primary health centers; ESI: Employees' State Insurance; CGHS: Central Government Health Insurance Scheme)

> **Points to Remember**
> - In **"mixed market"** healthcare systems, the government and private health services operate side-by-side. India has such system in place.
> - The public healthcare infrastructure in rural areas **has a three-tier system based on the population norms.**
> - World Health Organization norm for doctor patient population ratio is 1:1,000, while India has a ratio of 1:1,445.

## HEALTHCARE SYSTEM IN SOME OTHER COUNTRIES

### Healthcare System in United States

Health care in the *United States* is largely owned and operated by *private sector*. 58% of US community hospitals (which are private) are of non-profit, 21% (private) are for profit, and only 21% of hospitals are government owned. US though being top economic powered country in the world do not have universal health care coverage (The Atlantic, Fisher M, 2012).

US healthcare system is predominantly focused on curative care only and is heavily health insurance driven. The United States health system primarily depends on the employers to provide health insurance coverage to their employees and dependents. Government programs are only to the elderly, the disabled, and some of the poor. There is coordination between private and public programs so some people have both public and private insurance while others have neither.

- There is no system of government-owned medical facilities all over the nation.
- The defense and veterans have system like military hospital and veterans' hospitals.
- Health services for the terminally ill who are expected to live 6 months or less are subsidized by charities and government.

The US healthcare delivery system unevenly provides medical care of varying quality. There is underutilization of preventative measures so there is high prevalence of chronic disease. This suggests that the US healthcare system does not promote wellness but is only curative.

> *A concern for US health system is that the health gains are not equally distributed to the entire population.*

### Healthcare System in Canada

Canadian healthcare delivery system is mixed type healthcare delivery system with large contribution by the public healthcare delivery system. Also, it works on principles of primary and promotive health care but hugely dependents on the health insurance, which is funded by public sector. Some of the salient feature of Canadian healthcare delivery system is given here:
- The *Canadian government* ensures the quality of health care through federal standards and Medicare is cost effective.
- In each Canadian province, doctor is the one who handles the insurance claim, so the person who availed health care is free from billing or reclaim and level of care remains same to all.
- All essential basic care is covered by government which also includes maternity benefit.
- Canada (with the exception of the province of Quebec) is one of the few countries with a universal healthcare system but it does not include the coverage of medication prescription in its insurance system.

*Family physicians* (often known as general practitioners or GPs in Canada) are chosen by patient themselves. If a patient wishes to see a specialist or is counseled to see a specialist by their GP, a referral has to be made by a GP present in the local community to the hospital.

About 27.6% of Canadians' health care is paid by individual to private sector for not covered or partially covered care, like prescription of medication, dentistry and optometry. So, 75% of Canadians have some form of supplementary private health insurance; through their employers. 30% of health expenditures in Canada come from private sources (insurance and out-of-pocket payments) (Canada Health, Overview of Canada Health Act, 2009).

- Unlike USA, preventive care and early detection are considered as critical health issues in Canada.
- Unlike USA, Canada has a publicly funded medicare system though most of the services are provided by the private health care.

### Healthcare System in United Kingdom

United Kingdom's healthcare system is predominantly public healthcare system. It is a well knitted health system from bottom to top named as national health system.

*United Kingdom* differs in its healthcare system with respect to *England, Scotland, North Ireland and Wales,* as each of them have their own systems funded by and accountable to separate governments of those countries. The performance of the National Health System (NHS) across UK is ranked best healthcare system in the world by Commonwealth in 2014. The categories considered good were—*quality of care, access to care, efficiency, and equity* **(Flowchart 39.3)**.

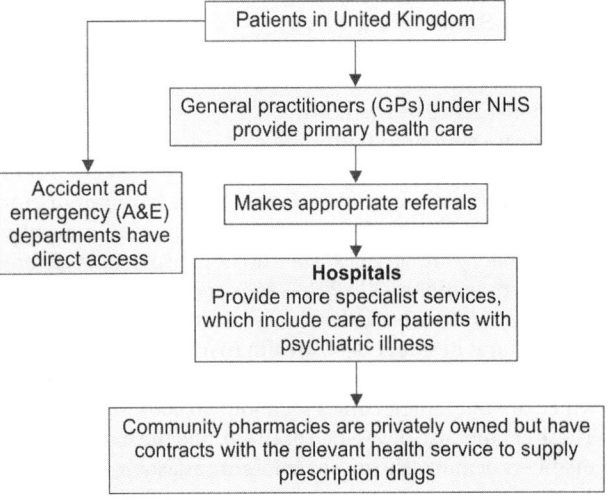

Flowchart 39.3: Healthcare system in United Kingdom.

- The NHS began in 1948 with the principle that good health care, should be available to all citizens, access to care should be based on clinical need of a person and not his ability to pay.
- "Putting patients first", is the core principle of NHS which is free of charge to patients in England.
- Though service's main focus was the diagnosis and treatment of disease, it plays an interesting role in preventing ill health and promoting good health.

*Public Health England (PHE)* is an operationally independent executive agency of the Health Department and it supports local authorities in their duty to improvise public health. It also has national responsibility for protecting the public against major health risks.

### Commissioning in NHS

When a GP refers a patient to a particular hospital for further investigation or treatment, the GP is by himself will be buying the care from referred hospital for that patient. This "secondary" provider (referred hospital) is paid to treat the patient through the NHS payment system. What care a GP can buy for his patient is determined by the commissioning organization (which is a local organization deciding on the GP to be part of NHS. This CCG constitutes other healthcare members and lay persons too within it). The services that CCGs commission include urgent and emergency care with planned hospital care and rehabilitative care.

The Care Quality Commission is responsible for assessing and makes judgments on safety and quality of care provided.

### The Chinese Healthcare System

*Traditional medicine in China* has been a practice for years, the western evidence-based medicine made its way to China in the beginning of 19th Century only. *Health care in China* consists of both public and private medical institutions and also insurance programs. 95% of the population in China have basic health insurance but it covers only about half of medical costs in China. Under the "Healthy China 2020" initiative government ensures insurance will be covering 70% of costs by 2018 and a total affordable health care to all by 2020 (Hoguard JL et al., Appl Health Econ Health Policy, 2011).

- Residents of urban areas in China are not provided with any free health care, they must either pay for treatment or purchase health insurance by their own.
- Healthcare system in both rural and urban areas are three-tiered system.
- In rural areas the first tier is made up of barefoot doctors working in village medical centers. They provide preventive and primary-care services. They do not have to be registered medical practitioners (*In 2014, there were 1.06 million village doctors and health workers*) (The State Council, Merging Urban-Rural Resident Basic Health Insurance, 2016).
- At the next level (second tier) are the township health centers, which are outpatient clinics for about 10,000–30,000 people. These centers also have a bed of 10–30, and the most qualified members of the staff in these centers are assistant doctors. The bare foot doctors and assistant doctors together make "rural collective health system".
- Only the most seriously ill patients will be referred to the third and final tier, the county hospitals, which serve 200,000–600,000 people and are staffed by doctors who hold 5-year medical school degree.
- GPs rarely practice alone, they work in a hospital with nurses and nonphysician clinicians.
- The central government in China is overall responsible and health authorities of China include National Health and Family Planning Commission along with local Health and Family Planning Commissions, who are responsible for healthcare delivery.

Fee for primary care in government-funded health institutions are regulated by local health authorities. Village doctors and health workers receive income through public health services reimbursement (e.g., immunizations and chronic disease screening) and the actual clinical services they provide. GPs at hospitals receive a base salary and payments based on their activities (e.g., surgeries performed). Hospital-based physicians always have strong financial incentives.

*Hospitals:* Hospitals can be public or private, non-profit or for-profit. Most township hospitals and community hospitals are public. The public and private secondary to tertiary care hospitals exist mainly in urban areas.

### Healthcare System in Bangladesh

The health system of Bangladesh relies mainly on the government for financing and for setting overall policies and service delivery mechanisms.

- The health system receive little priority in terms of national resource allocation so has a lot of problems.
- The health system of Bangladesh is a multiple health system in one way with four key system: (1) government, (2) private sector, (3) nongovernmental organizations (NGOs), and (4) donor agencies.
- The Ministry of Health and Family Welfare, manages this type of double health system, one of general health and family planning services through district hospitals, Upazila Health Complexes (with 10–50 beds) at subdistrict level. And administration is through Directorates General of Health Services (DGHS) and Family Planning (DGFP).
- According to the World Health Organization (WHO 2010) only about 3% of the gross domestic product (GDP) in Bangladesh is spent on health services.
- Government expenditure on health is just about 34% of the total health expenditure, the rest being out-of-pocket expenses (66%). Inequity is a serious problem in this health system (Ahmed SM et al., Dhaka University, 2015).
- The findings suggest that although the health system faces a lot of challenges, Bangladesh has demonstrated considerable progress in achieving the health-related *Millennium Development Goals (MDG)* especially MDG 4 and MDG 5.
- But Bangladesh does not have a comprehensive health policy.

## Healthcare System in Sri Lanka

Sri Lanka holds a unique position in South Asia as it is one of the first among the less developed nations to provide universal health, free education, strong gender equality, and better opportunity to social mobility.

- The health system in Sri Lanka is a mix of Allopathic, Ayurvedic, Unani and several other systems of medicine. Of all these systems allopathic medicine becomes dominant and is catering to the majority of the health needs of the people in the country.
- Sri Lankan health system consists of both public and private sector.
- The Health Ministry along with Provincial Health Services provide a wide range of promotive, preventive, curative and rehabilitative health care.
- Total expenditure on health is 3.6% of Sri Lankan GDP (Paskins Z et al., Postgrad Med J, 2001).
- The health policies in Sri Lanka were always in favor of PHC. Tertiary health care not very important in the public sector.
- The strength of the healthcare system in this country is a strong basic primary health care, and, not the high-tech intensive care units.
- The healthcare system is in reasonably well distributed throughout the country, within few kilometers of village too there is a health center.
- There is quite good road network to tertiary care in case of emergencies to be transported.
- Most importantly all health administrators were and are doctors.

## Healthcare System in South Africa

South Africa's Constitution guarantees every citizen to access the health services. However, everyone can access both public and private health services, depending on an individual's ability to pay **(Fig. 39.2)**.

- The healthcare system consumes 8.8% of the country's GDP (Mahlathi P, Geneva-WHO, 2015).
- The majority of patients access the public sector through District Health System.
- 16% of the population is served by private sector while the public sector serves 84%.
- Government mechanism is a primary health care approach with primary, secondary and tertiary healthcare system.
- In South Africa public health workers are permitted to work part time in the private sector since the early 1990s.

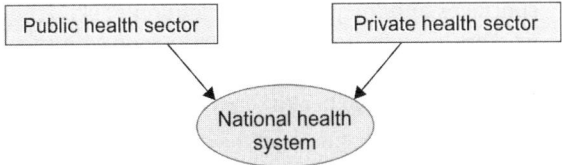

**Fig. 39.2:** Healthcare system in South Africa.

### Points to Remember

- **Health care in the United States** is largely owned and operated by *private sector*.
- The United States primarily **depends on employers to provide health insurance coverage to their employees and dependents**.
- The US healthcare delivery system **unevenly provides medical care of varying quality with no importance to wellness**.
- **Canada has cost-effective health care provided through province and the coverage is 100%**.
- Early detections are considered critical health issues and yearly checkups are recommended for everyone in Canada.
- UK is ranked best healthcare system in the world by Commonwealth in 2014.
- The NHS began in 1948 with access based on clinical need, not ability to pay.
- 95% of the population in China has basic health insurance coverage but covers only half of expenditure. Healthcare system is mixed.
- Health care was provided in both rural and urban areas through a three-tiered system. And 1st tier with bare foot doctors, 5 years medical degree doctors are found in 3rd and final tier.
- Government spends only 34% of total health care cost in Bangladesh.
- Healthcare system in Bangladesh is run by Bangladesh Government, private and NGOs in government dual administration is present.
- The strength of the Sri Lankan healthcare system is strong basic primary health care.
- The healthcare system is in reasonable distribution throughout the country in Sri Lanka.

## SUGGESTED READING

1. Ahmed SM, Alam BB, Anwar I, et al. Bangladesh Health System Review. In: Naheed A, Hort K (Eds). Health Systems in Transition. Dhaka: Dhaka University; 2015.
2. BBC. UK end-of-life care best in world. [online] Available from https://www.bbc.com/news/health-34415362.
3. Canada Health. (2009). Overview of the Canada Health Act.
4. Chokshi M, Patil B, Khanna R, et al. Health systems in India. J Perinatol. 2016;36(S3):S9-S12.
5. Dpeaflcio. The U.S. Health care System: An International Perspective. [online] Available from www.dpeaflcio.org.
6. Hoguard JL, Ostradeal JP, Yu Y. The Chinese healthcare system: structure, problems and challenges. Appl Health Econ Health Policy. 2011;9(1):1-13.
7. Isam A, Biswas T. Health systems in Bangladesh: Challenges and opportunities. Am J Health Res. 2014;2(6):366-74.
8. Jiang C, Ma J. Analyzing the Role of Overall Basic Medical Insurance in the Process of Universal Health Coverage. Chinese Health Ser Managt. 2015;2(320):108-10.
9. Mahlathi P, Dlamini J. South Africa's health system—A rapid analysis of stock and migration, minimum data sets for human resources for health and the surgical workforce in South Africa's health system. Geneva: WHO; 2015.
10. Samarage SM. Health care System: Sri Lanka; Migration and Human Resources for Health: From Awareness to Action. Geneva: CICG; 2006.
11. The Altantic. (2012). Fisher M. Here's a map of the countries that provide universal health care (America's Still Not on It).
12. The Guardian. (2011). How European nations run national health services: Belgium, France, Germany and Sweden. [online] Available from https://www.theguardian.com/healthcare-network/2011/may/11/european-healthcare-services-belgium-france-germany-sweden.
13. The State Council. The State Council's Suggestion on Merging Urban-Rural Resident Basic Health Insurance; 2016.
14. WHO. WHO health systems strategy. [online]. Available from http://www.who.int/healthsystems/strategy/en/.

# CHAPTER 40

# Human Resources for Health

*Sanjay Zodpey, Ritika Tiwari, Himanshu Negandhi*

## HEALTH SYSTEMS AND HUMAN RESOURCES FOR HEALTH

The health workforce has been highlighted as one of the key building blocks of World Health Organization (WHO)'s health system strengthening framework. The health workforce is not only a prerequisite to functioning of any health system but is crucial for achievement of global targets related to health and development. Implementation of efficient human resource management system improves health workforce outcome which in turn affects service delivery leading to better health outcomes. Establishing a competent heath workforce plays a vital role in building a robust, resilient, responsive health system.

The World Health Report 2006 considers that "health workers are all people primarily engaged in actions with the primary intent of enhancing health". The health workforce is characterized by its diversity and its complexity and includes people from a wide range of occupational backgrounds, e.g., doctors (allopathic and alternative medicine), nurses and midwives, public health professionals, pharmacists, dentists, allied health professionals (paramedical workers), grassroot workers, other health workers and support staff.

## GLOBAL HUMAN RESOURCES FOR HEALTH LANDSCAPE: NUMBERS AND CHALLENGES

- Lack of manpower in health in terms of skill and magnitude inhibits the proper implementation and monitoring of all health system responsibilities and delivery of quality healthcare services.
- In the year 2004, Chen et al., reanalyzed the data of an econometric cross-country study on human resources and health outcomes. Their analysis showed that HRH in aggregate terms accounts significantly for the three health outcome measures namely: maternal, infant, and under-five mortality rates (which speaks of the overall health system in the country).
- The study also suggested that number of health workers, i.e., doctors, nurses and midwives—lower the three mortality rates and controls these health outcomes significantly.

In the analysis of global workforce conducted by the Joint Learning Initiative—a consortium of more than 100 health leaders; it was proposed that mobilization and strengthening of human resources for health, is central to combating health crises in some of the world's poorest countries and for building sustainable health systems in all countries. Global HRH challenges were enumerated namely—global shortage, skill imbalances, maldistribution and migration, poor work environments and weak knowledge base. These global HRH challenges have been elaborated here:

- ***Global shortage:***
  - There is a strong global deficiency of HRH both in quality as well as in quantity.
  - Health service providers constitute about two-third of the global health workforce, while the remaining third is composed of health management and support workers.
  - As per the Global Health Workforce Alliance (GHWA) 2013 report; globally there is a deficit of about 7.2 million skilled health professionals. If this issue is not addressed now then the world will be short of 12.9 million healthcare workers by 2035. This may have serious implications over the health of billions of people across all regions of the world.
  - As stated in a recent study, by the year 2030, global demand for health workers may rise to 80 million workers, which would be double the current stock of health workers (2013) (Liu JX et al., Human Resource for Health, 2017).
  - While the supply of health workers is expected to reach 65 million over the same period, which may estimate into a worldwide net shortage of 15 million health workers.
  - As per this study by Liu et al. in 2017, efforts to scale-up health services to achieve universal health coverage (UHC) and health development goals are confronted by acute shortages and inequitable distribution of skilled health workers in many low and middle-income countries. This HRH shortage in turn translates into a constraint towards delivering essential health services.
- ***Skill imbalances:***
  - Nearly all countries have skill imbalances which create huge inefficiencies.
  - The skill mix depends too much on doctors and specialists. Thus, countries must revamp their health plans toward a workforce that more closely reflects the health needs of their populations.

- ***Maldistribution and migration***: Maldistribution exists nearly in all countries, which is gets worsened by unplanned migration. Health workers are more concentrated in urban areas everywhere. There is a need to improve within-country equity to attract and retain health workers to rural and marginal communities.

    Maldistribution between public and private sectors is severely affected by international migration. The brain drain of nurses and doctors is crippling health systems in many poor and developing countries.
- ***Poor work environments***: The countries must improve poor work environments by scaling up good practices and strengthen management of existing resources, assure adequate supplies and facilities, and create monetary and nonfinancial incentives to retain and motivate health workers. Also, there is a need to hear the voices of workers.
- ***Weak knowledge base***: The weak knowledge base on the health workforce hinders planning, policy development, and program operations. Deficiencies, such as less information, fragmentary data, and limited research must be remedied.

## ADDRESSING THE HUMAN RESOURCES FOR HEALTH ISSUE

To develop and implement strategies for effective and sustainable health workforce, WHO advocates an HRH Action Framework. It includes six action fields namely *HR management systems, leadership, partnership, finance, education and policy*; and four phases, i.e., *situational analysis, planning, implementation and monitoring and evaluation*. This HRH Action Framework is applicable globally, and it calls for review of the critical success factors of human resource management systems which include areas of intervention such as:

- ***Personnel systems***: Workforce planning (including staffing norms), recruitment, hiring, and deployment.
- ***Work environment and conditions***: Employee relations, workplace safety, gender equity, job satisfaction, and career development.
- ***HR information system*** integration of data sources to ensure timely availability of accurate data required for planning, training, appraising and supporting the workforce.
- ***Performance management***: Performance appraisal, supervision, and productivity.

In 2016, Global strategy on human resources for health: Workforce 2030 came into existence envisaging an accelerated progress in universal health coverage and accomplishment of UN Sustainable Development Goals. It was developed to ensure quality health workforce that is universally available, accessible, acceptable with optimal coverage through investment in health systems and implementation of effective policies to improve outcomes in health, social and economic development. It outlines global milestones to be achieved by the year 2020 and 2030 and provides policy option for WHO Member states and for other countries in order to achieve the four objectives with respect to human resources in health which are as follows:

- To improve health, social and economic development outcomes by ensuring universal availability, accessibility, acceptability, coverage and quality of the health workforce through adequate investments to strengthen health systems, and the implementation of effective policies at national, regional and global levels.
- Align investment in human resources for health with the current and future needs of the population and health systems, taking account of labor market dynamics and education policies, to address shortages and improve distribution of health workers, so as to enable maximum improvements in health outcomes, social welfare, employment creation and economic growth.
- Build the capacity of institutions at subnational, national, regional and global levels for effective public policy stewardship, leadership and governance of actions on human resources for health.
- Strengthen data on human resources for health for monitoring and accountability of national and regional strategies, and the Global Strategy.

> **Points to Remember**
> - HRH in aggregate terms accounts significantly for the three health outcome measures namely: Maternal, infant, and under-five mortality rates (which speaks of the overall health system in the country).
> - Global HRH challenges were enumerated namely—global shortage, skill imbalances, maldistribution and migration, poor work environments and weak knowledge base.
> - Strategies for effective and sustainable health workforce, WHO advocates an HRH Action Framework. It includes six action fields namely HR management systems, leadership, partnership, finance, education and policy; and four phases, i.e., situational analysis, planning, implementation and monitoring and evaluation.
> - Global strategy on human resources for health: Workforce 2030 provides policy options to Member states and other countries to accelerate progress in universal health coverage and UN Sustainable Development Goals.

## HUMAN RESOURCES FOR HEALTH SITUATION IN INDIA

In India, the health workforce is characterized by its diversity and its complexity. It includes people from a wide range of occupational backgrounds—doctors (allopathic and alternative medicine), nurses and midwives, public health professionals, pharmacists, dentists, allied health professionals (paramedical workers), grassroot workers, other health workers and support staff. In India, however, the biggest challenge for the provision of health care services and attaining the UHC is the acute shortage of health personnel and disproportionate skill mix of the existing staff.

As per an analysis undertaken by Sundararaman et al., in the year 2009, the trends of critical health indicators, such as infant mortality rate (IMR) and maternal mortality ratio (MMR) show a positive correlation with the availability of health personnel. Additionally, India in comparison to other countries (those with better availability of skilled health personnel) had higher mortality indicators. The shortage of nurses and midwives and physicians was as well reflected in some of the health indicators for India in comparison to countries, such as 5 in UK and 57 in India, IMR (2006); and 8 in UK, 4 in Australia and 450 in India, MMR (2005) (Sundararaman T et al., NHSRC—India, 2009).

A state-wise comparison of the HRH density with burden rates for leading infectious diseases depicts that states with low HRH density may show high burden rates of diarrheal and lower respiratory infections. However, apart from higher HRH density, other factors, such as better work quality and social determinants of health (education, gender equality, and higher income) also contribute toward improved population-based health outcomes.

Failure to sanction adequate number of public health facilities, absence of any uniform guidelines for the number of posts to be sanctioned for all the categories of health staff, financial constraints, and failure to attract and retain service providers against sanctioned posts in public health facilities have also been suggested as reason for HRH crisis in the country. Thus, a need for HRH reforms was felt to target various stages of the health workforce lifecycle. Since 2007, during the National Rural Health Mission (NRHM) addressing HRH issues has gained prominence. In order to attract and retain skilled service providers in rural and difficult areas several HRH reforms have been implemented such as: rural service as prequalification for admission in PG course, rotational posting in difficult areas, financial/nonfinancial incentives, preferential admission of those students who are likely to serve in under-serviced areas and multiskilling of existing staff such as AYUSH doctors.

## HUMAN RESOURCES FOR HEALTH CHALLENGES IN INDIA

As per study by the Indian Institute of Public Health, Delhi (IIPH, Delhi) and the Public Health Foundation of India (PHFI) in the year 2016, the total size of health workforce was estimated to be approximately 5 million in India. In these 5 million workers, approximately 1.2 million nonhealth workers are engaged in the health sector.

- *HRH density:* Estimates from National Sample Survey Office (NSSO) translates to approximately 29 health workers per 10,000 population if country's entire HRH is taken into consideration. If we considering the density of only doctors (including AYUSH) and nurses and midwives, the density of health workers is 20.6 per 10,000 population according the NSSO estimates. Estimates from NSSO are marginally below the WHO's minimum threshold of 22.8 workers per 10,000 population. However, if we consider ANM as part of the trained health workers then the density turns out to be close to 30 per 10,000 population. Thus, as per NSSO numbers there are 10 nurses and midwives per 10,000 population. This translates to 1.7 nurses and midwives per allopathic doctors as against the High Level Expert Group (HLEG) recommendation of two nurses and one ANM per allopathic doctor.
- *Inequitable geographical distribution:* There exists an enormous variation in density across states. Most of the central and eastern Indian states have low density of health workers ranging from approximately 23 per 10,000 population in Bihar and Northeast states other than Assam to as low as 7 per 10,000 population in Jharkhand. The only south Indian states reflecting lower density than the all India average is Andhra Pradesh and only eastern Indian state having higher density than the all India average is West Bengal. Highest concentration of health workers is in Delhi followed by Kerala, Punjab and Haryana. Considering only doctor, nurse and midwife density per 10,000 population, Delhi and Kerala numbers are far higher compared to other states with Bihar along with Jharkhand occupying the lowest position.

Density of physician and surgeon is also lower than five in states of Bihar, Jharkhand and Rajasthan. Delhi has the highest density of physician and surgeon but the density of nurses and midwives is the highest in Kerala. The HLEG recommendation for the doctor-nurse ratio in India is 1:3. Other states with acute adverse ratio (less than 1:1) of nurse to doctor are Bihar, Chhattisgarh, Goa, Haryana, Jammu and Kashmir, Karnataka, Madhya Pradesh, Maharashtra, Odisha, Punjab, Uttar Pradesh and West Bengal.

- *Rural-urban divide:* The uneven distribution of health workers is also reflected across rural-urban settings. Although rural India constituted approximately 71% of the total population in 2016, only 36% of all health workers are in the rural areas. This proportion is little lower for health associates and assistants and pharmacist. The proportion of physician and nurses in rural areas are 34% and 33% respectively.
- *Disparity between public and private sector:* Bulk of the total health workforce is employed in private sector. The proportion employed in private sector is far higher for doctors compared to nurse and midwife and other health workers. In case of AYUSH and dental practitioner, the share of public sector is <10%. However, approximately 45% of nurse and midwife are employed in public sector institutions. Further, private health sector in India consists of wide range of service providers ranging from "for-profit" hospitals, "not-for-profit" institutions (NGO, charitable institutions, trusts, etc.) and private individual practitioners. Distribution of all health workers by types of institutions reflect that overwhelming majority (53%) of these workers are self-employed in sole proprietorship or partnership entity. Only 6% of all health workers are employed in big corporate companies with public or private limited status.

> **Points to Remember**
> - The trends of critical health indicators like infant mortality rate (IMR) and maternal mortality ratio (MMR) show a positive correlation with the availability of health personnel.
> - Apart from higher HRH density, other factors, such as better work quality and social determinants of health (education, gender equality, and higher income) also contribute towards improved population-based health outcomes.
> - NSSO estimates there are approximately 29 health workers per 10,000 population if country's entire HRH is taken into consideration.
> - Most of the central and eastern Indian states have low density of health workers ranging from approximately 23 per 10,000 population in Bihar and Northeast states other than Assam to as low as 7 per 10,000 population in Jharkhand.
> - Rural India constituted approximately 71% of the total population in 2016, whereas only 36% of all health workers are in the rural areas.
> - Distribution of all health workers by types of institutions reflect that overwhelming majority (53%) of these workers are self-employed in sole proprietorship or partnership entity.

## SCENARIO OF HUMAN RESOURCES FOR HEALTH: INDIA VERSUS OTHER COUNTRIES

The World Health Report 2006 categorized India among the 57 countries facing most severe crisis in terms of availability of human resource for health. In 2014, the situation further deteriorated and 83 countries were short of the minimum thresholds of 22.8 skilled health professional per 10,000 population (Campbell J et al., WHO, 2013). In general, HRH in India is often characterized as inadequate and deficient, with inadequately qualified and poorly trained personnel and highly concentrated in major cities, leaving an acute gap in smaller towns and remote areas more often in rural areas.

Additionally, if we compare the HRH ratios for India with select countries, then it is evident that India is performing adequately.

- **Doctor-population ratio:** There is one doctor for every 834 Indians as per the country's current population estimate of 140 crore, which is better than WHO's prescribed norm of one doctor for 1,000 people. As per information provided by National Medical Commission (NMC), there are 13,08,009 allopathic doctors registered with the State Medical Councils and the National Medical Commission (NMC) as of June, 2022. Assuming 80% availability of registered allopathic doctors and 5.65 lakh active AYUSH doctors, the doctor-population ratio in the country is 1:834 (Press Information Bureau, MoHFW, GoI, July 2022). If we consider only allopathic doctors, current doctor population ratio is 1:1338 (in other words 0.75 per every 1,000 Indians)

  Cross country comparison of doctor-population ratio with some other countries is shown below **(Table 40.1)**.

**Table 40.1:** Cross country comparison of medical doctor-population ratio (WHO Global Health Observatory Report 2023).

| Country | Medical doctor-population ratio (WHO GHO 2023) |
|---|---|
| UK | 3.17 |
| USA | 3.55 |
| Brazil | 2.14 |
| China | 2.38 |
| Sri Lanka | 1.19 |
| India | 0.73 |
| Bangladesh | 0.67 |

- **Nurse-Population ratio:** The nurse to population ratio as recommended by WHO is 3:1,000 which is 2:1,000 for India. (adapted from National Health Profile 2022). There are 35.14 registered nurses, midwives, auxiliary nurse midwives and lady health visitors, Considering 80% availability, there are 498 nursing personnel available for every 1,000 Indians.

  Cross country comparison of nurse-population ratio is shown in **Table 40.2**.

**Table 40.2:** Cross country comparison of nurse-population ratio (WHO Global Health Observatory Report 2023).

| Country | Nurse-population ratio (WHO GHO 2023) |
|---|---|
| USA | 12.47 |
| UK | 9.16 |
| Brazil | 5.51 |
| China | 3.30 |
| Sri Lanka | 2.43 |
| India | 1.72 |
| Bangladesh | 0.61 |

Thus, it is evident that situation of HRH in India is evolving but remains inadequate.

## THE NATIONAL HEALTH POLICY 2017: INDIA'S CURRENT WAY FORWARD FOR HUMAN RESOURCES FOR HEALTH

Amidst the existing HRH challenges, the Government of India has been making attempts for attainment of the highest possible level of health and wellbeing for all at all ages. The recently announced National Health Policy (NHP) 2017—informs, clarifies, strengthens, and prioritizes the role of the government in shaping health systems in all its dimensions including development of human resources for health. The policy presents an indicative list of time bound quantitative goals aligned to ongoing national efforts as well as the global strategic directions. Some of the key HRH reforms as stated in the policy includes: "Better financing of professional and technical education, defining professional boundaries and skill sets, reshaping the pedagogy of professional and technical education, revisiting entry policies into educational institutions, ensuring quality of education and regulating the system to generate the right mix of skills at the right place".

Other proposed HRH reforms includes: Increasing the number of doctors and specialists, in states with large human resource deficit, attracting and retaining doctors in remote areas, specialist attraction and retention, establishing cadres like nurse practitioners and public health nurses to increase their availability in most needed areas, and creation of a public health management cadre in all states with a qualification in public health or related discipline as an entry criterion.

Thus, the NHP envisages an implementation framework which would provide a roadmap with clear deliverables and milestones for the government to achieve UHC through improved HRH policies and reforms.

## STRATEGIC OPTIONS FOR INDIA TO MEET HRH SHORTAGE AND CHALLENGES

In order to meet the existing HRH shortage and challenges there is a need to adopt strategic options which may include:
- **Continue with existing initiatives:** Continuing with existing initiatives, such as innovations under NHM, capacity building

and training initiatives and medical specialist training at District Hospital, should be continued to strengthen the country's HRH.

- **Set up professionally managed HR cell at state level:** For effective and efficient management of human resources at state level there is a need for overall HRH planning and management. Thus, the state HR cell could be set up to undertake tasks related to efficient and optimum use of human resources at state level.
- **Aligning "supply side" to the "need":** The supply side being on lower side and does not corresponds to the future need of trained health workforce in the country. Also, there is an imminent need to meet the gap of trained health professionals at every health facility as per Indian Public Health Standard (IPHS). Thus, the government policies need to align with the future need and link the growth of current supply capacity (of various health professionals) in accordance to the same.
- **Introducing mid-level service providers:** Introduction of mid-level service providers could be an imminent solution for meeting the current HRH crisis in the country. Development and integration of a cadre of mid-level care providers by introducing courses, such as BSc in Community Health, Competency-based bridge courses/Short courses, Nurse Practitioners and Public Health Nurses, etc., could help meet the current HRH shortage.
- **Leveraging technology for addressing HRH issues:** Adoption and integration of human resource management information system (HRMIS) can help in tackling the issues surrounding the availability and competence pertaining to the health professionals at state level. The increasing use of telemedicine (use of telecommunication and information technology to provide clinical health care from a distance) could prove to be helpful in meeting the requirement of health professionals in remote and resource–limited settings.
- **HRH needs for the future:** Effective policies at national level along with strong political commitment are needed to ensure availability and accessibility of quality of the health workforce in the future. Building the capacity of our state and national education institutions for developing a competent health workforce with decent employment opportunities would largely contribute towards meeting the HRH needs in the future.

## SUGGESTED READING

1. Anand S, Bärnighausen T. Human resources and health outcomes: cross-country econometric study. Lancet. 2004;364(9445):1603-9.
2. Campbell J, Dussault G, Buchan J, et al. A universal truth: no health without a workforce. Forum Report, Third Global Forum on Human Resources for Health, Recife, Brazil. Geneva, Global Health Workforce Alliance and World Health Organization; 2013.
3. Central Bureau for Health Intelligence. Directorate General of Health Services, Ministry of Health and Family Welfare, Government of India New Delhi 2017.
4. Chen L, Evans T, Anand S, et al. Human resources for health: overcoming the crisis. Lancet. 2004;364(9449):1984-90.
5. Indian Council of Medical Research, Public Health Foundation of India, and Institute for Health Metrics and Evaluation. India: Health of the Nation's States - The India State-level Disease Burden Initiative. New Delhi, India: ICMR, PHFI, and IHME; 2017.
6. Liu JX, Goryakin Y, Maeda A, et al. Global health workforce labor market projections for 2030. Human Res Health. 2017;15(1):11.
7. Ministry of Health and Family Welfare. National Health Policy. New Delhi: Ministry of Health and Family Welfare; 2017.
8. National Commission on Macroeconomics and Health. Report of the National Commission on Macroeconomics and Health. New Delhi: NCMH; 2005.
9. OECD. (2018). Nurses (indicator) Available from https://data.oecd.org/healthres/nurses.htm#indicator-chart.
10. OECD. (2018). Doctors (indicator). [Online] Available from https://data.oecd.org/healthres/doctors.htm.
11. Public Health Foundation of India. Strategic Framework on Human Resources for Health (HRH) in India. New Delhi: PHFI; 2016.
12. Sundararaman T, Gupta G. Human Resource for Health: The crisis, the NRHM response and the policy options. New Delhi: NHSRC India; 2009.
13. World Health Organization. (2016). Global strategy on human resources for health: Workforce 2030.
14. World Health Organization. Density of nursing and midwifery personnel (total number per 1000 population, latest available year—GHOG data). Geneva: WHO; 2018.
15. World Health Organization. The World Health Report 2006: working together for health. Geneva: World Health Organization; 2006.

# CHAPTER 41

# Health Financing

*Rashmi Kundapur, Sharon Baisal*

### PRE-READING ACTIVITY
- Visit different healthcare systems and talk to the people working there about the resources in system of health care
- Identify good system and bad system by talking to the clients attending the system finances
- Prepare a list of doubts/questions that you wish to clarify about healthcare system financing.

*Suggested environment and method for learning from the following text:*
- Silent, independent, at self-paced, reading followed by immediate mental recall.
- The students are also suggested to learn about the other locally relevant, practical aspects of the topic from his/her seniors and teachers.
- Self-directed learning or problem-based learning can also be used under the guidance of seniors, teachers, or mentors.

### HEALTHCARE FINANCING

*For successfully running healthcare system after human resource, another important resource is the finance. Adequate healthcare financing is the key for proper functioning of healthcare system.* The purpose of health financing is to make funding available, as well as to set the right financial incentives to providers, to ensure that all individuals have access to effective public health and personal healthcare [World Health Organization (WHO), 2000]. The aim of health system financing is "more money for health and more health for money".

## Healthcare Financing: An Overview

Healthcare financing is defined by WHO as function of a health system concerned with the mobilization, accumulation, and allocation of money to cover the health needs of the people, individually and collectively in the health system.

There is no fix norms about how much fund a health system requires. It depends upon the health needs of the community. Community with high disease burden or at greater threat of health risks will require more fund, while relatively healthy community requires lesser funds.

According to the Organization for Economic Cooperation and Development (OECD), in 2022, the health expenditure to GDP ratio remained by far the highest in the USA at 16.6% in 2022, followed by Germany at 12.7% and France at 12.1%. A further 14 high-income countries, including Canada and Japan, all spent more than 10% of their GDP on healthcare in 2022. For the year 2019–20, the total health expenditure (THE) for India was 3.27% of GDP and ₹ 4,863 per capita. However, public/government health expenditure (GHE) was low at 1.35% of GDP and ₹ 2,014 per capita (amounts to only 41% of THE).

## Sources of Healthcare Financing

- ***The tax-based public sector:*** Healthcare services provided by the government setup are largely funded from the fund received as a general taxation of the country. It is a huge fund for public healthcare system.
- ***Out-of-pocket expenditure (OOPE):*** It is the expenditure incurred by the community members for availing healthcare services. For betterment of people, OOPE in health should be reduced.
- ***External financing:*** Three important external sources are—(1) Donor international agencies [e.g. United Nations International Children's Emergency Fund (UNICEF), United States Agency for International Development (USAID), etc.], (2) Philanthropist (Bill and Melinda Gates Foundation, Rockefeller foundation, TATA, etc.), or (3) Fund from corporate sector responsibility (Azim Premji, Infosys, TCS, etc.). Small to huge amounts are funded by them for various activities especially for healthcare services for underdeveloped areas, unprivileged group of people, or problem of community health importance. Key building blocks for health system financing are as follow:
    - Raising sufficient funds for health
    - Improvement of financial risk protection and coverage for vulnerable groups
    - Improvement in the efficiency of resource utilization
    - Improved financial transparency and management.
- ***Pooling of resources:*** Pooling of the resources is the important strategy to meet country's health finance needs. It means to accumulate and manage financial resources to ensure that the financial risk of having to pay for health care is borne by all members of the pool and not by the individuals who fall ill. The main purpose of pooling is to spread the financial risk associated with the need to use health services. Countries with high out-of-pocket expenses have inefficient and insufficient

pooling of resources. Health insurance—social, community based, and private—are the important strategies under it. For the same, pooling of the fund (public and/or people) is carried out. Now, private health insurance has become huge part of health financing and the healthcare delivery systems of many countries are dependent on it.

> **History**
>
> The basic principle of health financing is of pooling of resources in order to manage the economic risks and it date back to ancient Greece. In medieval times, it was labor unions who established the welfare funds to assist sick and needy members of their unions. As the industrial revolution gathered its momentum later in 19th century, all workers and unions joined relief funds, which eventually became government regulation.
>
> In 1883, compulsory health insurance to all the workers in Germany came into being. This program proved to be highly successful and soon spread into other European countries. It eventually expanded into today's "social insurance".

## Health Financing in United States of America

The USA did not take any action in the past or in 20th century to either subsidize voluntary funds or make insurance for sickness mandatory.

*In nutshell, in US:*

- Private agencies have managed sickness care, private health insurance policies, and other private programs for those who were working in their agencies
- Senior citizens have Medicare and Medicare Supplementary Health Insurance (known as Medigap).

Health care in the US is technologically advanced, but expensive and was costing about $3.3 trillion dollars in 2016, which was 17.9% of its GDP. In 2016, the US spent almost $9,900 per capita, 25% greater than the next highest spending country (Pharmpress, Health economics, 2018). Consequences of increased US spending on health care include the following:

- Increased government spending on health
- Decline in workers' earnings per se due to higher payments for health insurance premiums
- Increased costs incurred by employers to buy a better insurance.

Even though US spends highest GDP in the world on health, many people in the US do not have health insurance, whereas many other developed countries with lower GDP expenditure, ensure universal access to health care. US health care spending is currently a major problem.

## Health Financing in United Kingdom

The National Health Service (NHS) is mainly funded from taxation and anyone who is resident in the UK is entitled to use it.
- The overall NHS spending is determined by UK government.
- For many years, NHS spending was within the range of 5.5–6.2% of GDP. In 2016, the health financing was 9.8% of GDP and in 2017, it was 9.9% (James JH et al., J R Soc Med, 2001).
- The NHS spending is mostly population-based allocations.

There are three other important sources of funding:
1. About 10 million people in the UK are covered by private insurance which equates to about 1% of GDP and insurance mainly purchases elective treatment.
2. Government supports older people requiring both clinical and social care.
3. Palliative care and acquired immunodeficiency syndrome (AIDS)/human immunodeficiency virus (HIV) treatment come from volunteer help.

## Health Financing in China

The Chinese health system has not been performing well since 1980s. The income gap between the rich and poor has widened and the "marketization" of medical services has led to a marked decline in equity and access.

- *The World Health Report* in 2000 showed Chinese health financing system was poor.
- The government spending was less than 20% and consumers themselves paid 60% of healthcare expenditure.
- Only 15% of the population is covered by social health insurance.
- The majority of residents, children, and immigrants were not covered by any health insurance system.
- Catastrophic medical expenditure is common in China.
- Although more than 95% of health facilities are public hospitals, 90% of them are on fees-for-service (China National Health Economics Institute, National Health Accounts Report, 2007).

Even in the field of preventive health services, 50% is paid as service charge. Therefore, health financing in China is extremely inequitable and coverage is very limited. The share of government spending in total health expenditure is less than 1% of GDP.

*Now China has put health financing on the political agenda to move toward universal coverage.*

## Health Financing in Bangladesh
(Islam A et al., Am J Econ Financ Manag, 2015)

Bangladesh spends only about 3.5% of its GDP on health. The per capita per annum health expenditure is about USD 27.
- About 63% of the total health expenditure is out-of-pocket expenses (OOPE).
- Government's share in the total health expenditure has declined considerably and it currently stands at around 35% of expenditure.
- Financial allocation for the health sector remained stagnant at 0.9% of the GDP.
- Evidence suggests that district and subdistrict level allocations for health are determined by the number of beds (for food and drugs) and staff in facilities (for salaries) and not on population size or other demographic sizes.

It is apparent that Bangladesh needs to spend more on health care and at the same time make every effort to use its existing healthcare resources more effectively and efficiently.

## Health Financing in Sri Lanka

Sri Lanka spends only 3–4% of its GDP on health. The private expenditure is 44% and government expenditure is 56%.

The five primary methods of funding in Sri Lanka—(1) general taxation to the state, country, or municipality; (2) social health insurance; (3) voluntary or private health insurance; (4) out-of-pocket payments; and (5) donations to charities.

## Health Financing in South Africa (Africana Agenda, the Beginner's Guide to Health Care in South Africa, 2002)

South Africa currently spends 8.8% of GDP on health care which is relatively high by international standards, still health inequalities lies throughout the country.

- The main sources of finance for health care are—government, households, employers, and nongovernmental organizations (NGOs).
- Government is the largest source of healthcare finance. Government also provides a tax benefit for those who purchase private healthcare through schemes.
- The second largest source of health finance is household spending. This takes place via contributions to medical schemes, direct OOPE, and to a limited extent to other forms of private insurance.
- Employers fund healthcare for their employees either directly through health services provided at the workplace or indirectly through contributions to medical schemes on behalf of their employees.
- Donors and NGOs provide only a small proportion of healthcare financing in South Africa which is increased since 1994 **(Table 41.1)**.

**Table 41.1:** Total health expenditure as percentage of gross domestic product for selected countries.

| Country | % |
|---|---|
| Afghanistan | 10.30 |
| Brazil | 8.91 |
| China | 5.32 |
| Ethiopia | 4.05 |
| Honduras | 7.59 |
| India | 3.89 |
| Myanmar | 4.95 |
| Nepal | 6.15 |
| Russian Federation | 5.56 |
| South Africa | 8.20 |
| Sudan | 6.31 |
| World | 9.90 |

*Source*: World Health Organization (WHO). (2015). Global Health Expenditure Database. [online] Available from: http://apps.who.int/nha/database.

### Points to Remember

- Pooling resources for economic risks started in Greece for funeral.
- In 2016, highest GDP on health was spent by USA (17.9% of GDP) and private system maintain health in USA which spent almost $9,900 per capita which was 25% greater than the next highest spender.
- For many years, NHS (UK) spending was within the range of 5.5–6.2% of GDP. In 2016, the health financing was 9.8% of GDP and in 2017, it was 9.9%. Total health financing is through NHS.
- More than 95% of Chinese health facilities are public hospitals, 90% of operational funds are dependent on fees-for-service. Chinese government share is less than 1%. There is a large gap between rich and poor for health access.
- Bangladesh spends only about 3.5% of its GDP on health and 35% only being government.
- Sri Lanka spends 3–4% of GDP and 56% is contributed by government.
- South Africa spends more with 8.8% on health but has lot of health inequality and the finance is managed mainly by government.

## Health Financing in India

Total Health care expenditure in India for 2019-20 was 3.27% of GDP. However, the Government Health Expenditure is only 41% (1.35% of GDP) and 47% of expenditure is the household OOPE (1.54% of GDP). Remaining was contributed from private health insurance and other donors.

Public support for healthcare system has been historically low in India; it was always less than 1% of the GDP. So, we had private health sector growing rapidly which accounted to about 3% of GDP in the beginning of 1990s to over 5% in 2012. This also means that the burden is on households and more so for the poorer sections as all of this is OOPEs. It is estimated that 20 million people each year fall below the poverty line for their expenditure in accessing the healthcare services 2007. (UNIDO, Taking Stock and Moving Forward).

Greater focus in health financing in recent years has made a larger allocation of money to health sector especially in the context of the National Rural Health Mission (NRHM).

- There is provision of some flexible funds to state governments under NRHM flexipool where they can make their own unique programs.
- The central government spelled out the strategy for achieving the goal through NRHM and mandated government health financing goal to 2–3% of GDP (Berman P et al., Gov. Health Financing in India, 2010).

After all that too, the problem exists—latest survey on health care said (WHO, Health Financing Profile in India, 2016):

- Private sector takes away about 80% of total outpatient treatment and 60% of total hospitalizations.
- The major source of funds for health care in private sector is household OOPE and that accounts to 72% of the total health expenditure.
- It revealed that 70% of all hospitals in the country are in the private sector and 80% of them in urban areas.
- Private health services provide almost entirely only curative care.
- Almost 60% of hospitalized treatment in rural areas and 42% in urban areas are financed by borrowings and sale of assets.

*The future strategies by Indian government in line with Universal health coverage are (WHO, Health Financing Profile in India, 2016):*

- "Increase in public funding of health to a minimum of 2.5% of GDP during the 12th five-year plan (2012–2017) and a minimum of 3% by year 2022".
- "Increased public expenditures thus leading to a sharp decline in the proportion of private out-of-pocket spending on health to 33% by year 2022".
- It is estimated that States' total funding on health will also increase to three times the Eleventh Plan levels involving a similar annual increase.
- The committee recommends introduction of specific health purpose transfers to equalize the levels of per capita public spending on health across different states. It also speaks on increasing public spending on procuring drugs and medicines.

### Points to Remember

- Public support for health care has been historically low in India and mainly *less than 1% of the GDP*.
- Increase in public funding of health to a minimum of *2.5% of GDP during the 12th five-year plan (2012–2017) and a minimum of 3% by year 2022*.
- Almost 60% of hospitalized treatment in rural areas and *42% in urban areas* are financed by borrowings and sale of assets.
- Private sector accounts for about *80% of total outpatient treatment and 60% of total hospitalizations*.
- *Greater focus in health in recent years* has made a larger allocation of money to health sector especially in the context of the *NRHM*.

## SUGGESTED READING

1. Berman P, Ahuja R, Tandon A, et al. (2010). Government Health Financing in India: Challenges in Achieving Ambitious Goals [online].
2. China National Health Accounts Report. Beijing: China National Health Economics Institute; 2007.
3. De Lew N, Greenberg G, Kinchen KH. A layman's guide to the US health care system. Health Care Financ Rev. 1992;14:151-69.
4. Duggal R. (2017). Financing healthcare in India—prospects for health insurance [online]. Available from http://www.cehat.org/cehat/uploads/files/A%20246%20Financing%20healthcare.pdf.
5. Health Economics. (2018). History of health care financing in the USA [online]. Available from: https://www.pharmpress.com/files/docs/health_economics_sample.pdf.
6. Himmelstein DU, Woolhandler S. The current and projected taxpayer shares of US health costs. Am J Public Health. 2016;106:449-52.
7. Islam A, Ahsan GU, Biswas T. Health System Financing in Bangladesh: A Situation Analysis. Am J Econ Financ Manag. 2015;1:494-502.
8. James JH. Healthcare financing for the under-served: UK. J R Soc Med. 2001;94:462-5.
9. Singh K. The growing out-of-pocket expenditure must be curtailed to enable a healthy society that is geared towards holistic development. Health Care Financ India. 2017;43:46.
10. United Nations Industrial Development Organization (UNIDO). (2007). Taking Stock and Moving Forward: The UNIDO–UNEP National Cleaner Production Centres.
11. World Health Organization (WHO). (2016). Health Financing Profile in India [online].

# CHAPTER 42

# Health Management

CM 16.1 Define and describe the concept of health planning
CM 16.2 Describe planning cycle
CM 16.3 Describe health management techniques

## A. BASICS OF MANAGEMENT

*Bhavesh Modi, Rashmi Kundapur, Sudhir Prabhu H, Shreyaswi Sathyanath M, Manjula R, Pranay Jadav, Kapil Gandha*

## INTRODUCTION

Health care is a complex and a multidisciplinary system. It has to have integration, coordination of a large number of people of varied interests. Typical management of patient requires a team; however small it may be. Treating doctor assumes a position of the leader in deciding course of patient management and instructs to team members and supervise their activities. When it comes to managing the health of a community consisting of thousands to millions of people [covered under one primary health center (PHC) area to entire country] requires bigger team. This team works through healthcare system and involved in the delivering various preventive, promotive, curative, palliative and rehabilitative care. Resources put in for managing healthcare system, are quite greater when compared to resources utilized in the management of one to few patients. Doctors involved in managing health of community also assume role of leadership as the case is with typical management of patients. This demands the understanding and skills of management amongst the doctor involved in healthcare delivery system, may be from Medical Officer of PHC to Director; up at state or country level. In these situation, role of doctors is expanded from mere healthcare providers to health manager of healthcare. Thus, with change in landscape in medical and health care over the time, understanding of basics of management science becomes integral part of medical education in modern days.

## MANAGEMENT SCIENCE

The word management simply means "getting things done." This is an oversimplification. But it is a science that encompasses many things. It started with commons sense built on experiences but over the period is developed as a science with borrowed principles from host of basic disciplines, such as Economics, Psychology, Mathematics, Statistics, Sociology, etc. Also, it has scope of applications in all kinds of organizations such as, corporate companies, engineering corporations, financial institutions, academic institutions and of course health care.

## Management Science has been Defined in Various Ways

- **According to FW Taylor**, Management is *"The art of knowing what you want to do and then seeing that it is done in the best and cheapest way."*
- **Henri Fayol** said: *"To manage is to forecast and plan, to organize, to command, to coordinate and control."*
- **Peter F Drucker** said that *"Management is a multipurpose organ that manages a business and manages managers and manages workers and work."*
- **According to Harold Koontz**, *"Management is the art of getting things done through and with people in formally organized groups."*

Thus management is defined as to attain effectively predetermined results (goals/objectives) by managing all available resources efficiently with changing external environment. It is about five "Rights". Getting "Right" works done by "Right" Persons, using "Right" amount of resources in "Right" time, with use of "Right" methods. Common understanding emerged from these definitions is "Management is facilitating coordinated efforts in a systematic way to accomplish common goals effectively and efficiently."

From the definition of management, certain aspects stand out quite prominently:
- Management is about managing resources and initiating actions.
- Primary purpose of management is to achieve predetermined results (objectives and goals) to its fullest extent that is effectiveness.
- Objectives and goals must be achieved with least expenditure of resources that is efficiency.

## RESOURCES

- *Manpower:* People are the essential driving force for any planned activity be it health related or not. Availability of skilled or trained workforce would decide how successfully we could conduct health activities.
- *Machines and materials:* Drugs, equipment, books, manuals, records, electronic resources, infrastructure, etc.
- *Money:* Can be considered as the most important resource in developing countries as health care needs to compete with other public services or goods. Money is also important as it is a resource which would be essential to procure other resources. Above three are classical resources which are to be managed. Few add following two as in the list of classical resource as their management is also important for attaining the desired results:
- *(Minutes) time:* Planning, scheduling and completing the activity without wastage of time.
- *Methods:* Techniques and approaches used to carry out the activities effectively and efficiently.

## EFFECTIVENESS AND EFFICIENCY

### Effectiveness

It is concerned with getting desired results (output, outcomes) following the processes. Focus on effective management brings in better results as it is result focused. This is not time focused but on idea focused. Measures of effectiveness are quality and quantity of output without considering the resource input.

### Efficiency

It is concerned with achieving desired result much faster and/or with lesser usages of resources. So, efficient management includes the concept of reaching the maximum with minimal resources and in less time. Measures of efficiency are resources spent versus output achieved.

### Balancing Effectiveness and Efficiency

Effective means achieving organizational goals and efficient *means* achieving goals with minimum waste of resources. Good management manages people and resources effective and efficiently to accomplish organizational goals. The pictorial presentation of management effort on two aspects, one is the means, i.e., resources and another is the ends, i.e., results-achievement is shown in **Figure 42A.1**, of management is directed towards controlling or reducing the use of resources at the same time increasing the outputs. But it is important to strike a balance between effective and efficiency.

Greater emphasis on effectiveness without focus on efficiency may result into over utilization of resources, while greater emphasis on efficiency can result in to reduced output, which may defeat the purpose. Balancing between effectiveness and efficiency acts in changing environment is a real art and science of management.

## THEORIES AND APPROACHES TO MANAGEMENT

The foundation of management sciences and approaches was mainly laid down during the industrial revolution. There are three common approaches to management (**Fig. 42A.2**).

### Classical Approach

This was developed during 1880–1920s. The focus here was to increase production by improving the organizational efficiency. They are as follow:
- Scientific management theory
- Bureaucratic management theory
- Administrative management theory

#### Scientific Management Theory

Historically, FW Taylor who is known as the father of scientific management, emphasized on the need for scientific approach to management of business organizations and the development of mutual trust between management and workers to increase productivity.

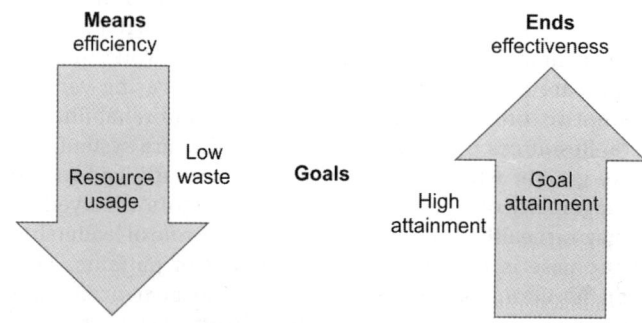

Fig. 42A.1: Effectiveness and efficiency.

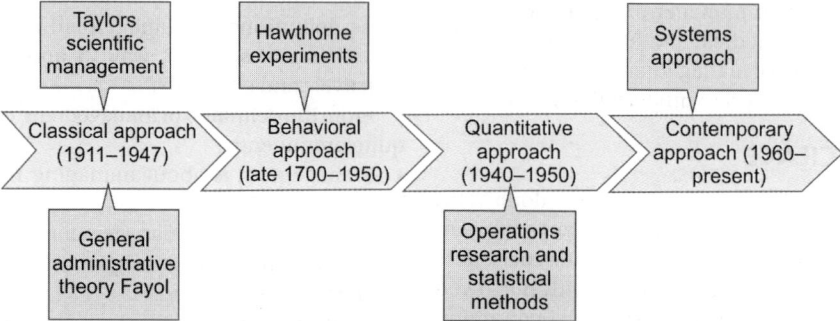

Fig. 42A.2: Evolution of management science.

### Bureaucratic Management

This was promoted by Max Webber, a German sociologist. He based formal organization on the principles given below:
- **Structure:** This means arrangement of positions within an organization based on a hierarchy, with each position having predetermined authority and responsibility.
- **Specialization:** Division of labor and tasks should be based on functions and specialization with its own chains of command.
- **Predictability and stability:** Formal rules and regulations form the basis of the system that operates the organization.
- **Rationality:** Impartial and rational recruitment of personnel should be followed.

### Administrative Management

It was believed that good managers are born, not made. Henri Fayol, the founder of classical management theory, dispelled this belief and focused on management as a skill that can be taught, learnt and mastered. He laid down the following principles:

*Principles of Management*
- **Division of work:** The work should be divided based on capabilities and aptitude among the members of the team to ensure productivity.
- **Authority:** As the managers work through the people, they should have the formal authority so that they can ask the subordinates to complete the task.
- **Discipline:** Fair codes of conduct and periodic supervision along with judicious use of rewards or punishments help develop a positive attitude towards discipline.
- **Unity of command:** It is ideal that an employee receives orders from one superior only.
- **Unity of direction:** All the functionaries of the organization work towards the same objective in one direction.
- **Subordination of individual interest to group interest:** The interest and goals of the organization comes first and receives emphasis over that of the individual.
- **Remuneration:** A satisfactory and predetermined remuneration to different personnel ensures productivity and avoids uncertainty.
- **Centralization of authority:** The important policy decisions and decisions regarding key matters should be centralized. Managers should be able to decide how much authority has to be retained and can be given to the subordinates for decision making.
- **Scalar chain:** Line of authority should be a well-defined and functional chain of senior-subordinate relationships from the top management to the lower levels.
- **Order:** Personnel and material should be in appropriate position to ensure efficiency.
- **Equity:** Absence of bias and just treatment of all individuals removes conflicts while ensuring cooperation and compliance among all.
- **Stability of tenure of personnel:** This ensures that the members find a sense of certainty and attachment to the job.
- **Initiative:** Personnel should be encouraged when they take initiative as it gives them a chance to build their confidence and hone skills.
- **Esprit de corps (team work):** Team spirit, feeling of kinship is essential for any organization to develop. There is strength in unity.

Though not all principles are mandatory and relevant to current management practices, but these are good guiding principles in many of the situations.

### Neoclassical Theory

Here, human relations and behaviors of individuals and groups is given importance. High morale increases productivity rather than working conditions alone.

Thus, an informal organization structure was introduced with the following principles:
- **The individual:** An individual in the organization is identified as a social entity with goals and aspirations.
- **The work group:** Social interactions within the group are also emphasized.
- **Participative management:** It also encourages participation of workers in the process of decision making.

This theory is widely applauded due to highlighting the role of human values and emotion in managing the organization, in compare to older one which were more focusing on task, methods and rules.

### Modern Approach

This approach recognized the organization as a system which may be multidisciplinary and dynamic, which means it should adapt to environmental changes. Some of the characteristics of this approach to management of organizations include: multimotivated, probabilistic, multidimensional and adaptive. There are three categories as given below:
1. Quantitative approach
2. Systems approach
3. Contingency approach

#### Quantitative Approach (Management Science Approach)

The focus is on managerial decision making and can further be studied under two areas:
1. **Operations research:** Advanced techniques such as linear programming, waiting line, routing and distribution models are used to improve the effectiveness of decisions.
2. **Management information system (MIS):** By providing meaningful information about its business processes using computerized information systems, organizations can bring about effective management.

#### Systems Approach

This uses an integrated approach wherein a system is defined as *"an entity made up of two or more interdependent parts that interact to form a functioning organism"* Subsystems that are interconnected and mutually dependent from a system. Components of a system include: individual, organization (formal or informal), physical environment and behaviors.

Three basic elements of the organization include:
1. A system-may consist of some functions, processes and components.

2. ***Linking processes:*** This ensures coordination and correlations of subsystems. The processes include "decision making, balance and communication".
3. ***Goals:*** There is a specific goal that every system is set to achieve.

### Contingency Approach

According to this, all types of problems in organizations cannot be solved by a single set of rules. It is important to analyze every problem individually, study the various aspects and then devise different ways to solve it. Hence, this approach is also known as situational approach. It is mixed of all theories and appropriate theory is used depending upon situation.

## MANAGEMENT FUNCTIONS

Management is all about carrying out some functions. They are known as management function. According to Luther Gullick, there are eight functions of management. They are:

- ***Planning:*** Planning is essential to decide how to go about achieving a certain task, breaking the job into several component activities, deciding the sequence in which the tasks will be done, entrusting the person who will do the task and when, etc.
- ***Organizing:*** Organizing the resources like personnel or man; material, money or finance, etc.
- ***Staffing:*** An appropriately trained person in the proper position will perform the planned activities. The responsibility of filling up the positions in the organization with such personnel lies with the senior management.
- ***Directing:*** The manager directs how the staff will work and instructs what or how the tasks will be performed. He also keeps a watch on the performance and provides guidance and ensures the appropriate quantity and quality of work.
- ***Coordinating:*** It is essential to ensure that all members of the team are working in an integrated manner to achieve the objective. The tasks should be done in a coordinated and mutually supportive way.
- ***Reporting or reviewing:*** It is important to periodically review the situation to know if the tasks are being done according to the plan or if some corrective measures have to be undertaken.
- ***Budgeting:*** Financial provisions have to be made and the expenditure has to be monitored, so as to remain within the grants that are sanctioned.
- ***Evaluation:*** Evaluation helps the management to determine how well the jobs have been done and what progress is being made towards the goals. The strategies being deployed is effective and efficient in getting desired results or any factor affecting it is periodically assessed to make necessary modification at top planning, policy, strategy, etc. level.

> **Management versus Administration**
> There is very thin line between management and administration. Administration is defined as "those functions in an organization, which are concerned with policy formulation, finance, production, distribution and ultimately control all key activities for meeting the organizational objectives" (Sheldon). Administration is more concerned with following the procedures and rules rather than results while management is focused on achieving the result hence flexible to change the methods and strategies. Nowadays term administration is restrictively used in government setting largely.

It is also remembered as POSDCORBE. Later on Mr Peter Drucker, the father of modern management has added "innovation" and "managing change" as another managerial function in the above list of eight functions.

Above mentioned functions are broadly clubbed in three functions:
1. **P**lanning
2. **I**mplementation
3. **E**valuation

Subsequently, with evolving of behavior theory, implementation is divided into two managerial functions "Organizing" and "Leading" and in place of evaluation, term "Controlling" is used which includes both; monitoring and evaluation. Thus as per modern management there are four broad managerial functions **(Fig. 42A.3)**:
1. Planning
2. Organizing
3. Leading
4. Controlling

> **Note**
> - Management is all about getting things done and achieving desired results.
> - It is about managing the resources.
> - The 5 Ms are important in resource management.
> - Effectiveness and efficiency are different concept. Efficiency is performing a task with minimal resources and cost and getting maximum output while effectiveness focuses on desired output following the processes.

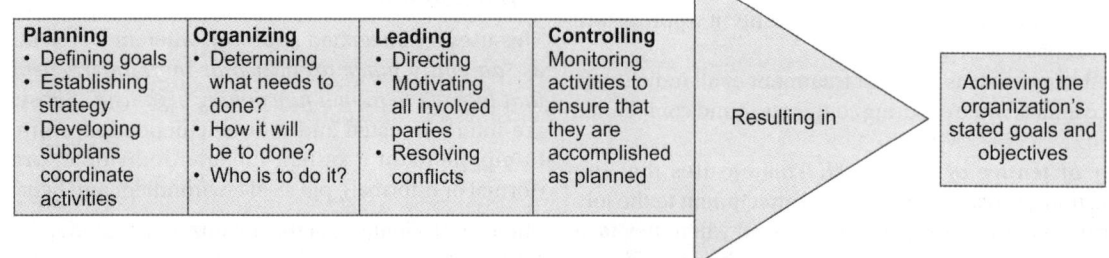

**Fig. 42A.3:** Broad functions of management.

# ORGANIZATION

Health system is a huge organization made of various big or small organizations. *An organization is a "deliberate arrangement of people to accomplish some specific purposes". Organization* is defined as "a rational combination of the activities of a number of people for the achievement of a common purpose or goal, by division of labor and functions and through a hierarchy of authority and responsibility." Any typical big organization or system is having three levels of managements performing various set of management functions to attain the desired results effectively and efficiently to achieve common goal understanding of hierarchy plan, hierarchy structure (level of management), management functions and managerial skills is necessary if one wishes to be good health managers.

## Definitions of the Terminologies used in the Hierarchy of Organization Plan (Fig. 42A.4)

### Vision

A well-informed and self-sustained view to achieve an ultimate state of affairs like health for all by 2,000. The purpose or intentions are directed towards overall societal purpose. A person or individual is called as "visionary," who always work towards bringing a change in the society to achieve this ultimate state, e.g., A Vision Statement for The National Rural Health Mission 2005-2012 says that "The National Rural Health Mission for the year 2005-2012 seeks to provide effective health care to rural population throughout the country and to raise public spending on health from 0.9% of *gross domestic product* (GDP) to 2-3% of GDP," with special focus on 18 states, which have weak public health indicators and/or weak infrastructure.

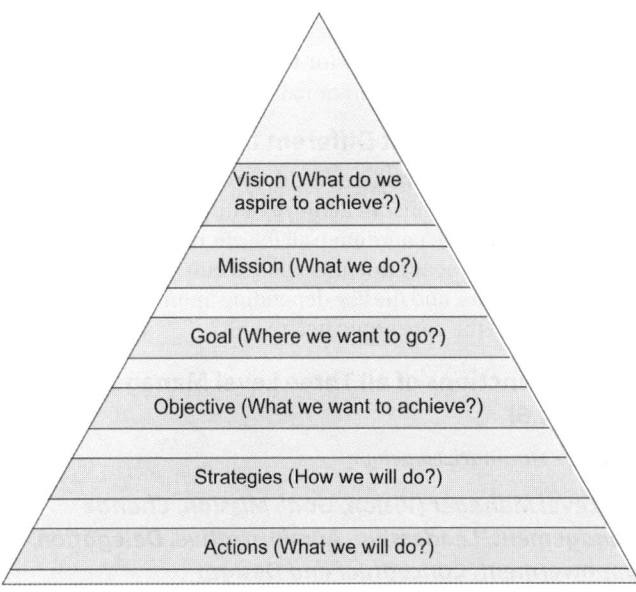

**Fig. 42A.4:** The hierarchy of organizational plans.

### Mission

The mission of an organization is described as the very reason why that organization exists. It states how its vision will be realized. The definition of mission must balance between present and future. The mission of the organization is described in its mission statement, e.g., the mission statement of department of community medicine in a medical college would be "To provide comprehensive training in community medicine to medical graduates and postgraduates, with the aim to make them better public health specialists."

If the mission statement is too narrow, it will limit the activities of the organization to the immediate present and prevent its growth and utilization of newer opportunities and technologies, whereas too broad definition of mission will not enable the organization to concentrate on any workable activity and opportunities at present.

### Goal

Goal is the ultimate state or results to be achieved. It can be broad or specific. It can be both qualitatively and quantitatively. Also, it may be time-bound or not. It is the point towards which all efforts, resources, activities, strategies and objectives are directed.

Goals play a major role in motivating people towards working in a coordinated fashion towards larger organizational objectives.

### Objectives

It would be the next step of translating the goal into smaller, specific, reliable, tangible, measurable and achievable activities. "Objectives are action orientation of the mission" and form the basis for taking action in appropriate direction and for measuring the performance. It will help the members of organization to know their job responsibilities. Objectives remain the statements of expected outcomes or output:
- Objectives are to be **S**pecific, **M**easurable, **A**chievable, **R**elevant and **T**ime-bound (**SMART**).
- Objectives form the benchmark and standards for measuring performances and progress towards achieving the larger organizational objectives.

### Strategies

Strategy is any decision, plan or action which takes into consideration the actions of competitors and other factors in external environment (external analysis), with the aim of, achieving the objectives. This strategy also deals with the most efficient use of the resources (internal analysis) that have been allocated for achieving the specific objective.

### Inputs

It is the resources put in the system, mainly money, manpower, machines and materials.

### Outputs

These are those results (effects) which are achieved immediately after implementing an activity. Usually, it is the net efforts "put out" from the system. It is concerned with target set for the specific tasks.

## Outcome

It is changes (effects) "coming out" (in the people) due to output. Evaluation measures the change that has occurred as a result of a program. They are not seen immediately after the end of the project activity. It is concerned with short-term (say around 2–5 years) objective of the organization or system.

## Impacts

These are the large changes (effects) that occur within the community, or within organization, society, or environment as a result of program outcomes. It is concerned with long-term objective (goal), of the organization or system.

The organizational hierarchy and steps of management with relationship can be understood as shown in **Figure 42A.5**.

## Organizational Structure

Organization of activities is easier, if there is an organizational chart describing the structure of the system viz. units, center and department. The goal and objectives of the organizations is clearly defined. Strategies of the program are specified. The program budget is decided prior. The relationships of the personnel are strengthened, if each one has a clear job description and knows to whom he is accountable for their action.

## Organizational Hierarchy Structure

It refers to "the arrangement of individuals into a series of superiors and subordinates. Individual workers are placed in a specific authority relationship, whose authority can be traced from the next level of authority, up to the top level of the hierarchy. This flow of authority constitutes a chain of command, the chain of direct authority from superior to subordinate."

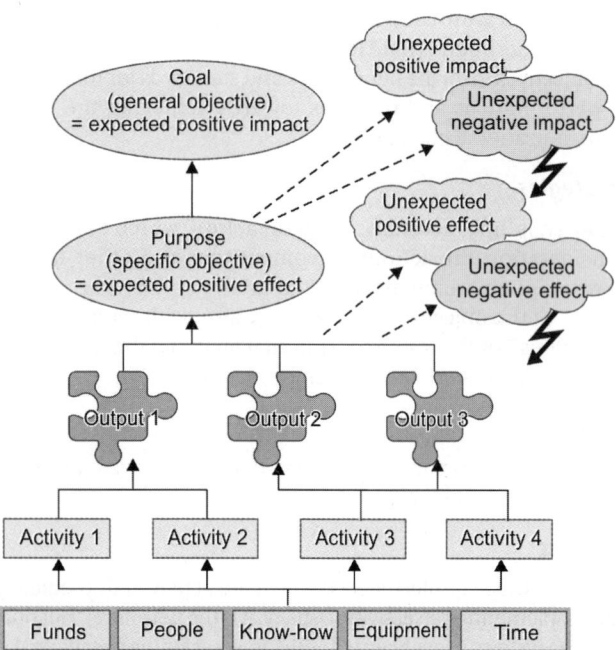

**Fig. 42A.5:** Management steps, their relationships and hierarchy.

The uninterrupted line of authority from superior to subordinate results in units of command so that each individual reports to one superior. This chain of command shows who reports to whom, who is responsible for the actions of an individual, who has authority over others, results in a pyramidal organizational structure (**Flowchart 42A.1**).

## Hierarchy-free Forms of Organization

This is a developing trend, during the last decade, and especially in French-based cultures. The term hierarchy-free is referred to all those organizations that decide to reduce or eliminate the number of hierarchical layers, implementing new forms of organizational design that grant employees more freedom and responsibility to undertake decisions that they, not their bosses decide are best. It has been studied in especially in information technology (IT) and computer technologies fields, that there are several benefits that affect the organization as well as the individuals. These benefits concern mostly engagement, innovation, flexibility and client proximity. Yet this hierarchy-free form of organization is yet to enter health care system, with lot of pilot testing and operational research.

## LEVELS OF MANAGEMENT

Basically, there are three ranks of management. Top level, middle level and lower level.

1. ***Top level management:*** It is also known as corporate management. They are involved with setting goal, finance, framing policy and strategy. They are called as top level managers, planners, policy makers, etc.
2. ***Middle level management:*** It is also known as strategic management. They are concerned with implementation, direction, control and monitoring and evaluation. They are called middle level managers, implementers, executives, etc.
3. ***First level or the lower level management:*** It is known as operational level management. They supervise day-to-day execution of the activities for the intended goals. They are called supervisors or operational manager, etc.

### Role and Functions at Different Level of Manager

The complexities of a modern health system call for joint effort by many people. To ensure achievement of the goals, system requires managers to coordinate all the efforts. These managers may be doctors, academicians, politicians, administrators, health supervisors, and the like depending upon the nature, size, and function of the concerned health unit.

### Various Functions of all Three Level Managers (Fig. 42A.6)

*These are summarized below:*

### Top Level Manager (Vision, Goal, Mission, Change Management, Leadership, Administrative, Delegation, Empowerment, Conceptual and Design)

- Determines the objective, plan and policies for overall organization direction

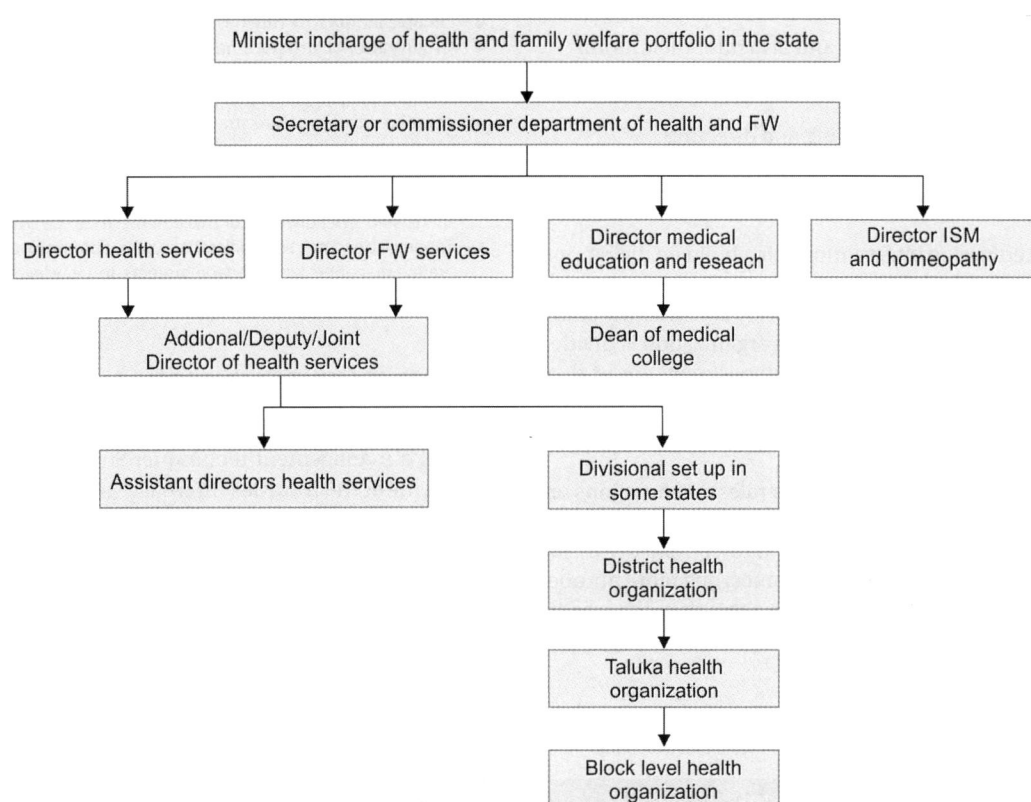

Flowchart 42A.1: Organizational structure of health services at state level.

(FW: family welfare; ISM: indian systems of medicine)

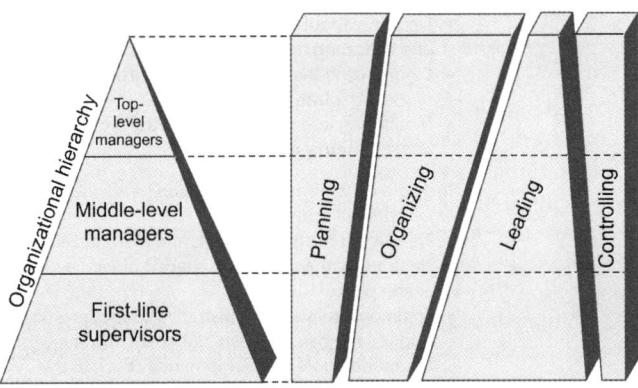

Fig. 42A.6: Time spent on management functions at different management levels.

- Mobilization of the available resources (assemble and bring together)
- Spend more time in planning and organizing
- More conceptual knowledge is required rather than technical skills
- Monitor middle level managers and responsible for performance of all departments (cross department responsibility too)
- Prepare long-term plan (5–20 years).

### Middle Level Manager (Problem Solving, Team Building, Interpersonal Skills)

- Working out strategies and plans to implement decisions and policies made by top level managers
- Job distribution and delegation to the subordinate staff
- Identify the workers according to the skills, aptitude, training and available time
- Coordinate, encourage and support subordinates
- Motivation and reward good work
- Bring the necessary change in the behavior of the subordinate through training or self-evaluation
- Evaluation of the work progress by holding staff meeting periodically
- Build a team spirit and avoidance or solution of conflict
- Make the decisions firmly but democratically
- Supervise lower level (first-line) managers and to find best way to use the resources to achieve goals
- Short-term plans quarterly and yearly.

### Lower Level Manager (Technical, Emotional Intelligence, Coaching for Performance, Supervisor)

- Ensure work done according to plan
- It directs the workers and employees on day-to-day production within the goals laid down by higher authorities

- Assign jobs to workers to make arrangements for their training and development
- Supervise and control workers and also raise their moral
- Maintains the link between lower level worker and middle level manager
- More time devoted for controlling and directing
- To arrange tools and materials, also advise and assist workers by explaining work procedures and solving their problems if any
- Rather than enforcing interventions, first build up the rapport with the intended beneficiaries
- Lower level managers make daily, weekly and monthly plans.

Though management structure of an organization is divided into three levels but there is no tight compartment about their roles and functions. Some overlapping of the functions and role or variation in the roles from organization to organization can be there.

Different levels of managers and their roles and functions are given in **Table 42A.1**.

As they move up the ladder, power and complexity of the duties increases. As far as numbers are concerned more number is required in first-line (lower level) managers then the middle level managers. And more number of middle managers are required than the top level managers.

> **Note**
> - Organizational structure has a hierarchy.
> - Organizational structure has vision, mission, goals and objectives following one after the other. Objectives need to be SMART.
> - Inputs, outputs, outcome and impact are very important as organizational structure strategy.
> - Management is in three levels, they are top, middle and lower level management.
> - Though three levels of management are important in public health, there is no strict division for this and there can be overlapping.
> - Top level becomes the think tanks and problem solvers, middle level are the managers who manage projects and low level are the people who build the projects.

## MANAGEMENT TECHNIQUES

A set of procedures is needed which has multiple activities which is called a management technique. Suitable and appropriate management techniques increase managerial capability, efficiency, effectiveness, and productivity of an organization.

### Classification of Management Techniques

Traditional or conventional techniques and modern management techniques.

**Table 42A.1:** Different level of managers and their roles and functions.

| Sr. No. | Level of management | Managers | Role and functions |
|---|---|---|---|
| 1. | Top | *Government settings:* Ministers and Secretaries<br>*Nongovernment settings:* Board of Directors, Trustees, Chairman, etc. | *Strategic role: Policy development and programming:*<br>• Developing the organization's goals, policy, plan, strategies with focus on long-term view<br>• Deciding about the need of resources, mobilizing and allocating them for implementation<br>• Emphasizing the growth and overall effectiveness of the organization<br>• Monitoring interaction between the organization and its external environment |
| 2. | Middle | *Government setting:*<br>• Commissioner<br>• Directors District Officials<br>• Block (Taluka) Health Officer<br>*Nongovernment settings:*<br>• Medical Director or superintendent<br>• Chief Executive Officers<br>• Managing Directors<br>• Chief Operating Officers<br>• Chief Finance Officers<br>• Divisional Head | *Tactical role: Implementing, and monitoring the organizational activities:*<br>• Translating the general goals and plans developed by strategic managers into specific objectives and action plan<br>• Traditional role an administrative controller who bridged the gap between higher and lower levels but modern role is developmental coach to the people who report to them who lead them with proper direction and motivation<br>• Coordination of resources |
| 3. | First or lower | *Government setting:* PHC-MO, Supervisors, Inspectors<br>*Nongovernment settings:* Assistant mangers, supervisors, team leaders, department heads, foremen, etc. | *Operational role: Supervising and directing nonmanagement team and controlling the activities:*<br>• Lower-level managers who supervise the operations of the organization<br>• Directly involved with nonmanagement employees<br>• Acting as a link between management and nonmanagement staff<br>• Implementing the specific plans developed with tactical managers |

### Traditional Methods of Management

These methods are based on behavioral sciences. It includes personnel selection, training and retraining, development of communication channels and skills, supervision, leadership development, motivational methods, team building and conflict resolution. These methods failed to meet the demand of today's projects. Therefore, better, effective and innovative managerial methods have been brought out.

### Modern Management Techniques

They are subdivided into:

| | |
|---|---|
| Statistical techniques | • Decision tree<br>• Time trends and forecasting |
| Activity analysis | • Work study<br>• Time motion studies<br>• Gantt chart |
| Mathematical techniques | • Simulation study or model<br>• System analysis<br>• Network analysis (Program evaluation and review technique, critical path method) |
| Financial techniques | • Cost benefit analysis<br>• Cost effective analysis<br>• Planning programming budgeting system<br>• Zero-base budgeting<br>• Input-output analysis |
| Miscellaneous | • Management by objectives<br>• Management by exception<br>• Strength, weakness, opportunities, challenges analysis |

#### Statistical Techniques

- **Forecasting:** It predicts future outcome of the activities-based on past experience. Two types of forecasting: *Wisdom-based (judgmental) and data-based (statistical)*.
  - *Forecasting-based on time trends:* It is used time series data which is plotted through line diagram (on *x*-axis-time and on *y*-axis event). Trend means the same series of events is happening over and over. For example, based on the occurrence of the disease in the area, an epidemiologist will plot a curve with all variation. This will show trend of that disease (seasonal trend or secular trends or any else) and based on this, we can forecast the probability of the occurrence of the potential diseases in the particular area (like mosquito-borne diseases in the post-monsoon time in urban slums). So, authority can be prepared and direct resources into the prevention of the potential outbreak.
- **Decision tree:** It is an algorithm which is made up of all the decisions and its possible outcomes (theory of choice or decision theory). Best decision comes from managers of any level of the organization. Best example of the decision tree is the flowchart of the diagnosing the pulmonary tuberculosis (TB) based on the algorithms.

#### Activity Analysis

- **Time motion studies:** In this technique, for allotted work or activity time is noted with stopwatch. The whole activities are subdivided into several tasks and for each task required time for each task will be noted. Based on this management can decide how the activity is completed rapidly yet efficiently.
- **Work-study or activity analysis or job analysis:** It is a management technique to check at what extent whether allocated job or work has been done (both qualitatively as well as quantitatively). Work-study is a procedure oriented. For a particular job systemic observation and recording of the activities are done. It gives conclusion about the appropriateness of the job for the person, job description, job rotation and training.
- **Gantt chart (Fig. 42A.7):** *A Gantt chart is a horizontal bar diagram. Gantt chart is used to assess the time duration and establish the sequence of activities for the completion of the project. In Gantt chart, x-axis represents total time duration of the project which may be fragmented in days, weeks or months. While on y-axis (Vertical axis in Gantt chart), tasks to be completed for the project are there. Bars are shaded as the project progresses, to show which tasks have been completed. People assigned to each task, resources, milestones and dependencies are also can be represented into Gantt chart. Gantt charts are simple to make and easy to appreciate so, they are used by any kind of complex projects.*

  *Uses of Gantt chart:*
  - *For scheduling and monitoring tasks within a project.*
  - *For communicating plans or status of a project.*
  - *Helps to manage time-based dependencies between activities.*
  - *It also helps to check how corrective measures can bring back the project on track.*

#### Mathematical Techniques

- **Systems analysis:** It is a management technique of finding out the cost-effectiveness of the available alternatives. A system is made up of independent subsystems, e.g., a huge system of hospital is made up subsystems, such as out-patient department (OPD), in-patient department (IPD), medical record, hospital supply, community health services, etc. Through system analysis, a manager can come to know the problems across the system which may lead to unnecessary wastage of money and resources. Therefore, it helps to find alternative solutions which are comparatively cheaper, than the usual one, which is beneficial to the organization.
- **Network analysis:** It is graphical representation of all operations and activities to be completed in order to reach an end objective. First, entire project or program is broken in to small events or activities. Then all the activities are arranged into the logical sequence and relation between all activities is described. First activity to be completed before other events is described. Linkage between two or more events is shown and time schedule for every event is also mentioned. Network analysis is done by two methods: **Program evaluation and review technique (PERT) and critical path method (CPM).**
  - ***Program evaluation and review technique:*** PERT is normally used in long-term projects, such as infrastructure, health policy programs, launching new products and services, etc. where exact time for execution

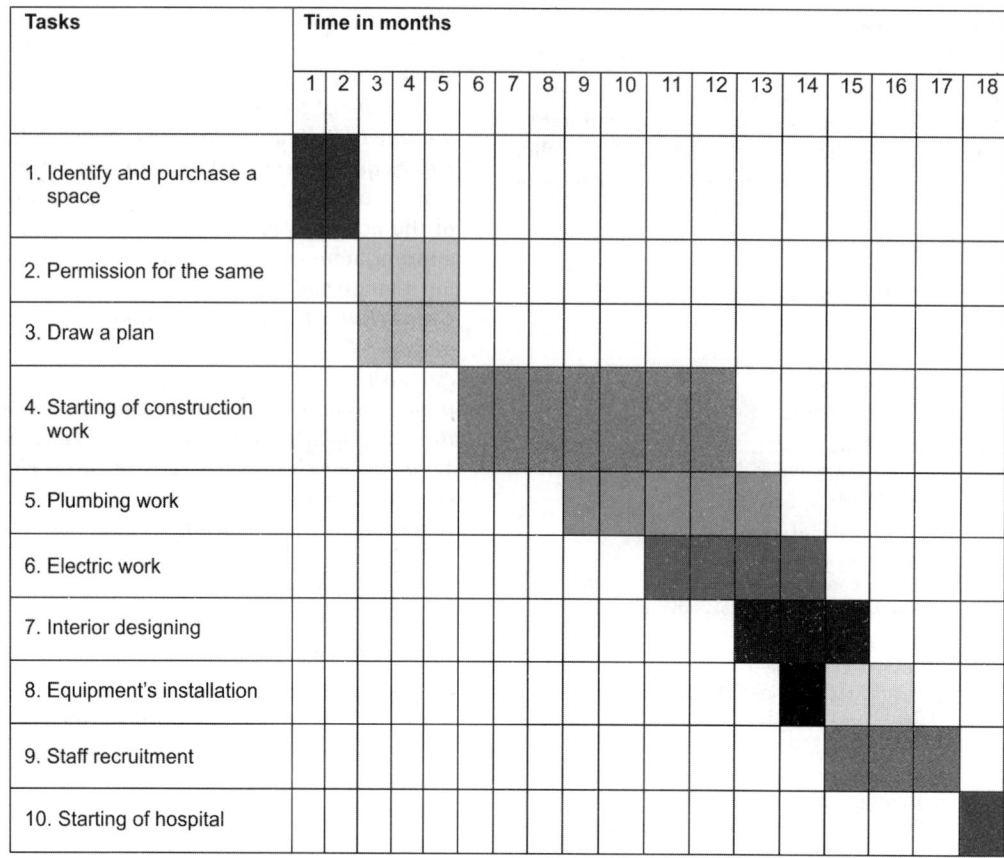

**Fig. 42A.7:** Gantt chart showing starting a surgical hospital in an area (hypothetical example).

of each phase in a project is uncertain. In PERT first, all necessary activates are arranged in logical sequence, through an arrow diagram (network). The PERT estimate is based on the best case scenario and worst case scenario of a task estimate. It also includes most likely time estimate that falls between the two. The expected activity time is then calculated by using the PERT formula. There are three estimation times involved in PERT; optimistic time estimate (TOPT), most likely time estimate (TLIKELY), and pessimistic time estimate (TPESS). ***The expected completion time (mean duration) of the project is calculated by E = (TOPT + 4\*TLIKELY + TPESS)/6. Variance is calculated by (TPESS-TOPT/6).***

– *Critical path method:* A project consists of many activities. Each activity takes certain time and has some cost. Critical path diagram maps the tasks in an orderly fashion with nodes joining certain activities. The longest path through the planned activities to the end of the project is the critical path. It dictates the overall time to complete the project, assuming that all the resources required are available at all the time. It allows prioritization of activities by taking corrective measures to meet the scheduled deadlines.

Steps in network analysis:
- Enlist all activities
- Arrange all activities in logical sequence (flowchart)
- Find the duration of each activity
- Know the dependencies between activities (by Gantt chart)
- Set logical endpoints (milestones) or nodes for each activity
- Identify critical path
- Calculate total time
- Replan.

A typical CPM diagram for the project "setting up nutrition counseling unit at RHTC" is illustrated.

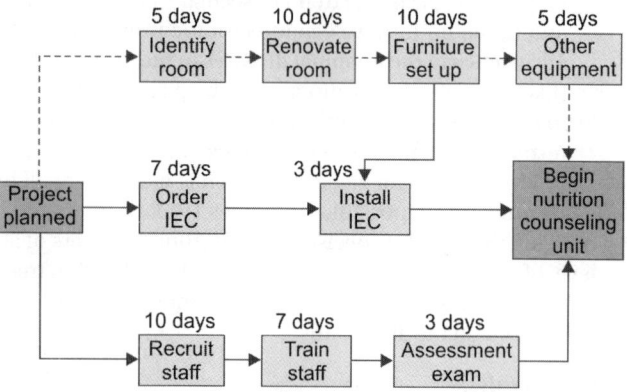

Critical path (dotted line): Start – identify room – renovate room – furniture –other equipment, 30 days

*Comparison between CPM and PERT:*

| CPM | PERT |
|---|---|
| Invented as industrial technique | Invented as military technique |
| It is activity oriented | It is event oriented |
| For the projects having predictable activities—deterministic model | For the projects having unpredictable activities—probabilistic model |
| Used for repetitive projects | Mainly used for nonrepetitive projects—research projects |
| Time of activities is well-known and precise (single time estimate) | Time of activities is uncertain—three time estimates |
| It considers cost analysis | Does not consider cost analysis |
| Critical and noncritical activates are differentiated | No such differentiation |

*Financial Techniques (Table 42A.2)*
- **Cost benefit analysis (CBA):** *In CBA,* benefits are measured in monetary terms so it helps to identify the programs which gives more benefits in terms of money. The major drawback of this technique is that, benefits may not be always expressed in monetary terms in the health field.
- **Cost effectiveness analysis (CEA):** It is superior technique than CBA in health management field. CEA is an expression of the desired effect of a program, service, institution or support activity in reducing a health problem. It compares total costs, and total effectiveness. Effectiveness is measured in natural units, (e.g., life years gained, heart attacks avoided). It is useful in balancing cost with patient's outcome. It helps to identify which modality alternative represents the best outcome per unit cost.

**Table 42A.2:** Financial management techniques.

| | Investment | Advantage | Result |
|---|---|---|---|
| Cost-benefit | Money | Money | Cost-benefit ratio |
| Cost effectiveness | Money | Services provided-life saved, disability avoided, blood pressure reduced, etc. | Cost per unit of advantage (e.g. cost per life saved) |
| Cost utility | Money | Multiple effects (quality as well as quantity)—money and/or life saved | Quality adjusted life year, disability adjusted life year, etc. |
| Input-output | Money, manpower, materials, time | Cases treated, life saved, vaccination done, money | Each input per unit of each output |

*Miscellaneous Techniques*
- **Management by objective:** It is a personnel management technique where managers and employee work together to set, record and monitor objectives for a specific periods of time. In this technique, every staff member is allotted a personal measurable objective to complete in a specific period of time. So, every individual objective works towards overall organizational goal.
- **Management by exception:** There are certain situations in which actual results significantly vary from planned results.

For these situations, management gives their time to check only those situations, e.g., if epidemic occurs in a particular area of a district, emergency medical officer (EMO). Taluka health officers (THO), medical officer (managers of different levels) and rapid response team (RRT) run to that area and give it to specific attention (active surveillance) and intervene. After the epidemic subside that area receive routine surveillance.
- **Strength, weaknesses, and opportunities threats or strength, weakness, opportunity and challenge analysis:** It is a technique to evaluate an organization. Sometimes, it is also called as SWOC analysis (Challenges instead threats). SWOT or SWOC analysis is used as a part of strategic planning. Strengths are the features of the organization that help to achieve goal and objective. Weaknesses decreases project's ability to achieve its objective. Opportunities come from external environment whose advantage can be taken for attaining the project's objective. Threats or challenges are also come from external environment which reduces the project's ability to achieve its objective. Strength and weaknesses are the internal factors which are controllable while opportunities and challenges are external factors over which there is no control.

> **Note**
> - Management techniques are traditional and modern methods and both are important. Traditional methods failed.
> - Modern management methods include statistical techniques, activity analysis, mathematical techniques and financial techniques.
> - Different level managers will be used different management techniques.

## MANAGEMENT AND MEDICINE SCIENCE

There are no much differences in adoption of medical science and management science. The analogy between management and management science can be better understood as given in **Table 42A.3**.

**Table 42A.3:** Analogy between medicine and management science.

| Medicine | Management |
|---|---|
| Organism | Organization |
| Anatomy | Structure |
| Physiology | Function |
| Biochemistry | Process |
| Pathology | Problem in attaining desired results |
| Investigations | Assessment (Monitoring and evaluation) |
| Diagnosis | Identification of problem |
| Treatment | Solution (Remedial actions) |

### Epidemiology and Health Management

The common understanding about the epidemiology is that it is a science to be used by specialist for epidemiological studies and research. But the fact is that epidemiology is the most powerful tool for Health Managers too, in health management. The principles, methods and tools of epidemiology can be applied at all different levels of management. In other words, large part of applied epidemiology has important role in health management.

Epidemiology is about health information. Information is needed for planning, implementation, monitoring and evaluation. The epidemiologists are the person looking for the answers of questions "what, why, who, where, when, how and Health Managers are also the person who have to keep on asking these questions."

The relationship between epidemiology and health management is summarized in **Table 42A.4**.

Table 42A.4: Summary epidemiological methods or tools, their application scopes.

| Epidemiological | Scope of application | By whom |
|---|---|---|
| Descriptive disease, description in terms of time plan and person | Health situation analysis what is the health programs and its frequency and who is affected where is present? | • Health worker<br>• PHC–MO<br>• District health manager |
| Analytical epidemiology confirmation of hypothesis and establishing cause-effect relationship | What causes the disease? Why it is continuing? What intervention can make the difference? | • Mid-level managers<br>• Top level managers |
| Intervention or experimental epidemiology | Effectiveness of the newer (methods) interventions for improving health situation | Top level management high level management |
| Evaluation epidemiology | Measure effectiveness of various health program and services | Top level and mid-level management (district health team) |

## SUMMARY

Management science along with epidemiological science is a need of healthcare providers in all level of management of health. As it is proven traditional method of health management has failed the understanding of basics of management and management techniques with organizational structure understanding will make the healthcare provider a perfect leader to bring change in health of the society.

## SUGGESTED READING

1. Baker SB. "Critical Path Method (CPM)" Archived June 12, 2010, at the Wayback Machine. University of South Carolina, Health Services Policy and Management Courses.
2. Drucker PF. The Practice of Management. New York: Harper Collins; 2010. p. 436.
3. Fayol, H. (1949). General and Industrial Management. (C. Storrs, Trans.). London: Sir Isaac Pitman & Sons, LTD. (Original work published 1918) [Internet]. [cited 2018 Oct 16].
4. Koontz H. The Management Theory Jungle. Acad Manage J. 1961;4(3): 174-88.
5. Kumar, Rajendra. Modeling and Simulation Concepts. Laxmi Publications; 2010.
6. Logframer. Output, outcome and impact. [online] Available from: https://logframer.eu/content/output-outcome-and-impact.
7. Sathe PV. Public Health Management. Epidemiology and Management for Health for All, 3rd edition. Mumbai: Vora Medical Publications; 2009. pp. 78-91.
8. Taylor FW. Shop Management. South Dakota: NuVision Publications, LLC; 2008. p. 112.
9. Taylor FW. The principles of scientific management. New York: Harper and Brothers; 1911. p. 156.
10. Weber M, Henderson AM, Parsons T. The theory of social and economic organization, New York: Oxford University Press; 1947.

# B. HEALTH PLANNING

*AM Kadri, Ankit Sheth, Nidhi Mangrola, Rajesh Chudasama, Bhavesh Modi*

## PLANNING

Planning is the most crucial and first step for any activity. Small task requires minimum planning but with increase in quantum of the activities, i.e., projects, program, organization or complex activities, importance of the methodological planning increases many folds. Success of any organization or system depends on quality of planning.

It is not possible for even wealthiest of wealthy country to meet all the needs, demands and expectations of its community because there is always a restriction on the available resources. Planning and managements is essential to maximize the use of available resources and achieve the desired goals and objectives. Planning is needed for effective program implementation and efficient use of resources.

Planning consists of deciding in advance what to do, how to do, when to do and who is to do it, and thus it bridges the gap between where we are presently and where we have to reach. Planning consists of taking conscious and well thought out decisions about which course of action to take out of the many available and most suitable methods to achieve these objectives. Planning ensures that predetermined objectives and goals are identified so that all resources can be allocated and dedicated in achieving these goals in the most optimal manner.

Plan must always precede action. Planning is a very scientific and systematic process which essentially visualizes as to where we are at present (present situation or baseline), where do we want to go (the future or "outcome"), why do we want to go there (logic) and how do we get there (process). It consists of a series of steps and we need accurate data at each of these steps. Planning is a process of analyzing a system or defining problems; assessing the extent of the problems prioritize the problems, formulating goals of objectives to meet them, examining and choosing strategies among alternate interventions, initiating the necessary actions for its implementation; monitoring the system to ensure proper implementations of the plan and evaluating the outcomes against the stated goals and objectives.

*We need planning to:*
- Match the limited resources
- To minimize wasteful of expenditures

- To develop the best course to define to attain goals or objectives in another word planning is for effective of efficient achievements of desired results.

Health manager depending upon his roles and responsibilities is often has to come across with the situation where he has to plan various health activities. The basics of planning process in the health sector can be remembered by answering the following key questions:
- Where are we at present? (situational analysis)
- Where do we finally want to reach? (objectives and goals)
- How do we will get there? (resources and constraints)
- How effectively we have performed the required activities? (evaluation, monitoring and feedback)
- What new problems do we face and how do we overcome them? (replanning).

# HEALTH PLANNING CYCLE

Health planning can be defined as an orderly process of defining community health problems, identifying unmet needs and surveying the resources to meet them, establishing priority goals that are realistic and projecting administrative action to accomplish the purpose of proposed program. Health planning has been there in some ways or others for many decades, but it is in recent past the thrust on using rational and scientific approach in health planning gas-gained momentum.

## Planning Process

Planning requires a critical analysis of the problem to be addressed. Problem analysis is important for developing a goal and objectives for the project that are realistic and achievable. Once the goal and objectives are set, strategies for achieving them can be determined. Resources needed in the project, and ways to obtain them, are then identified. The planning process also includes deciding how the project will be managed, sustained and evaluated.

## Elements of Planning

- ***Goals and objectives:*** It is planned end point of all activities and is concerned with the problem itself. They are talking about the ultimate results (impact or outcomes to be achieved).
- ***Policy:*** Guiding principles stated as an expectation. It is not binding but they are directive in nature.
- ***Program:*** Is a sequence of activities designed to implement plan and accomplish objectives.
- ***Schedule:*** Is a time sequence for the work to be done.
- ***Procedures:*** Is a set of rules for carrying out the work.
- ***Resources:*** Manpower, money, material, minutes (time), methods (skills-strategies)
- ***Target:*** Is discreet activity. It is degree of achievement, e.g., number of blood films, number of vasectomies. It is used of as operational level.

## Steps in Health Planning

Planning is a relational process which involves many steps. Also planning health services are to be carried out different level, i.e., national, state, district, below district or organizational level.

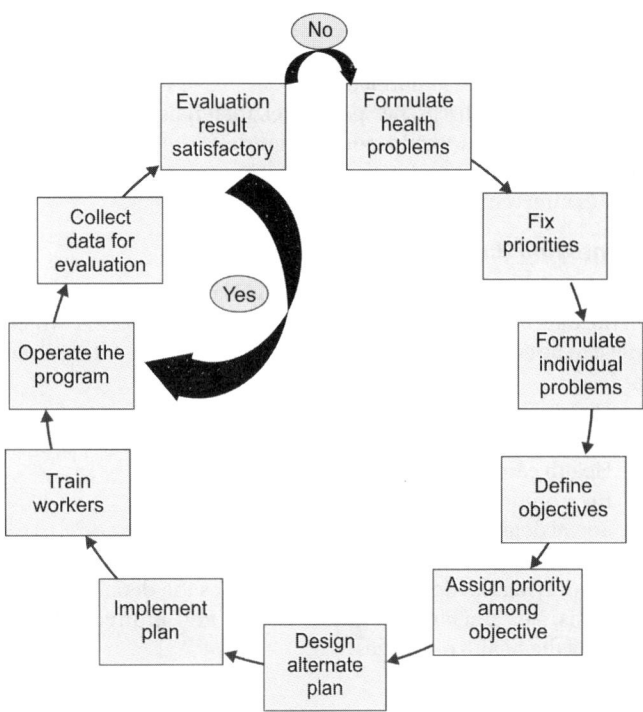

**Fig. 42B.1:** Planning cycle.

The planning steps may vary from level to level. However, the common steps for planning are as below **(Fig. 42B.1)**:
- Preplanning
- Identifying health problems
- Setting or selecting priorities
- Defining goals and objectives
- Strategy development
- Formulating the plan
- Implementation
- Monitoring and evaluation planning
- Replanning

### Preplanning

This is the stage where existing policies, legislation, health structure, institutes, political commitments, etc., are considered, assessed and based on that health planning units is created. The scope of planning for any particular health program should be limited to the general perimeters or "boundaries" in terms of place, time, population and disease condition(s).

### Analysis of Health Situation

This is the most important and crucial step in planning. Effective health planning and execution of health program depends only the reliable data. It is the assessing the health problems, direct and indirect factors in the occurrence of health problems, health and related institutes and services, opportunities for actions, availability of the resources.

Requirement of the data depends upon the broad purpose of the planning. In general, for health planning, following types of data would be required:

- Sociodemographic
- Epidemiological situation
- Health facilities and functioning
- Available resources, i.e., personnel, materials and finance.

Data collected would not only guide for the planning but would also act as baseline for monitoring and evaluation of the health interventions.

### Identifying the Health Problems

This can be equated with "Community Diagnosis." On the basis of the data analysis, enumeration of the health problems, which need to be addressed, can be done. Problems can be categorized as:
- Disease burden (medical)
- Behavior and custom culture, awareness
- Health care system related
- Environmental health management
- Social determination related
- Intersectorial related.

Identifying the health problems includes the detail problem analysis, i.e., tracking the direct causes and indirect factors leading the health outcomes.

### Setting the Priorities

The available resources are limited to meet the needs of people. Therefore, there is a need to select the pressing and urgent problems. For setting priorities, numbers of factors, i.e., economical, technical, financial, social, political, administrative, ethical, etc., must be taken into consideration. Three important aspects which is taken into considerations are as below:
1. Importance of public health problem. (How severely it is affecting the people? based on mortality, morbidity, suffering, cost of treatment and loss of productivity).
2. Availability of the effective interventions.
3. Cost of interventions (Treatment or preventive modality).

Some of the criteria used in prioritizing health problems in health planning are as below:
- Affecting large number of the people and their capacity.
- Associated with vulnerable groups.
- Largely prevalent in weaker sections of the community.
- Acute in nature.
- Having serious social and economic consequences.

### Defining the Goals and Objectives

Once priorities are set and it is decided to work on "identified" problem(s), next step is to set goal(s). Goal is the ultimate result, towards which all resources are diverted. They are generally broad and focusing on impact or long-term outcomes.

A goal is described in term of what to be attained, to what extent to be attained and when to attain.

Objectives are "broken down goal." They are precise (specific), more elaborative and may be further broken down in immediate, intermediate and ultimate objectives are focusing on output or short-term outcomes.

***Long-term objectives:*** Objectives can be defined as specific results that an organization, program or projects seeks to achieve in pursuing its basic mission or goal. Long-term means more than one year. Generally, they are organizational or program objectives. Objectives are essential for organizational success because they state direction; aid in evaluation; create synergy; reveal priorities; focus coordination; and provide a basis for effective planning, organizing, motivating, and controlling activities. Objectives should be specific, measurable, achievable, relevant, and time bound.

***Annual objectives (target):*** Annual objectives are short-term milestones that organizations must achieve to reach long-term objectives. Like long-term objectives, annual objectives should be specific, measurable, achievable, and relevant and time bound. We also use term "target" for such short-term objectives. A set of annual objectives is needed for each long-term objective. Short-term objectives are to be framed for all or important divisions, activities or outputs. Short-term objectives are especially important in strategy implementation, whereas long-term objectives are particularly important in strategy formulation. Annual objectives represent the basis for allocating resources.

Targets should not be confused with organizational or program objectives. Targets are mainly set at operational level (lower management level), focusing on performance.

### Deciding Strategies

Basically strategy is the part of plan write-up. It is the chosen approach out of available approaches and which would be taken for implementation.

Strategies are the means by which long-term objectives will be achieved. Strategies are potential actions that require top management decisions and large amounts of the organization, program or project's resources. In addition, strategies affect an organization's long-term prosperity, typically for at least 5 years, and thus are future-oriented. Strategies have multifunctional or multidivisional consequences and require consideration of both the external and internal factors facing the organization.

### Formulating the Plan

After setting the priorities and deciding the goal(s) and objectives; the next step is writing a plan. Plan means developing alternative ways of achieving the objectives and selection of a most appropriate way(s). There is not a single way to achieve the objectives. Hence, developing alternative ways requires both creativities and understanding. The planner should know the cause and effect relationship (applied epidemiology).

Along with identifying the most suitable ways, write-up should contain time sequence for the plan to be implemented, set of rules (procedures) for implementing the plan, use of resources, monitoring and evaluating, etc.

### Designing Implementation Plan

Implementation is also integral part of planning process. Before actual action to be occurred in the field, it requires to be thoroughly translated in to action(s). These action(s) should be directed towards specific objectives.

For instance, in a HIV prevention program, the strategy could be to only have health educational efforts, or else it could be a comprehensive strategy of combination of health education, blood safety, diagnosis and treatment, surveillance and prevention of parent to child transmission (PPTCT). Obviously, the choice of strategy will be strongly guided by the program objectives and your available or expected resources. If you do not have lot of resources, naturally you would select a strategy of limited activities which are likely to give you the best results. Now, having decided the strategy, write down a detailed action plan as to how the program will be executed. Do ensure that a "time-line" has been given for each objective, target and indicator, giving the date of each end point.

Place the required manpower, equipment, material and other logistics at the required places. If some more resources are expected, make a plan as to where they will be relocated and how. Make out detailed, written "operations manual" including the operative procedures for each activity, i.e., "who will do what to whom and in what manner." Ensure that your personnel have been centrally trained and tested for undertaking the procedures.

### Developing Monitoring and Evaluation Plan

For last many years, an emphasize is given to include monitoring and evaluation plan as an integral part of overall planning and a reasonable proportion of budget must be allocated along with a specific monitoring and evaluation frame work in planning.

#### Monitoring
Monitoring is a continuous process of observing, recording, reporting on various indicators (tasks and activities) and identifying any deviation from the desired. A frame work of monitoring and evaluation should be integral part of the planning, specifying what to be monitored, who will be monitor and how it will be monitored and how frequently it will be monitored, etc. The monitoring is used by operational level manager and middle level managers to early pick up any deviation and institute the corrective measures immediately.

#### Evaluation
While monitoring is for day-to-day control, evaluation is for validating the strategies and planning. It is done to know the relevance of the services, program, strategies or activities or to know the adequacy of the services, resources (inputs), to know the quality of the services, or efficacy, effectiveness and efficiency of services or program. Evaluation is used by top level management and some time by middle level management. It helps in replanning.

***Designing monitoring and evaluation framework:*** Monitoring or evaluation need may be different at different level of management. Different sets of indicators for different level of management may be created. Further indicators should be kept optimum in number, specific in nature and must cover all the three phases of management, inputs, process and outputs, outcomes or impact.

#### Deciding indicators:
- *Input indicators:* Manpower, material and supplies, financial resources.
- *Output indicators:* Task, activities, performance, target-related indicators.
- *Outcome or impact indicators:* Service utilization, knowledge and behavior change, reduction in mortalities or mortalities, change in health status.

### Replanning

Planning is continuous process and it requires constant watch through monitoring and evaluation. Due to change in health situation, advent of newer knowledge or technology in tackling the health problems or feedback on effectiveness, efficiency and efficacy of the interventions or strategies, replanning can be carried out.

The relationship between different planning activities and various level of management is shown below in the **Table 42B.1**.

However, there is interrelationship between different levels of managements and planning process and distinction between different may not be always clear.

**Table 42B.1:** Planning tasks at different levels of management.

| Level of management | Planning (with focus on) | Planning tasks |
| --- | --- | --- |
| Top | Strategic (outcome or impact) | • Prioritizing health problems<br>• Fixing goals<br>• Formulating polices<br>• Developing strategies<br>• Allocating resources<br>• Evaluation plan |
| Middle | Implementation (input-output) | • Planning for service delivery<br>• Output delivery<br>• Negotiating targets<br>• Logistic supports<br>• Human resource development<br>• Intersectoral coordination<br>• Monitoring plan |
| Lower | Operational (activities) | • Operational plan (microplanning of sessions, campaigns, activities, etc.)<br>• Supervision plan |

## STRATEGIC PLANNING

Planning activities are done at all three levels of management. At the top management level policies and strategies are formulated, resources are allocated and goals (health outcomes) are fixed. This is known as strategic planning.

Strategy is an action an organization takes to attain superior performance and *formulating, implementing and evaluating such strategies are strategic management.*

Strategy is management's overall plan and actions for deploying resources and skills taking into consideration opportunities and threats in the environment to achieve its mission, vision and objectives and to establish a favorable competitive position or success. Strategic plan is, in essence, a game plan for any project or program. Just as a cricket team needs a good game plan to have a chance for success, an organization must have a good strategic plan for complete success. A strategic plan results from tough managerial choices among numerous good alternatives, and it signals commitment to specific health situation, policies, procedures, and implementation in lieu of other, "less desirable" courses of action.

*Strategic planning* is an organization's process of defining strategies or directions and making decisions on allocating its resources to pursue this strategy including its capitals, and people. It involves the development of objectives and linking of these objectives with the resources which will be employed to action. Strategic planning is therefore concerned with overall all functions of management.

Strategic planning process is on-going and continuous cycle of situation analysis (internal evaluation and environmental scanning), establishing a mission, vision and objectives strategy formulation, strategy implementation, strategic control and performance evaluation.

## Strength Weakness Opportunities Threats (Challenges) Analysis

Strength, weakness, opportunities, threats (SWOT) (Challenges) analysis is a strategic planning tool used to evaluate the SWOT (C) of a project or program or services. It involves specifying the objectives of the program or services, or project and identifying and classifying the "internal factor" and "external factors" that are favorable and unfavorable to achieving these objectives. Internal factors are listed and classified as "Strengths" or "Weaknesses" and "external factors" are classified as "Opportunities" or "Threats (challenges)."

### Internal Strengths and Weaknesses

Based on internal analysis of organizations strive to pursue strategies that capitalize on strengths and improve weaknesses. They arise in the management, promotion, finance, accounting, production or operations, staff capacity, research and development, and management information systems. Identifying and evaluating organizational strengths and weaknesses in the functional areas of a business is an essential strategic management activity. Organizations strive to pursue strategies that capitalize on internal strengths and eliminate internal weaknesses.

### Environmental Analysis

It is one of the most important activities in the strategic management. It involves the evaluation of the "business" environment of the organization. All external influences that impact an organization's decision and performance. Environment consists of the international or national economy; changes in demographic structures; social, cultural and political trends; technology; legal, governmental and the natural environment, stakeholders, suppliers, clients or beneficiary; staff, unions and owners and shareholders, etc.

### External Opportunities and Threat (Challenges)

External opportunities and threats (C) are referred to benefit or harm to the organization, program or project due to any change in above factors in environment.

A basic tenet of strategic management is that organizations need to formulate strategies to take advantage of external opportunities and to avoid or reduce the impact of external threats.

Some of the examples in SWOT(C) analysis are shown below in typical general health system:

*Strength:*
- Well-defined goal, objectives, guidelines and targets
- A large network of healthcare institutes
- Political commitment
- Qualified, trained and motivated staff
- Decentralized planning flexibilities
- Computerized management information system

*Weaknesses:*
- Lack of local planning capacity
- Weak organizational leadership
- Irregular supplies and logistic support
- Overburden staff at field level
- Inadequate fund

*Opportunities:*
- High educational levels of communities
- Presence of active voluntary organizations
- Specialized private hospitals
- A good road connectivity
- Wide network of internet, electricity
- Good inter sectional collaboration

*Threats (challenges):*
- Rigid custom and cultural beliefs
- Nonacceptance of health insurance in community
- Low priority of health
- Inadequate safe drinking water and sanitation facilities in remote areas.

Thus, strategic planning is all about developing to strategies by using of the strength of the organization and minimizing the impacts of weaknesses, at the same time and tapping the opportunities looming out in the external environment and avoiding the threats or managing the challenges to the advantage of getting desired results. The process can be understood vide the schematic diagram given as **Figure 42B.2**.

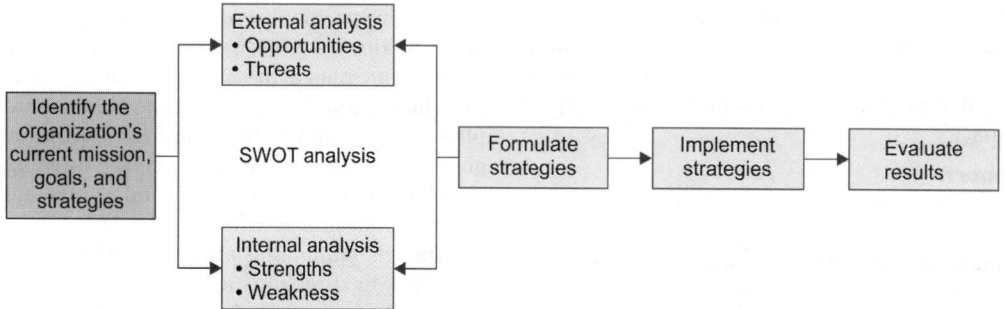

Fig. 42B.2: Strategic planning by using strength, weakness, opportunities, threats (SWOT) (challenges) analysis toll.

## OPERATIONAL PLANNING

It is a plan describing a how the organization will operate in practice to implement its action and monitoring plan, engage resources, deal risk, to obtain organizational objectives.

### Types of Operational Plan

At PHCs there are number of the activities and the range of operational responsibilities which requires a systematic approach in planning services. There are broadly two times of the activities:

#### Routine (Programmed) Type of Activities to be Performed Regularly

Routine preventive, promotive, curative activities, etc., immunizations, village health nutrition day (VHND), antenatal care (ANC), malarial surveillance, supervision of subcenter activities, etc., are the examples of the routine types of the activities. For such activities, fixing the job responsibilities, setting the rules for task or procedures, scheduling, and organizing the resources, realistic targets (workloads) are carried out. Organizational analysis, job description, job evaluation, work measurement, method studies, inventory control, value analysis, material handling, standardization, ABC or VED analysis (discussed in details in *Chapter 42E: Logistics and Finance Management*), etc., are some management techniques which can be used for such planning.

#### One Time Tasks which is not Routine but to be Performed on Special Occasions or for Special Purposes

National immunization day, camps, campaign, trainings are the examples of the onetime tasks. Apart from some of the management techniques mentioned above in programed (routine) activities, network analysis, Gantt chart, PERT, CPM are the management techniques very useful in one-time task plan.

For the best performance, operational plan should match program activities with community needs. Unmet need is one of the approaches, and gap analysis is the tool used in such planning. There are the situations where felt needs of the community and program objectives are matching hence better utilization of the services can be seen, but there are many examples where community felt needs and program objectives are not matching. Hence, for such instances along with planning for supply side demand side planning are also to be carried out.

### Steps in Operational (Program) Planning

The operational plan specified tasks, how this will be performed, who will perform them, when and where. There are three steps involved for these:
1. ***Developing list of all tasks with detail about description of the tasks and level of activities:*** All the activities to be carried out are thought about and exhaustive list of the all tasks are to be prepared. The salient descriptions of the tasks-activities are also noted. Against all the tasks level of activities are to be prepared. Level of activities is the answers to questions like how much? How many? Time required? Who will perform? etc.
2. ***Examining the task specifications:*** Every task has been defined and set of specific rules or guidelines are framed as a part of the program designing. Also there are the specific tasks which are prepared locally. They are to be critically reviewed one by one and examined for inconsistency, omission and feasibility and make necessary revisions.
3. ***Preparing a task schedules:*** It should contain the detail about time and resources to be used on time line or with specified period. Well thought of task scheduling will help:
   - Logical and rational sequencing of activities
   - Proper distribution of workload to staff by preventing overburdening or under work load to staff
   - Preventing overlapping of the task or involvement of same resources like man, machine, vehicle, etc.
   - Time slack or consumption of disproportionate resources for species task.
   - Supervision and review plan can be prepared accordingly.

### Advantage of Operational Planning

As program activities are planned in advance; better and efficient performances can be achieved because of following advantages:
- Wastage of staff and time and other resources could be avoided.
- Better clarity of role and coordinated efforts of team are elicited.
- Problems with unrealistic targets can go away.
- Locally prevalent challenges or constraints can be thought of in advance and plan can be prepared accordingly, thus their effects on performance can be minimized.
- Problems can be forecasted in advance hence innovative solutions can be thought of and used.
- Program activities can be matched with people's needs.
- Better intersectoral and intrasectoral coordination can be achieved.

### Cautions in Operational Planning

Though planning help in effective implementation, but some cautioned need to be kept in mind:
- ***Too much planning:*** Over planning becomes pure theoretical than the practical approach. Excessive concern with planning diverts attentions from implementation. It delays the implementation.
- ***Over reliance on targets:*** Many a times operational targets fixed at national level or state level are average targets of good performing and poorly performing units. Hence, for some PHC they become unrealistic, while for another unit it is already over passed targets. Though generalized targets are to be set at higher up, but local targets are to be fixed keeping local situations in mind. In case of unrealistic targets pressing too hard for the target will have rebound effects on performance. In case of better performing PHCs this will result in complacency.
- ***Institutionalizing of planning:*** A special team for planning are generally cannot relate themselves with field situations and such planning becomes unrealistic plan. Program or institutional (District, Taluka officers, PHC, MO, etc.) head and people are to be part of implementation should be part of the planning.
- ***Ignoring replanning:*** Planning is set of activities for future and some assumptions are used in preparing the plan. But there are substantial changes or wrong may be encountered. In such instances replanning is necessary.

# SUMMARY

Health planning is a managerial process to carry out health situational analysis, prioritize the health problems, fixes the health goals or objectives and formulates strategies, designs monitoring and evaluation framework and allocates resources. It is a systematic approach and uses for matching the limited resources with unlimited needs. There are different seven approaches and ten steps for planning. Planning is to be carried out at all levels of the health management. The purpose and planning tasks may be different at different levels of management. Strategic planning and operation planning are the two important planning process used at different level of management depending upon their role and needs. Strategic planning and management are one and same, they are used interchangeably. Strategic planning is the process of deciding on the objectives of the organization or changes in earlier specified objectives, on the resources used to attain these objectives and on the policies that are to govern the acquisition, sue and deposition of these resources. It is to get competitive advantage to other organizations or strategies or plan. It is linked with objectives and resources and takes into account the present and future internal as well as external environment.

SWOT analysis is tool used in the strategic planning, where internal strength and weaknesses and external opportunities and threats are analyzed. Based on that, strategies are developed linking with goals and objectives of the organization.

Strategic planning has certain benefits but there are some dangers to be taken care for its effective uses.

Strategic planning should be followed by operational planning. Operation planning increases the performance efficiency. It requires mainly three steps, task listing, task specification and task scheduling. There are two type of operational plan, one is routine (programmed) type and another is one-time task. For both the types; different management techniques can be used for preparing good operation plan.

# C. MANAGERIAL SKILLS

*Rivu Basu, Sanjib Bandyopadhyay, Kaushik Mitra, Saikat Bhattacharya, Bhavesh Modi*

## INTRODUCTION

Managerial skills are the personal ability put to use by the manager in specific position that she or he holds in organizational hierarchy. The most important skills required for managers are summarized by Robert Lukasz as technical skill, human skill (interpersonal skill), and conceptual skill. Different managerial positions require different sets of managerial skills. people. While technical skills are primarily concerned with doing job technically correct; human skills concern with emotions and intelligence and relations of persons involved in executing the jobs. For human skills, managers need to understand and work well with people. Capability to understand other people's emotions, pains, and agony, and to act in a manner that shows that you are really concerned and whatever you are saying is not only lip service.

- **Technical skills:** The job-specific knowledge required to perform the task. It is the ability to work in a particular area of expertise, ability to use the tools, techniques, and procedures for the particular job. These are specific abilities that people use to perform their jobs, perform a specialized task that involves a certain method or process, e.g., clinical, medical skills, accounting, statistical calculation, engineering, mechanical, typing, report writing, etc. Without technical skills, one is not able to manage the work effectively.

  These skills are most used by persons not in management and lower level management. Higher levels rely less on technical skills.

  *Example:* How to give subcutaneous vaccine to child of age 9 months to 15 years.

- **Conceptual skills:** Are the ability to visualize the organization as a whole and the ability to integrate the activities of the entire organization. These skills help managers understand how different parts of an organization relate to one another and to the organization as a whole. It is also useful in decision making, planning, and organizing, identifying problems, and resolve problems for the benefit of the organization. It requires logical thinking, reasoning powers, and analytical capabilities. These skills assume greater importance as manager acquires more responsibility. It is required the most by top level managers. Proportions of these three management skills vary from level to level **(Fig. 42C.1)**.

Managers are basically decision makers and take best decision out of available alternatives. Political and human relations skills (IPS-interpersonal skills) are most essential along with technical to establish health department as a leader in community health improvement.

- **Human skills:** An ability to understand, alter, lead, and control human behavior. It is the ability to work with individual and ability to understand their needs with empathy. At every managerial level, manager requires to interact with other in the mangers is the most important requirement for the good interpersonal skills.

  It includes interviewing job applicants, forming partnerships with other organizations, resolving conflicts, leading, negotiating, and motivating the staff. For a good human skill, manager

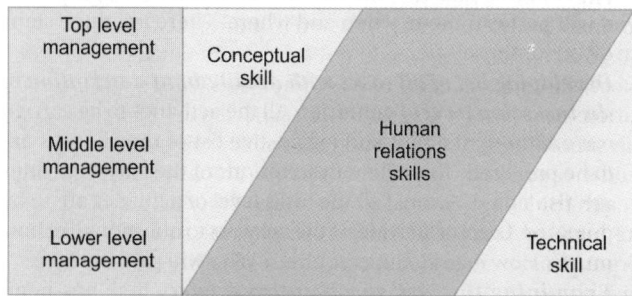

Fig. 42C.1: Managerial skills.

has to understand his own attitudes, beliefs, perceptions, and assumptions, and of other individual and group.

Health services organizations are human resource-intensive organizations. A congenial environment is conducive to productivity, satisfaction, and happiness. A health administrator must have good interpersonal skills to create such an environment. At the core of interpersonal relationships are communication and empathy. This skill helps understand and work well with people, interviewing job applicants, forming partnerships with other businesses, and resolving conflicts. Some of the important skills under interpersonal skills are:
- **Leadership skills**
- **Team building skills**
- **Motivational skills**
- **Communication skills**
- **Conflicts resolving skills**

Few of the important human skills are briefly described in this chapter.

## LEADERSHIP

Leaders are there in every sphere of our day-to-day lives. There are political leaders, organizational leaders, group leaders, community leaders, school leaders, and many more. But all of them have one common aspect; they have the ability to inspire, guide, and manage others to seek defined objectives. According to Keith Davis, "Leadership is the ability to persuade others to seek defined objectives enthusiastically. It is the human factor which binds a group together and motivates it toward goals." So, leaders have the ability to influence others and have managerial authority. What leaders do to achieve the objectives is leadership. Leadership may be defined as a process of inspiring and guiding a group and influencing that group to achieve its goals.

### Leadership and Management

Leadership goes beyond just managing people. Leaders do not require any managerial position for their activities. Leaders operate basically by virtue of their power possessed through their personal qualities and do not have to depend on their position in the organization. Now, the point is whether the reverse holds true or not. Do managers have to be leaders? By virtue of their positions, managers have to provide leadership to their groups and ideally, all managers should be leaders. Leading is one of the basic management functions, which a manager has to perform. So, leadership and managing are not synonymous. All managers are leaders, but all leaders are not managers.

The managers and leaders in an organization may be compared on the basis as depicted in **Table 42C.1**.

A successful leader ought not be a good manager but to be a successful manager one needs to be good leader. Managers at various levels in an organization are expected to be leaders so that the subordinates (or followers) are influenced and accept their guidance to reach the goals. In a block, Block Medical Officer of Health (BMOH) is in-charge and all the other doctors and staffs are his subordinates. If BMOH can play the role of a leader by virtue of his personal qualities, all the staffs will be willing to work with him and under his guidance and objectives will be achieved, that is, health indicators of the block will improve.

**Table 42C.1:** Differences between manager and leader.

| | Manager | Leader |
|---|---|---|
| Attainment of role | A person is a manager by virtue of his position in an organization | A person becomes a leader on basis of his personal qualities and charisma |
| Rights | Manager has formal rights in an organization | Leader has no formal rights in an organization |
| Followers | The subordinates of the manager in the organization are his followers | The group of employees whom the leader influences are his followers |
| Functions | A manager performs all basic management functions | Leader influences people to work for attainment of the objectives |
| Period | Managership is a stable post and has tenure | Leadership is temporary |
| Accountability for performance | Manager is accountable for self as well as subordinates' performance | Leaders have no accountability for performance |
| Concern | A manager's concern is attainment of the organizational goals | A leader's concern is attainment of group objectives as well as his followers' satisfaction |

### Theories of Leadership

Leadership has emerged since ancient times, when people gathered together and formed groups for accomplishment of their objectives. But study of leadership began in twentieth century, when theories related to leadership started to emerge.

#### University IOWA Model of Leadership (Fig. 42C.2)

The behavior presented by a leader during controlling of subordinates for achievement of objectives is known as leadership style. The University of IOWA studies explored three distinct leadership styles: Autocratic, democratic, and laissez-faire.

1. ***The autocratic leadership style*** described a leader who dictated his followers. This type of leadership is also known as authoritative or directive style of leadership. In this style, the entire authority is concentrated in the hands of the leader. He dictates work methods and policies and makes unilateral decisions. The group members have limited scope of decision making. So they cannot put forward their own views, even if, it is better for the organization. The leader demands complete obedience from his group members. The advantage of this autocratic style is speedy decision making and achievement of objectives as desired by the leader under his supervision. The disadvantage is that, this type of leadership may lead to loss of motivation among the group members, which in turn may lead to absenteeism and non-accomplishment of objectives.

2. ***Democratic leadership style*** involves group members or employees in decision making process. The members can put forward their own ideas, discuss among themselves, but the ultimate decision is taken by the leader based on these ideas. This type of leadership is also known as participative or consultative style of leadership. The leader guides the

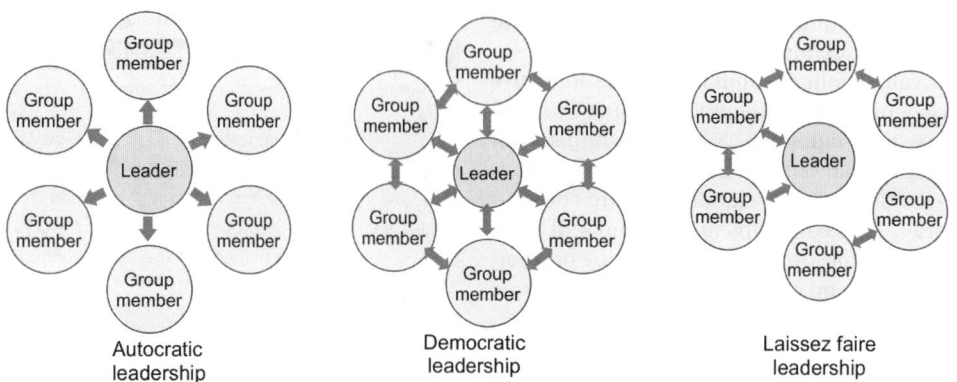

Fig. 42C.2: University of IOWA model of leadership.

members on what to perform and how to perform. The democratic leader has to accommodate, compromise and tolerate the views of the group members. The advantages of this democratic style of leadership are members get motivated; they are satisfied and objectives are attained. It leads to a good working environment. The main disadvantage is that this is time-consuming.

3. **Laissez-faire leadership style** of leadership is one in which the group members make their own decisions and their objectives. The group leader fully depends on the members to perform the job themselves. He allows them to set their own objectives and to achieve them. This leadership style works only when the employees/group members are skilled, loyal, and experienced.

### Managerial Grid (Fig. 42C.3)

The behavioral dimensions from the earlier studies provided the basis for the development of a two-dimensional grid for appraising leadership styles. The study was aimed at evaluating the leader's behavior along two variables, such as "concern for production" and "concern for people" plotted along the $x$-axis and $y$-axis, respectively. A leader with high concern for production is task-oriented and his basic emphasis is on reaching the desired objectives. A leader who has high concern for people avoids conflicting situations and endeavors for friendly relations with the group members. Both the variables "concern for production" and "concern for people" are plotted nine-point scale where 1 indicates low concern and 9 represents high concern.

The grid is divided into 81 categories into which a leader's behavioral style may fall. But, only five definite styles were named according to the position on the grid:
1. Impoverished management (1,1 or low concern for production, low concern for people)
2. Task management (9,1 or high concern for production, low concern for people)
3. Middle-of-the-road management (5,5 or medium concern for both production and people)
4. Country club management (1,9 or low concern for production, high concern for people)
5. Team management (9,9 or high concern for production, high concern for people).

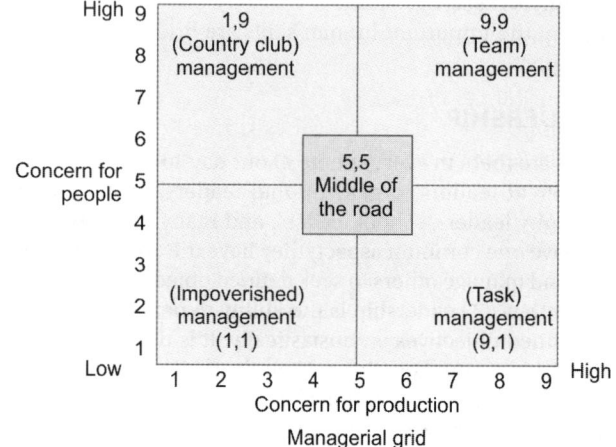

Fig. 42C.3: The managerial grid model of leadership.

### Situational Leadership—Best Leadership Style

The researchers are in a dilemma. Sometimes, autocratic style of leadership led to better group performance and attainment of group objectives. On the other hand, democratic style of leaders is more accepted by the group members. So, they may also work better with such types of leaders and yield better results. It is thought about that in different situation different style of leadership is to be adopted keeping the eye on the achieving the desired results, e.g., in case of emergency or urgent situation autocratic style of leaders gives better result, while in case of dealing with group of experienced or expert people democratic style of leadership may be adopted. If subordinates are competent and self-motivated then *Laissez-faire* style of leadership can work well. In short, no one leadership is best and successful leader uses different styles of leadership in different situation, which is known as situational leadership style.

## TEAM BUILDING

A team is defined as two or more interacting and interdependent individuals who come together to achieve specific organizational goals. Formal teams are work groups defined by the organization's structure and have designated work assignments and specific tasks directed at accomplishing organizational goals. The examples are committees, task forces, etc. They can be permanent groups or temporary groups. They are often developed according to strict hierarchy. Informal groups are social groups. They can be formed with any way like sharing the same transit to work.

A good manager ought to build team, because he/she does not work but get work through the people. Health care is a service oriented job which is highly dependent on human beings. Thus team building is important for better results. There are five stages of team building (group formation)—forming, storming, norming, performing, and often adjourning. It is also known as group dynamics.

1. *Forming* is the first stage of group development where the people join the team and decide its structure, function, and purpose.
2. The *storming* stage comes, when there is intragroup conflict, and there is tension regarding the leadership, roles, and responsibilities of each, etc.
3. *Norming:* In this stage, the cohesiveness begins to develop and the team members are able to unify to a common set of behaviors regarding the expectations of the group.
4. *Performing:* The next stage team starts to perform toward the given goal.
5. *Adjourning:* The last stage can be adjourning, when the group is dismantled after the task is done (in case of temporary team).

The few things that should be maintained in groups are— the role should be clearly defined (the expected behavior of a person occupying a particular position in a social structure), the norms (standard or expectations shared and supported by the group members), conformity to the norms and roles, and cohesiveness (the limit up to which group members are sharing the organizational goal).

Different teams spend different span of time in different stages of team building. Also it is not necessary that every team passes through each stage and every stage occurred in sequence. But once norming established, the effectiveness of the team improved at maximum. The good team leader takes the team to performing stage as early as possible with minimum or no storming stage and maintain that stage to yield maximum effectiveness.

## MOTIVATION

Motivation is the study of what makes people become more productive at work. In the early part of the twentieth century, it was believed that employees were motivated purely by money alone, that they did not enjoy work and needed close supervision. Later Elton Mayo noted social complexity of what motivated people, then came the work of Maslow and Herzberg. **Motivation is the study of the psychology of what makes people want to go to work and be productive when they get there.**

There are many important theories of motivation. In this small scope, it is impossible to discuss about all of them, thus the important theories shall be described.

## Early Theories of Motivation: Maslow's Hierarchy of Needs (Fig 42C.4)

Abraham Maslow (1908-1970) and Fredrick Herzberg (1923-2000) introduced their motivation theories in the 1950's that focused on the psychological needs of employees.

Though they are based on needs beyond the money but still they were quite simplistic. They only considered employees' expectation from the jobs and nothing else.

Maslow postulated that human beings are driven by some needs and those needs come in hierarchical manner. He identified five levels in this hierarchy of needs as shown in **Figure 42C.5**. He believed that once a given level of need is satisfied, it no longer motivates man. Then, the next higher level of need has to be activated in order to motivate the person. So when a person moves it is level by level upward or downward.

These needs are discussed one by one.

***Physiological needs:*** These needs are basic to human life and to be met first. They include food, clothing, shelter, air, water, and necessities of life. These needs remain at the base of the needs pyramid.

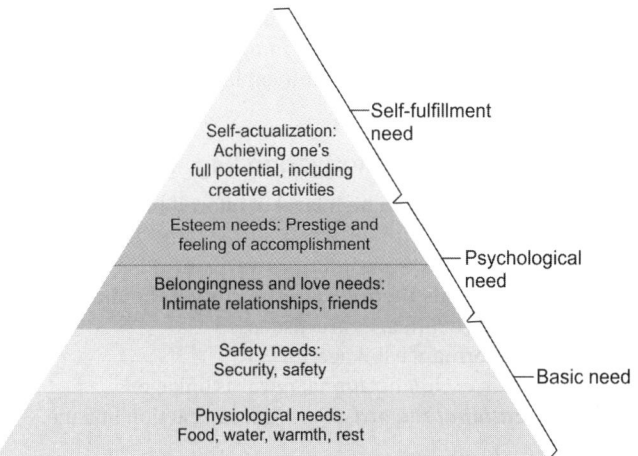

**Fig. 42C.4:** Maslow's hierarchy of needs models.
*Source:* Maslow AH. A Theory of Human Motivation. Psychological Review. 1943;50(4):370-96.

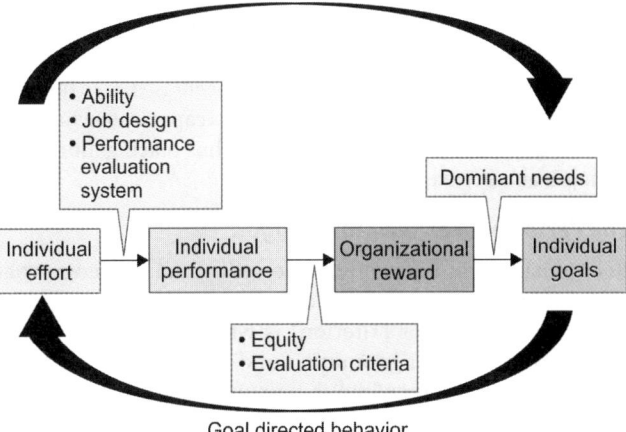

**Fig. 42C.5:** Integrated model of motivation.

***Safety needs:*** The next needs felt are called safety and security needs. Desires such as economic security and protection from physical dangers are examples. Meeting these needs requires more money so worker is prompted to work more.

***Social needs:*** As a social being, man is interested in social interaction, companionship, belongingness, etc. For this socializing and belongingness, individuals prefer to work in groups.

***Esteem needs:*** These needs refer to self-esteem and self-respect. They include such needs which indicate self-confidence, achievement, competence, knowledge and independence, ego satisfaction, and respect from others.

***Self-actualization needs:*** This level represents the pinnacle of need pyramid. This means to become actualized in what one is potentially good at. In effect, self-actualization is the person's motivation to transform perception of self-brilliance into reality.

*The main criticisms of the theory include the following:* The needs may or may not follow a definite hierarchical order and there may be overlapping in need hierarchy. For example, even if safety need is not satisfied, the social need may emerge or even be satisfied. Thus, though a classic theory, Maslow's need is considered to be partially true in today's age. Better models like the one discussed below can explain motivation in more concrete ways.

### Integrated Model of Motivation (Fig. 42C.5)

An employee will exert a high level of effort if he/she perceives a strong relationship between effort and performance, performance and rewards, and rewards and satisfaction of personal goals. This theory takes the core of the model. Thus here three kinds of linkages are discussed.
1. ***Effort:*** Performance linkage
2. ***Performance:*** Organizational rewards linkage
3. ***Organizational rewards:*** Personal satisfaction linkage.

### Effort: Performance Linkage

Level of individual performance is determined not only by the level of individual effort but also by the individual's ability to perform and by whether the organization has a fair and objective performance evaluation system. If someone perceives that she/he is not capable enough or his/her performance will go unnoticed due to favoritism, motivation decreases. Also training of the individual is required to increase his capacity to work. The person may also be not in the right job, thus placing him in the right job also increases performance.

### The Performance: Reward Linkage

Relationship will be strong if the individual perceives that performance (rather than seniority, personal favorites, equity of pay or some other criterion) is what is rewarded in the organization. A clear promotion and transfer policy, career development all comes into the picture. Rewards also play a key part in equity theory. Individuals will compare the rewards (outcomes) they have received from the inputs or efforts they made with the inputs–outcomes ratio of other individuals either from same or similar organizations. If inequities exist, the effort expended may be influenced.

### Rewards: Goal Relationship Linkage

The traditional need theories come into play here. Motivation would be high to the degree that the rewards an individual received for his/her high performance satisfied the dominant needs consistent with his/her individual goals. Rewards may be of two kinds—(1) intrinsic and (2) extrinsic rewards. Examples of intrinsic rewards are such as sense of accomplishment and self-actualization and extrinsic rewards may include working conditions and status. The intrinsic rewards are much more likely to produce attitudes about satisfaction that are related to performance.

Individual with high need for achievement is not motivated by the organization's assessment of his/her performance or organizational rewards; hence, the jump from effort to individual goals. High achievers are internally driven as long as the jobs they are doing provide them with personal responsibility, feedback, and moderate risks.

So overall this motivation model is a multivariate model to explain the complex relationship that exists between satisfaction and performance.

## CONFLICT MANAGEMENT

Conflict is the disagreement between two or more individuals or groups over an issue of mutual interest. Whenever two individuals or groups opine in two different ways, a conflict arises. In a layman's language, conflict is nothing but a fight either between two individuals or among group members. Every organization witnesses conflict more or less. While organization with good team performance enjoys higher effectiveness, conflicts drag it down. No organization can afford conflict.

Healthcare system wide high range of varied manpower, highly specialized to just skilled to semiskilled—gathered together under one roof. Sometimes, there are interpersonal conflicts in perceiving each other's performance or roles. Even client expectations, level of services, and neglect lead to conflict situations which adversely affect the quality of patient care and client satisfaction. The administrator is continually facing and attempting to solve individual or interpersonal or departmental conflicts. Different researches have shown that health managers spend 20% of their time dealing with conflicts. A good manager or leader should anticipate conflict early and try to resolve that before individuals take positions and freeze to them.

Not all conflicts are underproductive or unproductive. Positive conflicts are useful. Constructive conflict can promote innovation, creativity, and development of new ideas, which make organizational growth possible. In fact, it is seen that unless there is a low level of conflict, performance is not up to the mark. While looking at the types of conflicts, a usable classification can be made.

### Types of Conflict

- ***Task conflict:*** Conflicts over content and goals of the work. Suppose a particular job is to be done by the Medical Officer,

but he thinks that the ward sister should do the job. This kind of situations can lead to task conflicts.
- **Relationship conflict:** Conflict based on interpersonal relationships. A very common type of conflict that may occur due to maladjustments of two individuals in an organization. Like an issue due to common interests may occur between two visiting surgeons of the same department.
- **Process conflict:** Conflict over how work gets done. This is especially important in health care, when the process has not been planned and decided upon breaking into roles and responsibilities, like who is going to do a post-admission round of a surgical patient and up to what he can prescribe. Usually junior residents do this and thus come in conflict with the junior level faculties.

## Conflict Process

*To understand the pathology of conflict in an organization, it is imperative to have a look at the conflict process.* Conflict process consists of five stages that show how conflict begins, develops, and reveals among individuals or groups with different goals, interests or values of the organization **(Fig. 42C.6)**.

### Stage 1: Potential Opposition or Incompatibility
The first step in the conflict process is the presence of conditions that create opportunities for conflict to develop. These may due to lack of communications, ill-defined organizational structure, and due to personal factors such as differences in personalities and value systems may create conflict. People who are highly aggressive and authoritative and possess low self-esteem are more likely to be involved in conflict.

### Stage 2: Cognition and Personalization
If the antecedent conditions seem to have any negative impact on the interests of one party (individual/group), they will develop hostility toward the other party and the conflict reaches the second stage. It has been observed that so long one is unaware of conflict, for him it does not exist. It is at the felt level when the person is emotionally involved in a conflict creating anxiety, tension, frustration, anger, or hostility (explained later). Thus, we can define two kinds of conflict here like:
1. **Perceived conflict:** Awareness by one or more parties of the existence of conditions that create opportunities for conflict to arise.
2. **Felt conflict:** Emotional involvement in a conflict creating anxiety, tenseness, frustration, or hostility.

Like there may be long standing conflict between the two faculties of a department, and that did not hamper their functions. But suddenly one of them makes a scene for a trivial reason and that creates tension in the department. Thus the conflict becomes felt conflict.

### Stage 3: Intentions (Fig. 42C.7)
Intentions are decisions to act in a given way, intentions intervene between people's perception and emotions and their overt behavior.

As suggested by K Thomas, using two dimensions' cooperativeness (the degree to which one party attempts to satisfy the other party's concerns) and assertiveness (the degree to which one party attempts to satisfy his or her own concerns), five conflict-handling intentions can be identified.
- **Competing (Win–lose):** When one person seeks to satisfy his or her own interests regardless of the impact on the other parties to the conflict, he is competing. A strategy of win–lose is adopted to resolve the conflict. Therefore, group/individual stakes to win and makes others to lose.
- **Collaborating (Win–win):** A situation in which the parties to a conflict each desire to satisfy fully the concerns of all the parties. In collaborating, the intention of the parties is to solve the problem by clarifying differences rather than by accommodating various points of view.
- **Avoiding (Lose–lose):** A person may recognize that a conflict exists and wants to withdraw from it or suppress it. Avoiding included trying to just ignore a conflict and avoiding others with whom you disagree.

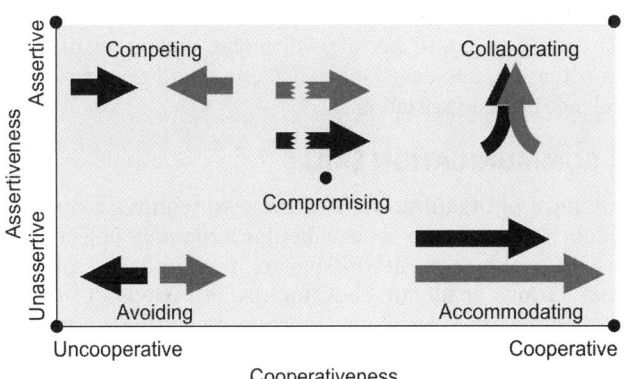

**Fig. 42C.7:** The intentions to resolve conflicts.
*Source:* Robbins SP, Judge T, Campbell T. Organizational Behavior. New York: Pearson; 2016.

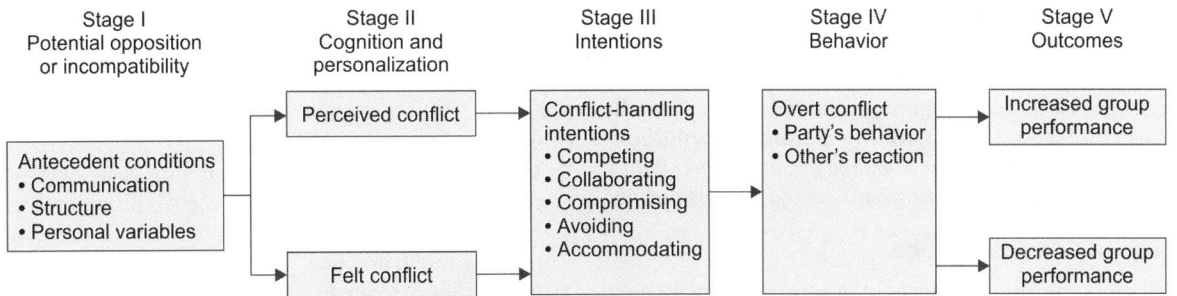

**Fig. 42C.6:** Stages of conflict management.
*Source:* Robbins SP, Judge T. Campbell T. Organizational Behavior. New York: Pearson; 2016.

- ***Accommodating (Lose–win):*** *A person may be* willing to place the opponent conflict ahead of her own. One party is willing to be self-sacrificing.
- ***Compromising:*** No clear win or lose situation. In this situation, each party to a conflict is willing to give up something.

A good manager has to help the conflicting parties to come to any intention to settle, else this may progress to the next stage that is conflict behavior.

### Stage 4: Behavior

This is a stage where conflict becomes visible. The behavior stage includes the statements, actions, and reactions made by the conflicting parties. These conflict behaviors are usually overt attempt to implement each party's intentions.

Disagreements, negative remarks, and challenging fall along the lower side of the continuum, while verbal attacks, threats, ultimatums, and physical attacks come on the upper side of the continuum.

### Stage 5: Outcomes

Outcomes are the consequences that result from interaction among conflicting parties.

These outcomes are functional when the constructive consequences of a conflict support the goals of the group or organization and improves its performance, or dysfunctional when the destructive consequences of a conflict hinder group performance.

Constructive consequences improve the quality of decisions, stimulate creativity or innovation, exploit hidden potential, encourage interest in group members, and foster environments of self-evaluation and change.

Destructive consequences could be devastating and disrupting. It could be large turnover, absenteeism, poor coordination, decreased job satisfaction, and even strikes or violence in an organization.

## COMMUNICATION SKILLS

Any form of organization, as a process, requires a multiple number of workers to act together for a common objective. In case of health care, the workers are often multidisciplinary, from various academic backgrounds, at various life stages. The team work is absolutely essential to get the work done. Obviously organizational structures are a very important part to this whole process, but one thing that acts as the software of the entire structure is flow of information, shared decisions, and participation. This cannot be done without communication. Thus communication acts as the tool by which the inorganic forms of the organization get life.

About 70–80% of manager's working time is spent in some kind of communication. Reading and writing memos, listening to our coworkers, or having one-to-one conversations with our supervisors are all forms of communication. It can be formally defined as *"a process of transforming message/information/advices/instructions/knowledge from one person to other with a view that both have common interpretation and understanding."*

### Functions of Communication

Effective communication enhances interpersonal relationships, builds trust and teamwork, prevents costly mistakes, motivates and gets things done. It is required:

- To make aware about
- To develop common understanding
- To condition mind so as to get right perception
- To motivate and support desired behavior
- To motivate and boost up morale
- To avoid doubts, misunderstanding, confusion, and biases.

### Modes of Communication

*There can be formal and informal ways of communication. Formal channels* are in-built in any organization and are an integral part of functioning of it. They are mandated, and are documented for future references. But organization studies reveal that for a smooth functioning of any organization, *informal communications are inevitable*. In fact, they are done more than formal communications that act as a way of smoothening systems, solve day-to-day problems, and may pave the way for agenda in formal communications, and hasten up decision making. They may be as nonformal as a chat in the cafeteria, or informal one-to-one meetings with principal, or peers.

Broadly classifying, *communication modes* can be:
- ***Verbal (Sounds, language):***
  - Written (journals, emails, blogs, and text messages)
  - Oral (speaking)
- ***Nonverbal (Facial expressions, body language, and posture)***
- ***Visual (Signs, symbols, and pictures).***

A very important skill to develop in communication is listening skills (Aural skills) that often get overlooked. This shall be discussed in details later.

> **Verbal Communications**
> Any communication where language is used. May be:
> - *Written:* Any form of writing is used, such as letters, emails, SMS, etc. Intended for one or many receivers. They have the advantage of having a permanent nature and ability to convey complex and detailed messages. Mostly formal communications, but can be informal too.
> - *Oral:* Spoken words. Intended for one or many receivers. They have the advantage of interactivity, feedback, control over receiver, and personal customization. Mostly informal communication.

Communication can be either *one-to-one* (Interpersonal communication) or *one-to-many* (Group communication or mass communication like in emails, meetings, etc.).

Interpersonal communication is the most important ways of communications for any successful manager. *Effective interpersonal communication requires three important skills:*
1. *Effective speaking*
2. *Effective listening*
3. *Showing appropriate emotions*

*Speaking skills has two elements (verbal and nonverbal components):*
1. ***Verbal component/language:*** It should be clear—simple, concise—short, comprehensive—covers all important aspects, candid—specific, and no ambiguity. This is an art in itself and requires much practice.
2. ***Nonverbal component:***
   - *Body language (kinesics):* Like use of facial expressions, eye movements, gestures, head movements, postures,

and physical appearances. Like a person asks you in the morning, "How do you do?" he replies "Fine" but with a sluggish appearance, that means maybe something is wrong with him, he may be trying to hide.
- *Touch (haptics):* Use of bodily contacts, greeting by handshake, and guiding with a pat all are under haptics. This is a very important technique for doctors. Even touching a patient properly can break many barriers in him and help in his management.
- *Use of space and time (proxemics and chronemics):* Being near to your patient helps him feel comfortable, also being near to a coworker who is in distress, also gives a sense of security to that person. Again, when a male person is too near a female person that may feel uncomfortable for both. So using space is a good managerial technique to communicate, as is being on time, and sticking to time schedules, i.e., using times properly.
- *Tone and voice modulation (paralanguage):* This is a term for various tonalities and modulation of voice while speaking. When in an emergency, if a leader speaks meekly, his subordinates will get the insecurity also. So the message has to be confident.

### Effective Listening

*There are some useful guidelines to be a good listener, a very important communication tool. These are:*
- Be patient, avoid trying to guess what someone is about to say
- Allow the speaker to finish their sentence
- Do not interrupt or talk over someone else when they are speaking
- Look at the person who is speaking, making eye contact
- Show that you are listening by using nonverbal reactions, such as nodding, smiling, and facial expressions
- Show curiosity by asking relevant probing questions
- Make a note of any questions you would like to ask after the speaker has finished
- Repeat what has been said to ensure understanding
- Do not fidget!

*Showing appropriate emotions:*
Three important feelings are reflected in the communication:
1. Empathy (when someone places at same level with the individual, understands his/her situation)
2. Sympathy (when one person is paternalistic toward another)
3. Apathy (no emotions at all, makes communication ineffective).
Appropriate emotions while speaking helps in communication of the message better.

### Communication Styles

Communication style is a way in which an individual interacts and exchanges information with others. Communication style is formed based on the mix of two concerns of a communication, (1) concern for self and (2) concern for others. In case of first, attitude of communication's concern is for own ideas, thoughts, opinions or wants while in case of second thought communicator is concerned for other's ideas, thoughts, and wants.

Based on the various amount of concern for self and others, communication styles can be divided into four.

1. *Assertive:* High concern for self + high concern for others
2. *Aggressive:* High concern for self + low concern for others
3. *Responsive:* Low concern for self + high concern for others
4. *Passive:* Low concern for self + low concern for others.

Above four styles can be better understood by a matrix based on two concerns as shown in **Figure 42C.8**.

Assertive and responsive are considered two better communication styles. But in different situation with different people; different styles can be used for effective communication. Use of communication skills and style is an art mastered by the many successful managers.

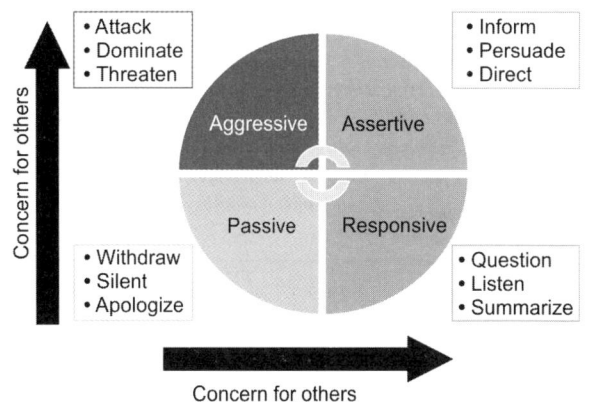

**Fig. 42C.8:** Communication style matrix based of two concerns.

## SUMMARY

Managerial skills are the abilities to be acquired by the manager to be effective manager. There are broadly three kinds of managerial skills—(1) conceptual, (2) human, and (3) technical. While conceptual and technical skills are major requirements for top and lower level managers, human skills are the most important skills, which are important for every level of managers. Mastering the human skills is the most important attribute of an effective manager.

## SUGGESTED READING

1. Hersey P, Blanchard KH. Management of Organizational Behaviour, Utilising Human Resources, 5th edition. New Delhi: Prentice Hall of India Pvt. Limited; 1988.
2. McMahon R, Barton E, Piot M, World Health Organization. (1980). On being in charge: a guide for middle level management in primary health care, 1st edition. [online] Available from: http://apps.who.int/iris/handle/10665/37015.
3. Ministry of Health and Family Welfare. Immunization Handbook for Medical Officer. 3rd edition; 2016.
4. Ministry of Health and Family Welfare. SOP for Hospital Management.
5. Murphy Herta A, Hildebrandt HW, Thomas JP. Effective Business Communication, 7th edition. Mcgraw-Hill; 1999.
6. NIHFW. Case Studies in Health Management; 1987.
7. NIHFW. Management Training Module for Medical Officer: Primary Health Care Centre; 1987.
8. Peddecord KM. Public health management tools. In: Robert B Wallace (Ed). Wallace/Maxcy–Rosenau-Last Public Health and Preventive Medicine, 15th edition. New York: McGraw-Hill; 2008. p. 1270.
9. Robbins SP, Coulter MA. Management. New York, NY: Pearson Education; 2017.
10. Robbins SP, Judge T, Campbell T. Organizational Behavior. New York: Pearson; 2016.
11. Sathe PV, Doke PP. Epidemiology and Management for Health Care, 3rd edition. Mumbai: Vora Medical Publications; 2011 (Reprint). pp. 86-7.

# D. MONITORING AND EVALUATION

*Sumit Malhotra, Manya Prasad*

### Case Scenario

*A designated first referral unit functioning at the subdivisional hospital within the district performed an audit to review the quality of emergency obstetric and newborn care provided by the hospital. It found that the percentage of deliveries performed by cesarean section was only 6% and there were 35% referrals from labor ward to the district hospital. This was a low cesarean section rate. At this level, 15% of delivery cases should undergo cesarean sections which were getting referred. Reasons for same were reviewed and changes were brought into the hospital for improving their emergency obstetric and newborn care services including emergency operation theater, blood storage facility, availability of services for managing hypertensive disorders and services within newborn care stabilization unit. A repeat audit after 6 months revealed an increase in cesarean sections within hospital.*

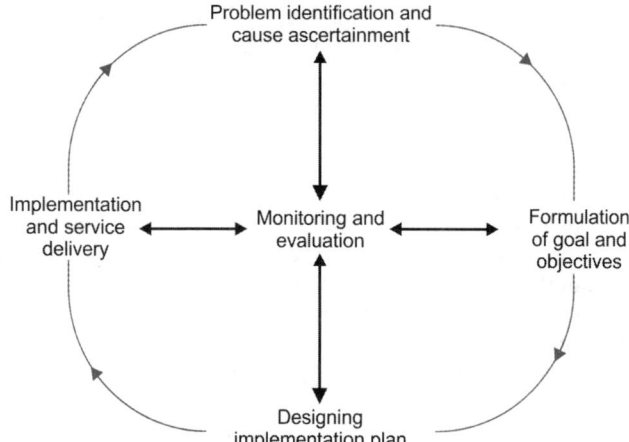

**Fig. 42D.1:** Program management cycle.

## INTRODUCTION

While managing the health of the community, various healthcare services are delivered. Monitoring and evaluation (M&E) are essential management tools which help to assess and ensure that healthcare services are implemented as planned and that desired results are being achieved. Monitoring progress and evaluating results are key functions in any healthcare delivery system for managing health of the community with the aim to improve the performance health services. It is similar to clinical practice, where a physician keeps an eye on the results of their intervention, modifying it to get the desired health outcome in the patient.

In an era where all decisions, whether for individual patients in clinical medicine, or for the masses in community health, are advocated to be evidence-based, M&E has the biggest role to play especially in managing community health where financial and human resources are put in. It is through these tools that evidence-based planning can be implemented. The data gathered from these tools provides the fodder for undertaking community-based projects in a scientific way.

Monitoring and evaluation shows whether a service/program is accomplishing its goals. It identifies program weaknesses and strengths, aspects that require an overhaul, and areas of the program at par with expectations. How M&E fits into the program management cycle is depicted in **Figure 42D.1**.

As depicted above, monitoring and evaluation is at the core of the program management cycle. It plays the key role in the identification of problem areas to guide the implementation of corrective action. Moreover, the nitty-gritty of the implementation plan is determined by monitoring progress and evaluating the impact. Thus, M&E activities form an integral component of all national health programs that you have already been exposed to.

## MONITORING

Monitoring is the continuous process of measuring, recording, collecting, and analyzing data on actual implementation of the program and communicating it to the program managers so that any deviation from the planned operations are detected, diagnosis for causes of deviation is carried out, and suitable corrective actions are taken.

### Example of Monitoring

A community health center during malaria endemic season continuously tracked number of fever cases presenting to an outpatient facility that were asked for slide preparation for malaria parasite detection. Minimum 15% of fever cases should have their slides prepared. Every month the facility checked how many fever cases were presumptively investigated for malaria so that no malaria case was missed out by healthcare providers.

Thus, routine data is collected and progress is measured. Whether program objectives are being met or not is a question that this exercise answers. As a by-product of this, the effectiveness of programs is assessed and whether resources are being efficiently used is also determined.

*The key questions that monitoring answers is:*
- Is the implementation of the program efficient? Efficiency refers to whether the input resources given into the work is appropriate in terms of the output produced.
- How is the implementation different at various points in time and geographical locations?
- Does the program achieve what was envisaged in terms of immediate gains/outputs?

Monitoring is a continuous and ongoing process. It requires contact with personnel and beneficiaries at various points. The results of this ongoing process is also compared to the situation in the beginning of the program.

### Approaches to Monitoring

The usual approaches that allow us continuous scrutiny and assessment of functioning of health systems in community medicine practice include:

- Health management information system (HMIS)
- Review meetings
- Supervision
- Audits and special studies

Let us understand now these approaches one by one:

### Health Management Information System

It is routine data capturing, generated as a part of healthcare delivery, and analyzing them for making managerial decisions about health services from ground action to governance level. This is conceptually analogous to the routine case file that is maintained to monitor a patient. It incorporates all the data needed by all the stakeholders, such as policy makers, clinicians, and health service users, at all levels, such as center, state, district, and sub district, to improve and protect population health.

Data obtained from HMIS could help to facilitate evidence-based decisions by all stakeholders at all levels for effective management of delivery of the healthcare services. Web-based HMIS portal captures data as per the HMIS formats at the district level. Some advantages of this system are:
- Primary data can be easily aggregated
- Information/reports flow quickly to the state headquarters and the ministry
- Meaningful analysis of the information available on the portal for policy interventions is possible.

The platforms for capture for routine data in health systems are currently undergoing digitization and information technology is utilized for reporting. The routine data can provide lots of information about how health systems are functioning and progress achieved in variety of indicators. Program managers and health personnel need to be properly trained in analyzing meaningful interpretation from routine health information system.

### Review Meetings

Periodic reviewing by the designated seniors is routinely undertaken to know the implementation status of the healthcare interventions. It is carried out from bottom to top at predefined periods (i.e., from primary health center to national level). It is similar to daily round taken by the ward medical officer to senior consultants. At the level below district, review meetings generally take place weekly to every month. To extend the analogy, this would be similar to the daily round that is taken by all doctors, senior or junior. A participatory discussion takes place during these meetings so that lacunae can be identified and timely corrective actions can be undertaken. This ensures that there is understanding between the ones making the policy and those implementing it, so that all move toward achieving a common vision. Often health workers encounter variety of bottlenecks in field settings, which can be understood while interacting with them during review meetings. Collective thinking can also be undertaken in finding solutions to these bottlenecks and thus problems can be solved in a participatory fashion which will influence worker's motivation and performance. This then can influence the results of the program activities. Meetings offer a platform for review of program activities and their function, concurrently giving a scope for altering the course of certain activities that were not performing as per expectations.

### Supervision

Supervision is the action or process of watching and directing what someone does or how something is done. **Supportive supervision and feedback** are the key to smooth program implementation and improvement. This serves as a way of ensuring staff competence, effectiveness, and efficiency through observation, discussion, support, and guidance.

There are range of grass root workers that are engaged in implementation of community health programs like Accredited Social Health Activists (ASHAs), Anganwadi Workers (AWWs), Auxiliary Nurse Midwives (ANMs), and health workers. These workers are expected to deliver range of interventions through adequate skills and competencies. Their work needs to be supervised and supported regularly to improve their work performance.

Supportive supervision utilizes standard check lists to supervise important and challenging tasks performed by health personnel and supervisors communicate the findings with an intention to improve systems. The feedbacks to personnel given are constructive, with focus accorded on solving problems. This is unlike the other form of supervision that is considered punitive and is merely fault finding exercise. Workers need to be motivated to perform efficiently and thus whenever supervision is to be done, it should be supportive in nature. When performing supervision, it is also important to recognize achievements, and offer praise for good practices observed.

Variety of methods can be adopted for doing supervision, contingent to objectives of supervision. These methods can be:
- Interaction with medical officers and health workers
- Observing interpersonal communication of service providers with patients
- Review of records for consistency: For example, TB notification register, laboratory register, treatment cards, register for drugs and consumables
- Use of protocols and checklists for different aspects of the program, e.g., diagnostic aspects, treatment, etc.
- Onsite observation of activities
- Patient home visits
- Examination of supplies (consumables; physical verification of drug/vaccine stock; within TB program—patient wise boxes, laboratory forms, treatment cards, transfer forms; functional status of equipment, date of preparation and expiry of reagents, etc.).

### Audits

Health facilities undertake quality improvement initiatives that utilize auditing. This is essentially required for certification and accreditation processes. Most of the health facilities that receive accreditation from an external agency signify that it provides quality service to its customers and beneficiaries. Performance standards at health facilities are monitored against certain benchmarks. There can be external audits performed by external/peer assessors; internal audits by internal team members, and clinical audits by clinical professionals within their clinics. All have a common agenda of improving quality at a health workplace. All health units can do audits as part of their routine functioning so as to review their performance and to achieve improvements incrementally.

## EVALUATION

The evaluation of the impact of the program is done to discern how much of the change in objectives can be attributed to the program. It is a measure of effectiveness that highlights the extent to which program achieves specific objectives. Largely broad gains, intermediate and long-term objectives can be scope of evaluation. Evaluation may be undertaken as a separate exercise during different stages of program implementation **(Table 42D.1)**.

**Table 42D.1:** Differences between monitoring and evaluation.

| Monitoring | Evaluation |
| --- | --- |
| It is the concurrent assessment of the healthcare services/programs | It is the periodic assessment of the healthcare services/programs |
| It aims to determine whether processes are proceeding as envisaged | It aims to ascertain attainment of results vis a vis set objectives |
| It is an integral part of implementation | Generally, it is done after some time has passed after implementation |
| It is carried out usually by internal members | It is carried out usually by external members. But may be carried out jointly by external and internal members |
| It gives ideas about current status and thus helps in immediate course correction, if required | It recommends change in strategies, revision of objectives aiming long-term perspective |
| It is concerned with healthcare system inputs, processes and outputs | It is concerned with health outcomes and impacts |
| It includes supervision, periodical review meetings, and analysis of routine programmatic data | It includes special data collection and analysis through more scientific methods |
| It has multiple points of data collection as routine | Data collection is done at intervals only |
| It focuses on healthcare implementation scenario and desired program results | It focusses on the relevance, and effectiveness and efficiency and sustainability of strategies being used to achieve desired objectives and goals |
| It helps in performance improvement through improved implementations | It helps in improving planning and strategies |
| It is more useful to lower level and middle level health managers | It is more useful to top level health managers (planners, policy makers) and all related stakeholders |

## STEPS IN DESIGN AND CONDUCT OF MONITORING AND EVALUATION

### Developing Frameworks and Appropriate Indicators

Frameworks highlight parts of program/project activities sequentially in a flow that helps us to understand their relationships. This advances knowledge on how these different components influence the final results to be achieved in a program/project cycle. Variety of frameworks can be designed to understand program/project components:

### Conceptual Framework

It identifies set of factors which can be proximal and distal determinants contributing to disease/risk factor which are targeted within the program/project activities. It is usually presented in form of a diagram. This is similar to web of causation that we usually depict while undertaking a clinic-psychosocial case study in community medicine practice. It helps us to know different factors that need to be tackled through program/project activities for obtaining maximum success in achieving results. An illustration presented below helps us in highlighting various factors that can influence one of the common community health problem in our country, i.e., iron deficiency anemia. Range of factors is presented below to highlight conceptually that these factors determine the occurrence of anemia in a community.

> *Factors affecting occurrence of iron deficiency anemia in a community:*
> - *Proximal determinants (Biomedical):* Nutritional iron content of food, iron availability, consumption of inhibitors and enhancers in diet, endemicity of malaria, and *H. pylori* infection.
> - *Intermediate determinants:* Food security, availability based on income and access, hygiene and sanitation, malnutrition, food fortification, healthcare access, and utilization.
> - *Distal determinants:* Agricultural output, health and economic policy framework and environment, inequity, poverty, and health insurance.

### Logical Framework

Logical frameworks or logic models provide a linear depiction of the inputs, activities, outputs, outcomes, and impacts **(Fig. 42D.2)**.

***Input indicators:*** Are resources provided for an activity, and include cash, supplies, personnel, equipment, and training.

***Process indicators:*** Transform inputs into outputs. These are activities that happen in programs such as training of health personnel, giving vaccines to children, holding village days, and village meetings are processes.

***Output indicators:*** Are the specific products or services that an activity is expected to deliver as a result of receiving the inputs. These are immediate effects produced as a result of processes in the programs. For instance, in a vaccination program, immediate output of vaccination days will be children vaccinated in an immunization session. For a health facility offering sterilization services to eligible couples, output would number of sterilization

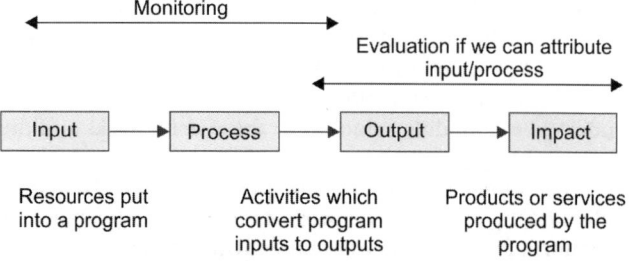

**Fig. 42D.2:** The M&E framework (Logic model).

acceptors in a month or a quarter, etc. Similarly, this would be the number of slides prepared in a month for malarial parasite detection.

***Outcome indicators:*** Refers to people prepared in a program and the effect it has on their actions. They are intermediate-term effects related to objectives. In an immunization program, outcome will be occurrence of diseases, such as measles and diphtheria, etc.

***Impact indicators:*** These are the effects of the service on the people and their surroundings. These may be economic, social, organizational, health, environmental, or other intended or unintended results of the program. Thus, impacts are long-term effects. In immunization program, child mortality averted due to vaccine preventable diseases will be the impact. Mortality parameters in maternal and child health programs are impacts. To take an example, in the Revised National Tuberculosis Program, inputs are staff trained in diagnosing TB cases and prescribing effective treatment and availability of new and effective TB drugs. The process is thus carried out where TB patients are identified and effective treatment is rendered to them. The output of these activities would be increase in the number of TB patients being cured. Thus, the impact is the improvement of the health status of the community **(Fig. 42D.3)**.

## Selecting Data Sources and Data Collection for Monitoring and Evaluation

Data sources are sources of information used to collect the data needed to calculate the indicators.

*Primary data collection methods* also fall into several broad categories. Among the most common are:
- Surveys, including personal interviews, telephone interviews, and instruments completed by respondent, received through the mail or e-mail
- Group discussions/focus groups
- Observations
- Document review, such as medical records, but also diaries, logs, minutes of meetings, etc.

**Special studies to monitor the health conditions:** Some of the examples of special studies that have been undertaken as part of M&E activities in India include:

*National Family Health Survey (NFHS):* It is a large-scale, health and demographic survey conducted in a representative sample of households throughout India. It is initiated in the year 1992. All NFHS have been conducted by the Ministry of Health and Family Welfare, Government of India, with the International Institute for Population Sciences, Mumbai, serving as the nodal agency. The main objective of NFHS is to provide essential data on health and family welfare and emerging issues. NFHS provides data that can be used for monitoring health and demography. Many indicators are reported in these survey results. Usually, it is to be carried out every 5 years. So far four rounds of NFHS were completed and preparation for fifth round is going on.

*Sample Registration System (SRS):* In order to strengthen the information pertaining to vital statistics, including births and deaths, every year, SRS bulletin and statistical report is released that carries information on birth rate, death rate, infant mortality rate, and fertility indicators. Periodically, special bulletin reports situation of maternal mortality in the country. Additionally, disease area specific surveys are undertaken that inform us about burden status of a particular disease/condition and trends in its occurrence.

*National Mental Health Survey:* During year 2015–2016 provides data on prevalence, pattern, and outcomes for mental disorders in the country.

*National NCD Monitoring Survey (2017):* It is conducted across different sites with a focus on noncommunicable disease risk

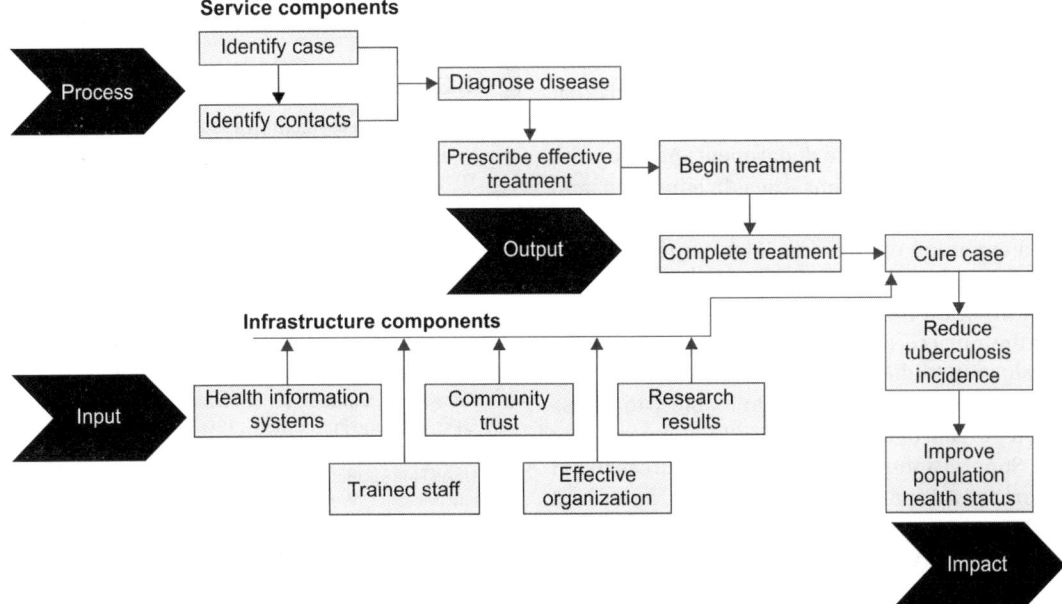

**Fig. 42D.3:** Logic model in Revised National Tuberculosis Control Program.

factors that include tobacco, alcohol, dietary salt intake, physical activity, body mass index, fasting blood sugar, and blood pressure.

*National Blindness Survey (2015-2018):* It is carried out to know the prevalence of blindness and visual impairment in the country.

*Secondary (routine) data collection methods:* It include those sources that generate and measure routine service delivery, such as clinic registers, patient records, program reports, etc. Variety of information can be gathered and analyzed using these data sources. HMIS under various health programs and at various hospitals are important source of such data.

### Analysis, Interpretation and Recommendations

Through appropriate analytic methods, data gathered is put for meaningful use and interpreted. Based on results of M&E, appropriate suggestions are made and future actions are decided.

Depending on the evaluation questions and indicators, some secondary data sources may be appropriate. Some existing data sources that often come into play in measuring outcomes of public health programs are produced below. This is an illustrative list, not exhaustive meant to highlight few available sources that are useful to lay hands that provide M&E related information.

## CHALLENGES AND PITFALLS IN MONITORING AND EVALUATION

Various challenges may arise in the implementation of M&E activities. Some are enlisted below:

- Poorly written or not written protocols: It is imperative that M&E activities be planned a priori and a stipulated proportion of the program budget be earmarked or these activities. Often project/programs are planned with poorly designed M&E structures in place.
- Major emphasis on program implementation/expansion: This, juxtaposed with inefficient planning, leads to wastage of resources.
- Coordination issues of resources planning and E struct, the various stakeholders often do not coordinate properly that results in mismanagement of the program and M/E activities. This especially occurs where two departments have to work together like in nutrition programs—health, education, and women and child development departments have to do joint planning and execution of programs. Monitoring activities suffer due to poor defined roles and joint responsibility.
- Incorrect information from beneficiaries—may under or overestimate the impact of the program. This is especially seen in special evaluation studies undertaken.
- Inadequate/no supervision—leading to inability to assess the competency of staff or the how efficiently input resources are utilized. Supervision requires special resources like if immunization activities need to be supervised, and travel support need to be provided to supervisors. Also, there should be availability of supervisors in the system to perform this role or appropriate manpower need to be assigned such role.
- This could be in data collection, entry or analysis. Also, there should be avn, entry or analysis. Systems also do not utilize the routinely collected data in HMIS portal and personnel are not trained to analyze it systematically.
- Choice of indicators inappropriate—this leads to erroneous estimates regarding the achievement of program results. Careful scrutiny of indicators needs to be done to draw meaningful conclusion based on their continuous tracking over time.
- *Data quality issues:* If data is not collected properly, it may compromise its quality in terms of completeness, accuracy, reporting, and thus limiting the utility of such data generated.

## CONCLUSION

Monitoring and evaluation are fundamental to program implementation and management cycles. They inform about the success and failures, return on investments made and way forward for implementing the programs to attain the desired objectives, outcomes, and impact.

## SUMMARY

- Monitoring is an ongoing continuous process of measuring, collecting, and analyzing data on actual implementation of the program that occurs throughout the life of the program.
- Evaluations are done usually at the end of program cycle, with due planning processes undertaken at the start of the program cycle.
- M&E plans are critical to design and conduct monitoring and evaluation.
- Frameworks and indicators are fundamental components in M&E plans.
- The five key components of logical frameworks include inputs, processes, outputs, outcomes, and impact.
- While selecting an indicator, care must be taken to ensure that it is one that affects program activities.
- Approaches to monitoring comprise of health management information system, review meetings, supervision, and audits.
- Examples of routine data sources include vital registration records, hospital clinical records, and reports.
- Examples of non routine data sources include special surveys, such as National Family Health Surveys, facility surveys, etc.

## SUGGESTED READING

1. Center for Disease Control and Prevention. Program performance and evaluation office. (online). [cited 2018 Sep 22]. Available from: https://www.cdc.gov/program/index.htm.
2. Connell JP, Kubisch AC, Schorr LB, et al. New approaches to evaluating community initiatives. New York, NY: Aspen Institute; 1995.
3. Fawcett SB, Paine-Andrews A, Francisco VT, et al. Evaluating community initiatives for health and development. In: Rootman I, Goodstadt M, Hyndman B, McQueen DV, Potvin L, Springett J, Ziglio E. (Eds). Evaluating Health Promotion Approaches. Copenhagen, Denmark: World Health Organization (Euro); 1999.
4. Fetterman DM, Kaftarian SJ, Wandersman A. Empowerment evaluation: Knowledge and tools for self-assessment and accountability. Thousand Oaks, CA: Sage Publications; 1996.
5. Frankel N, Gage A. M and E Fundamentals: A self-guided Mini-Course. USAID MEASURE Evaluation; 2016.
6. Hut-Mossel L, Welker G, Ahaus K, Gans R. Understanding how and why audits work: protocol for a realist review of audit programmes to improve hospital care. BMJ Open. 2017;7:e015121.
7. Patton MQ. Utilization-focused evaluation. Thousand Oaks, CA: Sage Publications; 1997.
8. Rossi PH, Freeman HE, Lipsey MW. Evaluation: A systematic approach. Newbury Park, CA: Sage Publications; 1999.

# E. LOGISTICS AND FINANCE MANAGEMENT

*Kapil Gandha, Umed Patel, Niravkumar Joshi, Bhavesh Modi*

*"Plans are nothing; planning is everything"*
—**Dwight D Eisenhower**

## LOGISTICS MANAGEMENT

### Introduction

To provide effective and quality healthcare at primary, secondary or tertiary level managerial skills amongst health personnel is very important. Items, such as drugs, vaccines, cleaning material, dressing material, etc., are the few of the examples which are needed for patient care, be it big hospital or small clinic. Stockout position at one place and excessive-stock at other, both situations are not uncommon but easily avoidable. Failing in proper logistic management can lead to economic losses in case of excessive stock and expiry of the drugs, vaccine, etc. At the same time, we fail to provide the service to the patients in case of stockout position. To provide care with quality management (optimum efficiency and effectiveness) few "*rights*" are important—right items, stored at right place, handled by right person, and available at right time. For example, Medical Officer—PHC should ensure one-month stock of vaccines to be stored in ice-lined refrigerator (ILR).

### Definitions

***Logistics:*** "The function of moving, storing, and distributing resources and goods".

***Logistics management:*** "The systematic and scientific process of planning, implementing, and controlling the efficient and effective flow and storage of resources (goods and services) from point of origin to the point of consumption in order to meet the customer's requirements."

***Inventory:*** "Usable but idle resource having an economic value".

### Importance of Logistics (Material) Management

- Based on available resources and morbidity pattern, any health institution can estimate and modify time-to-time requirement of the types and quantum of drugs and other material.
- Any organization would have to function with limited resources to get optimum results and that is the main theme of effective and efficient management.
- Logistic management is the key to management activities out of many management techniques. So the expected outcome would be constant supply of required items at lowest cost.
- Ensure minimum level of inventory so the money is not blocked. After all management is all about efficient and effective use of man, material, manpower, and money. To exercise logistics management in scientific way, two important techniques are ABC (**A**lways **B**etter **C**ontrol) and VED (**V**ital, **E**ssential, **D**esirable) analysis. Both these techniques are described in later part of the chapter.

### Supply Chain Management (Fig. 42E.1)

- Based on past experience and future forecasting requirement of drugs and other items is estimated.
- To get these items by tendering and procurement involves five activities:
  1. Rating of supplier
  2. Bids analysis
  3. Pricing
  4. Issue of orders
  5. Buying of goods.
- Inspection of the items on receiving
  - Quality and quantity
  - Documenting the receipts
- One-third of the total expenditure is used to buy material in hospital, so it is very important activity to run a hospital effectively.
- Supply of vaccines and contraceptive should be uninterrupted throughout the year and up to the last point of delivery all over country.
- Storage condition, e.g., cold chain maintenance is utmost priority.
- In many places, there is lack of management of material in scientific manner.
- Most of the procedures and operations heavily depend on the materials in organizations starting from PHC to district-level hospitals.

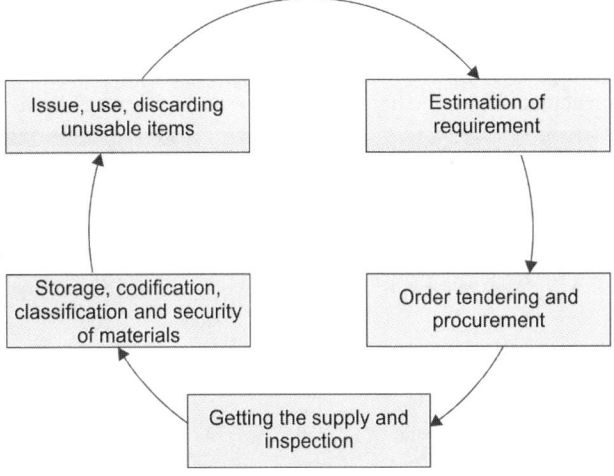

**Fig. 42E.1:** Supply chain.

### Inventory Control Techniques (Table 42E.1)

Many times various items are in usable state but because of the poor management it remains idle. This situation is because of the poor inventory technique. Scientific way of calculating the need of drugs and other items is very useful to save the money from various other costs like expiry of costly medicine without use, storage space, loss of items due to poor handling, etc.

Table 42E.1: Few important inventory control techniques.

| ABC | **A**lways **B**etter **C**ontrol |
|---|---|
| VED | **V**ital, **E**ssential or **D**esirable |
| SDE | **S**carce, **D**ifficult or **E**asy to obtain |

To prevent all these challenging situations, inventory control in a healthcare setting is the solution. Storing, controlling, and providing the items at a time of need in as easy as possible manner so that patient care should never suffer and at the same time cost borne by all these activities remains reasonably low as far as possible.

Out of above analysis, ABC and VED are most important and described next.

### Always Better Control Analysis

The cost and the quantity are two important criteria in relation to items used in day-to-day practice. According to *Pareto's law*— "*Vital few and trivial many*". Generally, a small proportion of items account for a large proportion of cost and vice versa. 70%, 20%, and 10% of the total items would cost 10%, 20%, and 70% respectively.

| Category A | Category B | Category C |
|---|---|---|
| Very strict control | Moderate control | Loose control |
| Frequent ordering | Ordering 3 monthly | 6 monthly ordering |
| Management by senior person | Middle level manager | Clerical staff can be delegated |
| Very short lead time period | Moderate efforts to reduce lead time | No issue of lead time |

**Steps to do ABC analysis:**
1. Based on the past experience and morbidity pattern list of the drugs/items is prepared. In table below for to learn the things list is limited to 10 items. Annual cost item wise can be calculated with the help of annul use and unit cost of item.

| Sr. No. | Item | Annual use (Quantity) | Unit cost (In ₹) | Annual cost (In ₹) |
|---|---|---|---|---|
| 1. | Capsule tetracycline | 40 | 1 | 40 |
| 2. | Capsule ampicillin | 1,500 | 3.86 | 5,800 |
| 3. | Syrup paracetamol | 5 | 8 | 40 |
| 4. | Spirit | 8 L | 100 | 800 |
| 5. | Tablet paracetamol | 40 | 1 | 40 |
| 6. | Tablet aspirin | 20 | 2 | 40 |
| 7. | Tablet diclofenac | 150 | 3 | 450 |
| 8. | Injection adrenalin | 5 | 16 | 80 |
| 9. | Injection ceftriaxone | 30 | 25 | 750 |
| 10. | Injection DNS | 05 | 30 | 150 |

2. Arrange the items based on the cost in descending order. Next step is to count the annual cost (as shown in the last column of the above table). Items wise cumulative percentage value then calculated. Based on the proportion category assigned, i.e., up to 70%—A: 70–90%, B and C for 90–100%.
In this example highest total costing (₹ 5,800) item is Sl. No. 2 so it comes first. next is Sl. No 4 (with ₹ 800) and so on we can arrange the items.
Total cost of the items is ₹ 8,190. Now if we calculate the percentage of Item A (5,800 × 100/8,190 = 70.81%). Likewise percentage is calculated as shown in the 4th column of the table.

| Sr. No. | Annual value (in descending order) | Cumulative annual value | Cumulative value % | Category |
|---|---|---|---|---|
| 2. | 5,800 | 5,800 | 70.81 | A |
| 4. | 800 | 6,600 | 80.58 | B |
| 9. | 750 | 7,350 | 89.74 | B |
| 7. | 450 | 7,800 | 95.23 | C |
| 10. | 150 | 7,950 | 97.06 | C |
| 8. | 80 | 8,030 | 98.04 | C |
| 1. | 40 | 8,070 | 98.53 | C |
| 3. | 40 | 8,110 | 99.02 | C |
| 5. | 40 | 8,150 | 99.51 | C |
| 6. | 40 | 8,190 | 100 | C |

3. Summary table establishing the principle of 70% money is needed for 10% item. Here in our example is cap ampicillin.

| Category | % items in inventory | Total money value | % of total money value |
|---|---|---|---|
| 2 | 10 | 5,800 | 70% |
| 4,9 | 20 | 1,550 | 20% |
| 1, 3, 5, 6, 7, 8, 10 | 70 | 840 | 10% |

In above example, we can conclude that ABC analysis is based on the quantity of items required in context of monetary terms only. Item like injection adrenalin has low capital investment and consumption but it is lifesaving.

*This limitation can be overcome by the VED analysis.*

### Vital, Essential or Desirable Analysis

It is based on "criticality" and importance rather than just on the cost of consumption.

Vital, essential, and desirable are three different categories in which items are classified as follows:
1. V = Vital lifesaving drugs. It should never be stockout.
2. E = Essential items. For brief period of time (one-two days) stockout can be tolerable.
3. D = Desirable. Stockout can be tolerable for longer period of time.

Quantity in proportion: V = 10%, E = 40%, D = 50%.

### How to do VED analysis

**Step 1:** Depend on the four important factors (stockout cost, lead time required to procure, nature of items, and source of supply) different drugs/items are assigned degree.

| Factor | First degree | Second degree | Third degree |
|---|---|---|---|
| Stockout cost | >Rs. X (30) | Between Rs. X and Y (60) | >Rs. Y (90) |
| Lead time to obtain | 1–4 weeks (30) | 4–8 weeks (60) | >8 weeks (90) |
| Nature of items | Made up to market std. (20) | Made up to suppliers design (40) | Made up to buyers design or proprietary items (60) |
| Source of supply | Locally available (20) | Out of city (40) | Imported and controlled supply (60) |

(Points assigned to the item types are shown in parenthesis).

**Step 2:** Based on the cumulative score, item is classified into three critical categories.

For example, injection adrenalin for health centers, Rampur. This center is 35 km away from district headquarter and 300 km away from state store. To simplify the things below an example of injection adrenalin is given.
- Stockout cost is 90 as stockout and unavailability cannot be acceptable so score is 90
- Lead time to obtain at center following order again considering geographic and other working condition—30
- Nature of item—20
4. Source of supply—40.
Total score = 90 + 30 + 20 + 40 = 180 and so injection adrenalin is essential item according to VED analysis.

| Points | Classification |
|---|---|
| 100–160 | Desirable |
| 161–230 | Essential |
| 231–300 | Vital |

By doing VED analysis still, we found limitation as shown in the example above as lifesaving item like adrenaline comes under essential category. To remove this limitation, we need to do combination of ABC and VED analysis as described below.

*Combination of ABC and VED analysis:* Cost vs. criticality

| | V | E | D | Combine category |
|---|---|---|---|---|
| A | AV | AE | AD | Cat I (15%) |
| B | BV | BE | BD | Cat II (40%) |
| C | CV | CE | CD | Cat III (45%) |

Category I: AV+BV+CV+AE+AD (*vital and costly item*) cover 15% of items.
Category II: BE+BD+CE (*essential but less costly*) cover 40% of items.
Category III: CD (*desirable but would not affect the functioning*) covers 45% items.

## Planning for Vaccines and Drugs at Health Center (Fig. 42E.2)

*Maximum/minimum inventory system:*
- **Buffer stock:** It is the emergency stock level which provides buffer against disaster situation, unusual transport delay or unexpected demand fluctuations, i.e., 25% of working stock

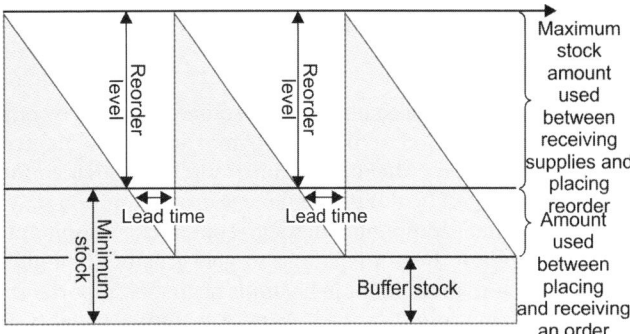

**Fig. 42E.2:** Maximum, minimum and buffer stock.

or 1-week stock. (At PHC, working stock is of 1 month, hence, 25% of 1 month working stock is 1 week stock).
- **Lead time:** Time period between putting order and reception of the supply for the use. Concept of lead time is important in calculation of minimum stock level. Geographic locations, road as well as weather condition, speed of deliveries, and transport system are few of the factors that can affect lead time, i.e., 1 week time (one fourth of the monthly requirement).
- **Working stock:** Whatever the stock used between two orders. In practice, it will be of 4 weeks' stock in case of a PHC.
- **Minimum stock level:** Sum total of buffer stock and stock used in between placing and receiving supply (lead time stock). It is also known as *reorder level* stock as when level reaches up to minimum stock level; there is a time to place the order. It can be expressed in terms of months/weeks or proportion of material out of total. Order should be placed to district vaccine store as soon as stock level falls to the reorder level. It will prevent the stockout situation. Minimum stock at PHC level is of 2 weeks (1 week buffer stock + 1 week lead time stock).
- **Maximum stock level:** Sum total of the minimum stock and that amount of stock used between orders (working stock). It is the largest amount of stock that is usually expressed as the number of months/weeks of supply. Maximum stock at PHC level is of 6 weeks (1 month working stock + 2 weeks minimum stock).

*Few more concepts for effective inventory control:*
- **FIFO = First in first out (*item received earlier should be first out to use*).**
- **EEFO = Early expired first out**
- **Push system** = Goods are supplied based on the decision from higher level regardless of the demand from the lower side where materials are used.
- **Pull system** = Materials are always obtained based on the demand from the lower side where materials are used.
- **Cyclic supply** = Periodic supply regardless of the knowledge of utilization pattern at lower side.
- **Electronic vaccine intelligence network (eVIN) initiative:** With the help of android-based app, we can measure real time stock up to last point of use. It enables cold chain handler (pharmacist) to enter data on issues, receipts, discards and demand. One gets real-time view into stock at the facilities along with notifications on a variety of events such as out-of-stock or batch expiry, as well as recommendations on optimal stocking.

## FINANCE MANAGEMENT

### Introduction

Finance is one of the most important resources required by any country or organization to run any program or project. Finance is the driving force of health administration as activities for the development of health need finances directly or indirectly. Health is essential component of socioeconomic development. The investment in health is bound to give greater dividends than investment. Investment in health is of greater importance in the developing countries, such as India, to improve quality of human life which eventually promotes economic development.

To efficiently utilize these financial resources, it is essential to plan, regarding the areas which require financial resources, and its proper utilization. This planning and assessment of efficient utilization of financial resources can be realized by budgeting and auditing.

### Budgeting

A budget can be defined as a quantitative expression of the operational plans of an organization for a future accounting period. It is a blue print of the projected plan of action expressed in financial terms for specified period of time. It is a plan expressed in terms of money. It is a plan that guides the allocation of financial and human resources to quantify goals and objectives of any program.

*The purpose of budget is generally:*
- To aid in financing the enterprises
- To clarify the operations of a program
- To help in future planning
- To measure efficiency.

It gives more importance to the cost aspects without any mention of the results. Preparation and approval of budget takes place before the actual budget period, during which it is to be utilized. It may detail income, expenditure, and the capital to be allocated for varied components of the program.

In any organization, there are number of activities that have to be performed to achieve the purpose for which the organization has been set up. Performing these activities needs resources, such as men, materials, and in some cases machinery. For procuring these resources you need money. Estimating the requirements of money to perform the activities during any particular period is budgeting.

One can use the budget together with periodic expenditure reports:
- To compare actual spending against expected costs
- To identify which programmers are more or less cost-effective
- To predict cash needs
- To determine where cost must be cut
- As input into difficult decisions such as which program to discontinue.

### Plan and Nonplan Budget

Plan and Nonplan budget are parts of the Government budget. The plan funds are utilized for developmental expenditure, such as schemes/project, which are included or are part of the 5-year plans. These schemes are mainly of capital nature. Capital expenditure means money spent by a business or organization on acquiring or maintaining fixed assets like setting up of new hospitals, new CHCs, modernization/expansion of existing hospitals, setting up of new specialty units, primary health centers, subcenters, etc.

If a project/scheme has been found to be useful, it may be transferred to nonplan budget on successful completion of 5 years. Nonplan funds are utilized to maintain and operate the facilities already established in the previous plan periods.

### Process of Budgeting in Health

The budget is prepared for a period of one financial year, i.e., April to March of the following year, which is a fiscal or financial year.

Under National Health Mission, bottom up approach has been adopted. The District Health Action plan is the main instrument for planning, intersectoral convergence, implementation, and monitoring of activities under the mission. It seeks to integrate all the related initiatives at the village, block and district levels. The head of the district (estimating officer) calls for a meeting of the doctors working in the district and invites their suggestions for any new requirement/new activities/need of any major replacements. He/she then asks accounts officer/accountant to prepare the requirements for the salaries, allowances, etc., for new activities/initiatives.

### Model Conventional Budget

In a conventional budget, objects of expenditure are of prime value, viz. pay of officers, pay of establishment, allowances, other expenditures, etc. as mentioned below:
- Wages and salaries
- Dearness allowances
- Other allowances
- Traveling allowances
- Office expenses
- Telephone expenses
- Rent, taxes, etc.
- Maintenance of vehicles including Petroleum, Oil and Lubricants (POL)
- Maintenance of machines/other equipment
- Medicine and supplies
- Contingencies.

The budget will be spent for capital expenditure and new items of work for:

*Example:* For setting up a training unit:
- Land acquisition
- Building
- Equipment
- Transport vehicles
- Furniture
- Telephones and internet
- Stationary and contingency

### Advantages of Budget

*The major advantages of a budget preparation are:*
- It cultivates the habit of planning—making careful study of the problems being faced by the organization and taking decisions

- It provides a clear opportunity to make budget provision as per objectives of the organization
- It assists in delegation of authority
- It is a tool for control over the activities of the organization
- Reduction in wastages and losses of all types.

### Conventional (Incremental) Budget versus Performance Budget

*The conventional (traditional) budget:*
- Emphasis on the items of expenditure without any corresponding indication of the results to be achieved
- It does not indicate the economics of operations
- It fails to provide an adequate link between the finances provided and spent, and the physical targets actually achieved. The traditional budget reveals what government purchases but not what the government does. In this type of budget, previous year's expenditure is applied to the next year with adding or removing components as per requirement. Only incremental amounts are added to the previous year's budget for estimating the next budget. Thus, it is easy to prepare in less time with lesser preparation cost.

As assessment of performance of last budget is not considered here, wasteful expenditure and priorities are not ascertained. It also can not include better alternatives for improved performance. Thus, the traditional budgeting would not be able provide adequate connection between the financial outlays and physical targets. Because of this shortcoming, the conventional budget has not been able to help the management either in planning or in control. It is to meet these shortcomings that performance budgeting was introduced by the government.

Government operations of functions, programs, activities, and projects can be better presented by performance budgeting. It gives emphasis on identifying relationship between financial input and physical output of government activities. Based on the relationship, performance can be compare to the money invested. For example, in case of an immunization program, government allocates XYZ amount for an immunization program under conventional budget. Whereas, in performance budget, number of immunized children are also taken into consideration along with expenditure on immunization program.

### Zero-based Budgeting

Zero-based budget is prepared considering the base as zero, i.e., without considering the budget of the previous year, whereas conventional budget where starting point for preparing budget is prior period's budget. While framing the budget for ensuing year an organization should start from ground "Zero". The concept requires that activities of an organization should be viewed afresh.

The old and the new activities of the program are ranked as per their importance. Based on that importance rank, resources are allocated to each activity without considering the past budgets or achievements.

### Outcome Budgeting

Development outcomes of government programs can be measured by outcome budget. The concept has been established to make budgets more cost-effective.

For example, in outcome budget, full immunization coverage (outcome) is compared with expenditure in immunization program.

### Difference between Performance-based Budget and Outcome Budget

Central Government Ministries started the system of performance budgeting in 1969. It has now been merged with the outcome budget. The concept of outcome budget was introduced by the Union Government in 2005–2006. It (outcome budget) is aimed at capturing the effectiveness of the financial allocations made in the budget and not just in terms of their physical output.

### Gender Budgeting

Gender budgeting looks at the government budget from gender perspective to assess how it addresses the needs of women in the areas, such as health, education, employment, etc. It does not seek to create a separate budget but seeks affirmative action to address specific needs of women.

## Accounting

Accounting is the measurement, processing, and communication of financial information about economic entities. Accounting means recording of the financial transactions that take place in a proper manner, classifying them periodically under pre-determined budget heads and at the end of a given period, aiding and collecting the information on how much has been received or spent under specific heads.

### Concept of Accounting

The American Institute of Certified Public Accountants has defined that "Accounting is the art of recording, classifying and summarizing in a significant manner and in terms of money, transactions and events which are, in part at least, of a financial character, and interpreting the results thereof."

*It helps in:*
- Finding out the actual receipts and disbursements made by an authorized organization in any given period.
- Know how much of these receipts and disbursements relate to the different activities based on the classification of the transactions into different heads and subheads.
- Ensuring that the actual receipts/disbursements relating to the different heads/subheads are as planned/budgeted for control purposes and planning for future.
- Analyzing the efficiency with which the operations are being performed in financial terms.
- Maintaining a record of the capital assets purchased or acquired during the period and the total of all such available capital assets with the unit/department at the end of the period.

## Financial Auditing

The practice of auditing accounts originated from the necessity of applying some system of checks upon persons whose business was to record the receipts and disbursements of money on behalf of others. Though the system was first introduced in charitable and government accounts, people soon realized its usefulness for their business accounts.

In public sector, audit plays a significant role as public money is involved and it should be seen that this money is utilized effectively and efficiently. Also, it is the duty of the auditor to check any cases of wasteful expenditure that could have been avoided.

### Test Audit

Test audit is conducted by the auditor to find out any shortcomings or errors in the accounts of an organization for carrying out detailed in depth audit.

### Internal Audit

The internal audit is a method that exists within the organization to ensure adequacy and propriety of transactions, the extent to which assets have been accounted for and safeguarded and level of compliance with the procedure and financial norms.

### External or Statutory Audit

The statutory audit of government department is compulsorily entrusted to the Controller and Auditor General of India who is the apex audit body and to the Director General of Audit at the state level. However, in case of business establishments and NGOs the annual accounts are sometimes, if required, compiled and audited by the professional Chartered Accountants.

### Principles of Auditing

Based on certain principles, audits are being carried out:
- The auditor should not be related to the organization being audited in any manner.
- The points dealt with an audit can be subjected to verification by evidence.

### Auditing Purposes

The broad objects of auditing are:
- Verification of accounts and financial records
- Detection of errors and frauds
- Prevention of error and frauds.

The knowledge of the fact, that the accounts will be audited, will prevent the clients/staff so inclined, from committing frauds and they will be more cautious while preparing accounts. The Companies Act requires an auditor to certify the books of accounts kept are adequate to give a true and fair view of State of affairs of the company and to explain its transactions.

### Types of Audit

Types of audits are as follows:
- Audit regarding rules and orders
- Audit regarding provision of funds
- Audit of revenue receipts
- Audit of sanctions
- Audit of expenditure
- Audit of stores and stock.

## SUGGESTED READING

1. Business Today. Insufficient allocation for the health sector. (2018). Available from: https://www.businesstoday.in/union-budget-2018-19/news/budget-2018-insufficient-allocation-health-sector-heathcare-scheme/story/269449.html.
2. Devnani M, Gupta AK, Nigah R. ABC and VED Analysis of the Pharmacy Store of a Tertiary Care Teaching, Research and Referral Healthcare Institute of India. J Young Pharm. 2010;2(2):201-5.
3. Indian Association of Preventive and Social Medicine, Post Graduate course in Health System and Management-2013, Module 6-Health Economics.
4. Kant S, Pandaw CS, Nath LM. A management technique for effective management of Medical store in hospitals. Medical store management technique. J Acad Hosp Adm. 1996–1997;8(9):41-7.
5. Mahatme MS, Dakhale GN, Hiware SK, Shinde A, Salve A. Medical store management: An integrated economic analysis of a tertiary care hospital in central India. J Young Pharm. 2012;4:114-8.
6. Ministry of Health & Family Welfare, Government of India. Immunization Handbook for Medical Officer, 3rd edition. (2016).
7. Ministry of Health and Family Welfare, Government of India. (2017). National Health Policy 2017.
8. Ministry of Health and Family Welfare, Government of India. (2018). Outcome Budget Archives.
9. National AIDS Control Organization. Ministry of Health & Family Welfare, Government of India. (2007). Operational guidelines for financial management.
10. Needles BE, Powers M. Principles of financial accounting, 12th edition. Boston: South-Western Cengage Learning; 2013.
11. Sathe PV. Epidemiology and Management for Health for All. Mumbai: Vora Medical Publications; 2005.
12. Soudarssanane MB. Drug inventory control as a method of teaching health economics—a six stage lecture discussion. Indian J Community Med. 1997;22(2):63-9.
13. State Health Society, Bihar. District Health Action Plan, Kaimur 2012-2013.
14. UNDP. Improving efficiency of vaccination systems in multiple states. (online). Available from: http://www.in.undp.org/content/india/en/home/operations/projects/health/evin.html.
15. World Health Organization. (2006). Vaccine stock management: guidelines on stock records for immunization programme and vaccines store managers. (online) Available from: http://apps.who.int/iris/handle/10665/69629.

# CHAPTER 43

# International Healthcare Agencies

*Viral Dave, Venu Shah, Arpit Prajapati*

CM18.1 Define and describe the concept of international health
CM18.2 Describe roles of various international health agencies

## INTRODUCTION

Health is an important fundamental human right and an international goal, which is essential to lead a better quality of life. According to Paul Russell, "Nothing on earth is more international than disease." Health and disease do not have any political or geological boundaries. Various health institutions are effectively needed for the betterment of health of the people across the globe.

Healthcare agencies can be defined as the agencies which mainly concerns for providing various healthcare facilities to the community and country, in order to prevent disease, promote health and empower the humanity as a whole.

### Contribution in Public Health

Healthcare agencies are providing different kind of supports to strengthen the public health systems. They provide technical guidance to the member countries regarding priority public health problem. They mainly function to reduce the burden of various infectious and noninfectious diseases. All the agencies work for strengthening the health system to achieve major public health goals.

## TYPES OF HEALTHCARE AGENCY

Healthcare agencies can be broadly classified as below:
- International agencies
- Government agencies
- Bilateral agencies
- Nongovernment organizations and donor agencies
- Voluntary agencies.

## INTERNATIONAL HEALTH AGENCIES

### Background

In the past, a series of international conferences and meetings were initiated from the year 1851 to 1938, in order to fight against several diseases such as cholera, yellow fever, and plague. Subsequently various organizations have been established one after the other namely, Pan American Sanitary Bureau (1902), the Office international d'Hygiene publique (1907), the Health Organization of the League of Nations, etc. United Nations have absorbed all the other health organizations to form the "WHO" after completion of World War II. Later on, international assistance was offered in different forms via different agencies such as multilateral agencies, bilateral agencies, nongovernmental organizations (NGOs), donor foundations and public-private partnership (PPP) **(Table 43.1)**.

### Importance in Public Health

All the international agencies function with core objective of improving overall health and development of the nations. Along with funding, they do provide technical expertise and evolve new strategies to improve the constantly changing public health needs. Most of the international agencies work towards achievement of sustainable development goals and universal

Table 43.1: International health agencies.

| Multilateral agencies | Bilateral agencies | Nongovernmental and other donor agencies |
|---|---|---|
| - World Health Organization<br>- United Nations International Children Emergency Fund (UNICEF)<br>- The United Nations Development Program (UNDP)<br>- World Bank (WB)<br>- Food and Agricultural Organization (FAO)<br>- International Labor Organization (ILO)<br>- United Nations Fund for Population Activities (UNFPA)<br>- Joint United Nations Program on HIV and AIDS (UNAIDS)<br>- Office of the UN High Commissioner for Refugees (UNHCR)<br>- UN Fund for Drug Abuse Control (UNFDAC) | - United States Agency for International Development (USAID)<br>- Colombo Plan<br>- Swedish International Development Agency (SIDA)<br>- Danish International Development Agency (DANIDA) | - International Red Cross<br>- The Rockefeller Foundation<br>- Ford Foundation<br>- Cooperative for Assistance and Relief Everywhere (CARE) International<br>- Aga Khan Foundation<br>- Bill and Melinda Gates Foundation |

health coverage. They help different countries to fight against the disease prevalent in their respective geographic areas. They focus mainly on resolving major public health problems like control of communicable diseases (HIV/AIDS, tuberculosis, malaria, etc.), emerging and re-emerging diseases and also various noncommunicable diseases.

## MULTILATERAL AGENCIES

### Definition

Institutions/agencies which pool resources from multiple donors (government as well as nongovernment) and offer technical and commodity assistance globally or country-wide through cash grants, commodity transfers, technical assistance, or loans.

Main focus of these institutes includes health and economic development. Multilateral health agencies involved in public health are described over here.

### World Health Organization

*Logo*

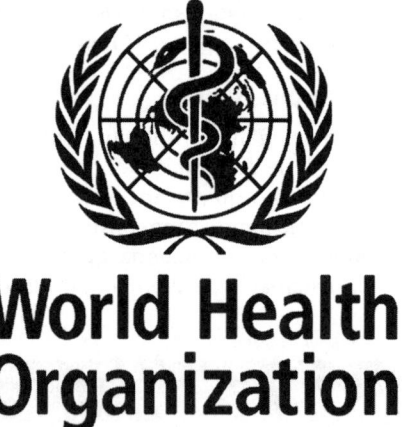

*Background*

Approval for establishment of WHO was set during International Health Conference which was organized in New York between 19th June and 22nd July 1946. The final constitution came into force on 7th April 1948. Every year 7th April is celebrated as "World Health Day" **(Box 43.1)**.

There are total 149 field offices and 6 regional offices of WHO **(Table 43.2)**. They give advice and provide technical assistance to ministries of health of respective countries regarding preventive and curative services. WHO jointly work with system of United Nation to achieve national priorities and improving health outcome. The WHO is responsible for conducting worldwide health surveys. It also prepares the World Health Report.

| Box 43.1: WHO at a glance. |
|---|
| • Member states: 194 |
| • Headquarters: Geneva |
| • Country offices: 150 |
| • Staff: More than 7,000 |
| • More than 700 institutions supporting WHO's work |
| • UN agencies, donors, foundations, NGOs and the private sector has close partnerships |

**Table 43.2:** Regional offices of WHO.

| Region | Headquarter |
|---|---|
| South-East Asian region | New Delhi, India |
| African region | Brazzaville, Republic of Congo |
| Region of Americas | Washington, DC (USA) |
| WHO European region | Copenhagen, Denmark |
| WHO Eastern Mediterranean region | Cairo, Egypt |
| WHO Western Pacific region | Manila, Philippines |

*Objective*

The prime objective of the WHO shall be the attainment by all peoples of the highest possible level of health.

Preamble of the WHO constitution is as below:
- As per the WHO, health can be defined as "a state of complete physical, mental and social well-being and not merely the absence of disease or infirmity".
- It states that achievement of the highest attainable standard of health is one of the basic rights of every human being without distinction of race, religion, political belief, economic or social condition.
- For attainment of peace and security, health of all people is fundamental and is dependent upon the fullest cooperation of individuals and states.
- WHO believes that the achievement of any state in the promotion and protection of health is of value to all. Regarding the promotion of health and control of disease, especially communicable disease, it is a common danger to have unequal development in different countries.
- WHO states that ability to live harmoniously in a changing total environment is essential for the healthy development of the child.
- As per WHO, extension to all people of the benefits of medical, psychological and related knowledge is essential to the fullest attainment of health.
- Government is responsible to provide adequate health and social measures, in order to improve the health of the people.

*Membership*

All member countries of the United Nation's have to accept the WHO's Constitution in order to become members of WHO. Members of WHO are grouped according to regional distribution. Total 194 Member States are there by the year 2017.

*Organization of WHO*

The WHO is working through:
- The World Health Assembly
- The Executive Board
- The Secretariat

***The World Health Assembly:*** Delegates representing from all the member states are the part of health assembly. In the beginning of annual meeting of the health assembly, president and other officers are being elected.

**Functions of the World Health Assembly:** It is the governing body of WHO which determines all the policies of organization including financial policies. The Director-General is appointed by the assembly. Performance of the board and of the Director-General is reviewed by health assembly.

***The Executive Board:*** It consists of 34 members, who are competent in the health field. Tenure of the elected members is three years. Board meetings are held twice a year. A chairman of the board is elected from the members who have participated in the board.

***Functions of the Executive Board:*** (1) to give result to the decisions and policies of the Health Assembly, (2) to accomplish the functions assigned by the Health Assembly, (3) submission of plans and program to the Health Assembly, (4) to make the agenda of summits of the Health Assembly, (5) to take urgent measures within the functions and financial resources of the organization to deal with events which necessitate immediate action.

***The Secretariat***

The secretariat comprises technical and administrative staff. The Director-General selected by the health assembly is the head of the secretariat. Director-General is supported by five assistant Director-Generals. Each of them is assigned responsibility of following divisions **(Box 43.2)**.

| Box 43.2: Administrative divisions. | |
|---|---|
| Epidemiological surveillance and health situation and trend assessment | Public information and education for health |
| Communicable diseases | Diagnostic, therapeutic and rehabilitative technology |
| Noncommunicable diseases | Strengthening of health services |
| Mental health | Personnel and general services |
| Family health | Information system support |
| Environmental health | Budget and finance |
| Vector biology and control | Health manpower development |

***Functions of the Secretariat:*** Administrative and technical support is offered to member states for planning of national health programs. Financial reports and budget estimates of the organization is prepared and submitted to the board, by the Director-General. Depending on the staff regulations of health assembly, staffs of the secretariat are appointed by the Director-General.

### Funding

WHO is funded in share by payments made by member states. Member states and partner organizations like civil society and other foundations contribute voluntarily. Recently, more than three quarters of organization's financing have come from voluntary donations.

### The South-East Asian Region of WHO

The WHO South-East Asian Region (SEAR) has 11 Member States namely; India, Bangladesh, Bhutan, Democratic People's Republic of Korea, Indonesia, Maldives, Myanmar, Nepal, Sri Lanka, Thailand, Timor-Leste.

***WHO works in the following fields related to public health (Fig. 43.1):***

- **Health systems:** WHO had initiated a drive to support countries in stirring towards Universal Health Coverage (UHC). With collaboration of WHO and other sectors including, civil society, global health partners, academia as well as private sectors, countries are being supported for the advancement, implementation and monitoring of concrete national health strategies.
- **Noncommunicable diseases (NCDs):** Worldwide, live of hundreds of millions of people are influenced by the four NCDs namely—cardiovascular and lung diseases, cancer and diabetes. WHO regularly updates guideline for management of above mentioned NCDs.
- **Promoting health through the life-course:** As a part of health promotion, WHO is addressing the issues of environment related risk, gender equality and human rights' protection. It tries to improve the social determinants of health.
- **Communicable diseases:** The organization is actively involved in care, treatment and prevention of tuberculosis, malaria, HIV as well as other neglected tropical diseases. All the vaccine-preventable diseases are under surveillance of WHO.

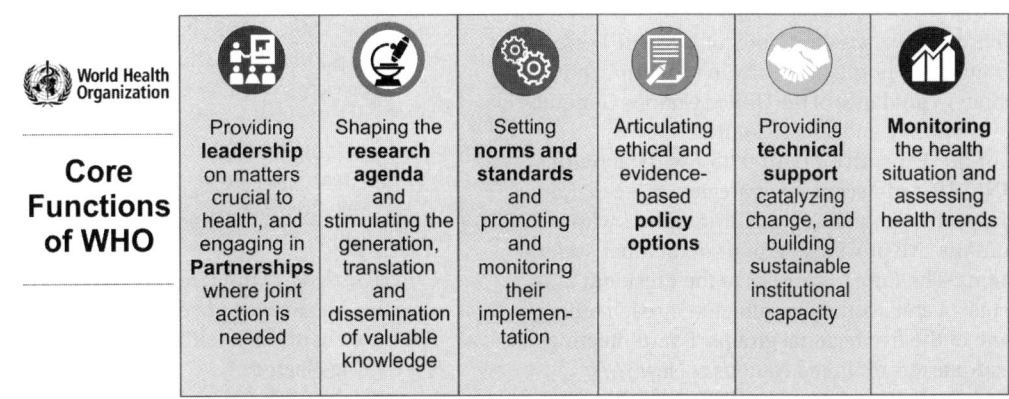

**Fig. 43.1:** Core functions of WHO.

*Source:* World Health Organization. WHO | What WHO does in countries [Internet]. WHO. World Health Organization; 2014 [cited 2018 Sep 19]. Available from: http://www.who.int/country-cooperation/what-who-does/en/

- **Preparedness, surveillance and response:** At the times of emergencies, WHO supports the countries in various tasks such as; risk assessments, deciding for the priorities, imparting crucial technical guidance, providing resources and financial support as well as monitoring of the health condition. Emergency preparedness and response capacity of each member states are strengthened by WHO.
- **Corporate services:** In order to achieve all the functions, WHO provides corporate services in the form of tools and resources.

## United Nations Children Fund

### Logo

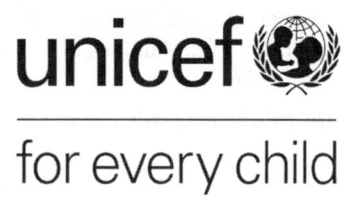

### Background

United Nations International Children's Emergency Fund (UNICEF) works in 190 nations for the protection of the rights of every child. UNICEF was established on 11th December 1946 by the United Nations General Assembly to deliver emergency food, clothing and to help children damaged by World War. In 1953, UNICEF became a permanent part of the United Nations system when its mandate was broadened to address the long-term needs of children and women in developing countries everywhere. Its name was shortened to the United Nations Children's Fund. However, UNICEF retained its original acronym.

The headquarter of UNICEF is at New York City, United States.

UNICEF has taken in account life cycle based approach with identification of specific importance of progress made in childhood and in adolescent age. UNICEF programs focus on the most deprived children, including disabled children, those having underprivileged circumstances as well as those influenced by ecological scarcity and rapid urbanization.

### Governance

The Executive Board (The governing body of UNICEF) offers the inter-governmental support to the body in synchronization with the general strategy guidance of the United Nations General Assembly and the Economic and Social Council.

The function of the Executive Board is to assess activities carried out by UNICEF and accept its strategies, budgets and national programs. Board comprises of total 36 members who are representative from the five provincial groups of member states at the United Nations. The Bureau consists of the President and four Vice-Presidents; overall work is coordinated by each officer who represents one of the five regional groups. Board meetings are held at the headquarters of United Nations at New York.

UNICEF works in collaboration with WHO, and the other external organizations such as UNDP, FAO and United Nations Educational, Scientific and Cultural Organization (UNESCO). In the early ages, UNICEF and WHO functioned together on vital problems such as tuberculosis, malaria and venereal diseases. Later, they also executed various health programs in the fields of maternal and child health, nutrition, environmental sanitation and health education.

### Functions of UNICEF (Fig. 43.2)

- **Health and nutrition**
  - UNICEF works to meet the essential health needs of the country's most vulnerable and susceptible women and children.
  - UNICEF supports for maternal nutrition during pregnancy and lactation. It takes measures for achieving optimal breastfeeding and complementary feeding for infants of 6 months or more. In addition to these, UNICEF also manages cases of severe acute malnutrition (SAM). It addresses the issue of micronutrient deficiencies among women and children by micronutrient fortification and supplementation.
  - For disabled children, UNICEF ensures provision of essential facilities at school, which include better physical accessibility, communication facilities as well as safe water and sanitation.
- **Education:** To complete the basic education cycle, quality learning is provided via educational program to all children, adolescents and girls, underprivileged children and those children who are debarred from society.
- **Disaster preparedness and response:** UNICEF helps in capacity building of the people in the field of disaster mitigation, preparedness and response, so that they can act promptly in cases of calamities and emergencies.
- **Child protection:** UNICEF is guarding children against violence, exploitation and abuse through child protection program. In this regard, it also builds the capacity of communities, civil society and nationwide organizations.
- **Youth and HIV/AIDS:** UNICEF provides platform to young people to improve their capacity of self-expression and social involvement. By initiatives related to sexual health, involvement of young persons will significantly help in sustaining a low prevalence of HIV/AIDS.

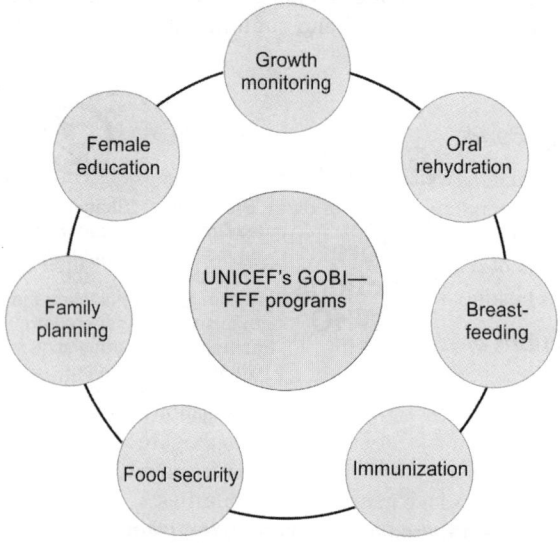

**Fig. 43.2:** UNICEF's GOBI—FFF programs.

## United Nations Development Program

### Logo

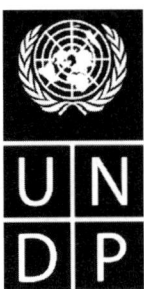

### Background

The United Nations Development Program (UNDP) is the United Nations' global development network. With the amalgamation of the Expanded Programme of Technical Assistance (EPTA) and the Special Fund, UNDP was established on 22nd November 1965. Its headquarters is in New York City.

### Functions of UNDP

- Provides funding for technical assistance and research activities pertaining to health problems affecting socioeconomic development.
- It offers expert advice, training and grants support to developing countries, with growing emphasis on support to the least developed countries.
- It emphasizes largely on sustainable development, democratic governance, peace building, environment and catastrophe resilience.

## World Bank

### Logo

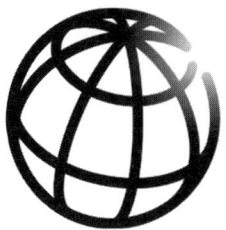

### Background

For financial as well as technical support, developing countries are mostly dependent on the World Bank. It is like a bank in the ordinary sense but with a distinctive partnership, it decreases poverty and supports development. The World Bank was established in 1944 and its headquarters is situated at Washington, DC.

### Functions of World Bank

- It provides loan for the projects related to the building of infrastructure such as road, dams, irrigation and electrical grids.
- Its work touches nearly all sectors that are vital for the fight against poverty, ensuring economic growth and improving the quality of life in developing countries.
- The World Bank Group assists in the government's efforts to reach universal health coverage (UHC) by the year 2030, which will change the health and well-being of individuals and societies.
- World Bank is working on health, nutrition and population strategy to improve the health outcomes at all national and international levels.

## Food and Agriculture Organization

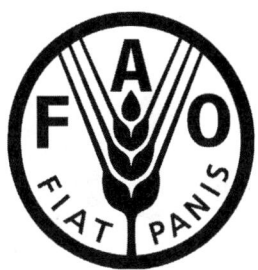

### Background

After established in 1945, the Food and Agriculture Organization (FAO) is the leading organization of the United Nations to defeat hunger. It is having its headquarters in Rome, Italy. Its goal is to reach food security for all and making the surety that people can live healthily by having uninterrupted access to food which is sufficient in quality as well as quantity. With a total of 197 members, it works in more than 130 countries all across world with belief of everybody can play a part in ending hunger.

### Functions of FAO

- It provides services to reduce hunger, food insecurity and undernourishment
- It makes farming, forestry and fisheries more productive and sustainable
- Assist in reducing rural poverty by social protection
- Supports in finding better techniques for rural people to deal with threats in their surrounding atmosphere and to increase the resilience of livelihoods in cases of emergencies.

## International Labor Organization

### Logo

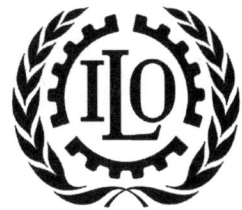

### Background

The International Labor Organization (ILO) was established in the year 1919 to accomplish worldwide peace and social justice. Labor commission has drafted the constitution of ILO during the peace conference, which was first held in Paris. The headquarters is in Geneva, Switzerland.

### Functions of ILO

- The ILO is devoted for social justice and human rights protection.

- It sets labor standards and develops policies as well as programs to improve working environment for all individuals.
- Organization has made strategy of social health protection to achieve the universal access to health care
- The organization runs the International Program on the Elimination of Child Labor (IPEC).

## United Nations Population Fund

### Logo

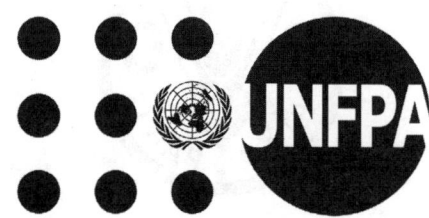

### Background

In the year 1969, The United Nations Population Fund (UNFPA) was created. Previously, it was known as United Nations Fund for Population Activities. It is the United Nations reproductive health and rights agency. Representatives from 36 nations assist the Executive Board of the UNFPA. Its primary task is to promote safe delivery and child birth throughout the world.

### Functions of UNFPA

- The organization works to improve access to family planning and helps to strengthen youth friendly and community oriented reproductive health services.
- Condoms are provided by which is one of the most effective forms of protection against STIs, including HIV.
- UNFPA along with the UNAIDS are committed to the vision of zero new HIV infections, zero discrimination and zero AIDS-related deaths.
- The organization is involved in promoting gender equality, reducing violence against females, eliminating child marriage as well as adolescent pregnancy.

## BILATERAL AGENCIES (TABLE 43.3)

### Definition of Bilateral Healthcare Agency

In addition to supporting multilateral agencies, industrialized nations offer grant in aids to the recipient countries under

Table 43.3: Bilateral agencies.

| Sr. No. | Bilateral agencies | Logo | Functions |
|---|---|---|---|
| 1. | United States Agency for International Development | USAID FROM THE AMERICAN PEOPLE | • Promote health and stability globally<br>• Works for the empowerment of women and girls and provides humanitarian assistance<br>• Assist for medical and nursing education, health education, sanitation, water supply, nutrition, family planning, control of communicable disease and agricultural programs |
| 2. | Colombo Plan | THE COLOMBO PLAN For Cooperative Economic and Social Development in Asia and the Pacific | • Working on four permanent programs:<br>  ➤ Drug Advisory Program (DAP)<br>  ➤ Programme for Public Administration and Environment (PPA & ENV)<br>  ➤ Program for Private Sector Development (PPSD)<br>  ➤ Long-term Scholarships Program (LTSP)<br>• Assist in industrial and agricultural development<br>• Help in promoting health through fellowships<br>• Financial support from New Zealand to set up AIIMS Delhi<br>• Cobalt therapy units available at various medical institutes of India |
| 3. | Swedish International Development Agency | Sida | • Provide assistance in the projects pertaining to primary health sector with chief focus on reproductive health and rights of females<br>• Help in environment and urban development with focus on water and sanitation and waste management, air and noise pollution<br>• Assist in research cooperation and mutual exchange in the field of knowledge and technology<br>• Assistance through UN agencies/NGOs in health, water and sanitation programs<br>• Assisting revised national tuberculosis control program with microscope, X-ray units and drugs including pilot project on short course chemotherapy in India |
| 4. | Danish International Development Agency | UDENRIGSMINISTERIET Ministry of Foreign Affairs of Denmark | • Focuses upon sustainable development and poverty eradication<br>• Provides support to government and nongovernment organizations<br>• Works for security and development of the nation<br>• Other areas of interest are migration, sustainable growth and development<br>• Assist for preventing leprosy, tuberculosis and blindness in countries like India |

bilateral agreement. Donor countries provide assistance depending on their objectives, technical expertise and geographical conditions. Agencies which receive funding from its native country's government and use it towards developing country are known as bilateral agencies.

## Funding of Bilateral Healthcare Agency

Aid provided by the donor country could be tied or untied. In case of tied aid, the recipient country must have to purchase the services and goods from the donor country and in case of untied funding they can buy the services on their own.

Key bilateral agencies with their service areas and contribution in public health are described below.

## NONGOVERNMENT ORGANIZATIONS AND DONOR AGENCIES (TABLE 43.4)

**Definition:** NGOs have been defined by the World Bank as "private organizations that pursue activities to relieve suffering, promote the interests of the poor, protect the environment, provide basic social services, or undertake community development".

**Importance in public health:** They constitute valuable resources in promoting health care. NGOs are contributing in fund raising, human resource development, capacity building, generation and utilization of knowledge, resource mobilization and research activities pertaining to public health. They often act as a supplement in activities conducted by government system. Brief description about activities of NGOs and various donor agencies working for public health are as follows:

Table 43.4: Nongovernment organizations and donor agencies.

| Sr. No | Nongovernment organizations and donor agencies | Logo | Functions |
|---|---|---|---|
| 1. | International Committee of the Red Cross | ICRC | • Helping people influence by armed conflict, respond to disasters in conflict zones<br>• Addressing sexual violence<br>• Building respect for law<br>• Economic security<br>• Enabling people with disability<br>• Helping detainee, humanitarian diplomacy<br>• Restoring family link, health care in danger |
| 2. | The Rockefeller Foundation | The ROCKEFELLER FOUNDATION | • In medical, health, and population sciences: Providing grants-in-aid for development of teachers and research workers<br>• Agricultural and natural sciences<br>• Arts and humanities<br>• Social disciplines<br>• International relationships<br>• It provides assistance to research institutes such as the All India Institute of Medical Sciences<br>• Funding for enhancement of farming, family planning and establishment of training and teaching centers including medical teaching in rural areas |
| 3. | Ford Foundation | FORD FOUNDATION | • Supports government agencies, civil society, academic and research institutions, and advocacy organizations<br>• Helps in research-cum action projects for overall improvement in the environment and for developing rural health services<br>• Provided fellowships to the Indian family planning officers to supplement National Institute of Health Administration and Education (NIHAE) training<br>• Sponsors health professionals to receive advanced training in other countries<br>• Provides grant in aid to selected institutes such as All India Institute of Medical Sciences (New Delhi), All India Institute of Hygiene and Public Health (Kolkata) and CMC, Vellore for conducting research and development of library |
| 4. | Cooperative for Assistance and Relief Everywhere (CARE) Renamed as "Centre for American Relief Everywhere" | care | • Focuses on developing the potential of women and girls<br>• Provides access to quality maternal and child healthcare among marginalized population<br>• Important projects run by CARE INDIA are "Axshya Project" which works to improve access to quality TB care, to support the efficacy of the Government's Integrated Child Development Services (ICDS) Program, improving maternal health through family and community involvement, Madhya Pradesh Nutrition Project, Bihar Technical Support Program, ICDS Systems Strengthening and Nutrition Improvement Project (ISSNIP), Strengthening Health and Nutrition Strategies in Community Platforms, Ensuring Newborn Survival through Intervention in the Community and Facilities |

## SUMMARY

Health, nowadays, is not a preview of only one agency, instead many agencies are working to promote health. The healthcare agencies provide support to the public health system to reduce the burden of various infections and non-infectious diseases. These international healthcare agencies include various multi-lateral agencies, bilateral agencies, NGOs, donor agencies and public-private-partnership.

*World Health Organization* plays a role in prevention and control of disease, family health, research and biomedical research and environmental health. *United Nations Children Fund* functions for mother and child health including nutrition, immunization and education. *Food and Agriculture Organization* which is mainly responsible for quantity and quality of food production, consumption including fisheries, farming and improving condition of farmers in the rural area. *International Labour Organization* promotes social justice and assists in economic and social stability among population. *United Nations Development Program* provide fund for population activities such as for family planning, and maternal and child health services. The *World Bank* is a UN agency that increases peace grant and improves living standards of population.

Other bilateral agencies such as *United States Agency for International Development* plays a role in controlling communicable diseases mainly malaria program and tuberculosis nutrition program. *Swedish International Development cooperation Agency* provides funds the Revised National Tuberculosis Programme (RNTCP). *Danish International Development Cooperation* initiated the National Programme for Control of Blindness and helps in control of leprosy and RNTCP.

Variaous nongovernmental organizations such as *International Committee of the Red Cross* responds to disasters and provides economic security. The *Rockefeller Foundation* which works for upliftment of rural areas by providing employement, electricity, water conservation, etc. *Ford Foundation* which supports governmental agencies and helps in projects for developing rural health services. *Care Foundation* which works for maternal and child health, women health, adolescents health child health and prevention of anemia.

## SUGGESTED READING

1. Home/Ford Foundation [Internet]. Available from: https://www.fordfoundation.org/
2. Home Page | Care International [Internet]. Available from: https://www.care-international.org/.
3. Home | Food and Agriculture Organization of the United Nations [Internet]. Available from: http://www.fao.org/home/en/.
4. International Committee of the Red Cross [Internet]. Available from: https://www.icrc.org/.
5. International Labour Organization [Internet]. Available from: https://www.ilo.org/global/lang--en/index.htm.
6. Miguel Angel Gonzalez'-Block ALOG–aJF. Oxford Textbook of Global Public Health. 6th ed. Oxford University Press. p. 327.
7. The Colombo Plan Secretariat [Internet]. Available from: http://www.colombo-plan.org/.
8. The Rockefeller Foundation [Internet]. Available from: https://www.rockefellerfoundation.org/.
9. U.S. Agency for International Development [Internet]. Available from: https://www.usaid.gov/.
10. UNDP - United Nations Development Programme [Internet]. Available from: http://www.undp.org/.
11. UNFPA - United Nations Population Fund [Internet]. Available from: https://www.unfpa.org/.
12. UNICEF. https://www.unicef.org/[Internet]. Available from: https://www.unicef.org/.
13. World Bank Group - International Development, Poverty, & Sustainability [Internet]. Available from: http://www.worldbank.org/.
14. World Health Organization. WHO | What WHO does in countries [Internet]. WHO. World Health Organization; 2014.

# CHAPTER 44

# Special Topics

## A. INTERNATIONAL CLASSIFICATION OF DISEASES

*Vaidehi S Gohil*

### INTRODUCTION

Morbid entities are assigned to a system of categories which is called as the "disease classification". The International Classification of Diseases and Related Health Problems (ICD) is a tool used for recording, reporting and grouping of the conditions and factors that influence health. It contains disease categories, health-related conditions and causes (external) of illness or death.

### PURPOSE

Main purpose of ICD coding is to permit the recording of the data systematically, data analysis, interpretation and to compare the mortality and morbidity data between different countries or areas and at different times. The ICD includes extensive variety of signs, symptoms, atypical findings, complaints and social factors that represent the health-related records. Health trends and statistics can be identified and compared globally by using ICD coding. It has the diagnostic classification standard used for both the clinical and research purposes. The unique alphanumeric code is given to all clinical entities so it can be easily stored and retrieved.

### THE WHO FAMILY OF INTERNATIONAL CLASSIFICATIONS

Main purpose of WHO Family of International Classifications (WHO-FIC) is to provide a concept-based framework of information which are related to health and its management and focuses to build the family of classifications in such a way that classifications become scientifically sound, culturally appropriate, and universally acceptable and applicable.

Currently, WHO-FIC family designates various integrated classification products that share similar features and can be used alone or jointly to provide information on different aspects of health and the healthcare system; e.g., the ICD as a reference classification which is mainly used for mortality and morbidity **(Flowchart 44A.1)**.

### HISTORICAL EVOLUTION OF ICD

Jacques Bertillon (1851–1922) (the Chief of Statistical Services of the City of Paris) was the chairperson of the committee held by the International Statistical Institute in Vienna in 1891 and the committee prepared a draft version of a classification of causes of death. The committee's report was presented and adopted at the meeting of the International Statistical Institute in Chicago in 1893. Bertillon adopted the classification based on anatomical site rather than the nature of disease. And it was called "Bertillon Classification of Causes of Death". The "Bertillon Classification of Causes of Death", received general approval and was adopted by several countries and cities. After that, in 1900 in Paris, the First International Conference was held for the revision of "Bertillon Classification of Causes of Death". Thus begins series of revision conferences approximately 10 years apart.

According to the WHO Nomenclature Regulations (adopted in 1967), most current ICD revision has to be used by Member States for mortality and morbidity statistics.

### INTERNATIONAL STATISTICAL CLASSIFICATION OF DISEASES AND RELATED HEALTH PROBLEMS, 10TH REVISION

The ongoing current version is "International Statistical Classification of Diseases and Related Health Problems, 10th revision" (ICD-10) since its initiation in 1989.

#### Structure

- ICD-10 comprises 3 major volumes and 22 major chapters.
- The chapters are subdivided into homogeneous blocks of three-character categories.

**Each block, includes sufficient three-character categories which are further subdivided by means of a fourth, numeric character after a decimal point that allows up to 10 subcategories.**

#### Coding Scheme

- The first character of the ICD code is a letter, and each letter is related with a particular chapter, except for the letter D

**Flowchart 44A.1:** Diagrammatic representation of three broad groups of WHO-FIC and its examples.

### Reference classifications
- It cover the main parameters of the health system, such as death, disease, functioning, disability, health and health interventions
- It is a product of international agreement
- It has achieved broad acceptance and official agreement for use and are approved and recommended as guidelines for international reporting of health

### Derived classifications
- It is based upon reference classifications
- It is prepared by adopting reference classification structure and classes, providing additional detail beyond that provided by the reference classification, or they may be prepared through rearrangement or aggregation of items from one or more reference classification

### Related classifications
- It is regarded as complementary to the reference and derived classifications
- Related classifications have their own sets of terms, but can also share terms as part of the WHO-FIC family

**Examples**

International Classification of Diseases (ICD)
International Classification of Functioning, Disability and Health (ICF)
International Classification of Health Interventions (ICHI)

International Classification of Diseases for Oncology, (ICD-O)
The ICD-10 classification of mental and behavioral disorders
Application of the ICD to dentistry and stomatology, (ICD-DA), etc.

International Classification of Primary Care (ICPC)
International Classification for Nursing Practice (ICNP)
International Classification of External Causes of Injury (ICECI), etc.

(WHO-FIC: World Health Organization Family of International Classifications)

(which is used in both Chapters II and III) and the letter H (which is used in both Chapters VII and VIII).
- More than one letter in the first position of their codes are used by four chapters (Chapters I, II, XIX, and XX).

*Examples*

Chapter XXI factors influencing health status and contact with health services (Z00–Z99):
Z58:    Problems related to physical environment
Z58.0:  Exposure to noise
Z58.1:  Exposure to air pollution
Z58.2:  Exposure to water pollution
Z58.3:  Exposure to soil pollution
Z58.4:  Exposure to radiation
Z58.5:  Exposure to other pollution
Z58.6:  Inadequate drinking-water supply
Z58.7:  Exposure to tobacco smoke
Z58.8:  Other problems related to physical environment
Z58.9:  Problem related to physical environment, unspecified

*"U" code in Chapter XXII:* New diseases of uncertain etiology are provisionally assigned by the code "U00–U49" by WHO codes. U50–U99 may be used in research. Currently, the range includes severe acute respiratory syndrome (SARS), and special codes for bacterial agents resistant to antibiotics.

*The "dagger and asterisk" system:* The dagger code (†) was used to describe the etiological condition for primary tabulation and asterisk code (*) for the clinical manifestation, relevant site, and or other aspects.

## ICD-11 FOR MORTALITY AND MORBIDITY STATISTICS (ICD-11 MMS)

International Classifications of Diseases, 11th revision for mortality and morbidity statistics (ICD-11 MMS) was released on 18 June 2018 allowing the Member States to prepare for implementation, including translation of ICD into their national languages. Reporting using ICD-11 will be started by Member States on 1st January 2022.

The ICD mainly includes categories for diseases, disorders, syndromes, foundation, symptoms, findings, injuries, external causes of morbidity and mortality, factors influencing health status, reasons for encounter of the health system and traditional medicine. Also additional details are included such as anatomy, substances, infectious agents or place of injury. ICD-11 has a set of rules and explanations, required reporting formats and necessary metadata **(Table 44A.1)**.

### Revision Steps

The revision of ICD-11 has taken place in several phases. First, a list of issues from the use of ICD-10 was identified and complied.

## Chapter 44: Special Topics

Table 44A.1: List of Chapter of ICD-11.

| Chapter number | Name of chapter | Code range |
|---|---|---|
| 01 | Certain infectious or parasitic diseases | 1A00–1H0Z |
| 02 | Neoplasms | 2A00–2F9Z |
| 03 | Diseases of the blood or blood-forming organs | 3A00–3C0Z |
| 04 | Diseases of the immune system | 4A00–4B4Z |
| 05 | Endocrine, nutritional or metabolic diseases | 5A00–5D46 |
| 06 | Mental, behavioral or neurodevelopmental disorders | 6A00–6E8Z |
| 07 | Sleep-wake disorders | 7A00–7B2Z |
| 08 | Diseases of the nervous system | 8A00–8E7Z |
| 09 | Diseases of the visual system | 9A00–9E1Z |
| 10 | Diseases of the ear or mastoid process | AA00–AC0Z |
| 11 | Diseases of the circulatory system | BA00–BE2Z |
| 12 | Diseases of the respiratory system | CA00–CB7Z |
| 13 | Diseases of the digestive system | DA00–DE2Z |
| 14 | Diseases of the skin | EA00–EM0Z |
| 15 | Diseases of the musculoskeletal system or connective tissue | FA00–FC0Z |
| 16 | Diseases of the genitourinary system | GA00–GC8Z |
| 17 | Conditions related to sexual health | HA00–HA8Z |
| 18 | Pregnancy, childbirth or the puerperium | JA00–JB6Z |
| 19 | Certain conditions originating in the perinatal period | KA00–KD5Z |
| 20 | Developmental anomalies | LA00–LD9Z |
| 21 | Symptoms, signs or clinical findings, not elsewhere classified | MA00–MH2Y |
| 22 | Injury, poisoning or certain other consequences of external causes | NA00–NF2Z |
| 23 | External causes of morbidity or mortality | PA00–PL2Z |
| 24 | Factors influencing health status or contact with health services | QA00–QF4Z |
| 25 | Codes for special purposes | RA00–RA26 |
| 26 | Traditional Medicine conditions—Module I | SA00–SJ3Z |
| V | Supplementary section for functioning assessment | VA00–VC50 |
| X | Extension codes | XS8HXD19J4 |

Possible solutions were formulated and input was received from many scientific groups, field testing, Member State comments, and ongoing submission and processing of proposals. Then, centralized editing occurred, with aimed to adjust imbalances in content and to ensure the overall structure is consistent and practicable for users.

## Structure

International Statistical Classification of Diseases and Related Health Problems, 11th revision is divided into three major volumes:
1. The tabular list (includes alphanumeric listing of diseases and disease groups, etc.)
2. The reference guide (an introduction and guidelines for certification, recording, rules for mortality and morbidity coding and lists for tabulation of statistical data)
3. The index (list of approximately 120,000 clinical terms).

## General Features of ICD-11

- **Both print and electronic (https://icd.who.int/)** versions are available and easily accessible by users.
- **Field trials:** Different types of field studies had done to test the fitness to the ICD-MMS like "line coding" (to assess whether both the system, i.e., ICD-10 and ICD-11 version yield the same code on the same case) and "inter coder reliability" (the information on a case will be coded by two different medical coders to assess whether they agree on the same code).
- **Governance structure of ICD-11:** For ICD-11, inputs from the experts and all the stakeholders were considered, such as Joint Linearization for Mortality and Morbidity Statistics (JLMMS) joint task force (JTF), the Classification and Statistics Advisory Committee (CSAC), Medical Scientific Advisory Committee (MSAC), Revision Steering Group (RSG), etc.
- **Language independent ICD entities:** ICD-10 has been translated into 43 languages and ICD-11 has been available in all six official languages since its publication (English, French, Spanish, Russian, Chinese, and Arabic). All entities have given the unique identifier (URI) and have a specific place in a hierarchy of groups, categories, and narrower terms. ICD-11 allows binding of any desired language to the elements of its foundation component. In this way, it facilitates translations or multilingual browsing.

## New Elements of ICD-11 (or Difference to ICD-10)

- **New chapters:** Some new added chapters are: Chapter 4: Disorder of immune system; Chapter 7: Sleep-wake disorder; Chapter 17: Conditions related to sexual health; Chapter 26: Traditional medicine; Section V: Supplementary section for functioning assessment and Section X: Extension codes.
- **New conceptual terms:** Some terms are added, such as foundation component (i.e., everything in ICD), entity (i.e., each element, such as diseases, disorders, injuries, external causes, signs and symptoms, etc.), linearization (i.e., classification hierarchy, such as chapter, block, category), stem code (i.e., category), extension code (i.e., additional information, such as severity scale value, temporality, etiology, specific anatomic details, histopathology, consciousness, etc.), multiple parents (i.e., an entity may be correctly classified in two different places, e.g., by site or by etiology).
- **Content model:** It is a structured framework in which each entity is defined in a standard way. Each ICD entity can be seen from different dimensions (property)s. For example, there are currently 12 defined main properties in the content model to describe an entity in the ICD: ICD entity title, classification properties, textual definitions, terms, body system/body part, temporal properties, severity of subtypes properties, manifestation properties (signs, symptoms or investigation findings), causal properties, specific condition properties, treatment properties, and diagnostic criteria.

## Salient Features of New Coding Scheme or Structure

- The chapter numbering is in *Arabic numbers* and not Roman numerals.
- There are *26 chapters* instead of 21 chapters in ICD-10.

- The coding scheme for categories now has *4 characters* and there are *2 levels of subcategories*.
- The coding always has a letter in the second position to differentiate from the codes of ICD-10.
- In ICD-11, the *first character of the code is always related to the chapter number*. It may be a number or a letter. For example, 2A00 is a code in Chapter 2 and AB00 is a code in Chapter 10.
- There are alphanumeric codes in ICD-11 and range from 1A00.00 to ZZ9Z.ZZ.
- Codes starting with "X" indicate an extension code.
- The inclusion of a forced number at the 3rd character position is to prevent spelling "undesirable words".
- The letters "O" and "I" are omitted to prevent confusion with the numbers "0" and "1".
- Asterisk codes become clinical forms or extension codes.

The terminal letter Y is reserved for the residual category "other specified" and the terminal letter "Z" is reserved for the residual category "unspecified".

Blocks are not coded within this code structure—each has its own. However, hierarchical relations are retained in the 4-digit codes. There is unused coding space allocated in all blocks to allow for later updates and to keep the codes stable.

### *Example*

- Chapter 06: Mental, behavioral or neurodevelopmental disorders
  - Disorders due to substance use or addictive behavior (Block L1-6C4)
  - Disorders due to substance use (Block L2-6C4)
- 6C40: Disorders due to use of alcohol:
  - 6C40.0: Single episode of harmful use of alcohol
  - 6C40.1: Harmful pattern of use of alcohol
  - 6C40.2: Alcohol dependence
  - 6C40.3: Alcohol intoxication
  - 6C40.4: Alcohol withdrawal
  - 6C40.5: Alcohol-induced delirium
  - 6C40.6: Alcohol-induced psychotic disorder
  - 6C40.7: Other alcohol-induced disorders
- 6C40.Y: Other specified disorders due to use of alcohol
- 6C40.Z: Disorders due to use of alcohol, unspecified

*Pre coordination, post coordination, and cluster coding*: The coding is represented with pre coordination (i.e., stem codes may contain all pertinent information about a clinical concept), post coordination (when additional detail pertaining to a single condition is described by combining multiple codes, i.e., stem codes and/or extension codes together) and cluster coding (when more than one code used together, e.g., stem code or stem codes and extension codes to describe a clinical concept).

For example, cluster coding for the diagnosis of gastric ulcer with acute hemorrhage associated with nicotine dependence is *DA60&XA2828/ME24.90/6C4A.2Z* where:

- *Condition:* DA60 is gastric ulcer.
- *Specific anatomy:* XA2828 indicates anatomy/location is gastric cardia.
- *Has manifestation:* ME24.90 indicates having acute gastro-intestinal bleeding, not elsewhere classified.
- *Associated with:* 6C4A.2Z is for nicotine dependence, unspecified.

### Applied Aspects

- ***ICD use in mortality statistics:*** ICD is widely used for medical research, evaluating health interventions, planning and follow-up of health care. Analysis of mortality data typically involves comparisons of data sets, e.g., those representing different regions or different points in time, provided data have been collected by same methods and same standards. Mortality coders must be familiar with the basic concept terms used to fill the death certificate, such as direct cause of death, causal relationship, sequence, starting point, duration, etc.
- ***ICD use in morbidity statistics:*** Morbidity data are used for statistical reporting mostly at national or local levels. ICD addresses the different levels of treatment (primary, secondary and tertiary) details primarily through multidimensional coding. It also uses in an academic research context; it is commonly conducted in applied settings to inform health system and public health agency to make the decision.
- ***ICD use in health information systems:*** Health information systems are increasingly based on digital (Electronic Health Record) e-reporting and coding. ICD-11 can be used more easily in such environments. Health facility-related data sources include public health surveillance (monitoring of the incidence and prevalence of diseases), health services data, and health system monitoring data (e.g., human resources, health infrastructure, financing) are recorded.

## SUGGESTED READING

1. World Health Organization. International Classifications of Diseases (ICD 11).

# B. QUALITY IN HEALTHCARE

*Ruchi Juyal, Vidisha Vallabh*

*"Quality means doing it right when no one is looking."*
—**Henry Ford**

## INTRODUCTION

The concept and vocabulary of quality are elusive. Different people have interpreted quality differently in different places and time periods. Quality can be understood as consistent delivery of a product or service according to expected standards. The idea of quality in business has existed since the barter system. The history goes back to the early 1900s when pioneers such as Frederick Winslow Taylor and Henry Ford acknowledged the value of quality control (QC) in business.

## EVOLUTION OF QUALITY IN HEALTHCARE

Although it is relatively a novel concept in health sector in our country, the notion of enforcing quality care in medical profession can be traced back to early 1900s in the form of "Medical Audit" in the United States of America (USA). As the transition to value-based care moved forward, the focus in patient care also has shifted toward quality and away from quantity.

> The Agency for Healthcare Research and Quality (AHRQ) defines quality healthcare as "doing the right thing for the right patient, at the right time, in the right way to achieve the best possible results".

The consensus on the importance of quality of care (QOC) in population programs emerged in the International Conference on Population and Development (ICPD) held in Cairo in 1994. QOC was perceived as an integral and major component of people's reproductive rights. India was a signatory to the proceedings of this conference and hence concept of quality in healthcare services was introduced in 1996 along with piloting of Reproductive and Child Health (RCH) program.

> **Saved by the Bell!**
> The district hospital in Nalgonda, Andhra Pradesh, was reporting an alarming 31% of the newborn suffering from birth asphyxia. The Quality Improvement team identified the possible reasons: Shortage of skilled staff and poor network connectivity between labor room staff and the sick newborn care unit (SNCU). A simple but unique initiative in form of a bell was placed between the SNCU and labor room to be rung as soon as the head of the baby was visible. This ensured that the nurses from the SNCU would rush to the labor room in time. This was strengthened by stamping all high-risk delivery case filed with high-risk stamp and quoting them in medical records during patient registration. The resultant reduction in birth asphyxia cases was dramatic. Adherence to these two practices resulted in over 25% reduction in asphyxia related admissions in the SNCU among inborn babies. Proper management of resources and an existing workforce can handle emergencies by setting up the right processes in place and using simple solutions.

## DEFINING QUALITY OF HEALTHCARE

The WHO definition of QOC is "the extent to which healthcare services provided to individuals and patient populations improve desired health outcomes. In order to achieve this, healthcare must be *safe, effective, timely, efficient, equitable, and people-centered*".

The Institute of Medicine (IOM) defines *healthcare quality* as "the degree to which healthcare services for individuals and populations increase the likelihood of desired health outcomes and are consistent with current professional knowledge".

## DIMENSIONS OF QUALITY IN HEALTHCARE

The six general dimensions of quality as described by IOM are:
1. *Safe*: Avoiding harm to people for whom the care is intended.
2. *Effective*: Providing evidence-based healthcare services to those who need them.
3. *People-centered*: Providing care that responds to individual preferences, needs, and values.
4. *Timely*: Reducing waiting times for the patients.
5. *Efficient*: Maximizing the benefit of available resources and avoiding waste.
6. *Equitable*: Providing care that does not vary in quality on account of age, sex, gender, race, ethnicity, geographical location, religion, socioeconomic status, linguistic or political affiliation.

> **Points to Remember**
> - With introduction of Medical Audits in USA since the 1900s, the focus of healthcare is transcending from quantity to quality.
> - *Quality of healthcare:* The degree to which healthcare services for individuals and populations increase the likelihood of desired health outcomes and are consistent with current professional knowledge (IOM).
> - Quality of care is a key component of the right to health, and the route to equity and dignity for the individuals and the community.
> - *Dimensions of healthcare:* Safe, effective, timely, efficient, equitable, and people-centered.

## IMPORTANCE OF QUALITY IN HEALTHCARE

Quality of care in health services is essential for achieving universal health coverage (UHC) and ambitious health-related targets for Sustainable Development Goals (SDGs). QOC is a key component of the right to health, and the route to equity and dignity for the individuals and the community.

In India, despite an escalating growth in the health sector, a sizeable gap still exists between the demand and supply of healthcare services, particularly in rural and difficult terrains. This is often filled by an informal network of care providers, which is still unregulated with no controls on the quality of services and no standardized protocols to measure the QOC. There are disparities in access to health services, which are further worsened by the poor functioning of public health system.

## QUALITY-OF-CARE FRAMEWORK IN HEALTH

Evaluating the effectiveness of a wide array of health policies and healthcare providers is futile, if the delivery of their services does not meet the standards. Donabedian in 1966 came out with three-component approach for evaluating the quality-of-care measurement for improvement in health services **(Fig. 44B.1)**.

## MEASUREMENT OF QUALITY IN HEALTHCARE

Measurement of quality in healthcare is essential to determine its effects on the desired outcomes. Rating of quality of healthcare services is a laborious task; however, widely employed patient satisfaction surveys expedite the understanding of critical areas in health care that require improvement.

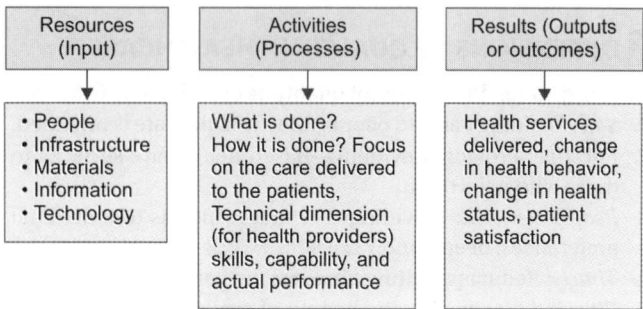

**Fig. 44B.1:** The Donabedian model for quality of care.

**Measuring health quality**

Measurement can show us a number of important pieces of information:
- How well our current process is performing?
- Whether we have achieved our aim(s).
- How much variation there is in our data and hence processes?
- Whether a small test of change is having the desired impact.
- Whether the changes made have resulted in an improvement.
- Whether a change has been sustained.

The first level (structural level) deals with the physical and staff characteristics of the healthcare system organization. The second level (process level) covers indicators that evaluate the interaction between the healthcare providers and the users (patients). The third level (clinical outcome) is directly associated with the patient's health status/satisfaction. A systems approach in quality of healthcare delineates the influence of these levels, independently as well as during their interaction on health outcomes **(Table 44B.1)**.

Quality of care can also be described in terms of inputs, processes, and outcome, where input includes availability of drugs and consumables, enabling work environment and adequate technical support; process may consist of good behavior by service providers, proper infection control practices, effective implementation of programs; and outcome may comprise of High-level of patient satisfaction, low mortality, morbidity, complications, referrals, and improvement in health indicators.

## MONITORING OF QUALITY IN HEALTHCARE

In any healthcare system, continuous measurement and analysis of data are required for monitoring the QOC being provided to the patients. There are many techniques by which monitoring can be done, which are as follows:

- ***Management information system (MIS):*** This recording and reporting system is a computerized information system consisting of patient database used for decision making. The indicators generated by this database can be used to monitor quality. For example, percentage of early registration of pregnant women, number of antenatal visit, completely immunized children, etc. indicate quality of the MCH services.
- ***Supervisory visits:*** Observation of ongoing healthcare activities by the supervisors can help in monitoring the quality, e.g., techniques of vaccination, health education sessions, etc.
- ***Health surveys:*** By these, we can assess various aspects of quality in healthcare, e.g., health-related behavior, knowledge and belief, etc.
- ***Patient satisfaction survey:*** These surveys provide good information on various aspects of quality as perceived by the patients, i.e., healthcare services, facility, interpersonal aspects, etc. These are usually conducted when patient comes out of the facility, hence, also known as *Exit Interviews*.

**Table 44B.1:** Quality of care in term of inputs, processes, and outcome.

| | *Input* | *Process* | *Outcome* |
|---|---|---|---|
| Patients' expectations | • Availability of services<br>• Availability of drugs and consumables<br>• Prompt and courteous services<br>• Clean and inviting environment at the health facility<br>• Barrier-free access<br>• No exclusion on the basis of caste and socioeconomic status | • Minimal waiting time and prompt referral, if required<br>• Good behavior by service providers<br>• Privacy and confidentiality<br>• Grievance redressal<br>• Access to information and involvement in decision making for the care | • No out of pocket expenditure<br>• Availability of guaranteed services<br>• High-patient satisfaction<br>• Treatment and cure |
| Service providers requirements | • Adequate and planned infrastructure<br>• Serviceable and calibrated equipment<br>• Availability of quality drugs<br>• Human resources—numerical adequacy with knowledge and skills<br>• Enabling work environment | • Adherence to clinical protocols<br>• Infection control practices<br>• Training and skill development<br>• Safe and effective nursing care | • Low mortality, morbidity, complications, referrals, etc.<br>• Efficiency in care in term of average length of stay, bed occupancy, etc.<br>• Adverse drug reactions and hospital-acquired infection<br>• High-staff satisfaction |
| Health systems requirements | • Allocation of adequate resources<br>• Facilities provide full range of services<br>• Adequate technical support | • Efficient logistics management<br>• Monitoring and supervision<br>• Effective implementation of programs | • Measurable deliverables of programs<br>• Improvement in health indicators<br>• Enhanced productivity in terms of volume |

> **Cheese for ease: Incorporating QI models in health care**
> The systems approach laid foundation for the birth of multiple theories, prominent principles being discussed in the chapter. The *Swiss cheese* model by James Reason in 2000 was one such model that propounded that hazards and losses in any system are separated by multiple barriers developed in processes stage. These barriers are never perfect in actual setting. Each barrier has certain holes (such as in Swiss cheese). The next barrier was so created to block any hazard from moving onto next stage thus translating into losses. Developed for the oil and airline industry, this model was soon adopted by the Royal College of Physicians. They developed an Endoscopy Global Rating Scale now used worldwide to save patients from catastrophic losses optimizing patient satisfaction.

> **Points to Remember**
> - Measurement of quality of healthcare is essential to determine its effects on the desired outcomes.
> - Avedis Donabedian, an American physician, in 1966 constructed a conceptual model for evaluation of quality in healthcare.
> - The framework based on the above model relied on structure, process, and outcome to gather information on quality in healthcare.
> - A systems approach to healthcare quality that measures the effectiveness, efficiency, and equity of the input, process, and outcome indicators is an important yet untapped tool to increase the value of healthcare quality.
> - Management information system, supervisory visit, health survey, and patient satisfaction survey are fruitful means for monitoring of the system.

## QUALITY CONTROL PROCESS

Quality control process is an eight-step process for monitoring and evaluating performance **(Box 44B.1)**.

> **Box 44B.1: Eight-step process for quality control.**
> 1. Establish control criteria
> 2. Identify the information relevant to the criteria
> 3. Determine ways to collect the information
> 4. Collect and analyze the information
> 5. Compare collected information with the established criteria
> 6. Make a judgment about quality
> 7. Provide information and, if necessary, take corrective action
> 8. Determine when there is a need for re-evaluation

### Quality Control

Quality control intends to ensure that the performed services are provided according to predefined standards or protocols. It is primarily aimed at the *prevention* of errors.

### Quality Assurance

American Society for Quality refers to Quality Assurance (QA) as "planned and systematic activities, which are implemented in a quality system, so that quality requirements of a product or service would be fulfilled". In health care, QA ensures constant vigilance of healthcare quality indicators that translates into maintenance of high-quality healthcare. It helps to identify the weaknesses/faults in the health services.

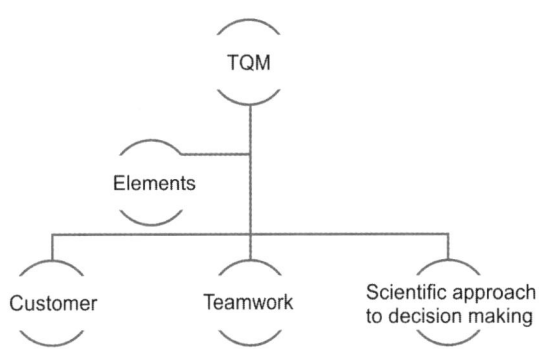

**Fig. 44B.2:** Total quality management (TQM).

The focus of QA is the discovery and correction of errors. These activities are carried out by QA personnel or department personnel.

### Quality Improvement

Quality improvement (QI) is an interdisciplinary process, aims at raising the quality of delivery of health services. The QI cycle identifies problem areas in a healthcare process and designs a sequence of step-wise solution for the problem, thus providing improvement at every opportunity. The newly designed solution is tested in practice and if not found satisfactory, the cycle is reinitiated.

### Total Quality Management

Total quality management (TQM), a much-favored management technique in the 1980s and 1990s, aims at success through achievement of customer satisfaction. It requires the participation of all members of the system in upgrading the process, services, and working environment of the organization. Since it assesses the overall quality of a system, hence, it is a multifaceted approach involving quality design and development, QC and maintenance, QI, and assurance **(Fig. 44B.2)**.

### Continuous Quality Improvement

Continuous quality improvement (CQI) was first used in manufacturing, and later expanded to business areas. Health insurance companies required justification to release funds to its beneficiaries and therefore were the forbearers of CQI in health care.

By building upon the framework of CQI, organizations could achieve the industry gold standards and showcase their achievements, inspiring many in their course. Since it entails a cycle of identifying problems, implementing a corrective system, and monitoring solutions, CQI not only imbibed from TQM and Lean Six Sigma but also from customer satisfaction. It propounds that all problems in achieving the ultimate aim of customer satisfaction arise from processes, not people.

#### Steps in Continuous Quality Improvement

Continuous quality improvement is a cyclical process. There are seven steps involved in implementing CQI cycle **(Table 44B.2)**.

**Table 44B.2:** Seven steps involved in implementing continuous quality improvement cycle.

| Steps | Activities |
|---|---|
| Step 1 | Identify an *area* where opportunities for improvement exist |
| Step 2 | Define a *problem* within that area, and outline the *sequence of activities* (the process) that should occur in that problem area |
| Step 3 | Establish the *desired outcomes* of the process and the *requirements* needed to achieve them |
| Step 4 | *Select specific steps* in the process; and for each step, list the factors that prevent the achievement of desired outcome |
| Step 5 | Collect and analyze data about the *factors that are preventing the achievement* of the desired outcomes of the desired steps |
| Step 6 | Take *corrective action* to improve the process |
| Step 7 | *Monitor* the results of the action taken |

> **Points to Remember**
> - Quality control processes standardize the quality of healthcare by harnessing and analyzing healthcare data and providing a prudent course of action.
> - Quality assurance by focusing on systems, processes, and team approach weeds out the weaknesses in a healthcare system. This is possible only through hierarchical organizational arrangements at national, state, and district level.
> - Total quality management is a management approach that enjoyed a widespread popularity in achieving long-term success through customer satisfaction at all levels of services.
> - The obstacles faced in customer satisfaction are rooted out by employing a quality improvement cycle that provided doable solution for improvement in quality process.

## HEALTHCARE QUALITY CONTROL IN INDIA

Quality improvement is linked to performance improvement, because improving quality tends to reduce the cost. Many nations have implemented customized guidelines to improve the quality of healthcare, e.g., Indian Public Health Standards (IPHS), National Quality Assurance Standards (NQAS), and National Accreditation Board of Health (NABH) in India, National Safety and Quality Health Service (NSQHS) Standards in Australia, and National Institute for Health and Care Excellence (NICE) guidelines in UK.

> Accreditation is a process by which healthcare organizations demonstrate their ability to meet the standards established by a recognized accreditation organization.

### Quality Council of India

Quality Council of India (QCI) came into existence in 1997 to establish and operate the National Accreditation Structure and promote quality through National Quality Campaign. It works towards assuring quality standards across all economic and social activities including Healthcare Establishments. One of the main objectives of QCI is to establish and operate national accreditation structure.

The QCI operation related to healthcare quality is carried out by its constituent boards namely NABH and National Accreditation Board for Testing and Calibration Laboratories (NABL).

> **Kayakalp: A Government of India initiative to Promote Hygiene and Sanitation in Public Health Facilities**
>
> With irregularities in health services reaching newfound depths, the Indian patient has found himself strapped for choice. The NFHS-4 data reveals that only 42% of the urban and 46% of the rural population opt for public health services, citing unavailable medical personnel, long-waiting time, and poor quality of healthcare services as the some of the causes.
>
> To gain trust of the beneficiaries in public health facilities, GOI launched "KAYAKALP" in 2015 to award public health facilities working relentlessly to set standards of excellence in patient care. This reflected not only in the high quality of cleanliness in the public health facility, but also the procedures developed and maintained for activities such as biomedical waste management. Team work and community participation with ventures like Swachh Swasth Sarvatra aim at capacity building and instilling assurance in public health services.
>
> The award scheme is intended to promote cleanliness, hygiene, and infection control practices in public healthcare facilities. Through an ongoing assessment of hygiene practices in various institutions, it aims to create sustainable practices related to improved cleanliness in public health facilities.
>
> Model public healthcare facilities replicating the set standards are recognized and incentivized on a public platform. Citation and cash prize are awarded to best district hospitals, CHC/subdistrict hospitals, and PHCs. Such practices are linked to positive health outcomes.

### National Accreditation Board for Hospitals and Healthcare Providers

National Accreditation Board for Hospitals and Healthcare Providers is a constituent board of Quality Council of India, which came into existence in 2006 with the vision to conceive and operate accreditation program for healthcare organizations. It works as an autonomous body and offers accreditation to hospitals, smaller health centers, laboratories, and testing centers. Gaining this accreditation is a momentous task, as it is the pinnacle of quality due the exhaustive and stringent list of 600 plus NABH quality objectives to be surmounted.

Its standards have been accredited by ISQua (International Society for Quality in Healthcare), hence making NABH accreditation at par with the world's most leading hospital accreditation.

### National Accreditation Board for Testing and Calibration Laboratories

National Accreditation Board for Testing and Calibration Laboratories is a constituent board of Quality Council of India. This autonomous body is only one of its kinds that assess laboratories in India for quality and consistency in the results. All the accredited laboratories have to follow ISO/IEC 17025 to maintain quality management system in testing and calibration. NABL also undertakes proficiency testing program for its accredited as well as applicant laboratories.

### Indian Public Health Standards

Indian Public Health Standards (IPHS) are in operation since 2006 under NRHM. These standards have been developed for different healthcare delivery points, viz subcenters, Primary Health Centers (PHCs), Community Health Centers (CHCs), Subdistrict and district hospitals. IPHS guidelines comprise of uniform standards designed to improve the quality of healthcare delivery in the country. Under this the services are grouped as "Minimum Assured Services or Essential services" and "Desirable Services". Essential Services include promotive, preventive, curative, referral services, and all the national health programs made available at the healthcare facility.

As per the changing protocols of the national health programs and launch of new programs, revised guidelines of IPHS have come up in 2012. Tailoring of guidelines to allow room for varied needs of a state is permissible. States and UTs are required to adopt these IPHS guidelines for strengthening the public healthcare institutions and put in their best efforts to achieve high quality of healthcare across the country. A diligent observation of these guidelines will not only improve the quality of healthcare delivery services but also will help to assess the functioning of a healthcare facility.

### Bureau of Indian Standards

Bureau of Indian Standards (BIS), the statutory National standards body of India, was constituted in 1987. It provides ISO certification in quality management systems to health centers. BIS has ensued guidelines for improvement in functioning of healthcare organizations and provision of quality healthcare services to consumers in a transparent manner.

### National Quality Assurance Standards

National Quality Assurance Standards (NQAS) were developed by the National Health Systems Resource Center (NHSRC) under Ministry of Health and Family Welfare (MoHFW), Government of India to improve service quality at different levels of Public Health Facilities. These standards set optimal benchmarks in terms of Patients' rights, service provision, clinical care, support services, infection control and quality management, etc.

Adoption of globally acclaimed best practices in Indian context as standards in Public Health for District Hospitals, CHCs, PHCs, and Urban PHCs has created a benchmark in public health delivery system. These standards are primarily meant for providers to evaluate their own system for QI. These standards are ISQua accredited and meet global benchmarks.

#### Points to Remember
- Quality of care in health services is essential for achieving universal health coverage and ambitious health-related targets for sustainable development goals.
- Various agencies in India, viz QCI, NABH, NABL, work tirelessly to improve the quality of healthcare provided by public as well as private institutions.
- BIS, NQAS, and IPHS are essential standards of paramount importance serving as an edifice to build upon and improve the services catered to the masses.

## SUMMARY

- Quality in anything means a distinctive attribute or characteristic possessed by someone or something. Quality of care according to WHO is the extent to which healthcare services provided to individuals and patient populations improve the desired health outcomes.
- In health care, quality has come a long way from an intangible idea adopted from management models to set standards and guideline to assess patient satisfaction. The Cairo conference (1994) and IOM report on patient care have now become milestones in health care, proposing guidelines for evaluation of health care, thereby shifting focus from quantity to quality.
- Quality of care in health services is essential for achieving universal health coverage and ambitious health-related targets for Sustainable Development Goals.
- In India, despite an escalating growth in the health sector, a sizable gap still exists between the demand and supply of healthcare services, particularly in rural and difficult terrains.
- Quality of care is a key component of the right to health, and the route to equity and dignity for the individuals and the community. This has expanded the dimensions of healthcare to be safe, effective, timely, efficient, equitable, and people-centered.
- The measurement of these dimensions utilizes the systems approach based on the Donabedian model of structure, process, and outcome; their monitoring employs management information system supervisory visits and surveys.
- Maintenance of the quality standards when once achieved is an ongoing cycle (continuous quality improvement) and is based on the management tenets of PDSA cycle, Lean Six Sigma, and TQM.
- These principles are active at each organizational hierarchy of public and private health system, from national to district levels. These organizations improve the quality of their services by matching them against various standards (IPHS, BSI, NQAS) recommended by CQI, NABL, and NABH. An institution accredited by the aforementioned processes instills a sense of pride, trust, and confidence in the beneficiaries.

## SUGGESTED READING

1. Approaches to Quality Improvement. Module 4. Agency for Healthcare Research and Quality, Rockville, MD. Available from: https://www.ahrq.gov/ncepcr/to ols/pf-handbook/mod4.html.
2. Ashton J. In: O'Neil M (Ed.). Health Manager's guide: Monitoring the quality of hospital care. Center for human services, Bethesda, USA: Quality assurance project; 2000. Available from: https://www.usaidassist.org/sites/assist/files/hspcarebook501.pdf.
3. Berwick DM. A user's manual for the IOM's 'Quality Chasm' report. Health Aff (Millwood). 2002;21:80-90.
4. Donabedian A. The quality of care. How can it be assessed? JAMA. 1988;260:1743-8.
5. Dubé C. Use of the endoscopy global rating scale by endoscopy services in Canada. Canadian Journal of Gastroenterology. 2013;27:684-5.
6. Government of India. (2018). Indian Public Health Standards.
7. Gupta I, Bhatia M. Indian Health Care System. In: Mossialos E (Ed). International Profiles of Health Care System. New York, NY: The Commonwealth Fund; 2017.
8. Jonge V, Nicolaas JS, van Leerdam ME, Kuipers EJ. 'Overview of the quality assurance movement in health care'. Best Practice and Research Clinical Gastroenterology. 2011;25(3):337-47.
9. National Accreditation Board for Hospitals & Healthcare Providers (NABH). (2018).
10. National Health Mission, Ministry of health and family welfare, GOI. Operational guidelines for quality assurance in public health facilities; 2013.
11. World Health Organization. (2006). Quality of care: a process for making strategic choices in health systems.
12. Yuan F, Chung KC. Defining quality in healthcare and measuring quality in surgery. Plast Reconstr Surg. 2016;137:1635-44.

# C. HEALTH ECONOMICS

*Abhik Sinha, Sukamal Bisoi*

## INTRODUCTION

The definition of health, as it suggest, has got a social part, or social well-being. Thus, the social part is integral to health. Health economics is an important part in this regard. At the end of the Bachelor of Medicine and Bachelor of Surgery (MBBS) curriculum a MBBS doctor is expected to learn some administrative and management skills. Thus knowledge regarding health economics, health financing is important in this regard.

The health sector consists of organized public and private health services and health-related nongovernment organizations and community groups, and professional associations. The concerned persons responsible for determining and managing different areas of a health sector are typically forced to consider questions such as: At what level should hospital fees be set? What should be the pay package for the doctors and nurses? Which treatments are the most cost-effective for people with HIV?

Thus these pertinent questions make all of us aware of the fact that we doctors also need an exposure of health economics.

### What is Economics?

Economics is the study of *scarcity* and the means by which we deal with this problem. Because resources are essentially limited, choices need to be made about how they are to be used. Economics, as a discipline, is concerned by and large with how we make these choices in the context of scarcity.

One of the key assumptions generally made in economics is that individuals will make these decisions *rationally*. This means that given good information they will choose to do things, such as utilize health services that will be in their best interests, where "best interests" is defined as maximizing their *utility* given the resources they have at their disposal:
- Economics is the social science that deals with weighing up of relative benefits of each course of action and choosing the best action in order to obtain maximum benefits.
- It consists of costs (resource use), benefits and efficiency.
- It differs from accountancy which deals with the monitoring of financial transactions.

## HEALTH ECONOMICS

- Health economics lies at the interface of economics and medicine and applies the discipline of economics to the topic of health (**Fig. 44C.1**).

- Health economics as a branch of economics concerned with issues related to efficiency, effectiveness, value and behavior in the production and consumption of health and healthcare.

## TYPE OF ECONOMICS

Basically, it is of two types: (1) Macroeconomics and (2) microeconomics.

### Macroeconomics

It deals with:
- **National output and income:** Indicators are gross national product (GNP), gross domestic product (GDP), net national product (NNP), etc.
- **Level of unemployment:** Indicator–unemployment rates
- **General price level:** Price indexes, e.g., consumer price index, producer price index, GDP deflator, etc.

*Gross National Product*

- Term denoting the total money value of the goods and services produced by a nation during a given year.
- It measures the overall importance of an economy.
- The most comprehensive measure of a nation's total output of goods and services.

*Gross Domestic Product*

- Similar to GNP except that it count all income produced within the borders of a country, including income earned by resident foreigners, but excludes income earned by citizens of the country who are residents abroad.
- GDP per capita is often considered an indicator of a country's *standard of living*.
  GDP = GNP – net income from abroad

### Microeconomics

- Microeconomics is a branch of economics that studies the behavior of *individual* households and firms in making decisions on the allocation of limited resources.
- Typically, it applies to markets where goods or services are bought and sold—consumers, resource owners and business firms.
- Microeconomics include: Industrial organization, labor economics, financial economics, public economics, political economics, *health economics*; urban economics, law and economics, etc.

*Efficiency*

Efficiency evaluates how well resources are used to achieve a desired outcome. It has a number of different aspects:
- *Allocative efficiency* measures the extent to which resources are allocated to the groups or individuals who can benefit most.
- *Technical efficiency* measures either the extent to which resources are combined to achieve maximum outcome, or

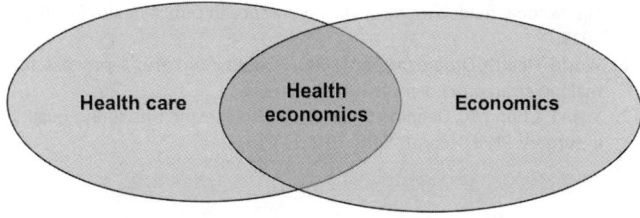

**Fig. 44C.1:** Health economics.

alternatively the minimum amounts of resources that are combined to achieve a given outcome, (e.g., identifying the least expensive way to effectively heal a peptic ulcer).

### Application Areas of Health Economics

- To formulate health services
- To establish the true costs of delivering health care and also estimate all real costs like the use of patients time, loss of output elsewhere in the system.
- To evaluate relative costs and benefits of particular policy.
- To identify determinants of growth and economic development elements of health expenditure by use of macroeconomics.
- To determine the economic characteristics of healthcare and health related activities.
- To find out the source of healthcare financing, social accounting system, self-financing insurance, etc.

## PER CAPITA INCOME AND PURCHASING POWER PARITY

### Per Capita Income

It measures the average income earned per person in a given area (city, region, country, etc.) in a specified year. It is calculated by dividing the area's total income by its total population.

This helps to ascertain a country's development status. It is one of the three measures for calculating the human development index of a country.

### Purchasing Power Parity

*Purchasing power parity* states that the exchange rate between two countries is equal to the ratio of the currencies' respective purchasing power.

The concept of purchasing power parity allows one to estimate what the exchange rate between two currencies would have to be in order for the exchange to be at par with the purchasing power of the two countries' currencies.

### What is a Cost?

Costs can be defined as the value of resources used to produce goods or services.

### Types of Costs

Costs may be:
- Health service costs
- Costs borne by patients and their families (out of pocket expenses)
- External costs borne by the rest of society. Costs can also be divided into:
- **Direct costs:** Where money actually changes hands, e.g., health service use, patient copayments and out of pocket expenses.
- **Indirect costs:** The value of lost productivity from time off work due to illness.
- **Intangible costs:** The "disvalue" to an individual of pain and suffering.
- **Opportunity cost:** The *New Oxford American Dictionary* defines it as "the loss of potential gain from other alternatives when one alternative is chosen." Opportunity cost is a key concept in economics, and has been described as expressing "the basic relationship between scarcity and choice."

### Benefits

Benefits are monetary values of desirable consequences of economic policies and decisions.

### Types

- **Direct**—values of desirable health and non-health outcomes directly related to the implementation of proposed interventions that can be estimated by using market based data.
- **Indirect**—the averted costs and savings resulting from the interventions but not related directly to them.
- **Intangible**—include the values of positive outcomes, (e.g., reduction in health risk, pain and suffering) which cannot be estimated from market data.

**Example:** Vaccination program against infectious disease with effect of herd immunity.
- Savings associated with preventing illness—direct benefit.
- Savings resulting from morbidity among unvaccinated persons due to herd immunity—indirect benefit.
- The reduced risks of catching the infection for those vaccinated and the peace of mind resulting from that risk reduction—intangible benefit.

### Economic Evaluation

Drummond et al. (1997) defines *economic evaluation as "the comparative analysis of alternative courses of action in terms of both their costs and consequences."* It considers both costs and consequences and is comparative.

### Methods of Economic Evaluation

- In *monetary* units: Cost-benefit analysis (CBA)
- In *natural* unit: Cost-effectiveness analysis (CEA)
- In units of *cardinal utility*: Cost-utility analysis
- *Only costs* are compared: Cost-marginal analysis

### Cost-benefit Analysis

The CBA assesses all effects, including health effects, in monetary units. The disadvantage of the CBA is that a monetary assessment of clinical results must be made even though methodologically this is difficult to perform. CBA may ignore many intangible but very important benefits that are difficult to measure in monetary terms, (e.g., relief of anxiety).

The final result is expressed as "cost-benefit ratio" (CBR) which can be calculated in the following way:

$$CBR = \frac{\text{Costs in monetary terms}}{\text{Benefits in monetary terms}}$$

For any intervention, CBR less than 1 is accepted.
An equivalent decision rule is:
Net benefit = Benefits in units of money – cost in units of money > 0

### Cost-effectiveness Analysis

The term "cost-effectiveness analysis" refers to an evaluation where the outcomes are one-dimensional. The costs are

expressed in monetary units and the results in nonmonetary units in CEA. Nonmonetary units may, e.g., be:
- Years of life gained
- Hospital days prevented.

Cost-effectiveness analysis is the most commonly applied form of economic analysis in the health economics literature, and is frequently used in drug therapy. However, it does not allow comparisons to be made between courses of action that have completely different therapeutic outcomes.

### Cost-utility Analysis

The cost-utility analysis (CUO) follows the same principle as the CEA. Costs are assessed in monetary units and the benefit is measured as a nonmonetary but utility-adjusted outcome, the quality-adjusted life year (QALY). The concept combines life expectancy and quality of life. If quality of life is an important aspect of therapy, this form of analysis should be chosen.

### Cost-minimization Analysis

Cost-minimization analysis (CMA) compares only costs of different interventions assuming to provide equal benefits. It is a partial evaluation because only the costs are compared not the benefits.

*Example:* Generic drug versus branded equivalent.

The cheaper intervention will provide the best value for the money. But it is rare for two healthcare interventions to provide exactly the same benefits.

## SUGGESTED READING

1. Basavanthapa BT. Nursing Administration, 2nd edition. New Delhi: Jaypee Brothers Medical Publishers; 2009. pp. 306-17.
2. Briggs A, Claxton K, Sculpher M. Decision modeling for health economic evaluation, 1st edition. New York: Oxford University Press; 2006.
3. Drummond MF, Sculpher MJ, Claxton K, et al. Methods for the Economic Evaluation of Health Care Programs, 4th edition. United Kingdom: Oxford University press; 2015.
4. Folland S, et al. The Economics of Health and Health Care, 4th edition. United Kingdom: Pearson Education; 2008.
5. Gottret P, Schieber G. Health Financing Revisited: A Practitioner's Guide. Washington: The World Bank; 2006.
6. Gupta I. (2013). Health Financing for Universal Coverage. Available from: http://www.nihfw.org/doc/Indrani%20Gupta.pdf.
7. Ministry of Finance. Union Budget 2016-17.
8. Murray CJ, Frenk J. A framework for assessing the performance of health systems. Bull World Health Organ. 2000;78(6):717-31.
9. National Institutes of Health. Health Economics Information Resources: A Self-Study Course. Available from: https:// www.nlm.nih.gov/nichsr/edu/healthecon/beginningend.pdf.

# D. HEALTH SYSTEM RESEARCH

*Pranab Chatterjee, Bhavna Seth, Abhimanyu Singh Chauhan*

## INTRODUCTION

For decades, health care has been structured by vertical programs, targeting specific diseases with disease-specific interventions. This was a viable approach, when a limited number of public health problems needed to be addressed in a short sequence of time, particularly with a focus on bringing down morbidity and mortality rapidly. This approach served India and some other developing nations well when the focus was on limiting deaths and disease counts. However, as these programs began to grow, it was noted that there were several activities, which led to cross-disease benefits, and many of these were either duplicated, or not conducted well, under the belief that it would be addressed by other programmatic approaches. For example, although interventions to improve access to water, sanitation, and hygiene (WaSH) may primarily be targeted for combating diarrheal diseases, they will have a positive impact on vector-borne diseases (by eliminating breeding sites), maternal and child health (by reducing morbidity and mortality), and gender issues (by providing women with safe access to WaSH). Moreover, from a clinical standpoint, patients do not pick and choose what diseases they shall have, and a health system must be robust enough to provide basic quality services that meet the needs of its population.

We are realizing the growing need and importance of investing in and planning for improved health systems, i.e., ensuring all parts of healthcare delivery are able to meet the needs of the population it serves, in a sustainable and resilient fashion.

## WHAT IS A HEALTH SYSTEM?

A system is an arrangement of parts and their interconnections, which are brought together to execute a common purpose. A system, which is concerned with the people's health, therefore, is the simplest way to view a health system.

The WHO describes a good health system as one that, "delivers quality services to all people, when and where they need them. The exact configuration of services varies from country to country, but in all cases requires a robust financing mechanism; a well-trained and adequately paid workforce; reliable information on which to base decisions and policies; well-maintained facilities and logistics to deliver quality medicines and technologies" (*Refer* also **Box 44D.1** for WHO definition of health systems).

**Box 44D.1: WHO definition of health systems.**

A health system consists of all organizations, people, and actions whose primary intent is to promote, restore, or maintain health. This includes efforts to influence determinants of health as well as more direct health-improving activities. A health system is, therefore, more than the pyramid of publicly owned facilities that deliver personal health services. It includes, e.g., a mother caring for a sick child at home; private providers; behavior change programmes; vector-control campaigns; health insurance organizations; and occupational health and safety legislation. It includes inter-sectoral action by health staff, e.g., encouraging the ministry of education to promote female education, a well-known determinant of better health.

## Components of Health Systems

### The 4-S Model

Dr Paul Farmer describes a 4-S model for components needed to deliver quality healthcare.
- Stuff (resources, e.g., medications, technology, and transport)
- Staff (physicians, nurses, community health worker—both appropriate numbers and competent and well-trained)
- Space (facilities—hospital)
- Systems (protocols and flow of care from contact to discharge from a healthcare system)

### Systems Thinking and the DEPLESET Framework

The "systems thinking" approach to health systems analysis framework incorporates the context within which the health system functions including the "demographic, economic, political, legal, regulatory, epidemiological, sociodemographic, and technological" contexts ("DEPLESET"). Additionally, complex interactions between health system elements and the contextual factors occur, to form the concept of "health system behavior", each of which are complex, dynamic interactions, working from the inputs, and processes to outcomes.

## WHY HEALTH SYSTEMS RESEARCH?

As the previous discussion highlights, health systems function through complex, multidisciplinary mechanisms, and can result into a wide spectrum of impacts, depending on the efficiency of the system. To ensure that improved outcomes are reached, it is essential to generate improved knowledge and evidence base, using which the systems may be informed or modified. To that end, it becomes essential to undertake health systems research to generate this information.

There has been a growing need to understand healthcare priorities and devise healthcare interventions, to enable healthcare improvements and to deliver equitable, quality healthcare with better outcomes. Research on these questions helps determine effective strategies to understand these complex interactions is needed to guide, "evidence-based-policy" recommendations are needed.

## WHAT IS HEALTH SYSTEMS RESEARCH?

Health systems research can address any or several components (service delivery, information and evidence, medical products and technology, healthcare workforce, health financing, leadership, and governance). The objective is to improve the coverage, quality, efficiency, and equity of health systems (i.e., enhance health outcomes and financial protection). **Figure 44D.1**, adopted from the guideline document developed by the WHO's Alliance for the Health Systems and Policy Research (AHSPR), demarcates the various domains of health systems research. **Box 44D.2** outlines the definition endorsed by them.

# Section 4: Community Health Management

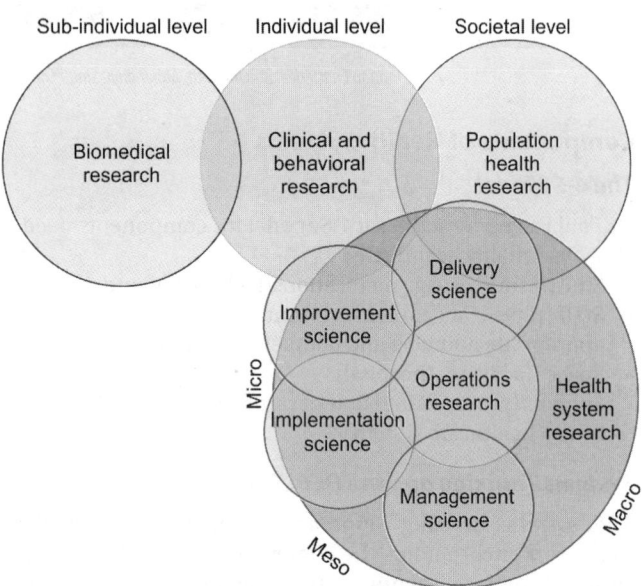

**Fig. 44D.1:** Domains of health systems research.
*Source:* Gilson, 2012.

> **Box 44D.2: Definition of health systems research (Gilson, 2012).**
> Health systems research is a multidisciplinary field of health research which studies governance, financial, and delivery arrangements for health care and public health services, implementation considerations for reforming or strengthening these arrangements, and broader economic, legal, political and social contexts in which these arrangements are negotiated and operated. The purpose of health systems research is to improve the understanding and performance of health systems. Health systems research includes all of health services research, most health policy research, and some clinical and population health research, but does not include any biomedical research.

## METHODS OF HEALTH SYSTEMS RESEARCH

Health systems research incorporates a wide range of study designs and methods. Health systems research has been classified into two major types by the WHO's AHSPR:

1. ***Fixed strategies:*** Designs fixed prior to initiation of data collection; and
2. ***Flexible strategies:*** Designs which evolve in course of the conduct of the study.

The basic tenets of these two strategies are summarized in **Table 44D.1**.

## DOMAINS OF HEALTH SYSTEMS RESEARCH

Though there is a diverse set of models characterizing health systems and health systems research, the common theme is that, broadly speaking, there are three domains under which health systems and policy research can be grouped:

1. Operational research
2. Implementation research
3. Health systems improvement research

**Table 44D.2** summarizes each of these domains with a specific research question as an example for each.

## BENEFITS OF HEALTH SYSTEMS RESEARCH AND USING HEALTH SYSTEMS RESEARCH OUTPUTS

Usage of health system research outputs is based on the domains of research described above. Research outputs may broadly include the following—publications highlighting the results; protocols; research posters; policy papers; reports, etc. Outputs from operational research would have the largest consumer base, with primary users being healthcare

**Table 44D.1:** Comparison of fixed and flexible study designs for health systems research.

| | *Fixed strategies* | *Flexible strategies* |
|---|---|---|
| A priori nature | Design fixed prior to initiation of data collection | Design may be evolved or modified based on intelligence obtained in course of data collection |
| Approach to study design | Positivist approaches preferred | Interpretivist approaches preferred |
| Usual objectives | To measure the effect or impact of a phenomenon (e.g., a healthcare intervention, a policy update, etc.) on specified health outcomes, in highly controlled and defined settings | To understand why an observed phenomenon is occurring |
| Nature of data collected | Generally quantitative | Generally qualitative |
| Statistical analyzes employed | Modeling and regressions for predictive analysis | Iterative and interpretive qualitative data analysis methods |
| Common data collection techniques | Surveys, structured and semi-structured interviews, routine vital statistics, epidemiological/ecologic data, record reviews, etc. | Qualitative methods, such as case study, grounded theory, ethnographic, life histories and phenomenological research |
| Example | Impact of the introduction of the Weekly Iron Folate Supplementation program on anemia in adolescent girls in a specific area | Reasons for discontinuation of DOTS in defaulter TB patients lost to follow-up in RNTCP in a specified area |

*Source:* Hoffman et al., 2012.

**Table 44D.2:** Domains of health systems research with examples.

| Domain | Characteristics | Examples |
|---|---|---|
| Operational research | • Develop solutions to ongoing issues in operational problems of a specific health program or a health service delivery unit<br>• Usually affect a localized area and needs to be addressed urgently<br>• Research needs often arise from issues identified through monitoring and evaluation activities | • Can the "communication for behavioral impact" (COMBI) strategy improve the poor compliance with mass drug administration for lymphatic filariasis elimination in Tamil Nadu? |

*Contd...*

Contd...

| Domain | Characteristics | Examples |
|---|---|---|
| | • Many types of study designs may be employed—from mathematical modeling, to operational experiments (RCTs), and analytical or descriptive studies | • Which locations should be targeted for providing HIV prevention services to adolescents and young adults in Mysuru district? |
| Implementation research | • Develop strategies/interventions to improve access of target population to existing programs and/or interventions<br>• Research needs arise from an existing program/intervention which is proven efficacious, but needs to be scaled up and integrated in existing systems<br>• Needs innovative approaches<br>• Usually conducted in two phases—in first phase descriptive and formative approaches used to identify the implementation challenges and devise interventions to address them; in second phase the developed interventions are then deployed and evaluated for efficacy<br>• Multidisciplinary research methods, with extensive use of social science techniques employed—such as stakeholder analysis, process mapping, qualitative research, critical pathway research, etc. | • Identify and evaluate strategies to improve vaccination coverage rates in children who are currently not reached by vaccination services under the universal immunization program<br>• Programmatic operationalization of oral cholera vaccines in hotspots of cholera outbreak using existing public health delivery systems to reduce outbreak frequency and case burden |
| Health systems improvement research | • Addresses research questions which are not disease or pathology specific but affect the systems as a whole and has implications on the performance of the system<br>• Highly multidisciplinary research, with a strong need for participation of experts from the social sciences, health economics, behavioral sciences, policy research, and anthropology<br>• Usually employ descriptive, comparative or evaluative approaches; may employ secondary data analysis plans<br>• According to the AHSPR, main goal is "The production of new knowledge to improve how societies organize themselves to achieve health goals" | • How effective are different incentive-based strategies to attract nurses to rural areas?<br>• What has been the impact of the Ebola Virus Disease epidemic on maternal and child health services and indicators in Western African countries? |

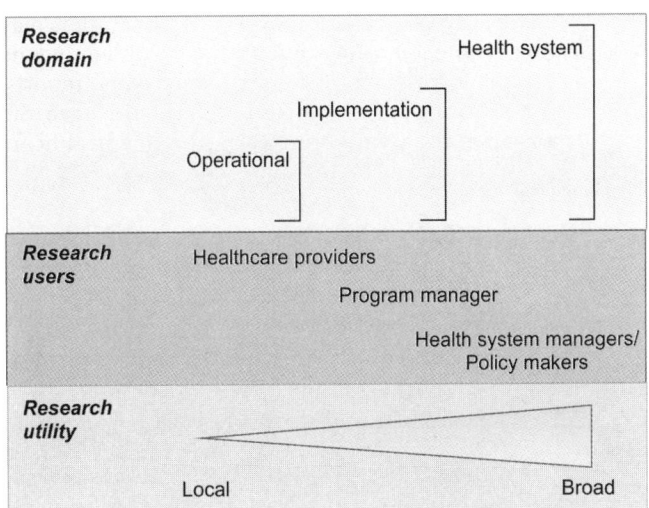

Fig. 44D.2: Health systems research and its users.

providers. Implementation research, by the dint of its nature, is of primary interest to program managers, especially those who are tasked with scaling up a program or an intervention. Research on health systems, either as a holistic whole or on some components of the system, are largely of interest to policy makers. The process of usage of health systems research outputs is summarized in **Figure 44D.2**.

# HEALTH SYSTEM RESILIENCE

"A resilient system has the capacity to absorb change due to external or internal shocks, maintain original functions and ensure long-term sustainability". Shocks, e.g., natural disasters (earthquakes, floods) or man-made disasters (such as wars, refugee migration) represent shocks to a health system, threatening the continuity of service delivery and destabilizing governance. A resilient health system is one designed and able to sustain such shocks, and prevent or contain disease outbreaks and maintain functional health institutions while sustaining achievements. Human resource, financing, governance, and service provision are key components that facilitate the creation of a resilient health system.

In the face of the changing global geopolitical scenario, emergent threats due to climate change and the ever-looming shadow of pandemics, it is more important now, than ever, to invest in resilient systems.

# SUGGESTED READING

1. Chang AY, Ogbuoji O, Atun R, Verguet S. Dynamic modeling approaches to characterize the functioning of health systems: a systematic review of the literature. Soc Sci Med. 2017;194:160-7.
2. Gilson L. Alliance for health policy and systems research. In: Gilson L (Ed). Health Policy and Systems Research: A Methodology Reader, 1st edition. Geneva: World Health Organization; 2012.
3. Health Systems and Services. (2007). Everybody's Business: Strengthening Health Systems to Improve Health Outcomes WHO's Framework for Action. Geneva: World Health Organization.
4. Hoffman SJ, Røttingen J, Bennett S, Lavis JN, Edge JS, Frenk J. Background Paper on Conceptual Issues Related to Health Systems Research to Inform a WHO Global Strategy on Health Systems Research. Ontario, Canada: World Health Organization; 2012.
5. Kruk ME, Myers M, Varpilah ST, Dahn BT. What is a resilient health system? Lessons from Ebola. Lancet. 2015;385(9980):1910-2.
6. Remme JH, Adam T, Becerra-Posada F, D'Arcangues C, Devlin M, Gardner C, et al. Defining research to improve health systems. PLoS Med. 2010;7(11):e1001000.

# SECTION 5

# Managing Community Health in India

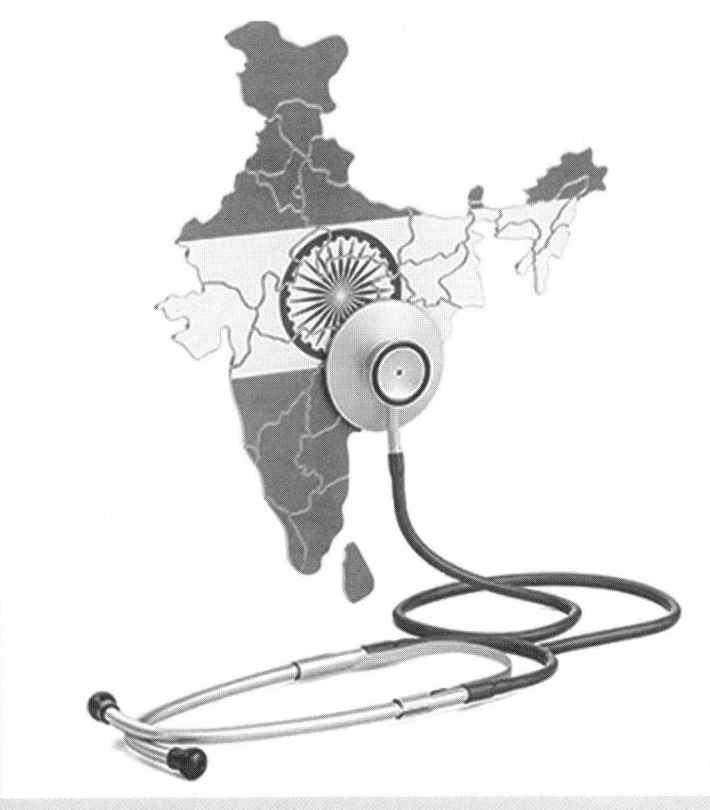

*"Healthy community makes healthy India."*

# SECTION OUTLINE

45. Health Situation in India
46. Indian Healthcare System
47. Health Policies and Programs in India
48. Monitoring and Evaluation System in India
49. Health Legislations in India
50. Indian Healthcare Agencies
51. Special Topics

# CHAPTER 45

# Health Situation in India

*Prakash Patel*

**CM10.1** Describe the current status of reproductive, maternal, newborn and child health

Numerous health problems are affecting the growth and development of India. Many people suffer and die because of many preventable and easily curable diseases. Health is the right of the people, and government of the country is responsible for looking after the health and health needs of the people living in the country. For managing health of the people, every country shall have health policy, health programs, healthcare delivery system, and health legislation. Under the constitutional provisions, the government of India owes protection of health of people and providing preventive, promotive, curative, and rehabilitative healthcare services to everyone. To bear these responsibilities, India has a huge network of healthcare delivery system. To manage the health of citizens, Government of India is framing various health policies, designing, and executing health programs as per the health needs of the people. It promulgates health legislations and enforces them to guard the health of Indians. Study of existing Indian healthcare delivery system, various health policies, health programs, and health legislations can give understanding about how the health of people are protected, and health problems affecting the people at a large are managed.

Despite having good economic progress in past few decades, India continues to face challenges of poverty and poor health. Though the country achieved remarkable progress in health-related indicators in past few decades, much still remains to be achieved.

## REPRODUCTIVE AND MATERNAL HEALTH

India has achieved a lot in improving the maternal health. The maternal mortality rate (MMR) is considered as a good indicator of maternal health as well as maternal healthcare services in the country. According to the special bulletin on maternal mortality in India 2018–20, sample registration system (SRS) report, the MMR in India declined from 167 in 2011–13 to 113 in 2016–18 and currently it is 97 in 2018–20 per 100,000 live births. The maternal healthcare services across the country showed significant progress in indicators like institutional deliveries and antenatal care (ANC) coverage. According to National Family Health Survey (NFHS-5, 2019–21) the institutional deliveries rate in India are 88.6% indicating that pregnant women coming to institutions for delivery are in good number. However, early antenatal registration (first ANC in first trimester) was only 58.6% in 2015–16 which has improved to 70.0% in 2019–21 and mothers who had 4 antenatal care visits was 58.1% in the year 2019–21.

As per NFHS-5 (2019–21), the contraceptive usage rate among the currently married women aged 15–49 using any of the modern methods was 66.7%. Adolescent fertility is not so uncommon. Adolescent birth rate is 43 per 1,000 women aged 15–19 years during 2019–21.

## CHILD HEALTH

Infant mortality rate (IMR) is a well-accepted proxy for quality of health system of a country. India was able to reduce IMR significantly to 28 per 1,000 live births in 2020 (SRS 2020 report, published in May 2022). India has very high burden of malnutrition among children. Approximately 36% of below 5 year children living in India are stunted (low height for age), 19% are wasted (low weight for height) and 32% are underweight (NFHS-5). Proportion of severely wasted children also went up from 6.4 to 7.7% from NFHS-3 to NFHS-5. India was placed at high end of "serious" category in global hunger index (GHI) severity scale, and ranked 107th out of 121 countries in 2022 (globalhungerindex.org). This was mainly due to the fact that under the age of 5 years, one out of every 5 children is "wasted" (low weight for height). Apart from the undernutrition, the important nutritional problems include xerophthalmia and iodine deficiency disorder.

## AGING

India reported exponential rise in elderly population which is mainly due to impressive increased life expectancy. Elderly population in actual number will reach to 17.3 crore in 2026 as projected by United Nations Population Fund. This data only shows the tip of the iceberg. This demographic transition marked with wide variation across the states and different social strata. Considering high rate of morbidity and mortality, rising elderly population in any society put extra pressure on available resources and it demands holistic approach including policy changes, social reform, and healthcare provision.

## INFECTIOUS DISEASES

Communicable diseases continue to be a major public health problem in India. Tuberculosis, malaria, and HIV are among the most important infectious disease in the country. **Tuberculosis** continues to pose threat to the health of people in the country and become lethal with concurrent HIV infection. Due to consistent TB surveillance effort in India, a record high notification of 24.2 lakh cases was seen in 2022; an increase of over 13% as compared to 2021 (India TB Annual Report 2023). A total of 63801 Multi Drug Resistant/Rifampicin Resistant (MDR/RR) TB cases were notified and 57,749 (91%) of them put on treatment. The HIV coinfection rate among incident TB patients is estimated to be 3.4%. TB comorbidities, especially HIV, Diabetes and Tobacco have been prioritized in NTEP. Over 94% of People Living with HIV (PLHIV) are being screened in ART centers for TB symptoms. Over 60% of the notified TB patients in the public sector have been screened for blood sugar.

Significant reduction has been observed in the **malaria** morbidity and mortality due to malaria in recent years. Cases declined from 2.03 million in 2000 to 1.13 million in 2015 and 0.17 million in 2022 and deaths declined by approximately 71% to 83 in 2022 from 287 in 2015. Proportion of *P. falciparum* cases remained approximately 57% during 2022. However, proportion of *P. falciparum* cases rose as time progresses which was contributed by increased Pf detection by widespread use of rapid diagnostic tests (NVDCP Official Website).

**HIV** prevalence in adult population, between 15 and 45 years was 0.21% (0.17–0.25%) in 2021. In the same year, HIV prevalence in adult male was estimated at 0.22% (0.18–0.28%) and in adult female was estimated at 0.19% (0.15–0.23%). The adult HIV prevalence in India has constantly declined from an estimated peak of 0.38% in the year 2001–03 through 0.34% in the year 2007 and 0.28% in the year 2012 to 0.21% in the year 2021. Similar consistent declines were recorded both in males and females in India. The total numbers of individuals infected with HIV in India were estimated to be 24.01 lakh (ranging from 19.92 lakh to 29.07 lakh) in 2021 whereas it was 22.26 lakh (ranging from 18.00 to 27.85 lakh) in the year 2007. There were 41.97 thousand (ranging from 26.50–67.45) deaths observed in 2021 (India HIV estimates 2021 factsheet).

**Diarrheal diseases** remain important cause of morbidity and mortality in children below 5 years of age. Around 10.76 million cases of diarrhea occur every year. Poor sanitary and hygienic condition continues to pose threat of diarrheal epidemic across the whole country. As reported by NFHS-5, 7.3% children under 5 years reported diarrhea in past 15 days in the year 2019–21. Another infection causing major mortality and morbidity in under-five children is acute respiratory infections (ARI) which caused 31.7 million episodes and 3,278 deaths in 2013. In 2019–21, according to NFHS-5, 2.8% children under 5 years reported ARI in past 15 days.

Along with these above mentioned infections, leprosy, filaria, Kala-azar, meningitis, viral hepatitis, Japanese encephalitis, dengue fever, enteric fever, and helminthic infestations are among the other important infectious diseases of public health importance in India.

## NONCOMMUNICABLE DISEASES

India is observing a significant rise in burden of noncommunicable disease (NCDs) in past few decades. NCDs cause increased morbidity and mortality across all the population subgroups leading to considerable loss in productive years of life. Now more than half (53%) death in India are accounted by NCDs mainly cardiovascular diseases, cancer, diabetes, and chronic respiratory diseases. Rising mortality due to NCDs place them ahead of other causes of mortality like injuries, communicable diseases, maternal, prenatal, and nutritional conditions. According to a recent estimate in 2016, probability of dying from any of cardiovascular diseases (CVD), cancer, diabetes or chronic respiratory disease in age group of 30 to 70 years is 23.3% in India (Global Health Estimates, 2016, WHO).

In comparison with the people of European origin, Indian develops CVD at least a decade earlier and during their highest productive period of life. According to the Global Burden of Disease study age-standardized estimates (2016), more than one forth (28.1%) of all deaths in India are caused by CVD.

According to NFHS-5 data, the estimated prevalence of hypertension (Systolic >140 mm of Hg and/or diastolic >90 mm of Hg or taking medicine to control blood pressure) amongst India's population aged more than 15 years is 21.3% in women and 24.0% in men. Earlier diabetes was considered as mild disease affecting mainly elderly, which, over the past thirty year, become one of the important cause of mortality and morbidity affecting young and middle aged people as well. According to NFHS-5 in population aged 15 and above prevalence of blood sugar level—high or very high (>140 mg/dL) or taking medicine to control blood sugar level is 13.5% in women and 15.6% in men, making it greatest noncommunicable epidemics.

Breast cancer, uterine cervical cancer, and cancer of lip/oral cavity are the three most commonly occurring cancers in India. They, together, account for nearly 33% of all cancers in India, and thus need to be tackled as a public health priority. Breast cancer is one of the leading causes of cancer among female (13.5%) with 1,78,361 new cases and 94,408 mortality as reported in 2020. Oral cancer accounts for around 10.3% of all cancers in India. Cervical cancer in India is the third most common cancer in India (9.4%). Every year, around 1.23 lakh new women are diagnosed with cervical cancer and 77348 of these women die of the disease in India. with 1,35,929 new cases and 75,290 deaths reported in 2020 (Globocan 2020). According to NFHS-5 (2019–21) 8.9% of women age 15 years and above and 38 % of men age 15 years and above use any kind of Tobacco. For Alcohol, 1.3% of women age 15 years and above and 18.8% of men age 15 years and above consume alcohol. Mental health is an important integral part of health and is more than just the absence of mental illnesses. In India, as per WHO estimate, mental health problems lead to 2,443 disability-adjusted life year (DALYs) per 100,000 populations. The age-adjusted suicide rate per 100,000 populations is 21.1. It is estimated that the economic loss due to mental health illnesses in India between the years 2012 and 2030 is 1.03 trillion dollars at 2010 currency exchange rate (Mental Health in India Factsheet, WHO).

## INJURIES AND VIOLENCE

Morbidity and mortality due to road traffic accident are one of the foremost and mounting public health problems in India. In India, reportedly, 153,972 people died and 384,448 people got injured in 2021 due to road accidents. These figures translate, on an average, into 1,130 accidents and 422 deaths every day or 47 accidents and 18 deaths every hour in the country (Road accidents in India Report 2021, MORTCH).

Apart from road traffic accidents, domestic accidents also put a great threat to health of the people in India. Drowning is the 3rd leading cause of unintentional injury/death; drowning is the third leading cause that accounts for 7% of all injury-related mortalities. According to an estimate, more than one million people in India are moderately or severely burnt every year. Fall, snakebite, unintentional poisoning, violence, and industrial accidents are other important causes of injury leading to death. Agriculture-related accidents are also important health issue. Agriculture workers are most vulnerable to occupational injuries having estimated incidence rate of 116/100,000 workers. Homicide and suicide are also fairly common in India. India reported mortality rate of 4.1/100,000 population in 2016 and in the same year suicide mortality rate of 16.3/100,000 population was reported (Global Health Estimates 2016).

## ENVIRONMENTAL RISKS

Exposures to environmental risk factors remain an important source of health risk in developing countries such as India, where weak environmental policies, poverty, and lack of infrastructure combine to cause high level of pollution. Environmental risk factors are one of the most difficult health issues to deal with in India.

In India, mortality rate attributed to exposure to unsafe water, sanitation, and hygiene (WASH) services was 18.6/100,000 population in 2016. Age-standardized mortality rate attributed to indoor and outdoor air pollution was 184.3/100,000 population in 2016 (Global Health Observatory data, WHO).

## OCCUPATIONAL HEALTH AND SAFETY

India is growing economy. Working age population in the country is above half billion. For the entire country, researcher have estimated approximately 45,000 occupational fatalities, another 17 Million occupational injuries and 1.9 million occupational diseases (NIHFW national portal for National Program for Prevention and Control of Occupational Diseases, 2014). This figure may be underestimate considering the fact that nearly 90% workers are working in unorganized sector where data are not properly maintained. Only around 10% engaged in organized sector and they are covered by existing health and safety legislation. There is enormous need for action to improve the health and safety of the workers requiring concerted national and local action.

## SUMMARY

| Sl. No. | Indicator | Current status |
|---|---|---|
| 1. | Crude death rate | 6.0/1,000 population (SRS 2020, Bulletin 2022) |
| 2. | Maternal mortality ratio | 97/100,000 live birth (SRS Special Bulletin 2018–20) |
| 3. | Percentage of institutional delivery | 88.6% (NFHS-5, 2019–21) |
| 4. | Infant mortality rate | 28/1,000 live birth (SRS 2020, Bulletin 2022) |
| 5. | Neonatal mortality rate | 20/1,000 live birth (SRS 2020 Report) |
| 6. | Under 5 mortality rate | 32/1,000 live birth (SRS 2020 Report) |
| 7. | Children under 5 years who are stunted (height-for-age) | 35.5% (NFHS-5, 2019–21) |
| 8. | Children under 5 years who are wasted (weight-for-height) | 19.3% (NFHS-5, 2019–21) |
| 9. | Children under 5 years who are severely wasted (weight-for-height) | 7.7% (NFHS-5, 2019–21) |
| 10. | Prevalence of diarrhea in under-5 children | 7.3% (NFHS-5, 2019–21) |
| 11. | Total fertility rate | 2.0 (SRS 2020 Report) |
| 12. | Incidence of TB | 188/100,000 population (2021) |
| 13. | Case fatality rate of TB | 4% (2019) |
| 14. | Malaria cases | 0.17 million (2022, NVBDCP Official Website) |
| 15. | Malaria death | 83 (2022, NVBDCP Official Website) |
| 16. | People living with HIV | 24.01 lakh (2021, India HIV Estimates 2021) |
| 17. | Adult HIV prevalence (15–45 years) | 0.21% (2021, India HIV Estimates 2021) |
| 18. | New HIV cases | 62.97 thousand (2021, India HIV Estimates 2021) |
| 19. | AIDS related deaths | 41.97 thousand (2021) |
| 20. | Deaths due to road traffic accidents | 1.53 lakh (2021) |
| 21. | Age-standardized mortality rate attributed to indoor and outdoor air pollution | 184.3/100,000 population (2016) |

## SUGGESTED READING

1. Global Health Estimates 2016: Deaths by Cause, Age, Sex, by Country and by Region, 2000-2016. Geneva: World Health Organization; 2018. Available from: https://www.who.int/healthinfo/ global_burden_disease/en/.
2. Srinath Reddy K, Shah B, Varghese C, Ramadoss A. Responding to the threat of chronic diseases in India. Lancet. 2005;366(9498):17449.
3. WHO (2018). In: WHO Global Report on Trends in Prevalence of Tobacco Smoking 2000-2025, 2nd edition. Geneva: World Health Organization.
4. World Health Organization. Mental Health in India. Available from: http://www.searo.who.int/india/topics/mental_health/about_mentalhealth/en/.
5. World Health Organization. Public Health and Environment. Global Health Observatory (GHO) Data. Geneva: World Health Organization. Available from: http://www.who.int/gho/phe/en/.

# CHAPTER 46

# Indian Healthcare System

*Kaushik Lodhiya, Dipesh Zalavadiya*

**CM17.5** Describe health care delivery in India

## HEALTH IN THE CONSTITUTION OF INDIA

Health is basic requirement of human being. Everyone has the right to the highest attainable standard of health which includes access to all medical services, proper housing, adequate sanitation, clean environment, adequate food, and healthy working conditions. A system of health protection for all is there guaranteed by human right to health. The human right to health care means that clinics, hospitals, medicines and doctors services must be available, accessible, acceptable, on an equitable basis, where and when needed.

Health is a fundamental human right as per Article 21. It is to be earned and maintained by the individual. There are many responsibilities which everyone should exercise in order to achieve optimum health. These are responsibilities regarding personal health, e.g. diet, care of teeth, skin, recreation, exercise, cultivation of healthful habits, immunization, and reporting early when falling sick. The responsibility for health rests also upon the community, society and state. As per the Constitution of India, health is a state responsibility. The state government is responsible for providing health services and implementation of health-related program. The Constitution also provides equal opportunity to citizens for employment to any state run healthcare institutions; not only the state, but also panchayat, and municipalities liable to improve and protect public health. Different components of right to health include: Right to appropriate healthcare; right to an adequate supply of water, food, nutrition and housing; right to healthy environment and healthy working condition; right to material, child and reproductive health; right to participate in health-related decision making; and right to access health-related information.

## EVOLUTION OF INDIAN HEALTHCARE SYSTEM

### Health Care During Ancient India

Ayurveda the oldest medical system in the world emphasized the need of healthy lifestyle including good diet, cleanliness, purity, proper behavior, mental, and physical discipline in ancient India. Around 100 BC Charaka has described the objectives of medicine in Charaka Samhita as of good health and combating disease. Medical education was started in the ancient universities of Taxshila and Nalanda during 600 BC–600 AD but with the passage of time, ancient universities disappeared.

**Health Care Before Independence**

**1881:** The first all India Census was taken, the first Indian Factories Act was passed.
**1897:** The Epidemic Disease Act was passed for the control and prevention of epidemic or spread of epidemic.
**1946:** Bhore Committee (The Health Survey Development Committee) submitted its report.

### Healthcare System in the Postindependence Era

Recommendations of Bhore Committee form the basis for future development of health in country. Major events in the healthcare system are as follows:

**1951:** The BCG vaccination programme was launched; first five-year plan began
**1953:** The National Malaria Control Programme and family planning programme initiated.
**1954:** The National Leprosy Control Programme and the National Water Supply and Sanitation Programme initiated; the Prevention of Food Adulteration Act was passed.
**1955:** The National Filaria Control Programme initiated.
**1958:** The National Malaria Control Programme was converted into National Malaria Eradication Programme.
**1962:** The National Smallpox Eradication Programme, The School Health Programme and The National Goitre Control Programme were launched. The District Tuberculosis Programme was formulated.
**1963:** The Applied Nutrition Programme, The National Trachoma Control Programme and Extended Family Planning Programme were launched
**1969:** The Central Births and Deaths Registration Act was passed.
**1971:** The Medical Termination of Pregnancy Act was passed by the parliament.
**1973:** The National Programme of Minimum Needs was incorporated in the fifth five-year plan.
**1975:** Integrated Child Development Service (ICDS) was launched on 2nd October, 1975.

**1976:** National Programme for Prevention of Blindness was formulated.
**1977:** Rural health scheme and Reorientation of Medical Education (ROME) was launched.
**1978:** Expanded Programme of Immunization was launched. Implementation of Oral Rehydration Therapy.
**1983:** National Leprosy Control Programme renamed to National Leprosy Eradication Programme. Guinea Worm Eradication Programme was launched.
**1985:** Universal Immunization Programme was launched. A separate Department of Women and Child Development was set up.
**1987:** National AIDS Control Programme and National Diabetes Control Programme initiated.
**1989:** Blood Safety Programme was launched.
**1992:** Child Survival and Safe Motherhood Programme (CSSM) was launched. The Infant Milk Substitute, Feeding Bottles and Infant Foods (Regulation of Production, Supply and Distribution) Act came into force.
**1993:** Revised National Tuberculosis Programme with DOTS introduced. National Nutrition Policy was formulated.
**1996:** Pulse Polio Immunization was initiated. Target free approach was adopted for Family Planning Programme.
**1997:** Reproductive and Child Health Programme (RCH) was launched.
**1998:** National Malaria Eradication Programme renamed as National Anti-Malaria Programme.
**2000:** National Population Policy 2000 was launched.
**2003:** National Vector Borne Disease Control Programme was approved. Cigarettes and other Tobacco Products (Prohibition, Regulation of Trade and Commerce, Production, Supply and Distribution) Act was passed.
**2004:** Mid-day meal scheme and Integrated Disease Surveillance Programme (IDSP) was launched.
**2005:** RCH II, National Rural Health Mission (NRHM), Janani Suraksha Yojana (JSY) were launched.
**2006:** Integrated Management of Neonatal and Childhood Illness (IMNCI) was launched.
**2008:** 108 Ambulance Project was launched. Noncommunicable Disease Programme was launched.
**2013:** National Health Mission (NHM), Reproductive Maternal Neonatal Childhood and Adolescent Health (RMNCH+A), Rashtriya Bal Swasthya Karykram (RBSK) were launched.
**2014:** Indian Newborn Action Plan, Mission Indradhanush and Swachh Bharat Abhiyan were launched.
**2015:** NITI Aayog replaced Planning Commission. Pradhan Mantri Jeevan Jyoti Bima Yojana and Pradhan Mantri Suraksha Bima Yojana were launched. Kayakalp initiative was started. Jan Aushadhi Yojana and Electronic Vaccine Intelligence Network (eVIN) started.
**2016:** Pradhan Mantri Surakshit Matritva Abhiyan launched.
**2017:** National Health Policy was launched.
**2018:** Ayushman Bharat—National Health Protection Mission initiated.

# NATIONAL HEALTH PLANNING

Provision of quality health services to the whole nation is difficult task. Expensive illness and high health care cost can drive nonpoor into poverty. Increasing demand of healthcare services with limited resources has led to health planning. World Health Organization has defined health planning as "The orderly process of defining health problems, identifying unmet needs and surveying the resources to meet them, establishing priority goals that are realistic and feasible, and projecting administrative action, concerned not only with the adequacy, efficacy and efficiency of health services but also with those factors of ecology and of social and individual behavior that affect the health of the individual and the community". Recommendations of Bhore Committee considered as a milestone for health planning in India. The various **national health committee, five-year plans and now NITI Aayog** are important for health planning in India.

# NATIONAL HEALTH COMMITTEES

The government has appointed various committees of experts starting from preindependence era to advocate about different health problems of the country. Their suggestions and reports are cornerstones for health planning in India. The important national health committees include:
1. Bhore Committee, 1946
2. Mudaliar Committee, 1962
3. Chadha Committee, 1963
4. Mukherjee Committee, 1965
5. Mukherjee Committee, 1966
6. Jungalwalla Committee, 1967
7. Kartar Singh Committee, 1973
8. Shrivastava Committee, 1975
9. Bajaj Committee, 1986

## Bhore Committee, 1946

The committee also known as The Health Survey and Development Committee was appointed by the Government of India in October 1943 under chairmanship of Sir Joseph Bhore to make survey of current position in regards to health conditions and healthcare organization and to give suggestions for future developments. The committee laid down many important recommendations in its final report in 1946.

### Important Recommendations of the Committee

- Integration of preventive, promotive and curative services at all administrative levels.
- Concept of primary health center (PHC) was given by the committee. Each PHC to cater 40,000 population including three subcenters (SCs). Each PHC to be manned by two doctors, one nurse, four public health nurses, four midwives, four trained dais, two sanitary inspectors, two health assistants, one pharmacist and 15 other class IV employees. Secondary health center [now called community health center (CHC)] was also proposed to provide support to PHCs in terms of referral, coordinating and supervisory institutions.
- In the long-term (3 million plan), the committee recommended one PHC with 75 beds and serving 10,000–20,000 populations and secondary level hospitals with 650 beds and District hospital (tertiary level hospital) with 2,500 beds.
- Three months training in preventive and social medicine to prepare "social physicians".
- Committee also proposed development of national health programmes.

## Mudaliar Committee, 1962

The Government of India in 1959 appointed a committee chaired by Dr AL Mudaliar. This committee also known as the "Health Survey and Planning Committee", was appointed for making recommendations for future expansion of health services.

### Important Recommendations of the Committee

- Strengthening of established PHCs before new ones are opened.
- Strengthening of district and subdivisional hospitals with specialist services.
- Regional organizations having in charge as Regional Deputy or Assistant Directors to be established in each state to supervise two to three district health and medical officers.
- Emphasis was given that a PHC should not serve to more than 40,000 population and that the preventive, promotive and curative services should be all provided at the PHC.
- Integration of medical and health services.
- An All India Health Service should be created to replace the Indian Medical Service.

## Chadha Committee, 1963

This committee was appointed under chairmanship of Dr MS Chadha, then the Director General of Health Services, to advise about the necessary arrangements for the maintenance phase of National Malaria Eradication Programme (NMEP).

### Important Recommendations of the Committee

- For every 10,000 population one basic health worker (multi-Purpose worker) was recommended.
- Strict vigilance and monitoring of implementation of NMEP is to be carried out by basic health workers.
- Basic health workers should visit house to house to implement malaria activities once in a month.
- Basic health worker to take additional duties of family planning, collection of vital statistics under supervision of the Family Planning Health Assistants (one per 3–4 basic health workers).

## Mukherjee Committee, 1965

After implementation of Chadha Committee's recommendations, it was observed that basic health workers could not function effectively due to multiple functions and could not do justice to malaria work or to family planning work. Under the chairmanship of the then Secretary of Health Shri Mukherjee, a committee was appointed to review the performance in the area of family planning.

### Important Recommendations of the Committee

- Separate staff for the family planning programme.
- The family planning assistants were to perform family planning duties only.
- The basic health workers were to be utilized for all purposes except for family planning.
- Delink the family planning from malaria activities so that the former would receive undivided attention of its staff.

## Mukherjee Committee, 1966

Shortage of fund led to difficulty to undertake effectively multiple activities of the mass programme, such as NMEP (maintenance phase), family planning, leprosy, smallpox, trachoma, etc. Under the chairmanship of the Union Health Secretary, Shri Mukherjee, a committee of state health secretaries was set up to look into this problem.

The committee worked out the details regarding Basic Health Service which should be provided at the block level, and some consequential strengthening required at higher levels of administration.

## Jungalwalla Committee, 1967

Under the chairmanship of Dr N Jungalwalla, the then Director of National Institute of Health Administration and Education (currently NIHFW) a committee known as the "Committee on Integration of Health Services" was set up in 1964 to look into various problems related to abolition of private practice by doctors in government services, integration of health services and the service conditions of doctors. The report was submitted in 1967. The committee defined "integrated health services" as:

a. A service with a unified approach for all problems instead of a segmented approach for different problems.
b. Medical care and public health programmes should be put under charge of a single administrator at all levels of hierarchy.

### Important Recommendations of the Committee

- Unified cadre
- Common seniority
- Improvement in their service conditions
- Equal pay for equal work
- Special pay for special work
- Recognition of extra qualifications
- Abolition of private practice by government doctors

## Kartar Singh Committee, 1973

This committee headed by then Additional Secretary of Health and titled the "Committee on multipurpose workers under Health and Family Planning" was constituted to study and make recommendations on the structure for integrated health and medical services at peripheral and supervisory levels.

### Important Recommendations of the Committee

Peripheral workers of various categories should be amalgamated into a single cadre of multipurpose workers (male and female). The auxiliary nurse midwives were to be converted into "Female health worker (FHW)" and the basic health workers, malaria surveillance workers, etc., were to be converted to "Male health worker (MHW)".

- The work of 3–4 FHWs and MHWs was to be supervised by one health supervisor (male or female respectively). The existing lady health visitors (LHV) were to be converted into female health supervisors (FHS).
- One PHC should cover a population of 50,000. It should be divided into 16 SCs (one for 3,000–3,500 population depending upon topography and means of communications) each to be staffed by a male and a FHW.
- The medical officer of PHC will be the overall in-charge of all peripheral staff.
- Training for all workers engaged in the field of family planning, health and nutrition should be integrated.

## Shrivastava Committee, 1975

This committee was set up in 1974 as "Group on Medical Education and Support Manpower" to determine steps needed to: (1) Reorient medical education in accordance with national needs and priorities and (2) Develop a curriculum for health assistants who were to function as a link between medical officers and MPWs.

### Important Recommendations of the Committee

- Creation of bands of semiprofessional and paraprofessional health workers from within the community itself (e.g., school teachers, postmasters, gram sevaks) to provide comprehensive preventive, promotive and curative health services.
- Establishment of three cadres of health workers namely—multipurpose health workers and health assistants between the community level workers and doctors at PHC.
- Development of a "Referral Services Complex."
- Establishment of a Medical and Health Education Commission for planning and implementing the reforms needed in health and medical education on the lines of University Grants Commission.

Acceptance of the recommendations of the Shrivastava Committee in 1977 led to the launching of the Rural Health Scheme. The major steps initiated were:
- Medical colleges involved in health care of selected PHCs with the objective of reorienting medical education according to rural population called Reorientation of Medical Education (ROME). It led to teaching and training of undergraduate students and interns at PHCs.
- Reorientation training of multipurpose workers engaged in the control of various communicable disease program into unipurpose workers.
- Training of village health guides and utilizing their services in the general health service system.

## Bajaj Committee, 1986

Under Dr JS Bajaj, the then professor at AIIMS an "Expert Committee for Health Manpower Planning, Production and Management" was constituted in 1985.

### Important Recommendations of the Committee

- National Medical and Health Education Policy formulation for training of teachers in health education science technology.
- Formulation of National Health Manpower Policy based on realistic survey.
- Educational Commission for Health Sciences (ECHS) is to be established on the lines of UGC.
- Establishment of Health Science Universities in various states and union territories for uniform standard of medical and health science education.
- Establishment of health manpower cells in the states and at center.
- Vocational course in paramedical sciences regarding health related fields with appropriate incentives to provide quality paramedical personnel in adequate numbers.
- Carrying out a realistic health manpower survey.

## PLANNING COMMISSION

After Independence, Planning Commission was established in 1950 by the government to make assessment of capital, material and human resources of the country and for the purpose of appropriate planning so that available resources could be utilized most effectively. The Planning Commission had been formulating successive Five-Year Plans. It gave recommendations and suggestions to the government on various issues of the country. The Planning Commission consisted of Chairman, Deputy Chairman and five members. It was chaired by the Prime Minister of the country. The Planning Commission worked through three major divisions—Programme Advisers, General Secretariat and Technical Divisions which were responsible for scrutinizing and analyzing various schemes and projects to be incorporated in Five-Year Plans. There were total 29 divisions in the Planning Commission, such as agriculture, health, environment, family welfare, housing, education, nutrition, water supply, manpower, rural development, science, and technology, etc.

Health sector was divided into the following subsectors:
- Communicable disease
- Medical education, training and research
- Family planning
- Water supply and sanitation
- Public health services
- Indigenous systems of medicine
- Curative service including PHCs, hospitals and dispensaries

### Five-Year Plans

The five-year plans were initiated for rebuilding of the country and balanced development of all sectors in the country by planning a long-term road map. It laid main emphasis on rural India, industrial development and health for all. The main objectives of health programs during the five-year plans were:
- Control and eradication of communicable diseases
- Development of health manpower resources
- Population stabilization
- Strengthening of basic health service through PHCs and SCs

### Health in Five-Year Plans

- The first five-year plan (1951–56) focused on control of communicable diseases especially malaria, family planning and population control, water supply and sanitation, education and training. The PHCs were established as per the recommendations of the Bhore Committee.
- The activities initiated in the first plan continued in the second five-year plan (1956–61). The specific objectives of the plan include: establishment of institutional facilities to improve service provision, development and employment of technical manpower, active campaign for environmental hygiene, family planning and other supporting programs to raise standard of people's health.
- The objectives of the third five-year plan (1961–66) were to expand health services, to provide minimum of physical well being and to create conditions favorable for greater efficiency

and productivity. The main emphasis was given on preventive Public Health Services (water supply and sanitation) and control of communicable diseases.
- The fourth five-year plan (1969–74) focused on strengthening of PHCs. High priority was given to preventive health services, control of malaria, TB, leprosy, trachoma, and eradication of smallpox.
- The fifth five-year plan (1974–79) saw launching of several schemes related to health. The urban health structure had expanded at the cost of the rural sectors in terms of health facilities, beds, etc. National Malaria Eradication Programme and National Leprosy Control Programme continued to receive more focus. The Family Planning was amalgamated with immunization and nutrition of children under the Minimum Needs Programme (MNP) to increase accessibility of health services in rural areas.
- Alma-Ata declaration of Health for All by 2000 AD (WHO, 1978) influenced the sixth five-year plan (1980–85). To provide Health for All, first ever health policy was formulated in 1983 keeping principles of primary health care. The plan focused on community involvement and universal primary health care to all sections of the society.
- During seventh five-year plan (1985–90) focus was given on decentralized planning and involvement of people in health planning. The expanded Programme of Immunization was converted into Universal Immunization Programme in 1985, and activities related to population control were also given focus.
- Massive economic crisis lead to delay of the eighth five-year plan (1992–97) by 2 years. To cope up with financial crisis, introduction of user fee, privatization of government run institution, and public private partnership were done.
- The ninth plan (1997–2002) focused on strengthening of PHCs and SCs. State specific strategies on health were evolved because states had different health scenarios and had different healthcare needs. The new initiatives include: Horizontal integration of vertical programs, development of disease surveillance and response mechanism, development and implementation of integrated noncommunicable disease control program, health impact assessment, development of management systems for disaster, emergency, accident, and trauma care.
- The tenth plan (2002–2007) focused on how to improve health status of the community by improving the coverage and quality of care by identifying and correcting the gaps in infrastructure and management. National Rural Health Mission was launched in 2005 to achieve this goal in rural area. The focus was on improving the accessibility of health services in rural areas reducing infant mortality rate (IMR), maternal mortality ratio (MMR) and total fertility rate (TFR), providing clean drinking water, reducing malnutrition among 0–3 years children, reducing anemia among women and girls and raising sex ratio for age group 0–6 years.
- Special attention was given to the health of marginalized groups, such as adolescents girls, women of all ages, children below the age of three, older persons, disabled and primitive tribal groups during eleventh five-year plan.

### Twelfth Five-Year Plan (2012–2017)

Twelfth five-year plan focused on Universal Health Coverage (UHC) in the country which to ensure assured access to essential medicines and treatment at an affordable price to each individual. High level expert group has defined UHC as follows: 'Ensuring equitable access for all Indian citizens in any part of the country regardless of income level, social status, gender, caste or religion, to affordable, accountable and appropriate, assured quality health services (promotive, preventive, curative and rehabilitative) as well as services addressing wider determinants of health delivered to individuals and populations, with the Government being the guarantor and enabler, although not necessarily the only provider of health and related services'. To achieve health goals cooperation between public and private sector had been strengthened. Medical education expanded in states which were under served during the plan. Prescription reform and universally available free of cost generic medicines were also given priority. The goal of UHC would be realized in two steps: (1) Clinical services at different levels which the government would finance and ensure provision through the public health system supplemented by contracted in private providers whenever required; (2) The universal provision of high impact, preventive and public health interventions which the Government would universally provide within the twelfth five-year plan **(Table 46.1)**.

### Outcome Indicators for Twelfth Plan

- Reduction of IMR to 25
- Reduction of MMR to 100
- Reduction of TFR to 2.1
- Prevention, and reduction of undernutrition in children under 3 years to half of NFHS-3 (2005-06) levels
- Prevention and reduction of anemia among women aged 15–49 years to 28%
- Raising child sex ratio in the 0–6 years age group from 914 to 950
- Reduction of poor households' out-of-pocket expenditure
- Prevention and reduction of burden of communicable and noncommunicable diseases (including mental illnesses) and injuries.

**Table 46.1:** Illustrative list of preventive and public health interventions to be funded and provided by government.

| 1. | Full immunization among children under 3 years of age, and pregnant women |
|---|---|
| 2. | Full antenatal, natal and postnatal care |
| 3. | Skilled birth attendance with a facility for meeting need for emergency obstetric care |
| 4. | Iron and folic acid supplementation for children, adolescent girls, and pregnant women |
| 5. | Regular treatment of intestinal worms, especially in children and reproductive age women |
| 6. | Universal use of iodine and iron fortified salt |
| 7. | Vitamin A supplementation for children aged 9–59 months |
| 8. | Access to a basket of contraceptives and safe abortion services |

*Contd...*

*Contd...*

9. Preventive and promotive health educational services including information on hygiene, handwashing, dental hygiene, use of potable drinking water, avoidance of tobacco, alcohol, high-calorie diet and obesity, need for regular physical exercise, use of helmets on two-wheelers and seat belts; advice on initiation of breastfeeding within 1 hour of birth and exclusively up to 6 months of age, and complimentary feeding thereafter, adolescent sexual health, awareness about RTI/STI; need for screening for NCDs and common cancers for those at risk
10. Home-based newborn care and encouragement for exclusive breastfeeding till 6 months of age
11. Community-based care for sick children with referral of cases requiring higher levels of care
12. HIV testing and counseling during antenatal care
13. Free drugs to pregnant HIV positive mothers to prevent mother to child transmission of HIV
14. Malaria prophylaxis, using long lasting insecticide treated nets (LLIN), and appropriate treatment
15. School check-up of health and wellness followed by advice and treatment if necessary
16. Management of diarrhea especially in children using oral rehydration solution (ORS)
17. Diagnosis and treatment of tuberculosis, leprosy including drug and multidrug resistant cases
18. Vaccines for hepatitis B and C for high-risk groups
19. Patient transport systems including emergency response ambulance services of the "dial 108" model

*Goals of communicable diseases in twelfth plan shall be as indicated as per below:*

- *Tuberculosis:* Reduce annual incidence and mortality by half
- *Leprosy:* Reduce prevalence to <1/10,000 population and incidence to zero in all districts
- *Malaria:* Annual malaria incidence of <1/1,000
- *Filariasis:* <1% microfilaria prevalence in all districts
- *Dengue:* Sustaining case fatality rate of <1%
- *Chikungunya:* Containment of outbreaks
- *Japanese encephalitis:* Reduction in mortality by 30%
- *Kala-azar:* Elimination by 2015, that is, <1 case per 10,000 population in all blocks
- *HIV/AIDS:* Reduce new infections to zero and provide comprehensive care and support to all persons living with HIV/AIDS and treatment services for all those who require it.

## NITI AAYOG

National Institution for Transforming India (NITI) was initiated by the government to replace Planning Commission on 1st January 2015 for fulfilling the needs of people of India. Prime Minister of the country is the chairperson of the Aayog. It works as a policy "Think Tank" to provide directional and policy inputs. It also provides technical advice to center and states along with designing policies and program for the government. It consists of two parts: (1) Team India Hub and (2) Knowledge and Innovation Hub. The first one works a bridge between states and central government while the later one works for building NITI's think-tank capabilities. NITI Aayog is developing itself as a state-of-the-art Resource Centre, with the necessary resources, knowledge and skills, that will enable it to act with speed, promote research and innovation, provide strategic policy vision for the government and deal with contingent issues.

### Members of NITI Aayog

- The Prime Minister as the chairperson
- Vice chairperson
- A chief executive officer
- A secretariat
- Five full-time members, two part-time members (from universities, research organizations), four ex-officio members of Union Council of Ministers
- A governing council consists of chief ministers of all states and union territories with legislatures and lieutenant governors of union territories (except Delhi and Puducherry)
- Regional councils consists of chief ministers of States and Lt. Governors of union territories in the region to address specific issues impacting more than one state or a region.
- Experts and specialists in various fields

NITI Aayog's entire gamut of activities can be divided into four main heads:
1. Design Policy and Programme Framework
2. Foster Cooperative Federalism
3. Monitoring and Evaluation
4. Think Tank and Knowledge and Innovation Hub

### Important Functions of the NITI Aayog (Fig. 46.1)

- To foster cooperative federalism through structured support initiatives and mechanisms with the States on a continuous basis, recognizing that strong States make a strong nation.
- To develop mechanisms to formulate credible plans at the village level and aggregate these progressively at higher levels of government.

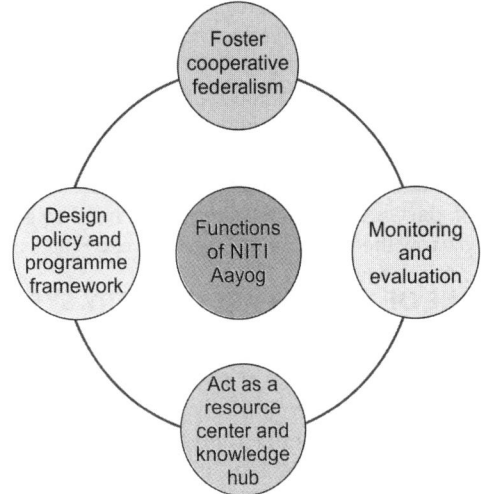

**Fig. 46.1:** Important functions of NITI Aayog.

- To design strategic and long-term policy and program frameworks and initiatives, and monitor their progress and their efficacy. The lessons learnt through monitoring and feedback will be used for making innovative improvements, including necessary mid-course corrections.

- To provide advice and encourage partnerships between key stakeholders and national and international like-minded think tanks, as well as educational and policy research institutions.
- To create a knowledge, innovation and entrepreneurial support system through a collaborative community of national and international experts, practitioners and other partners.
- To maintain a state-of-the-art Resource Center, be a repository of research on good governance and best practices in sustainable and equitable development as well as help their dissemination to stakeholders.
- To actively monitor and evaluate the implementation of programs and initiatives including the identification of the needed resources so as to strengthen the probability of success and scope of delivery.
- To focus on technology upgradation and capacity building for implementation of programs and initiatives.

## Health Index

NITI Aayog launched the Health Index to motivate States to improve population health and reduce disparities in the spirit of cooperative and competitive federalism and also to measure the performance of States and UTs. In February 2018, the first round of the Health Index (referred to as Health Index-2017) was released, which measured the annual and incremental performance of the States and UTs over the period of 2014-15 (base year) to 2015-16 (reference year). The indicators, methodology and categorization of States and UTs in the Health Index-2018 are consistent with the 2017 round with a total of 23 indicators grouped into domains of Health Outcomes, Governance and Information, and Key Inputs/Processes. The Health Index scores for 2017-18 (reference year) revealed large disparities in overall performance across States and UTs. Kerala championed the Larger States with an overall score of 74.01, while Uttar Pradesh was the least performing State with an overall score of 28.61. Among the Smaller States, scores varied between 38.51 in Nagaland and 74.97 in Mizoram. Among the UTs, the scores varied between 41.66 in Daman and Diu to 63.62 in Chandigarh. Overall, there is room for improvement in all States, even among the best-performing States there is substantial room for improvement. Among the least performing States/UTs, particularly, there is an urgent need to accelerate efforts to narrow the performance gap between States and UTs.

## OUTLINE OF HEALTHCARE DELIVERY SYSTEM IN INDIA

A healthcare system comprises of organization of administrative, management and service delivery components. The administrative components include the ministries and secretariats. The management components include the directorate level organizations. The service delivery components based on source of funding are represented in **Flowchart 46.1**.

## Organization of Public Health System in India

A health system is the coordinated functioning of all health-related organizations, responsible for delivery of all health-related services. In addition to curative services, health system also provides preventive, promotive, rehabilitative as well as administrative and managerial services.

In most of the countries health services are provided by union government through its health ministry. As per Indian Constitution, health is the state responsibility. So the responsibilities for provision of majority of health services in the states are delegated to the respective states. Therefore each state has their healthcare delivery system. However, the organizations and its functioning in various states are in line with the set-up at union level. For ease of understanding the organization of health system in India and its functioning, we have classified the health system at union level, state level, and at district level.

There are three different heads of organizations at different levels in health system according to the broad functions—political head, administrative head, and technical head.

### Political Head

A political head is the person appointed by the masses through democratic mechanism—election. He has broad vision on all relevant aspects and formulates health related policies in accordance with priorities of his political party and demands of masses, e.g., Union Health Minister, State Health Minister, and Cabinet Ministers.

### Administrative Head

He is an officer appointed by selection through Indian administrative services or respective states administrative services examinations. He functions as secretary to the government along with administration of all health related matters under his jurisdiction, e.g., Commissioner, Secretary, and Collector.

### Technical or Executive Head

He is a subject specialist with specific focus and concerned with planning, implementation, coordinating and monitoring of all health-related activities, e.g., directors of health and chief district health officers.

### Organization of Health System at the National Level

Health system at the national level comprises of (1) The Ministry of Health and Family Welfare, (2) The Directorate General of Health Services, and (3) The Central Council of Health and Family Welfare.

### The Ministry of Health and Family Welfare

The cabinet minister is the head of MoHFW and is assisted by a minister of state and deputy health minister. The ministry functions through the following four departments under its regulation **(Flowchart 46.2)**.
1. Department of Health and Family Welfare
2. Department of AYUSH
3. Department of Health Research
4. Department of AIDS Control

The Secretaries to government of India are the executive heads of these departments and are assisted by joint secretaries, deputy secretaries and other administrative staff.

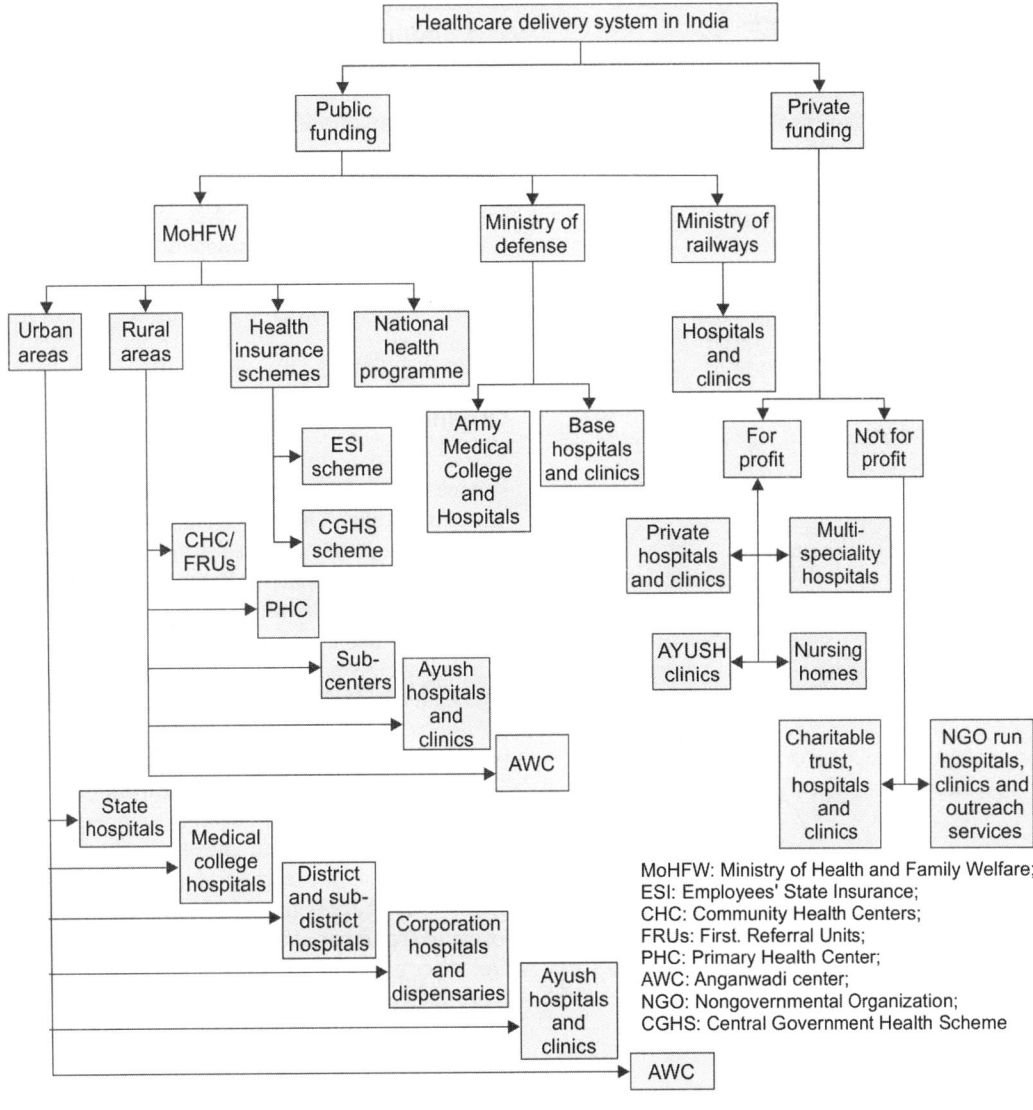

Flowchart 46.1: Healthcare delivery system in India.

The functioning of MoHFW is divided into Union Lists—functions exclusively of the union government and concurrent lists—functions which are joint responsibility of state and union government.

### Union List
- International health relations and administration of port quarantine
- Administration of central institutes
- Promotion of research through research centers and other bodies
- Regulation and development of medical, pharmaceutical, dental and nursing professions
- Establishment and maintenance of drug standards
- Census, collection and publication of other statistical data
- Immigration and emigration
- Regulation of labor in the working of mines and oil fields
- Coordination with states and with other ministries for promotion of health

### Concurrent List
- Prevention of extension of communicable diseases from one unit to another
- Prevention of adulteration of foodstuffs
- Control of drugs and poisons
- Vital statistics
- Labor welfare
- Ports other than major ones
- Economic and social planning, and
- Population control and family planning

### The Directorate General of Health Services

The directorate is headed by the Director General of Health Services (DGHS). DGHS acts as the *principal advisor* to the Union Government in medical and public health matters. There are additional directors, deputy directors, and administrative staff to support the DGHS. There are three units of the directorate viz. medical care and hospitals, public health and general administration.

# Section 5: Managing Community Health in India

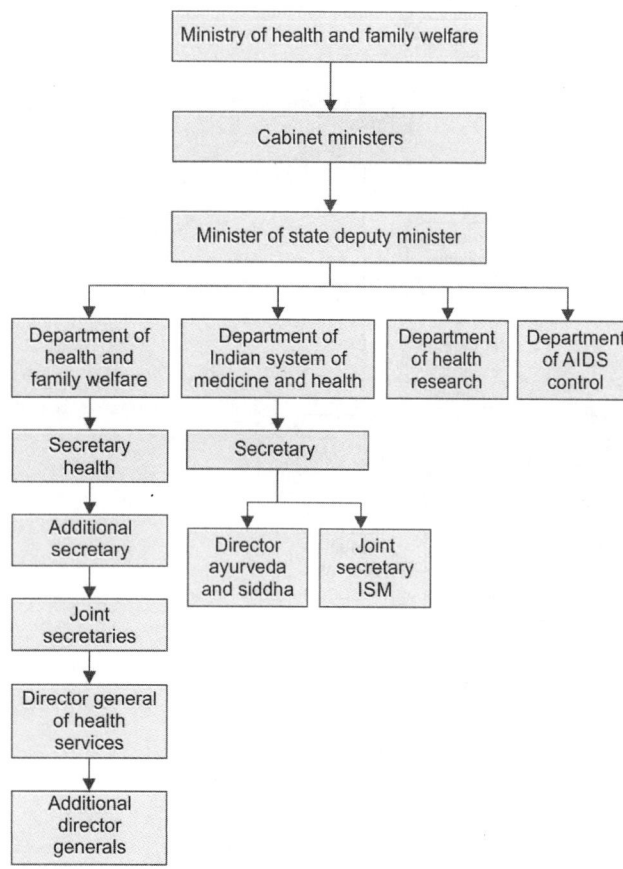

Flowchart 46.2: Chart for organization of health system at union level.

(ISM: Indian system of medicine)

Its functions are planning, programming, coordination, surveys and appraisal of all health matters.

### Specific Function
- International health relations and quarantine of all major ports in country and international airport
- Control of drug standards
- Maintain medical store depots
- Administration of postgraduate training programs
- Administration of certain medical colleges in India
- Conducting medical research through Indian Council of Medical Research (ICMR)
- Central Government Health Schemes
- Implementation of national health programmes
- Preparation of health education material for creating health awareness through Health Education Bureau
- Collection, compilation, analysis, evaluation and dissemination of information

### *The Central Council of Health and Family Welfare*

Since a concurrent list includes several joint responsibilities between states and union government, there is the formation of central council of health and family welfare. It is a council of all health ministers of states with union health minister as its chairman and State Health Ministers as its members. It makes broad outlines of policies and legislations in relation to medical and health services. It facilitates the distribution of central governments funds between the states and reviews the utilization of the same. It helps in promoting and maintaining cooperation between the Central and State Health administrations.

> **Key Note**
> Health system at national level consists of three bodies—the ministry, the directorate and the central council. The ministry is headed by cabinet minister and its work is executed by secretaries to the government. The DGHS is the main advisor to the Government in health issues. The central council ensures smooth coordination between states for execution of functions of concurrent list as well as equitable sharing of resources.

## Organization of Health System at the State Level

The ultimate accountability for delivery of all health related services to people within its jurisdiction lies with the state. The structure of health system at state level is same as that of union level with department of health and family welfare being headed by state health ministers. The health secretary/commissioner (IAS) acts as administrative head of department.

The State Directorate of Health Services is attached to and acts as a technical wing for department of health and family welfare. It is headed by various directors in-charge of independent health portfolios. The director of health is responsible for organization, planning and direction of all the health related activities. They are assisted by Additional directors, Joint directors, Deputy directors, Programme officers, etc., each of whom is in-charge of one or more program/subjects. These assistant directors are of two types—regional directors and functional directors. The regional directors look after all public health related matters at regional levels irrespective of their specialty. The functional directors look after particular areas of public health for entire state, e.g., reproductive and child health, family welfare activities, nutrition related activities, communicable and noncommunicable diseases related activities, etc. Usually specialists of particular branch are appointed as functional directors.

Although the states are overall responsible for all health related matters in the states, the union government can force state government to focus on implementation of particular schemes through its selected funding mechanisms. For example, Swachh Bharat Abhiyan which is centrally sponsored is implemented by all the states.

The directorate is accountable to the commissioner/health secretary. This structure is not uniform in all states and there are some variations in organization or nomenclature.

The organization of public health system at state level varies between states. Here, an organogram of Gujarat state is shown in **Flowchart 46.3** for reference.

> **Key Note**
> Organization of health system at state level is very similar to that at union level. The directors of the departments organize, plan and direct all the health programs of the state. The state is further divided into regions headed by regional deputy directors for smooth functioning.

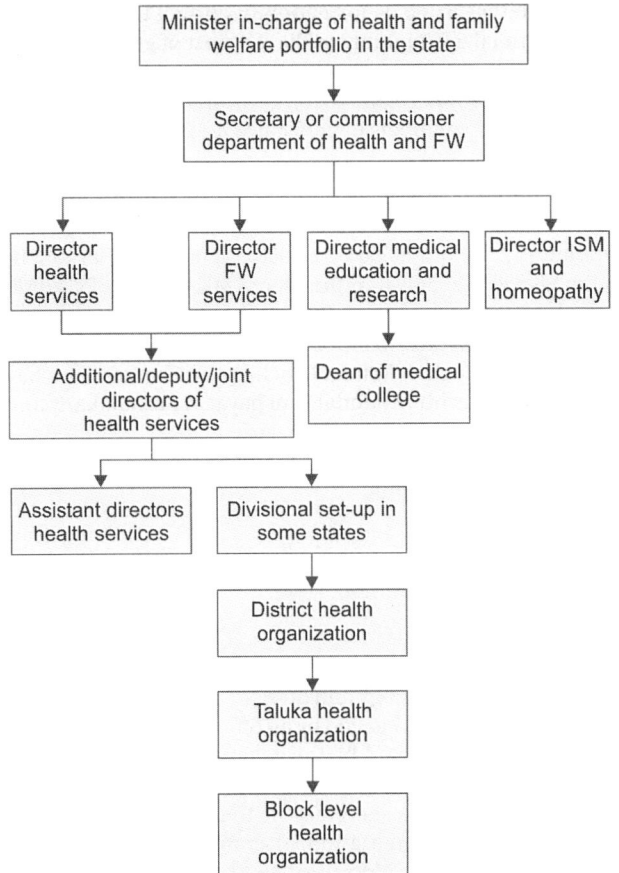

Flowchart 46.3: Organizational structure of health services at state level (Gujarat).

(FW: family welfare; ISM: Indian system of medicine)

## Organization of Health System at Regional Level

Some large states are divided into regions or divisions for administrative convenience. Each region covers about 3–5 districts. The officer in-charge at regional level is known as regional deputy director (RDD). The states have delegated authority to RDD supervise and monitor health and family welfare activities in their region through district authorities.

## Organization of Health System at the District Level

There are several healthcare programs implemented at district level. In order to bring them under unified control there was formation of district health society. The district health society acts as a middle level management organization with state and regional level on one side and rural health system on the other side. The information about healthcare programs implementation received from higher level is transmitted to the peripheral health set-up after amendment to suit the local requirement. Thus the district level authorities' act as managers and sorts out several issues regarding planning, logistics, implementation, monitoring as well as general administrative issues for provision of healthcare services to the district.

The district is the principle unit of administration with Collector (IAS) also known as District Magistrate as the administrative head. He is assisted by Assistant Collector in-charge of a section of a district and District Development Officer. For administrative convenience the districts are divided into the following six areas.

1. ***Subdivisions:*** Comprising of two or more divisions of the district and headed by an assistant collector
2. ***Tehsils (Talukas):*** Comprising of 200–600 villages and headed by a Tehsildar
3. ***Community development blocks:*** Comprising of around 100 villages and headed by block development officer. Blocks are the units for rural planning
4. ***Municipalities and corporations:*** A municipal corporation is an urban governing body for a big district with a population of 10 lakh or more, while a municipality is a governing body for a smaller urban district with a population of 100,000 or more
5. ***Villages***
6. ***Panchayats:*** For rural local self-governance

The officer in-charge of all the health and family welfare activities in the district is called Chief District Health Officer (CDHO) or Chief Medical officer (CMO) or District Medical and Health Officer (DM and HO) in different states. The CMO is assisted by Deputy CMO or Additional/Assistant District Health Officer (ADHO) and several programme officers, such as District Tuberculosis Officer (DTO), District Malaria Officer (DMO), Epidemic Medical Officer (EMO), Reproductive and Child Health Officer (RCHO), District Programme Officer (DPO) and Quality Medical Officer (QMO), etc. The number and specialization of these officers at district varies across different states of the country **(Flowchart 46.4)**.

> **Key Note**
>
> District health society headed by Collector is overall in-charge for decentralized administration of healthcare activities at district level. The CDHO acts as technical head for planning, implementing and monitoring health activities within the district.

Flowchart 46.4: Organization of health system at district level.

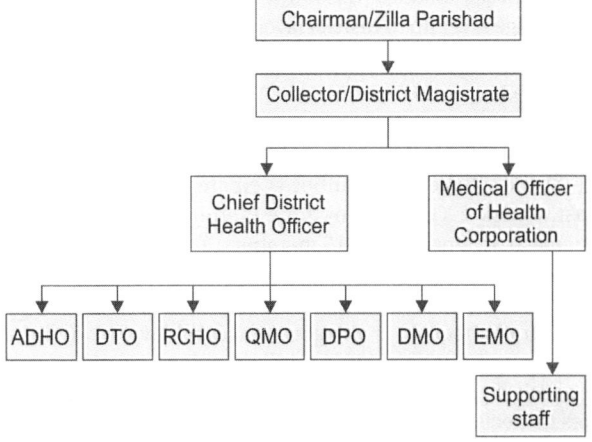

(ADHO: Assistant District Health Officer; DTO: District Tuberculosis Officer; RCHO: Reproductive and Child Health Officer; QMO: Quality Medical Officer; DPO: District Programme Officer; DMO: District Malaria Officer; EMO: Epidemic Medical Officer)

# DECENTRALIZED ADMINISTRATION THROUGH LOCAL SELF-GOVERNMENT FOR RURAL AND URBAN AREAS

## Local Self-Government for Rural Areas

Since Panchayati Raj Institutions (PRI) are involved in management of health services it is necessary to provide a short introduction about PRI.

The *Panchayat Raj* is one of the oldest political system of local governance in the south Asian countries viz. India, Pakistan, Bangladesh and Nepal. *Panch* means five and *ayat* means assembly. Panchayat means assembly of five persons elected by the local community. In olden days these assemblies were formed to settle dispute at local level. However with changing times the Indian government has empowered them by decentralizing several administrative functions to them. In 2009 the union government, has approved 50% reservation for women in PRIs. The panchayati raj strengthens the democracy and ensures participation of the people in governance. It is important to understand that gram panchayats are different from unelected Khap Panchayats or caste panchayats which are found in certain parts of India.

The Government of India in 1957 had appointed The Balwant Rai Mehta Committee to study the functioning of the Community Development Programme (1952) and the National Extension Service (1953) and to recommend improvement measures. The committee recommended formation of a system for "democratic decentralization". This led to establishment of the Panchayati Raj Institution. The Constitutional (73rd Amendment) Act 1992 provided constitutional status to the Panchayati Raj institutions. This Act provides for delegation of powers and responsibilities to the panchayats for the preparation of economic development plans and social justice. The panchayats can also levy and collect suitable taxes, fees, etc., as appropriate.

## Three-Tier Local Self-Government in Rural Areas

The rural local self-government in India popularly known as Panchayati Raj Institution is a three-tier administrative system from village level up to district level.

***Gram Panchayat:*** The Panchayati Raj institution at the village level is called *gram panchayat*. Gram means a cluster. Here it means cluster of villages. The Gram is again divided into a minimum of five constituencies depending on the population size of the villages. A member is elected from each of these constituencies. The body of these members constitutes Gram Panchayat. It consists of 5–15 members. The population catered by Gram Panchayat differs between states ranging from 3,000 to 20,000. One of them is elected as the Sarpanch/President. The Gram Panchayat is an agency for local level planning and development. It is involved in administration, sanitation, social, economic and public health related activities at village level. It takes its decisions through *gram sabha* which consists of all the adults/voters in the villages.

As per Constitution, the PRI is a three-tier structure and the *Gram Sabha* is not a tier of the PRI. It only acts as a recommending body. The Gram Sabha meets two to four times but can meet as and when necessary. A wide variety of issues are discussed in the meetings, such as formation of annual action plan and budget, annual account and audit of report of gram panchayat, selection of beneficiaries for different social service programs, such as Indira Awas Yojana (IAY), Pension Schemes, etc., along with election of members of panchayat and other schemes.

***Panchayat Samiti/Janpada Panchayat:*** The Panchayati Raj Institution at the block level is called Panchayat Samiti. It is representative of 100 villages of the block and covers a population of about 80,000–120,000. It consist of Sarpanch of all the village panchayat in the block; MLAs and MPs residing in the block area; representatives of women, scheduled castes, scheduled tribes and cooperative societies. It is known by various names such as Taluka Panchayat in Gujarat, Panchayat Samiti in Maharashtra, Mandal Panchayat in Karnataka, Mandal Praja Parishad in Andhra Pradesh, etc.

The Panchayat Samiti comprises of the following departments:
- General administration
- Finance
- Public work
- Agriculture
- Health
- Education
- Social welfare
- Information technology and others

Each department is headed by an officer. Block Development Officer (BDO), appointed by the government is the executive officer of the Samiti and is the chief of its administration. The BDO is the ex-officio secretary of the Panchayat Samiti. It functions for implementation of community development programs in the block **(Flowchart 46.5)**.

***Zilla Parishad:*** The Panchayati Raj Institution at the district level is called Zilla Parishad.

The Zilla Parishad comprises of all heads of Panchayat Samities of the district, MPs and MLAs of the district, representatives of scheduled castes, scheduled tribes. The number of members of Zilla Parishad vary from 40 to 70 in different states. One the member is elected as the chairperson of the Zilla Parishad. An IAS officer—collector is the chief of administration at the district level. The Chief District Health Officer is in-charge of all health and family welfare related activities in the district.

There are a wide variety of functions of Zilla Parishad which are divided among different committees (just as ministries are formed in state and union governments). These committees are called Standing Committees/Sthayee Samitis/Upa Samiti, etc., and are headed by a member of Zilla Parishad. The Chairperson of the Zilla Parishad has the over-all charge of the district.

## Local Self-Government for Urban Areas

The local self-government in urban areas is established as under:
- ***Nagar Panchayat or town area committee:*** The town area committee in areas with population of 5,000–10,000. Town area committee primarily provides sanitation related services.
- ***Nagar Palika or Municipalities (municipal council, municipal board, municipal committee):*** Municipal boards in areas with population ranging from 10,000 to 200,000.

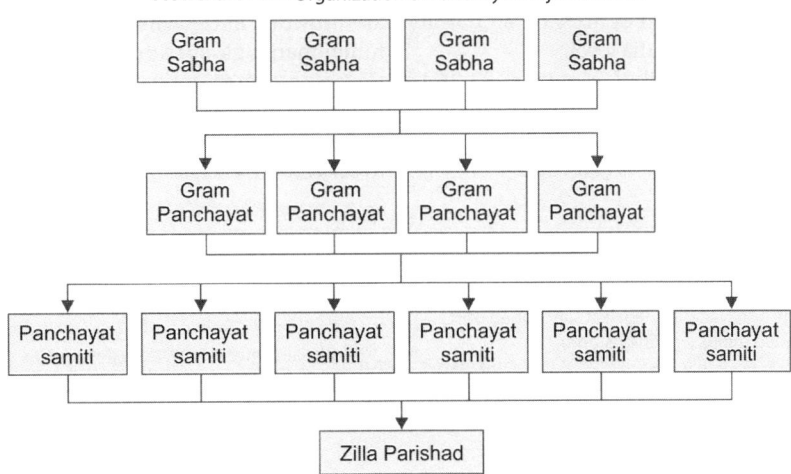

Flowchart 46.5: Organization of Panchayati Raj Institution.

The municipal boards are headed by president elected by members. Its main functions are:
- Construction and maintenance of roads
- Street lighting and water supply
- Sanitation and drainage
- Maintenance of hospitals and dispensaries
- Education and registration of births and deaths, etc.
- *Nagar Nigam or Municipal Corporation:* Corporations are for areas with more than 200,000 population. The corporation is headed by mayors elected from different wards of the city. The Commissioner (IAS), the Secretary, the Engineer and the Medical Officer Health form the executive body. It functions in the same way as a municipality but on a larger scale.

The municipal corporations have a higher amount of financial independence and have independent functioning as compared to municipality. The corporations deal directly with the state government while the municipalities have to approach the state government through director of Municipal Corporation or through the collector. The urban local governments function under supervision and guidance of local state government.

### Functioning of Urban Local Bodies

The ULBs are assigned several functions by the state government under the municipal legislation. However these functions of ULBs vary from state to state. Broadly the functions are classified as under:
- *Public health related activities*: Provision of water supply, sanitation related services, control of communicable diseases, etc.
- *Welfare activities*: Public facilities for education, recreation, parks and gardens, etc.
- *Public safety and regulatory functions*: Enforcement of building and construction related acts, issuing of birth and death certificates, collection of various taxes and fees, fire control services, etc.
- *Public infrastructure*: Construction and maintenance of roads of city, street lightings, etc.
- *Development activities*: Developing commercial markets, town planning, etc.

## STATUS OF HEALTHCARE SYSTEM IN INDIA

The urban health delivery system in India is grossly unorganized and non-uniform. The healthcare delivery in urban areas is dominated by private sector healthcare providers.

The status of rural health facilities as per Rural Health Statistics Report 2021-22 is given in **Table 46.2**.

**Table 46.2:** Table describing the norms and levels of achievement for rural health facilities as on March 2022.

| Sr. No | Indicator | National norms | | Status (2022) | |
|---|---|---|---|---|---|
| 1. | Rural population (mid-year population 2019) covered by a- | General | Tribal/hilly/desert | General | Tribal/hilly/desert |
| | Subcenter | 5,000 | 3,000 | 5,691 | 4,005 |
| | Primary health center (PHC) | 30,000 | 20,000 | 36,049 | 26,522 |
| | Community health center (CHC) | 120,000 | 80,000 | 164,027 | 105,893 |
| 2. | Number of subcenters per PHC | 6 | | 6 | 7 |
| 3. | Number of PHCs per CHC | 4 | | 5 | 4 |
| 4. | Rural population (mid-year population 2019) covered by a- | | | | |
| | HW (F) (at subcenters and PHCs) | | | 4,330 | |
| | HW (M + F) (at subcenters) | | | 3,850 | |

While the numbers of SC, PHC and CHCs have increased considerably under NRHM, the current numbers are still insufficient to meet their population norms. The shortfall in public health structures as per Rural Health Statistics 2021-22 is as follows:

| Health centers | % shortfall |
|---|---|
| Subcenter | 25 |
| PHC | 31 |
| CHC | 36 |

There was a shortfall of 3.5% of ANMs and 66.6% of HWM for the total requirement for ANM and HWM as per norms at SCs and PHCs **(Fig. 46.2)**.

At PHC levels, shortfall for the post of health assistant male + female was 74.2% There was a shortfall of 3.1% of allopathic doctors of the total requirement at all India level.

For CHC there was a huge shortfall of surgeons (83.2%), obstetricians and gynecologists (74.2%), physicians (79.1%) and pediatrician (81.6%). The overall shortfall of specialist at CHCs against the requirement for CHC was 79.5% **(Fig. 46.3)**.

**Note**
- Shortfall is defined as deficit/nonavailability against requirement for existing centers (staff required for the facility as per guidelines minus staff in position).
- Vacancy is defined as deficit/nonavailability against sanctioned posts (total posts of staff sanctioned minus staff in position).

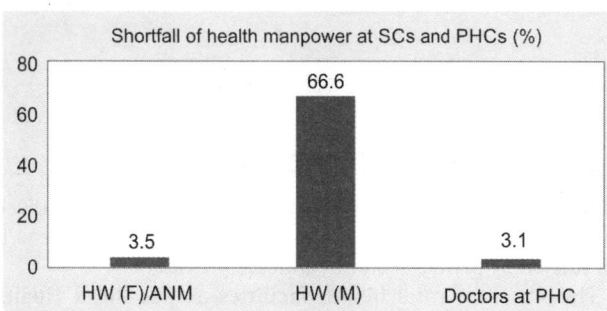

**Fig. 46.2:** Chart showing all India percentage deficit of health manpower in rural areas as on 31st march 2022.
(ANM: Auxiliary Nurse Midwife; HW(M): health worker male; HW(F): health worker female; PHC: primary health center)

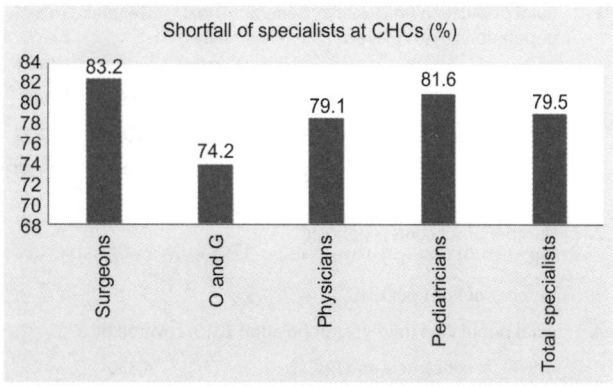

**Fig 46.3:** Chart showing all India percentage deficit of specialist at CHC at 31st March 2022.

## CONCEPT OF THREE-TIER HEALTHCARE SYSTEM

Public healthcare delivery system in India is divided into three levels—primary level, secondary level and tertiary level **(Fig. 46.4)**.

### Primary Level of Health Care (Primary Health Care)

The primary health care is provided at all levels of health care delivery systems, including SCs, anganwadi centers, PHC, CHC, subdistrict and tertiary care hospitals. However, SCs, anganwadi centers and PHC only provide primary level health care to the patients; while patients requiring secondary or tertiary level of health care are referred to higher facilities. The services are provided at the community level by grass root level health functionaries along with involvement of community volunteers. Community members, such as anganwadi workers, trained *dais*, village health guides, members of gram sabha, etc., provide assistance to the PHC staff in providing basic essential services to the remote villages in India.

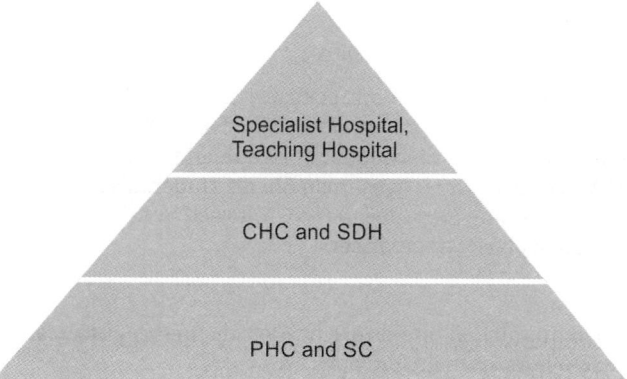

**Fig. 46.4:** Pictorial representation of three-tier rural healthcare system in India.
(CHC: community health centers; SDH: Subdistrict hospitals; PHC: primary health centers; SC: subcenter)

In the international health conference organized at Alma-Ata, USSR 1978 it was agreed upon by the participating nations to achieve basic level of health care for all by the year 2000 AD. It was projected as Health for All by 2000 AD. India is committed to achieving the health for all by 2000 goal. The key strategy of achieving health for all by 2000 AD was through primary health care.

### Secondary Level of Health Care

In addition to providing primary level of healthcare services, the secondary level health care provides services of specialist to its people, for higher quality healthcare services. The secondary level healthcare services are mostly provided at Taluka level and subdistrict level. The facility is called CHC. CHCs mostly provide curative services in addition to providing primary level services. A few of the CHCs have been upgraded to first referral unit (FRU) by addition of facility of blood bank, and services of anesthesia.

### Tertiary Level Health Care

These types of services are provided at district hospitals, medical college hospitals, AIIMS, etc. Services provided in these institutions are of speciality type and superspeciality type. In addition to providing healthcare services they also serve as the teaching and training centers for medical students along with medical and paramedical staff.

## ORGANIZATION OF RURAL PUBLIC HEALTH SYSTEM IN INDIA

The health care in India is provided by a mix of private service providers and public health system. The private providers are mostly concentrated in urban areas and focuses on provision of secondary and tertiary level of health care. The rural public healthcare system is well structured and organized into three-tier healthcare system based on population norms as described in **Table 46.3**.

Table 46.3: Population norms for various rural health facilities.

| Health centers | Plain areas | Hilly, tribal or difficult areas |
|---|---|---|
| Subcenter | 5,000 | 3,000 |
| Primary health center | 30,000 | 20,000 |
| Community health center | 120,000 | 80,000 |

In order to provide comprehensive primary level health care and to expand the provision of services, the Government of India announced the establishment of Health and Wellness Centers (HWC) in 2017 under Ayushman Bharat. Under this scheme the subcenters were upgraded to HWC followed by urban and rural PHCs in a phase wise manner.

## IPHS Guidelines 2022

In comparison with the IPHS guidelines of 2012, the revised IPHS 2022 guidelines classify the HWCs as:
1. **Health and Wellness Centres—Primary Health Centre:**
   a. HWC-PHC in rural areas
   b. HWC-UPHC in urban areas
2. **Health and Wellness Centers–Subhealth Center:**
   a. Health and Wellness Center–Subhealth Center in rural areas
   b. Urban Health and Wellness Center in urban areas

## Subhealth Center (also Known as Subcenter)/Health and Wellness Centers–Subhealth Center

### Concept and Norms

A SC is the peripheral structure of healthcare delivery system in the rural areas. It is the first point of contact between the primary healthcare system and the rural community. A SC serves a population of about 5,000 in plain areas and 3,000 in hilly, tribal and backward areas. In urban areas one Urban-HWC per 15,000–20,000 population caters predominantly to poor and vulnerable populations, residing in slums or other such pockets There are about 157,935 and 3894 rural SC functioning in the rural and urban areas of country as on 31st March 2022 as per Rural Health Statistics bulletin, 2021–22.

### Structure and Staffing

As per IPHS Standards 2022, the type of staff viz Community Health Officer (CHO), Auxiliary Nurse Midwife (ANM) and a Multi-Purpose Worker (MPW) (Male) or two ANMs, and support staff as mentioned in **Table 46.4** has been selected taking into consideration services and program requirements of the HWC-SHC. The Urban-HWC is to be staffed with a Medical Officer, a Staff Nurse/Pharmacist, Male-MPW and one support Staff. The SC building consists of Screening and holding area, Registration area, Waiting area, consultation room, Health and Wellness area, Clinical laboratory, Day care beds, record keeping, Store, Teleconsultation area and Residential Quarters. The staff pattern in each of the SCs is presented in **Table 46.4**.

Table 46.4: The staff pattern in each of the SCs.

| Subcenter staff | HWC-SHC | UHWC |
|---|---|---|
| Medical officer | | 1 |
| Community health officer | 1 | |
| Staff nurse | | 1 |
| Multi-purpose health worker | 1 Male + 1 Female | 1 |
| MPW male | | 1 |
| Sanitary staff* | | 1 |
| Security staff* | | 1 |

*can be hired/outsourced.

### Functions

The expected services to be provided at HWC are as follows:
- Complete care during pregnancy and childbirth
- Neonatal and infant health related services
- Childhood and adolescents health services
- Family planning and contraceptive services along with other reproductive healthcare services
- Management of communicable diseases and services under national health programmes
- OPD services for acute simple illness and management of common communicable diseases
- Screening and management of noncommunicable diseases
- Screening and management of mental health disorders
- Management of common ophthalmic and ENT problems
- Basic dental care
- Geriatric and palliative healthcare services
- Emergency medical services and trauma care (that can be managed at the level)

### Monitoring Mechanism at Subcenters

*Internal mechanisms:* Internal monitoring is done by health staff at higher level. The health supervisors—male and female have to visit the SC every week and MO-PHC has to visit the SC every month for supportive supervision and record checking.

*External mechanisms:* External monitoring is done by PRI and gram panchayats of the village. The following aspects are monitored:
- Regularity in attending clients
- Referral and transportation of emergency cases
- Appropriate utilization of fund
- Behavior of staff members
- Facilities available at the SC, such as waiting area, drinking water, toilets, etc.

List of furniture, equipment and consumables, newborn corner in labor room, suggested list of drugs at SC, standards for deep burial pit and biomedical waste (management and handling) rules, records, reports and registers, IDSP format, checklist for external monitoring, proforma for facility survey of SCs on Indian Public Health Standard (IPHS), model citizen's charter for SCs are provided in revised IPHS standards for SC. Readers may refer to them for in-depth knowledge about SC.

> **Key Note**
> Subcenter is the first point of contact between the community and the health system, with only health workers as primary level service providers.

## Primary Health Center

### Concept and Norms

*Primary health center is the rural hospital and first point of contact for the rural population and the doctor in public health system (medical officer). The PHCs were established to provide preventive health care integrated with curative services, rural population with emphasis on preventive and promotive aspects of health care. It caters a population of about 30,000 in plain areas and 20,000 in hilly/tribal/hard to reach areas. Urban PHCs are for 50,000 population and polyclinic is for 2.5–3.0 lakh population. There are about 24,935 and 6,118 PHCs functioning in rural and urban areas of the country as on 31st March 2022 as per Rural Health Statistics bulletin, 2021–22. The development and maintenance of the PHCs is through state government under the Minimum Needs Programme (MNP)/Basic Minimum Services (BMS) Programme.*

IPHS 2022 guidelines classify the rural and urban PHC as:
- **HWC-PHCs:** Ideally, for rural areas, the states should aspire to make all PHCs functional as 24 × 7 facilities. However, there is a need to prioritize PHCs conducting deliveries to function as 24 × 7 HWCPHCs. All other PHCs should continue to provide routine care along with preventive and promotive health interventions and function as PHCs-HWCs.
- **Urban HWC-PHCs:** In urban areas, assured round-the-clock emergency and secondary care services are readily available, owing to the presence of higher level health care facilities. Thus primary health centres are expected to provide routine OPD care along with preventive and promotive health interventions and function as UPHCs-HWCs. However, the UPHCs with indoor beds already conducting deliveries can continue to function as 24 × 7 UPHCs-HWCs.
- **Specialist UPHC/Polyclinic (Urban):** "Multispecialty UPHC/Polyclinics" in urban areas should be established with the aim to further reduce morbidity and mortality by providing specialist services on ambulatory/day care basis, closer to the urban community. Such poly clinic services would be limited to outpatient care.

### Structure

A PHC building should have the following areas of appropriate size: waiting area, outpatient department, wards—separate for male and female patient, labor room, operation theater (optional), minor OT/dressing room/injection room, laboratory, general store, dispensing cum store area, infrastructure for AYUSH doctor, waste disposal pit—in line with central pollution control board (CPCB) guidelines, cold chain room, logistics room, generator room, office room, dirty utility room for dirty linen, and used items. Health and wellness room, Medical Imaging and Residential Quarters. For training purposes/IEC activities/meetings, an auditorium or a lecture hall for about 30 persons should be available.

### Staff

Staff of a PHC comprises of an MO along with paramedical staff and other staff (**Table 46.5** for IPHS norms).

**Table 46.5:** Indian Public Health Standards (IPHS) norms.

| Staff | PHC Essential | PHC Desirable | 24 × 7 PHC Essential | 24 × 7 PHC Desirable |
|---|---|---|---|---|
| Medical officer—MBBS | 1 | 1 | 2 | 1 |
| Medical officer—AYUSH | | 1 | | 1 |
| Medical officer—Dental | | 1 | | 1 |
| Pharmacist | 1 | | 1 | 1^ |
| Nurse-midwife (staff-nurse) | 2 | 1 | 7** | |
| Health worker (female)/ANM | 1* | | 1* | |
| Health assistant (male) | 1 | | 1 | |
| Health assistant (female)/lady health visitor | 1 | | 1 | |
| Health educator/Counsellor | | 1 | | 1 |
| Laboratory technician | 1 | | 2 | 1 |
| Dental assistant | | 1 | | 1 |
| Physiotherapist | | | | 1 |
| Ophthalmic assistant | | 1 | | 1 |
| Cold chain and vaccine logistic assistant | | 1 | 1 | |
| Accountant | 1 | | 1 | |
| Dressor | 1 | | 1 | |
| Data entry operator | 1 | | 1 | |
| Sanitation staff | 1 | | 4*** | |

*For subcenter area of PHC.
**1 in IPD in each shift including FP services + 1 for labor deliver recovery in each shift + 1 for OPD including NCD screening
***Shift duty.
^1 allopathy pharmacist + 1 storekeeper

### Functions

It has 4–6 beds for inpatient treatment. It is the referral center for about six subcenters. It provides preventive, promotive as well as curative services with emphasis on MCH services. It provides supportive supervision to the functioning of SC which falls under the PHC.

The services of all eight essential elements of primary health care are to be provided at PHC level. The broad services to be provided at PHC level are enumerated as follows:
1. Medical care
2. Maternal and child health including family planning services
3. Safe water supply and sanitation
4. Prevention and control of locally endemic diseases
5. Recording and reporting vital events
6. Health education
7. Services under national health programmes
8. Referral services
9. Training of health staff and health volunteers
10. Basic laboratory services

### Monitoring of PHC Functioning

Monitoring is essential to maintain quality and make suitable changes timely. PHC is monitored by internal as well as external monitoring mechanisms.

Internal monitoring is done by checking of records and periodic supervision, patient satisfaction surveys, medical audit, death audit by health staff at higher level and medical officer of PHC.

Various aspects of functioning of PHC are externally monitored by Village Health Sanitation and Nutrition Committee (VHSNC), Rogi Kalyan Samiti (RKS), Panchayati Raj Institution (PRI), and community monitoring framework as per strategies of GOI/State Government.

List of suggested equipment and furniture including reagents and diagnostic kits, facilities at newborn corner in labor room/OT, essential drugs list for PHC, check list for monitoring by external mechanism, description of job responsibilities of medical officer and other staff at PHC, charter of patients' rights for PHC, proforma for facility survey for PHC as per IPHS, facility based maternal death review form, integrated disease surveillance project reporting formats, list of statutory and regulatory compliances for PHC are provided in revised IPHS standards for PHC. Readers may refer to them for in-depth knowledge about PHC.

### 24 × 7 Primary Health Centers

The existing PHCs are upgraded in several states to provide continuous and round the clock delivery services. The criteria/requirements for declaring a PHC as 24 × 7 PHC are described below. However, these requirements are in addition to the primary services which a PHC is routinely expected to provide.

Essential additional services to be provided by a PHC to be considered as a 24 × 7 PHC are:
1. Provision of uninterrupted 24 × 7 delivery service, both assisted and normal*
2. Essential newborn care
3. Immediate referral for mother and child health emergencies to appropriate predetermined referral centers*
4. Routine antenatal care and routine immunization services for children and pregnant women (in addition to fixed day services).
5. Postnatal care
6. Early and safe services for medical termination of pregnancy (including manual vacuum aspiration)
7. Family welfare services
8. Prevention and management of reproductive tract infections
9. Essential laboratory services related to pregnancy, newborn care and children

For providing these services the technical staff of PHC particularly the medical officers and the staff nurses will be provided training on basic emergency obstetric care.

The ultimate goal of the union government is to upgrade all PHC to 24 × 7 PHC. However, it is not immediately possible. Hence, the government has formulated a checklist to rank and prioritize the PHCs to be upgraded for continuous functioning. The checklist essentially grades the PHC based on scoring of the following elements: location of the facility and its accessibility, population size, presence of technical staff at the facility and staff quarters, number of deliveries conducted annually, functional labor room, availability of referral services, other health facilities in the locality, etc.

> **Key Points**
> Primary health center is the first point of contact between doctor and the community, mainly providing primary level services in addition to curative services. It has 4–6 beds for indoor patients. A few of the PHCs are upgraded for providing 24 × 7 basic emergency obstetric care services.

## Community Health Centers

### Concept and Norm

The secondary level healthcare services are provided by CHCs, FRUs and the subdistrict and district hospitals. The CHCs are 30 bedded hospitals, established to provide referral services to patients referred from PHCs and SC as well as cases requiring specialist services and visiting directly to the center. It provides specialist care in medicine, surgery, obstetrics and gynecology, pediatrics, dental and AYUSH.

As per IPHS 2022 Guidelines CHCs can be divided into:
A. **Non-FRU CHCs (rural):** Non-FRU CHCs are those that provide essential services including preventive, promotive, curative, palliative, and rehabilitative services, etc. Curative services include normal delivery, stabilization of common emergencies, etc. Non-FRU CHCs in rural areas will have 30 essential beds.
B. **FRU CHCs (rural and urban):** FRU CHCs, in addition to the above services, provide specialized care which can be rendered through specialists (physicians, surgeons, obstetricians, pediatricians, and anesthesiologists) and the accompanying infrastructure (functional operation theatre and blood storage unit). Both elective and emergency surgical services of secondary level care shall be provided. FRU-CHCs will provide surgical services and go beyond obstetric services.

One CHC serves as a referral center for about four PHCs and caters to a population of about 80,000 for tribal/hilly/desert areas and 120,000 for plain areas. According to RHS 2021–22, 5,480 CHC in Rural and 584 CHCs in Urban area were functional as of March 2022.

All CHCs at block headquarters level (in rural and urban areas) are to be developed as Block Public Health Units (BPHU).

### Structure

The CHC building should provide the following facilities—minimum 30 indoor beds, X-ray, ECG and other laboratory facilities one operation theater and labor room. These facilities are provided through CHC building in seven different zones described as follows:
1. *Entrance zone:* Registration/record room, queue area outside registration room, pharmacy cum store, pharmacy cum store for AYUSH, public utilities and free space.
2. *Ambulatory zone (OPD):* Space for four General Doctor room, space for two AYUSH doctors room, eight specialist rooms with attached toilets, treatment room, refraction room, nursing station, casualty, dress room, injection room, female injection room, common toilets, public utility areas, waiting area, vaccine and logistics room, cold chain room.
3. *Diagnostic zone:* Pathology laboratory (optional), sample collection space, disinfectants storage, imaging room, preparation room, change room, public utilities, and toilet.

4. ***Intermediate zone (inpatient nursing units)***: Nursing station, four wards with six beds each (two female wards and two male wards), four private rooms (two each for male and females) with toilets, two isolation rooms with toilet (one for male and one for female)
5. ***Critical zone (operational theater/labor room)***: Patient area (preanesthesia and postoperative resting), staff rooms (changing, resting), supplies area (trolley bay, equipment storage, sterile storage), operating/labor room area (scrub, instrument sterilization, disposal), public utilities, free space
6. ***Service zone***:
   - Dietary (dry store, day store, preparation, cooking, delivery, pot wash, utensil wash, utensil store, and trolley park)
   - Central sterilization supply department (CSSD)
   - Laundry
   - Civil engineering
   - Electrical engineering
   - Mechanical engineering, waste disposal, fire protection, telephone, and intercom
   - Mortuary
7. ***Administrative zone***: General administration area and general store for public utilities.

### Staff

The staff pattern of CHC is described in **Table 46.6**.

Considering the shortage of specialist in the country any MBBS doctor who has received short-term training or have experience of at least 2 years in the particular speciality can be utilized against the speciality post. One ophthalmologist is recommended for every five CHCs.

### Functions

Non-FRU CHCs are envisaged to deliver services related to maternal and child health (including normal delivery), infectious diseases, nutritional disorders including iron-deficiency anemia, mental health conditions, noncommunicable diseases, Eye, Oral and ENT care. Early identification and treatment of these diseases coupled with prevention, promotion and risk reduction at community level is the only way to address disease burden at the population level.

**Table 46.6:** Medical staff pattern of community health center (CHC).

| Personnel | Non FRU-CHC | | FRU-CHC | |
|---|---|---|---|---|
| | E | D | E | D |
| Specialists and medical officers | | | | |
| General surgeon | | | 1 | 1 |
| Physician | 1 | | 1 | 1 |
| Obstetrician and gynecologist | | | 1 | 1 |
| Pediatrician | | | 1 | 1 |
| Anesthetist | | | 1 | 1 |
| Microbiologist | | | | 1 |
| General duty medical officer | 3 | 1 | 6 | 2 |
| Medical officer—AYUSH | | | 1 | 1 |
| Medical officer—Dental | 1 | | 1 | |

In addition supporting staff includes a team of nurses and paramedical staff, administrative staff and class 4 staff.

Services at FRU CHCs include specialist care, operative services and blood transfusion facilities in addition to maternal and child health care services.

The following services are provided at CHC:
- Routine and specialist OPD services and IPD services
- Emergency services
- Services of eye specialist (one for every five CHCs)
- Laboratory services
- Services under all the National Health Programmes

### First Referral Unit

A CHC/subdivisional hospital/district hospital can be declared as FRU only if it satisfies the following three criteria in addition to providing routine and emergency services that it is required to provide:
- Availability of emergency obstetric care with facilities of cesarean section;
- Care for sick newborns; and
- 24 × 7 blood storage facility.

> **Key Note**
> Community health centers are 30 bedded hospitals established to provide secondary level services at taluka level. It is staffed with specialists, medical officers and team of paramedics. It serves as a referral center for PHCs and SCs. A few of the CHCs are upgraded to first referral units.

## Subdistrict Hospitals

### Concept and Norms

Subdistrict hospitals (SDHs) also called as subdivisional hospitals play a very important role in reducing the burden of district hospitals on one side and acting as a referral center for SC, PHC, and CHC on other side. Since it provides specialist services, it also acts as a FRU and helps in preventing maternal and infant mortality. The number of beds of SDH varies from 31 to 100 depending on the catchment population and rate of admission in the hospital. It serves a population of about 5–6 lakhs. Around 1,275 SDH were functional in the country as on 31st March 2022.

### Structure and Staffing for SDH and DH

The National Health Policy, 2017 recommends two beds per 1,000 population. It is therefore proposed that the provision of one bed per 1,000 population is an 'Essential' norm for every district while two beds per 1,000 is a target they should aspire towards 'Desirable'. Districts with less than 5 lakh population with a functional DH do not need a Sub District hospital. Districts with populations between 5–10 lakh can have one SDH. Thereafter, one SDH for every 10 lakh population can be considered for the provision of comprehensive secondary care health services.

The 'Essential' number of beds in a district should be provided through the public health system of tertiary care (Medical Colleges), secondary care (DH, SDH and selected CHCs) and primary care (PHCs and remaining CHCs).

To achieve the 'Desirable' number of beds, the contribution of the private sector (based on the access to private health care in the local area), Railways, Armed Forces, Power Grid, Coal fields, Employees' State Insurance (ESI) and other Public Sector

Undertaking (PSU) hospitals may also be considered while continuing to strengthen and increase bed provision at public health facilities

Rough estimates of required essential and desired bed for SDH and DH are described in **Table 46.7.**

**Table 46.7:** Population wise requirement of essential and requited beds in district.

| Population | Essential beds | Desirable beds |
|---|---|---|
| Less than 2 lakh | 50 beds + 15 additional (Emergency and day care beds) | 100 |
| Between 2–5 lakh | 100 beds + 25 additional (Emergency and day care beds) | 200 |
| Between 5–10 lakh | 50 beds + 15 additional (Emergency and day care beds) | 300 |
| Between 10–20 lakh | 300 beds + 49 additional (Emergency and day care beds) | 400 |
| Between 20–30 lakh | 400 beds + 60 additional (Emergency and day care beds) | 500 |
| More than 30 lakhs | 500 beds + 65 additional (Emergency and day care beds) | 700 |

The details about structure, facilities, and manpower requirement of a SDH are provided in Revised IPHS standards for SDHs and DHs in 2022.

### Functions

The functions of a SDH are as follows:
- It provides specialist services to the population of the subdivision area of the district.
- It provides referral services to the health centers below Taluka level.
- It conducts training activities for the health-center staff.

## District/Specialist Hospital

### Concept and Norms

District hospital provides secondary level healthcare services as well as referral services to its district population. It serves not only people living in district headquarters and adjoining areas but also to people living in rural areas of the district. There must be one district hospital in every district as per norm to serve as a referral center for hospitals and/or health centers below the district level. However, the bed strength of the district hospital may vary depending on the population of the district, geographic size, and terrain of the district. In 2022, 767 district hospitals were functional in the country.

**Table 46.8:** Total medical and paramedical manpower required as per bed strength of district hospital.

| Cadre | SDH (100 Beds) | | DH (50 Beds) | | DH (200 Beds) | |
|---|---|---|---|---|---|---|
| | E | D | E | D | E | D |
| Doctors | 43 | 52 | 36 | 49 | 70 | 88 |
| Staff nurse | 72 | | 33 | | 135 | |

Total medical and Nursing manpower required as per bed strength of district hospital is given in **Table 46.8**.

The details about structure, facilities, and manpower requirement of a district hospital are provided in Revised IPHS standards for SDHs and DHs 2022.

### Functions

District hospital provides curative, preventive, and promotive healthcare service. In addition to routine OPD, indoor and emergency services the district hospital should also provide all basic speciality services. Larger hospital of more than 300 beds strength should aim to provide superspeciality services as well.

District hospitals must also have epidemic cell and disaster management units for rapid response in epidemic situations.

District hospitals should also provide skill based trainings to health staff.

> **Key Note**
> Roughly there are 1.6 lakh SC, 31,000 PHC, 6,064 CHC, 1,270 SDH and 767 DH functional in the country.

## JOB RESPONSIBILITIES OF STAFF OF HEALTH CENTERS

### Job Responsibilities of Medical Officer

A medical officer is the team leader of the staff at PHC. He is responsible for providing administrative, managerial, as well as healthcare service delivery activities in the PHC. He is responsible for functioning of PHC, implementation of all the programs in PHC areas, functioning of subcenters under PHC in addition to provision of curative services. A brief description of responsibilities of Medical Officer PHC is as follows:

### Curative Services

- He organizes routine OPD services for the patients. He will distribute the duties to the PHC staff for smooth functioning of PHC. He also manages for patients requiring curative services to patients outside the OPD timings.
- He cooperates and coordinates with other healthcare facilities providing curative services in PHC area.
- He also makes periodic visits at least once a month to SCs, under the PHC for supervision along with provision of curative services to community.

### Preventive and Health Promotive Activities

He will ensure proper implementation of various National Health and Family Welfare Programmes in the PHC area through his support staff. He will assist in formulation of various plans form implementation, provide supportive supervision to his team, perform monitoring activities, and provide guidance and direction to his health team. He will establish and maintain liaison with various key persons, such as block development officer, various social welfare agencies and community leaders and ensure their support in implementation of various health programs.

### Reproductive and Child Health Programme

- He acts as the leader of the PHC team to provide antenatal, intranatal and postnatal services. He will ensure motivation of women for institutional deliveries.
- He will supervise his team in implementation of special programs on nutrition, prophylaxis for vitamin A deficiency amongst children (1-5 years), prophylaxis for nutritional anemia amongst mothers, children and adolescent girls.

- He will coordinate with ICDS functionaries in provision of MCH services.
- He will ensure early detection and proper management of diarrhea, ARI and pneumonia cases in PHC area.
- He will periodically visit schools and conduct health check-up of school students.
- He will receive necessary trainings in tubectomy, NSV and IUCD insertion and organize vasectomy or tubectomy camps.
- He will ensure adequate supply of drugs, equipment, and logistics for the uninterrupted service delivery.

### Universal Immunization Programme
- He will ensure correct implementation of Universal Immunization Programme (UIP) as per latest policy.
- He will ensure adequate supplies and proper storage of vaccines through maintenance of cold chain at all levels.

### National Vector Borne Disease Control Programme
- He will provide administrative managerial and technical support to the PHC team for implementation of National Vector Borne Disease Control programs (NVBDCP) (Malaria, filaria, kala-azar, acute encephalitis syndrome (AES)/Japanese encephalitis (JE), dengue/chikungunya). He is responsible for all the operations under NVBDCP in PHC area.
- He will provide trainings and guide his team on implementation of latest treatment schedules under NVBDCP.
- He will ensure adequate supply of drugs, diagnostic test kits, equipment, chemicals and other logistics for continuous operations under NVBDCP.
- He will help in preparing line listing of cases and classifying high-risk areas as per NVBDCP guidelines.
- He conducts all NVBDCP IEC activities in the PHC area.
- He will ensure regular reporting of activities under NVBDCP to the District Malaria Officer/Civil Surgeon, CDHO.

### Control of Communicable Diseases
- He will initiate and take appropriate actions for the control of any outbreak or epidemic in his area.
- He will ensure regular weekly reporting under the Integrated Disease Surveillance Project.
- He will ensure chlorination of the wells and form liaison with appropriate agency for the same.
- He will ensure implementation of leprosy control activities, RNTCP and NACP in his PHC area.

### Other National Health Programmes
He will be entirely responsible for implementation and operationalization of all the health programmes including National Programme for Control of Blindness, Noncommunicable Disease Control Programme, etc., in his area.

### Training Activities
- He will update and maintain a database for trainings taken by staff, send them for appropriate trainings and use their skills accordingly.
- He will conduct or organize trainings for the staff of PHC and ASHA and arrange for retraining whenever needed.

### Administrative Work
- He will update and maintain all the inventory and stock register.
- He has to get the indents prepared and submit them timely for drugs, logistics and other consumables for uninterrupted functioning of all programs in his PHC.
- He will conduct review meetings monthly with the PHC staff to monitor and guide their activities.
- He will collect all the reports from the periphery to submit them to higher authority timely.

## Job Responsibilities of Health Educator
Currently health educator is available at block level PHC. He is under administrative control of the MO-PHC.

### Duties and Functions
- He will prepare and maintain the records of educational activities, tour programs, daily dairies, and other registers.
- He will assist in preparation of appropriate maps and charts of the PHC.
- He will facilitate the MO-PHC in conduction of trainings of health workers and ASHAs.
- He will celebrate important health days in the block area.
- He will make liaison with opinion leaders, local medical practitioners, school teachers, community, and religious leaders to orient them about the family welfare programme, and secure their assistance for the same.
- He will conduct IEC activities—film shows, exhibition, lecturers and dramas with regard to various national health programmes.
- He will provide various logistics for IEC activities by PHC staff.
- He will supervise the IEC activities by health staff and guide them.
- While on tour he will verify the records, reports, and stock registers of peripheral health staff particularly in relation to family welfare programme.
- He prepares report on IEC activities in the area and sends it monthly to district authorities.

## Job Responsibilities of Health Assistant Female (Lady Health Visitor) (Female Supervisor)
The job responsibilities of health assistant female are as follows:

### Supervision and Guidance
- The LHV supervises ANM of the subcenters under the PHC. In addition to the ANM she also provides supervision and guidance to *dais* and ASHAs in the area.
- She visits the SC weekly on a fixed day to observe and provide supportive supervision and training.

### Teamwork
- She facilitates building of team spirit among health workers.
- She coordinates health activities with other health staff, health assistant male, *dais* and ASHAs.
- She coordinates health activities with activities of school, sanitation and other departments.

- She attends the review meetings at PHC and provides inputs.
- She assists the medical officer in planning and distribution of work to the staff.

### Supplies, Equipment and Maintenance of Subcenters

- She ensures timely supply and maintenance of drugs and logistics to the subcenter.
- She ensures the cleanliness of the SC premises.

### Records and Reports

- Examines the records and registers by ANM and provides guidance for their proper maintenance.
- She collects and reviews the reports of work done by ANMs and submits it to MO-PHC every month.

### Training

- She will conduct the trainings of ASHAs and *dais* with the support of ANM.
- She will provide the required support to the MO-PHC in organizing various training activities for different categories of health personnel.

### Function Specific to Health Assistant Female

The HAF supervises the work of HWF with focus on programmatic aspects of Reproductive and Child Health Programme and Family Welfare Programme.

## Job Responsibilities of Health Assistant Male

### Supervision and Guidance

- The health assistant male supervises health workers male of the subcenters under the PHC.
- He visits the SC weekly on a fixed day to observe and provide supportive supervision and training to HWM.

### Teamwork

- He facilitates building of team spirit amongst health workers.
- He coordinates health activities with activities of female health supervisor, other health staff, village health guide and ASHA.
- He coordinates health activities with activities of school, sanitation and other departments.
- He attends the review meetings at the PHC and provides inputs.
- He assists the medical officer in planning and distribution of work to the staff.

### Supplies, Equipment and Maintenance of Subcenters

- He ensures timely supply and maintenance of drugs and logistics to the subcenter.
- He ensures the proper maintenance of HWM kit.

### Records and Reports

- Examines the records and registers by ANM and provides guidance for their proper maintenance.
- He collects and reviews the reports of work done by ANMs and submits it to MO-PHC every month.

### Training

He will provide the required support to the MO-PHC in organizing various training activities for different categories of health personnel.

### Function Specific to Health Assistant Male

The HAM supervises the work of HWM with focus on programmatic aspects of communicable and noncommunicable disease control programs and environmental sanitation programs.

## Job Responsibilities of Laboratory Technician

The laboratory technician functions under MO-PHC. The functions of laboratory technician are as under:
- General sanitation of the laboratory.
- Proper handling and maintenance of laboratory equipment.
- Following of biomedical waste management rules.
- Record keeping for laboratory test done and submit monthly reports to MO-PHC.
- Submit timely indent reports for laboratory consumables to MO-PHC.

He will have to perform laboratory investigations advised by the medical officer. The lists of minimum laboratory investigations to be performed at PHC are given in IPHS standards for PHC.

## Job Functions of Health Worker Female (ANM)

She will carry out the following activities in SC area villages:

### Maternal and Child Health

- Early registration of all pregnancies and provide a minimum of 4 ANC visits
- Perform urine sugar and albumin testing along with hemoglobin estimation of pregnant woman
- Refer them to higher centers for RPR testing for syphilis and if any danger signs of pregnancy are identified
- Conduct deliveries in subcenter, supervise and assist deliveries conducted by *dais* and refer difficult cases of labor to higher centers
- Provide at least two postnatal home visits, screen the newborn for birth defects, advice mother on postnatal care, and counsel her for early initiation of breastfeeding and immunization.
- She will provided health education to mothers in group as well as individually on IYCF, family planning and immunization.
- Track the growth and development of the children up to 5 years, manage for minor sickness as per IMNCI strategy, and refer difficult cases.

## Job Functions of Health Worker Male

The health worker male has to visit each house at least once a fortnight and record his visit on the main entrance of the house as per guidelines. His duties for different National Health Programme are:

### National Vector Borne Disease Control Programme

***Malaria:*** During his fortnightly visit to each house he shall inquire about any fever cases and if found he will collect the blood smears.

- He will maintain the record of the blood smears collected and send the blood smears to PHC laboratory twice weekly.
- He will provide radical treatment to positive cases and verify radical treatment provided by ASHA or FTD based on results obtained by RDK.
- He will assist health assistant male in planning of spraying operations in pre and post monsoon season.

### Family Planning

- Maintain and update eligible couple register
- Motivate eligible couples to accept family planning methods
- Build rapport with village leaders, female leaders, *dais*, ASHA and promote family planning activities
- Participate in Mahila Mandal meetings and conduct awareness activities on family planning.

#### Medical Termination of Pregnancy

- Guide the community of the harms of unsafe methods of abortion; provide them information about the availability of services for medical termination of pregnancy.
- Refer the women requiring pregnancy termination services to nearest approved institution.

#### Nutrition

- Growth monitoring of children and provide appropriate advice thereby. Referral of severe cases of malnutrition to higher centers.
- Provide IFA tablets to ANC, PNC adolescents and syrup to less than 5 years children as per guidelines.
- Administer vitamin A solution to under 5 children as per the guidelines.
- Provide health education to community about the locally available foods and the importance of nutritious diet for mothers and children.
- Coordinate with Anganwadi workers in growth monitoring and distribution of food supplements to the beneficiaries.

#### Universal Programme on Immunization

- Ensure complete immunize pregnant women and children as per immunization schedule.
- Prompt reporting of all AEFI and management of minor cases at SC level.
- ANM is responsible for maintenance of cold chain at the facility and outreach level.
- She prepares the work plan, due list of beneficiaries with the help of ASHA and AWW. She indents for required vaccines and logistics weekly.
- She tracks the dropouts, left-outs and motivates them for immunization.

#### Communicable and Noncommunicable Diseases

- She will assist the health worker male in notifying the medical officer and informing health supervisors about any abnormal increase in cases of any disease.
- Along with health worker male she will screen, identify, provide health education and counseling wherever required, treat and refer difficult cases of communicable and noncommunicable diseases.
- She will maintain all the records of all events and do periodic reporting to the PHC.
- She will conduct all relevant health education activities.
- She will assist health worker male, coordinate the activities carried out by VHSNC and guide AHSA and village health guide to provide various services under various National health programmes for communicable and noncommunicable diseases.

#### Record-keeping

- Prepare and maintain maps of areas highlighting facilities and other landmarks.
- Prepare and maintain charts of SC villages highlighting important demographic indicators.
- Record all vital events like births and deaths and report to the PHC.
- Maintain all the records and registers related to mother, child health and family planning.
- Submission of weekly and monthly reports in required formats to the health supervisor female.

#### Team Activities

- Participate in sector meetings monthly at PHC and or at block level.
- Coordinate activities with health worker male, health volunteers, ASHA, *dais*, etc.
- Coordinate with PRI and VHSC in implantation of various programs.

- Distribute contraceptives to the needy couples
- If she is trained in IUCD insertion, she can even insert IUCD

***In areas endemic for Kala-azar or Japanese encephalitis or filariasis:*** During his home visits he will ask for any fever or encephalitis case or lymphedema/hydrocele in last 15 days. Identify them, record them and refer to PHC/CHC for further investigations and treatment.

- He will ensure their follow up and complete treatment.
- He will plan and conduct health education activities in such areas.
- Provide follow-up services for female clients on accepting family planning services

***RNTCP and Leprosy eradication programme:*** Screen for tuberculosis or leprosy cases and refer them to PHC for diagnosis and treatment.

- Identify positive cases for leprosy or tuberculosis (TB). Arrange for their regular follow-up to check for compliance with treatment, side effects to drugs. Motivate defaulters to complete the treatment.
- Update and maintain the records of leprosy and tuberculosis patients.
- Provide health education to the community on various aspects of TB and leprosy.

#### Universal Immunization Programme

- Assist or cooperate with health worker female in implementation of UIP and delivery of various services under it.
- Assist health assistant male for monitoring and supervision.

#### Reproductive and Child Health Programme

- Assist or cooperate with health worker female in implementation of RCH programme and delivery of various services of the program.
- Identify male community leaders and provide them orientation training on family welfare programme.
- Screen for STI among male and refer them to PHC.
- Assist health assistant male for monitoring and supervision.

#### Communicable Disease

- Continue surveillance and weekly reporting under IDSP.
- Notify Medical Officer for any abnormal increase in cases of communicable diseases and implement control measures under the supervision of health assistant male.
- Conduct health education activities.

#### Environmental Sanitation

- Coordinate with VHSC to ensure chlorination of drinking water sources regularly and motivation for the use of latrines.
- Conduct health education activities for methods of disposal of solids and liquid wastes, use of smokeless Chula's, use of sanitary latrines, and sanitation in and around the house.

#### Record-keeping

- Prepare and maintain maps of areas highlighting facilities and other landmarks.
- Prepare and maintain charts of SC villages highlighting important communicable disease indicators, such as for malaria, tuberculosis, leprosy, etc.
- Record all vital events like births and deaths and report to the PHC.
- Maintain all the records and registers related to communicable diseases and family planning.
- Submit the weekly and monthly reports in required formats to the health supervisor male.

> **Key Note**
> Medical officer is the team leader of the staff at PHC and its SCs. He does administrative and managerial activities at PHC along with monitoring and supervision of services provided by paramedics, in addition to providing curative services himself. Health educator is responsible for preparation and dissemination of IEC logistics along with participation in IEC activities of various health programs. He monitors and supervises IEC activities by other paramedics. HAF supervises the health activities by ANM along with coordination of other health activities. HAM supervises the health activities by HWM along with coordination of other health activities. ANM provides all the primary level healthcare services as per various health programs particularly maternal and child health related services to people living in the catchment area of the SC. HWM provides all the primary level healthcare services as per various health programs particularly noncommunicable and communicable disease related services to people living in the catchment area of the SC.

# ORGANIZATION OF URBAN HEALTH SYSTEM IN INDIA

Most of the Indian cities have their hospitals or dispensaries constructed by Urban Local government—Municipal Corporation. However, they are usually inadequate to meet the demand of the public. There are also state governments hospitals and health centers along with industrial hospitals, Employees State Insurance Schemes (ESIS) hospitals, Urban Health and Family Welfare Centers (UHFWCs), in addition to a huge and varied private sector to cater to the health needs of urban population. These institutes focus on providing curative services and coverage on urban slums is neglected. There have been efforts to provide primary healthcare through various schemes sponsored by central and state governments which are described here. Despite it there is no uniform public health structure across the urban areas of India till date.

## Urban Family Welfare Centers

The urban family welfare centers (UFWCs) were established since the first five-year plan. They are supposed to provide primary healthcare services, maternal and child health related services, family welfare services along with outreach services with special focus on urban slums. The UFWCs are classified into three types based on population covered by them. Type 1 covers 10,000–25,000 population, type 2 covers 25,000–50,000 and type 3 covers more than 50,000 urban populations.

The National Health Policy 2002 (NHP 2002) made recommendations to establish a uniform structure to provide primary health care to the urban population. NHP 2002 proposed establishment of a two-tier structure. Tier 1 comprising of a PHC catering to 1 lakh population that provides OPD services along with provision of services under all national health programmes. Tier 2 comprises of public hospitals that act as referral centers for Urban Primary Health Centers. The expenditure for establishment and maintenance of Urban Health Center is to be borne jointly by the state and union government.

## National Urban Health Mission

These urban public health structures described above will be upgraded to urban health centers. The existing human resources will be reorganized. In addition to public health structures, NUHM focuses on intersectoral coordination, involvement of NGO and self-help groups and public-private partnerships for providing health services to urban people.

The urban health centers will provide OPD services, maternal and child health including family welfare services, basic laboratory services, provision of essential drugs, counseling, besides facilitating referral to the second tier health facilities. The second tier hospitals include medical college hospitals, corporation hospitals, district hospitals or any public or private hospital identified and capable for handling referral cases. *More details is provided in Chapter 47: Health Policies and Programs in India.*

# COMMUNITY PARTICIPATION IN PROVISION OF HEALTHCARE SERVICES—RURAL AND URBAN

In addition to the public health system, the primary health care is also provided by community members as per the recommendations of Rural Health Scheme, 1977. In order to achieve health for all by 2000 AD, the strategy was to implement primary health care through community participation. As a result various functionaries were appointed at village level.

The village level functionaries form the first line of contact for the community to the health system. These are non-medical personnel having a will for healthcare service delivery. They are voluntary persons from the community and willing to donate two to three hours a day to community health services. They receive an honorarium in return.
- ICDS functionaries
- Mahila Swasthya Sangh (MSS)
- Accredited Social Health Activities (ASHA)
- Various strategies/measures under NRHM to strengthen community participation.

## Anganwadi Center Scheme

*Angan* is a Hindi word which means courtyard. Anganwadi worker is a voluntary part time worker selected by the community for which she works. She caters to the population of about 1,000 in urban slums and 700 in hilly tribal backward areas (i.e., around 200 households, approx. 150–200 children <6 years, 30–45 pregnant and lactating mothers and 200 women in 15–45 years age group). Her primary focus is on mother and child health. Her beneficiaries include children <6 years of age, pregnant and lactating mothers, and adolescent girls. Her duties includes providing non-formal preschool education, *Balbhog* and other nutritional supplements, growth monitoring and basic health facilities for children and pregnant mothers, referral of high-risk cases, assist in conduction of Mamta Divas activities, and maintains records. She functions in liaison with other health workers. She is trained for 4 months by ICDS department. She is assisted by a helper at the AWC. For every 20–25 AWC there is one supervisor called Mukhya Sevika. Every 3–4 Mukhya Sevika are supervised by Child Development Project Officer.

## Mahila Swasthya Sangh

It is an organization of group of women consisting of ANM, AWW, Gram Sevika and other female volunteers. Their main activity is supporting the ANM in providing maternal and child healthcare services.

## Accredited Social Health Activities

ASHA is an honorary volunteer who acts as a link between the community and the public healthcare system. She is provided performance based incentives for various healthcare activities. The counterpart of ASHA for urban areas is called Urban Social Health Activities (USHA). *More about criteria and functions of ASHA is described in Chapter 47: Health Policies and Programs in India.*

## Various Strategies/Measures under NRHM to Strengthen Community Participation

### Village Health Sanitation and Nutrition Committee

There was a need for collective decision making regarding health priorities as well as health determinants at village level. The formation of Village Health Sanitation and Nutrition Committee under NRHM supported decentralized community level planning and decision making process. The committee addresses the local needs and serves the purpose of community involvement in planning and monitoring mechanisms regarding health services.

The VHSNC acts as a subcommittee of Gram Panchayat. It should have a minimum of 15 members which includes elected members of Panchayat, health workers and health volunteers, representations from all community subgroups along with ASHA who will be the member secretary and convener of the committee.

### The Rogi Kalyan Samitis (Patient Welfare Society/Hospital Development Committee)

There has been a growing demand to improve the quality of services provided by the public health facilities. However, the funding of the public sector is unable to meet these demands. Hence, there came the concept of Rogi Kalyan Samiti. Rogi Kalyan Samitis (RKS) is a registered society that essentially performs management and regulatory functions for the health facility. It is set up in all district hospitals, SDHs, FRUs and CHCs. It basically functions to improve quality of services with accountability, people's involvement and transparency.

It consists of the following members:
- Peoples representatives—MLA/MP
- Leading members of the community
- Health officials (including an AYUSH doctor)
- Local district officials
- Local CHC/FRU in-charge
- Representatives of the Indian Medical Association
- Members of the local bodies and Panchayati Raj representative
- Leading donors

Rogi Kalyan Samitis functions as an NGO and not as a government body. It will raise funds primarily by imposing user charges for utilization of various hospital services, collecting funds from donor agencies, donations, and loans from financial agencies along with grants from government.

Private agencies can be permitted to provide high tech services of MRI, CT scan, sonography, pathology services, etc., or setup their units in hospital premises in return of a fixed fee to the RKS society.

The funds collected will be used for providing quality services to the public by the hospital, hiring of staff as per need, procurement of drugs and equipment locally, general maintenance of the hospital, etc.

### The Panchayati Raj Institution

The Panchayati Raj Institution (PRI) has strengthened the representation and participation of community in establishing health priorities and providing rural health services.

## OTHER MECHANISMS FOR PROVIDING HEALTH CARE IN INDIA

### Health Insurance in India

Health Insurance in India is still in its early stages of development. A few of the insurance schemes operated by union and state government such as Rashtriya Swasthya Bima Yojana (RSBY) which is being replaced by Pradhan Mantri Jan Arogya Yojana or National Health Protection Scheme *(This is further described in Chapter 47: Health Policies and Programs in India)*, Employees State Insurance Scheme (ESIS) and the Central Government Health Scheme (CGHS) *(This is further described in Chapter 49: Health Legislations in India)*. In addition, there are also public and private insurance companies along with community based organizations providing health insurance facilities to individuals and families. The CGHS and ESIS cover a large group of salary earners in India. In India a total of around 300 million people are under cover of some kind of health insurance. Among them over 243 million people are under cover of different forms of government sponsored insurance schemes. The dependence on commercial insurance is merely in only about million. Health insurance can be looked upon as a step towards nationalizing health services.

### Public Private Partnerships

It is a known by surveys that a large majority of rural population (78%) as well as urban population (81%) were treated from private sector for any sickness in 2004. The reasons as per 60th NSSO mainly include nonavailability of services, long waiting period, unsatisfied with public health services, nonaccessibility of public health services. (MOHFW, NSSO: 42nd, 52nd, and 60th round, 2007).

When it comes to utilization of inpatient services, again the private sector has dominated as compared to public sector. So it is need of hour to utilize the facilities of large private sector through public private partnerships.

### Partnership with Rural Medical Practitioners

There are several Rural Health Practitioners formally or informally trained and providing healthcare services to 6.5 lakh villages in India. The rural masses have trust in them and are often the first point of contact whenever any health need arises. These RMPs can be contacted, trained in various interventions under NRHM to provide desired services to the rural masses. They can play a crucial supplementary role in achieving universal health coverage.

### *Partnership with Non-Governmental and Civil Organizations*

GOI has made recommendations for cooperation and collaboration with NGOs and civil organizations to supplement the public health system in healthcare delivery. These agencies can be involved in training activities of health staff and volunteers, implementation of various National Health Programmes as per their capacities, IEC activities, etc., provisions are made under NRHM to make partnerships at local levels with NGOs for supplementing health service delivery.

### *Partnerships with Private Practitioners for Speciality Services*

There are several schemes such as Chiranjivi Yojana and Bal Sakha Yojana in Gujarat which provide complete package of maternal and child healthcare services to the beneficiaries in private institutions. The government will identify such private institutions and reimburse them for service provided by them to the beneficiaries. Several such schemes are also in operation in other states by other names.

## OTHER AGENCIES PROVIDING HEALTH SERVICES

### Defense Medical Services

Defense employees are provided comprehensive health services through their own organization of dispensaries and hospitals. Ministry of Defense funds the operationalization and maintenance of these services.

### Health Services for Railway Employees

Railway employees are provided comprehensive health services through their own organization of dispensaries, clinics and railway hospitals. The health services for a railway division are supervised by a chief health inspector. The employees are provided health check-up upon joining the services and routinely every year thereafter. In order to provide complete package of maternal and child health services there are lady medical officers, health visitors and midwives. The Ministry also provides specialist services to its employees and their families at divisional levels.

### Private Agencies

In a large country such as India, the government is unable to provide complete package of services to all. As a result there is a boom of private medical practice in India. There are a variety of private practitioners ranging from a small dispensary to state of art multispecialty hospitals. Amongst all the practitioners of medicine, the allopathic providers have dominated the service delivery. About 70% of the private practitioners are general practitioners. It also includes the services offered by various trust hospitals, religious hospitals or caste hospitals. It purely relies on out of pocket expenditure of the public resulting in gross variations in services charges from providers to providers.

The private sector is unorganized and the private practitioners are free to charge any amount of service fees. There are a few of the regulatory bodies such as Medical Council of India and Indian Medical Association which regulate some of the activities of private practitioners.

### Voluntary Agencies in India

A voluntary health agency is any organized not for profit organization concerned with providing health related services. It is governed by non-medical and/or professionals and its organization varies from national to local levels. They collect funds from private sources for delivery of services. These agencies usually provide specific kind of services depending on the mission of the organization, e.g., cancer-related services or disability-related services, etc. The main advantage of voluntary agencies is that their services are not limited by the public health system and can initiate or implement a new program/strategy on their own for the betterment of the public.

A few of the well-known voluntary health agencies functional in India are enumerated here:
- Indian Council for Child Welfare
- All India Women's Conference
- Family Planning Association of India
- The Kasturba Memorial Fund
- Indian Red Cross Society
- Bharat Sevak Samaj
- Tuberculosis Association of India
- Hind Kusht Nivaran Sangh
- Central Social Welfare Board
- Professional bodies, such as the Indian Medical Association, All India Dental Association, The Trained Nurses Association of India
- International agencies, such as Rockefeller Foundation, Ford Foundation and CARE

A few of the functions of voluntary health agencies are described below
- ***Provision of services to the needy:*** This includes patient care and nursing, home visits, OPD services, outreach services, training and supervision of voluntary workers, IEC related activities, etc.
- ***Supplementing the work of official agencies:*** Since there is always scarcity of resources and several other restrictions in public sector, the voluntary agency can supplement them by providing the support of skilled human resource or providing funds for purchase of special equipments or necessary logistics.
- ***Research and implementations of new innovative technology or ideas:*** Since implementation of any new idea for improved service delivery will require approval from government bodies, it will take years to implement the same. Voluntary agencies can pioneer the same and provide results to the government for its implementation as a project or program. It can guide the work of official agencies and provide evidence-based constructive ideas, e.g., the demonstration by Rockefeller Foundation regarding bore-hole latrine and implementation of the idea played a lead role in solving the problem of hookworm in

India. RCA latrines are widely accepted and promoted in environmental sanitation program.
- **Grants/scholarships:** It can provide financial assistance through scholarships or grants for research and development or training.
- **Epidemics/disasters:** During disasters these agencies come forward and share the responsibility to solve the problem.
- **Policy formation:** It can affect policy formulation through interpretation of public demands.

## SUGGESTED READING

1. Borkar G. Health in Independent India. New Delhi: Ministry of Health.
2. Chadha MS. Report of the Special Committee on the preparation for entry of the NMEP into the Maintenance Phase, Ministry of Health, Government of India; 1963.
3. Directorate General of Health Services, New Delhi. Report of The Committee on Integration of Health Services; 1967.
4. Government of India, Ministry of Health and Family Welfare, Statistics Division, Rural Health Statistics; 2018.
5. Government of India. Government of India's Resolution setting up the Planning Commission. New Delhi; 1950.
6. Guidelines for Operationalizing a Primary Health Centre for Providing 24-Hour Delivery and Newborn Care under RCH-II. Maternal Health Division, Department of Family Welfare, Ministry of Health and Family Welfare, Government of India.
7. Hogarth J. Glossary of healthcare terminology. Copenhagen, World Health Organization, Regional Office for Europe; 1975. [online] Available from http://whqlibdoc.who.int/publications/9290201231.pdf.
8. Islam B. Right to health: A constitutional mandate in India. IJARIIE. 2017;3(3):2627-38.
9. Ministry of Health, Government of India, New Delhi. Report of The Health Survey and Planning Committee (August 1959–October 1961).
10. Ministry of Health and Family Planning, Government of India. New Delhi. Health Services and Medical Education: A Programme for Immediate Action. Report of the group on Medical Education and Support Manpower. Allied Publishers Private Limited; 1975.
11. National Health Mission, Government of India, Ministry of Health and Family Welfare, Guidelines for Rogi Kalyan Samitis. [online] Available from http://nhm.gov.in/nhm/nrhm/guidelines/nrhm-guidelines/constitution-of-rogi-kalyan-samities.html.
12. National Health Mission, Government of India, Ministry of Health and Family Welfare, Guidelines for Village Health Sanitation and Nutrition Committee.
13. National Health Mission, Government of India, Ministry of Health and Family Welfare, Indian Public Health Standards (IPHS). Guidelines for Sub-Centres, Revised 2022. New Delhi: NHM; 2022.
14. National Health Mission, Government of India, Ministry of Health and Family Welfare, Indian Public Health Standards (IPHS): Guidelines for District Hospitals, Revised 2022. New Delhi: NHM; 2022.
15. National Health Mission, Government of India, Ministry of Health and Family Welfare, Indian Public Health Standards (IPHS): Guidelines for Sub-District/Sub-Divisional Hospitals Revised; 2022.
16. National Health Mission, Government of India, Ministry of Health and Family Welfare, Indian Public Health Standards, Guidelines for Primary Health Centres, Revised 2022. New Delhi: NHM; 2022.
17. National Health Portal, India. Bajaj Committee, 1986. NHP CC DC. April 03, 2015. [online] Available from https://www.nhp.gov.in/bajaj-committee-1986_pg.
18. National Health Portal, India. Bhore Committee, 1946. NHP CC DC; 2015. [online] Available from https://www.nhp.gov.in/bhore-committee-1946_pg.
19. National Health Portal, India. Kartar Singh Committee, 1973. NHP CC DC. April 03, 2015. [online] Available from https://www.nhp.gov.in/kartar-singh-committee-1973_pg.
20. National Health Portal, India. Mukherjee Committee; 1965. NHP CC DC. April 03, 2015. [online] Available from https://www.nhp.gov.in/mukherjee-committee-1965_pg.
21. National Health Portal, India. Mukherjee Committee; 1966. NHP CC DC. April 03, 2015. [online] Available from https://www.nhp.gov.in/mukherjee-committee-1966_pg.
22. NITI Aayog (National Institution for Transforming India), Government of India. Constitution of NITI: Functions. [online] Available from http://niti.gov.in/content/functions.
23. NITI Aayog. Healthy States Progressive India Report on the Ranks of states and Union Territories. Health Index June; 2019.
24. Planning Commission, Government of India, New Delhi. Social Sectors Twelfth Five Year Plan (2012–2017) Vol III.
25. Report of the Task Force on Comprehensive Primary Healthcare Rollout. Ministry of Health and Family Welfare, Government of India.
26. World Health Organisation, Select Health Parameters: A comparative analysis across the National Sample Survey Organisation (NSSO) 42nd, 52nd and 60th Rounds, 2007, Ministry of Health and family Welfare, Government of India, in collaboration with WHO, Country Office India.
27. National Health Mission, Government of India, Ministry of Health and Family Welfare, Indian Public Health Standards (IPHS): Guidelines for Community Health Centres, Revised 2022. New Delhi: NHM; 2022.

# CHAPTER 47

# Health Policies and Programs in India

*Bratati Banerjee, Rupsa Banerjee, Bhargav Dave, Nidhi Mangrola, Ankit Sheth*

| | |
|---|---|
| CM 3.6 | Discuss National Vector Borne disease Control Program |
| CM 5.6 | Enumerate and discuss the National Nutrition Policy, important National Nutritional Programs including the Integrated Child Development Services Scheme (ICDS), etc. |
| CM 8.3 | Enumerate and describe disease specific National Health Programs including their prevention and treatment of a case |
| CM 9.6 | Describe the National Population Policy |
| CM 10.4 | Describe the Reproductive, Maternal, Newborn and Child Health (RMNCH); child survival and safe motherhood interventions |
| CM 10.5 | Describe Universal Immunization Program; Integrated Management of Neonatal and Childhood Illness (IMNCI) and other existing Programs. |
| CM 10.7 | Enumerate and describe the basis and principles of the Family Welfare Program including the organization, technical and operational aspects. |
| CM 12.4 | Describe national program for elderly |
| CM 15.3 | Describe National Mental Health programme |
| CM 16.4 | Describe national policies related to health and health planning |
| CM 17.4 | Describe national policies related to health and health planning |

## INTRODUCTION

To guide health care in the country, health policies are needed, which outline the priority areas, the specific achievements desired in terms of goals and objectives, and the measures required to realize these goals, as per expectations of the government. A policy is a set of guiding principles or statement of intentions or objectives, along with a description of the measures to be taken and the resources to be utilized, to achieve the stated objectives. Government of India has formulated various policies from time to time, for improving health status of people of India, the key policies being National Health Policy (NHP), National Population Policy, National Nutrition Policy, etc.

While policies are the wish lists that state the intentions about what to achieve, health programs are the definite strategies and set of actions with instructions, aiming to achieve the desired objectives. Health programs focus on specific community health problems or specific vulnerable groups. It contains goal, objectives, strategies, and list of activities, along with set of instructions or guidelines for implementation. Thus, a program can be said to be a "prescription" written by community medicine practitioners to promote the health of the people of a country and protect them against health threat. India has designed and is implementing numerous health programs, since as early as the year of independence.

## HEALTH AND HEALTH-RELATED POLICIES

### NATIONAL HEALTH POLICY 2017

The first NHP was framed in 1983 to provide comprehensive and decentralized health care, accessible to all. NHP 2002 focused on achieving an acceptable standard of good health for the population and ensuring an equitable access to health services across all strata. NHP 2017 addresses various changes in the health scenario in the country that have occurred since the previous health policy, viz., increasing burden of noncommunicable diseases (NCDs), growing healthcare industry, increasing out-of-pocket expenditure on health that contributes to poverty, and enhanced fiscal capacity of the country due to rising economic growth.

### Goal

- The attainment of the highest possible level of health and well-being for all at all ages, through a preventive and promotive healthcare orientation in all developmental policies.
- Universal access to good quality healthcare services without anyone having to face financial hardship as a consequence.

### Key Policy Principles

- Professionalism, integrity and ethics
- Equity
- Affordability
- Universality

- Patient centered and quality care
- Accountability
- Inclusive partnerships
- Pluralism
- Decentralization
- Dynamism and adaptiveness.

## Objectives

To improve health status of the population and achieve equity through universal health coverage, reinforcing trust in public healthcare system and align the growth of the private health sector with public health goals.

## Specific Quantitative Goals and Objectives

### Health Status and Program Impact

*Life expectancy and healthy life:*
- Increase life expectancy at birth from 67.5 to 70 by 2025.
- Establish regular tracking of disability adjusted life years (DALY) index as a measure of burden of disease and its trends by major categories by 2022.
- Reduction of total fertility rate (TFR) to 2.1 at national and subnational level by 2025.

*Mortality by age and/or cause:*
- Reduce under-five mortality to 23 by 2025 and maternal mortality rate (MMR) from current levels to 100 by 2020.
- Reduce infant mortality rate to 28 by 2019.
- Reduce neonatal mortality to 16 and still birth rate to "single digit" by 2025.

*Reduction of disease prevalence/incidence:*
- Achieve global target of 2020 which is also termed as target of 90:90:90, for HIV/AIDS, i.e., 90% of all people living with HIV know their HIV status; 90% of all people diagnosed with HIV infection receive sustained antiretroviral therapy (ART); and 90% of all people receiving ART will have viral suppression.
- Achieve and maintain elimination status of leprosy by 2018, kala-azar by 2017, and lymphatic filariasis in endemic pockets by 2017.
- Achieve and maintain a cure rate of more than 85% in new sputum positive patients for tuberculosis (TB) and reduce incidence of new cases, to reach elimination status by 2025.
- Reduce the prevalence of blindness to 0.25/1,000 by 2025 and disease burden by one-third from current levels.
- Reduce premature mortality from cardiovascular diseases, cancer, diabetes or chronic respiratory diseases by 25% by 2025.

### Health Systems Performance

*Coverage of health services:*
- Increase utilization of public health facilities by 50% from current levels by 2025.
- Antenatal care (ANC) coverage to be sustained above 90% and skilled attendance at birth above 90% by 2025.
- More than 90% of the newborn are fully immunized by 1 year of age by 2025.
- Meet the need of family planning above 90% at national and subnational level by 2025.
- About 80% of known hypertensive and diabetic individuals at household level maintain "controlled disease status" by 2025.

*Cross sectoral goals related to health:*
- Relative reduction in prevalence of current tobacco uses by 15% by 2020 and 30% by 2025.
- Reduction of 40% in prevalence of stunting of under-five children by 2025.
- Access to safe water and sanitation to all by 2020 (Swachh Bharat Mission).
- Reduction of occupational injury by half from current levels of 334 per lakh agricultural workers by 2020.
- National/State level tracking of selected health behavior.

### Health Systems Strengthening

*Health finance:*
- Increase health expenditure by government as a percentage of gross domestic product (GDP) from the existing 1.15 to 2.5% by 2025.
- Increase state sector health spending to more than 8% of their budget by 2020.
- Decrease in proportion of households facing catastrophic health expenditure from the current levels by 25%, by 2025.

*Health infrastructure and human resource:*
- Ensure availability of paramedics and doctors as per Indian Public Health Standards (IPHS) norm in high priority districts by 2020.
- Increase community health volunteers to population ratio as per IPHS norm, in high priority districts by 2025.
- Establish primary and secondary care facility as per norms in high priority districts (population as well as time to reach norms) by 2025.

*Health management information:*
- Ensure district-level electronic database of information on health system components by 2020.
- Strengthen the health surveillance system and establish registries for diseases of public health importance by 2020.
- Establish federated integrated health information architecture, health information exchanges and National Health Information Network by 2025.

## NATIONAL POPULATION POLICY

Efforts for family planning in India started as early as 1952 when it was the first country in the world to launch the National Family Planning Program. It focused on encouraging people to adopt the small family norm. The first National Population Policy was framed in 1976 which increased legal age of marriage for both girls and boys and emphasized on small family norm. The NHP in 1983 set the target of achieving replacement level of TFR by the year 2000.

The National Population Policy was drawn in the year 2000 with the goal of population stabilization in India. It aims to achieve net replacement levels of TFR by 2010 and offers a comprehensive package of reproductive and child health (RCH) services through both government and nongovernment sectors.

Net replacement level is the amount of fertility needed to keep the population the same from generation to generation. It refers to the TFR that will result in a stable population without it increasing or decreasing. It is expressed as the total number of live births a woman would need to have over her childbearing years, which is typically ages 15–44.

## Objectives

***Immediate:*** To address the unmet needs for contraception, healthcare infrastructure and health personnel and to provide integrated service delivery for basic RCH care.

***Medium-term:*** To bring TFR to replacement levels by 2010, through vigorous implementation of intersectoral operational strategies.

***Long-term:*** To achieve a stable population by 2045, at a level consistent with the requirement of sustainable economic growth, social development, and environmental protection.

## National Sociodemographic Goals for 2010

- Address the unmet needs for basic RCH services, supplies, and infrastructure.
- Make school education up to age 14 free and compulsory and reduce dropouts at primary and secondary school levels to below 20% for both boys and girls.
- Reduce infant mortality rate to below 30 per 1,000 live births.
- Reduce MMR to below 100 per 100,000 live births.
- Achieve universal immunization of children against all vaccine preventable diseases.
- Promote delayed marriage for girls not earlier than age 18 and preferably after 20 years of age.
- Achieve 80% institutional deliveries and 100% deliveries by trained persons.
- Achieve universal access to information/counseling and services for fertility regulation and contraception with a wide basket of choices.
- Achieve 100% registration of births, deaths, marriage, and pregnancy.
- Contain the spread of acquired immunodeficiency syndrome (AIDS) and promote greater integration between the management of reproductive tract infections (RTI), sexually transmitted infections (STI) and the National AIDS Control Organization (NACO).
- Prevent and control communicable diseases.
- Integrate Indian systems of medicine (ISM) in the provision of RCH services and in reaching out to households.
- Promote vigorously the small family norm to achieve replacement levels of TFR.
- Bring about convergence in implementation of related social sector programs so that family welfare becomes a people-centered program.

## Strategic Themes

- ***Decentralized planning and program implementation:*** This is achieved through Panchayati Raj Institutions who will identify unmet needs of contraception in their area and provide services at the village level.
- ***Convergence of service delivery at village level:*** Village self-help groups will provide basic RCH services at the village level in conjunction with Integrated Child Development Services (ICDS).
- ***Empowering women for improved health and nutrition:*** This will help them make improved choices regarding family planning as well as maintain health and nutrition for herself and her children.
- ***Child health and survival:*** It is an important predictor of family planning and adoption of small family norms.
- ***Meeting unmet needs for family welfare services:*** To be achieved by strengthening health infrastructure and referral services and ensuring supply of contraceptives and equipment.
- ***Underserved populations:*** Population in slums, tribal areas, and hard-to-reach areas are to be provided with basic health and RCH services including contraception, with focus on avoiding teenage pregnancies and on men for undergoing non-scalpel vasectomies.
- ***Diverse health providers:*** Involving private practitioners to provide RCH services and involvement of nonmedical fraternity counseling and advocacy.
- ***Collaboration with NGOs and private sector:*** For increasing clinic outlets and mobile clinics, strengthening management information system, conducting information, education and communication (IEC) activities and social marketing of contraception.
- ***Mainstreaming ISM and homeopathy:*** To fill up the manpower gaps, ISM and H institutions may be utilized to provide RCH services.
- ***Contraceptive technology and research on RCH:*** To be promoted.
- ***Provisions for older population:*** National policy on older persons will promote old age care and support which will reduce the incentive to have large families.
- ***Information, education and communication:*** This is central to the success of the family welfare program.

The government provides certain measures to promote small family norm such as rewards to Panchayats for universalizing small family norm, reducing infant mortality, and promoting completion of primary schooling, for promoting girl child survival, cash incentives for first two births only, cash incentives, and insurance coverage for couples who undergo sterilization after two living children, and who marry after legal age and practice proper birth spacing.

## NATIONAL NUTRITION POLICY

The National Nutrition Policy was formulated in 1993 to improve the nutritional status of the Indian population, through various direct and indirect interventions.

### Direct (Short-term) Interventions

- Nutrition interventions especially for vulnerable groups:
  - Expansion of ICDS cover to remaining half of the blocks by 2000 AD.
  - Inclusion of adolescent girls within the ambit of ICDS. All girls in community development blocks and 50% in urban slums to be included by 2000 AD and providing them iron

supplementation and skill upgradation in health and nutrition, so as to prepare them for safe motherhood.
- In order to reduce the incidence of low-birth-weight babies to 10% by 2000 AD, supplementary nutrition to expectant mothers right from 1st trimester. This should continue for the 1st year after pregnancy.
- Improving growth monitoring in 0-3 years. This is to be with close involvement of mothers by triggering appropriate behavioral changes among the mothers along with adequate health and nutrition education so as to empower them to manage the nutrition needs of their children effectively.
- Fortification of essential food with appropriate nutrients, e.g., salt with iodine and/or iron. Research in iron fortification of rice and other cereals to be intensified. Iodized salt should cover all the endemic areas.
- Efforts to produce and popularize low-cost nutrient foods from indigenous and locally available raw materials to be intensified and to involve women in this activity.
- Control of micronutrient deficiencies, e.g., vitamin A, iron, folic acid and iodine, amongst the vulnerable groups, by intensification of existing programs, so as to completely eliminate nutritional blindness and reduce anemia in expectant women to 25% by 2000 AD.

### Indirect (Long-term) Interventions

- To ensure aggregate food security, a per capita availability of 215 kg per person/year of food grains needs to be attained with target of at least attaining 230 million tons of food grains production by 2000 AD.
- Improving the dietary pattern by promoting the production and availability of nutritionally rich foods.
- Ensuring an equitable food distribution through the expansion of the public distribution system. It should also ensure availability of coarse grains, pulses and jaggery besides cereals, sugar and oil at reasonable prices, particularly to those living below poverty line.
- Implementing measures to increase income of those below poverty line by restructuring of poverty alleviation and employment generation programs, land reforms, ensuring minimum wages, women's employment and education, equal remuneration to women for work, thus improving status of women.
- Implementing other measures that have a bearing on nutrition such as increasing education and status of women, improving health particularly immunization, maternal care, small family norm, and adequate birth spacing.
- Extensive basic health and nutrition education. It shall be included in school curricula and all nutrition programs.
- Strengthening of prevention of food adulteration.
- Strengthening of nutrition surveillance by strengthening National Nutrition Monitoring Bureau (NNMB) and National Institute of Nutrition (NIN).
- Community participation through increased awareness, involvement of Panchayats and women. Given the problem of mounting delivery cost of various nutrition interventions, mobilize resources within the community.
- Enhancing communication and research in field of nutrition are essential aspects of the strategy.
- For administration and monitoring National Nutrition Council under chairpersonship of Prime Minister and a coordination committee, under the Secretary, Department of Women and Child Development, have been recommended. Nutrition surveillance shall be the task of NIN and NNMB. Similar set up has been suggested at the state level.

### Strategy during Twelfth Five-Year Plan

The focus shifted from food security to nutrition security and emphasized on prevention of micronutrient deficiencies such as iron, iodine and vitamin A.

*Strategies for twelfth plan included:*

- Strengthening and restructuring of the ICDS.
- Preparing a multisectoral program to address maternal and child malnutrition.
- Launching nationwide IEC campaign against malnutrition.
- Bringing strong nutritional focus to the programs of the ministries that deal with health, drinking water supply and sanitation, school education, agriculture, food and public distribution.

## SUGGESTED READING

1. MoHFW. National Health Policy 2017. Ministry of Health and Family Welfare, Government of India, New Delhi.
2. MoHFW. National Population Policy 2000. Ministry of Health and Family Welfare, Government of India, New Delhi.
3. MoHRD. National Nutrition Policy 1993. Department of Women and Child Development, Ministry of Human Resource Development, Government of India, New Delhi.
4. Planning Commission. Nutrition. Women's Agency and Child Rights. Twelfth Plan (2012–2017), Vol. III, Planning Commission, Government of India, New Delhi; 197-214.

# NATIONAL HEALTH MISSION

## INTRODUCTION

India registered significant progress in improving life expectancy at birth, reducing mortality due to malaria, as well as reducing infant and maternal mortality by end of 20th century. In spite of the progress made, a high proportion of the population, especially in rural areas, continued to suffer and die from preventable diseases, pregnancy, and childbirth-related complications as well as malnutrition. The rural public healthcare system in many states and regions was in an unsatisfactory state leading to pauperization of poor households due to expensive private sector health care. In the beginning of 21st century, India was in the midst of an epidemiological and demographic transition—with the attendant problems of increased chronic disease burden and a decline in mortality and fertility rates leading to an ageing of the population. Another major problem was low public health expenditure, which was reduced from 1.3% of GDP in 1990 to 0.9% of GDP in 1999.

Thus, the National Rural Health Mission (NRHM) was launched by Government of India in 2005 to combat certain existing problems such as centralized planning, fragmented disease specific approach, gross regional inequalities, lack of action in areas of safe water, sanitation, hygiene, and nutrition, etc. The policy aimed to provide universal access to equitable, affordable and accountable quality health care, responsive to the needs of the people. It also aimed at reduction of child and maternal deaths, achieving population stabilization, gender, and demographic balance.

National Rural Health Mission was launched on 12th April 2005 to cover the entire country with special focus on 18 states including 8 Empowered Action Group (EAG) states, viz. Bihar, Chhattisgarh, Jharkhand, Madhya Pradesh, Odisha, Rajasthan, Uttarakhand, Uttar Pradesh.

While NRHM was formulated for rural areas, it was further proposed to launch a similar mission for the health care needs of urban poor, through a National Urban Health Mission (NUHM). Accordingly, on 1st May 2013, NUHM was launched under the ambit of National Health Mission (NHM), which thus combined under its overall umbrella its two submissions, NRHM and NUHM.

## NATIONAL HEALTH MISSION

National Health Mission was launched by the Government of India in 2013 subsuming the NRHM and NUHM. It is both flexible and dynamic and is intended to guide States towards ensuring the achievement of universal access to equitable, affordable, and quality healthcare services that are accountable and responsive to people's needs. The main programmatic components include health system strengthening in rural and urban areas, reproductive, maternal, neonatal, child and adolescent health (RMNCH+A) and communicable and NCDs **(Fig. 47.1)**.

The framework for implementation of NHM draws on several sources. First, it builds on the framework for implementation for the first phase of the NRHM initiated in 2005. The second is the learning from NRHM implementation over the past 7 years, and third from the twelfth five-year plan **(Table 47.1)**.

### Vision

Attainment of universal access to equitable, affordable and quality healthcare services, accountable and responsive to people's needs, with effective intersectoral convergent action, to address the wider social determinants of health.

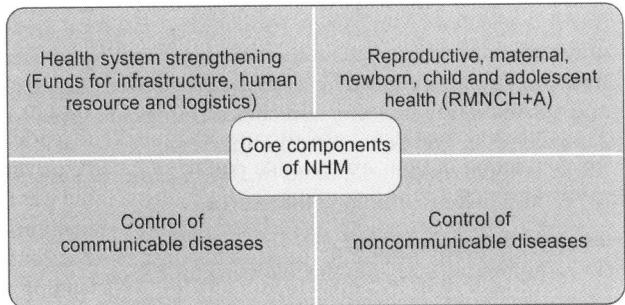

**Fig. 47.1:** Core components of the National Health Mission (NHM).

**Table 47.1:** NHM framework.

| NHM ||
|---|---|
| **NRHM** | **NUHM** |
| NRHM seeks to provide quality healthcare to the rural population, especially the vulnerable groups. Under the NRHM, the Empowered Action Group (EAG) States as well as North Eastern States, Jammu and Kashmir and Himachal Pradesh have been given special focus. The thrust of the mission is on establishing a fully functional, community owned, decentralized health delivery system with intersectoral convergence at all levels, to ensure simultaneous action on a wide range of determinants of health such as water, sanitation, education, nutrition, social and gender equality | NUHM seeks to improve the health status of the urban population, particularly urban poor and other vulnerable sections by facilitating their access to quality primary healthcare. NUHM covers all state capitals, district headquarters and other cities/towns with a population of 50,000 and above (as per census 2011) in a phased manner. Cities and towns with population below 50,000 will continue to be covered under NRHM |

(NHM: National Health Mission; NRHM: National Rural Health Mission; NUHM: National Urban Health Mission)

| Indicators | Expected outcome of NHM by 2017 | Current status |
|---|---|---|
| MMR | <1/1,000 live births | 0.97/1,000 live birth (SRS Special Bulletin 2018–20) |
| IMR | 25/1,000 live births | 28 /1,000 live birth (SRS 2020, Bulletin 2022) |
| TFR | 2.1 | 2.0 (SRS 2020 Report) |
| Anemia | Prevent and reduce anemia in women aged 15-49 years | 57% women are anemic (NFHS 5) |
| TB | Reduce annual incidence and mortality by half | Incidence: 188/1,00,000 population (2021) |
| Prevalence of leprosy | <1/1,000 population and incidence to zero in all districts | Only 5 stated have prevalence >1/10,000 population as of January 2023 |
| Annual incidence of malaria | <1/1,000 population | 0.17 million (2022, NVBDCP Official Website) |

### Institutional Mechanisms

***Center:*** Mission Steering Group (MSG), chaired by The Union Minister of Health and Family Welfare. NHM is headed by a Mission Director and a team of Joint Secretaries, and is responsible for planning, implementing and monitoring of the mission activities. Technical support is provided by National Health Systems Resource Centre (NHSRC), and National Institute of Health and Family Welfare (NIHFW) is the apex body for training.

***State:*** The State Health Mission (SHM) is headed by the State Chief Minister. The State Health Society (SHS) carries out its functions under the mission and is headed by the Chief Secretary. The State Program Management Unit (SPMU), State Health System Resource Centers (SHSRC), and the State Institutes of Health and Family Welfare (SIHFW) carry out similar functions for the state, as at the center. The SPMU acts as the main secretariat of the SHS.

***District:*** District Health Mission (DHM)/City Health Mission (CHM) is headed by the chief of the local self-government, i.e., Chair Person Zila Parishad/Mayor, depending upon whether the district is predominantly rural or urban. District Health Society (DHS) is headed by the District Collector. Urban Health Committee is headed by the Municipal Commissioner/District Magistrate/Deputy Commissioner/District Collector/Subdivisional Magistrate/Assistant Commissioner, based on whether the city is the district headquarter or a subdivisional headquarter. For the seven mega cities of Delhi, Mumbai, Chennai, Kolkata, Bengaluru, Hyderabad and Ahmedabad, NHM will be implemented by the City Health Mission.

***Community participation and decentralized planning:*** For ensuring public control and accountability of public health institutions towards the public, Rogi Kalyan Samitis/Hospital Management Committees have been formed for management of public health institutions at the level of primary health center (PHC) and above. Village Health, Sanitation and Nutrition Committees (VHSNC) function at the level of the village. These have representatives from elected bodies like Panchayats, Panchayat Samitis, and Zila Parishad.

***Village health, sanitation and nutrition committees:*** The VHSNC is a subcommittee or a standing committee of the Gram Panchayat, and focuses on social determinants of health, and access to health services, especially of the more marginalized sections in the village.

## Strategies

### Integration
There is horizontal integration of all existing vertical programs except National AIDS Control Program at state, district and block levels.

### Decentralized Planning
Village health, sanitation and nutrition committee prepares intersectoral village health plan. The village, block and city health plans are consolidated by the District Program Management Unit (DPMU) to make the intersectoral district health plan, which are then merged to form state program implementation plan (PIP) that has to be approved by the center for implementation.

### Facility-based Service Delivery
***Norms:*** Norms, guided by the IPHS, are to be followed, with appropriate provisions for increased caseloads.

***Quality:*** Quality assurance of all services provided at every facility are to be ensured through developing a quality management system, with recognition and rewards for facilities that meet standards of quality certification. Every facility is required to display prominently the citizen's charter and develop a grievance redressal mechanism.

***Cleanliness:*** The Ministry of Health and Family Welfare has launched a national initiative "Kayakalp" in May 2015, to ensure cleanliness in health facilities. Under this, awards are given to those public health facilities that demonstrate high levels of cleanliness, hygiene and infection control.

***District hospital and knowledge center (DHKC):*** This is responsible for providing all secondary and some extent of tertiary care to manage most morbidities within the district; adequate referral support; skill-based in-service training of various categories of health personnel; district planning, data management and analysis.

***District public health resource center:*** This center functions through a team comprising of public health managers, epidemiologists, medical entomologist, (optional), microbiologist, data management and analysis or health informatics specialists, public health administrator, and hospital manager. It provides technical inputs, support and handholding for planning, data analysis, and knowledge management.

***District education and training center:*** This is developed in the district to provide pre-service training for nurses of all categories, provide training for trainers and where feasible skill-based, in-service training for all categories.

### Outreach Services
Outreach services are provided by subcenter through auxiliary nursing midwife (ANM), anganwadi worker (AWW), and accredited social health activist (ASHA) in rural area and by Urban Primary Health Centre (UPHC) through ANMs in urban area.

Healthcare delivery facilities should be within 30 minutes of walking distance from habitation. In remote, far flung, difficult to reach areas and urban slums, services are provided through mobile medical units (MMUs).

### Accredited Social Health Activist
To relieve the burden of work of the health worker female (HWF) a new band of community-based functionaries, named ASHAs has been introduced under the NRHM (in 2005), and subsequently continued under the NHM, to work as an interface between the community and the public health system. Initially, it was proposed to have one ASHA per 1,000 population, but later it was increased depending on the workload, to more than one ASHA per habitation in tribal, hilly and desert areas. In the urban areas there is one ASHA for 200–500 households.

#### Key features of ASHA
- ASHA is a woman resident of village—"Married/Widow/Divorced" and preferably in the age group of 25–45 years, has minimum formal education up to eighth class, with effective communication skills and leadership qualities.
- ASHA is selected by the village Panchayat in the rural areas, under the supervision and guidance of block medical officer. Induction training is given for 23 days, spread over 12 months and subsequently periodic refresher trainings are given for 2 days, once in every alternate month.
- ASHA is supervised and guided by HW (F) who, along with AWW, also helps in training other ASHAs.

#### Roles and responsibilities of ASHA
ASHA is required to carry out the following functions:
- Create awareness on health and its social determinants.
- Counsel women on issues of RCH.

- Facilitate accessing health and health related services at Anganwadi center/subcenter/PHC.
- Mobilize the community to take action in convergent areas like water supply and sanitation, health and hygiene education programs.
- Help AWW in the field activities.
- Arrange escort/accompany seriously ill children/women with pregnancy related complications to nearest pre-identified health facility.
- Provide primary medical care for minor ailments, for which she is provided a drug kit that includes AYUSH and allopathic formulations. She can also be a provider of directly observed treatment short course (DOTS) for TB.
- Act as a depot holder for oral rehydration solution (ORS) packets, iron folic acid (IFA) tablets, chloroquine, disposable delivery kits (DDK), oral pills, condoms, etc.
- Inform about the births, deaths, and any unusual health problems/disease outbreaks in her village, to the subcenter/PHC.
- Promote construction of household toilets under total sanitation campaign.
- Work with village health and sanitation committee to develop a comprehensive village health plan.
- Work for other national health programs under NHM.

*Honorarium*

ASHA is an honorary worker and she is entitled for performance-linked incentives/compensation for her work, so that she can earn at least ₹ 3,000 per month. She is also compensated for her work under different health programs and for attending trainings. Other incentives are certificate of acknowledgment for good work preference in admission to ANM/GNM schools.

## Indian Public Health Standards

Indian Public Health Standards, formulated under the NRHM, for sub-centers, primary health centers, community health centers, Sub-District and District Hospitals, were published in 2007 and revised in 2012 as the reference point to provide standardized public health care services and general principles for infrastructure planning and up-gradation of health facilities as per the population of the States and UTs. Since the last revision of the IPHS in 2012, a number of new initiatives, interventions and programs have been introduced in the public health system of India. To account for these developments and in light of newer advances in health, science, and technology, the IPHS standards were revised in IPHS 2022. These standards indicate minimum requirements and cover infrastructure, staff, equipment, drugs, and investigation facilities. Additionally, the 2022 revised guidelines emphasize on the services to be delivered at each level of facility.

**Broad objectives of the IPHS:**
- To define uniform benchmark to ensure high quality services that are accountable, responsive, and sensitive to the needs of the community.
- To specify the minimum assured (essential) and achievable (desirable) services that are expected to be provided at different levels of public health facilities.
- To provide guidance on health systems strengthening components which includes architectural design of facilities, human resources for health, drugs, diagnostics, equipment, administrative and logistical support services to improve the overall health related outcomes
- To achieve and maintain an acceptable standard of quality of care at public health facilities
- To facilitate monitoring and supervision of the facilities
- To provide guidance and tools for governance, leadership and evaluation

*IPHS standards for subcenters, PHC, CHC, district hospitals have already been covered in Chapter 46: Indian Healthcare System.*

## Mainstreaming of AYUSH

Interventions for mainstreaming AYUSH initiated under NHM are as follows:
- AYUSH practitioners are being trained in SBA, IUCD insertion, RMNCH, IMNCI and preventive, promotive activities, and screening for NCD.
- Integrated AYUSH hospitals with 50/100 bed capacity along with specialty clinics, specialized therapy centers, and AYUSH wings have been set up in district hospitals.
- AYUSH facilities are co-located in all government healthcare facilities providing primary and secondary care, up to the block level. AYUSH doctors and AYUSH paramedics have been deployed in the health facilities.
- Standard treatment guidelines and a model drugs list of AYUSH drugs for community health workers, is being developed.
- Clinical research on AYUSH medicines will be promoted and also a web-based "AYUSH Research Portal" has been launched.
- AYUSH modules have been included in training of ASHA, along with inclusion of Ayurvedic and Unani medicines in the ASHA kit.
- AYUSH Gram will be promoted, wherein one village per block will be selected for implementation of integrated primary care through AYUSH and modern system of medicine.

## Services Delivery Programs

- *RMNCAH+N services*: All schemes and programs under Reproductive and Child Health Program Phase II (RCH-II) would be absorbed into the NHM. The NHM provides an opportunity to build on past work and renew the emphasis on strategies for improving maternal and child health (MCH) through a continuum of care and the life cycle approach. There is additional focus on adolescence as a distinct "life stage" and the strategy is to increase knowledge and access to reproductive health services and information for adolescents and to address nutritional anemia.
- *Control of communicable diseases*: The NHM will continue to focus on communicable disease control programs and disease surveillance. The strategies, interventions and activities will be appropriately adapted and fine-tuned to meet the distinct challenges of urban settings. The Flexipool fund for communicable diseases will facilitate the states in preparing state, district and city specific PIPs.

- *NCD:* NCDs account for 53% of the total deaths (10.3 million) and 44% (291 million) of DALYs lost in India (MoHFW, Framework for implementation, NHM 2012–2017). By 2030, NCDs are projected to cause up to 67% of all deaths in India. Most NCDs have common risk factors such as tobacco use, unhealthy diet, physical inactivity, alcohol use and require integrated interventions targeting these risk factors. The rising burden of NCDs calls for concerted public health action. In addition to clinical approaches, preventive action and policy responses involving multiple stakeholders are required, and the NHM will need to address the growing burden of NCDs. The programs for addressing burden of NCDs are: National Programme for Prevention and Control of Non-Communicable Diseases (NP-NCD), National Program for the Control of Blindness (NPCB), National Mental Health Program (NMHP), National Program for the Healthcare of the Elderly (NPHCE), National Program for the Prevention and Control of Deafness (NPPCD), National Tobacco Control Program (NTCP), National Oral Health Program (NOHP), National Program for Palliative Care (NPPC), National Program for the Prevention and Management of Burn Injuries (NPPMBI) and National Program for Prevention and Control of Fluorosis (NPPCF).

Health programs related to control of communicable and NCDs are discussed in next sections of this chapter.

### New Initiatives

*ANMOL:* ANMOL, meaning ANM online, is a tablet-based application, which will facilitate maintaining integrated RCH register; standardizing the maternal and child care services provided; planning work schedule thus saving time; planning Village Health and Nutrition Day (VHND) as per the date specified, along with the vaccines and logistics required. Audio and video counseling can also be done through ANMOL, thus helping to create awareness among beneficiaries.

*Kilkari:* Kilkari, meaning "a baby's gurgle," is a service that delivers 72 weekly, free, time-appropriate, audio messages, about pregnancy, childbirth and child care, directly to family's mobile phones, starting from second trimester of pregnancy till the child is 1 year old. Average duration of one call is approximately 1 minute.

*Mobile academy:* It is a free, audio training course for ASHAs, to expand and refresh their knowledge base, improve their communication skills, reducing their need to travel, while providing them the flexibility to learn at their own pace and at their convenient time.

*Addressing social determinants:* Focus is on important issues like levels of malnutrition through the ICDS scheme; outbreaks of water-borne diseases through Swachh Bharat Mission; health of preschool and school children and out of school adolescents through the ICDS scheme and education department; gender, age at marriage of girls, and women empowerment through SABLA scheme.

### Financing of NHM

The Government of India has a policy commitment to increase public expenditure on health to at least 2.5% of the GDP. Attaining a public expenditure of 2.5% of the GDP cannot be achieved without a major effort from the states, which currently account for nearly two-thirds of total public health expenditure. State governments would contribute to 25% of the share under the NHM, except for the North-East states and the special category states (J&K, Himachal Pradesh, and Uttarakhand) where the state share would be 10%. This requires creating the necessary political and administrative will in the states through active advocacy and incentives. With both central and state government increasing their health spends; the immediate objective of reducing out of pocket expenditure should be more attainable.

NHM would have six financing components, namely:
1. *NRHM/RCH flexi-pool*—to be utilized for health systems strengthening including infrastructure, MMUs, Patient transport systems (for referral and emergency), procurement of equipment and drugs, AYUSH mainstreaming and drugs, support to ASHAs and VHSNC, MCH interventions, adolescent health interventions, and immunization.
2. *NUHM flexi-pool*—to be utilized to meet the health needs of urban population particularly the poor and vulnerable sections.
3. *Flexible pool for communicable disease*—to be utilized for interventions under Communicable Disease Control Programs.
4. *Flexible pool for NCD including injury and trauma*—to be utilized for interventions under noncommunicable disease control programs.
5. *Infrastructure maintenance*
6. *Family welfare central sector*—to be utilized to support Management Information System, such as Health Management Information System (HMIS) and Mother and Child Tracking Scheme (MCTS), Population Research Centers, NIHFW, International Institute of Population Sciences (IIPS), National Commission on Population, and National Health System Resource Centre (NHSRC).

### Monitoring and Evaluation of NHM

There will be four major approaches to monitoring and evaluation. They include:
1. Use of data from large scale population surveys—through using the periodic Population Health Surveys, Sample Registration Surveys (SRS), Death statistics, National Sample Survey Organization (NSSO) data on cost of care and morbidity, District Level Household Survey (DLHS), and National Family Health Survey (NFHS).
2. Commissioning implementation research or evaluation studies.
3. Use of HMIS data and field appraisals and reviews.
4. Monitoring of health outcomes, output and process indicators. Other than the outcome measures above, monitoring and evaluation also includes progress with respect to other dimensions of achieving the goal of universal health care.

## NATIONAL URBAN HEALTH MISSION

As per Census 2011, population of India has crossed 121 crores with the urban population at 37.7 cores which is 31.16% of the total population. Urban growth has led to rapid increase in number of urban poor population, many of whom live in slums and other squatter settlements. As per United Nations projections, 53% of the total population of India will be in urban regions by 2050 (UN, World Urbanization Prospects, 2018). While the Jawahar Lal Nehru Urban Renewal Mission is beginning to tackle the urban infrastructure issues, urban health issues need immediate attention, especially in the context of the urban poor. It also needs attention from a public health perspective.

Despite the supposed proximity of the urban poor to urban health facilities their access to them is severely restricted. This is on account of their being "crowded out" because of the inadequacy of the urban public health delivery system. Ineffective outreach and weak referral system also limits the access of urban poor to health care services. Social exclusion and lack of information and assistance at the secondary and tertiary hospitals makes them unfamiliar to the modern environment of hospitals, thus restricting their access. The lack of economic resources inhibits/restricts their access to the available private facilities. Further, the lack of standards and norms for the urban health delivery system when contrasted with the rural network makes the urban poor more vulnerable and worse off than their rural counterpart.

In order to effectively address the health concerns of the urban poor population, the Government of India launched a NUHM in May 2013 that covers all state capitals, district headquarters and cities/towns with a population of more than 50,000. Towns with population less than 50,000 will continue to be covered under NRHM.

The NUHM would have high focus on:
- Urban poor population living in listed and unlisted slums
- All other vulnerable population such as homeless, rag-pickers, street children, rickshaw pullers, construction and brick and lime kiln workers, sex workers, and other temporary migrants.
- Public health thrust on sanitation, clean drinking water, vector control, etc.
- Strengthening public health capacity of urban local bodies.

## Goal

The National Urban Health Mission would aim to improve the health status of the urban population in general, but particularly of the poor and other disadvantaged sections, by facilitating equitable access to quality health care through a revamped public health system, partnerships, community-based mechanism with the active involvement of the urban local bodies.

## Core Strategies

- Improving the efficiency of public health system in the cities by strengthening, revamping and rationalizing existing government primary urban health structure and designated referral facilities
- Promotion of access to improved health care at household level through community-based groups: Mahila Arogya Samitis (MAS) and ASHA
- Strengthening public health through innovative preventive and promotive action
- Increased access to health care through creation of revolving fund
- IT-enabled services (ITES) and e-governance for improving access improved surveillance and monitoring
- Capacity building of stakeholders
- Prioritizing the most vulnerable amongst the poor
- Ensuring quality health care services.

## Institutional Mechanism for Implementation of NUHM

The NUHM would leverage the institutional structures of the NRHM at the national, state and district level for operationalization of the NUHM. The MSG of the NRHM will be expanded to work as the apex body for NUHM also. Every Municipal Corporation, Municipality, Notified Area Committee, and Town Panchayat will become a unit of planning with its own approved broad norms for setting up of health facilities.

The National urban health service delivery model would make a concerted effort to rationalize and strengthen the existing public healthcare system in urban areas and promote effective engagement with the non-governmental sector (profit/not for profit) for expanding reach to urban poor, along with strengthening the participation of the community in planning and management of the healthcare service delivery.

Components of the proposed urban health service delivery model have been shown in **Figures 47.2 and 47.3**. Essential health services at community, U-PHC and U-CHC levels are described in **Table 47.2**

### Finance Management

The Government of India is committed to increase public expenditure on health to at least 2.5% of GDP, with the objective of reducing out-of-pocket expenditure. The center:state funding pattern is 60:40 for all the states except for the North-East states and the special category states (J&K, Himachal Pradesh, and Uttarakhand) where the state share is 10%.

Funding to states shall be based on the approved PIPs, under following components:
- NRHM RCH flexi-pool
- NUHM flexi-pool
- Flexible pool for communicable diseases
- Flexible pool for NCDs including injury and trauma
- Infrastructure maintenance
- Family welfare central sector component—all funds are from center.

Funds for NHM are managed by the Financial Management Group (FMG), which transfers funds for all the programs under NHM to State Health Societies (SHS) electronically through the RBI approved banks.

### Monitoring and Evaluation

#### Health Management Information System

The web-based HMIS under NHM facilitates the flow of physical and financial performance from the district level to the state HQ and the center. Information regarding the health indicators of India is available at the HMIS website *http://nrhm-mis.nic.in*. GIS-enabled HMIS application provides visual/spatial depiction of HMIS data on dynamic maps.

#### Mother and Child Tracking System

A software e-MAMTA has been developed by statistics division of Ministry of Health and Family Welfare, Government of

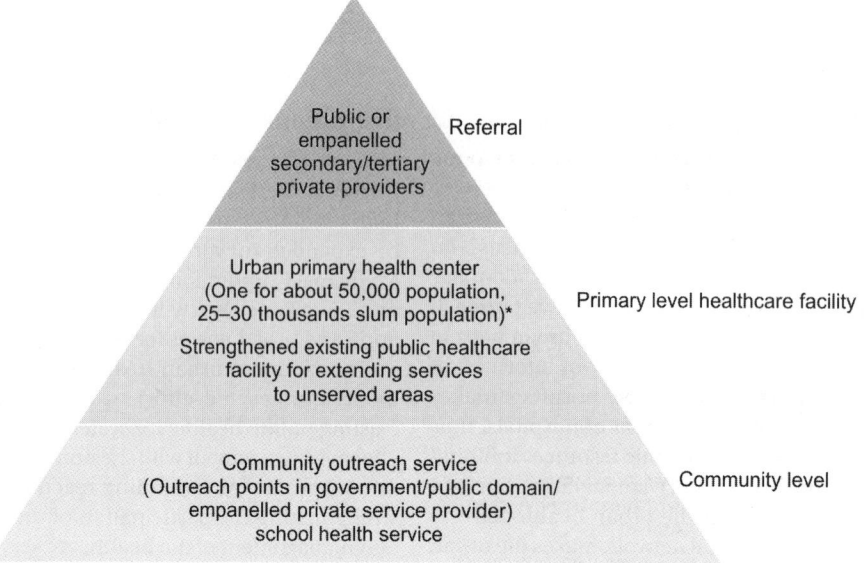

**Fig. 47.2:** Urban healthcare delivery model.

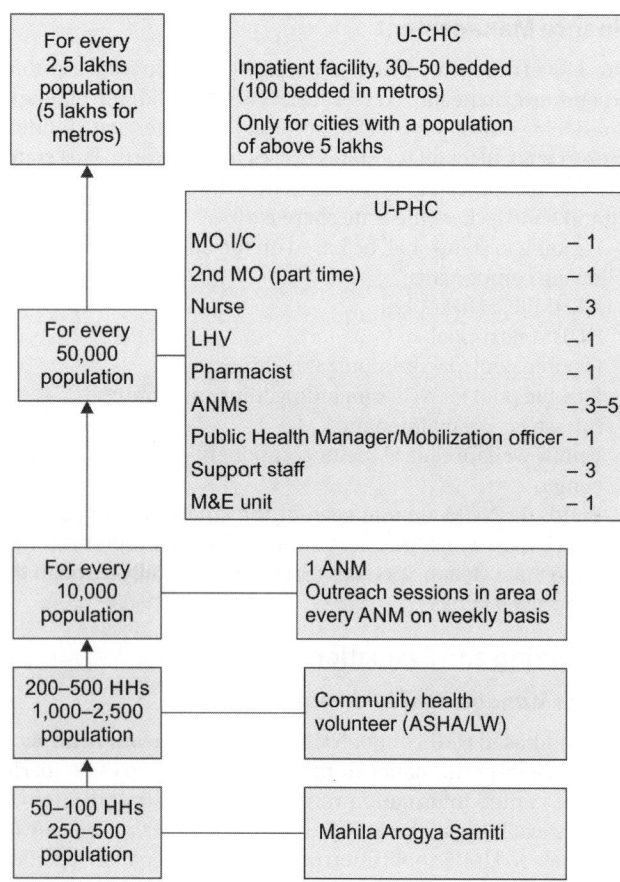

**Fig. 47.3:** Level of urban healthcare facilities.
(HHs: households; PHC: primary health center; CHC: community health center; LW: link worker; MO I/C: medical officer incharge; LHV: lady health visitor)

India for tracking of antenatal mothers and children under web-enabled name-based MCTS, along with tracking and monitoring severely anemic women, low birth weight babies, and sick neonates. MCTS is used for sending appropriate health promotion messages on mobile phone of the beneficiaries according to month of pregnancy or age of the child and also for direct transfer of Janani Suraksha Yojana (JSY) benefits into bank accounts of the pregnant women, after delivery. Mother and Child Tracking Facilitation Centre (MCTFC) has been set up at NIHFW, to support MCTS.

### Other Mechanisms for Monitoring and Evaluation

These include maternal death review, perinatal and child death review, common review mission (CRM), death statistics, National Sample Survey Organization (NSSO) data on cost of care and NFHS, District Level Household Survey (DLHS), SRS, and census.

### District/City Level Vigilance and Monitoring Committees (D/CLVMC)

These have been established at district/city level (for seven megacities of India, viz. Delhi, Mumbai, Kolkata, Ahmedabad, Hyderabad, Chennai and Bengaluru), to monitor the progress of implementation of NHM, and review intersectoral convergence, community monitoring mechanisms, management information system, etc.

### Governance and Accountability Framework

This consists of MSG at the national level; SHM and Governing Body (GB) of SHS at the state level; District/City Health Society at the district level and Rogi Kalyan Samiti (RKS) at the facility level.

**Table 47.2:** Levels of service delivery.

| Services* | Levels of service delivery | | |
|---|---|---|---|
| | Community (Outreach) | First point of service delivery (U-PHC) | Referral center-U-CHC (Specialist service) |
| **A. Essential health services** | | | |
| A1. Maternal health | • Registration, ANC, identification of danger signs, referral for institutional delivery, follow-up<br>• Counseling and behavior promotion | ANC, PNC, initial management of complicated delivery cases and referral, management of regular maternal health conditions, referral of complicated cases | Delivery (normal and complicated), management of complicated gyne maternal health condition, hospitalization and surgical interventions, including blood transfusion |
| A2. Family welfare | Counseling, distribution of OCP/CC, referral for sterilization, follow-up of contraceptive related complications | Distribution of OCP/CC, IUD insertion, referral for sterilization, management of contraceptive related complications | Sterilization operations, fertility treatment |
| A3. Child health and nutrition | Immunization, identification of danger signs, referral, follow-up, distribution of ORS, pediatric cotrimoxazole postnatal visits/counseling for newborn care | • Diagnosis and treatment of childhood illnesses, referral of acute cases/chronic illness<br>• Identification and referral of neonatal sickness | Management of complicated pediatric/neonatal cases, hospitalization, surgical interventions, blood transfusion |
| A4. RTI/STI (including HIV/AIDS) | Referral, community level follow-up for ensuring adherence to treatment regime of cases undergoing treatment | Symptomatic diagnosis and primary treatment and referral of complicated cases | Management of complicated cases, hospitalization (if needed) |
| A5. Nutrition deficiency disorders | • Height/weight measurement, Hb testing, distribution of therapeutic doses of<br>• IFA, promotion of iodized salt, nutrition supplements to identified children and pregnant/lactating women<br>• Promotion of breastfeeding, complementary feeding for prevention of undernutrition | Diagnosis and treatment of seriously deficient patients, referral of acute deficiency cases | • Management of acute deficiency cases, hospitalization<br>• Treatment and rehabilitation of severe undernutrition |
| A6. Vector-borne diseases | • Slide collection, testing using RDKs, DDT<br>• Counseling for practices for vector control and protection | Diagnosis and treatment, referral of terminally ill cases | Management of terminally ill cases, hospitalization |
| A7. Mental health | | Initial screening and referral | Psychiatric and neurological services, including hospitalization, if needed |
| A8. Oral health | | Diagnosis and referral | Management of complicated cases, hospitalization (if needed) |
| A9. Hearing impairment/Deafness | | | Management of complicated cases, hospitalization (if needed) |
| A10. Chest infection (TB/Asthma) | Symptomatic search and referral, ensuring adherence to DOTs, other treatment | Diagnosis and treatment and referral of complicated cases | Management of complicated cases |
| A11. Cardiovascular disease | BP measurement, symptomatic search and referral, follow-up of under-treatment patients | Diagnosis and treatment and referral during specialist visits | Management of emergency cases, hospitalization and surgical interventions (if needed) |
| A12. Diabetes | Blood/urine sugar test (using disposable kit), symptomatic search and referral | Diagnosis and treatment referral of complicated cases | Management of complicated cases, hospitalization (if needed) |
| A13. Cancer | Symptomatic search and referral, follow-up of under-treatment patients | Identification and referral, follow-up of under-treatment patients | Diagnosis, treatment, hospitalization (if needed) |
| A14. Trauma care (burns and injuries) | First aid and referral | First aid, emergency resuscitation, documentation for MLC (if applicable) and referral | Case management and hospitalization, physiotherapy and rehabilitation |
| A15. Other surgical interventions | Not applicable | Identification and referral | Hospitalization and surgical interventions |
| **B. Other support services** | | | |
| B1. IEC/BCC | IPC, health camps/fairs, performing arts, wall/poster writing, events (in schools, women's groups) | Distribution of health education material | Distribution of health education material |
| B2. Counseling | Individual and group/family counseling | Patient/attendant counseling | Patient/attendant counseling |
| B3. Personal and social hygiene | IEC on hygiene, community mobilization for cleanliness drives, disinfection of water sources, etc. | Not applicable | Not applicable |

*Services based on situational analysis.

(IEC: information, education and communication; IPC: interprocess communication; PNC: postnatal care; BCC: behavior change communication; ANC: antenatal care; DDT: dichlorodiphenyltrichloroethane; OCP: oral contraceptive pill; IUD: intrauterine device; IFA: iron folic acid; RTI: reproductive tract infections; STI: sexually transmitted infection; CC: condom counseling)

## Section 5: Managing Community Health in India

### Outcome Indicators

Goal is to reduce out-of-pocket expenditure by improving quality of primary care, increasing accessibility of all to these services; ensuring availability of care within the golden hour and the full package of assured services within the district.

*Some of the outcome indicators are as follows:*
- Reduction in out-of-pocket expenditure to less than 20% of total health expenditure.
- Percentage of population in need of specific services, which is actually able to access these services, which should be 100% access.
- List of assured services that are available on cashless basis and the time/difficulty to access these services.

### Common Review Mission

Common review mission is being carried out annually since November 2007, to review changes in the health system since the launch of the NRHM, examine and document progress, identify the constraints and recommend policy measures for implementation. The seventh CRM held in November 2013 was the first review mission for NHM with its two sub-missions. The most recent one is the 14th CRM, held in 2021 in covered twelve states and one Union Territory. Evaluation teams comprised of government officials, public health experts, representatives of the development partners and civil society organizations.

Report of the 14th CRM 2021 observed that all the states reviewed have reported better adequacy of health infrastructure, increased availability and improved utilization of services, as compared to previous CRMs. Of the 13 states visited, all states/UTs have made significant progress in operationalization of Ayushman Bharat—Health and Wellness Centers to provide Comprehensive Primary Health Care.

The primary health care facilities visited were largely providing Reproductive, Maternal and Child Health and Communicable disease services including ANC care, immunization, family planning and TB identification and treatment follow-up. The roll-out of newer services such as oral, eye, ENT, elderly, and palliative care had to yet pick up pace.

Routine immunization (RI) services are improving across all states, with increase in use of IT enabled platforms such as eVIN, ANMOL, etc. review of the programs showed consistent decline in incidence of most of the vector-borne diseases (VBD). Multidrug-resistant TB (MDR) and extensively drug-resistant TB (XDR) cases of TB were found to be rising. The various NCD-related national Programs are at varying stages of implementation across states.

Community processes and convergence showed ASHAs are in place in most of the states and ASHA program under the NUHM is also being implemented. Availability of Smart phones with ASHAs and ASHA facilitators was reported in some states. Many states reported use of IT applications to streamline ASHA payments. Considering upgradation of Primary Health Centers as Health and Wellness Centers and increase in scope, Rogi Kalyan Samiti at PHC has been reformed as Jan Arogya Samiti-PHC (JAS-PHC).

Regarding NUHM, States have prioritized upgradation of urban Primary Health Centers to HWCs. In some states constraints were noted on account of high proportion of vacant positions of MBBS Medical officer at PHCs. In most states visited, absence of Mahila Arogya Samitis (MAS) in urban areas was seen to be a major concern.

### SUGGESTED READING

1. MoHFW, Government of India. Annual Report (2014–15). Ministry of Health and Family Welfare, Government of India, New Delhi.
2. MoHFW. Annual Report 2016–17. Ministry of Health and Family Welfare, Government of India, New Delhi.
3. MoHFW. Framework for Implementation, National Health Mission 2012–2017. Ministry of Health and Family Welfare, Government of India, New Delhi.
4. MoHFW. Framework for implementation, National Urban Health Mission 2012–2017. Ministry of Health and Family Welfare, Government of India, New Delhi.
5. MoHFW. Indian Public Health Standards (IPHS) guidelines for community health centers revised 2012, Directorate General of Health Services, Ministry of Health and Family Welfare, Government of India, New Delhi.
6. MoHFW. Indian Public Health Standards (IPHS) guidelines for primary health centers revised 2012, Directorate General of Health Services, Ministry of Health and Family Welfare, Government of India, New Delhi.
7. MoHFW. Indian Public Health Standards (IPHS) guidelines for subcenters revised 2012, Directorate General of Health Services, Ministry of Health and Family Welfare, Government of India, New Delhi.
8. MoHFW. Tenth Common Review Mission 2016. Ministry of Health and Family Welfare, Government of India, New Delhi.
9. NRHM. Accredited Social Health Activist (ASHA) guidelines, National Rural Health Mission. Ministry of Health and Family Welfare, Government of India, New Delhi.
10. NRHM. Award to public health facilities: Kayakalp. NRHM. Ministry of Health and Family Welfare, Government of India, New Delhi; May 2015.
11. NRHM. Mission Document, National Rural Health Mission. Ministry of Health and Family Welfare, Government of India, New Delhi.
12. Planning Commission. Health and FW in 12th Five-Year Plan (2012–17), Vol. II, Planning Commission, Government of India, New Delhi.

## REPRODUCTIVE AND CHILD HEALTH PROGRAM

### INTRODUCTION

The Reproductive and Child Health Program was launched in its first phase in 1997 (RCH-I) which integrated all ongoing programs on MCH and focused on child survival and safe motherhood, along with implementation of target free approach, training, IEC activities, RTI/STI clinics, facilities for safe abortions, enhanced community participation and adolescent health and reproductive hygiene. In addition to this, the program focused on districts with high crude birth rate and low female literacy **(Box 47.1)**.

> **Box 47.1: The Reproductive and Child Health Programs.**
> 1880 – Establishment of Training of Dais in Amritsar
> 1902 – 1st Midwifery Act to promote safe delivery
> 1930 – Setting up of advisory committee on maternal mortality
> 1946 – Bhore Committee Recommendation on Comprehensive and Integrated Health Care
> 1952 – Primary Health Center Network and Family Planning Program
> 1956 – MCH centers become integral part of PHCS
> 1961 – Department of Family Planning created
> 1971 – MTP Act
> 1974 – Family planning services incorporated in MCH care
> 1977 – Renaming Family Planning to Family Welfare
> 1978 – Expanded program on immunization
> 1985 – Universal Immunization Program
> 1992 – Child Survival and Safe Motherhood Program
> 1997 – RCH Program Phase-1 (15-10-1997)
> 2005 – RCH Program Phase-2 (01-04-2005)

(MCH: Maternal and Child Health; RCH: Reproductive and Child Health)

The major interventions under RCH-I were:
- Essential obstetric care including early registration of pregnancy, provision of minimum antenatal check-ups, safe delivery and minimum of three postnatal check-ups.
- Emergency obstetric care including strengthening of first referral units (FRUs).
- 24-hour delivery services at PHCs/CHCs.
- Medical termination of pregnancy.
- Control of RTI and sexually transmitted disease (STD).
- Immunization, bringing Universal Immunization Program (UIP) under the RCH program.
- Essential newborn care including resuscitation of newborn, prevention of hypothermia, exclusive breastfeeding, prevention of infections, and referral of sick newborns.
- Control of diarrheal diseases and acute respiratory infections in infants.
- Prevention and control of anemia and vitamin A deficiency in children.
- Training of Dais, with the objective of making deliveries safe. To bring about outcomes as envisioned in the Millennium Development Goals (MDGs), the National Population Policy 2000 (NPP 2000), the Tenth Plan, the NHP 2002 and Vision 2020 India, the second phase of the program.

(RCH-II) started in 2005 with the following strategies:
- Essential obstetric care including increasing institutional deliveries and ensuring skilled attendance at delivery.
- Emergency obstetric care including operationalizing of FRUs to provide round-the-clock delivery services, newborn care, emergency care of sick children, safe abortion services, treatment of RTI/STI, essential laboratory services and referral services. The three criteria for FRU were availability of surgical interventions, newborn care and blood storage facility on a 24-hour basis.
- Strengthening of referral system.

RCH-II focused on minimizing the regional variations in the areas of reproductive child health and population stabilization through an integrated, focused, participatory program meeting the unmet needs of the target population, and provision of assured, equitable, responsive quality services.

# A STRATEGIC APPROACH TO REPRODUCTIVE, MATERNAL, NEWBORN, CHILD AND ADOLESCENT HEALTH PLUS NUTRITION (RMNCAH+N) IN INDIA

Reducing maternal and child mortality are central to achievement of National Health Goals, MDGs 4 and 5 as well as Sustainable Development Goal 3. Huge and strategic investments are being made by Government of India to achieve these goals. At various global platforms, India has reaffirmed its commitment to make every effort towards achieving these goals. The National Call to Action: Child Survival and Development, 2013, was an iteration of this commitment, where the Government with all its partners launched the strategic roadmap for accelerating child survival and improving maternal health.

In order to bring greater impact through the RCH program, it is important to recognize that reproductive, MCH cannot be addressed in isolation as these are closely linked to the health status of the population in various stages of life cycle. The health of an adolescent girl impacts pregnancy while the health of a pregnant woman impacts the health of the newborn and the child. High maternal and child mortality in adolescent young mothers and a smaller but significant contribution of adolescents to total fertility brings the focus back on the need to address adolescents as an integral part of the strategy. Therefore, any effort to improve the survival of mothers and children requires intervention at various stages of life including the adolescence phase, pre pregnancy period, during pregnancy and delivery, after childbirth and then in the newborn period and childhood.

Just as different stages in the life cycle are interdependent, so are the aspects of where and how healthcare is provided. Household or community education contributes to preventing health complications, quality care provided at the community level helps avoid the need for hospitalization, and sound referral systems at primary care level support early identification of risks and better treatment for acute and complicated conditions.

Thus, there are two dimensions to healthcare: (1) stages of the life cycle and (2) places where the care is provided. These together constitute the "Continuum of Care." **(Fig. 47.4)** This strategic approach to RMNCH+A was initiated in 2013. Recently, it has been renamed as RMNCAH+N. The strategic approach denotes:
- Inclusion of adolescence as a distinct "life stage" in the overall strategy, where key interventions should be made
- Linking the nutrition related strategies and schemes to all the life stages to improve the overall health outcome and thus cater the nutrition related causes leading to morbidity and mortality in these age groups **(Fig. 47.5)**.

RMNCAH+N approach to improving MCH describes the most essential health *preventive, promotive and curative* interventions and packages of services across various life stages which when delivered to scale will provide maximum gains in terms of saving lives and improving overall health status of the community **(Fig. 47.6)**.

The strategic interventions under RMNCAH+N **(Fig. 47.7)**.

# Section 5: Managing Community Health in India

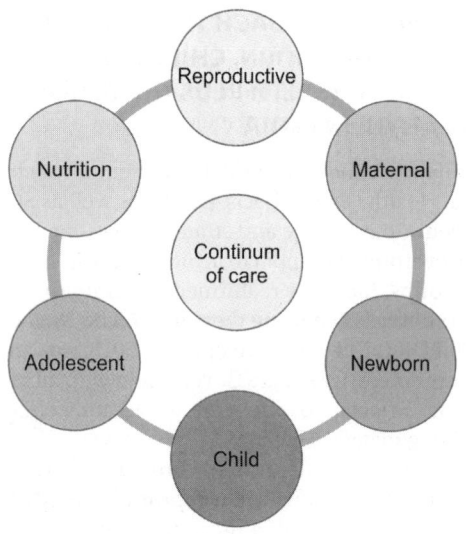

Fig 47.4: Continuum of care.

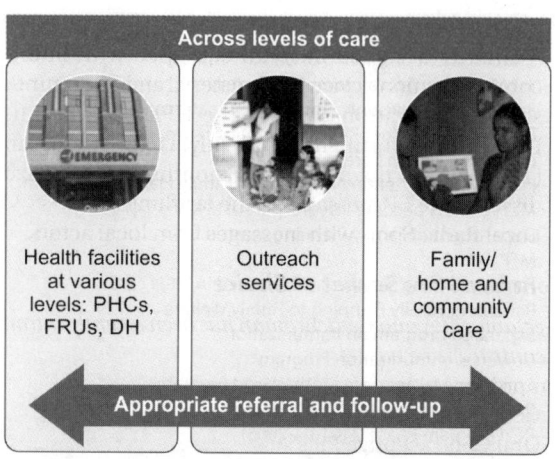

Fig. 47.6: Referral and follow up across levels of care.

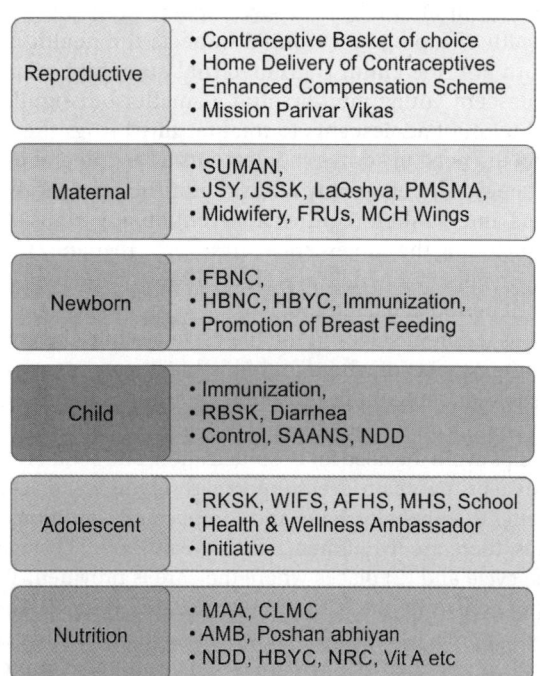

Fig 47.5: Schemes related to all life stages.

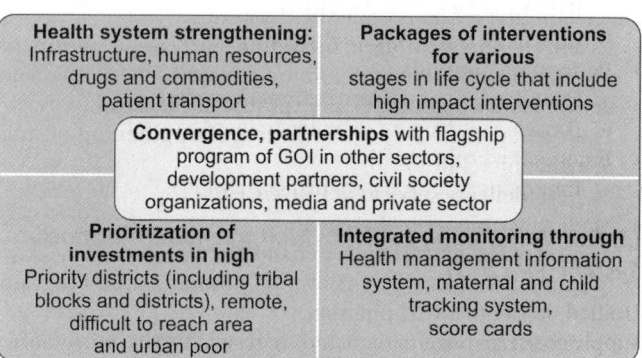

Fig. 47.7: Key components essential to improve the health of the mother and the baby.

*Key strategic actions:*
- Delivering assured services:
  - Roll out of Injectable Contraceptive DMPA (Antara) at one go till Sub center level
  - Augmentation of Post Partum IUCD (PPIUCD) Services to all delivery points
  - Augmentation of Sterilization services through High Fertility District compensation scheme
  - Condom Boxes at strategic locations (like Heath Facilities, Gram Panchayat Bhavan
  - Social Marketing of condoms and pills: Social Marketers under the government's scheme
  - Mission Parivar Vikas' Campaigns: (4 per year)

HFD districts may organize Mission Parivar Vikas Campaign in April, July, October and January (11 to 25 of the designated months). In July and October, the activity will be clubbed with WPD and Vasectomy Fortnight. For April and January, the activity is proposed to be divided into 7 days preparatory work and client mobilization activities; 7 days-service delivery.

- Promotional Schemes:
  - *"NAYI PAHEL"*—an FP KIT for "Newly Weds"
  - *Saas Bahu Sammelan*

It is aimed to facilitate improved communication between mothers-in-law and daughters-in-law through interactive games and exercises and building on their experiences.

## REPRODUCTIVE HEALTH

There are total 9 key interventions:

### (1) Mission Parivar Vikas

India was the first country in the world to have launched a National Programme for Family Planning in 1952. Mission Parivar Vikas was launched in 2016 initially for 146 high priority districts in the 7 high focus states (Bihar, Uttar Pradesh, Assam, Chhattisgarh, Madhya Pradesh, Rajasthan and Jharkhand), is scaled up in all districts of the seven high focus states as well as six north-eastern states of the country with an aim to ensure availability of contraceptive products to the clients at all the levels of health systems.

- SAARTHI-Awareness on Wheels
  - A smartly designed bus/van equipped with interactive communication devices, IEC material and FP commodities shall be operationalized in the HFDs during Mission Parivar Vikas fortnight (April, July, October and January (11" to 25" of the designated months)) to sensitize and disseminate FP messages in the far-flung areas.
  - Local Radio Spots with messages from local actors.

### (2) Contraceptive Basket of Choice

- *Injectable MPA and Centchroman has been recently introduced in contraceptive basket*
- Temporary Methods
  - Condoms (Nirodh)
  - Oral Contraceptive Pills
  - Combined Oral Contraceptives (Mala N)
  - Centchroman (Chhaya)
  - IUCD 380 A and Cu IUCD 375
  - Injectable MPA (Antara Program)
- Permanent Methods
  - Male Sterilization (Conventional Vasectomy/NSV)
  - Female Sterilization (Minilap/Laparoscopic)
- Emergency Contraception
  - Emergency Contraceptive Pills (Ezy Pill)

### (3) Family Planning Logistics Management Information System (FP-LMIS)

Unified Software for FP logistics to streamline FP logistics and supply chain management. It is Web based, App based and SMS based application. Instant access to stock information from National level to ASHA level can be obtained.

### (4) National Family Planning Indemnity Scheme (NFPIS)

There has been growing concern about the quality of sterilization services being offered, particularly at the camp facilities. The continuing high number of complications, failures and deaths following sterilizations also results in increased litigation being faced by the providers, which is another barrier in scaling up the sterilization services. To address this issue, the Government of India had introduced the "National Family Planning Insurance Scheme" since 25th November, 2005 which has now been modified into "Family Planning Indemnity Scheme" with effect from 1st April, 2013. Under this scheme compensation is provided for death/failure/complications cases arising out of sterilization failures for acceptors as well as service providers.

### (5) Enhanced Compensation Scheme

It initiated in 2014 to provide sterilization services in 11 high focus states. Under this scheme monetary compensation is provided depending upon the procedure and the center where the procedure is done.

### (6) 'Home Delivery of Contraceptive Scheme'

To deliver contraceptives including condoms to the beneficiaries by ASHA

### (7) Vasectomy Fortnight

Observation of 'Vasectomy Fortnight' in the month of November every year in all States of India to raise awareness on male participation and promotion of male sterilization.

### (8) World Population Day Campaign

The campaigns conducted every year increases the knowledge and skills of the people worldwide towards their reproductive health and family planning.

### (9) Quality Assurance Committees at State and District Levels

To monitor the quality of Family Planning services including adverse events.

## MATERNAL HEALTH

Quality antenatal care, essential obstetric care and postnatal care for mother and newborn is provided under the program to reduce mortality.

Quality and comprehensive ANC incorporates at least four antenatal visits including early registration and first ANC with first trimester. The ANC package includes physical and abdominal examinations, Hb estimation, screening for Gestational Diabetes Mellitus, Thyroid disorders, HIV/Syphilis and urine investigation, TT/Td, Immunization, distribution of IFA tablets and Calcium (6 months during antenatal period and 6 months during postnatal period) and counselling for nutrition etc. Early detection of high-risk pregnancies, follow up and management are important component of antenatal care.

Government of India provides free institutional delivery at its network of health facilities including sub-center, primary health centers, community health centers, sub-district hospital, districts hospital etc., to reduce maternal and neonatal morbidity and mortality. To provide essential obstetric care services, Government of India is operationalizing the 24 × 7 PHCs services and providing training to SNs/LHVs/ANMs under skilled attendance at birth.

Ensuring postnatal care within first 24 hours of delivery and subsequent home visits on 3rd, 7th, 14th and 42nd day is the important components for identification and management of emergencies occurring during postnatal period. The ANMs, LHVs, and staff nurses are being oriented and trained for tackling emergencies identified during these visits.

There are total 12 key interventions for maternal health under this new program:

### (1) Strengthening of First Referral Units (FRUs) for Provision of Emergency Obstetric and Neonatal Care

While operationalizing the FRUs, the thrust is on the critical components such as manpower, blood storage units and referral linkages etc., as well as managing life-threatening complications and include facilities for obstetric surgery, blood transfusion, anesthesia, specialist pediatric care, operation theater and required equipment, in addition to facilities for MTP, tubectomy, vasectomy and pediatric care for high-risk neonates and other severe problems of early childhood availability of trained manpower (skill based training for health care providers) is linked with operationalization of FRUs.

### (2) Operationalizing MCH Wings and Obstetric High Dependency Unit (HDU)/ICUs

Maternal and child health wings are proposed to be set up in high case load facilities which will be comprehensive units with adequate beds, antenatal waiting rooms, labor wing, essential newborn care room, special newborn care units, operation theater, blood storage units, postnatal ward, and academic wing. This is to ensure provision of emergency maternal and newborn care services including 48-hour stay and postnatal care.

### (3) LaQshya Initiative

In 2017, Ministry of Health and Family Welfare launched program 'LaQshya'—quality improvement initiative in labor room and maternity OT. LaQshya program will benefit every pregnant woman and newborn delivering in public health institutions. Program will improve quality of care for pregnant women in labor room, maternity operation theatre and obstetrics intensive care units (ICUs) and high dependency units (HDUs).

Following facilities are being taken under LaQshya initiative on priority:
- All government medical college hospitals.
- All district hospitals and equivalent healthy facilities.
- All designated FRUs and high case load CHCs with over 100 deliveries/60 (per month) in hills and desert areas.

Under the initiative, multi-pronged strategy has been adopted such as improving infrastructure upgradation, ensuring availability of essential equipment, providing adequate human resources, capacity building of health care workers and improving quality processes in labor room.

*LaQshya Web portal*—All LaQshya related data will be uploaded on the portal for prompt report generation as well as visualization of dashboard to monitor progress in key maternal newborn indicators at various levels (facility, district, state and national)

*Safe delivery App*—Job aid as well as training tool for health workers.

Quality Improvement in labor room and maternity OT will be assessed through national quality assurance standards (NQAS). Every facility achieving 70% score on NQAS will be certified as LaQshya certified facility. Furthermore, branding of LaQshya certified facilities will be done as per the NQAS score. Facilities scoring more than 90%, 80% and 70% will be given platinum, gold and silver badge accordingly. Facilities achieving NQAS certification, defined quality indicators and 80% satisfied beneficiaries will be provided incentive of ₹ 6 lakhs, ₹ 3 lakhs and ₹ 2 lakhs for medical college hospital, district hospital and FRUs respectively.

### (4) Janani Suraksha Yojana

Janani Suraksha yojana, which is a modification of national maternity benefit scheme (NMBS), is a safe motherhood intervention under NRHM, where cash assistance is provided to pregnant women, which is linked to ANC during pregnancy, institutional care during delivery and immediate postpartum care in a health center. JSY is a 100% centrally sponsored scheme under implementation in all states and union territories (UTs), with special focus on low-performing states (LPS).

*Goal*

To reduce maternal and neonatal mortality by promoting institutional deliveries among poor pregnant women.

*Category of states*

Under the scheme states have been categorized as LPS which have institutional delivery 25% or less that includes eight EAG states and the states of Jammu and Kashmir and Assam, and high-performing states (HPS) which have institutional delivery rate more than 25% applicable for rest of states/UTs **(Table 47.3)**.

Eligibility for financial assistance for institutional delivery is as follows:
- LPS—all pregnant women delivering in government health facilities
- HPS—all BPL/SC/ST women delivering in government health facility
- LPS and HPS—all BPL/SC/ST women delivering in accredited private health facilities.

Cash assistance of ₹500/- per delivery is given to all BPL pregnant women, preferring to deliver at home irrespective of age and parity, in both LPS and HPS states. Each beneficiary registered under this yojana should have a JSY card, a MCH card, Aadhar number and an Aadhar-linked bank account.

ASHA or link worker should identify pregnant women from BPL households; ensure registration of pregnancy, three antenatal check-ups; counsel for institutional delivery, escort the woman to the predetermined health facility and stay with her till woman is discharged after delivery; get the birth/death of child/mother registered, make postnatal home visits; counsel for breastfeeding; arrange to immunize the child; counsel for family planning services and for availing benefits under the scheme.

Government healthcare facilities will provide emergency obstetric services free of cost. If specialists are not available in government health facilities, financial assistance is available for hiring services of specialists from private sector, or to empaneled specialist doctors working in other government institutions.

Monitoring and evaluation is done through monthly report submitted by HW (F) to PHC, which is consolidated at each level and submitted to higher level, through district and state to center. Evaluation of the scheme is done by independent institutions.

### (5) Janani Shishu Suraksha Karyakram

Janani Shishu Suraksha Karyakram (JSSK) was launched in June 2011 to provide all expenses related to delivery in a public institution, including caesarean section. Entitlements for the mother include free drugs and consumables, free diagnostics,

**Table 47.3:** Pattern of cash assistance under JSY for institutional delivery (₹).

| Category | Rural area | | | Urban area | | |
| --- | --- | --- | --- | --- | --- | --- |
| | Mother | ASHA | Total | Mother | ASHA | Total |
| Low-performing states | 1,400 | 600 | 2,000 | 1,000 | 400 | 1,400 |
| High-performing states | 700 | 600 | 1,300 | 600 | 400 | 1,000 |

(ASHA: accredited social health activist; JSY: Janani Suraksha Yojana)

free blood wherever required and free diet for the duration of the woman's stay in the facility, expected to be 3 days in case of a normal delivery and 7 days in case of a caesarean section. All sick newborns till 30 days of birth and all sick infants accessing public health institutions for treatment are also entitled to similar free services. Free transport is also provided both ways and in between facilities in case of a referral.

### (6) Pradhanmantri Surakshit Matritva Abhiyan

Pradhan Mantri Surakshit Matritva Abhiyan (PMSMA) was launched to provide fixed-day assured, comprehensive and quality ANC universally to all pregnant women (in 2nd and 3rd trimester) on the 9th of every month.

While ANC is routinely provided to pregnant women, special ANC services are provided by OBGY specialists/radiologist/physicians at government health facilities under PMSMA. As part of the campaign, a minimum package of ANC services is provided to pregnant women in their 2nd/ 3rd trimesters at Government health facilities (PHCs/ CHCs, DHs/urban health facilities, etc.) in both urban and rural areas. Using the principles of a single window system, it is envisaged that a minimum package of investigations and medicines such as IFA and calcium supplements etc. would be provided to all pregnant women attending the PMSMA clinics. One of the critical components of the Abhiyan is identification and follow-up of high-risk pregnancies and red stickers are added on to the mother and child protection cards of women with high-risk pregnancies.

### (7) Surakshit Matritva Aashwasan

Surakshit Matritva Aashwasan (SUMAN) is a multipronged and coordinated policy approach that subsumes all the existing initiatives under one umbrella in order to create a comprehensive initiative for addressing the existing inequalities in maternal and newborn health care services and move towards zero preventable maternal and newborn deaths. It was launched on 10th October 2019.

This initiative focuses on assured delivery of maternal and newborn healthcare services encompassing wider access to free, and quality services, zero tolerance for denial of services, assured management of complications along with respect for women's autonomy, dignity, feelings, choices and preferences, etc. **(Fig. 47.8)**.

Under the scheme, the beneficiaries visiting public health facilities are entitled to several free services. The services available are shown in the figure. However, since all services cannot be provided at all facilities, each health facility is expected to notify the service guarantee package on the basis of their current resources and service availability with measures put in place to reach 100% of the expected service standards for the level of that facility. The packages under SUMAN has been divided into Basic, BEmONC and CEmONC for both maternal and newborn services.

### (8) Midwifery Services Initiative

Guidelines on Midwifery services were released in December 2018 with the aims to create a cadre of nurse practitioners in

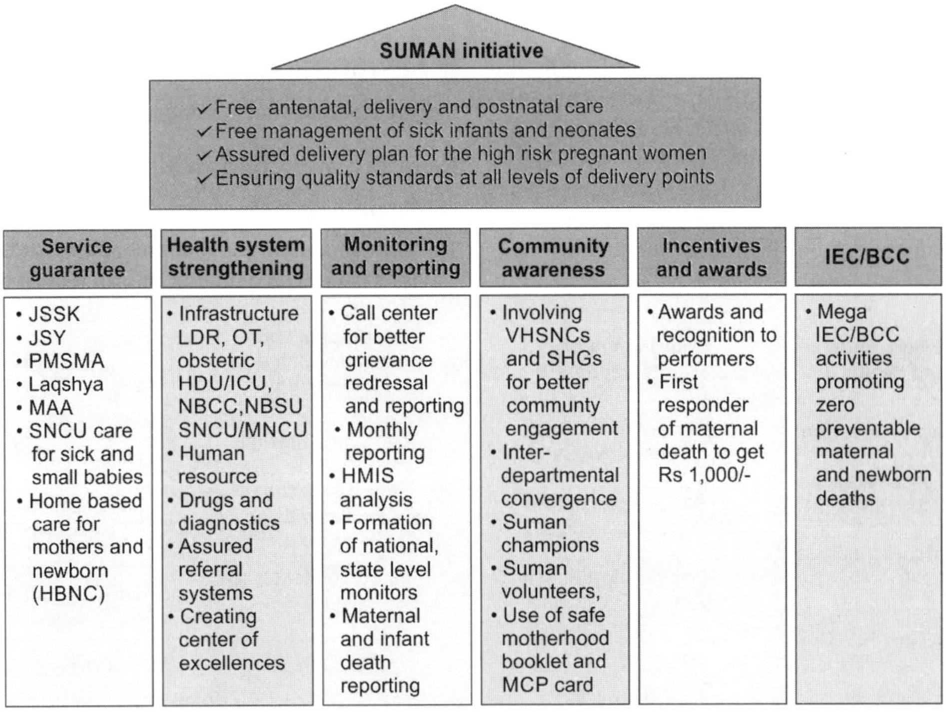

---

**SUMAN initiative**

- ✓ Free antenatal, delivery and postnatal care
- ✓ Free management of sick infants and neonates
- ✓ Assured delivery plan for the high risk pregnant women
- ✓ Ensuring quality standards at all levels of delivery points

| Service guarantee | Health system strengthening | Monitoring and reporting | Community awareness | Incentives and awards | IEC/BCC |
|---|---|---|---|---|---|
| • JSSK<br>• JSY<br>• PMSMA<br>• Laqshya<br>• MAA<br>• SNCU care for sick and small babies<br>• Home based care for mothers and newborn (HBNC) | • Infrastructure LDR, OT, obstetric HDU/ICU, NBCC,NBSU SNCU/MNCU<br>• Human resource<br>• Drugs and diagnostics<br>• Assured referral systems<br>• Creating center of excellences | • Call center for better grievance redressal and reporting<br>• Monthly reporting<br>• HMIS analysis<br>• Formation of national, state level monitors<br>• Maternal and infant death reporting | • Involving VHSNCs and SHGs for better community engagement<br>• Inter-departmental convergence<br>• Suman champions<br>• Suman volunteers,<br>• Use of safe motherhood booklet and MCP card | • Awards and recognition to performers<br>• First responder of maternal death to get Rs 1,000/- | • Mega IEC/BCC activities promoting zero preventable maternal and newborn deaths |

**Fig. 47.8:** Components of Surakshit Matritva Aashwasan (SUMAN).

(LDR: labor, delivery, recovery and postpartum room; HDU: high dependency unit; SNCU: special newborn care unit; HMIS: health management information system; VHSNC: village health sanitation and nutrition committee; IEC: information, education and counseling; MCP: mother and child protection; MNCU: maternal and newborn care unit; SHG: self help groups; BCC: behavior change communication; NBSU: newborn stabilization unit; PMSMA: Pradhanmantri Surakshit Matritva Abhiyan)

midwifery who are skilled in accordance to ICM competencies, knowledgeable and capable of providing compassionate women-center, reproductive, maternal and newborn health care services and also develop an enabling environment for integration of this cadre into the public health system, in order to achieve the SDGs for maternal and newborn health.

It will help to decongest higher level of healthcare facilities and expand access to quality maternal and neonatal services in remote areas including pockets of high home delivery rates and urban slums.

### (9) Comprehensive Abortion Care Services (CAC)

WHO issued technical guidance in 2003 to strengthen the capacity of health systems to provide safe abortion care (SAC) and postabortion care (PAC). Comprehensive abortion care (CAC) includes all of the elements of PAC as well as safe induced abortion for all legal indications (i.e. as allowed by national law). It aims to provide holistic knowledge in all aspects of abortion care including counselling, legal issues, abortion provision and post abortion contraception.

The following components of care should be ensured at all these facilities to have an enabling environment for the women coming for abortion care services:
- Privacy and confidentiality maintained for all clients
- Respectful, courteous and nonjudgmental health staff
- Reproductive rights respected while providing services
- Clean and hygienic surroundings
- Availability of 24 × 7 running water supply, uninterrupted power supply (including power back-up), and clean toilets (separate for male and female)
- Assured referral linkages

Different levels of health facilities in the public health system have different cadres of health care workers who can provide different abortion-related services. It ranges from informing and educating the women about the availability and legality of abortion care; helping them to recognize early pregnancy and confirming it; providing abortion care; and referring them to an appropriate facility for the management of complications.

### (10) Capacity Building of Human Resource

- *'Dakshata'* (means adroitness) is an initiative by MoHFW to improve the quality of care at the delivery points of the country through a focused program which includes a concise training package for competency enhancement for medical officers, Nurses and ANMs; developing a system of post-training follow-up and mentoring; ensuring availability of essential commodities, supplies and equipment in the labor rooms; and strengthening the capacity of the facilities and the system to measure quality of care on a regular basis.
- An 18-week training module in *life saving anesthesia skills (LSAS)* and a16-week training module for *Emergency Obstetric Care* is developed for MBBS doctors.
- *Skilled Birth Attendant (SBA)* Training is a part of technical strategy for reduction of maternal mortality by giving universal access to skilled attendance at birth and timely access to quality services for timely management of life-threatening obstetric complications.

### (11) Universal screening for Gestational Diabetes Mellitus, HIV and Syphilis

### (12) Maternal, Perinatal and Child Death Surveillance and Response (MPCDSR)

### Other Models of Public Private Partnership for Maternal Care

These include Chiranjeevi Yojana in Gujarat, Saubhagyawati Scheme in Uttar Pradesh, Janani Suvidha Yojana in Haryana, Janani Sahyogi Yojana in Madhya Pradesh, Ayushmati Scheme in West Bengal and Mamta Friendly Hospital Scheme in Delhi.

## NEWBORN AND CHILD HEALTH

Key strategic interventions under child health are shown in **Fig. 47.9**:

### Newborn and Child Health Related Interventions

### (1) Home-based Newborn Care

The Government of India launched the HBNC program in 2011 (revised 2014) which mainly aims to reduce neonatal morbidity

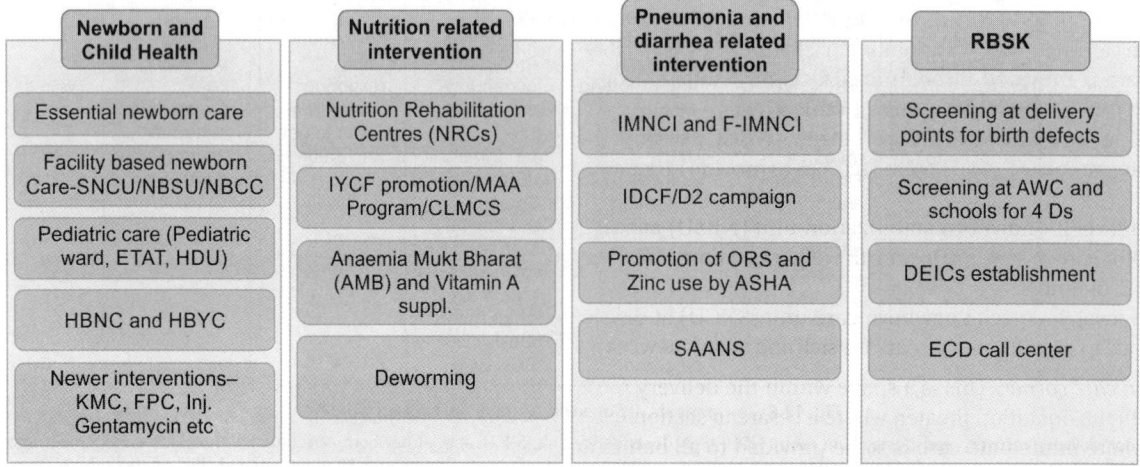

**Fig. 47.9:** Interventions under child health.

and mortality through home visits by ASHAs and ANMs in the postnatal period both in case of home deliveries and institutional deliveries, for providing essential newborn care, detection of preterm and LBW newborns, identification of illness and prompt referral, supporting family to adopt healthy practices and counseling for family planning.

Six visits are made in case of institutional delivery (on days 3, 7, 14, 21, 28, and 42) and seven visits in case of home delivery (on days 1, 3, 7, 14, 21, 28 and 42) where the ASHA takes weight and temperature of the newborn, ensures warmth, provides skin, cord and eye care, identifies illness and refers promptly, and counsels mother on exclusive breastfeeding, newborn care and against unhealthy practices.

### (2) Home-based Care for Young Child (HBYC)

Home-Based Care for Young Child Programme (HBYC) was launched in 2018 for promotion of health and nutrition of young children (3–15 months), for reducing child morbidity and mortality and for promotion of growth and early childhood development. Under HBYC, ASHA provides incentivized five home visits on 3rd, 6th, 9th, 12th and 15th months. ASHAs are being paid incentive of ₹ 250/- per HBYC category child for five scheduled home visits.

During the visit, ASHA will do the following activities:
- Counseling for exclusive breast feeding till 6 months and continued breast feeding with adequate complementary feeding afterward.
- Counseling of mothers and caregivers and support to identify and manage problems related to nutrition and health in their child.
- Facilitate for early identification of delay in growth and development of children by using the MCP card.
- Support in prevention and management of common childhood illnesses
- Assist in prompt referral of sick children to health facilities for management of complications and follow ups.

### (3) Facility-based Newborn Care (FBNC)

With momentum of increased institutional deliveries stimulated by JSY and JSSK under NHM, operational guidelines of FBNC were laid out in 2011 for improving the quality of services for newborn care at the delivery points. For sick newborns, facility-based care is provided through fixed facilities at different levels of health care at special care units. **(Table 47.4)**
- MCH level 1—newborn care corner (NBCC) within the delivery room/OT of all health facilities to provide immediate care.
- MCH level 2—newborn stabilization unit (NBSU) at CHC/FRU for care of sick and low birth weight newborns for short period of time.
- MCH level 3—special newborn care unit (SNCU) at district hospital to provide special care for sick and at-risk newborns.

*Newborn care corner:* This is a space within the delivery room or within the operation theater, where a cesarean section takes place where immediate care is to be provided to all babies at birth. It is now mandatory that at every facility where a baby is born, there should be a NBCC. The essential list of equipments that should be available at each NBCC includes a radiant warmer, a hand operated resuscitator, a weighing scale, pump suction, thermometer, light for examination, and a syringe hub cutter. Each NBCC should have at least a designated doctor and staff nurse to ensure proper functioning of the NBCC. All doctors, staff nurses, and ANMs engaged in conducting deliveries must be trained in NSSK. This is a 2 day training program addressing importance of "at-birth" essential care interventions like basic newborn resuscitation, prevention of hypothermia, prevention of sepsis, early initiation of breastfeeding, etc.

**Table 47.4:** Newborn care services matrix.

| | NBCC | NBSU | SNCU |
|---|---|---|---|
| Services | • Prevention of infection<br>• Thermal care<br>• Resuscitation<br>• Early initiation of breastfeeding and sustained support<br>• Weight monitoring<br>• Identification and prompt referral of "at-risk" and "sick" newborns | • Management of LBW ≥1,800 and <2,500 g<br>• Phototherapy for newborns with hyperbilirubinemia<br>• Management of sepsis<br>• Referral services | • Management of LBW <1,800 g<br>• Management of all sick newborns except those requiring ventilation and major surgery<br>• Follow-up of all high-risk newborns<br>• Referral services |
| Training of health staff | NSSK | F-IMNCI | FBNC |

(FBNC: facility-based newborn care; F-IMNCI: facility-based integrated management of neonatal and childhood illness; LBW: low birth weight; NBSU: newborn stabilization unit; NBCC: newborn care corner; NSSK: Navjat Shishu Suraksha Karyakram; SNCU: special newborn care unit)

*Newborn stabilization unit:* All first referral units (FRUs) or community health centers (CHCs) with less than 3,000 deliveries per year should have an NBSU (in addition to the NBCC at the place of delivery) within or in close proximity of the maternity ward where sick and/or LBW babies can be cared for shorter periods. Each NBSU should have one trained doctor and at least one trained nurse per shift, i.e., at least four staff nurses trained in facility-based integrated management of neonatal and childhood illness (F-IMNCI).

The F-IMNCI is a standard 11 day skill-based training combining classroom sessions with hands-on training.

*Special newborn care unit:* All CHCs or FRUs where more than 3,000 deliveries occur annually should have a 12-bedded SNCU to provide special care by trained health staff to small and sick newborns—all except ventilation and major surgery. For every additional 1,000 deliveries, four more beds are recommended. Also, each SNCU should have an associated "step-down unit" with adult beds for rooming-in of the babies with mothers after the acute phase of the illness is over. The step-down unit should have 30% of the SNCU beds.

The 12-bedded SNCU (with four-bedded step-down) in each shift should have at least one pediatrician, three medical officers trained in FBNC with 12 trained staff nurses.

All staff should be trained in the FBNC which is 4 day training along with a 2 weeks observership at designated SNCUs. It includes a skill-based training in essential and special care along with housekeeping and management of special equipment.

*Criteria for admission to SNCU:*
- Birth weight less than 1,800 g or more than 4,000 g
- Period of gestation less than 34 weeks
- Perinatal asphyxia
- Apnea or gasping
- Refusal to feed
- Respiratory distress (RR >60 or grunting or retractions)
- Severe jaundice (appears <24 hours or stains palms and soles or lasts >2 weeks)
- Hypothermia less than 35.4°C or hyperthermia more than 37.5°C
- Central cyanosis
- Shock (capillary filing time >3 minutes, weak pulse, and cold periphery)
- Coma or convulsions or encephalopathy
- Abdominal distension
- Diarrhea or dysentery
- Bleeding
- Major malformations.

All babies requiring ventilator support or major surgery will require tertiary care management at an NICU with highly trained health staff.

**Triage of a sick newborn:** Newborns with following "emergency signs" require immediate admission and prompt treatment at SNCU:
- Hypothermia (temperature <36°C)
- Gasping or apnea
- Severe respiratory distress (RR >70 per minute, severe retractions, and grunting)
- Central cyanosis
- Shock (capillary filing time >3 minutes, weak pulse, and cold periphery)
- Coma, convulsions, or encephalopathy.

Newborns with following "priority signs" will need rapid assessment and admission to SNCU:
- Cold stress (temperature between 36.4° and 35°C)
- Respiratory distress (RR >60, no retractions or grunting)
- Irritable or restless
- Abdominal distension
- Severe jaundice
- Severe pallor
- Bleeding from any site
- Major congenital malformations
- Weight less than 1,800 g or >4,000 g.

Newborns with following "nonurgent signs" do not require urgent attention but will need further assessment and counseling:
- Transitional stools
- Posseting
- Minor birth trauma
- Superficial infections
- Minor malformations
- Jaundice
- All cases not categorized as emergency or priority.

## Pneumonia and Diarrhea related Interventions

### (1) Integrated Management of Neonatal and Childhood Illnesses (IMNCI)

Everyday many caregivers all around the world bring their sick children to primary level health centers where healthcare providers use symptoms and signs to provide best care. But due to limited comprehensive diagnostic and treatment infrastructure, providing quality primary care is a serious challenge. In response to this challenge, WHO and UNICEF developed a preventive and curative strategy called "IMCI" in 1995 which was renamed to "Integrated Management of Neonatal, Childhood Illness" (IMNCI) in 2003 to include newborns in India. The term "integrated" implies that whenever any child reports for any illness, the healthcare provider should always examine for a list of symptoms which can contribute to morbidity and mortality. More than 100 countries have adopted the IMCI strategy and have started implementing its three components—(1) improving skills of health worker, (2) strengthening of health systems, and (3) improving family and community childcare practices. IMNCI is an integrated child health approach focusing on the well-being of the whole child. It has been pegged as an essential component for primary healthcare and universal health coverage. This strategy has shown to reduce child mortality by about 15%.

IMNCI plus includes (1) skilled care at birth, (2) IMNCI including inpatient care, and (3) immunization.

For syndromic diagnosis and treatment, children are divided into two age categories:
1. Young infants up to 2 months
2. Children 2 months up to 5 years

A combination of symptoms and signs helps in arriving at a child's classification rather than a diagnosis. Classification indicates the severity of the condition, based on which specific actions need to be taken as to whether the young infant or the child should be urgently referred to another level of care/given specific treatment at the OPD or may be safely managed at home. The classifications are color-coded—"pink" suggests hospital referral or admission, "yellow" indicates initiation of treatment, and "green" calls for home management.

All sick young infants up to 2 months of age (excluding care at birth) must be always assessed for "possible bacterial infection or jaundice" and the major symptom "diarrhea". All sick children age 2 months up to 5 years must be examined for "general danger signs" which indicate the need for immediate referral or admission to a hospital. They must then be routinely assessed for major symptoms—cough or difficult breathing, diarrhea, fever, and ear problems. Also warranted is routine assessment for nutritional and immunization status, feeding problems, and other potential problems.

The various steps under IMNCI are shown in **Flowcharts 47.1 and 47.2**:
- **Step 1: assess**—all sick young infants and children should be assessed for:
  - Symptoms and signs of serious illness that may require urgent referral
  - Symptoms and signs of common health conditions
    ♦ Nutrition status, immunization status, and other problems.

## Chapter 47: Health Policies and Programs in India

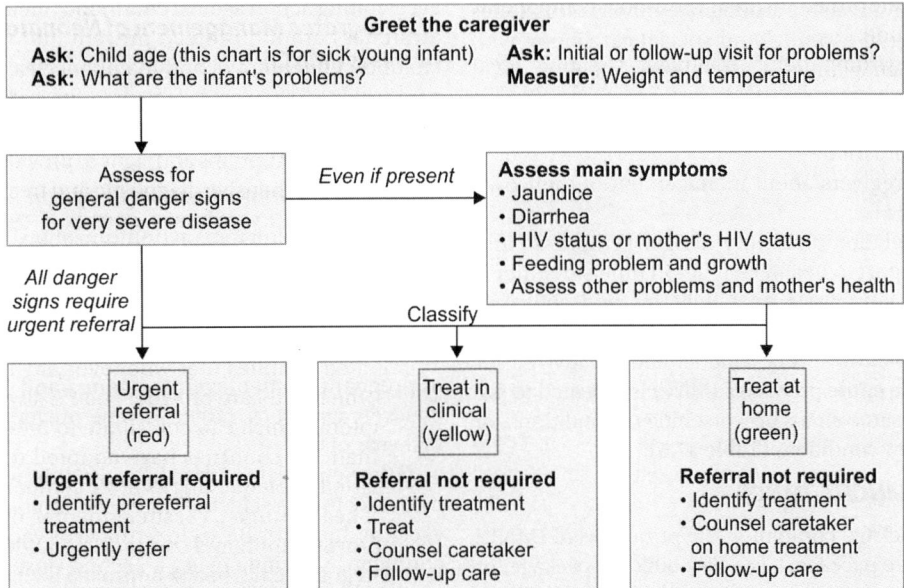

Flowchart 47.1: IMNCI case management in the outpatient health facility, first-level referral facility, and at home for the sick young infant up to 2 months of age.

(IMNCI: Integrated Management of Neonatal and Childhood Illnesses; HIV: human immunodeficiency virus)

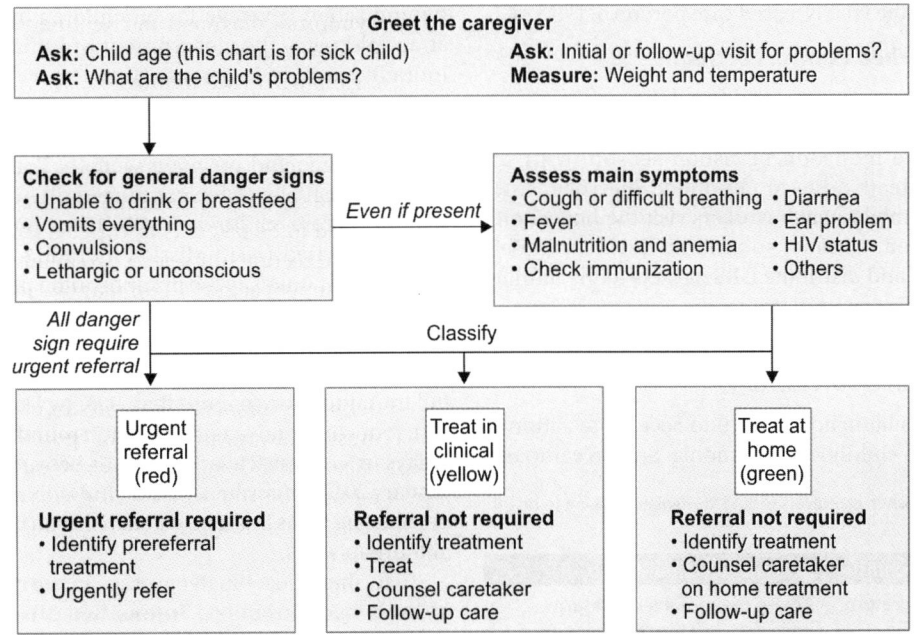

Flowchart 47.2: IMNCI case management in the outpatient health facility, first-level referral facility and at home for the sick child from age 2 months up to 5 years.

(IMNCI: Integrated Management of Neonatal and Childhood Illnesses; HIV: human immunodeficiency virus)

- ***Step 2: Classify***—the severity of clinical symptoms and signs is color coded as—"red or pink" suggests hospital referral or admission, "yellow" indicates initiation of specific treatment, and "green" calls for home management.
- ***Step 3: Treat***—an integrated treatment plan should be developed based on all the symptoms and signs. For example, a mother may bring the child only for diarrhea but it is also essential to treat any accompanying malnutrition and/or fever, which may have been missed by mother. In case of presence of multiple conditions, use treatment option for the most serious classified illness.
  - Those requiring urgent referral (red category) should be given essential initial treatment before referral.
  - Yellow category children can be managed by treatment at the health facility.
  - All should be advised about treatment at home by caregivers.

- **Step 4: Counsel**—it is critical to counsel caregivers about management and care of their children. The various components of counseling include:
  - Counseling regarding home treatment (treating local infections and giving oral drugs)
  - Counseling regarding breastfeeding, complementary feeding, and fluid intake
  - Counseling caregivers about management of their own health
  - Teaching caregivers to identify danger symptoms and signs and to report to health facilities in timely manner
  - Counseling to emphasize on follow-ups and complete immunization.
- **Step 5: Follow-up care**—every child should be advised for follow-up when the entire process of IMNCI is repeated to see for improvement, same status or worsening of conditions, or development of new conditions **(Table 47.5)**.

### (2) Facility-based IMNCI (F-IMNCI)

It is an integrated package combining the principles of IMNCI with facility-based care package. It is a skill-building package for medical officers and nurses working in 24 × 7 PHCs, FRUs, CHCs and District Hospitals which do not have trained pediatricians. Skill-based training is given to MOs and nurses. Those who are not trained in IMNCI will get the full package of training on F-IMNCI for 11 days and those who are already trained in IMNCI will receive 5 days of training, on the facility-based care portion of F-IMNCI.

### (3) Intensified Diarrhea Control Fortnight

To increase awareness about use of ORS and Zinc in diarrhea—an Intensified Diarrhoea Control Fortnight (IDCF) is being observed during pre-monsoon/monsoon season, with the aim of 'zero child deaths due to childhood diarrhea' since 2014. During the fortnight health workers visit the households of under five children, conduct community level awareness generation activities and distribute ORS packets to the families with children under five years of age.

### (4) SAANS (Social Awareness and Action to Neutralize Pneumonia Successfully)

SAANS Initiative was launched in 2019 to accelerate action to reduce deaths due to childhood pneumonia. SAANS campaign is rolled out in the States/UTs every year with the aim of accelerating action against childhood pneumonia by generating awareness around protect, prevent and treatment aspects of childhood pneumonia and to enhance early identification and care seeking behaviors among parents and caregivers.

## Immunization

### (1) Universal immunization Program

The Expanded Program on Immunization (EPI) was launched in 1978, to decrease morbidity and mortality from the six common vaccine preventable diseases in childhood and also to achieve self-sufficiency in vaccine production. In 1985, the UIP was started, which included two components—(1) immunization of pregnant women against tetanus and (2) immunization of children against six target vaccine preventable diseases in the first year of life.

Other changes in the UIP schedule were introduction of new vaccines in selected states, viz. Japanese encephalitis (JE) vaccine, hepatitis B vaccine, rotavirus vaccine, pneumococcal conjugate vaccine; giving a second dose of measles vaccine; pentavalent vaccine replacing DPT vaccine; switch from tOPV to bOPV; introduction of IPV, etc. **(Table 47.6)**.

### (2) Mission Indradhanush

To strengthen and re-energize the program and achieve full immunization coverage for all children and pregnant women at a rapid pace, the Government of India launched "Mission Indradhanush" in December 2014.

The goal of Mission Indradhanush is to ensure full immunization with all available vaccines for children up to 2 years of age and pregnant women. Four phases of Mission Indradhanush have been conducted till August 2017 and more than 2.53 crore children and 68 lakhs pregnant women have been vaccinated (NHP, Mission Indradhanush).

To further intensify the immunization program, Government of India launched the **Intensified Mission Indradhanush (IMI)** on October 8, 2017. The focus of special drive was to improve immunization coverage in select districts and cities to ensure full immunization to more than 90% by December 2018. Under IMI, four consecutive immunization rounds were conducted for 7 days in 173 districts every month between October 2017 and January 2018. Intensified Mission Indradhanush has covered low performing areas in the selected districts (high priority districts) and urban areas.

To further boost the RI coverage in the country, Government of India had introduced **Intensified Mission Indradhanush 2.0 (IMI 2.0) from** December 2019 to March 2020, IMI 3.0 in February 2021 and IMI 4.0 launched in February 2022 to ensure reaching the unreached with all available vaccines and accelerate the coverage of children and pregnant women. Three rounds of Intensified Mission Indradhanush 5.0 (IMI 5.0) under the theme "A big leap towards measles and Rubella Elimination" has been recently conducted in August 2023—with an objective to identify and vaccinate all unvaccinated and under vaccinated children till five years of age. Post MI and IMI Campaigns, the estimates showed a remarkable improvement in FIC, reflecting these as key drivers in boosting immunization coverage in the

**Table 47.5:** Danger signs when caregivers should immediately report to health facility.

| Sick young infant (0–2 months) | Sick child (2 months–5 years) |
|---|---|
| Advise the caregiver to return immediately if the young infant has any of the following:<br>• Breastfeeding poorly<br>• Reduced activity<br>• Becomes sicker<br>• Develops a fever<br>• Feels unusually cold<br>• Fast breathing<br>• Difficult breathing<br>• Palms and soles appear yellow | Advise the caregiver to return immediately if the child has any of the following:<br>• Any sick child:<br>  ➤ Not able to drink or breastfeed<br>  ➤ Becomes sicker<br>  ➤ Develops a fever<br>• If child has no pneumonia:<br>  ➤ Cough or cold:<br>  ➤ Fast breathing<br>  ➤ Difficult breathing<br>• If child has diarrhea, also return if:<br>  ➤ Blood in stool<br>  ➤ Drinking poorly |

Table 47.6: Current immunization schedule under universal immunization program (UIP).

| Vaccine | When to give | Dose | Route | Site |
|---|---|---|---|---|
| *For pregnant women* | | | | |
| Td-1 | Early in pregnancy | 0.5 mL | Intramuscular | Upper arm |
| Td-2 | 4 weeks after TT-1 | 0.5 mL | Intramuscular | Upper arm |
| Td-Booster | If received 2 TT doses in a pregnancy within the last 3 years | 0.5 mL | Intramuscular | Upper arm |
| *For infants* | | | | |
| BCG | At birth or as early as possible till 1 year of age | 0.1 mL (0.05 mL until 1 month age) | Intradermal | Left upper arm |
| Hepatitis B | At birth or as early as possible within 24 hours | 0.5 mL | Intramuscular | Anterolateral side of left mid-thigh |
| OPV-0 | At birth or as early as possible within the first 15 days | 2 drops | Oral | Oral |
| OPV 1, 2 and 3 | At 6 weeks, 10 weeks and 14 weeks | 2 drops | Oral | Oral |
| RVV (rotavirus vaccine) | At 6 weeks, 10 weeks and 14 weeks | 5 drops | Oral | Oral |
| Pentavalent | At 6 weeks, 10 weeks and 14 weeks | 0.5 mL | Intramuscular | Anterolateral side of left mid-thigh |
| F-IPV (1st and 2nd dose) | At 6 weeks and 14 weeks | 0.1 mL | Intradermal | Right upper arm |
| PCV*(pneumococcal conjugate vaccine) | At 6 weeks, 14 weeks and 9 months | 0.5 mL | Intramuscular | Anterolateral side of right mid-thigh |
| MR 1st dose (Measles Rubella) | At 9 completed months to 12 months | 0.5 mL | Subcutaneous | Right upper arm |
| Japanese encephalitis*** (1st dose) | 9 completed months to 12 months | 0.5 mL | Subcutaneous | Left upper arm |
| f-IPV 3rd dose | 9 completed months to 12 months | 0.1 mL | Intradermal | Left upper arm |
| Vitamin A (1st dose) | 9 months with measles | 1 mL (1 lakh IU) | Oral | Oral |
| *For children* | | | | |
| DPT booster-1 | 16–24 months | 0.5 mL | Intramuscular | Anterolateral side of left mid-thigh |
| OPV booster-1 | 16–24 months | 2 drops | Oral | Oral |
| MR 2nd dose | 16–24 months | 0.5 mL | Subcutaneous | Right upper arm |
| Japanese encephalitis* (2nd dose) | 16–24 months with DPT/OPV booster | 0.5 mL | Subcutaneous | Left upper arm |
| Vitamin A (2nd to 9th dose) | 16 months with DPT/OPV booster Then, one dose every 6 months, up to age of 5 years | 2 mL (2 lakhs IU) | Oral | Oral |
| DPT booster-2 | 5–6 years | 0.5 mL | Intramuscular | Upper arm |
| Td | 10 years and 16 years | 0.5 mL | Intramuscular | Upper arm |

* Rotavirus vaccine in entire country except Uttar Pradesh supported through domestic budget; UP through Gavi support
** PCV is currently in 26 States/UTs
*** JE vaccine has been introduced in routine immunization in 276 districts across 21 states.
(DPT: diphtheria pertussis tetanus; OPV: oral polio vaccine; BCG: bacille Calmette-Guerin)

country. During these drives, around 3.39 crore children and 87 lakh pregnant women were vaccinated. Moreover, an average increase of 18.5% points in FIC was noted as compared to NFHS-4 in the 190 districts and urban areas covered under IMI.

## Nutrition Related Interventions

### (1) MAA—"Mother's Absolute Affection"

It is a nationwide program launched in 2016 by MoHFW in an attempt to bring undiluted focus on promotion of breastfeeding and provision of counselling services for supporting breastfeeding through health systems. The program has been named 'MAA' to signify the support a lactating mother requires from family members and at health facilities to breastfeed successfully.

### (2) Infant and Young Child Feeding (IYCF)

is a set of well-known and recommended appropriate feeding practices for newborn and children up to two years of age.

Optimal IYCF Practices:
- Early initiation of breastfeeding; immediately after birth, preferably within one hour.
- Exclusive breastfeeding for the first six months of life.

- Timely introduction of complementary food (maintaining adequate diet and dietary diversity) beyond six months along with continued breastfeeding. Breastfeeding should be continued minimum for 2 years and beyond.
- Mother should communicate, look into the eyes, touch and caress the baby while feeding. Practice responsive feeding.

Under MAA program, promotion of IYCF services is done at health facilities, community level (outreach) and through home visits.

### (3) Lactation Management Centre (CLMC)

National Health Mission has taken the initiative to establish lactation management centers at secondary and tertiary level public health facilities to provide lactation support for mothers who can, or can eventually, breastfeed. This facility-based lactation management strategy adopting the procedures of collection, processing, storage and dispensing of donor human milk and mother's own milk along with provision of lactation support to the mothers would be a key component for protecting, promoting, and supporting breastfeeding.

The lactation management centers would be established at three levels:

i. At medical colleges and district hospitals: Comprehensive lactation management centres (CLMCs) for donor human milk collection, storage, processing and dispensing for babies admitted in health facilities.
ii. Sub-district hospitals and FRUs: Lactation management units (LMUs) for collecting, storing and dispensing of mother's breast milk, expressed and stored for consumption by her own baby.
iii. All delivery points: Lactation support units (LSUs) for providing lactation support to mothers at all delivery points.

### (4) Nutritional Rehabilitation Center

#### Introduction

Undernutrition is one of the most concerning health and development issues in India as in other parts of the world. Undernutrition encompasses stunting (chronic malnutrition), wasting (acute malnutrition) and deficiencies of micronutrients (essential vitamins and minerals). The high mortality and disease burden resulting from undernutrition call for urgent implementation of interventions to reduce their occurrence and consequences and this would include determined action on the social determinants of undernutrition.

Prevalence of undernutrition in urban and rural areas (NFHS-5, 2019–21)

| Indicators | Urban | Rural | Total |
|---|---|---|---|
| Children under 5 years who are stunted (height-for-age) (%) | 30.1 | 37.3 | 35.5 |
| Children under 5 years who are wasted (weight-for-height) (%) | 18.5 | 19.5 | 19.3 |
| Children under 5 years who are severely wasted (weight-for-height)(%) | 7.6 | 7.7 | 7.7 |
| Children under 5 years who are underweight (weight-for-age) (%) | 27.3 | 33.8 | 32.1 |

#### What are the types of undernutrition?

The three indices—(1) weight-for-age, (2) height-for-age, (3) weight-for-height are used to identify three nutrition conditions: underweight, stunting and wasting, respectively. Each of the three nutrition indicators is expressed in standard deviation units (Z-scores) from the median of the reference population.

#### Severe acute malnutrition

Severe acute malnutrition (SAM) is defined by very low weight-for-height (Z-score below-3SD of the median WHO child growth standards), a mid-upper arm circumference <115 mm, or by the presence of nutritional edema.

Severe acute malnutrition increases significantly the risk of death in children under 5 years of age. It can be an indirect cause of child death by increasing the case fatality rate in children suffering from common illnesses such as diarrhea and pneumonia. Children who are severely wasted are 9 times more likely to die than well-nourished children.

#### Addressing SAM in children under-five years

Programmatically, it is helpful to categorize children with SAM into "complicated and uncomplicated" cases based on clinical criteria.

WHO and UNICEF in their joint statement have recommended two major approaches to address children with SAM:
1. Facility/hospital-based care for children with SAM and medical complications.
2. Home/community-based care for children with SAM but without medical complications.

In other words, effective management of SAM must be based on the basic principle of "Continuum of Care"—from the home and community, to the health center/health facility and back again.

#### Nutrition rehabilitation center (facility-based care for children with SAM and medical complications)

Nutrition rehabilitation center (NRC) is a unit in a health facility where children with SAM are admitted and managed. Children are admitted as per the defined admission criteria and provided with medical and nutritional therapeutic care. Once discharged from the NRC, the child continues to be in the nutrition rehabilitation program till she/he attains the defined discharge criteria from the program.

#### Objectives of NRC

- To provide clinical management and reduce mortality among children with severe acute malnutrition, particularly among those with medical complications
- To promote physical and psychosocial growth of children with SAM
- To build the capacity of mothers and other caregivers in appropriate feeding and caring practices for infants and young children
- To identify the social factors that contributed to the child slipping into severe acute malnutrition.

#### Services provided at the facility

The services and care provided for the inpatient management of SAM children include:
- 24-hour care and monitoring of the child
- Treatment of medical complications

- Therapeutic feeding
- Providing sensory stimulation and emotional care
- Social assessment of the family to identify and address contributing factors
- Counseling on appropriate feeding, care and hygiene
- Demonstration and practice-by-doing on the preparation of energy dense child foods using locally available, culturally acceptable and affordable food items
- Follow-up of children discharged from the facility.

*Screening for SAM cases in community (Flowchart 47.3)*
*Principles of Hospital-based Management at NRC*

Each SAM child should be immediately screened to identify medical complications and its severity. Triage is the process of rapidly screening sick children. Triage must be done for all pediatric patients coming to the health facility. The first step is to check every child for emergency signs and provide emergency treatment as necessary keeping in mind the ABCD steps: Airway, Breathing, Circulation, Coma, Convulsion, and Dehydration.

At the same time, SAM child is managed appropriately for feeding and weight gain.

The principles of management of SAM are based on three phases: (1) Stabilization phase, (2) Transition phase and (3) Rehabilitative phase.

1. **Stabilization phase:** Children with SAM without an adequate appetite and/or a major medical complication are stabilized in an in patient facility. This phase usually lasts for 1–2 days. The feeding formula used during this phase is starter diet which promotes recovery of normal metabolic function and nutrition- electrolytic balance. All children must be carefully monitored for signs of overfeeding or over hydration in this phase.
2. **Transition phase:** This phase is the subsequent part of the stabilization phase and usually lasts for 2–3 days. The transition phase is intended to ensure that the child is clinically stable and can tolerate an increased energy and protein intake. The child moves to the transition phase from stabilization phase when there is:
   – At least the beginning of loss of edema
   – Return of appetite
   – No nasogastric tube, infusions, no severe medical problems
   – Is alert and active.

The ONLY difference in management of the child in transition phase is the change in type of diet. There is gradual transition from starter diet to catch-up diet (F 100). The quantity of catch-up diet (F 100) given is equal to the quantity of starter diet given in stabilization phase.

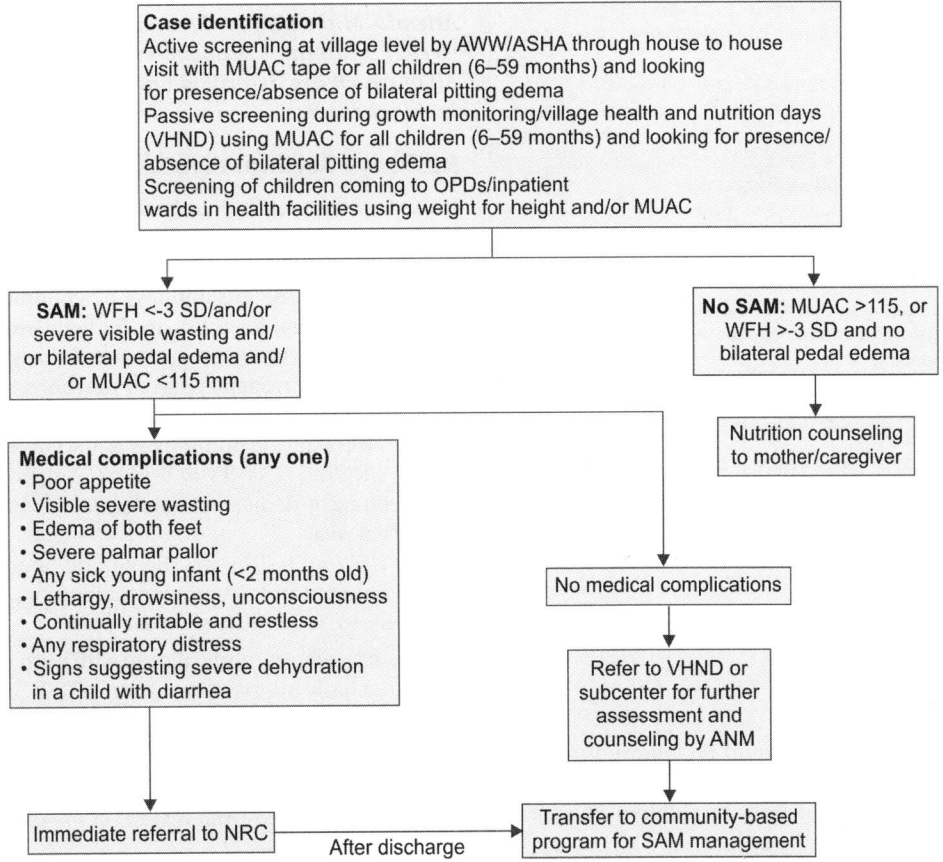

Flowchart 47.3: Screening for SAM Cases in Community.

(NRC: nutritional rehabilitation center; MUAC: mid upper arm circumference; WFH: weight for height; SAM: severe acute malnutrition)

3. **Rehabilitation phase:** Once children with SAM have recovered their appetite and received treatment for medical complications they enter rehabilitation phase. The aim is to promote rapid weight gain, stimulate emotional and physical development and prepare the child for normal feeding at home. The child progresses from transition phase to rehabilitation phase when:
   - She/he has reasonable appetite; finishes >90% of the feed
   - that is given, without a significant pause
   - Major reduction or loss of edema
   - No other medical problem.

> *Criteria for discharge*
> - Discharge criterion for all infants and children is 15% weight gain and no signs of illness.
> - This should be achieved through facility-based care in NRC when community-based program is not in place.
>
> **Discharge from nutrition rehabilitation center**
> *Child*
> - Edema has resolved
> - Child has achieved weight gain of >15% and has satisfactory weight gain for 3 consecutive days (>5 g/kg/day)
> - Child is eating an adequate amount of nutritious food that the mother can prepare at home
> - All infections and other medical complications have been treated
> - Child is provided with micronutrients
> - Immunization is updated
>
> *Mother/caregiver*
> - Knows how to prepare appropriate foods and to feed the child
> - Knows how to give prescribed medications, vitamins, folic acid and iron at home
> - Knows how to make appropriate toys and play with the child
> - Knows how to give home treatment for diarrhea, fever and acute respiratory infections and how to recognize the signs for which medical assistance must be sought
> - Follow-up plan is discussed and understood
>
> Where community-based program is well functioning, child can be transferred from facility-based care to community-based care for achieving target weight gain of 15%, based on the following criteria:
> - Child has completed antibiotic treatment
> - Has good appetite (eating at least 120–130 cal/kg/day)
> - Has good weight gain (of at least 5 g/kg/day for three consecutive days) on exclusive oral feeding
> - No edema
> - Caretakers sensitized to home care and education has been completed
> - Immunization is up-to-date
>
> If the child has not recovered in 4 months, she/he is classified as a "non-responder".
>
> **Failure to respond**
> | Criteria | Approximate time after admission |
> |---|---|
> | Failure to regain appetite | Day 4 |
> | Failure to start to lose edema | Day 4 |
> | Edema still present | Day 10 |
> | Failure to gain at least 5 g/kg/day for 3 successive days after feeding freely on catch-up diet | |

*Follow-up*
Children discharged from NRC should be followed up at the community level to ensure appropriate feeding, follow-up at NRC for scheduled visit and to identify the children who are not responding to the treatment.

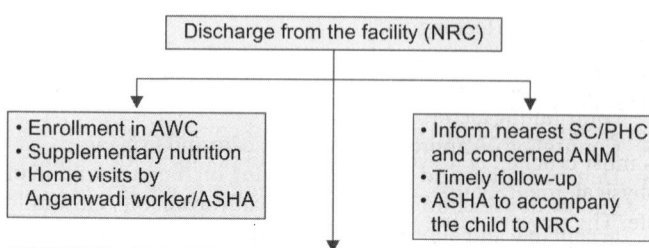

*Conclusion*
The establishment of NRC is justified at tertiary level hospital as prevalence of SAM is high in community. But at the same time, community linkage for home-based management is necessary to sustain the nutritional status of individual.

It must be recognized that although treatment is urgently needed for those who are severely undernourished, preventing child undernutrition in community as a whole is also critical. NRCs will reduce child mortality but will not improve the general nutritional status of children in the community. From the perspective of health sector, the most important intervention is promotion of appropriate infant and young child feeding and nutrition practices and related maternal undernutrition, which will in turn help to achieve improved nutritional status in the community.

***Other nutrition interventions under child health are Anemia Mukt Bharat Strategy, National Deworming Day (NDD), Vitamin A supplementation and POSHAN Abhiyan, all of which are described under nutrition related programs in this chapter.***

### Rashtriya Bal Swasthya Karyakram (RBSK)

It was launched in 2013 for health screening and early intervention services through early detection and management of 4 Ds (birth defects, deficiencies, childhood diseases, and developmental delays and disabilities) in children and adolescents 0–18 years of age, for a list of 30 identified health conditions. Implementation of the program is as follows:
- *For newborns:* Facility-based newborn screening at public health facilities and community-based newborn screening by ASHAs during home visits as part of HBNC.
- *For children 6 weeks to 6 years:* Anganwadi center-based screening by dedicated mobile health teams, to be conducted twice a year.
- *For children 6–18 years:* Screening of children enrolled in Government and Government aided schools, by mobile health teams, to be conducted once a year.

***Referral:*** Newborns and children with birth defects are referred to District Early Intervention Centres (DEIC) in district hospitals *for confirmation, further assessment and as referral linkage to appropriate health facility.*

***Management:*** *Free of cost management of children identified with ailment in DEIC and referral at pre identified tertiary level institutions for surgery.*

## Journey of First 1,000 Days

The **"First 1,000 Days"** refers to the period that begins with pregnancy planning and goes up to when the child reaches her second birthday. The first thousand days in a person's life is most crucial, as it establishes a solid platform for a child's physical, mental and social health, leading to the rest of their life. The power of first thousand days encompasses the right nutrition, stimulation, love and support; beginning with the pre-conception period and continuing in the first two years of a child's life. Rastriya Bal Swashthya Karyakram (RBSK), has shifted the focus from **"only survival to healthy survival"** through timely screening and early management to improve the quality of life from birth till 18 years of age. This program is designed to focus on the children at-risk and intervene during the critical years of brain development through medical, surgical and therapeutic interventions, at zero cost to the families. The **document "Journey of First 1,000 Days"** is an initiative to help the parents and families to best utilize their potential in good child rearing practices during the first thousand days. The objective of this document is to provide parents and health care providers with the most recent and up-to-date knowledge regarding the most important factors that can impact a child's cognitive development.

## Strengthening Facility Based Paediatric Care

It has the potential to reduce childhood deaths in sick children and is an integral part of the service delivery package under National Health Mission.

The vision for pediatric care at district hospital is to set up a comprehensive unit comprising of the following sub-units:

- Paediatric Outpatient Facility (including immunization and counselling services)
- Emergency Triage Assessment and Treatment (ETAT) Facility
- Pediatric Inpatient Facility
  - High dependency unit
  - Pediatric ward
  - Diarrhea treatment unit
  - Isolation room
- Ancillary (eg; laboratory, imaging, pharmacy) and Auxiliary Facilities (eg; play area, hospital kitchen)

The general pediatric care facility will function in close coordination with specialized units of Newborn care facilities, NRC and DEIC.

## ADOLESCENT HEALTH

The priority interventions in adolescent healthcare are:

### (1) Iron and Folic Acid Supplementation

Under the **National Iron Plus Initiative**, the *Weekly Iron and Folic Acid Supplementation (WIFS) scheme* has been launched to address nutritional anemia among adolescent girls and boys in both rural and urban areas. ***Both the programs are further explained in detail under the heading Nutrition related programs in this chapter.***

### (2) Nutrition Program for Adolescent Girls

It aims to address nutritional needs of adolescent girls. Under this scheme, 6 kg of ration is to be given to under nourished adolescent girls, as per their weight through the public distribution system free of cost to the families identified in this scheme. The scheme targets girl children between 11 and 19 years who are less than 35 kg.

### (3) Adolescent Reproductive and Sexual Health Program

Adolescent Friendly Health Clinics (AFHC) provides clinical and counseling services to adolescents on fixed days, through existing health system. Counseling for adolescents on puberty, RTI/STI prevention, contraception, abortion, sexual abuse, mental health problems, nutrition, substance abuse, etc., are done by dedicated trained counselors, at fixed facilities on fixed day and fixed time. Outreach activities including counseling services are conducted in schools, colleges and vocational training centers, during village health and nutrition days.

### (4) Menstrual Hygiene Scheme

The activities under the scheme are:
- Community-based health education to promote menstrual health
- Ensure regular and uninterrupted supply of good quality sanitary napkins to adolescent girls
- Sourcing, procurement, storage and distribution of sanitary napkins to adolescent girls
- Training of ASHAs and teachers in menstrual health; and
- Providing safe disposal mechanisms for sanitary napkins. Sanitary napkins are provided under NHM's brand "Freedays," available at a cost of ₹ 1 for BPL and ₹ 6 for APL girls, for a pack of six napkins.

### (5) Rashtriya Kishor Swasthya Karyakram (RKSK)

The Rashtriya Kishor Swasthya Karyakram was launched on 7th January, 2014 for adolescents in the age group 10–19 years. The key principle of this program is adolescent participation and leadership, equity and inclusion, gender equity and strategic partnerships with other sectors and stakeholders. The program envisions enabling all adolescents in India to realize their full potential by making informed and responsible decisions related to their health and well-being and by accessing the services and support they need to do so.

*Objectives*

| Improve nutrition: | Improve sexual and reproductive health: |
|---|---|
| • By reducing malnutrition<br>• By reducing iron deficiency anemia | • Reduce teenage pregnancies<br>• Provide early parenting support for adolescent parents |
| **Enhance mental health:** Address the psychological needs of adolescents | **Prevent injuries and violence:** Promote positive attitude among adolescents for the prevention of injuries and violence |
| **Prevent substance misuse:** Increase awareness on the ill effects of substance misuse | **Address NCDs:** Promote healthy lifestyle at a younger age in order to prevent NCDs, i.e. hypertension, stroke, cardiovascular diseases, and diabetes |

## Strategies

- **Strategies/interventions to achieve objectives can be broadly grouped as:**
  - Community based interventions
  - Peer Education (PE)
  - Quarterly Adolescent Health Day (AHD)
  - Weekly Iron and Folic Acid Supplementation Programme (WIFS)
  - Menstrual Hygiene Scheme (MHS)
- **Facility based interventions**
  - Strengthening of Adolescent Friendly Health Clinics (AFHC)
- **Convergence**
  - **Within Health and Family Welfare**—FP, MH (incl VHND), RBSK, NACP, National Tobacco Control Programme, National Mental Health Programme, NCDs and IEC
  - **With other departments/schemes**—WCD (ICDS, KSY, BSY, SABLA), Youth Affairs and Sports
- **Social and Behavior Change Communication with focus on Inter Personal Communication**

### (6) School Health Program

The school health program was launched to address the health needs of school going children and adolescents in the 6–18-year-age groups in the Government and aided schools.

The program entails biannual health screening of students for early management of disease, disability, and common deficiency and linkages with secondary and tertiary health facilities as required **(Fig. 47.10)**.

### (7) School Health and Wellness Programme

As a part of the Health and Wellness component of the Ayushman Bharat Programme, School Health and Wellness Programme (launched in Feb 2020) is being implemented in government and government aided schools in districts (including aspirational districts). Two teachers in every school designated as "Health and Wellness Ambassadors", will be trained to transact health promotion and disease prevention information in the form of interesting activities for one hour every week. 24 hour sessions will be delivered through weekly structured interactive classroom based activities.

### Monitoring

Monitoring of RMNCAH+N program is done through:

- HMIS-based Dashboard Monitoring System for Various MCH Indicators; and
- Web-enabled Mother and Child Tracking System (MCTS)
- Maternal Death Review,
- Child Death Review,
- Joint Review Mission,
- National Surveys Including SRS, NFHS and DLHS, and
- Survey-based Score Card using Data Available from National Health Surveys.

## SUGGESTED READING

1. Guideline for management of Severe Acute Malnutrition Children at Nutritional Rehabilitation Centre. National Rural Health Mission, 2012. Ministry of health and Family welfare. GOI.
2. Indian Newborn Action Plan. Ministry of Health and Family Welfare. September 2014. Available from: https://www.newbornwhocc.org/INAP_Final.pdf
3. International Institute of population science and macro international. National Family Health Survey 4, 2015–2016: India fact sheet. Mumbai: IIPS; 2017.
4. MoHFW. Annual report (1999–2000). Ministry of Health and Family Welfare, Government of India, New Delhi.
5. MoHFW. Annual Report (2003–04). Ministry of Health and Family Welfare, Government of India, New Delhi.
6. MoHFW. Annual Report (2005–06). Ministry of Health and Family Welfare, Government of India, New Delhi.
7. MoHFW. Annual Report (2014–15). Ministry of Health and Family Welfare, Government of India, New Delhi.
8. MoHFW. Annual Report (2016–17). Ministry of Health and Family Welfare, Government of India, New Delhi.
9. MoHFW. A Strategic Approach to Reproductive, Maternal, Newborn, Child and Adolescent Health (RMNCH+A) in India, February 2013. Ministry of Health and Family Welfare, Government of India, New Delhi.
10. MoHFW. Facility Based Newborn Care Operational Guide, Guidelines for Planning and Implementation, 2006. Ministry of Health and Family Welfare, Government of India, New Delhi.
11. MoHFW. Intensified Mission Indradhanush Operational Guidelines. National Health Mission, Ministry of Health and Family Welfare, Government of India, New Delhi.
12. MoHFW. Operational Guidelines Rashtriya Bal Swasthya Karyakram (RBSK), Child Health Screening and Early Intervention Service under NRHM 2013. Ministry of Health and Family Welfare, Government of India, New Delhi.
13. MoHFW. Student's Handbook, Integrated Management of Neonatal and Childhood Illness, 2003. Ministry of Health and Family Welfare, Government of India, New Delhi.

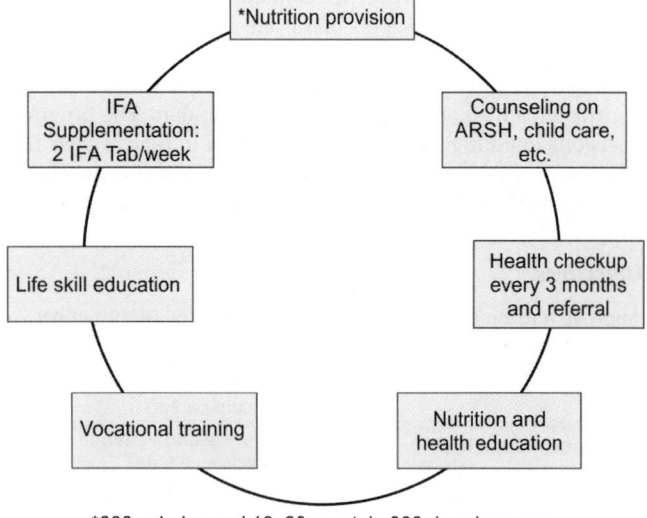

*600 calories and 18–20g protein 300 days in a year

**Fig. 47.10:** Components of School Health Program.

# PROGRAMS FOR COMMUNICABLE DISEASES

The programs for prevention and control of major communicable and NCDs are covered under the umbrella of NHM.

## NATIONAL VECTOR-BORNE DISEASE CONTROL PROGRAM

National Malaria Control Program was launched in 1953 which was merged with the ongoing programs against filariasis and kala-azar in 2003–04 to form the National Vector Borne Disease Control Program (NVBDCP) along with dengue, chikungunya, and JE.

Since 2005, NVBDCP has been a part of NHM and presently the program aims to control these six major vector-borne diseases.

The Directorate of NVBDCP, which is the nodal agency for the planning, implementation and monitoring of the program, is under the Directorate General of Health Services, Ministry of Health and Family Welfare, Government of India.

*Strategies for prevention and control of vector-borne diseases under NVBDCP:*

- Disease management including early case detection with active, passive and sentinel surveillance and complete effective treatment, strengthening of referral services, epidemic preparedness, and rapid response.
- Integrated vector management including indoor residual spraying (IRS) in selected high-risk areas, long-lasting insecticidal nets (LLINs), use of larvivorous fish, antilarval measures in urban areas including biolarvicides and minor environmental engineering including source reduction.
- Supportive interventions that include, behavior change communication (BCC), intersectoral convergence, human resource development, Public Private Partnership (PPP), operational research, monitoring, and evaluation.
- Vaccination, only against JE.
- Annual mass drugs administration, only against lymphatic filariasis.

## MALARIA

### National Framework for Malaria Elimination in India (2016–2030)

It was launched in February 2016 with a vision to eliminate malaria nationally and contribute to improved health, quality of life, and alleviation of poverty.

### Goals

- Eliminate malaria (zero indigenous cases) throughout the entire country by 2030
- Maintain malaria-free status in areas where malaria transmission has been interrupted and prevent reintroduction of malaria

### Objectives

The framework has four objectives:
1. Eliminate malaria from all 26 low (Category 1) and moderate (Category 2) transmission states/union territories (UTs) by 2022.

**Table 47.7:** Classification of states/union territories (UTs) for malaria elimination in India (2014).

| Category | Definition |
|---|---|
| Category 0: Prevention of re-establishment phase | States/UTs with zero indigenous cases of malaria (currently no state/UT) |
| Category 1: Elimination phase | States/UTs with API<1, and all their districts reporting API<1 (15 states/UTs) |
| Category 2: Pre-elimination phase | States/UTs with API<1, but some of their districts reporting API>1 (11 states) |
| Category 3: Intensified control phase | States/UTs with API>1 (10 states/UTs) |

(API: Annual Parasite Incidence)

2. Reduce the incidence of malaria to less than 1 case per 1,000 population per year in all states and UTs and their districts by 2024.
3. Interrupt indigenous transmission of malaria throughout the entire country, including all high transmission states and union territories (UTs) (Category 3) by 2027.
4. Prevent the re-establishment of local transmission of malaria in areas where it has been eliminated and maintain national malaria-free status by 2030 and beyond **(Table 47.7)**.

### Strategies

The strategies of the malaria elimination framework are broadly as following:
- Early diagnosis and radical treatment
- Case-based surveillance and rapid response
- Integrated vector management (IVM)
  - Indoor residual spray (IRS)
  - LLINs/Insecticide treated bed nets (ITNs)
  - Larval source management (LSM)
- Epidemic preparedness and early response
- Monitoring and evaluation
- Advocacy, coordination and partnership
- Behavior change communication and community mobilization
- Program planning and management.

### The Specific Objectives and Key Interventions Recommended for Each Category are Detailed here

#### Category 3 (intensified control phase)

| Specific objectives | Key interventions |
|---|---|
| - Achieve universal coverage with malaria preventive and curative services<br>- Establish an efficient system to reduce ongoing transmission of malaria | - Massive scaling up of existing disease management and preventive approaches and tools, aimed at a significant reduction in the prevalence and incidence of malaria as well as associated deaths |

*Contd...*

*Contd...*

| Specific objectives | Key interventions |
|---|---|
| • Reduce malaria specific morbidity and mortality<br>• Contain and prevent possible outbreaks of malaria, particularly among non-immune high risk mobile and migrant population groups<br>• Emphasize reducing malaria morbidity and mortality in high transmission pockets such as tribal, hilly, forested and conflict affected areas | • Screening of all fever cases suspected for malaria<br>• Classification of areas as per local malaria epidemiology and grading of areas as per risk of malaria transmission followed by implementation of tailored interventions<br>• Strengthening of intersectoral collaboration<br>• Special interventions for high-risk groups such as tribal populations and populations residing in conflict affected or hard-to-reach areas<br>• One-stop centers or mobile clinics on fixed days in tribal or conflict affected areas to provide malaria diagnosis and treatment, and increasing community awareness with the involvement of other agencies and service providers as required<br>• Timely referral and treatment of severe malaria cases to reduce malaria-related mortality<br>• Strengthening all district and subdistrict hospitals in malaria endemic areas as per Indian Public Health Standards with facilities for management of severe malaria cases<br>• Establishment of a robust supply chain management system<br>• Maintenance of an optimum level of surveillance using appropriate diagnostic measures<br>• Equipping all health institutions (primary healthcare level and above), especially in high-risk areas, with microscopy facilities and rapid diagnostic tests (RDTs) for emergency use and injectable artemisinin derivatives for treatment of severe malaria |

### Category 2 (Pre-elimination phase)

The states/UTs in pre-elimination phase are those close to entering the elimination phase.

Therefore, malaria elimination interventions will be introduced with particular focus on setting up an elimination surveillance system and initiating elimination phase activities in those districts where the annual parasite incidence (API) has been reduced to less than 1 case per 1,000 population at risk per year. The planning of elimination measures will be based on epidemiological investigation and classification of each malaria case and focus.

### Category 1 (Elimination phase)

| Specific objective | Key interventions |
|---|---|
| • Interrupt transmission of malaria<br>• Immediately notify each detected case | • In elimination areas, where transmission is focal and incidence/risk has become extremely low, all efforts will be directed at interrupting local transmission in all active foci of malaria |

*Contd...*

*Contd...*

| Specific objective | Key interventions |
|---|---|
| • Detect any possible continuation of malaria transmission<br>• Determine the underlying causes of residual transmission<br>• Forecast and prevent any unusual situations related to malaria, ensure epidemic preparedness and respond in a timely and efficient manner to outbreak situations<br>• Prevent re-establishment of local transmission of malaria<br>• Ascertain elimination of malaria | • Mandatory notification of each case of malaria from the private sector, other organized government sectors or any other health facility<br>• Adequate case-based surveillance and complete case management established and fully functional across the entire country to handle each case of malaria<br>• Investigation and classification of all foci of malaria<br>• A strict total coverage of all active foci by effective vector control measures<br>• Early detection and treatment of all cases of malaria by means of active and/or passive case detection to prevent onward transmission<br>• State and national level malaria elimination database established and operational<br>• Implementation of interventions for effective screening, management and prevention of malaria among mobile and migrant populations<br>• Establishment of an effective epidemic forecasting and response system<br>• Ensuring rigorous quality assurance of all medicines and diagnostics<br>• Setting up a national-level reference laboratory which will serve the following two functions.<br>  1. All positive and a fixed percentage of negative slides will be referred to this laboratory for confirmation of diagnosis and cross-checking. After elimination has been achieved in each state/UT, 100% of cases will be notified to this laboratory for confirmation of diagnosis. The laboratory will be notified immediately on all positive cases of malaria by each state/UT through either SMS, e-mail or telephone with information on name, gender, address (village and district), date and type of testing and type of parasite for each positive case of malaria so that a national level database can be maintained.<br>  2. Training of master trainers and accreditation/certification of microscopists as per Indian Public Health Standards shall also be undertaken at this laboratory.<br>• During investigation of foci, all suspected cases of malaria are to be screened for malaria. These could include household members, neighbors, schoolchildren, workplace colleagues and relatives<br>• Surveillance of special groups, migrant populations or populations residing in the vicinity of industrial areas is also to be covered under surveillance operations. |

### Category 0 (Prevention of re-establishment phase)

The probability of malaria becoming re-established in a malaria free area varies with the level of receptivity and vulnerability of the area. If either of these factors is zero, the probability of malaria becoming re-established is zero even if the other factor has a high value. When importation of malaria due to the arrival of migrants from a malaria area coincides with increase in receptivity because of halted vector control measures or socioeconomic development of an area, for example, re- establishment of malaria transmission is possible. In the absence of appropriate action, the area is likely to become malarious again and the duration is determined by the level of receptivity and vulnerability.

When any area, whether a state/UT or a district within a state/UT, has achieved malaria elimination, the specific objectives will be as follows:
- Detect any re-introduced case of malaria;
- Notify immediately all detected cases of malaria;
- Determine the underlying causes of resumed local transmission;
- Apply rapid curative and preventive measures;
- Prevent reintroduction and possible re-establishment of malaria transmission; and
- Maintain malaria-free status in these areas.

## National Strategic Plan for Malaria Elimination (2017–2022)

### Vision
It focuses on strategic policies to provide universal intervention package, paving the way for malaria elimination by 2030.

### Goal
- Eliminate malaria (zero indigenous cases) by 2022 in all the districts of 22 states/UTs of existing category 1 and 2, and in districts having API less than 1 of category 3 states.
- All remaining districts (having API >2), to be brought into elimination and pre-elimination phase.
- Maintain malaria free status in areas where malaria transmission has been interrupted and prevent reintroduction of malaria by strengthening surveillance.

### Objectives
- Achieve universal coverage of case detection and treatment services in endemic districts, to ensure 100% parasitological diagnosis of all malaria cases and complete treatment of all confirmed cases.
- Strengthen surveillance to detect, notify, investigate, classify and respond to all cases.
- Near universal coverage of population at risk by vector control intervention.
- Near universal coverage of population at risk by appropriate BCC activities.
- Effective program management and coordination at all levels to deliver a combination of targeted interventions for malaria elimination.

### Strategies
- ***Surveillance, diagnosis and case management:*** Surveillance of malaria is done by active case detection (ACD) where blood smears are collected by MPWs during fortnightly house visits and by passive case detection (PCD) where fever cases reporting to peripheral health volunteers/ASHA, subcenters and PHCs are diagnosed by rapid diagnostic tests (RDTs) and examination of blood smears.
  Case management is done according to the national malaria drug policy guidelines: *(These is already discussed in Chapter 17E: Epidemiology of Vector-borne Diseases and its Prevention and Control.)*
- ***Strengthening of referral services:*** Referral of severe malaria cases to the nearest health facility requires transport facilities. Transport available under NHM will be used, and if not available, it will be provided by the program.
- ***Epidemic preparedness and rapid response:*** An outbreak is confirmed if there is doubling of slide positivity rate as compared to the same period of previous year, if there is increasing trend of malaria incidence compared to the corresponding months of the previous year or if there is increasing vector density and positive findings of other supportive factors. On confirmation of outbreak, rapid response team (RRT) is constituted which conducts urgent epidemiological investigation. Confirmed and suspected cases of malaria are treated, and antivector and antiparasitic measures are undertaken. Close surveillance of the affected area is continued for 1 month after the outbreak has been contained.
- ***Integrated vector management:*** This is done by anti-larval methods (chemical larvicides, LSM and biological control using larvivorous fish), anti-adult measures (chemical insecticides used for indoor residual spray/space spray and genetic control measures) and personal protective measures (use of mosquito repellants, insecticide treated bed nets/long-lasting insecticidal nets and protective clothing). Effective epidemiological surveillance for entomological parameters such as vector density, seasonal prevalence, susceptibility status to insecticides, feeding behavior, quality of indoor residual spray, and effectiveness of insecticides is required to complement vector control activities. Civic by-laws to prevent mosquitogenic conditions are in place in a few states.
- ***Supportive interventions:*** These include behavior change communication, PPP and intersectoral convergence, human resource development through capacity building, operational research including studies on drug resistance and insecticide susceptibility, monitoring and evaluation of the program through periodic reviews/field visits and web-based management information system. The Swachh Bharat and Digital India missions have helped in creating an enabling environment for malaria elimination. A robust logistics management information system including procurement of drugs and equipment, and supply chain monitoring is required to ensure uninterrupted availability of commodities essential to run the program.

## Urban Vector-borne Disease Scheme 2016

Urban malaria is on the rise because of increase in urban population due to migration, unplanned growth of towns and cities, unhygienic water storage practices due to water shortage, unrestricted land use, development project activities along with inadequate trained manpower to carry out vector control activities.

This scheme is implemented in urban areas with API ≥2 where population is at least 40,000. The local administrative bodies run

the scheme under supervision of the state health authority. The control strategies under this scheme are:
- Source reduction
- Antilarval measures
- Aerosol space spray
- Early diagnosis and complete treatment
- Legislative measures.

### Funding

The Government of India provides technical assistance and logistics support. State governments bear the operational costs and ensure implementation of the program. North-Eastern states are provided 100% central assistance for program implementation that includes operational cost. Organizational structure is shown in **Figure 47.11**.

## FILARIASIS

National Health Policy envisages to achieve and maintain elimination status of lymphatic filariasis in endemic pockets by 2017. Global target for elimination of filariasis is by 2020. Elimination of lymphatic filariasis (LF) is defined as cessation of lymphatic filariasis as a public health problem when the number of microfilaria carriers in the community is less than 1% and children born after initiation of elimination of lymphatic filariasis are free from circulating antigenemia, i.e., presence of adult filarial worm in human body.

### Elimination of Lymphatic Filariasis Program

#### Objectives

- To reduce and eliminate transmission of lymphatic filariasis by Mass Drug Administration of DEC in endemic areas.
- To reduce and prevent morbidity in affected persons.
- To strengthen the existing health care services.

### Strategies for Elimination of Lymphatic Filariasis

- Twin Pillar Strategy for Elimination of Lymphatic Filariasis:
  1. ***Single day mass drug administration annually with DEC and albendazole:*** Annual Mass Drug Administration (MDA) with diethylcarbamazine citrate (6 mg/kg body weight) and albendazole, to all eligible population in endemic areas is done to interrupt transmission of the disease, for a minimum of 5 years or more aiming at minimum 85% actual drug compliance. MDA is not given to pregnant women, children below 2 years of age, and seriously-ill persons. Single day supervised drug administration by door-to-door visit, supplemented with drug administration at booths and groups, followed by two-day mopping up is recommended.
  2. ***Morbidity management:*** Filariasis damages lymphatic vessels causing lymphedema which is managed by washing, elevation of affected limb, exercise, use of proper footwear and surgery. Acute attacks are managed by antibiotics. Scaling up of hydrocele operations in identified CHCs/district hospitals/medical colleges is also done.
- ***Transmission Assessment Survey (TAS):*** The World Health Organization (WHO) guidelines 2011 recommend conducting TAS in every implementation unit after minimum of five effective rounds of MDA with more than 65% coverage and microfilaria rate less than 1% in each of the sentinel and random sites, in the last round of microfilaria survey. TAS is done after a minimum of 6 months after the last MDA using immunochromatographic test (ICT) card with finger-tip blood in the field.
- ***Vector control measures:*** Even though breeding sites of culex mosquitoes are difficult to control, antilarval measures including source reduction, use of larvivorous fish and personal protective measures is encouraged.
- ***Behavior change communication:*** It focuses on vector control, compliance to MDA and home-based management of morbidity in lymphedema patients.

Organizational structure is shown in **Figure 47.12**.

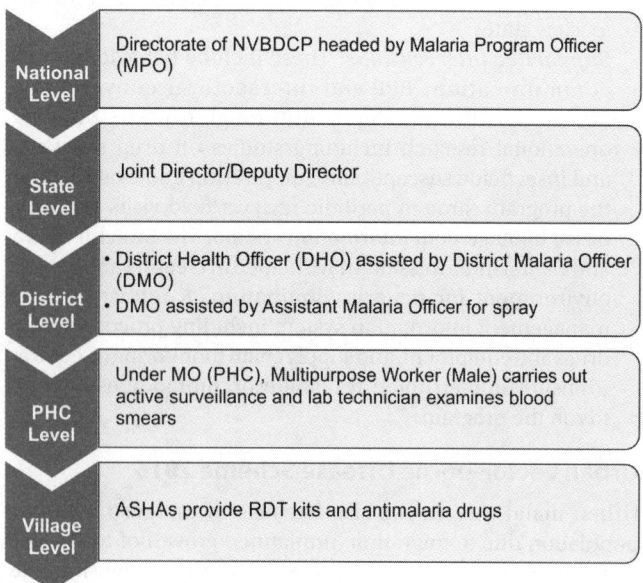

**Fig. 47.11:** Organization of NVBDCP (Malaria).
(ASHA: accredited social health activist; NVBDCP: national vector borne disease control program; RDT: rapid diagnostic tests)

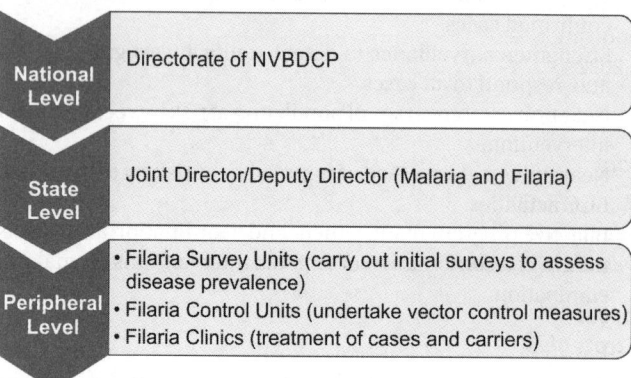

**Fig. 47.12:** Organization of NVBDCP (filaria).
(NVBDCP: national vector borne disease control program).

## Newer Initiatives

### Triple-Drug Therapy

In 2017, following successful drug trials, World Health Organization endorsed a *new Triple-Drug Therapy* to fight LF using I*vermectin with DEC and albendazole (IDA).* In June 2018, India made new commitments to accelerate their program to eliminate LF and initiated the new IDA protocol in five districts in the country. Initially in 2018 only in 5 districts the IDA therapy was implemented. Later in 2019, 11 more districts of Uttar Pradesh were added and as of 2020, it has been implemented in 21 districts of 6 states.

### DEC-fortified Salt

It appears to be the most viable and proven solution to reduce the transmission and thus eliminate filaria. As per the DEC-fortified salt strategy, a low dose of DEC (0.1–0.4% w/w) is added to the regular cooking salt consumed by the endemic communities for 12–24 months. DEC-fortified salt strategy is a simple, inexpensive, prompt and efficient way to eliminate LF. The strategy can be run on the existing countrywide deployment of iodized salt under the National Iodine Deficiency Disorders Control Programme.

## KALA-AZAR

Concerned with the increasing incidences of Kala-azar in the country, the GoI launched a Centrally Sponsored Kala-azar Control Programme in the endemic states in 1990–91. The National Health Policy (2002) set the goal of Kala-azar elimination in India by the year 2010 and later revised in 12th Five Year Plan document to 2015 and then to 2017.

India has been making consistent strides in its fight for the elimination kala-azar by 2023, from interventions like pucca houses through Pradhan Mantri Awas Yojana (PMAY), rural electrification, timely testing, treatment, periodic high-level review, to incentivizing through award distribution for states/districts/blocks, government along with its stakeholders are ensuring a robust ecosystem for early detection of the disease and its timely treatment. India has now confined the disease to only four districts in Bihar and Jharkhand with currently reporting a 98.7% decline in cases from 44,533 in 2007 to 834 in 2022.

### National Kala-azar Elimination Program

#### Goal

To improve the health status of vulnerable groups and at-risk population living in kala-azar endemic areas, by the elimination of kala-azar so that it no longer remains a public health problem.

#### Target

To reduce the annual incidence of kala-azar to less than 1 per 10,000 population at block PHC level.

#### Objectives

- Reducing the incidence of kala-azar in the endemic communities including the poor, vulnerable, and hard to reach population.
- Reducing case fatality rate due to kala-azar.
- Treatment of post-kala-azar dermal leishmaniasis (PKDL) to reduce the parasite reservoir.
- Prevention and treatment of kala-azar and HIV, TB coinfections.

### Strategies for Elimination

- *Early diagnosis and complete treatment:* Kala-azar is diagnosed using rapid diagnostic kits at PHC and district hospital level. Parasitological diagnosis includes spleen, bone marrow and lymph node aspiration procedures. PKDL is diagnosed using slit skin biopsy.

  **Case definition**
  **Visceral leishmaniasis (VL)/Kala-azar (KA)**
  - *A "suspect" case:* History of fever of more than 2 weeks and enlarged spleen and liver, not responding to anti-malarial and antibiotic treatment, in a patient from an endemic area.
  - Or a patient with above symptoms clinically examined by doctor and found positive on screening with rapid diagnostic test.
  - Or in cases with past history of kala-azar or in those with high suspicion of kala-azar but with negative RDT test result but found positive by examination of bone marrow/spleen aspirate for LD bodies at appropriate level (district hospital).

  **Post-kala-azar dermal leishmaniasis**
  - *Probable PKDL:* A patient from a KA-endemic area with multiple hypopigmented macules, papules, plaques or nodules, who are RDT positive.
  - *Confirmed PKDL:* A patient from a KA-endemic area with multiple hypopigmented macules, papules, plaques or nodules, who is parasite positive in slit-skin smear (SSS) or biopsy.

  Treatment for visceral leishmaniasis under the program is with single day single dose of 10 mg/kg body weight of intravenous liposomal amphotericin B (LAMB). Alternatively, miltefosine capsules of 10 mg (children) or 50 mg (adults) can be given for 28 days to patients 2–65 years of age. Other treatment options are IV amphotericin B deoxycholate @ 1 mg/kg body weight on alternate days for 15 doses, and combination of paromomycin injection intramuscular and miltefosine at a dose of 11 mg/kg body weight for 10 days, together with miltefosine for 10 days. For PKDL, drug of choice is miltefosine 100 mg orally per day for 12 weeks, others being amphotericin B deoxycholate and LAMB.

- *Integrated vector management including indoor residual spraying:* IRS up to a height of 6 feet with 50% dichlorodiphenyltrichloroethane (DDT) at a dose of 1g/$m^2$ of wall surface, is done twice a year, including complete coverage of cattle sheds in kala-azar endemic areas, to limit sand fly population. Recently DDT was replaced with synthetic pyrethroid (SP) in districts reporting DDT resistance.

- *Surveillance:* Kala-azar surveillance is through passive case reporting and quarterly active case search. VL and PKDL cases are reported to the center since kala-azar has been declared a notifiable disease in West Bengal and Bihar. Vector surveillance is also carried out.

- **Capacity building:** Capacity building is done in the form of induction training, on the job training, along with reorientation training of program staff, done regularly.
- **Supervision, monitoring and evaluation of program and program management:** Monitoring indicators used are detection rate, treatment completion rate, coverage rate of vector control, final cure rate, treatment failure rate, loss to follow-up rate, etc.

## JAPANESE ENCEPHALITIS

Japanese encephalitis presents as acute encephalitis and is classified under a group of encephalitic conditions known as acute encephalitis syndrome (AES).

### National Program for Prevention and Control of JE/AES

#### Goal

To reduce morbidity, mortality, and disability in children due to JE/AES.

#### Objectives

- To strengthen and expand JE vaccination in affected districts.
- To strengthen surveillance, vector control, case management and timely referral of serious and complicated cases.
- To increase access to safe drinking water and proper sanitation facilities to the target population in affected rural and urban areas.
- To estimate disability burden due to JE/AES, and to provide for adequate facilities for physical, medical, neurological and social rehabilitation.
- To improve nutritional status of children at risk of JE/AES.
- To carry out intensified IEC/BCC activities regarding JE/AES.

#### Strategies

The program aims at prevention and control, as there is no specific cure for the disease, through vaccination along with public health measures for prevention of the disease, case identification and symptomatic and early case management, to minimize risk of death and complications.

- **Vaccination against JE:** JE vaccination was started with a campaign in 2006, to vaccinate all children 1–15 years of age with single dose of live attenuated SA-14-14-2 vaccine. Currently JE vaccine is given under UIP in endemic states. Two doses of JE vaccine, at 9 months, and at 16–24 months have been included under RI since 2013.
- **JE/AES surveillance:** It includes epidemiological surveillance for AES, entomological surveillance, and veterinary based surveillance to monitor all factors influencing the transmission and effective control of the disease, and to detect early warning signals of impending outbreaks.
  
  **Case definition**
  
  **Suspect case**
  - Acute onset of fever, not more than 5–7 days duration
  - Change in mental status with/without
    - New onset of seizures, excluding febrile seizures
  - Other early clinical findings, which may include irritability, somnolence or abnormal behavior, greater than that seen with usual febrile illness.
  
  **Probable case**
  - Suspected case in close geographic and temporal relationship to a laboratory confirmed case of AES/JE in an outbreak.
  - AES due to other agent—a suspected case in which diagnostic testing is performed and an etiological agent other than AES/JE is identified.
  - AES due to unknown agent—a suspected case in which no diagnostic testing is performed/no etiological agent is identified/test results are indeterminate.
  
  **Laboratory confirmed case**
  - Presence of immunoglobulin G (IgM) antibody in serum and/or cerebrospinal fluid (CSF)
  - Four fold difference in immunoglobulin G (IgG) antibody titer in paired sera
  - Virus isolation from brain tissue
  - Antigen detection by immunofluorescence/polymerase chain reaction (PCR).
- **Case management:** Management of JE/AES is done in PHC/district hospital. Complicated cases are referred to nearest higher center for further management. The steps for management of JE/AES are:
  - Management of airways and breathing
  - Management of circulation
  - Control of convulsion and intracranial pressure
  - Control of temperature
  - Fluid, electrolytes and calories/nutrition
  - General management
  - Specific treatment of any treatable cause
  - Investigations, sample collection and transportation
  - Reporting of a case
  - Rehabilitation
- **Vector control:** Because of the exophilous habit of culex mosquitoes, vector control is aimed at outdoor space spray with ultra-low volume fogging, along with use of repellants and protective clothing especially for outdoor workers is recommended.
- **Information, education and communication:** IEC activities focus on keeping pigs away from human dwellings since it is a reservoir host for JE, using bed nets and protective clothing, awareness regarding signs and symptoms of the disease, and encouraging early reporting of cases to health facilities.

## DENGUE AND CHIKUNGUNYA FEVER

Both dengue and chikungunya fever are transmitted by *Aedes* mosquito and hence both the diseases are more prevalent in the postmonsoon period, when vector breeding is most likely to occur. NVBDCP mandates the same prevention and control strategies for both the febrile illnesses.

### Long-term Strategies for Prevention and Control

#### Early Case Reporting and Management

Detection of outbreak is done through fever alert surveillance where health workers at all levels including grass-root level are trained to report cases of fever directly to the District VBDC Officer. This is supplemented by a call center under Integrated Disease Surveillance Project (IDSP) to report outbreaks. Sentinel surveillance sites with laboratory support have been set up all over the country in public health facilities as well as private clinics/nursing homes.

## Case Definition

### Dengue

**Probable DF/DHF:** A case compatible with clinical description of dengue fever during outbreak OR non-ELISA based NS1 antigen/IgM positive.

**Clinical description:** Acute febrile illness of 2–7 days duration, with 2 or more of the following manifestations: Headache, retro-orbital pain, myalgia, arthralgia, rash, and hemorrhagic manifestations.

**Confirmed dengue fever:** A case compatible with clinical description of dengue fever with at least one of the following:
- Isolation of the dengue virus (virus culture positive) from serum, plasma, leukocytes
- Demonstration of IgM antibody titer by ELISA positive in single serum sample
- Demonstration of dengue virus antigen in serum sample by NS1-ELISA
- IgG seroconversion in paired sera after 2 weeks with four-fold increase of IgG titer
- Detection of viral nucleic acid by PCR.

### Chikungunya
- **Probable or suspected case:** A patient meeting the clinical criteria only
- **Confirmed (definitive) case:** A patient meeting both the clinical and laboratory criteria
- **Clinical criteria:** Acute onset of fever and severe arthralgia/arthritis with or without skin rash and residing or having left an epidemic area 15 days prior to onset of symptoms
- **Laboratory criteria:** At least one of the following tests done in the acute phase of illness:
  - *Direct evidence*: Virus isolation/presence of viral RNA by RT-PCR.
  - *Indirect evidence:*
    - Presence of virus specific IgM antibodies in single serum sample, collected in acute or convalescent stage.
    - Four-fold increase in IgG values in samples collected at least three weeks apart.

Management of dengue and chikungunya cases is supportive and symptomatic. However, cases of dengue should be followed up for hemorrhagic symptoms. Pain management is done for cases of chikungunya fever.

Epidemic preparedness and rapid response plan in case of outbreaks include availability of treatment facilities with beds, equipment and diagnostic materials, drugs, intravenous volume expanders, and whole blood.

## Integrated Vector Management

It includes entomological surveillance along with larval surveys, and vector control. Emergency vector control during outbreaks is done by immediate targeted source reduction program, along with periodic household spraying with pyrethrum and ultra-low volume (ULV) malathion fogging of the entire ward/village.

## Supportive Interventions

It includes capacity building and training of health personnel, behavior change communication for vector control, intersectoral collaboration and partnership between the health and non-health sectors-government, private and NGOs, and legislative support in the form of civic by-laws.

# NATIONAL TUBERCULOSIS ELIMINATION PROGRAM

India has the highest burden of TB in the world and accounts for 24% of TB cases worldwide. The efforts to reduce the prevalence of TB began back in 1951 with the launch of BCG vaccination program in India with the support of WHO and UNICEF (The United Nations International Children's Emergency Fund). After that in 1962, the National Tuberculosis Program (NTP) became operational. However, the treatment success rates remained low and the death rates remained high. Therefore, along with WHO and Swedish International Development Cooperation Agency (SIDA), Government of India reviewed the TB situation in the country and came to following conclusion:
- NTP, though technically sound, suffered from managerial weakness
- Inadequate funding
- Over-reliance on X-ray for diagnosis
- Frequent interrupted supplies of drugs
- Low rates of treatment completion.

In 1993, in order to overcome these lacunae, NTP was revised to Revised National Tuberculosis Control Program (RNTCP).

Revised National Tuberculosis Control Program adopted the DOTS (directly observed treatment, short-course chemotherapy) strategy.

The revised strategy was introduced in the country in a phased manner
- Phase I 1992-2006
- Phase II 2006-2012
- Phase III 2012-2017.

At the start of 2020, the central government renamed the RNTCP as the National Tuberculosis Elimination Program (NTEP). It emphasizes on achieving the sustainable development goal of ending TB by 2025, five years ahead of the global targets.

## GOALS

- To reduce mortality and morbidity from TB.
- To interrupt chain of transmission until TB ceases to be a public health problem in India.

## OBJECTIVES

Revised national tuberculosis control program was launched with the following objectives.
- To cure at least 85% of all newly detected infectious cases of pulmonary TB (new sputum smear-positive).
- To detect at least 70% of estimated new smear positive pulmonary TB cases.

Newer objectives have currently been framed to achieve a TB free India as follows:
- To reduce incidence of TB and mortality due to TB.
- To prevent emergence of drug resistance and effectively manage drug-resistant TB.
- To improve outcomes among HIV-infected TB patients.
- To involve private sector.
- To decentralize and align NTEP management units with NHM block level units within general health system.

## EVOLUTION OF WHO GLOBAL TB STRATEGIES

In 2006, WHO released **stop TB strategy** with six principal components, to realize the global TB-related MDGs by 2015 (**Fig. 47.13**). The targets linked to the MDGs and endorsed by the stop TB partnership were to be achieved by the following timelines:
- *By 2005:* Detect at least 70% of new sputum smear-positive TB cases and cure at least 85% of these cases.
- *By 2015:* Reduce TB prevalence and death rates by 50% relative to 1990.
- *By 2050:* Eliminate TB as a public health problem (1 case per million population).

Many initiatives were under this strategy like developing and piloting National Airborne Infection Control Guidelines and developing and piloting strategy for Practical Approach to Lung Health.

### End TB Strategy

In 2014, the World Health Assembly approved to end global TB epidemic by "End TB Strategy".

### Vision

A world with zero death, disease and suffering due to TB.

### Goal

End the global TB epidemic (**Table 47.8**).

Table 47.8: Indicators, milestones and targets for ending TB.

| Indicators | Milestones | | Targets | |
|---|---|---|---|---|
| | 2020 | 2025 | SDG 2030 | End TB 2035 |
| Reduction in number of TB deaths compared with 2015 (%) | 35% | 75% | 90% | 95% |
| Reduction in TB incidence rate compared with 2015 (%) | 20% <85/100,000 | 50% <55/100,000 | 80% <20/100,000 | 90% <10/100,000 |
| TB-affected families facing catastrophic costs due to TB (%) | Zero | Zero | Zero | Zero |

(SDG: Sustainable Development Goals)

### Principles

- Government stewardship and accountability, with monitoring and evaluation.
- Strong coalition with civil society organizations and communities.
- Protection and promotion of human rights, ethics and equity.
- Adaptation of the strategy and targets at country level, with global collaboration.

### Pillars and Components

See **Figure 47.14**.

## ORGANIZATION OF NTEP

Restructuring of the TB program management system—changes envisaged in the National Surveillance Program (NSP) include the following (**Flowchart 47.4**):
- *National level:* Creation of four divisions each in charge of key programmatic areas, with a commensurate increase in

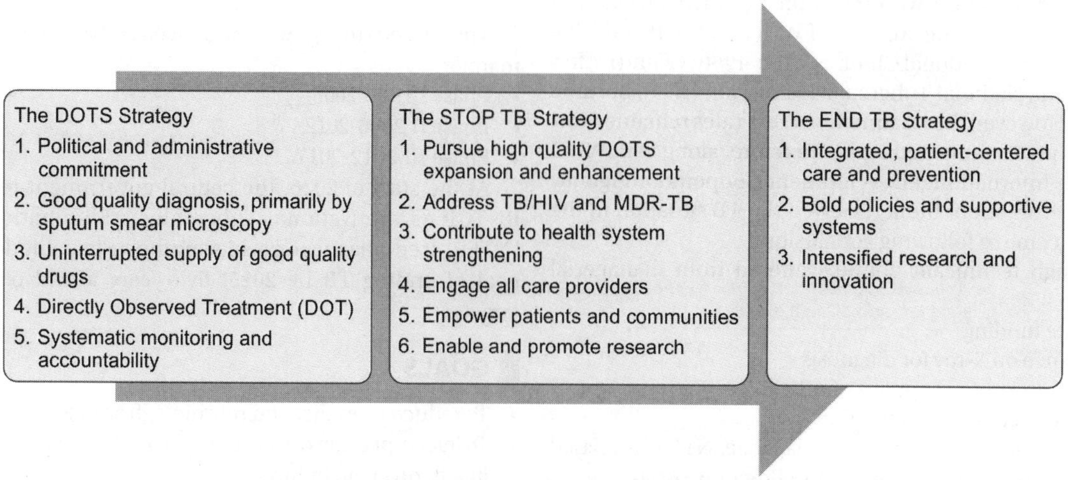

---

**The DOTS Strategy**
1. Political and administrative commitment
2. Good quality diagnosis, primarily by sputum smear microscopy
3. Uninterrupted supply of good quality drugs
4. Directly Observed Treatment (DOT)
5. Systematic monitoring and accountability

**The STOP TB Strategy**
1. Pursue high quality DOTS expansion and enhancement
2. Address TB/HIV and MDR-TB
3. Contribute to health system strengthening
4. Engage all care providers
5. Empower patients and communities
6. Enable and promote research

**The END TB Strategy**
1. Integrated, patient-centered care and prevention
2. Bold policies and supportive systems
3. Intensified research and innovation

Fig. 47.13: World Health Organization (WHO) global TB strategy.

| | |
|---|---|
| **Integrated, patient-centerd care and prevention** | • Early diagnosis of tuberculosis including universal drug-susceptibility testing, and systematic screening of contacts and high-risk groups<br>• Treatment of all people with tuberculosis including drug-resistant tuberculosis, and patient support<br>• Collaborative tuberculosis/HIV activities and management of comorbidities<br>• Preventive treatment of persons at high risk, and vaccination against tuberculosis |
| **Bold policies and supportive systems** | • Political commitment with adequate resources for tuberculosis care and prevention<br>• Engagement of communities, civil society organisations, and public and private care providers<br>• Universal health coverage policy, and regulatory frameworks for case notification, vital registration, quality and rational use of medicines, and infection control<br>• Social protection, poverty alleviation and actions on other determinants of tuberculosis |
| **Intensified research and innovation** | • Discovery, development and rapid uptake of new tools, interventions and strategies<br>• Research to optimise implementation and impact, and promote innovations |

**Fig. 47.14:** Pillars and components.

**Flowchart 47.4:** Organization of NTEP (National TB Elimination Program).

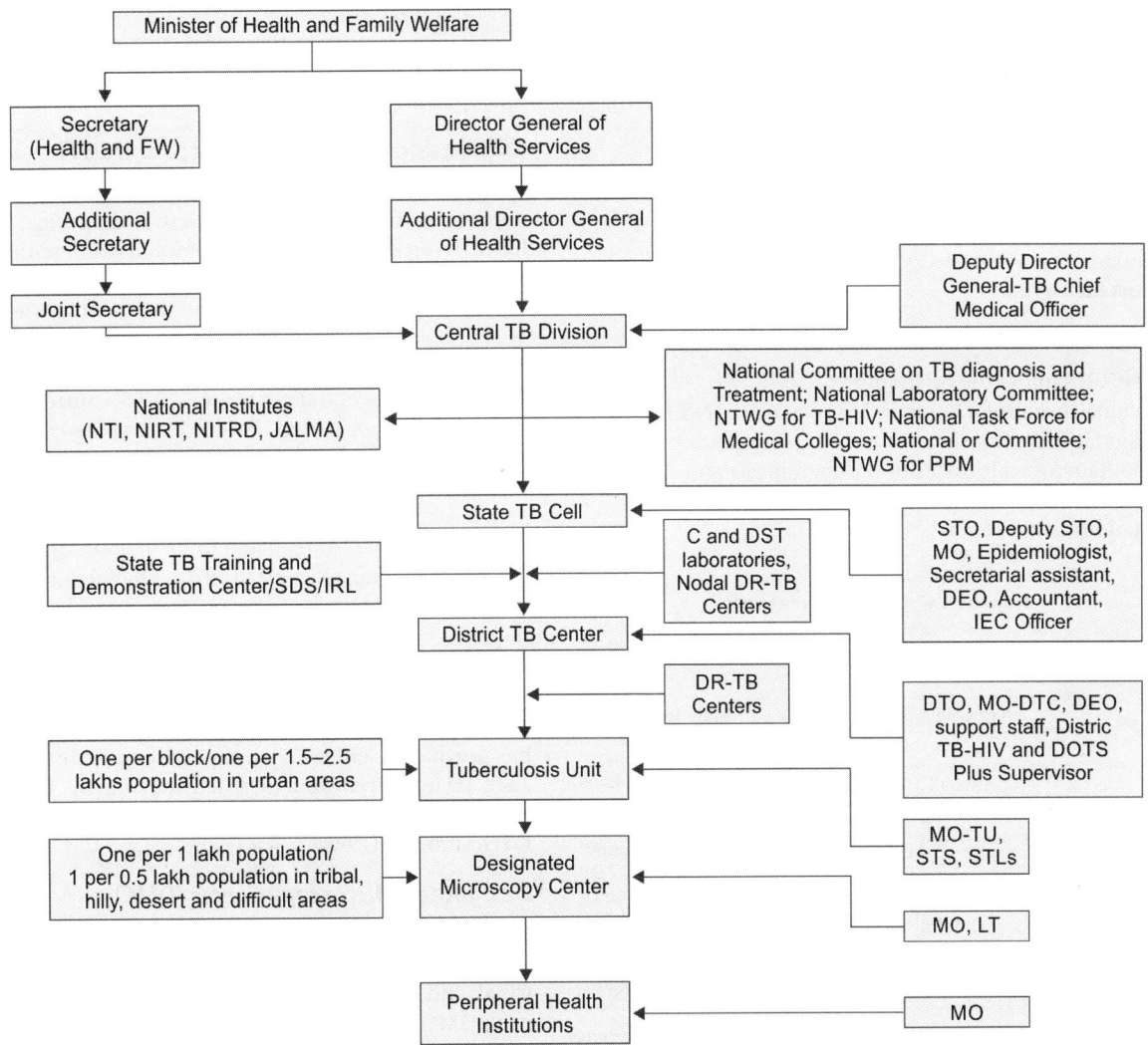

(DR-TB: drug-resistant TB; DST: drug-sensitive testing; DTO: District TB Officer; IRL: intermediate reference laboratory; JALMA: Japanese Leprosy Mission for Asia; LT: laboratory technician; NIRT: National Institute for Research in TB; NITRD: National Institute of TB and Respiratory Disease; NTI: National Tuberculosis Institute; NTWG: National Technical Working Group; SDS: State Drug Store; STLSs: senior TB laboratory supervisors; STO: State TB Officer; STS: senior treatment supervisor; PPM: public private mix; MO: medical officer)

staff strength including technical and operations staff. The key areas will be:
- Surveillance, monitoring and evaluation, research, human resource development
- Partnership, advocacy communication and social mobilization (ACSM), patient support system
- Finance, procurement, supply chain
- Diagnosis, treatment.

- *State level:* Creation of four divisions similar to the structure at the national level.
- *District level:* Unified cadre for supervision to provide one TB supervisor for every block.
- *Block level:* One community volunteer for communicable disease for every 1,000 population to undertake community focused functions like active case finding, treatment support, etc. Program-specific honorarium will be available to these functionaries.

## LABORATORY NETWORK

***Quality assured laboratory services:*** NTEP has established a nationwide laboratory network, with a defined hierarchy for carrying out sputum microscopy with external quality assessment (EQA). The quality assurance activities of NTEP include:
- Internal quality control
- On site evaluation (OSE)
- External quality control
    - Panel testing
    - Random blinded rechecking.

The structure of laboratory network at different levels is shown in **Flowchart 47.5**.

### National Reference Laboratory (NRL)

The six NRLs under the program are:
- National Institute for Research in Tuberculosis (NIRT), Chennai
- National Tuberculosis Institute (NTI), Bengaluru
- Lala Ram Swarup Institute of Tuberculosis and Respiratory Diseases (LRS), Delhi
- JALMA Institute, Agra
- Regional Medical Research Center, Bhubaneswar
- Bhopal Memorial Hospital and Research Center, Bhopal.

NIRT, Chennai, in addition to being one of the NRLs is also one of the WHO designated supranational reference laboratory for the South-East Asia Region. The NRLs work closely with the intermediate reference laboratories (IRLs), monitor and supervise the ILRs activities and also undertake periodic training for the IRL staff in EQA, culture and drug-sensitive testing (DST), line probe assay (LPA), and cartridge-based nucleic acid amplification test (CBNAAT) activities. As per NSP 2017–2025 establishment of two additional NRLs (West and North-East) will be done.

### Intermediate Reference Laboratory

One IRL has been designated in the state TB training and demonstration centers. IRL carries out monitoring and supervision of EQA activities, mycobacterial culture and DST and drug-resistance surveillance (DRS). The IRL conducts on-site evaluation visits to districts for sputum microscopy at least once a year. The IRL undertakes panel testing of senior TB laboratory supervisors (STLS) at each district TB center (DTC). The IRL ensures the proficiency of staff performing NTEP smear microscopy activities by providing training to laboratory technicians and STLS.

### Culture and DST Laboratories (C and DST)

In additional to IRLs, the program also involves the microbiology department of medical colleges for providing diagnostic services for drug-resistance TB, extrapulmonary tuberculosis (EP-TB), and research. The NTEP provides additional human resources, equipments and, training to C and DST laboratories.

### District TB Center

The DTC is the nodal center for all TB control activities of a district. All reports from the subdistricts are consolidated and sent to the next level from DTC. The District TB Officer (DTO) is responsible for all TB activities in the district including EQA activities-mainly Random Blinded Rechecking (RBRC) procedure and maintenance of regular supply of good quality laboratory consumables and reagents to all designated microscopy centers (DMCs) in the district.

### Tuberculosis Unit (TU)

The TB unit is a subdistrict supervisory unit, established for 500,000 population (250,000 in tribal and hilly areas). Program has provided a senior TB lab supervisor, on contractual basis, to each TU for carrying out EQA activities-on-site evaluation visits to DMCs and RBRC of routine DMC slides coordinated by the DTO at the DTC level.

### Designated Microscopy Center (DMC)

The most peripheral laboratory under the NTEP network is the DMC which serves a population of around 100,000 (50,000 in tribal and hilly areas). A binocular microscope is supplied for each DMC and is manned by a trained laboratory technician (LT) of the state health system.

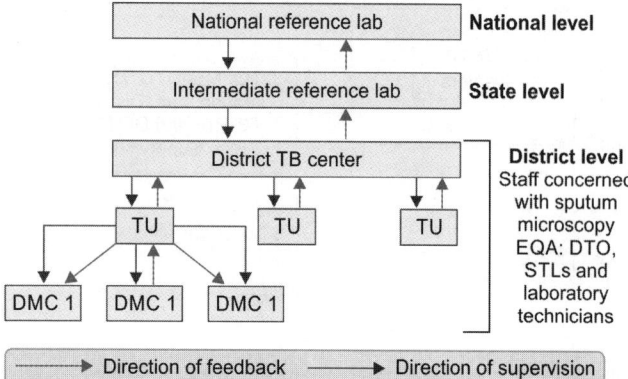

**Flowchart 47.5:** Laboratory network.

(DTO: DTO: District TB Officer; STLs: senior TB laboratory supervisors; EQA: external quality assessment; TU: tuberculosis unit; DMC: designated microscopy centers)

*NTEP endorsed TB diagnostics:*

| Pulmonary and extrapulmonary | Drug-resistance TB (DR-TB) |
|---|---|
| *Smear microscopy (for AFB):* Sputum smear stained with Ziehl-Neelsen staining or fluorescence stains and examined under direct or indirect microscopy with or without LED.<br>*Culture:*<br>• Solid (Lowenstein Jansen) media<br>• Liquid media (Middle Brook) using manual, semiautomatic or automatic machines, e.g., BACTEC, MGIT, etc.<br>*Rapid diagnostic molecular test:*<br>• Conventional PCR-based line probe assay (LPA) for *Mycobacterium tuberculosis* (MTB) complex<br>• Real-time PCR-based nucleic acid amplification test (NAAT) for MTB complex, e.g., GeneXpert or cartridge-based nucleic acid amplification test (CB-NAAT) | • Rapid molecular test (LPA/CB-NAAT)<br>• Liquid culture and DST<br>• Solid culture and DST |

## NATIONAL STRATEGIC PLAN FOR TB ELIMINATION (2017–2025)

### Vision

Tuberculosis-free India with zero deaths, disease and poverty due to TB.

### Goal

To achieve a rapid decline in burden of TB morbidity and mortality while working towards elimination of TB in India by 2025.

### Pillars

There are four pillars of National Strategic Plan "Detect-Treat-Prevent-Build" (DTPB) **(Fig. 47.15)**.

### (A) Detect

This aims at early identification of presumptive TB cases, targeted toward improving laboratory systems and diagnosis, case finding, and catering to patients in the private sector.

*Laboratory systems and diagnosis*

Strategies include using high efficiency diagnostic tools for early and accurate diagnosis linked treatment across the country; strengthening surveillance systems; purchasing services from the private sector, ensure notification through laboratories from the private sector and link to laboratory surveillance; promoting and fostering research in conjunction with the TB Research Consortium for new diagnostic tools; building capacity for diagnosis of latent TB infection (LTBI).

*Case finding*

Strategies include implementation of the revised diagnostic algorithm with expanded definitions of TB symptomatics, using chest X-ray (CXR) as a screening test and subsequent use of rapid molecular test. For early diagnosis of drug resistance, DST will be offered to all diagnosed TB patients. For improvement of early and quality diagnosis focus will be on engagement of the private sector, awareness generation campaigns, use of extrapulmonary TB (EPTB) guidelines, active case finding through screening.

Active case finding (ACF) activity in vulnerable groups will be focused over the next 5 years to reach the vulnerable groups through community and institutional screening activities **(Table 47.9)**.

*Private sector involvement*

Private providers will be involved in case detection by increasing private health provider engagement; providing free diagnostic tests and drugs to TB patients in private sector; increasing support for patients seeking care in private sector; enhancing surveillance and quality improvement; expanding ICT support; building management capacity; strengthening regulatory approaches; involving corporate hospitals.

**Table 47.9:** Vulnerable groups according to priority to be screened for TB.

| Priority | Urban area | Rural area | Tribal area |
|---|---|---|---|
| 1. | Slum | Difficult to reach villages | Difficult to reach villages and hamlets |
| 2. | Prisons inmates | Mine workers | Villages with known higher case load |
| 3. | Old age homes | Stone crusher workers | Tribal school hostels |
| 4. | Construction site workers | Population groups with known high malnutrition | Areas with known high malnutrition |
| 5. | Refugee camps | Populations known to drink raw milk | Villages seeking care from traditional healers |
| 6. | Night shelters | Populations known to eat uncooked meat | Populations known to drink raw milk |
| 7. | NACO/SACS identified HRG for HIV | NACO/SACS identified HRG for HIV | Populations known to eat uncooked meat |
| 8. | Homeless | Weaving and glass industrial workers | Tribal areas with little ventilated huts |
| 9. | Street children | Cotton mill workers | |
| 10. | Orphanages | Unorganized labor | |
| 11. | Homes for destitute | Tea garden workers | |
| 12. | Asylums | Villages largely seeking care from traditional healers | |

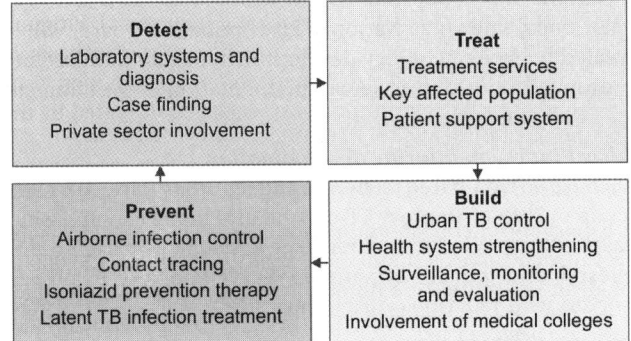

**Fig. 47.15:** Strategic pillars: Detect-Treat-Prevent-Build strategy.

### (B) Treat

The strategies for this are providing treatment services, mapping of key affected population, and developing a patient support system.

#### Treatment services—strategies include

- Initiation of appropriate treatment for all diagnosed TB patients.
  - Provision of daily regimen for all TB patients.
  - Introduction of shorter regimen for MDR TB.
  - Incorporation of new treatment strategies with newer drugs.
  - Effective strategy to ensure standards for TB care in India (STCI) for patients treated by private providers.
- Implementation of TB treatment services in health facilities and communities.
  - Decentralization of treatment services through ICT support.
  - Promote appropriate treatment adherence mechanism including provision of mobility support to workers, patient enablers and insurance to TB patients, social support systems, nutrition support, ICT mechanisms, pharmacovigilance, etc.
  - Extend patient support services for patients in private sector.
  - Roll out of DST-guided treatment for DRTB.
- Regular and long-term follow up and rehabilitation of all treated TB patients.

#### Key affected population

Strategies include mapping of key affected population; screening of population in vulnerable groups for symptoms and signs suggestive of TB; campaign approach to address TB in key population, which may be undertaken by national campaign against TB, to achieve widespread awareness for identifying TB symptomatics, or by community campaign by symptom screening in vulnerable population.

#### Patient support systems

This includes linking Pradhan Mantri Jan Dhan Yojana, Aadhar and Nikshay for direct cash benefit to patients; reducing out-of-pocket expenditure for TB patients; providing financial support to provide nutrition; patient-centered approach to treatment.

#### Drug regimen

*Already discussed in Chapter 17A: Epidemiology of Airborne Diseases and its Prevention and Control.*

### (C) Prevent

Goal is to prevent the emergence of TB in susceptible population. This is aimed to be achieved through airborne infection control, contact tracing and treatment of LTBI.

#### Airborne infection control

Measures to be undertaken in healthcare settings include providing separate inpatient facility for bacteriologically positive DS/DR TB patients and other airborne infectious patients; proper infection control measures in ART centers; proper disposal of sputum and infected materials; wet mopping and disinfection; proper ventilation, renovation if necessary; provision of N95 masks and periodic screening for concerned staff.

#### Contact tracing

All close contacts, especially household contacts of a TB patient will be screened for TB using Chest X-ray (CXR). Reverse contact tracing for search of any active TB case in the household must be undertaken in case of pediatric TB patients.

#### Latent TB infection treatment

In clinical situations, the most obvious group for LTBI treatment will include high-risk patients. The risk groups that will be prioritized for screening and further investigation to rule out TB and treatment, will include people living with HIV; child PTB contacts; patients with silicosis; all patients who are clinically indicated or at high risk, e.g., patients on immunosuppressive drugs; high-risk adult contacts.

### (D) Build

This strategy aims to build and strengthen enabling policies, empowered institutions and human resources to respond to the TB epidemic.

#### Urban TB control systems

A separate City/Urban TB Control Mission will be constituted under the SHS headed by the administrative head of the city. ACF will be undertaken in urban slums, utilizing the services of female health worker. The primary place for getting TB services will be the Urban-PHC near a slum. Specialist services in case of complications for TB patients will be provided at Urban-CHC, along with C&DST and DR-TB services. The strategic interventions for TB control in urban areas during the NSP period include:

- **Private sector engagement:** Incentives, free drugs and diagnostic tests
- **Social mobilization campaign:** Special focus on women, children and youth
- **Primary healthcare services:** U-PHC near slum area, diagnosis of presumptive TB
- **Referral services:** U-CHC for every 4–5 U-PHCs, government hospitals and medical colleges.

#### Health system strengthening

A National TB Policy and TB Bill will be formulated, and an apex body, known as National TB elimination board, will be created to facilitate policy development, ensure multisectoral coordination, and overview implementation of the strategies for TB elimination.

#### Surveillance, monitoring and evaluation

Case-based web-based recording and reporting (**NIKSHAY**) was set up in 2012, to improve TB surveillance in the country, which has been extended to include drug-resistant TB cases, online referral and transfer of patients. Surveillance of healthcare workers with rapid molecular testing, and surveillance of migrants have also been started.

### Involvement of medical colleges in NTEP
- Selected medical colleges will be designated centers of excellence (COE)
- Decentralized drug resistant TB services
- Culture service support
- Air-borne infection control measures in healthcare facilities in districts
- Private provider engagement
- Research.

### TB Notification

Tuberculosis has been declared a notifiable disease in India on 7th May 2012, with an objective to improve diagnosis and case management, to accelerate reduction of TB transmission and to prevent further drug resistance.

### 99 DOTS

It was initially started in 2015 as an ICT-enabled system to improve compliance to medication in patients receiving daily fixed dose combination (FDC) medications in high burden ART centers for HIV-TB coinfected patients. In 2016, it expanded to include all HIV-TB patients at all ART centers in India. The blister pack of FDC-antituberculosis therapy (ATT) contains hidden toll-free numbers which are revealed once the patient takes the tablets. Once the patient takes a tablet he calls the toll-free number from any phone as evidence that he has consumed the medicine. The number sequence for every patient is unique and can be used to track the treatment adherence of the patient from the platform by any healthcare worker.

### Standards for TB Care

The International Standards for TB Care, formulated in 2009, is a set of 21 standards to monitor TB diagnosis, treatment, public health and prevention. Similarly, Standards for TB Care in India were released in 2014, which is a set of 27 standards that govern the diagnosis and treatment of both PTB and EPTB and HIV-TB coinfection and other comorbid conditions, public health, and prevention.

### Nikshay Poshan Yojana

All notified TB patients on Nikshay portal will get financial incentive of ₹ 500/month for duration of anti-TB treatment through direct benefit transfer (Aadhar enabled bank accounts).

### Direct Benefit Transfer Schemes

- Honorarium to treatment supporters: For provision of treatment support to TB patients (Adherence, ADR monitoring, counselling ₹ 1,000/- to ₹ 5,000/-).
- Patient support to tribal TB patients: (Financial patient support ₹ 750/-).
- Nutritional support to all TB patients: (Financial support to patients ₹ 500/-month).
- Incentives to private providers: (₹ 500/- for notification and ₹ 500/- for reporting of treatment outcome.
- Incentives to informant: (₹ 500/- is given on diagnosis of TB among referrals from community to public sector health facility).

### TB-Mukt Panchayat Initiative

- Aims to measure and appreciate the efforts of the Gram Panchayats at the village level to make India TB-free.
- To receive the TB-Mukt Panchayat status, Panchayats should provide support to patients with TB and monitor their progress quarterly based on certain pre-requisite indicators.

### Family-centric Model for TB

One family member for every confirmed patient with TB will be enrolled under NIKSHAY, making them a trained primary caregiver. This ensures timely recovery, proper nutrition, and reduction in social stigma to the patient.

A caregiver should be >14-years-old, spend maximum time with the patient, consented to take responsibility, and is acceptable to the patient.

## NATIONAL AIDS CONTROL PROGRAMME

The National AIDS Control Programme was first launched in 1987 and focused on HIV screening and educational activities. National AIDS Control Project (NACP)-I launched in 1992 introduced national HIV surveillance system, prevention activities among high-risk groups (HRGs), information on HIV and the blood safety program. NACP-II launched in 1999 scaled-up targeted interventions for HRGs, greater involvement of people living with HIV (PLHIV), community networking and treatment program. NACP-III launched in 2007 continued prevention, care, support and treatment efforts with a focus on increasing service access points through institutional scale-up and out-reach. NACP-IV launched in 2012, focused on the process of reversal of the AIDS epidemic. The NACP Phase-IV (Extension) was first approved for the period of 2017–2020 and then further extended for one more year, i.e., 2020–21. The NACP Phase-V (2021–26) aims to reduce annual new HIV infections and AIDS-related mortalities by 80% by 2025–26 from the baseline value of 2010. The NACP Phase-V also aims to attain dual elimination of vertical transmission, elimination of HIV/AIDS related stigma while promoting universal access to quality STI/RTI services to at-risk and vulnerable populations. In 2017 the National Strategic Plan for HIV/AIDS and STI 2017–24 was formulated, for paving the way to an AIDS free India.

### NACP-V (2021–26)

The unprecedented momentum of the national AIDS response under NACP Phase-IV and Extension would be sustained to anchor the country progress as newer challenges emerge in the form of expanding epidemic in many States, very high level of HIV/AIDS epidemic in north-eastern States, more and more of HRG population using virtual platforms to solicit clients and rising prevalence of high-risk behaviors among the general population. The HIV and STI epidemic response will be at a very crucial stage in the NACP Phase-V given the national commitment of achieving the end of the AIDS epidemic by 2030. While the tenets of Test and Treat, Viral Suppression, Prevention and Enabling Environment complying to the HIV/AIDS Act and Rules will remain the backbone of the program, the recent initiatives of community systems strengthening and differentiated models of treatment and prevention will continue to be built upon.

## Goal

To reduce annual new HIV infections and AIDS-related death by 80% since the baseline value of 2010; Eliminate Vertical Transmission of HIV and Syphilis; Eliminate HIV/AIDS-related Stigma and Discrimination; Promote Universal Access to Quality STI/RTI Services.

## Objectives

- HIV/AIDS prevention and control
  - 95% of people who are most at risk of acquiring HIV infection use comprehensive prevention
  - 95% of HIV positive know their status, 95% of those who know their status are on treatment and 95% of those who are on treatment have suppressed viral load
  - 95% of pregnant and breastfeeding women living with HIV have suppressed viral load towards attainment of elimination of vertical transmission of HIV
  - Less than 10% of people living with HIV and key populations experience stigma and discrimination
- STI/RTI prevention and control
  - Promote universal access to quality STI/RTI services to at-risk and vulnerable populations;
  - Attainment of elimination of vertical transmission of syphilis

## Strategies

| Strategic interventions | | | |
|---|---|---|---|
| New generation communication strategy | Reaching the missing million—the virtual approach | Promoting integrated service delivery through one-stop centers | Provision of comprehensive package of services through "Sampoorn Suraksha" |
| Augmenting contact tracing and index testing promoting early detection of undiagnosed infections | Leveraging dual test kits (HIV and syphilis) for dual elimination and integrated service package to the people who are at higher risk | Addressing linkage loss at all levels | Differentiated care model augmenting adherence |

*Contd...*

| Strategic interventions | | | |
|---|---|---|---|
| Prioritize sexual and reproductive health services for women at increased risk of HIV infection and women living with HIV | Adapting new approaches to expand the reach of viral load testing services | Enhancement of private sector engagement | IT enabled client centric integrated monitoring, evaluation, and surveillance system |
| Enhancement of community support through community system strengthening | Building and augmenting synergies | Anchoring the response through focused program management and review | Enhancing the strategic information systems to meet the evidence needs in ever evolving and dynamic epidemiological and programmatic context |

Leveraging technology to bring efficiency and expand the reach of the services.

Consolidation and expansion of existing interventions across prevention-testing-treatment continuum with critical enablers of IEC, laboratory services and strategic information management.

## Package of Services

While the existing interventions will be sustained, optimized, and augmented, newer strategies will be adopted, piloted, and scaled-up under the program to respond to the geographic and community specific needs and priorities. The HIV and AIDS (Prevention and Control) Act, 2017 will continue to be the cornerstone of the national response to HIV and STI epidemic in NACP Phase-V. The Act will be the enabling framework to break down barriers driving delivery of a comprehensive package of services in an ecosystem free of stigma and discrimination. These include prevention services; care, support and treatment services; IEC services; capacity building; and SIMS.

### A. Prevention Services

- **Targeted interventions for high-risk groups and bridge population:** Targeted Interventions are preventive interventions for HRGs in a defined geographic area. HRGs include female sex workers/commercial sex workers (FSW/CSW), men who have sex with men (MSM), transgenders (TG) and injecting drug users (IDU). Bridge population includes long distance truck drivers (LDT) and single male migrants (SMM).
  Specific interventions available for IDUs are:
  - Distribution of clean needles and syringes
  - Abscess prevention and management
  - Opioid substitution therapy (OST), and
  - Linkage with detoxification/rehabilitation services. MSMs and TGs are provided with lubricating materials and FSWs are distributed female condoms.

Interventions for bridge population are important to prevent the infection from entering the general population. For migrants, services like distribution of condoms and IEC are provided at source (their villages), at transit point (rail or bus stations) and at destination (places of work). For truckers, clinics for preventive, diagnostic and treatment services are conducted at trans-shipment locations and are co-branded as Khushi-Suraksha clinic.

- *Link worker scheme:* In this scheme link workers, who are trained members of the community, provide information and skills on HIV/AIDS prevention to vulnerable members of the community like youth, PLHIV, women having casual sex partners and also to members belonging to HRG and bridge population. Currently this scheme is active in high prevalence districts of selected endemic states.
- *Management of STI/RTI:* Strategies for STI/RTI control are (1) Strengthen STI/RTI control and prevention, and (2) Eliminate parent to child transmission of HIV and syphilis.
    - **Strengthen STI/RTI control and prevention**
    This is done by provision of standardized services and treatment for STI/RTI, convergence of sexual and reproductive health (SRH) services with NHM and private sector, focusing on "at risk" population. Strategy followed is syndromic case management (SCM) with appropriate laboratory test at all levels of care, for general as well as at risk populations, along with partner management, counseling services and free supply of condoms. There are designated STI/RTI clinics (DSRC) supported by Department of AIDS Control all over the country, at least one center per district, for case management. Collaboration between organized public and private sector is ensured varied modes of service delivery like static and mobile clinics, health camps, and hybrid models are utilized.
    SCM is based on the principle that STIs present with a gamut of symptoms and signs which are similar yet distinctive, and frequently more than one infection occurs together. Prepacked color-coded STI/RTI kits are available for syndromic management of STIs/RTIs. ***Details about syndromic management are discussed in Chapter 17G: Epidemiology of Contact Diseases and its Prevention and Control.***
    - **Eliminate parent-to-child transmission of syphilis**
    In accordance with UN SDGs, India has set the goal to eliminate parent-to-child transmission of syphilis by 2017 with a target to reduce the incidence of congenital syphilis to less than 0.3 cases per 1,000 live births by 2017. The objectives are to:
        ♦ Ensure universal and early registration of pregnant women at first ANC visit in first trimester.
        ♦ Ensure early screening of pregnant women for both syphilis and HIV at least once during the pregnancy.
        ♦ Identify and provide prompt treatment to all seroreactive pregnant women.
        ♦ Promote institutional delivery, and
        ♦ Follow up the newborn up to 18 months of age.
    Guidelines for diagnosis have been given along with criteria for suspect and confirmed cases. Management is by giving injection benzathine penicillin to the mother or alternatively oral erythromycin or azithromycin. Prophylactic or curative treatment is given to the baby as required.
    - **STI surveillance**
    STI surveillance in India includes passive syndromic case reporting from designated STI/RTI clinics and TI sites, STI/RTI etiological reporting from reference and research laboratories, and HIV sentinel surveillance which reports prevalence of serosyphilis.
- *Management of sexual violence:* After a sexual assault, the following preventive and supportive measures are mandated:
    - **Prevention of unwanted pregnancy:** Emergency contraception with levonorgestrel or combined oral contraceptive pill Mala D.
    - **Postexposure prophylaxis against STI:** This is different for adults and children and is done as per Department of AIDS Control guidelines **(Tables 47.10 and 47.11)**.
    - **Postexposure prophylaxis against HIV:** Done as per Department of AIDS Control guidelines.
    - **Postexposure prophylaxis against Hepatitis B:** If the victim is not vaccinated against Hepatitis B, both vaccine and Hepatitis B immunoglobulin should be administered within 24 hours, followed by completion of vaccine schedule.
    - **Follow-up services:** The victim should be told whom to contact in case of any subsequent problems related to the incident.
    - **Psychological support:** Both immediate and long-term.
- *Condom promotion:* Condom Social Marketing Programme was launched under NACP-III to increase condom acceptance and use. Under this program, condoms were made available in non-conventional shops such as petrol pumps, wine-shops, PDS shops, dhabas, lodges, etc.
- *Blood safety:* The blood safety program was also launched under NACP-III to provide safe and quality blood and blood products with the objective of ensuring reduction in the transfusion associated HIV transmission to 0.5%. Testing for

**Table 47.10:** Postexposure prophylaxis against sexually transmitted infection for adults, adolescents and older children, weighing >45 kg.

| For protection against | Drug |
| --- | --- |
| Gonorrhea, chlamydia | Tablet azithromycin 1 g orally, single dose under supervision plus tablet cefixime 400 mg orally single dose |
| Trichomonas, bacterial vaginosis | Tablet metronidazole 2 g single dose or tablet tinidazole 2 g single dose |

**Table 47.11:** Postexposure prophylaxis against sexually transmitted infection for children.

| For protection against | Drug |
| --- | --- |
| Gonorrhea | Cefixime 8 mg/kg of body weight as a single dose or ceftriaxone 125 mg by intramuscular injection |
| Chlamydia | Erythromycin 12.5 mg/kg body weight orally 4 times a day for 14 days or azithromycin 20 mg/kg body weight orally once a day for 3 days |
| Trichomonas | Metronidazole 5 mg/kg body weight orally 3 times a day for 7 days |

HIV along with hepatitis B, hepatitis C, malaria and syphilis is mandatory for all blood units collected at blood banks. Professional blood donation was banned w.e.f. 1st January 1998.

- **HIV counseling and testing services (HCTS):** HCTS is important for early diagnosis of HIV in clinically suspected individuals; safety of blood, blood products, organs and tissues; prevention of parent to child transmission; voluntary testing of high risk groups; monitor epidemiological trends of infection and identify population groups requiring specific interventions. Individuals can access HCTS in through self-initiated or voluntary approach or by provider-initiated approach. Rapid test kits are recommended by NACO for screening, which are more than 99.5% sensitive and more than 98% specific.

  The HIV counseling and testing services include the following components:
  - Integrated counseling and testing centers (ICTC)
  - Prevention of parent-to-child transmission of HIV (PPTCT)
  - HIV/TB collaborative activities

- **Integrated counseling and testing centers:** These centers provide diagnostic facilities, counseling services, referrals for STI treatment, condom promotion, care and support for opportunistic infections and referrals to designated centers for ART. ICTCs have been classified into two types: (1) Facility-based HIV testing and (2) community-based HIV testing centers.

  Facility-based HIV testing approaches include standalone ICTCs (SA-ICTC) which are located at tertiary healthcare facility and have full time counselor and laboratory technician; facility ICTCs (F-ICTC) which are run below the block level at 24 × 7 PHCs by existing paramedical staff of the health facility; and public-private partnership ICTCs (PPP-ICTC) run in private facilities with the support of District AIDS Prevention Control Units/State AIDS Control Societies (DAPCU/SACS) similar to F-ICTCs.

  Community-based HIV testing approaches include Mobile ICTC in hard-to-reach areas; screening by ancillary healthcare providers; screening by NGO-led targeted intervention program; HCTS for prison inmates and at workplace for both organized and unorganized sector.

- **Prevention of parent-to-child transmission of HIV:** The primary route of transmission of HIV in children is mother-to-child transmission which occurs during pregnancy, childbirth and breastfeeding with equal frequency. PPTCT is a four-pronged program:
  - *Prong 1:* Primary prevention of HIV, especially among
  - women of child bearing age.
  - *Prong 2:* Preventing unintended pregnancies among women living with HIV.
  - *Prong 3:* Prevent HIV transmission from pregnant women infected with HIV to their child.
  - *Prong 4:* Provide care, support and treatment to women living with HIV, her children and family.

  The essential package of PPTCT services in India consists of HIV counseling and testing, diagnosis and treatment of mother and child, pregnancy management and care of other conditions **(Fig. 47.16)**.

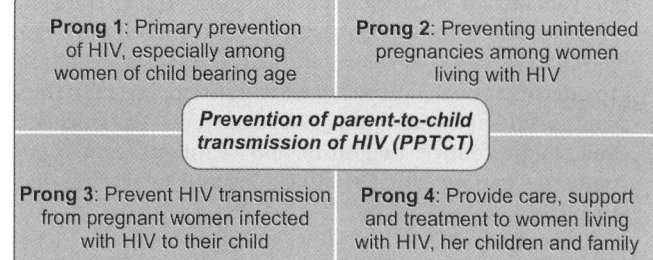

Fig. 47.16: Approaches to prevention of parent-to-child transmission of HIV under National AIDS Control Project.

- **HIV/TB collaborative activities:** TB is the most common opportunistic infection among HIV-infected individuals. A four-pronged approach with the involvement of both NACP and NTEP for prevention and control of HIV-TB is in place **(Table 47.12)**.

- **Prevention and management of occupational exposure to blood borne infections:** Standard precautions which guide the prevention of blood-borne infections in high risk workplace settings are as follows:
  - Hand-washing before and after all medical procedures.
  - Use of protective barriers such as gloves, masks, goggles, aprons and boots to prevent direct contact with blood and body fluid.
  - Safe handling and immediate safe disposal of sharps: Not recapping needles, using special containers and needle cutters/destroyers for sharp disposals, using forceps for guiding sutures, using vacutainers where possible.
  - Respiratory hygiene and cough etiquette.
  - Environmental cleaning by routine cleaning and disinfection.
  - Safe decontamination and disposal of contaminated waste or patient care equipment.

- **Postexposure prophylaxis:** In any case of exposure to blood and/or body fluid, the following steps are mandated for post-exposure prophylaxis against blood-borne infections **(Tables 47.13 and 47.14)**.

Table 47.12: HIV/TB collaborative activities National AIDS Control Project and Revised National Tuberculosis Control Programme.

| Prevention | Early detection of TB/HIV |
|---|---|
| • Isoniazid preventive treatment<br>• Air borne infection control<br>• Awareness generation | • 100% coverage of provider initiated testing and counseling (PITC) in TB patients<br>• PITC in presumptive TB cases<br>• Rapid diagnosis of TB and DR-TB in PLHIV<br>• Intensified case finding (ICF) activities at all HIV settings—ICTC, ART, LAC and TI settings |
| **Prompt treatment of TB/HIV** | **Management of special TB/HIV cases** |
| • Early initiation of ART regardless of CD4 count<br>• Prompt initiation of TB treatment | • TB/HIV patients on protease inhibitor-based ARV<br>• TB/HIV in children<br>• TB/HIV in pregnant women<br>• Drug-resistant TB/HIV |

(ART: antiretroviral therapy; ARV: antirabies vaccine; ICTC: integrated counseling and testing centers; PLHIV: people living with HIV)

**Table 47.13:** Categorization of exposure.

| Category of exposure | Definition and example |
|---|---|
| Mild exposure | Mucous membrane/non-intact skin with small volumes, e.g., a superficial wound (erosion of the epidermis) with a plain or low-caliber needle, or contact with the eyes or mucous membranes, subcutaneous injections following small-bore needles |
| Moderate exposure | Mucous membrane/non-intact skin with large volumes or percutaneous superficial exposure with solid needle, e.g.: a cut or needle stick injury penetrating glove |
| Severe exposure | Percutaneous with large volume, e.g.:<br>• An accident with a high caliber needle (>18 G) visibly contaminated with blood;<br>• A deep wound (hemorrhagic and/or very painful wound);<br>• Transmission of a significant volume of blood;<br>• An accident with material that has previously been used intravenously or intra-arterially |

**Table 47.14:** Postexposure prophylaxis (PEP) regimen.

| Exposure | Status of source | | | |
|---|---|---|---|---|
| | HIV positive and asymptomatic | HIV positive and clinically symptomatic | HIV status unknown | HIV negative |
| Mild | Consider 2-drug PEP | Start 2-drug PEP | Consider 2-drug PEP | No PEP is required if the source blood is confirmed HIV negative |
| Moderate | Start 2-drug PEP | Start 3-drug PEP | Consider 2-drug PEP | |
| Severe | Start 3-drug PEP | Start 3-drug PEP | Consider 2-drug PEP | |

A negative test in the source patient does not exclude the risk of infection since "window period" for HIV extends for a period of 6 weeks when the infection is not detectable.

HIV PEP should be started ideally within 2 hours and not later than 72 hours of exposure. Initially 2-drug therapy should be started. PEP should be continued for 4 weeks. In case the source patient is on ART and is considered to have drug resistance, expert physicians should be consulted. PEP for Hepatitis B includes vaccination and administration of immunoglobulin. All healthcare personnel should be vaccinated against hepatitis B.

### B. Information, Education and Communication Services

IEC is an important part of HIV/AIDS control. The services include promotion of safe behavioral practices, reduction of stigma and discrimination, promotion of services for counseling and testing, ART, increasing condom use. Services are focused on youth and women who are more vulnerable to HIV infection.

The various channels of communications used are mass media, exhibitions, film shows, folk troupes, hoardings, bus panels, kiosks, adolescent education programs and formation of Red Ribbon Clubs in schools. Recently an app has been launched by NACO that helps assess the risk of a person for contracting HIV/AIDS, locate nearby health facilities and to access toll free helpline number 1097.

### C. Care, Support, and Treatment Services

The objective of these services is to improve the survival and quality of life of people living with HIV/AIDS. Services provided are ART, prevention and treatment of opportunistic infections, psychosocial support, home-based care, and reduction of stigma.

- *Antiretroviral therapy:* Free ART initiative had been launched in 2004 under NACP-II through ART centers. From 2016, guidelines for eligibility for ART were changed as per WHO recommendations, to treat all PLHIV with ART regardless of CD4 count, clinical stage, age or population. Adequate counseling for treatment compliance should be done in all PLHIV, especially for those with higher CD4 count as they are likely to be asymptomatic and more likely to default. ***ART has been discussed in 17G: Epidemiology of Contact Diseases and its Prevention and Control.***
- *HIV comorbidities:* Comorbidities such as TB, hepatitis, leishmaniasis, etc., should be managed as per guidelines.
- *Service delivery mechanism:* Care, support and treatment services are provided through ART and ART Plus centers overlooked by Centers of Excellence (CoE). Pediatric ART centers and CoE are also in place for providing pediatric ART. Decentralization is achieved through Link ART centers and Link ART Plus centers at subdistrict and CHCs to reduce case load and waiting time in ART centers and increase treatment adherence. The ART centers are also linked to ICTCs, STI clinics, PPTCT services in various institutions. There is cross referral with the NTEP program as well to tackle the burden of TB/HIV. Care and support centers (CSCs) are run at the district level by NGOs and provide as a link between PLHIV families and ART centers.

### D. Capacity Building

It involves training of manpower and technical staff. These training programs are held in the COE and other designated training centers across the country. A PG Diploma course in HIV medicine has been started along with various national and regional distance learning courses. Apart from training, intersectoral collaboration is an important part of capacity building. Involving the private sector in care, support and treatment of PLHIV has effectively aided HIV/AIDS control efforts.

### E. Strengthening Strategic Information Management

Strategic Information Management under NACP-IV is a system for data generation through surveillance, monitoring and research, and translation of this data to guide program management and policy making. The Strategic Information Management Unit has four divisions: (1) Monitoring and evaluation, (2) Research, (3) Surveillance and epidemiology, and (4) Data analysis and dissemination.

The SIMS is a web-based reporting, data management and decision support system run by the Monitoring and Evaluation Division where data is collected monthly from over 30,000 reporting units. A system for web-based data storage has also been developed by the name of NACO Cloud—Meghraj.

### Surveillance of HIV/AIDS

Under the program, components of surveillance are: (1) AIDS case surveillance, (2) HIV sentinel surveillance, (3) STD surveillance, and (4) Behavioral surveillance.

- ***AIDS case surveillance:*** It is done by all medical institutions identifying the suspected cases and referring them to the referral hospitals for confirmation.
- ***HIV sentinel surveillance (HSS):*** First conducted by ICMR in 1985, it was subsequently taken over by NACO in 1993–94 with an objective to determine the geographical spread of HIV infection and important routes of transmission. Sentinel sites were used to screen high-risk groups, bridge population and antenatal clinic (ANC) women (proxy indicator for general population) for HIV infection. The surveillance was done bi-annually and the 14th round of HSS was held in 2017 in 1,323 sentinel sites—829 sites among ANC clinic attendees and 494 sites among high-risk groups and bridge populations.
- ***STD surveillance:*** It was started recently to estimate the magnitude of STD in the country. Data will be collected from STD clinics with laboratory support along with syndrome based information from peripheral institutions and community surveys.
- ***Behavioral surveillance:*** The National Integrated Biological and Behavioral Surveillance (NIBBS) was initiated to strengthen the high risk group surveillance activities and integrate the biological and behavioral surveillance efforts which were being carried out separately. National IBBS 2014–15 has been completed in all the regions for all study groups and report has been published.

## NATIONAL STRATEGIC PLAN FOR HIV/AIDS AND SEXUALLY TRANSMITTED INFECTION (STI) 2017–2024

Based on the recommendations of a mid-term appraisal of NACP-IV held in 2016, the National Strategic Plan was proposed to steer the program forward.

### Vision

Paving the way for an AIDS free India.

**Table 47.15:** Objectives and outcomes of NACP under NSP 2017–24.

| Sl. No. | Objectives | Outcomes |
|---|---|---|
| 1. | Reduce new infections by 80% by 2024 (Baseline 2010) | New infections reduced from >100,000 to <21,000 |
| 2. | Link 95% of estimated PLHIV to services by 2024 | 2.01 million PLHIV know their status |
| 3. | Ensure ART initiation and retention of 90% of PLHIV for sustained viral suppression by 2024 | 1.90 million PLHIV on ART are retained and have sustained viral suppression |
| 4. | Eliminate mother-to-child transmission of HIV and syphilis by 2020 | Attain dual elimination by 2020 |
| 5. | Eliminate HIV-related stigma and discrimination by 2020 | HIV/AIDS considered as a chronic manageable disease |
| 6. | Facilitate sustainable NACP service delivery by 2024 | • Integration of identified components of NACP with NHM<br>• Domestic funding for NACP is 100% |

(NACP: National AIDS Control Project; NHM: The National Health Mission; NSP: National Surveillance Programme; PLHIV: people living with HIV)

### Mission

Attain universal coverage of HIV prevention, universal care, continuum of services that are effective, inclusive, equitable and adapted to needs.

### Goal

Achieving zero new infections, zero AIDS related deaths and zero discrimination **(Table 47.15)**.

### Priorities

- Accelerating HIV prevention in "at risk group" and key population.
- Expanding quality assured HIV testing with universal access to comprehensive HIV care.
- Elimination of mother to child transmission of HIV and syphilis.
- Addressing the critical enablers in HIV programming.
- Restructuring the strategic information system to be efficient and patient-centric.

## NATIONAL LEPROSY ERADICATION PROGRAMME

The National Leprosy Control Programme was launched in 1955 which aimed at early detection of leprosy cases and treatment with dapsone monotherapy. Multidrug therapy was started in 1982 thus shortening the duration of treatment, and the program was renamed National Leprosy Eradication Programme in 1983.

Elimination of leprosy is denoted by a prevalence of less than 1 case per 10,000 population. Elimination was achieved at the national level by 2005, but the disease is still endemic in some states, viz. Chandigarh, Odisha, Delhi, Goa, Chhattisgarh, Dadra and Nagar Haveli, and Lakshadweep.

### Vision

"Leprosy-free India" is the vision of the NLEP.

### Objectives

- To reduce prevalence rate less than 1/10,000 population at subnational and district level.
- To reduce Grade II disability % <1 among new cases at national level
- To reduce Grade II disability cases <1 case per million population at national level.

- Zero disabilities among new child cases.
- Zero stigma and discrimination against persons affected by leprosy.

## Achievements during 2020

- Percentage of Grade II disability (G2D)/visible deformity among new cases decreased from 3.05% in 2018–19 to 2.39% (2019–20).
- The G2D amongst new cases/million population decreased from 2.65/million population as on 31st March, 2019 to 1.94/million population as on 31st March 2020.
- Child cases percentage has reduced from 7.67% as on 31st March 2019 to 6.86 % as on 31st March 2020.
- Prevalence rate of leprosy has come down from 0.69/10,000 population (2014–15) to 0.45 (2021–22).
- Annual new case detection rate per 100,000 population has come down from 9.73 (2014–15) to 5.52 (2021–22).

India can achieve the target of *"Leprosy Mukt Bharat"* by 2027, 3 years ahead of the sustainable development goals (SDGs) with the whole of government approach and the society's support.

## Strategies

### Case Detection and Management

*Early case detection:* Early case detection is essential in leprosy to prevent progression of the disease to disability. Enhanced active and early case detection strategy has been introduced through *Active Case Detection and Regular Surveillance strategy* (ACD and RS) throughout the year.

Three-Pronged strategy was used:

1. **Leprosy case detection campaign (LCDC):** 14 day active case detection campaign in high endemic districts in the form of house-to-house visits were made by teams comprising of one ASHA and one male volunteer/field level worker (FLW) for search of leprosy cases. Intensive IEC activities were undertaken through miking and display of banners/posters during and before LCDC. Community leaders/representatives were involved to resolve issues faced during campaign.

   Case detection is done mainly on clinical grounds. Leprosy is classified into paucibacillary (PB) and multibacillary (MB) based on clinical presentation in the field **(Table 47.16)**.

   ASHAs, AWWs and other community volunteers are given incentives to detect suspected cases of leprosy from villages and confirm their diagnosis at PHCs and follow up of confirmed cases for treatment completion. Incentive being paid after leprosy case confirmation is ₹ 250. In addition, they are supposed to follow up the confirmed case for treatment completion and incentives being given for same are ₹ 400 for PB case and ₹ 600 for MB case follow up. Inspite of this, they spend less time on low incentive-based programs.

   Hence, in order to interrupt the transmission of leprosy in the community ***ASHA Based Surveillance for Leprosy Suspects (ABSULS) was introduced in 2017.*** Under this unique approach a*ctive surveillance of leprosy suspects* or nil suspect identified during previous month is reported by ASHA with signature. This active surveillance by the community itself and validation even of nil cases by health system is the gold standard to ensure early detection of leprosy cases.
2. **Focused leprosy campaign (FLC)** in low endemic districts
3. **Special plan for hard-to-reach areas**

### Leprosy screening

Convergence of leprosy screening for targeting different age groups
- Rashtriya Bal Swasthya Karyakram (RBSK) to screen children (0–18 years) at Anganwadi Centers and Government schools.
- Rashtriya Kishor Swasthya Karyakram (RKSK) for screening and counselling the children of teen age group (13–19 years) at Adolescent Friendly Clinics.
- Comprehensive Primary Health Care Programme of Ayushman Bharat, to screen 30+ years population at HWCs.

### Treatment

Treatment for leprosy by multidrug therapy (MDT) is as follows:
- **Multibacillary patients (adult)** *(course of 12 months to be completed by 18 months)*
  - *Supervised once a month:* Rifampicin 600 mg, clofazimine 300 mg, dapsone 100 mg PLUS
  - *Unsupervised daily (self-administered):* Clofazimine 50 mg (if not available, 100 mg capsule on alternate days), dapsone 100 mg.
- **Paucibacillary patients (adult)** *(course of 6 months to be completed by 9 months)*
  - *Supervised once a month:* Rifampicin 600 mg, dapsone 100 mg PLUS
  - *Unsupervised daily:* dapsone 100 mg
  - For children and adults with weight less than 35 kg dose of rifampicin is reduced to 450 mg once a month, dapsone 50 mg every day and clofazimine 150 mg once a month and 50 mg on alternate days **(Box 47.2)**.
  - MDT drugs are supplied in *blister calendar packs* each containing 4 weeks treatment to ensure that all the required drugs are available and consumed on a regular basis. Post-treatment surveillance is done by clinical examination at the time of completion of treatment and subsequently annually for 2 years in PB and 5 years in MB cases to detect relapse.

MoHFW with approval of WHO has revised the treatment of Leprosy. It has introduced a 3-drug regimen for Pauci-bacillary (PB) cases in place of 2-drug regimen for 6 months. This revised treatment will be implemented all over the country from 1st April 2025.

***Further details of classification and treatment of leprosy is explained in Chapter 17G: Epidemiology of Contact Diseases and its Prevention and Control.***

**Table 47.16:** Classification of leprosy.

|  | Paucibacillary | Multibacillary |
|---|---|---|
| Skin lesions | ≤5 lesions | 6 and more lesions |
| Nerve involvement | No/only one nerve trunk involved | More than one nerve trunk involved |
| Skin smear | Negative at all sites | Positive at any site |

**Box 47.2:** Directly observed rifampicin supervised.
- \>35 kg: 600 mg
- 20–35 kg: 450 mg
- <20 kg: 10–156 mg/kg

### Disability Prevention and Medical Rehabilitation (DPMR)

For prevention and management of disability, dressing material, supportive medicines and micro-cellular rubber (MCR) footwear are provided to leprosy patients. The patients are also empowered with trainings in self-care procedure for preventing aggravating disability to the insensitive hands/feets. Emphasis is also being placed on correction of permanent disability through reconstructive surgeries (RCS). DPMR activities are carried out in a three-tier system, i.e., primary (up to sub-district level), secondary (district headquarter hospitals and district nucleus units) and tertiary level care (central institutions), supported by medical colleges and NGOs. Government of India has recognized 115 institutions (61 government and 54 NGO institutions) for conducting RCS. ₹ 8,000 is given as incentive to the leprosy affected person undergoing RCS in identified government/NGO institution. For prevention of disability, the patients are given dressing material, medicines, and microcellular rubber (MCR) footwear.

### Information, Education and Communication (IEC) Including Behavior Change Communication (BCC)

Intensive IEC activities are conducted for awareness generation and reduction of stigma and discrimination against leprosy affected persons. These activities are carried through mass media, outdoor media, rural media, advocacy meetings and inter personnel communication organizing camps at schools, colleges, and in community.

Special annual mass awareness campaigns *named Sparsh Leprosy Awareness Campaigns (SLAC)* were launched on 30th January, 2017, i.e., Anti Leprosy Day, to reduce stigma and discrimination against persons suffering from leprosy. Since then, every year, nationwide Gram Sabhas in villages across the country are being organized in cooperation and coordination with allied sectors of health department. Village community is encouraged to participate in these meetings, and school children are encouraged to spread awareness about the disease through plays, posters, etc.

*"Sapna"* is a concept (mascot) designed and developed using a common girl living in community, who will help spread awareness in the community, through key IEC messages. Sapna can be local school going girl who is willing to be 'Sapna'. There can be any number of Sapna's in a village.

In 2020, convergence of NLEP was made with Rashtriya Kishor Swasthya Karyakram (RKSK) for counselling the children of teen-age group (13–19 years) about leprosy at Adolescent Friendly Clinics.

### Human Resource and Capacity Building

- Training of general health staff like medical officer, health workers, health supervisors, laboratory technicians and ASHAs are conducted every year to develop adequate skills for diagnosis and management of leprosy cases.
- **Leprosy and kala-azar:** A flow chart has been developed to guide the staff to differentiate between leprosy and kala-azar, both of which may present with skin lesions which may be for long duration. So cases of kala-azar are suspected to have leprosy also they should bent for confirmation, and vice versa.

### Planning, Supervision and Monitoring

Decentralized planning through district health plans, formulated through bottom-up process and Programme Implementation Plan (PIP) should be prepared as a result-oriented process. Programme is being monitored at different level through analysis of monthly progress reports, through field visits by the supervisory officers and program review meetings held at central, state and district level. For better epidemiological analysis of the disease situation, emphasis is put on assessment of New Case Detection and Treatment Completion Rate and proportion of grade II disability among new cases. Visits by joint monitoring teams with members from GOI, ILEP and WHO have been as integral part of NLEP.

*NIKUSTH:* A software introduced in 2019 for real time monitoring of leprosy patients across the country and facilitating better monitoring and evaluation of NLEP. This software was upgraded and named as Nikusth 2.0 in January 2023 to develop a complete database of leprosy patients, proper tracking and follow-up of individual case.

**NGO services under SET scheme:** NGOs are getting grants from Government of India under Survey, Education and Treatment (SET) scheme. Various activities undertaken by the NGOs are IEC, Prevention of Impairments and Deformities, Case Detection and MDT Delivery. From Financial year 2006 onwards, grant-in-aid is being disbursed to NGOs through State Health Societies. The Leprosy Mission Trust India (TLMTI), is the largest leprosy-focused nongovernmental organization (NGO) in India.

### Post Exposure Prophylaxis

*Administration of Single Dose of Rifampicin (SDR)*

### Eligibility Criteria for PEP

*Inclusion criteria*

- A person who has been living/working/having social activities for more than 3 months and 20 hours/week with a newly detected case of leprosy in the last 1 year.
- Age older than or equal to 2 years.

*Exclusion criteria*

- Pregnant women (PEP can be given after delivery).
- People receiving rifampicin therapy for any reason in the last 2 years (e.g., for TB or leprosy treatment, or as a contact from another index case).
- People with a history of liver disorders or renal disorders.
- People who have possible signs and/or symptoms of leprosy.
- People who have possible signs and/or symptoms of TB.
- Person with acute febrile illness.

*Activities to be carried out during postexposure prophylaxis are shown in* **Figure 47.17**.

### Immunoprophylaxis

***Mycobacterium indicus pranii (MIP) vaccine:*** Made-in-India leprosy vaccine launched in 2017 on pilot basis in five districts of Bihar and Gujarat. It is approved by the Drug Controller General of India and the FDA in the US. Vaccine to be given to the people living in close contacts with the infected. It is to be given along with a dose of rifampicin. By the use of this vaccine the cases can be brought down by 60% in 3 years.

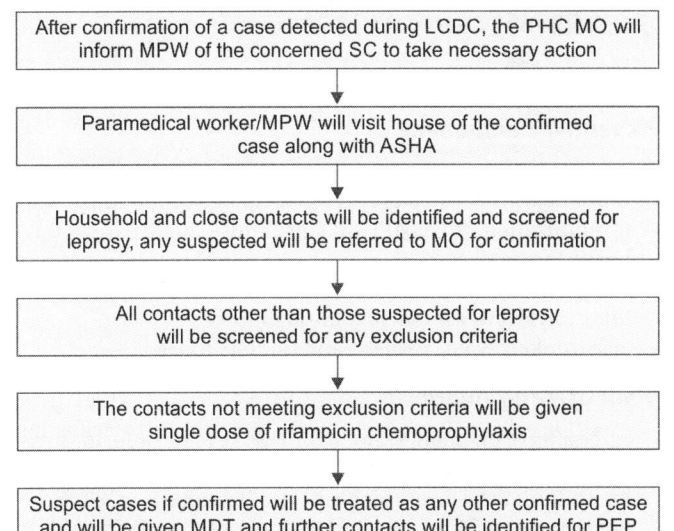

Fig. 47.17: Activities during postexposure prophylaxis for leprosy.
(ASHA: accredited social health activist; LCDC: leprosy case detection campaign; MDT: multidrug therapy; PHC: primary health center; MO: medical officer; SC: subcenter; PEP: postexposure prophylaxis)

## NATIONAL STRATEGIC PLAN AND ROADMAP FOR LEPROSY (2023–27)

The Government of India has launched National Strategic Plan (NSP) and Roadmap for Leprosy (2023–27) on 30th January, 2023, to achieve zero transmission of leprosy by 2027, i.e., 3 years ahead of the Sustainable Development Goal (SDG) 3.3. The NSP and Roadmap contains implementation strategies, year-wise targets, public health approaches and overall technical guidance for the program. The strategy and roadmap focus on awareness for zero stigma and discrimination, promotion of early case detection, prevention of disease transmission by prophylaxis (Leprosy Postexposure prophylaxis) and roll out of web-based information portal (Nikusth 2.0) for reporting of leprosy cases.

## GLOBAL PERSPECTIVE

The Global Leprosy Strategy 2016–2020 (**Fig. 47.18**) aims at early detection of leprosy disease and prompt treatment to prevent disability and reduce transmission of infection in the community. The strategy is designed to achieve a long-term goal of a 'leprosy-free world', which refers to a situation wherein the community is free of morbidity, disabilities and social consequences due to leprosy.

Elimination of leprosy as a public health problem at the global level was achieved in the year 2000. Over 16 million patients have been diagnosed and treated since the introduction of MDT over the past three decades.

### Strategic Pillars

- Strengthen government ownership, coordination and partnership
- Stop leprosy and its complications
- Stop discrimination and promote inclusion

### Global Targets for 2030

- 120 countries reporting zero new autochthonous cases
- 70% reduction in annual number of new cases detected
- 90% reduction in rate (per million) of new cases with grade 2-disability
- 90% reduction in rate (per million children) of new child cases with leprosy

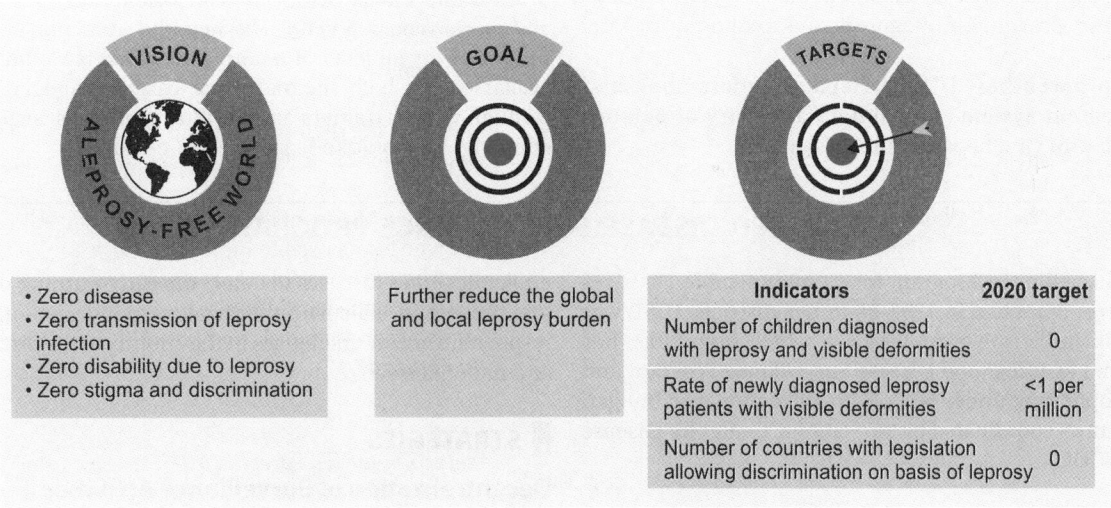

Fig 47.18: Global Leprosy Strategy 2016–2020.

## NATIONAL VIRAL HEPATITIS CONTROL PROGRAM

On the occasion of the World Hepatitis Day, 28th July 2018 Ministry of Health and Family Welfare, Government of India has launched the National Viral Hepatitis Control Program (NVHCP). It is an integrated initiative to achieve Sustainable Development Goal (SDG) 3.3 which aims to ending viral hepatitis by 2030. This is a comprehensive plan covering the entire gamut from Hepatitis A, B, C, D and E, and the whole range from prevention, detection and treatment to mapping treatment outcomes.

### Aim

- To achieve country wide elimination of Hepatitis C by 2030;
- Achieve significant reduction in the infected population, morbidity and mortality associated with Hepatitis B and C viz. Cirrhosis and Hepato-cellular carcinoma (liver cancer);
- Reduce the risk, morbidity and mortality due to Hepatitis A and E.

### Key Objectives

- Enhance community awareness on hepatitis and lay stress on preventive measures among general population especially high-risk groups and in hotspots.
- Provide early diagnosis and management of viral hepatitis at all levels of health care
- Develop standard diagnostic and treatment protocols for management of viral hepatitis and its complications.
- Strengthen the existing infrastructure facilities, build capacities of existing human resources and raise additional human resources, where required, for providing comprehensive services for management of viral hepatitis and its complications in all districts of the country.
- Develop linkages with the existing national programs towards awareness, prevention, diagnosis and treatment for viral hepatitis.
- Develop a web-based "Viral Hepatitis Information and Management System" to maintain a registry of persons affected with viral hepatitis and its sequelae.

### Components

#### Preventive Component

This is the cornerstone of the NVHCP. It includes:
- Awareness generation and behavior change communication
- Immunization of Hepatitis B (birth dose, high-risk groups, healthcare workers)
- Safety of blood and blood products
- Injection safety, safe sociocultural practices
- Safe drinking water, hygiene and sanitary toilets

#### Diagnosis and Treatment

- Screening of pregnant women for HBsAg to be done in areas where institutional deliveries are < 80% to ensure their referral for institutional delivery for birth dose Hepatitis B vaccination.
- Free screening, diagnosis and treatment for both hepatitis B and C would be made available at all levels of health care in a phased manner.
- Provision of linkages, including with private sector and not for profit institutions, for diagnosis and treatment.
- Engagement with community/peer support to enhance and ensure adherence to treatment and demand generation.

#### Monitoring and Evaluation, Surveillance and Research

Effective linkages to the surveillance system would be established and operational research would be undertaken through Department of Health Research (DHR). Standardized monitoring and evaluation framework would be developed and an online web based system is established.

#### Training and Capacity Building

This will be a continuous process and will be supported by NCDC (National Centre for Disease Control), ILBS (Institute of Liver and Biliary Sciences) and state tertiary care institutes and coordinated by NVHCP. The hepatitis induction and update programs for all level of health care workers would be made available using both, the traditional cascade model of training through master trainers and various platforms available for enabling electronic, e-learning and e-courses.

## INTEGRATED DISEASE SURVEILLANCE PROGRAM

National Surveillance Program for Communicable Diseases (NSPCD) was launched in 1997–98 in five districts. IDSP was launched in India in November 2004, which from 2012, has been named as Integrated Disease Surveillance Program and has been operating under NHM with 100% domestic budget. The program is coordinated by the National Center for Disease Control (NCDC).

### OBJECTIVE

To strengthen the disease surveillance in the country by establishing a decentralized state-based surveillance system for epidemic prone diseases to detect the early warning signals, so that timely and effective public health actions can be initiated in response to health challenges in the country at the district, state and national level.

### STRATEGIES

#### Decentralization of Surveillance Activities

Surveillance activities under IDSP are run through decentralized surveillance units at the district, state and central level, as shown in **Figure 47.19**.

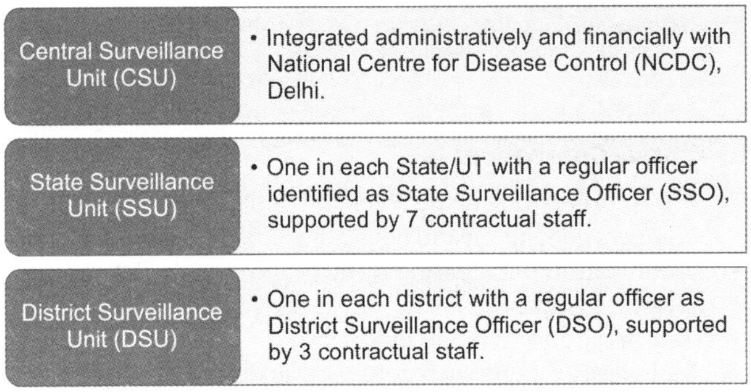

| | |
|---|---|
| Central Surveillance Unit (CSU) | • Integrated administratively and financially with National Centre for Disease Control (NCDC), Delhi. |
| State Surveillance Unit (SSU) | • One in each State/UT with a regular officer identified as State Surveillance Officer (SSO), supported by 7 contractual staff. |
| District Surveillance Unit (DSU) | • One in each district with a regular officer as District Surveillance Officer (DSO), supported by 3 contractual staff. |

**Fig. 47.19:** Decentralization of surveillance activities under Integrated Disease Surveillance Project (IDSP).

## Human Resource Development

The National Project Officer (NPO) coordinates the activities of the program at the CSU, through a team of staff of NCDC that includes epidemiologist, microbiologist, statistician, along with a team of contractual staff comprising of consultants, statistician, data manager, etc. The SSUs are run by state surveillance officers and DSUs by district surveillance officers. All the project officers and staff in both public and private sectors are trained on a regular basis. District Surveillance Officers are trained under the Field Epidemiology Training Program (FETP).

## Information and Communication Technology

A nation-wide information and communication technology (ICT) network was started under NCDC connecting all DSUs, SSUs, major Medical Colleges and CSU and an IDSP portal (www.idsp.nic.in) has been set up. A 24 × 7 call center was established in 2008 with a toll free number 1075 (1800-11-4377) where people can report disease alerts from anywhere across the country. The information received is provided to the SSUs/DSUs through e-mail and telephone for investigation and response.

## Data Management

Data on epidemic prone diseases is collected under IDSP on a weekly basis (Monday-Sunday) on prescribed formats from various reporting units. There are broadly three types of surveillance under IDSP, to be reported as follows:
- "S" (suspected cases) for syndromic surveillance to be reported by health worker, village volunteers or nonformal practitioners.
- "P" (presumptive cases) for presumptive surveillance reported by medical officer.
- "L" (laboratory confirmed cases) for laboratory surveillance.

The reporting units which are identified under IDSP for specific forms are:
- "S" form—Subcenter
- "P" form—PHC, CHC, other government hospitals and identified private hospitals
- "L" form—PHC labs, district public health labs, other government hospital labs, referral labs and identified private hospital labs.

**Table 47.17:** List of diseases under surveillance.

| Diseases under surveillance: Presumptive (P form) | Diseases under surveillance: laboratory confirmed (L form) |
|---|---|
| • Acute diarrheal disease (including acute gastroenteritis)<br>• Bacillary dysentery<br>• Viral hepatitis<br>• Enteric fever<br>• Malaria<br>• Dengue/DHF/DSS<br>• Chikungunya<br>• Acute encephalitis syndrome<br>• Meningitis<br>• Measles<br>• Diphtheria<br>• Pertussis<br>• Chickenpox<br>• Fever of unknown origin (PUO)<br>• Acute respiratory infection (ARI)/ influenza like illness (ILI)<br>• Pneumonia<br>• Leptospirosis<br>• Acute flaccid paralysis <15 years of age<br>• Dog bite<br>• Snake bite<br>• Any other state specific disease (Specify)<br>• Unusual syndromes NOT captured above (specify clinical diagnosis) | • Dengue/DHF/DSS<br>• Chikungunya<br>• JE<br>• Meningococcal meningitis<br>• Typhoid fever<br>• Diphtheria<br>• Cholera<br>• *Shigella* dysentery<br>• Viral hepatitis A<br>• Viral hepatitis E<br>• Leptospirosis<br>• Malaria |

(DHF: dengue hemorrhagic fever; DSS: dengue shock syndrome; JE: Japanese encephalitis).

*Source:* Integrated Disease Surveillance Programme" Ministry of Health and Family Welfare GOI; https://idsp.nic.in.

All the data collected are forwarded to DSUs and SSUs and compiled at CSU, and also made available in the IDSP portal on weekly basis. All outbreaks are investigated by the rapid response teams (RRT). There are 20 syndromes/diseases under surveillance **(Table 47.17)**.

## Laboratory Component

Laboratories also provide weekly data on the total number of samples tested and number of samples found positive. The laboratory form has 12 specific diseases and provision for reporting of any other disease.

## SUGGESTED READING

1. Central Leprosy Division. Guidelines of ASHA Based Surveillance for Leprosy Suspects, National Leprosy Eradication Programme, Central Leprosy Division, Ministry of Health and Family Welfare, Government of India, New Delhi.
2. Central Leprosy Division. National Leprosy Eradication Programme. Training Manual for Medical Officers 2013. Central Leprosy Division, Ministry of Health and Family Welfare, Government of India, New Delhi.
3. Central Leprosy Division. Operational Guidelines for Leprosy Case Detection Campaign, National Leprosy Eradication Programme, Central Leprosy Division, Ministry of Health and Family Welfare, Government of India, New Delhi.
4. Central Leprosy Division. Post Exposure Prophylaxis, National Leprosy Eradication Programme, Central Leprosy Division, Ministry of Health and Family Welfare, Government of India, New Delhi.
5. Central TB Division. RNTCP. National Strategic Plan for Tuberculosis Control 2017–2025. Central TB Division, DGHS, Ministry of Health and Family Welfare, Government of India, New Delhi.

6. Central TB Division. TB India 2016. Revised National Tuberculosis Control Programme. Annual Status Report. Unite to End TB. Central TB Division, DGHS, Ministry of Health and Family Welfare, Government of India, New Delhi.
7. Central TB Division. Technical and Operational Guidelines for TB Control in India 2016. Central TB Division, Ministry of Health and Family Welfare, Government of India, New Delhi.
8. Common Flow Chart for Leprosy and Kala-azar Workers. (2018). [online] Available from: http://nlep.nic.in/pdf/Common%20 Flow%20chart%20 for%20Leprosy%20and%20Kala%20Azar%20 workers.pdf.
9. Health Programmes/Wellness. National Health Portal of India [internet]. Nhp.gov.in. 2020. Available from: https://www.nhp.gov.in/healthprogramme/national-health-programmes.
10. MoHFW. Annual Report (2016–17), National AIDS Control Organization, Ministry of Health and Family Welfare, Government of India, New Delhi.
11. MoHFW. Japanese Encephalitis, Annual Report (2016–17), Ministry of Health and Family Welfare, Government of India, New Delhi.
12. MoHFW. Malaria in National Vector Borne Disease Control Programme. Annual Report 2016–17. Ministry of Health and Family Welfare, Government of India, New Delhi; pp. 56-61.
13. MoHFW. National Leprosy Eradication Programme, Annual Report (2016– 17). Ministry of Health and Family Welfare, Government of India, New Delhi.
14. MoHFW. National Leprosy Eradication Programme. Programme Implementation Plan (PIP) and Guidelines for Continuation of NLEP during 12th Plan Period (2012–13 to 2016–17). Ministry of Health and Family Welfare, Government of India, New Delhi.
15. MOHFW. Revised National Tuberculosis Control Programme. Annual Report 2018. Ministry of Health and Family Welfare, Government of India, New Delhi.
16. MOHFW. Yaws Eradication Programme. National Centre for Disease Control. Ministry of Health and Family Welfare, Government of India, New Delhi.
17. NACO. Antiretroviral Therapy Guidelines for HIV Infected Adults and Adolescents, May 2013. Department of AIDS Control, Ministry of Health and Family Welfare, Government of India, New Delhi.
18. NACO. HIV Sentinel Surveillance 2016–17 Technical Brief December 2017. National AIDS Control Organization, Ministry of Health and Family Welfare, Government of India, New Delhi.
19. NACO. Link Worker Scheme: Operational Guidelines April 2015. National AIDS Control Organization, Ministry of Health and Family Welfare, Government of India, New Delhi.
20. NACO. National AIDS Control Programme Phase IV (2012–2017): Strategy Document. Department of AIDS Control, Ministry of Health and Family Welfare, Government of India, New Delhi.
21. NACO. National Guidelines for HIV Testing, July 2015. National AIDS Control Organization, Ministry of Health and Family Welfare, Government of India, New Delhi.
22. NACO. National Guidelines on Prevention, Management and Control of Reproductive Tract Infections and Sexually Transmitted Infections. Department of AIDS Control, Ministry of Health and Family Welfare, Government of India, New Delhi.
23. NACO. National HIV Counseling and Testing Services (HCTS) Guidelines, December 2016, National AIDS Control Organization, Ministry of Health and Family Welfare, Government of India, New Delhi.
24. NACO. National Integrated Biological and Behavioral Surveillance (2014–15). National AIDS Control Organization, Ministry of Health and Family Welfare, Government of India, New Delhi.
25. NACO. National Strategic Plan for HIV/AIDS and STI 2017–24. December 2017. National AIDS Control Organization, Ministry of Health and Family Welfare, Government of India, New Delhi.
26. NACO. Post Exposure Prophylaxis (PEP) November 2015, National AIDS Control Organization, Ministry of Health and Family Welfare, Government of India, New Delhi.
27. NACO. Sankalak: Status of National AIDS Response December 2017. National AIDS Control Organization, Ministry of Health and Family Welfare, Government of India, New Delhi.
28. NACO. Updated Guidelines for Parent to Child Transmission (PPTCT) of HIV using Multi Drug Antiretroviral Regimen in India, December 2013, National AIDS Control Organization, Ministry of Health and Family Welfare, Government of India, New Delhi.
29. NCDC. (2018). Integrated Disease Surveillance Programme, India, [online]. National Centre for Disease Control, DGHS, MOHFW, GOI, New Delhi. Available from http://idsp.nic.in. [Last accessed January 2019].
30. NCDC. Eradicating Guinea Worm Disease, Indian scenario, National Centre for Disease Control, Ministry of Health and Family Welfare, Government of India, GOI, New Delhi.
31. NCDC. Guinea Worm Eradication Programme. National Centre for Disease Control, Ministry of Health and Family Welfare, Government of India, New Delhi.
32. NCDC. National Guidelines for Diagnosis, Case Management, Prevention and Control of Leptospirosis. 2015. National Centre for Disease Control, Ministry of Health and Family Welfare, Government of India, New Delhi.
33. NCDC. National Rabies Control Programme. National Centre for Disease Control Portal, DGHS, Government of India, New Delhi.
34. NICD. Yaws Eradication Programme in India, Programme Strategy and Operational Guidelines 1996, NICD, Ministry of Health and Family Welfare, Government of India.
35. NVBDCP. Elimination of Lymphatic Filariasis. Annual Report (2016–17). NVBDCP, Ministry of Health and Family Welfare, Government of India, New Delhi. pp. 70-2.
36. NVBDCP. Guidelines for Filaria Control in India and its Elimination 2009. NVBDCP, Ministry of Health and Family Welfare, Government of India, New Delhi.
37. NVBDCP. Long-term Action Plan for Prevention and Control of Dengue and Chikungunya 2007. Directorate of NVBDCP, DGHS, Ministry of Health and Family Welfare, Government of India, New Delhi.
38. NVBDCP. National Framework for Malaria Elimination in India (2016–2030). Directorate of National Vector Borne Disease Control Programme, Directorate General of Health Services, Ministry of Health and Family Welfare, Government of India, New Delhi.
39. NVBDCP. National Guidelines for Transmission Assessment Survey for Elimination of Lymphatic Filariasis India 014 (for District and State level health officials). NVBDCP, Ministry of Health and Family Welfare, Government of India, New Delhi.
40. NVBDCP. National Road Map for Kala-azar Elimination 2014. Directorate of NVBDCP, DGHS, Ministry of Health and Family Welfare, Government of India, New Delhi.
41. NVBDCP. Operational Guidelines. National Programme for Prevention and Control of Japanese/Acute Encephalitis Syndrome 2014. Directorate of NVBDCP, DGHS, Ministry of Health and Family Welfare, Government of India, New Delhi.
42. NVBDCP. Operational guidelines for Urban VBD Control Scheme 2016. Directorate of NVBDCP, DGHS, Ministry of Health and Family Welfare, Government of India, New Delhi.
43. NVBDCP. Operational Guidelines on Kala-azar Elimination in India 2015. Directorate of NVBDCP, DGHS, Ministry of Health and Family Welfare, Government of India, New Delhi.
44. NVBDCP. Strategic Plan for Malaria Control in India 2017–2022. Directorate of NVBDCP, DGHS, Ministry of Health and Family Welfare, Government of India, New Delhi.
45. Planning Commission. Report of the Working Group on Disease Burden for the 12th Five-Year Plan, Planning Commission, GOI, pp. 194–7.
46. Planning Commission. Report of the Working Group on Disease Burden for the 12th Five Year Plan, Planning Commission, Government of India, pp. 202-12.
47. Preparatory activities for Post Exposure Prophylaxis (PEP). (2019). [online] Available from: http://www.nlep.nic.in/pdf/OG_PEP_FF. pdf.
48. WHO. (2015). The End TB Strategy. Global strategy and targets for tuberculosis prevention, care and control after 2015. WHO, Geneva. [online] Available from: http://www.who.int/tb/post2015_TBstrategy.pdf.
49. WHO. (2017). Rabies Vaccines and Immunoglobulins: WHO Position Summary of 2017 Updates 2018. [online] Available from: http://apps.who. int/iris/bitstream/handle/10665/259855/WHO-CDS-

NTD-NZD-2018.04-eng. pdf;jsessionid=4CA0B3A5230D7DA8D321B158107CEBF5?sequence=1.
50. WHO and Stop TB Partnership. (2006). The Stop TB Strategy 2006. [online] WHO, Geneva. Available from http://www.who.int/tb/publications/2006/stop_tb_strategy.pdf.
51. World Bank. Integrated Disease Surveillance Project, India, World Bank Joint Implementation Review Mission Reports. Available from: http:// www.worldbank.org/projects/P073651/inte-grated-disease-surveillance- project?lang=enandtab=overview.

## ERADICATION STRATEGIES FOR VARIOUS COMMUNICABLE DISEASES

### ERADICATION OF POLIOMYELITIS

In 1988, when the World Health Assembly declared its commitment to eradication and the Global Polio Eradication Initiative (GPEI) was formed in pursuit of this goal, there were 350,000 annual cases of WPV in 125 countries. By the end 2018, only 33 cases were identified—all from two neighboring countries (Afghanistan and Pakistan).

India achieved polio elimination certification in March 2014 after maintaining polio-free status for 3 years since the last case of wild polio in 2011. On 27 March 2014 the South-East Asia Region of WHO was declared polio-free and was the fourth WHO region to achieve this status. The strategies adopted for polio eradication involve universal immunization and included RI with coverage level of more than 90%; supplementary immunization (Pulse Polio Immunization) conducted country-wide on a single day on National Immunization Days (NID) and in selected districts at high risk of polio transmission on Sub-National Immunization Days (sNID); enhanced surveillance of Acute Flaccid Paralysis (AFP); targeted mop-up campaigns.

### Polio Endgame Strategy 2019–2023 (Fig. 47.20)

The *Polio Eradication and Endgame Strategic Plan* (PEESP) addressed the GPEI program period from 2013 to 2018. It identified four objectives towards the goal of achieving eradication: (1) to detect and interrupt all poliovirus transmission; (2) to strengthen immunization systems and withdraw OPV; (3) to contain poliovirus and certify the interruption of transmission; and (4) to begin to plan for the responsible transition of the polio eradication effort.

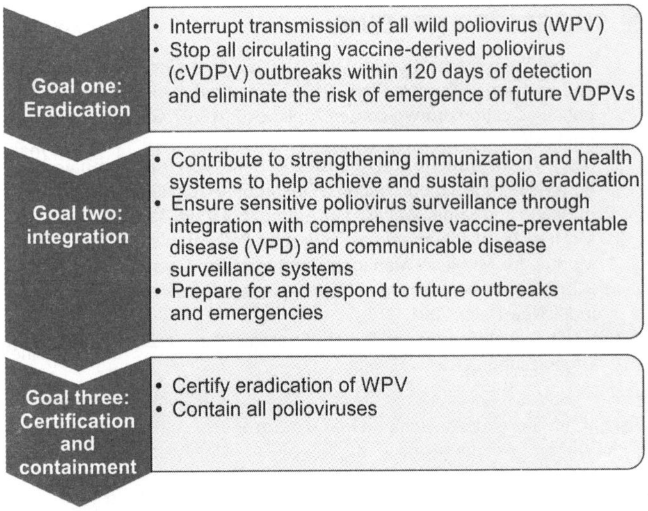

Under the PEESP, the GPEI achieved many remarkable successes:
- Wild poliovirus type 2 (WPV2) declared eradicated in 2015;
- Wild poliovirus type 3 (WPV3) last reported in November 2012, giving high confidence that global circulation has ceased;
- Overall reduction in wild poliovirus type 1 (WPV1) cases since 2013:
  - No WPV detection anywhere outside of the three endemic countries since 2014;
  - No WPV detection outside of Afghanistan/Pakistan since 2016; and
- Major circulating vaccine-derived poliovirus type 2 (cVDPV2) out-break in the Syrian Arab Republic controlled despite ongoing war.

The *Polio Endgame Strategy 2019–2023* is not intended to supersede the *Polio Eradication and Endgame Strategic Plan* (PEESP), as the four objectives and the core strategies to achieve eradication have proven effective around the world. Rather, the current strategy offers a review of what activities should continue, what improvements will be implemented, and what innovations will be introduced to ensure that the GPEI successfully addresses the risks to eradication.

The strategy also supports the *Strategic Action Plan on Polio Transition* and provides a bridge to the *Polio Post-Certification Strategy* (PCS). As such, it lays the groundwork for both the transition currently under way in polio-free countries and the post-certification period of a polio-free world yet on the horizon.

The current challenges faced by India are the risk of international importation of wild polio virus and subsequent spread from neighboring countries and the development of circulating vaccine derived polio virus (cVDPV). To maintain polio-free status activities to continue are maintaining immunity by both supplementary immunization activities (SIA) and enhanced RI; annual seroprevalence surveys to determine immunity levels; AFP surveillance; continued environmental surveillance; immunization of travelers.

### EFFORTS TO ELIMINATE MEASLES

The Global Measles and Rubella Strategic Plan 2012–2020 aims at elimination of measles and rubella. The goal of the strategic plan was to reduce the global measles mortality at least by 95% compared with 2000 estimates and achieve regional measles and rubella/CRS elimination goals by the end of 2015; and to achieve measles and rubella/congenital rubella syndrome (CRS) elimination in at least five WHO regions by the end of 2020. The

**Goal one: Eradication**
- Interrupt transmission of all wild poliovirus (WPV)
- Stop all circulating vaccine-derived poliovirus (cVDPV) outbreaks within 120 days of detection and eliminate the risk of emergence of future VDPVs

**Goal two: integration**
- Contribute to strengthening immunization and health systems to help achieve and sustain polio eradication
- Ensure sensitive poliovirus surveillance through integration with comprehensive vaccine-preventable disease (VPD) and communicable disease surveillance systems
- Prepare for and respond to future outbreaks and emergencies

**Goal three: Certification and containment**
- Certify eradication of WPV
- Contain all polioviruses

Fig. 47.20: Goals of the *Polio Endgame Strategy 2019–2023*.
*Source:* WHO.

Measles–Rubella (MR) 2020 program had the goal to eliminate measles by 2020, but due to the COVID-19 outbreak, it was revised to 2023.

India targeted a vaccination coverage of 95% with two doses of MR vaccine to achieve measles and rubella elimination by 2023. Measures that have strengthened India's MR elimination strategy include the development and implementation of the National Strategic Plan for MR elimination; introduction of rubella-containing vaccine into the routine immunization program; launching a nationwide MR supplementary immunization catch-up campaign; transitioning from outbreak-based surveillance to case-based acute fever and rash surveillance; expansion of MR Laboratory network to 27 labs across the country and implementation of the roadmap plan for MR elimination across the country.

### Roadmap to Measles and Rubella Elimination in India by 2023

The roadmap is for charging and enabling each district to set goals towards achieving at least 95% MRCV2 coverage by age 2 years, or at the latest age 5 years and achieving and maintaining sensitive fever and rash surveillance.

### Goal

Achieving and Sustaining Measles and Rubella Elimination in India

### Strategies

- Achieve and maintain high population immunity with at-least 95% vaccination coverage of two doses of measles and rubella containing vaccine in every district of every state of India. Ensure that all children receive MRCV2 by 24 months of age and that missed doses are provided up to 5 years of age, with two doses given 4 weeks apart. Vaccination card retention should be promoted.
- Sustain a sensitive and timely case-based Fever and Rash and Congenital Rubella Syndrome (CRS) surveillance.
- Ensure adequate outbreak preparedness and respond rapidly to measles and rubella outbreaks. IV. Developing and maintaining a proficient laboratory network.
  - Building capacity of laboratory network for existing and new methodologies to support surveillance program
  - Strengthening the laboratory network for high quality of MR diagnosis (serology and virology)
  - Under the MR campaign, the MR vaccine is to be introduced targeting all children from 9 months to <15 years, irrespective of their prior vaccination status and history of measles/rubella illness, to be completed in 3-4 weeks' time. Subsequently, the MR vaccine will be introduced in the RI, replacing the two doses of measles vaccine.

In case of a measles outbreak, investigation and control measures should be initiated simultaneously by immunization of children in the neighboring PHCs/districts and vitamin A to eligible children, along with management of diarrhea and ARI cases following measles.

## ELIMINATION OF MATERNAL AND NEONATAL TETANUS

Maternal and neonatal tetanus elimination (MNTE) in India, i.e., less than one case of neonatal tetanus per 1,000 live births across the entire country, was achieved in May 2015. The strategies used for elimination were:

- Increase and sustain high coverage levels with two doses or a booster dose of TT in pregnant women
- Increase proportion of deliveries by trained personnel; intensify skilled birth attendants' training
- Supply DDKs to ensure clean practices for domiciliary deliveries
- Implement essential newborn care, including cord care, to reduce risks of neonatal tetanus
- Strengthen surveillance system and undertake follow-up action in areas from where cases are reported
- Continue IEC activities in the community to promote clean deliveries with special focus in areas from where cases have been reported and in areas where the proportion of deliveries by untrained personnel is high.

## SUMMARY

Health policies and programs play a major role in prevention and control of public health problems, in respect of major diseases and their determinants. With enormous efforts many public health achievements have been successful, beginning from eradication of Smallpox to disease free status of Guinea worm and Yaws, elimination of maternal and neonatal tetanus, and most recently South-East Asia Region being declared free of polio. The journey is ongoing and many more diseases have been taken up or are under consideration for eradication/elimination/control, which are also expected to show landmark achievements in the near future.

## SUGGESTED READING

1. Global Polio Eradication Initiative. (2013). Fact File: Polio Eradication and Endgame Strategic Plan 2013–18. [online] Available from: http://polioeradication.org/wp-content/uploads/2016/07/GPEI_Plan_FactFile_EN-1.pdf.
2. MoHFW. Introduction of Measles-Rubella Vaccine (Campaign and Routine Immunisation). National Operational Guidelines 2017. Ministry of Health and Family Welfare, Government of India, New Delhi.
3. MoHFW. Special Programmes for Vaccine Preventable Diseases, Training Module for Mid-level Managers, Immunisation Strengthening Project; RCH Programme, Ministry of Health and Family Welfare, Government of India, New Delhi; 2001.
4. WHO. Global Measles and Rubella Strategic Plan 2012–20. World Health Organization; 2012

# PROGRAMS FOR NONCOMMUNICABLE DISEASES

## NATIONAL PROGRAMME FOR PREVENTION AND CONTROL OF NON-COMMUNICABLE DISEASES

National Programme for Prevention and Control of Cancer, Diabetes, Cardiovascular Diseases, and Stroke (NPCDCS) was launched in 2010 which was merged with the ongoing National Cancer Control Programme to form the NPCDCS in 2011-12. The program aimed at controlling the common modifiable risk factors for cancer, cardiovascular diseases and diabetes (tobacco use, unhealthy diet, physical inactivity, and harmful use of alcohol); promoting healthy lifestyles, early diagnosis, and disease management. In the last few years, many new diseases or disease groups have been added to NPCDCS such as nonalcoholic fatty liver, chronic kidney disease, ST-elevation myocardial infarction (STEMI), etc. To this effect, NPCDCS has been renamed by MoHFW in May 2023 as **"National Programme for Prevention and Control of Non-Communicable Diseases (NP-NCD)"**.

### OBJECTIVES

- Prevent and control common NCDs through behavior and lifestyle changes.
- Provide early diagnosis and management of common NCDs.
- Build capacity at various levels of healthcare for prevention, diagnosis and treatment of common NCDs.
- Train human resource within the public health set up, viz. doctors, paramedics and nursing staff, to cope with the increasing burden of NCDs.
- Establish and develop capacity for palliative and rehabilitative care.
- Support for development of database of NCDs through surveillance system and to monitor NCD morbidity, mortality and risk factors.

### MANAGEMENT STRUCTURE

NP-NCD is implemented through the national, state and district NCD cells, which are responsible for overall planning, implementation, monitoring and evaluation of the different activities at their respective levels, under the program **(Fig. 47.21)**.

The program is to be implemented through existing public health infrastructure and systems by establishment of NCD clinic at CHCs and district level, trained manpower and strengthening of tertiary level health facilities. The NP-NCD program has two components, viz. (1) cancer (2) diabetes, cardiovascular diseases (CVDs), stroke and other newly added diseases. All the activities at state, districts, CHC and subcenter level will be planned under the program and will be closely monitored through NCD cell at different levels **(Fig. 47.22 and Table 47.18)**.

| National NCD division | • Program-in-charge (MoHFW) and identified DGHS Officers<br>• Operational guidelines, monitoring and evaluation, training, capacity building |
|---|---|
| State NCD division | • State Program Officer (NCD) and identified DHS Officers<br>• State action plan, develop information on NCDs, training and capacity building, monitoring, raise public awareness |
| District NCD division | • District Program Officer (NCD) and Officers of District health system<br>• District action plan, district database of NCDs, program implementation, training and capacity building |

Fig. 47.21: Management structure of NP-NCD (National Programme for Prevention and Control of Non-Communicable Diseases)

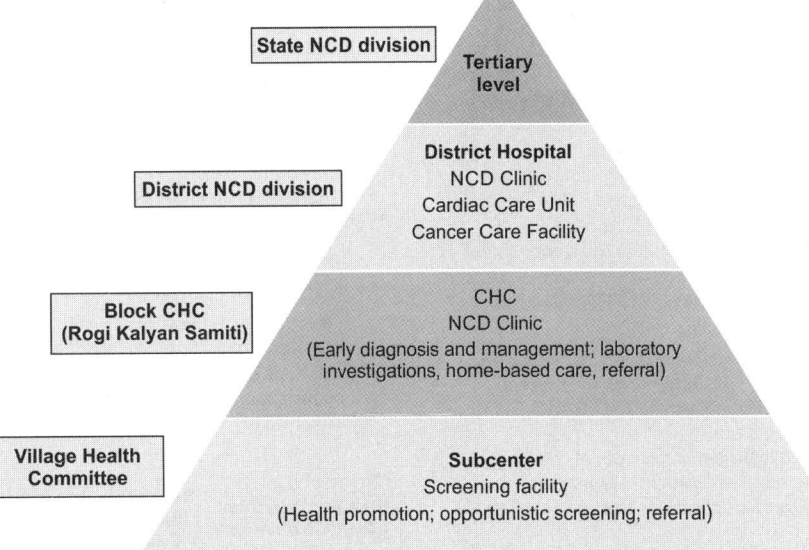

Fig. 47.22: Management structure of noncommunicable disease (NCD) cell.
(CHC: community health center)

**Table 47.18:** Packages of services to be made available at different levels under NP-NCD (National Programme for Prevention and Control of Non-Communicable Diseases).

| Level | Services |
|---|---|
| Community level | • Active enumeration of the eligible population and registration of the families, risk assessment of NCDs using community based assessment checklist (CBAC), mobilization of community for screening of NCDs at nearest AB-HWC<br>• Health promotion, lifestyle modification, follow up for treatment compliance and lifestyle modification |
| Subcentre/ SHC-HWC | • Health education for awareness generation and behavior change, organising wellness activities<br>• Screening of diabetes, hypertension, three common cancers (oral, breast and cervical)<br>• Referral of suspected cases to PHC/PHC-HWC or nearby health facility for diagnosis confirmation and management. SHC-HWC team to also facilitate the referrals and follow up on referred suspected patients<br>• Dispensing of prescribed medicines and follow up of patient for treatment compliance and lifestyle modification<br>• Teleconsultation services from SHC-HWC to HWC-PHC/UPHC<br>• Maintaining electronic health records (EHR) and generation of ABHA IDs |
| PHC/PHC-HWC/ UPHC-HWC | • Health promotion activities including wellness activities for behavior change<br>• Screening of diabetes, hypertension, three common cancers (oral, breast and cervical), COPD and asthma, CKD, NAFLD among OPD attendees<br>• Confirmation of diagnosis, treatment initiation, and management of common NCDs as per standard management protocol and guidelines<br>• Referral of complicated NCD cases to higher facilities. Bi-directional referral linkages to be established and follow up to be ensured<br>• Teleconsultation services and counselling services<br>• Maintaining electronic health records (EHR) and generation of ABHA IDs |
| CHC/SDH | • Health promotion including counselling<br>• Opportunistic screening of diabetes, hypertension, three common cancers (oral, breast and cervical)<br>• Screening of COPD and asthma, CKD, NAFLD, STEMI among suspected cases<br>• Confirmation of diagnosis, treatment initiation, and management of common NCDs as per standard management protocol and guidelines<br>• Teleconsultation services and counselling services<br>• Maintaining electronic health records (EHR) and generation of ABHA IDs<br>• Management of cases of common NCDs and regular follow-up<br>• Referral of complicated cases to District Hospital/ higher healthcare facility |
| District Hospital | • Opportunistic screening of diabetes, hypertension, three common cancers (oral, breast and cervical)<br>• Screening of COPD and asthma, CKD, NAFLD, STEMI among suspected cases<br>• Diagnosis and management of cases of common NCDs: outpatient and inpatient care, including emergency care particularly for cardiac and stroke cases<br>• Management of complicated cases of common NCDs, or referral to higher healthcare facility |
| | • Follow-up cancer chemotherapy and palliative care services for cancer cases, physiotherapy services for NCDs including stroke patients, dialysis facilities for CKD patients, etc<br>• Health promotion for behavior change and counselling for NCD cases. IEC activities on important Health Days<br>• Bidirectional referral linkages and follow up mechanism to be established and ensured<br>• Teleconsultation services and counselling services<br>• Maintaining electronic health records (EHR) and generation of ABHA IDs |
| Medical College/ Tertiary Cancer Centers | • Diagnosis and management of complicated cases of common NCDs acts as tertiary referral facility<br>• Comprehensive cancer care including prevention, early detection, diagnosis, treatment, palliative care and rehabilitation at Tertiary Cancer Centers<br>• Support program in capacity building of health staff<br>• Support program in preparing standard guidelines and protocols<br>• Support in supervision, monitoring, evaluation and operational research<br>• Bidirectional referral linkages and follow up mechanism to be established and ensured<br>• Teleconsultation services and counselling services<br>• Maintaining electronic health records (EHR) and generation of ABHA IDs |

## STRATEGIES (FIG. 47.23)

Following are the strategies of the program:
- Health promotion for prevention of NCDs and reduction of risk factors.
- Screening, early diagnosis, management, referral and follow up of common NCDs.
- Capacity building of healthcare providers.
- Evidence based standard treatment protocols.
- Uninterrupted drug and logistics supply.
- Task sharing and people-centered care.
- Information system for data entry, longitudinal patient records.
- Monitoring, supervision, evaluation and surveillance including technology enabled interventions.

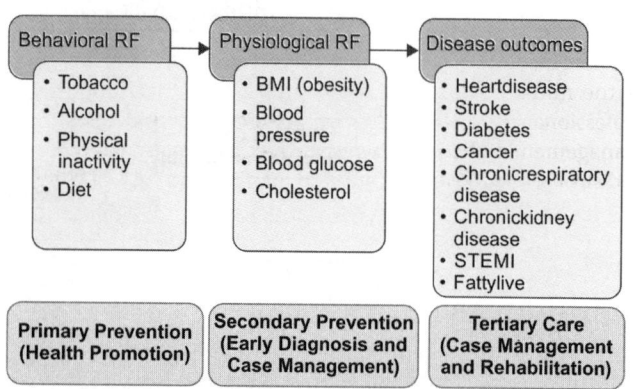

**Fig. 47.23:** Level of noncommunicable diseases (NCD) prevention and management.

- Multi-sectoral coordination and linkages with other National Programmes.
- Implementation research and generation of evidences.

### Health Promotion

Modification of the behavioral risk factors, viz., tobacco use, unhealthy diet, physical inactivity and harmful use of alcohol through promotion of healthy lifestyle, is the mainstay of preventing the common NCDs. The common messages for behavior change are aimed at intake of healthy diet with restriction of salt and saturated fats, regular moderate to vigorous physical activity, prohibition of smoking and alcohol intake, reduction of obesity, stress management, and awareness about early warning signs of cancer.

### Early Diagnosis

Early detection of NCDs by means of screening before the appearance of symptoms is important to prevent advanced disease and disability. Screening for NCDs is done by means of two strategies:

- *Opportunistic screening:* It will be done in population aged 30 years and above attending any level of healthcare facility for hypertension, diabetes mellitus and common cancers (breast, cervical and oral). All suspected cases from the periphery will be referred to district hospitals or tertiary care centers.
- *Population-based screening:* It will be done for hypertension, diabetes mellitus, and the three common cancers among all men and women aged 30 years and above by peripheral health workers. ASHAs will use a community-based assessment checklist for screening the NCDs. ANMs and staff nurses will be trained in oral visual examination (OVE), clinical breast examination (CBE), and visual inspection using acetic acid (VIA). All suspected cases will be referred to higher centers. Follow-up screening will be done every year for hypertension and diabetes mellitus and every 5 years for cancers.

### Treatment

Treatment for NCDs, along with other services, is available at PHC, CHC, district hospitals, tertiary care hospitals, and tertiary cancer centers.

### Capacity Building of Human Resource

National Institute of Health and Family Welfare has been identified as the nodal agency under the program, for training health professionals on health promotion, prevention, early detection and management of diabetes, hypertension, cardiovascular diseases and stroke, and in cancer care, and management of CCU.

### Newer Initiatives

Some new initiatives included in the program are as follows:
- **Observance of NCD Week/Fortnightly (Swasth Nagrik Saptah/Pakhwada):** Observance of World Stroke Day, i.e., 29th October, National Cancer Awareness Day, i.e., 7th November and World Diabetes Day, i.e., 14th November every year.
- **m-Health Strategies:** m-Diabetes and m-Cessation interventions.
- **K4H:** Knowledge for health for NCDs.
- Advocacy and network with people living with NCDs (PLNCDs)
- Linkages with other programs: Joint TB-diabetes collaborative activities, National Programme for Palliative care (NPPC), Integration with National Urban Health Mission (NUHM), National Oral Health Programme (NOHP), National Tobacco Control Programme (NTCP), National Programme for Health Care of Elderly (NPHCE), National Programme for Control of Blindness and Visual Impairment (NPCB and VI), National Mental Health Programme (NMHP, Ayushman Bharat—Pradhan Mantri-Ayushman Bharat Health Infrastructure Mission (PM-ABHIM), Ayushman Bharat-PM-JAY Rashtriya Bal Swasthya Karyakram (RBSK), Rashtriya Kishor Swasthya Karyakram (RKSK), Rashtriya Arogya Nidhi (RAN) and with AYUSH for utilizing Yoga, Homeopathy, Ayurveda, and Unani as interventions for NCD control.

## FINANCIAL MANAGEMENT

Financial management groups (FMG) of program management support units at state and district level, which are established under NRHM, will be responsible for maintenance of accounts, release of funds, expenditure reports, utilization certificates and audit arrangements.

State NCD cell will submit monthly statement of expenditure in the prescribed format to the SHS and national NCD cell. The funds will be released to states/UTs under two separate components of the NP-NCD, i.e., (1) cancer and (2) diabetes, cardiovascular diseases and stroke (DCS) through the SHS to carry out the activities at different levels. Funds released from state to DHS would include the funds for CHCs and subcenters to cover the entire district.

## NATIONAL CANCER REGISTRY PROGRAMME

The National Cancer Registry Programme (NRCP) was started in 1982 by ICMR. There are two types of registries: Population-based cancer registry and hospital-based cancer registry. There are 29 population-based and 7 hospital-based cancer registries in the country.

# NATIONAL PROGRAMME FOR HEALTH CARE OF THE ELDERLY

National Programme for Health Care of the Elderly (NPHCE) was launched in 2010 during the eleventh plan period in 100 districts of 21 states, in order to address the health-related problems in elderly people in the country and was expanded to other districts in a phased manner during the twelfth plan.

The elementary objective of the NPHCE is to offer distinct, specialized and comprehensive healthcare to the elderlies at various healthcare delivery system level including services through outreach approach. The program is funded and its enactment is supervised by the MoHFW, Government of India. After initial thrust to fully implement the program all over the country, the responsibility of running the program will be on the State Governments. Through this initiative, the elderly person gets free, specialized health care facilities through the state health care delivery system. Initially the program was launched in 100 selected districts but over a period of time more districts have been added to provide geriatric out-patient department (OPD), in-patient department (IPD) and physiotherapy and laboratory services. Presently out of the 716 districts of the country the program has already been sanctioned in 600 districts of 36 states or union territories (UTs). 20 medical colleges have established RGCs. Both NCAs (National Centres for Ageing) are in various stages of development.

> **The vision of the NPHCE is:**
> - To provide accessible, affordable, and high-quality long-term, comprehensive and dedicated care services to an aging population
> - Creating a new "architecture" for aging
> - To build a framework to create an enabling environment for "a society for all ages"
> - To promote the concept of active and healthy aging
> - Convergence with National Rural Health Mission (NRHM), AYUSH and other departments like Ministry of Social Justice and Empowerment

## OBJECTIVES

- To provide an easy access to promotional, preventive, curative and rehabilitation services to the elderly, through community-based primary healthcare approach.
- To identify health problems among the elderly and provide appropriate health interventions in the community, with a strong referral back up support.
- To build capacity of the medical and paramedical professionals as well as caretakers within the family, for providing health care to the elderly.
- To provide referral services to the elderly patients through district hospitals and regional medical institutions.

The program has three components:
1. Dedicated primary care through district hospital, community health center (CHC), primary healthcare center (PHC), subcenter (SC).
2. Secondary and tertiary care through RGCs at selected medical colleges
3. Centers of excellence—National Centers for Aging—AIIMS Delhi and Madras Medical College, Chennai.

## CORE STRATEGIES

- *Preventive and promotive care:* The preventive and promotive healthcare services such as regular physical exercise, balanced diet, stress management, avoidance of smoking or tobacco products and prevention of fall, etc. are provided by expanding access to health practices through domiciliary visits by trained health workers. They will impart health education to the elderly and their caregivers. Besides, regular monitoring and assessment for any infirmity or illness by organizing weekly clinic at PHCs. Community-based primary healthcare approach including domiciliary visits by trained healthcare workers.
- *Management of illness:* Dedicated outdoor and indoor patients services have been developed at PHCs, CHCs, district hospitals (dedicated 10 bedded ward) and RGCs for management of chronic and disabling diseases by providing central assistance to the state governments.
- *Health manpower development for geriatric services:* To overcome the shortage of trained medical and paramedical professionals in geriatric medicine, in service training through specific modules developed for training of medical officers, nurses and community-based workers is being conducted. Postgraduate (PG) course–MD (geriatric medicine) which is presently imparted through four medical colleges (two private and two governments) is targeted to be initiated at all RGCs.
- *Medical rehabilitation and therapeutic intervention:* By arranging therapeutic modalities like therapeutic exercises, training in activities of daily life (ADL) and treatment of pain and inflammation through physiotherapy unit at CHC, district hospital and RGC levels for which necessary infrastructure, medicine and equipment have been provided to these identified units.
- *Information, education and communication (IEC):* Health education programs using mass media, folk media and other communication channels are being promoted to reach out to the target community for promoting the concept of healthy aging, importance of physical exercise, healthy habits, and reduction of stress. Camps for regular medical check-up are being organized at various levels where IEC activities are also specifically promoted.
- Continuous monitoring and independent evaluation of the program and research in geriatrics.
- *Longitudinal Ageing Study of India (LASI):* 2016 is a long-term study being carried out by International Institute for Population Sciences (IIPS) Mumbai along with international partners to assess medical and social characteristics of Indian elderly. The study follows 60,000 individuals across 36 states or UTs for at least 5 years and is proposed to extend to 25 years.

## SUPPLEMENTARY STRATEGIES

- Promotion of PPP in geriatric health care.
- Mainstreaming AYUSH, revitalizing local health traditions and convergence with programs of Ministry of Social Justice and Empowerment in the field of geriatrics.
- Reorienting Medical Education to support geriatric issues.

NPHCE is implemented at various levels of healthcare under the NP-NCD framework. There are two National Centers for Ageing (NCA), at AIIMS New Delhi and Madras Medical College, Chennai, which provide specialized geriatric care through a 200 bedded facility along with training of professionals and undertaking research activities. Geriatric clinics at several superspeciality medical college hospitals have 30 beds for geriatric care. Geriatric units at district hospitals, CHCs and PHCs and activities related to geriatric health at subcenters, form the remaining tiers of NPHCE service delivery.

Given below are the various levels of implementation of the program and the activities carried out at each level of health care. The monitoring and supervision of the program is done by the state and district NCD cells. The expenditure is shared by central and the state government on 80:20 basis.

***Subcenter:*** Services provided at the subcenter include domiciliary visits by ANM/male health care workers to home bound/bedridden elderly persons and provide training to the family care providers in looking after them; health education related to healthy ageing; providing suitable calipers and supportive devices from the PHC to the elderly persons to make them ambulatory.

***PHC (in select 100 districts):*** Weekly geriatric clinic run by a trained medical officer conducting routine health assessment of the elderly persons; provision of medicines; maintenance of records; public awareness on different aspects of geriatrics; referral for diseases when needed, to CHC or district hospital.

***CHC/FRU for the elderly from PHCs and below:*** Geriatric clinic for the elderly twice a week; rehabilitation unit for physiotherapy; domiciliary visits by the rehabilitation worker for bedridden elderly; referral of difficult cases to district hospital/higher healthcare facility.

***District hospital:*** Geriatric clinic for regular dedicated OPD services to the elderly; 10-bedded geriatric ward for inpatient care of the elderly; facilities for laboratory investigations; provision of medicines for geriatric patients; existing health care services to continue; conducting camps for geriatric services in PHCs/and other sites; referral services for severe cases to tertiary level hospitals.

***Regional geriatric centers:*** These are located in the department of medicine in 15 selected medical institutions of the country. Services provided include geriatric clinic (specialized OPD for the elderly) 30 bedded geriatric ward for inpatient care and dedicated beds for the geriatric patients in various specialties; laboratory investigations for elderly; tertiary health care for cases referred from medical colleges, district hospitals, and lower health facilities **(Fig. 47.24)**.

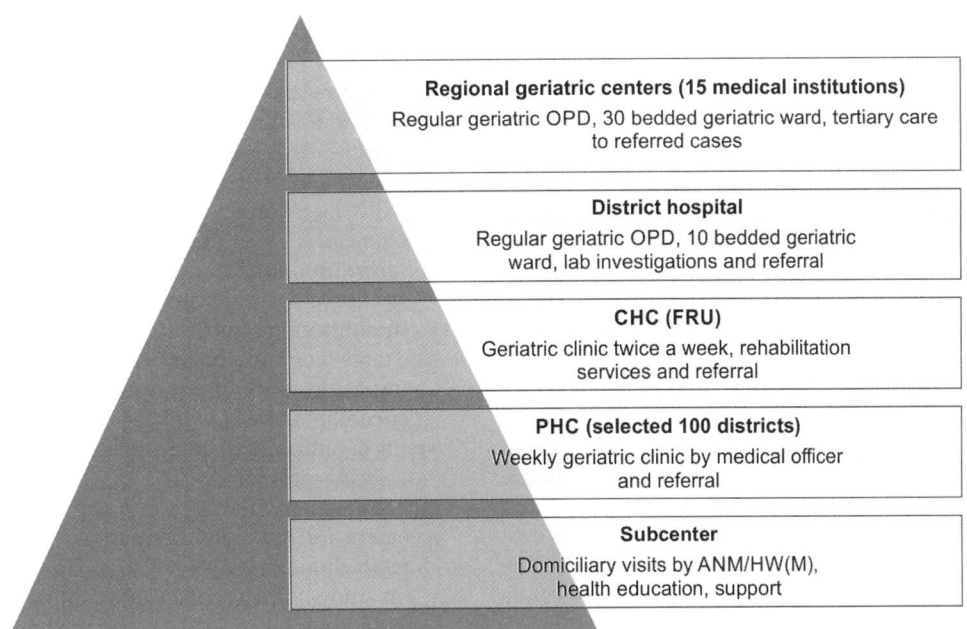

**Fig. 47.24:** Healthcare delivery under NPHCE (National Program for Health Care of the Elderly).
(ANM: auxiliary nursing midwife; CHC: community health center; FRU: first referral unit; PHC: primary health center)

## NATIONAL TOBACCO CONTROL PROGRAMME

The National Tobacco Control Programme was launched in 2008-09, for implementation of The Cigarettes and Other Tobacco Products (Prohibition of Advertisement and Regulation of Trade and Commerce, Production, Supply and Distribution) Act (COTPA) of 2003, in response to the WHO Framework Convention on Tobacco Control guidelines. It was initially started in 18 districts of 9 states and gradually up-scaled to operate in all states of India.

### OBJECTIVES

- To bring greater awareness about the harmful effects of tobacco use and tobacco control laws.

- To facilitate effective implementation of the tobacco control laws.

## COMPONENTS

The activities under the program are carried out at various levels of health care as follows:

*National level:* Campaigns to create public awareness against tobacco; establishing tobacco testing laboratories; integration of the program with NHM; research and training on alternative crops and livelihoods; monitoring and evaluation of the program, including surveillance.

*State level:* Dedicated tobacco control cells for anti-tobacco activities; training of stakeholders; state level campaigns to create public awareness against tobacco; integrating tobacco control with other health programs and activities; monitoring enforcement of tobacco control laws and reporting.

*District level:* Training of stakeholders; local IEC activities; school awareness programs; tobacco cessation centers (TCC); monitoring enforcement of tobacco control laws.

*Block level:* Block development committee meetings twice a year with tobacco control as special agenda; orientation and sensitization of the elected representatives and officials; organizing awareness campaigns, in synergy with the NCD programs; activities for tobacco free schools and offices in the block.

*Village level:* Developing an annual village action plan towards making the village tobacco free; sensitization of village level officials, Gram Panchayat members and community-based organizations about health hazards of tobacco use; organizing special IEC campaigns involving school children; special meetings of Gram Sabha for sensitizing villagers on laws against tobacco use; reporting violations of COTPA; developing tobacco control volunteers in every village (at least one per village).

Tobacco cessation centers are located in health facilities and carry out activities for tobacco cessation. They are usually located in medical colleges, dental colleges, specialty hospitals, private hospitals, district hospitals, CHCs, PHCs, subcenters, DOTS centers, etc. The manpower situated in the TCC can be any health care professional with training on tobacco cessation. ANMs and counselors can also be trained to provide tobacco cessation services. Only medical practitioners can carry out pharmacological interventions. Tobacco cessation activities include behavioral counseling along with pharmacologic approach, if necessary.

## MANAGEMENT STRUCTURE

Management structure of the program is depicted in the **Figure 47.25**.

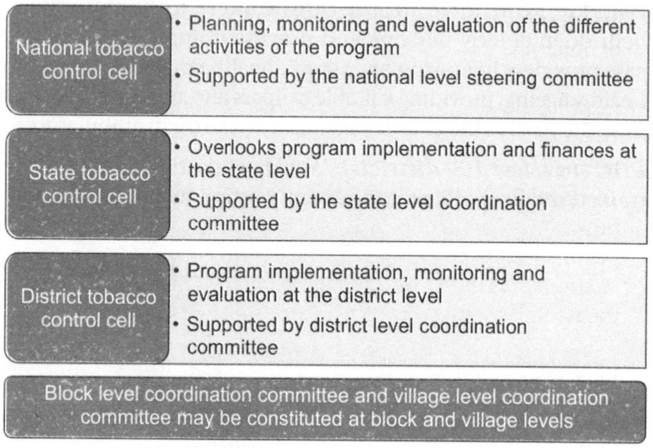

| | |
|---|---|
| National tobacco control cell | • Planning, monitoring and evaluation of the different activities of the program<br>• Supported by the national level steering committee |
| State tobacco control cell | • Overlooks program implementation and finances at the state level<br>• Supported by the state level coordination committee |
| District tobacco control cell | • Program implementation, monitoring and evaluation at the district level<br>• Supported by district level coordination committee |
| Block level coordination committee and village level coordination committee may be constituted at block and village levels | |

Fig. 47.25: Management structure of NTCP (The National Tobacco Control Programme).

## DRUG DE-ADDICTION PROGRAMME

Drug de-addiction measures can broadly be divided into supply reduction activities and demand reduction activities. The supply reduction activities, which aim at reducing the availability of illicit drugs, come under the purview of Ministry of Home Affairs and Ministry of Revenue and include raising taxes and imposing ban on illicit drugs. Demand reduction measures deal with awareness generation, treatment and rehabilitation of drug using patients and is dealt with by Ministry of Health and Family Welfare.

The National Drug De-Addiction Programme was launched in 1987 and modified in 1992 and had the following objectives:
- Demand reduction by providing treatment services including preventive health care and after care.
- To develop human resources for providing treatment to addicts.
- To improve quality of services and delivery.
- To secure participation of the local government body/institution. The National Drug Dependence Treatment Centre (NDDTC) was established in Ghaziabad under AIIMS, New Delhi with 50 beds, offering both inpatient and outpatient services for drug-dependent people. Drug de-addiction centers were established in NIMHANS, Bengaluru; PGI, Chandigarh; Dr. RML Hospital, New Delhi; JIPMER, Puducherry; and Smt. SK Hospital, New Delhi. Currently 122 drug de-addiction centers are operational across the country.

In 2014 the National Policy for Drug Demand Reduction was formulated under Ministry of Social Justice and Empowerment, under two broad areas—illicit drugs and pharmaceutical and chemical preparations. The policy has the following objectives:
- To undertake drug demand reduction efforts.
- To create awareness and educate people about the ill-effects of drugs abuse.
- To provide for a range of community-based services.
- To alleviate the consequences of drug dependence.
- To facilitate research, training, documentation and collection of relevant information.
- To develop human resources and build capacity.
- To ensure that stigmatization and discrimination of individuals' dependent on drugs is actively discouraged.

## NATIONAL PROGRAMME FOR PREVENTION AND CONTROL OF DEAFNESS

The National Programme for Prevention and Control of Deafness (NPPCD) was launched in 2007 to tackle the burden of preventable hearing loss through all levels of prevention. Most common causes of preventable childhood deafness are infections, complications at the time of birth and use of ototoxic medicines. Other causes that affect at any age are injury, noise induced hearing loss and wax in the external ear canal.

### GOAL

To prevent and control major causes of hearing impairment and deafness, so as to reduce the total disease burden by 25% of the existing burden, by the end of twelfth five-year plan.

### OBJECTIVES

- To prevent the avoidable hearing loss on account of disease or injury.
- Early identification, diagnosis and treatment of ear problems responsible for hearing loss and deafness.
- To medically rehabilitate persons of all age groups, suffering from deafness.
- To develop institutional capacity for ear care services by providing support for equipment, material and training of personnel.
- To strengthen the existing intersectoral linkages for continuity of the rehabilitation program, for persons with deafness.

### LEVELS OF PREVENTION OF HEARING LOSS

- *Primary prevention:* Immunization against measles, mumps and rubella; treatment of upper respiratory infections; appropriate breast feeding practices, treatment for antenatal infections like syphilis and toxoplasmosis, genetic counseling, careful use of ototoxic drugs, protection against loud noise.
- *Secondary prevention:* Screening for early detection and treatment; surgery.
- *Tertiary prevention:* Hearing aids and cochlear implants.

### STRATEGIES

- Strengthening of the service delivery including rehabilitation.
- Human resource development for ear care.
- Promoting outreach activities and public awareness through appropriate and effective IEC strategies with special emphasis on prevention of deafness.
- Developing institutional capacity of the district hospitals, CHCs and PHCs.

### COMPONENTS OF THE PROGRAM

- *Prevention through behavior change communication:* Awareness generation through different channels of communication regarding prevention of hearing loss and seeking prompt treatment.
- *Capacity building:* This includes training of health professionals at various levels of health care, provision of specialists and equipment for diagnosis and treatment, stepping up rehabilitation and hearing aid provision, screening for hearing impairment and referral to appropriate higher centers.
- Monitoring and supervision at state and central levels.
- Public private partnership.
- Operational research and evaluation.

## NATIONAL PROGRAMME FOR CONTROL OF BLINDNESS AND VISUAL IMPAIRMENT

The National Programme for Control of Blindness was launched in 1976 as a continuation of National Programme for Trachoma control when causes of preventable blindness other than trachoma came into focus. In 2017, it was redesignated as National Program for Control of Blindness and Visual Impairment and the definition of blindness was modified by WHO to "presenting distance visually acuity less than 3/60 (20/4,000) in the better eye and limitation of field of vision to be less than 10 degrees from the center of fixation".

### GOAL

To reduce the prevalence of blindness to 0.3% by 2020. According to the National Blindness and Visual Impairment Survey 2015-2019, prevalence of blindness in all age groups is 0.36% and that of visual impairment is 2.55%.

### OBJECTIVES AND TARGETS

- To reduce the backlog of blindness through identification and treatment of blind at primary, secondary and tertiary levels based on assessment of the overall burden of visual impairment in the country.
- To continue three ongoing signature activities under NPCB:
  - Performance of 66 lakhs cataract surgeries per year;
  - School eye screening and distribution of 9 lakhs free spectacles per year to school children suffering from refractive errors;
  - Collection of 50,000 donated eyes per year for keratoplasty.
- Develop and strengthen the strategy of NPCB for "Eye Health" and prevention of visual impairment; through provision of comprehensive eye care services and quality service delivery.
- Strengthening and upgradation of Regional Institutes of Ophthalmology (RIO) to become center of excellence in various subspecialties of ophthalmology and also other partners like medical college, district hospital, subdistrict hospital, vision center, NGO eye hospital.
- Strengthening the existing infrastructure facilities and developing additional human resources for providing high quality comprehensive eye care in all districts of the country.
- To enhance community awareness on eye care and lay stress on preventive measures.
- Increase and expand research for prevention of blindness and visual impairment.

- To secure participation of voluntary organizations/private practitioners in delivering eye care.

## ACTIVITIES

The main activities under the program are:
- Cataract surgery by intraocular lens (IOL) implantation
- School eye screening and free spectacles to school children
- Eye banking and free keratoplasty
- Eye care education
- Diagnosis and treatment of diabetic retinopathy, glaucoma, childhood blindness
- Training of eye surgeons, paramedical ophthalmic assistants.

## IMPLEMENTATION OF THE PROGRAM

Decentralization of the program is done through the District Blindness Control Societies (DBCS) which, along with the State Blindness Control Societies (SBCS), are responsible for implementation of program activities in the states and districts. The SBCS and DBCS are merged with state and district health societies respectively under the NHM.

The functions of the DBCS include planning and implementation of the program activities through government and private sector, involvement of NGOs and community participation; monitoring and quality control; financial and material management; social mobilization and creating public awareness; orientation and training of health functionaries; arrangement of screening and cataract surgery camps; and monitoring and providing financial assistance to eye banks and eye donation centers.

## VISION 2020: THE RIGHT TO SIGHT

It aims to reduce avoidable (preventable and curable) blindness by 2020 in India as well as globally. It targets six diseases, i.e., cataract, refractive errors, childhood blindness, corneal blindness, glaucoma and diabetic retinopathy. The infrastructure for implementation includes a four-tier structure comprising 20 COE for laying of standards, research and training; 200 training centers for retinal and corneal surgeries and training; 2,000 service centers for common eye surgeries, and 20,000 vision centers for primary eye care **(Fig. 47.26)**.

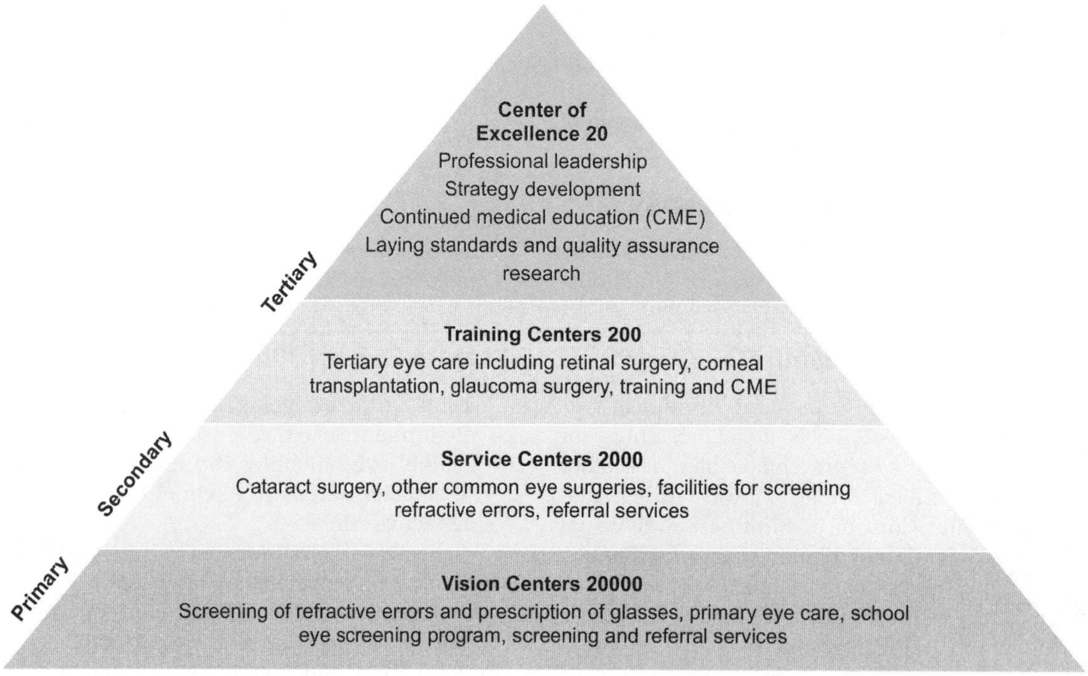

**Fig. 47.26:** Proposed structure for Vision 2020.

## NATIONAL MENTAL HEALTH PROGRAMME

The National Mental Health Programme was started in 1982 with the aim of making minimum mental healthcare available and accessible to all, by integrating mental health with primary health care services. In 1996, a community-based approach named District Mental Health Programme (DMHP) was started under the National Mental Health Programme (NMHP) to decentralize mental health services and to provide mental health service at the community level by integrating mental health with the general healthcare delivery system. It was launched on a pilot basis in Karnataka and in four districts in Andhra Pradesh, Tamil Nadu, Assam and Rajasthan by NIMHANS, Bengaluru. It provided training in basic mental health care, proposed the formation of mental health team at the district level, provided essential psychotropic drugs, and ensured review of the program every month at the district level during monthly meetings with Medical Officer Primary Health Centers (MO-PHCs).

The NMHP was re-strategized in the year 2003 (in X Five Year Plan) with the following components:
- Extension of DMHP to 100 districts
- Up gradation of psychiatry wings of government medical colleges/general hospitals
- Modernization of state mental hospitals
- IEC
- Monitoring and evaluation

## DISTRICT MENTAL HEALTH PROGRAMME (DMHP)

The District Mental Health Programme (DMHP) started as a component of the NMHP with the following objectives:
- Provision of comprehensive mental healthcare services at community settings.
- Defining strategies for promotion of mental health and prevention of illness.
- Conducting IEC activities for stigma reduction and community participation.
- Integration of mental health with general health services.
- Strengthening of information system and research.
- Special focus on underprivileged section of the society.

DMHP envisages provision of basic mental healthcare services at the community level:
- **Service provision:** Provision of mental health out-patient and in-patient mental health services with a 10 bedded inpatient facility.
- Out-reach component:
  - Satellite clinics: 4 satellite clinics per month at CHCs/PHCs by DMHP team
  - Targeted interventions:
    ♦ Life skills education and counselling in schools,
    ♦ College counselling services,
    ♦ Work place stress management, and
    ♦ Suicide prevention services
- **Sensitization and training of health personnel:** At the district and sub-district levels
- **Awareness camps:** For dissemination of awareness regarding mental illnesses and related stigma through involvement of local PRIs, faith healers, teachers, leaders, etc.
- Community participation:
  - Linkages with self-help groups, family and caregiver groups and NGOs working in the field of mental health
  - Sensitization of enforcement officials regarding legal provisions for effective implementation of Mental Health Act.

The team of workers at the district under the program consists of a psychiatrist, a clinical psychologist, a psychiatric social worker, a psychiatry/community nurse, a program manager, a program/case registry assistant and a record keeper. **Up gradation of psychiatry wings of government medical colleges/general hospitals**

Every medical college should ideally have a department of psychiatry with minimum of three faculty members and inpatient facilities of about 30 beds as per the norms laid down by the Medical Council of India. The aim of the scheme is to strengthen the training facilities for Under-Graduates and Post-Graduates at psychiatry wings of government medical colleges/hospitals. The grant covers construction of new ward, repair of existing ward, procurement of items like cots, tables and equipments for psychiatric use such as modified ECTs.

The DMHP envisages a community-based approach to the problem, which includes:
- Training of mental health team at identified nodal institutions.
- Increase awareness and reduce stigma related to mental health problems. Promote community participation in the mental health service development and to stimulate efforts towards self-help in the community.
- Provide service for early detection and treatment of mental illness in the community (OPD/Indoor and follow up.
- Increase access to preventive services to the population at risk, in particular, addressing the risk of suicide and attempted suicide.
- Inform the person with mental illness, their caregivers, professionals and other stakeholders of the rights of persons with mental illness and ensure that rights are respected during the provision of care and services.
- Broad base mental health into other related programs such as RCH, Sarva Shiksha Abhiyan (SSA), work place intervention and similar programs.
- Ensure a motivating and empowering work place for staff by allowing an opportunity to improve their skills and recognition of their work.
- Improve the infrastructure for mental health service delivery.

## ORGANIZATION OF MENTAL HEALTH SERVICES

National Mental Health Programme is implemented through the following organizational structure.

### Day Care Centre

- Provides rehabilitation and recovery services to persons with mental illness so that the initial intervention with drug and psychotherapy is followed up and relapse is prevented.
- Helps in enhancing the skills of the family/caregiver in providing better support care.
- Provides opportunity for people recovering from mental illness for successful community living.

### Residential/Long-Term Continuing Care Centre

- Chronically mentally ill individuals, who have achieved stability with respect to their symptoms and have not been able to return to their families and are currently residents of the mental hospitals, will be shifted to these centers.
- Residential patients in these centers will go through a structured program which will be executed with the help of multidisciplinary team consisting of psychologists, social workers, nurses, occupational therapists, vocational trainers and support staff.

**District level:** Specialist psychiatry services are available in the form of mental health teams for consultation of referred cases, occupational therapy, behavioral therapy, training, research, supervision, medical education and development.

### Community Health Centers

- Outpatient services and inpatient services for emergency psychiatry patients and counseling services.
- **PHC level:** The medical officer-PHC is to oversee outpatient services, counseling services in accessing social care benefits and pro-active case findings and mental health promotion activities
- **Village level:** The multipurpose worker and health supervisor refer mental health cases to the PHC, conduct counseling for alcohol and drug abuse victims, follow up cases undergoing treatment, liaison with parents for management of mentally ill children, etc.

### Tertiary Level Activities

#### Manpower Development Schemes

- **Centers of Excellence in Mental Health:** Up- gradation of 10 existing mental hospitals/institutes/Medical Colleges will be taken-up to start/strengthen courses in psychiatry, clinical psychology, psychiatric social work and psychiatric nursing.
- **PG Training Departments of Mental Health facilities:** Government Medical Colleges/Government Mental Hospitals will be supported for starting/increasing intake of PG courses in Mental Health.

## MENTAL HEALTH POLICY

It was launched in October 2014 to promote mental health, prevent mental illnesses, enable recovery, and ensure socioeconomic inclusion of persons affected by mental illness, by providing accessible, affordable and quality health and social care to all persons through their life-span, within a rights-based framework. The goal is to reduce stress, disability, exclusion, morbidity and premature mortality associated with mental health problems.

## MENTAL HEALTHCARE ACT 2017

This Act provides for mental healthcare and services for persons with mental illness and protects, promotes, and fulfills the rights of such persons during delivery of mental healthcare and services. It requires central and state governments to establish central and state mental authority as well as Mental Health Review Board.

## NATIONAL ORAL HEALTH PROGRAMME

The National Oral Health Policy was drafted in 1995 by the Indian Dental Association, to address the issue of oral health. Following this, a pilot project on oral health was initiated in 1999 with AIIMS, New Delhi as the nodal agency. The NOHP was approved in the twelfth five-year plan for implementation in 200 districts in the country. The program runs under the national, state and district oral health cells, in liaison with the existing NCD cells.

### OBJECTIVES

- To improve the determinants of oral health, e.g., oral hygiene, diet, etc., and to reduce disparity in oral health accessibility in rural and urban population.
- To reduce morbidity from oral diseases by strengthening oral health services at subdistrict/district hospital, to start with.
- To integrate oral health promotion and preventive services with general healthcare system and other sectors that influence oral health, namely various National Health Programs.
- To encourage promotion of PPPs model for achieving better Public Health goals.

### STRATEGIES

- IEC/BCC to create public awareness on oral hygiene, prevention of oral health problems, dietary counseling, prevention of tobacco use, early identification of oral diseases and referral, oral health screening of children in schools, etc.
- Training of healthcare staff at all levels.
- Human resources including dental surgeons, dental hygienist, and dental assistants.
- Logistic support including dental chairs with supportive equipment and consumables.
- Program management by the oral health cells.
- Monitoring, supervision and evaluation of the program.

### PROGRAM IMPLEMENTATION

The program functions at two levels—(1) activities up to district level under NHM, (2) tertiary level activities at state and central levels.

- *NHM component:* Dental unit at health facilities (district level and below) with the following components: Manpower support (dentist, dental hygienist, dental assistant); equipment, including dental chair; consumables for dental procedures.
- *Tertiary component:* At tertiary level health care facilities, include the following activities: Designing IEC materials; organizing national/regional nodal officers' training programs; preparing state/district level trainers by conducting workshops, to train the paramedical health functionaries associated in health care delivery.

## NATIONAL PROGRAMME ON PREVENTION AND MANAGEMENT OF BURN INJURIES

A pilot program was initiated by MoHFW in six districts of three states in 2010 to ensure prevention of burn injuries, provide timely and adequate treatment in case burn injuries do occur, reduce mortality, complications and ensuing disabilities, and provide effective rehabilitative interventions, if disability has set in. In 2014, the National Program on Prevention and Management of Burn Injuries (NPPMBI) was approved to be expanded to another 67 state government medical colleges and 19 district hospitals.

### OBJECTIVES

- To reduce incidence, mortality, morbidity and disability due to burn injuries.
- To improve awareness among the general masses and vulnerable groups especially the women, children, industrial and hazardous occupational workers.
- To establish adequate infrastructural facility and network for BCC, burn management, and rehabilitation interventions.
- To carry out research for assessing behavioral, social and other determinants of burn injuries in our country for effective need-based program planning for burn injuries, monitoring, and subsequent evaluation.

### COMPONENTS

Components of the program include: (1) Prevention program (IEC); (2) Treatment; (3) Rehabilitation; (4) Training; (5) Monitoring and evaluation; (6) Research.

The program will be currently implemented in the designated burns units of 70 state government medical colleges and 25 district hospitals. Operational guidelines for establishment of burns units have been finalized along with list of equipment, manpower and architectural design required, along with a practical manual on burn injury management. A burns data registry along with software has been developed to collect, compile, and analyze burns data. Training of manpower and research on burn injuries has also been started.

## NATIONAL SICKLE CELL ANAEMIA ELIMINATION PROGRAM

An estimated 7% of the world's population carries an abnormal hemoglobin gene, while about 300,000–500,000 are born annually with significant hemoglobin disorders. They consist of two major groups: Thalassemia and Sickle cell syndromes. Sickle cell syndromes are more frequent and constitute 70% of affected births worldwide. Sickle Cell Disease (SCD) is a hemoglobin disorder that requires lifelong management and contributes to infant, childhood as well as adult morbidity and mortality. SCD, as a genetic condition, is widespread among the tribal population in India where about 1 in 86 births among STs have SCD. At present there is no permanent cure for the disease. However, with good management of the disease, severity, and complications can be curtailed to improve the quality of life and life span of the people suffering from the disease. With this focus, The National Sickle Cell Anaemia Elimination Program, was introduced in the Union Budget 2023, focuses on addressing the significant health challenges posed by sickle cell disease, particularly among tribal populations of the country.

### GOAL

Eliminate sickle cell disease as a public health problem in India before 2047.

### OBJECTIVES

- Provision of affordable, accessible, and quality care to all SCD patients.
- To reduce the prevalence of SCD and sickle cell trait.

### STRATEGIC PILLARS

- **Primary prevention strategies:**
  - Primary prevention strategies focus on awareness generation and premarital and preconceptional counselling to prevent the conception of a child with homozygous genotype.
  - Prevention requires setting up genetic counselling and testing interventions in high prevalence districts to prevent sickle cell disease in the offspring. Genetic counselling and health promotion activities can lead to substantial reduction in the number of children born with the disease.
  - Widespread community involvement and support are essential as there are existing diversity of cultures and opinions about a number of issues relevant to genetics, such as human reproduction issues.
- **Secondary prevention and screening:** Secondary prevention focuses on the following components related to early diagnosis and care of sickle cell disease.
  - Screening for detection of sickle cell trait to reduce the birth of children affected with sickle cell disease and screening for early detection of sickle cell disease to achieve a reduction in mortality and morbidity with improvement in quality of life of the affected.
- **Holistic management and continuum of care**
  - Management of persons with sickle cell disease at primary, secondary, and tertiary health care levels
  - Advanced diagnostic and treatment modalities at tertiary health care facilities
  - Integration with AYUSH
  - Patient support system
  - Community Adoption
  - Rehabilitation

The program shall be carried out in a mission mode covering the entire population from zero to 40 years of age. In the first year the priority will be given to population between zero to eighteen years of age which will be followed by screening of the entire population up to 40 years of age in the second and third year. The program shall be a part of the National Health Mission and shall focus on universal population-based screening, prevention, and management of sickle cell disease in all tribal and other highly prevalent areas of India. A targeted approach for screening may be adopted in nontribal districts based on prevalence of the Sickle Cell Disease as assessed during routine facility-based testing of antenatal mothers in the 1st trimester, at the primary health care facilities in the State. The program would be integrated with existing mechanisms and strategies under NHM to ensure the utilization of existing resources and also minimize the duplication of efforts. For example, the established platform of Rashtriya Bal Swasthya Karyakram (RBSK), Pradhan Mantri Surakshit Matritva Abhiyan (PMSMA), and Anemia Mukt Bharat would be leveraged to achieve the targets for the Sickle Cell mission.

## SICKLE CELL CARDS

Every individual who is screened for SCD will be provided a sickle cell card. The card will show the status of the individual viz, normal, carrier or diseased. The cards are color coded separately for male (blue) and female (pink). Based on the card's status, the individual will receive treatment and counselling services. Counsellors at the primary health care centers shall be using sickle cell cards for the purpose of premarital and pre-conceptional counselling by matching the cards of prospective matches. Matching of the cards will show the chances of their children being born with SCD or SCT.

## TELE MEDICINE FACILITY

At AB-HWCs, roll-out of telemedicine services through e-Sanjeevani-HWC will be strengthened. Specialists at e-Sanjeevani-HWC Telemedicine hubs shall be trained on all aspects of SCD. Ministry of Tribal Affairs in collaboration with ICMR/AIIMS or similar reputed institutes would open a Helpline and also facilitate Tele Medicine facility at center of excellences for sickle cell disease. Public awareness regarding both variants of e-Sanjeevani application viz., e-Sanjeevani HWC and e-Sanjeevani OPD shall be undertaken.

## INTEGRATION OF AYUSH IN SICKLE CELL DISEASE CARE

Yoga is an integral component of comprehensive primary healthcare provided through Ayushman Bharat Health and Wellness Centres (AB-HWC). Ministry of AYUSH, Ministry of Health and Family Welfare, Ministry of Tribal Affairs in coordination shall support epigenetic and clinical research on the role of Yoga in the prevention and cure of sickle cell disease complications.

## SUGGESTED READING

1. ICMR. (2018). National Cancer Registry Programme, National Centre for Disease Information and Research, ICMR, Government of India. [online]. Available from http://www.ncrpindia.org/. [Last accessed January 2019].
2. MoHFW. (2018). National Programme for Control of Blindness. Ministry of Health and Family Welfare, Government of India, New Delhi. [online] Available from: http://npcb.nic.in/. [accessed January 2019].
3. MoHFW. Drug De-Addiction Programme, Annual Report (2010–11), Ministry of Health and Family Welfare, Government of India, New Delhi.
4. MoHFW. Drug De-Addiction Programme. Report of Working group for the 11th Five Year Plan. Ministry of Health and Family Welfare, Government of India, New Delhi.
5. MoHFW. National Mental Health Programme, Annual Report (2015–16). Ministry of Health and Family Welfare, Government of India, New Delhi.
6. MoHFW. National Oral Health Programme, Annual Report (2014–15), Ministry of Health and Family Welfare, Government of India, New Delhi.
7. MoHFW. National Oral Health Programme, Annual Report (2016–17), Ministry of Health and Family Welfare, Government of India, New Delhi.
8. MoHFW. National Programme for Control of Blindness, Annual Report (2015–16), Ministry of Health and Family Welfare, Government of India, New Delhi.
9. MoHFW. National Programme for Control of Blindness, Annual Report (2016–17), Ministry of Health and Family Welfare, Government of India, New Delhi.
10. MoHFW. National Programme for Prevention and Control of Cancer, Diabetes, Cardiovascular diseases and Stroke (NPCDCS). Ministry of Health and Family Welfare, Government of India, New Delhi. Last updated on 13.07.2017.
11. MoHFW. National Programme for Prevention and Control of Cancer, Diabetes, Cardiovascular diseases and Stroke, Annual Report (2016–17), Ministry of Health and Family Welfare, Government of India, New Delhi.
12. MoHFW. National Programme for Prevention and Control of Cancer, Diabetes for Prevention and Control of Cancer, Cardiovascular diseases and Stroke: Broad Guidelines, 2013. Ministry of Health and Family Welfare, Government of India, New Delhi.
13. MoHFW. National Programme for Prevention and Control of Deafness (NPPCD), Operational Guidelines for 12th Five-Year Plan, Ministry of Health and Family Welfare, Government of India, New Delhi.
14. MoHFW. National Programme for Prevention and Control of Deafness, Annual Report (2016–17), Ministry of Health and Family Welfare, Government of India, New Delhi.
15. MoHFW. National Programme for the Health Care of the Elderly, Annual Report (2016–17), Ministry of Health and Family Welfare, Government of India, New Delhi.
16. MoHFW. National Programme for the Health Care of the Elderly. Operational Guidelines 2011–12, Ministry of Health and Family Welfare, Government of India, New Delhi.
17. MoHFW. National Programme on Prevention and Management of Burn Injuries, Annual Report (2015–16), Ministry of Health and Family Welfare, Government of India, New Delhi.
18. MoHFW. National Tobacco Control Cell, MoHFW, GOI. National Tobacco Control Programme, Operational Guidelines 2012. Ministry of Health and Family Welfare, Government of India, New Delhi.
19. MoHFW. National Tobacco Control Programme, Annual Report (2016–17). MoHFW, GOI, New Delhi.
20. MoHFW. New Pathways New Hope. National Mental Health Policy of India. October 2014. Ministry of Health and Family Welfare, Government of India, New Delhi.
21. MoHFW. Tobacco Control Legislation and National Tobacco Control Programme, Annual Report (2011–12), MoHFW, GOI, New Delhi.
22. MoLJ. The Mental Health Care Act, 2017. The Gazette of India, Ministry of Law and Justice, Government of India, New Delhi.
23. MoSJE. National Policy for Drug Demand Reduction, 2014. Policy, Ministry of Social Justice and Empowerment, Government of India, New Delhi.
24. Planning Commission. Twelfth Plan. District Mental Health Programme: Policy Group DMHP dated 29 June 2012. Planning Commission, Government of India, New Delhi.
25. WHO. (2013). Universal Eye Health: A Global Action Plan 2014–2019 [online] Available from http://www.who.int/blindness/AP2014_19_English.pdf.
26. WHO. (2017). Deafness and hearing loss. [online] Available from: http://www.who.int/mediacentre/factsheets/fs300/en/. [Last accessed January 2019].

# NUTRITION-RELATED PROGRAMS

Nutrition is the most important direct determinant of health and hence a major focus of welfare measures. To combat the problem of malnutrition several measures are being taken, at the outset of which lies the National Nutrition Policy formulated in 1993 and most recently the National Nutrition Mission (NNM) established in 2017. There are several national programs to combat both macro- and micronutrient deficiency in the vulnerable sections of the population. *National Nutrition Policy has been discussed at the beginning of this chapter.*

## NATIONAL NUTRITION MISSION (POSHAN ABHIYAAN)

National Nutrition Mission, also named as POSHAN that stands for "PM's Overarching Scheme for Holistic Nourishment," was launched in March 2018 in Jhunjhunu district of Rajasthan. The NNM, as an apex body under Ministry of Women and Child Development, will monitor, supervise, and targets to reduce level of under-nutrition, stunting, anemia (among young children, women and adolescent girls) and low birth rate by ensuring convergence of various nutrition related schemes.

### Goal

The goal of NNM is to improve nutritional status of children (0–6 years), adolescent girls, pregnant and lactating mothers in a time bound manner during the next three years, with the following targets:
- Prevent and reduce stunting in children (0–6 years) @ 2% per annum
- Prevent and reduce undernutrition in children (0–6 years) @ 2% per annum
- Reduce low birth weight @ 2% per annum
- Reduce the prevalence of anemia among children, adolescent girls and women (15-49 years) @ 3% per annum.

### Components

- *Information Communication Technology Enabled Real Time Monitoring of Schemes (ICT-RTM):* It includes mobile application for field functionaries preloaded on mobile phones and a dashboard for desktops to be used at block, state and national level. It enables collection of information on Anganwadi service delivery and its impact on nutrition outcomes of beneficiaries on a regular basis. This information is available to the States/UTs and MWCD on real time basis on web-based dashboards. A mobile application for AWWs is also made available for recording daily AWC activities, registration of beneficiaries, and sending daily photographs to ensure delivery of services.
- *Training and capacity building:* Capacity enhancement of frontline functionaries has been planned through "incremental learning by doing approach" (ILA) which has been structured across 21 modules and will be implemented in states/UTs at the following levels—(1) State resource groups (SRG)—Quarterly; (2) District resource groups (DRG)— Quarterly; (3) Block resource groups (BRG)—Monthly; (4) Sector level (AWWs)—Monthly.
- *Community mobilization and behavior change communication:* It will include (1) community-based events (CBE) for critical milestones in the 1,000 days period; (2) IEC and advocacy to support nutrition behavior change; and (3) *Jan Andolan* to improve nutrition by various activities involving participation of children at AWCs, delivering nutrition messages through folk songs, cultural activities, promoting yoga at AWCs, display of nutrition promotional messages at AWCs, SMS to beneficiaries, etc.
- *Innovation:* Funds will be earmarked for the development and implementation of innovations and pilots, particularly showing the convergent nutrition action to achieve one or more desirable nutritional results. The successful pilots may be taken up later on for scaling up on a broader platform.
- *Performance incentives:* The Mission intends to give annual monetary incentives to states/UTs which achieve the goals in improving the nutritional status of the targeted beneficiaries. Cash awards will be given to frontline functionaries such as AWW, ASHA, ANM for achieving desired targets and/or contributing significantly in other child health and development activities reducing the level of undernutrition.
- *Flexi activities:* A separate flexi-fund has been created which will be available to the state/UT for utilization at its discretion to address specific regional needs.

### Events Under POSHAN Abhiyaan

*Community Based Events (CBE):* In order to strengthen processes for community engagement, empowerment of beneficiaries and behavioral change towards better nutrition, CBEs will be organized twice per month (8th and 22nd) by each Anganwadi Centre and supported with an amount of ₹ 250/- each. Under Community Based Events, Annaprashan Diwas, Suposan Diwas (specifically focused on orienting husbands), celebrating coming of age-getting ready for pre-school at AWC, messages related to public health for improvement of nutrition and to reduce illness, importance of hand-wash and sanitation, prevention of anemia, importance of nutritious food, diet diversity etc. will be covered.

*Village Health Sanitation Nutrition Day (VHSND)* is conducted regularly on 15th of the month in convergence with Health Department of Gram Panchayat.

### Jan Andolan

Since the launch of POSHAN Abhiyaan in March 2018, these events have helped in reaching out to communities through the nation's biggest nutrition-centric annual Jan Andolans. The month of September is celebrated as Rashtriya Poshan Maah across the country. Similarly, in/around March every year, Poshan Pakhwada is celebrated.

### Monitoring and Implementation

The National Council on India's Nutritional Challenges will: (1) Provide policy directions to address India's nutritional challenges through coordinated intersectoral action; (2) Coordinate and review convergence between Ministries; and (3) Review programs for nutrition on a quarterly basis. An Executive Committee will report to the National Council on India's Nutrition Challenges and will be the apex body for nutrition related activities providing guidance for implementation of various programs/schemes under the NNM.

It is aimed to initiate convergent action plans at state, district, and block levels and through Village Health Sanitation and Nutrition Day (VHSND) at village level, to achieve synergy and desired results.

## Poshan 2.0

It is an Integrated Nutrition Support Programme initited in 2022 by aligning the Supplementary Nutrition Programme under Anganwadi Services, Scheme for Adolescent Girls and Poshan Abhiyaan. It seeks to address the challenges of malnutrition in children, adolescent girls, pregnant women and lactating mothers through a strategic shift in nutrition content and delivery and by creation of a convergent ecosystem to develop and promote practices that nurture health, wellness and immunity.

Poshan 2.0 shall focus on Maternal Nutrition, Infant and Young Child Feeding Norms, Treatment of MAM/SAM and Wellness through AYUSH. It will rest on the pillars of Convergence, Governance, and Capacity-building. Poshan Abhiyan will be the pillar for Outreach and will cover innovations related to nutritional support, ICT interventions, Media Advocacy and Research, Community Outreach and Jan Andolan.

It focuses to reduce wasting and under-weight prevalence besides stunting and anemia, supported by the *'Poshan Tracker'*, a new, robust ICT centralized data system which is being linked with the RCH Portal (Anmol) of MoHFW. The POSHAN Tracker will enable real-time monitoring and tracking of all AWCs, AWWs and beneficiaries on defined indicators.

With a view to address various gaps and shortcomings in the on-going nutrition program and to improve implementation as well as to accelerate improvement in nutrition and child development outcomes, the existing scheme components have been re-organized under Poshan 2.0 into the primary verticals given below:
- Nutrition Support for POSHAN through Supplementary Nutrition Programme (SNP) for children of the age group of 06 months to 6 years, pregnant women and lactating mothers (PWLM); and for Adolescent Girls in the age group of 14 to 18 years in Aspirational Districts and North Eastern Region (NER);
- Early Childhood Care and Education (3-6 years) and early stimulation for (0–3 years);
- Anganwadi Infrastructure including modern, upgraded Saksham Anganwadi; and
- Poshan Abhiyaan.

For leveraging convergence for food and nutrition, **POSHAN Vatikas** (kitchen gardens and nutri-gardens) shall be set up at or near Anganwadi Centres, wherever possible and in Government led schools and Gram Panchayat lands where benefits can easily be provided to women and children.

## Saksham Anganwadi

Under Saksham Anganwadi, 2 lakh AWCs @ 40,000 AWCs per year shall be strengthened, upgraded and rejuvenated across the country for improving nutrition delivery including Poshan Vatikas for stimulating the creative, social, emotional, cognitive and intellectual development of children under 6 years of age in convergence with education development programs, providing/adding more services with better infrastructure including internet/wifi connectivity, LED screens, water purifier/installation of RO machine and Early Childhood Care and Education with smart learning aids, audio-visual aids, child-friendly learning equipment and art work (educational painting, practice board for children, information board), etc.

# INTEGRATED CHILD DEVELOPMENT SERVICES SCHEME

The ICDS scheme was launched in 1975 as a pilot project in 33 districts. In the sixth five-year plan, it was further expanded and converted into a program, covering the entire country. The scheme is implemented by the Ministry of Women and Child Development through Anganwadi Centers (AWC). Repositioning the AWC as a "vibrant Early Childhood Development (ECD) center" is under consideration. Currently, it is named as "Umbrella ICDS Scheme" that comprises of several subschemes, viz. Anganwadi services, Scheme for Adolescent Girls (SAG), Pradhan Mantri Matru Vandana Yojana (PMMVY), National Nutrition Mission, Child Protection Services, and National crèche Scheme.

## Objectives

- To improve the nutrition and health status of the children in the age group 0–6 years.
- To lay the foundations for proper physical, social, and psychological development of the child.
- To reduce the incidence of morbidity, mortality, malnutrition and school drop outs.
- To achieve effective coordination and implementation of policy amongst the various departments to promote child development.
- To enhance the capability of the mother to look after normal health and nutritional needs of the child through proper nutrition and health education.

## Services and Beneficiaries

The ICDS scheme includes a package of six services: Supplementary nutrition, preschool nonformal education, nutrition and health education, immunization, health check-up, and referral services, for the following beneficiaries **(Table 47.19 and Fig. 47.27)**.

The ICDS scheme is implemented at the village level through the Anganwadi and mini AWC according to population norms as follows:
- **For rural/urban projects:** 1 AWC for 400–800, 2 AWCs for 800–1,600, 3 AWCs for 1,600–2,400 and thereafter 1 AWC for every 800 population
- **For mini AWC:** 1 mini AWC for 150–400 population

**Table 47.19:** Services provided at Anganwadi center.

| Children less than 6 years | Pregnant and lactating women |
|---|---|
| • Supplementary nutrition<br>• Pre-school non-formal education (children 3–5 years)<br>• Nutrition and health education (to mothers)<br>• Immunization<br>• Health check-up<br>• Referral services | • Supplementary nutrition<br>• Immunization against tetanus<br>• Health check-up<br>• Referral services<br>• Nutrition and health education |

- *For tribal and other difficult areas:* 1 AWC for 300–800, 1 mini AWC for 150–300 population
- *Anganwadi on demand (AOD):* Settlements with at least 40 children under 6 years but no AWC.

Every AWC at the village level is supervised by an AWW. A group of 20–25 AWCs are supervised by a Mukhya Sevika or Supervisor and constitute a Sector. At the block level, the Child Development Project Officer (CDPO) overlooks the program.

### Functions of Service Providers

*Anganwadi worker:* She is responsible for enlisting the beneficiaries in her village and providing all services in the ICDS package, maintaining records, treating common ailments and referring to PHC/higher center and enrolling children into schools. There is a helper to AWW at each AWC, who cooks and serves food to children and mothers, ensures cleanliness of the children, keeps the AWC clean and brings small children from their homes to the AWC.

*Mukhya Sevika:* She is responsible for guiding, supporting and supervising the AWWs in her sector, organizing monthly meetings for AWWs to discuss operational problems if any, and maintaining liaison and developing linkages between AWWs and other functionaries.

*Child development project officer:* He/she is the leader of the program at the block level and supervises its implementation, allocates targets, ensures maintenance of records, arranges training and educational programs, keeps account of equipment and materials and prepares and dispatches periodic reports of the project.

*Role of PHC and health infrastructure:* Health check-up, referral services, immunization, health and nutrition education, continuing education of ICDS and health functionaries, monitoring of the health component of ICDS, support the AWW and supply additional medicines to the kit of AWW, training of AWW.

### Package of Services in Detail

- *Supplementary nutrition:* Calorie as well as financial norms are set as follows for provislon of supplementary nutrition to the beneficiaries **(Table 47.20)**.

  For children aged 3–6 years, the supplementary nutrition is given in the AWC in the form of a morning snack followed by a hot cooked meal. For children below 3 years of age, pregnant and lactating mothers take home ration is provided. For malnourished children, food items are given in the form of micronutrient fortified and/or energy dense food as take-home ration in addition to meals served in the AWC. Supplementary nutrition is to be provided 300 days a year or 25 days a month.

- *Prophylaxis against anemia and vitamin A deficiency (VAD):* IFA tablets and vitamin A supplementation is done for all children registered at AWCs according to national guidelines.

**Table 47.20:** Supplementary nutrition to Integrated Child Development Services beneficiaries.

| Beneficiary | Energy (calories/day) | Protein (g/day) |
|---|---|---|
| Children 6–72 months | 500 | 12–15 |
| Severely underweight children 6–72 months | 800 | 20–25 |
| Pregnant women and nursing mothers | 600 | 18–20 |
| Adolescent out-of-school girls 11–14 years | 600 | 18–20 |

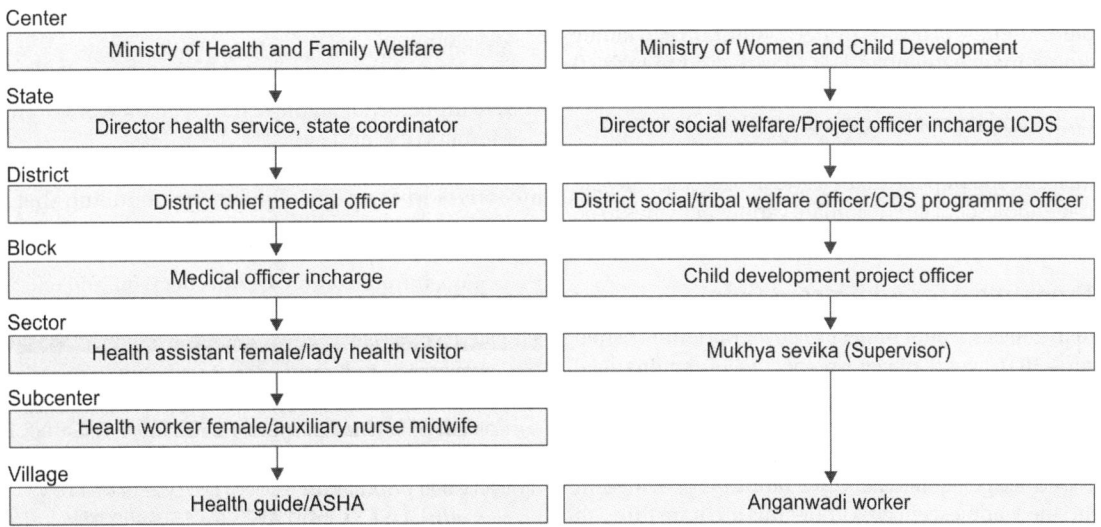

**Fig. 47.27:** Organization structure of Integrated Child Development Services scheme.

- **Immunization:** It is done by the health worker (F) as per the National Immunization Schedule. The AWW is responsible for registration, identification and follow up of the children and pregnant women for immunization.
- **Health check-up and referral:** Health check-up of the registered children is done once in 1–3 months by the HWF or LHV or a medical officer to detect and treat early any disease, malnutrition or infection. Any child with severe disease or malnutrition is immediately referred to the PHC or higher center. Antenatal check-up of pregnant women is done by HWF/LHV and delivery and postnatal care are provided by trained personnel.
- **Non-formal preschool education:** It aims at proper physical, social, psychological and cognitive development of the children, by innovative methods of learning. Children 3–5 years of age are engaged by the AWW for about 2 hours a day in play, group work, e.g., singing rhymes, and development of healthy habits, e.g., cutting nails, washing hands before meals. Materials used for activities include chalks, crayons, paints, cut papers, blocks, models, toys, clay and mud, etc. non-formal pre-school education has also shown to enhance school enrollment and reduce school drop-outs.

Other schemes implemented through ICDS are Kishori shakti yojana (KSY), nutrition program for adolescent girls (NPAG), SAG and PMMVY, which are described below.

## Kishori Shakti Yojana

*Kishori Shakti Yojana (KSY)* has been introduced by Ministry of Women and Child Development. This scheme aims to empower adolescent girls (age) of 11–18 years with focus on out-of-school girls.
- To improve nutritional and health status of girls includes IFA supplementation along with deworming.
- To provide the required literacy and numeracy skills through the nonformal stream of education, to stimulate a desire for more social exposure and knowledge and to help them improve their decision-making capabilities.
- To train and equip the adolescent girls to improve/upgrade home-based and vocational skills.
- To promote awareness of health, hygiene, nutrition and family welfare, home management and child care, and to take all measure as to facilitate their marrying only after attaining the age of 18 years and if possible, even later.
- To gain a better understanding of their environment related social issues and the impact on their lives.
- To encourage adolescent girls to initiate various activities to be productive and useful members of the society.

## Nutrition Programme for Adolescent Girls

It was started in 2006 as a pilot project to cover undernourished adolescent girls 10–19 years of age irrespective of the financial status of the family. Cut offs for weight in relation to age are used to define undernourishment (weight <30 kg for girls 11–15 years and weight <35 kg for girls 15–19 years). Free food grains @ 6 kg per beneficiary per month is provided to all undernourished adolescent girls under this program through the public distribution system.

## Scheme for Adolescent Girls

This scheme was launched in 2010 as Rajiv Gandhi Scheme for Empowerment of Adolescent Girls (RGSEAG)—SABLA and replaces KSY and NPAG. In non-SABLA districts, KSY and NPAG function as per guidelines. SAG focuses on out of school adolescents who are not covered by school health program and aims to improve their health and nutrition status and equip them with knowledge and skills on family welfare, health, hygiene, etc. The scheme has the following objectives:
- Enable the adolescent girls for self-development and empowerment.
- Improve their nutrition and health status.
- Promote awareness about health, hygiene, nutrition, ARSH and family and child care.
- Upgrade their home-based skills, life skills and tie up with National Skill Development Program (NSDP) for vocational skills.
- Mainstream out of school adolescent girls into formal/nonformal education.
- Provide information/guidance about existing public services such as PHC, CHC, post office, bank, police station, etc.

The scheme includes nutrition component (take home ration or hot cooked meal providing 600 calories, 18–20 g of protein per beneficiary per day for 300 days a year) and non-nutrition component (includes IFA supplementation, health check-up and referral, nutrition and health education, counseling on family welfare, ARSH, child care practices and home management, life skills education and vocational training). Nutritional component is given to out of school girls 11–14 years age and all girls 14–18 years age. Non-nutrition component is given twice or thrice a week to all out of school girls 11–18 years age except for vocational training which is given to girls 16–18 years age.

## Pradhan Mantri Matru Vandana Yojana

The Indira Gandhi Matritva Sahyog Yojana (Conditional Maternity Benefit Scheme), which was started in 2010 was renamed as PMMVY in 2017 and had the following objectives:
- Providing partial compensation for the wage loss in terms of cash incentives so that the woman can take adequate rest before and after delivery of the first living child.
- The cash incentive provided would lead to improved health seeking behavior amongst the Pregnant Women and Lactating Mothers (PW and LM).

All eligible pregnant and lactating women receive cash incentives in three installments on condition that they fulfill specific conditions relating to MCH as given in **Table 47.21**.

Table 47.21: Cash benefit under Pradhan Mantri Matru Vandana Yojana.

| Installment | Condition | Amount |
| --- | --- | --- |
| First installment | Early registration of pregnancy | ₹ 1,000 |
| Second installment | Received at least one ANC (can be claimed after 6 months of pregnancy) | ₹ 2,000 |
| Third installment | Childbirth is registered Child has received first cycle of BCG, OPV, DPT and Hepatitis-B or its equivalent/substitute | ₹ 2,000 |

# NATIONAL NUTRITION PROGRAMS

Under-nutrition prevalent in India is both macronutrient deficiency (protein-energy malnutrition) as well as micronutrient deficiency (notably deficiencies in iron, iodine, vitamin A and zinc). Nutrition programs in India are directed against general malnutrition and at specific nutritional deficiencies.

*Programs directed against general malnutrition:*
- Integrated Child Development Services Scheme
- Nutrition program for adolescent girls which runs under ICDS platform
- PM POSHAN Scheme
- Antyodaya Anna Yojana
- Annapurna Scheme
- Applied Nutrition Program
- Special Nutrition Programme, Balwadi Nutrition Programme, Tamil Nadu Integrated Nutrition Programme and Wheat based Supplementary Nutrition Programme, which are now part of ICDS.

*Programs directed against specific nutritional deficiencies:*
- Vitamin A Prophylaxis Programme
- National Nutritional Anemia Prophylaxis Programme
- Anemia Mukt Bharat
- National Iodine Deficiency Disorders Control Programme.

## PM POSHAN Scheme Mid-Day Meal Scheme

It was started in India from 1995 under the name of 'National Programme of Nutritional Support to Primary Education (NP-NSPE)'. In 2007, NP-NSPE was renamed as 'National Programme of Mid-Day Meal in Schools,' which is popularly known as Mid-Day Meal Scheme. In September 2021, the Mid-Day Meal Scheme was renamed 'PM POSHAN' or Pradhan Mantri Poshan Shakti Nirman. Under the scheme, there is provision of hot cooked meal to children of pre-schools or Bal Vatika (before class I) in primary schools also in addition to the children of classes I to VIII studying in 11.20 lakh schools.

### Objectives

The main objectives of the PM POSHAN Scheme are to address two of the pressing problems for majority of children in India, viz. hunger and education by improving the nutritional status of eligible children in Government and Government-aided schools as well as encouraging poor children, belonging to disadvantaged sections, to attend school more regularly and help them concentrate on classroom activities.

### Implementation

The PM POSHAN scheme provides cooked meal with the specific amount of calorific values along with adequate quantities of micronutrients **(Table 47.22)**.

Meal is also provided during summer vacation in drought affected areas. Norms for engagement for cook-cum-helpers are as follows:
- One cook-cum-helper for schools up to 25 students;
- Two for schools with 26–100 students;
- One additional for every 100 students thereafter.

Table 47.22: Amount of calories and protein provided under PM POSHAN scheme.

| S. No. | Items | Primary | Upper primary |
|---|---|---|---|
| **Nutrition norm per child per day** | | | |
| 1. | Calorie | 450 | 700 |
| 2. | Protein | 12 g | 20 g |
| **Food norms per child per day** | | | |
| 1. | Food grains | 100 g | 150 g |
| 2. | Pulses | 20 g | 30 g |
| 3. | Vegetables | 50 g | 75 g |
| 4. | Oil and fat | 5 g | 7.5 g |
| 5. | Salt and condiments | As per need | As per need |

Monitoring is done daily to ensure: (1) Regularity and wholesomeness of the mid-day meal served to children; (2) Cleanliness in cooking and serving of the mid-day meal; (3) Timeliness in procurement of good quality ingredients, fuel, etc.; (4) Implementation of varied menu; and (5) Social and gender equity.

## Antyodaya Anna Yojana (under Ministry of Agriculture, Consumer Affairs, Food and Public Distribution)

It was launched in December 2000 with the provision to provide food grains in highly subsidized rates to 1 crore poorest families out of the BPL families identified under the Targeted Public Distribution System. Each family will get 35 kg of food grains per month at ₹ 2/kg for wheat and ₹ 3/kg for rice. It was extended to include all eligible BPL families in 2009 with priority to families of HIV-positive persons in the AAY list.

## Annapurna Scheme (Under Ministry of Agriculture, Consumer Affairs, Food and Public Distribution)

This scheme covers the destitute senior citizens 65 years and above who should be getting pension under the Indira Gandhi National Old Age Pension Scheme but are not getting. These individuals are given 10 kg of food grains per person per month free of cost.

## Applied Nutrition Program (under Ministry of Rural Development)

This program was started in 1963 with the objective of encouraging people to be aware of their nutritional needs, produce of nutritious food themselves and supplement their diets to improve their own nutritional status. The beneficiaries included children 3–6 years old and pregnant and lactating women. Main activities included education and support for kitchen gardening, providing seeds and seedlings, poultry farming, pisciculture, beehive keeping and nutrition education. The program, however, did not succeed.

## Vitamin A Prophylaxis Programme (Under Ministry of Health and Family Welfare)

The program was started in 1970 with the objective to reduce the prevalence of vitamin A deficiency disorders from 0.6 to 0.5%.

## Strategies

- Health education to encourage appropriate infant and young child feeding practices including feeding of colostrum.
- Early detection and treatment of infections.
- Administration of nine mega doses of vitamin A to children every 6 months, starting from 9 months till 5 years of age (1 lakh IU at 9 months with measles immunization, 2 lakhs IU at 16–18 months with DPT booster, followed by 2 lakhs IU every 6 months till 5 years of age). In some states there are 2 months in the year fixed for vitamin A administration along with other child health services.

Activities for sick children:
- All children with xerophthalmia to be treated at health facilities.
- All children having measles, to be given one dose of vitamin A if they have not received it in the previous month.
- All cases of severe malnutrition to be given one additional dose of vitamin A.

## National Iron Plus Initiative (NIPI) Programme

National Nutritional Anemia Prophylaxis Programme was launched in 1972 with the aim to prevent nutritional anemia in children and pregnant and lactating women. In 2011, MoHFW expanded the NNACP and renamed it as a National Iron Plus Initiative (NIPI) Programme. Currently the program is part of RMNCAH+N, and provides iron and folic acid supplementation to various age groups as given in **Table 47.23**.

**Table 47.23:** Iron folic acid supplementation to beneficiaries.

| Beneficiaries | Formulation doses | Frequency and duration |
|---|---|---|
| Children 6–59 months | 1 mL Iron and Folic Acid syrup. (Each mL of Iron and Folic Acid syrup containing 20 mg elemental Iron + 100 mcg of Folic Acid) Bottle (50 mL) to have an 'auto-dispenser' | Biweekly throughout the period of 6–60 months |
| Children 5–10 years | 45 mg elemental iron + 400 µg folic acid (pink color tablet) | Weekly throughout the period of 5–10 years |
| Adolescents 10–19 years | 100 mg elemental iron + 500 µg folic acid (Blue color tablet) | Weekly throughout the period of 10–19 years |
| Pregnant women | 100 mg elemental iron + 500 µg folic acid (red color tablet) | • Prophylactic: 1 tablet daily, starting after the first trimester<br>• Clinically anemic: 2 tablets daily for 6 months |
| Nursing mothers | 100 mg elemental iron + 500 µg folic acid (red color tablet) | Daily for 6 months |
| Acceptors of family planning | 100 mg elemental iron + 500 µg folic acid (red color tablet) | Daily for 100 days |
| Women in reproductive age group | 100 mg elemental iron + 500 µg folic acid (red color tablet) | Weekly throughout the reproductive period |

**Table 47.24:** Dose and regime for deworming.

| Age group | Dose and regime |
|---|---|
| Children 12–59 months of age | Biannual dose of 400 mg albendazole (½ tablet to children 12–24 months and 1 tablet to children 24–59 months) |
| Children 5–9 years of age<br>School-going adolescent girls and boys 10–19 years of age<br>Out-of-school adolescent girls 10–19 years of age<br>Women of reproductive age (non-pregnant, non-lactating) 20–49 years | Biannual dose of 400 mg albendazole (1 tablet) |
| Pregnant women | One dose of 400 mg albendazole (1 tablet), after the first trimester, preferably during the second trimester |

## Deworming

Along with iron and folic acid supplementation, nutrition education to improve overall dietary intake as well as consumption of iron and folate rich foods is also done under the program. Also, deworming is done to control helminthic infestation in children and pregnant women **(Table 47.24)**.

## Weekly Iron and Folic Acid Supplementation (WIFS)

The WIFS is a national scheme launched in 2012 which aims to cover all children studying in classes I to XII of government, government aided and municipal schools and out of school adolescent girls. Objective of WIFS is to reduce the prevalence and severity of anemia in adolescent population (10–19 years).

IFA tablet has been made blue ('Iron ki nili goli') to distinguish it from the red IFA tablet for pregnant and lactating women **(Fig 47.28)**.

The main activities in this scheme are:
- Supervised administration of weekly iron and folic acid supplements
- Screening of target groups for moderate and severe anemia and referral to an appropriate health facility

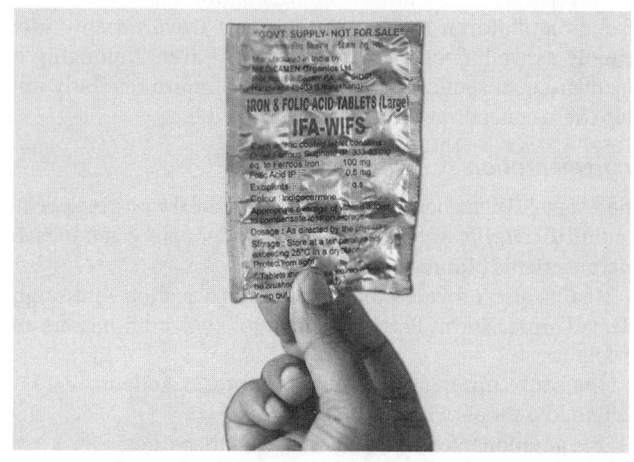

**Fig. 47.28:** Iron and folic acid tablet (Iron ki nili goli).

- Biannual deworming six months apart, for control of helminthic infestation and
- Information and counseling for improving dietary intake and preventive actions for intestinal worm infestation.

### Anemia Mukt Bharat (Fig. 47.29)

The Anemia Mukt Bharat—intensified Iron-plus Initiative launched in 2018 aims to strengthen the existing mechanisms and include newer strategies for tackling anemia. It focuses on six target beneficiary groups, through six interventions and six institutional mechanisms to achieve the envisaged target under the POSHAN Abhiyan. The Anemia Mukt Bharat strategy will be implemented in all villages, blocks, and districts of all the States/UTs of India through existing delivery platforms as envisaged in the National Iron Plus Initiative (NIPI) and Weekly Iron Folic Acid Supplementation (WIFS) Programme. The dosage, frequency and duration of prophylactic iron folic acid supplementation and deworming in this initiative are similar to that mentioned in **Tables 47.23 and 47.24**.

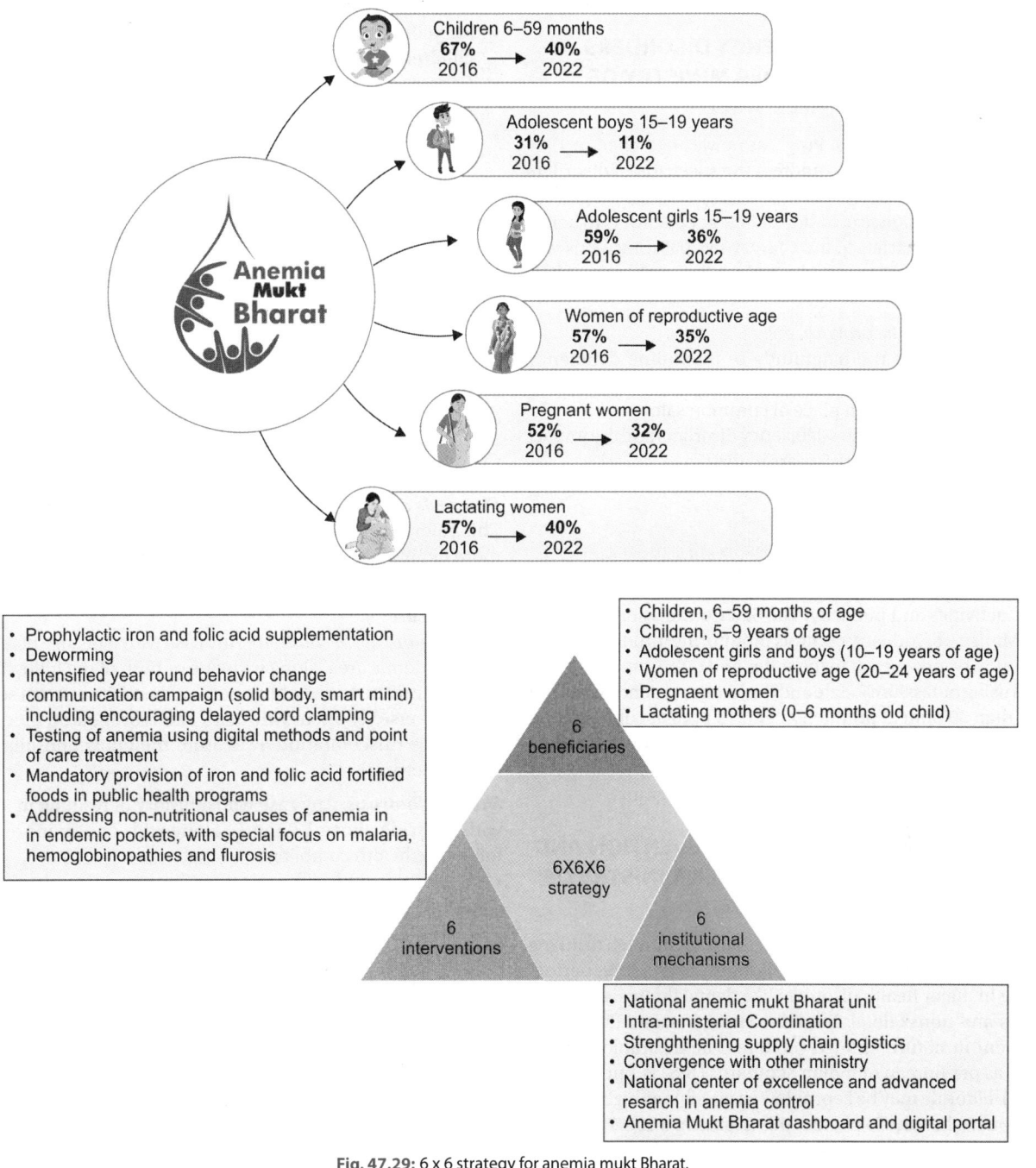

Fig. 47.29: 6 x 6 strategy for anemia mukt Bharat.
*Source:* https://anemiamuktbharat.info/home/6x6x6-strategy/.

### Objectives

To reduce prevalence of anemia by 3% point among children, adolescents and women in reproductive age group (15-49 years), between the year 2018-2022.

### Beneficiaries and Target

The strategy is estimated to reach out to 450 million beneficiaries with specific anemia prevalence targets for year 2022 to be achieved among various population groups.

*Strategies are shown in Figure 47.29.*

## NATIONAL IODINE DEFICIENCY DISORDERS CONTROL PROGRAM (UNDER MINISTRY OF HEALTH AND FAMILY WELFARE)

The National Goitre Control Programme was launched in 1962 and was renamed in 1992 to address the spectrum of disorders that are caused by iodine deficiency. The goal of the program is to reduce the prevalence of iodine deficiency disorders to below 10% in endemic districts of the country by 2000. Since this was achieved, the goal was modified to reduce the prevalence of IDD to below 5%.

*The activities under the program are:*
- Surveys to assess the magnitude of the iodine deficiency disorders in districts.
- Supply of iodized salt in place of common salt.
- Resurveys to assess iodine deficiency disorders and the impact of iodized salt after every 5 years in districts.
- Laboratory monitoring of iodized salt and urinary iodine excretion.
- Health education and publicity.

The MoHFW is responsible for the overall functioning of the program including conducting assessment surveys and carrying out IEC activities and publicity. The Salt Commissioner's Office under Ministry of Industry controls monitoring, production and distribution of iodized salt to the states and UTs. Common salt is iodized using potassium iodate and the iodine content should not be less than 30 ppm at production and 15 ppm at consumption levels under the Food Safety and Standards Act. IEC regarding the importance of consumption of iodized salt in prevention of iodine deficiency disorders is central to the program.

## NATIONAL PROGRAMME FOR PREVENTION AND CONTROL OF FLUOROSIS (UNDER MINISTRY OF HEALTH AND FAMILY WELFARE)

Fluorosis is caused by excess intake of fluorides through drinking water/food products/industrial pollutants, over a long period, resulting in major health disorders like dental fluorosis, skeletal fluorosis and nonskeletal fluorosis. These harmful effects are permanent in nature and irreversible. The desirable limit of fluoride as per Bureau of Indian Standards (BIS) is 1 ppm (1 mg per liter). Fluoride may be kept as low as possible as high fluoride is injurious to health. To combat this problem, a 100% centrally approved NPPCF was launched in 2008-09.

### Goal

Prevention and control of fluorosis cases in the country.

### Objectives

- To collect, assess and use the baseline survey data of fluorosis of Ministry of Drinking Water Supply for starting the project.
- Comprehensive management of fluorosis in selected areas.
- Capacity building for prevention, diagnosis and management of fluorosis cases.

### Strategies

- Surveillance of fluorosis in the community including school children.
- Capacity building (Human Resource) in the form of training and manpower support.
- Establishment of diagnostic facilities in the district/medical hospitals.
- Management of fluorosis cases including treatment, surgery and rehabilitation.
- Health education for prevention and control of fluorosis cases.

### Surveillance of Fluorosis in a Community

At the national level the nutrition cell coordinates and monitors all administrative and technical issues related to implementation of the program. For surveillance of fluorosis, case definitions, sampling, and survey methodology have been given.

### Case Definition

#### Fluorosis endemic area

This refers to a habitation/village/town having fluoride level more than 1.5 ppm in drinking water or the population has all health complaints of fluorosis.

#### Suspect case

*Dental fluorosis (in children):* Any case with a history of residing in an endemic area, along with one or both of the following:
- Chalky white teeth/white spots on the white enamel surface.
- Transverse yellow, brown/black bands or spots on the enamel surface (discoloration away from the gums and bilaterally symmetrical).

*Skeletal fluorosis:* Any case with a history of residing in an area with fluoride above 1.0 mg/L, along with one or more of the following health complaints:
- Severe pain and stiffness in neck, back bone (lumbar region), shoulder, knee and hip region. Pain may commence either in 1 or 2 or more joints. Patient has restricted mobility of cervical and/or lumbar spine and has to turn the whole body towards that side to see.
- Knock knee/bow leg (in children, adolescents).
- Inability to squat (advanced stage of skeletal fluorosis).
- Ugly gait and posture (advanced stage of skeletal fluorosis).

*Nonskeletal fluorosis:* Any case with a history of residing in an endemic area, along with one or more of the following health complaints:

- *Gastrointestinal problems:* Consistent abdominal pain, intermittent diarrhea/constipation, bloated feeling, nausea, loss of appetite.
- *Neurological manifestations:* Nervousness and depression, tingling sensation in fingers and toes, excessive thirst and tendency to urinate frequently (polydipsia and polyuria).
- *Muscular manifestations:* Muscle weakness and stiffness, pain in the muscle and loss of muscle power, unable to walk or work.

### Confirmed case

Any suspected case can be confirmed after retrieval of a clinical history, by the following tests:
- Any suspected case with high level of fluoride in urine (>1 mg/L).
- Any suspected case with interosseous membrane calcification in the forearm confirmed by X-ray radiograph.
- Any suspected case, if kidney ailment is prevailing, serum fluoride needs to be tested, besides urine fluoride.

### Sampling Procedure

Based on the level of fluoride content, the villages can be identified in the following categories:

| Strata | Fluoride level |
|---|---|
| I | Up to 1.0–3.0 ppm |
| II | 3.1–5.0 ppm |
| III | >5.0 ppm |

All children in the age group 6–11 years from primary schools in the randomly selected villages are surveyed for dental fluorosis. In randomly selected 20 households of the sample villages where dental fluorosis is prevalent in school children, survey is conducted for skeletal and nonskeletal fluorosis.

### Prevention and Control

Preventive measures include defluoridated water, rainwater harvesting, restrict intake of fluoride rich items, e.g., tobacco, supari, black tea, lemon tea and black/rock salt; avoid use of fluoride-rich cosmetics/drugs, e.g., fluoridated toothpastes, mouthwashes and use of foods rich in calcium and vitamin C. Clinically suspected cases are confirmed and managed by supplementation with vitamin C, D, antioxidants, calcium, treatment of malnutrition and treatment of deformities. Awareness is generated about the disease, safe and unsafe sources of drinking water and promotion of rainwater harvesting.

## ZINC SUPPLEMENTATION (UNDER MINISTRY OF HEALTH AND FAMILY WELFARE)

Zinc supplementation has been shown to reduce the duration and severity of episodes of acute diarrhea. Zinc supplementation is used as an adjunct to ORS under the national program, to control acute diarrheal diseases. The dose of zinc administration is 10 mg per day in infants 2–6 months of age (dispersible tablet to be given in expressed breast milk) and 20 mg per day in 6 months to 5 years of age, for 14 days.

## SUGGESTED READING

1. Department of Women and Child Development, Ministry of Human Resource Development, GOI.
2. Guidelines for implementation for adolescent girls' scheme as a component under centrally sponsored ICDS (general scheme) September 2000.
3. Guidelines for operationalizing Nutrition Programme for Adolescent Girls (NPAG). [online] Available from: http://wcd.nic.in/ npag/guidelines. htm.
4. Integrated Child Development Services Scheme Portal. (2018). Ministry of Women and Child Development, GOI, New Delhi. [online] Available from: http://icds-wcd.nic.in.
5. Lal S. Integrated Child Development Services, National Health Programme series No. 7, NIHFW, New Delhi; 1988.
6. Ministry of Women and Child Development. (2018). National Nutrition Mission Administrative Guidelines 2018. M/o Women and Child Development, GOI, New Delhi.
7. MoHFW. A Strategic Approach to Reproductive, Maternal, Newborn, Child and Adolescent Health (RMNCH+A) in India. Ministry of Health and Family Welfare, Government of India, New Delhi. 2013; pp.14, 15, 19, 26.
8. MoHFW. Guidelines for Control of iron Deficiency Anaemia. National Iron+ Initiative: Towards infinite potential in an anaemia free India. NRHM, Adolescent Division. Ministry of Health and Family Welfare, Government of India, New Delhi. 2013; pp. 17-22.
9. MoHFW. Immunization Handbook for Medical Officers 2011. MOHFW, Ministry of Health and Family Welfare, Government of India, New Delhi, p. 26.
10. MoHFW. National Iodine Deficiency Disorders Control Programme, Annual Report (2016–17). Ministry of Health and Family Welfare, Government of India, New Delhi.
11. MoHFW. National Programme for Prevention and Control of Fluorosis, Revised Guidelines (2014). Ministry of Health and Family Welfare, Government of India, New Delhi.
12. MoHFW. Special Programmes for Vaccine Preventable Diseases, Training Module for Mid-level Managers, Immunisation Strengthening Project; RCH Programme, Ministry of Health and Family Welfare, Government of India, New Delhi; 2001.
13. MoHRD. (2018). Mid-Day Meal Scheme. Department of School Education and Literacy, Ministry of Human Resource Development, Government of India, New Delhi. [online]. Available from: http:// mhrd.gov.in/mid-day- meal.
14. MoRD. Guidelines for Annapurna Scheme 2000. Ministry of Rural Development, Government of India, New Delhi.
15. NIHFW. (2014). Applied Nutrition Programme. National Institute of Health and Family Welfare, Ministry of Health and Family Welfare, Government of India, New Delhi. [online]. Available from: http://www. nihfw.org/ NationalHealthProgramme/ APPLIEDNUTRITIONPROGRAMME. html.
16. PIB. Antyodaya Anna Yojana. (2013). Press Information Bureau, Government of India, New Delhi. [online] Available from: http:// pib.nic.in/newsite/ efeatures.aspx?relid=95141.
17. Pradhan Mantri Matru Vandana Yojana, Scheme implementation guidelines 2017. Ministry of Women and Child Development, GIO, New Delhi.
18. WHO. Global Measles and Rubella Strategic Plan 2012–20. World Health Organization; 2012.

# PROGRAMME FOR UNIVERSAL HEALTH COVERAGE

## AYUSHMAN BHARAT PROGRAMME

- Over 50 crore Indians to be covered
- Families identified as per socioeconomic Caste Census, 2011
- Beneficiaries: Poor, deprived rural families and identified occupational category of urban workers' families
- Cover of ₹5 lakhs per family per year for secondary and tertiary care hospitalization in all empaneled public and private hospitals
- There will be no cap on the family size and age
- Funded 60:40 by center and state
- To be merged with other state schemes

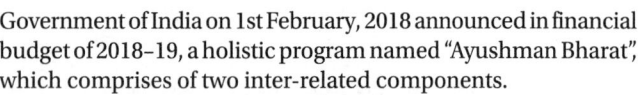

Government of India on 1st February, 2018 announced in financial budget of 2018–19, a holistic program named "Ayushman Bharat", which comprises of two inter-related components.
1. Health and Wellness Center (HWC)
2. National Health Protection Scheme

The first component involves upgradation of all the Sub Health Centres (SHCs), Primary Health Centres (PHCs) and Urban Primary Health Care Centres (UPHCs) to Health and Wellness Centres (HWCs) for the delivery of comprehensive primary healthcare. The second component comprises of Ayushman Bharat Pradhan Mantri Jan Arogya Yojana (PMJAY) which aims to provide financial protection for secondary and tertiary care to socially vulnerable and low-income households. This was aimed at making path breaking interventions to address health holistically in primary, secondary and tertiary healthcare systems, covering health promotion as well as health prevention.

## NATIONAL HEALTH PROTECTION SCHEME

India's health sector faces immense challenges. Healthcare in India is largely underpenetrated, with government expenditure at around 1.25% of the GDP and an underperforming public healthcare ecosystem. It continues to be characterized by high out-of-pocket expenditure, low financial protection, low health insurance coverage amongst both rural and urban population.

Approximately 62 of our population has to pay for their own health and hospitalization expenses and are not covered through any form of health protection. Besides using their income and savings, people borrow money or sell their assets to meet their healthcare needs. Nearly 5-6 crore Indians are pushed into poverty every year because they are unfortunately compelled to spend half of their annual household expenditure to meet medical needs, especially for hospitalization. Various state level government insurance schemes already exist in India, but still 80% of population are not covered under any insurance scheme.

To overcome this situation, on September 23, 2018, the Prime Minister of India launched "Ayushman Bharat", world's largest government-funded healthcare scheme, in Jharkhand's capital Ranchi. This health protection scheme was named as Pradhan Mantri Jan Arogya Yojana (PMJAY) also known as Ayushman Bharat-National Health Protection Scheme (AB-NHPS). It will subsume the existing Rashtriya Swasthya Bima Yojana (RSBY), launched in 2008 and senior citizen health insurance scheme.

### Beneficiaries

| | |
|---|---|
| **Rural area:** The beneficiaries are identified based on the deprivation categories (D1, D2, D3, D4, D5, and D7) identified under the SECC database | **Rural area categories:** The different categories in rural areas include<br>• D1: Families having only one room with kuccha walls and kuccha roof<br>• D2: Families having no adult member between the ages of 16 and 59 years<br>• D3: Female-headed households with no adult male member between the ages of 16 and 59 years<br>• D4: Disabled members and no able-bodied adult member in the family<br>• D5: SC/ST households<br>• D7: Landless households deriving major part of their income from manual casual labor<br>Families in rural areas having any one of the following will be automatically included:<br>• Households without shelter<br>• Destitute/living on alms<br>• Manual scavenger families<br>• Primitive tribal groups<br>• Legally released bonded labor |
| **Urban area:** 11 defined occupational categories are entitled under the scheme | **Urban area categories:**<br>• Beggars<br>• Rag-pickers<br>• Domestic workers<br>• Street vendors/cobblers/hawkers/other service providers working on the streets<br>• Construction workers/plumbers/masons/labor/painters/welders/security guards/coolies and other head-load workers<br>• Sweepers/sanitation workers/malis<br>• Home-based workers/artisans/handicrafts workers/tailors<br>• Transport workers/drivers/conductors/helpers to drivers and conductors/cart pullers/rickshaw pullers<br>• Shop workers/assistants/peons in small establishments/helpers/delivery assistants/attendants/waiters<br>• Electricians/mechanics/assemblers/repair workers; washer-men/chowkidars<br>• Other work/nonwork (Pension/Rent/Interest, etc.) |

In addition, Rashtriya Swasthya Bima Yojana (RSBY) beneficiaries in states where it is active are also included.

### Benefits of PM-JAY for Indian Health System

- Help India progressively achieve Universal Health Coverage (UHC) and Sustainable Development Goals (SDG).
- Ensure improved access and affordability of quality secondary and tertiary care services through a combination of public hospitals and well measured strategic purchasing of services in healthcare deficit areas, from private care providers, especially the not-for profit providers.
- Significantly reduce out of pocket expenditure for hospitalization.
- Align the growth of private sector with public health goals.
- Enable creation of new health infrastructure in rural, remote and under-served areas.
- More than 1 lakh long-term and 80 lakhs short-term jobs will be created.
- Increase health expenditure by government as a percentage of GDP.
- Enhanced patient satisfaction.
- Improved health outcomes.
- Improvement in population-level productivity and efficiency.
- Improved quality of life for the population.

## AYUSHMAN AROGYA MANDIR (HEALTH AND WELLNESS CENTER)

Under the aegis of Government of India's flagship program of Ayushman Bharat-Health and Wellness Centres (AB-HWCs), more than 1.6 lakhs AB-HWCs have been successfully established across the States/UTs over the last 5 years. These AB-HWC's are equipped with the required resources including infrastructure, human resources, drugs and diagnostics, IT framework, etc.

The AB-HWCs are being recognized by the weakest section of society as facility which are not only near to their doorstep but also can be approached for consultation about majority of the primary healthcare needs These centres have been successful in taking the thinking and health care delivery from illness to wellness.

At present Health and Wellness Centre term is replaced by "AYUSHMAN AROGYA MANDIR" with the tagline "Arogyam Parmam Dhanam".

### Need

The subcenter (SC) and primary healthcentre (PHC) are the peripheral outpost and the first hope of healthcare for the remote population. They fulfil the basic primary healthcare needs of the families surviving in difficult circumstances in the remote areas. Optimum utilization of SCs and PHCs is hindered due to factors like poor infrastructure, lack of manpower, geographical barriers, weak monitoring and supportive supervision. The under-utilization has also affected the health seeking behavior of rural population negatively. They either refrain from seeking healthcare services or resort to alternate solutions which includes unskilled practitioners (quacks, traditional faith healers). When treatment fails, they travel to cities and private healthcare facilities for better quality of care, which leads to over-burdened hospitals and unaffordable out of pocket expenses.

### Proposed infrastructure

- Branding/Color coding of all sub health centers and PHCs will be done and citizen charter will be displayed.
- Space for examination room with adequate privacy.
- Diagnostics and medicine dispensation room.
- Wellness room and waiting area.
- Labor room at delivery points.

To ensure delivery of Comprehensive Primary Health Care (CPHC), existing Sub Health Centres (SHCs) covering a population of 3,000 5,000 are being transformed to Health and Wellness Centres (AB-HWCs). Primary Health Centres (PHCs) in rural and urban areas are also being converted into AB-HWCS. On 14th April 2018, Honorable Prime Minister launched the first HWC at Jangla, Bijapur, Chhattisgarh.

The AB-HWCS at the Sub Health Centre (SHC) level would be equipped and staffed by an appropriately trained Primary Health Care team led by a Community Health Officer (CHO) who will be a Mid-level Health Provider (MLHP) with BSC nursing/GNM degree or Ayurveda practitioner trained in 6 months certificate program and comprising of Multi-Purpose Workers (male and female) and ASHAs. A PHC that is linked to a cluster of AB-HWCs at the SHCS would serve as the first point of referral for many disease conditions for the AB-HWCs in its jurisdiction In addition, it would also be strengthened as a AB-HWC to deliver the expanded range of primary health care services. The Medical Officer at the PHC would be responsible for ensuring that CPHC services are delivered through all SHC Level AD-HWCs in her/his area and through the PHC.

CPHC is complemented by outreach services. Mobile Medical Units and Home and Community based care, enabling a seamless continuum of care that ensures the principles of equity, universality and removing any financial hardship.

### Package of 13 Comprehensive Services

See **Figure 47.30.**

## CONCLUSION

The two pillars of Ayushman Bharat are—HWCs, and PM-JAY (world's largest health insurance scheme). PM-JAY aims to provide a free insurance cover to approximately 50 crore Indians, and hence requires tremendous resources. On the other hand, HWCs are focused towards strengthening of healthcare delivery system, which is of primary importance and hence more resources should be directed towards it. In conclusion, without strengthening of HWC, if more resources are directed towards PM-JAY, then it may not be cost-effective in long-term.

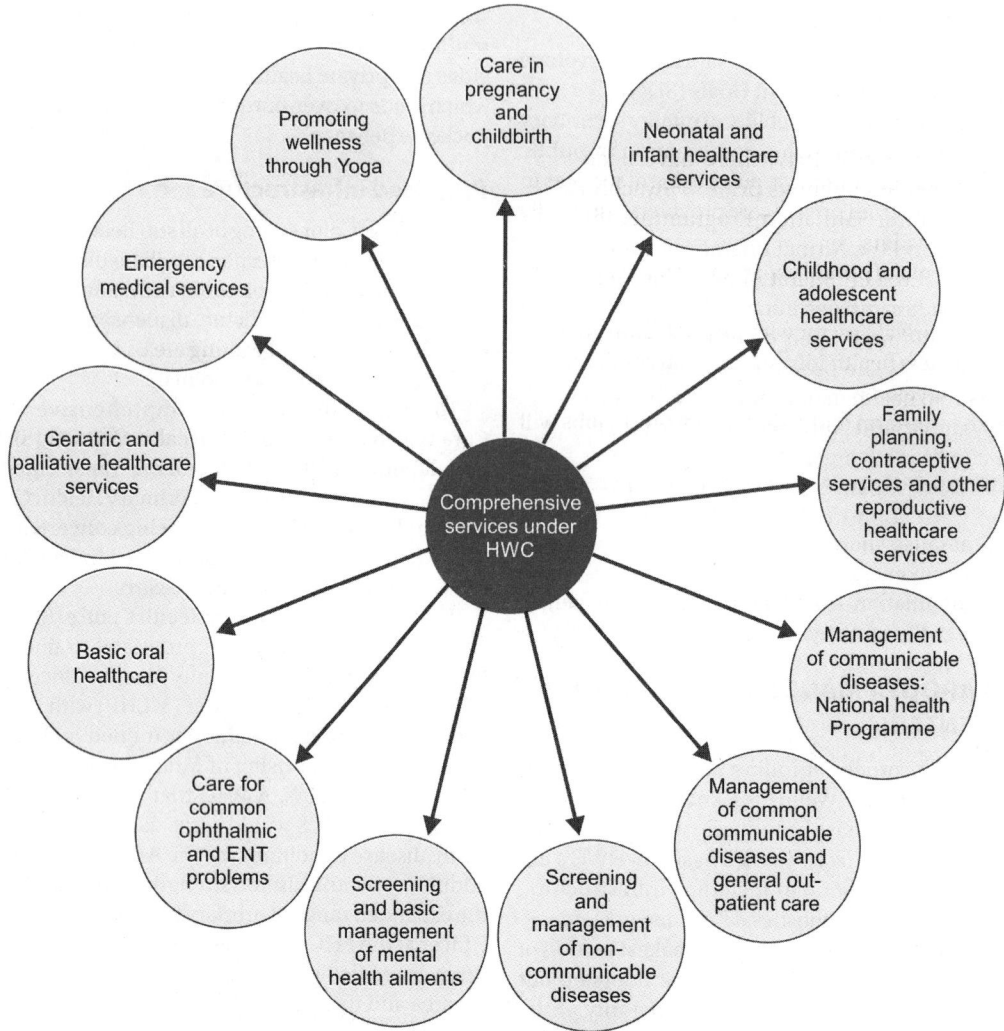

**Fig. 47.30:** Package of 13 comprehensive services.
(HWC: Health and Wellness Center)

## SUGGESTED READING

1. Home Ayushmaan Bharat [Internet]. Pmjay.gov.in. 2019 [cited 6 February 2019]. Available from: https://www.pmjay.gov.in/.
2. Ministry of Health and Family Welfare. Comprehensive primary health care—Government of India [Internet]. [cited 2018 Jun 4]. Available from: http://nhm.gov.in/nrhm-components/health-systemsstrengthening/comprehensive-primary-health-care.html.

# PROGRAMS ADDRESSING SOCIAL DETERMINANTS OF HEALTH

## SWACHH BHARAT MISSION

Since India's independence in 1947, there have been three rural sanitation intervention attempts prior to Swachh Bharat Mission: the Central Rural Sanitation Programme, the Total Sanitation Campaign, and the Nirmal Bharat Abhiyan. Swachh Bharat Mission (SBM), Swachh Bharat Abhiyan, or Clean India Mission is a country-wide campaign initiated by the Government of India in 2014 to eliminate open defecation and improve solid waste management. The program also aims to increase awareness of menstrual health management. It is a restructured version of the Nirmal Bharat Abhiyan launched in 2009 that failed to achieve its intended targets.

Initiated by the Government of India, the mission aimed to achieve an "open-defecation free" (ODF) India by 2 October 2019 through construction of toilets. An estimated 89.9 million toilets were built in the period. The objectives of the first phase of the mission also included eradication of manual scavenging, generating awareness and bringing about a behavior change regarding sanitation practices, and augmentation of capacity at the local level. The second phase of the mission aims to sustain the open defecation free status and improve the management of solid and liquid waste, while also working to improve the lives of sanitation workers.

The mission was split into two: rural and urban. In rural areas "SBM-Gramin" was financed and monitored through the Ministry of Drinking Water and Sanitation (since converted to the Department of Drinking Water and Sanitation under the Ministry of Jal Shakti) whereas "SBM-urban" was overseen by the Ministry of Housing and Urban Affairs.

As part of the campaign, volunteers, known as *Swachhagrahi*, or "Ambassadors of cleanliness", promoted the construction of toilets using a popular method called Community-Led Total Sanitation at the village level. Other activities included national real-time monitoring and updates from non-governmental organizations such as The Ugly Indian, Waste Warriors, and SWACH Puné (Solid Waste Collection and Handling).

### Planned Initiatives Under SBM

- The Government appointed CPWD with the responsibility to dispose of waste from Government offices.
- The Ministry of Railways planned to have the facility of cleaning on demand, clean bed-rolls from automatic laundries, bio-toilets, dustbins in all non-AC coaches.
- The Swachh Bharat Swachh Vidyalaya campaign was launched by the Minister of Human Resource Development, Government of India by participating in the cleanliness drive along with the school's teachers and students. Separate toilet facilities for male and female students have been established in schools under the 'Swachh Bharat Swachh Vidyalaya' scheme.

## KAYAKALP AWARD SCHEME

The Swachh Bharat Abhiyan focuses on promoting cleanliness in public space. Same way cleanliness and hygiene in healthcare facilities is critical in preventing infections and also provide patients with a positive experience and encourages molding behavior related to clean environment. 'Kayakalp Award Scheme' was launched on May 15, 2015 as an extension of Swachh Bharat Abhiyan to improve and promote the cleanliness, hygiene, waste management and infection control practices in public healthcare facilities and incentivize the exemplary performing facilities. It was initiated from district hospitals in 2015 and expanded to PHC level (2016) and then it covered all Urban Health Facilities by 2017.

### OBJECTIVES

- To promote cleanliness, hygiene and infection control practices in public healthcare facilities.
- To incentivize and recognize such public healthcare facilities that show exemplary performance in adhering to standard protocols of cleanliness and infection control.
- To inculcate a culture of ongoing assessment and peer review of performance related to hygiene, cleanliness and sanitation.
- To create and share sustainable practices related to improved cleanliness in public health facilities linked to positive health outcomes.

### SELECTION OF FACILITIES

The awards for individual public health facility will be given to those that score the highest based on a set of defined criteria. There will be three subcategories:

#### Best District Hospitals

In every state the two top ranked district hospitals will receive an award. The first and second best district hospital level facilities will receive cash award of ₹ 50 and ₹ 20 lakhs respectively.

For small states only the first ranking facility in this category will be awarded.

#### Best CHC/SDH Award

In every state, the top two ranked CHCs/SDHs will receive an award. The first and second ranked CHCs/SDHs will receive cash awards of ₹ 15 and 10 lakhs respectively. For small states there will be only one award for the best facility in this category.

### Best PHC Award

In every district, the best PHC (24 × 7) will receive a cash award of ₹ 2 lakhs.

In order to motivate, sustain and improve performance in facilities that score over 70%, but do not make it to the list of top two/one in a particular year, a certificate of commendation plus cash award would be given as follows:.
- District hospital ₹ 300,000
- CHC/SDH ₹ 100,000
- Primary health centers ₹ 50,000

## AWARDS CRITERIA

The awards would be distributed based on the performance of the facility on the following parameters.

Following are the prerequisites for applying for an award:
- Constituted a Cleanliness and Infection Control Committee.
- Instituted a mechanism of periodic internal assessment/peer assessment based on defined criteria.
- Achieved at least 70% score in the criteria during the peer assessment process.

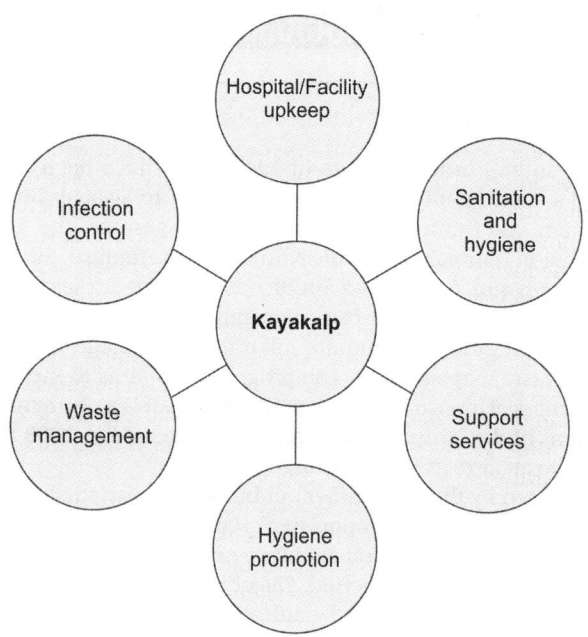

## SWACHH SWASTH SARVATRA

To complement efforts of Swachh Bharat Mission and Kayakalp towards achieving clean India and healthy India, the Ministry of Health and Family Welfare (MoHFW) and Ministry of Drinking Water and Sanitation (MoDWS) have started an integrated scheme named as "Swachh Swasth Sarvatra" (SSS) on December 29, 2016. The aim of this scheme is to strengthen CHCs in open defecation free (ODF) blocks across the country along with behavioral change to enable them achieve higher levels of cleanliness and hygiene with the goal of making India free of open defecation.

Three broad objectives of this scheme are:
1. Enabling Gram Panchayat where Kayakalp awarded PHCs are located to become ODF.
2. Strengthening CHC in ODF blocks to achieve higher level of cleanliness to meet Kayakalp standards through a support of ₹ 10 lakhs under NHM.
3. Build capacity through training in Water, Sanitation and Hygiene (WASH) of nominees from covered PHC and CHC.

## ACTIVITIES UNDER SWACHH SWASTH SARVATRA

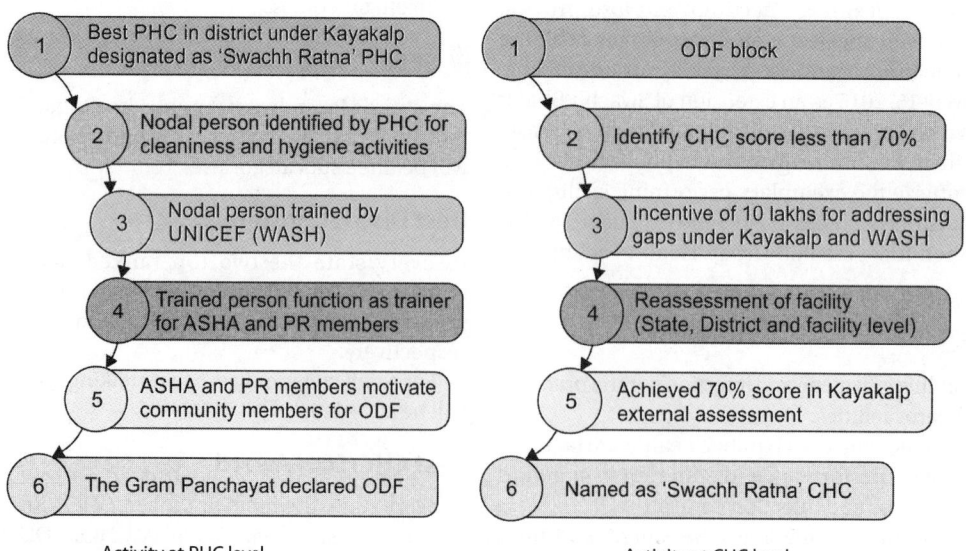

Activity at PHC level    Activity at CHC level

## SUGGESTED READING

1. National Health System Resource Centre. Kayakalp and Swach Swasth Sarvatra. Available from: http://qi.nhsrcindia.org/kayakalp-swachh-swasth-sarvatra.

## MISSION SHAKTI

(Integrated Women Empowerment Programme) Umbrella Scheme for Safety, Security and Empowerment of Women.

Mission Shakti has two sub-schemes 'Sambal' and 'Samarthya'. In the "*Sambal*" sub-scheme, which is for safety and security of women, the existing scheme of One Stop Centre (OSC), Women Helpline (WHL), Beti Bachao Beti Padhao (BBBP) have been included with modifications and a new component of Nari—women collective has been added.

In the 'Samarthya' sub scheme, which is for empowerment of women, existing schemes of Ujjawala, Swadhar Greh and Working Women Hostel have been included with modifications. In addition, the existing schemes of National Creche Scheme and PMMVY under umbrella of ICDS have now been included in Samarthya.

The components under Mission Shakti have the broad objectives of either protecting or assisting women who are victims of violence or in difficult circumstances or for empowering women. The objectives of the mission are as under:

- Provide immediate and comprehensive continuum of care, support and assistance to women affected by violence and for those in distress;
- To put in place quality mechanisms for rescue, protection and rehabilitation of women in need of assistance and victims of crime and violence;
- To improve accessibility to various government services available for women at various levels;
- Making people aware about Government schemes and programs as well as legal provisions to fight social evils like dowry, domestic violence, sexual harassment at workplace and to promote gender equality etc.
- Capacity building and training of functionaries/duty bearers under various schemes/legislations.
- Collaboration with partner Ministries/departments/states/UTs for convergence of policies, programs/schemes and to create an enabling environment for public private partnership for safety and empowerment of women across sectors.
- Create awareness among masses for inducing positive behavioral change towards women and girls.
- To prevent gender-biased sex selective elimination; to ensure survival, protection, education and development of the girl child.

### SUGGESTED READING

1. Ministry of Women and Child Development. Scheme Implementation Guidelines: Mission Shakti. Available from: https://wcd.nic.in/sites/default/files/Mission%20Shakti%20Guidelines%20for%20implementation%20during%2015th%20Finance%20Commission%20period%202021-22%20to%202025-26_1.pdf

## PRADHAN MANTRI UJJWALA YOJANA 2.0: SWACHH INDHAN BEHTAR JEEVAN

In May 2016, Ministry of Petroleum and Natural Gas (MOPNG), introduced the 'Pradhan Mantri Ujjwala Yojana' (PMUY) as a flagship scheme with an objective to make clean cooking fuel such as LPG available to the rural and deprived households which were otherwise using traditional cooking fuels such as firewood, coal, cow-dung cakes etc. Usage of traditional cooking fuels had detrimental impacts on the health of rural women as well as on the environment.

The target under the scheme was to release 8 crore LPG connections to the deprived households by March 2020, which was achieved in September 2019.

Ujjwala 2.0: Additional allocation of 1.6 crore LPG connections under PMUY scheme with special facility to migrant households.

### SUGGESTED READING

1. About PMUY [Internet]. [cited 2023 July 19]. Available from: https://www.pmuy.gov.in/about.html

# CHAPTER 48

# Monitoring and Evaluation System in India

*Kedar Mehta, Paragkumar Chavda*

| | |
|---|---|
| **CM4.3** | Demonstrate and describe the steps in evaluation of health promotion and education program |
| **CM8.5** | Describe and discuss the principles of evaluating control measures for disease at community level bearing in mind the public health importance of the disease |
| **CM8.7** | Describe the principles of management of information systems |
| **CM9.7** | Enumerate the sources of vital statistics including census, SRS, NFHS, NSSO, etc. |

## INTRODUCTION

Monitoring and evaluation (M and E) are ongoing activities that helps all the concerned people specially policymakers and planners of the country to know the status of health and related aspects. M and E also helps to know whether activities planned are progressing as per desired direction and speed, and whether the strategies adopted, and intervention carried out are effective to achieve desired results. Every country is having its own monitoring and evaluation system. India is also having monitoring and evaluation system to keep eye on the health condition of the people of India as well as know the progress and impacts of health programs and interventions. Monitoring is being carried out internally by its own inbuilt mechanism of health system by Ministry of Health, while evaluation is carried out by external agency or sometimes using internal system. Routine reporting system also known as Management Information System is sheet-anchor in monitoring system, while various special surveys carried out periodically or based on need; are part of evaluation mechanism in India.

## MONITORING SYSTEM

### Health Management Information System

In India monitoring of the health program is being carried out by regular reporting system known as Management Information System (MIS) focusing on various process and output indicators as inbuilt part of healthcare delivery system. MIS is the most common reporting and feedback system used for monitoring performance of government health system and health program. The statistics (Monitoring and Evaluation) division in the Ministry of Health and Family Welfare is responsible for monitoring and evaluation of the National Family Welfare Programmes in India.

Health management information system (HMIS) is a web-based monitoring system developed by Ministry of Health and Family Welfare under National Health Mission (NHM). Its purpose is to monitor the performance of programs and the services provided through the large network of health facilities across rural and urban areas by use of information technology and provide timely feedback to improve the performance **(Flowchart 48.1 and Table 48.1)**. Earlier, this reporting system was running as paper-based system, but with advent of the information technology, web-based electronic reporting system is used now.

### Methods

Information is reported on a monthly frequency using specific reporting format by Primary Health Centers/Community Health Centers under the NHM. Similarly, there are reporting formats from village to national level institutes. It contains both, process and output indicators.

Around 300+ process and output indicators are monitored through HMIS. These indicators are reviewed against desired level of performance to know the progress. Also, further intelligences are drawn by creating composite index by use of combined indicators. For example, in RMNCAH+N (Reproductive, Maternal, Neonatal, Child & Adolescent Health + Nutrition) health program, a composite index is calculated based on 16 RMNCAH+N indicators covering the following 4 stages of life cycle:
1. Pre-pregnancy/reproductive age
2. Pregnancy care
3. Childbirth/delivery
4. Postnatal, maternal and newborn care.

Based on the composite scores of the states/districts, they are divided into 4 parts (for individual category) using quartiles. The lowest ranking (lowest quartile) states/ districts (D)—depict very low performance, (C)—low performing, (B)—promising and (A)—good performance. Thus, information gathered through HMIS system is used to not only grading the level of achievement of individual performance but it is also used to categorize geographical areas to monitor overall performance of identified individual institute or geographical area.

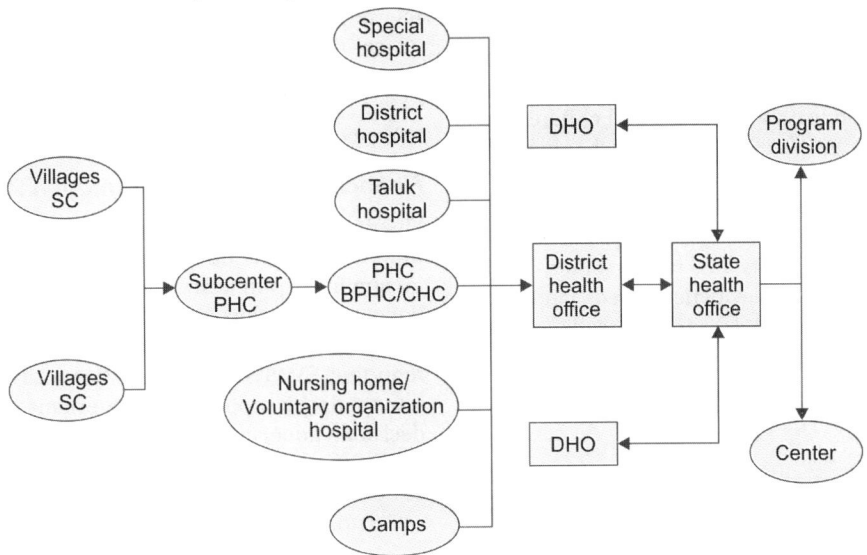

Flowchart 48.1: Hospital management information system (HMIS) reporting and feedback system.

Table 48.1: Some important content included in the monthly reports under HMIS to have an idea about activities, services and facilities being monitored in India.

| From-to | Content |
|---|---|
| Subcenter to PHC/CHC | *Performance report:* Report on all aspects of performance Family planning, immunization, diarrheal diseases, malaria, leprosy, blindness, deaths of all types<br>*Inventory report:* Malaria drugs, family planning aids, vaccines, ORS, basic drugs and others |
| PHC/hospital to district | *Consolidated information* collected from subcenter level<br>*Family welfare:* Sterilizations, IUDs, OP, condom users, MTP, etc.—stock position and the details of the above staff wise and unit wise, etc.<br>*Vital statistics:* Births, stillbirths, deaths, maternal deaths, infant deaths, neonatal deaths<br>*FW performance* like – Antenatal care (ANC) cases, institutional deliveries, vaccination, cold chain equipment, surveillance on diphtheria, measles, etc. Medical intelligence data on 41 identified diseases from general fever to ulcer of stomach to snakebites.<br>*Hospital IP and OP* statistics<br>*Inventory report:* Malaria drugs, family planning, vaccines, ORS, basic drugs and others<br>*Vacancy position*<br>*IEC reports* on contacts, group activities, TB, Malaria, Leprosy monthly reports |
| District to DHS | *Consolidated report* of all information collected from lower level institutions under the DMO<br>Monthly summary of *program statistics* for each program: Malaria, TB, leprosy, blindness, etc.<br>*Summary statistics* for Family Welfare Services (presently RCH)<br>*Inventory report:* Malaria drugs, family planning, vaccines, ORS, basic drugs and others<br>*Vacancy position*<br>*IEC reports* on contacts, group activities, TB, malaria, leprosy—monthly reports |
| DHS to Center | Monthly summary of *program statistics* for each program—Malaria, TB, leprosy, blindness, etc.<br>*Summary statistics* for Family Welfare Services (presently RCH) |

## Program Specific Management Information System

Though, HMIS, is developed as a comprehensive monitoring system in India covering vide range of information for various health programs and services, many vertical programs have their own data reporting system with program-specific data formats from peripheral institutes to national level institutes.

They include National AIDS Control Programme, Integrated Disease Surveillance Project (IDSP), National Tuberculosis Elimination Programme (NTEP), National Vector Borne Disease Control Programme (NVBDCP), etc.

Most health programs have identified indicators for yearly or quarterly monitoring of their performance. For example, in RNTCP, the indicators are monitored on quarterly basis include proportion of patients cured of tuberculosis, proportion of patient's relapse/default/failure, proportion of patients on drug resistant tuberculosis. The indicators monitored on yearly basis include annual incidence rate of infection, prevalence rate, treatment cure rate, failure rate, relapse rate.

> **Note**
> - Health information system is from primary health center to state and nation
> - Programme-oriented health information system for individual program
> - NACO, RNTCP, NVBDCP all have separate health information system

## Additional Systems

Besides HMIS, there are additional reporting system at national level as well as many states have developed their own monitoring system to monitor special needs. Many of them monitoring process indicators, while few are monitoring output indicators. Few of the key mechanism created as a monitoring system are as follows:

## Mother and Child Tracking System

Mother and child tracking system (MCTS) is an initiative of Ministry of Health and Family Welfare to leverage information technology for monitoring and tracking the healthcare and immunization services to pregnant women and children up to 5 years of age. Here, as a first step a pregnant mother is enrolled in this online tracking system. This system generates reminders/alerts for all the next due services. These reminders go to the service providers as well as beneficiaries. This system also helps in generating work plan for ANMs. It is implemented in all 36 states of the country. It will help in evidence-based planning and continuous assessment of service delivery to pregnant women and children. *(http://nrhm-mcts.nic.in/Home.aspx).*

## Drug Logistics Information and Management System (DLIMS), Gujarat

Drug logistics information and management system (DLIMS) is an online web-based application system developed by National Informatics Center to monitor entire logistic and supply chain, right from procurement processes starting from tender processing, to placing purchase orders and for stock monitoring and drug distribution. This system integrates various inter-related activities of the Central Medical Stores. The objectives of DLIMS are:
- To improve efficiency and effectiveness of drug logistics and warehousing system.
- Use latest information and communication technology to improve various functions like procurement; indenting, placing order, bill payment, etc. to serve in a better and effective manner.
- Facilitate continuous online monitoring of all activities.
- Integrate all inter-related activities through common database to avoid redundancy, increase accuracy and enhance transparency.

## Electronic Vaccine Intelligence Network

Electronic vaccine intelligence network (eVIN) is an indigenously developed technology system in India that digitizes vaccine stocks and monitors the temperature of the cold chain through a smartphone application. eVIN aims to support the Government of India's Universal Immunization Programme by providing real-time information on vaccine stocks and flows, and storage temperatures across all cold chain points in selected twelve states of India currently. The technological innovation is implemented by the United Nations Development Programme (UNDP).

It provides an integrated solution to address widespread inequities in vaccine coverage by supporting state governments in overcoming constraints of infrastructure, monitoring and management information systems and human resources, often resulting in overstocking and stock-outs of vaccines in storage centers.

## Training Management Information System

Training management information system (TMIS) is visualized as a "Single Window" for all static database related to training, i.e. documents related to trainings like training guidelines, training manuals, course content, training calendars, circulars and other relevant material and the dynamic database which would capture all real-time trainings, nominations, certificate generation, post-training evaluation and post-training deployment. The purpose of the TMIS is to have a centralized database of trained human resource to strengthen the public sector health delivery system.

## Finance Management Information System

Financial management information system (FMIS) is to monitor fund flow and its utilization. It supports the automation and integration of public financial management processes including budget formulation, execution (e.g. commitment control, cash/debt management, and treasury operations), accounting, and reporting. FMIS is used to track financial events and summarizes information. It supports adequate management reporting, policy decisions, fiduciary responsibilities, and preparation of auditable financial statements. It is designed with good relationships between software, hardware, personnel, procedures, controls and data.

# EVALUATION

Evaluation is aimed to know the effectiveness of the strategies or innovations. For evaluation of outcome or impact of different health programs in India, special surveys are being carried out. Some of the important mechanisms created to evaluate the health outcomes and impact of health programs are described briefly here under five broad headings.

> **Note**
> - Mother and child tracking system is important in RCH care.
> - Electronic vaccine intelligence gives an idea of vaccine coverage in the community.
> - Training management and Electronic management system manages the system approach.

## Evaluation of Health Program for Family Welfare

The following two mechanisms provide data on birth rate, fertility rate and death rate. They serve as impact indicators for the family welfare program.

1. **Census:** Census survey is conducted by Office of the Registrar General and Census Commissioner under Ministry of Home Affairs, Government of India every 10 years. Though census is a huge exercise with multiple objectives, the information gained through it helps in evaluating the impact of family welfare and other health programs as it provides annual birth rate, death rate, and total fertility rate by studying entire population of the country. Other details of census, India is available from this link: *http://censusindia.gov.in.*
2. **Civil registration system (CRS):** Civil registration system is primarily designed to issue birth and death registration certificate to the citizens of India. For an individual, records emanating from CRS provide her/his legal identity and access to the rights of a citizen including entitlements (social benefits provided by the Government). For the system, it provides information on birth registrations, death registrations, infant death registrations, sex ratio at birth, age-specific mortality rates, etc. Civil registration records are the best source of *vital*

*statistics* for planning and evaluation of many health programs related to primary health care, family planning, maternal and child health. At the national level it is under Office of the Registrar General and Census Commissioner, India, Ministry of Home Affair; Government of India. More details about CRS is available from this link: *http://www.censusindia.gov.in/2011-Common/CRS.html*.

## Evaluation of Impact of Health Program on Reproductive, Maternal and Child Health

- **Sample registration system (SRS):** It is also carried out by Office of the Registrar General and Census Commissioner under Ministry of Home Affairs; Government of India. The main objective of SRS is to provide reliable estimates of birth rate, death rate and infant mortality rate at the natural division level for major states and at the State level for smaller states. It also provides data for other measures of fertility and mortality including total fertility, infant and child mortality rate at higher geographical levels. Thus, it gives idea about effectiveness of various health programs, viz. family welfare, maternal and child health, epidemic control. Average time to publication of SRS annual reports is about 2 years. SRS estimates are generally valid and reliable for the country as a whole and for bigger states with more than 10 million population. Thus, its importance in evaluating the effectiveness of various health programs is considerable, especially, maternal health, child health and fertility.

  *Following demographic statistics are available from SRS:*
  - **Population distribution:** Population by 5-year age sex groups 0-4, to 70+ until 1994, and to 85+ since 1995.
  - **Fertility:** Population by marital status, age-specific and marital fertility rates, age-specific fertility rates by education, birth order and interval wise distribution of births.
  - **Mortality:** Age-specific death rates by 0, 1-4, and 5-year age groups from 5-9 until 85+, crude death rate, child mortality, IMR, MMR, U5MR, % distribution of deaths by age.
  - Access to medical care at birth and death.

  More details about SRS is available from this link: *http://www.censusindia.gov.in/Vital Statistics/SRS/Sample Registration System*.

- **National family health survey (NFHS):** The NFHS are nationwide surveys conducted with a representative sample of households throughout India by The Ministry of Health and Family Welfare (MOHFW), Government of India (GOI). NFHS was established with primary purpose of evaluation of impact of health programs. Also, it is established as system with periodic study. An important objective of the NFHS surveys has been to provide national and state estimates of fertility, family planning, infant and child mortality, reproductive and child health, nutrition of women and children, the quality of health and family welfare services, and socioeconomic conditions.

  While earlier rounds of NFHS were targeted to evaluate the impact of maternal, child and family welfare programs, in the subsequent rounds, its scope expanded to include evaluation of some areas of effect of health programs related with infectious diseases, and non-communicable disease. Additional information on various health determinants are also collected through NFHS.

  The NFHS surveys use standardized questionnaires, sample designs, and field procedures to collect data. Four NFHS surveys have been conducted till date. NFHS-1 in 1992-93, NFHS-2 in 1998-99, NFHS-3 in 2005-06, NFHS-4 in 2015-16 and NFHS-5 in the year 2019-20. All these serve as a major landmark in the development of a demographic and health database for India.

  More information about NFHS and its reports is available from this link: *http://rchiips.org/NFHS/index.shtml*.

- **District Level Household Survey (DLHS):** The earlier rounds of NFHS were designed to provide the evaluation picture at state level. But it was felt that within the state, impact of program is not similar in all districts. Also, district is the basic nucleus of planning and implementation of the health programs. Hence, it was decided to have special studies to evaluate the health programs at district level to know the utilization of services provided by government health facilities, people's perceptions on quality of services.

  DLHS was a household survey at the district level. International Institute for Population Sciences (IIPS), Mumbai was the nodal agency for conducting the District Level Household and Facility Survey. DLHS-1 was done in 1998-99, DLHS-2 in 2002–04, DLHS-3 in 2007–08 (in all states) and DLHS-4 in 2012-13 (in certain states only). Though, it was developed as a system of periodical survey, but with expansion of the scope of NFHS from state to district level, now no more DLHS is planned.

- **Coverage Evaluation Survey (CES):** Apart from Government Health Organizations, some international organizations like UNICEF also conducts special survey like CES. Its main objective is to assess the immunization coverage in children, indicators of maternal, newborn and child health. First coverage evaluation survey was carried out in year 2009. Second was carried out in the year 2018.

> **Note**
> - Evaluation system like census, sample registration system, NFHS evaluation all are important data sets of the country to collect many information
> - These data can give multiple monitoring and evaluation gives multiple analysis for managing system in general

## Evaluation of Impact of Health Program for Disease Control

National programs also carry out periodic evaluation exercises that come out with suggestions about the changes required in programs as per the changing needs. We take example of HIV surveillance here.

**HIV surveillance:** National AIDS Control Programme (NACP), India, has one of the world's largest and most robust *HIV sentinel surveillance (HSS)* systems. Since 1998 it has helped the national government to monitor the trends, levels and burden of HIV among different population groups in the country and craft effective responses to control HIV/AIDS. This survey is carried out amongst STD clinics as representative of high-risk group. Till year 2010, HIV sentinel surveillance was carried out annually thereafter it is done every 2 years. Till date 17 rounds are completed and 17th round was completed in 2021.

Data from HSS is instrumental in district re-categorization and subsequent decentralized evidence-based planning and implementation. The data is used to estimate HIV prevalence, incidence and burden. It gives ideas about impact of interventions under NACP.

For high-risk groups (HRGs) and Bridge Populations, a nationwide *integrated biological and behavioral surveillance (IBBS)* is being carried out as a strategic shift to strengthen the surveillance system among these groups. While HSS is clinic based the IBBS is community-based survey. First nationwide IBBS was carried out in the year 2014-15. It is more robust study designed to evaluate the impacts of NACP in High-Risk Groups. It evaluates HIV related knowledge and behavior as well as HIV and STI prevalence. It provides crucial evidence base for planning and implementation of programmatic initiatives under NACP besides giving information about impact of program.

***Non-communicable diseases:*** Some health programs on non-communicable diseases, conduct baseline survey to generate the data on current practices. For example, in National Tobacco Control Programme, "Global Adult Tobacco Survey" (GATS) India was conducted in 2009–2010 as a household survey of persons aged 15 years and above. A nationally representative probability sample was used to provide national and regional (North, West, East, South, Central and North-East) estimates by residence (urban and rural) and gender, and state estimates by gender. The survey was designed to produce internationally comparable data on tobacco use and other tobacco control indicators using standardized questionnaires, proper sample designs, and effective data collection and management procedures. GATS-2 survey has been conducted in 2016-17 and reports are available from WHO website.

### Evaluation of Impact of Program on Nutrition

National nutrition monitoring bureau (NNMB) was established under the aegis of Indian Council of Medical Research in the year 1972 in 10 states of India the Bureau carries out special nutrition related surveys (as and when required) and the objective of such special surveys is to collect, on a continuous basis, data on diet and nutritional status of the communities in the urban, rural and tribal areas using a standard and uniform methodology by adopting statistically valid study design and sample size; and to periodically evaluate the ongoing national nutrition programs to identify their strengths and weaknesses, and to recommend appropriate corrective measures.

**Important findings (indirect indicators)** from such special surveys of NNMB: Survey showed that in about 40% of households, the dietary energy intake by preschool children was inadequate, while that of adult men and women were adequate, reflecting inappropriate child feeding practices prevailing in the community. About 55% of the preschool age children were underweight, 52% were stunted and 15% were wasted. The prevalence of underweight and stunting was considerably high even among adolescents. Prevalence of Bitot spots, an objective sign of vitamin A Deficiency among 1–5 years' children was more than 0.5% in 6 out of 8 States surveyed indicating public health significance of the problem. The prevalence of central obesity was about 33% in men (WHR 0.95) and 77% in women (WHR 0.80). The prevalence of hypertension was about 25% among adult men and women. The prevalence of diabetes mellitus was about 4% in men and 3% in women in rural Andhra Pradesh.

### Evaluating the Socioeconomic Impact of Health and Health Services

**National sample survey office (NSSO):** The surveys on social consumption relating to health is conducted by national sample survey office to provide basic quantitative information on health sector like morbidity, hospitalization, extent of prenatal and postnatal care by women, expenditure incurred on treatment received from health services in public and private sectors, etc. While the other surveys mentioned here are conducted mainly by the Ministry of Health in Government of India, the NSS are carried out by the Ministry of Statistics and Programme Implementation of Government of India.

The last NSS survey on health (71st round) was conducted in 2014 with an objective to study the self- reported morbidity rates, the utilization of public and private health services by various sections of the population to address these morbidities, and out-of-pocket expenditure incurred on health care. This survey report mentioned that more than 70% of ailments were treated in private sector in India and almost 63% patients preferred to get admitted in private institutions. More information related to NSS are available on *http://www.mospi.gov.in/national-sample-survey-office-nsso*.

## SUMMARY

The finances required and man-days spent for implementation of health programs and services for a large country like India are enormous. The policymakers need to know whether the health programs and services are working as planned and the extent to which they are successful in achieving desired result. For that country needs a strong monitoring and evaluation system.

In India, there is an inbuilt system of routine reporting and feedback for monitoring the health program and services. With advent of IT, and expansion of network of internet, IT enabled reporting and feedback system is established. HMIS is such comprehensive monitoring mechanism in India. But besides that many vertical programs are having their own routine reporting and feedback system. Also, to monitor specific area of operation like logistics and supply, finance, etc. many other monitoring mechanisms are in place in India.

Evaluation is to know the outcome and impact of the health programs. There are quite a few mechanisms to monitor impact of reproductive, maternal and child health but still a regular system of evaluation especially for disease control and other programs are not adequate in India. However, many special surveys are being carried out to evaluate specific health situation or impact.

## SUGGESTED READING

1. Electronic Vaccine Intelligence Network (eVIN). National Health Mission, Ministry of Health and Family Welfare, Government of India, 2016.
2. Global Adult Tobacco Survey (GATS): fact sheet, India 2016-17; 2017. [online] Available from http://www.who.int/tobacco/surveillance/survey/gats/GATS_India_2016-17_FactSheet.pdf.

3. Gujarat Medical Services Corporation Limited. Drug Logistics Information and Management System (DLIMS), Gujarat. [online]. Available from: http://www.cips.org.in/documents/DownloadPDF/ downloadpdf.php?id=436andcategory=Health
4. International Institute for Population Sciences (IIPS) Mumbai. District Level Household and Facility Survey. [online] Available from: http://rchiips.org/.
5. International Institute for Population Sciences (IIPS) Mumbai. National Family Health Survey, India. [online] Available from: http:// rchiips.org/NFHS/index.shtml.
6. Ministry of Health and Family Welfare - Government of India. Mother and Child Tracking System. [online] Available from: http:// nrhm-mcts.nic.in.
7. Ministry of Health and Family Welfare - Government of India. National Nutrition Monitoring Bureau. [online] Available from: http://nnmbindia.org/default.html.
8. Ministry of Health and Family Welfare - Government of India. Training Management Information System. [online] Available from: http://tmis-mohfw.gov.in/.
9. Ministry of Health and Family Welfare. Health Management Information system [online] Available from: https://nrhm-mis.nic.in/SitePages/Home.aspx.
10. Ministry of Statistics and Programme Implementation - Government of India. National Sample Survey Office. [online] Available from: http://www.mospi.gov.in/national-sample-survey-office-nsso.
11. National AIDS Control Organisation, Ministry of Health and Family Welfare. HIV Sentinel Surveillance. [online] Available from: http://naco.gov.in/surveillance-epidemiology-0.
12. Office of the Registrar General and Census Commissioner, Ministry of Home Affairs, Government of India. Census, India. [online] Available from: http://censusindia.gov.in/.
13. Office of the Registrar General and Census Commissioner, Ministry of Home Affairs, Government of India. Civil Registration System. [online] Available from: http://www.censusindia.gov.in/2011-Common/CRS.html.
14. Office of the Registrar General and Census Commissioner, Ministry of Home Affairs, Government of India. Sample Registration System. [online] Available from: http://www.censusindia.gov.in/2011-Common/Sample_Registration_System.html.

# CHAPTER 49

# Health Legislations in India

*Priya Arora, Gurmeet Kaur*

| CM11.2 | Describe the role, benefits and functioning of the employees state insurance scheme |
|---|---|

## INTRODUCTION

Public health laws are an important tool to empower the state to create conditions for healthy populations. Although individual autonomy and privacy are of paramount importance in a democratic society, yet sometimes, coercive power of public health rules and laws is needed to maintain public health and safety. These laws and policies authorize, obligate and control government and private action concerning health. Measures to handle emergency response in a health crisis (e.g., outbreak control) is just one facet of these public health laws. These laws are also an important tool for promotion and protection of health of individuals and populations (e.g., improve road safety and reduce tobacco use). Sometimes, these laws may seem to be impinging on individual rights and freedom (e.g., social distancing and quarantine), therefore, a fine and delicate balance has to be maintained to achieve the greater good for the society and respecting individual rights at the same time.

The public health laws may either be directly related to some health action or may be indirectly having an influence on the health of the population.

As medical professionals, most of us will have some brush with the law, either during clinical practice in the form of medicolegal cases or during public health practice to educate people and report violations of public health laws. And, therefore, knowing about these laws is important for health professionals.

The laws can take two forms:
1. **Acts**: Act means statute or laws adopted (enacted) by a national or state legislative assembly or any other governing body. These are the laws passed by legislature. They describe the applicability, definitions for governance, and penalties for violation of the Act.
2. **Rules**: Rules are explicit statements that describe the standard methods and procedures, i.e., tell the people what is to be done (or not). Rules help in application and enforcement of the provisions specified by the Act.

## CLASSIFICATION OF HEALTH LAWS

The various laws related to public health can broadly divided into following groups:
- **Disease prevention and control**:
  - Epidemic Disease Act, 1897
  - Narcotic Drugs and Psychotropic Substances Act, 1985
  - The Drugs and Cosmetics Act 1940 and The Drugs and Cosmetics Rules, 1945
  - COTPA, 2003
  - Disaster Management Act, 2005.
- **Protecting vulnerable group**:
  - *Women*:
    - Domestic Violence Act, 2005
    - Indecent Representation of Women (Prohibition) Act, 1986
    - The Dowry Prohibition Act, 1961
    - The Immoral Traffic (Prevention) Act, 1956.
  - *Children*:
    - The Infant Milk Substitutes, Feeding Bottles and Infant Foods (Regulation of Production, Supply and Distribution) Act, 1992
    - The Child Labor (Prohibition and Regulation) Act, 1986
    - The Child Marriage Restraint Act, 1929
    - The Juvenile Justice (Care and Protection of Children) Act, 2000
    - Right to Education Act, 2009
    - Protection of Children from Sexual Offences Act (POCSO), 2012
  - *Aged:* Persons Maintenance and Welfare of Parents and Senior Citizens Act, 2007.
  - *Disabled:* Person with Disabilities (Equal Opportunities, Protection of Rights and Full Participation) Act, 1995.
  - *Occupational workers*:
    - Employee State Insurance Act, 1948
    - Factory Act, 1948
    - Workmen Compensation Act, 1923
    - Maternity Benefit Act, 1961
    - Minimum Wages Act, 1948
    - The Bonded Labor System (Abolition) Act, 1976
    - The Mines Act 1952
  - *Menatally Ill:* The Mental Health Act, 1987.

- *Environmental health safety laws:*
  - Environment Protection Act, 1986
  - Water (Prevention and Control of Pollution) Act, 1974
  - Biomedical Waste Management Act, 1998 and 2016
  - The Municipal Solid Waste (Management and Handling) Rules, 2000
- *Food safety laws:*
  - Food Safety and Standards Regulation Act, 2006
  - Prevention of Food Adulteration Act, 1954
- *Public health services related laws:*
  - The Census Act, 1948
  - Birth, Death and Marriage Registration Act, 1969
  - Medical Termination of Pregnancy (MTP) Act, 1971
  - Preconception and Prenatal Diagnostic Techniques Act, 1994

Some of the important Public Health Laws are described in this chapter.

## DISEASE PREVENTION AND CONTROL

### Epidemic Diseases Act, 1897

"An Act to provide for the better prevention of the spread of dangerous epidemic diseases".

The Act was introduced to control the plague epidemic that broke out in the 1890s, in the then Bombay state, by the colonial government. It gives the power to the central and state governments for prevention and control of the spread of epidemic diseases.

The Act empowers the authorities to make temporary regulations or issue public notices for inspection and temporary isolation of persons suspected to be infected with any such disease.

When it is felt that there is a threat of an outbreak of any dangerous epidemic disease, any ship or vessel leaving or arriving at any port can be inspected and any person intending to sail therein, or arriving thereby, can be detained, as considered essential for outbreak control. The Act also has similar provisions for travel by railways.

Furthermore, the expenses incurred in compensation, traveling, temporary accommodation, segregation of infected persons, etc. by the concerned officers are compensable by the authorities empowered by the government.

### *Punishment under the Act*

Violation of the Act is punishable under Section 188 of the Indian Penal Code (IPC).

No definition or description of a "dangerous epidemic disease" is given in the Act, so it can be used as per the discretion of the public health authorities of the region.

### The Epidemic Diseases (Amendment) Bill, 2020

The Bill amends the Epidemic Diseases Act (1897) to include protections for healthcare personnel combatting epidemic diseases and expands the powers of the central government to prevent the spread of such diseases.

Under the Bill, an 'Act of violence' includes any of the following Acts committed against a healthcare service personnel: (i) harassment impacting living or working conditions, (ii) harm, injury, hurt, or danger to life, (iii) obstruction in discharge of duties, and (iv) loss or damage to the property or documents of the healthcare service personnel. Property includes: (i) clinical establishment, (ii) quarantine facility, (iii) mobile medical unit, and (iv) any other property in which a healthcare service personnel has direct interest, in relation to the epidemic.

The Bill specifies that no person can: (i) commit or abet the commission of an Act of violence against a healthcare service personnel, or (ii) abet or cause damage or loss to any property during an epidemic. Contravention of this provision is punishable with imprisonment between 3 months and 5 years, and a fine between ₹ 50,000 and 200,000. Further, if an Act of violence against a healthcare service personnel causes grievous harm, the person committing the offence will be punishable with imprisonment between 6 months and 7 years, and a fine between ₹ 100,000 and 500,000. These offences will be cognizable and non-bailable.

### Narcotic and Psychotropic Substance Act, 1985

- The Opium Act, 1857 was earlier used to exercise control over illegal drugs.
- The Narcotic Drugs and Psychotropic Substances Act, 1985 prohibits the production, manufacture, cultivation, possession, sale, purchase, transport, storage, and/or consumption of any narcotic drug or psychotropic substance. The Act applies to the whole of India and also to all Indian citizens outside India and to all persons aboard ships and aircrafts that are registered in India.
- The law regulates use and possession of drugs, makes trafficking in drugs illegal and punishable, and allows the government to exercise control over the cultivation, production and use of some drugs, for medicinal purposes.

### *Punishment under the Act*

Punishment for production, manufacture, possession, sale, etc. of illegal drugs and substances depends on the quantity of drugs and the kind of drug. The quantity has been classified into small, small but less than commercial and commercial. The maximum punishment for these offences varies from 6 months to 10 and 20 years, respectively along with fine.

There is provision for rigorous imprisonment for up to 30 years or death penalty in extreme cases for repeat offenders (usually those involved in trafficking).

*The Narcotic Drugs and Psychotropic Substances (Amendment) Act, 2014* amended the Act to relax restrictions on essential narcotic drugs (morphine, fentanyl, and methadone), which have medicinal use for pain relief and palliative care. The amendment removed mandatory death penalty in case of a repeat conviction for trafficking large quantities of drugs and the punishment for "small quantity" offences has been increased from a maximum of 6 months to 1 year imprisonment.

### Drugs and Cosmetics Act 1940

Blood transfusion services including setting up of blood banks are regulated by the Drugs and Cosmetics Act 1940. The Act specifies about the accommodation, equipment, manpower, reagents, and supplies, practices to be followed in blood transfusion services. National AIDS Control Organization (NACO) acts as a facilitator for these services. The Act ensures the availability of safe blood by mandatory testing of blood for various diseases, phasing out of professional blood donors, and prohibits selling of blood or blood components for profit. The Act also provides for standards to be followed by blood banks and blood transfusion services including guidelines for blood transfusions. The permission to set-up blood banks is granted by the Drugs Controller General of India (DCGI).

The license of the blood banks not adhering to the guidelines may be cancelled.

## Cigarettes and Other Tobacco Products (Prohibition of Advertisement and Regulation of Trade and Commerce, Production, Supply, and Distribution) Act or COTPA, 2003

The Act aims to regulate advertisement, trade and commerce in, and production, supply, distribution, and sale of cigarettes and other tobacco products in India.

*Provisions under the Act include:*
- Prohibition of smoking at public places except in separate designated smoking areas in hotels, restaurants, airports, and in open spaces.
- Prohibition of advertisement of tobacco products, including surrogate advertisement, via leaflets, documents, video films, hoardings, etc.
- Sale of tobacco to minors and in an area within a radius of one hundred yards of any educational institution is forbidden.
- Packaging of tobacco products must contain pictorial warnings and nicotine and tar content.

### Punishment under the Act

For manufacturers who fail to adhere to provisions of the Act regarding display warnings on packages, first conviction is punishable with up to 2 years in imprisonment or with fine, which can extend to ₹5,000. Subsequent conviction is punishable with up to 5 years in imprisonment or with fine, which can extend to ₹10,000.

Smoking in public places, selling tobacco products to minors, or selling tobacco products within a radius of 100 m from any educational institution is punishable with a fine of up to ₹200 and all offences are compoundable.

Advertisement of tobacco products, on first conviction is punishable with up to 2 years in imprisonment or with fine, which can extend to ₹1,000. Subsequent conviction is punishable with up to 5 years in imprisonment or with fine, which can extend to ₹5,000.

## Disaster Management Act, 2005

The Disaster Management Act was passed in 2005 and extends to the whole of India. The aim of the Act is to provide statutory structure and functions for effective management of disasters. The Act gives a new multidisciplinary focus on disaster mitigation, prevention, preparedness and response, and move away from just relief-centric activities.

*The Act mandated the creation of the following bodies:*
- National Disaster Management Authority with the Prime Minister of India as Chairperson.
- National Executive Committee composed of Secretary level officers of the Government of India from various Ministries.
- State disaster management authorities with Chief Minister as the Chairperson.
- National Disaster Response Force for the purpose of specialist response to a threatening disaster situation or disaster.

These institutions are responsible for disaster preparedness, risk reduction, and disaster response at their respective levels. It also takes into consideration the need for capacity building at various levels for disaster management. The role of the central government is to ensure guidelines are in place for integration of disaster mitigation and prevention with the development plans at all levels, implementation and monitoring the disaster management plans, cooperation with international agencies and other countries, coordinating disaster response activities between states, and identifying nodal ministries for different disasters.

At the local level, the Act mandates the creation of response plans and procedures for allocation of responsibilities, prompt relief measures, procurement of supplies for effective response, establishment of communication links, and dissemination of information to public.

The Act further contains the provisions for financial mechanisms such as the creation of funds for the response, National Disaster Mitigation Fund, and similar funds at the state and district levels.

### Punishment under the Act

Whosoever, without reasonable cause, obstructs any authorized person in discharge of his duties for disaster management or refuses to comply with any direction given by authorities, is liable to be punished with imprisonment of up to 1 year. If such refusal or obstruction leads to loss of lives or imminent danger thereof, it is punishable with imprisonment up to 2 years.

### National Disaster Management Plan, 2016

The National Disaster Management Plan (NDMP) is in accordance with Sendai Framework adopted by UN for disaster risk reduction. It covers all phases of disaster management—prevention, mitigation, preparedness, response, and recovery. It provides for coordination among all the agencies and departments of the government by assigning roles and responsibilities of all levels of administration right up to Panchayat and Urban Local body level in a matrix format.

# PROTECTING VULNERABLE GROUPS

## Women

### Domestic Violence Act, 2005

The Act aims to provide for protection of the rights of women who are victims of violence of any kind occurring within the family.

The Act specifies definition of "domestic violence" that includes not only physical violence, but also other forms of violence such as emotional or verbal, sexual, and economic abuse. "Domestic violence" not only includes actual abuse but also the threat of abuse. Any kind of behavior by husband or male partner or their relatives that falls in the above categories is termed as domestic violence. Demanding dowry from the woman or her relatives is also covered under this definition.

The Act covers relationships by consanguinity, marriage, or a relationship in the nature of marriage (which includes live-in relationships) or adoption. The relationships with family members of the husband or partner, living together as a joint family, are also included. The Act also provides legal protection to sisters, widows, mothers, single women, or women living with them.

The Act ensures the woman's right to secure housing by providing residence in the matrimonial or shared household, whether or not she has any rights in the household, by means of a residence order passed by a court.

The Act directs the government to appoint Protection Officers and nongovernmental organizations (NGOs) for providing assistance to women for medical examination, legal aid, safe shelter, etc.

### Punishment under the Act
- Under the provisions of the Act, through court orders, the abuser can be prevented from aiding or committing an act of domestic violence, entering the any specified place, attempting to communicate with the abused, isolating any assets used by both the parties, and causing violence to the abused or her relatives.
- Breach of protection order or interim protection order by the accused is a cognizable and nonbailable offence, which is punishable with imprisonment up to 1 year or with fine which up to ₹20,000 or with both.

## Dowry Prohibition Act, 1961

It applies to the whole of India except the State of Jammu and Kashmir. "Dowry" refers to any property or valuable security given or agreed to be given either directly or indirectly by one party to a marriage to the other party to the marriage; or by the parents of either party to a marriage before or any time after the marriage but does not include Mehr.

### Punishment under the Act
- According to provisions of the Act, demanding (directly or indirectly), giving, taking, or abetting dowry is punishable with imprisonment and fine.
- Where the death of a woman is caused by burns or bodily injury within 7 years of marriage and it is shown that soon before death, she was subjected to cruelty or harassment by husband or relatives is known as dowry deaths and punishment for this is for 7 years and may extend up to life.
- The offences committed against this Act are cognizable, nonbailable, and non-compoundable.

## Immoral Traffic (Prevention) Act, 1956 and Immoral Traffic Prevention Act, 1986

The Act intends to combat trafficking and sexual exploitation for commercial purposes. While according to the 1951 Act, prostitution is not an offence, practicing it in a brothel or within 200 m of any public place is illegal. The Act lays down rules and regulations regarding the sensitive issue of prostitution and protects women and children from forceful flesh trade.

The Act was amended in 1986 to comply with the United Nations Declaration on the Suppression of Trafficking, for prevention and prohibition of prostitution by criminalizing sex work.

## Children

### Infant Milk Substitutes, Feeding Bottles and Infant Foods Act, 1992 and Amendment 2003

The Infant Milk Substitutes, Feeding Bottles, and Infant Foods Act, 1992 and its 2003 amendment aims to promote breastfeeding and regulate production, supply, marketing, and use of infant foods. The Act applies to whole of India.

Infant food refers to the food that is marketed, or represented as complementary to mother's milk to provide the nutritional needs of the infant after 6 months up to 2 years while infant milk substitute is any food being marketed or represented as partial or full replacement for mother's milk for the infant up to 2 years of age. The products have to meet the standards of the Prevention of Food Adulteration Act, 1954, or the Bureau of Indian Standards.

This Act prohibits the advertisement, promotion, or misleading people to believe that infant food, feeding bottles, and infant milk substitutes are an acceptable replacement of mother's milk. The Act forbids contacting expecting mothers and mothers of infants to offer inducement or sell or promote these products.

The Act mandates labels on these products that emphasize mother's milk is the best food for an infant and provide instructions for usage, nutritional information, ingredients used, expiry, etc. Pictures of babies or mothers are not permitted and its likeness to human milk is not to be mentioned by using words like humanized, maternalized, etc.

Promotion of infant milk substitutes, feeding bottles or infant food is not permitted in any healthcare facility and no bribing is to be done to health workers for the purpose of promoting the use of such substitutes/bottles/foods.

### Punishment under the Act
- Conviction under the provisions of this act can result in a maximum jail sentence of 3 years and/or a maximum fine of ₹5,000.
- Under this Act, companies can also be charged for an offence, by charging all those who were aware of the violation and are in a position of responsibility. Offences under this Act are bailable and cognizable.

## The Child Labor (Prohibition and Regulation) Act, 1986

The Act prohibits the engagement of children in certain stipulated employments and regulates the conditions of work of children in others. It extends to the whole of India. "Child" means a person who has not completed 14th year of age.

The Act prohibits children from working in any occupation listed in Part A of the Schedule, e.g., catering at railway establishments, construction work on the railway, plastics factories, automobile garages, etc. Part B of the Act enlists certain processes where children are prohibited to work, e.g., beedi making, tanning, soap manufacture, brick kilns, etc. These provisions do not apply to a workshop where the occupier is working with the help of his family or in a government recognized or aided school.

The Act fixes the hours, timings, and rest intervals for children during their work and prohibits overtime for working children. The total number of hours of work on any day for children will not exceed 6 hours, with an hour rest period after 3 hours of work. Children are prohibited to work between 7 PM and 8 AM. It is compulsory to give one weekly off to children. The Act also gives directions regarding safe working conditions for children.

### Punishment under the Act

Violation of the provisions of the Act, by persons who employ or permit children to work, is liable to be punished with imprisonment for a term of not be less than 3 months and extendable up to 1 year or with fine of not be less than ₹10,000 but which may extend to ₹20,000 or with both. Repeat offence under the Act is punishable with imprisonment for a term of not be less than 6 months but which may extend to 2 years. Employees who fail to keep a correct record of children are also liable to be punished.

### Child Marriage Restraint Act, 1929 and Prohibition of Child Marriage Act, 2006

Child Marriage Restraint Act, 1929 fixed the age of marriage for girls at 14 years and boys at 18 years. It is popularly known as the Sarda Act, after its sponsor Har Bilas Sarda. The age for marriage was later raised to 18 years for girls and 21 years for boys in 1978. The Act extends to the whole of India except Jammu and Kashmir.

"Child" means any male, who has not completed 21 years of age; and any female, who has not completed 18 years of age. "Child marriage", according to the Act, means a marriage to which either of the contracting parties is a child.

### Punishment under the Act:

- Any male, above 18 but below 21 years of age, who contracts a child marriage, is liable to be punished with simple imprisonment up to 15 days or with fine up to ₹1,000 or with both. Any male, above 21 years of age, who contracts a child marriage, is liable to be punished with simple imprisonment up to 3 months or with fine or both.
- In case of child marriage of minors, parent or guardian, or any person having charge of minor, who does any act to promote, permits child marriage is liable for 3 months imprisonment and/or fine.
- *Prohibition of Child Marriage Act, 2006* aims at prohibition of solemnization of child marriages rather than just restraining them.
- Every child marriage is voidable at the option of the contracting party who was a child at the time of the marriage by filing a decree of nullity in the district court. The male contracting party or his parent or guardian may also be directed to pay maintenance to the female party till she gets remarried. Male partners above 18 years are liable for rigorous imprisonment up to 2 years and fine up to ₹1 lakh.
- Whoever performs, conducts, directs or abets, promotes child marriage or permits it to be solemnized, or negligently fails to prevent it from being solemnized, including attending or participating in a child marriage, is liable to be punished with rigorous imprisonment up to 2 years and fine which may extend to ₹1 lakh.

### The Juvenile Justice (Care and Protection of Children) Act, 2000

The Act deals with issues related to juveniles in conflict with law and children in need of care and protection, and their social integration and rehabilitation through various institutions established under this enactment. Under the provisions of the Act, "juvenile" or "child" means a person who has not completed 18th year of age. The three broad areas covered by the Acts are:

1. *Juveniles in conflict with law*: Anyone less than 18 years of age who has committed any offence as per the law of the land. The Act mandates state governments to set up Juvenile Justice Boards for matters pertaining to juveniles in conflict with law or offences committed by juveniles. The board consists of a Magistrate and two social workers, including a woman, who have been involved in health, education, or welfare activities pertaining to children for a minimum of 5 years.
2. Children in need of care and protection including destitute, orphaned, abandoned, and surrendered children. The Act provides for the creation of Child Welfare Committees, institutions such as shelter homes, aftercare organizations, etc., are established and child protection officers are appointed.
3. Rehabilitation and social integration of children including their adoption from care homes.

### Juvenile Justice (Care and Protection of Children) Act, 2015

The amended Act allows for juveniles in conflict with law in the age group of 16–18, who have committed Heinous Offences, to be tried as adults. It came into force in 2016.

### Right of Children to Free and Compulsory Education Act, 2009

The Right of Children to Free and Compulsory Education Act or Right to Education Act (RTE), is an Act of the Parliament of India enacted on 4 August 2009, which describes the modalities of the importance of free and compulsory education for children between 6 and 14 in India under Article 21a of the Indian Constitution. India became one of 135 countries to make education a fundamental right of every child when the Act came into force on 1 April 2010.

The RTE Act provides for the right of children to free and compulsory education till completion of elementary education in a neighborhood school. It clarifies that "compulsory education" means obligation of the appropriate government to provide free elementary education and ensure compulsory admission, attendance and completion of elementary education to every child in the 6–14 age group. "Free" means that no child shall be liable to pay any kind of fee or charges or expenses which may prevent him or her from pursuing and completing elementary education.

The Act makes education a fundamental right of every child between the ages of 6 and 14 and specifies minimum norms in elementary schools. It requires all private schools to reserve 25% of seats to children (to be reimbursed by the state as part of the public-private partnership plan). Children are admitted in to private schools based on economic status or caste-based reservations. It also prohibits all unrecognized schools from practice, and makes provisions for no donation or capitation fees and no interview of the child or parent for admission. The Act also provides that no child shall be held back, expelled, or required to pass a board examination until the completion of elementary education. There is also a provision for special training of school drop-outs to bring them up to par with students of the same age.

The Right to Education of persons with disabilities until 18 years of age is laid down under a separate legislation—the Persons with Disabilities Act. A number of other provisions regarding improvement of school infrastructure, teacher-student ratio and faculty are made in the Act.

## Protection of Children Against Sexual Offences Bill (POCSO), 2012

The act was enacted to provide a robust legal framework for the protection of children from offences of sexual assault, sexual harassment and pornography, while safeguarding the interest of the child at every stage of the judicial process. The framing of the Act seeks to put children first by making it easy to use by including mechanisms for child-friendly reporting, recording of evidence, investigation and speedy trial of offences through designated Special Courts. The act is gender-neutral for both children and for the accused. With respect to pornography, the Act criminalizes watching or collection of pornographic content involving children also. The Act makes abetment (encouragement) of child sexual abuse an offence. After the 2019 Amendment Act, the POCSO Act punishment is even stricter. A violation of the POCSO Act carries a maximum punishment of life imprisonment and in some cases death penalty. It also provides for various procedural reforms, making the tiring process of trial in India considerably easier for children. A Victim of Child Sexual Abuse can file a complaint at any time irrespective of his/her present age.

## Aged

### Persons Maintenance and Welfare of Parents and Senior Citizens Act (2007)

This act provides assured services for the maintenance and welfare of parents and senior citizens. This Act is applicable in entire India except Jammu and Kashmir. Certain descriptions include children, i.e., son, daughter, grandson, and granddaughter who are not minor. Maintenance is providing food, clothing, residence and medical attendance, and treatment. Parents include father or mother whether biological, adoptive, or stepfather or stepmother whether the parents are senior citizens (more than 60 years) or not. If they cannot support themselves in terms of food, clothing, and residence from their income (pension and income from property) then the requirements are looked after by their children. Such parents can apply to the court regarding the complaint against the children and court can ask the children to give monthly allowance even if the court has not settled the case. On failure of compliance, the court can issue the warrants or levy fine or issue imprisonment for a month. The monthly allowance may not be more than ₹10,000. Apart from this, State governments are directed to open old age homes and ensuring special services for senior citizens in all government funded or aided hospitals to provide such as separate queue, separate clinics, special preference for beds for admission, and impart research work on diseases among older persons.

## Disabled

### Persons with Disabilities (Equal Opportunities, Protection of Rights and Full Participation) Act, 1995

The aim of this Act is to provide for a legal framework for protection of rights and ensuring justice for persons with disabilities. The Act is applicable to the whole of India.

The Act describes disability as blindness, low vision, leprosy-cured, hearing impairment, locomotor disability, mental retardation, and mental illness. Disabled person is one who is suffering from not less than 40% of any of the disability as certified by a medical authority.

The Act gives fundamental right to all disabled people for equal opportunity. There is provision in the Act to create a central level and state level coordination committees and an executive committee; the duties being to formulate policies, to assess and direct the activities of government and NGOs, and to appraise the programs and policies for the disabled.

The Act stipulates the direction to government and local bodies for following activities:
- ***Prevention of disabilities:*** This is done by screening children for identification of "At Risk" cases, prenatal, perinatal, and postnatal care of mother and child and awareness campaigns for the public.
- ***Education:*** Each disabled child shall have the right to free education till the age of 18 years with free books, uniform and scholarships, suitable transportation, and barrier free environment.
- ***Occupations:*** 3% vacancies in government educational institutes and jobs shall be reserved for blindness or low vision, hearing impairment, locomotor disability, and cerebral palsy. No employee can be terminated from service or demoted if s(he) becomes disabled during the service.
- ***Easy access:*** All the places shall be made barrier free to give easy access of public utilities public buildings, rail compartments, buses, ships, etc. to facilitate their use by the disabled.
- ***Social security:*** Financial assistance at NGOs, insurance coverage to employees with disability and preferential allotment of land at concessional rates are some schemes for social security cover to the disabled.

### Punishment under the Act

Those who avail or attempt to avail benefits meant for the disabled in a fraudulent manner are punishable with imprisonment up to 2 years or a fine up to ₹20,000.

## Occupational Workers

### Employee State Insurance Act, 1948

Employees' State Insurance (ESI) Scheme of India is a multidimensional social security system tailored to provide socioeconomic protection to worker population and their dependents covered under the scheme.

The ESI Scheme is an integrated measure of Social Insurance embodied in the ESI Act and it is designed to accomplish the task of protecting "employees" as defined in the ESI Act, 1948 against the impact of incidences of sickness, maternity, disablement, and death due to employment injury (EI) and to provide medical care to insured persons (IPs) and their families. The ESI Scheme applies to factories and other establishment's viz. road transport, hotels, restaurants, cinemas, newspaper, shops, and educational or medical institutions wherein 10 or more persons are employed. However, in some states threshold limit for coverage of establishments is still 20. Employees of the aforesaid categories of factories and establishments, drawing wages up to ₹15,000 a month, are entitled to social security cover under the ESI Act. ESI Corporation has also decided to enhance wage ceiling for coverage of employees under the ESI Act from ₹15,000 to ₹21,000.

The ESI Scheme is financed by contributions from employers and employees. With effect from 1st July 2019, the rate of contribution by employer is 3.25% of the wages payable to employees. The employees' contribution is at the rate of 0.75% of the wages payable to an employee. Employees, earning less than ₹137 a day as daily wages, are exempted from payment of their share of contribution.

### Coverage

In the beginning, the ESI Scheme was implemented at just two industrial centers in the country in 1952, namely Kanpur and Delhi. Keeping pace with the process of industrialization, the Scheme today, stands implemented at over 843 centers in 33 States and Union Territories. The Act now applies to over 7.83 lakhs factories and establishments across the country, benefiting about 2.13 crores IPs or family units. As of now, the total beneficiary stands at over 8.28 crores.

### Infrastructure

Ever since its inception in 1952, the infrastructural network of the Scheme has kept expanding to meet the social security requirements of an ever increasing worker population. ESI Corporation has so far set up 151 hospital and 42 hospital annexes for inpatient services. Primary and outpatient medical services are provided through a network of about 1,450/188 ESI dispensaries or AYUSH (Ayurveda, Yoga, Unani, Siddha and Homeopathy) units, and 954 panel clinics.

The Corporation has also set up five Occupational Disease Centers, one each at Mumbai (Maharashtra), New Delhi, Kolkata (West Bengal), Chennai (Tamil Nadu), and Indore (Madhya Pradesh) for early detection and treatment of occupational diseases prevalent amongst workers employed in hazardous industries.

### Security Benefits

The Section 46 of the Act envisages following six social security benefits:

1. *Medical benefit:* Full medical care is provided to an IP and his family members from the day he enters insurable employment. There is no ceiling on expenditure on the treatment of an IP or his family member. Medical care is also provided to retired and permanently disabled IPs and their spouses on payment of a token annual premium of ₹120.
   - **System of treatment:** Generally, the allopathic system of medicine is used for providing medical benefit. However, where a substantial number of workers' demand treatment by Indian system of medicine and Homoeopathy (ISM & H) other than Allopathy and where the State Government has recognized the qualifications in such system, treatment facilities may be provided under the ISM & H as well. The various ISM & H systems of treatment in vogue are—Ayurvedic, Unani, Siddha, Yoga therapy, and Homeopathy.
   - **Scale of medical benefit:**
     - *To IPs:* IPs are entitled to avail treatment in ESI dispensary/hospital/diagnostic center and recognized institutions, to which he is attached such as:
       - Outpatient treatment
       - Domiciliary treatment by visits at their residences
       - Specialists consultation
       - Inpatient treatment (hospitalization)
       - Free supply of drugs dressings and artificial limbs, aids, and appliances
       - Imaging and laboratory services
       - Integrated family welfare, immunization and Maternal and Child Health (MCH) program and other national health program, etc.
       - Ambulance service or reimbursement of conveyance charges for going to hospitals, diagnostic centers, etc.
       - Medical certification
       - Special provisions.
     - *To family members of IPs:* Members of a family of an IP are entitled to one or other of the following scales of medical benefits:
       - "FULL" Medical Care, i.e., all facilities as for IPs including hospitalization.
       - "EXPANDED" Medical Care, i.e., all facilities as for IPs except hospitalization. A small number of IPs in the States of Gujarat and Bihar fall under this category.
   - **Benefits to retired IPs:** On payment of ₹10 PM in lump sum for 1 year in advance, medical benefit can be provided to an IP and his or her spouse who leaves insurable employment on attaining the age of superannuation after being insured for not less than 5 years, till the period for which contribution is paid. And to an IP and his/her spouse who ceases to be in insurable employment on account of permanent disablement due to EI shall be entitled to medical benefit.
   - **Administration of medical benefit in a state:** The administration of Medical Benefit under the ESI Scheme is the statutory responsibility of the State Government except in the Union Territory of Delhi where the ESI corporation has taken over direct responsibility to administer the same with effect from 1.4.1962. The corporation has also taken

the responsibility of directly administering the existing Occupational Disease Centers at Delhi. Mumbai, Calcutta, Chennai and Nagda as well as the Scheme in the Industrial pocket of Uttar Pradesh, i.e., Noida and Greater Noida.
- **Domiciliary treatment:** An IP and his family members are entitled to free medical attendance by IMO/IMP (Insurance Medical Officer/Insurance Medical Practitioner Panel) at their residence when the condition of the patient is such that he/she cannot reasonably be expected to attend the dispensary or clinic.
- **Specialist consultation:** The standard of Medical Care under the ESI Scheme provides for specialist consultation to IP in all cases and to members of their families in areas with "expanded" and "full" medical care. Arrangements for specialist consultation may be provided at specialist or diagnostic centers, ESI Hospitals, or at such other institutions by appointing specialists or super specialists on full time or part-time basis where suitable arrangements exist.
- **Inpatient treatment:** Inpatient treatment is provided at hospitals constructed by ESI corporation or by reservation of beds in the hospitals owned by the State Government, Local Fund Organization or Private Bodies, or by constructing annexes to such institutions. The ESI Scheme pays for these beds on the basis of occupied bed days. The corporation has framed standard plans for construction of different sizes of hospitals or annexes mainly with a view to achieving uniformity and standardization all over the country.
- **Imaging services:** Imaging and investigations including computed tomography (CT) scan, magnetic resonance imaging (MRI), echocardiography, and laboratory facilities are provided free of cost to IPs and their families at state level specialty hospitals or other institutions having tie up with ESI Scheme.
- **Special provisions:** Other special provisions are like no bar on benefits under other enactments, no reduction of wages during sickness, no termination/dismissal/discharge/reduction during sickness, etc.
- **Reimbursement:** Under Regulation 69, every employer has to arrange for first aid medical care and transport of accident cases till the injured IP is seen by the IMO/IMP and such employer is entitled to reimbursement of expenses incurred in this regard up to the maximum of scale prescribed from time to time. However, reimbursement is not permissible, if the employer is required to provide such medical aid free of charge under any other enactment. The cost of provision of such emergency treatment would be reimbursed to the employer by the Director/Administrative Medical Officer (AMO) (ESI Scheme) of the respective state and, therefore, all claims duly supported by relevant receipts and vouchers should be sent to him for verification and payment.

2. ***Sickness benefit:***
   - Sickness benefit represents periodical cash payments made to an IP during the period of certified sickness occurring in a benefit period when IP requires medical treatment and attendance with abstention from work on medical grounds. Sickness benefit is 70% of the average daily wages and is payable for 91 days during 2 consecutive benefit periods.
   - To become eligible to sickness benefit, an IP should have paid contribution for not less than 78 days during the corresponding contribution period. A person who has entered into insurable employment for the first time has to wait for nearly 9 months before becoming eligible to sickness benefit, because his corresponding benefit period starts only after that interval.
     ♦ *Extended sickness benefit (ESB):* The rate of Extended Sickness Benefit works out to about 80% of the average wages at the maximum, which is initially payable for a period of 124 days, in addition to 91 days' of Sickness Benefit, which may be extended to 309 days. In fit cases, Extended Sickness Benefit for an additional period of 330 days is also admissible, on recommendation of the Special Medical Board. A few uncommon diseases, over and above 34 diseases listed, can also qualify for the same benefit under discretion of the competent Medical Authority of ESI. Corporation, New Delhi. In addition to list, Director General/ Medical Commissioner are authorized to sanction ESB for a maximum period up to 730 days in cases of rare but treatable diseases or under special circumstances, such as, adverse reaction to drugs which have not been included in the above list, depending on the merits of each case, on the recommendations of RDMC/AMO, or either authorized officers running the medical scheme. To be entitled to the ESB, an IPs should have been in continuous employment for 2 years or more at the beginning of a spell of sickness in which the disease is diagnosed and should also satisfy other contributory conditions.
     ♦ *Enhanced sickness benefit:* It was introduced w.e.f. 1.8.1976 as an incentive to IPs/insured woman (IW) for undergoing vasectomy or tubectomy. IPs eligible to ordinary sickness benefit are paid enhanced sickness benefit at 100% of average daily wages for undergoing sterilization operations for family welfare. Duration of enhanced sickness benefits is up to 7 days in the case of vasectomy and up to 14 days in the case of the tubectomy from the date of operation or from the date of admission in the hospital as the case may be. The period is extendable in case of postoperative complications.

3. ***Maternity benefit:*** Maternity benefit rate is 100% of average daily wages. Maternity benefit for confinement or pregnancy is payable for a period of 26 weeks. Miscarriage or MTP-payable for 6 weeks (42 days) from the date following miscarriage. Sickness arising out of pregnancy, confinement, and premature birth-payable for a period not exceeding 1 month. In the event of the death of the IW during confinement leaving behind a child, maternity benefit is payable to her nominee.

4. ***Disablement benefit:***
   - **Temporary disablement benefit (TDB):** TDB is payable to an employee who suffers EI or occupational disease and is certified to be temporarily incapable to work. "EI"

has been defined as a personal injury to an employee caused by accident or occupational disease arising out of and in the course of his employment, being in insurable employment, whether the accident occurs or the occupational disease is contracted within or outside the territorial limits of India. The benefit is not subject to any contributory conditions. An IP is eligible from the day he joins the insurable employment. TDB rate is 90% of average daily wages. There is no prescribed limit for the duration of TDB. This is payable as long as temporary disablement lasts and significant improvement by treatment is possible. If a temporary disablement spell lasts for less than 3 days (excluding day of accident), IP will be paid sickness benefit, if otherwise eligible.

- **Permanent disablement benefit (PDB):** PDB is payable to an IP who suffers permanent residual disablement as a result of EI (including occupational diseases) and results in loss of earning capacity. The proper authority for assessing loss of earning capacity for injuries is the medical board and for occupational diseases, special medical board. The duration of PDB may be for the period given by medical board, if assessment is provisional or for entire life if assessment is final. The PDB rate is calculated as percentage of loss of earning capacity as assessed by the Medical Board/Medical Appellate Tribunal (MAT)/EI Court in relation to TDB. Hence, the maximum rate of PDB can be equal to the rate of TDB. PDB amount is revised by the ESI Corporation from time to time to adjust for inflation.

5. *Dependents benefit (DB):* DB paid at the rate of 90% of wage in the form of monthly payment to the dependents of a deceased IP in cases where death occurs due to EI or occupational hazards.
6. *Other benefits:*
   - *Funeral expenses:* An amount of ₹10,000 is payable to the dependents or to the person who performs last rites from day one of entering insurable employment.
   - *Confinement expenses:* An insured women or an IP in respect of his wife in case confinement occurs at a place where necessary medical facilities under ESI Scheme are not available.

In addition, the scheme also provides some other need-based benefits to insured workers.

- *Vocational rehabilitation (VR):* To permanently disabled IP for undergoing VR training at VR services (VRS).
- *Physical rehabilitation:* In case of physical disablement due to EI.
- *Old age medical care:* For IP retiring on attaining the age of superannuation or under VRS/ERS and person having to leave service due to permanent disability IP and spouse on payment of ₹120 per annum.

### *Rajiv Gandhi Shramik Kalyan Yojana*

This scheme of unemployment allowance was introduced w.e.f. 01.04.2005. An IP who becomes unemployed after being insured for 3 or more years, due to closure of factory or establishment and retrenchment or permanent invalidity is entitled to unemployment allowance equal to 50% of wage for a maximum period of up to 2 years, medical care for self and family from ESI hospitals or dispensaries during the period IP receives unemployment allowance and vocational training provided for upgrading skills—expenditure on fee or traveling allowance borne by ESI Corporation.

### *Factories Act, 1948 (Amended in 1987)*

This is an Act to consolidate and amend the law regulating labor in factories. It came into force on the 1st day of April, 1949 as the Factories Act, 1948 and extends to the whole of India (Government of India, 1948). Later on, it was amended by the Factories (Amendment) Act, 1987 (Act 20 of 1987).

This act was enacted with the prime objective of protecting workmen employed in factories against industrial and occupational hazards. With that intent, it imposes upon owners and occupier certain obligations to protect unwary as well as negligent workers and to secure employment for them, which is conducive and safe. The Act's objective is to protect human beings from being subjected to unduly long hours of bodily strain and manual labor. This serves to assist in formulating national policies in India with respect to occupational safety and health in factories and docks in India. It deals with various problems concerning safety, health, efficiency, and well-being of the persons at work places.

The Act is administered by the Ministry of Labor and Employment in India through its Directorate General Factory Advice Service and Labor Institutes (DGFASLI) and by the State Governments through their factory inspectorates. DGFASLI advises the Central and State Governments on administration of the Factories Act and coordinating the factory inspection services in the States. Various provisions of the Act are described in the following 11 chapters.

#### *Chapter I—Preliminary*

According to this Act, the interpretation of the word "factory" means any premises whereon 10 or more workers are working, or were working on any day of the preceding 12 months, and in any part of which a manufacturing process is being carried on with the aid of power, or is ordinarily so carried on. Or whereon 20 or more workers are working, or were working on any day of the preceding 12 months, and in any part of which a manufacturing process is being carried on without the aid of power, or is ordinarily so carried on.

#### *Chapter II—The Inspecting Staff*

The State Government may, by notification in the Official Gazette, appoint such persons as possessing the prescribed qualification to be inspectors for the purposes of this Act and may assign to them such local limits as it may think fit. Those inspectors can enter with assistants, being persons in the service of the government, or any local or other public authority or with an expert, as he thinks fit, any place which is used, or which he has reason to believe, is used as a factory and can make examination of the premises, plant, machinery, article or substance, and inquire into any accident or dangerous occurrence.

The State Government may appoint qualified medical practitioners to be certifying surgeons for the purposes of this Act within such local limits or for such factory or class or description of factories as it may assign to them, respectively. These certifying surgeons shall carry out such duties as may be prescribed in connection with the examination and certification of young persons under this Act and examination of persons engaged in factories in such dangerous occupations or processes as may be prescribed.

### Chapter III—Health

This chapter deals with following sections:

- *Section 11—cleanliness:* Every factory shall be kept clean and free from effluvial arising from any drain, privy, or other nuisance.
- *Section 12—disposal of wastes and effluents:* Effective arrangements shall be made in every factory for the treatment of wastes and effluents due to the manufacturing process carried on therein, so as to render them innocuous, and for their disposal.
- *Section 13—ventilation and temperature:* Effective and suitable provisions shall be made in every factory for securing and maintaining in every workroom the adequate ventilation by the circulation of fresh air, and such a temperature as will secure to workers therein reasonable conditions of comfort and prevent injury to health. Walls and roofs shall be of such material and so designed that such temperature shall not be exceeded but kept as low as practicable. Where the nature of the work carried on in the factories involves, or is likely to involve, the production of excessively high temperature, such adequate measures as are practicable, shall be taken to protect the workers therefrom, by separating the process, which produces such temperature from the workroom, by insulating the hot parts or by other effective means.
- *Section 14—dust and fume:* Effective measures shall be taken to prevent its inhalation and accumulation in any workroom, and if any exhaust appliance is necessary for this purpose, it shall be applied as near as possible to the point of origin of the dust, fume or other impurity, and such point shall be enclosed so far as possible. In any factory, no stationary internal combustion engine shall be operated unless the exhaust is conducted into the open air.
- *Section 15—artificial humidification:* The State Government may make rules for prescribing standards of humidification and regulating the methods used for artificially increasing the humidity of the air after prescribing tests for determining the humidity of the air.
- *Section 16—overcrowding:* No room in any factory shall be overcrowded to an extent injurious to the health of the workers employed therein. There shall be in every workroom of a factory in existence on the date of commencement of this Act at least 9.9 cubic meters and of a factory built after the commencement of this Act at least 14.2 m³ of space for every worker employed therein.
- *Section 17—lighting:* In every part of a factory, where workers are working or passing, there shall be provided and maintained sufficient and suitable lighting, natural or artificial, or both. In every factory, all glazed windows and skylights used for the lighting of the workroom shall be kept clean on both the inner and outer surfaces. In every factory effective provision shall, so far as is practicable, be made for the prevention of glare and formation of shadows.
- *Section 18—drinking water:* In every factory, effective arrangements shall be made to provide and maintain at suitable points conveniently situated for all workers employed therein a sufficient supply of wholesome drinking water. All such points shall be legibly marked "drinking water" in a language understood by a majority of the workers employed in the factory and no such points shall be situated within 6 m of any washing place, urinal, latrine, spittoon, open drain carrying sullage or effluent, or any other source of contamination unless a shorter distance is approved in writing by the Chief Inspector. In every factory, wherein more than 250 workers are ordinarily employed, provisions shall be made for cooling of drinking water during hot weather by effective means and for distribution thereof.
- *Section 19—latrines and urinals:* In every factory, sufficient latrine and urinal accommodation of prescribed types (separate for male and female) shall be provided conveniently situated and accessible to workers at all times while they are at the factory. Such accommodation shall be adequately lighted and ventilated and maintained in a clean and sanitary condition at all times.
- *Section 20—Spittoons:* In every factory, there shall be provided a sufficient number of spittoons in convenient places and they shall be maintained in a clean and hygienic condition.

### Chapter IV—Safety

No young person shall be required or allowed to work at any machine, unless he has been fully instructed as to the dangers arising in connection with the machine and the precautions to be observed, and has received sufficient training in work at the machine, or is under adequate supervision by a person who has a thorough knowledge and experience of the machine. No woman or child shall be employed in any part of a factory for pressing cotton in which a cotton-opener is at work. No person shall be employed in any factory to lift, carry, or move any load so heavy as to be likely to cause him an injury. No person shall be required or allowed to enter any chamber, tank, vat, pit, pipe, flue, or other confined space in any factory in which any gas, fume, vapors, or dust is likely to be present to such an extent as to involve risk to persons being overcome thereby, unless it is provided with a manhole of adequate size or other effective means of egress. In every factory, all practicable measures shall be taken to prevent outbreak of fire and its spread, both internally and externally, and to provide and maintain safe means of escape for all persons in the event of a fire, and the necessary equipment and facilities for extinguishing fire.

### Chapter IVA—Provisions Relating to Hazardous Processes

The State Government may appoint a Site Appraisal Committee for grant of permission for the initial location or for the expansion of a factory involving a hazardous process. The Site Appraisal Committee shall examine an application for the establishment of a factory involving hazardous process and make its recommendation to the State Government within a period of 90 days of the receipt of such application in the prescribed form.

The occupier of every factory involving a hazardous process shall disclose in the manner prescribed, all information regarding dangers including health hazards and the measures to overcome such hazards arising from the exposure to or handling of the materials or substances in the manufacture, transportation, storage, and other processes, to the workers employed in the factory, the Chief Inspector, the local authority, within whose jurisdiction the factory is situate, and the general public in the vicinity. Every occupier of a factory involving any hazardous process shall maintain accurate and up-to-date health records or, as the case may be, medical records, of the workers in the factory who are exposed to any chemical, toxic, or any other harmful substances which are manufactured, stored, handled, or transported and such records shall be accessible to the workers.

### Chapter V—Welfare

In every factory, adequate and suitable facilities for washing (separate or screened for both male and female) shall be provided and maintained for use of the workers therein. Such facilities shall be conveniently accessible and shall be kept clean. Besides that, there should be a suitable place for keeping clothing not worn during working hours and for the drying of wet clothing. In every factory, suitable arrangements for sitting shall be provided and maintained for all workers obliged to work in a standing position, in order that they may take advantage of any opportunities for rest, which may occur in the course of their work. There shall, in every factory, be provided and maintained so as to be readily accessible during all working hours first-aid boxes or cupboards equipped with the prescribed contents, and the number of such boxes or cupboards to be provided and maintained shall not be less than 1 for every 150 workers ordinarily employed at any one time in the factory. In every factory wherein more than 500 workers are ordinarily employed, there shall be provided and maintained an ambulance room of the prescribed size, containing the prescribed equipment, and in the charge of such medical and nursing staff as may be prescribed and those facilities shall always be made readily available during the working hours of the factory.

The State Government may make rules requiring that in any specified factory wherein more than 250 workers are ordinarily employed, a canteen or canteens shall be provided and maintained by the occupier for the use of the workers. In every factory wherein more than 150 workers are ordinarily employed adequate and suitable shelters or rest-rooms and a suitable lunch-room, with provision for drinking water, where workers can eat meals brought by them, shall be provided and maintained for the use of the workers. In every factory, wherein more than 30 women workers are ordinarily employed there shall be provided and maintained a suitable room or rooms for the use of children (crèches) under the age of 6 years of such women. In every factory, wherein 500 or more workers are ordinarily employed the occupier shall employ in the factory such number of welfare officers as may be prescribed.

### Chapter VI—Working Hours of Adults

No adult worker shall be required or allowed to work in a factory for more than 48 hours in any week or more than 9 hours in any day. The periods of work of adult workers in a factory each day shall be so fixed that no period shall exceed 5 hours and that no worker shall work for more than 5 hours before he has had an interval for rest of at least half an hour. There should be provisions of weekly and compensatory holidays as per the norms. Where a worker works in a factory for more than 9 hours in any day or for more than 48 hours in any week, he shall, in respect of overtime work, be entitled to wages at the rate of twice his ordinary rate of wages. No adult worker shall be required or allowed to work in any factory on any day on which he has already been working in any other factory. There shall be displayed and correctly maintained in every factory, a notice of periods of work for adults, showing clearly for every day the periods during which adult workers may be required to work. No woman shall be required or allowed to work in any factory except between the hours 6 AM and 7 PM.

### Chapter VII—Employment of Young Persons

No child who has not completed his 14 years shall be required or allowed to work in any factory. A child who has completed his 14th year or an adolescent shall not be required or allowed to work in any factory, unless a certificate of fitness granted with reference to him by a certifying surgeon. This certificate should be in the custody of manager of the factory. No child shall be employed or permitted to work in any factory for more than four and a half hours in any day and during the night.

### Chapter VIII—Annual Leave with Wages

Every worker who has worked for a period of 240 days or more in a factory during a calendar year shall be allowed during the subsequent calendar year, leave with wages for a number of days calculated at the rate of if an adult, one day for every 20 days of work performed by him during the previous calendar year and if a child, 1 day for every 15 days of work performed by him during the previous calendar year.

Chapters IX, X, and XI deals with special provisions, penalties and procedure and other supplemental procedures, respectively.

## The Workmen's Compensation Act, 1923 (Amended in 1984 and 2000)

The Act specifies the compensation for which any worker, employed in any hazardous occupation, is eligible in case of injury. In case of death of the worker, his dependents can claim the benefits provided by the Act. The compensation can be claimed for an injury that disables him for more than 3 days, totally or partially.

The disablement means the loss in the earning capacity of a workman in every employment which he was capable of doing at the time of the accident. The disablement may be temporary or permanent. A workman must have been employed in the specified occupation for a continuous period of at least 6 months to be eligible for claiming compensation. For any delay in paying compensation by the employer beyond 1 month, interest is to be paid on the arrears as per the rules specified.

## Maternity Benefit Act, 1961 (Amended 1995, 2017)

The Maternity (Amendment) Bill 2017, an amendment to the Maternity Benefit Act, 1961. The Maternity Benefit Act 1961 protects the employment of women during the time of her maternity and entitles her of a "maternity benefit", i.e., full paid absence from work—to take care for her child. The Act is applicable to all establishments employing 10 or more persons.

The Act is applicable to all establishments, which are factories, mines, plantations, Government establishments, shops and establishments under the relevant applicable legislations, or any other establishment as may be notified by the Central Government.

As per the Act, to be eligible for maternity benefit, a woman must have been working as an employee in an establishment for a period of at least 80 days in the past 12 months. Payment during the leave period is based on the average daily wage for the period of actual absence.

The Maternity Benefit Amendment Act has increased the duration of paid maternity leave available for women employees from the existing 12 to 26 weeks. Under the Maternity Benefit Amendment Act, this benefit could be availed by women for a period extending up to a maximum of 8 weeks before the expected delivery date and the remaining time can be availed post childbirth. For women who are expecting after having two children, the duration of paid maternity leave shall be 12 weeks (i.e., 6 weeks pre- and 6 weeks post-expected date of delivery).

Maternity leave of 12 weeks to be available to mothers adopting a child below the age of 3 months from the date of adoption as well as to the "commissioning mothers". The commissioning mother has been defined as biological mother who uses her egg to create an embryo planted in any other woman.

The Maternity Benefit Amendment Act has also introduced an enabling provision relating to "work from home" for women, which may be exercised after the expiry of the 26 weeks of leave period. Depending upon the nature of work, women employees may be able to avail this benefit on terms that are mutually agreed with the employer.

The Maternity Benefit Amendment Act makes crèche facility mandatory for every establishment employing 50 or more employees. Women employees would be permitted to visit the crèche four times during the day (including rest intervals).

### *The Minimum Wages Act, 1948*

An Act for fixing minimum rates of wages in certain employments for skilled and unskilled workers to protect them from exploitation and ensure a basic standard of living to the workers and their families.

The Central or State Government would appoint a competent authority to decide about minimum wages and keep on revising it every 5 years according to the change in economic growth and the cost of living.

### *Central Government Health Scheme, 1954*

The Central Government Health Scheme (CGHS) was started under the Indian Ministry of Health and Family Welfare in 1954 with the objective of providing comprehensive medical care facilities to Central Government employees, pensioners, and their dependents residing in CGHS covered cities (360). CGHS caters to the health care needs of eligible beneficiaries covering all four pillars of democratic set up in India namely (1) Legislature, (2) Judiciary, (3) Executive, and (4) Press. CGHS is the model healthcare facility provider for Central Government employees and pensioners, and is unique of its kind due to the large volume of beneficiary base, and open-ended generous approach of providing health care. CGHS provides health care through Allopathic, Homoeopathic, Ayurveda, and Unani systems of medicine.

- *Eligibility for joining CGHS:*
  - All Central Government employees drawing their salary from Central Civil Estimates and their dependent family members residing in CGHS covered areas
  - Central Government pensioners or family pensioners receiving pension from Central Civil Estimates and their eligible dependent family members
  - Sitting and ex-members of Parliament
  - Ex-Governors and Lieutenant Governors
  - Freedom Fighters
  - Ex-vice Presidents
  - Sitting and retired Judges of Supreme Court
  - Retired Judge of High Courts
  - Journalists accredited with Press Information Bureau (PIB) (in Delhi)
  - Employees and pensioners of certain autonomous or statutory bodies, which have been extended CGHS facilities in Delhi.
- *Facilities available under CGHS:*
  - Outpatient department (OPD) treatment including issue of medicines
  - Specialist Consultation at Polyclinic/Government Hospitals
  - Indoor treatment at Government and Empaneled Hospitals.
  - Investigations at Government and Empaneled Diagnostic Centers.
  - Cashless facility available for treatment in empaneled hospitals and diagnostic centers.
  - Reimbursement for treatment availed in Government or Private Hospitals under emergency.
  - Reimbursement of expenses incurred for purchase of hearing aids, artificial limbs, appliances, etc., as specified.
  - Family Welfare, Maternity, and Child Health Services.
  - Medical consultation and dispensing of medicines in Ayurveda, Homeopathy, Unani and Siddha system of medicines.

## Mentally Ill Persons

### *Mental Health Act, 1987 (For Care and Rehabilitation of Mentally Ill Persons)*

The Mental Health Act, 1987 repeals Indian Lunacy Act, 1912 and Lunacy Act, 1977 (Jammu and Kashmir) and extends to whole of India. Under this Act 1987, a "Mentally Ill person" means a person who is in need of treatment by reason of any mental disorder other than mental retardation.

The Act provides for licensing and regulating psychiatric hospitals and nursing homes. The Act provides for regular, thorough supervision of mental hospitals and nursing homes by monthly joint inspection of three visitors designated by the Central or State authority for health services.

Any person aged 18 and above can voluntarily get admission for inpatient treatment. In case of minor (less than 18 years of age) mentally ill, can be presented for admission by the guardian as a voluntary patient. Admission to psychiatric hospital under special circumstances can also be made on request of a relative or a friend of the patient, if the patient is not in a position to express willingness for admission as a voluntary patient, provided the medical officer in charge is satisfied that it is in the interest of the patient to do so. The rules for keeping or discharge of admitted patients have also been made explicit depending on the state of mental health of the patient. Patients admitted on voluntary basis, if they request for discharge, are obliged to be discharged by the medical officer in charge within 24 hours of receiving the request, no person admitted on the request of another person can be kept in the mental hospital for more than 90 days unless admitted under a reception order. The Act also provides for legal intervention for the same through reception orders passed by a magistrate.

Physical or mental cruelty to mentally ill patients is forbidden. Similarly, conduct of research on a mental patient is forbidden, unless voluntarily consent from patient or relatives is obtained. The human rights of a mentally ill person are protected under the Act. Penalties and fines for contravening the provisions of the Act have been discussed.

## ENVIRONMENT HEALTH AND SAFETY LAWS

### The Environment (Protection) Act, 1986

The Environment (Protection) Act, 1986 was enacted to provide for the protection and improvement of environment. This Act is applicable to the whole of India.

The Act provides powers to make rules to regulate environmental pollution, to notify standards and maximum limits of pollutants of air, water, and soil for various areas and purposes; prohibition and restriction on the handling of hazardous substances and location of industries. The Central Government is empowered to constitute authority or authorities for the purpose of exercising or performing such of the powers and functions, appoint a person for inspection, for analysis of samples, and for selection or notification of environmental laboratories.

The government shall establish or recognize one or more environmental laboratories and analysts for the purpose of analysis who shall give report in specified manner.

According to the Act, the Central Government may issue directions in writing to any person or officers or any authority to comply. There could be closure, prohibition of the supply of electricity or operation or process; or stoppage or regulation of the supply of electricity or water or any other service.

#### Punishment under the Act

The owners or occupier of companies, factories, institutions, etc. found to be the cause of pollution are liable for punishment and/or fine or both.

### Air (Prevention and Control of Pollution) Act, 1981

The Air (Prevention and Control of Pollution) Act is an Act to provide for the prevention, control, and abatement of air pollution, for the establishment of central and state level boards that would be entrusted with this duty. It extends to the whole of India.

The main functions of the Central Board shall be to improve the quality of air and to prevent, control, or abate air pollution in the country. The board shall advise government, plan the program for prevention, coordinate, perform, and organize all the activities or delegate, lay down standards of air and collect compile, and publish technical and statistical data needed for achieving the goal. The state boards are concerned with monitoring the air quality and taking action for the same.

#### Punishment under the Act

Failure to comply with the provisions is punishable with imprisonment for a term of not less than 1 year and 6 months but may extend to 6 years and with fine, and in case the failure to comply continues, an additional fine may be imposed.

### Water (Prevention and Control of Pollution) Act, 1974

The Water (Prevention and Control of Pollution) Act is an Act to provide for the prevention and control of water pollution and the maintaining or restoring of wholesomeness of water for the establishment, The Act mandates the creation of Central and State Pollution Control Boards for this purpose. The board(s) lay down, modify or annul, the standards for water bodies.

Apart from water safety, the boards also give specification for sewage and trade effluents. Monitoring of adherence to standards by various establishments or individuals and setting up laboratories is also the duty of these boards.

#### Punishment under the Act

Failure to comply with the direction on conviction, is punishable with imprisonment for a term of up to 3 months or with fine up to ₹10,000 or with both and in case the failure continues, with an additional fine.

### Biomedical Waste Management Rules, 2016

Due to concerns about biomedical waste generated at national and international level, the Union Ministry of Environment and Forest, Government of India has notified "Biomedical Waste (Management and Handling) Rules, 1998" amended on 2nd June 2000 and draft amended 2011 and Biomedical Waste Management Rules 2016 under the provision of Sections 6, 8, and 25 of the Environment (Protection) Act.

These rules shall apply to all persons who generate, collect, receive, store, transport, treat, dispose, or handle biomedical waste in any form including hospitals, nursing homes, clinics, dispensaries, veterinary institutions, animal houses, pathological laboratories, blood banks, AYUSH hospitals, clinical establishments, research or educational institutions, health camps, medical or surgical camps, vaccination camps, blood donation camps, first aid rooms of schools, and forensic laboratories and research laboratories.

Biomedical waste means any waste, which is generated during the diagnosis, treatment or immunization of human beings or animals, or research activities pertaining thereto or in the production or testing of biological or in health camps.

The rules shall not apply to radioactive waste, hazardous chemicals (manufacture and storage import), municipal solid waste, lead acid batteries, hazardous waste (management, handling, and transboundary), e-waste, and hazardous microorganisms that are covered under various other rules.

The Act defines duties for occupiers and operators of biomedical waste managers.

*Duties of the occupier:*
- "Occupier" means a person having administrative control over the institution and the premises generating biomedical waste, which includes a hospital, nursing home, clinic, dispensary, veterinary institution, animal house, pathological laboratory, blood bank, healthcare facility, and clinical establishment, irrespective of their system of medicine.
- The rules define the duties of occupier with reference to handling, segregation, transport, treatment, and disposal of biomedical waste so that there is no adverse effect to humans and environment. This also includes pretreatment through disinfection and sterilization as per the WHO/NACO guidelines. Liquid chemical waste needs to be pretreated or neutralized prior to mixing with other effluent generated from healthcare facilities. It is also the duty of the occupier to get the authorization from Central Pollution Control Board (CPCB) or State Pollution Control Board.
- Occupier shall phase out use of chlorinated plastic bags, gloves, and blood bags within 2 years from the date of notification of these rules and establish a Bar-Code System for bags or containers containing biomedical waste to be sent out of the premises or place for any purpose within 1 year from the date of notification of these rules. Also daily records have to be maintained and monthly report to be made available on the website.
- It is the duty of the occupier to ensure safety of the healthcare workers and waste handlers by organizing training (and retraining annually), immunization (hepatitis B), and annual health check-ups. The details of training programs conducted, number of personnel trained, number of personnel not undergone any training, and any accidents shall be provided in the Annual Report.
- He/she has to ensure treatment and disposal of liquid waste in accordance with the Water (Prevention and Control of Pollution) Act, 1974. Untreated human anatomical waste, animal anatomical waste, soiled waste, and biotechnology waste shall not be stored beyond a period of 48 hours.
- Incinerators should be according to specification given in rules. But will not establish such facilities on-site, if common treatment facilities are available within 70 km. A committee should be constituted which should meet 6 monthly and minutes should be submitted along with annual report.

*Duties of the operator of a common biomedical waste treatment and disposal facility:*
- "Operator" of a Common Biomedical Waste Treatment Facility (CBMWTF) means a person who owns or controls a CBMWTF for the collection, reception, storage, transport treatment, disposal, or any other form of handling of biomedical waste.
- The duties of the operator are similar to the occupier except that he also has to inform the prescribed authority immediately regarding the occupiers, which are not handing over the segregated biomedical waste in accordance with these rules; provide training and assist occupier for conducting workers.
- The handling and disposal of all the mercury waste and lead waste shall be in accordance with the respective rules and regulations.
- Advisory and monitoring bodies to be established for proper compliance and implementation of these rules.

*Punishment under the Act*
The occupier or operator of a facility shall be liable for all the damages caused to the environment or the public due to improper handling of biomedical wastes.

Penalty is imposed on whosoever person or owners or occupier found to be the cause of pollution. Punishment is for a term, which may extend to 5 years or with fine which may extend to ₹1 lakh or both. If not complied with, a fine of ₹5,000 per day extra and if not comply for more than 1 year then imprisonment may extend up to 7 years. Head of the department or in-charge of small unit may be liable for punishment, if the owner or occupier produces enough evidence of innocence. The CPCB and state boards have power to close or cancel or deny the authorization to run hospital or any biomedical waste treatment facility whichever is causing pollution.

## Municipal Solid Waste (Management and Handling) Rules, 2000

Under the EPA 1986, to safeguard the environment and human health, Government of India has laid down Municipal Solid Waste Management Rules.

These rules lay down the responsibility of management of solid waste disposal and various standards for disposal of treated leachate (liquid that seeped through solid waste and other medium and has extracted dissolved or suspended material from it).

The management of the solid waste has been made the responsibility of municipal authority and the overall responsibility of enforcement being given to District Magistrate or Deputy Commissioner.

Solid Waste Management Rules, 2015 draft has been published with more provisions and putting responsibility on generator of solid waste who could be individual household, institution, etc. The focus is currently on segregation of waste at source of generation, i.e., at the household level and use of waste for generation of energy.

# FOOD SAFETY LAWS

## Food Safety and Standards Act, 2006 (The Food Safety and Standards Act, 2006)

The aim of Food Safety and Standards Act is to lay down standards for articles of food and to regulate their manufacture, storage, distribution, sale, and import, to ensure availability of safe and wholesome food for human consumption. The Act extends to the whole of India.

Food means any substance, whether processed, partially processed, or unprocessed, which is intended for human consumption and includes primary food, genetically modified or engineered food, or food containing such ingredients, infant food, packaged drinking water, alcoholic drink, chewing gum, and any substance, including water used into the food during its manufacture, preparation, or treatment.

The Act mandates the creation of a body to be known as the Food Safety and Standards Authority of India (FSSAI) to exercise the powers conferred under this Act. The FSSAI will have representatives from the government departments, i.e., agriculture, commerce, consumer affairs, food processing health, legislative affairs, etc., and also from small scale and food industries and eminent food technologists.

### Enforcement of the Act

The Food Safety Officers shall enforce and execute within their area the provisions of this Act. His functions will be—(1) prohibit in the interest of public health, the manufacture, storage, distribution, or sale of any article of food, which could be toxic, injurious, and unsafe; (2) carry out survey of the industrial units; (3) conduct or organize training programs; (4) ensure an efficient and uniform implementation of the standards and other requirements as specified and also ensure a high standard of objectivity, accountability, practicability, transparency, and credibility; and (5) sanction prosecution for offences punishable with imprisonment under this Act.

The Act directs the appointment of Food Analysts and setting up of laboratories for the same.

*Punishment under the Act has been defined for various offences like:*

- Penalty for selling food not of the nature or substance or quality demanded, substandard food or misbranded food or food with extraneous matter, misleading advertisement, unhygienic process, possession of adulterant, carrying out a business without license, etc.
  - Compensation in case of injury or death of consumer—if any person manufactures or distributes or sells or imports any article of food causing injury to the consumer or his death, he is liable to pay compensation to the victim or the legal representative of the victim, a sum—(1) not less than ₹5 lakh in case of death; (2) not exceeding ₹3 lakh in case of grievous injury; and (3) not exceeding ₹1 lakh, in all other cases of injury.

### Prevention of Food Adulteration Act, 1954 (PFA Act)

The PFA Act was enacted in 1954 with the aim of ensuring pure and wholesome quality food to the consumers, to protect their health from the fraudulent practices of traders and to encourage fair trade-practices. The Act has been amended in 1965, 1976, and 1986. The enforcement of the Act is responsibility of state governments.

The Act provides protection to the consumers against adulteration or contamination of food that may have deleterious effects on the health. The Act also deals with the frauds that can be perpetrated by the dealers by supplying cheaper and adulterated foods. The Act regulates the use of chemicals, pesticides, flavors, and other additives in food preparation. Provision is made under this Act for enrichment and fortification of foods.

As defined under the Act, an article is deemed to be adulterated:

- If it is sold by a vendor and is not of the nature demanded by the purchaser and is not of the quality, which it purports to be
- If the article contains any other substance so as to affect injuriously the nature or quality there of
- If it is substituted wholly or partially by an inferior substance
- If the constituent of the article is abstracted partially or wholly, as to affect its quality
- If the article has been prepared, packed, or kept under insanitary conditions and has become contaminated as to cause injury to the health
- If the article consists of filthy, rotten, putrid, or decomposed substance and is unfit for consumption
- If the article is obtained from a diseased animal
- If the article contains any poisonous substance
- If the article contains prohibited preservative or coloring matter in excess of the prescribed limits
- If the quality of the article falls below the prescribed limits. The rules are framed by the "Central Committee for Food Standards" and any food that does not conform to the specified minimum standards is said to adulterated.

The State Governments appoint Public Analyst and Food Inspectors, who control the food supply, storage, and marketing of foods. A chain of 82 State Food Laboratories and four Central (Regional) Food Laboratories are working in the country for the purpose of the PFA Act.

The food inspectors draw and dispatch the sample of suspected food article to the laboratory for testing. If the adulteration is proved, the trader is awarded a minimum imprisonment of 6 months and a fine of ₹1,000. If the adulteration results in grievous health problem or even death, the punishment will go up to life imprisonment and a fine of ₹5,000. With the amendment in 1986, the consumer and the voluntary organizations have been empowered to take the samples of food.

## PUBLIC HEALTH SERVICES RELATED LAWS

### The Census Act, 1948

Census is an enumeration of a population, which records identities of all persons in every place of residence, with age, or birth date, sex, occupation, national origin, language, marital status, income, and relationship to head of household in addition to information on the dwelling place. Many other items of information may be included, e.g., educational level (or literacy), and health-related date such a permanent disability.

A de facto census assigns according to their location at the time of enumeration.

A de jure census assigns persons according to their usual place of residence at the time of enumeration.

The Constitution of India has made this exercise mandatory for the Union Government and the legal basis for this exercise is provided for by the Census Act 1948. The Census Organization has been set up under the Ministry of Home in 1961, which provides a vital continuity to conceive, plan, and implement the program of census in the country. The organization is headed by the Registrar General and Census Commissioner, and the deemed authorities in the central and State Governments have the power to appoint census officers for conduct of the census operations in any territory or part thereof.

During the course of the census operations, all persons in the area are legally bound to answer the questions asked to them to their best possible knowledge except for the provisions given to women regarding names of certain relations forbidden by caste or tradition.

### Punishment under the Act

Any person who refuses access to census officers as specified in the Act, who gives false information to census officers, damages marks or letters affixed for census purpose, trespasses into census office or any census officer not complying to his duty directions shall be punishable with a fine of up to ₹1,000 and the latter may also be punished with imprisonment of up to 3 months.

## The Registration of Births and Deaths Act, 1969

The Registration of Births and Deaths Act was enacted with the aim to collect and compile vital statistics. The Registrar General, India is the chief authority for coordinating the work of civil registration throughout the country. At the state level, Directors of Health Services, or Health Economic and Statistics maybe designated as Chief Registrars. The local registrars are mainly drawn from Panchayat, police, health or revenue, departments in rural area while in urban areas, Health Officers of the Municipalities or corporations, or the executive officers are the registrars.

Every registrar has to register births and deaths occurring within his/her administrative area. The information regarding occurrence is to be given within 21 days in both the events of deaths and births. Registration for delayed events may be done on payment of prescribed fee, if done within 1 month. In case of delay more than 30 days but within a year, besides late fee, an affidavit is required from a notary public. For registration of events beyond 1 year, an order from class I officer or magistrate is necessary. The data is sent periodically from every local registrar to the Chief Registrar who sends reports to the Registrar General, India. On the basis of the annual vital statistics returns received from the states, the Registrar General, India brings out a comprehensive annual report entitled, "Vital Statistics of India".

The Act also provides for medical certification of cause of death. As per the provisions of the Act, a medical practitioner who is attending the deceased during his last breath or illness, is liable to certify free of cost and in the prescribed format, the cause of death.

## The Medical Termination of Pregnancy Act, 1971 and the MTP Rules and Regulations, 2003

Abortion means termination of pregnancy before the fetus becomes viable (before 28 weeks of gestation). It can be spontaneous or induced and legal or illegal.

Abortion leads to legal, ethical and moral quandary. It is a matter of serious concern that unsafe abortion is the third leading cause of maternal deaths in India, contributing 8% of all such deaths annually (India Today, 2018). In 1971, the increasing cases of maternal morbidity and mortality due to unsafe abortions, as well as the notion that abortions could be used as a method of population control, encouraged the government to enact the MTP Act. It was amended in 2002 with an aim to facilitate better coverage and implementation by adopting strategies such as devolution of regulatory power to states, punitive action against those performing unsafe abortions, formulation of guidelines for physical infrastructure and approval of Medical Methods of Abortion (MMA). The Medical Termination of Pregnancy (Amendment) Act, 2021 (MTPA 2021) was approved on the 16th of March 2021 thereby amending the provisions of the Medical Termination of Pregnancy Act, 1971 (MTPA 1971). The Amendment raises the upper gestation limit from 20 to 24 weeks for particular groups of women, and would include rape survivors, incest victims, and other vulnerable women (such as differently-abled women, minors), among others.

*Medical Termination of Pregnancy Act specifies:*
- Conditions (indications) under which termination of pregnancy can be done
- Person who is authorized to perform MTPs
- Place where MTP can be performed.

### Indications for Termination of Pregnancy

Pregnancy can be terminated in the following situations:
- Where continuance of the pregnancy poses a grave physical or mental risk to life of the pregnant woman, e.g., woman suffering from mitral stenosis, viral hepatitis, etc.
- Where there is a risk of the child being born with serious handicap, e.g., German measles, maternal X-ray exposure, teratogenic drugs exposure, etc. leading to congenital anomalies.
- In case of rape victims where pregnancy can have a grave injury to the health of pregnant woman.
- Where pregnancy occurs as a result of failure of any contraceptive device used by married woman or her husband.
- The pregnant woman's actual or reasonably foreseeable environment, e.g., extreme poverty.

### Person Who can Perform MTP

After commencement of MTP Act, only RMPs are authorized to perform MTP whose name has been entered in State Medical Register and possess one or more of the following experience:
- Has completed 6 months of house surgery in gynecology and obstetrics.
- Has experience in obstetrics at any hospital for not less than 1 year.
- Has assisted an RMP in performing 25 cases of MTP of which at least 5 have been performed independently.
- Has a postgraduate degree or diploma in gynecology and obstetrics.

### Place Where MTP can be Performed

No termination of pregnancy shall be made in accordance with this Act at any place other than:
- A hospital established or maintained by the Government.
- A place approved for the purpose by Government.

- Nongovernmental institutions which have obtained a license from the chief medical officer of the district.

Medical Termination of Pregnancy rules amended in 2003 allows termination of early pregnancy up to 7 weeks using MMA with the key requirements of:
- Provided only by certified abortion providers
- Can be provided from approved sites as well as nonapproved clinics with referral linkages to an approved MTP site provided a certificate of access to a registered place is displayed in the clinic of the owner.

To ensure comprehensive abortion care accessible to women, the Ministry of Health and Family Welfare (MoHFW) is promoting safer technology like electrical vacuum evacuation (EVA) and manual vacuum aspiration (MVA) and with the introduction of MMA using a combination of drugs mifepristone and misoprostol (1 tablet of mifepristone 200 mg and 4 tablets of misoprostol 200 µg each), women access to safe abortion services has been strengthened globally and in India. MMA drugs need to be a part of the essential drug lists for all states.

**Key Provisions of the MTP Amendment Act, 2021**

|  | MTP Act 1971 | MTP Amendment Act, 2021 |
| --- | --- | --- |
| Indication (Contraceptive failure) | Only applies to married women | Unmarried women are also included |
| Gestational age limit | 20 weeks for all indications | 24 weeks for rape survivors. Beyond 24 weeks for fetal abnormalities |
| Medical practitioners opinion required before termination | One RMP till 12 weeks. Two RMPs till 20 weeks | One RMP till 20 weeks. Two RMPs for 20–24 weeks. Medical board approval after 24 weeks |
| Breach of woman's confidentiality | Fine upto ₹ 1,000 | Fine and/or imprisonment of 1 year |

> No pregnancy can be terminated without consent of the pregnant woman except if she is a minor or mentally ill (guardian permission required in such case) as per MTP Act.

### The Preconception and Prenatal Diagnostic Techniques (Prohibition of Sex Selection) Act, 1994

This Act was enacted for regulation of use of prenatal diagnostic techniques for the purposes of detecting genetic abnormalities or metabolic disorders or chromosomal abnormalities or certain congenital malformations or sex-linked disorders and for the prevention of misuse of these techniques for sex determination leading to sex selective abortions and female feticide. This Act extends to the whole of India except Jammu and Kashmir.

As per the provisions of the Act, it is mandatory for every genetic or prenatal diagnostic center or laboratory or clinic to be registered. No prenatal diagnostic tests can be performed at a place other than a place registered under this Act. No person or specialist or team of specialists would conduct sex selection on a woman or man. No ultrasound or any machine or equipment capable of detecting sex of the fetus can be sold to any persons or center that is not registered under the Act. No person or place or center shall be used or caused to be used by any person for conducting prenatal diagnostic techniques except for the purposes of detection of certain specified abnormalities, viz. chromosomal abnormalities, genetic metabolic diseases, sex-liked genetic diseases, etc.

The Act prohibits any person, including a relative or husband of the pregnant woman, to seek or encourage the conduct of any prenatal diagnostic techniques except in conditions where qualified persons satisfied with the following reasons in writing:
- Age of the pregnant woman is above 35 years;
- The pregnant woman has undergone two or more spontaneous abortions or fetal loss;
- The pregnant woman had been exposed to potentially teratogenic agents, such as drugs, radiation, infection, or chemicals;
- The pregnant woman or her spouse has a family history of mental retardation or physical deformities, such as spasticity or any other genetic disease.

The pregnant woman must be explained the side effects of the test and written consent has to be obtained. No person shall communicate to the pregnant woman concerned or her relatives or any other person the sex of the fetus by words, signs, or in any other manner. No person shall conduct or cause to conduct in any genetic counseling center or laboratory or clinic, prenatal diagnostic techniques including ultrasonography, for the purpose of determining the sex of fetus.

The Act mandates the constitution of supervisory boards by the Central and State governments to enforce the provisions of the Act and to investigate and prosecute violations of the same. The Act also prohibits publication, distribution, and communication of any advertisement for sex determination in any form including internet. Violation of this is punishable with imprisonment for a term, which may extend to 3 years and with fine which may extend to ₹10,000.

Any medical geneticist, gynecologist, RMP, or person who owns center, or employed in such center and provides his professional or technical services, and who violates any of the provision of the Act shall be punishable with imprisonment for a term which may extend to 3 years and with fine which may extend to ₹10,000 and on any subsequent conviction, with imprisonment which may extend to 5 years and with fine which may extend to ₹50,000 and their registration can be suspended for 2 years.

Any person including pregnant woman (unless she was compelled to undergo such diagnostic test) who seeks the aid of a medical or genetic professional or center for the purpose other than specified by the Act, shall be punished with imprisonment for a term which may extend to 3 years and with fine which may extend to ₹10,000 and on any subsequent conviction with imprisonment which may extend to 5 years and with fine which may extend to ₹50,000.

The offences under the violation of this Act are cognizable, nonbailable, and non-compoundable.

## SUGGESTED READING

1. Central Government Health Scheme, Government of India. About CGHS. [online] Available from: https://cghs.gov.in/index1.php?lang=1&level=1&sublinkid=5783&lid=3656.

2. Employees' State Insurance Corporation, Ministry of Labour & Employment, Government of India. Information-Benefits. [online] Available from: https://www.esic.nic.in/information-benefits.
3. Gazette of India. The Cigarette and other Tobacco Products (Prohibition of Advertisement and regulation of trade and commerce, production, supply and distribution) Act, 2003 (34 of 2003) Govt. of India. [online] Available from: https://indiacode.nic.in/bitstream/123456789/2053/1/200334.pdf.
4. Gazette of India. The Dowry Prohibition Act, 1961. Gazette of India Act No. 28 of 1961 and amended in 1986. [online] Available from: http://www.lawsindia.com/Advocate%20Library/C083.HTM.
5. Gazette of India. The Environment (Protection) Act No. 29 of 1986 GSR 1198(E) dated 12 Nov, 1986. Available from: www.moef.nic.in/sites/default/files/eprotect_act_1986.pdf.
6. Gazette of India. The Immoral Traffic Prevention Act (1956) [Act No 104 of 1956] as amended upto Act No 44 of 1986.
7. Gazette of India. The Juvenile Justice (Care and Protection of Children) Act, 2000 (56 of 2000). [online] Available from: http://khoyapaya.gov.in/mpp/resources/Juvenile%20Justice%20Act%20 2000.pdf.
8. Gazette of India. The Narcotic Drugs and Psychotropic Substances Act, 1985 [Act No 61 of 1985 dated 16th September 1985, Act No. 2 of 1989).
9. Gazette of India. The Pre-conception and Prenatal Diagnostic Techniques (Prohibition of Sex selection) Act, 1994 (Act No. 57 of 1994) [As amended by Prenatal diagnostic Techniques (Regulation and Prevention of Misuse) Act, 2002.
10. Gazette of India. The Registration of Births and Deaths Act 1969. [online] Available from: https://indiacode.nic.in/ bitstream/123456789/1682/1/196918.pdf.
11. Gazette of India. Workman's Compensation Act. [Act No. 6 of Year 1974]. Available from: https://labour.gov.in/sites/default/files/TheWorkmenAct 1923%281%29.pdf.
12. Government of India. Business Portal of India : Legal Aspects : Key Regulations: Manpower: Laws relating to Working Hours, Conditions of Service & Employment : Factories Act, 1948. [online] Available from: https://archive.india.gov.in/business/legal_aspects/ factories_act.php.
13. Government of India. The Mental Health Act, 1987. New Delhi: Delhi Law House; 2002
14. Govt of India. Municipal Solid Waste (Management and Handling) Rules, 2000. New Delhi: Min of Environment and Forests; 2000.
15. Govt of India. The Child Labour (Prohibition and Regulation) Act, 1986 (61 of 1986). [online] Available from: https://www.ilo.org/dyn/natlex/docs/WEBTEXT/27803/64848/E86IND01.htm.
16. Govt of India. The Child Marriage Restraint Act, 1986 (19 of 1929). [online] Available from: http://wcd.nic.in/child-marriage-restraint-act-1929-19-1929.
17. Govt of India. The Infant Milk Substitutes, Feeding Bottles and Infant Foods (Regulation of Production, Supply & Distribution) Act, 1992 (Act No 41 of 1992). [online] Available from: http://www.wcd.nic.in/sites/default/files/infantmilkpact1.pdf.
18. Govt of India. The Persons with Disability (Equal Opportunities, Protection of Rights and Full Participation) Act, 1995 (1 of 1996). [online] Available from: http://niepmd.tn.nic.in/documents/PWD%20ACT.pdf.
19. India. The Factories Act. [online] Available from: https://www.ilo.org/dyn/natlex/docs/WEBTEXT/32063/64873/E87IND01.htm.
20. National Health Portal of India. Employment State Insurance Scheme (ESIS). [online] Available from: https://www.nhp.gov.in/employment-state-insurance-scheme-esis-_pg.
21. National Portal of India. Employees' State Insurance Scheme. [online] Available from: https://www.india.gov.in/spotlight/employees-state-insurance-scheme#tab=tab-4.
22. Occupational Health and Safety: Legal and Operational Guide. Unit 6 Occupational Health and safety Legislation in India. [online] Available from: https://pria-academy.org/pdf/OHS/unit6/OHS_Unit-6_Course%20 Content_OHS%20Legislation%20in%20India.pdf.

# CHAPTER 50

# Indian Healthcare Agencies

*Viral Dave, Venu Shah, Bhavik Rana, Arpit Prajapati*

## INTRODUCTION

Each country has its own unique system of healthcare delivery. As per the Constitution of India, state government is responsible for the health of the people. The direct healthcare services are delivered via three-tier system (primary, secondary, and tertiary), in each state. Additionally, there are certain institutes which do not provide direct health services but they give a strong support to the structure of healthcare system in India. They offer resources and technical guidance pertaining to training, research, policy making, program management, monitoring and evaluation. Present section provides an overview of such government and non-government institutes which are backbones of Indian Health System which may not be visible directly to general community **(Table 50.1)**.

**Table 50.1:** List of important government health institutes.

| Institute | Main functional area |
|---|---|
| National Centre for Disease Control (NCDC) | Surveillance, control and research in the field of communicable diseases |
| National Institute of Health and Family Welfare (NIHFW) | Development of technical guidelines, IEC material and provision of postgraduate courses in the field of public health |
| Indian Council of Medical Research (ICMR) | Research and training in the field of medical science |
| National Institute of Disaster Management (NIDM) | Development of resources, training and policy framing for disaster management |
| National Tuberculosis Institute (NTI) | Research for the tuberculosis, coordination and implementation of Revised National Tuberculosis Control Programme |
| International Institute for Population Sciences | Training and Research in Population Studies for developing countries in the Asia and Pacific region |
| Pasteur Institute of India, Coonoor | Research and development of vaccine |
| Central Research Institute (CRI), Kasauli | Research and development of vaccines and antisera |

(IEC: Information, Education, and Communication)

## National Centre for Disease Control

Previously, this institute was known as National Institute of Communicable Diseases (NICD).

National Centre for Disease Control (NCDC) is administered by Directorate General of Health Services, Ministry of Health and Family Welfare, Government of India.

**Location:** New Delhi, India

**Organogram:**

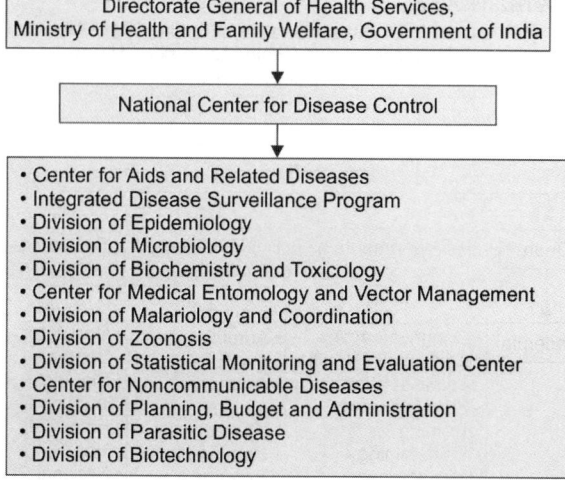

## Functions

The functions of NCDC broadly cover three areas: (1) health services, (2) training, and (3) research.
- This institute provides health services like:
  - Surveillance of communicable diseases
  - Outbreak investigations and recommendations on control measures
  - Referral, diagnostic services for various communicable diseases of microbial origin
  - Quality control of biological substances, storage and supply of reagents, test kits and vaccines
  - Entomological investigations of public health importance
  - Evaluation of chemical compounds and assessment of biochemical parameters to establish clinical diagnosis, e.g., thyroid function tests, etc.

- It plays a major role by developing human resources in the health sector of India through trainings. It offers post-graduation courses like Master in Public Health (Field Epidemiology) and Epidemic Intelligence Service (India), Medical Entomology and Vector Management, and Postgraduate Advanced Diploma in Public Health Entomology. It caters as a vital training center for other government organizations dealing in entomology, epidemiology, and services related to laboratory.
- National Centre for Disease Control is involved in conducting research in various fields like epidemiology including surveillance of epidemic prone disease, entomology with advanced research related to insecticides and applied research in the field of public health.

## National Institute of Health and Family Welfare

Administered by Department of Health and Family Welfare, Government of India, National Institute of Health and Family Welfare (NIHFW) is one of the most important technical institutes working for improvement of health and family welfare in the country.

**Location:** New Delhi, India

**Organogram:**

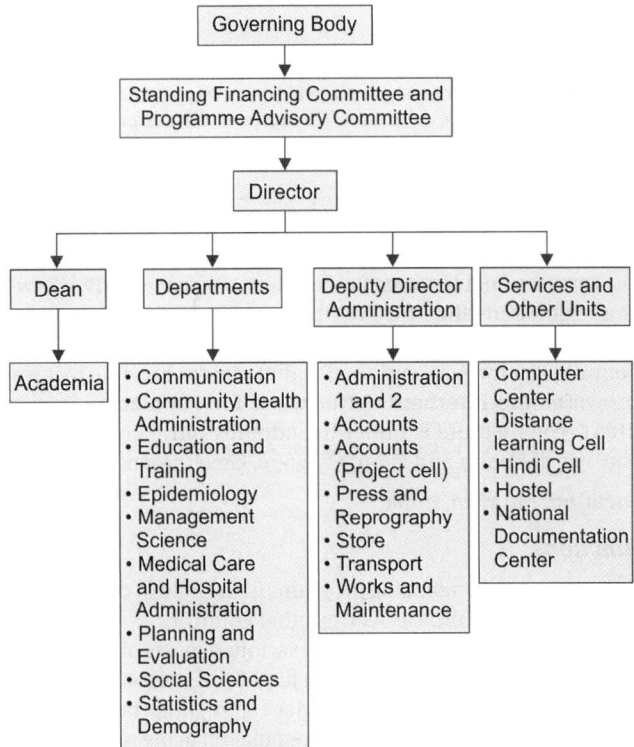

### Functions
- Offers postgraduate courses in subjects pertaining to health administration, biomedical science, social sciences, demography, communication health economics, statistics, population education and management sciences, population sciences, etc.
- Conducts and promotes research in various fields related to health and family welfare.
- Develops tools and guidelines for evaluation of health services and programs.
- Publication of monographs, journals, research papers, technical reports, bulletins, newsletters, and books.
- Prepares and disseminates Information, Education, and Communication (IEC) about health and family welfare.

## Indian Council of Medical Research

### Introduction
Indian Council of Medical Research (ICMR) is one of the premium institutes in the world which actively participates in formulation, promotion, and coordination of biomedical research. The headquarter of ICMR is situated at New Delhi.

### Administration
Union Health Minister is the president of governing body and source of funding is Department of Health Research, Ministry of Health and Family Welfare, Government of India.

### Functions
- ***Intramural research:*** Indian Council of Medical Research has made outstanding contribution as a knowledge generating agency. ICMR has total 26 research institutes/centers including 21 mission-oriented national institutes and 5 regional centers (**Table 50.2**). They are dealing with various communicable diseases of national importance. Additionally, ICMR has made extensive contributions in the areas of nutrition, reproductive and child health, occupational and environmental health and research complimenting health systems. ICMR's regional medical research institutes/centers have been contributing in tackling regional health problems.
- ***Training and capacity building:*** Indian Council of Medical Research is involved in training and capacity building of young investigators, medical and allied health professionals and providing funding support for research projects to investigators from all over the country.
- ***Extramural research:*** Indian Council of Medical Research provides extramural funding to strengthen research capabilities within the institutes of the council as well as other research institutes, medical colleges and non-governmental organizations (NGOs) for various research projects.
- ***Miscellaneous:*** Indian Council of Medical Research offers fellowship programs and financially assists symposia, seminars, workshops, training courses, and conferences. Emeritus Scientist scheme is offered by council for experienced senior medical scientists and teachers which empower them to carry out research on specific biomedical topics.

> **Key Points**
> - National Health and family welfare is a body which render health services
> - ICMR is the body which promote and practice health research.

## National Tuberculosis Institute

National Tuberculosis Institute (NTI) was established in 1959 by Government of India for formulating and coordinating the implementation of Revised National Tuberculosis Control Programme

Table 50.2: List of Indian Council of Medical Research (ICMR) institutes (21) and regional institutes (5) situated across the country.

| Institute of ICMR | Place |
|---|---|
| National JALMA Institute for Leprosy and Other Mycobacterial Diseases (NJILOMD) | Agra |
| National Institute of Occupational Health (NIOH) | Ahmedabad |
| National Institute of Traditional Medicine | Belgaum |
| National Centre for Disease Informatics and Research | Bengaluru |
| National Institute for Research in Environmental Health (NIREH) | Bhopal |
| National Institute for Research in Tuberculosis (NIRT) | Chennai |
| National Institute of Epidemiology (NIE) | Chennai |
| National Institute of Malaria Research (NIMR) | New Delhi |
| National Institute of Pathology (NIP) | New Delhi |
| National Institute of Medical Statistics (NIMS) | New Delhi |
| National Institute of Nutrition (NIN) | Hyderabad |
| National Animal Resource Facility for Biomedical Research (NARFBR) | Hyderabad |
| National Institute of Research in Tribal Health (NIRTH) | Jabalpur |
| National Institute of Cholera and Enteric Diseases (NICED) | Kolkata |
| National Institute for Research in Reproductive Health (NIRRH) | Mumbai |
| National Institute of Immunohaematology (NIIH) | Mumbai |
| National Institute of Cancer Prevention and Research (NICPR) | Noida |
| Rajendra Memorial Research Institute of Medical Sciences (RMRIMS) | Patna |
| Vector Control Research Centre (VCRC) | Puducherry |
| National Institute of Virology (NIV) | Pune |
| National AIDS Research Institute (NARI) | Pune |
| *Regional Medical Research Centers:* Bhubaneswar, Dibrugarh, Gorakhpur, Port Blair and Jodhpur. | |

(RNTCP) which is National Tuberculosis Elimination Program (NTEP) now. It is governed by Directorate General of Health Services, Ministry of Health and Family Welfare, Government of India.

**Location:** Bengaluru, Karnataka, India

## Functions

*Following activities are undertaken at National Tuberculosis Institute:*

- National level training for personnel involved with NTEP.
- Monitoring, supervision, coordination and evaluation of NTEP.
- Research on various aspects of epidemiology, treatment and preventive strategies of tuberculosis.
- Publication of training modules, annual reports, guidelines and dissemination of information.
- Health education and communication about tuberculosis in the community.

## National Institute of Disaster Management

This institute was set up with vision to develop resources, provide trainings, frame policies and conduct researches in the subject of disaster management which includes preparedness and mitigation of disasters. National Institute of Disaster Management (NIDM) is functioning under the aegis of Ministry of Home Affairs, Government of India.

**Location:** New Delhi, India

## Functions

They are defined by Section 42(9) of National Disaster Management Act, 2005, as below:

- Create modules for training, undertake and promotes research and record keeping in disaster management, and organize training programs.
- Prepare and execute human resource development plan regarding every aspect of disaster management.
- Provide assistance in national level policy formulation.
- Provide assistance to the state governments and state training institutes in the preparation of policies, framework, strategies, and any other assistance.
- Create awareness among concerned personnel which also includes school teachers or students and college, those associated with various aspects of disaster management.
- Achievement of above-mentioned objectives is dealt by undertaking various activities in the field of disaster prevention, mitigation, and management across various states of India and abroad.

> **Key Points**
> - National Institute of Tuberculosis works on Tuberculosis exclusively to bring down the mortality and morbidity in every day of life
> - National Institute of Disaster Management creates preparedness and mitigation of disaster occurrence only and works for emergency situation.

## International Institute for Population Sciences (IIPS)

The International Institute for Population Sciences (IIPS) serves as a regional institute for Training and Research in Population Studies for ESCAP (United Nations Economic and Social Commission for Asia and the Pacific) region. Previously it was known as the International Institute for Population Studies (IIPS). The Institute is under the administrative control of the Ministry of Health and Family Welfare, Government of India.

**Location:** Mumbai, India

## Functions

- It offers regular teaching programs in the field of demography to students of India as well as other countries.
- Conduct scientific research on various aspects of population in India and other countries in the ESCAP region.
- It provides consultation services and undertakes special studies on problems related to population at the request of the Government, the United Nations and other specialized agencies.
- Institute maintains an excellent library with most recent books on population and related topics.

## Pasteur Institute of India

It was established in the year 1907, as Pasture Institute of Southern India, now working as an autonomous body under Ministry of Health and Family Welfare, Government of India.

**Location:** Coonoor, Tamil Nadu, India

## Functions

- Institute produces the DPT group of vaccines and Vero cell-derived rabies vaccine. It provides vaccines to the Expanded Programme on Immunization renamed as Universal Immunization Programme run by Government of India.
- It is involved in research and development of tissue culture rabies vaccine.
- The institute conducts academic and training program for the postgraduate students and other scientists in the field of vaccine production.
- It conducts research for development of cost-effective newer vaccines.
- Institute has rabies diagnostic laboratory. It is also providing 24-hour emergency services for the treatment of animal/dog bite cases.

## Central Research Institute

Central Research Institute (CRI) serves national health programs in India since 1905, through its contribution in research and production of vaccines, surveillance, training, and teaching in the subject of microbiology. It is governed by Director General of Health Services, Ministry of Health and Family Welfare, Government of India.

**Location:** Kasauli, Himachal Pradesh, India

## Functions

- It is a research center of international level which produces vaccines (DPT, tetanus toxoid, and yellow fever), antisera (anti-snake venom, tetanus toxoid), and diagnostic reagents.
- It is a national reference center for *Salmonella* and *Escherichia coli*, providing research, diagnostic and training facilities.
- This institute functions as Rabies Research Center and a tertiary level healthcare facility with referral center for animal bites/snake bites and rabies.
- Major contribution is given by CRI, in elimination of polio from India by isolation and identification of poliovirus from the cases of acute flaccid paralysis, through its WHO accredited "National Polio Laboratory".
- World Health Organization (WHO) approved national influenza center of CRI is involved in surveillance and research of influenza.
- It is also a yellow fever and polio vaccination center for international travel with a well-equipped clinical laboratory.
- The institute also offers postgraduate training in microbiology and certificate course in immunology.

> **Key Points**
> International Institute of Population Science, Pasteur Institute of India and Central Research Institute all are specialized institutes one for demography and population science and other two for vaccines exclusively.

## VOLUNTARY HEALTH AGENCIES IN INDIA (TABLE 50.3)

In India, voluntary health organizations as well as autonomous bodies are directly or indirectly involved in the public health system. They are kind of NGOs who mainly function in the field of health. All of them provide support and technical guidance in the field of research, development, and interventions related to health care.

**Table 50.3:** Contribution of voluntary health agencies in India.

| Voluntary health agency | Functions/activities |
|---|---|
| Hind Kusht Nivaran Sangh | • Production and distribution of health education material on leprosy<br>• Conducting training courses for physiotherapy technicians at leprosy training centers<br>• Providing aid to voluntary organizations and leprosy patients<br>• Publication of quarterly Indian Journal of Leprosy |
| Indian Council for Child Welfare | • Advocating children's rights, crèches for children of working and ailing mothers and education of underprivileged children<br>• Education centers and support services |
| Tuberculosis Association of India | • Train the doctors, give quality diagnostic and treatment services<br>• Promote health education by providing consultations and arranging seminars<br>• Fund raising by organizing a tuberculosis (TB) seal campaign every year |
| Bharat Sevak Samaj | • Enhancement in rural sanitation and cleanliness<br>• Promotion of reaching health by people through their own efforts |
| Kasturba Gandhi National Memorial Trust | Involved in conducting various programs in the fields of health care, education, vocational training and employment generation |
| Family Planning Association of India | Engaging men and boys to promote gender equality and empowerment for all including the poor and vulnerable group |
| All India Women's Conference | • Working energetically for freedom, education and empowerment of women and children<br>• Family planning clinics |
| The All India Blind Relief Society | • Organizes the eye camps for the relief of the blind<br>• Providing teaching and training to the visually challenged, aiding them to recognize their power |
| Professional bodies (Indian Medical Association and its state branches) | • Conducting national and state conferences, publish and circulate scientific journals and newsletters<br>• Promote research work<br>• Setup ethics and standard of professional education and organize medical camps during natural disasters |

## Indian Red Cross Society

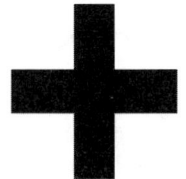

**Indian Red Cross Society**

### Background

India did not have any society for relief services for the soldiers at the time of First World War in 1914. Later on, a branch of the St John Ambulance Association and a Joint Committee of the British Red Cross have initiated relief services during war for the soldiers and civilians who were affected during the war. Indian Legislative Council had introduced a bill to constitute the Indian Red Cross Society (IRCS), independent of the British Red Cross on 3rd March 1920. The act was last amended in 1992, and rules were created in 1994. The society works with the objective of executing programs for the health promotion disease prevention and alleviation of suffering among the people.

### Administration

The IRCS has 35 state/union territories branches and 700 districts branches. The Honorable President of India is the leader of the society and it is chaired by the honorable Union Health Minister.

### Functions

- *Relief work:* The prime function of the society is to provide disaster response and thereby it assists millions of people ranging from refugees to victims of natural disasters.
- *Milk and medical supplies:* Many hospitals, dispensaries, maternity and child welfare centers, institutes, and orphanages receive aid from the society in the form of milk powder, medicines, vitamins, and other materials.
- *Armed forces:* Indian Red Cross Society provides service for the injured and sick soldiers. In Bengaluru, there is a center, which provides various facilities without any charges including facility of operation theater, physiotherapy, library, and recreation facilities for all the servicemen.
- *Maternal and child welfare services:* It extends maternal and child development activities for the weaker section of the community.
- *Family welfare:* These are run by different branches of the states and districts. They provide contraceptives and other family planning devices and encourage eligible couples to accept small family norms.
- *Blood bank and first aid:* Since 1962, the Indian Red Cross remains one of the largest voluntary blood banks in India. Motivational campaigns are conducted regularly for organization of voluntary blood donation camps.
- *Vocational training center (VTC):* The IRCS offers opportunities to increase vocational skills among low-income groups.
- *HIV/AIDS:* The IRCS is actively involved in the prevention of HIV/AIDS. Through youth peer education program, youth are given training for disseminating information about the prevention of HIV/AIDS.

### Central Social Welfare Board

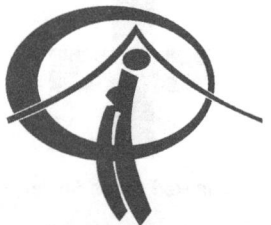

### Background

The Central Social Welfare Board is an independent organization established in the year 1953 under the general administrative control of the Ministry of Education. It provides technical and financial assistance to the voluntary organizations for the welfare of women, children, and families. It works with the objective of linking the government and the people.

The Central Social Welfare Board has implemented many projects like Grant-in-Aid, Mahila Mandals, Welfare Extension Projects, Dairy Scheme, Socio-economic Programme, Condensed Courses of Education Programme for adolescent girls and women, Awareness Generation Programme, Vocational Training Programme, National Creche Scheme, Integrated Scheme for Women's Empowerment for North Eastern States, Short Stay Home Programme and Family Counseling Center Programme.

### Functions

- Board surveys the necessity of voluntary welfare organizations in the nation and provides financial support to existing organizations.
- It has initiated "Family and Child Welfare Services" in the rural area which is involved in teaching of craft, social education, literacy classes, maternity aid for women, milk distribution, balwadis, and organization of play centers for children.
- For the urban area, board has started a scheme of industrial cooperatives which provide support to the women of lower-middle class to earn by doing paid work.

## NON-GOVERNMENTAL ORGANIZATION WORKING UNDER NATIONAL HEALTH MISSION

Government of India promotes the NGOs for effective implementation of various health programmes, especially in underserved areas. Various types of NGOs working under Reproductive and Child Health (RCH) Programme are mother NGO (MNGO), field NGO (FNGO), and service NGO (SNGO). Each district has one MNGO whose prime objective is to improve RCH indicators. Under MNGO, 3–4 FNGOs are working with intention of identifying unserved and high priority areas. Service NGOs provides clinical services and other specialized services like training of dai, medical termination of pregnancy (MTP) services, family planning services, and male involvement in MCH care. Each SNGO covers 100,000 population and contribute in achieving objectives of RCH.

### Public Health Concerns where International Organizations are Helping and there is Need to Focus by Indian Government

- Bridging the gaps between various stakeholders in identifying, quantifying and dealing with common health problems in India. The strategies of implementing various components of different National Health Programmes should follow the principle of equitable distribution.
- Community involvement in terms of identifying the need and planning the solution feasible to local circumstances with special emphasis to partnership between practitioners of indigenous system of medicine and government.

- Use of appropriate technology, adopting novel and multiple approaches in providing services including various social media which can reach easily to youth as well as to other vulnerable population.
- Capacity building of the key persons at community levels like school teachers, peers in youth and also of grassroot level health workers by sensitization, orientation, hands on trainings and workshops; continued education by various means.
- Provision of services in terms of treatment, resources, counseling in a phase of critical requirement by community with main focus to high priority areas.
- Government institutes/organization may face their own limitations in certain aspects which NGO or private healthcare providers may not. Implementation of some facets of national health programs may be handed over to such stakeholders with freedom in decision making whenever required.

## SUCCESS STORY

Elimination of poliomyelitis from India is a success story of coordinated efforts between Government Agencies, International Health Agencies, and NGOs. Although, the list of agencies which have contributed in this achievement is exhaustive, few of them are mentioned herewith. ICMR first established a Polio Research Unit (currently known as Enterovirus Research Centre) in 1949 at Mumbai. A surveillance unit for polio was also set up. Polio vaccine testing unit was started in NCDC in 1968. WHO provided technical and financial support and initiated National Polio Surveillance Project in 1997 in collaboration with Government of India. Pasteur Institute of India was the first Government agency to manufacture oral polio vaccine in India. The field unit, National Institute of Virology also serves as center for surveillance of acute flaccid paralysis. NCDC harbors Regional Reference Laboratory for Polio for South East Asia Region (established in 1991).

## SUGGESTED READING

1. Central Social Welfare Board, Ministry of Women and Child Development. (2019). [online]. Available from http://cswb.gov.in/.
2. ICMR at a glance. Activities and achievements. Available from https://www.icmr.nic.in/file_download/document/Imp_achievements.pdf.
3. Indian Red Cross Society. (2019). Education and training Programmes. [online]. Available from http://www.indianredcross.org/.
4. Lahariya C. A brief history of vaccines and vaccination in India. Indian J Med Res. 2014;139(4):491-511.
5. Ministry of Health and Family Welfare. (2017). Directorate General of Health Services. [online]. Available from http://dghs.gov.in/content/1407_3_NationalCentreforDiseaseControl.aspx.
6. Ministry of Health and Family Welfare. (2018). Central Research Institute. [online]. Available from http://www.crikasauli.nic.in/index.php.
7. National Institute of Health and Family Welfare. (2014). About NIHFW. [online]. Available from http://www.nihfw.org/WAboutUS.aspx.
8. National Institute of Virology. J Postgrad Med. 2000;46(4):299-302. [online]. Available from http://www.ncbi.nlm.nih.gov/pubmed/11435663.
9. National Tuberculosis Institute, Bangalore. (2012). Scientific Gallery on Tuberculosis. [online]. Available from http://ntiindia.kar.nic.in/.
10. NIDM, Ministry of Home Affairs, Government of India. (2018). Role of Media in disaster management. [online]. Available from https://nidm.gov.in/.
11. Pasteur Institute of India, Coonoor. (2005). An overview. [online]. Available from http://pasteurinstituteindia.com/.
12. The International Institute for Population Sciences (IIPS). [online]. Available from http://www.iipsindia.ac.in/about-iips

# CHAPTER 51

# Special Topics

**CM 7.9** Describe and demonstrate the application of computers in epidemiology
**CM 8.7** Describe the principles of management of information systems
**PE 19.4** Define cold chain and discuss the methods of safe storage and handling of vaccines (vertical integration with pediatrics department)

## A. VILLAGE HEALTH AND NUTRITION DAY: PLANNING AND PREPAREDNESS

*Bharatkumar M Gohel*

### INTRODUCTION

Maternal mortality ratio (MMR) and infant mortality rate (IMR) are very crucial indicators for any nation. They reflect not only the health situation of the country but also socioeconomic development of the nation. Initial Family Planning Programme was expanded as CSSM (Child Survival and Safe Motherhood) Programme in 1992. Later on the same got various revisions from MCH (Maternal and Child Health) Programme, RCH (Reproductive and Child Health) Programme phases I and II, RMNCH (Reproductive Maternal Neonatal Child Health) Programme, RMNCH+A (Reproductive Maternal Neonatal Child Health Plus Adolescent) to RMNCAH+N (Reproductive Maternal Neonatal Child Adolescent Health Plus Nutrition) Programme under the umbrella of NHM (National Health Mission). For effective service delivery with universal coverage all the services of RMNCAH+N components are provided under Village Health and Nutrition Day (VHND).

Village Health Sanitation and Nutrition Committees (VHSNCs), one of the key interventions introduced by NRHM, are an important mechanism to ensure community participation at all levels. The VHND is organized once every month at the fixed site in the village. It serves as an interface between the community and the health system. On the appointed day, Accredited Social Health Activists (ASHAs) and Anganwadi Workers (AWWs) mobilize the villagers, especially women and children to assemble at the VHND site. The auxiliary nurse midwife (ANM) and other health personnel attend the session to provide basic services and information about the preventive, promotive and curative aspects of health care along with referral services, which create awareness among the villagers to seek health care at appropriate facilities. Health services are to be provided at the doorsteps by the VHND which is held at the sites very close to their habitation so that villagers would not have to spend time or money on travel.

### CONCEPT OF VILLAGE HEALTH AND NUTRITION DAY

Concept of VHND is based on provision of all the services related to RMNCAH+N:
- On fixed day
- At fixed site
- At the doorstep of community.

Village health and nutrition day is run and made successful by ANM, ASHA, AWW, the Panchayati Raj Institution's (PRI's) representative and if possible multipurpose health worker (MPHW) male, ASHA facilitator and volunteers.

### OBJECTIVE OF VILLAGE HEALTH SANITATION AND NUTRITION COMMITTEES

- Inform the community about health programs and enable them to participate in their planning and implementation.
- Take action on social determinants and all public health services directed toward improved health outcomes.
- Facilitate community to voice health needs.
- Equip panchayats with understanding to play their role in governance of health.
- Facilitate work of ASHA and other healthcare providers.

### SERVICES PROVIDED ON VILLAGE HEALTH AND NUTRITION DAY

- Registration of all pregnant women, adolescent girls and eligible children.
- Vaccination to all eligible children, adolescent girls and pregnant women.
- Antenatal services [antenatal care (ANC) registration, basic laboratory investigations, screening for high-risk pregnancies, general and obstetric examination, prophylactic and

therapeutic iron folic acid (IFA) and calcium supplements, nutritional diet supplements, counseling, etc.].
- Postnatal services (general and obstetric examination, prophylactic and therapeutic IFA and calcium supplements, nutritional diet supplements, counseling, etc.).
- Prophylactic vitamin A solution and IFA supplementation to children less than 5 years of age.
- Weighing and recording of weight of children less than 5 years.
- Adolescent girls' care (measurement of height, weight and BMI, dietary counseling, health education on menstrual hygiene and reproductive health, etc.).
- Distribution of condoms and oral contraceptive pills (OCPs) to all eligible couples as per their choice.
- Supplementary nutrition to underweight children and pregnant women.
- Tracking of drop-out beneficiaries and service provision.
- Awareness about prevention and control of communicable diseases like leprosy, TB, water-borne diseases, vector-borne disease, etc.
- Referral services as and when needed.

## ISSUES TO BE DISCUSSED ON VILLAGE HEALTH AND NUTRITION DAY

- Birth preparedness and registration for Janani Suraksha Yojana (JSY)
- Danger signs during pregnancy
- Emphasis on institutional delivery and postnatal care
- Counseling on essential newborn care, exclusive breastfeeding and complementary feeding
- Care during diarrhea, ARI (acute respiratory infection) and home management of these illnesses
- Prevention of malaria, TB, leprosy, STIs, RTIs including HIV/AIDS and other communicable diseases
- Prevention of non-communicable diseases
- Identification of referral transport
- Importance of nutrition, safe drinking water and basic sanitation
- Health education of children and adolescent girls.

*Identification of cases needing special attention like:*
- Children with birth defects
- Children with disabilities
- Children with danger signs
- Children with grade III and grade IV malnutrition for referral
- High-risk pregnancies
- Pay special attention to the SC, ST, minorities and weaker sections.

To conduct VHND effectively proper microplanning, unbroken supply of vaccines and logistics, skilled human resources, adequate infrastructure, effective IEC and BCC activities, community participation and supportive supervision are required.

## MICROPLANNING OF VILLAGE HEALTH AND NUTRITION DAY

Microplanning is very important and essential step toward the success of service delivery at VHND. The final coverage of various services depends on the quality of microplanning and its skillful prosecution. Various steps of microplanning are mentioned below:
- Preparing an area map
- Baseline population survey
- Calculation of beneficiaries
- Calculation of vaccines and logistics required
- Planning the time, place and person for service delivery
- Infrastructure requirement for VHND
- Human resources and their job at VHND
- Post-VHND preparations.

### Preparing an Area Map

The microplanning is initiated at the village level—a very basic unit of the community. A precise map of village (ward for urban area) is prepared showing clear cut boundaries with proper landmarks so the issue of bordering area can be minimized. The map must include all faliyas, high-risk areas, construction sites, nomadic settlements, etc. The microplan is to be evaluated quarterly and updated every year. The map can be prepared with the help of google map or other applications.

### Baseline Population Survey

While preparation of map decides work area, baseline population survey decides the type and load of beneficiaries. Yearly family health survey (FHS) is the tool to retrieve baseline statistics like: total population, eligible couples, adolescent population, birth rate, death rate, under five population, number of pregnant women, etc.

The record is uploaded and updated with mother and child tracking system (MCTS) software. All the targets, indicators and indents for supply are calculated on the base of these data. So it is very crucial to gather and feed authenticated data in the system. It is a duty of female health worker (FHW) with the help of ASHA/USHA to carry out family health survey in their areas using standard prescribed format.

### Calculation of Beneficiaries

Family health survey gives actual number of pregnant women (PW) at a time of survey. At any point of time we may be able to have data of only 6 months of pregnancy. It is assumed that pregnancies during first trimester might be missed because of low early registration. Furthermore, chances of medical termination of pregnancy (MTP) for unplanned accidental pregnancies and chances of miscarriages are also high during first trimester. So it is presumed that practically surveyor would get only 6 months' duration pregnancies captured during survey. Doubling the same data would give annual number of pregnant women. For infants (I), actual number of infants is the annual number of infants, because at any time all the infants (from day-0 to day-365) would be captured by surveyor.

### Calculation of Vaccines and Logistics Required

Having handy information on number of pregnant and infants, requirement of vaccines and logistics are calculated as shown in **Table 51A.1**.

**Step 1**: Monthly target of pregnant women or infants is calculated dividing yearly target by 12. To determine required doses of

Table 51A.1: Vaccines and logistics requirement calculation.

| Steps → | Step 1 | Step 2 | Step 3 |
|---|---|---|---|
| Name of vaccine | Doses required A = (No. of beneficiaries) × (No. of doses) | Vaccine vials required B = A/No. of doses per vial | Actual vaccine vials required C = B × Wastage Multiplication Factor (WMF) |
| Td | =(PW × 2) | =(PW × 2)/10 | =[(PW × 2)/10] × 1.11 |
| BCG | =(Infant × 1) | =(Infant × 1)/10 | =[(Infant × 1)/10] × 2 |
| OPV | =(Infant × 5) | =(Infant × 5)/20 | =[(Infant × 5)/20] × 1.11 |
| Pentavalent | =(Infant × 3) | =(Infant × 3)/10 | =[(Infant × 3)/10] × 1.11 |
| f-IPV | =(Infant × 3) | =(Infant × 3)/25 | =[(Infant × 3)/25] × 1.11 |
| PCV* | =(Infant × 3) | =(Infant × 3)/54 | =[(Infant × 3)/54] × 1.11 |
| RVV* | =(Infant × 3) | =(Infant × 3)/1 | =[(Infant × 3)/1] × 1.33 |
| MR | =(Infant × 2) | =(Infant × 2)/10 | =[(Infant × 2)/5] × 1.33 |
| JE* | =(Infant × 2) | =(Infant × 2)/5 | =[(Infant × 2)/5] × 1.33 |
| DPT | =(Infant × 2) | =(Infant × 2)/10 | =[(Infant × 2)/10] × 1.11 |

*Applicable to selected states where these vaccines are used
(Td: tetanus toxoid + diphtheria toxoid in adult concentration; BCG: Bacillus Calmette–Guérin; DPT: diphtheria + pertussis + tetanus; IPV: inactivated polio vaccine; JE: Japanese encephalitis; MR: measles + rubella; OPV: oral polio vaccines; PCV: pneumococcal conjugate vaccine; RVV: rotavirus vaccine)

each vaccine, number of beneficiaries (pregnant women or infant) is multiplied by the number of doses required for full immunization.

**Step 2**: Monthly doses when divided by the number of doses each vial contains, will give number of vials required for particular vaccine during the month.

**Step 3**: However, it is not possible to utilize all the doses in vaccine vial. Wastage of vaccines by one or other mean is always observed. Few drops of vaccine remaining in vial, cold chain break and color change of VVM from usable to non-usable, reconstituted vaccines remaining unutilized after 4 hours to be discarded, accidental breaking of vials, unutilized vaccine vials after 28 days under open vial policy, etc. are the reasons.

That is the reason why one should demand vaccines considering wastage multiplication factor (WMF) while asking for indent. WMF can be calculated on the base of wastage rate (WR). Formula of WMF is, WMF = 100/(100−WR). Acceptable WR and WMF as per official guidelines for various vaccines and logistics are mentioned in **Table 51A.2**.

Table 51A.2: Acceptable WR and WMF for vaccines and logistics.

| Vaccine/Logistics | Acceptable WR | Acceptable WMF |
|---|---|---|
| BCG | 50% | 2.00 |
| MR, JE*, RVV | 25% | 1.33 |
| Tetanus Toxoid, Hepatitis-B, OPV, f-IPV, Pentavalent, DPT, PCV*, Vitamin A | 10% | 1.11 |
| 0.1 mL AD syringe, 0.5 mL AD syringe, 5.0 mL reconstitution syringe | 10% | 1.11 |

*Applicable to selected states where these vaccines are used
(BCG: Bacillus Calmette–Guérin; DPT: diphtheria + pertussis + tetanus; IPV: inactivated polio vaccine; JE: Japanese encephalitis; MR: measles + rubella; OPV: oral polio vaccines; PCV: pneumococcal conjugate vaccine; RVV: rotavirus vaccine)

## Planning the Time, Place and Person of the Session

The workload is calculated on the base of total population of the area or total injection load. Total population gives crude idea about number of sessions required, while the number of injections is more specific indicator to determine the number of sessions to be held. Both are given in **Table 51A.3**.

Table 51A.3: Criteria to decide number of sessions in a given area.

| Frequency of session | Total population of area | Injection load |
|---|---|---|
| Twice a month | >1,500 | 51–100 |
| Once a month | 500–1500 | 26–50 |
| Alternate month | 300–500 | 1–25 |
| Quarterly | <300 | Hard to reach area |

After determining the number of sessions required per month in a particular village, appropriate place should be selected. It may be sub-center, anganwadi center, panchayat house, school building or a hired building. ANM/FHW is the key person of VHND session. Anganwadi worker, anganwadi helper, ASHA/USHA, MPW, volunteer, etc. are supporting the session.

***Session sites are of four types:*** **(1) Fixed session sites**: These are the session sites where vaccine storage facility is available: [urban health center (UHC)/primary health center (PHC)/community health center (CHC)/district hospital (DH)]. **(2) Outreach session sites**: These are the session sites where vaccine storage facility is not available and workers do session carrying vaccines in vaccine carriers from the vaccine storage facility. **(3) Tagged session site**: These are the session sites having identified pockets which are tagged to the nearby session. Beneficiaries are called for service utilization by active mobilization. **(4) Mobile session sites**: These are the sessions done by mobile van team. In the areas of scattered population mobile sessions are helpful.

These sessions are held on fixed days, usually on every Monday at fixed session sites and on Wednesday at outreach session sites.

## Infrastructure and Logistics Requirement for VHND

The place should be spacious enough having clinic room, examination portion, waiting area and toilet block. There should be a clinic room with examination table and curtain to maintain privacy during ANC check-ups. There must be adequate waiting area because after immunization the child is supposed to be there for 30 minutes. Toilet block is needed for urine sample collection. Weighing scales for adult, children and young infants, scale to measure height, sphygmomanometer, stethoscope, fetoscope, thermometer, necessary medicines, laboratory equipment, vaccines, registers, etc. should be available.

## Responsibility of Accredited Social Health Activist

Accredited social health activist acts as convener of VHSNC and ensures regular organizing VHN days. She visits all households and coordinates with the AWW, FHW and MPHW.

She makes the list of—(1) pregnant women for registration and antenatal check-ups; (2) women who need ANC for the first time or for repeat visits; (3) children who need immunization, who were left out or drop out; (4) children who need care for malnutrition; (5) children with special needs; and (6) target couples for family planning services.

She ensures that all the enlisted beneficiaries take the services provided on VHN day.

### Responsibility of Anganwadi Worker

She ensures the (1) cleanliness of AWC and availability of clean drinking water, (2) ensures a place with privacy at the AWC for ANC, (3) measures weight of children, pregnant and keep records, (4) coordinate activities with ASHA and FHW.

### Responsibilities of ANM/FHW

She ensures that (1) VHND is held without fail, (2) adequate supply of drugs, instruments, IEC materials, etc., (3) provides the required services to all the beneficiaries in coordination with ASHA and AWW, (4) reporting of VHND to medical officer in-charge, and (5) organizing group discussions on providing social and health issues.

*Post-VHND preparations:* After VHND session ASHA and ANM updates the due list of beneficiaries. It includes addition and deletion of beneficiaries as per the factual situation.

## SUMMARY

Village health and nutrition day, if organized regularly and effectively, can bring about much needed behavioral changes in the community and can also induce health-seeking behavior in the community leading to better health outcomes.

## SUGGESTED READING

1. Ministry of Health and Family Welfare, Government of India. (2014). National Health Mission, Handbook for members of Village Health Sanitation and Nutrition Committee. [online]. Available form http://www.nhm.gov.in/communitisation/village-health-sanitation-nutrition-committee.html.
2. Ministry of Health and Family Welfare, Government of India. (2017). Immunization Handbook for Medical Officers. [online]. Available from https://mohfw.gov.in/basicpage/immunization-handbook-medical-officers.
3. National Health Mission, Ministry of Health and Welfare, Govt. of India. (2013). Village Health Nutrition Day. [online]. Available from http//nhm.gov.in/communitisation/village-health-nutrition-day.html.

# B. COLD CHAIN MANAGEMENT

*Hitesh M Shah, Darshan Mahyavanshi*

## INTRODUCTION

Immunization is one of the most cost-effective weapons of preventing childhood diseases with high mortality and morbidity. Universal Immunization Programme (UIP) launched in 1985 aimed to protect children against various vaccine preventable diseases (VPDs) in our country. On December 25th, 2014, Government of India (GoI) launched Mission Indradhanush (MI) in selected districts to increase coverage of immunization in India by 2020. Mission Indradhanush was intensified as Intensified Mission Indradhanush (IMI) with an objective to accelerate full immunization coverage to more than 90% by December 2018. Measles rubella (MR) vaccine campaign was launched in 2017 with objectives to eliminate measles and control rubella in phased manner. GoI added Rotavirus, adult Japanese encephalitis, inactivated polio vaccine and pneumococcal conjugate vaccine in UIP in phased manner. As spectrum of UIP is broadening, logistic management of vaccines including cold chain management is becoming priority to maintain potency of vaccines.

## DEFINITION

Cold chain consists of a series of storage and transport links, all of which are designed to keep the vaccine at the recommended temperature from the point of manufacture until it reaches the target beneficiary.

The *cold chain* is a system of storing and transporting vaccines at recommended temperatures from the point of manufacture to the point of use **(Fig. 51B.1)**.

In this chapter, vaccine storage and distribution from peripheral Cold Chain Point (CCP), mainly PHC is discussed.

## VACCINE SAFETY

Vaccines lose their potency due to exposure to **(Tables 51B.1 and 51B.2)**.
- Heat (temperature above + 8°C)—all vaccines under UIP
- Cold (temperature below + 2°C)—hepatitis B, pentavalent, IPV, DPT, TT, Td and Rota vaccine (liquid)
- Light—BCG, Measles and Measles Rubella (MR).

### Heat Damage

Heat can damage all UIP vaccines if temperature rises above + 8°C. Temperature range for storage of vaccine at *cold chain points* like PHC at periphery should be + 2 to + 8°C. To ascertain the usability of vaccines against heat damage, vaccine vial monitor (VVM) is an important indicator. All UIP vaccines are having VVM on the vial **(Fig. 51B.2)**.

### *Vaccine Vial Monitor (VVM)*

Vaccine vial monitor is an indicator to know the usability of vaccine. Based on VVM readings, vaccines can be labeled as in usable stage and unusable stages. Previously VVM reading was done in four stages. In that case, stages I and II are usable and III and IV are considered as unusable stages.

*Usable stage:* If the inner square is lighter than outer circle color, the vaccine can be used.

*Unusable stage:* If the inner square color is similar or darker to outer circle, the vaccine cannot be used.

### *Expiry Date*

Before opening the vial, always check for expiry date of vial. The vial should be within the expiry date.

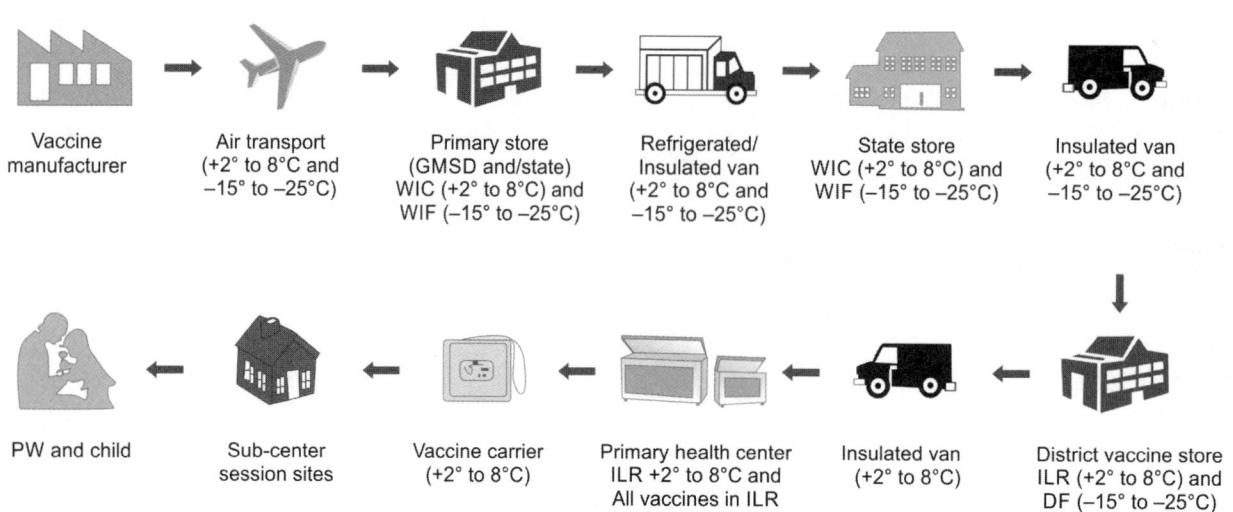

**Fig. 51B.1:** Immunization supply chain levels in India.
*Source:* Handbook of Vaccine and Cold Chain Handlers. New Delhi: Ministry of Health and Family Welfare (GoI); 2016.

**Table 51B.1:** Vaccine safety.

| Vaccine | Exposure to heat/light | Exposure to cold | Recommended temperature at PHC |
|---|---|---|---|
| *Heat and light sensitive vaccines* | | | |
| BCG | Relatively heat stable, but sensitive to light | Not damaged by freezing | +2°C to +8°C |
| OPV | Sensitive to heat | Not damaged by freezing | +2°C to +8°C |
| Measles, MR | Sensitive to heat and light | Not damaged by freezing | +2°C to +8°C |
| Rota virus (Liquid and freeze dried) | Sensitive to heat | Can be damaged by freezing (liquid only) | +2°C to +8°C |
| Japanese encephalitis | Sensitive to heat | Not damaged by freezing | +2°C to +8°C |
| *Freeze sensitive vaccines* | | | |
| Pentavalent vaccine | Relatively heat stable | Freezes at −3°C (Should not be frozen) | +2°C to +8°C |
| DPT | Relatively heat stable | Freezes at −3°C (Should not be frozen) | +2°C to +8°C |
| Hepatitis B | Relatively heat stable | Freezes at −0.5°C (Should not be frozen) | +2°C to +8°C |
| DT | Relatively heat stable | Freezes at −3°C (Should not be frozen) | +2°C to +8°C |
| TT / Td | Relatively heat stable | Freezes at −3°C (Should not be frozen) | +2°C to +8°C |

*Source:* Immunization Handbook for Medical Officers, 2016, Ministry of Health and Family Welfare, GoI.

**Table 51B.2:** Most vaccines to least vaccines.

| Vaccines sensitive to heat | Vaccines sensitive to freezing |
|---|---|
| **Most** | |
| BCG (after reconstitution) | Hep-B |
| Oral Polio Vaccine | Pentavalent/DPT |
| Inactivated Polio Vaccine | DT |
| Japanese encephalitis (live) | TT/Td |
| Measles, MR, Rotavirus (freeze dried and liquid) | Rotavirus (liquid) |
| Pentavalent/DPT | |
| BCG (before reconstitution) | |
| Japanese encephalitis (inactivated) | |
| DT, TT, Td, Hep-B | |
| **Least** | |

Reconstituted BCG, measles/MR, opened liquid freeze Rota or reconstituted freeze dried Rota vaccine and JE are most heat sensitive vaccines. The vaccines should be used within four hours of reconstitution. That is why all the vaccinators are trained to write the date and time of reconstitution of vaccine on vaccine vial with special marker pen.

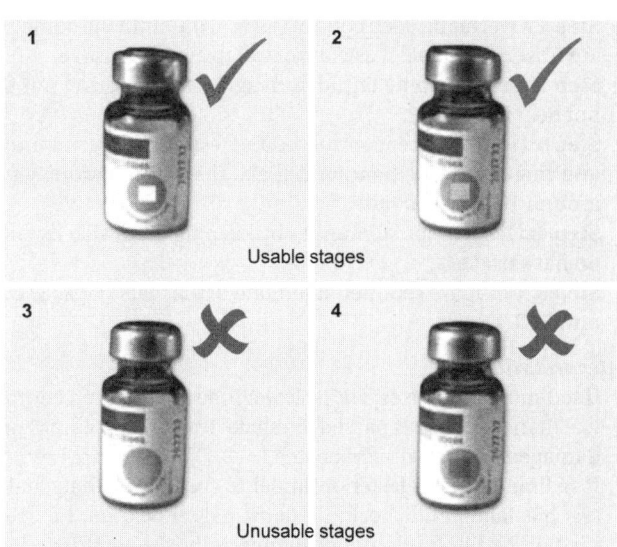

**Fig. 51B.2:** Vaccine vial monitor usable and unusable stages.
*Source:* Immunization Handbook for Medical Officers, 2016, Ministry of Health and Family Welfare, GoI.

### Electronic Vaccine Intelligence Network

Electronic Vaccine Intelligence Network (eVIN) is an indigenously developed technology system in India that digitizes vaccine stocks and monitors the temperature of the cold chain through a Smartphone application. In partnership of Ministry with Health and Family Welfare, GoI and United Nations Development Programme (UNDP), eVIN was launched to manage vaccine stocks and monitor the temperature of all cold chain points (PHCs mainly) through installed temperature loggers. Electronic Vaccine Intelligence Network aims to provide real time data on vaccine stock and temperature monitoring of cold chain points. eVIN is now operational in 19 states and 2 union territories covering 521 districts in India.

## Cold Damage

Hepatitis, Pentavalent/DPT, IPV, TT/Td and Rotavirus (liquid) vaccines as well as diluents are liable to damage due to freezing. Shake test is an important test to find out whether the vials are frozen or not. The shake test should be performed only when health staff suspect freezing of freeze sensitive vials. It is not done on routine basis.

### Checking for Cold Damage

***The shake test:*** Test is used to check whether freeze sensitive vaccine has been damaged by exposure to temperature below 0°C.

***Procedure of shake test:*** Take two vials, one test vial (which is suspected that may have been frozen), and one frozen control vial. Take a vaccine vial with batch, antigen, and manufacturer same as suspected vial.

- **Step 1**: Overnight, keep control vial at –20°C until the contents are frozen and label it as control vial to avoid its usage.
- **Step 2**: Let it become liquid form again after freezing but do not heat it.
- **Step 3**: Hold together control vial and test vial between thumb and finger of same hand and shake the vials vigorously for around 10 to 15 seconds.
- **Step 4**: Observe for 30 minutes by keeping them side by side on flat surface.
- **Step 5**: Compare sedimentation rate of the vials (**Figs. 51B.3 and 51B.4**).

*Interpretation*
- If sedimentation of test vial is slower than in the frozen control vial than test vial has passed the shake test. The vaccine is not damaged and can use that batch.
- If sedimentation is faster or similar to control vial than shake test has failed and vaccine is damaged and cannot be used further. Notify in-charge or higher authority for corrective actions.

*Note:* Some vials have large labels which conceal the vial contents. This makes it difficult to see the sedimentation process. In such cases, turn the control and test vials upside down and observe sedimentation taking place in the neck of the vial.

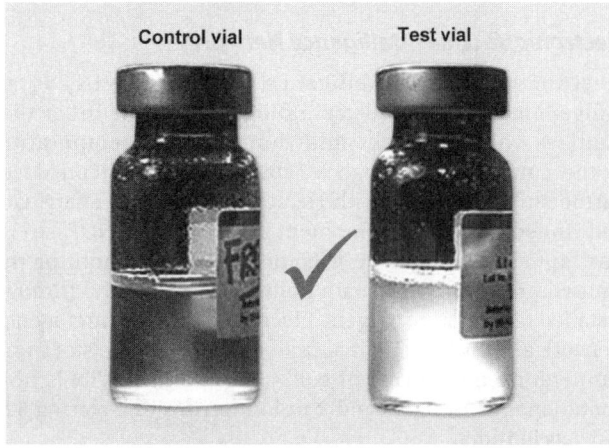

Fig. 51B.3: Passed shake test.

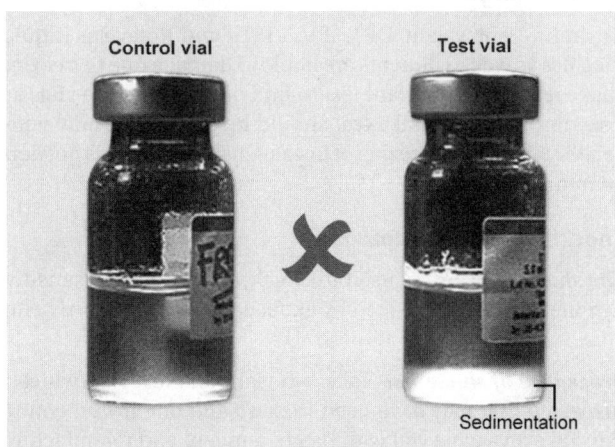

Fig. 51B.4: Failed shake test.

### Light Damage

BCG and Measles/MR vaccines are light sensitive vaccines. Direct exposure to sunlight can damage the vaccine. So BCG and Measles are supplied in Amber colored vials to protect direct sunlight.

## KEY ELEMENTS OF COLD CHAIN MAINTENANCE

At PHC (CCP) level, proper planning and infrastructure are needed for cold chain maintenance.

### Key Elements at PHC (CCP) Level

1. *Personnel:* To manage vaccines storage, distribution and cold chain maintenance.
2. *Equipment:* To store and transport vaccine.
3. *Procedures:* To ensure that vaccines are stored and transported at appropriate temperature range.

### *Personnel*

- Pharmacist is designated as vaccine and cold chain handler (VCCH) at PHC level.
- Second VCCH is also identified per PHC by Medical Officer (MO) to observe cold chain in absence of Pharmacist.
- VCCHs are responsible for management of stock of all UIP vaccines and their cold chain maintenance.
- Temperature monitoring of cold chain equipment should be done twice daily. The temperature should be recorded in temperature logbook twice daily and MO should supervise it and sign the temperature log book at a periodic interval.
- Medical Officer PHC is the overall in-charge of cold chain management at PHC level.

### *Cold Chain Equipment and Procedures*

Cold chain infrastructure includes a network of Vaccine Stores along with requisite Walk-in-coolers (WIC), Walk-in-freezers (WIF), Deep Freezers (DF), Ice Lined Refrigerators (ILR), Refrigerated Vans, Insulated Vaccine Vans, Cold Boxes, Vaccine Carriers and Ice packs from national level to states up to the outreach sessions.

- ***Walk in cold rooms (WIC):*** They are located at regional level for storage of vaccines up to 3 months.
- ***Deep freezer (large) and Ice lined refrigerator (large)***: Deep freezers are supplied at district level and used for making icepacks and to store OPV and measles or MR vaccine. Rest of the vaccines should be stored at Ice Lined Refrigerators (ILRs) at district level.
- ***Deep freezer (small):*** It is distributed at PHCs, Urban Family Planning center and postpartum centers. The temperature of deep freezer is between –15 and –25°C. Deep freezers at PHC should be used for making ice packs for cold box and vaccine carrier for storage in emergency situation as well as transportation to session site. No vaccine should be stored at deep freezer at sub-district level. Ice packs should be arranged in criss cross manner to allow passage of air in between (**Fig. 51B.5**).
- ***Ice lined refrigerator (small):*** It maintains the temperature between +2 and +8°C. It is distributed at PHCs, Urban Family Planning center and postpartum centers. All the vaccines at

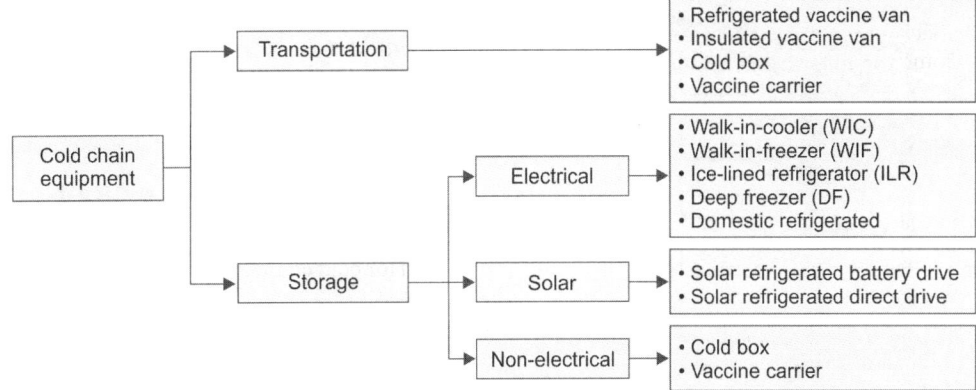

**Cold Chain Equipment and Procedures.**

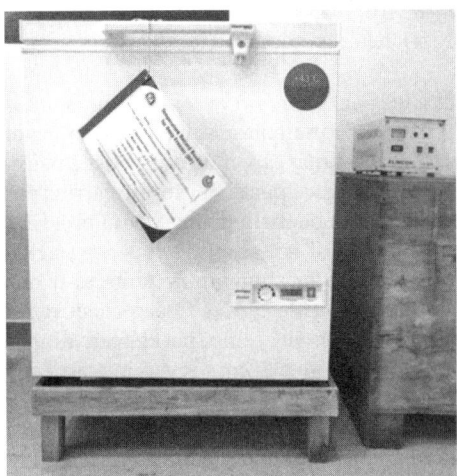

Fig. 51B.5: Deep freezer.

PHC level should be stored at ILR only. All the vaccines should be stored in the baskets provided with ILR. OPV, Measles/ MR, BCG and Rotavirus vaccine should be stored at bottom of the basket while Pentavalent, DPT, TT/Td and hepatitis B should be stored at upper part of basket **(Fig. 51B.6)**. Vaccine should never be kept on the floor of ILR.
- **Do's and Don'ts for ILR/DFs**: The equipment should be kept in cool room away from direct sunlight and at least 10 cm away from the wall. The equipment should be leveled and voltage stabilizer should be used to stabilize the voltage. "Do not switch off" label should be marked on socket. Temperature monitoring should be done as per guidelines at PHC level. Always keep the equipment locked and do not open it frequently. Defrost the equipment periodically. Do not keep any drug in equipment. Do not keep more than one month requirement at PHC level.
- The diluents supplied along with vaccine must be used to reconstitute the vaccine. They should be at same temperature of vaccine to avoid thermal shock. They should be stored in ILR to maintain the temperature. If storage capacity is less, the diluents should be placed in ILR at least 24 hours before of supply to session site. This is known as "Bundling" of diluents.

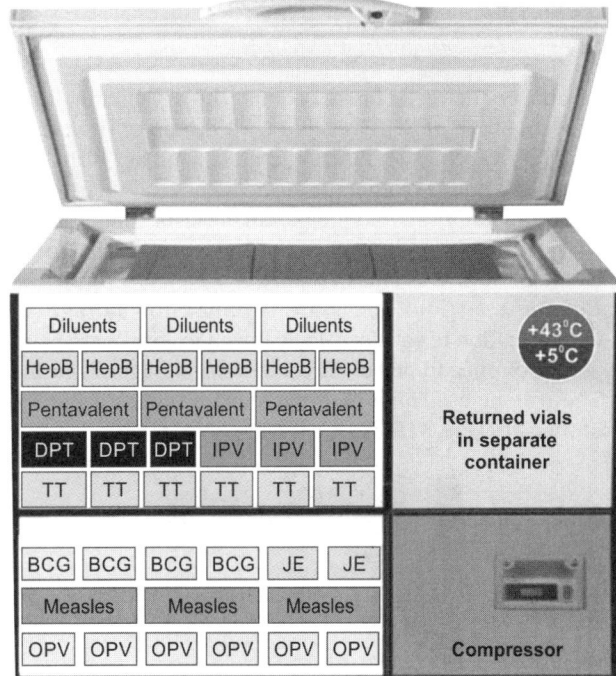

Fig. 51B.6: Arrangement of vaccines inside ILR.

- **Domestic refrigerator**: Domestic refrigerator can maintain temperature within recommended temperature range of +2 to +8°C. It can be used for storage of vaccine at private clinics and nursing homes but the prerequisite is that continuous power supply should be there and they are dedicated to store vaccines only. In domestic refrigerator, ice packs should be stored at freezer compartment while all the vaccines and diluents should be stored at refrigerator compartment. Measles/MR, BCG, OPV and Rota vaccine should be stored on the top shelf. DPT, Pentavalent, TT/Td, IPV, Hep-B and JE should be stored in middle shelves, and diluents should be stored near vaccines with which they are supplied **(Fig. 51B.7)**.

It is important to ensure Birth doses of vaccines—BCG, hepatitis B birth dose and OPV 0 dose as early as possible after birth. Keeping in view, the importance of birth doses, a domestic refrigerator should be placed in recovery room

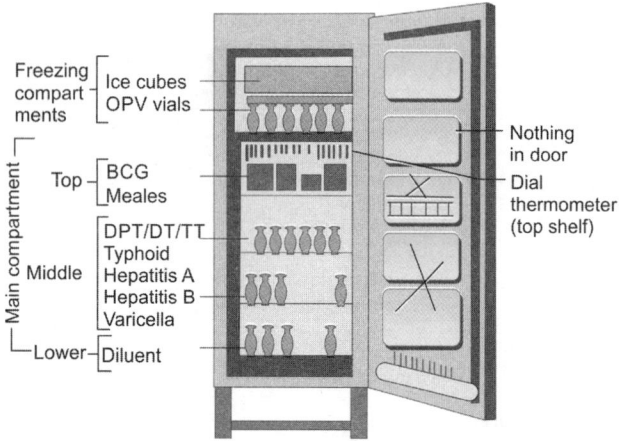

Fig. 51B.7: Arrangement of vaccines in domestic refrigerator.

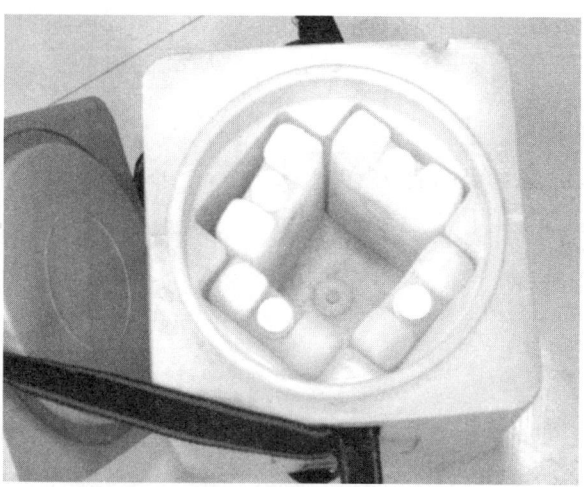

Fig. 51B.9: Vaccine carrier.

of labor room at all delivery points. The refrigerator should contain stock of BCG vaccine with diluents, Hepatitis B and OPV vaccines and it should be labeled as "Birth Dose vaccine" boldly. No other drugs/medicines should be kept in this refrigerator to avoid programmatic error. The birth dose vaccines should be given to all neonates before discharge from hospital within 24 hours of birth.

- *Cold boxes*: Cold boxes are supplied for storage and transportation of vaccines. Fully frozen ice packs are placed at the bottom and side of the cold box for storage of vaccines. They can be used for emergency storage and transportation of vaccines **(Fig. 51B.8)**.

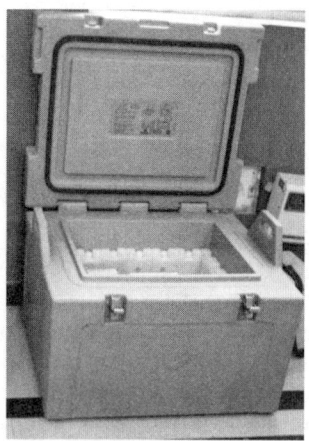

Fig. 51B.8: Cold box.

- *Vaccine carriers (with four conditioned ice packs):* Vaccine carrier can maintain the temperature between +2 and +8°C for 12 hours, if properly handled. They used to transport vaccines and diluents from PHC to session site. Vaccines and diluents should be kept in a zipper bag in vaccine carrier to avoid freezing of freeze sensitive vaccines and spillage of label of vaccine. Never use two ice packs containing day carrier or thermos flask for transportation of vaccine to session site **(Fig. 51B.9)**.

- *Ice packs:* Ice packs contain water and they should be frozen in deep freezer. No salt should be added in water to freeze it. The water level marking indicated on ice packs to fill the water. Before using ice packs in vaccine carrier, conditioning of ice packs should be carried out at PHC level **(Fig. 51B.10)**.
  a. **Conditioning of ice packs**: When ice packs are taken from deep freezer, they are frozen and if kept in same condition in vaccine carrier, freeze sensitive vaccine may be frozen accidentally. So, ice packs need to be kept at room temperature before placing it in vaccine carrier. This process is known as "conditioning of ice packs". The ice pack is considered as adequately "conditioned" when the beads of water covers ice packs surface and "crackling sound" heard of water/ice on shaking. Four conditioned ice packs should be placed in vaccine carrier for transportation of vaccines.
  b. Ice packs have two pits. They should be used to keep reconstituted BCG and Measles/ MR vaccine during session. No vaccine should be stored at sub-center level. PHC is the last point of storage for vaccines in rural area **(Tables 51B.3 and 51B.4)**.

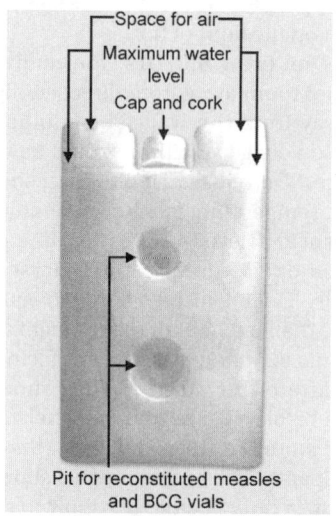

Fig. 51B.10: Ice pack.

In case of emergency situation like power failure, the following alternative arrangements should be followed.

**Table 51B.3:** Cold chain equipment summary.

| Equipment | Temperature | Storage capacity | Holdover time |
|---|---|---|---|
| *Electric based cold chain equipment* | | | |
| Deep freezer (Large) | −15°C to 25°C | 200 ice packs or OPV stock for 3 months (120,000–180,000 doses) | 43°C for 18 hours 32°C for 22 hours |
| ILR (Large) | +2°C to +8°C | BCG, DPT, DT, TT, measles, Hep-B vaccine stock for 3 months (60,000 doses) | At 43°C for 62 hours At 32°C for 78 hours |
| Deep freezer (Small) | −15°C to 25°C | 100 ice packs | At 43°C for 18 hours At 32°C for 22 hours |
| ILR (Small) | +2°C to +8°C | BCG, OPV, DT, DPT, TT, measles, Hep-B vaccine stocks for one month (25,000 doses) | At 43°C for 62 hours At 32°C for 78 hours |
| *Non-electric cold chain equipment* | | | |
| Cold box (Large) | +2°C to +8°C | All vaccines stored for transport Or in case of power failure (6,000 doses of mixed antigen with 50 ice packs/ 72–96 ice packs) | At 43°C for 6.5 days At 32°C for 10 days |
| Cold box (Small) | +2°C to +8°C | All vaccines stored for transport Or in case of power failure (1500 doses of mixed antigen with 24 ice packs/36 ice packs) | At 43°C for 6.5 days At 32°C for 10 days |
| Vaccine carrier (1.7 liters) | +2°C to +8°C | All vaccines carried for 12 hours (4 ice packs and 16–20 vials) | At 43°C for 34 hours At 32°C for 51 hours |

An emergency plan of action as per guideline has to be displayed on ILR/DF as well as on the entrance of facility.

## OPEN VIAL POLICY

According to open vial policy 2015, to minimize the vaccine wastage, policy allows reuse of partially used multidose vials of applicable vaccines under UIP in subsequent sessions—fixed and outreach. All open vials should be returned to cold chain point at the end of the session and segregated by reusable and non-reusable vials according to following:

**Table 51B.4:** Alternative storage arrangements for emergencies.

| Equipment | Options |
|---|---|
| ILR | Store vaccines in cold boxes with conditioned ice packs. Place thermometer inside the cold box. OR Transfer to nearby PHC or other vaccine storage facility. |
| Deep freezer | Freeze ice packs in domestic refrigerator/s or in commercial ice factory. OR Collect required quantity of frozen ice packs from nearby PHC in cold boxes on session days (hold over time may not be same). |
| | At the district level, transfer OPV to available ILR or refrigerator. OR Store OPV in cold box lined with frozen ice packs or commercial ice in polythene bags. |
| Voltage stabilizer | Disconnect the stabilizer and obtain replacement immediately from float assemblies from District/Regional HQ and reconnect. |

> Reusable vaccine can be used for 4 weeks (28 days) and non-reusable vaccines can be used maximum for 4 hours after open or partially used by maintaining proper recommended temperature and conditions.
> In case of any AEFI reported, all open vials (usable and non-usable) should not be discarded or used. All open vials should be stored under proper cold chain till investigation is complete.

- ***Reusable***: DPT, TT/Td, Hep-B and Pentavalent vaccine vials. All reusable vaccines should be used within 28 days of opening the vial provided that VVM is in usable stage and vial within expiry date.
- ***Non-reusable***: Measles, BCG, Rotavirus and JE (should be discarded after 48 hours or before subsequent sessions whichever is earlier).

## REVERSE COLD CHAIN

Reverse cold chain is maintaining the cold chain in the reverse direction from the point of use to the vaccine testing laboratory or to maintain from the outreach/session sites to back at cold chain point.

## SUGGESTED READING

1. Government of India. Handbook of Vaccine and Cold Chain Handler, 2nd edition. New Delhi: Ministry of Health and Family Welfare; 2016.
2. Government of India. Immunization Handbook for Medical Officers. New Delhi: Department of Health and Family Welfare; 2016.
3. Government of India. Operational guidelines for introduction of Rota virus vaccine in the Universal Immunization Programme (UIP) in India; 2019.
4. Government of India. Operational guidelines for introduction of Rota virus vaccine in the Universal Immunization Programme (UIP) in India; 2015.
5. UNDP, INDIA. Improving efficiency of vaccination systems in multiple states. [online]. Available from: http://www.in.undp.org/ content/India/en/home/operations/projects/health/evin.html.

# C. ADVERSE EVENTS FOLLOWING IMMUNIZATION AND ITS MANAGEMENT AT COMMUNITY LEVEL

*Nilesh Fichadiya, RB Jain*

## INTRODUCTION

You learnt about the Universal Immunization Programme of India in previous chapters. Vaccines used in India's Universal Immunization Programme are extremely safe and effective. However, adverse events may occasionally occur following immunization. People have become more concerned about the risks associated with vaccines because of their wider use and due to continuous decline in the vaccine preventable diseases. Moreover, newer vaccines are also being added up in the existing pool year after year. Furthermore, technological advances and continuously increasing knowledge about vaccines have led to investigations focused on the safety of existing vaccines.

Adverse event following immunization (AEFI) is defined as: *"Any untoward medical occurrence which follows immunization which does not necessarily have causal relationship with immunization."*

The adverse event may be any unfavorable or unintended symptom, sign, or disease, or any abnormal laboratory finding. If not rapidly and effectively dealt with, it can undermine confidence in a vaccine and ultimately have dramatic consequences for immunization coverage and disease incidence.

## CATEGORIZATION OF AEFI (CIOMS/WHO, 2012)

The Council for International Organizations of Medical Services (CIOMS) and WHO have given five categories of AEFI. **Table 51C.1** shows these five types of AEFI with their definitions.

**Table 51C.1:** Cause-specific categorization of AEFIs.

| Sr. No. | Cause-specific type of AEFI | Definition |
|---|---|---|
| 1. | Vaccine product related | An AEFI that is caused or precipitated by a vaccine due to one or more of the inherent properties of the vaccine product |
| 2. | Vaccine quality defect-related reaction | An AEFI that is caused or precipitated by a vaccine that is due to one or more quality defects of the vaccine product, including its administration device as provided by the manufacturer |
| 3. | Immunization error-related reaction (formerly "program error") | An AEFI that is caused by inappropriate vaccine handling, prescribing or administration and thus it is preventable |
| 4. | Immunization anxiety-related reaction (formerly "injection reaction") | An AEFI arising from anxiety about the immunization (or injection) |
| 5. | Coincidental event | An AEFI that is caused by something other than the vaccine product, immunization error or immunization anxiety |

## Vaccine Product-related Reaction

*Case Scenario*

A 2-month-old infant received 1st dose of pentavalent vaccine. The infant developed fever and painful induration at the site of injection in the late evening. The mother brought the baby to the health center, where the doctor prescribed paracetamol syrup 2.5 mL every 6–8 hours and advised application of a clean cold cloth at the site of induration.

This type of AEFI develops due to individual's response to the inherent properties of vaccine product.

Developing fever and induration after a dose of pentavalent is an example of *vaccine product-related AEFI*. It happened due to baby's immune response to the antigens present in the vaccine. This is quite common as around 50% of vaccinees develop this type of reaction after a dose of pentavalent vaccine. This type of reaction subsides within a day or two, so it is not a matter of concern.

Let's consider another very common "vaccine product related AEFI". Almost 90–95% vaccinees will develop a papule two or more weeks after administration of BCG vaccine, which will progress to pustule followed by ulceration and heals after several months, leaving a permanent scar.

## Vaccine Quality Defect-related Reaction

Very rarely, AEFI happens due to quality defect in vaccine production. For example, in 1955 in the United States, 40,000 people developed abortive polio and 200 people were paralyzed after being vaccinated by inactivated polio vaccine which was manufactured by Cutter Laboratory. The investigations revealed that the manufacturing process was defective and the vaccine contained live virus (Fitzpatrick M, J R Soc Med, 2006).

This type of AEFI is known as "Vaccine quality defect-related reaction". They used to occur more frequently in early days of immunization program, however, with the introduction of good manufacturing process (GMP) and regulatory authorities, such occurrences are *extremely rare*.

## Immunization Error-related Reactions (*Formerly* "Program Error")

*Case Scenario*

In 1992, in a clinic of country A, BCG immunization was conducted for neonates. Five neonates collapsed after immunization. Four of them, were resuscitated and survived, but one died. Investigation revealed administration of muscle relaxant instead of BCG vaccine, which was stored in the same refrigerator where BCG was kept.

An adverse event can also occur as a result of inappropriate handling, prescribing or administration of a vaccine.

This is an example of "immunization error related reaction" which happened due to lack of training, negligence or mistake of the vaccinator. An immunization error-related reaction may lead to a cluster of events associated with a particular provider, health facility, or even a single vial of vaccine that has been inappropriately prepared or contaminated.

Other examples of immunization error-related reaction are:
- Several vaccinees developed suppuration at the site of vaccination after getting vaccine from a particular vaccinator.
  *Reason*: This can happen if the vaccinator fails to follow sterile practices and the needles were contaminated or the reconstituted vaccine vial was used beyond the stipulated period of 4 hours.
- After getting measles vaccine, an 8-year-old girl developed anaphylaxis, collapsed and died.
  *Reason*: The girl was allergic to measles vaccine. She reported the history of allergy to the previous doses of vaccines but the vaccinator ignored the history and gave the vaccine in spite of contraindication.
- Five infants developed sterile abscess after getting DPT vaccine.
  *Reason*: The DPT vaccine was stored at sub-zero temperature and frozen. The vaccinator saw precipitate inside the vaccine vial but still had given that vaccine instead of discarding it.

As you might have already realized, that immunization error-related reaction is *potentially preventable by following immunization best practices and guidelines*.

### Immunization Anxiety-related Reactions (*Formerly* "Injection Reactions")

> *Case Scenario*
>
> In 2012, measles catch-up campaign was conducted in district A, where children of 9 months to 9 years were vaccinated at anganwadis and schools. In a school of district A, 8 girls had syncope and collapsed. They were given recombinant position and monitored closely. Out of them, 4 recovered within short time while 4 were admitted to the nearby hospital for further management. They were discharged on the same day after recovery.
>
> The incidence happened because the vaccine preparation and administration were done in front of the students which caused immunization anxiety-related reaction.

Let's consider the next type of AEFI which is known as *immunization anxiety-related reaction*. Following are salient points of this type of reaction.
- These types of AEFIs occur as a result of anticipation or fear of injection or pain of injection rather than the vaccine itself.
- The reaction is unrelated to the content of the vaccine.
- These types of reactions are more common in children over 5 years of age. The common reaction is fainting.
- Younger children tend to react differently, with vomiting being a common symptom of anxiety. They may also scream.
- Anxiety about immunization can also cause hyperventilation, leading to specific symptoms such as light-headedness, dizziness, and tingling around mouth and hands.

To prevent immunization anxiety-related reaction, proper planning should be done to avoid overcrowding at the immunization sessions and the vaccine should be prepared out of recipient's view.

### Coincidental Events

> *Case Scenario*
>
> A one and half year-old child was administered booster dose of DPT and polio, and 2nd dose of measles with vitamin A. The mother reported that the child developed high fever, breathing difficulty, cough and sore throat within a few days of vaccination, and had to be hospitalized.
>
> Further investigation of this AEFI revealed that the child had developed pneumonia which was not a known vaccine-product related AEFI of any given vaccine. Most likely, the child was in incubation period of pneumonia when vaccinated and his pneumonia was falsely attributed to vaccination.

The fifth type of AEFI is known as "coincidental event". Such events occur coincidentally after immunization and are attributed falsely to the administration of vaccine. In other words, a chance temporal association, i.e. an event happening after immunization is falsely considered to be caused by immunization.

Coincidental events are not uncommon because infections and other illnesses are more likely to happen early in life when many doses of vaccines are also given.

## VACCINE REACTIONS

**Table 51C.2** shows categorization of reported adverse reactions by frequency of occurrence.

**Table 51C.2:** Categorization of reported adverse reactions by frequency of occurrence (WHO, Global Manual on Surveillance of AEFI, 2014).

| Frequency category | Frequency (%) |
|---|---|
| Very common | ≥10% |
| Common (frequent) | ≥1% and <10% |
| Uncommon (infrequent) | ≥ 0.1% and <1% |
| Rare | ≥ 0.01% and <0.1% |
| Very rare | <0.01% |

### Common Minor Vaccine Reactions

**Table 51C.3** shows proportion of reaction occurrences likely to be observed with the UIP vaccines.

### Severe Reaction

"Severe" is used to describe the intensity of a specific event (as in mild, moderate or severe).

### Serious Reactions

An AEFI will be considered "serious" if it meets any of the following criteria:
- Results in death
- Leads to permanent impairment or damage
- Requires inpatient hospitalization
- Results in a congenital anomaly/birth defect

Table 51C.3: Proportion of reaction occurrences likely to be observed with the UIP vaccines.

| Vaccine | Local adverse events (pain, swelling, redness) | Fever (>38°C) | Irritability, malaise and systemic symptoms |
|---|---|---|---|
| BCG | 90–95% | — | — |
| OPV | None | Less than 1% | Less than 1% |
| IPV | Up to 29% | — | — |
| Hepatitis B | Adults: Up to 15% Children: Up to 5% | 1–6% | — |
| Hib | 5–15% | 2–10% | — |
| Pertussis (DwPT) | Up to 50% | Up to 50% | Up to 55% |
| Tetanus | ~10% | ~10% | ~25% |
| Measles/MR/MMR | ~10% | 5–15% | 5% (Rash) |
| JE live-attenuated | <1% | — | — |

- Clustering of cases
- Raises community concern.

## AEFI PREVENTION

### At Vaccination Site

- Maintenance of cold chain throughout the activity.
- Recording of details including manufacturer details, date of expiry, batch number, and time of opening vial.
- Check for transparency, flocculation, VVM of vaccine and temperature of diluents.
- Maintain sterile non-touch method while handling and administering vaccines keeping in mind contraindications and vaccine guidelines.
- Ensuring sufficient post-vaccination wait period (30 minutes) and avoiding crowding at vaccination center.

### At Cold Chain Point

- Maintaining cold chain and temperature logbook.
- Ensure proper stacking of vaccine and ice packs as per guidelines.
- Record maintenance of vaccine stock, AEFI reporting.
- Ensuring safe transportation and maintenance of cold chain during transportation.
- Ensuring cold chain maintenance for open vial vaccines received back from session sites.

## AEFI MANAGEMENT

- All medical officers acting as supervisors will carry an emergency *AEFI treatment kit* with them during field visit of immunization sessions **(Table 51C.4)**.
- All vaccinators will also carry an *emergency AEFI treatment kit*.
- AEFI kit should be available at the session site during mass vaccination campaign, like measles-rubella vaccination campaign.
- All *AEFI management centers* will be provided with AEFI treatment kits and AEFI reporting forms.
- The *AEFI management centers* will display AEFI action plan with referral transportation system and phone numbers of referral centers.
- The AEFI management centers will report the AEFI as per laid out procedures in the national guidelines.
- The private sector management centers will be reimbursed for treatment costs of AEFI cases as per standard protocol.

Table 51C.4: AEFI management kit.

| 1. Injection adrenaline (1:1000) solution | 2 ampule |
|---|---|
| 2. Injection hydrocortisone (100 mg) | 1 vial |
| 3. Disposable syringe-tuberculin syringes (1 mL) OR insulin syringe (without fixed needle of 40 units) | 3 |
| 4. Disposable syringes (5 mL) and 24/25 G IM needle | 2 sets |
| 5. Scalp vein set 22/24G | 2 sets |
| 6. Tab Paracetamol (500 mg) | 10 tab |
| 7. IV fluids (Ringer lactate/normal saline) | 1 unit |
| 8. IV fluid (5% dextrose) | 1 unit |
| 9. IV drip set | 1 set |
| 10. Cotton wool, adhesive tape | 1 each |
| 11. AEFI case reporting form (CRF) | 1 form |
| 12. Label showing date of inspection, expiry date of injection adrenaline and shortest expiry date of any of components | 1 label |
| 13. Drug dosage table for injection adrenaline and hydrocortisone | 1 table |
| 14. In hospital settings, oxygen support and airway intubation facility should be available | |

## RECOGNITION AND TREATMENT OF ANAPHYLAXIS

Anaphylaxis after immunization needs special mention as it is a very rare but severe and potentially fatal allergic reaction. Anaphylaxis can be prevented by asking the vaccinees about known allergies and previous adverse reactions to vaccines before immunization. Anaphylaxis may be confused with syncopal attack/fainting and vice versa. The health-workers should be trained to distinguish anaphylaxis from other common benign reactions like fainting (vasovagal syncope), anxiety and breath-holding spells. Such differentiation is of vital importance in saving life of a vaccinee who has developed anaphylaxis. **Table 51C.5** shows the differences between the two.

Table 51C.5: Distinguish anaphylaxis from fainting (vasovagal reaction).

| | Fainting | Anaphylaxis |
|---|---|---|
| Onset | Usually at the time or soon after the injection | Usually after some delay, between 5 and 30 minutes, after injection |
| Skin | Pale, sweaty, cold, and clammy | Red, raised, and itchy rash; swollen eyes, face, generalized rash |
| *Systemic symptoms* | | |
| Respiratory | Normal to deep breaths | Noisy breathing from airways obstruction (wheeze or stridor) |
| Cardiovascular | Bradycardia, transient hypotension | Tachycardia, hypotension |
| Gastrointestinal | Nausea, vomiting | Abdominal cramps |
| Neurological | Transient loss of consciousness, relieved by supine posture | Loss of consciousness, not relieved by supine posture |

Generally, severe reactions have rapid onset. Most life-threatening reactions begin within 10 minutes of immunization.

That is why it is advised that the beneficiary be kept under observation for at least 30 minutes after the injection.

Unconsciousness is rarely the only manifestation of anaphylaxis—it only occurs as a late event in severe cases. An important feature of anaphylaxis is weak carotid pulse (as opposed to fainting, in which carotid pulse is strong). Anaphylaxis usually involves multiple body systems. However, symptoms limited to only one body system (e.g. skin itching) can also occur, leading to delay in diagnosis. Occasionally, reaction symptoms may recur 8 to 12 hours after onset of the original attack and there can be prolonged attacks lasting up to 48 hours.

The progression of mild early signs to late life-threatening symptoms is listed in **Table 51C.6**.

Table 51C.6: Progression from mild early signs to late life-threatening symptoms in case of anaphylaxis.

| Mild, early warning signs | • Itching of the skin, rash, and swelling around injection site<br>• Dizziness and general feeling of warmth<br>• Painless swellings in parts of the body, e.g. face or mouth<br>• Flushed, itching skin, nasal congestion, sneezing, tears<br>• Hoarseness, nausea, vomiting<br>• Swelling in the throat, difficult breathing, and abdominal pain |
|---|---|
| Late, life-threatening symptoms | Wheezing, noisy and difficult breathing, collapse, low blood pressure, irregular weak pulse. |

## Treatment

Points to remember while managing a patient of anaphylaxis **(Flowchart 51C.1)**:
- Anaphylaxis is an emergency. So, begin treatment immediately; and at the same time, plan should be made to transfer the patient immediately to the nearest hospital.

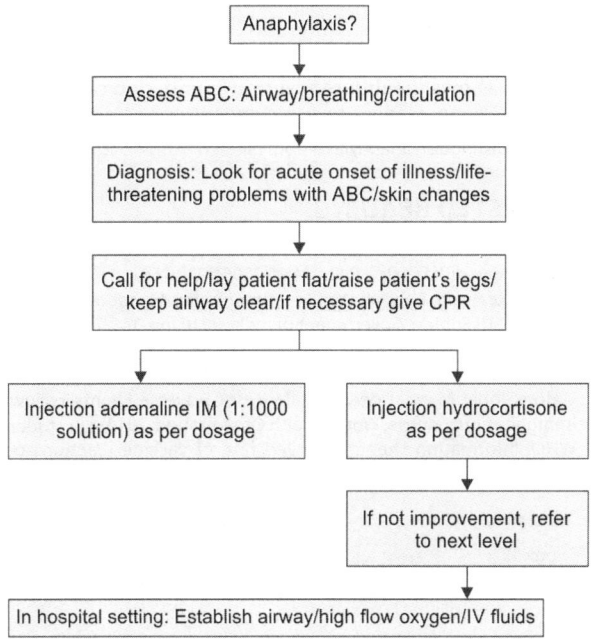

Flowchart 51C.1: Protocol for management of anaphylaxis.

- Adrenaline (epinephrine) stimulates the heart, reverses the spasm in the lung passages, and reduces edema and urticaria, thus it has countering effect against anaphylaxis. But this is a very potent agent which can cause irregular heartbeat, heart failure, severe hypertension, and tissue necrosis if used in inappropriate doses. So it must be used with caution in appropriate doses.
- Adrenaline is a drug with short expiry, thus it is necessary to ensure that all adrenaline ampules are checked for expiry dates regularly.
- If the patient is conscious, place his/her head lower than the feet. If already unconscious, place the patient in the recovery position (pronate) and ensure that the airway is clear. Assess heart rate and respiratory rate (if the patient has a strong carotid pulse, he/she is probably not suffering from anaphylaxis).
- If there is no heartbeat, begin cardiopulmonary resuscitation (CPR).
- Give adrenaline 1:1000 solution at a dose of 0.01 mL/kg up to a maximum of 0.5 mL injected deep intramuscularly (or subcutaneously in very mild cases). Also, give an additional half dose around the injection site (deep intramuscular injection) to delay antigen absorption **(Table 51C.7)**.
- Give injection hydrocortisone IM or slow IV as per dosage shown in **Table 51C.8**.
- Give oxygen by facemask, if available.
- Call for professional assistance but never leave the patient alone. Call an ambulance.
- If there is no improvement in the patient's condition within 10–20 minutes of the first injection, repeat the dose of adrenaline up to a maximum of three doses in total.
- Recovery from anaphylactic shock is usually rapid after adrenaline.
- Mark the immunization card clearly so that the individual never gets a repeat dose of the offending vaccine.

Table 51C.7: Injection adrenaline (1:1000 solution) dosage chart IM (0.01 mg/kg) with 24/25G needle.

| Age group | 0–1 year | 1–6 years | 6–12 years | 12–18 years | Adults |
|---|---|---|---|---|---|
| Dosage (in mL) using 1 mL tuberculin syringe | 0.05 | 0.1 | 0.2 | 0.3 | 0.5 |
| Dosage (in units) using 40 units insulin syringe | 2 | 4 | 8 | 12 | 20 |

Table 51C.8: Injection hydrocortisone (IM or slow IV) dosage chart.

| Age | Less than 6 months | 6 months to 6 years | 6–12 years | >12 years |
|---|---|---|---|---|
| Dose | 25 mg | 50 mg | 100 mg | 200 mg |

## AEFI REPORTING SYSTEM

### In Rural Areas

- The primary responsibility of AEFI reporting lies with the MPHW (F)/FHW/ANM at each sub-center who provides immunization services.
- All minor AEFI cases are to be entered in AEFI register at PHC level on weekly basis and to be submitted in monthly HMIS report.

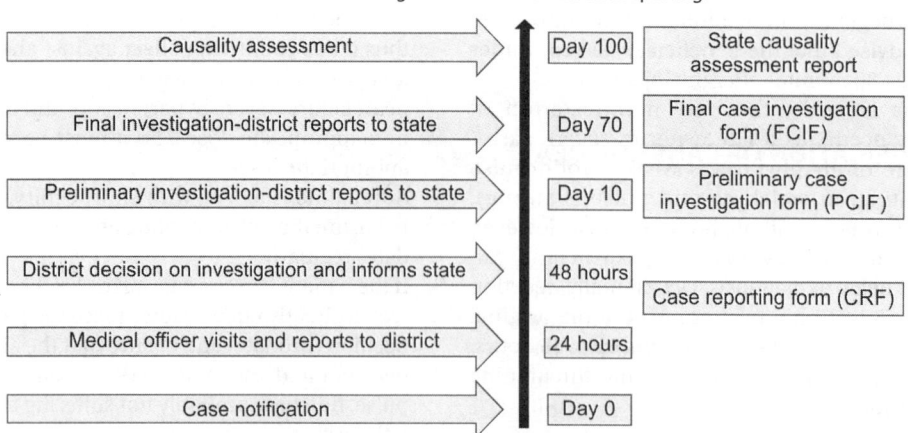

Flowchart 51C.2: AEFI guidelines—timelines and reporting.

- All serious and severe AEFI are to be reported as shown in **Flowchart 51C.2**.

### In Urban Areas

- AEFI reporting is primarily the responsibility of the health workers and the medical officers of the corporations, municipalities, and towns who provide immunization services through urban health facilities, MCH centers, and DH (district hospital).
- It is also mandatory that private practitioners both in rural and urban areas who administer vaccines report AEFI to the district health authorities.
- *Immediate notification of serious and severe AEFI.*
- All severe and serious AEFI are to be immediately notified by the first person who identifies the event.
- This "first" person should notify the case to the nearest government PHC, CHC or the District Immunization Officer (DIO) by quickest means of communication, e.g. telephone, messenger, etc.
- All people involved in reporting AEFI should be aware of the timeline and channels of reporting.

### Causality Assessment

Causality assessment is the systematic evaluation of the information obtained about an AEFI to determine the likelihood of the event having been caused by the vaccine/s received. It is a critical part of AEFI monitoring and enhances confidence in the national immunization program. The AEFI report must have investigation formats, relevant documents, and a diagnosis for being eligible for causality assessment. The causality assessment process has four steps:

1. *Eligibility*: To determine if the reported AEFI case satisfies the minimum criteria for causality assessment.
2. *Checklist*: To systematically review the relevant and available information to address possible causal aspects of the AEFI.
3. *Algorithm*: To obtain a direction as to the causality with the information gathered in the checklist.
4. *Classification*: To categorize the AEFI's association to the vaccine/vaccination based on direction determined in the algorithm.

All the cases being investigated by the district should be assessed by the causality assessment experts of the state AEFI committee after discussing all the investigation formats and reports available. It is recommended to disseminate the results so that others can learn from the experience. Immunization errors will need to be corrected and for coincidental incidents, communication to maintain confidence is necessary. Thus, it is important to have a monitoring system for AEFI.

## SUMMARY

All healthcare providers should be aware of the different aspects of AEFI and be prepared to respond to public concerns. Timely response to public concerns about the safety of vaccines as well as prompt communication will preserve the trust in the immunization program. The objectives of AEFI guidelines are to improve the efficiency of surveillance and quality of immunization services at all levels. This will ensure immunization safety of all vaccine recipients leading to achievement of goals of national immunization program.

## SUGGESTED READING

1. Fitzpatrick M. The cutter incident: How America's first polio vaccine led to a growing vaccine crisis. J R Soc Med. 2006;99(3):156.
2. Ministry of Health & Family Welfare. Immunization Handbook for Medical Officers, 3rd Edition. Government of India; 2016. pp. 149-72.
3. Ministry of Health and Family Welfare. AEFI Surveillance and Response: Operational Guidelines. Government of India; 2015.
4. WHO. Global Manual on Surveillance of Adverse Events Following Immunization. Geneva: World Health Organization; 2014.
5. WHO. Information sheet: observed rate of vaccine reactions polio vaccines. Geneva: World Health Organization; 2014.

… Chapter 51: Special Topics

# D. MEDICAL CERTIFICATION OF CAUSE OF DEATH (MCCD), MATERNAL DEATH SURVEILLANCE AND RESPONSE (MDSR), CHILD DEATH REVIEW (CDR)

*Sudhir Prabhu H, Saurabh Kumar*

## MEDICAL CERTIFICATION OF CAUSE OF DEATH (MCCD)

Mortality indicators though available, may not be a reliable source of health information on most occasions. Accurate and complete mortality records may help policy makers and program managers to plan effective health interventions for reducing the prevalence or plan preventive strategies. Hence not only declaring but also ascertaining and certifying the cause of death becomes a very important responsibility of a doctor. Ascertaining the correct cause will contribute to the legal record and will also be a vital source for mortality statistics required for planned health interventions at the local and global contexts.

International classification of diseases (ICD)—6th revision, 1948 first advocated for a single cause of death and termed it as underlying cause of death which was defined as "(a) disease or injury which initiated the train of morbid events directly leading to death, (b) circumstances of accident or violence which produced the fatal injury". Currently, ICD-X is being used for coding the underlying cause of death, which will soon be replaced by ICD-XI.

ICD-XI originally published in 2019 is now officially in effect for the national and international recording and reporting of causes of illness, death- and more. As of 2022, 35 countries are using ICD-XI.

Registration of Births and Deaths Act, 1969 states every death should be medically certified whether at the hospital or in the community. Medical certification of cause of death is not the same as the death certificate, while the former is to be issued by a registered allopathic medical practitioner, a death certificate can be issued only by Registrar. Only when MCCD is submitted along with death report registrar will issue death certificate. Tracing back the natural history for establishing the cause of death, especially for deaths that are not in a health care establishment may not be easy. The medical certifier is obliged to see not only completeness of the certificate but also to accurately describe the precise diagnosis for the underlying cause of death which is with his best medical knowledge. Causes if according to ICD code will simplify for vital statistics records. Certification although it follows a standard format, filling is not uniform on most occasions and tends to be more difficult for chronic than acute diseases.

### Parts of an International Death Certificate

**Part I:** Disease or condition directly leading to death
- *Immediate cause (Line 1a):* Disease, injury or condition directly leading to death.
- *Antecedent cause/s (Line 1b, 1c):* Morbid condition, if any, giving rise to the above cause (underlying conditions).

**Part II:** Other significant conditions contributing to death, but not related to cause of death.

### Filling an MCCD (Fig. 51D.1)

- Arrange the sequence of events leading to death in a chronological order
- Identify the underlying COD (cause of death): that would be the condition which would have started the chain of events which lead to the death of the person.
- Fill the sequence of events in reverse order in the death certificate, i.e. immediate/direct cause should be written first and what led to direct cause below it till underlying COD is entered.

A correctly filled MCCD will have a single underlying cause of death at the bottom part of Part I of MCCD with consequences that it leads to in the part above it in order until the immediate cause which would be the top upper most part of Part I. The doctor completes the MCCD form in India called FORM No. 4 (institutional deaths) and FORM No. 4A (non-institutional deaths) to certify the cause of death.

A physician who has seen the patient in the last 14 days should be the one who should fill out the MCCD. Under Registration of Births and Deaths Act, 1969, no money should be collected for issuing an MCCD and declining to certify death may entertain a fine of upto ₹ 50. In case of suspicious deaths, a registered medical practitioner should only certify the death and not fill the cause of death in the MCCD form, meanwhile inform the police who will decide whether post-mortem is needed or not.

### Errors done While Filling in Death Certificate

- Commonest error made is the immediate cause being filled as mode of dying (e.g.: choking, gagging, etc.). It is important to

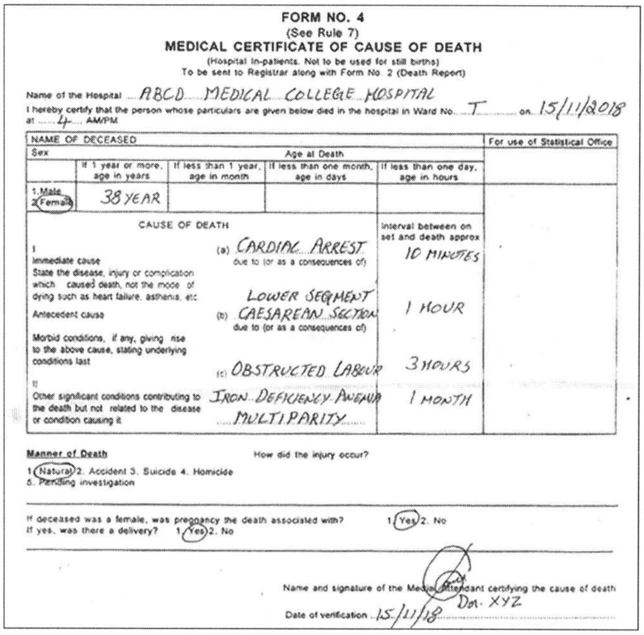

Fig. 51D.1: Filling of Indian MCCD (Form 4 for hospital deaths).

remember that asphyxia, coma, syncope, heart failure is the mode and should never be filled in part I or part II of MCCD.
- Leaving few parts empty or filling only one part of death certificate.
- Filling in a wrong cause of death, when no reliable information is available (e.g.: Myocardial infarction for all deaths).
- Not filling the manner of dying. Manner of dying includes natural or unnatural. Unnatural deaths include accident, suicide, homicide.

*Example 1:* A 38-year-old grand multipara (G6P5) a case of iron deficiency anemia with Hb of 6 g% was referred to ABCD medical college hospital with obstructed labor for 3 hours, she was taken for emergency LSCS, one hour into surgery, she developed cardiac arrest and died within 10 minutes although all necessary resuscitative measures were tried.

## MATERNAL DEATH SURVEILLANCE AND RESPONSE (MDSR)

The MDSR system is a continuous cycle of identification, notification, and review of maternal deaths followed by actions to improve quality of care and prevent future deaths.

The maternal death surveillance and response was born out of the gap analysis of maternal death review of the last 5 years.

The maternal death review process was initiated by government of India in 2010 with the goal of reducing maternal mortality and morbidity by improving the quality of obstetric care and by exploring the deficiencies in health system. But in the gap analysis of maternal death review of the last few years, it was observed that there were varying levels of reporting, lack of capacity of even established institutions in conducting effective death reviews and delays in reporting the key findings.

In view of the India's failure to achieve the indicator of Maternal Mortality ratio of 109 by 2015 of MDG Goal 5 (Improve Maternal Health), the maternal death surveillance and response becomes more meaningful as the process of annual decline in MMR needs to be accelerated. MDSR is a form of continuous surveillance and supports all the three processes—monitoring, reviewing and action. It enables routine identification and timely notification of maternal deaths, thereby linking health information systems and quality improvement systems from ground level to state and national level. This helps in quantification and determination of major causes of maternal deaths and also in giving us the information whether the maternal deaths were preventable or not. The information about the untimely deaths, if acted upon, will help prevent future deaths. MDSR links the information system with specific responses, i.e. improvement in maternal health by reducing maternal mortality.

### Process of Maternal Death Review Surveillance and Response

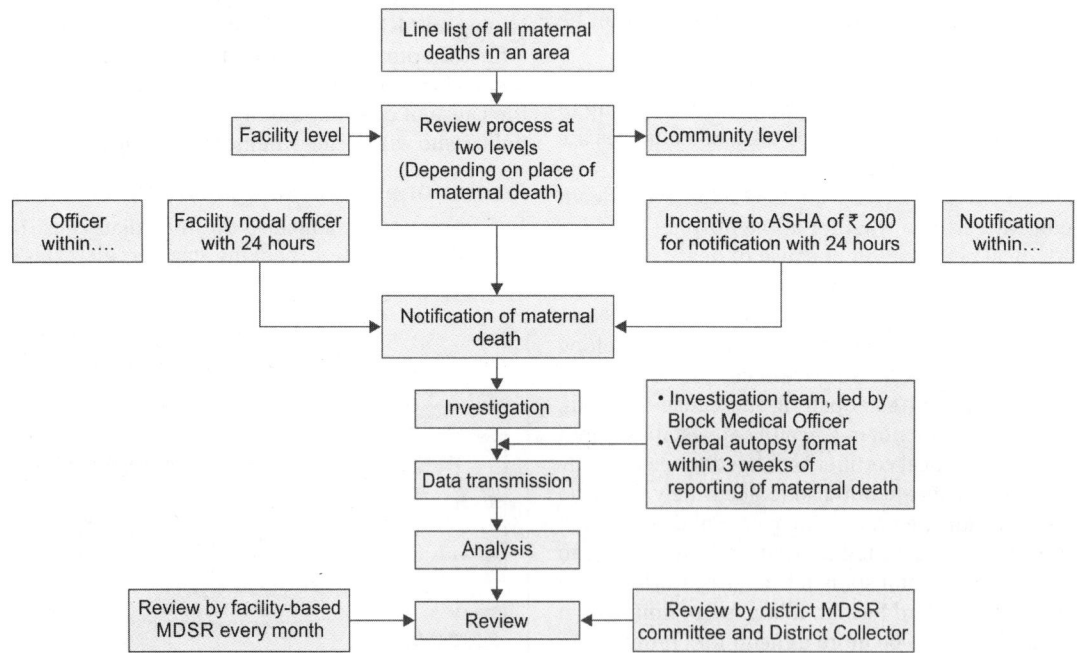

### Summary of Maternal Death Review Surveillance and Response Timelines

| Steps | Person responsible | Community based MDSR (Timeline) | Person responsible | Facility Based MDSR (Timeline) |
|---|---|---|---|---|
| Notification | ASHA/Link worker (primary Informant) | Within 24 hours of maternal death to ANM/ Urban Health worker/ Block Medical Officer (BMO) | Treating Medical Officer (MO) | Immediately to Facility Nodal Officer (FNO) (Form 3) should be maintained |
| Reporting | a. ASHA (Primary Informant) –Incentive of Rs 200 for ASHA<br>b. BMO office | Within 24 hours of maternal death to ANM in Form 1<br>Prepare line list of all women deaths (Form 2) and maternal deaths (Form 3)- To be sent to DNO by 5th of every month | FNO-Should ensure completion of Form-1,3,4 | Within 24 hours of maternal death, Form-1 to be sent to District Nodal Officer<br>Within 48 hours of maternal death, Form 4 should be received by DNO<br>Form 3 electronically to DNO every month. |

*Contd...*

Contd...

| Steps | Person responsible | Community based MDSR (Timeline) | Person responsible | Facility Based MDSR (Timeline) |
|---|---|---|---|---|
| Verification | LHV/ANM/Urban ANM/ Urban Health worker | Within 1 week Countersigned Form 1 submitted to BMO | | |
| Investigation | 3 member Team by BMO/ Urban health Officer – Verbal Autopsy (Incentive of Rs 150 for each member) | Within 3 weeks of reporting maternal death in Form 5 and submitting to District Nodal Officer (DNO) | Treating Medical Officer under the Guidance of FNO | Within 24 hours using the Facility-based Maternal Death Review (FBMDSR) format (Form 4) |
| Case Summary | BMO | Within 24 hours after completing CBMDR in Form 6 to DNO | | |
| Analysis | BMO | Present in the District Level review Meeting being conducted by CMO | | All deaths to be analyzed on a monthly basis. |
| Review | District MDSR Committee Chaired by CMO/DC | | FBMDSR Committee every month | Minutes to be send to DNO |

Progress of MDSR has varied amongst various states. Today states can be divided into three categories depending upon the maternal mortality ratio, and the following approaches need to be taken:
- State with high MMR
  - Focus on tracking of maternal deaths
  - The facility and community-based MDSR should be institutionalized in all the districts
  - Identification of gaps
- States with moderately high MMR (predicted to achieve the target MMR within five years at the current progress)
  - Identification of gaps
  - Appropriate facilities to manage indirect cause of maternal deaths
- States with low MMR (where MMR is below the National average)
  - Addressing indirect causes of maternal deaths
  - MDSR and maternal near miss implementation should be ensured at all hospitals
  - Perinatal death reviews should be introduced
  - Obstetric high dependency unit in all district hospitals should be started.

## CHILD DEATH REVIEW

"Child Death Review (CDR) is a strategy to understand the geographical variation in causes of child deaths and thereby initiating specific child health interventions". Moreover, we can also get key information about the key health care delivery services and also social factors if any for preventive actions by analyzing the underlying cause of death among children.

Before conducting child death review it is important to define the child deaths by age categories, as etiological and preventable factors may be different for each. Definitions for age categories include:
- **Neonatal deaths:** Neonatal deaths are deaths occurring during the neonatal period, commencing at birth and ending 28 completed days after birth.
- **Post-neonatal deaths:** Deaths occurring from 29 days of life to under one year are called post-neonatal deaths.
- **Infant deaths:** Deaths of children less than 1 year of age.
- **Child deaths:** Deaths of children less than 5 years of age.
- **Stillbirth:** Stillbirth is the birth of a newborn after 20th completed week of gestation, weighing 500 g or more, when the baby does not breath or show any sign of life after delivery.

### Importance

All maternal and child deaths are reviewed at district collectors' office with emphasis on identifying the problems at social, medical or health system level, so that appropriate interventions and preventive measures could avert further deaths. Major focus will be
- Issues pertaining to the health care delivery system providing child health care services, especially at the local level.
- Performing a gap analysis would help reproductive and child care officers/program managers to identify priority areas and execute prompt corrective measures.
- Child mortality data can be useful for policy makers, health administrators, medical professionals to evaluate mortality trends over time so as to evaluate the impact of ongoing programs and thereby plan effective allocation of health resources for preventing and managing neonatal and childhood illnesses.

### Key Points

All the child deaths (from birth to 5 years) would have to be reported and reviewed irrespective of the place of death, which can be at a health facility, home or during transit. Review would take place under two age categories: (1) 0–28 days and (2) 29 days–5 years.

District nodal officer (RCHO/DHO/MOH) is overall incharge for planning and implementation of child death review process in the district. All the records and formats including notification cards/investigation/verbal autopsy forms should reach him within stipulated time (or on monthly basis). The implementation of the Child Death Review requires that a nodal person is identified and designated at Block, District and State to support and monitor the processes, ensure quality of data collected and compiled and transmit data to the next level.

## Child Death Review Process

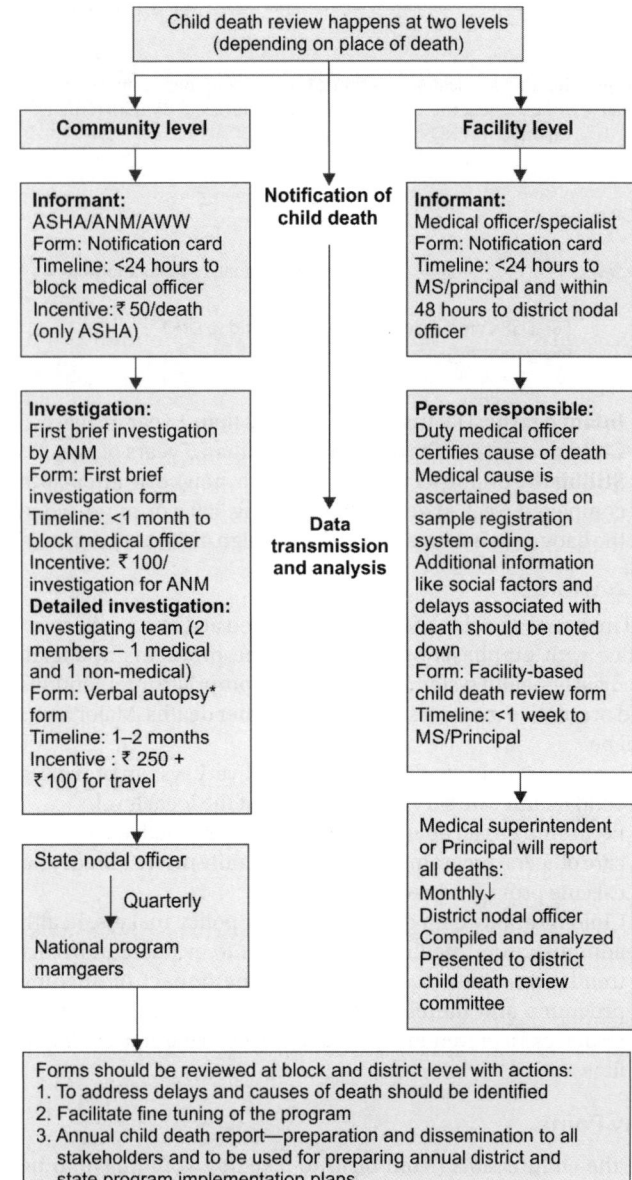

*Verbal autopsy (an investigation of train of events, circumstances, symptoms and signs of illness leading to death through an interview of the relatives or associates of the deceased) and Social autopsy (identifying social, behavioral, and health systems contributors to neonatal and child deaths). It should be completed within 1-2 months of the death.

## MDSR AND CDR COMMITTEES

The Maternal and CDR Committee should be assigned the responsibility of reviewing Child Death Reports:
- District Magistrate/District Collector (Chairperson)
- Chief Medical Officer (Member Secretary)
- District Nodal Officer (for Child Death Review)
- Pediatrician/MD Pediatrics degree holder from the district, one or two in number
- District Project Officer for ICDS
- Representative/s from recognized professional bodies (IAP, NNF, IAPSM)
- Expert from medical college/development agency
- Any other official or person deemed important for providing a specific technical input (at the discretion of the Chairperson).

The Child Death Review meeting should be conducted simultaneously with the Maternal Death Review, every month, with the purpose of reviewing the causes and trend of child deaths in the district.

**State level taskforce:** A single State Level Taskforce will be constituted for review of both maternal and child deaths. The meeting of the taskforce is to be convened every 6 months.

*Members*
- Principal Secretary Health and Family Welfare
- Mission Director
- Commissioner Health
- Director General of Health Services
- Deputy Director/Director Child Health under NRHM
- State Nodal Officer, Child Death Review
- Pediatricians and Public Health Experts from State Govt. and Private Medical Colleges (Maximum 3)
- Obstetric Specialists from State Govt. and Private Medical Colleges (Maximum 1)
- State ICDS Officer
- Deputy Director/Director Nursing
- Deputy Director/Director MSD (materials/supplies and disposables)
- Any other expert, official, person deemed important for discussion on a particular issue (at the discretion of the Chairperson).

## SUMMARY

To summarize the case summaries of child deaths (both CBCDR & FBCDR) will be reviewed at district and block level by the designated officials and action will have to be taken accordingly.

In addition, there is a need for in-depth analysis of the filled-up formats to identify the trends in different factors associated with child deaths. For the in-depth analysis of data, states may take support from experts from Medical Colleges, Universities and other specialized agencies at state and/or district level. The analyzed data will be used for developing the Annual Child Death Report for the state.

## SUGGESTED READING

1. Child death review operational guidelines [Internet] New Delhi: National health mission, Ministry of Health and Family Welfare, Government of India; 2014.
2. Commission on Information and Accountability for Women's and Children's Health: keeping promises, measuring results. Geneva, World Health Organization; 2011.
3. Medical certification of cause of death, 4th ed. Geneva: WHO; 1979. Available from: http://apps.who.int/iris/handle/10665/40557.
4. National Health Mission. Guidelines for Maternal Death Surveillance & Response. Available from: http://nhm.gov.in/nrhm-components/rmnch-a/maternal-health/guidelines.html.
5. Sample Registration System, Office of Registrar General, India. Special Bulletin on Maternal Mortality in India 2014-16.
6. WHO, FIGO, UKaid, E4A, UNFPA, CDC, ICM. Maternal Death Surveillance and Response: Technical Guidance. Information for Action to Prevent Maternal Death 2013.

# E. USE OF INFORMATION TECHNOLOGY IN COMMUNITY HEALTH CARE

*Pradeep Aggarwal, Rakesh Kakkar*

## INTRODUCTION

In today's world of digital era, no sector has been left untouched with the involvement of technology, the same stands true for healthcare sector. Information technology (IT) can be defined as "the study or use of systems (especially computers and telecommunications) for storing, retrieving, and sending information". Simply stating it is the utilization of electronic media for storing digital information that can be easily retrieved from its stored format at the time of transmission intended for ease in its communication and rapidity in its utilization.

Use of IT in health has facilitated in reducing the cost borne by the families, the accessibility and services for their health care have been improved. Appropriate use of e-health initiatives has enabled in addressing all the components of universal health care, thus achieving health goals in terms of accessibility, high quality, affordability at individual level, reduction in disease burden, and effective monitoring. m-health (mobile health) further expand the vision of Universal Health Coverage (UHC) to address the vastly underserved healthcare needs when combined with current ongoing mobile phone reach in underserved areas and rapidly growing smart phone adoption.

The concept of use of IT in community health care (CHC) has been strengthened with the launch of Digital India campaign by the government of India on 1st of July 2015. In the modern digitized world, the relevance of this topic is self-explanatory to medical undergraduates who cannot think of separating themselves from their smart devices even during daily activities of living like toileting, mouth care, bathing, dressing, grooming, and eating. Specifically, this topic will attempt to lay ground for how they can utilize modern electronic media during their professional roles as community healthcare providers.

The overall success of "Digital India" program and "Ayushman Bharat" program warrants that community healthcare professionals irrespective of the stage in their professional career must understand, imbibe, and endorse "Use of IT in CHC".

Utility of IT in CHC can be elaborated on the following subtopics:
- e-Health and m-Health: Concepts and scope
- Telemedicine and community health
- Health care: Health education, training, monitoring, epidemic forecasting
- Electronic health records (EHR)
- Health management information system (HMIS)
  - RMNCAH+N (Reproductive, Maternal, Newborn, Child and Adolescent Health Plus Nutrition)
  - CMIS/SIMS (Computerized Management Information System/Strategic Information Management System) in NACP (National AIDS Control Programme)
- Reporting in integrated disease surveillance program
- Mother and child tracking system (MCTS)
- 99 DOTS and Nikshay in National Tuberculosis Elimination Programme (NTEP)

## E-HEALTH AND M-HEALTH

Gunther Eysenbach (2001) defined e-Health as "an emerging field in the intersection of medical informatics, public health and business, referring to health services and information delivered or enhanced through the Internet and related technologies" and "not only a technical development, but also a state-of-mind, a way of thinking, an attitude, and a commitment for networked, global thinking, to improve healthcare locally, regionally, and worldwide by using information and communication technology".

As per World Health Organization (2011) m-Health is defined "m-Health or mobile health" being "component of e-Health" as "medical and public health practice supported by mobile devices, such as mobile phones, patient monitoring devices, personal digital assistants (PDAs), and other wireless devices" with "use and capitalization on a mobile phone's core utility of voice and short messaging service (SMS) as well as more complex functionalities and applications including general packet radio service (GPRS), third and fourth generation mobile telecommunications (3G and 4G systems), global positioning system (GPS), and Bluetooth technology".

In term of concepts and scope of e-Health and m-Health for CHC, the definitions are self-explanatory. Simply stating, whenever electronic media is being used to develop, document, and communicate for the sake of achieving, ensuring and bettering CHC, it is e-Health; and whenever smart devices are further enhancing this opportunity to besting CHC by on-the-go mobility, it is m-Health.

When decoding "10 e' sine-Health" as documented by Gunther Eysenbach (2001), e-Health envisages efficiency, enhancing quality evidence based, empowerment, encouragement, education, enabling, expansive, ethical, and equitable CHC. As far as decoding m-Health and its utility, there are and will be no dearth of opportunities to pursue and to innovate when delivering CHC especially when CHC is going to fall on the shoulders of budding physicians who all are already becoming dependent on mobile smart devices constantly downloading or developing new apps to make both personal and professional lives easier and smoother for themselves. Moreover, even if the inflexible physicians will want to remain within their shells when limiting themselves to living in predigital era, the leaders and managers of social systems are evolving communities, societies, and populations toward total dependence on digital and mobile media systems wherein the older generation of physicians will have no option but to give into the likes of e-Health and m-Health to practice all health care including CHC.

To name a few among scores of e-Health initiatives from National Health Portal, the self-explanatorily named e-Health initiatives are "e-Aushadhi", "Family Planning Logistics MIS", "Poshan Tracker", and "Chirayu". Similarly, to name a few among almost nearing a hundred of m-Health initiatives (websites and apps) from National Health Portal, the mobile apps with self-explanatory names are "Safe Pregnancy and Birth", "Mobile-Family Planning Tool: CycleTelTM, "TB Detect", "Malaria Early Epidemic Detection System (MEEDS)", "Cardiopulmonary Resuscitation (CPR)", "NewBornCare" and "HealthPhone Poshan-Nutrition".

> **Initiatives in e-Health and m-Health**
>
> *Vital events*
>
> **Vital registration:** Vital statistics at a community level related to data regarding live births, deaths, marriages, etc. The most common way of collecting information on these is through civil registration and later data entry is being done to convert it into electronic form by entering in computer, by the use of IT we can capture the real time data from the set location.
>
> **Birth and death entry application system:** This system is being used in Gujarat to capture and monitor statistical data of birth, death, and stillbirth. It has a capability to analyze the demographic and personal information that has been stored in the system. The main aim is to maintain data base of birth and death records.
>
> **E-Olakh:** This is another example of effective use of information and communication technology (ICT) that is client oriented and has been developed for birth, death, stillbirth records. It not only maintains real time database of vital registration but also facilitates issuing of birth and death certificates.
>
> *Maternal and child health*
>
> **Maternal child tracking system (MCTS):** This has been developed by Government of India and is being used Pan India under NRHM (National Rural Health Mission) web portal. The aim is to tackle the issue of maternal deaths that could be prevented if by addressing the issues of healthcare accessibility during antenatal, intrapartum, and postpartum period.
>
> **e-Mamta (MCTS):** It is an interactive provider cum beneficiary-oriented name-based registration platform, that accounts for tracking of every pregnant woman and children that gives village level work plan to the healthcare provider and SMS to the beneficiary.
>
> *Child Health—Rashtriya Bal Swasthya Karyakram (RBSK)*
>
> Under RBSK the early identification and early intervention for children from birth to 18 years to cover 4 "D"s viz. defects at birth, deficiencies, diseases, development delays including disability is screening by healthcare providers. This program has been enabled through a cloud-based, tablet PC system, providing dashboard-based reports for various levels of administrators or doctors at all levels which is named as **Chirayu**.

## TELEMEDICINE AND COMMUNITY HEALTH

Telemedicine has reduced geographical barriers like difficult to reach hilly terrains, deserts, underdeveloped rural, and tribal areas by reducing the cost and providing accessible, affordable care where people gain not only economically as well as in terms of time and travel for specialty care services. World Health Organization (1998, 2010) defined telemedicine as "the delivery of healthcare services, where distance is a critical factor, by all healthcare professionals using information and communication technologies for the exchange of valid information for diagnosis, treatment, and prevention of disease and injuries, research and evaluation, and for the continuing education of healthcare providers, all in the interests of advancing the health of individuals and their communities."

Telemedicine is able to provide safe, timely, cost-effective, and qualitative health care to even individual patients in spite of their physicians being located far away from them in very remote locations. Therefore, it is a no-brainer that telemedicine can and will guide CHC for managing, documenting, monitoring and educating communities' health care including prevention of their diseases and health promotion activities among them with early recognition and management of epidemics and pandemics. The modern world is a globalized one wherein telemedicine can overcome geographical and corresponding economic barriers as far as the availability of educational, awareness, communication, and referral resources to one-and-all through "safe-and-protected internet" but only after the community leaders, their local managers and on-site care-delivery equipment may have been arranged with the resources from among the communities being served. To name a few from National Health Portal, the telemedicine initiatives in India are "e-Hospital", "National Health Helpline" and "National Telemedicine Network (NTN)".

## HEALTH CARE: HEALTH EDUCATION, TRAINING, MONITORING, AND EPIDEMIC FORECASTING

Information technology is also playing vital role in health care, health education, training, monitoring, and epidemic forecasting. World Health Organization states health education in CHC being "any combination of learning experiences designed to help individuals and communities improve their health, by increasing their knowledge or influencing their attitudes" and training in health care is an essential part of "knowledge transfer and training for outbreaks".

World Health Organization annually document "World Health Statistics series" as quantification of global health's status as per the monitored "Sustainable Development Goals" as defined, refined, and revised from time to time.

Epidemic forecasting in CHC World Health Organization is all for "anticipating epidemics" on the lines of anticipating disasters and weathers by calling out for collaboration among closely related multifaceted fields so that epidemic forecasting does not remain in the state of infancy any longer than it has already been.

Myers et al. (2000) called for forecasting as an essentiality for preparedness against diseases and Shawn Dolley (2018) reiterated the essential role of "Big Data" for delivering CHC with astute precision. Not only for forecasting for bettering care delivery during CHC, IT will definitely be indispensable for CHC education and training programs and IT-based monitoring of CHC programs. Without question, the budding and aging physicians must or will have to imbibe the core user-friendly concepts of IT if they will want to survive as a deliverer of modern CHC that is slowly and surely becoming dependent on the evolving systems of IT-based healthcare education, training, monitoring, and forecasting. The sooner the physicians' community realizes the essentiality for "being digitally literate" and "being IT literate", the sooner they will break their barriers to sustain and grow in fast-evolving digitalized and globalized world irrespective of whether they are limited to just delivering CHC or overall healthcare-in-toto.

## ELECTRONIC HEALTH RECORDS

Electronic medical records (EMR) are "everything" contained within "a paper chart, such as medical history, diagnoses, medications, immunization dates, allergies" but their utility is "limited because they do not easily travel outside the practice" and may "even have to be printed out and mailed for another provider to see it".

Comparatively, per practice fusion, Electronic Health Records (EHR) "are digital records of health information" and "contain all" that's there in EMR "— and a lot more" such as "past medical history, vital signs, progress notes, diagnoses, medications, immunization dates, allergies, laboratory data and imaging reports" and additional information like "insurance information, demographic data, and even data imported from personal wellness devices" which are "instantly accessible to authorized providers across practices and health organizations, helping to inform clinical decisions and coordinate care" among "all clinicians and organizations involved in a patient's care such as laboratories, specialists, imaging facilities, pharmacies, emergency facilities, and school and workplace clinics."

Considering the requirements for transparency, accountability, and continuity of patient care, they are morally, ethically, and legally essential for all health care including CHC. Therefore, it can never be stressed enough that EHR must be part and parcel of all modern CHC to ensure fast, smooth, affordable, and accessible CHC to all components of the community. EHR being IT-based modality also create banks of extractable data to audit the delivered CHC thus self- reflecting on its efficacy to recognize if there is any further need to innovate when trying to remain up-to-date as well as closing the gaps if any in the currently delivered CHC.

## HEALTH MANAGEMENT INFORMATION SYSTEM: RMNCAH+N AND CMIS/SIMS IN NACP

World Health Organization (1993, 2004) defined HMIS as "an information system specially designed to assist in the management and planning of health programs, as opposed to delivery of care". Under "Digital India" initiative, "Health Statistics Information Portal" and online "Health Management Information System interface" play the above-mentioned role.

As per Ministry of Health and Family Welfare, Government of India (2013), RMNCAH+N is "a strategic approach to reproductive, maternal, newborn, child and adolescent health plus nutrition in India" which includes role of HMIS for "tracking of stocks" of medicines, for "monitoring and review" of RMNCAH+N "to strengthen this system and improve the quality of data" and "improved decision-making" via "HMIS-based dashboard monitoring system".

As per National AIDS Control Organization, the "National AIDS Control Programme Phase III (2007–2012)" had initially depended on "an offline Computerized Management Information System (CMIS) introduced in 2002 to capture and maintain the database of HIV/AIDS control program across the country" to eventually integrate with "Strategic Information Management System (SIMS), an integrated web-based reporting and data management system launched in 2008 to replace CMIS" with "real time data entry and access to the user" via "online Data Item Report" for "analysis and evidence-based action, timely corrective measures for program managers and policy makers which help in monitoring at the grassroot level".

The above-mentioned quotes directly from the original sources are self-explanatory that without IT-based HMIS, the quality of delivered CHC can be neither quantified transparently nor corrected timely to effectively manage the quantity of delivered CHC whether it is for reproductive health or maternal health or newborn health or child health or adolescent health or AIDS control within the communities.

## REPORTING IN INTEGRATED DISEASE SURVEILLANCE PROGRAMME

Integrated Disease Surveillance Programme (IDSP) initiated in 2004 by Ministry of Health and Family Welfare with objective "to strengthen decentralized laboratory-based IT-enabled disease surveillance system for epidemic prone diseases to monitor disease trends and to detect and respond to outbreaks in early rising phase through trained Rapid Response Team" through "Integration and decentralization of surveillance activities through establishment of surveillance units at Center, State and District level", "Human Resource Development—Training of State Surveillance Officers, District Surveillance Officers, Rapid Response Team and other medical and paramedical staff on principles of disease surveillance", "Use of Information Communication Technology for collection, collation, compilation, analysis, and dissemination of data", "Strengthening of public health laboratories", and "Inter sectoral co-ordination for zoonotic diseases".

Essentially, IDSP cannot function without IT-based interfaces if it wants to first decentralize so as to monitor the needs as well as the adequacy of CHC delivery at remotest independent units of communities.

## MOTHER AND CHILD TRACKING SYSTEM

As per Ministry of Health and Family Welfare, Mother and Child Tracking System is "an innovative, web-based application" utilizing "information technology for ensuring delivery of full spectrum of health care and immunization services to pregnant women and children up to 5 years of age" so as "to facilitate and monitor service delivery as well as to establish a two-way communication between the service providers and beneficiaries."

At the core of all communities formed of human populations is "mother and child", and if their health and welfare is not tracked, it destabilizes the core of communities formed of human populations wherein the future of such communities becomes bleaker to no future at all. Without IT-based communication systems, this tracking cannot be envisaged in timely, accessible and attainable fashion to make any immediate and long-term impact on "mother and child" and their communities being served with delivered CHC.

## 99 DOTS AND NIKSHAY IN NTEP

Central Tuberculosis Division of Ministry of Health and Family Welfare adopted strategies to strengthen NTEP by envisaging National Strategic Plan for Tuberculosis Elimination 2017–2025.

99 DOTS is innovative Directly Observed Treatment, short-course strategy for reaching to 99% tuberculosis (TB) patients as "a low-cost approach for monitoring and improving TB medication adherence" wherein "each anti-TB blister pack is wrapped in a custom envelope, which includes hidden phone numbers that are visible only when doses are dispensed" and thereafter "patients make a free call to the hidden phone number, yielding high confidence that the dose was "in-hand and has been taken" because enrollees "receive a series of daily reminders (via SMS and automated calls)" and "missed doses trigger SMS notifications to care providers, who follow up with personal, phone-based counseling".

Recently 99 DOTS integrated with Nikshay that is "a web-enabled and case-based monitoring application" so as to ensure "monitoring of TB patients" when "used by health functionaries at various levels across the country" wherein it "covers various aspects of controlling TB using technological innovations" using "SMS services" along with "web-based technology" ensuring "communication with patients and monitoring the program on day to day basis".

In a nutshell, TB being one of the major communicable diseases disabling Indian population eats into major economic resources allotted by Government of India for health care. Vision for eliminating TB by strategically planning during 2017–2025 cannot be realized without IT-based monitoring of TB patients receiving DOTS that in turn is aiming to prevent development of multidrug resistant TB strains because development of multidrug resistant TB strains will surely push the time frame for eliminating TB much beyond the year 2025.

## NIKUSTH

A real time leprosy reporting software was introduced in 2019 across India. It is an integrated ICT application for leprosy data management and patient tracking under NLEP. Nikusth 2.0 was recently launched on 30th January 2023 to develop a complete database of leprosy patients, proper tracking and follow-up of individual case, to facilitate program monitoring, evaluation, action and policy modification.

## AYUSHMAN BHARAT DIGITAL MISSION

It aims to develop the backbone necessary to support the integrated digital health infrastructure of the country. It will bridge the existing gap amongst different stakeholders of Health-care ecosystem through digital highways. A unique ABHA (Ayushman Bharat Health Account) Number will be used for the purposes of identifying persons, authenticating them, and threading their health records (only with the informed consent of the patient) across multiple systems and stakeholders. Health professional and health facility registries will be developed and ABHA Mobile App for easy access of data to the individual.

## DAKSHATA-ONLINE LEARNING PROGRAM

Empowering workforce to get fully skilled in hiv/aids supply chain management. It offers highly interactive content, based on adult learning principles and developed in consultation with supply chain experts which you can access anywhere, at any time, at your convenience. With this flexibility, you will be able to finish each module easily and will also enjoy various activities, quizzes and games.

### eVIN-Co-WIN-U-WIN

**eVIN:** Innovative technology based, health system strengthening tool which was rolled out in 2015 with technical support from UNDP under GAVI HSS support evin is rolled out in 36 states and UTs and digitizing the vaccine stocks and storage temperatures in more than 29,500 cold chain points in the countries.

**Co-WIN:** It is a state of the art digital solution from the government of India to achieve universal vaccination against COVID-19. It has been developed for empowering both citizens and healthcare workers.

**U-WIN:** Digital solution for Universal Immunization Programme-facilitate tracking of every pregnant woman, new born, child and adolescent vaccination.

Planning vaccination sessions, updating vaccination status on real time basis from the last mile of service delivery by the vaccinator.

## LIMITATIONS

In context to potential scope of IT in underexplored areas of health care, it is difficult to imagine future health care without IT support. In future itself, only the applications will vary but health care will not be delivered without IT-based interfaces and applications except for "tender loving care (TLC)" which will always need humans' humane touch.

Certain limitations cannot be overlooked with the use of technologies like for implementation of technologies availability of trained manpower is essential. Technical constraints, including connectivity, bandwidth provision, and reliability, also need to be taken care of along with availability of health professionals for correct diagnosis and treatment.

Cost consideration and affordability need to be taken into account for the development and implementation of national plan for e-Health along with its integration into the health system. People residing in rural and remote areas need to be made aware of the existence of such e-Services in their areas; their ethical and social issues also need to be addressed.

As far as problems of IT encroaching our healthcare including CHC, the major immediate problem is the safety of data and exploitation of data to breach the patients' expectations of privacy leading to dangerous outcomes. Essentiality of education and training of modern CHC providers and professionals in protecting the data and ensuring the confidentiality will go a long way to achieving the sanctity of data's oceans which can then safely ensure governance of communities' health care without putting their privacy or them at risk.

There is no escaping "Use of IT in CHC" just like human existence seeming impossible without smart devices today and it is better to surrender to the flow of time and imbibe IT in CHC before the time changes again for better or worse depending on the change in our needs and the tools we will need to deal with them as the future of human existence unfolds.

## SUGGESTED READING

1. 99DOTS. [online]. Available from https://www.99dots.org/.
2. About IDSP. [online]. Available from https://idsp.nic.in/index4.php?lang=1&level=0&linkid=313&lid=1592.
3. ADL/IADL Checklist. [online]. Available from https://www.seniorplanningservices.com/files/2013/12/Santa-Barbara-ADL-IADL-Checklist.pdf.
4. A health Telematics Policy. [online]. Available from http://apps.who.int/iris/bitstream/handle/10665/63857/WHO_DGO_98.1.pdf?sequence=1&isAllowed=y.
5. Ayushman Bharat-National Health Protection. [online]. Available from https://www.india.gov.in/spotlight/ayushman-bharat-national-health-protection-mission.
6. Computerized Management Information System (CMIS) [online]. Available from http://www.cortindia.in/STRC%5CPM%5CNACO's%20CMIS.pdf.
7. Developing Health Management Information Systems. [online]. Available from http://www.wpro.who.int/health_services/documents/developing_health_management_information_systems.pdf.
8. Digital India. [online]. Available from http://digitalindia.gov.in/content/about-programme.
9. E-Health Initiatives from States across India. [online]. Available from https://www.nhp.gov.in/e-health_initiatives_from_states_across_india_mtl.
10. G Eysenbach. What is e-health? [online]. Available from https://www.ncbi.nlm.nih.gov/pmc/articles/PMC1761894/.
11. Global Health Observatory (GHO) data. [online]. Available from http://www.who.int/gho/publications/world_health_statistics/2018/en/.
12. Guidelines for the Development of Health Management Information Systems. [online]. Available from http://iris.wpro.who.int/bitstream/handle/10665.1/5449/9290611065_eng.pdf.
13. Knowledge transfer and training for outbreaks. [online]. Available from http://www.who.int/knowledge-transfer/health-training/en/.
14. m-Health new horizons for health through mobile technologies. [online]. Available from https://www.who.int/goe/publications/goe_mhealth_web.pdf.
15. Monitoring and Evaluation. [online]. Available from https://nrhm-mis.nic.in/SitePages/HMIS-AboutUS.aspx.
16. Myers MF, Rogers DJ. Forecasting Disease Risk for Increased Epidemic Preparedness in Public Health. [online]. Available from https://www.ncbi.nlm.nih.gov/pmc/articles/PMC3196833/.
17. NACO. Strategic Information Management System (SIMS) – An Overview. [online]. Available from http://naco.gov.in/sites/default/files/SIMS%20Wall%20Chart.pdf.
18. National Strategic Plan for Tuberculosis Elimination 2017–2025. [online]. Available from https://tbcindia.gov.in/WriteReadData/ NSP%20Draft%2020.02.2017%201.pdf.
19. Nikshay. [online]. Available from http://nikshay.gov.in/AboutNikshay.htm.
20. NRHM. Mother & Child Tracking System. [online]. Available from http://nrhm-mcts.nic.in/.
21. NRHM. Mother and Child Tracking System (MCTS). [online]. Available from http://apps.nic.in/apps/government/mother-and-child-tracking-system-mcts.
22. Telemedicine Opportunities and Developments in Member States. [online]. Available from http://www.who.int/goe/publications/goe_telemedicine_2010.pdf.

# F. ESSENTIAL MEDICINES

*Anusha Rashmi*

| | |
|---|---|
| CM 19.1 | Define and describe the concept of essential medicine |
| CM 19.2 | Describe the role of essential medicine in primary health care |
| CM 19.3 | Describe counterfeit medicine and its prevention |

## INTRODUCTION

As per World Health Organization (WHO), Essential Medicines are those that satisfy the priority health care needs of any person. These medicines should have established safety, efficacy, and comparative cost effectiveness. The aim behind formulating essential medicine list (EML) is to ensure that these medicines are available in adequate amounts, in appropriate dosage forms and strengths with assured quality. EML is expected to aid in improving quality and accessibility of health care while ensuring cost effective use of resources. This also helps in satisfying the Alma Ata Declaration of 'health for all' by providing essential medicines at low costs thus paving the way for healthcare as a fundamental right. This has obvious importance for resource limited country like India. Further, EML is intended to promote rational use of medicines.

## Evolution of Essential Medicines List

Tanzania was the first country to compose its own country specific EML in 1970. In 1975, the World Health Assembly requested WHO to assist member states in identifying essential medicines specific to them and assuring their availability, assuring good quality at reasonable cost. WHO published first model list of essential medicines in 1977 which contained 186 medicines. It was intended to be used as a template by member countries. It stated that *essential medicines* were "of utmost importance, basic, indispensable and necessary for the health and needs of the population" and criteria for selection were based on efficacy, safety, quality, and total cost. The emphasis was laid on disease burden and treatment guidelines as basis for selecting essential medicines.

In 1985, the list of essential medicines of the WHO was recognized as important, mainly for the public sector and its scope was to guide the procurement, distribution, rational use, and quality assurance of medicines. As the disease diversity and burden grew, the number of medicines in the WHO EML increased over the years, a trend that has also been seen with National List of Essential Medicines (NLEM) of India. The 23rd list of essential medicines has been released on July 2023 by WHO.

## Requirement for Country Specific EML

The essential medicines list prepared by WHO is a prototype list that can be used as a template by individual countries. Since priority health care needs of countries differ, it is logical that each country shall have its own country specific EML. Socio-demographic factors and economy are other factors that are likely to influence composition of EML for any country.

## National List of Essential Medicines (NLEM) India

India as a country adopts the guidelines from WHO and has come up with a country list called National List of Essential Medicines (NLEM). The country brought out its first essential drug list 1n 1996. Subsequently, the list has been revised in 2003, 2011, 2015 and 2022. The changes made in NLEM from 2011 till 2022 are shown in **Table 51F.1**.

The NLEM may serve multiple purposes as under:
- Promote the rational use of medicines.
- Guide safe and effective treatment of priority disease conditions of a population and optimize the available health resources of the country.
- It can also serve as a guiding document for:
  - State governments to prepare their list of essential medicines.
  - Developing Standard Treatment Guidelines to Help in preparing hospital formularies.
  - Procurement and supply of medicines in the public sector as well as private sector hospitals
  - Reimbursement of cost of pharmaceutical products by employers
  - Reimbursement by insurance companies
- Identifying the 'MUST KNOW' domain for the teaching and training of health care professionals (medical, dental, pharmacy and nursing).

## Some Salient features of NLEM 2022

- The NLEM 2022 contains 384 medicines as compared to 376 in NLEM 2015. Maximum numbers of medicines, i.e., 108 (including duplications) are in anti-infective therapeutic category of medicines. The second maximum numbers of medicine 63 (including duplication) are in anti-cancer agents including immunosuppressive and medicines used in palliative care therapeutic category.
- In NLEM 2022, 34 medicines have been added and 26 medicines have been deleted.
- In India, the healthcare system is categorized as a three-tier system with primary, secondary, and tertiary levels having different health care concerns and medicine requirements. While a primary health care level setup may require medicines prescribed in an outpatient setup like basic antibiotics, analgesics, and anti-inflammatory drugs; a tertiary level setup might need more parenteral medicines, medicines for critical care settings, for specialized treatments like organ transplantation and for inpatient setup. In NLEM, the medicines have been categorized as P – Primary healthcare facilities, S – Secondary healthcare facilities, T – Tertiary healthcare facilities. Over the years, the drugs which were only used in tertiary care are now being increasingly used in secondary care setups **(Table 51F.1)**.
- In general, fixed dose combinations (FDCs) have not been included unless; the combination has unequivocally

proven advantage over individual ingredients administered separately, in terms of increasing efficacy, reducing adverse effects and/or improving compliance. The committee recommends continued medical education to physicians for judiciously using fixed dose combinations and recommends pharmaceutical industry to critically assess the benefit and rationality of FDC before introducing such formulations in the market.

**Table 51F.1:** National List of Essential Medicine in 2022 categorized according to the level of healthcare (P – Primary healthcare facilities, S – Secondary healthcare facilities, T – Tertiary healthcare facilities).

### Section 1: Medicines used in Anesthesia

| Sr. No. | Medicine | Level of Healthcare |
|---|---|---|
| 1. | Halothane | S, T |
| 2. | Isoflurane | S, T |
| 3. | Ketamine | P, S, T |
| 4. | Nitrous oxide | P, S, T |
| 5 | Oxygen | P, S, T |
| 6. | Propofol | P, S, T |
| 7. | Sevoflurane | S, T |
| 8. | Thiopentone | P, S, T |
| 9. | Bupivacaine | S, T |
| 10. | Lignocaine | P, S, T |
| 11. | Lignocaine (A) + Adrenaline (B) | P, S, T |
| 12. | Atropine | P, S, T |
| 13. | Glycopyrrolate | S, T |
| 14. | Midazolam | P, S, T |
| 15. | Morphine | P, S, T |
| 16. | Atracurium | S, T |
| 17. | Baclofen | S, T |
| 18. | Neostigmine | S, T |
| 19. | Succinylcholine | S, T |
| 20. | Vecuronium | S, T |

### Section 2: Analgesics, Antipyretics, Non-steroidal Anti-inflammatory Drugs (NSAIDs), Medicines used to treat Gout and Disease Modifying Agents used in Rheumatoid Disorders

| Sr. No. | Medicine | Level of Healthcare |
|---|---|---|
| 1. | Acetylsalicylic acid | P, S, T |
| 2. | Diclofenac | P, S, T |
| 3. | Ibuprofen | P, S, T |
| 4. | Mefenamic acid | P, S, T |
| 5. | Paracetamol | P, S, T |
| 6. | Fentanyl | S, T |
| 7. | Morphine | P, S, T |
| 8. | Tramadol | S, T |
| 9. | Allopurinol | P, S, T |
| 10. | Colchicine | P, S, T |
| 11. | Azathioprine | S, T |
| 12. | Hydroxychloroquine | P, S, T |
| 13. | Methotrexate | P, S, T |
| 14. | Sulfasalazine | S, T |

### Section 3: Antiallergics and Medicines used in Anaphylaxis

| Sr. No. | Medicine | Level of Healthcare |
|---|---|---|
| 1. | Adrenaline | P, S, T |
| 2. | Cetirizine | P, S, T |
| 3. | Dexamethasone | P, S, T |
| 4. | Hydrocortisone | P, S, T |
| 5. | Pheniramine | P, S, T |
| 6. | Prednisolone | P, S, T |

### Section 4: Antidotes and Other Substances used in Management of Poisonings/Envenomation

| Sr. No. | Medicine | Level of Healthcare |
|---|---|---|
| 1. | Activated Charcoal | P, S, T |
| 2. | Atropine | P, S, T |
| 3. | Calcium gluconate | P, S, T |
| 4. | D-Penicillamine | P, S, T |
| 5. | Desferrioxamine | S, T |
| 6. | Methylthioninium chloride (Methylene blue) | S, T |
| 7. | N-acetylcysteine | P, S, T |
| 8. | Naloxone | P, S, T |
| 9. | Neostigmine | P, S, T |
| 10. | Pralidoxime chloride (2-PAM) | P, S, T |
| 11. | Snake venom antiserum | P, S, T |
| 12. | Sodium nitrite | S, T |
| 13. | Sodium thiosulphate | S, T |

### Section 5: Medicines used in Neurological Disorders

| Sr. No. | Medicine | Level of Healthcare |
|---|---|---|
| 1. | Carbamazepine | P, S, T |
| 2. | Clobazam | S, T |
| 3. | Diazepam | P, S, T |
| 4. | Levetiracetam | S, T |
| 5. | Lorazepam | P, S, T |
| 6. | Magnesium sulphate | S, T |
| 7. | Midazolam | P, S, T |
| 8. | Phenobarbitone | P, S, T |

*Contd...*

*Contd...*

### Section 5: Medicines used in Neurological Disorders

| Sr. No. | Medicine | Level of Healthcare |
|---|---|---|
| 9. | Phenytoin | P, S, T |
| 10. | Sodium Valproate | P, S, T |
| 11. | Acetylsalicylic acid | P, S, T |
| 12. | Ibuprofen | P, S, T |
| 13. | Paracetamol | P, S, T |
| 14. | Sumatriptan | P, S, T |
| 15. | Amitriptyline | P, S, T |
| 16. | Flunarizine | P, S, T |
| 17. | Propranolol | P, S, T |
| 18. | Levodopa (A) + Carbidopa (B) | P, S, T |
| 19. | Trihexyphenidyl | P, S, T |
| 20. | Donepezil | S, T |

### Section 6: Anti-infective Medicines

| Sr. No. | Medicine | Level of Healthcare |
|---|---|---|
| 1. | Albendazole | P, S, T |
| 2. | Mebendazole | P, S, T |
| 3. | Albendazole | P, S, T |
| 4. | Diethylcarbamazine (DEC) | P, S, T |
| 5. | Ivermectin | P, S, T |
| 6. | Praziquantel | S, T |
| 7. | Amoxicillin | P, S, T |
| 8. | Amoxicillin (A) + Clavulanic acid (B) | P, S, T |
| 9. | Ampicillin | P, S, T |
| 10. | Benzathine benzylpenicillin | P, S, T |
| 11. | Benzylpenicillin | P, S, T |
| 12. | Cefadroxil | P, S, T |
| 13. | Cefazolin | P, S, T |
| 14. | Cefixime | S, T |
| 15. | Cefotaxime | S, T |
| 16. | Ceftazidime | S, T |
| 17. | Ceftriaxone | S, T |
| 18. | Cloxacillin | P, S, T |
| 19. | Piperacillin (A) + Tazobactam (B) | T |
| 20. | Meropenem | T |
| 21. | Azithromycin | P, S, T |
| 22. | Cefuroxime | P, S, T |
| 23. | Ciprofloxacin | P, S, T |
| 24. | Clarithromycin | S, T |
| 25. | Clindamycin | P, S, T |
| 26. | Co-trimoxazole Sulfamethoxazole (A) + Trimethoprim (B)] | P, S, T |
| 27. | Doxycycline | P, S, T |
| 28. | Gentamicin | P, S, T |
| 29. | Metronidazole | P, S, T |
| 30. | Nitrofurantoin | P, S, T |
| 31. | Phenoxymethylpenicillin | P, S, T |
| 32. | Procaine Benzylpenicillin | P, S, T |
| 33. | Vancomycin | S, T |
| 34. | Clofazimine | P, S, T |
| 35. | Dapsone | P, S, T |
| 36. | Rifampicin | P, S, T |
| 37. | Amikacin | S, T |
| 38. | Bedaquiline | T |
| 39. | Clofazimine | S, T |
| 40. | Cycloserine | S, T |
| 41. | Delamanid | T |
| 42. | Ethambutol | P, S, T |
| 43. | Ethionamide | S, T |
| 44. | Isoniazid | P, S, T |
| 45. | Levofloxacin | P, S, T |
| 46. | Linezolid | P, S, T |
| 47. | Moxifloxacin | P, S, T |
| 48. | Para-aminosalicylic acid | S, T |
| 49. | Pyrazinamide | P, S, T |
| 50. | Rifampicin | P, S, T |
| 51. | Streptomycin | P, S, T |
| 52. | Amphotericin B | S, T |
| 53. | Clotrimazole | P, S, T |
| 54. | Fluconazole | P, S, T |
| 55. | Griseofulvin | P, S, T |
| 56. | Itraconazole | S, T |
| 57. | Mupirocin | P, S, T |
| 58. | Nystatin | S, T |
| 59. | Terbinafine | P, S, T |
| 60. | Acyclovir | P, S, T |

*Contd...*

*Contd...*

### Section 6: Anti-infective Medicines

| Sr. No. | Medicine | Level of Healthcare |
|---|---|---|
| 61. | Valganciclovir | S, T |
| 62. | Abacavir | S, T |
| 63. | Abacavir (A) + Lamivudine (B) | S, T |
| 64. | Lamivudine | S, T |
| 65. | Tenofovir Disoproxil Fumarate (TDF) | S, T |
| 66. | Tenofovir Disoproxil Fumarate (A) + Lamivudine (B) | S, T |
| 67. | Tenofovir Disoproxil Fumarate (A) + Lamivudine (B) + Dolutegravir (C) | P, S, T |
| 68. | Tenofovir Disoproxil Fumarate (A) + Lamivudine (B) + Efavirenz (C) | S, T |
| 69. | Zidovudine | S, T |
| 70. | Zidovudine (A) + Lamivudine (B) | S, T |
| 71. | Zidovudine (A) + Lamivudine (B) + Nevirapine (C) | S, T |
| 72. | Efavirenz | S, T |
| 73. | Nevirapine | P, S, T |
| 74. | Dolutegravir | S, T |
| 75. | Raltegravir | S, T |
| 76. | Atazanavir (A) + Ritonavir (B) | S, T |
| 77. | Darunavir | S, T |
| 78. | Darunavir (A) + Ritonavir (B) | S, T |
| 79. | Lopinavir (A) + Ritonavir (B) | S, T |
| 80. | Ritonavir | S, T |
| 81. | Daclatasvir | S, T |
| 82. | Entecavir | S, T |
| 83. | Ribavirin | S, T |
| 84. | Sofosbuvir | S, T |
| 85. | Tenofovir Alafenamide Fumarate (TAF) | S, T |
| 86. | Tenofovir Disoproxil Fumarate | S, T |
| 87. | Miltefosine | P, S, T |
| 88. | Paromomycin | P, S, T |
| 89. | Artemether (A) + Lumefantrine (B) | P, S, T |
| 90. | Artesunate | P, S, T |
| 91. | Artesunate (A) + Sulfadoxine Pyrimethamine (B) | P, S, T |
| 92. | Chloroquine | P, S, T |
| 93. | Primaquine | P, S, T |
| 94. | Quinine | P, S, T |
| 95. | Mefloquine | T |

### Section 7: Anticancer agents including Immunosuppressives and Medicines used in Palliative Care

| Sr. No. | Medicine | Level of Healthcare |
|---|---|---|
| 1. | 5-Fluorouracil | T |
| 2. | 6-Mercaptopurine | T |
| 3. | Actinomycin D | T |
| 4. | All-trans retinoic acid | T |
| 5. | Arsenic trioxide | T |
| 6. | Bendamustine hydrochloride | T |
| 7. | Bleomycin | T |
| 8. | Bortezomib | T |
| 9. | Calcium folinate | T |
| 10. | Capecitabine | T |
| 11. | Carboplatin | T |
| 12. | Chlorambucil | T |
| 13. | Cisplatin | T |
| 14. | Cyclophosphamide | T |
| 15. | Cytosine arabinoside | T |
| 16. | Dacarbazine | T |
| 17. | Daunorubicin | T |
| 18. | Docetaxel | T |
| 19. | Doxorubicin | T |
| 20. | Etoposide | T |
| 21. | Gefitinib | T |
| 22. | Gemcitabine | T |
| 23. | Hydroxyurea | T |
| 24. | Ifosfamide | T |
| 25. | Imatinib | T |
| 26. | Irinotecan HCl trihydrate | T |
| 27. | L-Asparaginase | T |
| 28. | Lenalidomide | T |
| 29. | Melphalan | T |
| 30. | Methotrexate | S, T |
| 31. | Oxaliplatin | T |
| 32. | Paclitaxel | T |
| 33. | Rituximab | T |
| 34. | Temozolomide | T |
| 35. | Thalidomide | T |
| 36. | Trastuzumab | T |
| 37. | Vinblastine | T |
| 38. | Vincristine | T |
| 39. | Bicalutamide | T |
| 40. | Letrozole | T |
| 41. | Leuprolide acetate | T |
| 42. | Prednisolone | S, T |

*Contd...*

### Section 7: Anticancer agents including Immunosuppressives and Medicines used in Palliative Care

| Sr. No. | Medicine | Level of Healthcare |
|---|---|---|
| 43. | Tamoxifen | T |
| 44. | Azathioprine | T |
| 45. | Cyclosporine | T |
| 46. | Mycophenolate mofetil | T |
| 47. | Tacrolimus | T |
| 48. | Allopurinol | S, T |
| 49. | Amitriptyline | S, T |
| 50. | Dexamethasone | S, T |
| 51. | Diazepam | S, T |
| 52. | Filgrastim | T |
| 53. | Fluoxetine | S, T |
| 54. | Haloperidol | S, T |
| 55. | Lactulose | S, T |
| 56. | Loperamide | S, T |
| 57. | Metoclopramide | S, T |
| 58. | Mesna | T |
| 59. | Midazolam | S, T |
| 60. | Morphine | S, T |
| 61. | Ondansetron | S, T |
| 62. | Tramadol | S, T |
| 63. | Zoledronic acid | T |

### Section 8: Medicines affecting Blood

| Sr. No. | Medicine | Level of Healthcare |
|---|---|---|
| 1. | Erythropoietin | S, T |
| 2. | Ferrous salts: (a) Iron Dextran (b) Iron sorbitol citrate complex | P, S, T |
| 3. | Ferrous Salt (A)+ Folic acid (B) | P, S, T |
| 4. | Folic acid | P, S, T |
| 5. | Hydroxocobalamin | P, S, T |
| 6. | Hydroxyurea | S, T |
| 7. | Iron sucrose | S, T |
| 8. | Enoxaparin | S, T |
| 9. | Heparin | S, T |
| 10. | Phytomenadione (vitamin $K_1$) | P, S, T |
| 11. | Protamine sulphate | S, T |
| 12. | Tranexamic acid | P, S, T |
| 13. | Warfarin | S, T |

### Section 9: Blood products and Plasma substitutes

| Sr. No. | Medicine | Level of Healthcare |
|---|---|---|
| 1. | Fresh frozen plasma | S, T |
| 2. | Platelet rich plasma/Platelet concentrates | S, T |
| 3. | Red blood cells/Packed RBCs | S, T |
| 4. | Whole blood | S, T |
| 5. | Dextran-40 | S, T |
| 6. | Coagulation factor IX | S, T |
| 7. | Coagulation factor VIII | S, T |
| 8. | Cryoprecipitate | S, T |

### Section 10: Cardiovascular Medicines

| Sr. No. | Medicine | Level of Healthcare |
|---|---|---|
| 1. | Diltiazem | P, S, T |
| 2. | Glyceryl trinitrate | P, S, T |
| 3. | Isosorbide dinitrate | P, S, T |
| 4. | Metoprolol | P, S, T |
| 5. | Adenosine | S, T |
| 6. | Amiodarone | S, T |
| 7. | Digoxin | S, T |
| 8. | Esmolol | S, T |
| 9. | Lignocaine | S, T |
| 10. | Verapamil | S, T |
| 11. | Amlodipine | P, S, T |
| 12. | Enalapril | P, S, T |
| 13. | Hydrochlorothiazide | P, S, T |
| 14. | Labetalol | P, S, T |
| 15. | Ramipril | P, S, T |
| 16. | Sodium nitroprusside | S, T |
| 17. | Telmisartan | P, S, T |
| 18. | Dobutamine | S, T |
| 19. | Dopamine | S, T |
| 20. | Noradrenaline | S, T |
| 21. | Spironolactone | P, S, T |
| 22. | Acetylsalicylic acid | P, S, T |
| 23. | Clopidogrel | P, S, T |
| 24. | Dabigatran | S, T |
| 25. | Enoxaparin | S, T |
| 26. | Heparin | S, T |
| 27. | Streptokinase | S, T |
| 28. | Tenecteplase | S, T |
| 29. | Atorvastatin | P, S, T |

*Contd...*

*Contd...*

### Section 11: Dermatological Medicines (Topical)

| Sr. No. | Medicine | Level of Healthcare |
|---|---|---|
| 1. | Clotrimazole | P, S, T |
| 2. | Framycetin | P, S, T |
| 3. | Fusidic acid | P, S, T |
| 4. | Silver sulphadiazine | P, S, T |
| 5. | Betamethasone valerate | P, S, T |
| 6. | Calamine | P, S, T |
| 7. | Benzoyl peroxide | P, S, T |
| 8. | Coal tar (A) + Salicylic Acid (B) | P, S, T |
| 9. | Podophyllin resin | S, T |
| 10. | Salicylic acid | P, S, T |
| 11. | Permethrin | P, S, T |
| 12. | Glycerin/glycerol | P, S, T |

### Section 12: Diagnostic Agents

| Sr. No. | Medicine | Level of Healthcare |
|---|---|---|
| 1. | Fluorescein | S, T |
| 2. | Proparacaine | S, T |
| 3. | Tropicamide | S, T |
| 4. | Barium sulphate | S, T |
| 5. | Gadobenate dimeglumine | T |
| 6. | Iohexol | S, T |
| 7. | Meglumine diatrizoate | S, T |

### Section 13: Dialysis Components (Hemodialysis and Peritoneal Dialysis)

| Sr. No. | Medicine | Level of Healthcare |
|---|---|---|
| 1. | Hemodialysis fluid | S, T |
| 2. | Peritoneal dialysis solution | S, T |

### Section 14: Antiseptics and Disinfectants

| Sr. No. | Medicine | Level of Healthcare |
|---|---|---|
| 1. | Chlorhexidine | P, S, T |
| 2. | Ethyl alcohol (Denatured) | P, S, T |
| 3. | Hydrogen peroxide | P, S, T |
| 4. | Methylrosanilinium chloride (Gentian Violet) | P, S, T |
| 5. | Povidone iodine* | P, S, T |
| 6. | Glutaraldehyde | S, T |
| 7. | Potassium permanganate | P, S, T |

### Section 15: Diuretics

| Sr. No. | Medicine | Level of Healthcare |
|---|---|---|
| 1. | Furosemide | P, S, T |
| 2. | Hydrochlorothiazide | P, S, T |
| 3. | Mannitol | P, S, T |
| 4. | Spironolactone | P, S, T |

### Section 16: Ear, Nose and Throat Medicines

| Sr. No. | Medicine | Level of Healthcare |
|---|---|---|
| 1. | Budesonide | P, S, T |
| 2. | Ciprofloxacin | P, S, T |
| 3. | Clotrimazole | P, S, T |
| 4. | Xylometazoline | P, S, T |

### Section 17: Gastrointestinal Medicines

| Sr. No. | Medicine | Level of Healthcare |
|---|---|---|
| 1. | Omeprazole | P, S, T |
| 2. | Pantoprazole | S, T |
| 3. | Domperidone | P, S, T |
| 4. | Metoclopramide | P, S, T |
| 5. | Ondansetron | S, T |
| 6. | 5-aminosalicylic acid (Mesalazine/Mesalamine) | S, T |
| 7. | Dicyclomine | P, S, T |
| 8. | Hyoscine butyl bromide | P, S, T |
| 9. | Bisacodyl | P, S, T |
| 10. | Ispaghula | P, S, T |
| 11. | Lactulose | S, T |
| 12. | Oral rehydration salts | P, S, T |
| 13. | Zinc sulfate | P, S, T |
| 14. | Somatostatin | T |

### Section 18: Hormones, other Endocrine Medicines and Contraceptives

| Sr. No. | Medicine | Level of Healthcare |
|---|---|---|
| 1. | Dexamethasone | S, T |
| 2. | Fludrocortisone | S, T |
| 3. | Hydrocortisone | P, S, T |
| 4. | Methylprednisolone | S, T |
| 5. | Prednisolone | P, S, T |
| 6. | Ethinylestradiol (A)+ Levonorgestrel (B) | P, S, T |
| 7. | Levonorgestrel | P, S, T |
| 8. | Ormeloxifene (Centchroman) | P, S, T |
| 9. | Hormone releasing IUD | T |
| 10. | IUD containing Copper | P, S, T |
| 11. | Condom | P, S, T |
| 12. | Glimepiride | P, S, T |
| 13. | Insulin (Soluble) | P, S, T |
| 14. | Insulin Intermediate Acting (NPH) | P, S, T |
| 15. | Insulin Glargine | P, S, T |
| 16. | Insulin Premix Injection 30:70 (Regular: NPH) | P, S, T |

*Contd...*

### Section 18: Hormones, other Endocrine Medicines and Contraceptives

| Sr. No. | Medicine | Level of Healthcare |
|---|---|---|
| 17. | Metformin | P, S, T |
| 18. | Teneligliptin | P, S, T |
| 19. | Glucose | P, S, T |
| 20. | Clomiphene citrate | T |
| 21. | Human chorionic gonadotropin | S, T |
| 22. | Medroxyprogesterone acetate | P, S, T |
| 23. | Norethisterone | P, S, T |
| 24. | Carbimazole | P, S, T |
| 25. | Levothyroxine | P, S, T |

### Section 19: Immunologicals

| Sr. No. | Medicine | Level of Healthcare |
|---|---|---|
| 1. | Tuberculin, Purified Protein derivative | P, S, T |
| 2. | Anti-rabies immunoglobulin | P, S, T |
| 3. | Anti-tetanus immunoglobulin | P, S, T |
| 4. | Anti-D immunoglobulin | S, T |
| 5. | Diphtheria antitoxin | P, S, T |
| 6. | Hepatitis B immunoglobulin | S, T |
| 7. | Human normal immunoglobulin | T |
| 8. | Snake Venom Antiserum | P, S, T |
| 9. | BCG vaccine | P, S, T |
| 10. | DPT+ Hib+ Hep B vaccine | P, S, T |
| 11. | DPT vaccine | P, S, T |
| 12. | Hepatitis B vaccine | P, S, T |
| 13. | Japanese encephalitis vaccine | P, S, T |
| 14. | Measles vaccine | P, S, T |
| 15. | Oral poliomyelitis vaccine | P, S, T |
| 16. | Rotavirus vaccine | P, S, T |
| 17. | Tetanus toxoid | P, S, T |
| 18. | Rabies vaccine | P, S, T |

### Section 20: Medicines for Neonatal Care

| Sr. No. | Medicine | Level of Healthcare |
|---|---|---|
| 1. | Alprostadil | S, T |
| 2. | Caffeine | S, T |
| 3. | Surfactant | S, T |

### Section 21: Ophthalmological Medicines

| Sr. No. | Medicine | Level of Healthcare |
|---|---|---|
| 1. | Acyclovir | P, S, T |
| 2. | Ciprofloxacin | P, S, T |
| 3. | Natamycin | P, S, T |
| 4. | Povidone iodine | P, S, T |
| 5. | Prednisolone | P, S, T |
| 6. | Proparacaine | P, S, T |
| 7. | Acetazolamide | P, S, T |
| 8. | Latanoprost | P, S, T |
| 9. | Pilocarpine | P, S, T |
| 10. | Timolol | P, S, T |
| 11. | Atropine | P, S, T |
| 12. | Homatropine | P, S, T |
| 13. | Phenylephrine | P, S, T |
| 14. | Tropicamide | P, S, T |
| 15. | Carboxymethyl cellulose | P, S, T |
| 16. | Hydroxypropyl methylcellulose | T |

### Section 22: Oxytocics and Antioxytocics

| Sr. No. | Medicine | Level of Healthcare |
|---|---|---|
| 1. | Dinoprostone | S, T |
| 2. | Methylergometrine | P, S, T |
| 3. | Mifepristone | P, S, T |
| 4. | Misoprostol | P, S, T |
| 5. | Oxytocin | P, S, T |
| 6. | Betamethasone | P, S, T |
| 7. | Nifedipine | S, T |

### Section 23: Medicines used in treatment of Psychiatric Disorders

| Sr. No. | Medicine | Level of Healthcare |
|---|---|---|
| 1. | Clozapine | T |
| 2. | Fluphenazine | P, S, T |
| 3. | Haloperidol | S, T |
| 4. | Risperidone | P, S, T |
| 5. | Amitriptyline | P, S, T |
| 6. | Escitalopram | P, S, T |
| 7. | Fluoxetine | P, S, T |
| 8. | Lithium | S, T |
| 9. | Sodium valproate | P, S, T |
| 10. | Carbamazepine | P, S, T |
| 11. | Clonazepam | P, S, T |
| 12. | Zolpidem | P, S, T |
| 13. | Clomipramine | P, S, T |
| 14. | Fluoxetine | S, T |
| 15. | Buprenorphine | P, S, T |
| 16. | Buprenorphine (A) + Naloxone (B) | P, S, T |
| 17. | Nicotine (for nicotine replacement therapy) | P, S, T |

*Contd...*

*Contd...*

**Section 24: Medicines Acting on the Respiratory Tract**

| Sr. No. | Medicine | Level of Healthcare |
|---|---|---|
| 1. | Budesonide | P, S, T |
| 2. | Budesonide (A) + Formoterol (B) | P, S, T |
| 3. | Hydrocortisone | P, S, T |
| 4. | Ipratropium | P, S, T |
| 5. | Montelukast | S, T |
| 6. | Salbutamol | P, S, T |
| 7. | Tiotropium | P, S, T |

**Section 25: Solutions correcting Water, Electrolyte Disturbances and Acid-base Disturbances**

| Sr. No. | Medicine | Level of Healthcare |
|---|---|---|
| 1. | Glucose | P, S, T |
| 2. | Glucose(A) + Sodium chloride (B) | P, S, T |
| 3. | Oral rehydration salts | P, S, T |
| 4. | Potassium chloride | P, S, T |
| 5. | Ringer lactate | P, S, T |
| 6. | Sodium bicarbonate | P, S, T |
| 7. | Sodium chloride | P, S, T |
| 8. | Water for injection | P, S, T |

**Section 26: Vitamins and Minerals**

| Sr. No. | Medicine | Level of Healthcare |
|---|---|---|
| 1. | Ascorbic acid (vitamin C) | P, S, T |
| 2. | Calcium carbonate | P, S, T |
| 3. | Calcium gluconate | P, S, T |
| 4. | Cholecalciferol | P, S, T |
| 5. | Pyridoxine | P, S, T |
| 6. | Riboflavin | P, S, T |
| 7. | Thiamine | P, S, T |
| 8. | Vitamin A | P, S, T |

**Section 27: Medicines for COVID–19 management**

| Sr. No. | Medicine | Level of Healthcare |
|---|---|---|
| 1. | Dexamethasone | P, S, T |
| 2. | Enoxaparin | S, T |
| 3. | Methylprednisolone | S, T |
| 4. | Paracetamol | P, S, T |
| 5. | Oxygen | P, S, T |

## Counterfeit Medicine

The WHO defines counterfeit medicines as the one which is "deliberately and fraudulently mislabelled with respect to identity or source." They have been named as SSFFC by the WHO which stands for "substandard, spurious, falsely labelled, falsified and counterfeit (SSFFC) medicines". This can include both generic or branded medicines. The medicines may have active ingredients or may have them in wrong or in doses not sufficient as required.

For any country to curb the production of counterfeit medicines there should be strict policies in place and appropriate implementation. The important factors required for keeping the counterfeit medicines at bay are a strong political commitment, drug regulatory bodies, trade policies, health literacy, cooperation among various stakeholders, having adequate and appropriate legislations.

## SUMMARY

- Essential drugs play an important component of healthcare delivery.
- The concept of essential drugs is mainly focussed on provision of drugs of importance at a cost every individual can afford.
- Along with quality of drugs, essential drugs mainly focus on the public health impact based on priority of diseases thus allowing for flexibility at national level for selection of drugs of essential needs.

## SUGGESTED READING

1. Essential Medicines—an overview | ScienceDirect Topics. https://www.sciencedirect.com/topics/pharmacology-toxicology-and-pharmaceutical-science/essential-medicines.
2. Executive summary: the selection and use of essential medicines 2021: report of the 23rd WHO Expert Committee on the selection and use of essential medicines. Accessed August 1, 2023. https://www.who.int/publications-detail-redirect/WHO-MHP-HPS-EML-2021.01
3. Kar SS, Pradhan HS, Mohanta GP. Concept of Essential Medicines and Rational Use in Public Health. Indian J Community Med. 2010;35(1):10-13.
4. National List of Essential Medicines (NLEM), 2022 | Ministry of Health and Family Welfare | GOI.
5. Shrivastava SRB, Shrivastava PS, Ramasamy J. Public Health Measures to Fight Counterfeit Medicine Market. Int J Prev Med. 2014;5(3):370-371. https://www.ncbi.nlm.nih.gov/pmc/articles/PMC4018649/
6. The National List of Essential Medicines of India 2022 (NLEM 2022): Tommy, Toe the Line - The Lancet Regional Health - Southeast Asia. https://www.thelancet.com/journals/lansea/article/PIIS2772-3682(23)00062-8/fulltext
7. Verma S, Kumar R, Philip P. The Business of Counterfeit Drugs in India: A Critical Evaluation. Published online January 1,2014:141-8.
8. WHO Model List of Essential Medicines - 23rd list, 2023. https://www.who.int/publications-detail-redirect/WHO-MHP-HPS-EML-2023.02

# Index

Page numbers followed by *b* refer to box, *f* refer to figure, *fc* refer to flowchart, and *t* refer to table.

## A

Aam Aadmi Bima Yojana 230
Abacavir 480
Abortion 667, 678
  illegal 705
  induced 678
  rate 224
  spontaneous 678, 1056
  unsafe 679
Abruptio placentae 677
Accidents 694, 705, 719
  deaths 588*f*
  epidemiology of 587
Acclimatization 104, 722
Accredited Social Health Activist 580, 618, 636, 682, 742, 889, 950, 958, 968, 984, 1001, 1064, 1066
Acellular pertussis vaccine 328
Acetic acid 576, 620
Acetylsalicylic acid 1089
Acid rain 79
Acid-base disturbances 1092
Acid-fast bacilli 310, 313
Acquired immunodeficiency syndrome 471, 474, 475, 475*t*, 487, 490, 817, 860, 902, 955
  case surveillance 998
  clinical features of 474
  cocktail therapy 480
  control of 476
  epidemic 472*f*
  epidemiology of 473
  history of 471
  prevention of 476
  symptoms of 474*f*
Actinomycosis 347
Active immunization 256, 378
  agents 256*fc*
Acute diarrheal diseases
  control 365
  epidemiology of 365
  prevention 365
Acute respiratory distress syndrome 694
Acute respiratory infection 261, 265, 268, 685, 694, 748, 752, 759
  burden of 265
  control of 270
  epidemiology of 264, 265
  management of 270
  prevention of 270
Adenovirus 366
Adenylate cyclase 325
Adolescence Education Program 479
Adolescent friendly health
  initiatives 688
  services 688
Adolescent reproductive and sexual health 707, 708
  program 979
Adrenaline 894, 1077*t*
Adverse event following immunization 1074
  categorization of 1074
  cause-specific type of 1074
*Aedes aegypti* 119, 121, 429, 436, 438
  eggs of 121
  index 123, 430
  mosquito breeds 121
*Aedes albopictus* 119
*Aedes vittatus* 119
Aerosols 117, 405
Aflatoxins 652
Agglutinogens 325
Agoraphobia 741
Air (Prevention and Control of Pollution) Act 1052
Air 786
  pollution 78, 79, 79*f*, 83, 748, 908
    carcinogenic effects of 80*fc*
    control of 82, 82*t*
    effects of 80*fc*, 81
    health effects of 80
    interpret measurements of 78
    measuring 81
    prevention of 82, 82*f*
    types of 79
  pressure 72, 73
    knowledge of 73
  quality 720
    index 81, 81*f*, 83
    monitoring 82
  temperature 101
Airborne disease 260*b*, 261, 261*b*, 261*f*, 261*t*, 262, 264*b*, 332
  characteristic of 260
  epidemiology of 261
  general epidemiology of 260
  notification of 264
  prevention of 264
  transmission 260
    dynamics of 262*t*
    prevent 262, 263
Airborne infection control 264, 992
Airborne transmission 252, 260, 403
Airway 322
  management 324
Alanine aminotransferase 453, 462
Albendazole 394, 398, 984, 985
Alcohol 310, 551, 565, 572, 579, 581, 706, 744
  abuse 742
  consumption 547
    trends, worldwide level of 818
  harmful use of 542, 611
  rehabilitation 138
  use 154, 705
    disorders 741
    tackling 575
Alkaline phosphatase 453
Allergy, history of 198
Allethrin 118
Allicin 38
Allopathic medicine 854
Alpha-fetoprotein 769
Alpha-thalassemia 768
Alteplase 615
Altitude 422
  sickness 760
Alveolar infiltrates 336
Alzheimer's disease 713, 766
Amantadine 292, 296, 303
Ambient air quality 100
Amenophis 338*f*
American Cancer Society 576
American College of Cardiology 541
American Diabetic Association 562
American Heart Association 541, 558
American Psychiatry Association 740
American Water Works Association 810
Amino acid 29, 30
  essential 30
  requirement of 29*t*
  score 30
Amlodipine 615
Ammonia 719
Amniotic membranes, condition of 681
Amoebiasis 128, 387, 487
  control 387
  epidemiology of 387
  life cycle of 389*f*
  prevention 387
Amoebic dysentery 115, 761
Amoxicillin 270, 615
  high dose 270
Amphixenoses 403
Ampicillin 270, 894
Amylase rich foods 46
Analgesics 1089
Anaphylaxis 1076, 1076*f*, 1077*t*, 1089
  protocol for management of 1077*fc*
  treatment of 1076
Ancylostoma 396
  *caninum* 397
  *duodenale* 396, 397
Ancylostoma, life cycle of 397*f*
Ancylostomiasis
  control 396
  epidemiology of 396
  prevention 396
Anemia Mukt Bharat 1023, 1025, 1025*f*
  strategy 978

Anemia 153, 517, 630, 635, 678, 728
    classification of 637t, 678t
    effects of 706f
    iron deficiency 635
    nutritional 706
    prevalence of 188, 637, 755
    prophylaxis against 1021
    vicious cycle of 707f
Aneuploidy 766
Anganwadi 687, 1021
    center 160, 708
        scheme 949
    worker 632, 889, 958, 1021, 1064, 1067
Angina, membranous 320
Angiotensin inhibitor 615
Anicteric leptospirosis 417
Animal bites 405
Annapurna Scheme 1023
Annual blood examination rate 425
*Anopheles* 119
    *culicifacies* 120, 121, 422
    *dirus* 422
    *epiroticus* 422
    *fluviatilis* 422
    *minimus* 422
    *stephensi* 422
Anorexia 327
Antara Program 669
Antenatal care 680, 963
    objectives of 680
    registration 1064
    rise of 153
Antenatal healthcare services 688, 1064
Anthocyanins 37
Anthracosis 729
Anthrax 147, 333, 347, 796
    bacillus 795
    endospores 333
    mode of transmission in 334f
Anthrophilism, degree of 426
Anthropometric methods 642
Anthropometry 642
Anthropozoonoses 403
Anti-tuberculosis drugs 314
Antibiotic 324, 328, 457
    penicillin G 324
    prophylactic 328
    prophylaxis 511
    role of 511
    treatment 504
Antibody, protective 378f
Anticancer agents 1090
Antigen
    detection 425
    types of 473
    viral 296
Antigenic drift process, sequence of 298f
Anti-hepatitis C virus 466
Anti-larval operations 446
Antileprosy drugs, second line of 499
Anti-lice shampoos 125
Antimalarial drugs, doses of 427t
Antioxidants 36, 37, 37t
    cellular effects of 37

Antipyretics 1089
Antirabies vaccine 996
Antiretroviral drugs 476, 479, 480
Antiretroviral regimens 481
Antiretroviral therapy 471, 478, 479, 481, 481t, 844, 996
    initiation of 480
    regimens 480
    register 314
Anti-rodent measures 129
Antisepsis 784
Antiseptic 255, 784, 1091
Antitetanus serum 511
Antitoxin, dosage of 323
Anti-tubercular drugs
    classes of 316t
    first line 315t
Antiviral drugs 292, 303
Antyodaya Anna Yojana 1023
Anuria 418
Anxiety disorder, generalized 741
Aorta, diseases of 549
Apathy 740
Appetite
    lack of 457
    loss of 728
Applied Nutrition Program 1023
Aqua privy 96
Aqueous suspensions 117
Arachnida 116
Arenaviridae 531
Argasidae 126
Argemone poisoning 653
Arrhythmias 418
Artemisinin-combination therapy 523
Artery, diseases of 549
Arthralgia 287
Arthritis 246, 287, 558
Arthropod
    borne diseases 115, 115t, 833
    characteristic of 115, 116t
    control of 115, 127
    prevention of 115, 127
Arthrosclerosis, cerebral 742
Artificial finger-nails 784
Asafoetida 41
Asanas 55, 56, 56t
    advantages of 56
Asbestos fibers, types of 728f
Asbestosis 728, 729f, 735
Ascariasis
    control 392
    epidemiology of 392
    prevention 392
*Ascaris lumbricoides* 366, 392
    life cycle of 393f
Ascorbic acid 34, 35
Asepsis 784
Ashtanga yoga 55, 56t
Asian flu 290
Asian tapeworm 347
Aspartate aminotransferase 453
Aspirin 615, 894
Assisted reproductive technology 672

Assman's psychrometer 75
Asthma 609, 767
    childhood 744
    development of 198
Astrovirus 366
Atal Mission for Rejuvenation and Urban Transformation 749
Atal Pension Yojana 230
Atazanavir 480
Atenolol 615
Atmosphere 774
Atmospheric pressure, measurement of 73
Atracurium 1089
Atrial fibrillation 547
Atropine 1089
Attack rate 156, 168, 250
Attention-deficit hyperactivity disorder 741
Attitudes 722
Audit 889
    internal 898
    principles of 898
    types of 898
Auditoria 72
Autism 742
Autoclave 791, 791f
    standards for 792
Autopsy tissues 335
Auxiliary nurse midwife 580, 889, 940, 958, 1011, 1064
Avian flu 261
    control measures for 292
    outbreaks 298
Avian influenza 147, 289, 290, 290t, 291-293, 293t, 296
    groups for 291b
    natural reservoir of 291
    virus, subtypes of 291
Axilla 272
Ayurveda 928
AYUSH
    integration of 1018
    mainstreaming of 959
    research portal 959
    units 1046
Ayushman Arogya Mandir 1029
Ayushman Bharat 929
Ayushman Bharat Digital Mission 1086
Ayushman Bharat Pradhan Mantri Jeevan Jyoti Bima Yojana 230
Ayushman Bharat Program 1028
Azadirachtin 117
Azidothymidine 471
Azithromycin 268, 504

# B

Baby-friendly hospital initiative 698
Bacillary dysentery 115, 339
Bacilli harbors 325, 326
Bacillus Calmette-Guerin 695, 975, 997, 1066
    adverse events with 317
    immune reconstitution inflammatory syndrome 317

vaccination 494
    impact of 316
    vaccine 316, 317
*Bacillus*
    *anthracis* 248, 333-335
    *cereus* 366
    *sphaericus* 446
    *thuringiensis* 446
Backache 454, 455
Baclofen 1089
Bacteria 88, 366, 384, 474, 487
    free water 88
    gram-negative 325
Bacterial meningitis epidemics, elimination of 331
Bacteriological index 497
Bagassosis 730
Bajaj committee 929, 931
*Balamuthia mandrillaris* 339
Balanced mechanical ventilation system 71
Balanitis 487
*Balantidium coli* 90
Balsakha 850
Band neutrophils 270
*Bandicota*
    *bengalensis* 419
    *indica* 419
Barbados diabetes reversal study focus areas 566
Barium carbonate 129
Baroda development screening test for infants 699
Barometers, types of 73
Barometric pressure 725
Barrier method 660
Basal body temperature 668
Basal metabolic rate 55
Baseline population survey 1065
Bat rabies 405
Bayley infant neurodevelopment screen 699
B-cell non-Hodgkin lymphoma 475
Becquerel 77
Beef tapeworm 347
Behavior 168, 466, 886
    change communication 236, 963, 969, 984, 1000, 1013, 1019
    disorders 740
    health problems 154
    interventions 478
    surveillance 148, 998
    unusual 740
Below poverty line 68, 641
Bendiocarb 118
Benzene hexachloride 413
Beta-blockers 615
Beta-carotene 37
Beta-endorphin, release of 53
Beta-glucans 38
Beta-thalassemia 768
Beti Bachao Beti Padhao 231, 1033
BG Prasad classification, modified 68
Bhore Committee 850, 929
Bictegravir 480

Bifenthrin 118
Bilateral healthcare agency 904
    funding of 905
Billing's method 668
Biolarvicides 446
Biological agents 20, 720
Biological disease, categories of 795
Biological integrated detection system 797
Biological weapons 795
    convention 798
Biomedical waste 94, 788, 789
    management 788
        adverse consequences of 788
        benefits of 788
        rules 789, 1052
        segregation of 789$f$
        treatment facility 792
Biopsy 335
    bronchial 335
Biostatistics 198$b$
Bioterrorism 400, 794
    clinical laboratories in 797
Biphasic clinical presentation 333
Bipolar disorders 741
Bird
    flu 291
    influenza viruses 291
Birth
    asphyxia 694
    attendants, training of 512
    defects 689
        cause of 288
        congenital 689
        prevention of 689
        injury 694
    preparation for 697
    preparedness 681, 695
    rate 217, 218
        high 220, 659
        low 220
    unwanted 679
    weight 266
        low 48, 630, 674, 686, 694, 971
Bisphenol A 635
Biting density 426
Bitot's spots 638
Black water fever 424
Bladder cancer 731, 731$t$
Bleaching powder 786
Bleeding 697
    severe 816
Blind trial, triple 178
Blinding glare 110
Blindness 474, 599
    absolute 599
    causes of 600, 600$f$
    control of 601
    curable 599
    epidemiological determinants of 600
    manifest of 599
    nutritional 601
    prevention of 601
Block development officer 938

Blood 434, 728
    agar 323
    bank 473, 1062
    borne diseases
        control 459
        epidemiology of 459
        prevention 459
    borne route, prevention of 477
    cholesterol assay 615
    count, complete 453
    donors, male 146$t$
    forming organs 77
    glucose
        estimation 715
        test strips 615
    pressure 187, 618, 619, 680
        elevated 551
        measure 545$b$
        measurement 546$f$, 615
        recording of 715
        systolic 188
        tracking of 541
    products 1090
    safety 995
        program 929
    sample 418
    separation of 349
    sugar testing 544, 626
    transfusion 761
    urea 544
Bloodstream infection 329
Body
    divisions 116
    fluids 292
    language 886
    mass index 634, 642
    systems 713$f$
    temperature, raised 269
    weight 28, 31, 35, 642
Bone 310
    densitometry 715
Borderline
    lepromatous 496
    tuberculoid 496, 497
*Borrelia*
    *hermsii* 457
    *parkeri* 457
    *turicatae* 457
Botulism 347, 796
Boulogne sore throat 320
Box and Whisker diagram 196
Brain neoplasms 742
Brainstem dysfunction, stage of 406
Breast 574
    cancer 170$f$, 207, 580, 715, 926
        advanced 582
        control of 581, 582$f$
        early detection of 582
        epidemiology of 580
        prevention 581, 582$f$
        problem statement of 581$t$
        screening for 582

disease, benign 581
examination 682
    clinical 582, 620
milk 46
self-examination 582
Breastfeeding 153, 630, 632, 634, 664, 682, 695
    advantages of 696b
    exclusive 153, 368
    practices 630
Breath, shortness of 292, 728
Breathing 695
    noisy 269
Breeding
    habits 423, 423t, 449
    places 120, 121
Breteau index 122, 430
Bristol stool chart 367f
British ability scales 699
Broca index 634
Broken family 66
Bronchial mucosa 289
Bronchiolitis 269
Bronchitis 266
Bronchoalveolar lavage 729
Bronchoscopy 728
Brown dog tick 457
*Brucella*
    *abortus* 345
    *melitensis* 345
Brucellosis 345
*Brugia malayi* 438, 439
Bubonic plague 243f, 412
Buccal mucosa 276
Budget
    advantages of 896
    preparation, major advantages of 896
    purpose of 896
Build healthy public policy 238
Building Construction Regulation Act 122, 229
Bunyaviridae 451
Bupivacaine 1089
Bureau of Indian Standards 915
Bureaucratic management 865
Burnout 733, 733t
Buruli ulcer 93
Butylatedhy droxyanisole 648, 649
Byssinosis 729
Bystanders, role of 592

## C

Caffeine 744
Calcium 36, 38, 40, 41, 43
    channel blocker 615
    supplementation 680
Calendar rhythm method 667
Calf muscle tenderness 418
Calicivirus 366
*Calymmatobacterium granulomatis* 487
*Campylobacter* 366
    *coli* 380
    *enteritis* 381
    *jejuni* 339, 366, 367, 380, 381
    *laridis* 380
    *upsaliensis* 380

Campylobacteriosis 570
    control of 380, 570
    epidemiology of 380
    prevention of 380, 570
Canada for General Public Heat Stress Assessment 103
Cancer 50, 474, 577, 609, 611, 719, 748, 755, 766, 767, 819, 926, 1007
    cervical 472, 483, 585, 715, 744
    cervix
        natural history of 583f
        screening for 584
    colorectal 715
    control 574
        measures for 577f
    diagnosis 576
    education 575
    modifiable risk factors in 574t
    occupational 726, 731
    oral 580
    patterns 571
    prevention 574, 577, 577f, 575t
    prostate 715
    registry program 577
    risk factors for 572
    screening 576
        methods of 576
    types of 574
*Candida*
    *albicans* 474, 487
    *krusei* 345
    *tropicalis* 345
Candidiasis 345
    esophageal 474
Cane sugar 347
Cannabinoids 744
Capacity building 986, 1013, 1033
Carbamates 118
Carbohydrate 29, 38, 40, 41-43, 48, 565
    type of 29, 29t
Carbon
    dioxide 774
    monoxide 79
        levels of 81
Carcinogenic effects 80, 81
Carcinoma 570
    hepatocellular 466
    invasive cervical 475
Cardamom 41
Cardiac rehabilitation 138
Cardiomyopathy 475
Cardiovascular control 433, 549
Cardiovascular diseases 49, 204, 536, 549, 553, 554f, 555, 611, 612, 617, 618f, 619, 620, 669, 766, 926, 1007
    causation of 550f
    classification of 549, 549f
    death rates of 246
    epidemiology of 549, 556
    management of 484
    mortality rates 549b
    prevention of 549, 551
    risk factors for 550, 550b, 551f
Cardiovascular risk prediction chart 619f
Cardiovascular system 80fc

effects on 80
involvement 418
Carditis 558
Carotene 38, 40, 41, 43
Carotenoids 38, 572
Cartridge-based nucleic acid amplification test 311-313
Case based surveillance system 515
Case-control study 170, 170t, 172
    advantages of 172t
    data of 172
    design of 170fc
    disadvantages of 172t
Case-fatality rate 158, 250, 435, 507, 527
Cat cry syndrome 766
Cataract 601, 715
    development of 170
Catarrhal stage 326
Ceftriaxone 894
Cefuroxime 270
Cell
    culture
        derived 446
        vaccines 408
    modification of 768
    wall antigens 382
Cellular extract vaccine 369
Census population, trend of 217f
Centchroman 667, 669
Centers for Disease Control and Prevention 141, 471, 822
Central Births and Deaths Registration Act 928
Central Council of Health and Family Welfare 936
Central Food Technological Research Institute 39
Central Government Health Scheme 737, 1051
Central nervous system 77, 310, 383, 404, 418, 445, 508, 767
    dysfunction 285
    toxoplasmosis 475
Central Pollution Control Board 81, 82
Central Research Institute 1061
Central Social Welfare Board 1062
Cerebral palsy 690, 1045
Cerebrospinal fluid 284, 418, 445, 473, 796, 986
Cerebrovascular disease 549
Cervical
    cap after insertion 662f
    lymph nodes enlargement 300
    mucus secretions 668
    pap smear 715
Cervical cancer 472, 483, 585, 715, 744
    advanced 585
    control of 584, 585f
    early detection of 585
    epidemiology of 582
    prevention 584, 585f
    problem statement of 583t
    risk factors of 583
Cervicitis 487
Cervix uteri 574
Chadha Committee 929, 930
Chagas disease 128
Chancroid 487

Chandipura virus 524
Chandler's index 398
Chemical 720
    agents 20, 720
    biological, radiological and nuclear threats 798
    composition 25
    control 116, 122, 127
    disinfectants 256$t$
    factors 765
    hazards 719, 720
    waste 788
Chemoprophylaxis 259, 294, 296, 301, 303, 414, 419, 427, 498
    long-term 427, 761
    short-term 427
Chemosterilants 129
Chemotherapy 368
Chest
    pain 310
    X-ray 313, 728
Chhaya 667
Chickenpox 261, 274$f$
    epidemiology of 272
Chiggerosis 116
Chikungunya 115, 140, 420, 433, 513, 524, 933, 987
    epidemiology of 433
    fever 986
    life cycle of 434$f$
    prevention 433
    virus 433
Chilblains 723
Child death 1081, 1082
    review 1079
        process 1082
Child development project officer 1021
Child Labor (Prohibition and Regulation) Act 1043
Child Marriage Restraint Act 233, 1044
Child mortality 685, 691, 693, 808$f$, 844
    rate 817$f$
Child survival and safe motherhood 694, 1064
    program 512, 929
Childhood disability 690
    prevention of 690
Childhood infections 688
    prevention and control of 689
Childhood mortality 692$f$, 695$f$
    rate 691$f$
Chinese Healthcare System 852
Chiranjeevi Yojana 850
Chi-square
    distribution table 208
    test 207, 208
Chitta vritti nirodha 55
Chlamydia trachomatis 487, 501, 502
Chloramines 88
Chloramphenicol 457
    doxycyclline 457
Chlorination 86, 88
Chlorine 88, 719
    amount of 88, 89
    solution 86
    tablets 86
    treatment 246
Chloroquine 426, 761
Cholangiopancreatography, endoscopic retrograde 394
Cholera 116, 245, 258, 339, 345, 359, 360, 362, 364$f$, 513, 519$f$, 524, 804
    classification of 362$t$
    control of 140
    deaths 804$t$
    epidemic, investigation of 362
    epidemiology of 359
    impact of 244
    kit, contents of 364$f$
    management of 362$t$
    outbreak of 518$f$
    rapid test for 362$f$
    toxin, mechanism of action of 361$f$
    vaccine
        oral 363, 363$f$, 369
        parenteral 369
Cholesterol 49, 551, 565
    total 626
Chorea 560
Chromosomal disorders 16
Chromosome 765
Chronic obstructive pulmonary disease 19, 604, 604$f$, 605, 609, 616, 726, 751
    control of 604
    epidemiology of 604
    prevention of 604
*Chrysanthemum cinerariaefolium* 116
Cigarettes and Other Tobacco Products Act 575, 580
Ciprofloxacin 761
Cirrhosis 50
City Health Mission 958
Civil registration system 225, 1036
Civil war 840
Clarithromycin 499
Clavulanic acid 270
Climate change 748, 773, 776
    causes of 773, 773$fc$
    impact of 775
    magnitude of 774
    mechanism of 774, 774$f$
Climatic exposure 779
Clonorchiasis 402$f$
*Clostridium*
    *botulinum* 344
    *tetani* 505, 507, 508
Cocaine 744
*Coccidioides* 474
Coccidioidomycosis 474, 475
Cochlear implants 1013
Cognitive behavioral intervention 733
Cohort study 174
    advantages of 175$t$
    design of 173$fc$
    disadvantages of 175$t$
    types of 173
Cold 105
    box 1072, 1072$f$
    common 266
    damage 1069
    effect of 100, 100$fc$
    rooms, walk in 1070
    stress 723
    weather, management of 105
Cold chain
    equipment 1070, 1071, 1073$t$
        procedures 1070, 1071, 1073$t$
        summary 1073$t$
    maintenance 1070
    management 1068
    reverse 1073
Colitis, hemorrhagic 384
Collapse, stage of 361
Colocasia 40
Colombo plan 904
Coma, stage of 406
Common minor vaccine reactions 1075
Communicable diseases 22$t$, 152, 249, 536$f$, 694, 705, 706, 755, 779, 815, 901, 926, 948, 1005
    control of 946, 955, 959
    flexible pool for 960
    goals of 933
Communication 232, 350, 504, 797
    channels of 233
    formal 233
    functions of 886
    impact of 235
    medium of 233
    modes of 886
    nonverbal 233
    one-way 233
    process 232, 232$f$, 233
    purposes 292
    skills 881, 886, 887, 887
    two-way 233
Community 796, 963
    awareness 498$f$
    capacity of 778
    care 67
    diagnosis 150, 152, 154, 162, 830, 834
        methods of 161
        process 162$fc$
        technique of 160
    empowerment 479
    genetics 771, 713
    health 79, 243, 821, 830, 833, 834, 834$t$, 836, 923, 1084
        activities 821
        center 481, 515, 914, 940, 943, 944$t$, 962, 1007, 1011, 1016, 1083
        importance 95, 332
        interventions 152, 810
        management 801, 833, 836
        measurement 824$t$
        needs assessment process 826, 826$f$
        problem 152, 241
        professionals 78
        programs 821
        status of 161
    healthcare seeking behavior of 161
    influences 821
    intervention trial 176, 834

involvement 836
level 633
medicine 6, 6t, 803, 832
    experts 9
    practice 6, 9, 146
    specialists 7, 8, 8f
    triad of 832f
members
    behavior of 232
    practice of 232
mobilization 8, 369, 1019
nutrition 160
ophthalmology 602
organization 822
oriented healthcare 8, 833
participation 123, 610, 823, 839, 949, 958
prolonging longevity of 832
promoting health of 832
Component bar diagram 197
Comprehensive abortion care services 970
Comprehensive cohort
    study 178
    trials 178
Computing air quality index 81
Condom 661f, 669
    counseling 963
    efficacy of 476
    female 476, 661, 662f
    male 476, 660
    programming 478
    promotion 995
    use 476
    vending machines 476
Conflict management, stages of 885f
Congenital anomalies 690, 693, 694
Congenital birth defects
    causes of 689
    risk factors for 689
Congenital disorders 768
Congestion, nasal 268
Conjunctival suffusion 417, 418
Conjunctivitis 287, 1091
    neonatal 490
Connective tissue 909
Constipation 50
Contact diseases 471
    control of 471
    epidemiology of 471
    prevention of 471
Continuous flow method 346
Contraceptive 682
    basket of choice 967
    benefits of 660
    combined injectable 667
    combined oral 664
    counseling for 669
    hormonal 664, 666f, 667
    methods 658f
        effectiveness of 670
    pill
        combined hormonal 664
        emergency 664, 665, 669
        hormonal oral 667
    non-hormonal oral 667
    oral 581, 664, 669, 963
    scheme, home delivery of 967
    technology 955
Convulsions 280, 696
Copenhagen climate change conference 776
Copper T 375 663f
Copper T 380a 663f
Cord traction 681
Core
    disciplines 6
    information 545
    population 487f
    strategies 961, 1010
Corneal clouding 279
Corneal scar 638
Corneal ulceration 638
Corneal xerosis 638
Coronary artery disease 549, 715
Coronavirus disease 2019 (COVID-19) 261, 366, 524, 527, 532
    management, medicines for 1092
    pandemic 308, 741
    testing protocol 534f
    vaccine 534, 535
Corpulence index 634
Corpus uteri 574
Corticosteroid treatment, early 268
*Corynebacterium diphtheriae* 321, 324, 345
Coryza, acute 266
Cosmic radiation 76
Cost-benefit analysis 873, 917
Cost-effectiveness analysis 873, 917, 918
Co-trimoxazole 477
    prophylaxis therapy 476, 483
Cough 292, 327
    classic symptoms of 310
    etiquette 263, 319
    exhaustive paroxysms of 325
Couple protection rate 224, 670
Covaxin 535
Covishield 535
Cowpox lesion 831
*Coxiella burnetii* 345
Crash protective vehicle design 592
C-reactive protein 559
Cresol 786
Crimean-Congo hemorrhagic fever 147, 451, 454, 514, 524, 527
Critical path method 871
Cross ventilation 71
Cross-sectional study 175
    design of 175fc
Croup, malignant 320
Crude birth rate 217
    pattern of 217
    trend of 218f
Crude death rate 158, 217, 810f
Crude phenol 786
Crustacea 116, 126
Cryosphere 774
Cryptococcal disease 483
Cryptococcosis, extrapulmonary 475
Cryptococcus 474
Cryptosporidiosis 474, 475
*Cryptosporidium* 86, 366, 474, 525
Crystalline silica 727f
*Ctenocephalides*
    *canis* 116t
    *felis* 116t
Cubic space 112
*Culex* 119, 121, 121t
    *fatigans* 439
    *quinquefasciatus* 439, 441
    *tritaeniorhynchus* 443
    *vishnui subgroup* 121
Cushing's syndrome 541
Cyanosis 269
    central 697
Cyclone 774, 780
Cyclops 126
    transmitted diseases 116
*Cyclospora* 366
    *cayetanensis* 339
Cyclozoonoses 400
Cyfluthrin 118
Cypermethrin 118
Cysteine 29
    stones 50
Cystic fibrosis 766
Cystitis 487
Cytomegalovirus 251, 259, 366, 474, 573
    infection 474, 475
Cytotoxic waste 788

## D

Dagger and asterisk system 908
*Dai* 681
Dairy farms, sanitation of 345
Dakshata-online learning program 1086
Danger signs 681, 682
Dangerous epidemic disease 1041
Danish International Development Agency 904
Darunavir 480
Data
    collection
        methods 192, 892
        system, types of 625
        tool 192
    documentation sheet 193
    entry tools 193
    management, planning for 185
    presentation 194
        methods of 194, 194fc
    types of 188f
    utilization of 644
Day care centre 1015
Dead, burial of 782
Deafness 285, 288, 715
Death 406, 519f
    Bertillon classification of causes of 907
    causes of 693f, 747, 747t, 759f, 1079
    certificate 1079
    child 1081, 1082
    infant 1081

medical certification of cause of 1079
neonatal 819, 1081
post-neonatal 1081
pregnancy-related 676
premature 714f
rate 217, 218, 246
   age-specific 159, 160
   high 244
   low 659
   specific 158
statistics 960
Deep burial, standards for 792
Deep trench latrine 97f
Deep vein thrombosis 549
Defense medical services 951
Defibrillator 615
Dehydration 327, 367
Delirium 712
Delivery 510, 969
  expected date of 680
Delphi technique 828
Delta variant 533
Deltamethrin 118
Dementia 246, 715
  development of 187
Demographic health survey 68, 645
Demographic transition model 218f
Dengue 133, 140, 420, 933, 986, 987
  control 428
  epidemiology of 428
  fever 115, 122, 418, 428, 431t, 513, 525, 987
    treatment of 431
  hemorrhagic fever 115, 147, 418, 428, 431, 513, 1003
  prevention 418
  shock syndrome 513, 1003
  virus infections, manifestations of 430f
Dental fluorosis 1026
Deoxyribonucleic acid 460, 473, 635, 769
Depression 195, 705
  management of 484
Dermatitis 116
  allergic contact 730
  occupational 730
Dermatolymphangioadenitis, acute 440
Detergent 255
Dew point 74, 75
Deworming 636, 707, 1024
  dose and regime for 1024t
Dextrose infusion 615
Dhyana 57
Diabetes mellitus 48, 310, 319, 542, 551, 562, 567, 569, 601, 611, 613, 613t, 616, 669, 715, 755, 766, 767, 926, 1007
  control 562
  epidemiology of 562
  gestational 562, 970
  insulin resistance 712
  malnutrition-related 562
  management of 565
  prevention 562
  tuberculosis with 319
  types of 16

Diabetic eye complications 601
Diagnostic test 142, 142t, 452
Diaphragm 661
Diarrhea 50, 133, 153, 279, 292, 345, 365-367, 367b, 368, 382, 384, 418, 475, 613, 613t, 693, 972
  acute
    bloody 365
    watery 365
  bloody 366, 366t
  childhood 368f
  control of 369f, 370, 974
  diseases 367b, 694, 926
    chronic 384
    control of 367
    prevention of 367
  osmotic 367, 367t
  persistent 365, 366
  prevention of 369f, 370
  secretory 367, 367t
  traveler's 366, 384, 760, 761
  types of 342t
Diatoms 88
Diazepam 615
Dichlorodiphenyltrichloroethane 91, 413, 421, 573, 963
Diclofenac 894, 1089
Didanosine 480
Diet 551, 611
Dietary
  advice 680
  assessment 643, 644
  cholesterol consumption 32
  factor 27, 581
  fat 32
    intake 170f
  fiber 37, 37t, 49
  folate 34
  goals 27
  practices 630, 636
  sources 33
Dietetics 25
Diethylstilbestrol 666
Differential leukocyte count 453
Digenetic parasite 448
Digestive disorders 366
Digestive system, diseases of 909
Diltiazem 615
Diphtheria 261, 320, 321, 321b, 323, 324, 345, 513, 524, 680, 699, 1066
  antitoxin 323
    dosage of 323t
  cutaneous 322, 323
  epidemiology of 320
  malignant 323
  outbreak of 321
  pertussis tetanus 257, 695, 975
    replacement of 510f
  toxoid 323
Dipylidium caninum 116
Direct Benefit Transfer Schemes 993
Direct Healthcare Services 1058
Directly observed therapy 320

Directorates General of Health Services 852
Disability 138, 547, 588
  adjusted life year 396, 542, 595, 804, 824, 849, 926
  alleviation of 442
  limitation 138, 606, 770
  prevention 138, 499, 1045
    and medical rehabilitation 499, 1000
  rate 157
  reduction of 332
  types of 690
Disaster
  classification of 778t
  management 778
    Act 1042
    cycle 780, 780f
  manmade 778
  natural 778, 815
  phase 781
  types of 778, 780t
Discomfort index 101
Disinfectants 255, 256, 786, 1091
  effects of 461, 467
  mass distribution of 781
Disinfection 783
  efficacy of 255f
  procedures 786
  prophylactic 255
  terminal 255
Disposable delivery kit, ensuring adequate supply of 512
Disseminated endemic mycosis 475
Distance vision impairment 600
District Blindness Control Societies 1014
District Health Mission 958
District Level Household Survey 161
District Malaria Officer 937
District Mental Health Program 742, 745, 1015
District Program Management Unit 958
District Tuberculosis Center 990
District Tuberculosis Officer 937
District Tuberculosis Program 928
Diuretics 1091
Dizziness 454, 455, 543
Doll and Hill study 246
Dolutegravir 480, 481
Domestic
  accidents 927
  rodents 128
  tourist visits 759
  violence 1043
    Act 1042
Donor agencies 905t
Donovanosis 487
Double blind trial 178
Double chamber incinerator 791f
Double pyramid model 44f
Down's syndrome 764, 766
Dowry Prohibition Act 1043
Doxycycline 336, 427, 457, 761
Dracontiasis 116
Dracunculiasis 385
  control of 385

epidemiology of 385
prevention of 385
*Dracunculus medinensis* 90, 385
life cycle of 386*f*
Drinking water 751, 1049
acceptability parameters of 90*t*
bacteriological quality of 90*t*
boiling of 127
chemical parameters of 91*t*
facilities 85
filtration of 127
quality, surveillance of 90
sources of 85*f*
supply 90
surveillance 90
Droplet transmission 260
Dropsy, epidemic 653
Drowning 594, 595
Drowsy 696
Drugs 315, 316, 551, 563, 761, 995
abuse 705
and Cosmetics Act 1041
class 545
de-addiction Program 1012
dosage of 482
logistics information and management system 1036
regimen 992
sensitive testing 989
susceptibility testing 313
therapy, triple 985
use 705
Dry bulb thermometer 100, 102, 103, 103*f*
Dug well 96
Dumb rabies 407
Dust powders 117
Dyscalculia 690
Dysentery 345, 384
Dysgraphia 690
Dyslexia 690
Dyslipidemia 52, 542, 715
Dyspnea 336

# E

Ear
nodular infiltration of 496*f*
nose and throat medicines 1091
Earthquakes 780
Eating disorders 705
Ebola 254, 796
virus
disease 147, 514, 527
ecology of 528*f*
*Echinococcus granulosus* 401
Eclampsia 677
management of 677
Ecological studies 169, 170, 645
advantages of 169
Economic growth 844
Ectoparasites 487
Edema 631
Education 168, 223, 504, 633, 855, 902
Efavirenz 476, 477, 480

Effective couple protection rate 671
Efficient human resource management system, implementation of 854
Egg, nutritive value of 43*t*
E-health 1083, 1084
Eight Millennium Development Goals 843*f*
Electric discharge 109
Electrical hygrometer 75
Electrocardiogram 715
Electrolyte disturbances 1092
Electronic
health records 1085
scale 631
vaccine intelligence network 839, 1036, 1069
initiative 895
Elek immunoprecipitation test 323
Elephantiasis 438
Elvitegravir 480
E-Mamta 1084
Embolic stroke 547
Emergency medical system 592
Emerging diseases 523
epidemiology of 526
impact of 523
Emesis 457
Emotional intelligence, Daniel Goleman dimensions of 705
Emotional support therapy 548
Employees Compensation Act 229
Employees Provident Funds and Miscellaneous Provisions Act 229
Employees State Insurance 850
Act 229, 1046
Scheme 737, 850, 1046
Employment Exchange Act 229
Emtricitabine 480
Enalapril 615
Encephalitis 128, 406, 474, 524
End tuberculosis strategy 319, 988
Endemic typhus 451
Endocrine system, disorders of 541, 633
Energy 28, 1021
expenditure 54*t*
Enfuvirtide 480
Engineering method 107
*Entamoeba histolytica* 90, 342, 345, 366, 388, 487
Enterovirus 366
Entomological index 430, 441
Entomology 115
Environmental (Protection) Act 1052
Environmental health 7, 901
Act 122
management 876
problem 153
safety Laws 1041, 1052
Environmental Hygiene Committee 111
Environmental management 122
Environmental pollution 573
reducing 575
Environmental protection 844
Environmental risk 819, 927
factors 722

Environmental sanitation 948
improvement of 363
Environmental tobacco smoke 81
Enzyme-linked immunosorbent assay 279, 280, 284, 288, 334, 388, 407, 445, 452, 475, 527, 531, 796
technique, rabies specific 407
E-Olakh 1084
Epidemic Diseases Act 1041
Epidemic intelligence service 526
Epidemic Medical Officer 937
Epidemic prone diseases 513
diagnosis of 516
Epidemic typhus 116
Epidemiological studies, classification of 164*t*
Epidemiological triad 322
Epidemiology 6, 151, 277, 726, 873
concept of 150
role of 514
triangle of 22*f*
uses of 152
Epididymitis 487
Epididymo-orchitis 284, 440
Epiglottitis, acute 266
Epinephrine 615
Episiotomy, site of 682
Epizootic 249
Epornithic disease 291, 296
Epstein-Barr virus 474, 573
Equine
antitoxin 511
rabies immunoglobulin 259
Equity 865, 953
Ergonomics 733
hazards 720
Ergot 652
Erythema nodosum leprosum 498*f*
Erythematous skin patch 496
Erythrocyte sedimentation rate 433, 559
Erythrocytic schizogony 423
Erythromycin 324, 457
Eschar, triad of 457
*Escherichia coli* 89, 366, 382-384, 387
enteroaggregative 342, 366, 383, 384
enterohemorrhagic 383
enteroinvasive 366, 383
enteropathogenic 366, 382
enterotoxigenic 382, 383
infection
control 382
epidemiology of 382
prevention 382
types of 384*t*
Estimated delivery date 680
Estriol 769
Ethambutol 315
Ethinyl estradiol 666
Ethionamide 499
Ethnicity 168, 466
Etravirine 480
Eugenics 768, 769
European Society of Cardiology 541
European Society of Hypertension 541
Excreta disposal, methods of 96

Exercise 30, 52, 55, 565
  aerobic 53
  regimes 54
  regular 54
Extrinsic incubation period 253, 420
Eye
  diseases 246
  donation 602
  medical examination of 715
  protection 263
  seeking flies 502

# F

Face, swelling of 728
Facial expressions 886
Factories Act 737, 1048
Fainting 1076
Falciparum
  incidence, annual 425
  malaria 418
    treatment of 427t
Falls 595
Family 65
  cycle 65
  functions of 66
  health 901
  income 69
  life education 709
  physicians 851
  planning 223, 659, 660, 672, 852, 931, 948
    commissions 852
    logistics management information system 967
    method 669
    postpartum 669
    program 1064
  redefining of 66
  size 222
  types of 65
  welfare 659, 660, 869, 937, 1062
    central sector 960
    services 689
Farmer's lung disease 729
Fasciola hepatica 347
Fascioliasis 402f
Fastidious growth hampers 327
Fasting glucose, impaired 565
Fat 30, 31, 565
  visible 31
Fatal cardiovascular diseases, risk stratification of 552t
Fatigue 728
Fatty acids 31
  saturated 31
  types of 31t
  unsaturated 31
Fatty liver disease, non-alcoholic 609
Fecal
  laboratory studies 367
  occult blood test 576
  streptococci 90
Feces 786
  disease from 95f
  disinfection of 786t
  examination 342
Feeding
  bottles 1043
  complementary 47
  habits 121
  practices 639
Fentanyl 1089
Fertility 222, 1037
  control 225
  indicators 222, 222t, 223
  rate 223
    total 153, 224, 658
Fetal
  loss 1056
  movements 677
  tissue sampling 770
Fetoscope 1066
Fever 268, 269, 285, 386, 417, 454, 455, 457, 558, 1076
  dengue 115, 122, 418, 428, 431t, 513, 525, 987
  enteric 345, 371
  epidemic relapsing 116
  filarial 440
  hemorrhagic 128
  high-grade 292, 296
  louse-borne relapsing 451, 457
  relapsing 116
  rheumatic 555, 556, 560
  surveillance 431
  triad of 457
  typhoid 246, 339, 370, 372
  viral hemorrhagic 796
Fiber 565
  foods, moderate 37
Field epidemiology training program 525
Filaria 984f
Filariasis 115, 441f, 933, 984
  acute 440
  control 438, 441
  epidemiology of 438
  prevention 438, 441
Finance
  auditing 897
  management 896, 961, 1009
    information system 1036
    techniques 871, 873, 873t
First aid 1062
First referral unit 677, 944, 1011
Fitness 54
Five-year plans 931
Fixed-dose combinations drugs 315t
*Flavivirus* 451, 528
  *fibricus* 435
Flavonoids 37, 38
Flea 124
  bites, protection against 337
  borne typhus 451, 457
  index, specific 124
  life cycle of 124f
  percentage incidence of 124
  types of 124
Floods 780
Fluid
  balance 677
  inoculation of 831
Fluorescence
  angiography 715
  light-emitting diode microscope 313
  microscopy 425
Fluoride level 1027
Fluoroquinolone 316
Fluorosis
  endemic area 1026
  surveillance of 1026
Fly
  borne diseases 115
  life cycle of 123
Fogging 446
Folic acid 34, 963
  supplementation 680, 979, 1024, 1024t
  tablet 702, 1024f
Fomite 252, 502
Food 25, 35, 38, 40
  additives 366, 648
  adulteration 48, 650
    Act, prevention of 25, 650, 1054
  allergy 50, 744
  and nutrition surveys, large-scale 645
  and water, safety of 363
  articles 648
  bacterial contamination of 342, 342t
  balance sheets 644
  borne diseases 342, 775
    epidemiology of 342
    outbreak, investigation of 350
    transmission of 342
  borne infections 342, 342t
    control of 344
    prevention 344
  classification of 25
  contaminants 572
    points of 343f
  economics 634
  establishments, investigation of 351
  fortification 636, 649, 707
    advantages of 650
  frequency questionnaire 643
  group 36-38, 45, 544
    balance of 43, 44t
  handlers 351
    hygiene 344
  hygiene 759
  ingested 342
  intake 567
  item 44, 48, 650
  low fiber 37
  phytochemicals in 38t
  plate 44
    concept of 43
  poisoning 345, 347, 514
    bacterial causes of 342, 342t
  preservatives 48, 648
    toxic effects of 649t
  processing techniques 343, 343t

pyramid, concept of 43
quality of 630
rainbow 40
records 643
safety 343, 781
    and standards Act 1053
    Laws 1041, 1053
sampling 351
security 630
stuffs 42, 651
toxicants 48, 650
Foot care program 441
Ford foundation 905
Formalin 786
Fostering disease awareness 332
Fragile X syndrome 766
Framingham Heart Study 175, 246
*Francisella tularensis* 339
Freedom, degrees of 205, 206
Frost nip 105
Frostbite 105, 723
Fumigation 129
Fundamental human right 899
Funding 901, 984
    agencies 539
    audit regarding provision of 898
    primary methods of 860
Fundoscopic examination 715
Funeral expenses 1048
Fungal
    agents 487
    infections 345
Fungi 474
Funiculitis 440
Furious rabies 407
Furosemide 615
Fusarium toxins 654

## G

Galactosemia 50
Gallbladder disease 50
Gamete intrafallopian transfer 672
Gamma variant 533
Gamma-aminobutyric acid 57
Gantt chart 871, 872$f$
Garbage 94, 112
Gaseous emissions 790
Gastroenteritis 115, 373, 761
Gastrointestinal problems 50, 1027
Gastrointestinal system 77
Gender related development index 17
Gene 765
    multiple 766
    therapy 768
General fertility rate 223
General flea index 124
General random blood sugar 553
Generic antiretrovirals 480$t$
Genetic 633, 764
    constitution 765
    control 118, 122
    counseling 16, 769
    disorder 689, 764, 766, 771

effects 724
engineering, use of 795
factors 550, 563
heritage 767
inheritance, types of 766
susceptibility 310
Geneva protocol 798
Genital
    hygiene, lack of 584
    molluscum contagiosum 487
    scabies 487
    ulcer 490
    warts 487, 584
Genitourinary system 310
    diseases of 909
Genotype 765, 765$f$
Gerber's test 347
Geriatric 711
    assessment, comprehensive 714
    health 711
        problems 712
    healthcare
        centers 715
        includes 714$b$
        services 715
    services 1010
Germ theory 19, 245, 248
    concept of 248
    discovery of 831
    limitations of 19
Get2020 505
*Giardia* 90, 366
    *intestinalis* 366, 390, 391
    *lamblia* 366, 487
Giardiasis 347, 390, 487
    control of 390
    epidemiology of 390
    life cycle of 391$f$
    prevention of 390
Glare 110
Glaucoma 601, 715
Glimepiride 615
Global Adult Tobacco Survey 744, 1038
Global cholera epidemic 243
Global Dengue Situation and Strategy for Prevention and Control 432
Global health 842
    level of 838
    security 285
    situation 815
Global leprosy strategy 1001$f$
Global noncommunicable disease network 539
Global polio eradication initiative 357
Globe thermometer 100
Glucometer 615
Glucose 368
    injectable solution 615
    tolerance, impaired 562, 565
Glycemic index 29, 48
Glyceryl trinitrate 615
Glycogen 29
Glycopyrrolate 1089

Goiter 641
Gonorrhea 487
Good Health Financing System 849
Gram Panchayat 938
Gram Sabha 938
Granular activated carbon 86
Granules 117
Granuloma inguinale 487
Gravity flow autoclave 792
Greenhouse gases, sources of 774$t$
Gross domestic product 17, 852, 867, 916
Gross national product 916
Gross reproduction rate 224
Group communication 236
Growth 685
    chart 701$f$
    monitoring of 630, 632, 645, 698
    rate 751
Guillain-Barré syndrome 381
Guinea worm
    disease 90, 93, 126, 385
    larvae of 126

## H

H antigen 289
H1N1 influenza 254, 524
    virus 244
Haddon matrix 589
    phases in 589$f$
*Haemaphysalis* 452
    *spinigera* 451, 452
*Haemophilus*
    *ducreyi* 487
    *influenzae* 325, 510, 688
    *influenzae B* 148, 270, 699
        *epiglottitis* 323
        *meningitis* 810
Hallucinogens 744
Halogenic acids 790
Halothane 1089
Hand arm vibration syndrome 724, 724$f$
Hand hygiene 262, 263
    major forms of 784$t$
Handicap 138, 138$f$
Handwashing 245, 262, 784
    steps of 785$f$
Hantavirus pulmonary syndrome 261
Hard tick 125, 125$f$, 126$t$
Hardy-Weinberg
    equilibrium 765
    law 765, 766$f$
Harmful agents
    elimination of 735
    substitution of 735
Harmful hazards, elimination of 735
Hazard 720
    analysis 349
    respiratory 719
Head injury 172
Headache 417, 454, 455, 457, 543, 677
    sudden onset of 336
Health 14, 25, 55, 74, 93, 105, 150, 368$f$, 702, 852, 902, 928

adjusted life expectancy 824
and Wellness Center 1029, 1030
assistant
    female, job responsibilities of 946
    male, job responsibilities of 947
belief model 67
centers 619, 939, 941
challenges, human resources for 856
child 153, 685, 816, 925, 947
communication 232
    application of 236
    methods in 233
    types of 233
concept of 13, 14
concerns 649
conditions, measurement of 834
consequences 596, 748
department 852
determinants of 16, 16f
development 833
dimensions of 14, 14f, 15
economics 227, 916, 916f
education 123, 125, 136, 237, 390, 394, 396, 409, 419, 478, 489, 544, 708, 823, 839, 1084
    approach 237
    level for 238
    principles of 237
educator, job responsibilities of 946
equity 64, 226
    assessment 749
facilities 876, 889, 974t
finance 859-861, 954
for all by 2000 842
goal 831
hazards 84, 718, 720f
human resources for 854
impact 537
    assessments 123
index 934
indicators 747b, 755
information
    digital records of 1085
    systems 910
infrastructure and human resource 954
insurance 230, 841, 950
issues 705, 705t
laws, classification of 1040
legislations 1040
magazines 235
major determinant of 7
management 7, 863, 873
    information system 161, 889, 954, 960, 961, 969, 1034, 1085
manager 875
manpower development 1010
planning 874
    cycle 875
    steps in 875
plus nutrition 684
policies 853
    and programs 324, 953
problems 152, 153, 154, 183, 710, 876

specific approach 835
program 464, 960
    evaluation of 152
promotion 57, 67, 136, 237, 270, 538, 564, 606, 612, 706, 713, 1009
    activities 612, 612f, 945
research
    domains of 183t
    uses of computer in 214
risk during travel, determinants of 759
schemes 464
screening 702
sector reforms, four sets of 840f
seeking behavior 60
service 17, 400, 825, 951
    availability of 161
    coverage of 954
    evaluation trial 176
    research, conduction of 8, 152
situation 925
    analysis of 875
    human resources for 855
social determinants of 62, 62f, 63f
spectrum of 15, 16f
status 751, 754, 954
surveillance, use of 147
survey 912
    and Development Committee 850
system 226, 687, 796, 797, 835, 848, 854, 901, 919
    components of 919
    functions 848
    organization of 934, 936, 937
    performance 954
    reform, concept of 840
    research 919, 920, 920b, 920f, 920t, 921f
    resilience 921
    strengthening 954, 992
    structure 848
    WHO definition of 919b
worker 854
    current stock of 854
    female 940, 947, 958
    male 940, 947
    protection of 414
workforce 854
Healthcare 73, 75, 231, 852, 853, 863, 928, 1084
    agencies 899
    types of 899
    delivery 756
    facilities 958
    indicators 160
    system 6, 7, 848, 850fc, 934, 935fc, 1058
    financing 859
    sources of 859
    level of 1089, 1089t, 1090, 1092
    medicalization of 838
    poor coverage of 154
    professionals 332
    quality control 914
    radiation in 78
    responses 183

secondary level of 940
services 8, 225, 331, 363, 464, 558, 683, 709, 737, 851, 851fc, 852, 853f, 853, 928
system 850, 876
    concept of three-tier 940
    hospital-based 837
    mixed 850
    proper functioning of 859
    public support for 861, 862
    status of 939
    types of 849
tertiary level 940
workers 263b, 821
    control 318
Healthy community 823
    characteristic of 823f
Healthy dietary habits and lifestyle, promoting 690
Hearing 699
    aids 1013
    disorders 246
    impairment 690, 1045
    loss
        noise-induced 107, 719, 723
        prevention of 1013
Heart
    attack 134
    disease 748, 819
        congenital 549
        coronary 174, 609
        ischemic 52, 549
        rheumatic 549, 556–558, 558f, 559, 559t, 560, 560t, 561
    involvement 558
    muscle, damage 323
Heat 718
    action plan 750
    cramp 102, 722
    damage 1068
    disorders, prevention and management of 722
    effects of 100, 461
    exhaustion 102, 102t, 722
    health action 105
    illnesses, development of 722
    index 74, 75, 103
    rash 101, 722
    stress 101, 719, 721, 722
        effects of 101
        indices 102
    stroke 102, 102t, 723
    syncope 722
    syndrome 74
    waves 774
*Helicobacter pylori* 525, 572, 573
Helmet wearing, mandatory laws on 592
Helminth 397, 474
Hemagglutination inhibition 445
Hemagglutinin, filamentous 325
Hematopoietic system 77
Hemochromatosis 766

Hemoglobin 194, 635*t*
   disorders
      severe 764
         trait genes for 764
   glycated 565
   level 199, 453
Hemoglobinopathy, gene-related 767
Hemolytic uremic syndrome 376, 383
Hemophilia 768
*Hemophilus influenzae* 463
Hemoptysis 310
Hemorrhage 417, 677
   antepartum 677
   postpartum 677, 681
Hemorrhagic manifestations 288, 418
Hendra virus infection 514
Henipaviral diseases 527
Heparin 615
Hepatitis 50, 147, 492, 682, 699, 705
   A 257, 339, 345, 760
      virus 345, 377, 378
   acute 168*t*, 520*f*, 521*f*
   B 257, 459, 460, 464, 472, 510, 818
      birth dose 697
      coinfection 483
      control of 459
      core antigen 460
      diagnosis of 462*f*
      epidemiology of 459
      prevention of 459
      surface antigen 477
      vaccine 369
      virus 461, 487, 572, 575
   C 465, 472, 477
      characteristic of 465
      coinfection 483
      control of 465
      epidemiology of 465
      natural history of 466
      prevention of 465
      virus 572, 818
   E 339, 378, 379, 379*t*
      virus 345
   vaccination 478
   viral 116, 345, 379, 418, 469, 818
Herd immunity 137, 258, 259
   concept of 137*f*
   levels 259*t*
Herpes
   genitalis 487
   simplex virus 486
   virus 251, 474
Hexachlorocyclohexane 91
High efficiency particulate air systems 787
High fever headache 457
High test hypochlorite 86
High-density lipoprotein-cholesterol 626
Hill cultivation type 754
Hindu Marriage Act 223
Histidine 29
Histocompatibility complex 563
Histogram 196
*Histoplasma* 474

Histoplasmosis 402*f*, 474
   extrapulmonary 475
Hoarseness 728
Hodgkin's disease 574
Holder method 346
Holistic management 1017
Homelessness 705
Homeopathy 955
Homicide 705
Hong Kong flu 290
Honorarium 959
Hookworm 396
Hormonal methods 660
Hormone 563, 573, 1091
   replacement therapy 573
Hospital infection control 294
Hospital management information system 1035*fc*
Hospital waste, types of 788
Hospital-acquired infections 783
   epidemiology of 783
Host 249
   characteristics of 21*f*
   defense mechanisms 253
House flies 123
   diseases transmitted by 123
House index 122, 430
House mouse mite 457
Housefly, life cycle of 123*f*
Household food record method 644
Household noise 106
Household water treatment and safe storage 86
   methods 86
Household wealth 693
Human acquire inhalational anthrax 333
Human artificial chromosomes 768
Human blood index 426
Human chorionic gonadotropin 769
Human development
   historical index of 805*f*
   index 17, 805, 824, 825
      components 825*t*
Human disease, risk factors for 170
Human genome project 768
Human health 105, 400
Human herpesvirus 487, 572
Human immunodeficiency virus 145, 146, 307, 310, 318, 319, 319*fc*, 459, 471, 472*t*, 475, 475*t*, 483, 487, 495, 572, 615, 674, 680, 682, 687, 705, 706, 748, 817, 860, 902, 973
   care setting 318
   control of 471, 476
   counselling 478
   early detection of 996
   encephalopathy 475
   epidemic 472*f*
   epidemiology of 471, 473
   history of 471
   infected syringe of 478
   infection 482
      prevention of 476, 481

   substantial risk of 482
   treatment of 481
   needle transmission of 478
   nephropathy 475
   positive tuberculosis 314
   prevalence 926
   prevention 471, 476
   prompt treatment of 996
   screening 146*t*
   sentinel surveillance 998
   status, classification on 314
   structure of 473*f*
   syndrome, acute 474
   testing 478
      strategy for 475*f*
   treatment service, three-tier model of 481
Human immunoglobulin 281
Human infections 290
   viruses 290
Human leukocyte antigen 557
Human papillomavirus 257, 485, 487, 572, 575, 616
   infection 583
Human poverty index 17, 18
Human protein requirements 30
Human rabies 407
   immunoglobulin 259
   prevention of 407
Human resource development 1003
Human respiratory
   syncytial virus 265
   tract 265
Human T-cell lymphotropic virus 471
Human tetanus immunoglobulin 511
Human waste 91
Humidex 74, 75, 103
Humidification, artificial 1049
Humidifier 74
   types of 74
Humidity 74, 75, 422, 467, 722
   absolute 74, 75
   low 74, 74*t*
   measuring 74
   relative 74, 75, 262
Huntington's disease 766
Hyalomma anatolicum 451
Hydatid disease 339
Hydatidosis 401*f*
Hydrocele 440
Hydrochlorothiazide 615
Hydrocortisone 615, 1077*t*
Hydrogen sulfide 719
Hydrophobia 404, 407
Hygiene 505, 830
   services 927
Hygrometer 74, 75
*Hymenolepis diminuta* 116, 128
Hyperglycemic effects 319
Hypertension 49, 541, 541*t*, 544*f*, 544*t*, 551, 601, 609, 616, 669, 715, 766
   chronic 677
   classification of 541
   clinical features of 543

complications of 543
epidemiology of 541
essential 541
gestational 677
pharmacotherapy for 545t
prevention of 541
risk factors for 542
secondary 541
surveillance in 545
Hypertensive disorders 677
classification of 677t
Hyperthermia 269, 696
Hyperthyroidism 541
Hypochlorite ions 88
Hypochlorous acid, formation of 88
Hypothermia 105, 694, 696, 723
Hypothesis 169
facts 520
stating alternate 204
testing 204
two-tailed 205
Hypothyroidism, congenital 770
Hypoxia, result of 327

# I

Ibalizumab 480
Ibuprofen 615, 1089
Ice pack 1072, 1072f
conditioning of 1072
Iceberg, tip of 24
Ice-lined refrigerator 194, 893, 1070
basket of 270
Icteric leptospirosis 417
Iliotibial band injuries 58
Illiteracy 742
Illness 18, 18t, 295
duration of 373t
phase of 452
Illumination, level of 109
Imidazole 761
Immersion foot 105
Immoral Traffic Act in Women and Girls Act 229
Immoral Traffic Prevention Act 489, 1043
Immune response 253, 557
Immunity 261, 278, 283, 287, 291, 325, 330, 353, 359, 372, 422, 460, 466, 494, 502, 507
cell mediated 494
herd 137, 258, 259
status 20
types of 253fc
waning 259
Immunization 137, 263, 281, 328, 363, 374, 378, 511, 632, 680, 708, 806, 852, 974, 1022
activities, supplementary 355
agenda 281
anxiety 1075
childhood 699
passive 258, 280, 281, 378, 409, 511
program 288

routine 354, 355
status 266
supply chain levels 1068f
Immunochromatographic card test 441
Immunofluorescent antibody titer 445
Immunoglobulin 46
A 142
G 142, 378
M 378, 796
antibody 287
Immunohistochemistry, pleural biopsy for 335
Immunoprophylaxis 1000
Impulse noise 107
In vitro fertilization 672
In vivo
gene therapy 768
technique 768
Inactivated polio vaccine 355, 356, 1066
Inanition 712
Incineration 94, 789
advantages of 791
disadvantages of 791
principles of 790
Incisional vasectomy 668
scalpel incisions 668
Incontinence 712
Incubation period 249, 300f, 796
uses of 253
Indecent Representation of Women (Prohibition) Act 1040
India Newborn Action Plan 690
India Population Trajectory 219f
Indian Council of Medical Research 183, 556, 560, 577, 1059
Indian Healthcare Agencies 1058
Indian Healthcare System 850, 928
evolution of 928
Indian Public Health Standard 858, 914, 959
Indian Red Cross Society 1061
Indian tick typhus 451, 457
Indinavir 480
Indira Awaas Yojana 114
Indira Gandhi National Old Age Pension Scheme 716
Indoor air pollution 310
sources of 80fc
Industrial anthrax, incidence of 335
Industrial wastes 94
Industrial workers, consumer price index for 68
Infant and young child feeding 695
practices 153
promotion of 636
Infant milk substitutes 1043
Infant mortality 691, 694
causes of 694
control of 694
prevention of 694
rate 692, 824, 855, 1064
Infections 249, 270, 345, 563, 630fc, 689, 696b, 742, 816
bacterial 345, 347, 483
chain of 274, 326

childhood 688
control 318
committee 786
practices 303
elimination of 140
emerging of 523
gastrointestinal 152, 167
hospital-acquired 783
latent 250
maternal 690
mode of 439, 449
nosocomial 786
parasitic 345
prevention 696
rate 441
reservoir of 250, 262, 360, 366, 372, 377, 385, 388, 391, 393, 395, 397, 405, 429, 439, 473, 502
respiratory 294, 705
risk 783, 784
reduction for 455
source of 250, 253, 254, 262, 291, 322, 372, 384, 405, 414, 422, 461, 467, 473, 495
transmission of 436
treatment of mixed 427
viral 345
Infectious agent 249, 573
Infectious diseases 249, 254, 514f, 759-761, 808f, 811f, 817, 926
acute 613t
affecting brain 742
control of 809
epidemiology of 248, 260
Infective material 262, 273, 278, 330, 354, 377, 461, 467
Inflammatory bowel disease 50
Influenza 257, 261, 290, 291, 296, 298, 300, 514
A 290t
pandemics of 523
viruses 296
B 300
virus 300
C virus 300
clinical features 300
communicability period of 292
complications 300
control 301
disease burden of 290
epidemiology of 289, 297
immunity against 291
isolation of 294
management 300
pandemic 290, 295f
prevention 301
season 298
surveillance 295t, 304
network 294
vaccine, inactivated 291, 303
virological surveillance 294
virus 291, 297, 300, 304
different strains of 291
spreads 291

Information technology 1083
　use of 1083
Information, education and communication 498, 641, 955, 963, 986, 1000, 1010, 1058
　services 997
Inguinal bubo 490
Inhalational anthrax 332
　cases of 335
Inhalers, spacers for 615
Injury 705, 760, 819, 927
　epidemiology of 587, 588
　exercise-induced 58
　prevention 592
　types of 587
Inoculation rate 426
Insecticides 122, 122t
　classification of 116, 117fc
　control of 124, 126
　group of 118
　natural 116
　synthetic 117
　use of 449
Institutional delivery 506
　promotion of 512
Institutional Ethics Committee 212
Institutional Review Board 212
Insulin 615
Integrated child development services 231, 374, 928
　scheme 1020
　　organization structure of 1021f
Integrated disease surveillance
　program 148, 285, 525, 1002, 1085
　project 161, 304, 332
Integrated vector control 127
　approach 119
Integrated vector management 127, 127f, 426, 431, 983, 985, 987
Integrated Women Empowerment Program 1033
Intensity 106
Intensive care units 783
Interferon-gamma release assays 314
Intermittent noise 107
International Committee of Red Cross 905
International concerns, public health emergencies of 762
International Dark-Sky Association 109
International Day of Yoga 55
International Health Agencies 899t
International Health Regulations 264, 525, 761, 762f
　principles of 762
International Healthcare Agencies 899
International Institute of Population Sciences 960, 1060
International Labour Organization 737, 903
International Poverty Line 824
International Statistical Classification of Diseases and Related Health Problems Revision 907
Interventions Under Child Health 970f
Intestinal diseases, epidemiology of 338, 341
Intestinal worms 366

Intestines 418
Intimate partner violence 596
Intoxications 342t
Intracytoplasmic sperm injection 672
Intradermal rabies vaccination 408
Intramural research 1059
Intramuscular mumps immunoglobulin, treatment with 285
Intramuscular rabies vaccination 408
Intranasal vaccine 294, 294t, 296
Intraocular pressure, tonometry for 715
Intrauterine contraceptive devices 660, 662, 663, 667, 669, 682, 963
　insertion of 663
Intrauterine growth retardation 674
Invasive screening test 770
Inventory control techniques 893
Iodine 35, 36, 36t, 639
　deficiency
　　disorders 639, 640t, 641t
　　health consequences of 640
　requirement 640
　status, community assessment of 641
　test 347
Iodized salt 702
Iron 35, 38, 40, 41, 43, 680, 682, 963
　absorption 635
　deficiency anemia 635
　　treatment of 707
　functions of 635
　requirements 35t
　supplementation 398, 636, 979, 1024t
　tablet 702, 1024f
　therapy
　　oral 707
　　parenteral 707
Irradiation, ultraviolet 86
Irritable bowel syndrome 50
Irritant contact dermatitis 730
Isoflavones 38
Isoflurane 1089
Isolation 254, 263
　techniques 327
Isoleucine 29
Isoniazid 315, 483
　preventive therapy 318, 319
Isosorbide dinitrate 615
Isosporiasis 475
Itch mite 126
Ivermectin 985
Ixodidae 126

**J**

Jai Vigyan Mission 560
James Lind's experiment 244f
Jan Andolan 1019
Janani Shishu Suraksha Karyakaram 231, 512, 684, 688, 968
Janani Suraksha Yojana 512, 684, 688, 968
Janpada Panchayat 938
Japanese encephalitis 115, 258, 420, 443, 514, 699, 760, 933, 986, 1003, 1066
　Control of 443

　epidemiology of 443
　history of 443
　incidence, trend of 444f
　prevention of 443
　vaccination against 986
Japanese Leprosy Mission 989
Jaundice 418, 521t, 697
Jawaharlal Nehru National Urban Renewal Mission 749
Jet lag 760
Job stress 732
Joint 310
　aches 457
　family 65
　involvement 558
Joint Monitoring Program 85, 96
Jungalwalla Committee 929, 930
Juvenile Justice (Care and Protection of Children) Act 1044

**K**

K antigens 382
Kala-azar 115, 140, 448, 450, 933, 985, 1000
　control of 447
　epidemiology of 447
　prevention of 447
Kaposi's sarcoma 471, 474, 475
Kartar Singh Committee 929, 930
Kata thermometer 103, 103f
Kayakalp 914
　Award Scheme 1031
Keratomalacia 638
Ketamine 1089
Kidney
　disease, chronic 49, 609
　disorders 541
Kilkari 960
Kishori Shakti Yojana 1022
Kleb-Loefflers bacilli 321
Klinefelter syndrome 766
Koch's postulates 19, 246
Koplik's spots 276, 278
Kuppuswamy's classification 68
Kuppuswamy's method 69t
Kyasanur forest disease 116, 451
　virus 451
Kyoto protocol 776

**L**

Labor
　force participation rate 718
　progress of 681
　third stage of 681
Laboratory technician, job responsibilities of 947
Lactation period 45
Lactational amenorrhea method 668
Lactoferrin 46
Lactoperoxidase 46
Laissez-Faire leadership style 882
Lamivudine 476, 477, 480
Language 699, 886
Laparoscopic tubal occlusion 668

LaQshya initiative 968
Larva 119
    migrans, cutaneous 398, 402f
Laryngeal diphtheria 322, 323
Laryngotracheobronchitis 279
Lassa fever 128, 527, 531, 796
    transmission 531f
Latent tuberculosis 313
    infection
        cases of 307
        treatment 992
Lathyrism 651
    prevention and control of 652
Latrines 751
    and septic tank, types of 96f
    pour flush-type of 96
    service type 96
Leber's hereditary optic atrophy 766
Legs 116
*Leishmania* 449
    *donovani* 447, 448
    *promastigotes* 448
Leishmaniasis 420
    atypical disseminated 475
    cutaneous 128, 448
    visceral 115
Leonine facies 496f
Lepra reaction 497
    treatment of 499
    type 1 498f
Lepromin test 497
    interpretation of 497fc
Leprosy 495, 500, 933, 1000
    case detection campaign 999, 1001
    classification of 497, 497fc, 999t
    control 492
    epidemiology of 492
    immunological classification of 496, 496fc
    Mukt Bharat 999
    pathogenesis of 496fc
    prevention 492, 498f
    screening 999
*Leptospira*
    *biflexa* 416
    *interrogans* 416
Leptospirosis 128, 416, 418, 514, 524
    control of 416
    epidemiology of 416
    prevention of 416
    severe 417
*Leptotrombidium deliense* 126
Leucine 29
Leukemia 570, 732
    acute myelogenous 766
Levofloxacin 336
Lice 125
    life cycle of 125f
Life index, physical quality of 17, 805, 824, 825
Life table methods 670
Light emitting diodes 109
Light pollution 109
    prevention of 110
    types of 109

Lignocaine 1089
Limbs 56
Link worker 962
    scheme 995
Lipid metabolism 551
Lipid profile 615, 715
    fasting 544
*Liponyssoides sanguineus* 457
Liposomal amphotericin B 985
Liquefied petroleum gas 751
Liquid waste disposal 98
*Listeria* 345
    *monocytogenes* 345
Listeriosis 347
Literacy rate 222, 222f, 751
Live vaccine 369, 378
Liver
    diseases 50
    failure, acute 379
    flukes 347
    function tests 453
Loa loa 439
Locomotor
    disability 1045
    impairment 690
    system, effect of 724
Loeffler's serum slope 323
Logistics 893, 1066
    management 893
        importance of 893
London's water supply system 245
Lopinavir 480
Louse-borne
    diseases 116
    epidemic typhus 451, 457
Low birth weight 48, 630, 674, 686, 694, 971
    management of 688
    prevention of 687
Low body temperature effects 105
Lower respiratory tract infections, acute 265
Low-traffic dispensing outlet 476
Luminous flux 109
Luminous intensity 109
Lung 418
    biopsy 728
    cancer 172, 174, 715, 726, 731, 731t, 744
        operating for 170
    diseases 246
    function test 728
    ultrasonography of 728
Lycopene 37, 38
Lymph nodes 310
    enlarged 454
Lymphadenitis, tubercular 310
Lymphadenopathy 287, 454
    associated virus 471
Lymphangitis, acute filarial 440
Lymphatic filariasis 140, 420, 438
    elimination of 984
Lymphatic tissue 38
Lymphedema 440
Lymphogranuloma venereum 487
Lymphoma 475, 570
Lysine 29

## M

Macroangiopathy 562
Macrolide 457, 499
Macronutrients 25, 29, 47
Macular degeneration, age-related 601
Maculopapular rash, generalized 287
Magnesium 34, 36
    sulfate 615
Mahatma Gandhi National Rural Employment Guarantee Act 231
Mahila Aarogya Samiti 839
Mahila Swasthya Sangh 949
Maintenance and Welfare of Parents and Senior Citizens Act 715, 716
Malaise 336, 1076
Malaria 115, 133, 420-422, 483, 513, 517, 682, 688, 693, 755, 761, 818, 933, 981, 984f
    control of 420, 426
    diagnosis of 424
    epidemiology of 420
    incidence of 519f
    manmade 422
    milestones of 421
    parasite 477
        life cycle of 423, 424f
    prevention of 420, 426, 483
    prophylaxis of 761t
    severe 424
    technical strategy for 427
    treatment of 426, 426f, 427
    tribal 422
    urban 422
    vector of 120, 422
Malathion 117
    dosage of 118
Malformation, congenital 172, 172t
Malignancy 310
Malnutrition 48, 153, 269, 448, 601, 628, 630fc, 694, 705, 712
    acute 629
    covariates of 633
    moderate acute 629
    proxy markers of 636
    severe acute 629, 693, 902, 976, 977
Mammography 582, 715
Management information system 865, 912, 960, 1034
Mandatory seatbelt use laws 592
Manmade radiation 76
    sources of 76t
Manpower Development Schemes 1016
*Mansonella perstans* 439
*Mansonia annulifera* 439, 446
Mansonia mosquito 123
Mansonides 123
Mantoux tuberculin skin test 313
Marburg virus disease 527
Marfan syndrome 766
Marital fertility rate 223, 224
Maslow's hierarchy of needs models 883, 883f
Mason's hygrometer 74, 75f
Mass
    deworming 702
    drug administration 440, 443

media 236
  campaigns 478
  communication 235
  vaccination campaigns 813
Massachusetts Sanitary Commission 93
Massive economic crisis 932
Mastoid process 909
Mastoiditis 280
Maternal and child health 752t, 756, 1064
  situation 815
Maternal and Child Welfare Services 1062
Maternal child tracking system 1084
Maternal death 674, 676, 819
  late 676
  lifetime risk of 676
  process of 1080
  surveillance and response 683, 1079, 1080
    community based 683, 1080
Maternal education 266
Maternal health 153, 674, 684, 947, 967
  current status of 674
  indicators of 683, 683t
Maternal mortality 675, 678, 679, 806
  causes of 676, 679, 679f
  indices of 676
  prevention of 679
  rate 676, 806
  ratio 675f, 676, 806f, 816f, 824, 1064
Maternal nutritional status 689
Maternal tetanus 506
  elimination of 1006
Maternity Benefit Act 229, 737, 1050
Mathematical techniques 871
Matrilineal family 66
Maximum inventory system 895
Measles 261, 276, 279, 280, 513, 699, 742, 1066
  and rubella
    laboratory network 281
    partnership 281, 288
    surveillance data 276
  care of 279
  control of 280b
  diagnosis of 280b
  disease transmission of 278t
  epidemiology of 276
  fatality rate of 279
  incidence rate 277f, 277t
  management of 280b
  mumps, rubella 283, 287
  pathogenic phase of 278f
  prevention of 280b
  second dose of 280
  treatment for 279
  uncomplicated 279
  vaccine 270, 276, 280, 281, 282
Mebendazole 394
Mechanical negative pressure ventilation 72
Mechanical ventilation 71, 72
Medical
  benefit, administration of 1046
  doctor-population ratio 857, 857t
  entomology 115
  genetics 16

interventions 804
officer, job responsibilities of 945
Research Council 102
sociology 60
surveillance 737
Medical Termination of Pregnancy Act 1055, 1056
Medicine
  affecting blood 1090
  alternative 854
  anti-infective 1089, 1090
  cardiovascular 1090
  community 6, 6t, 803, 832
  counterfeit 1092
  dermatological 1091
  endocrine 1090
  essential 615, 1088
  gastrointestinal 1091
  Indian system of 869, 936, 937, 955
  indigenous systems of 931
  institute of 911
  ophthalmological 1091
  preventive 831
Medina worm 385
Meditation 57
Medium-traffic dispensing outlet 476
Mefenamic acid 1089
Mefloquine 427, 761
Melanoma 172
Memory 171
Mendelian disorders 766
Mendelian inheritance 766f
Meningeal irritation 418
Meningitis 474, 475
  acute bacterial 330
  cerebrospinal 330
  vaccine-preventable, bacterial 331
Meningococcal disease
  diagnosis 331
  outbreaks 332
  treatment 331
Meningococcal infection pneumonia, presentations of 329
Meningococcal meningitis 261, 329, 330, 514, 760
  clusters 329
  epidemiology of 329
  risk factors for 330
Meningococcal sepsis 329
Meningococcemia 329, 330
Meningococcus 148, 330
Menstrual disorder 705
Menstrual hygiene 707
  management guidelines 98
  scheme 979
Menstrual induction 667
Menstrual period 680
Menstrual regulation 667
Mental dimension 15
Mental disorder 705, 741
  diagnostic and statistical manual for 742
  prevalence of 706
Mental health 706, 740, 779, 818, 901
  Act 1051

gap action program 745
literacy 743
policy 1016
problems 748
promotion of 745
services, organization of 1015
Mental Healthcare Act 1016
Mental illness 19, 690, 742, 767, 775
  causes of 742b
  classification of 740
  epidemiology of 741
  occurrence of 742f
  prevention of 743
  risk factors of 741, 742b
  treatment of 742
Mental retardation 16, 690
Mentally ill persons 1051
  rehabilitation of 1051
Mesothelioma 731
Metabolic diseases 742
Metabolism, inborn errors of 16
Metaplasia, keratinizing 638
Metazoonosis 401
Metformin 615
Methadone maintenance treatment 478
Methane 774
Methionine 29
Methylene blue test 347
Metoprolol 615
M-health 1083, 1084
Microfilaremia, asymptomatic 440
Microfilaria survey 442
Microfiltration, advanced membranes for 87
Micronutrient 25, 47, 572
  deficiency 48, 635
  supplementation 702
Micro-pill 665
Microsporidia 366
Microwave 792
Midazolam 1089
Mid-day Meal
  Program 702
  Scheme 231
Middle east respiratory syndrome 261, 760
  coronavirus 514, 527
Mid-upper arm circumference 977
Miliary tuberculosis 307
Milk 34, 42, 43t
  borne infections 345t
  hygiene 345
  pasteurization, tests for 347
  products 42
    nutritive value of 43t
  tests for 347
Millennium Development Goal 830, 842-844
Mineral 26, 35, 38, 40-43, 117, 565, 755, 1092
Mini pill 665
Minilap tubectomy 668
Minimental state examination 715
Minimum adequate diet 644
Minimum inventory system 895
Minimum meal frequency 644
Minimum Wages Act 1051
Minocycline 499

Missed pills 664
　management of 664t
Mission Indradhanush 281, 289, 974
Mission Parivar Vikas 966
Mission Shakti 1033
Mission Steering Group 957
Mission Vatsalya 231
Mite 126
　borne diseases 116
Mitigation 776
Mitochondrial inheritance 766
Mitral regurgitation, mild 559
Modern management techniques 871
Molecular genetics 768
Molluscum contagiosum virus 487
Monitor vaccine storage temperature 839
Monogamous family 66
Monogenic disorders 766
Monosomy 766
Monovalent tetanus toxoid 509
Mood changes 740
Morbidity 541, 547, 579, 581, 583, 588, 686
　causes of 819
　childhood 695b
　management 984
　maternal 675
　occupational 734
　statistics 910
　surveillance 624
Morbillivirus 276, 278
Morning-after pill 665
Morphine 615, 1089
Morphological index 497
Mortality 542, 547, 579, 581, 583, 588, 954, 1037
　causes of 692, 819
　childhood 692f, 695f
　indicators 158
　infant 691, 694
　maternal 675, 678, 679, 806
　neonatal 691, 694
　occupational 734
　perinatal 691
　pertussis related 327
　post-neonatal 691
　rate 216, 796
　　proportional 158
　statistics 910
　surveillance 624
　under-five children 690
Mosquito 119, 121
　bites
　　prevent 690
　　protection against 122
　borne diseases 115
　density 426
　life cycle of 119, 119f
　net 122
　types of 120f
Mother and child tracking
　scheme 960
　system 961, 1036, 1085

Motion
　range of 53
　sickness 760
Motivation 237, 883
　early theories of 883
　integrated model of 883f, 884
Motor vehicle traffic, reducing 592
Mucocutaneous leishmaniasis 448
Mucous membranes 300
Mukhya Sevika 1021
Mukhyamantri Amrutam Yojana 850
Multicentre growth reference study 631
Multidimensional poverty index 18, 68, 824, 826, 826t
Multidrug therapy 385, 493, 1001
Multifactorial causation, theory of 19
Multifocal leukoencephalopathy, progressive 475
Multiple bar diagram 197
Multivariate regression, types of 210
Mumps 261, 282-284, 286
　attack of 283
　control of 282
　epidemiology of 282
　infection 285, 286
　　clinical presentations of 284t
　　presumptive diagnosis of 284
　rubella
　　and varicella vaccine 280
　　vaccines 280
　vaccine 285
　　characteristics of 286t
Municipal Board 938
Municipal Committee 938
Municipal Corporation 939
Municipal Council 938
Municipal Solid Waste (Management and Handling) Rules 1053
Murine typhus 116, 128, 451, 457
*Musca sorbens* 502
Muscle 457
　pain 457
Musculoskeletal system, diseases of 909
Mutagens 765, 766
Mutations, combination of 766
Myalgia 417, 454, 455
Mycobacteria
　atypical 474
　growth indicator tube 313
　nontuberculous 310
Mycobacterial infection, disseminated nontuberculous 475
*Mycobacterium* 86
　*indicus pranii* vaccine 1000
　*tuberculosis* 307, 309, 310, 312, 313, 345, 474, 494, 533
　　characteristics of 315
　　discovery of 306
*Mycoplasma hominis* 487
Mycosis, disseminated 475
Myelomas 570
Myocardial infarction 134

Myocarditis 323
Myoclonus epilepsy 766

# N

N95 mask 292
*Naeglaria fowleri* 339
Nagar Nigam 939
Nagar Palika 938
Nagar Panchayat 938
Nairovirus 451, 454
Nanofiltration 87
Narcotic Drugs and Psychotropic Substances (Amendment) Act 1041
Nasal diphtheria, anterior 322
Nasopharyngitis 330
National Accreditation Board of Health 914
National Accreditation Board of Testing and Calibration Laboratories 914
National Action Plan Combating Viral Hepatitis 466
National Action Plan on Climate Change 777
National Aeronautics and Space Administration 349
National AIDS Committee 484
National AIDS Control Organization 141, 476, 484, 993, 955
　Acts 1042
National AIDS Control Program 929, 1037
National Air Monitoring Program 82
National Air Quality Index 81
National Air Quality Monitoring Program 82
National Blindness Survey 892
National Blood Transfusion Council 477
National Cancer Control Program 577
National Cancer Registry Program 577, 1009
National Center of Disease Control 304, 332, 1058, 1059
National Center of Health Statistics 631
National Commission on Population 960
National Creche Scheme 1033
National Crime Record Bureau Report 588, 743
National Deworming Day 978
National Diabetes Control Program 929
National Disaster Management Authority 782, 798, 1042
National Disaster Management Plan 1042
National Environmental Engineering Research Institute 82
National Family Health Survey 161, 192, 225, 542, 629, 658, 670, 687, 828, 891, 925, 960, 1037
National Family Planning Indemnity Scheme 967
National Family Planning Program 664
National Family Welfare Program 225
National Filaria Control Program 442, 928
National Food Security Act 229
National Framework of Malaria Elimination 428, 981
National Guidelines of Control of Iron Deficiency Anemia 678

National Health and Family Planning Commission 852
National Health and Family Survey 265
National Health Committees 929
National Health Helpline 1084
National Health Mission 822, 929, 956, 957, 998, 1034, 1062
　core components of 957f
　evaluation of 960
National Health Policy 842, 857, 953, 984
National Health Programs 946
National Health Protection Scheme 842, 1028
National Health Service 860
National Health System 851
　Resource Centre 957, 960
National Heart Institute 246
National Heart, Lung, and Blood Institute 246
National Housing Bank 114
National Immunization Schedule 510
National Institute of Cholera and Enteric Diseases 359
National Institute of Communicable Diseases 1058
National Institute of Disaster Management 1058, 1060
National Institute of Health and Care Excellence 914
National Institute of Health and Family Welfare 957, 1058, 1059
National Institute of Mental Health and Neurosciences 741
National Integrated Biological and Behavioral Surveillance 998
National Iodine Deficiency Disorder Control Program 140, 641, 1023, 1026
National Iron Plus Initiative Program 636, 1024
National Kala-Azar Elimination Program 985
National Leprosy Control Program 928, 929
National Leprosy Eradication Program 998
National Medical and Health Education Policy 931
National Mental Health Program 742, 745, 960, 1014
National Mission of Green India 777
National Mission of Strategic Knowledge for Climate Change 777
National Mission of Sustainable Agriculture 777
National Mission of Sustaining Himalayan Ecosystem 777
National Nutrition Mission 1019
National Nutrition Monitoring Bureau 1038
National Nutrition Policy 955
National Nutrition Programs 1023
National Nutrition Survey 645
National Nutritional Anemia Prophylaxis Program 707, 1023
National Oral Health Program 960, 1016
National Pension Scheme 230
National Policy on Older Persons 715
National Population Policy 225, 929, 954
National Population Surveillance 147

National Program of Control of Blindness 505, 599, 960
　and Visual Impairment 505, 1013
National Program of Healthcare of Elderly 715, 716, 960, 1010
National Program of Hypertension 545
National Program of Minimum Needs 928
National Program of Palliative Care 960
National Program of Prevention and Control of Cancer, Diabetes, Cardiovascular Diseases, and Stroke 539
National Program of Prevention and Control of Deafness 960, 1013
National Program of Prevention and Control of Diabetes, Cardiovascular Disease and Stroke 577, 618
National Program of Prevention and Control of Fluorosis 960, 1026
National Program of Prevention and Control of Non-communicable Diseases 548, 560, 564, 618, 621, 960, 1007, 1007f
National Program of Prevention and Management of Burn Injuries 960, 1017
National Program of Prevention of Blindness 929
National Program of Stroke 548
National Quality Assurance Standards 914, 915
National Rural Drinking Water Program 341
National Rural Health Mission 512, 856, 861, 957
National Safai Karamcharis Finance and Development Corporation 230
National Safety and Quality Health Service 914
National Sample Survey Office 718, 856, 1038
National Sickle Cell Anemia Elimination Program 1017
National Smallpox Eradication Program 928
National Social Assistance Program 230
National Sociodemographic Goals 955
National Solar Mission 777
National Strategic Plan and Roadmap for Leprosy 1001
National Strategic Plan of HIV/AIDS and Sexually Transmitted Infection 998
National Strategic Plan of Malaria Elimination 983
National Strategic Plan of Tuberculosis Elimination 991
National Stroke Registry Program 548
National Surveillance Program 988, 998
National Technical Working Group 989
National Telemedicine Network 1084
National Tobacco Control Program 960, 928, 1011, 1012f, 1038
National Tuberculosis Elimination Program 140, 319, 987, 1060
　organization of 988
National Tuberculosis Institute 989, 1058, 1059
National Urban Health Mission 949, 957, 960

National Urban Housing and Habitat Policy 749
National Urban Livelihood Mission 749
National Validation Day 355
National Vector Borne Disease Control Program 140, 929, 946, 947, 981, 984
National Viral Hepatitis Control Program 469, 1002
National Water Mission 777
Nausea 386, 418, 457
Navjat Shishu Suraksha Karyakram 971
Near vision impairment 600
Nebulizer 615
*Necator americanus* 396, 397
Neck
　pain 454, 455
　swelling of 728
Needle and Syringe Program 478
Neglected tropical disease 93, 394, 404, 438
*Neisseria*
　*gonorrheae* 487
　*meningitidis* 329, 330, 708
Nelfinavir 480
Nelson's column 244f
Neonatal and childhood illness, management of 265, 271, 929
Neonatal tetanus 505, 506, 509, 694
　cases, trend of 507f
　elimination of 1006
Neonicotinoids 118
Neostigmine 1089
Nephelometric turbidity unit 86
Nephrotic syndrome 49
Nerve damage 323
Nervousness 740
Neural tube defect 764, 770
Neuraminidase 303
　inhibitors 292, 296
Neurological diseases 742
Neurosis 740
Nevirapine 477t, 480
New information technologies 236
Newborn and child health 970
Newborn care services matrix 971t
Newborn stabilization unit 969, 971
Niacin 34, 43
Nicotine
　dependence 910
　use 705
Night
　blindness 638
　sweats 310
Nikshay Poshan Yojana 993
Nikusth 1086
Nipah 524, 527
　virus 529, 530f
　virus infection 514
NITI Aayog 933
　important functions of 933, 933f
Nitrogen oxide 79
Nitrous oxide 774, 1089
*Nocardia*
　*asteroids* 345
　*brasiliensis* 345

Nocardiasis 345
Noise 719, 723, 748
    continuous 107
    dosimeter 107f
    exposure 106t
        types of 107
    health effects of 107
    industrial 106
    measurement
        instruments for 107
        methods for 107
    pollution 106, 107
    properties of 106
    sound levels of 106t
    vehicular 106
Noncommunicable disease 22t, 23, 29, 152, 536, 536f, 552t, 553, 609, 609t, 610, 612, 612f, 613-617, 618t, 619, 624, 625t, 628, 690, 705, 748, 755, 815, 818, 901, 926, 948, 1038
    cell, management structure of 1007f
    challenge of 133
    control of 539f, 610f, 611b, 612b, 1008t
    epidemiology of 536, 541
    essential 615t
    impact of 537t
    level of 1008f
    management of 613, 615
    prevention of 137, 610f, 611b, 612, 612b, 1008t
    programs 612, 616, 929
    progression of 611f
    risk factors for 52, 537f
    screening for 617
    surveillance 624, 624b, 625f
        system, components of 625f
Non-fatal cardiovascular diseases, risk stratification of 552t
Non-formal preschool education 1022
Nongovernment organizations 160, 632, 852, 861, 905t, 1062
    and donor agencies 905
Non-governmental and civil organizations 951
Non-Hodgkin's lymphoma 474
Noninvasive screening test 769
Nonnucleoside reverse transcriptase inhibitors 480
Nonskeletal fluorosis 1026
Non-steroidal anti-inflammatory drugs 1089
Nontetanus prone injuries, management of 511
Nontyphoidal *Salmonella* 366, 475
Norfloxacin 761
Norovirus 339, 347, 524
Norwalk virus 366
No-scalpel vasectomy 668, 669, 669f
Nosocomial infection 786
    categorization of 784t
    prevention of 783
    risk 783t
    since prevention of 786
    surveillance of 786
Novel coronavirus 261

Nucleic acid amplification test 468
Nucleic acid tests 527, 529
Nucleoside reverse transcriptase inhibitor 480, 481
Null hypothesis 203
Nutrients 25, 28, 565
    analysis systems 645
    proportions of 27t
Nutrition 20, 25, 45, 223, 246, 278, 279, 368f, 565, 633, 752, 948
    and health 25
    committees 958
    education 702
    epidemiology of 628
    global targets for 646
    in health, role of 25
    Monitoring Bureau 638
    program 646, 979
    program for adolescent girls 1022
    rehabilitation center 978
    related disorders 628
    sociocultural aspects of 47
    supplementary 1021, 1021t
Nutritional anemia 706
    prevention of 706
Nutritional assessment 641
    methods of 642, 642fc
Nutritional deficiency 153, 775
Nutritional disorders 48, 755
Nutritional epidemiology 628
Nutritional problems 706, 748
Nutritional rehabilitation center 976, 977
Nutritional status 48, 266
    indicators 159, 646
Nutritional support 279
Nutritional surveillance 48, 148, 645
Nutritive agents 20
Nutritive losses 39
    preventing 39
Nutritive value 26, 40

# O

O antigens 382
Obesity 207, 208, 542, 547, 551, 563, 705
    assessment of 634
    classification of 634t
    consequences of 634
    control of 634
    epidemiology of 633
    prevalence of 755
    prevention of 634
Obligatory cyclozoonoses 400
Obstetric care 680
    comprehensive 683
    emergency 682
    essential 682
Obstructed labor 678, 694
Obstruction, life-threatening 322
Occupational cancer 726, 731
    prevention of 732
Occupational disease 725, 726
    centers 1046
    list of 726t

Occupational environment 720f
    and health hazards 720
Occupational exposure 333, 573
Occupational health 717
    safety 819, 927
        legislation 737
Occupational injuries and accidents 732
    prevention of 733
Occupational situation 72
Occupational stress and burnout, prevention of 733
Occupational therapy 548
Occupational workers 1040, 1046
Old age medical care 1048
Old Age Pension Scheme 230
Oliguria 418, 677
Omicron variant 533
*Onchocerca volvulus* 439
Open vial policy 1073
Operational planning 879
    steps in 879
    types of 879
Ophthalmia neonatorum 487
Ophthalmic diseases 775
Opioid 744
    substitution therapy 478, 994
Opisthotonus 508, 509f
Opportunistic infections 474
    prevention of 484
Oral cancer
    control of 580, 580f
    early detection of 580
    epidemiology of 579
    prevention of 580, 580f
    problem statement of 579t
    screening for 580
Oral glucose tolerance test 565, 626
Oral polio vaccine 355, 695, 697, 975, 1066
Oral rehydration
    solution 362, 689
    therapy 153
Oral visual examination 620
Orchitis 284, 285
Organ 74, 76, 77
Organic dust toxic syndrome 719
Organochlorine 573
    compounds 117
Organophosphorus compounds 117
Organosulfur compounds 38
Ormeloxifene 669
Ornithodoros species 457
Orthomyxoviridae family 297
Orthotoluidine
    arsenite 89
    test 89
Oryzanol 32
Oseltamivir 292, 296
Osmolarity ORS-composition 368t
Osmosis, reverse 87
Osteoporosis 246, 715
Otitis media 266, 279, 327
Ottawa Charters health promotion emblem 237f
Outdoor air pollution, sources of 80fc

Ovaries 574
Overnutrition 563, 628
Overweight
    childhood 630
    prevalence of 755
Oxygen 615, 1089
Oxytocics 1091
Ozone 718, 719

## P

Pain 728, 1076
    abdominal 418
    burning 386
    epigastric 677
    lower abdominal 490
Paired T-test 205, 206
Palliative care 139, 484, 538, 577, 860
Paludrine 761
Panchayat Samiti 938
Panchayati Raj Institution 612, 950
    organization of 939fc
Pancreatic disorders 563
Pandemic flu 296
    control measures for 292
Pandemic influenza 244, 290, 290t, 292-293
    develops, novel strain of 291
    viral strains 291
    virus 291f
Panic disorder 741
Pantothenic acid 33
Pap cytology test 576
Paracetamol 615, 894, 1089
Paradox, prevention 622
Paragonimiasis 402f
Parainfluenza viruses 298
Paralytic poliomyelitis 354
    vaccine-associated 354
Parameters 751
Paramyxoviridae 278
Parasite 266
    demonstration of 425, 425t
    density index 425
    incidence, annual 425, 981
    rate 425
Parasitic infestations 347
Paratyphoid 116
    fever 339
Parboiling, advantages of 39
Parent-to-child transmission, prevention of 476, 479
Parotitis 284, 285
Partograph 681
Passive immunization 258, 280, 281, 378, 409, 511
    agents 259fc
Pasteurization 345, 346
    methods of 346
    process 346t
        supervision of 346
Patient support systems 992
Patrilineal family 66
Paucibacillary 497f, 999
Payment of Gratuity Act 229

Pelvic inflammatory diseases 487
Penicillin 615
    allergy 324
    G 457
Penicilliosis 475
Pentavalent vaccine 270, 323, 510f
Peptic ulcer 50
Perineal hygiene 682
Periodic health check-up 714
Periodic medical examinations 736
Peripheral arterial disease 549
Peripheral pulses palpation 544
Permanent Disablement Benefit 1048
Permethrin 118
Personal hygiene 575, 682
Personal protective equipment 292, 785
    serves 785
    use of 294, 736
Persons with Disabilities (Equal Opportunities, Protection of Rights and Full Participation) Act 1045
Pertactin 325
Pertussis 261, 325, 326, 699, 1066
    clinical course of 326f
    complications 327
    diagnosis of 327
    diagnostic test 327f
    diseases, stages of 327f
    exhibits seasonal trend 326
    infections of 326f
    laboratory diagnosis 327
    toxin 325
    treatment of 328
    vaccines 323
Pesticide exposure 722
Pfizer-Biontech and Moderna vaccines 535
Pharyngeal diphtheria 322, 323
Pharyngitis 268
    acute 266
    progresses with severe 268
Phenothrin 118
Phenotype 765, 765f
Phenyl pyrazoles 118
Phenylalanine 29
Phenylketonuria 16, 50
    screening for 770
Pheochromocytoma 541
Philosophical dimension 15
*Phlebotomus argentipes* 448
Phosphatase test 347
Phosphorus 36, 38, 40, 41, 43
Photophobia 454, 455
Physical activity 31, 52, 543, 573, 575
    moderate 211
Physical environment 21, 269, 502, 507, 590, 594, 634
Physical exercise 56, 56t
    types of 53
Physical fitness 722
    components of 52
Physical health hazards 721
Physical therapy 548
Physical work environment 735

Phytic acid 38
Pie diagram 197
Pinta 487t
Piped natural gas 751
*Pistia stratiotes* 439
Pit latrine 96
Placenta
    pathological changes in 424
    previa 677
Plague 128, 243, 336, 401f, 413, 415f, 514, 796
    control of 411
    distribution of 412f
    epidemiology of 411
    manifestation of 336, 336fc
    natural foci of 336
    outbreak, management of 337t
    prevention of 411
    treatment of 336
Planning Commission 931
Plantar
    fascia 58
    fasciitis 58
Plasma
    protein A, pregnancy-associated 769
    pyrolysis 791
        treatment technology 791
    substitutes 1090
*Plasmodium*
    *falciparum* 423, 483, 517, 755
        malaria 423, 427
    *ovale* 423
    *vivax* 423
        malaria 426
Platelet
    counts 453
    ratio index 468
Plenum ventilation 71
Pleura 310
Pleural fluid 334
Pluralism 954
Pneumococcal conjugate vaccine 257, 271, 1066
Pneumococcal pneumonia 699
Pneumococcal polysaccharide vaccine 257, 271
Pneumococcal vaccine 271
Pneumococcus 148
Pneumoconiosis 726
*Pneumocystis carinii* pneumonia 471, 474
Pneumonia 261, 266, 267, 269, 322, 474, 693, 839, 972
    bacterial 270
    causes of 266t
    classification of 267, 267t, 268
    control of 369, 370
    early detection of 336
    prevention of 369, 370
    severe 267
Pneumonic plague 335, 336, 413, 414
    epidemiology of 336f
    outbreak of 336
    primary 336
    secondary 336

Poisoning 595
Polio 138f, 254, 258, 345, 352, 699
   end game strategy 357, 1005
   eradication strategy 357
   information system 357
   trends globally 352f
   vaccine 354
   virus, vaccine derived 353, 357
Poliomyelitis 116, 254, 339, 352, 814
   control 352
   elimination of 1063
   epidemiology of 352
   eradication of 1005
   paralytic 354
   prevention 352
Poliovirus 339, 345
   wild 254, 353f
Pollution Control Committees 82
Polyandrous family 66
Polyandry behavior 487
Polycyclic aromatic hydrocarbons 718
Polygamy behavior 487
Polygenic disorders 766
Polygon, frequency 196
Polygynous family 66
Polymerase chain reaction 323
Polyneuropathy 323
Polyphenols 37
Polysaccharide vaccines 331
Polyvalent vaccines, manufacturing of 839
Ponderal index 634
Poor environmental sanitation 679
Poor hand hygiene 630
Population
   based cancer registries 577, 578f
   based stroke registry 548
   criteria 747
   density 220, 220f
   displacements 779
   distribution 216, 1037
   explosion 219, 220, 658
      consequences of 220
   growth 153, 216, 343, 774
   health surveys 960
   heterogeneity 259
   high-risk 354
   mobility 448
   pyramid 219, 219f, 220f
   research centers 960
   risk 174
   specified 151
   strategy 564, 584
Pork tapeworm 347
Poshan 2.0 1020
   Abhiyaan 978, 1019
   Scheme 1023t
   tracker 1083
   Vatikas 1020
Positive predictive value 145, 146
Positive pressure system 71
Positive serologic test 287
Positive skin smear 497
Postcoital contraception 665
Post-conception methods 660, 667
Post-diphtheritic paralysis 323
Post-disaster phase 781
Post-exposure prophylaxis 137, 280, 407, 409, 482, 511, 761, 995, 995t, 996, 1000
   against hepatitis B 995
   regimen 997t
Post-exposure vaccination 275
Post-kala-azar dermal leishmaniasis 449
Postmortem examination 348
Postnatal care 681, 963
Postpartum 46
Post-travel illness surveillance information 759
Potassium chloride 368
Pott's disease 310
Pot-type ceramic filter 87f
Pour flush latrine 96f
Poverty 62, 262, 467, 742
Pradhan Mantri Adarsh Gram Yojana 231
Pradhan Mantri Awas Yojana 114, 749, 985
Pradhan Mantri Gramin Awaas Yojana 114, 231
Pradhan Mantri Jan Arogya Yojana 230, 850
Pradhan Mantri Jan Dhan Yojana 231
Pradhan Mantri Kaushal Vikas Yojana 231
Pradhan Mantri Matru Vandana Yojana 231, 1022, 1022t
Pradhan Mantri Sahaj Bijli Har Ghar Yojana 231
Pradhan Mantri Shram Yogi Maan-Dhan 230
Pradhan Mantri Suraksha Bima Yojana 230
Pradhan Mantri Surakshit Matritva Abhiyan 688, 929, 969
Pradhan Mantri Surakshit Matritva Yojana 231
Pradhan Mantri Ujjwala Yojana 231, 1033
Pradhan Mantri Vaya Vandana Yojana 230, 716
Pranayama 56
   advantages of 56
Pre-Conception and Pre-Natal Diagnostic Techniques Act 225, 822, 1056
Predisaster phase 780
Prednisolone 615
Pre-eclampsia 677
Pre-exposure prophylaxis 137, 409, 481
Pre-exposure vaccination 761
Pregnancy 422, 722
   effects on 81
   medical termination of 221, 948
   period 45
   rate 224
   termination of 1055
   unwanted 995
Pre-Natal Diagnostic Techniques (Prohibition of Sex Selection) Act 225
Preterm birth
   causes of 687
   complications 693
Prevacuum autoclave 792
Primaquine 426, 427
Primary care trust 341
Primary data collection
   methods 891
   technique 161
Primary health center 84, 515, 850, 863, 940, 942, 943, 962, 1001, 1011
   concept of 929
   level of 958
Primary healthcare 237, 609, 610, 613, 614, 682, 833, 837, 838, 940
   center 160
   eight elements of 839
   movement 840
   philosophy of 850
   principles of 838
   reforms, four sets of 840
   role of 611f
Primary school enrolment rate 844
Prion diseases 347
Proctocolitis 487
Prodromal stage 406
Progesterone-only pill 665
Progestin-only contraceptive pills 664, 667, 669
Program specific management information system 1035
Proguanil 761
Prohibition of Child Marriage Act 1044
Propofol 1089
Propoxur 118
Prostate specific antigen 576
Prostitution 487
Protease inhibitors 480
Protection of Children against Sexual Offences Bill 1045
Protein 29, 38, 40-43, 565, 1021
   digestibility 30
   energy ratio 30, 30t
   quality, quantitative assessment of 30
   requirement of 29t, 30, 31t
   supplementary action of 30
Proteinuria 418
Protozoa 474
Prudent diet 27
Pruritis 386
Pseudomembrane, obstructive effects of 322
*Pseudomonas*
   *aeruginosa* 166
   *mallei* 795
Psychiatric disorders, treatment of 1091
Psychological health 760
Psychosis 740
Psychosocial environment 21
Psychrometer 74, 75
*Pthirus pubis* 487
Puberty, early onset of 220
Public distribution system 630
Public health 232, 831
   Act 831
   action 523, 525, 831
   challenge 771
   communications 232
   concept of 830
   concerns 1062
   facilities 856
   Foundation 150, 856
   hypertension of 541
   importance 638, 764
      arthropods of 119

interventions 244
issues, emergence of 243
Laws 1040
management competency 9
measures 304
  breakdown of 525
nutrition 7
problem 748
  severity of 641
professionals 854
services 931
  reimbursement 852
  related laws 1041, 1054
significance, category of 637
surveillance 737
  uses of 147
system, organization of 934
Public information 82
Public policy reforms 840, 1013
Public private partnership 850, 950
  development of 841
Pull system 895
Pulmonary embolism 549
Pulse 34, 39
  nutritive value of 40
  oximeter 615
  polio immunization 354, 356, 929
Punishment Under Act 1041-1045, 1052, 1053, 1055
Pupa 119
  index 122, 430
Purified duck embryo vaccine 408
Push system 895
P-value 211, 520
Pyramid, second level of 822
Pyrazinamide 315
Pyrethroids, synthetic 118
Pyrethrum 116
Pyridoxine 34, 316

## Q

Q-fever 345
Qualitative data 188, 203
  simple table presenting 195
Quality assurance 213, 913
Quality control 911, 913
  process 913
Quality in healthcare
  measurement of 912
  monitoring of 912
Quality medical officer 937
Quality of life 17, 825
  after stroke 548
  improvement of 332
Quality-adjusted life year 824, 918
Quantitative buffy coat method 425
Quantitative data 203, 188
  simple table presenting 195
Quantitative goals and objectives, specific 954
Quantitative research 184
Quarantine 255
Quinolones 499

## R

Rabies 258, 404, 407, 760
  control of 403, 409
  epidemiology of 403
  immunoglobulin, administration of 409
  pathogenesis of 406f
  prevention 403
  virus particles 405f
Radiation 76, 573, 581, 908
  absorbed dose 77
  annual limit of 76t
  effects of 77, 77t
  exposure 742
    protection against 77
  hazards 724
  internal 76
  ionizing 76
  manmade 76
  nonionizing 76
  sickness
    acute 77
    chronic 77
  types of 76
  units of 76, 76t
Rajiv Awas Yojna 749
Rajiv Gandhi Shramik Kalyan Yojana 1048
Raltegravir 480, 481
Randomized control trials 176
Rapid diagnostic test 984
  kits 425
Rapid fluorescent focus inhibition test 407
Rapid plasma reagin 489, 680
Rapid sand filter 87, 87t, 88, 88f
Rash, triad of 457
Rashtriya Bal Swasthya Karyakram 560, 690, 771, 929, 978
Rashtriya Kishor Swasthya Karyakram 636, 979
Rashtriya Swasthya Bima Yojana 230, 850
Rashtriya Vayoshri Yojana 716
Rat
  bite fever 128
  flea borne diseases 116
*Rattus*
  *norvegicus* 412, 419
  *rattus* 128, 412
Raynaud's phenomenon, secondary 724
Real time-polymerase chain reaction 292, 296, 300, 313, 334
Red blood cells 678
Red ribbon clubs 479
Reduviid bugs 116
Re-emerging diseases 523
  impact of 523
Refractive errors 601
Registration of Births and Deaths Act 1055
Regression 210
Rehabilitation 53, 138, 357, 499, 548, 566, 593, 606, 715, 770
  care 538
  community based 138, 139, 744
  medical 499
  neurological 138
  physical 138, 1048
  psychological 499
Rehydration 368
Reiter's syndrome 381
Relief work 1062
Renal diseases 49
Renal failure
  acute 49
  end-stage 310
Renal stones 50
Re-orient health services 238
Repellents 122, 124
Reproductive and child health 153, 161, 694
  program 945, 948, 964, 965b, 1062
  piloting of 911
Reproductive and maternal health 815, 925
Reproductive health 656, 657f, 670, 966
  and family welfare 656
  care 656
  current status of 658
  twelve pillars of 656
Reproductive life cycle 657f
Reproductive maternal neonatal child health 1064
Reproductive tract infection 472, 490t, 682, 955, 963
  management of 489, 995
Reservoir 115, 250, 273, 291, 327, 331, 339, 354, 362, 376, 412, 417, 436, 449, 452, 454, 462, 469
  source of 422, 461, 467
Respiratory diphtheria 322
Respiratory disease, chronic 926
Respiratory failure 292
Respiratory protection devices 263
Respiratory rate 269
Respiratory syncytial virus 259, 265
Respiratory system 80fc, 260
  diseases of 909
  effects on 80
Respiratory tract 265
  anatomy of 265
  infection, lower 265, 292, 744
  medicines acting on 1092
Reston virus 527
Resuscitation, cardiopulmonary 723
Reticuloendothelial system 448
Retinitis 474, 475
Retinol 638
Retinopathy, diabetic 715
Reverse transcriptase polymerase chain reaction 279, 280, 285, 287, 379, 452, 527, 531, 796
Revised National Tuberculosis Control Program 320, 929, 996t, 891f
Reye's syndrome 300
Rhabdomyolysis 722
Rheumatic fever 555, 556, 560
  acute 556, 558, 559t, 560
  iceberg phenomenon of 557f
  natural history of 558, 558f
  pathogenesis of 557f

prevention of 559f
treatment of 560t
Rheumatic heart disease 549, 556-558, 558f, 559f, 559t, 560, 560t, 561
diagnosis of 558
iceberg phenomenon of 557f
pathogenesis of 557, 557f
Rheumatoid disorders 1089
Rhinitis, allergic 268
*Rhipicephalus sanguineus* 457t
Riboflavin 33, 34, 43, 292, 296
Ribonucleic acid 280, 473
*Rickettsia* 457
*conori* 457
*prowazekii* 86
Rickettsial diseases 456
prevention and control of 457
Rickettsial pox 116, 128, 451, 457
Rifampicin 307, 315
Rift valley fever 527
Right of Children to Free and Compulsory Education Act 1044
Right to Education Act 1044
Rilpivirine 480
Rimantadine 292, 296, 303
Ritonavir 480
Road traffic
accidents 748, 927
collisions and injuries, prevent 761
injuries 590, 591f
Rockefeller foundation 905
Rocky mountain spotted fever 451, 457
Rodent 128, 128f, 128t
borne diseases 833
control 124, 419
infestation rate 125
Rodenticides 129
Roentgen 77
Rogi Kalyan Samitis 950
Rotator cuff injuries 58
Rotavirus 339, 366, 699
vaccine 369, 1066
Rothman causal pies 249f
Roundworm 392
Rubella 251, 261, 280, 286, 288, 289, 699, 742, 1066
acquired 287
classification of 287
complications of 287
elimination 289
epidemiology of 286
infection 288
specific treatment for 288
syndrome, congenital 286, 288
transmission 287
vaccination 690
vaccine 288t
doses of 288
virus
isolation of 287
specific nucleic acid, detection of 287
Rule of Halves 542, 542f
Rural and Village Development 231

Rural health 746, 750
facilities 941t
Rural housing standards 112
Rural malaria 422
Rural medical
practitioners 950
services, experience of 837
Rural Public Health System, organization of 940

## S

Sabin 355
Sabka Sath Sabka Vikas, principle of 846
Safe and wholesome water 84
concept of 84
Safe disposal 98
Safe drinking water 360, 394
availability of 825
supplies, installation of 127
Safe water and sanitation, programs for 341
Safe-and-protected internet 1084
Saksham Anganwadi 1020
Salbutamol 615
Saliva 473
Salk 355
*Salmonella*
*abortus* 371
*cholerasuis* 371, 373
*enteritidis* 371
*gallinarum* 371
*incidence of* 775
*paratyphi* 371-374
*typhi* 339, 369, 371, 372, 374
chloramphenicol resistant 373
*typhimurium* 371, 795
Salmonellosis 128, 370
epidemiology of 370
Salpingitis 487
Salt reduction 543t
broad strategies for 543
strategies 543
Sample registration
survey 658
system 225, 676, 891, 925, 1037
Sandfly 123
borne diseases 115
diseases transmitted by 124
fever 115
life cycle of 124f
Sanitary waste disposal 98
methods 98
Sanitation 93, 262, 344, 360, 374, 389, 391, 394, 395, 450, 467, 505, 759, 927, 958
barrier 374f
impact of 93
managing 98
measures 129
services, classification of 96t
special event 98
Sanitizer 255
Saponins 38
Saproamphixenoses 401
Saproanthropozoonoses 401

Saprometa-anthropozoonoses 402
Saprozoonoses 401
Saquinavir 480
Sarcomas 570
Sardonic smile 508
Scabies 116
Scalar chain 865
Scars 639
Scatter diagram 196, 208
*Schistosoma*
*flatworms* 339
*haematobium* 573
Schistosomiasis 93
Schizophrenia 742
School Health Program 702, 980
components of 702, 980f
Scientific management theory 864
Screening test 142, 142t, 475
properties of 143
Scrotal swelling 490
Scrub typhus 116, 128, 418, 525
Scurvy 244
Seasonal flu strains 301
Seasonal influenza 290, 290t, 297, 300f
communicable period for 300f
prevention of 302f
surveillance system 294
vaccine 303
Seasonal variation 417, 634
Sedatives 744
Sedentary 44, 48
Sedimentation 87
Selected potential bioterrorism agents, features of 796
Semantic barrier 235
Senile dementia 713
Senior Citizen Welfare 230
Sensitivity 144-146, 740
Sentinel site surveillance 645
Sentinel surveillance system 148
Sepsis 678, 696b
neonatal 693
Septic sore throat 345
Septic tank 96, 96f
Septicemia 373
recurrent 475
*Sergentomyia punjabensis* 449
Serological test 145, 334, 457
Serotypes 360
Serpent worm 385
Serum antibody 294
response 294
Serum bilirubin 453
Serum cholesterol level 199
Serum creatinine 544
assay 615
Serum hepatitis 487
Serum neutralization test 527
Serum rubella immunoglobulin G antibody level 287
Service delivery
first point of 963
levels of 963, 963t
programs 959

Severe acute respiratory syndrome 147, 254, 261, 305, 514, 527, 532, 908
Severe malaria
    pathogenesis of 424
    pathology of 424
Sevoflurane 1089
Sewage 94
    treatment 94, 96
        plant 97, 97*f*
Sex ratio 220, 752, 754
    trend of 220, 221*f*
Sex specific death rates 158
Sex worker
    commercial 473, 487, 994
    female 994
Sexual and intimate partner 596
Sexual health 656, 657*f*, 909
Sexual violence, management of 995
Sexually transmitted diseases
    control 485
    epidemiology of 485
    prevention 485
    surveillance 998
Sexually transmitted infection 148, 154, 202, 463, 472, 483, 485, 486, 486*f*, 487, 487*f*, 488*f*, 489, 490, 490*t*, 492, 664, 682, 688, 705, 706, 955, 963, 995*t*
    advantages of 490*t*
    complications of 488
    disadvantages of 490*t*
    drugs kits of 491*f*
    management of 489, 995
    prevention of 476, 478
    surveillance 995
    syndromes 490
Shake test
    failed 1070*f*
    passed 1070*f*
    use of 839
Shakir's tape 839
Shallow trench latrine 97*f*
Sherman traps 129
*Shigella* 345
    *boydii* 375
    *dysenteriae* 375, 383
    *flexneri* 375
    *sonnei* 375
    vaccine 369
Shigellosis
    control of 375
    epidemiology of 375
    prevention of 375
Shin splints 58
Shock 418, 428
Short range biological standoff detection system 797
Sick building syndrome 71
Sickle cell
    anemia 16, 766, 767
    disease 764
        care 1018
    trait, prevalence of 202
Sickness 18, 18*t*
    absenteeism 725
    benefit 1047

Silicosis 310, 726
    compensation for 728
    diagnosis of 727*f*
Simple bar diagram 197
Simvastatin 615
Single blind trial 178
Single gene
    disorders 766
    inheritance 766
Sinusitis
    acute 266
    acute bacterial 268
Skeletal fluorosis 1026
    advanced stage of 1026
Skill development 231
Skilled birth attendant 510, 681
Skin 418
    cancers 732
    diseases 775
    disorders 719
Slaughterhouse sanitation 349
Sleep
    disorders 541
    wake disorders 909
Sling psychrometer 75, 75*f*
Slit-skin smear 985
Slow sand filter 87, 87*t*, 88*f*
Smallpox 147, 245, 254, 261, 276, 796, 831
    eradication 831
        advisory group 141
        program 813
Smear
    thick 425
    thin 425
Social
    activism 61
    and health system factors 678
    behavior 699
    blindness 599
    cognitive theory 67
    defense 61, 229
    deviants 61
    diagnosis 227
    dimension 15
    distancing 534
    economic classes 68
    environment 502, 590
        type of 60
    epidemiology 64, 226
    evils 61
    groups 613, 693, 755
    insurance 229
    interventions 228
    mapping 228, 228*f*
    marketing in family welfare, role of 670
    medicine 226, 831
    mobility 68
    network 235
    pathology 61
    phobia 741
    psychology 227
    reaction 779
    rehabilitation 499
    security 228, 1045
        schemes 230*t*

    status 62
    stratification 67
    structures 61
    surveys 227
    therapeutics 228
    welfare 229
        measures 489, 672
        schemes 231*t*
Sociodrama 234, 235
Socioeconomic status 68, 298, 486, 495, 502, 557, 584, 679, 824
    scales 68
Sociogram 227*f*
Socio-politico-developmental model 742*f*
Socratic method 233
Sodium 36, 565
    chloride 368
        infusion 615
Soft
    helminths 833
        control 385
        epidemiology of 385
        prevention 385
    pollution 908
    reservoir 251
    salinization 417
    sore 487
    temperature 417
    tick 125, 125*f*, 126*t*, 457
    transmitted helminth 395, 396
Solar water disinfection 86, 86*f*
Solid waste
    concept of 93
    disposal 98
    impact of 94
    management 94, 95
Sore throat, presence of 323
Sound level 106
    meters 107*f*
Spanish flu 289, 290
Sparsh leprosy awareness campaigns 1000
Spasmodic croup 323
Special newborn care unit 969, 971
Speech 699
    interference levels 107
    therapy 548
Spermicides 661
Sphygmomanometer 1066
Spine 310
Spiritual dimension 15
Spirochete, bacterial 457
Spironolactone 615
Spittoons 1049
Spleen
    crises 767
    rate 425
Splenomegaly 517
Split vaccines 303
Sponge 661
Sporogony 423
Sporozoite rate 426
Sporulating bacilli 322
Sputnik V COVID-19 vaccine 535
Sputum 728, 786
    examination 728

microscopy 311
  smear microscopy 311
Sri Lankan Health System 853
Stakeholders, training of 1012
Standard deviation 26, 193, 200
Stanford Binet intelligence scale 699
Staphylococcal pharyngitis 323
*Staphylococcus aureus* 345, 525
State Blindness Control Societies 1014
State Health Mission 957
State Health Society 957
State Health System Resource Centers 957
State Institutes of Health and Family Welfare 957
State Pollution Control Boards 82
State Program Implementation Plan 958
State Program Management Unit 957
Statin 615
Statistical inference
  procedure, elements of 204
  steps of 205
Statistical methods, usage of 198
Statistical test 203$t$, 205, 210
Stavudine 480
Steam disinfection 125
ST-elevation myocardial infarction 540, 554
Sterile water 285
Sterilization 255, 346, 783
  efficacy of 255$f$
  female 660, 668
  laparoscopic 669
  male 660, 668
  processes 346$t$
Stethoscope 615, 1066
Sthira Sukham Asanam 55
Stiffness 454, 455
Stigma Reduction Program for Mental Health 743$f$
Stillbirth 1081
Stochastic effect 77
Stool sample collection 356, 361
Strain 278, 325, 380
Strategic health authority 341
*Streptococcus*
  *pneumoniae* 268, 300
  *pyogenes* 345
Streptomycin 315, 336
Stress 169, 733, 733$t$
  persistent 542
  psychological 551
  role of family in 67
Strict Implementing Motor Vehicle Driving Law 744
Stroke 246, 609, 744, 767, 819, 1007
  epidemiology of 541, 546
  hemorrhagic 547, 548
  ischemic 546, 548
  prevention of 139, 546
  risk factors for 547
  symptoms of 547
  thrombotic 547
  types of 546
*Strongyloides stercoralis* 474
Strongyloidiasis 474

Substance
  regulate availability of 744
  use 743
    disorder 478
    harmful effect of 744
    prevention of 744
Sub-unit vaccines 303
Succinylcholine 1089
Suicide 595, 705, 743
  prevention 819
Sulfadoxine pyrimethamine 426
Sulfamethoxazole 761
Sulfonamides 336
Sulforaphanes 38
Sulfur dioxide 79, 719
Supplemental suckling technique technique 697
Surakshit Matritva Aashwasan 969
  components of 969$f$
Surveillance 797
  cycle 340$f$
  specific objectives of 786
  systems 340, 341$f$, 786
  types of 147
Sustainable development goals 746; 831, 842, 845$b$, 846, 988
  achieve 815
  birth of 844
Sustainable financing system 841
Swachh Bharat Abhiyaan 341
Swachh Bharat Mission 1031
Swachh Indhan Behtar Jeevan 1033
Swachh Swasth Sarvatra 1032
Swan neck flask 246
  experiment 245
Swedish International Development Agency 904
Swelling 1076
Swine flu 261, 290, 291
Sydenham's chorea 558
Sylvatic yellow fever 436
Symposium 234
Syphilis 477, 487, 674, 688, 970
  parent-to-child transmission of 489, 995
Syrian ulcer 320
Syringe service program 478
Systemic lupus erythematosus 728

### T

Tachycardia 454
*Taenia*
  *asiatica* 347
  *saginata* 347
  *solium* 342, 347, 401, 401$f$
Taeniasis 345, 347
Tapioca 40
Tax-based public sector 859
T-distribution table 205
Team building skills 881
Telecommunication 233, 1083
Telemedicine 1084
  facility 1018
Temperature 262, 722, 1049, 1073

greater 287
inversion 79
variation poses 100
Temporary disablement benefit 1047
Temporary settlements and camps 782
Teneligliptin 615
Tenofovir 476, 477, 480
Teratogenic effects 725
Terpenoids 38
Testicular inflammation 284
Tetanospasmin 508
Tetanus 323, 680, 699, 1066
  control of 505, 509
  epidemiology of 505
  maternal 506
  neonatal 505, 506, 509, 694
  pathogenesis of 508$fc$
  prevention of 505, 509
  prone injuries 511
  spores 507$f$
  toxoid 506, 509, 680
    vaccine 506, 509, 510$f$
  types of 509
Tetracycline 336, 457, 499, 894
  chloramphenicol 336
Thalassemia 764, 767
  gene 756
Thalidomide study 172
Therapeutic exercises 1010
Thermal
  comfort 75, 100
  indices 100
Thermometer 615, 1066
Thiamin 33, 34, 42, 43
Thiopentone 1089
Thoracic syndrome, acute 767
Threadworm 339
Threonine 29
Thyroid 77
  hyperplasia 641
  stimulating hormone 641
Tick 125, 126, 451, 457
  borne
    diseases 116, 451$t$, 453
    encephalitis 402$f$
    relapsing fever 451, 457
    viral disease 452$t$
  life cycle of 125$f$
  typhus 116
Tobacco 572, 579, 611, 706, 744, 818
  consumption 551
  control of 575
  harmful effect of 744$f$
  smoke 908
  usage survey 193$t$
  use 705
Tocilizumab 534
Tocopherols, quantities of 32
Toilet 113
  and hand washing facilities 98
Tokyo subway 795
Torch light model 837$f$
Total leukocytic count 453
Total quality management 913, 913$f$

Total sanitation campaign 99, 341
Tourniquet test 430
Toxic ingredients 651*t*
Toxin 563, 652
    detection of 653
    mediated disease 326
*Toxoplasma gondii* 251, 345, 474
Toxoplasmosis 345, 347, 474
Tracheal cytotoxin exhibit 325
Tracheobronchial
    diphtheria 322
    pseudomembranes, mechanical removal of 324
Trachoma 93, 116, 501, 601
    active 503
    control 501
    elimination of 504
    epidemiology of 501
    infection 503*f*
    prevention 501
Traditional birth attendants 681
Training management information system 1036
Transect walk 228
Transgenders 994
Transient ischemic attack 547
Transmission assessment survey 984
Trauma Care and Physical Resources, organization of 593
Travel
    epidemiology 759
    health risks 760
    notice 763, 763*t*
    purpose of 759
Traveler
    behavior of 759
    health 758
    treatment of 762
    under public health observation 762
Trench
    fever 116, 451, 457
    foot 105, 723
*Treponema pallidum* 487
Tribal health 746, 752
*Trichinella spiralis* through pork 347
Trichinosis 128
*Trichomonas vaginalis* 487
Trichomoniasis 487
Trichuriasis 366, 394
    control 394
    epidemiology of 394
    life cycle of 395*f*
    prevention 394
*Trichuris trichiura* 394
Triglycerides 31, 626
Trimethoprim 761
Triple-drug therapy 985
Trismus 508, 508*f*
Trisodium citrate 368
Trisomy 766
Trivalent inactivated influenza vaccine 303
Trivandrum developmental screening chart 699

Trombiculid mite 126
Troponin test strips 615
Trypanosomiasis 116
Tsetse flies 116
T-test
    one-sample 205
    unpaired 206
Tubal embryo transfer 672
Tubal ligation 668*f*
Tuberculosis 133, 152, 261, 307, 309, 310, 312, 314*b*, 317-320, 345, 347, 472, 483, 615, 682, 705, 748, 755, 815, 933
    active 310
    adult drug sensitive 315*t*
    antibiotic resistant 307
    bacilli 310
    care, standards for 993
    childhood 699
    control 319, 320*b*
    diagnosis and treatment 478
    diagnostic tool for 313*b*
    disseminated 310
    drug resistant 314, 316, 991
    early detection of 996
    epidemiology of 306
    extrapulmonary 310, 312, 312*fc*, 314
    first line drugs for 315*t*
    history of 306
    incidence of 307
    infections control for 318
    latent 313
    microbiological confirmation of 313*b*, 314
    multidrug-resistant 308, 319
    mycobacterium 307, 309, 310, 312, 313, 345, 474, 494, 533
    natural history of 311*f*
    notification 993
    prevention of 316
    preventive treatment 318
        contraindications of 318
    prompt treatment of 996
    pulmonary 178*fc*, 312*f*, 314, 474, 726, 871
    retreatment case of 314
    risk factors for 310*b*
    sabin drugs for 315*t*
    salk drugs for 315*t*
    second line drugs for 315*t*
    treatment of drug-resistant 316
    unit 990
    urogenital 310
Tuberculous meningitis 310
Tularemia 116, 128, 147, 796
Tumor
    markers 576
    necrosis factor 310, 424
*Tungapenetrans* 116
Tuning fork 615
Turner syndrome 766
Tuskegee syphilis study 211
Twenty-four hour recall technique 643
Typhoid 115, 258, 339, 418, 760
    carriers of 373
    fever 246, 339, 370, 372

    diagnosis of 373*t*
    epidemiology of 370
    serologic diagnosis of 373*f*
    sangli outbreak of 371
    vaccines 369
Tyrosine 29

# U

Udai Pareekh's classification 68
Udai Pareekh's scale 69*t*
Ujjawala Scheme 489, 1033
Ulcer 279
    care of 499
    mouth 279
Ultra-low volume malathion fogging 987
Ultrasonography 582
Ultraviolet irradiation lamp 86, 86*f*
*Uncinaria stenocephala* 397
Under-five mortality rate 685, 686*f*
Undernutrition 310, 628, 705
    prevalence of 629*f*
    risk factors for 629
    types of 976
Underweight 565, 628, 629, 755
United Kingdom's Healthcare System 851
United Nations Children Fund 902
United Nations Development Group's 844
United Nations Development Program 842, 903, 1036
United Nations Framework Convention on Climate Change 773
United Nations International Children's Emergency Fund 85, 96, 641, 688, 859
United Nations Millennium Development Goals 694
United Nations Population Fund 683, 904
United States Agency for International Development 859
Universal Coverage Reforms 840
Universal Health Coverage 841, 842, 903, 911
    strategy 841
Universal Immunization Program 323, 324, 328, 446, 511, 929, 946, 948, 974, 975*t*
Universal Program on Immunization 948
Universal Thermal Climate Index 103
Upper respiratory tract infections 265
    acute 265
Urban Family Welfare Centers 949
Urban Health System, organization of 949
Urban healthcare
    delivery model 962*f*
    facilities, level of 962*f*
Urban heart, core indicators of 749*t*
Urban primary health centre 958
Urban rural poverty alleviation 230
Urban tuberculosis control systems 992
Urban Vector-Borne Disease Scheme 983
*Ureaplasma urealyticum* 487
Urethral discharge 490
Urethritis 487
    nongonococcal 487
Uric acid stones 50

# Index

Urinary iodine excretion 641
Urinary tract infection 49, 688
Urine 786
    analysis of 544
    disinfection of 786t
    examination 626
    ketones test strips 615
    microalbuminuria test strips 615
    protein test strips 615
    sample 418
Urticaria 386
Uterine cervical cancer 926

## V

Vaccination 280, 282, 296, 414, 437, 446, 453, 489, 781
    primary course of 328
    routine 760
    schedule 446, 708
    status 261
    Under Universal Immunization Program 446
Vaccine 257, 258, 280, 288, 294, 300, 303, 331, 498, 708, 760, 781, 975, 1066, 1069, 1076
    and drugs, planning for 895
    arrangement of 1072f
    carrier 1072, 1072f
    characteristics 355
    conjugate 331
    effectiveness 259
    preventable diseases 357
    product-related reaction 1074
    quality defect-related reaction 1074
    reactions 1075
    safety 1068, 1069t
    sensitive 1069
    type 257, 286
        irrespective of 303
    vial monitor 839, 1068
Vagabond's disease 125
Vaginal
    candidiasis 487
    diaphragm 662f
    discharge 490
    sponge 662f
Vaginitis 487
Vaginosis, bacterial 487, 688
Valvulitis, echocardiographic 559
Varicella 257, 272
    vaccine against 275
    zoster 273
Vasectomy
    fortnight 967
    incisional 668
Vasovagal reaction 1076t
Vector 115, 128, 250, 388
    bionomics 436, 448
    borne
        diseases 152, 252, 339, 420, 451, 457t, 745, 748
        transmission 403
    control 446, 449, 453, 781
        measures 128, 426, 431, 434, 437, 441, 984
    remote sensing in 123
    density 420
    feeding habits 420
    indices 426
    infectivity rate 441
Vecuronium 1089
Vehicle borne 252
    transmission 403
Venereal disease 485
    research laboratory 680
Venous plasma glucose 565
Ventilated pit latrine 96f
Ventilation 71, 72, 262, 1049
    adequate 263
    and lighting condition 112
    lack of 495
    mechanical 318
    mode of 72t
    natural 318
    standards of 72t
    types of 71, 72
Verbal communication 233, 886
Vibramycin 761
Vibration white fingers 724, 724f
*Vibrio cholerae* 245, 339, 345, 359, 523, 524
*Vibrio parahaemolyticus* 339
Village Health and Nutrition Day 960, 1064
    concept of 1064
    microplanning of 1065
Village Health and Sanitation Committee 839
Village Health Sanitation and Nutrition Committee 822, 950, 969, 1064
Village Health Sanitation and Nutrition Day 1019
Vincent's angina 323
Violence 760, 819, 927
    act of 1041
    against children 819
Viral agents 487
    range of 265
Viral disease 276, 347
Viral hepatitis 116, 345, 379, 418, 469, 818
    child transmission of 818
    control 376
    epidemiology of 376
    prevention 376
Viral vectors 768
Viremia 434
Virulence 20, 250
Virus 366, 451, 474
    isolation of 434
    strain 290
Vis-à-vis sustainable development goals 845t
Visceral leishmaniasis 448, 985
Vision 699, 867, 957, 983, 988, 991, 998
    2020 1014
    Impairment
        causes of 600t
        moderate-to-severe 600
    proposed structure for 1014f
    statement 844
Visual acuity, presenting distance 599
Visual blindness 599
Visual communication 233
Visual disturbances 677
Visual impairment 599, 690
    categories of 599t
Visual system, diseases of 909
Vital events 1084
Vital registration 1084
Vital statistics 645, 747, 747t
Vitamin 26, 32, 38, 40, 41, 43, 565, 755, 1092
    A 32, 34, 42, 46, 637, 638, 639t, 702
        administered 280
        dosage of 281t, 639
        prophylaxis program 1023
        rich food 639
        supplementation 280, 368, 978
    A deficiency 279, 37, 638, 1021
        indicators of 638t
        prevalence of 637f
    administering supplemental dose of 639
    $B_1$ 33
    $B_{12}$ 34
    $B_6$ 33
    C 35, 35t, 37, 572
    D 32
        precursor of 32
        deficiencies 310
    E 33, 37, 572
    fat-soluble 32
    K 33
        deficiency 33
    water-soluble 33, 46
Vocational rehabilitation 139, 500, 1048
Volatile organic compounds 79
Voluntary blood donation 477, 479
Voluntary Health Agencies 1061, 1061t
Voluntary medical male circumcision 476
Vomiting 386, 418, 677
Vulnerable groups 22, 152, 487, 1040, 1042

## W

Waist
    circumference 544
    hip ratio 634
Warm chain 695b
Waste
    agricultural 94
    and effluents, disposal of 1049
    biodegradable 94
    disposal 349
    genotoxic 788
    infectious 788
    management
        methods of 94
        options 95t
        process 95f
    nonbiodegradable 94
    noncontrolled 93
    nonhazardous 94
    pathological 788
    pharmaceutical 788
    quantum of 788
    radioactive 94, 788
    type of 93, 790, 791
    water, collection of 833

Water (Prevention and Control of Pollution) Act 1052
Water 104, 505
  and sanitation 779
  bodies, mapping of 419
  borne diseases 339, 340, 775
    agents 339, 339$t$
    epidemiology of 338, 339
    historical perspective of 338
    preventing 340
  borne 85, 338
    outbreak, investigation of 340
    pathogens 100
  carriage system 96
  chlorination principles and practices 810
  collection of 833
  conservation 91
    and rainwater harvesting, concept of 84
  diseases 85, 339
    classification of 339$t$
  dispersible
    granules 117
    powder 117
  hardness of 89
  health hazards of 84
  pollution 91, 908
  prior, pH level of 88
  quality 100
    standards 84
    surveillance 90
  requirement of 84
  samples, collection of 91
  sanitary sources of 84
  seal 96
  soluble granules 117
  sources of 520
  supply 112, 113, 389, 392, 781
    and sanitation 931
  surrounding iceberg 24
  treatment 86
    plants, community based 87
  vapor 774
Waterhouse Friderichsen syndrome 330
Weaknesses 878
Wealth index 68
Weighed-food records 643
Weighing
  machine 615
  scales 1066

Weight
  control 575
  gain 677, 680
    gestational 31
  loss 54, 55, 728
Weil's disease 339
Weil-Felix reaction 457
Well-functioning health information system 849
Wet bulb
  globe temperature 102, 103$f$
  thermometer 100
Wheeze 269, 728
Whisper test 715
Whole cell
  killed vaccine 363
  vaccine 328
Whole-body vibration 724
Whooping cough 261, 325, 514
  epidemiology of 325
Wild life rabies 405
Woolsorter's disease 332
Work stress 720
Workmen's Compensation Act 737, 1050
Workplace violence 718
Work-study 871
World AIDS Day 471
World Bank 903
  functions of 903
World Glaucoma Awareness Week 602
World Health Assembly 900
  functions of 900
World Health Organization 203, 624, 627, 740, 805, 900
  family of international classifications 908
  global tuberculosis strategy 988$f$
  health system framework 849$f$, 849$fc$
World Population Day Campaign 967
World Sight Day 602
Wound
  care 408, 499
  management 408$t$
  treatment 408
*Wuchereria bancrofti* 438, 439, 441
*Wuchereriasis*, diagnosis of 441$f$

## X

Xerophthalmia, classification of 638$t$
Xerophthalmic fundus 638
Xerosis, conjunctival 638

## Y

Yaws 116, 487
Yellow fever 115, 147, 420, 435, 514, 760
  control of 435, 437
  epidemics 437
  epidemiology of 435
  intermediate 436
  prevention of 435, 437
  urban 436
  virus, transmission of 436$f$
*Yersinia pestis* 243, 336
  orientalis strain of 243$f$
Yoga 55
  history of 55
  role of 57
Yogasanas 55
Yogic diet 57

## Z

Z score 191
Zalcitabine 471
Zanamivir 292, 296
Zidovudine 480
Ziehl-Nielsen stain 313
Zika 527
  virus 254, 451, 528, 529, 690, 718
    disease 514
    ecology of 529$f$
    infection 689
    outbreak 529$b$
Zinc 34, 36
  phosphide 129
  supplementation 368, 1027
Zonal blood testing centers 477
Zooanthroponoses 403
Zoonosis, impact of 400
Zoonotic disease 333, 400, 719
  control 400
  epidemiology of 400
  prevention 400
  transmission of 403
  virus 289
Zoonotic plague 337
Zooprophylaxis 128
Z-score 203
Z-tests 206
Z-value 521
Zygote intrafallopian transfer 672